BMA

BRITISH MEDICAL ASSOCIATION

COMPLETE FAMILY HEALTH GUIDE

BMA

BRITISH MEDICAL ASSOCIATION

COMPLETE FAMILY HEALTH GUIDE

Medical Editor
DR TONY SMITH

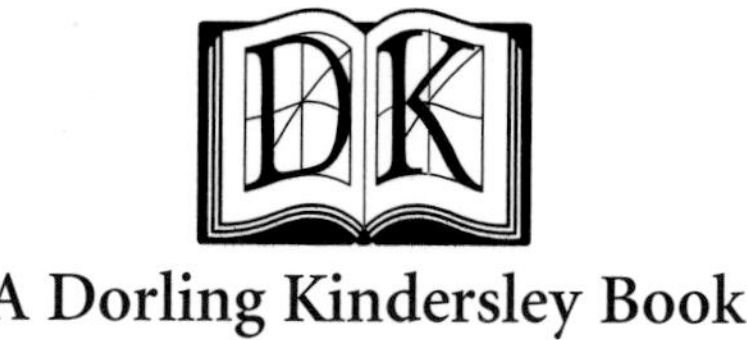

A Dorling Kindersley Book

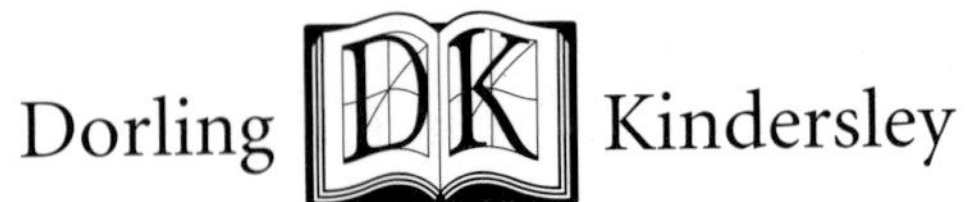

LONDON, NEW YORK, MUNICH,
MELBOURNE, AND DELHI

First UK Edition, 2000
4 6 8 10 9 7 5 3

Published in the United Kingdom by Dorling Kindersley Limited,
80 Strand, London, WC2 0RL
A Penguin Company

The British Medical Association Complete Family Health Guide provides general information on a wide range of health and medical topics. The book is not a substitute for medical diagnosis, however, and you are advised always to consult your doctor for specific information on personal health matters. The naming of any organization, product, or alternative therapy in this book does not imply BMA endorsement; the omission of any such names does not indicate BMA disapproval.

A CIP catalogue record for this book is available
from the British Library

ISBN 0-7513-2722-0

Colour reproduction by GRB Editrice, Verona, Italy
Printed and bound in Spain by AGT, Toledo

FOREWORD

THE SECOND HALF OF THE 20TH CENTURY saw dramatic changes in medicine. Deaths from infections became rare in western countries. Advances in science began to find the causes of many illnesses and explain why they affected some people but not others. New techniques became able to visualize the interior of the body. Surgery was transformed by "keyhole" and microsurgical methods.

As we enter the third millennium people can live longer in good health than ever before. Nevertheless, many will die prematurely or become disabled by injury or long-term disease. Much of this illness can be prevented by a healthy lifestyle, having a few simple screening tests, and being aware of the early symptoms of disease.

The aim of the *Complete Family Health Guide* is to provide people with the information they need to take full advantage of these recent advances. It explains how the body works, what can go wrong, and what can be done to preserve and restore health. Charts give practical guidance to help you assess any symptoms you may have and give clear advice on when to see a doctor. The *Complete Family Health Guide* sets out the important features of a healthy lifestyle and explains why we should try to identify our own health priorities by taking account of the disorders that have affected previous generations and older members of our families.

Health information is now available from telephone help lines, self-help organizations, and the internet. These new sources have not, however, made medical books like this redundant. The flood of novel data is often contradictory and of variable quality and usefulness. By contrast, the *Complete Family Health Guide* is based on advice from a panel of medical consultants chosen by the BMA, and their experience provides an unrivalled assurance of quality and reliability.

Tony Smith

DR TONY SMITH MA BM BCh

MEDICAL EDITOR

British Medical Association

Chairman of the Council Dr. Ian Bogle

Treasurer Dr. W. J. Appleyard

Chairman of the Journal Committee Sir Anthony Grabham

Medical editors and reviewers

Medical Editor Tony Smith MA BM BCh

Deputy Medical Editor Sue Davidson MB BS MRCP MRCGP DRCOG

Michael Adler MD FRCP FFPHM
Robert N. Allan MD FRCP
Sir Peter Beale KBE FRCP FFCM FFOM DTM&H
A. Graham Bird FRCP FRCPath
Robin L. Blair MB FRCS(Ed.) FRCS(C.) FACS
Fiona Boag MB BS FRCP
Charles G. D. Brook MA MD FRCP FRCPCH
Christopher Davidson MA(Cantab.) MB FRCP FESC
J. Michael Dixon MD FRCS
Andrew Doble MS FRCS(Urol.)
Terry Hamblin DM FRCP FRCPath
Bruce Hendry MD PhD
S. R. Iliffe MRCGP
Paresh Jobanputra DM MRCP MRCGP
W. F. Kelly MD FRCP
P. Kendall-Taylor MD FRCP
Peng T. Khaw PhD MRCP FRCS FRCOphth
Helen Kingston MD FRCP DCH
Leslie Klenerman ChM FRCS
George T. Lewith MA DM MRCP MRCGP
David Mabey BM BCh DM FRCP
H. Manji MA MD MRCP
G. Keith Morris MD FRCP
Guy Neild MD FRCP FRCPath
Noel D. L. Olsen MSc FRCP FFPHM
A. Parshall BSc MB BS PhD MRCPsych
M. R. Partridge MD FRCP
R. C. Peveler DPhil MRCPsych
Rosalind Ramsay MA MB BS MRCPsych
T. M. Reynolds MB ChB BSc MD
T. J. Ryan DM FRCP
P. J. Sanderson MB PhD FRCPath
J. A. Savin MA MD FRCP DIH
Julian Shah MB ChB LRCP MRCS FRCF
David V. Skinner FRCS FFAEM
David Sutton MD FRCP FRCR DMRD MCAR
Roy Taylor BSc MB ChB MD FRCP FRCPE
Martin Thornhill MB BS BDS MSc PhD FDSRCS(Ed.) FFDRCSI
James Walker MD FRCP(Glas.) FRCP(Edin.) FRCOG FRSM
Chris Williams DM FRCP
Jennifer A. Young MA MD FRCPath RCPI

Contributors

Samir Alvi BSc MB BS PhD DFFP DRCOG
Ursula Arens
Helen Barnett BPharm
Jeffrey L. Barron MB ChB MSc MMed FRCPath
Sue Bosanko
Jane de Burgh RGN
Helen Byrt PhD
Nancy Duin
Martin Edwards BDS SDSRCS PhD
Helen Epstein PhD
Marie Fallon MB ChB DRCOG
Mary Fogarty MSc MB BCh BAO NUI
Philip Gaut PhD
Bruce George MS FRCS
Jennifer Glasspool PhD
Sandra Goldbeck-Wood MB ChB
Katherine Heimann
Chris Higgins
Kate Hope MB BS MRCS LRCP
Amanda Jackson-Russell PhD
Marion Jowett
Ann Kramer
Lynne Low MB ChB
Theresa McCrone RGN
Ian McKee MB ChB DRCOG DFFP
Chris McLaughlin
Sheena Meredith MB BS LRCP MRCS
Sanjida O'Connell
J. Pearce
D. A. Pearson MA MRCGP
Elliot Philipp MMA FRCS FRCOG
Paulette Pratt
Punit S. Ramrakha MA BM BCh MRCP PhD
Rosalind Ramsay MA MB BS MRCPsych
Michael J. Rennie PhD FRSE
Mike Rogers BPharm MRPharmS
Omar Sattaur
Christine Scott-Moncrieff MB ChB MFHom
Anne Slavotinek MB BS FRCP PhD
Patricia Spallone PhD
Jane Stirling PhD
Joanna Thomas
Lindy Van den Berghe BMedSci BM BS
Richard Walker PhD
Robert Whittle MB BS
Sam Wilde
Robert Youngson MB ChB DTM&H DO FRCOphth

Dorling Kindersley

Project Managing Editors Maxine Lewis, Janet Mohun

Project Editor Jolyon Goddard

Editors Ann Baggaley, Katie John, Alyson Lacewing, Esther Ripley

Editorial Assistance Jane de Burgh, Sue Cooper, Heather Jones, Nicki Lampon, Mukul Patel, Teresa Pritlove, Hazel Richardson

Assistant Medical Editor Penny Preston MB ChB MRCGP

Project Administration Delyth Hughes

Project Managing Art Editor Louise Dick

Design Assistance Kirsten Cashman, Janice English, Marianne Markham, Chris Walker

DTP Design Jason Little

Production Michelle Thomas

Senior Managing Editor Martyn Page

Deputy Art Director Bryn Walls

Editorial Director Jackie Douglas

Art Director Peter Luff

First US edition

Project Managing Editor Andrea Bagg

Deputy Managing Editor Maxine Lewis

Senior Editors Paul Docherty, Jill Hamilton, Nicki Lampon, Mary Lindsay, Andrew Macintyre, Janet Mohun

Deputy Senior Editor Jolyon Goddard

Editors Ann Baggaley, Judith Bettesworth, Edda Bohnsack, Martin Bryant, Jane de Burgh, Alan Byrne, Louise Clairmonte, Sue Cooper, Patricia Davis, Kim Dennis-Bryan, Patricia Dent, Kathy Fahey, Francesca George, Peter Harrison, Fiona Hunter, Katie John, Sarah Keer-Keer, Jo Lankester, Alyson McGaw, Ben Morgan, Sean O'Connor, Mukul Patel, Hazel Richardson, Esther Ripley, Nikki Taylor, Stephen Taylor, Gaia Vince, John Watson

Editorial Assistance Judit Z. Bodnar, Peter Frances, Angeles Gavira, Rachel Hutchinson, Robert Johnston, Heather Jones, Nancy Lieberman, Donna Loh, Rebecca Marsland, Ann Mummery, Irene Pavitt, Andrew Pine, Jennifer Quasha, Teresa Pritlove, Juliet Roberts

Indexer Sue Bosanko

Medical Editor-in-chief David Goldman MD FACP

Associate Medical Editor David A. Horowitz MD

Medical Editor Tony Smith MA BM BCh

Deputy Medical Editor Sue Davidson MB BS MRCP MRCGP DRCOG

Assistant Medical Editors Naomi Craft BSc MB BS MRCGP, Gabrielle Murphy BA BSc MB ChB, Fiona Payne MB BS, Penny Preston MB ChB MRCGP, Amanda Rouse BSc MB BS MRCP MRCGP, Frances Williams MA MB BChir MRCP DTM&H MRCPCH

Project Managing Art Editor Louise Dick

Project Deputy Managing Art Editor Marianne Markham

Senior Designer Mark Batley

Designers Amanda Carroll, Janice English, Sara Freeman, Spencer Holbrook, Johnny Pau, Chris Walker

Design Assistance Kirsten Cashman, Nicola Hampel, Elaine Hewson, Richard Horsford, Sasha Howard, Anne Renel, Mark Wilde

DTP Design Jason Little

DTP Assistance Zirrinia Austin, Louise Waller

Anatomy Visualizer Richard Tibbitts

Illustrators Evi Antoniou, Debbie Maizels, Patrick Mulrey, Richard Tibbitts, Halli Verrinder

Picture Researchers Andrea Sadler, Suzanne Williams

Production Michelle Thomas

Project Administration Delyth Hughes, Vicky Wilks, Anna Youle

Project Researcher Claire Isaac BSc MB ChB

Senior Managing Editor Martyn Page

Senior Managing Art Editor Bryn Walls

Editorial Director Jackie Douglas

Art Director Peter Luff

Editorial Development Director (US) Jeanette Mall

Editorial Director (US) LaVonne Carlson

Publisher (US) Chuck Lang

CONTENTS

HOW TO USE THIS BOOK.....11

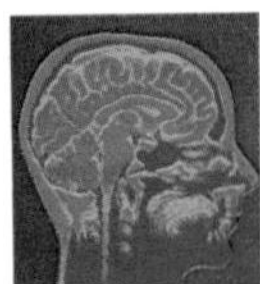

TAKING CONTROL OF YOUR HEALTH
15–86

INTRODUCTION.....16

INHERITANCE, AGE, AND HEALTH.....20
- Understanding inheritance.....24
- Health at different ages.....27
- Health care throughout life.....38

LIFESTYLE AND HEALTH.....46
- Diet and health.....48
- Exercise and health.....55
- Alcohol, tobacco, and drugs.....62
- Sex and health.....67
- Psychological health.....72
- Safety and health.....77

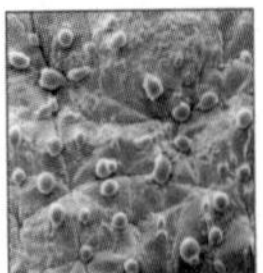

ASSESSING YOUR SYMPTOMS
87–210

INTRODUCTION.....88

GENERAL CHARTS.....92
- Feeling unwell.....92
- Tiredness.....94
- Loss of weight.....96
- Being overweight.....98
- Difficulty sleeping.....100
- Fever.....102
- Excessive sweating.....104
- Lumps and swellings.....106
- Feeling faint and passing out.....108
- Headache.....110
- Vertigo.....112
- Numbness and/or tingling.....114
- Twitching and tremor.....116
- Facial pain.....118
- Difficulty speaking.....119
- Forgetfulness and/or confusion.....120
- Feeling depressed.....122
- Anxiety.....124
- Itching.....125
- General skin problems.....126
- Rash with fever.....128
- Hair and scalp problems.....130
- Painful or irritated eye.....132
- Disturbed or impaired vision.....134
- Hearing loss.....136
- Earache.....138
- Sore throat.....139
- Hoarseness and/or voice loss.....140
- Coughing.....142
- Shortness of breath.....144
- Wheezing.....146
- Difficulty swallowing.....147
- Vomiting.....148
- Recurrent vomiting.....150
- Abdominal pain.....152
- Recurrent abdominal pain.....154
- Swollen abdomen.....156
- Anal and rectal problems.....157
- Diarrhoea.....158
- Constipation.....160
- Chest pain.....162
- Palpitations.....164
- Poor bladder control.....165
- Frequent urination.....166
- Painful urination.....168
- Back pain.....170
- Neck pain or stiffness.....172
- Painful arm or hand.....174
- Painful leg.....175
- Painful joints.....176
- Swollen ankles.....178

MEN'S CHARTS.....180
- Impotence.....180
- Testes and scrotum problems.....181
- Problems with the penis.....182

WOMEN'S CHARTS.....184
- Breast problems.....184
- Absent periods.....186
- Painful periods.....188
- Heavy periods.....189
- Abnormal vaginal bleeding.....190
- Lower abdominal pain in women.....192
- Abnormal vaginal discharge.....194
- Genital irritation in women.....195
- Painful intercourse in women.....196

CHILDREN'S CHARTS.....198
Vomiting in children.....198
Diarrhoea in children.....200
Fever in children.....202
Breathing problems in children.....204
Coughing in children.....206
Abdominal pain in children.....208
Weight problems in children.....210

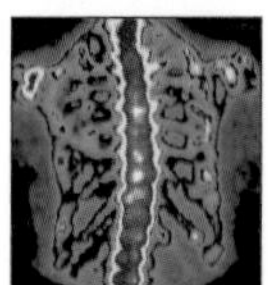

LOOKING FOR DISEASE
211–256

INTRODUCTION.....212

VISITING YOUR DOCTOR.....216
Medical history and examination.....218
Obtaining samples for testing.....221

TESTING SAMPLES.....224
Tests on blood structure and function.....226
Chemical tests.....229
Tests for microorganisms.....234
Cell and tissue tests.....236
Genetic tests.....238

VISUALIZING INTERNAL ORGANS.....242
Imaging techniques.....244
Viewing techniques.....254

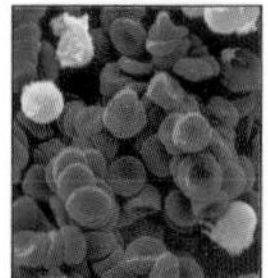

YOUR BODY AND DISEASE
257–872

INTRODUCTION.....258

GENES AND INHERITANCE.....264
Genetic disorders.....270

CANCER.....274
Living with cancer.....278

INFECTIONS AND INFESTATIONS.....284
Viral infections.....288
Bacterial infections.....299
Protozoal and fungal infections.....305
Worm infestations.....310

SERIOUS INJURIES AND ENVIRONMENTAL DISORDERS.....314
Serious injuries.....316
Poisoning and environmental disorders.....321

SKIN, HAIR, AND NAILS.....328
Generalized skin conditions.....332
Localized skin conditions.....340
Skin infections and infestations.....351
Minor skin injuries.....356
Hair and nail disorders.....358

MUSCULOSKELETAL SYSTEM.....362
Bone disorders.....368
Joint and ligament disorders.....374
Muscle and tendon disorders.....388
Musculoskeletal injuries.....391

CARDIOVASCULAR SYSTEM.....396
Major cardiovascular disorders.....402
Heart rate and rhythm disorders.....415
Heart valve and muscle disorders.....421
Peripheral vascular disorders.....430

BLOOD AND THE LYMPHATIC AND IMMUNE SYSTEMS.....440
Blood disorders.....446
Disorders of the lymphatic system.....458
Immune disorders.....460
Allergies.....466

RESPIRATORY SYSTEM.....470
Nose and throat disorders.....474
Lung disorders.....482

NERVOUS SYSTEM AND MENTAL FUNCTION.....508
General nervous system disorders.....516
Disorders of the brain and spinal cord.....521
Peripheral nervous system disorders.....543
Mental health disorders.....551

EYES AND VISION.....566
Eye disorders.....570
Eyelid and tear system disorders.....583
Vision disorders.....586

EARS, HEARING, AND BALANCE.....592
Outer- and middle-ear disorders.....596
Hearing and inner-ear disorders.....599

TEETH AND GUMS.....606
Disorders of the teeth.....608
Gum disorders.....617

DIGESTIVE SYSTEM.....620
General digestive and nutritional problems.....626
Disorders of the mouth, tongue, and oesophagus.....632
Disorders of the stomach and duodenum.....639
Disorders of the liver, gallbladder, and pancreas.....643
Disorders of the intestines, rectum, and anus.....655

HORMONES AND METABOLISM.....670
Pituitary gland disorders.....676
Thyroid and parathyroid gland disorders.....679
Adrenal gland disorders.....684
Metabolic disorders.....687

URINARY SYSTEM.....694
Kidney disorders.....698
Disorders of the bladder and urethra.....709

MALE REPRODUCTIVE SYSTEM.....716
Disorders of the testes, scrotum, and penis.....718
Prostate disorders.....724
Male hormonal disorders.....728

FEMALE REPRODUCTIVE SYSTEM.....730
Menstrual, menopausal, and hormonal problems.....734
Disorders of the female reproductive organs.....741
Breast disorders.....754

SEX AND REPRODUCTION.....762
Sexually transmitted infections.....764
Sexual problems.....769
Infertility.....774

PREGNANCY AND CHILDBIRTH.....778
Problems in pregnancy.....784
Problems in labour.....800
Problems after childbirth.....806

INFANCY AND CHILDHOOD.....810
Problems in babies.....816
Chromosome and gene disorders.....821
Skin and hair disorders.....828
Musculoskeletal disorders.....832
Disorders of the cardiovascular and respiratory systems.....836
Disorders of the nervous system.....844
Developmental and psychological disorders.....851
Eye and ear disorders.....856
Disorders of the digestive system.....862
Endocrine and metabolic disorders.....866
Disorders of the reproductive and urinary systems.....870

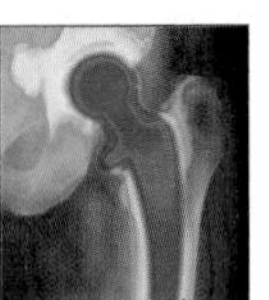

TREATING DISEASE
873–998

INTRODUCTION.....874

DRUG TREATMENT.....878
Understanding drugs.....880
Drugs for infections and infestations.....883
Drugs acting on the skin.....890
Drugs for musculoskeletal disorders.....894
Drugs for cardiovascular disorders.....897
Drugs for blood and immune system disorders and cancer.....903
Drugs for respiratory disorders.....909
Drugs acting on the brain and nervous system.....912
Drugs for eye and ear disorders.....919
Drugs for digestive disorders.....922
Vitamin and mineral supplements.....927
Drugs acting on the endocrine system and metabolism.....930
Drugs acting on the reproductive and urinary systems.....936

SURGERY.....940
Having an operation.....942
Types of surgery.....947

CARE AND THERAPIES.....954
Care of the sick.....956
Rehabilitation therapies.....961
Death and dying.....964
Psychological therapies.....968
Complementary therapies.....972

FIRST AID.....976
First-aid procedures.....978
Dressings and bandages.....996

DRUG GLOSSARY, USEFUL ONLINE SITES AND ADDRESSES, AND INDEX
999–1104

Drug glossary.....1000
Useful online sites and addresses.....1026
Index.....1038
Acknowledgments.....1103

HOW TO USE THIS BOOK

This book is arranged into thematic sections that deal with all aspects of health, disease, and medicine. The following pages explain this structure and supply detail on special features in each section. To locate a specific topic, use the contents list at the beginning of the book or the comprehensive index at the end, which direct you to sections, articles, boxes, and charts. Extensive cross-references in the text direct you to information on related topics and to carefully selected online sites giving further information to help you to manage your health.

STRUCTURE OF THE BOOK

HOW THE BOOK IS ORGANIZED

This book contains six sections. The first five are arranged around themes of health and disease and deal with a healthy lifestyle, symptoms, diagnosis, diseases, and treatments. The sixth section contains additional information and an index.

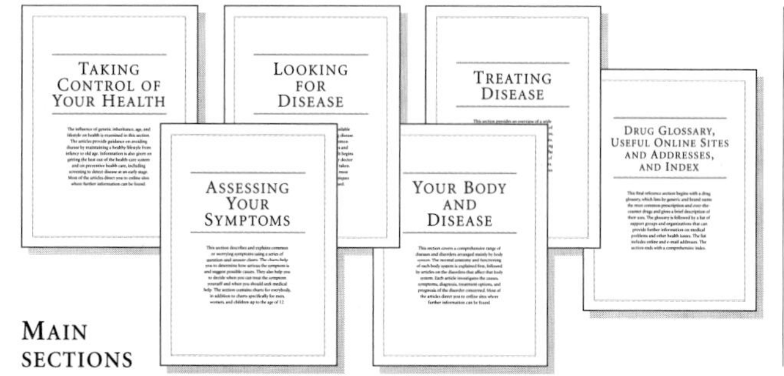

Arthritis Care
Online: www.arthritiscare.org.uk
18 Stephenson Way
London NW1 2HD
Tel: (020) 7916 1500
E-mail: info@arc.org.uk

Further information
The final section has a drug glossary, a list of useful online sites and addresses, and an index.

HOW EACH SECTION IS ORGANIZED

Each section has an introduction and contains two or more subsections with their own introductions. The subsections cover their subjects in a series of articles, which are accompanied by feature boxes that highlight and illustrate key information.

Section opener
A single page at the beginning of each section displays the section title

Section introduction
These pages provide an overview of the entire contents of the section

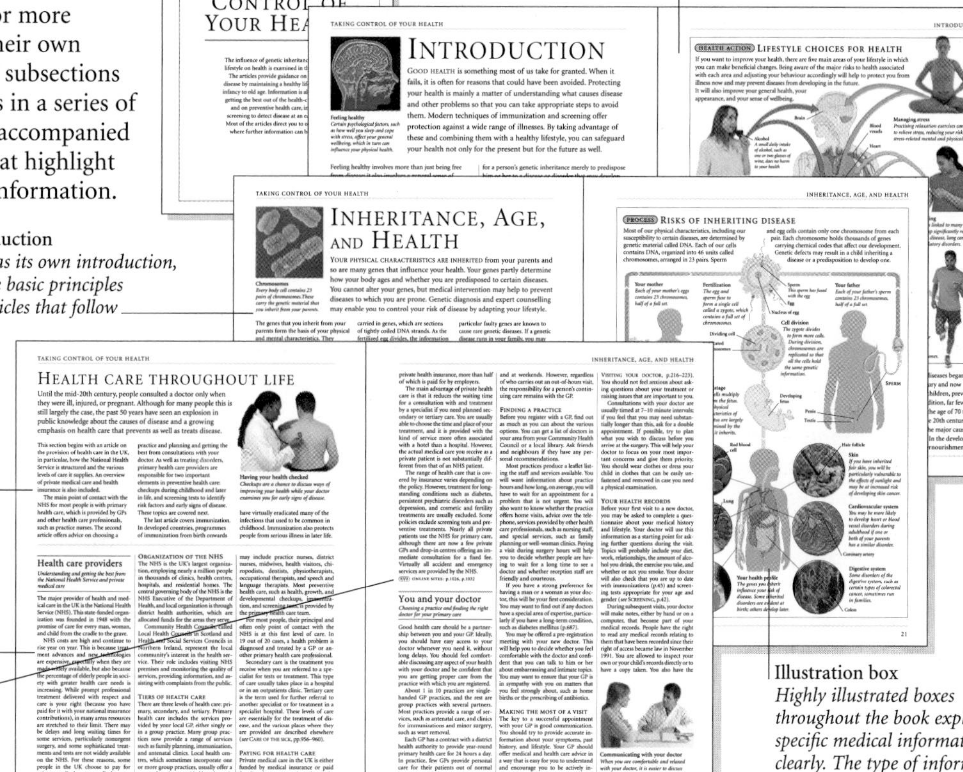

Subsection introduction
Each subsection has its own introduction, which explains the basic principles underlying the articles that follow

Articles introduction
The articles in each subsection are outlined in a brief introduction, which may provide cross-references to related subsections

Article
Each article deals with a specific subject, such as a disease, a type of drug, or another aspect of health care

Online symbol
Articles that end with this symbol direct you to useful online sites and addresses listed at the back of the book

Illustration box
Highly illustrated boxes throughout the book explain specific medical information clearly. The type of information in each box is indicated by a label in the top left corner

WHAT EACH SECTION CONTAINS

TAKING CONTROL OF YOUR HEALTH

Articles in this section help you to assess your current and potential health status by looking at aspects of your genetic inheritance and lifestyle. The articles also examine the influence of aging and environment on health. In addition, this section provides guidance on following a healthy lifestyle as well as information on certain other preventive health-care measures, such as immunization and screening programmes.

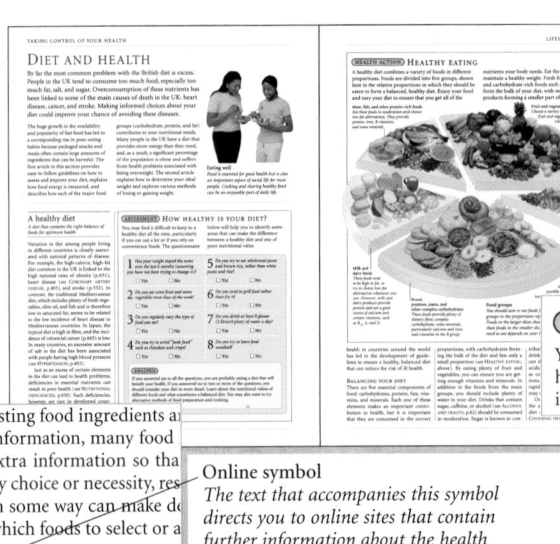

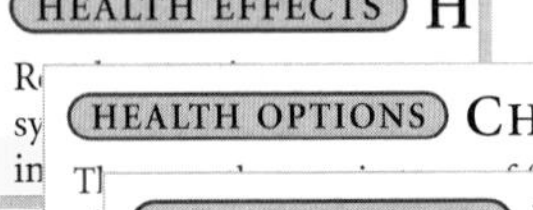

Feature boxes
Boxes in this section have various roles, including: helping you to assess your health; looking at the effects of lifestyle on health; presenting health-maintenance options; and focusing on practical action that you can take to improve your health

Online symbol
The text that accompanies this symbol directs you to online sites that contain further information about the health issue in which you are interested

ASSESSING YOUR SYMPTOMS

In this section, 70 charts cover the most common symptoms experienced by men, women, and children. Each chart focuses on one main symptom, explores possible causes, and advises on whether you should use self-help measures or seek medical help. For detailed instructions on how to use the charts, *see* p.90.

Colour-coding
The charts are grouped in four colour-coded sections, which respectively contain charts that apply to everyone, to men, to women, and to children

Questions and answers
Each chart contains a series of questions. Your answers to these lead you from a starting point to a finishing point, where you will be advised on what action to take

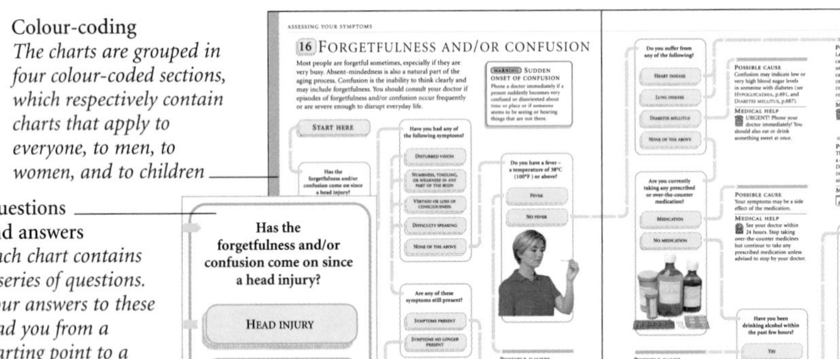

LOOKING FOR DISEASE

This section explains the principles of commonly used screening and diagnostic tests and investigations, including laboratory tests and techniques for looking inside the human body, such as endoscopy and scanning. The method used in each test or investigation is explained and illustrated.

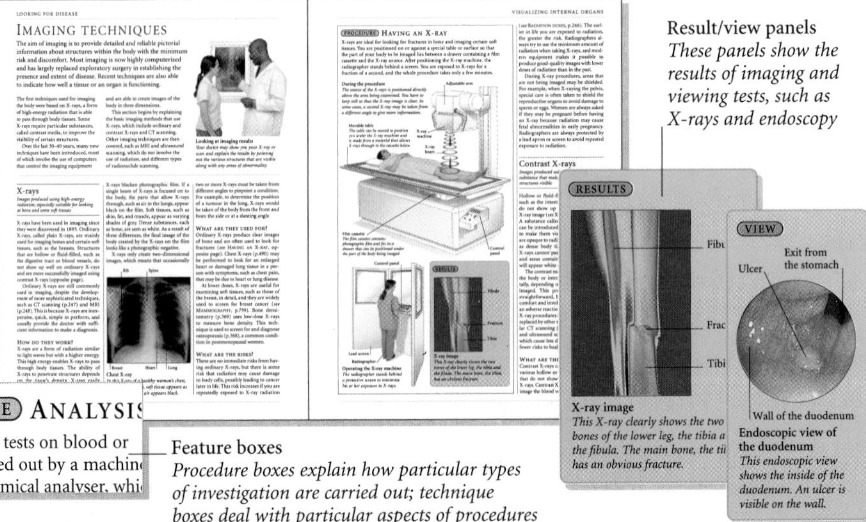

X-ray image
This X-ray clearly shows the two bones of the lower leg, the tibia a the fibula. The main bone, the ti has an obvious fracture.

Endoscopic view of the duodenum
This endoscopic view shows the inside of the duodenum. An ulcer is visible on the wall.

PROCEDURE H
X-rays are ideal for lo
tissues. You are positi
the part of your body to be image

Result/view panels
These panels show the results of imaging and viewing tests, such as X-rays and endoscopy

Feature boxes
Procedure boxes explain how particular types of investigation are carried out; technique boxes deal with particular aspects of procedures

YOUR BODY AND DISEASE

This section examines more than 750 disorders, ranging from minor conditions, such as warts, to serious diseases, such as lung cancer. The section contains 21 subsections, generally arranged by body system. There are special subsections on genetic disorders, cancer, infections and infestations, serious injuries, disorders during pregnancy and childbirth, and disorders in infants and children.

ANATOMY AND PHYSIOLOGY INTRODUCTIONS

These highly illustrated subsection introductions explain the normal anatomy (structure) and physiology (function) of a particular body system. They both stand on their own as detailed guides to the body and provide background information to the disorders considered in the articles that follow them.

Photographic detail
Magnified photographs show the detailed structure of crucial parts of the anatomy

Overview illustration
Large illustrations identify the main anatomical components of each body system

Location
Where useful, the location in the body of various parts of the anatomy is illustrated

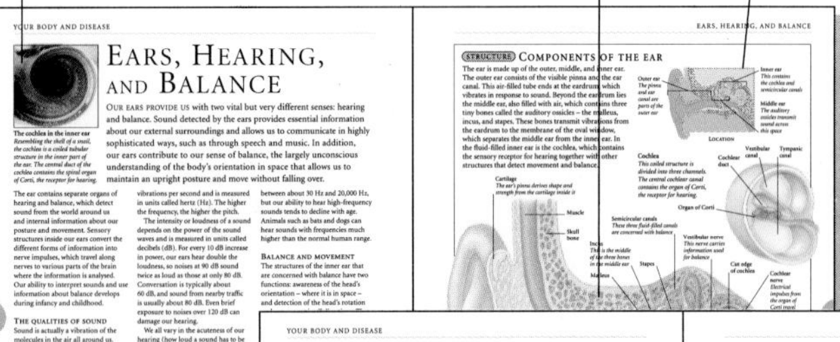

Detail illustration
The structure and function of each main anatomical component of the body system is illustrated and explained

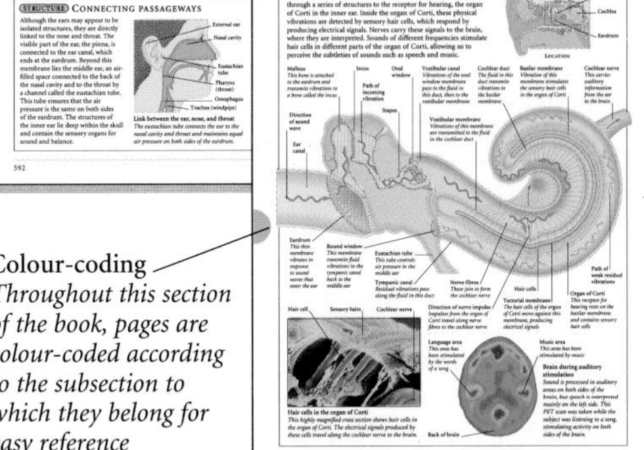

Colour-coding
Throughout this section of the book, pages are colour-coded according to the subsection to which they belong for easy reference

DISORDER ARTICLES

Each article covers the causes and symptoms of a disorder, the methods used to diagnose it, treatment choices, and the likely prognosis. Particular factors that either increase the risk of developing the disorder or are not significant are listed for each article.

Key anatomy
The key parts of the anatomy affected by the disorders covered in each group of articles are clearly illustrated

Online symbol
Text accompanying this symbol, at the end of an article, cross-refers you to online sites giving information on the disorder covered in that article

with a probe or suction device ear may be gently flushed o warm water from a syringe. Wa age sometimes recurs after treat
(WWW) ONLINE SITES: p.1031

Risk factor information
Factors that increase the risk of developing a particular disorder are highlighted at the beginning of each article. When factors are variable or not significant, this is also indicated

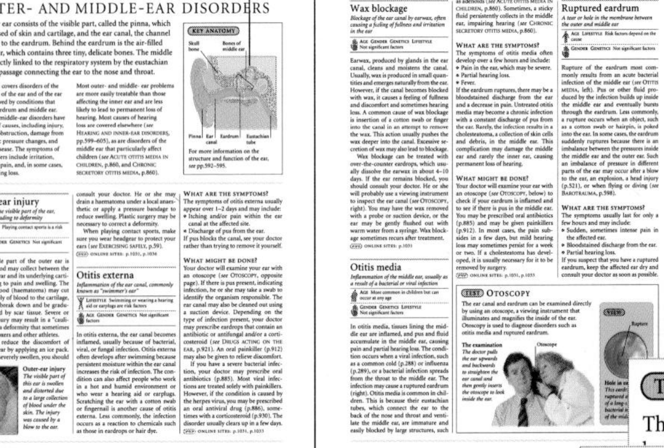

Feature boxes
Test boxes explain and illustrate particular test procedures; self-help boxes detail measures that you can take at home; treatment boxes describe and illustrate how a treatment for a particular disorder is carried out

(TEST) OTOSCOPY
The ear canal and eardrum car

(SELF-HELP) PROTEC
Excessive noise can damage the

(TREATMENT) STAPED
This operation is carried out t a disorder in which the stapes becomes immobilized by bony hearing loss. Under local or ge of the stapes are removed and

Age symbol
Any ages at which a disease or disorder is more likely to develop are listed here

AGE

Gender symbol
Text accompanying this symbol tells you if a disorder affects only or mostly males or females

GEN

Genetics symbol
Text accompanying this symbol indicates if a disease or disorder has an inherited component

GEN

Lifestyle symbol
Lifestyle factors that may increase the risk of developing a condition are listed here

LIF be s

Variable risk factors symbol
When a condition has various forms or causes, this symbol indicates that risk factors depend on the cause or type of disorder

Not significant symbol
If age, gender, genetics, or lifestyle are not risk factors for a condition, they are listed here

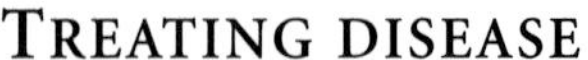

TREATING DISEASE

This section gives an overview of patient care and the wide range of medical treatments in current use, including drugs, surgery, and various therapies. The final part of the section covers the main first-aid techniques.

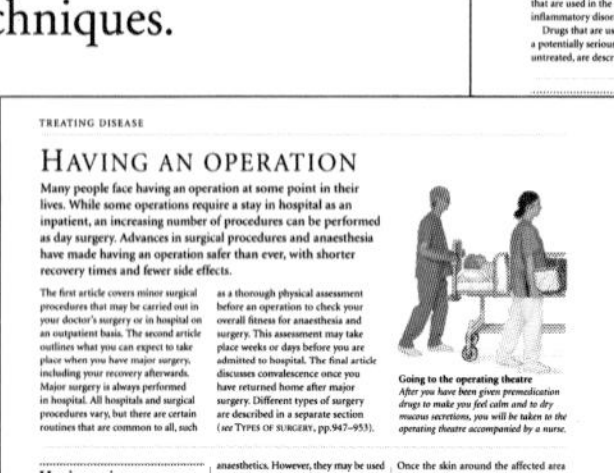

SURGERY

These articles describe the experience of having an operation, including preparations for surgery and postoperative care. They also explain how types of surgery work.

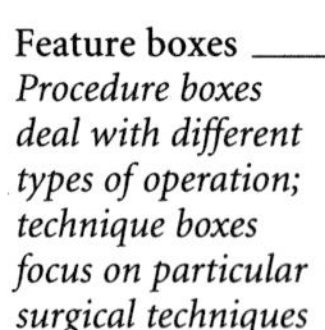

Feature boxes
Procedure boxes deal with different types of operation; technique boxes focus on particular surgical techniques

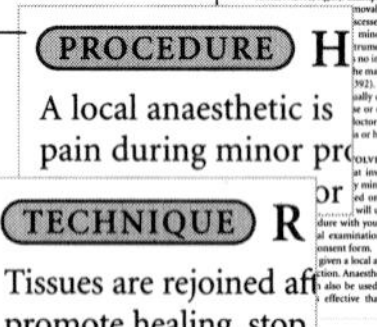

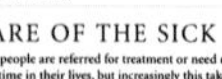

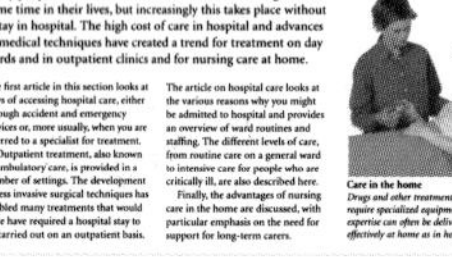

CARE AND THERAPIES

This part of the treatments section covers different types of care, from critical care to home nursing. It also looks at rehabilitation, psychological, and complementary therapies.

Online symbol
Articles in the surgery and care and therapies sections that finish with this symbol direct you to online sites

FIRST AID

These articles tell you what to do in an emergency. They illustrate the general principles of first aid for a range of injuries and disorders and list the essential components of a first-aid kit for the home.

Warning box
These boxes detail key information that should be read before using certain first-aid techniques

DRUGS

Each article deals with a group of drugs, such as antibiotics. Articles are grouped by the body system or the type of disorder the drugs are used to treat.

Warning boxes
Precautions that apply when using certain drugs, and situations in which certain drugs should not be used, are detailed here

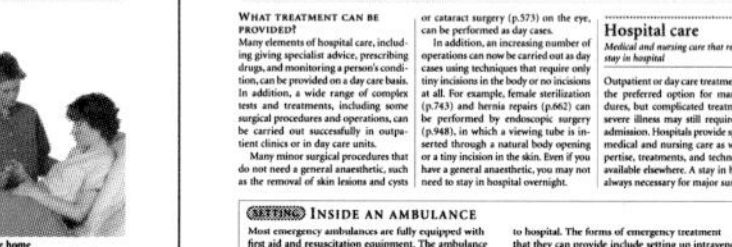

Feature boxes
Drug action boxes illustrate how particular drugs work; self-administration boxes give instructions on how to take certain drugs

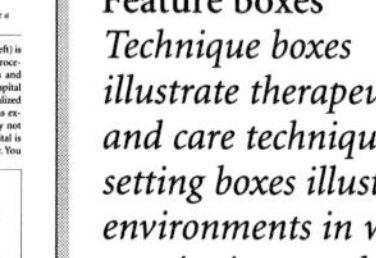

Feature boxes
Technique boxes illustrate therapeutic and care techniques; setting boxes illustrate environments in which care is given, such as inside an ambulance

Feature boxes
Technique boxes look at techniques that are needed in many first aid situations; special case boxes outline variations on certain techniques that may be used when treating particular injuries

DRUG GLOSSARY, ONLINE SITES, AND INDEX

This final section of the book provides additional information, including a drug glossary and a list of organizations that provide information related to medical conditions. The section ends with a comprehensive index.

DRUG GLOSSARY

This glossary provides a guide to many common prescription and over-the-counter drugs.

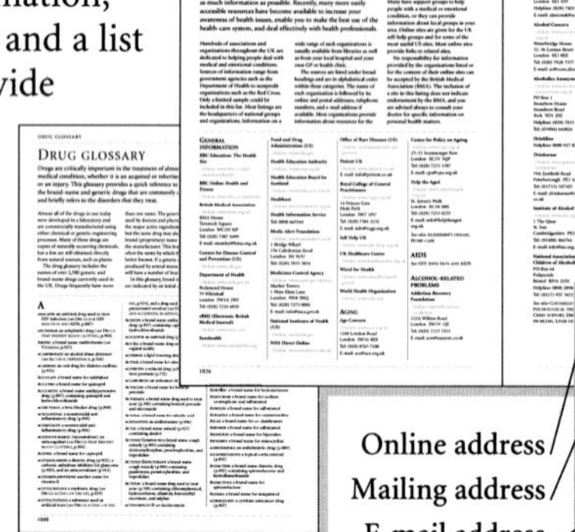

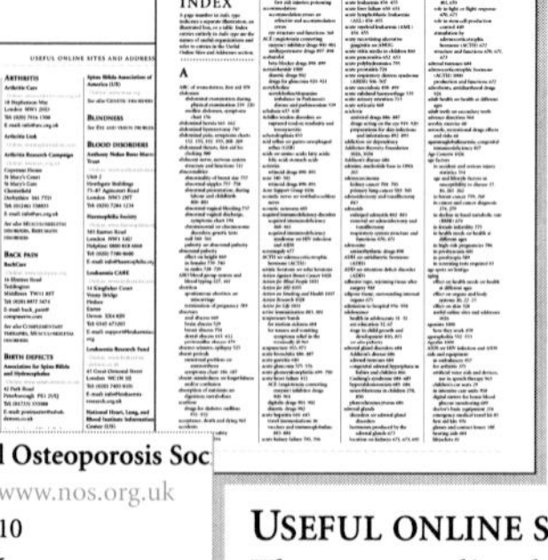

Online address
Mailing address
E-mail address

INDEX

This detailed 65-page index contains 13,000 entries and lists all the book's articles, feature boxes, and illustrations.

USEFUL ONLINE SITES AND ADDRESSES

These pages list the contact addresses of organizations that provide further information about specific medical conditions and other health issues.

Taking Control of Your Health

The influence of genetic inheritance, age, and lifestyle on health is examined in this section. The articles provide guidance on avoiding disease by maintaining a healthy lifestyle from infancy to old age. Information is also given on getting the best out of the health-care system and on preventive health care, including screening to detect disease at an early stage. Most of the articles direct you to online sites where further information can be found.

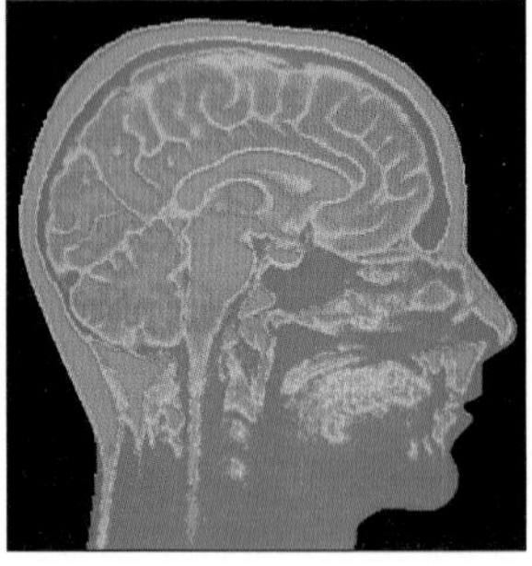

Feeling healthy
Certain psychological factors, such as how well you sleep and cope with stress, affect your general wellbeing, which in turn can influence your physical health.

INTRODUCTION

GOOD HEALTH is something most of us take for granted. When it fails, it is often for reasons that could have been avoided. Protecting your health is mainly a matter of understanding what causes disease and other problems so that you can take appropriate steps to avoid them. Modern techniques of immunization and screening offer protection against a wide range of illnesses. By taking advantage of these and combining them with a healthy lifestyle, you can safeguard your health not only for the present but for the future as well.

Feeling healthy involves more than just being free from disease; it also involves a general sense of wellbeing. Your health and wellbeing depend in part on factors that are often beyond your control, such as the amount of pollution in your environment and the security of your employment. However, there are many aspects of your lifestyle that you can change or adapt to improve your physical and mental health and reduce your chance of becoming ill. This part of the book explores a number of strategies that help you to take control of your health. It also explains the health-care system in the UK and screening programmes that help to identify potential health problems.

WHAT DETERMINES HEALTH?

Your health is partly determined by your genes, but it is also inextricably linked with your environment and lifestyle. Your chance of developing many diseases is determined at the moment of conception by the mix of genetic material that you inherit from your parents. If you inherit a specific faulty gene, such as the gene that causes cystic fibrosis, this will inevitably lead to the development of a disease. However, it is more common for a person's genetic inheritance merely to predispose him or her to a disease or disorder that may develop later in life, such as diabetes mellitus.

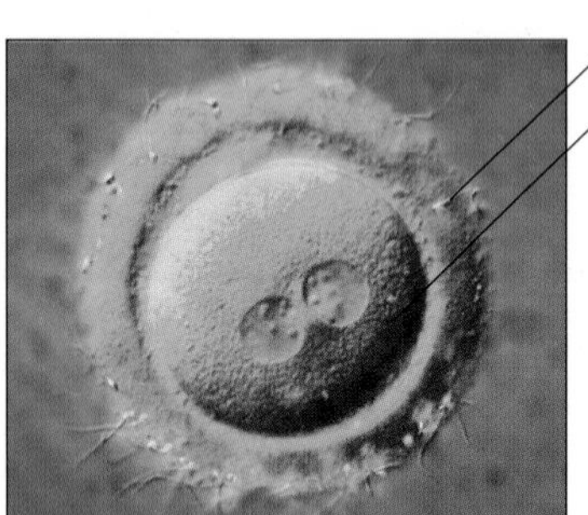

The moment of conception
Your susceptibility to many diseases is programmed at conception when the sperm and egg cells fuse, bringing together half a set of genes from each parent.

Even if you are genetically susceptible to a disease, your chance of developing it can be influenced by a number of other factors, many of which are related to the way you live. For example, lifestyle factors such as diet, exercise, smoking, and alcohol consumption are important determinants of health. If you adopt a healthy lifestyle and have appropriate screening tests, you may be able to reduce your risk of developing the diseases that are common in your family.

Your environment can also influence your health and susceptibility to certain diseases. For example, living at high altitudes where the atmosphere is thinner may pose problems for people who have respiratory diseases. In towns and cities, high levels of atmospheric pollution may worsen the symptoms of respiratory diseases such as asthma. Regardless of where you live, excessive exposure to the sun for even short periods of time increases the risk of skin cancer.

Other determinants of health include age, gender, ethnicity, and occupation. For example, the risk of heart disease increases with age and is more common in men, Asian people, and people with sedentary jobs.

ARE PEOPLE GETTING HEALTHIER?

At the beginning of the 20th century, many people died before they reached the age of 50, and a large number of deaths occurred in childhood. Most people now survive well into adulthood, and the average life

HEALTH ACTION LIFESTYLE CHOICES FOR HEALTH

If you want to improve your health, there are five main areas of your lifestyle in which you can make beneficial changes. Being aware of the major risks to health associated with each area and adjusting your behaviour accordingly will help to protect you from illness now and may prevent diseases from developing in the future. It will also improve your general health, your appearance, and your sense of wellbeing.

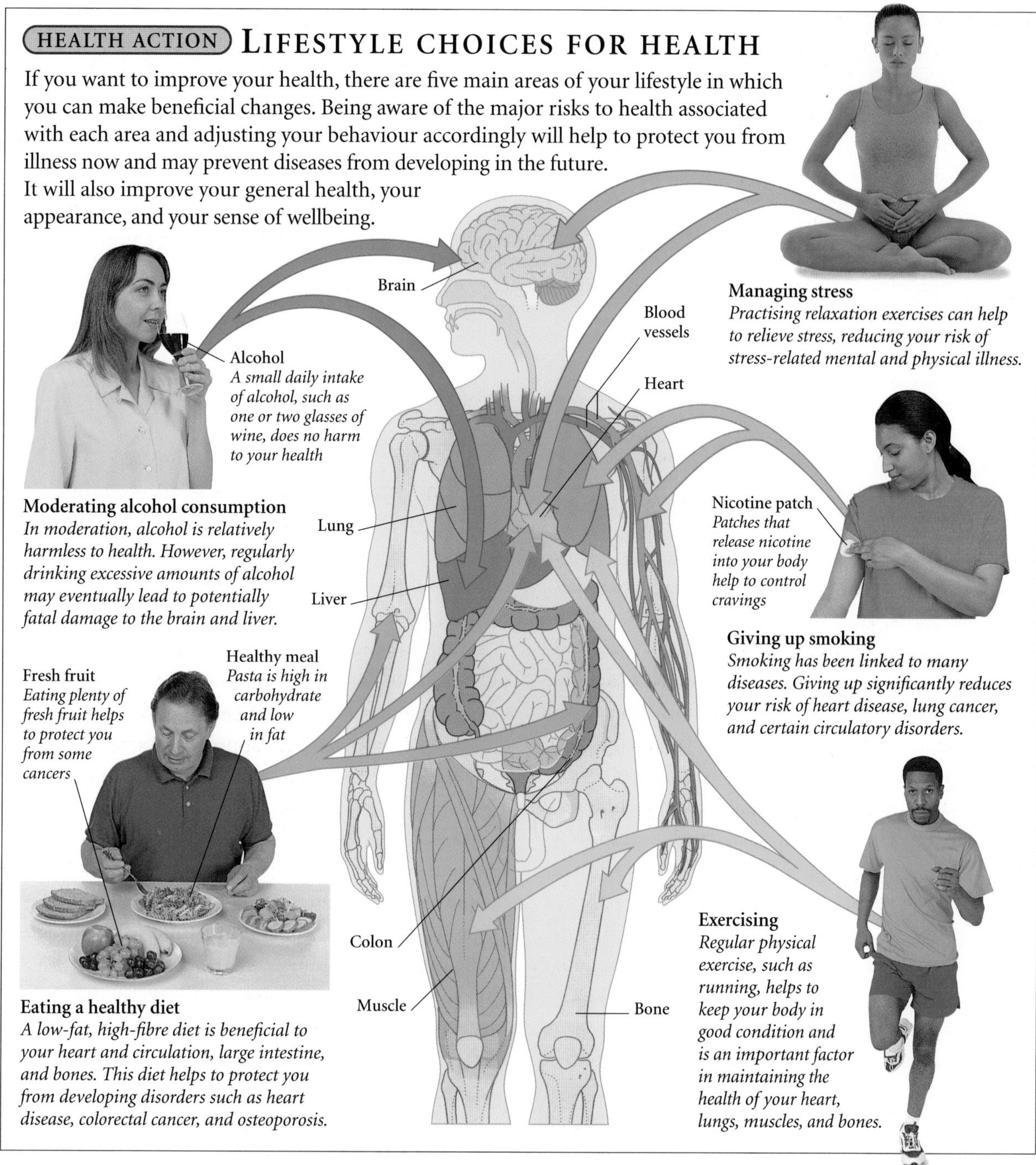

Managing stress
Practising relaxation exercises can help to relieve stress, reducing your risk of stress-related mental and physical illness.

Moderating alcohol consumption
In moderation, alcohol is relatively harmless to health. However, regularly drinking excessive amounts of alcohol may eventually lead to potentially fatal damage to the brain and liver.

Giving up smoking
Smoking has been linked to many diseases. Giving up significantly reduces your risk of heart disease, lung cancer, and certain circulatory disorders.

Eating a healthy diet
A low-fat, high-fibre diet is beneficial to your heart and circulation, large intestine, and bones. This diet helps to protect you from developing disorders such as heart disease, colorectal cancer, and osteoporosis.

Exercising
Regular physical exercise, such as running, helps to keep your body in good condition and is an important factor in maintaining the health of your heart, lungs, muscles, and bones.

expectancy for a child born in the UK today is over 74 years. A man who has reached the age of 70 can expect to live to the age of 81 or more, and a woman of 70 to live to at least the age of 84. Life expectancy began to rise towards the end of the 19th century as improvements in nutrition and public hygiene took effect. The discovery of antibiotics in the first half of the 20th century further increased life expectancy by reducing deaths caused by infection. Immunization programmes for many infectious diseases began around the middle of the last century and now protect 80 per cent of the world's children, preventing millions of deaths each year. In addition, far fewer adults become seriously ill before the age of 70 than was the case at the beginning of the 20th century.

However, as people live longer, the major causes of ill health and death have changed. In the developed world, infectious disease and undernourishment have

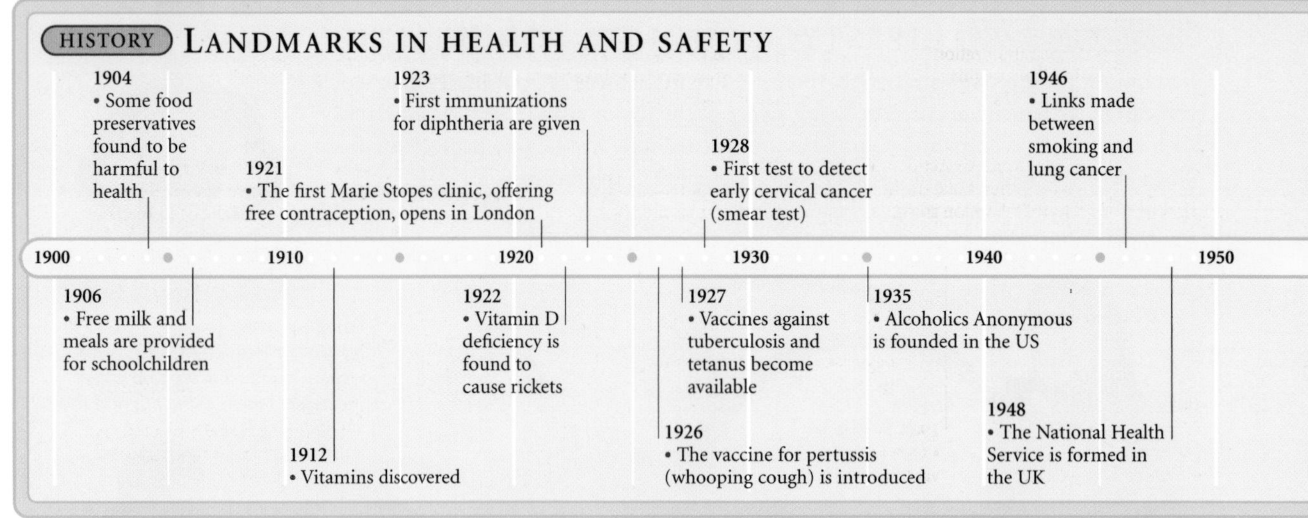

Advances in prevention and protection
A better understanding of the mechanisms of disease led to the discovery that lifestyle factors such as smoking and a high-fat diet contribute to major illnesses. The response was an emphasis on people living healthily to reduce their chance of disease and safety legislations and immunizations to protect the population.

been superseded by heart disease, cancer, stroke, and smoking-related lung disease. Factors such as a high-fat diet and a sedentary lifestyle contribute to many of these disorders and are strongly associated with the way people live in an affluent society. Another major cause of death and disability in developed countries is accidents, particularly traffic accidents.

Disorders such as poor vision, deafness, arthritis, and loss of memory, tend to develop with increasing age. Although people enjoy more years of good health than formerly, elderly people can still expect a period of on average 10 years of disability from mental or physical illness. As more people live beyond the age of 80, this period of impaired health is likely to lengthen.

Assessing your health

To understand your inheritance and reduce your risk of disease, you need to know as much as possible about conditions that run in your family. There may be certain disorders, especially types of cancer or heart disease, that have occurred in several family members under the age of 50. You can create a family medical tree of disorders that run in your family and then discuss them with your doctor. He or she will check your state of health and advise you about changes to your lifestyle, such as cutting down on high-fat foods or taking more exercise, that help to reduce your risk of developing these diseases.

At certain times in your life, particularly as you get older, you will be offered screening tests for early signs of diseases, such as breast cancer or glaucoma. Your doctor may suggest extra screening to detect at an early stage any disorders that run in your family.

Choosing a healthy lifestyle

In recent years, there has been clear evidence that people can reduce their susceptibility to disease by targeting unhealthy aspects of their lifestyle. The fall in the numbers of deaths before the age of 65 from stroke, coronary artery disease, and certain types of cancer in the past 20 years has been largely attributed

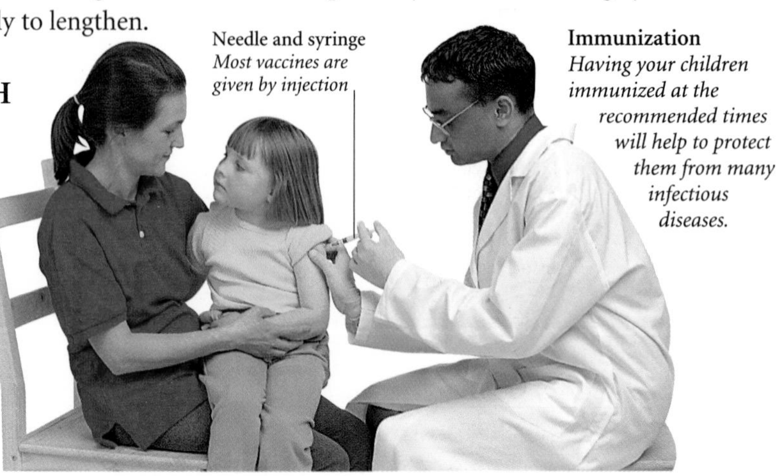

Needle and syringe
Most vaccines are given by injection

Immunization
Having your children immunized at the recommended times will help to protect them from many infectious diseases.

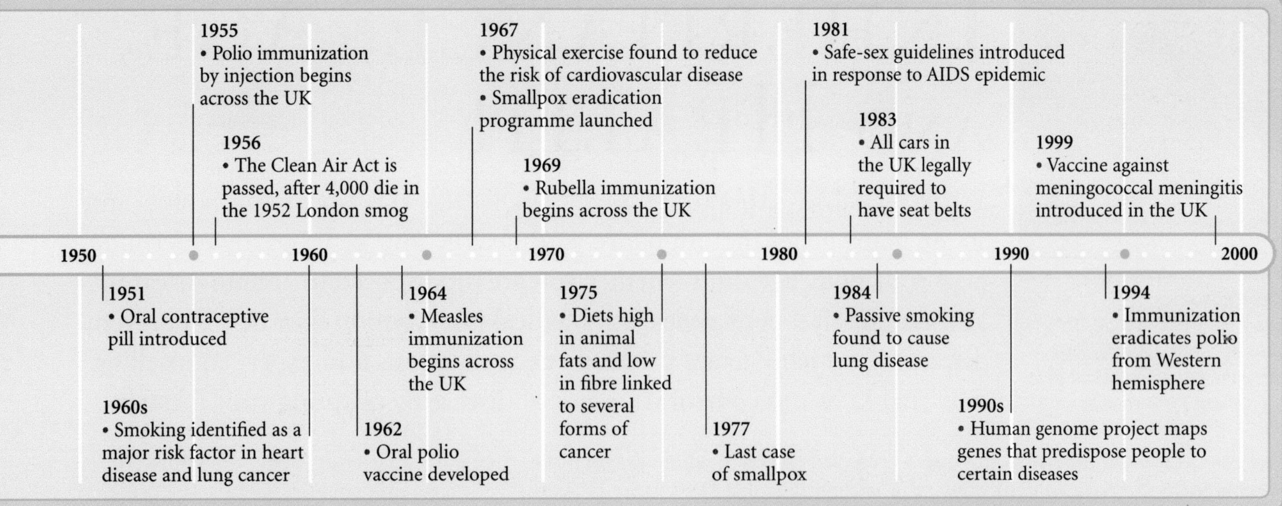

to a fall in the number of smokers and a better understanding of what makes a healthy diet. By contrast, the strains of modern living, such as the break-up of relationships, long working hours in stressful jobs, and loss of contact with family and friends, can affect mental and physical wellbeing.

Nearly everyone is aware of the features that make up a healthy lifestyle, but too few people manage to act on this information. By adopting a healthy diet, exercising regularly, not smoking, and limiting your alcohol intake, you can bring about an almost instant improvement in your general health and reduce the risk of diseases developing in the future. You will also find that you look and feel better.

Unhealthy habits can be difficult to break, especially if they do not seem to cause immediate damage to your health. Committing yourself to long-term changes such as giving up smoking or losing weight takes considerable willpower; you may find it easier if you seek support from family and friends. You will benefit whatever your age because it is never too late to make lifestyle changes to improve your health.

ORGANIZATION — HOW THIS PART OF THE BOOK IS ORGANIZED

This part of the book begins by looking at how your genetic inheritance influences your health and risk of disease and the way in which your health priorities change with increasing age. Whatever your genetic inheritance or age, changing certain aspects of your lifestyle can have a significant effect on your health and wellbeing and reduce your risk of disease. Practical guidance is given on how to make health-promoting changes to your lifestyle.

INHERITANCE, AGE, AND HEALTH p.20
How genetic make-up influences health and health priorities change with age.

Understanding inheritance p.24
How your genetic background causes or increases the risk of certain disorders.

Health at different ages p.27
How health risks and priorities change over your lifetime.

Health care throughout life p.38
Using the health service and finding a GP plus screening tests and immunizations.

LIFESTYLE AND HEALTH p.46
The influence that various lifestyle factors have on your health and wellbeing.

Diet and health p.48
Advice on the foods that make up a healthy diet, understanding food labelling, and controlling your weight.

Exercise and health p.55
The health benefits of exercise, choosing an exercise plan, and exercising safely.

Alcohol, tobacco, and drugs p.62
The effects on health of smoking, alcohol, and the use of recreational drugs.

Sex and health p.67
The positive health benefits of sexual relationships plus guides to safe sex and different forms of contraception.

Psychological health p.72
Lifestyle factors that affect psychological health, particularly the influence of stress on health, advice on sleeping well, and coping with loss and bereavement.

Safety and health p.77
Safety in a variety of environments: at home, at work, on the roads, around water, and on holiday, as well as guidelines for travel immunizations.

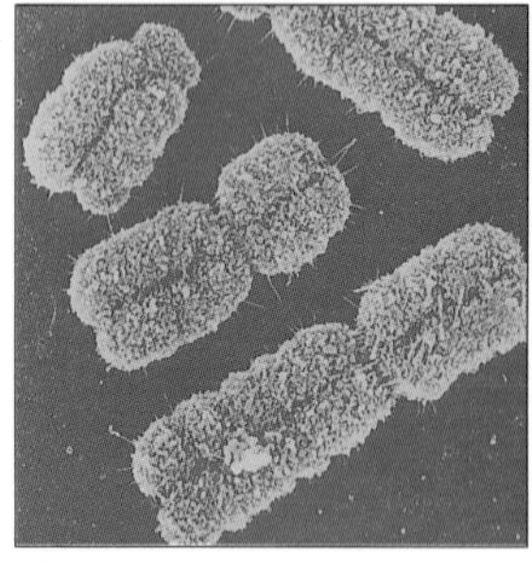

Chromosomes
Every body cell contains 23 pairs of chromosomes. These carry the genetic material that you inherit from your parents.

INHERITANCE, AGE, AND HEALTH

YOUR PHYSICAL CHARACTERISTICS ARE INHERITED from your parents and so are many genes that influence your health. Your genes partly determine how your body ages and whether you are predisposed to certain diseases. You cannot alter your genes, but medical intervention may help to prevent diseases to which you are prone. Genetic diagnosis and expert counselling may enable you to control your risk of disease by adapting your lifestyle.

The genes that you inherit from your parents form the basis of your physical and mental characteristics. They determine many aspects of your appearance, such as the colour of your eyes and hair. They direct the striking bodily changes that are brought about by growth and aging, noticeably during infancy and puberty. Genes also affect your body chemistry, which may influence your risk of disease.

YOUR INHERITANCE

At conception, the fertilized egg, or zygote, is a single cell that contains all the information necessary to make a new human being. This information is unique to each individual and is carried in genes, which are sections of tightly coiled DNA strands. As the fertilized egg divides, the information is duplicated so that a copy exists in every cell of the growing baby's body.

There are about 35,000 pairs of genes in each body cell, but only certain ones are active, depending on the cell's specialized function. Genes direct the activity of every cell by controlling the production of proteins. For example, some genes are responsible for the production of proteins that cause cells to form tissues, such as skin, hair, and muscle; others give rise to proteins that control body organs or fight infection.

Faulty genes may cause an organ to develop or function abnormally, and particular faulty genes are known to cause rare genetic diseases. If a genetic disease runs in your family, you may decide to have tests to find out if you have inherited the faulty gene. More common disorders, such as heart disease, have also been shown to have a genetic component. Screening tests to detect these diseases early on are particularly important if your family history suggests that you are at risk.

CHANGING HEALTH NEEDS

As you age and pass through distinct life stages, your body's needs and your health concerns change accordingly. For example, infants need high-energy diets to promote rapid growth, whereas elderly people require less energy and eat proportionately less.

Young adults are most at risk from accidents, but later in life people are increasingly susceptible to degenerative disease as the functioning of their body organs and major body systems gradually declines. Natural healing processes also tend to become less efficient as the immune system's resistance to disease is reduced with age. The body's systems tend to age at different rates and are affected by genetic and lifestyle factors that vary from one person to the next.

Although life expectancy has risen dramatically in the UK over the past century (*see* LENGTHENING LIVES, left), your personal good health throughout life and during old age is inevitably the result of the genes you have inherited and the way you live your life.

DATA LENGTHENING LIVES

In the UK during the last 100 years, life expectancy has risen dramatically due to improvements in nutrition, sanitation, and health care. As a result, the proportion of older people in the population has grown. This trend has led to changing demands on the health-care system because there are now more people experiencing long-term illness and the effects of aging.

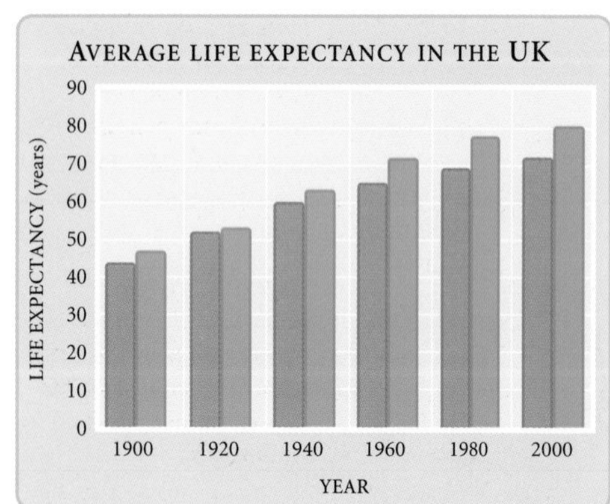

Life expectancy
At the beginning of the 20th century, average life expectancy at birth in the UK was only about 45 years. One hundred years later, it has risen by two-thirds to about 75 years. Females continue to live longer than males.

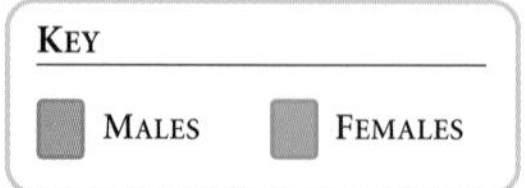

(PROCESS) RISKS OF INHERITING DISEASE

Most of our physical characteristics, including our susceptibility to certain diseases, are determined by genetic material called DNA. Each of our cells contains DNA, organized into 46 units called chromosomes, arranged in 23 pairs. Sperm and egg cells contain only one chromosome from each pair. Each chromosome holds thousands of genes carrying chemical codes that affect our development. Genetic defects may result in a child inheriting a disease or a predisposition to develop one.

Your mother
Each of your mother's eggs contains 23 chromosomes, half of a full set.

Fertilization
The egg and sperm fuse to form a single cell called a zygote, which contains a full set of chromosomes.

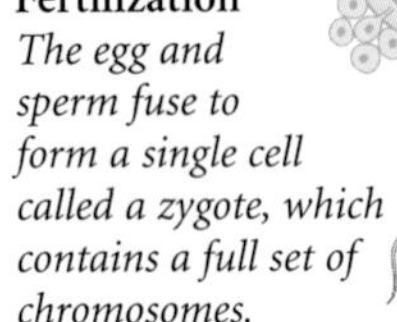

Your father
Each of your father's sperm contains 23 chromosomes, half of a full set.

Cell division
The zygote divides to form more cells. During division, chromosomes are replicated so that all the cells hold the same genetic information.

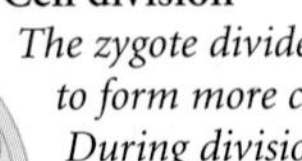

Fetal stage
The cells multiply to form the fetus. The physical characteristics of the fetus are largely determined by the genes it inherits.

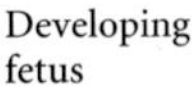

Blood
Some blood disorders are inherited. These include thalassaemia, which affects the ability of red blood cells to carry oxygen, and haemophilia, which affects blood clotting.

Red blood cell

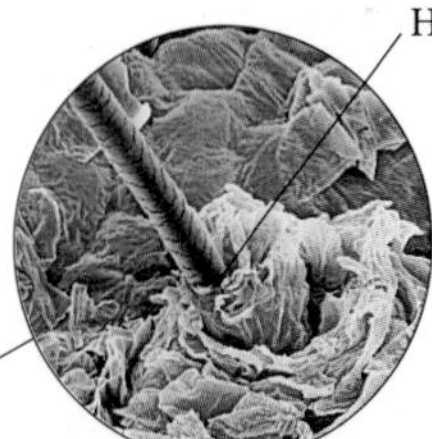

Skin
If you have inherited fair skin, you will be particularly vulnerable to the effects of sunlight and may be at increased risk of developing skin cancer.

Respiratory system
You are more likely to develop an allergic breathing disorder, such as asthma, if either of your parents has asthma, hay fever, or eczema.

Lung

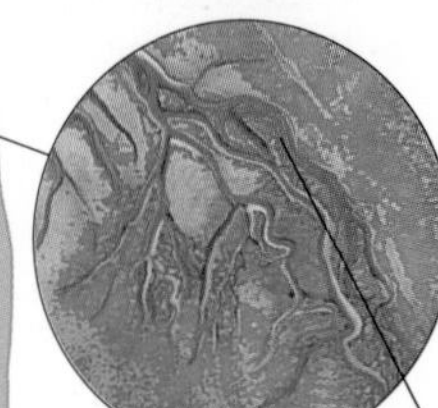

Cardiovascular system
You may be more likely to develop heart or blood vessel disorders during adulthood if one or both of your parents has a similar disorder.

Joints
Many joint disorders, such as osteoarthritis and rheumatoid arthritis, have an inherited element, but do not usually develop until adulthood.

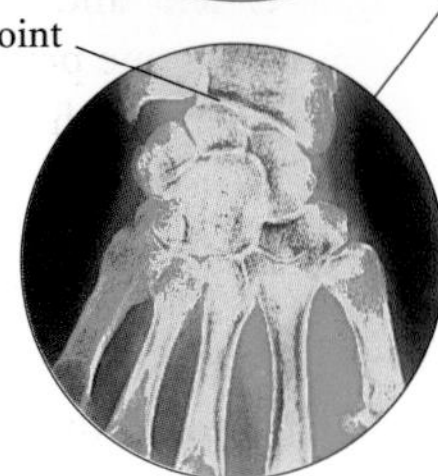

Your health profile
The genes you inherit influence your risk of disease. Some inherited disorders are evident at birth; others develop later.

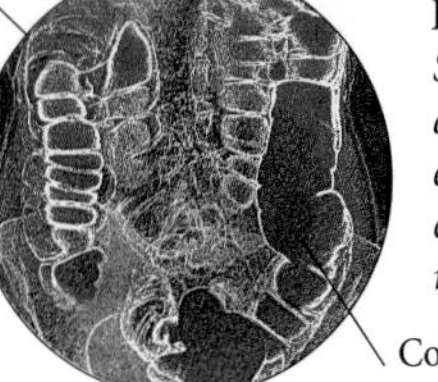

Digestive system
Some disorders of the digestive system, such as certain types of colorectal cancer, sometimes run in families.

PROCESS GROWTH AND AGING

The process of growth begins in the developing embryo and continues throughout childhood until early adulthood. By adulthood, the organs have fully developed, and the individual is capable of having children. After a peak at around the age of 30, the functioning of almost every body system gradually begins to decline. The rate of decline and its consequences for the individual are determined by a complex interaction of genetic characteristics and lifestyle factors. The chart below describes some specific changes that occur in the body's organs during each life stage.

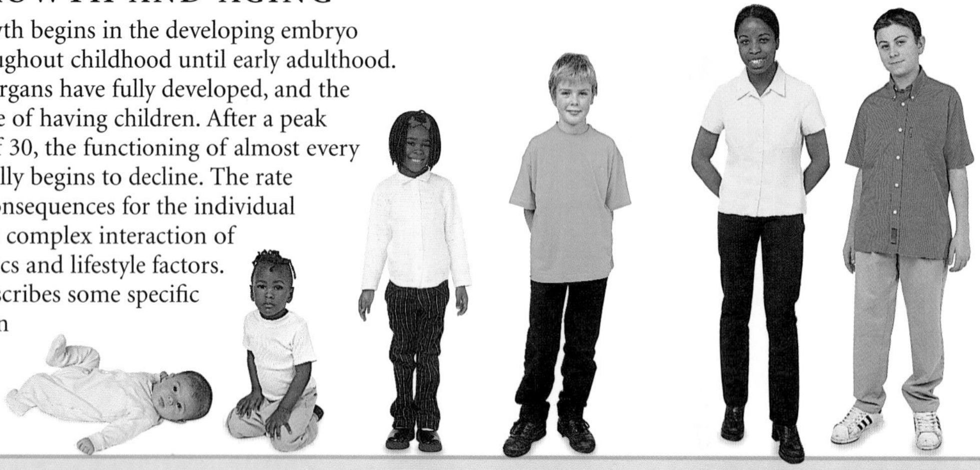

Body System	Birth–1 year	1–12 years	12–18 years
Bones, muscles, and joints	• Long bones are two-thirds cartilage at birth but gradually become harder. • Muscles gradually become able to support body weight.	• During childhood, bones grow larger and stronger as areas of cartilage are gradually replaced by bone, which is harder.	• Bone growth stops when all the cartilage has been replaced by bone. • By the age of 18, muscles have become fully developed.
Digestive organs and daily energy needs	• Newborns digest only liquids, then semi-solid food at about 4 months. • A high-energy diet is needed to provide energy for rapid growth.	• Digestive system is now mature and child can digest most foods. • Energy needs decrease because rate of growth slows after the age of 1.	• Adolescents need a balanced diet that is high in energy to fuel rapid growth; boys need more energy from food than girls.
Brain and nerves	• All nerve cells are present at birth; nerve connections continue to form. • A newborn baby has several basic reflexes, such as sucking.	• Connections between nerve cells develop fastest before the age of 6 enabling walking, talking, and bowel and bladder control by the age of 3.	• By 18 years, the nervous system is fully developed; intellectual abilities are still developing. Puberty signals major psychological changes.
Eyes and ears	• By 4 months, an infant can see a full range of colours and shades. • By 6 months, an infant can distinguish voices from other noises.	• Vision becomes sharper and hearing becomes more acute as nerve connections continue to form up until the age of 7.	• Shortsightedness, which is often inherited, tends to become apparent in adolescence.
Heart and blood vessels	• A newborn baby has a relatively fast resting heart rate of about 120 beats per minute; this rate will gradually decrease.	• Resting heart rate continues to slow down as a child grows older.	• Average resting heart rate is about 60–80 beats per minute; the rate is slowest in people who are athletic and physically fit.
Lungs and airways	• The trachea (windpipe) is softer and more easily compressed in a newborn baby than in an adult. A baby takes 40–50 breaths a minute.	• As the lungs mature during childhood, breathing rate decreases. • In children under the age of 5, airways are small and easily irritated.	• As the lungs become more efficient at taking in oxygen, the average breathing rate falls to 12–15 breaths a minute by adulthood.
Reproductive organs	• Ovaries contain over one million eggs at birth, and testes contain primitive sperm, which mature at puberty.	• At puberty, hormonal changes stimulate sexual development. Puberty begins in girls from the age of 10 and in boys from the age of 12 onwards.	• Most adolescents have reached sexual maturity by the age of 18.
Urinary organs	• Blood flow to the kidneys is low in the first few months, creating a potential risk of a build-up of toxins normally excreted by the kidneys.	• Urine becomes more concentrated as the kidneys become more efficient at retaining water needed by the body.	• No significant changes.
Skin, hair, and teeth	• First primary teeth appear: lower central incisors erupt at 6–10 months, upper central incisors at 8–12 months.	• Full set of primary teeth present by the age of 33 months. Adult incisors and first molars appear at 6–9 years, canines and premolars at 9–12 years.	• Hormones stimulate oil and sweat production in skin. • Second molars appear at 11–13 years, third molars after 17 years.

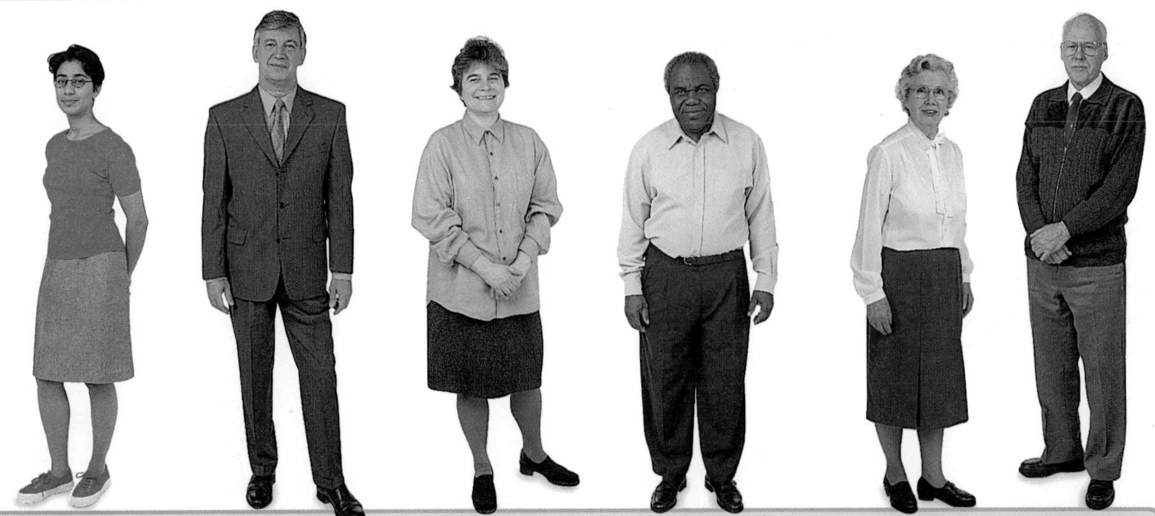

18–50 YEARS	50–70 YEARS	OVER 70 YEARS
• Bones are at maximum density during early adulthood. • After the age of 25, muscle bulk and strength start to decrease.	• Bones become weaker, particularly in postmenopausal women. • Muscle strength and bulk continue to decrease.	• Wear and tear on joints leads to increasing stiffness and pain. • Muscle strength at the age of 85 is about half the strength at the age of 25.
• After the age of 30, energy needs drop by 5 per cent every decade. Decreasing energy needs cause many people to gain weight in middle age unless diet is adjusted.	• The volume of digestive fluids decreases and the intestines work less efficiently, leading to harder faeces that may require straining to expel.	• Sense of taste becomes less acute as fewer than half the taste buds remain active. Chewing and swallowing may be more difficult due to tooth loss and gum disease.
• Ability to learn gradually declines, but life experiences accumulate and intellectual abilities continue to develop.	• Short-term memory and ability to concentrate may become less efficient. • Physical reactions become slower.	• By the age of 90, the brain has lost up to a tenth of its tissue, making it less efficient and leading to some loss of intellectual ability and physical coordination.
• By the age of 40, the lenses of the eyes may become less elastic, leading to difficulty in focusing on close objects. • Loss of hearing begins in the 30s.	• After the age of 50, it may be harder to see in low light or to see moving objects. • By the age of 70, it may be difficult to hear faint or high-pitched sounds.	• Ability to distinguish fine visual detail continues to decline. • Deterioration in hearing may make a hearing aid necessary.
• After the age of 40, artery walls lose elasticity, causing a rise in blood pressure. High blood pressure is one factor that may potentially lead to heart disease.	• Heart muscle becomes less elastic; the heart pumps harder but is less able to respond to increased effort.	• By the age of 85, the heart is unable to support long periods of strenuous activity. As stamina decreases, elderly people become tired more easily.
• Peak lung function is reached at 20–30 years. By 45 years, the lungs may not expand fully due to loss of some alveoli (air sacs) and weakening of rib muscles.	• By the age of 65, lung efficiency has decreased to about three-fifths of its optimum level.	• By the age of 80, the lungs function only half as effectively as the lungs of a young adult, and moderate exertion may cause shortness of breath.
• Women usually go through the menopause at 45–55 years and afterwards are no longer fertile. In men, testosterone levels start to decline at the age of 40–50.	• In men, the prostate gland usually starts to enlarge after the age of 50; it may constrict the bladder outlet, making the passing of urine difficult.	• A decreasing level of testosterone in men reduces sexual desire. Fewer viable sperm are produced.
• Women who have given birth may have reduced pelvic muscle strength and tone, which may cause problems with urination.	• In women, falling oestrogen levels also reduce pelvic muscle strength and tone. This may cause further difficulty in controlling urination.	• After the age of 75–80, kidneys become less efficient, and it takes longer for them to clear toxic chemicals from the blood.
• By the late 40s, the skin is less elastic and wrinkles appear. • Half of people over 40 years have grey hair. Some men begin to lose their hair.	• Surface of the skin becomes drier. • Hair may become considerably thinner, especially in men. • Teeth may begin to fall out.	• Skin becomes less able to regulate body temperature by retaining or losing heat, making people more susceptible to the effects of cold or hot weather.

UNDERSTANDING INHERITANCE

Only recently has evidence emerged showing the importance of inherited factors in determining our risk of developing disease. We take for granted the fact that children resemble their parents and other relatives and that families typically share physical and behavioural characteristics. It is this shared biological inheritance that also accounts for certain diseases "running in families".

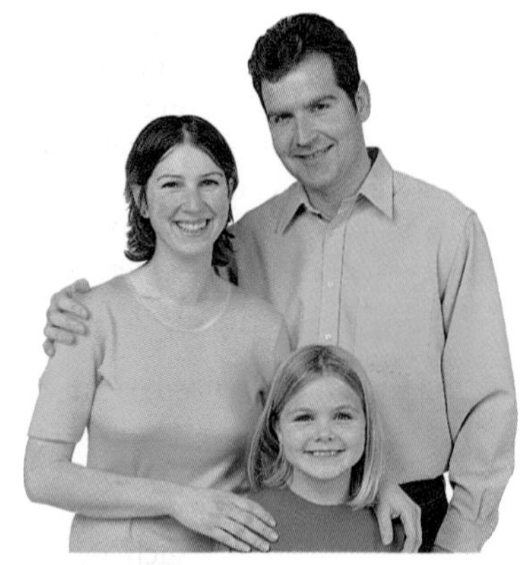

Family similarities
Children resemble their parents not only in appearance and personality but also in susceptibility to certain diseases.

Many of our physical and behavioural characteristics are determined by our genes. An explanation of the structure and function of genes and how they are inherited is given elsewhere (*see* GENES AND INHERITANCE, pp.264–269).

Genetic factors, along with lifestyle factors, contribute to many common diseases. The genes that you inherit from your parents help to explain why susceptibility to certain diseases varies from one family to the next, although only a few rare disorders are directly caused by abnormal genes.

By collecting information on your family's medical history, you may be able to identify diseases that appear to be particularly common in your family. This type of information can provide a valuable early indication of genetic tendencies to particular diseases.

The range of genetic tests used to determine whether either partner in a couple has inherited specific faulty genes (*see* GENETIC TESTS, pp.238–241) is increasing all the time. Geneticists can assess the risk of the couple's children inheriting the faulty genes and give advice on the likely effects on their health. In many cases, this allows the symptoms of a genetic disorder to be treated early or relieved effectively.

You and your inheritance

Understanding how the genes you inherit may influence your health

The genes you inherit from your parents programme your development from a single fertilized cell at the moment of conception to adulthood. In each body cell, you have about 35,000 pairs of genes arranged on 23 pairs of chromosomes. One chromosome from each pair is inherited from your mother, the other from your father. The mix of genes is slightly different in each sibling.

Each gene provides instructions for a cell to carry out a single chemical process, which in most cases involves building a protein. Genes also control the growth and reproduction of cells. They are responsible for the development of the embryo, first into a baby, then a child, and eventually an adult. Throughout your life, genes control cell functions and the repair and replacement of dead or damaged cells.

Blood relatives have many genes in common, and these genes help to determine family physical characteristics and other traits. Most of these traits, such as the shape of the nose, are trivial and have no significance for your health. Other traits, such as being abnormally tall or short or having a tendency to be overweight, can be associated with an increased risk of certain diseases.

Some diseases, such as haemophilia (p.452) and cystic fibrosis (p.824), are directly caused by a fault or mutation in a single gene or pair of genes. These rare diseases follow a predictable pattern of inheritance, and this means that families in which the gene is present can usually be given clear, reliable information regarding the risk of the disease affecting future generations.

More common than these genetic disorders are those in which genes, along with other factors, contribute to a family's susceptibility to certain diseases. For example, some disorders, such as coronary artery disease (p.405), tend to run in families, but lifestyle factors such as a high-fat diet, smoking, and lack of exercise also play a part in determining whether these diseases develop.

In some diseases that have a genetic component, including asthma (p.483), environmental factors, such as living in a polluted area, also play a crucial role. The complex interplay between genetic susceptibility and environment makes it difficult to predict the risks in adult life for children who are born into families affected by disorders of this kind.

(WWW) ONLINE SITES: p.1032

Your family medical history

Assessing your risk of developing a genetic disorder or passing one on to your children

You may have noticed that some diseases seem to "run in your family". These disorders may have a genetic basis or be due to lifestyle factors or a combination of the two. You can create a record of the disorders that have affected your family by making a medical family tree (opposite page), which may help you to assess your own risk of disease.

GATHERING INFORMATION

Information on your parents, brothers, and sisters is the most important, but you can provide a fuller picture by finding out about as many generations as possible, including your uncles, aunts, and grandparents. It is also helpful to

ASSESSMENT MAKING A MEDICAL FAMILY TREE

To make your medical family tree, you need key pieces of information about your relatives. You should research at least as far back as your grandparents because a genetic predisposition to a certain disease may be masked in one generation but nevertheless passed on to succeeding generations. Key facts include date of birth and, if the person is deceased, cause of death and the age at which it occurred. If possible, you should find out about lifestyle factors, such as smoking, body weight, alcohol consumption, and exercise.

YOUR PATERNAL GRANDFATHER (1906–1968)

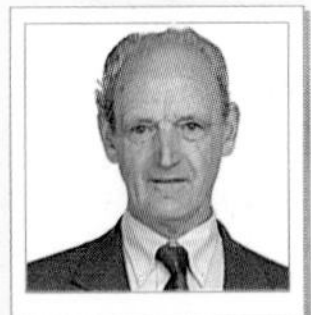

MEDICAL HISTORY
Angina
LIFESTYLE FACTORS
Nonsmoker
CAUSE OF DEATH
Heart attack at the age of 62

YOUR PATERNAL GRANDMOTHER (1909–1965)

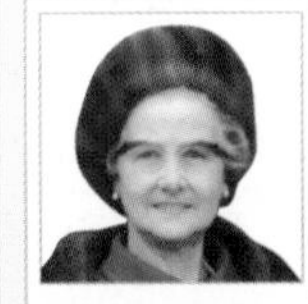

MEDICAL HISTORY
None
LIFESTYLE FACTORS
Nonsmoker
CAUSE OF DEATH
Colorectal cancer at the age of 56

YOUR MATERNAL GRANDFATHER (1912–)

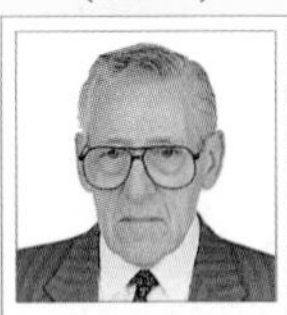

MEDICAL HISTORY
None
LIFESTYLE FACTORS
Active, nonsmoker
HEALTH STATUS
In good health

YOUR MATERNAL GRANDMOTHER (1915–1985)

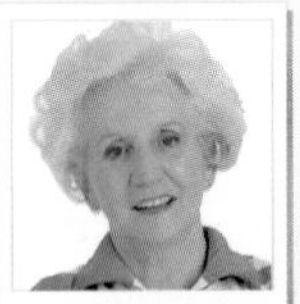

MEDICAL HISTORY
Diabetes mellitus
LIFESTYLE FACTORS
Smoker
CAUSE OF DEATH
Stroke at the age of 70

YOUR PATERNAL UNCLE (1932–)

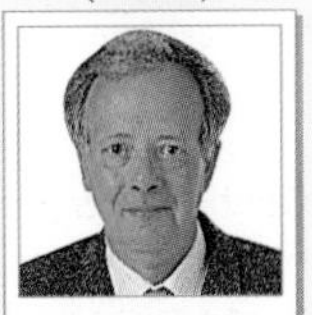

MEDICAL HISTORY
None
LIFESTYLE FACTORS
Active, nonsmoker
HEALTH STATUS
In good health

YOUR PATERNAL UNCLE (1929–)

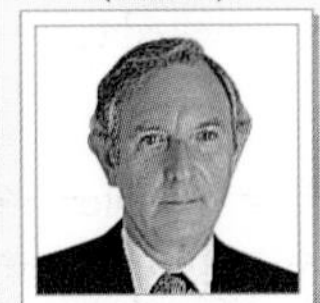

MEDICAL HISTORY
Coronary artery disease
LIFESTYLE FACTORS
Sedentary, smoker
HEALTH STATUS
In poor health

YOUR FATHER (1928–)

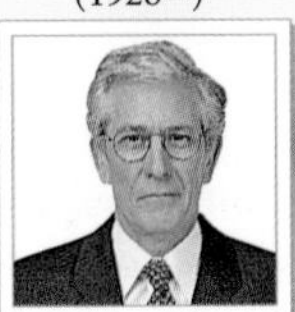

MEDICAL HISTORY
Treated for polyps in the colon
LIFESTYLE FACTORS
Active, nonsmoker
HEALTH STATUS
In good health

YOUR MOTHER (1936–)

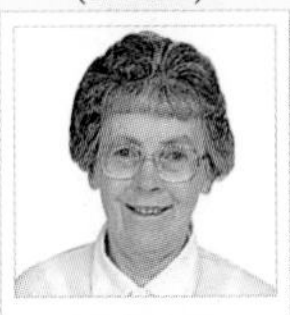

MEDICAL HISTORY
Diabetes mellitus
LIFESTYLE FACTORS
Nonsmoker
HEALTH STATUS
Overweight

YOUR MATERNAL UNCLE (1938–1950)

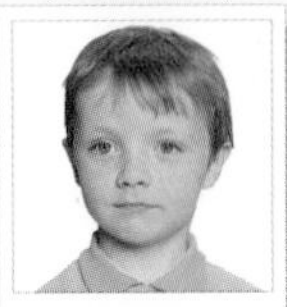

MEDICAL HISTORY
None
LIFESTYLE FACTORS
Was active
CAUSE OF DEATH
Polio at the age of 12

YOUR MATERNAL UNCLE (1940–)

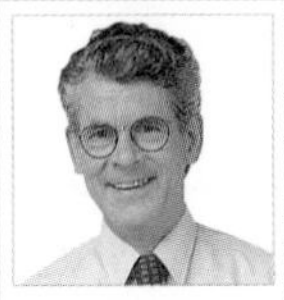

MEDICAL HISTORY
None
LIFESTYLE FACTORS
Nonsmoker
HEALTH STATUS
In good health

SISTER (1964–)

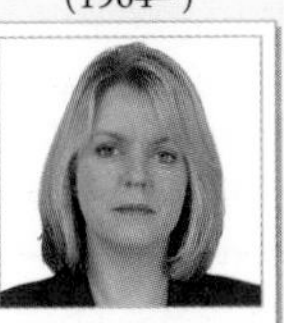

MEDICAL HISTORY
None
LIFESTYLE FACTORS
Active, smoker
HEALTH STATUS
Overweight

SISTER (1966–)

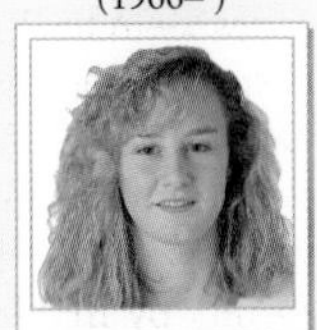

MEDICAL HISTORY
Kidney failure, aged 12 years. Kidney transplant at 14
LIFESTYLE FACTORS
Smoker
HEALTH STATUS
In good health

BROTHER (1968–)

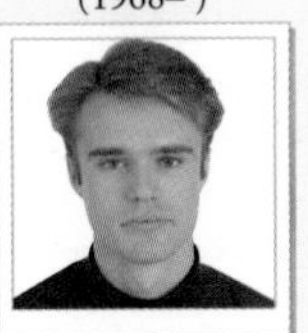

MEDICAL HISTORY
None
LIFESTYLE FACTORS
Nonsmoker
HEALTH STATUS
In good health

YOU (FEMALE) (1970–)

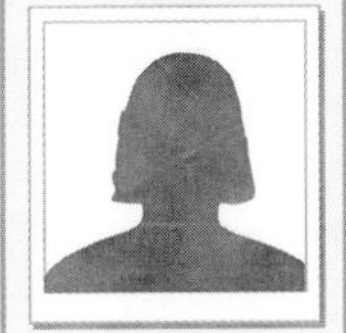

MEDICAL HISTORY
None
LIFESTYLE FACTORS
Nonsmoker
HEALTH STATUS
In good health

PARTNER

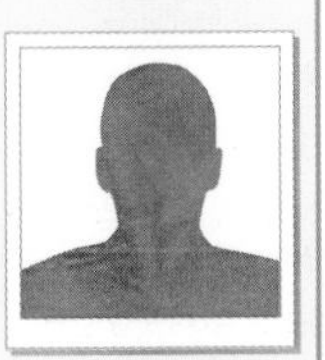

Example of a family tree
A family tree enables you to detect disease trends, but you will need your doctor's help to interpret your risk of disease. This example assumes that you are female and were born in 1970. From this record, the doctor would conclude that you and your siblings are at risk of polyps in the colon, which may lead to colorectal cancer, and diabetes mellitus. If you are planning to have a child, you should look at both your own and your partner's family trees to assess possible health risks for the child.

know something about your relatives' lifestyles to help you and your doctor to assess whether any diseases were largely due to behaviour or inheritance.

You may want to find out about your medical family tree out of curiosity, but you will find this information useful whenever a doctor needs to ask questions about illnesses in your family. You are likely to be asked about your family medical history when you first see a new doctor; you are expecting a baby; if you are admitted to hospital; and if you develop symptoms of a disorder with a genetic component, such as asthma.

Assessing the information

You may be able to come to some conclusions about your risk of disease by looking at your medical family tree. If your investigation suggests that a particular disease has affected more than one member of your family, you should consult your doctor. In some cases, you may be referred for genetic counselling to assess your risk of developing a disorder or passing it on to your children.

DRAWING YOUR OWN CONCLUSIONS Longevity runs in families, and, if many of your relatives lived beyond the age of 80, you have a good chance of doing the same, especially if you adopt a healthy lifestyle. If many of your relatives died young, you should try to find out the causes of death. You may be susceptible to disorders that have occurred more than once in your family.

You should suspect an inherited disorder if more than one child in your family was stillborn or died in childhood; if more than one adult died from heart disease or cancer before the age of 60; if more than two people in the family had a long-term disorder, such as arthritis (p.374); or if more than one family member had the same disabling or fatal disease. Deaths before the age of 60 are especially relevant, unless they were caused by accidents or by an infection, such as tuberculosis, that occurred before effective treatment was available.

PROFESSIONAL INTERPRETATION Genetic counsellors are trained to assess your risk of disease and determine whether you are a carrier of a faulty gene that causes a genetic disorder. Carriers do not have the disorder because the faulty gene is masked by a normal gene, but children of carriers can inherit the faulty gene. The counsellor will try to find out whether the high frequency of a disease in your family is due more to genetics or lifestyle. For example, if colorectal cancer (p.665) runs in your family, this could be due to eating habits shared by family members, since the disease may be associated with a high-fat, low-fibre diet. However, there may still be an inherited component.

CONSIDERING THE OPTIONS Your family medical history may suggest that you are at risk of an inherited disorder. In this case, the counsellor will tell you whether a specific gene abnormality for the disorder has been identified and whether there is a diagnostic test to see if you have the gene (*see* GENETIC TESTS, pp.238–241). If a test is available, the counsellor can provide information that will help you to decide whether or not to have the test. For example, you may be told whether the disease develops in everyone who inherits the faulty gene and whether preventive treatment is available. You may be told whether antenatal testing of the embryo or fetus is possible and what the implications are for any children you might have.

Some people decide not to proceed with genetic tests for a variety of reasons. Prospective parents may feel there is no point in worrying about a disorder that would not necessarily affect them or their child, or they may choose to carry on with a pregnancy even if there is an increased risk of their child being affected by a genetic disease. They may also be concerned by the stigma associated with "labelling" someone as having or being a carrier of a disorder. Other people want to know the results of a test even if they would not act on them. Bear in mind that the test result for one family member may have implications for other family members who may not want to know the outcome.

Members of some ethnic groups are susceptible to particular genetic disorders, and individuals may be offered a screening test based on this fact alone. For example, 1 in 10 black people carries the gene for sickle-cell disease (p.448), a disorder of red blood cells. If you are Jewish, a genetic counsellor may recommend that you be screened for the metabolic disorder Tay–Sachs disease (p.868) because 1 in 30 Ashkenazi Jews, compared with only 1 in 300 of the general population, carries the faulty gene that causes the disease.

What you can do

If tests show that you have a faulty gene, your course of action will depend on whether you already have the symptoms of a genetic disorder or whether you are at high risk of developing the disorder. If you carry a faulty gene and you are planning a family, there are several options to consider.

PEOPLE WITH A GENETIC DISORDER Certain genetic disorders can be treated. For example, a person who has inherited a tendency to high levels of cholesterol in the blood (*see* INHERITED HYPERLIPIDAEMIAS, p.692) may be treated with a low-fat diet and lipid-lowering drugs (p.935). Children with the genetic disorder haemophilia (p.452) may be given regular transfusions of Factor VIII, a protein that helps the blood to clot.

PEOPLE AT RISK If you find that you have a gene that predisposes you to a particular disorder, such as breast cancer (p.759), you can be screened regularly to detect cancerous changes at an early stage. You may also be able to make lifestyle changes to help to reduce the risk of developing a disease. For example, if your family history suggests that you are at increased risk of developing diabetes mellitus (p.687), you should keep your weight within the normal range.

CARRIERS If you carry a faulty gene that could be passed on to your children, you and your partner may decide not to have children or may consider various family planning options such as adoption or artificial insemination (p.775). You may be able to take advantage of advances in assisted conception (p.776), in which fertilization is carried out in the laboratory and the embryo is tested for the faulty gene. Only an embryo that does not have the genetic fault is then implanted into the uterus. If you are already expecting a baby and are told that your baby is affected by a genetic abnormality, you may want to consider terminating the pregnancy (p.789).

(WWW) ONLINE SITES: p.1026, p.1032

HEALTH AT DIFFERENT AGES

Your susceptibility to health hazards changes over your lifetime, and your health priorities should change accordingly. During childhood and early adult life, accidents claim the most lives, but after the age of 50, cancer and heart disease are leading causes of death. Falls, strokes, and dementia are major threats in later life.

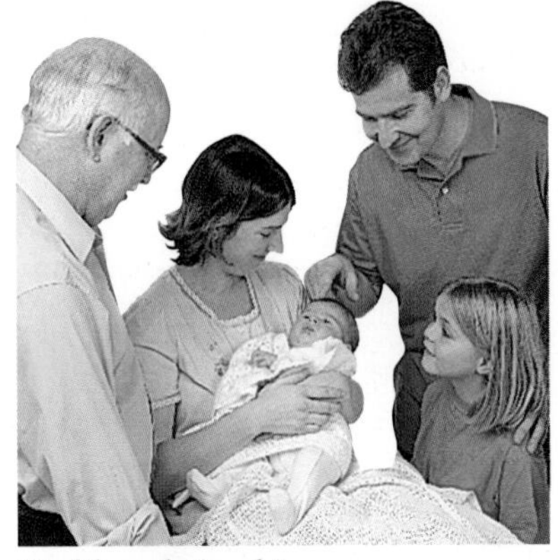

Healthy relationships
Involving the whole family in major life events strengthens family relationships and contributes to psychological health.

People born today can expect to live, on average, for about 77 years, but thousands of people will die before they reach the age of 65. Some of these premature deaths will be the result of unavoidable accidents or of disorders present at birth, but most will be due to preventable conditions.

People of all ages can reduce their risk of illness and premature death by adopting a three-pronged strategy. The first priority is a healthy lifestyle; the second is immunization; and the third is to identify disease early on by having appropriate screening tests (*see* HEALTH CARE THROUGHOUT LIFE, pp.38–45).

For many people, the most crucial determinant of health is their lifestyle. People who exercise regularly, eat a healthy selection of foods, and do not smoke can substantially reduce their risk of disease. Within any country, regional variations in the rate of premature mortality are due mostly to variations in these risk factors.

The articles in this section describe normal physical and emotional development and examine the factors that promote continued good health at each of the major stages of life. These stages include infancy, the preschool years, the school years, adolescence, adulthood, older adulthood, and old age. In addition, there are separate articles on important health issues during pregnancy, following childbirth, and during the menopause.

Health in infants

Taking care of your baby from birth until the age of 1 year

A baby's physical growth is rapid after birth: during the first year of life, your baby will triple his or her weight and double in height. Changes in the child's internal organs are equally dramatic. During the first year, there is rapid development of the brain and nervous system, which enables the baby to begin to make sense of and explore his or her environment. Mental skills, such as the beginnings of language, and physical skills, such as mobility and hand–eye coordination, start to develop.

Thanks to improvements in hygiene, immunization programmes, and the use of antibiotics, serious threats to health in the first year of life are relatively few in developed countries. With the exception of some problems that cannot be prevented, such as those associated with prematurity, congenital abnormalities (those present at birth), and genetic diseases, the major risks at this age are sudden infant death syndrome (p.820) and accidents.

DIET AND TOOTH CARE

An average baby has doubled his or her birth weight by about 6 months of age. Babies need more calories in proportion to their body weight than adults do, more even than adults involved in heavy manual work, and therefore need to be fed frequently. Both bottle- and breast-feeding provide the correct balance of nutrients and allow you to form a close bond with your baby. However, breast milk has additional benefits (*see* FEEDING YOUR INFANT, p.28).

By the age of 7 months, your baby's milk teeth may have begun to break through the gums. As soon as they appear, you should brush them twice a day and follow advice from your dentist on fluoride supplements, which may be recommended in areas where fluoride is not present in the water supply.

PREVENTING ILLNESS

Infections are uncommon in the first months of life because babies have some immunity given by their mothers' antibodies and, if they are breastfed, from breast milk. Later in infancy, babies become vulnerable to minor bacterial and viral illnesses, including coughs, colds, and diarrhoea. Your baby will gradually acquire immunity to the organisms that cause these disorders, but you can reduce the risk of infection by keeping him or her away from people who have an infectious illness, and by regularly cleaning toys and maintaining hygiene.

Infections such as pertussis (p.492) and measles (p.293) can be prevented by having your baby immunized (*see* ROUTINE IMMUNIZATIONS, p.45). Most

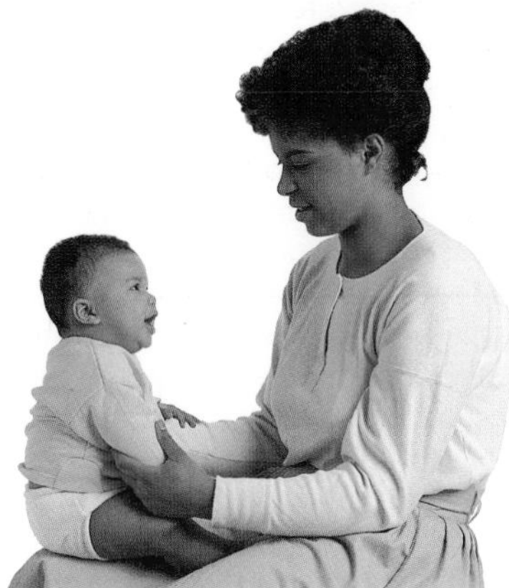

Interacting with your baby
You can encourage healthy psychological development by interacting with your baby from early infancy.

HEALTH OPTIONS FEEDING YOUR INFANT

Doctors advise that breast-feeding should be continued for at least 6 months and ideally for a year. Breast milk is better for your baby than milk formula, but, as long as the formula is prepared according to the instructions, bottle-feeding is a satisfactory alternative feeding method. By about 4–6 months of age, your baby can digest increasingly complex foods, and you can gradually introduce solid foods into his or her diet. However, your baby should also continue to receive breast milk or formula throughout the first year of life.

BREAST- OR BOTTLE-FEEDING

If possible, all mothers should breast-feed for the first month. Every extra month brings more benefits, but bottle-feeding may be a solution if you are taking drugs that pass into breast milk and might pose a danger to your baby or if there are other considerations (*see* HEALTH IN PREGNANCY AND AFTER CHILDBIRTH, p.33). Breast-fed babies are less susceptible to nappy rash (p.829) and to sudden infant death syndrome (p.820), and are less likely to become overweight as adults.

Natural protection from breast milk
Breast milk contains natural antibodies that protect against intestinal and respiratory infections and reduce the risk of allergies developing.

Nutritious formula
When milk formulas are made up correctly, they are as digestible and nutritious as breast milk but do not contain protective antibodies.

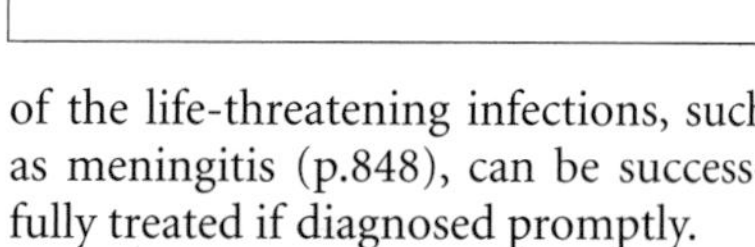

WEANING

During weaning, gradually introduce solid foods, first as purées and later in mashed or minced form. To reduce the risk of allergies and digestive upsets, do not give wheat-based foods, eggs, cows' milk, citrus fruits, fatty foods, or strong spices before the age of 6 months, and avoid nut products and honey before a year. Avoid sweet foods and do not add salt to your baby's food.

Diet at 4–6 months
Start with baby rice or purées of vegetables or fruit during or after a milk feed. Slowly increase the amount of solid food, including puréed meat, fish, poultry, and pulses.

Diet at 6–9 months
You can now give mashed or minced food before the milk. Diluted fruit juices may be given. At 9 months, peeled apple and bread encourage self-feeding and provide chewing practice.

of the life-threatening infections, such as meningitis (p.848), can be successfully treated if diagnosed promptly.

Although sudden infant death syndrome (p.820), known as SIDS, is one of the greatest risks for babies in the first few months, the number of deaths from this condition is decreasing. To reduce the risk of SIDS, babies under 6 months should sleep on their backs on a firm, well-ventilated mattress with their feet near the bottom of the cot. Do not let your baby get too warm because babies cannot effectively regulate their body temperature, and overheating is known to be a risk factor in SIDS.

Babies who are regularly exposed to tobacco smoke are at increased risk of respiratory infections, asthma (p.483), ear infections, and SIDS. Ideally, parents should give up smoking or, at the very least, minimize the risk by restricting smoking to outside the home.

A SAFE ENVIRONMENT

Accidents are one of the major causes of injury and death in infants under the age of 1 year. Many serious accidents could be avoided by taking safety precautions (*see* HOME SAFETY AND HEALTH, p.77). It is also wise for you and your babysitters to take a first-aid course.

Never leave a baby unattended on a raised surface such as a bed; in the bath or near a pool of water (*see* SAFETY IN AND AROUND WATER, p.81); or with a dog or a cat, even if the pet is well trained (*see* PETS AND HEALTH, p.82).

From the age of 6–8 months, a baby may be sufficiently mobile to get hold of potentially dangerous objects. An older sibling's toys may have small parts that pose a choking hazard, and playing with plastic bags puts your baby at risk of suffocation. Lock away all chemicals and drugs, and store matches and sharp or fragile objects out of reach.

In the car, your baby should travel in an appropriate car seat (*see* CHILDREN'S CAR SEATS, opposite page).

PSYCHOLOGICAL HEALTH

Bonding between you and your baby begins at birth and is important for your child's emotional development. A regular routine and consistent emotional care from a limited number of adults is essential for your baby to develop trust and self-confidence.

Maintaining eye contact and talking to your baby encourages communication. Your child will become accustomed to brief separations by spending time with other carers, such as grandparents and babysitters. Interacting with different people will also help to encourage your baby's social development.

(WWW) ONLINE SITES: p.1028, p.1035

Health in preschool children

Taking care of your child's health between 1 and 5 years of age

Between the ages of 1 and 5 years, your child continues to grow and to develop in four important areas: movement and coordination; vision and manipulative skills; hearing and speech; and play and social skills. The most important preventable health threats during this time are accidents and infections.

Diet and tooth care

During the preschool years, children are growing rapidly and developing complex skills and need high-energy food that is rich in nutrients, vitamins, and minerals (*see* A HEALTHY DIET, p.48). Their diet should include plenty of calcium-rich food, such as milk, cheese, and yogurt, to build strong bones and teeth. A pint of milk each day provides the recommended daily amount of calcium. Semi-skimmed milk can be given after the age of 2, but skimmed milk is low in protein and vitamin A and does not provide enough energy for children under 5. Fats in foods such as cheese and yogurt are important for growth and development, so these foods should not be replaced by low-fat equivalents.

Preschool children should eat plenty of fruit and vegetables because these provide vital vitamins and minerals and help to prevent constipation. Children who eat a balanced diet do not usually need vitamin or mineral supplements, but liquid drops of vitamins A, C, and D can be given to those who eat a poor diet. Although iron-deficiency anaemia (p.447) is relatively common, you should consult your doctor before giving your child iron supplements.

Your child may prefer to have several smaller meals than to eat three main meals a day. Offer healthy snack foods, such as fruit, bread, and cheese. The preschool years are the time to promote healthy eating habits that should last a lifetime. Mealtimes can also provide a focus for social development.

By the age of 3, all of your child's primary (milk) teeth should have appeared, and he or she should start to have regular dental checkups. These visits help a child to become familiar with the experience in case treatment is needed later for cavities as a result of tooth decay (*see* DENTAL CARIES, p.609). You can help to prevent tooth decay by limiting the number of occasions when your child has sweets and fizzy drinks and by brushing his or her teeth afterwards and each morning and night. If the water supply in your area does not contain fluoride, your dentist may suggest that your child has fluoride drops or tablets.

Preventing illness

Preschool children tend to have frequent minor infections, such as coughs, colds, and diarrhoea. These will become less common as your child acquires

HEALTH ACTION — Children's car seats

An unrestrained child can be killed by being thrown forwards at a speed of only 8 kph (5 mph). Even on a short trip, your child should be safely secured in a car seat complying with current UK or European safety standards. Your child's weight and age determine whether the car seat should be forward- or rear-facing and when a new, larger one is needed. Never place a child in a passenger seat that is fitted with an airbag. You should never use second-hand children's car seats.

Car seat-belt *The safety seat is secured by the car seat-belt*

Safety harness *The harness can be adjusted for a snug fit*

Carrying handle *If it has a carrying handle, the seat can double as a convenient carrier for your baby*

Rear-facing position *The rear-facing seat position is the safest for infants under the age of 1 year*

Infant seat
You must use a seat that faces to the rear, secured with the car seat-belt, for infants that weigh less than 10 kg (22 lb) and are under the age of 9 months.

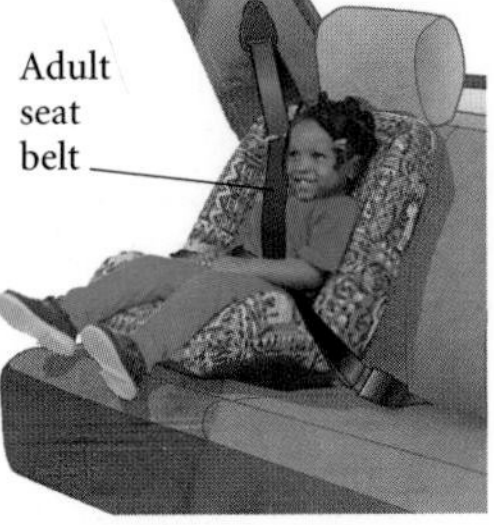

Forward-facing seat
You can use an adult seat-belt to secure a child of 9–18 kg (20–40 lb) in a forward-facing child seat.

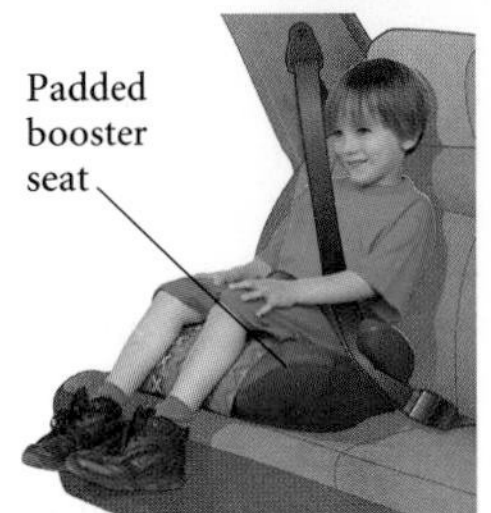

Booster seat
A booster seat elevates a child of about 15–25 kg (33–55 lb) so that the seat-belt fits correctly.

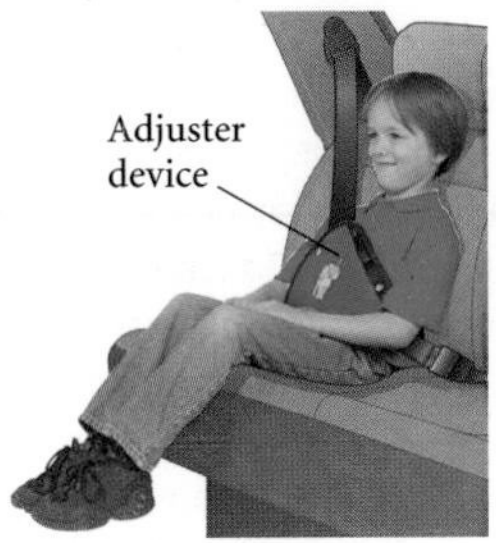

Seat-belt adjuster
An adjuster device can be used to position an adult seat-belt correctly for an older child.

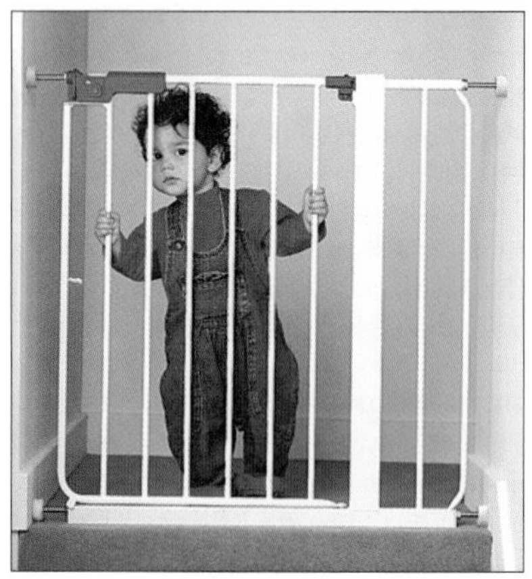

Stair safety gate
If you have a young child, install safety gates with a childproof lock at the top and bottom of staircases. Bars on the gate should be vertical to prevent climbing.

immunity to the bacteria and viruses to which he or she is exposed. Immunization can help to prevent some of the more serious infections (*see* ROUTINE IMMUNIZATIONS, p.45).

A SAFE ENVIRONMENT

Accidents in the home, such as poisoning, falls, and drowning, are the major causes of injury at this age. A child's natural curiosity makes an occasional minor injury unavoidable, but you can reduce the chance of serious injury by making your environment as safe as possible (*see* HOME SAFETY AND HEALTH, p.77) and by encouraging your child to be responsible for his or her own safety. If you learn simple first aid, you may be better able to deal with accidents. Make sure that carers and babysitters know how to deal with emergencies.

HOME SAFETY Hazardous items such as detergents, bleaches, alcohol, medicines, and matches should be stored in locked cupboards or out of reach. Cover unused electrical sockets, especially those near the floor, with safety plugs; fit safety locks on your windows; ensure that glass doors and tables are made of shatterproof glass; and put protective corner devices on furniture.

SAFETY OUTSIDE THE HOME As toddlers become more active and able to understand simple instructions, parents can help them to be aware of and negotiate potential hazards outside the home. At this age, safety is learned most easily by example so, wherever possible, use pelican crossings and explain when it is safe to cross the street. In the garden or the park, teach your child never to eat berries, leaves, or seeds, and never leave him or her unattended near water. At the playground, make sure that the apparatus is mounted on a safe surface such as bark or rubber. Show your child how to climb safely and take turns, and talk about the danger of running in front of swings and stepping off moving roundabouts. In the car, make sure that your child is securely fastened in a safety seat of the appropriate type and size (*see* CHILDREN'S CAR SEATS, p.29).

PSYCHOLOGICAL HEALTH

Playing forms an important part of your child's emotional and social development. You can stimulate your baby by offering interesting things to look at and touch, and activities to practise and think about. These will encourage your child to explore his or her own capabilities, develop new skills, and learn about the world and other people. By praising your child's achievements during play, you can boost his or her self-esteem and self-confidence. Play groups and nursery schools offer organized play and provide the opportunity to make friends with other children and adults.

(WWW) ONLINE SITES: p.1026, p.1028

Health in school-age children

Your child's physical and emotional health between the ages of 5 and 12

Physical growth and development are slow and steady during the school years, in contrast to the rapid changes that occur during the preschool years and adolescence. Your child's motor skills are refined between the ages of 5 and 12, and running, jumping, and throwing steadily improve. School significantly influences your child's intellectual and emotional development, and he or she becomes noticeably better at logic, reasoning, and problem-solving.

Just as during the preschool years, the major preventable threats to a child's health while he or she is at school are accidents and infections. During the school years, your child becomes more independent and should continue to be taught to take responsibility for his or her own health and safety.

DIET AND TOOTH CARE

You can establish good eating habits at home by giving your child a healthy breakfast, incorporating fruit and vegetables into the diet, and limiting the amount of food and drinks containing sugar (*see* A HEALTHY DIET, p.48). Iron-deficiency anaemia (p.447) may become a problem because many children of school age are particular about what they eat. Try to ensure an iron-rich diet by encouraging your child to eat lean red meats, egg yolks, and leafy green vegetables. Calcium is also essential in the diet for bones to grow normally and increase in strength and density.

About 1 in 50 children at primary school, and 1 in 10 at secondary school, are overweight. Dieting without medical advice is not appropriate because an overweight child has the same nutritional needs as all children, but he or she can be encouraged to cut out high-calorie snacks and drinks and to take more exercise. If your child is very overweight, consult your doctor who may suggest that you see a dietitian.

Good dental hygiene is important because your child's permanent teeth emerge during the school years. Your child may still need help with toothbrushing, and can be shown how to use dental floss (*see* CARING FOR YOUR TEETH AND GUMS, p.610). Keeping sweet snacks and fizzy drinks to the minimum will reduce the chance of tooth decay. Orthodontic problems, in which teeth grow irregularly or are overcrowded may become apparent, and regular dental checkups are essential. If the fluoridation of your water supply is inadequate, your dentist may recommend fluoride supplements.

EXERCISE

Whenever possible, encourage your child to walk rather than ride in a car because weight-bearing exercise such as walking helps to build strong bones. Activities such as cycling and swimming strengthen the heart and lungs (*see* THE BENEFITS OF EXERCISE, p.55). Organised sports and team games help to improve motor and social skills.

PREVENTING ILLNESS

By the time your child starts school, he or she should have had most routine immunizations (p.45). A child who has an infectious disease, such as influenza (p.289), should be kept at home because infections spread rapidly at school.

A SAFE ENVIRONMENT

Your child's susceptibility to accidents increases as he or she develops physically and becomes more adventurous. About half of all deaths in children aged 5–12 years are caused by accidents that might have been prevented by providing a safe environment and teaching children a few simple, common-sense rules.

HOME SAFETY Encourage your child to put away toys that could cause an accident and teach him or her what to do in a home emergency, such as a fire (*see* HOME SAFETY AND HEALTH, p.77).

To help to prevent accidents, particularly burns, keep electrical appliances such as kettles and irons out of reach of younger children and place saucepans at the back of the cooker with their handles turned away from the front. Teach older children how to handle electrical appliances and cooking equipment safely. In addition, keep matches, cigarettes, and lighters in a safe place.

SAFETY OUTSIDE THE HOME When children begin to venture out alone, make sure they know their own address and phone number. Talk about what your child would do if approached by a "stranger" and which adults to contact for help. Make sure your child knows about road safety (*see* SAFETY ON THE ROAD, p.83) and uses safety equipment in vehicles (*see* CHILDREN'S CAR SEATS, p.29). Teach your child to swim as soon as possible (*see* SAFETY IN AND AROUND WATER, p.81) and make sure he or she uses the proper safety equipment during sports. A child who has a medical condition, such as asthma (p.483) or a food allergy (p.467), should be encouraged to take some responsibility for his or her own medicines or foods.

Find out what health education your child is receiving at school so that you can reinforce messages about addictive substances such as alcohol, tobacco, and drugs (pp.62–66), and basic sex education. You can begin to talk about the importance of not keeping secrets in certain circumstances and how to resist pressure to engage in irresponsible activities from peers or older people.

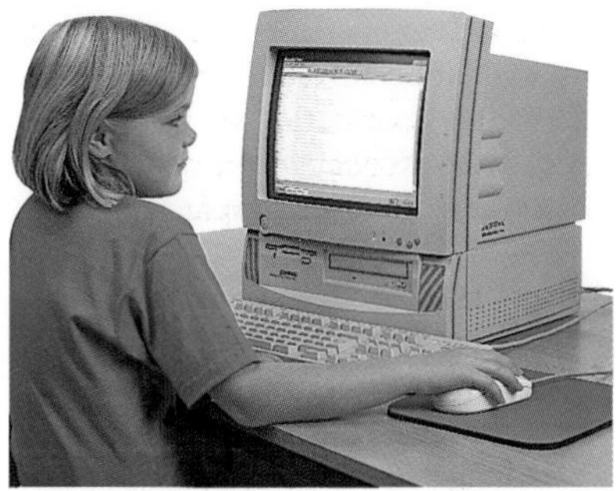

Using home computers wisely
Computers are a good learning tool, but time spent at the computer should not be at the expense of outdoor and physical activities and socializing with friends.

PSYCHOLOGICAL HEALTH

School helps your child to become more independent and build new social skills. School-age children begin to rely on friends for companionship and support, and to share advice and feelings. Your child's need for independence and privacy should be respected, but firm guidance and clear boundaries continue to be necessary for healthy growth.

Children with siblings, particularly a newborn brother or sister, may experience feelings of rivalry and jealousy. Set aside time to listen to each child alone and acknowledge his or her feelings. All children need to recognize their individual strengths and to feel that they are valued members of the family.

(WWW) ONLINE SITES: p.1026, p.1028

Health in adolescents

Special health needs between the ages of 12 and 18

The physical changes of adolescence, known as puberty, usually begin between the ages of 10 and 14 and can continue for 3–4 years. Girls generally start puberty earlier than boys, and the first sign in most girls is breast enlargement, followed by growth of underarm and pubic hair. Menstruation usually starts at around 12–13 years; consult your doctor if it has not started by the age of 15. By about 16–17 years, body fat has increased around the hips and thighs, and the pelvis has broadened. In boys, the first signs of puberty are underarm and pubic hair. The testes and penis enlarge, the chest and shoulders broaden, and the voice deepens. These changes are usually obvious by 13–15 years; facial hair is usually well established by the age of 17.

Emotional changes during adolescence can be difficult and may strain family relationships unless communication is maintained. These emotional changes may cause insecurity, boredom, moodiness, and withdrawal, and lead to participation in high-risk activities. Major health risks in the teenage years include accidents, sexually transmitted infections, pregnancy, and suicide.

DIET

Weight may double during adolescence due to increases in height, muscle development, and fat deposition. During puberty, teenagers require more calories in proportion to their body weight than at any other period in their lives apart from infancy. They need to eat regularly and often, and should be offered well balanced and healthy family meals (*see* A HEALTHY DIET, p.48) and a ready supply of healthy snacks.

Many teenagers feel physically unattractive and are preoccupied with their appearance. In some cases, this concern may become an obsession with food. Up to 1 in 100 teenage girls suffers from an eating disorder such as anorexia nervosa (p.562) or bulimia (p.563).

EXERCISE

Regular aerobic activities, such as jogging and swimming, help to keep the cardiovascular, respiratory, and musculoskeletal systems healthy (*see* THE BENEFITS OF EXERCISE, p.55). As well as promoting physical and psychological health, team sports are a good way for a teenager to make friends and learn about dedication, discipline, and teamwork.

PREVENTING ILLNESS

Many adolescents have acne (p.340), a skin condition that is associated with raised hormone levels during puberty. Early treatment of this problem can prevent teenagers from losing confidence and forming a negative self-image at a stage when appearance and peer relationships are crucially important.

Parents should be alert to signs that a teenager may be suffering from depression (p.554) or even feeling suicidal (*see* ATTEMPTED SUICIDE AND SUICIDE, p.556). About 1 in 5 deaths of people under the age of 25 is a suicide. Changes in behaviour may also be an indication of drug abuse (*see* DRUGS AND HEALTH, p.65) or alcohol abuse (*see* ALCOHOL AND HEALTH, p.62). More bizarre personality changes or signs of paranoia may indicate a serious psychiatric illness, such as schizophrenia (p.560).

Most schools provide education on alcohol, tobacco, and drugs, but it is important for parents to reinforce these messages at home and create an atmosphere in which teenagers are able to ask questions and discuss issues freely. Your child should then be better equipped to make safe, informed choices.

A SAFE ENVIRONMENT

Accidents are the greatest single threat to life for young people. Many accident-related deaths result from participation in high-risk activities by teenagers, who may feel that they are invulnerable to injury. Young people may be more likely to take steps to protect their health if they understand that seemingly harmless activities may put them and other people in serious danger.

The risk of sports injury is reduced by physical preparation, such as warming up and cooling down (p.60), and by appropriate equipment and training.

All teenagers need to be made aware of the risks of drinking, drug abuse, and driving (*see* SAFETY ON THE ROAD, p.83), whether they are car drivers or passengers, and should be aware of the importance of safety equipment such as motorcycle helmets and car seat-belts.

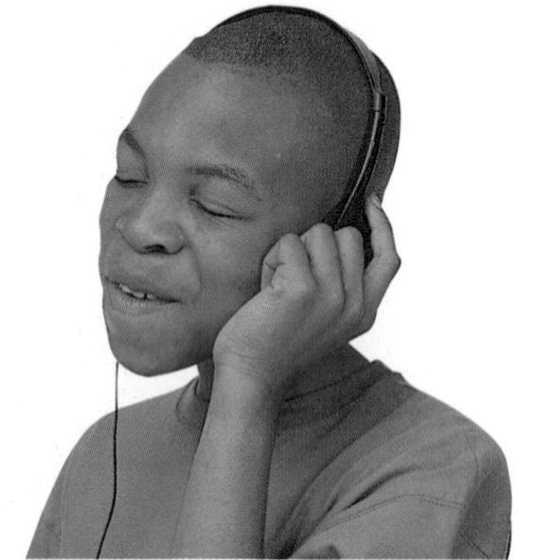

Loud music

*Teenagers should be warned that regularly listening to music at high volumes can lead to permanent hearing loss (*see *NOISE-INDUCED HEARING LOSS, p.601).*

SEXUAL SAFETY

The UK has the highest rate of teenage pregnancy in Western Europe, with 1 in 8 women having a baby in her teens. Most often, these are unplanned pregnancies that might have been prevented by improved education about sex and contraception (*see* SEX AND HEALTH, pp.67–71). There are many books available that can be used as a backup for conversations on these subjects. Topics should include homosexuality, sexual fantasies, and masturbation. Teenagers may also need to be shown how to use a condom to help to prevent pregnancy and the spread of sexually transmitted infections, such as HIV infection (*see* HIV INFECTION AND AIDS, p.297).

PSYCHOLOGICAL HEALTH

Many adolescents experiment with new friends, appearance, and behaviour. At this time, relationships between parents and teenagers may change, and maintaining good communication can be difficult. Poor communication can make teenagers and their families feel frustrated. To prevent this, try to listen to each other and express your point of view without blame or judgment.

Teenagers should bear in mind that achieving independence does not mean cutting themselves off from others. It is important for them to know when and how to access support. If they feel unable to discuss problems with parents, a grandparent, teacher, or counsellor may be a source of guidance and support.

(WWW) ONLINE SITES: p.1026, p.1028

Health in adults

Factors most likely to affect your health between the ages of 18 and 50

By the age of 25, all of your body systems have fully matured and should be functioning well. Towards the end of your 20s, the strength and bulk of your muscles start to decrease as part of the normal aging process. The strength and density of bone continue to increase steadily until your mid-30s and then begin to gradually decrease. Generally, early adulthood is the time of life when people are at their healthiest.

For young adults, accidents and suicide are greater risks to life than illness. However, women in their 30s and 40s, are more likely to die from illness than from injury. Breast cancer (p.759) is the leading single cause of death in women aged 35–54 years in the UK. The major causes of death in men under the age of 45 are accidents, followed by cardiovascular diseases and suicide. Cancer of the testis (p.719) is the most common cancer in men aged 25–34. However, advances in the treatment of this cancer have allowed most affected men to be cured, usually by a combination of surgery and chemotherapy.

DIET

Try to follow a healthy diet (p.48). Eating less fat and more fibre protects against heart disease and may reduce your risk of developing colorectal cancer (p.665) in later life. Vitamins A, C, and E may help to protect against cancer. To ensure an adequate intake, try to eat plenty of citrus fruit and vegetables, which contain large amounts of these vitamins.

EXERCISE

Any weight-bearing exercise, such as walking or running, slows down the deterioration of muscle and bone that is a normal part of aging (*see* THE BENEFITS OF EXERCISE, p.55). You are less likely to develop heart disease and osteoporosis (p.368) when you are older if you build up the strength of your skeleton while you are young. However, it is important to maintain a regular exercise routine throughout your life (*see* TAKING REGULAR EXERCISE, p.57). Research has shown that athletes who exercise vigorously when they are young but who stop completely when they are older are even less likely to stay healthy than those who have never exercised.

PREVENTING ILLNESS

In addition to modifying your diet and exercising regularly, you can reduce the chance of developing illnesses such as AIDS, cancer, and heart disease by changing other aspects of your lifestyle if they are not healthy. Safe sex (p.68) protects against HIV infection and, if you are female, may also lower your risk of cancer of the cervix (p.750).

If you are careful about exposure to the sun (*see* SAFETY IN THE SUN, p.80), you can significantly reduce your risk of developing skin cancer (p.344).

Drinking alcohol to excess (*see* ALCOHOL AND HEALTH, p.62) and smoking or chewing tobacco (*see* TOBACCO AND HEALTH, p.63) are risk factors for lung cancer (p.503), mouth cancer (p.634), stomach cancer (p.642), and cancer of the oesophagus (p.638). Smoking causes about 1 in 3 deaths from cancer, 1 in 4 deaths from heart disease, and more than 4 in 5 deaths from chronic obstructive pulmonary disease (p.487). Giving up smoking, even if you have smoked heavily until your 40s, is the single most important preventive measure for all of these diseases. After giving up, health improvements are rapid, especially in the case of heart disease. You can also reduce your risk of accidents and liver disease by keeping your alcohol consumption within safe limits.

A SAFE ENVIRONMENT

Men are about three times more likely than women to be killed in accidents and about one and a half times more likely to be seriously injured. This difference is probably due to the fact that men tend to take greater risks than women. For example, young men are more likely to drive after drinking alcohol. Avoid alcohol and always take safety precautions (*see* VEHICLE SAFETY, p.84) when you drive. Many sports and leisure activities, such as mountain climbing and skiing, carry risks. Make sure that you have the correct training before taking part and use recommended safety equipment.

PSYCHOLOGICAL HEALTH

During this stage of your life, you may embark on a long-term sexual relationship. At their best, relationships are loving and mutually supportive, but if you are having problems, it is important to discuss your feelings with your partner or, if necessary, consult a counsellor (*see* SEX THERAPY, p.773).

If you and your partner wish to have a baby, you will need to prepare yourselves physically before attempting to conceive (*see* HEALTH IN PREGNANCY AND AFTER CHILDBIRTH, right). If you have been trying to conceive for over a year and have been unsuccessful, consult a doctor (*see* INFERTILITY, pp.774–777).

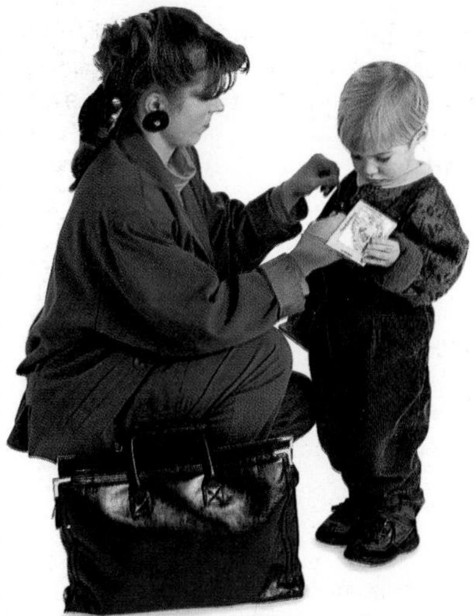

Balancing family and work pressures
Keeping a balance between the demands of your family life and your working life can sometimes be difficult.

In your working life, you may sometimes be subject to high levels of stress (p.74). Try to address difficulties at work early on and learn to relax in your free time. Enrolling on a course to learn a new skill, such as another language, or trying out a new sport or activity can help to boost your self-esteem.

If you are combining being a parent with work, try to make free time for yourself in your routine. If you feel generally anxious, especially if there is no apparent cause, you should consult a doctor or therapist (*see* PSYCHOLOGICAL THERAPIES, pp.968–971).

(WWW) ONLINE SITES: p.1026, p.1034, p.1037

Health in pregnancy and after childbirth

Health during pregnancy and following the birth of your baby

Having a baby is a major event and it is difficult for a couple to prepare emotionally for the way it will change their life. As a mother-to-be, you can influence the health of your unborn child by trying to stay healthy before and during pregnancy. Preparing for the birth and postnatal period can help you to adapt more easily to rapid changes in your body and make your pregnancy much more enjoyable (*see* PREGNANCY AND CHILDBIRTH, pp.778–809).

HEALTH BEFORE CONCEPTION

Ideally, you and your partner should see your doctor at least 3 months before you begin to try conceiving because the health of both parents affects the health of the child. For example, if either of you has a family history of genetic disease, there may be a risk of passing the disease on to your child. In this case, your doctor may suggest investigation and genetic counselling (p.272). Your doctor will advise you both to follow a healthy diet (p.48), not to smoke, and to avoid alcohol and drugs that could affect fertility and general health (*see* ALCOHOL, TOBACCO, AND DRUGS, pp.62–66).

Your doctor can check that you are immune to rubella (p.294) and not a carrier of a virus such as hepatitis B (*see* CHRONIC HEPATITIS, p.645) or HIV infection (p.297) that could affect your baby. To reduce the risk of neural tube defects (p.844), such as spina bifida, you should take at least 400 micrograms of folic acid daily, starting at least 3 months before you try to conceive. If you have a pre-existing disease that could influence your pregnancy, such as asthma (p.483), it should be well controlled beforehand.

A HEALTHY PREGNANCY

Pregnant women can provide a healthy environment for their growing babies and make the pregnancy more comfortable by eating a nutritious diet and exercising regularly (*see* EXERCISE AND RELAXATION IN PREGNANCY, p.34).

DIET Pregnant women need to obtain about twice as much protein, iron, calcium, and folic acid from their diet as women who are not pregnant (*see* GOOD SOURCES OF VITAMINS AND MINERALS, p.52). A healthy diet that incorporates an extra 300 calories per day, plus 6–8 glasses of fluid, should provide the recommended levels of most nutrients. You should continue to take daily supplements of folic acid until week 12 of pregnancy to reduce the risk of your child developing neural tube defects. Many pregnant women also need to boost their intake of iron by eating iron-rich foods. Your doctor will advise you whether or not you need to take additional supplements.

To protect your baby from the damaging effects of listeriosis (p.301) or toxoplasmosis (p.307), you should avoid eating pâté, raw shellfish, foods that contain raw eggs, and unpasteurized food such as certain types of soft or blue-veined cheese. You can also help to prevent food poisoning (p.629) by making sure that meat and poultry are cooked until they are no longer pink inside and by washing vegetables and salads thoroughly. You should avoid all contact with cat faeces and cat litter and wear gloves when gardening to prevent contact with harmful organisms.

ALCOHOL, TOBACCO, AND DRUGS Fetal growth can be affected by alcohol, so ideally, you should avoid it altogether during pregnancy or, at the very least, restrict your intake to safe amounts (*see* SAFE ALCOHOL LIMITS, p.62). It is especially important that you and your partner do not smoke during and after your pregnancy. Smoking during pregnancy increases the risk of premature labour (p.798), miscarriage (p.791), and growth retardation (*see* INTRA-UTERINE GROWTH RETARDATION, p.796). Being in a house where people smoke increases a baby's risk of sudden infant death syndrome (p.820), known as SIDS. During pregnancy, consult your doctor before you take over-the-counter preparations, although it is safe to use paracetamol for a headache. Your doctor will also advise you about taking prescribed drugs for a disorder such as epilepsy (p.524). These drugs are, in most cases, less harmful to the fetus than the disorder would be if it were uncontrolled.

HEALTH ACTION EXERCISE AND RELAXATION IN PREGNANCY

Antenatal and other gentle exercises help to keep you fit, prepare you for the physical demands of labour, and speed recovery after the birth. Relaxation exercises relieve stress and conserve energy to allow you to cope more effectively with labour.

EXERCISE

You can maintain your previous level of exercise during pregnancy, but you may need to modify some exercises because you are more vulnerable to injury, especially to your back. Drink lots of water and try not to push your heart rate over 140 beats per minute.

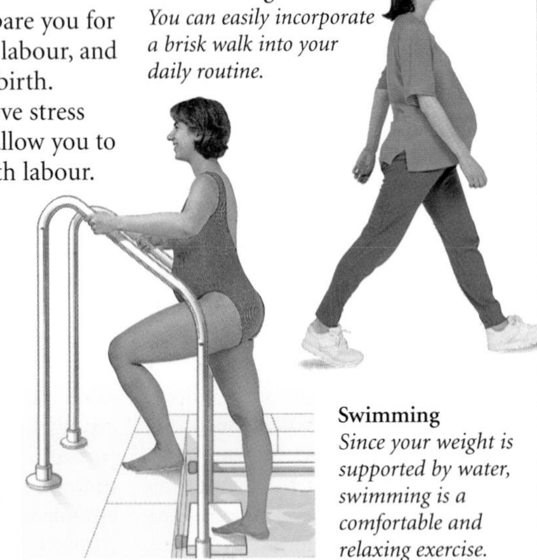

Brisk walking
You can easily incorporate a brisk walk into your daily routine.

Swimming
Since your weight is supported by water, swimming is a comfortable and relaxing exercise.

ANTENATAL EXERCISES

Exercises can help to relieve some of the discomforts of pregnancy, such as backache, and in most cases are very beneficial for both mother and baby. For example, pelvic tilt exercises are an excellent way to improve posture. Antenatal exercise classes can teach you how to exercise safely.

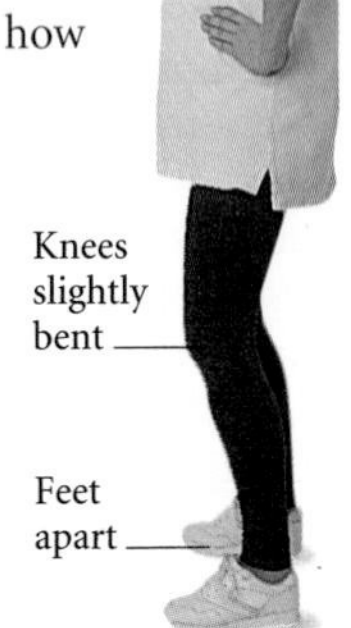

Pelvic tilt exercises
Tighten your buttocks and tuck your pelvis under, then relax the buttocks and rock the pelvis back; repeat several times. Do this a number of times a day.

RELAXATION

Certain breathing and relaxation techniques, such as massage, can help you to cope better with labour. Antenatal or yoga classes may teach you how to contract and relax muscle groups all over your body (*see* RELAXATION EXERCISES, p.75).

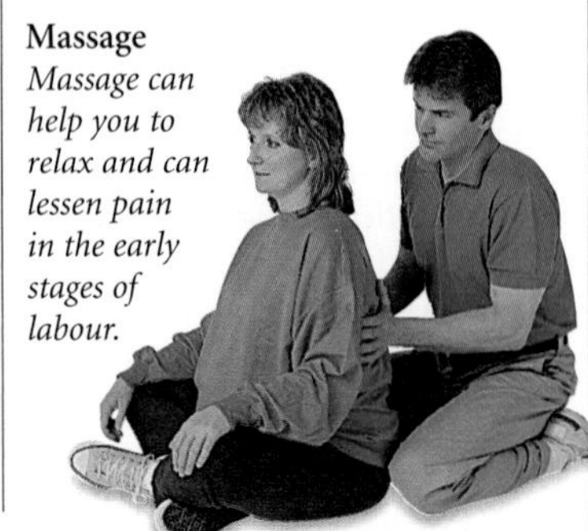

Massage
Massage can help you to relax and can lessen pain in the early stages of labour.

RELATIONSHIPS Expectant parents may feel excited, nervous, or frightened by the prospect of having a baby. Men sometimes describe feelings of alienation because their partner's attention is focused on the new baby. Sexual relationships often change. Some couples experience an increase in libido, but, especially during the first 3 months, nausea and tiredness in the woman may decrease her interest in sex. Some men find their partner's new shape disturbing or worry about hurting the baby during intercourse. You may find it helpful to experiment with different sexual positions that avoid putting pressure on the uterus. Whatever your feelings about sex during pregnancy, it is important to talk about them with your partner so you can find mutually acceptable ways of showing your love for each other.

PREPARING FOR THE BIRTH

Discuss with your doctor or midwife the risks and benefits of home and hospital birth, and ask about suitable pain relief during labour and delivery. A birth plan may help to clarify your expectations, but try to remain open-minded in case things do not go as planned.

Breast-feeding has many advantages over using milk formula (*see* FEEDING YOUR INFANT, p.28). Breast milk needs no preparation and is sterile and at the right temperature. In addition, the hormones your body produces during breast-feeding tighten the uterus and help you to get back into shape after the birth. Breast-feeding also reduces your long-term risk of breast cancer (p.759).

Drawbacks include having to be available day and night for feeding, unless you can express and store your milk. Breast-feeding may be painful at first, but good advice can often prevent

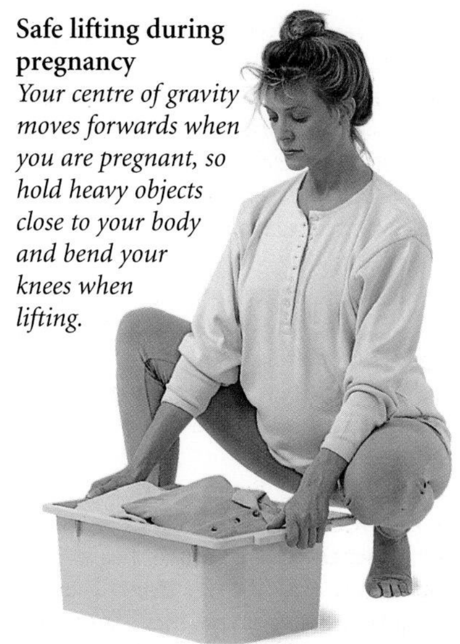

Safe lifting during pregnancy
Your centre of gravity moves forwards when you are pregnant, so hold heavy objects close to your body and bend your knees when lifting.

early problems such as cracked nipples (*see* AVOIDING CRACKED NIPPLES, p.809). You can prepare for breast-feeding during pregnancy by reading books and attending antenatal classes.

If you plan to return to work, you may choose to bottle-feed, perhaps after a short period of breast-feeding. In addition to reducing dependence on you, bottle-feeding gives your partner an opportunity to bond closely with the baby. It is important to maintain good hygiene when preparing formula.

AFTER THE BIRTH

Caring for a baby can be very demanding on your energy, patience, time, and finances. There is a lot to learn at a time when you may feel exhausted and uncomfortable. Most new mothers experience a few days of depression after childbirth (p.807). If your depression is severe or persistent, discuss it with your doctor or midwife. Although it may be difficult, try to take care of yourself by maintaining a healthy diet, exercising gently, and getting enough rest. Enlist the support of friends and family to help you. Be aware that the emotional upheaval a baby brings can put a strain on relationships with your partner and other children, who may feel left out.

After a vaginal delivery, the mother's vulva may feel tender, especially after an episiotomy (*see* ASSISTED DELIVERY, p.805). Most doctors recommend waiting at least 3 weeks before you resume sexual intercourse. If you were using a cap or a diaphragm as contraception before pregnancy, it will need to be refitted. An intrauterine device should not be inserted until at least a month after the birth. The progestogen-only pill can be used while breast-feeding, but avoid combined oral contraceptives. Breast-feeding reduces fertility, but it is not a reliable contraceptive method.

(WWW) ONLINE SITES: p.1035

Health in older adults

Taking care of your health between the ages of 50 and 70

You may notice the first signs of aging during your middle years even if you are fit and healthy. Wrinkles and grey hair are common, and your face and extremities look thinner because fat moves to your trunk and abdomen. Your muscles lose some bulk and strength; your heart becomes less efficient; and blood vessels lose elasticity. Bones continue to decrease in strength and density.

By the age of 50, diseases rather than accidents are the major threat to life. The greatest health risk for women is cancer, followed by cardiovascular and respiratory diseases. Men are most at risk of cardiovascular disease, followed by cancer and respiratory diseases.

Although all cancers become more common with increasing age, some can be treated successfully if they are detected early. The most common cancers in older women are lung cancer (p.503), breast cancer (p.759), cancer of the uterus (p.748), and colorectal cancer (p.665). Older men are more likely to develop lung cancer, prostate cancer (p.726), bladder tumours (p.715), colorectal cancer, and stomach cancer (p.642). Women are offered screening for breast and cervical cancer, and screening for colorectal cancer in both sexes is becoming more common (*see* COMMON SCREENING TESTS, p.44).

Aging is inevitable, but, by following a healthy lifestyle, you can maintain a good level of fitness and delay or minimize some of the associated changes.

DIET AND TOOTH CARE

A diet that is low in saturated fat can slow the deposition of fat on the walls of the arteries (*see* ATHEROSCLEROSIS, p.402), preventing coronary artery disease and stroke. Women may be able to prevent osteoporosis (p.368) by making sure that they obtain enough calcium in their diet (*see* HEALTH AT THE MENOPAUSE, p.36). High-fibre foods should form a substantial part of your diet to prevent constipation. A high intake of fruit and vegetables may also help to reduce your risk of colorectal cancer.

Good dental hygiene and tooth care (*see* CARING FOR YOUR TEETH AND GUMS, p.610) and regular visits to the dentist can help to prevent problems such as dental caries (p.609), gingivitis (p.617), and periodontitis (p.618), a condition that affects many older people and is a major cause of tooth loss. Losing teeth was once seen as an inevitable part of aging, but modern dentistry helps most people to avoid the need for dentures.

EXERCISE

Regular exercise plays a major role in preventing coronary artery disease (*see* THE BENEFITS OF EXERCISE, p.55). Osteoarthritis (p.374), in which the protective cartilage at the ends of bone wears away, often begins during the middle years, but exercise can prevent stiffness and keep joints mobile (*see* LIVING WITH ARTHRITIS, p.375). However, age-related bone and muscle loss can make you susceptible to injury, even if you follow your usual exercise routine. If you have been inactive for a while, seek medical advice before starting to exercise (*see* EXERCISING SAFELY, p.59).

PREVENTING ILLNESS

By the age of 65, the efficiency of the immune system has started to decline in most people, increasing their vulnerability to infections and cancer. You should take advantage of screening, such as eye tests and blood pressure measurement (*see* SCREENING, p.42), which can pick up early signs of diseases. You can reduce your risks of developing cancer and heart disease by not smoking and not drinking excessive amounts of alcohol. It is never too late to change bad habits and reap the health benefits (*see* HEALTH IN ADULTS, p.32).

By the age of 50, most people have difficulty in focusing on nearby objects (*see* PRESBYOPIA, p,589). Many other eye conditions become more common with increasing age, including glaucoma (p.575) and cataract (p.573). If such disorders are not detected and treated,

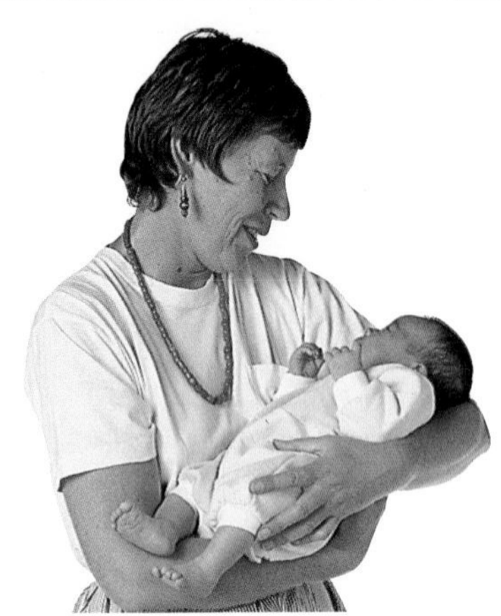

The joy of being a grandparent
As a grandparent, you can enjoy a child's company without the responsibilities associated with being a parent.

deteriorating vision can make activities such as driving dangerous. Many problems can be prevented by making sure that you have regular eye examinations.

PSYCHOLOGICAL HEALTH

Most people look forward to retiring during this time. Although this transition can be a rewarding experience, it can also generate feelings of isolation and loss of status and worth. Preparing for retirement by taking up new activities can help to ease the way.

For many people, this is a period of change and loss in their personal relationships, sometimes as a result of illness or death. Some will be coming to terms with their children reaching adulthood and moving away from home. Many people move house at this stage of life, perhaps to a smaller home or to an area where the pace of life is slower. For many couples, this can be a time to renew their relationship and to rediscover old pastimes and shared experiences.

Sex can be more rewarding in this stage of life, although women may find that they need to use a vaginal lubricant jelly after the menopause (*see* MENOPAUSAL PROBLEMS, p.737), and men may find that erections are less firm or long-lasting than in their youth. Although the frequency and prevalence of impotence (p.770) increases with advancing age, it is not an inevitable consequence of getting older. Men who experience more than an occasional episode of impotence should consult their doctor.

(WWW) ONLINE SITES: p.1026, p.1034, p.1037

Health at the menopause

Health considerations at the time when a woman stops menstruating

The menopause is the stage in a woman's life when her menstrual periods cease and she is no longer fertile. At the menopause, the ovaries no longer release eggs or produce the hormone oestrogen. The menopause usually takes place between the ages of 45 and 55 and may be sudden or may take several years.

Although some women experience unpleasant symptoms, more than 3 in 4 have only mild problems or none at all. Common symptoms include fluid retention, hot flushes, night sweats, aches and pains, and mood swings. All of these problems are linked to fluctuating levels of hormones (*see* MENOPAUSAL PROBLEMS, p.737), but most effects are only temporary. Other symptoms, such as vaginal dryness as a result of low oestrogen levels, will persist but can be managed relatively easily.

Before the menopause, women have a lower risk of coronary artery disease (p.405) than men because oestrogen has a protective effect. During and after the menopause, the fall in oestrogen levels increases a woman's risk of heart disease and speeds up the age-related process of osteoporosis (p.368), in which bones become more vulnerable to fracture.

Some women experience problems linked with the psychological impact of the menopause. The knowledge that you are no longer fertile may cause negative feelings, as may visible signs of aging.

POSITIVE STEPS

The symptoms and health risks associated with the menopause can be greatly reduced by modifying your lifestyle. Hormone replacement therapy (p.937) or other drug treatment may be advisable for some women. Support from your friends and relatives can also help you to cope better with the menopause.

LIFESTYLE CHANGES Regular aerobic exercise, such as swimming and running, helps to reduce the risk of heart disease. The earlier you start the better, but it is never too late. Stopping smoking (*see* TOBACCO AND HEALTH, p.63) and eating a healthy diet (p.48) also help to protect you against heart disease and cancer. You can reduce the risk of osteoporosis by not smoking, keeping your alcohol intake within the recommended limits (*see* SAFE ALCOHOL LIMITS, p.62), and taking regular weight-bearing exercise such as low-impact aerobics and walking. A calcium-rich diet is vital because it stimulates healthy bone growth and helps to prevent the progression of osteoporosis. If your diet is not high in calcium, you may wish to take a daily supplement of 1,000–1,500 mg of calcium with added vitamin D.

DRUG TREATMENT Women may wish to consider hormone replacement therapy (HRT) to reduce symptoms such as hot flushes and vaginal dryness. HRT usually involves taking a combination of the hormones oestrogen and progesterone. Oestrogen boosts levels that have fallen during the menopause, reduces the rate of bone loss, and provides protection against osteoporosis. Progesterone is included in HRT because oestrogen taken alone may increase your susceptibility to cancer of the uterus (p.748).

Treatment with HRT is usually continued for at least 5 years and may be continued indefinitely. Taking HRT for 10 years or more increases the risk of breast cancer developing. For this reason, HRT may not be appropriate for women who are already at increased risk of breast cancer. However, for most women, the beneficial effects of the treatment on the heart and bones outweigh this slight risk. Alternatives to HRT that help to prevent osteoporosis (p.368) are available, but none seems to have the same beneficial effect on the heart. Some women add soya products, such as tofu, to their diet because these have a natural oestrogenic effect.

PSYCHOLOGICAL SUPPORT If you are having psychological problems associated with the menopause, it is important to talk about your feelings with your partner or with another woman who is also going through the menopause. Relaxation (*see* RELAXATION EXERCISES, p.75) and other natural treatments may also help. If psychological problems persist, consult your doctor, who may prescribe antidepressant drugs (p.916).

(WWW) ONLINE SITES: p.1026, p.1037

Health in old age

Maintaining health and fitness when you are over the age of 70

Many people maintain good health and remain fit into old age. With fewer responsibilities and more leisure time, this can be an enjoyable stage of life. However, some of the physical changes that started during your middle years continue. You may not be able to move as quickly and easily as you once did. Recovery from illness and injury will take longer. Failing eyesight and hearing, urinary incontinence (p.710), an enlarged prostate gland (p.725) in men, and prolapse of the uterus and vagina (p.747) in women are some of the common concerns among older people.

The most serious health risks in this age group are accidents, heart disease, cancers of the respiratory and digestive tracts, diabetes mellitus (p.687), pneumonia (p.490), and stroke (p.532).

Diet and exercise

You should continue to follow a healthy diet (p.48) and drink plenty of water. You may find that you need fewer calories as you get older, and should avoid gaining excess weight. Making changes to your diet may add years to your life.

In the UK, 1 in 2 women will have developed osteoporosis (p.368) by the age of 80, making them vulnerable to fractures. To prevent bone thinning, eat plenty of calcium-rich foods, such as dairy products, and exercise regularly (*see* Keeping physically active, right). If you have a specific disorder, such as diabetes mellitus, your dietitian or doctor will be able to provide dietary advice.

Preventing illness

It is never too late to stop smoking, and doing so will slow the deterioration of many organs, particularly the heart and lungs. Giving up smoking will also reduce your chance of developing heart disease and some types of cancer. You should have regular health checkups (p.40). If you are taking medication for more than one condition, you should review your medicines with your doctor on a regular basis. This enables him or her to identify potential interactions between your prescribed drugs and any over-the-counter drugs you are taking.

HEALTH ACTION Keeping physically active

It is important to stay active as you get older because it keeps you fit and delays problems associated with aging. Regular exercise improves strength, muscle tone, and coordination, increases your alertness and reaction time, and can help to prevent falls. It is never too late to begin enjoying the benefits of regular exercise, as long as you start gradually. You should try to exercise at least 3–4 times a week.

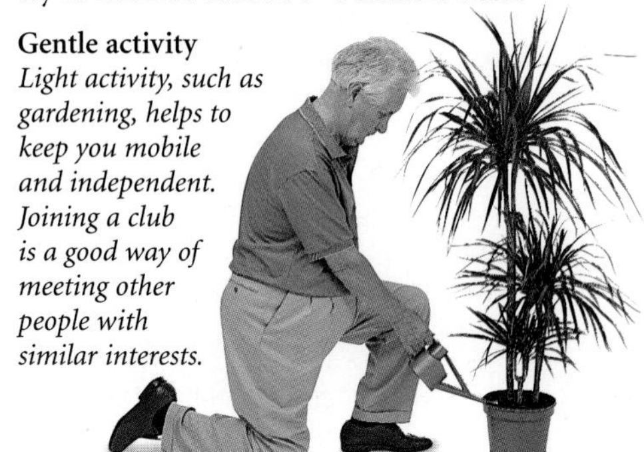

Gentle activity
Light activity, such as gardening, helps to keep you mobile and independent. Joining a club is a good way of meeting other people with similar interests.

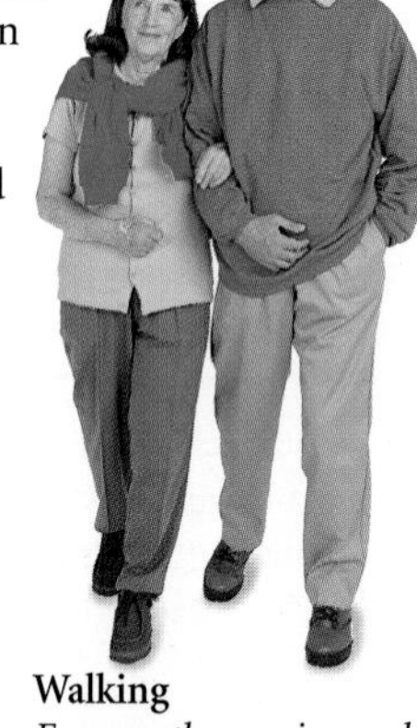

Walking
Even gentle exercise, such as walking at least 3 km (2 miles) each day, can significantly improve your health.

Avoiding accidents

People over the age of 70 may have an especially high risk of falls if they have mobility problems or attacks of fainting or dizziness. You can help to avoid falls by getting up slowly to reduce feelings of faintness and using a walking stick or frame. If you are on long-term medication, ask your doctor whether it can affect balance and coordination, and have your vision and hearing checked regularly because the eyes and ears help you to keep your balance. You can also have your home adapted to make it safer (*see* Home safety and health, p.77).

As you age, your body becomes less able to adjust to changes in temperature. Even when you are indoors, cold may aggravate heart and respiratory problems. To avoid becoming cold, keep the room you are in at a temperature of 19°C (68°F), even if you do not feel cold.

Psychological health

As you grow older, your memory may become less efficient, but you can stimulate your mind with activities such as solving crossword puzzles, taking up a new hobby, or learning a new language. Dementia (p.535), a general impairment of intellect, memory, and personality, is a serious condition that affects 1 in 20 people aged 70–80 and 1 in 5 people of 80 plus. About half of all dementia cases are caused by Alzheimer's disease (p.536), a progressive disorder of the brain. You should seek medical advice if you are worried about memory loss.

Another possible problem is depression (p.554), which is thought to affect 1.5 million people over the age of 65 in the UK. A major cause is the loss of a partner or other close companion (*see* Loss and bereavement, p.76). Other causes include prolonged, painful illness; loss of mobility; and a move to sheltered accommodation or a residential home. Activities can relieve feelings of isolation and provide opportunities for friendship. The potential for fulfilling sexual relationships is no less at this age than at earlier stages of adulthood.

(WWW) ONLINE SITES: p.1026, p.1034, p.1037

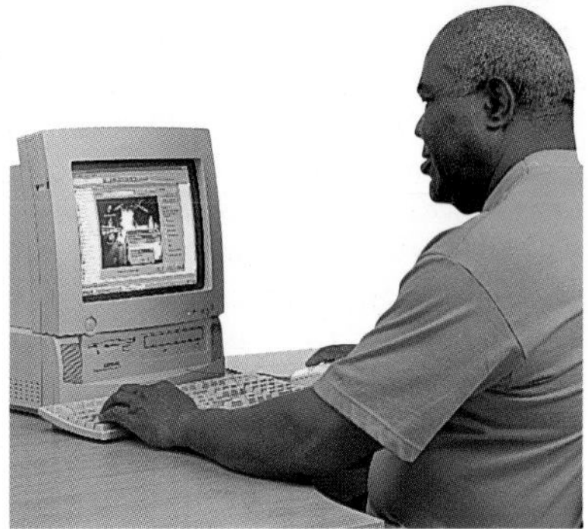

Stimulating your mind
Learning to use a home computer can stimulate your mind and give you access to a wide range of interesting information.

HEALTH CARE THROUGHOUT LIFE

Until the mid-20th century, people consulted a doctor only when they were ill, injured, or pregnant. Although for many people this is still largely the case, the past 50 years have seen an explosion in public knowledge about the causes of disease and a growing emphasis on health care that prevents as well as treats disease.

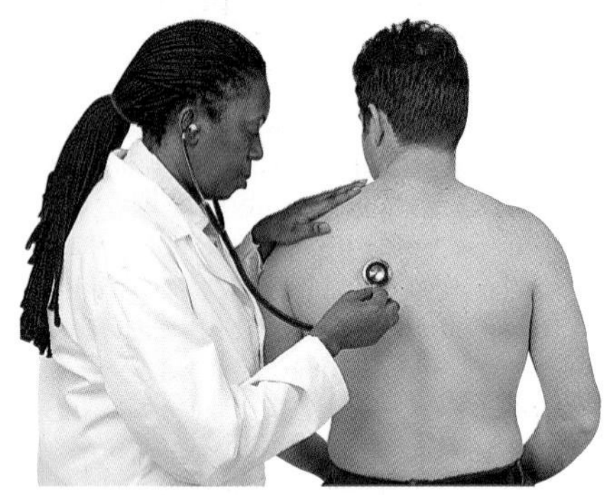

Having your health checked
Checkups are a chance to discuss ways of improving your health while your doctor examines you for early signs of disease.

This section begins with an article on the provision of health care in the UK, in particular, how the National Health Service is structured and the various levels of care it supplies. An overview of private medical care and health insurance is also included.

The main point of contact with the NHS for most people is with primary health care, which is provided by GPs and other health care professionals, such as practice nurses. The second article offers advice on choosing a practice and planning and getting the best from consultations with your doctor. As well as treating disorders, primary health care providers are responsible for two important elements in preventive health care: checkups during childhood and later in life, and screening tests to identify risk factors and early signs of disease. These topics are covered next.

The last article covers immunization. In developed countries, programmes of immunization from birth onwards have virtually eradicated many of the infections that used to be common in childhood. Immunization also protects people from serious illness in later life.

Health care providers

Understanding and getting the best from the National Health Service and private medical care

The major provider of health and medical care in the UK is the National Health Service (NHS). This state-funded organization was founded in 1948 with the promise of care for every man, woman, and child from the cradle to the grave.

NHS costs are high and continue to rise year on year. This is because treatment advances and new technologies are expensive, especially when they are made widely available, but also because the percentage of elderly people in society with greater health care needs is increasing. While prompt professional treatment delivered with respect and care is your right (because you have paid for it with your national insurance contributions), in many areas resources are stretched to their limit. There may be delays and long waiting times for some services, particularly nonurgent surgery, and some sophisticated treatments and tests are not widely available on the NHS. For these reasons, some people in the UK choose to pay for private medical care, usually by contributing to a medical insurance plan.

ORGANIZATION OF THE NHS

The NHS is the UK's largest organization, employing nearly a million people in thousands of clinics, health centres, hospitals, and residential homes. The central governing body of the NHS is the NHS Executive of the Department of Health, and local organization is through district health authorities, which are allocated funds for the areas they serve.

Community Health Councils, called Local Health Councils in Scotland and Health and Social Services Councils in Northern Ireland, represent the local community's interest in the health service. Their role includes visiting NHS premises and monitoring the quality of services, providing information, and assisting with complaints from the public.

TIERS OF HEALTH CARE

There are three levels of health care: primary, secondary, and tertiary. Primary health care includes the services provided by your local GP, either singly or in a group practice. Many group practices now provide a range of services such as family planning, immunization, and antenatal clinics. Local health centres, which sometimes incorporate one or more group practices, usually offer a range of services provided by other primary care specialists. These specialists may include practice nurses, district nurses, midwives, health visitors, chiropodists, dentists, physiotherapists, occupational therapists, and speech and language therapists. Most preventive health care, such as health, growth, and developmental checkups, immunization, and screening tests, is provided by the primary health care team.

For most people, their principal and often only point of contact with the NHS is at this first level of care. In 19 out of 20 cases, a health problem is diagnosed and treated by a GP or another primary health care professional.

Secondary care is the treatment you receive when you are referred to a specialist for tests or treatment. This type of care usually takes place in a hospital or in an outpatients clinic. Tertiary care is the term used for further referral to another specialist or for treatment in a specialist hospital. These levels of care are essentially for the treatment of disease, and the various places where they are provided are described elsewhere (*see* CARE OF THE SICK, pp.956–960).

PAYING FOR HEALTH CARE

Private medical care in the UK is either funded by medical insurance or paid for directly at some private hospitals. About 6 million people in the UK have private health insurance, more than half of which is paid for by employers.

The main advantage of private health care is that it reduces the waiting time for a consultation with and treatment by a specialist if you need planned secondary or tertiary care. You are usually able to choose the time and place of your treatment, and it is provided with the kind of service more often associated with a hotel than a hospital. However, the actual medical care you receive as a private patient is not substantially different from that of an NHS patient.

The range of health care that is covered by insurance varies depending on the policy. However, treatment for long-standing conditions such as diabetes, persistent psychiatric disorders such as depression, and cosmetic and fertility treatments are usually excluded. Some policies exclude screening tests and preventive treatments. Nearly all private patients use the NHS for primary care, although there are now a few private GPs and drop-in centres offering an immediate consultation for a fixed fee. Virtually all accident and emergency services are provided by the NHS.

(WWW) ONLINE SITES: p.1026, p.1032

You and your doctor

Choosing a practice and finding the right doctor for your primary care

Good health care should be a partnership between you and your GP. Ideally, you should have easy access to your doctor whenever you need it, without long delays. You should feel comfortable discussing any aspect of your health with your doctor and be confident that you are getting proper care from the practice with which you are registered.

About 1 in 10 practices are single-handed GP practices, and the rest are group practices with several partners. Most practices provide a range of services, such as antenatal care, and clinics for immunizations and minor surgery, such as wart removal.

Each GP has a contract with a district health authority to provide year-round primary health care for 24 hours a day. In practice, few GPs provide personal care for their patients out of normal hours. Instead, they use cooperative or agency arrangements for cover at night and at weekends. However, regardless of who carries out an out-of-hours visit, the responsibility for a person's continuing care remains with the GP.

Finding a practice

Before you register with a GP, find out as much as you can about the various options. You can get a list of doctors in your area from your Community Health Council or a local library. Ask friends and neighbours if they have any personal recommendations.

Most practices produce a leaflet listing the staff and services available. You will want information about practice hours and how long, on average, you will have to wait for an appointment for a problem that is not urgent. You will also want to know whether the practice offers home visits, advice over the telephone, services provided by other health care professionals, such as nursing staff, and special services, such as family planning or well-woman clinics. Paying a visit during surgery hours will help you to decide whether people are having to wait for a long time to see a doctor and whether reception staff are friendly and courteous.

If you have a strong preference for having a man or a woman as your doctor, this will be your first consideration. You may want to find out if any doctors have a special area of expertise, particularly if you have a long-term condition, such as diabetes mellitus (p.687).

You may be offered a pre-registration meeting with your new doctor. This will help you to decide whether you feel comfortable with the doctor and confident that you can talk to him or her about embarrassing and intimate topics. You may want to ensure that your GP is in sympathy with you on matters that you feel strongly about, such as home births or the prescribing of antibiotics.

Making the most of a visit

The key to a successful appointment with your GP is good communication. You should try to provide accurate information about your symptoms, past history, and lifestyle. Your GP should offer medical and health care advice in a way that is easy for you to understand and encourage you to be actively involved in maintaining your health and in any treatment you may require (*see* VISITING YOUR DOCTOR, p.216–223). You should not feel anxious about asking questions about your treatment or raising issues that are important to you.

Consultations with your doctor are usually timed at 7–10 minute intervals; if you feel that you may need substantially longer than this, ask for a double appointment. If possible, try to plan what you wish to discuss before you arrive at the surgery. This will help your doctor to focus on your most important concerns and give them priority. You should wear clothes or dress your child in clothes that can be easily unfastened and removed in case you need a physical examination.

Your health records

Before your first visit to a new doctor, you may be asked to complete a questionnaire about your medical history and lifestyle. Your doctor will use this information as a starting point for asking further questions during the visit. Topics will probably include your diet, work, relationships, the amount of alcohol you drink, the exercise you take, and whether or not you smoke. Your doctor will also check that you are up to date with immunizations (p.45) and screening tests appropriate for your age and gender (*see* SCREENING, p.42).

During subsequent visits, your doctor will make notes, either by hand or on a computer, that become part of your medical records. People have the right to read any medical records relating to them that have been recorded since their right of access became law in November 1991. You are allowed to inspect your own or your child's records directly or to have a copy taken. You also have the

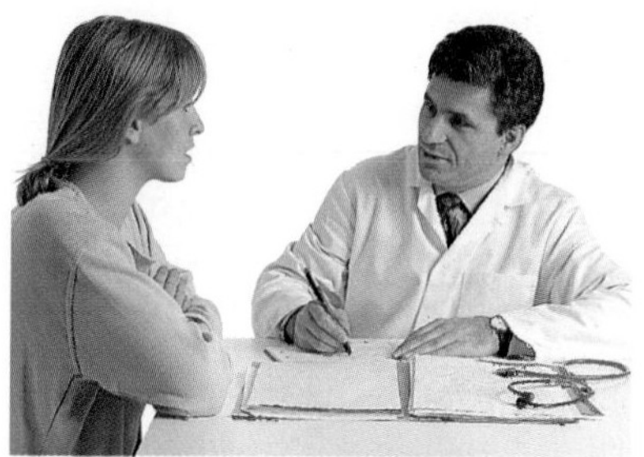

Communicating with your doctor
When you are comfortable and relaxed with your doctor, it is easier to discuss problems openly. You should always try to discuss important issues first.

(ASSESSMENT) GROWTH CHARTS FOR BABIES

During regular checkups in the first 2 years of life, a baby's growth is monitored to detect problems at an early stage. Weight, length, and head circumference (measured around the largest part of the head) are plotted against the baby's age on growth charts. Your baby's growth curves can then be compared with the range of typical measurements for babies of the same age, shown as shaded bands on the charts. If a growth curve falls outside the shaded area or displays an erratic pattern, it indicates a possible problem.

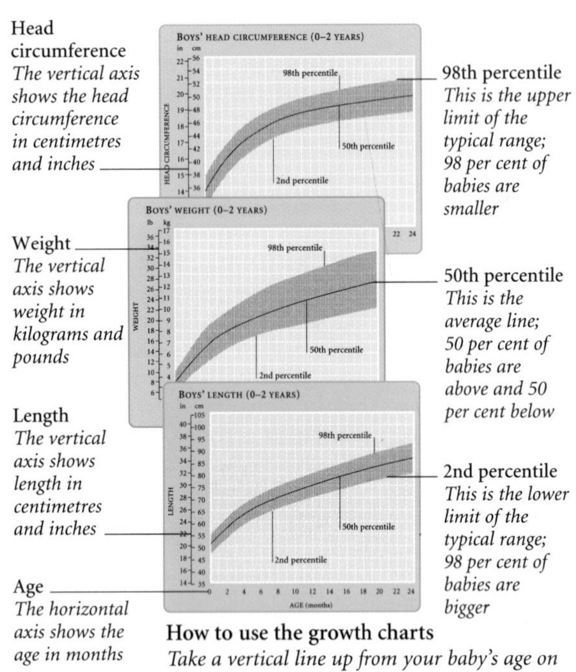

How to use the growth charts
Take a vertical line up from your baby's age on the bottom of the chart and a horizontal line from the measurement of length, weight, or head circumference on the left and plot the point at which they cross.

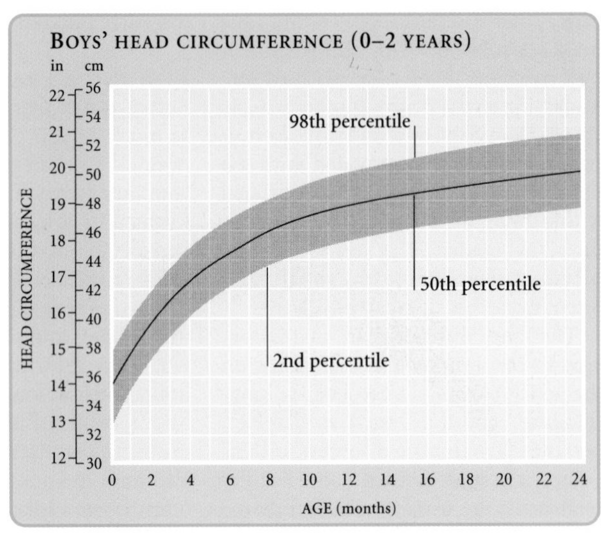

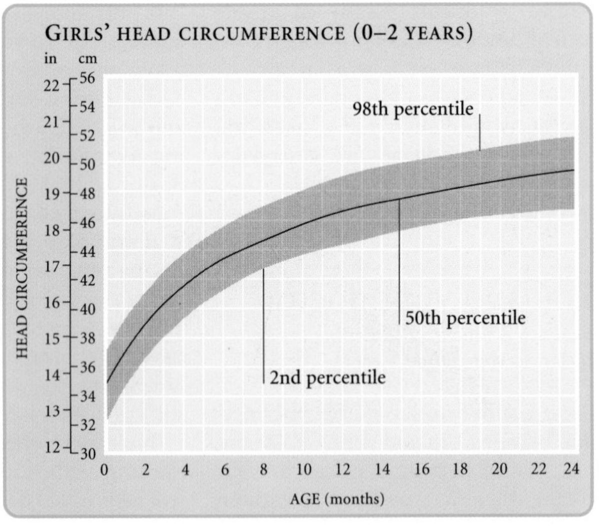

right to read letters and notes if you are referred for secondary or tertiary care. Your doctor may be asked to report on your medical history and state of health for life insurance purposes, welfare benefits, private medical schemes, for a new employer, or for evidence in court. He or she must have your written consent before passing on this information.

Your complete health records, including letters to and from consultants, details of any hospital admissions and summaries of any treatment you have received, are transferred with you if you change your GP or sign on with a new doctor when you move to another area.

(WWW) ONLINE SITES: p.1026, p.1032

Health checkups

Visits to the doctor or a health clinic to check on your state of health, or to monitor a child's growth and development

Health checkups are an opportunity to talk about your or your child's general health with a primary health care specialist, such as a doctor or health visitor, when there are no immediate medical problems to be dealt with.

In babies and infants, health checks tend to focus on healthy growth and development. Checkups in adults usually include a physical examination (*see* PHYSICAL EXAMINATION, p. 219) in order to establish your current state of health and tests, such as blood pressure measurement, to look for factors that increase your risk of disorders (*see* COMMON SCREENING TESTS, p.44). Later in life, health checks are designed to detect potential problems or assess your general functions as you age.

In the UK, regular checkups are only offered routinely in childhood and after the age of 70. Pregnant women have regular health checks with their doctor or midwife as part of their antenatal care. You may also have a health check when you join a new practice or be required to have checkups for insurance purposes or when you begin a new job.

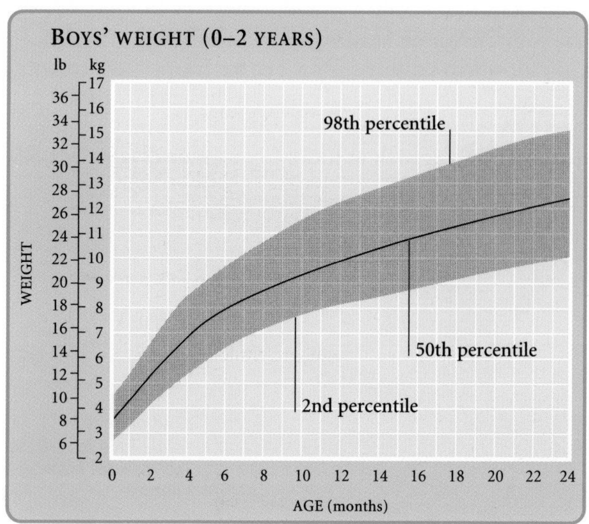

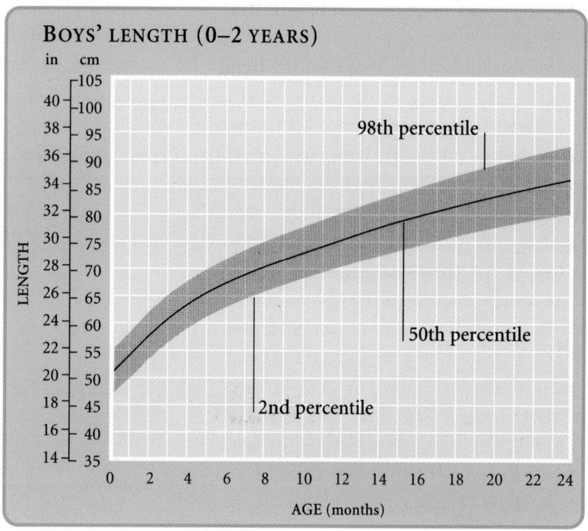

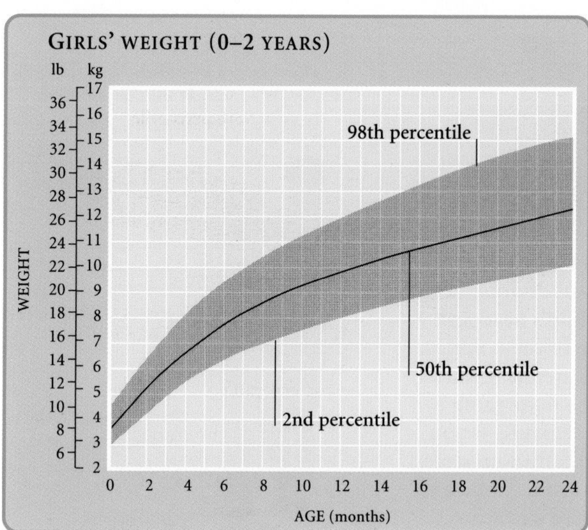

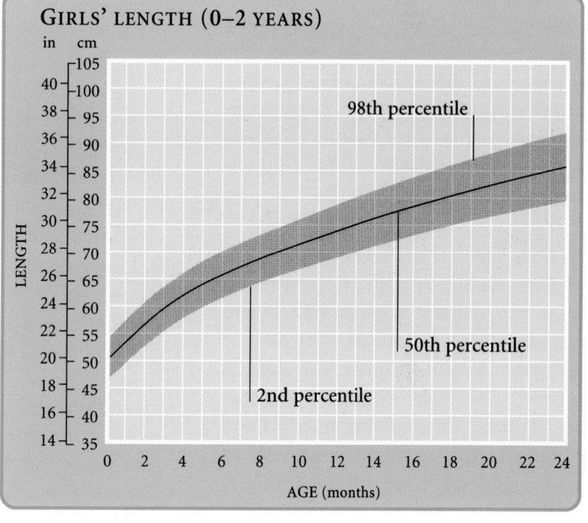

Some employers and private health care providers offer regular health checks as part of their general provision, although the value of these is disputed.

CHECKUPS IN CHILDHOOD All newborn babies have a complete physical examination within 24 hours of their birth to identify potential problems. During the examination, the doctor listens to the baby's heart for problems such as a heart murmur (*see* CONGENITAL HEART DISEASE, p.836) and checks the eyes for abnormalities such as cataracts (p.573). Until a child reaches school age, subsequent checkups are carried out at regular intervals by your doctor or a health visitor at your local health clinic. After your child starts school, checkups are not routine, but children who need special monitoring may be seen regularly by community paediatricians.

The purpose of health checks in childhood is to ensure that the child's physical, social, and intellectual development are progressing satisfactorily. Although the exact age at which children reach developmental milestones varies (*see* GAINING SKILLS DURING THE FIRST FIVE YEARS, p. 814), the doctor or health visitor will check that the child has gained certain skills within predicted age ranges. These include gross motor skills, such as the ability to sit up; fine motor skills, such as picking up a small object; and social skills, such as using language. Your child will also have regular hearing and vision tests.

Physical growth is monitored by measuring a baby's weight and length and also head circumference, which is an accurate indicator of general growth during the first 2 years. These measurements are recorded on a chart (*see* GROWTH CHARTS FOR BABIES, above).

At key intervals in childhood, such as before starting school and around the time of puberty, a child's growth, development, and physical and social skills are checked so that any problems can be dealt with promptly. Measuring height and weight is an essential part of checkups, and many parents like to keep their own record of their child's growth (*see* GROWTH CHARTS FOR CHILDREN, right).

CHECKUPS IN ADULTS Health checks in adult life rely partly on questionnaires about lifestyle and partly on a few basic tests such as measurement of blood pressure. Your doctor may also measure your height and weight to make sure that they are within a healthy range (*see* ARE YOU A HEALTHY WEIGHT?, p.53). Excess weight increases the risk of many disorders, particularly atherosclerosis (p.402), in which arteries are narrowed by fatty deposits. Underweight women may have reduced fertility (*see* FEMALE INFERTILITY, p.775), and, in either sex, being underweight increases the risk of osteoporosis (p.368) in later life.

Your GP will decide from your medical history whether you need particular screening tests (p.44). As you get older, health checks are used to detect the early stages of disease and assess factors that are important to your future independence, such as your mobility, muscle strength and coordination, hearing, vision, and mental health.

ACTING ON YOUR CHECKUP

Using the results of your checkup, your doctor will suggest ways in which you can maintain and promote your own or your child's health. You can also discuss any particular health concerns you may have. You may need further tests if there are factors that increase your risk of disease, such as your lifestyle, family history, occupation, or travel abroad.

(WWW) ONLINE SITES: p.1026, p.1032

ASSESSMENT GROWTH CHARTS FOR CHILDREN

Growth charts are used to record a child's growth from 2 to 18 years. During health checks, your doctor or health visitor measures your child's weight and height and plots them against age on a chart. Your child's growth curve can then be compared with the typical range, represented by the shaded part of the chart, for all children of the same age. You may want to measure and record your child's growth at more frequent intervals yourself.

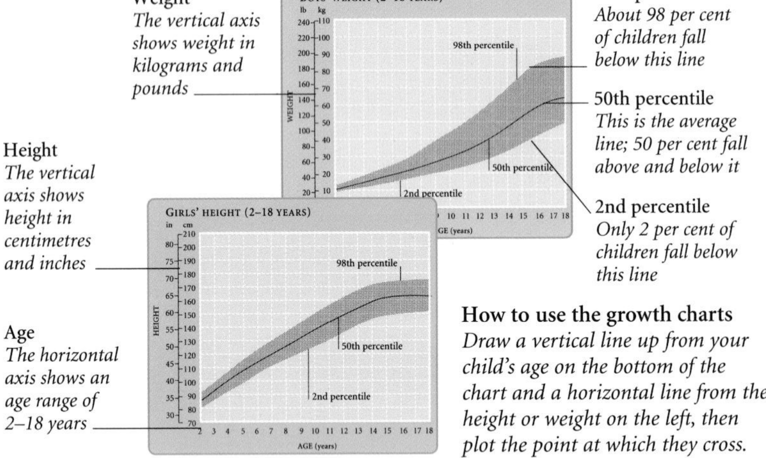

Weight
The vertical axis shows weight in kilograms and pounds

Height
The vertical axis shows height in centimetres and inches

Age
The horizontal axis shows an age range of 2–18 years

98th percentile
About 98 per cent of children fall below this line

50th percentile
This is the average line; 50 per cent fall above and below it

2nd percentile
Only 2 per cent of children fall below this line

How to use the growth charts
Draw a vertical line up from your child's age on the bottom of the chart and a horizontal line from the height or weight on the left, then plot the point at which they cross.

MEASURING YOUR CHILD

To measure your child's height, ask the child to stand up straight, with his or her back against a wall or door. Lower a book on to your child's head and mark where the base of the book meets the wall. Measure the distance from this mark to the floor using a lockable metal tape measure. If you weigh your child on bathroom scales, make sure that they are accurate and standing on a flat, hard surface.

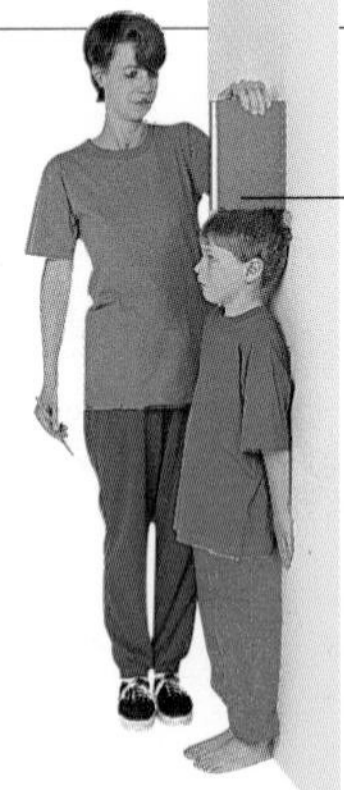

Marker guide
To get an accurate measurement, use a book or cereal box as a guide

Measuring height
Make sure your child is barefoot and is standing up straight.

Screening

Detecting disease or risk factors for a disease before symptoms develop

Screening is an important element of preventive medicine. Most screening tests are used to detect risk factors associated with disease or to make an early diagnosis of a treatable condition. Less commonly, if there is a rare inherited disease in your family history, screening may be carried out to find out if you have an abnormal gene that could cause a disorder in you or your children (*see* TESTS FOR ABNORMAL GENES, p.239).

You may be offered screening tests at different stages of your life. A few tests are offered to women as part of national screening programmes, while others are available on request or are suggested if there are risk factors which predispose you to a particular disease.

Before accepting a test, you should ask your doctor what it involves, if it carries risks, and how reliable it is. You should also consider the possible implications of the test results. No test is completely accurate, and sometimes a test can miss disease or suggest disease when it is not present. An abnormal result may lead to further investigations for which you might not be prepared.

WHY PEOPLE ARE SCREENED

It is not possible or even worthwhile to screen for every risk factor or disease. Tests are useful only if they detect a disease or risk factor that can be treated effectively, and which benefits from early treatment. For example, women are screened for cervical abnormalities such as cervical dysplasia (p.750) that can be treated before cancer of the cervix (p.749) develops.

Some screening tests are offered to adults at stages of life when the risk of certain diseases increases (*see* COMMON SCREENING TESTS, p.44). You may be offered other tests if you have a higher than normal risk of a disorder due to

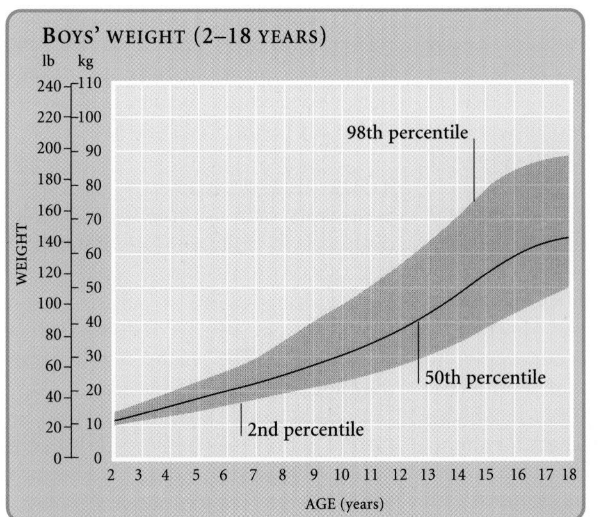

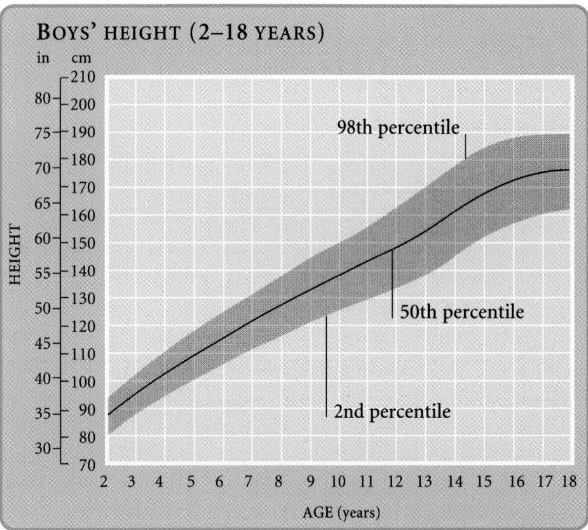

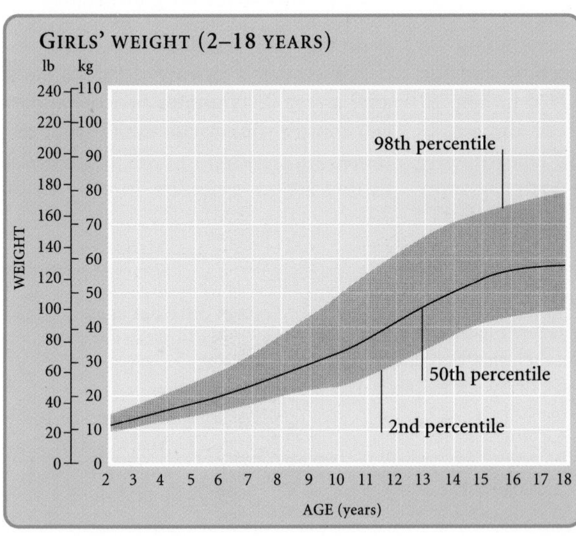

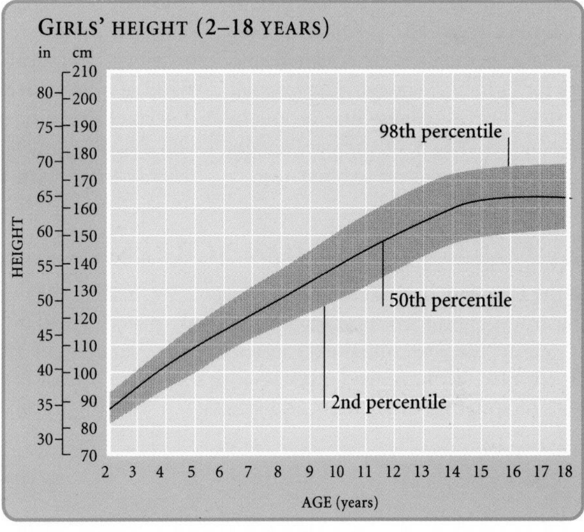

factors in your lifestyle such as heavy smoking, your age, family history of disease, or a pre-existing illness that increases the risk of other disorders.

STAGE OF LIFE Your risk of developing certain disorders depends on your age. For this reason, the type and frequency of screening tests that your doctor may recommend will change as you grow older. Women are offered a specific programme of tests during pregnancy (*see* ROUTINE ANTENATAL CARE, p.786), in which they are tested regularly for conditions such as pre-eclampsia (*see* PRE-ECLAMPSIA AND ECLAMPSIA, p.794) or diabetes mellitus (p.687) that can be harmful to the mother or the baby or both. The fetus may also be screened by ultrasound (*see* ULTRASOUND SCANNING IN PREGNANCY, p.793) for abnormalities such as heart disorders that may require treatment after birth.

ADULT SCREENING Screening for early signs of breast cancer (p.759) and cervical cancer is offered on the NHS to women in specific age groups. Cervical cancer screening is offered to sexually active women every 3–5 years until the age of 65, and breast cancer screening is offered every 3–5 years to women aged 50–65. Screening tests for other cancers, such as colorectal cancer (p.665) and prostate cancer (p.726) are available, but these are not yet offered routinely in the UK. One of the most common screening tests is blood pressure measurement. The reason is because high blood pressure (*see* HYPERTENSION, p.403) itself is symptomless but is a major risk factor for heart disease and stroke. Blood pressure is usually measured in the doctor's surgery, often when you see the doctor for another health problem.

INHERITED DISORDERS A number of disorders, including abnormally high levels of cholesterol and other lipids in the blood (*see* INHERITED HYPERLIPIDAEMIAS, p.692), colorectal cancer, and breast cancer, tend to run in families. If any members of your family have been affected by one of these disorders, your doctor may suggest that you undergo screening tests to look for early disease. For example you may be offered regular faecal occult blood tests (p.233) that detect blood in the stools if you have a family history of colorectal cancer. A woman with a family history of breast cancer, may be offered breast X-rays (*see* MAMMOGRAPHY, p.759) earlier or more often than is usual. Particular forms of breast cancer are known to be caused by inherited faulty genes. Although there are tests that can identify specific abnormal genes (*see* TESTS FOR ABNORMAL GENES, p.239), these are not yet widely available in the UK.

CHRONIC CONDITIONS If you have a long-term disorder, you may be offered regular screening to detect early signs of complications. For example, people with diabetes mellitus are screened routinely for kidney disease, cardiovascular disorders, nerve damage, and problems in the blood vessels of the eye, which, left untreated, may lead to blindness.

HAZARDOUS OCCUPATIONS In some occupations, workers are exposed to dust or toxic chemicals that can increase the risk of some diseases. If your occupation carries known health risks, make sure that you take appropriate safety measures (*see* SAFETY AND HEALTH AT WORK, p.82) and take part in screening programmes offered by your employer.

WHO CARRIES OUT SCREENING?

Most screening is carried out at your doctor's surgery, and at special clinics such as well-woman clinics, or is organized by your employer. However, it may be necessary for your doctor to refer you to a specialist for certain tests such as colonoscopy (p.661), in which a viewing tube is used to check for abnormalities in the colon.

There are a number of simple health checks that you can carry out regularly yourself. Self-screening includes breast self-examination (p.755), examining the testes (p.720), and inspecting skin for signs of skin cancer (p.344) to help to detect early indications of disease. If you discover any signs of abnormality, discuss them with your doctor as soon as possible. Although it is now possible to buy screening test kits for some disorders over the counter, you should always consult your doctor if you are concerned about a health risk. He or she will arrange for you to have appropriate tests, interpret the results, and advise about any further tests you may need.

YOUR TEST RESULTS

Some tests, such as those for metabolic disorders in children (*see* SCREENING FOR METABOLIC DISORDERS, p.867), produce a clear positive or negative result that does not usually require further investigation. The results of other tests may not be as easy to interpret.

If your test results are negative, no further action may be needed until the next screening test is due. No screening test is 100 per cent accurate, and, rarely, a disorder may be present even though test results were negative. When this happens, the result is called a false-negative.

Sometimes a disease develops soon after a test: if symptoms become apparent, consult your doctor even if your test result was negative. You will be advised if further action is needed. In most cases,

ASSESSMENT COMMON SCREENING TESTS

In the UK, only heel prick tests, cervical smear tests, and mammography are offered as nationwide screening programmes. Your doctor may recommmend other tests on the basis of your age, occupation, and genetic and lifestyle factors. Some tests may be performed by your GP while others are carried out in hospital clinics. Screening for eye disease is carried out by your optician during routine eye tests.

Tests at different ages
Most tests to detect early signs of disease begin in adulthood. Extra tests are added after the age of 50.

SCREENING TEST	DISEASE	WHEN RECOMMENDED	COMMENTS
Heel prick blood test (*see* SCREENING FOR METABOLIC DISORDERS, p.867)	Hypothyroidism (p.680) Phenylketonuria (p.867)	Soon after birth	Blood sample is taken for analysis from the heel of all newborn babies
Blood pressure measurement (p.404)	Hypertension (p.403)	Every 5 years from about the age of 20	Blood pressure is often checked during visits to the doctor. High blood pressure is a risk factor for heart disease and stroke
Blood cholesterol tests (p.231)	Hypercholesterolaemia (p.691)	Every 5 years from about the age of 20	High cholesterol levels are a risk factor for heart disease and stroke
Cervical smear test (p.749)	Cervical dysplasia (p.750) Cancer of the cervix (p.750)	Every 3–5 years from first sexual activity to 65 years	Test is offered every 5 years, but 3-year intervals between tests are recommended
Faecal occult blood (p.233)	Colorectal cancer (p.665)	Every year from the age of 50	Test is available on request from your GP and is becoming standard practice
Mammography (p.759)	Breast cancer (p.759)	Every 3–5 years from the age of 50	Offered to women aged 50–65, the test may continue after 65 years on request
Eye pressure measurement (*see* TONOMETRY, p.576)	Glaucoma (p.575)	Every 2 years from the age of 40	Eye tests by an optician are free for people over 65 or those at high risk of glaucoma

regular screening tests pick up diseases before symptoms develop.

If your test result is positive, your doctor may want to repeat the test or arrange for additional investigations to confirm the result and perhaps provide more information. For example, if a breast X-ray reveals an abnormality, an additional test, in which a sample of cells is collected using a needle and syringe (*see* ASPIRATION OF A BREAST LUMP, p.756), may be needed to find out what is causing the abnormality.

(WWW) ONLINE SITES: p.1026

Immunization

A method of producing artificial immunity to infectious diseases, usually involving a course of injections

Immunization is a way of boosting the body's defences against infectious diseases. Most immunizations use a vaccine containing a tiny amount of a weakened or inactivated form of a disease-causing organism (*see* VACCINES AND IMMUNOGLOBULINS, p.883). When the vaccine is introduced into your body, it stimulates your immune system to produce antibodies against the disease so that you are protected if you are exposed to the organism at some time in the future. Most vaccines are given by injection, although a few, such as poliomyelitis, can be given orally. For most immunizations, several injections are given over a period of months or years to build up adequate protection.

TIMING OF IMMUNIZATIONS

Most routine immunizations (right) are given during infancy and childhood according to an immunization schedule. In addition, people who are at particular risk, because of the nature of their work or travel, may be offered extra immunizations during their adult life. Keep records of all your immunizations and those of your children in case a doctor other than your GP needs to know about your immune status.

BABIES AND CHILDREN Immunizations are given to babies during their first year, when infectious diseases are most likely to be serious. A baby has some natural protection from antibodies that pass through the placenta during pregnancy, but this immunity wears off by about 6 months after birth. Premature babies are immunized routinely after birth because they are at high risk of serious illness if they develop an infection.

By the time children start school, most will have completed the first part of their schedule of immunizations. A BCG vaccination against tuberculosis is given around puberty, and booster doses of some vaccines are given to school leavers aged 16–18 years. Timings can be adjusted if a child misses immunizations or starts the schedule late.

SPECIAL CIRCUMSTANCES Adults sometimes need a booster dose in special circumstances. For example, you may need an extra injection against tetanus (p.302) if you sustain a deep or dirty cut.

Influenza (p.289) and pneumococcal pneumonia (p.490) can be serious disorders, particularly in people over the age of 65 or in those who have reduced immunity because of long-term conditions such as diabetes mellitus (p.687) or HIV infection and AIDS (p.297). Both children and adults in these high-risk groups are offered immunization against these diseases. You may also need to have extra immunizations if you plan to travel to a country that has a high incidence of infectious diseases, such as hepatitis and yellow fever (*see* TRAVEL IMMUNIZATIONS, p.86).

RISKS OF IMMUNIZATION

Immunizations have few side effects, although there may be some inflammation around the injection site or a mild fever. If you have any reactions to initial doses, tell your doctor so that he or she can advise you about subsequent doses. Serious side effects are extremely rare. Concern that immunization with the measles, mumps, rubella (MMR) vaccine may be associated with autism and Crohn's disease have not been substantiated. Research has shown that, in general, the risks to children from routine immunizations are substantially lower than the risks associated with the diseases against which they protect.

Homeopathic types of vaccine have been shown to be ineffective. If you rely on them, you could be putting yourself or your children at risk.

(WWW) ONLINE SITES: p.1028, p.1033, p.1037

(HEALTH ACTION) ROUTINE IMMUNIZATIONS

Immunizations give protection against several infectious diseases and are scheduled during childhood. Serious reactions to immunizations are rare; consult your doctor if you are worried.

Routine schedule

Timing of immunizations can be adjusted if some doses are missed. Most immunizations are given by injection.

DISEASE	TIMING OF IMMUNIZATIONS						
	AGE (MONTHS)				AGE (YEARS)		
	2	3	4	12–15	3–5	10–14	16–18
Diphtheria*	✓	✓	✓		✓		✓
Tetanus*	✓	✓	✓		✓		✓
Pertussis*	✓	✓	✓				
Poliomyelitis	✓	✓	✓		✓		✓
Haemophilus influenzae type b (Hib)	✓	✓	✓				
Meningitis C (Meningococcus C)	✓	✓	✓				✓†
Measles, mumps, rubella (MMR)				✓	✓		
Tuberculosis (BCG)						✓	

*given as one vaccine to babies up to 4 months

†if not given previously

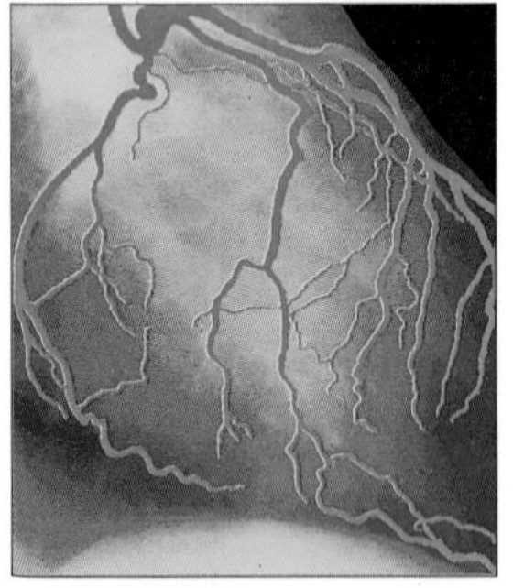

Healthy heart
Lifestyle factors such as diet can affect the coronary arteries and thus the health of your heart.

LIFESTYLE AND HEALTH

YOUR HEALTH IS INFLUENCED by two major factors: your genetic make-up, which determines your predisposition to disease, and your lifestyle. You cannot change inherited factors, but you can adapt your behaviour to control your risk of disease or injury. You have some control over what you eat and drink and whether you smoke, exercise, or practise safe sex. Your lifestyle choices affect your present and future health.

In the developed world, life expectancy has risen greatly over the last century due to improvements in public health. However, every year in the UK almost 90,000 people die before the age of 65, often from long-term diseases such as cancer or heart disease. You can reduce your risk of developing some of these diseases by adopting a healthy lifestyle.

UNDERSTANDING THE RISKS

It is important to be aware of the lifestyle factors associated with certain diseases so that you can make informed choices. For example, tobacco smoking is a critical factor in a third of all deaths from cancer. Several lifestyle factors, including smoking and a high-fat diet, are known to contribute to the development of heart disease.

In order to make informed decisions about your health priorities, you need to take into account your individual circumstances. Your doctor can help you to do this. Your age is one of the most important factors and greatly influences the lifestyle decisions that you need to make. For example, young adults are statistically more likely to experience illness or injury associated with risk-taking behaviour, such as sexually transmitted infections or reactions to recreational drugs, than to suffer from ill health due to long-term disease. Another consideration is work: if you have a dangerous occupation, such as construction work, paying close attention to safety could be the most important factor in protecting your health in the short term. Nevertheless, it is important to recognize that some lifestyle choices, such as tobacco smoking, do not carry an immediate and obvious threat but can ultimately cause serious damage to your health (*see* ASSESSING HEALTH RISKS, left).

MAKING LIFESTYLE CHANGES

Most health habits, such as food choices and taking exercise, are formed in our families when we are children. Giving children a healthy lifestyle from birth maximizes their chances of growing into healthy adults and establishes habits that they may find easier to maintain in later life. Some families may find it difficult to make healthy lifestyle choices. For example, they may not be able to afford good food or housing. However, everyone can do something to improve health.

The first step towards a healthier lifestyle is to identify activities that pose significant risks to your health. It is easier to change these activities if you can see immediate benefits. Long-term changes, such as giving up smoking, increasing the amount of exercise that you take, or changing your diet, are often more difficult to make and maintain, especially if they involve overcoming social pressure. You may need to seek support from family, friends, and health professionals.

(ASSESSMENT) ASSESSING HEALTH RISKS

Some activities, such as hang-gliding, are clearly dangerous and carry a significant risk every time you do them. For other types of behaviour, the risks to health may not be as obvious. Eating one high-fat meal does not damage your health, but consistently including too much fat in your diet may increase your risk of developing heart disease over time.

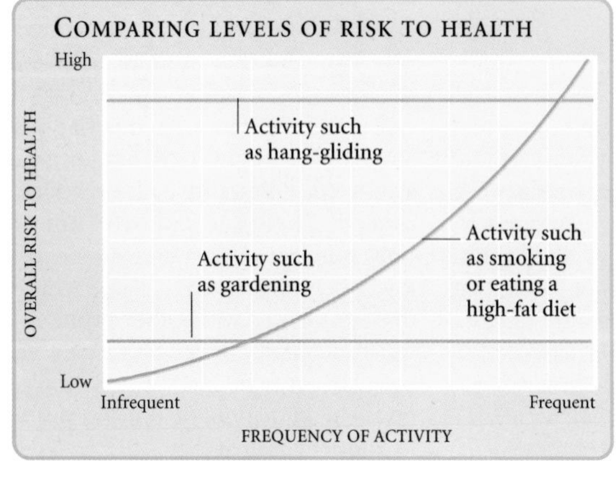

Cumulative risk
Some activities, such as gardening, carry the same risk each time you do them. With other activities, such as smoking, the risk to health tends to be cumulative; they are likely to damage your health only if they are carried out repeatedly over a period of time.

HEALTH OPTIONS MAKING LIFESTYLE CHOICES

All aspects of life, including work, travel, home, and leisure, carry risks and benefits to health. Some of these risks differ from one person to another. For example, a high-fat diet may be more harmful for a middle-aged man than for a young girl. You need to balance these risks and benefits so that you can enjoy your life while staying healthy.

Work and travel
Some occupations, such as construction work, carry a much greater risk of injury than sedentary occupations. Your method of transport also involves specific health benefits and risks.

Home
Activities that take place in the home, such as eating, sleeping, and being with your family, have a major influence on physical and mental health. As children, we learn healthy or unhealthy habits in the home environment.

Leisure
You should consider the health benefits and risks of different activities when deciding how to spend your free time. Sports, hobbies, and social activities can all benefit your physical and mental health, but some carry a risk of injury or harm.

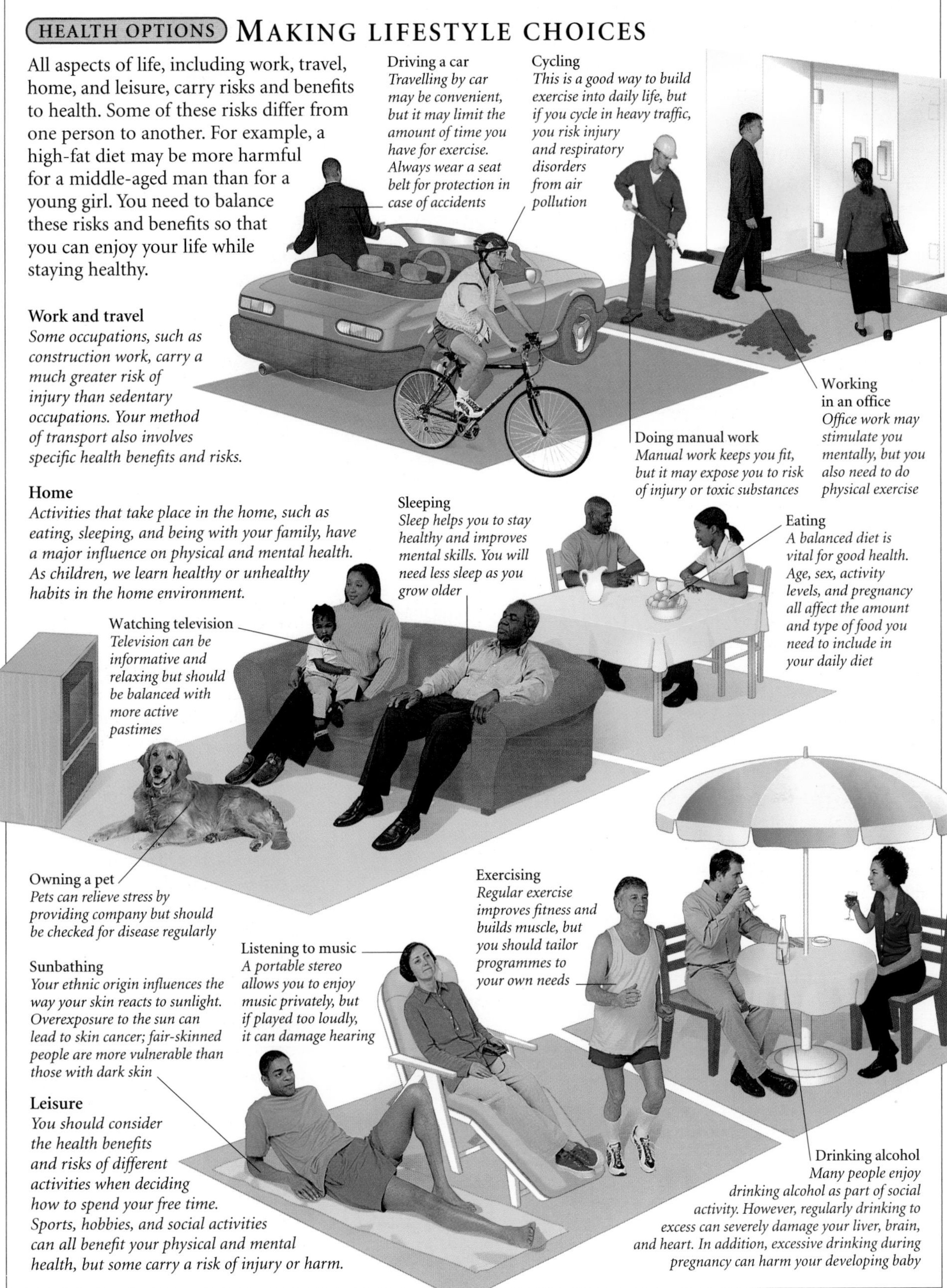

DIET AND HEALTH

By far the most common problem with the British diet is excess. People in the UK tend to consume too much food, especially too much fat, salt, and sugar. Overconsumption of these nutrients has been linked to some of the main causes of death in the UK: heart disease, cancer, and stroke. Making informed choices about your diet could improve your chance of avoiding these diseases.

The huge growth in the availability and popularity of fast food has led to a corresponding rise in poor eating habits because packaged snacks and meals often contain large amounts of ingredients that can be harmful. The first article in this section provides easy-to-follow guidelines on how to assess and improve your diet, explains how food energy is measured, and describes how each of the major food groups (carbohydrate, protein, and fat) contributes to your nutritional needs. Many people in the UK have a diet that provides more energy than they need, and, as a result, a significant percentage of the population is obese and suffers from health problems associated with being overweight. The second article explains how to determine your ideal weight and explores various methods of losing or gaining weight.

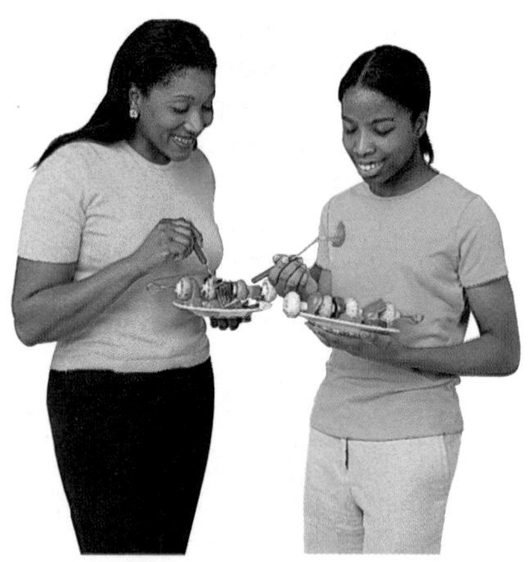

Eating well
Food is essential for good health but is also an important aspect of social life for most people. Cooking and sharing healthy food can be an enjoyable part of daily life.

A healthy diet

A diet that contains the right balance of foods for optimum health

Variation in diet among people living in different countries is closely associated with national patterns of disease. For example, the high-calorie, high-fat diet common in the UK is linked to the high national rates of obesity (p.631), heart disease (*see* CORONARY ARTERY DISEASE, p.405), and stroke (p.532). In contrast, the traditional Mediterranean diet, which includes plenty of fresh vegetables, olive oil, and fish and is therefore low in saturated fat, seems to be related to the low incidence of heart disease in Mediterranean countries. In Japan, the typical diet is high in fibre, and the incidence of colorectal cancer (p.665) is low. In many countries, an excessive amount of salt in the diet has been associated with people having high blood pressure (*see* HYPERTENSION, p.403).

Just as an excess of certain elements in the diet can lead to health problems, deficiencies in essential nutrients can result in poor health (*see* NUTRITIONAL DEFICIENCIES, p.630). Such deficiencies, however, are rare in developed countries such as the UK.

The knowledge gained by nutritionists from studying the effects of diet on

ASSESSMENT HOW HEALTHY IS YOUR DIET?

You may find it difficult to keep to a healthy diet all the time, particularly if you eat out a lot or if you rely on convenience foods. The questionnaire below will help you to identify some areas that can make the difference between a healthy diet and one of poor nutritional value.

1 *Has your weight stayed the same over the last 6 months (assuming you have not been trying to change it)?*
☐ YES ☐ NO

2 *Do you eat some fruit and some vegetables most days of the week?*
☐ YES ☐ NO

3 *Do you regularly vary the type of food you eat?*
☐ YES ☐ NO

4 *Do you try to avoid "junk food" such as chocolate and crisps?*
☐ YES ☐ NO

5 *Do you try to eat wholemeal pasta and brown rice, rather than white pasta and rice?*
☐ YES ☐ NO

6 *Do you tend to grill food rather than fry it?*
☐ YES ☐ NO

7 *Do you drink at least 8 glasses (2 litres/4 pints) of water a day?*
☐ YES ☐ NO

8 *Do you try to leave food unsalted?*
☐ YES ☐ NO

ANALYSIS

If you answered yes to all the questions, you are probably eating a diet that will benefit your health. If you answered no to two or more of the questions, you should consider your diet in more detail. Learn about the nutritional values of different foods and what constitutes a balanced diet. You may also want to try alternative methods of food preparation and cooking.

HEALTH ACTION HEALTHY EATING

A healthy diet combines a variety of foods in different proportions. Foods are divided into five groups, shown here in the relative proportions in which they should be eaten to form a balanced, healthy diet. Enjoy your food and vary your diet to ensure that you get all of the nutrients your body needs. Eat the correct amount to maintain a healthy weight. Fresh fruit and vegetables and carbohydrate-rich foods such as potatoes should form the bulk of your diet, with meat, fish, and dairy products forming a smaller part of your daily intake.

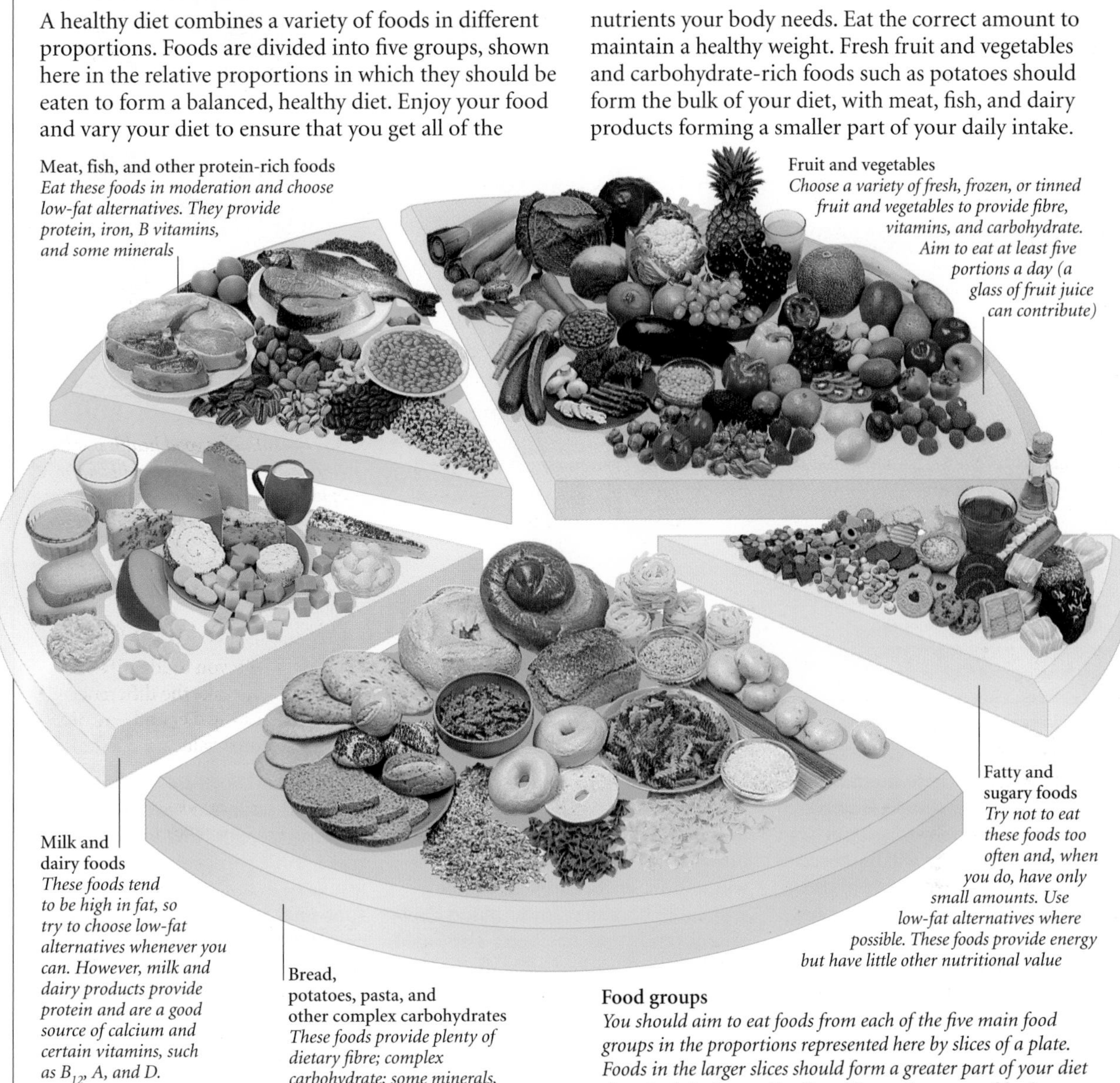

Meat, fish, and other protein-rich foods
Eat these foods in moderation and choose low-fat alternatives. They provide protein, iron, B vitamins, and some minerals

Fruit and vegetables
Choose a variety of fresh, frozen, or tinned fruit and vegetables to provide fibre, vitamins, and carbohydrate. Aim to eat at least five portions a day (a glass of fruit juice can contribute)

Fatty and sugary foods
Try not to eat these foods too often and, when you do, have only small amounts. Use low-fat alternatives where possible. These foods provide energy but have little other nutritional value

Milk and dairy foods
These foods tend to be high in fat, so try to choose low-fat alternatives whenever you can. However, milk and dairy products provide protein and are a good source of calcium and certain vitamins, such as B_{12}, A, and D.

Bread, potatoes, pasta, and other complex carbohydrates
These foods provide plenty of dietary fibre; complex carbohydrate; some minerals, particularly calcium and iron; and vitamins in the B group.

Food groups
You should aim to eat foods from each of the five main food groups in the proportions represented here by slices of a plate. Foods in the larger slices should form a greater part of your diet than foods in the smaller slices. The total amount of food you need to eat depends on your body size, age, and activity levels.

health in countries around the world has led to the development of guidelines to ensure a healthy, balanced diet that can reduce the risk of ill health.

BALANCING YOUR DIET

There are five essential components of food: carbohydrates, protein, fats, vitamins, and minerals. Each one of these elements makes an important contribution to health, but it is important that they are consumed in the correct proportions, with carbohydrates forming the bulk of the diet and fats only a small proportion (*see* HEALTHY EATING, above). By eating plenty of fruit and vegetables, you can ensure you are getting enough vitamins and minerals. In addition to the foods from the main groups, you should include plenty of water in your diet. Drinks that contain sugar, caffeine, or alcohol (*see* ALCOHOL AND HEALTH, p.62) should be consumed in moderation. Sugar is known to contribute to tooth decay. Carbonated drinks, even those that are low in sugar, can damage the teeth because they are acidic. Excess caffeine from drinks such as coffee and cola can cause palpitations (a feeling that the heart is beating rapidly) and insomnia, and caffeine may worsen symptoms of anxiety.

Other important health factors are the amount of salt you have in your diet and the types of fat you eat (*see* CHOOSING HEALTHY FATS, p.50).

HEALTH OPTIONS CHOOSING HEALTHY FATS

There are three main types of fat found in foods and oils: saturated, monounsaturated, and polyunsaturated. Too much fat in the diet, particularly saturated fat, is unhealthy. Your total fat consumption should be under 35 per cent of your daily calorie intake, with most of the fat as monounsaturates and polyunsaturates.

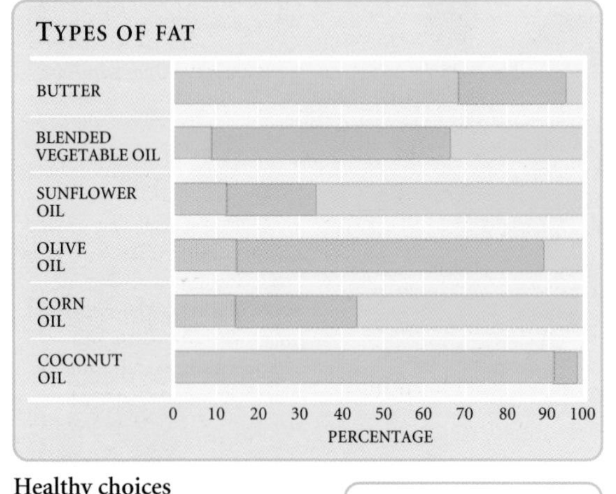

Healthy choices
The amount and type of fat in foods varies greatly. Red meat, most dairy products, and some oils have a fairly high saturated fat content. Lean meat, white fish, and olive oil are healthier choices.

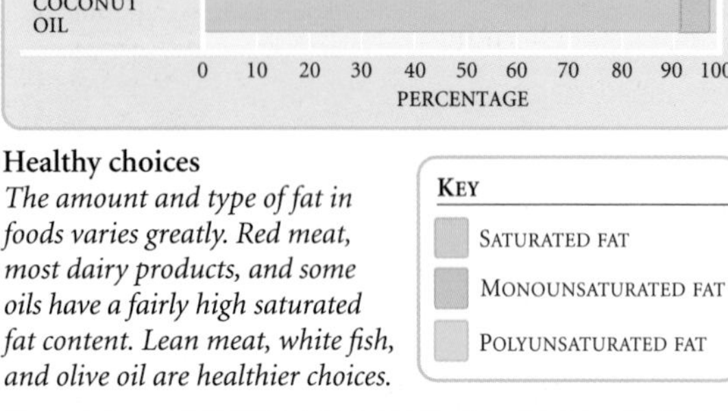

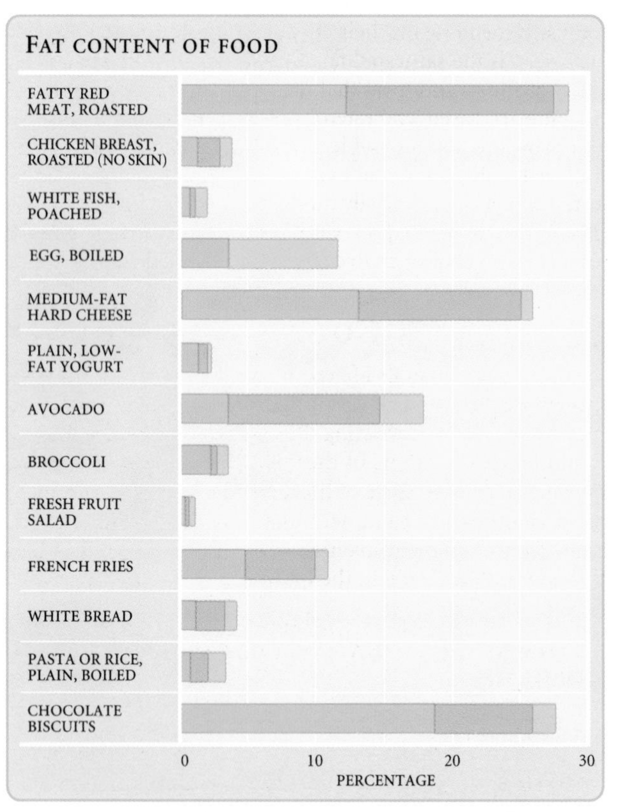

CARBOHYDRATES These should be the body's main energy source. However, if you eat more carbohydrate than your body needs, the excess will be stored as fat. There are two main types of carbohydrate in food: simple and complex.

Simple carbohydrates are made up of sugars. They provide your body with a quick energy boost but can be harmful to the teeth. Foods such as biscuits, cakes, and sweets contain large quantities of simple carbohydrates.

Complex carbohydrates have a more complicated structure than simple carbohydrates and are made up of starches and dietary fibre. Starches are digested slowly and therefore provide sustained energy. Pasta, bread, vegetables such as potatoes, and rice contain high levels of starch. Dietary fibre consists of the fibrous parts of plants that are not completely broken down during digestion. Fibre can be divided into two kinds: soluble fibre and insoluble fibre.

Insoluble fibre adds bulk to faeces, aiding the passage of material through the intestines. People who have plenty of this type of fibre in their diet seem to have a reduced risk of colorectal cancer. Major sources of insoluble fibre include brown rice, fruits, pulses, vegetables, wheat bran, seeds, and whole grains.

Soluble fibre may lower blood cholesterol levels and has been associated with a reduced risk of heart disease and stroke. Good sources include fruits, oats, beans and pulses, and vegetables.

Complex carbohydrates should form the major part of your daily diet. Simple carbohydrates should be kept to a minimum because, although they provide energy, they are low in vitamins and minerals and contain little fibre.

PROTEIN Protein is essential for building and repairing cells in the body. Insufficient protein in the diet causes serious health problems, but such deficiency is largely restricted to developing countries where the availability of food is limited. A more common problem in the UK is too much protein, particularly animal protein. Excess protein is converted into fat in the body. Many protein-rich foods are also high in calories and saturated fat. A high-protein diet may therefore lead to obesity. Foods that are high in protein include meat, fish, cheese, and nuts. About a sixth of your total calorie intake should ideally be obtained from protein.

FATS Fats are a source of energy and are essential for the absorption of certain vitamins. The amount and type of fat in your diet are important in determining your general health. Your intake of fat also affects your risk of developing coronary artery disease or of having a stroke. The link here is cholesterol, a fat-like substance that is essential for normal body functioning but can be a risk to health in excess. The higher the level of cholesterol in your blood (*see* HYPERCHOLESTEROLAEMIA, p.691), the greater your risk of developing atherosclerosis (p.402), the narrowing of the arteries that may eventually lead to cardiovascular disease.

An individual's level of blood cholesterol depends partly on genetic factors, but in many cases the main influence is the amount and type of fat in the diet. Fats can be either saturated or unsaturated, depending on their chemical structure; it is the saturated fats found in dairy products and meat that mainly contribute to raised cholesterol levels in the body. It is also advisable to avoid hydrogenated fats, sometimes known as transfats, which are artificially produced and have properties that are similar to saturated fats. Hydrogenated fats are often found in butter substitutes and manufactured food items such as biscuits and cakes. In contrast, unsaturated fats seem to provide some protection against cardiovascular disease, with polyunsaturates having a greater protective effect than monounsaturates.

For a healthier diet, make sure that no more than a third of your daily calorie are obtained from fat and choose foods that contain unsaturated rather than saturated fats. You should also try to limit your intake of foods that are high in cholesterol, such as shellfish and eggs. However, the fat intake of young children should not be restricted (*see* HEALTH IN PRESCHOOL CHILDREN, p.29).

VITAMINS AND MINERALS Vitamins and minerals both play vital roles in growth and metabolism (*see* GOOD SOURCES OF VITAMINS AND MINERALS, below). Apart from vitamin K, which is formed by intestinal bacteria, and vitamin D, which

HEALTH ACTION GOOD SOURCES OF VITAMINS AND MINERALS

Vitamins and minerals are essential for growth and health, and certain vitamins play a key role in preventing disease. Requirements for some of these elements depend on gender, stage of life, and age. Most vitamins and all minerals have to come from food or supplements because they are not produced in the body.

Recommended daily allowances (RDAs) serve as a guide to minimum requirements for the main vitamins and minerals. Some vitamins are toxic if consumed in excess. For example, pregnant women should avoid foods that contain high levels of vitamin A because of potential harmful effects on the developing fetus.

Eating for health
RDAs are based on the needs of a healthy adult with an average energy output; 1 milligram (mg) equals 1,000 micrograms (mcg). Requirements for certain vitamins and minerals may differ according to factors such as stage of life and gender.

VITAMINS AND MINERALS	RDA	GOOD SOURCES	EFFECTS
Vitamin A	1 mg	Calves' liver, eggs, carrots, melon	• Important for healthy eyes, hair, skin, and bones • Can be toxic in excess
Vitamin B_1 (Thiamine)	1 mg	Meat, whole grains, peas, fortified cereals and breads	• Helps in energy production • Essential for the proper functioning of the nervous system
Vitamin B_2 (Riboflavin)	1.5 mg	Eggs, meat, milk products, leafy vegetables	• Involved in the release of proteins from nutrients • Helps to maintain the nervous system and muscles
Vitamin B_3 (Niacin)	15–20 mg	Fish, whole grains, peanuts, peas	• Essential for the utilization of energy from food • Helps to maintain healthy skin
Vitamin B_6	1.5 mg	Meat, fish, whole grains, bananas	• Necessary for blood formation • Helps to regulate the cells in the nervous system
Vitamin B_{12}	1 mcg	Milk, fish, meat, eggs, yeast	• Vital for the growth of blood cells in the bone marrow • Essential for a healthy nervous system
Vitamin C	40–60 mg	Many fruits and vegetables	• Strengthens tissues • Helps the body to use iron • May help the immune system to fight disease
Vitamin D	5 mcg	Dairy products, oily fish, also formed in the skin by sunlight	• Enhances calcium absorption for strong teeth and bones • Can be toxic in excess
Vitamin E	10 mg	Vegetables, eggs, fish, margarine	• Protects tissues and organs against degenerative disease • Can be toxic in excess
Vitamin K	70 mcg	Leafy green vegetables, pigs' liver, also formed by intestinal bacteria	• Essential for proper blood clotting • Necessary for bone formation • Can be toxic in excess
Folic acid	200 mcg†	Leafy green vegetables, organ meats, whole grains, fortified bread, nuts	• Helps to prevent neural tube defects (p.844) in fetuses • Contributes to healthy cells and blood
Calcium	at least 800 mg	Dairy products, eggs, peas, dry beans, edible fish bones	• Necessary for healthy bones, teeth, and muscles • Helps with conduction of nerve impulses
Iron	14 mg	Eggs, meat, milk products, leafy green vegetables	• Aids formation of red blood cells and certain proteins • Maintains healthy muscles

† Women planning a pregnancy and pregnant women in the first 12 weeks of pregnancy should take 400 mcg of folic acid a day

HEALTH OPTIONS UNDERSTANDING FOOD LABELS

Manufacturers of most prepacked foods are required to provide items of important information on food labels. Labels must give the name of the food; a list of ingredients; its weight; how long the food can be kept and how to store it; how to cook and prepare it; the name and address of the maker, packer, or seller of the food; sometimes the place of origin.

NUTRITION INFORMATION

Typical values per	100g	Portion
Energy	1741kJ 414kcal	1219kJ 290kcal
Protein	3.5g	2.5g
Carbohydrate	65.8 g	46.1g
of which sugars	49.1g	14.4g
Fat	15.2g	10.6g
of which saturates	3.6g	2.5g
Fibre	2.3g	1.6g
Sodium	0.1g	0.1g

Based on 8 portions per cake

INGREDIENTS:
Raisins, glacé cherries, wheatflour, egg, partially hydrogenated vegetable oil, pecan nuts, sugar, glucose syrup, honey, flavourings, emulsifiers (E471, E435), spices, salt, preservative (E202), gelling agent (E440), acidity regulator (E330), colours (E127, E133, E102, E129)

- **THIS PRODUCT CONTAINS NUTS**
- **SUITABLE FOR VEGETARIANS**

Typical or average values
The figures are given for 100 g or 100 ml of the food. Some labels also list quantities per average portion or serving

Fat
The fat content is broken down to show how much of the fat is saturated

Sodium
This shows how much salt is included

Energy
The energy content is measured in kilojoules (kJ) and kilocalories (kcal)

Protein
The protein content must be shown even when there is very little or none

Carbohydrate
The total carbohydrate content is broken down to give the amount of sugars

Fibre
This shows the amount of roughage in the food

Portions
A normal portion size helps you to assess your intake of nutrients

Ingredients
The ingredients must be listed on the label in order of weight, beginning with the heaviest. Additives and preservatives are often shown by their E (European) numbers

Additional information
A label may show if the food is suitable for people with dietary restrictions

Making choices
A food label should give a list of ingredients along with a breakdown of the nutrients so that you can see exactly what the food contributes to your diet. This information enables you to compare similar products and to choose foods according to your dietary needs.

is produced in the skin by the action of sunlight, all vitamins and minerals must be obtained from your diet.

The majority of people in the UK obtain adequate amounts of vitamins and minerals from their diet. Some vitamins, including vitamins A, D, E, and K, are harmful if they are consumed in excess. However, some people may need to take vitamin and mineral supplements (pp.927–929). For example, women who regularly lose iron through heavy menstrual bleeding may be prescribed iron supplements. Children who are reluctant to eat a normal range of foods may be given vitamins A, C, and D in the form of drops. Elderly people who have a low or restricted intake of food may also need supplements. Older women should make sure they have adequate calcium in their diet to help to prevent the bone disorder osteoporosis (p.368).

People who eat a vegetarian diet usually have an adequate intake of vitamins and minerals, but vegans, who eat no animal products, are at risk of vitamin B_{12} deficiency and should also ensure that they get enough calcium in their diet.

FLUIDS Water is essential for life, and makes up almost four-fifths of the body. Water is lost by sweating and passing urine and must be replaced. Inadequate water intake may lead to kidney problems, such as kidney stones (p.701), and constipation (p.628). Some water is obtained from solid foods, but you should also drink plenty of fluids. Try to drink at least 8 glasses (2 litres/3½ pints) of nonalcoholic fluid a day. In hot weather or during exercise, you may need more. The need for water is also increased by diarrhoea, vomiting, diuretics (drugs that increase urine output), and caffeine.

YOUR ENERGY REQUIREMENTS

The body needs a constant reserve of energy to function properly. Energy from food is measured in units called kilojoules (kJ) or kilocalories (kcal), which are usually referred to simply as calories.

The number of calories you need to obtain from your diet depends on how much energy your body uses. This depends partly on how efficiently your body cells use energy, which is genetically determined, and partly on your level of physical activity. The rate at which your body uses energy simply to maintain basic processes such as breathing and digestion is called your basal metabolic rate (BMR). Extra calories are needed for all your day-to-day activities. Energetic activities, such as sports, increase the calorie requirement. Most of these extra calories should come from complex carbohydrates, such as bread. However, people who have physically demanding jobs also require extra fat and sugar, which are rich sources of energy.

Your stage of life also has an influence on your energy requirements. For example, a growing, active teenager usually needs more calories than an adult. Calorie requirements tend to decrease as you get older because BMR declines with age and activity may be reduced. A pregnant woman needs more calories than a nonpregnant woman.

CHOOSING NUTRITIOUS FOOD

Fresh foods tend to be healthy, but they often have a short shelf life. Processing techniques are used to increase shelf life. Many processed foods have as many vitamins and minerals as fresh food. Food preservatives prevent the growth of microorganisms, which could cause food poisoning (p.629).

Labels on packaged food (*see* UNDERSTANDING FOOD LABELS, left) provide information about the content, allowing you to compare similar products and make healthy choices. In the UK, regulations are in place concerning how food is labelled and the type of nutritional information that is given. In addition to listing food ingredients and nutritional information, many food labels provide extra information so that people who, by choice or necessity, restrict their diet in some way can make decisions about which foods to select or avoid.

WWW ONLINE SITES: p.1035

Controlling your weight

Maintaining your weight within a healthy range for your height

An essential part of a healthy lifestyle is maintaining your body weight within the range considered normal for your height. In recent decades, the number of overweight people in developed countries has risen significantly. For example, between 1980 and 1997, the number of overweight men in the UK rose from around 1 in 16 to around 1 in 6, and the number of overweight women has increased from around 1 in 12 to 1 in 5. Approximately 1 in 50 primary school children and 1 in 10 children of secondary school age are above the healthy weight range for their height.

Excess weight amounting to obesity (p.631) is a major threat to health. Disorders associated with being obese, such as coronary artery disease (p.405), high blood pressure (*see* HYPERTENSION, p.403), and stroke (p.532), rank among the leading causes of illness and death in developed countries such as the UK. Being underweight can also cause health problems, including an increased risk of infertility (pp.774–777) and the bone disorder osteoporosis (p.368).

Causes of weight problems

In the UK, the main factor contributing to the general weight gain of the population is lack of exercise combined with overeating. Children's pastimes are far more sedentary than those of former generations, and many adults do not exercise at all. In addition, an increasing number of people rely on convenience foods, which tend to be high in saturated fat and simple carbohydrates, both of which are high in calories.

There are various reasons why someone may be underweight. Some people are naturally thin and find it difficult to gain weight no matter what they eat. Others start within the normal weight range but then develop an eating disorder, such as anorexia nervosa (p.562) or bulimia (p.563), and lose a great deal of weight, eventually becoming abnormally thin. Weight loss can also result from loss of appetite due to long-term illness such as depression (p.554), tuberculosis (p.491), or rheumatoid arthritis (p.377).

Finding your ideal weight

Height and weight charts offer a quick and easy way to find out whether you are within the recommended weight range for your height. Your ideal body weight depends on both your height and on the amount of muscle tissue you have. For example, an athlete should weigh more than a healthy but relatively sedentary person of the same height. This is because exercise increases muscle, which is heavier than other types of body tissue. For this reason, the charts provide healthy ranges for height and not precise measurements.

Recent research indicates that the distribution of fat around the body is an important determinant of health. Excess fat around the abdomen is more closely linked to cardiovascular diseases than fat elsewhere in the body. To find out whether you are a healthy weight, you should both check if your weight falls within the recommended range for your height and measure your waist size (*see* ARE YOU A HEALTHY WEIGHT?, below).

Doctors and nutritionists use weight and height measurements to calculate body mass index (BMI). This is a widely accepted and more precise method of

ASSESSMENT Are you a healthy weight?

You can check whether you are a healthy weight by using the height/weight graph below. Height and weight measurements can be used to calculate your body mass index (BMI), an indicator of body fat.

Even if the graph indicates that you are a healthy weight, you are still at increased risk of cardiovascular disease if your waist measurement is greater than 89 cm (35 in) for women and 102 cm (40 in) for men.

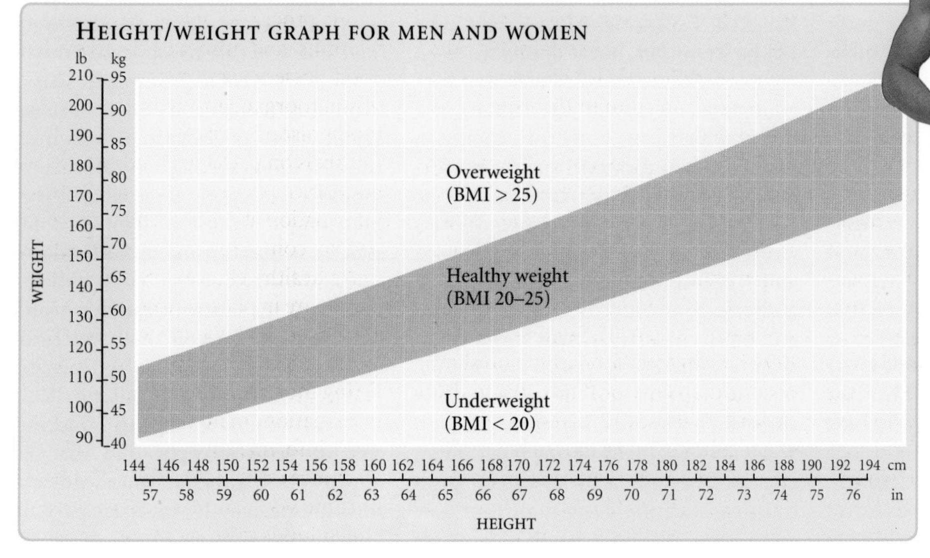

Measuring your waist
Your waist measurement indicates whether you have excess abdominal fat.

Using the graph
Find your height and weight on the axes. Trace a vertical line from your height and a horizontal line from your weight. The point at which the lines cross on the graph indicates whether or not you are within a healthy range.

checking if you are over- or underweight by providing an indication of total body fat content. The BMI is calculated by dividing a person's weight in kilograms by the square of his or her height in metres. A BMI figure under 20 means that you are underweight, while a figure of 25 or more is an indication that you are overweight.

LOSING WEIGHT

If the height/weight chart confirms that you are overweight, you can lose excess weight by following a slimming diet and taking exercise. In rare circumstances, a doctor may advise drug treatment or surgery as well as a slimming diet to aid weight loss in a very obese person.

Before you attempt to lose weight, you should try to identify why you may be overweight. The most likely cause is a combination of overeating and lack of exercise, but you may find it helpful to look at your reasons for overeating. For example, do you tend to eat when you feel unhappy or is overeating a habit that has become established in your family?

The best way to lose weight is to combine calorie reduction with regular exercise. Plan what you need to do to succeed. For example, if you need more exercise, arrange a time each day to take a brisk walk. If you are tempted by the wrong foods, make a list of healthy foods before going to the supermarket.

Success in dieting also depends on being realistic about how much weight you can lose. Set yourself a practical, short-term target, revising it as you go along. About 2–4 kg (4.5–9 lb) a month is sensible. If you want to lose more than this or have any health problems, consult your doctor before you start.

You also need to consider what you hope to achieve by losing excess weight. It is important for you to accept that weight loss may not solve all your problems. It may make you feel better and more confident, will certainly improve some aspects of your health, but it is unlikely to help a failing relationship or make you more popular. However, the health benefits are worth any effort and lifestyle changes you may have to make.

SLIMMING DIETS If your diet does not provide you with enough calories for all your energy needs, your body will start to use up excess fat as an energy source. Therefore, you should begin to lose weight if you make changes to your diet to include fewer calories than before. Publications that list the calorie content of a variety of foods, both natural and processed, are widely available, and this information can also be found on the labels of most packaged food (*see* UNDERSTANDING FOOD LABELS, p.52). A good starting point for most people is to try to reduce their daily calorie intake by about 500 calories. This can be achieved by cutting down on high-fat foods, such as cakes, pastries, cheese, and fried dishes, and replacing them with healthy, low-calorie foods, such as fruit, vegetables, and grilled dishes.

If your normal diet already consists mainly of low-calorie foods, you simply need to cut down on the quantity of food you eat. The best type of slimming diet is one that is low in calories but balanced so that you stay well nourished (*see* HEALTHY EATING, p.49).

Alcohol contains no healthy nutrients and is high in calories. It is therefore advisable to reduce your alcohol consumption as much as possible when you are trying to lose weight.

Rapid weight-loss plans and fasting to lose weight should be avoided. They can damage your health by forcing your body to function on insufficient energy supplies and depriving it of the range of nutrients it needs to function well. Such plans do not produce sustainable weight loss or encourage you to adopt sensible, long-term healthy eating habits.

EXERCISE Exercising to lose weight need not be strenuous, but it does have to be regular. Sustained regular exercise raises your basal metabolic rate (BMR), the rate at which your body uses energy to maintain basic processes such as breathing, digestion, and the heartbeat. If your BMR rises, you use up more calories (*see* EXERCISE AND HEALTH, pp.55–61) and will lose weight if you also follow a calorie-controlled diet. Exercise tones and builds muscles, which weigh more than fat. Therefore, as you become fitter, you may find that the scales initially register a few more kilograms, although you will not actually be any fatter. Exercise can also stimulate your appetite; you must resist eating more than your new diet allows. As you become older, your metabolism slows down, and therefore your body uses up fewer calories. It is important to remain as active as possible to prevent the gradual weight gain that is common among older people.

DRUGS AND SURGERY Weight-reducing drugs are usually recommended only for people whose weight is a serious threat to health, and such treatment should never take the place of a balanced, low-calorie diet. A few drug treatments for weight loss, such as bulking agents that make you feel full, are available over the counter. However, most weight-reducing drugs are available only on prescription, and regular monitoring is required during treatment. Certain drugs, notably appetite suppressants, are now rarely prescribed because of their potential side effects. Amphetamines have been found to be addictive and are no longer recommended for weight loss. The newer drugs that act by blocking the absorption of fat should be combined with a slimming diet and should not be taken long term.

Generally, surgical procedures, such as stomach-stapling and jaw-wiring, are considered only as a last resort for a person who is extremely obese.

GAINING WEIGHT

Many people think that being underweight is not a health risk. It can be just as unhealthy as being overweight and requires careful treatment. If you are more than 15 per cent under the lowest normal weight for your height according to the chart, are excessively tired, and unable to keep warm, you should see your doctor to exclude an underlying condition that requires treatment.

It is important to gain weight sensibly to build up muscle and bone and achieve a healthy level of body fat. Although fatty and fast foods are high in calories, you should avoid eating large quantities to gain weight because of their unhealthy effects, such as causing high blood pressure and increasing risk of heart disease. Put on weight slowly by eating a healthy, balanced diet. Several small, nutritious meals each day provide a better supply of energy than one or two large meals.

Regular exercise helps to build muscles, increases strength, and may also improve your appetite. You should start slowly, especially if you tire easily, and build up the amount you do gradually.

(WWW) ONLINE SITES: p.1031, p.1035

EXERCISE AND HEALTH

Exercise is an essential part of any healthy lifestyle. This idea is not a new one; the fact that physical activity is linked to good health can be traced back to the Greeks in the fifth century BC. Since then, research has proven that exercise prolongs life, protects health, and can reduce the risk of disease. Taking part in team sports also provides the opportunity for social contact.

Developments in mechanization and computerization over the past century have meant that people in developed countries now lead a more sedentary lifestyle, and too few people exercise regularly. By making a concerted effort to incorporate physical activity into your daily life, you can become significantly healthier.

The first article in this section outlines the overwhelming physical and psychological benefits of being active.

Exercise also has an effect on other aspects of your lifestyle. For example, people who exercise tend to smoke less than those who do not. Developing a habit of regular physical activity may encourage you to give up smoking.

The second article provides practical guidelines for assessing how fit you are and improving your level of fitness.

The last article explores safe habits and routines to adopt when exercising to minimize the risk of injury.

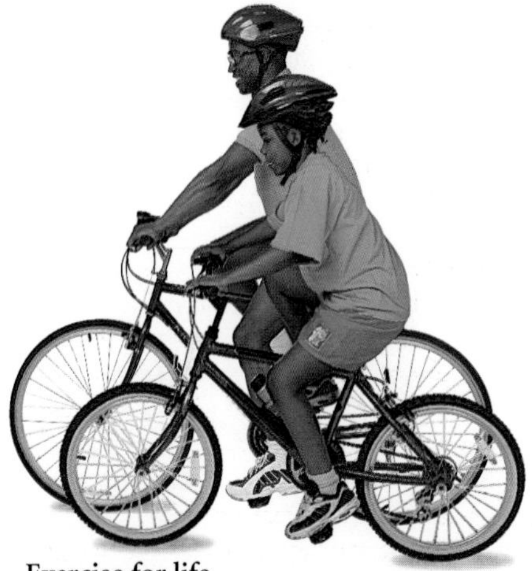

Exercise for life
Exercising on a regular basis can improve the quality of your life by improving your strength, stamina, and psychological health and by providing you with the opportunity to socialize with other people.

The benefits of exercise

How regular exercise benefits your physical and psychological health

Most people know that exercise is part of a healthy lifestyle. In recent decades, the number of people in the UK taking regular exercise has increased, but many still do too little exercise. For example, only 1 in 5 women and about 1 in 3 men takes enough exercise to protect themselves against coronary artery disease.

Exercise protects physical and mental health. It has a particularly positive effect on the respiratory, cardiovascular, and musculoskeletal systems (*see* HOW EXERCISE BENEFITS HEALTH, p.56).

By taking regular physical exercise, you can reduce your risk of developing long-term disease, increase your life expectancy, and improve your quality of life in later years. When you make exercise a part of your daily routine, you will probably find it a lot easier to perform ordinary tasks, such as shopping, gardening, doing housework, and climbing stairs. In addition to the more obvious physical benefits, exercising regularly can improve your psychological well-being. Developing a habit of exercising with other people can also help you to make new friends.

CARDIOVASCULAR HEALTH

Research has shown that people who do little or no exercise are at increased risk of coronary artery disease (p.405) and heart attack (*see* MYOCARDIAL INFARCTION, p.410). However, for exercise to give you effective protection against heart disease, it has to be regular and sustained over your lifetime. Exercising only in your youth is no guarantee of benefits later in life.

When you exercise regularly, your heart becomes stronger and more efficient and can pump more blood with every heartbeat, making it able to cope with extra demands. The amount of regular exercise that you take also influences your chance of surviving a heart attack if you should ever have one; people who have exercised regularly are more likely to survive.

Regular exercise helps to reduce blood cholesterol levels and lowers blood pressure. Both of these factors reduce the risk of developing fatty plaques in your arteries (*see* ATHEROSCLEROSIS, p.402). Research shows that people who already have coronary artery disease or lower limb ischaemia (p.434) may benefit from exercise because of the improvement that it makes to the blood supply. These benefits may be experienced within 2 months of starting regular exercise.

RESPIRATORY HEALTH

Regular exercise improves the efficiency of your respiratory muscles and increases the usable volume of the alveoli (air sacs) in the lungs. It also increases the efficiency of the exchange of oxygen and carbon dioxide in the lungs. Active people are able to extract more oxygen from a single breath and have a slower breathing rate. If you have a respiratory disease, such as chronic obstructive pulmonary disease (p.487), regular exercise may help to improve the amount of activity that you can do on a daily basis without feeling breathless.

MUSCULOSKELETAL HEALTH

Exercising improves the condition of your bones, joints, and muscles. Taking regular exercise helps you to keep yourself flexible and mobile for longer and improves your quality of life.

MAINTAINING STRONG BONES Weight-bearing exercises, such as walking and running, help to improve bone strength, density, and development. This kind of exercise is particularly important for physical development during childhood and adolescence, when the bones are still growing. It is also important for women of all ages to do weight-bearing exercises regularly because they help to

HEALTH EFFECTS How exercise benefits health

Regular exercise protects your health by benefiting different body systems. It may be planned and structured, such as going for a run, or incidental, such as cycling to work. Below is a selection of exercises, both structured and part of daily living, that benefit different parts of your body; many exercises are beneficial to more than one part. For example, tennis is aerobic and benefits your heart, lungs, and muscles; it is weight-bearing and improves bone strength; and it requires a range of movements that improves joint mobility.

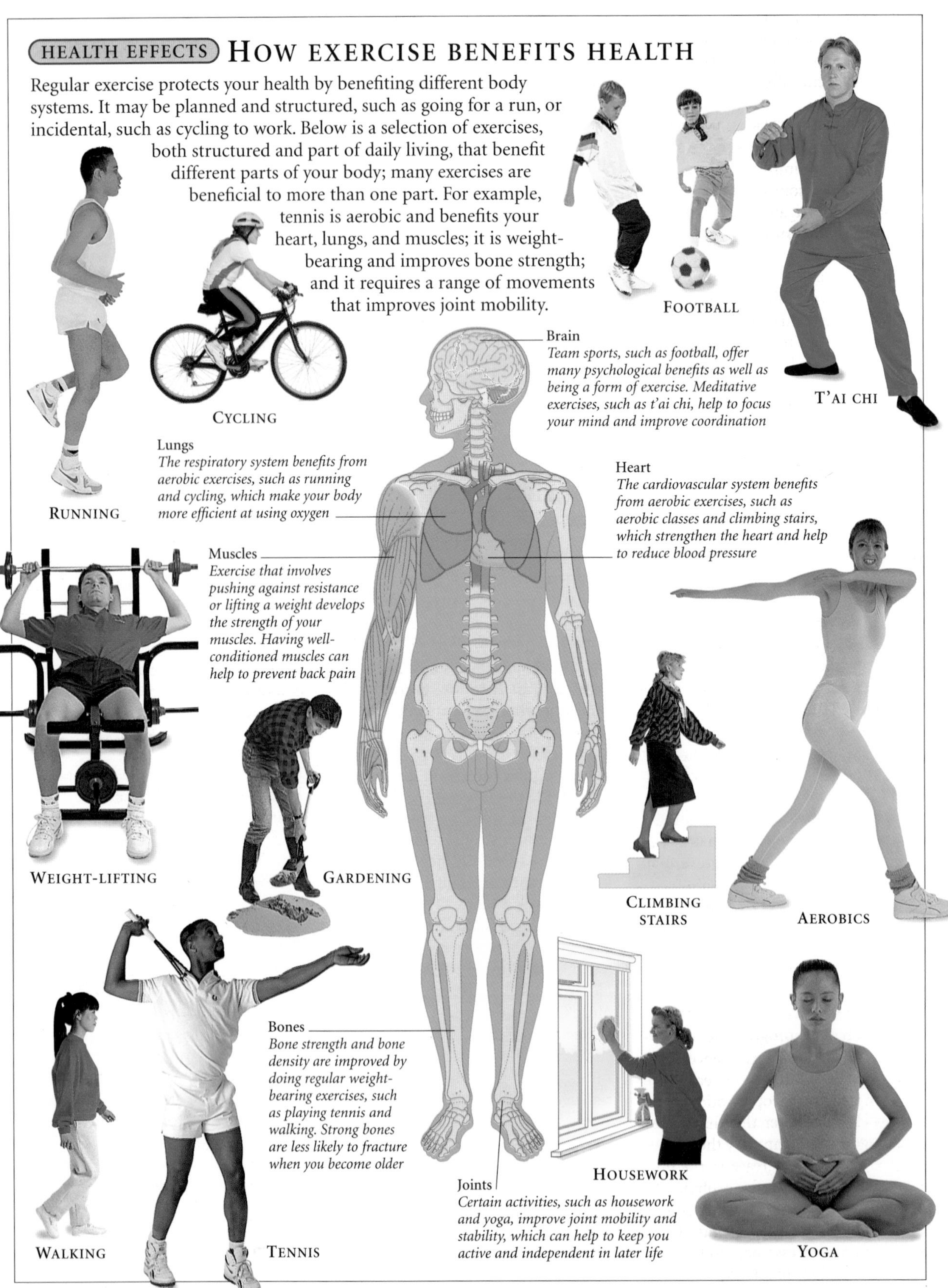

slow down the accelerated bone loss caused by the decline in levels of the hormone oestrogen (*see* OSTEOPOROSIS, p.368) that occurs after the menopause.

MOBILIZING AND STABILIZING JOINTS Regular exercise improves the flexibility of joints and minimizes stiffness. It also helps to stabilize joints by strengthening the muscles and ligaments surrounding them. By maintaining joint mobility, exercise can help you to remain independent and able to do more in later life. If you have a joint disease, such as rheumatoid arthritis (p.377), strength-building exercises may stabilize affected joints and reduce further damage.

INCREASING MUSCLE STRENGTH You should exercise your muscles regularly to keep them in good condition. Muscle size and strength can be increased with exercises that work against resistance, such as lifting moderate weights. Aerobic exercises that build stamina, such as running and cycling, make the muscles more efficient so that they can work for longer periods of time. Stronger muscles, and the increased confidence that often comes from feeling and looking fit, also improve your posture.

After about the age of 25, you lose a small amount of muscle each year as part of the normal aging process. If you keep your muscles strong and healthy, this loss of muscle bulk and strength can be kept to a minimum.

Lower back pain (p.381) is often a result of poor muscle strength and lack of flexibility. Regularly doing exercises that concentrate on strengthening particular muscle groups and improving overall flexibility can help to prevent back pain (*see* PREVENTING BACK PAIN, p.382) and keep you mobile.

PSYCHOLOGICAL WELL-BEING

When you begin a programme of regular exercise, you may experience some psychological benefits from early on. For example, many people notice a feeling of well-being after they have been exercising; this is commonly thought to be the result of an increase in the production by the brain of morphine-like chemical compounds known as endorphins. These chemical compounds act as natural antidepressants, and they can help you to feel more relaxed.

Mildly anxious or depressed people may notice a marked improvement in their mood after exercising regularly for some time. For this reason, exercise is increasingly being incorporated into psychological therapies. You may find that exercise helps you to cope with stress (p.74). It also promotes regular, deep, and refreshing sleep (p.73).

By exercising regularly, you are more likely to look and feel healthy, which can increase your confidence and self-esteem. You may also experience a sense of achievement when you meet short-term goals in your exercise routine.

Taking part in a team sport or joining a health club or gym can be a way of expanding your circle of friends. Team sports foster mutual respect, shared responsibility, and self-discipline. These benefits are widely recognized and are particularly important for children.

Research into the effects of exercise among people who work in offices has found that regular exercise generally leads to a more productive workforce.

(WWW) ONLINE SITES: p.1031

Taking regular exercise

Taking steps to increase the amount of physical activity in your daily life

For exercise to be beneficial (*see* THE BENEFITS OF EXERCISE, p.55), it has to be regular and consistent. The type and amount of activity you can incorporate into your lifestyle depends on the time you have available to exercise. The best form of exercise is one that you enjoy doing and can fit into your daily routine. Exercise should be tailored to your age, state of health, and lifestyle.

RECOMMENDED LEVEL OF EXERCISE

Recent evidence has shown that even gentle exercise has measurable positive effects on life expectancy; consequently, everyone should try to lead an active life. If your life is fairly active already, there are guidelines on the amount and the frequency of additional exercise you can take to gain the maximum benefit to your general health. Current

ASSESSMENT HOW FIT ARE YOU?

When trying to assess how much exercise you do in your everyday life, it is important to be as honest as possible. Completing the simple questionnaire below can give you an indication of whether or not you need to increase the amount of regular exercise that you take.

1 *Can you climb one or two flights of stairs without shortness of breath or heaviness or tiredness in your legs?*

☐ YES ☐ NO

2 *When you have the choice, do you take the stairs rather than the escalator or lift?*

☐ YES ☐ NO

3 *Do you have plenty of energy to enjoy your leisure time at the end of the working day?*

☐ YES ☐ NO

4 *Would you walk for 10 minutes rather than drive?*

☐ YES ☐ NO

5 *Can you carry out a conversation during light to moderate exercise, such as brisk walking?*

☐ YES ☐ NO

6 *Do you do moderate exercise that makes you sweat and breathe harder for 15 minutes or more at least three times a week?*

☐ YES ☐ NO

ANALYSIS

If you answered yes to all of the questions above, you are reasonably fit and are exercising to a level that will benefit your health. If you answered no to any of the questions, you should consider incorporating more physical exercise into your daily routine. If you do not already follow a regular exercise routine, you could consider starting to do so after consultation with your doctor.

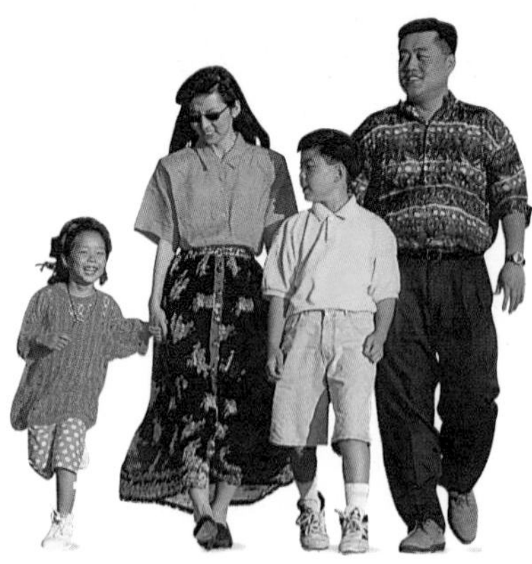

Walking is for everyone
People of all ages can enjoy walking. Walking briskly for 3 km (2 miles) a day will significantly benefit your health.

recommendations are that you should do at least 30 minutes of exercise at moderate intensity on at least 5 days of the week. A brisk 30-minute walk will provide a healthy amount of exercise for the day. However, if you want to change your appearance by improving your muscle tone or losing excess body fat, or if you want to become even more fit, you will have to exercise harder and for longer periods of time.

STARTING OUT

If your life is sedentary, begin by taking simple steps to become more active in your daily routine. For example, you could make a habit of climbing the stairs instead of taking the lift. However, if your life already includes some physical activity, think about starting a regular exercise routine, such as swimming, brisk walking, or jogging.

Make sure that your exercise routine is realistic for you, that you slowly build up the amount of exercise you take, and that you learn safe techniques in order to protect yourself from injury (*see* EXERCISING SAFELY, opposite page). You may be encouraged to continue exercising on a regular basis once you begin to experience its positive physical and psychological effects. If you begin an exercise programme with a friend, you can motivate each other.

CONSULT YOUR DOCTOR If you have never exercised regularly before, or if you think you may be at particular risk from exercise, you should consult your doctor before starting a regular exercise programme. You should consult your doctor if you have a chronic medical condition, such as coronary artery disease (p.405), high blood pressure (*see* HYPERTENSION, p.403), diabetes mellitus (p.687), chronic kidney failure (p.706), or asthma (p.483). You should ask your doctor for advice if you are overweight or if you are over age 35 and have not exercised regularly for several years.

Your doctor may recommend certain types of exercises that are appropriate for you. For example, if you are overweight and have not exercised for some years, your doctor may suggest gentle exercise, such as walking or cycling, to avoid putting too much strain on your heart and to reduce the risk of injury to your knees, feet, or ankles. If you have asthma, your doctor may suggest that you start swimming. You may need to take your usual medication beforehand. He or she may also tell you to avoid exercising in a cold environment, which can trigger asthma.

ASSESS YOUR FITNESS Overall fitness is a combination of three factors: stamina, flexibility, and strength. To improve your level of fitness, you need to do regular exercise that works your heart and lungs (builds stamina), improves your joint mobility (increases flexibility), and increases your muscle strength.

Before starting regular exercise, it is a good idea to estimate your overall fitness (*see* HOW FIT ARE YOU?, p.57). Think about the activity you do in a normal day or week. You may be surprised to find that you already do some exercise most days, such as playing with your children or walking to work.

HEALTH OPTIONS CHOICES FOR FITNESS

Different exercises benefit different aspects of fitness (stamina, flexibility, or strength) to a greater or lesser extent. Some types of exercise, such as swimming, offer benefits in all of these aspects. You can choose the best activity to improve a specific aspect of fitness or review the overall fitness benefits of activities that you already do or are considering taking up.

FITNESS BENEFITS OF DIFFERENT ACTIVITIES

ACTIVITY	FITNESS BENEFITS		
	STAMINA	FLEXIBILITY	STRENGTH
Aerobics	★★★★	★★★	★★
Basketball	★★★★	★★★	★★
Cycling (fast)	★★★★	★★	★★★
Climbing stairs	★★★	★	★★★
Dancing (aerobic)	★★★	★★★★	★
Golf	★	★★	★
Hiking	★★★	★	★★
Jogging	★★★★	★★	★★
Swimming	★★★★	★★★★	★★★★
Tennis	★★	★★★	★★
Walking (briskly)	★★	★	★
Yoga	★	★★★★	★

Using the chart
The activities above have been graded according to their benefit to each aspect of fitness. By comparing the benefits of each activity, you can tailor an exercise programme to your own fitness needs.

KEY

★ Small effect ★★★ Very good effect
★★ Good effect ★★★★ Excellent effect

(ASSESSMENT) YOUR PULSE RECOVERY TIME

The time it takes for your pulse to return to its resting rate after exercise can be used to monitor improvements in your fitness. As you become fitter, your pulse recovery time decreases. You should be able to notice a difference in how quickly your pulse recovers within 4 weeks of starting regular exercise that makes your heart and lungs work hard.

Neck pulse *Find your pulse on the side of the neck with your first and second fingers*

Watch *Use a watch to time beats per minute*

Taking your neck pulse after exercise *Count the number of beats for 10 seconds and multiply the result by 6 to calculate beats per minute. Continue taking your pulse every minute until it returns to its resting rate.*

Your resting pulse can be used as an indication of your general cardiovascular fitness. A fairly slow pulse indicates that your heart is fit. If you stop exercising regularly, you will lose the level of fitness you have attained. However, you can regain your fitness by restarting an appropriate exercise programme.

CHOOSING THE RIGHT EXERCISE

Exercise needs vary depending on age, lifestyle, and fitness. Individual sports and activities improve different aspects of fitness (*see* CHOICES FOR FITNESS, opposite page). You should choose exercises that help you to develop a balance of stamina, suppleness, and strength and that you can do all year round. Decide what your fitness goal is and choose an activity that will help you to achieve it.

GETTING THE MOST FROM YOUR EXERCISE PROGRAMME

If your goal from regular exercise is to achieve an optimal level of fitness, you might set yourself a target heart rate. It is a good idea to monitor and record improvements in your fitness at regular intervals, such as once a month. This evidence of the benefits from exercise should encourage you to continue your programme. You can monitor your fitness level by taking your pulse while at rest and then measuring how quickly it returns to its resting rate after exercising vigorously (*see* YOUR PULSE RECOVERY TIME, above). As you become fitter, your pulse recovery time decreases.

TARGET HEART RATE To calculate this, first estimate your maximum heart rate, which is normally about 220 minus your age. Your target heart rate during exercise is 60–80 per cent of your maximum heart rate. You can measure your pulse to monitor your heart rate during exercise, but wearing an electronic heart-rate monitor is easier and gives a more accurate measurement. At first, it may be hard to exercise at this rate, but it will become easier as you become fitter.

PLANNING YOUR PROGRAMME When you start to increase the amount of exercise that you take, you must build up gradually (*see* EXERCISING SAFELY, right). Initially, increase the number of times each week that you exercise and do not be too concerned about how long you exercise or how hard you work. When you are exercising more frequently, you can then focus on increasing the length of time for which you exercise. Finally, you should increase the intensity of your exercise so that you eventually achieve your target heart rate. To obtain maximum benefit, you should aim to exercise every day for at least 30 minutes at your target heart rate.

(WWW) ONLINE SITES: p.1031

Exercising safely

Taking all sensible precautions to avoid injury from exercise

Each type of exercise has its own potential hazards and may require the use of specialized equipment. Be sure to set yourself realistic goals in order to avoid overexertion or injury. If you are not fit or have exercised only sporadically, you should begin slowly and build up gradually. Sudden strenuous exercise could result in injury (*see* SPORTS INJURIES, p.391). You may need advice from your doctor before you start exercising (*see* TAKING REGULAR EXERCISE, p.57).

SPECIALIZED EQUIPMENT AND PROTECTION

Some activities, such as walking and swimming, require little or no specialized equipment. However, for sports such as cricket, cycling, and skiing, having appropriate equipment is essential. Proper footwear and clothing is very important; for example, badly designed or poorly fitting shoes may result in injury to the Achilles tendon and may aggravate hip and back problems. Make sure that you always wear the right amount and type of clothing. If you are exercising outside, it is important to protect your skin and eyes from the sun (*see* SAFETY IN THE SUN, p.80). If you are using exercise equipment at home, follow the instructions carefully so that you do not harm yourself by using it incorrectly. If you work out at a gym, ask an instructor to show you how to use the equipment safely if you are unsure.

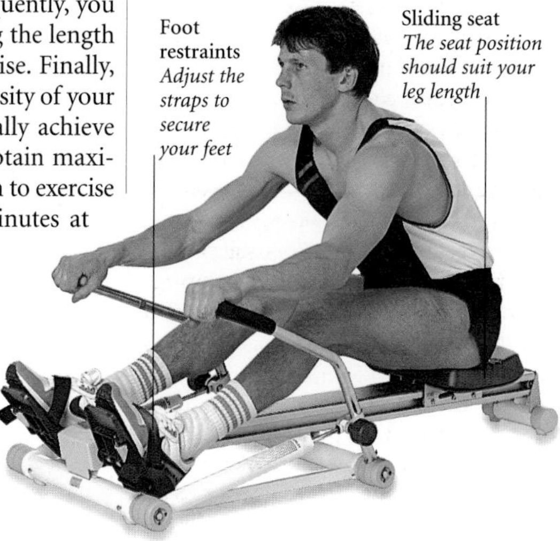

Using equipment safely *To prevent physical injury through misuse, any type of exercise equipment, such as this rowing machine, should be used according to the manufacturer's instructions.*

GOOD EXERCISE HABITS

Develop a simple routine of warming up and cooling down (right) to minimize the risk of injury while exercising, and repeat it every time you exercise.

Knowing when to stop is a vital part of exercising safely. Common sense and your body will tell you what your upper limit is and when not to push yourself above it. If you notice signs that suggest overexertion, you should stop at once. Serious warning symptoms include:

- Chest pain.
- Pain in the neck, jaw, or arms.
- Awareness of an irregular heartbeat (palpitations).
- Nausea.
- Severe shortness of breath.
- Dizziness and light-headedness.

If you have any of these symptoms, you should discuss them with your doctor.

Resting between exercise sessions is essential to allow your body to recover. Mild muscle stiffness is common if you exercise regularly, and a gentle walk may relieve it. However, if your muscles are very stiff and your joints are painful, rest until you feel able to exercise again.

DANGERS OF OVEREXERTION

Exercising too often or too hard, which is often called overtraining, seems to undo the benefits of moderate exercise (*see* THE BENEFITS OF EXERCISE, p.55). The most common injuries due to overtraining include severe muscle stiffness, joint sprains, and stress fractures.

You may be exercising too much if you develop any of the following symptoms:

- Reduced appetite.
- Difficulty sleeping.
- Feeling constantly exhausted.
- Waking up tired and listless.
- Unintentional loss of weight.
- Loss of desire to keep fit.
- Recurrent infections or injuries.

In females, overtraining may disrupt the levels of sex hormones. In women, this disruption can cause periods to stop (*see* AMENORRHOEA, p.735), and in girls, it can delay the start of menstruation. It may also contribute to female infertility (p.775) and osteoporosis (p.368).

You may need to make small adjustments to include physical activity in your life. However, if you find that you are rearranging your life around exercise, you are doing too much.

(WWW) ONLINE SITES: p.1031

(HEALTH ACTION) WARMING UP AND COOLING DOWN IN YOUR EXERCISE ROUTINE

You should follow a routine to stretch your muscles, tendons, and ligaments before and after exercise to prevent cramping and stiffness and to minimize the risk of injury. Your warm-up should involve aerobic exercise followed by a series of stretches. After exercise, use a cool-down routine to slow the pace so that you are still warm while you stretch out your muscles. Repeat the stretches on both sides of the body and hold each stretch for at least 10 seconds. Some suitable warm-up and cool-down exercises are shown here.

AEROBIC EXERCISES

Aerobic activity increases the flow of blood through the soft tissues of the body. This increased blood flow raises their temperature and makes them more flexible. You should aim to do gentle aerobic exercises for between 8 and 10 minutes as part of both your warm-up and your cool-down routines.

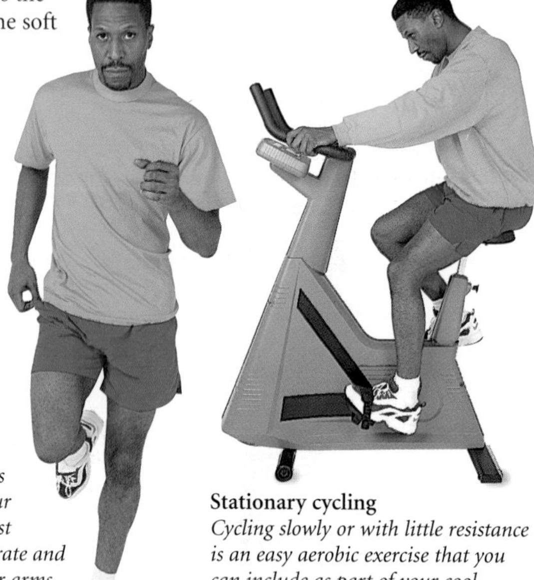

Jogging
Gentle jogging or running is a good way to warm up your muscles. You need to run fast enough to raise your heart rate and breathing rate. Moving your arms helps to raise your heart rate and create momentum.

Stationary cycling
Cycling slowly or with little resistance is an easy aerobic exercise that you can include as part of your cool-down routine. This exercise allows the heart rate to decrease gradually.

UPPER BODY STRETCHES

Stretching your chest and neck can help to relieve tension across the top of your back. Stretching your upper back by holding your arms out in front of you, clasping your hands, and rounding your back may also help. Upper body stretches improve your shoulder mobility.

Hands clasped behind back

Chest stretch
Clasp your hands behind you, and, while keeping your shoulders down, slowly move your arms up as far as they will go.

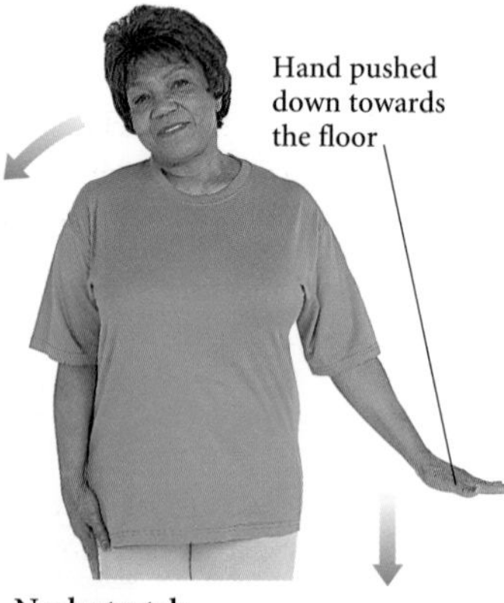

Hand pushed down towards the floor

Neck stretch
While holding your arm out to one side, push your hand downwards. Then let your head fall to the opposite side.

ARM STRETCHES

Like the upper body stretches, stretching your arms can help to relieve tension across the top of your back. You may find stretching easier on one side, depending on whether you are right- or left-handed. You should stretch your arms and shoulders before playing racket sports.

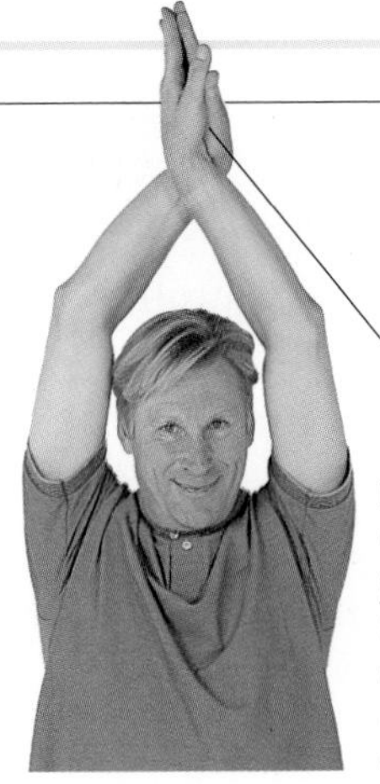

Full arm stretch
Cross your arms and put your hands together. Raise your arms overhead, behind your ears, and stretch upwards.

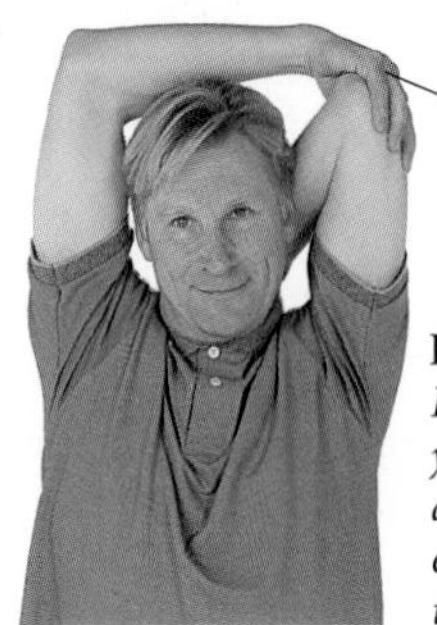

Back of arm stretch
Put one hand between your shoulder blades and pull gently on the elbow to stretch the muscle.

LEG STRETCHES

Many sports injuries affect the legs, so making sure that you stretch your leg muscles is especially important. You should always perform a series of leg stretches before taking part in activities that rely heavily on using your legs, such as brisk walking, running, jogging, and cycling.

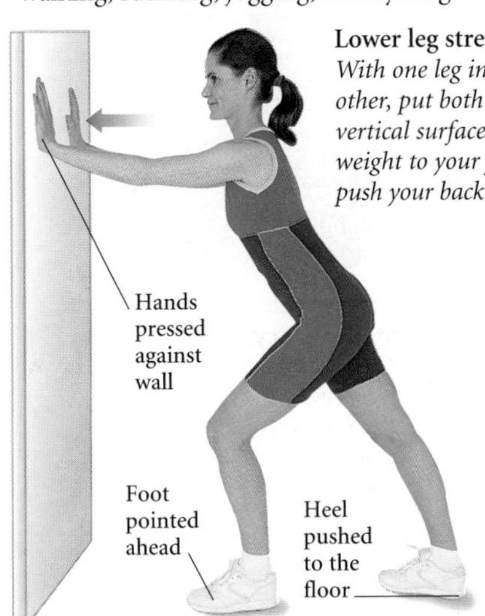

Lower leg stretch
With one leg in front of the other, put both hands on a vertical surface. Transfer your weight to your front leg and push your back heel to the floor.

Trunk of body held upright

Inner thigh muscles stretched

Knee slightly bent

Inner thigh stretch
With your feet wide apart, bend one knee and lean your body weight to that side. Keep your back straight; avoid twisting.

Knee bent at about 90°

Hip and thigh stretch
Kneel with one knee directly above its ankle and stretch the other leg back so that the knee touches the floor. Place your hands on your front knee for stability.

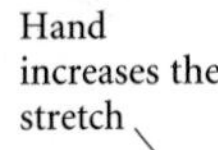

Hand increases the stretch

Back of thigh stretch
In a lying position, bend both legs and bring one knee towards your chest. Grasp your toes with one hand and gently pull on the back of the thigh with the other.

TRUNK STRETCHES

Do not forget to stretch muscles in your trunk. For example, by stretching out your back and the sides of your body before and after working in the garden, you may prevent back pain.

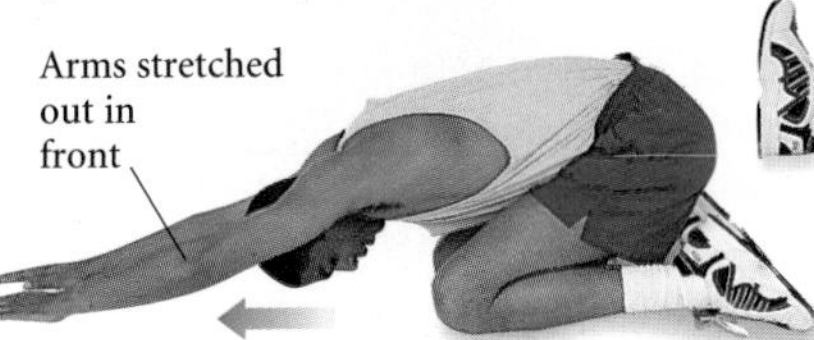

Lower back stretch
While kneeling, place your head on the floor in front of you and stretch your arms above your head, away from your body.

Knee pushed back by the arm

Trunk turned past bent knee

Trunk-twisting stretch
Sit with one leg straight and the other bent and crossed over it. Turn towards the knee that is bent, place your arm in front of the knee, and push against that leg while turning your body towards your other arm.

Shoulders in line with each other

Side stretch
With your feet shoulder-width apart, stand up straight. Then put one arm over your head, lean from the waist, and reach slowly to the side with your upper hand to feel the stretch.

ALCOHOL, TOBACCO, AND DRUGS

Many people use alcohol, tobacco, or recreational drugs for pleasure. However, all of these substances may cause severe health problems. Knowledge of their harmful effects can help you to make informed choices about whether or not to use them.

Alcohol is safe in moderation, but having more than two or three drinks a day can pose short-term risks, from alcohol poisoning to traffic accidents. In the long term, excessive alcohol consumption causes serious problems, such as heart, liver, and brain disease, and can lead to alcohol dependence.

Tobacco smoke contains over 4,000 chemicals, including nicotine, which is addictive, and other chemicals that increase susceptibility to cancer and to narrowing of the arteries, a cause of heart disease and stroke. The smoke may also have adverse effects on the health of people, particularly children, who live around a smoker.

All recreational drugs alter your state of mind; many, such as LSD and marijuana, can impair judgment and increase the risk of accidents. Drugs may be highly addictive and may cause death from overdose or side effects. Most recreational drugs are illegal.

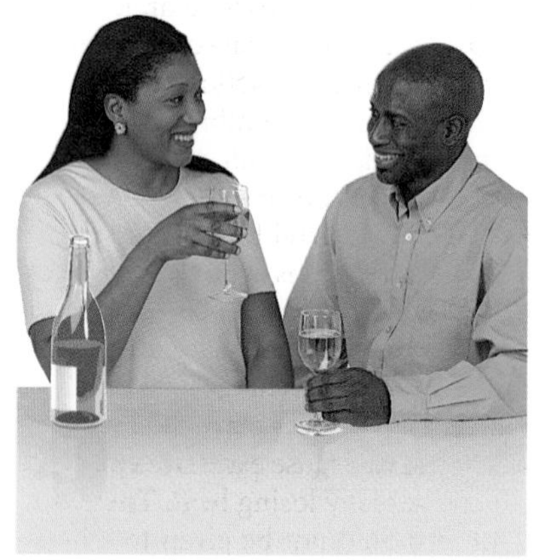

Social drinking
Alcohol consumption can be an enjoyable part of your social life, but you should keep your consumption within safe limits.

Alcohol and health

How alcohol affects health and how to use alcohol responsibly

Alcohol has been used for centuries at celebrations and social occasions. It is a drug that alters a person's mental and physical state, reducing tension and facilitating social interaction, but it may also cause loss of control over behaviour. Although moderate alcohol consumption (*see* SAFE ALCOHOL LIMITS, right) promotes a feeling of relaxation and has a beneficial effect on health, excessive use of alcohol over a long period can result in serious physical, psychological, and social problems.

Excessive long-term drinking severely reduces life expectancy and is a significant cause of preventable death. In the UK, excessive consumption of alcohol is thought to cause up to 28,000 deaths each year from disease and accidents. About 1 in 6 deaths on the road is due to drink–driving (*see* SAFETY ON THE ROAD, p.83), and 1 in 4 accidents at work is related to excessive drinking.

HEALTH ACTION SAFE ALCOHOL LIMITS

Alcohol intake is measured in units. Current UK guidelines set by the medical profession state that, in general, men should drink no more than 3 units a day and women no more than 2 units of alcohol each day. You should try to keep within these limits and have at least one or two days each week when you do not consume any alcohol.

Units of alcohol
The number of units in a drink is calculated on the basis of the volume of the drink and the percentage of alcohol by volume (ABV). Measures served in bars or at home do not always correspond to those shown here.

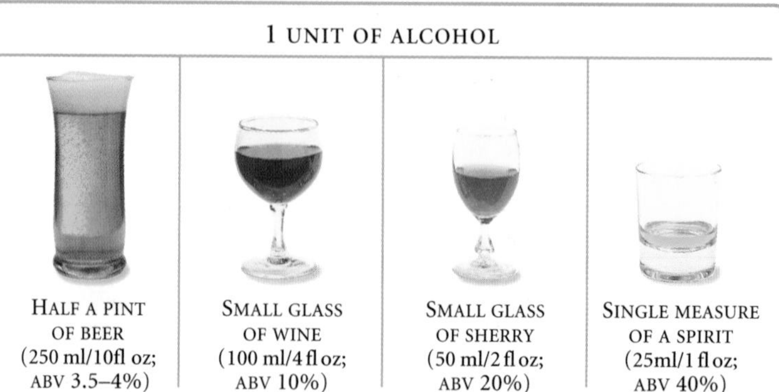

EFFECTS OF ALCOHOL USE

When you drink alcohol, it is absorbed into the blood from the stomach and small intestine. It is carried to the liver, where it is broken down by enzymes to be used for energy or stored as fat. A small amount is eliminated unchanged in urine and in exhaled breath. Alcohol reaches its maximum concentration in the blood about 35–45 minutes after intake. The actual concentration depends on various factors, such as the weight of the individual and whether the alcohol has been drunk with food or on an empty stomach.

The rate at which alcohol is broken down (metabolized) in the liver also varies between individuals, and heavy drinkers can metabolize it more quickly. The average rate is about 1 unit per hour. On any occasion, your body cannot alter the rate at which it breaks down alcohol, so that the more you drink, the longer it will take for your blood alcohol concentration to return to normal. If you drink heavily at night, you may still be intoxicated the next morning.

SHORT-TERM EFFECTS Alcohol is a sedative, depressing the action of the central nervous system. In particular, it affects the part of the brain that controls movement, impairing reaction times and coordination. Your inhibitions are suppressed, and, although you may feel more confident, your judgment may be impaired for several hours after drinking. Just one drink is enough to have this effect, making it dangerous for you to drive or operate machinery. Alcohol causes blood vessels in the skin to dilate. Although this effect may make you feel warm and can cause excessive sweating, you are actually losing heat. Therefore, alcohol should not be given to anyone chilled from exposure to the cold.

Alcohol causes increased urine production, and you may feel dehydrated if you have several drinks in quick succession. Heavy drinking often leads to a hangover, with headache, nausea, dizziness, and a dry mouth. Hangovers are the result of adverse reactions to alcohol itself and to chemical additives, which are found particularly in dark-coloured drinks such as red wine and whisky. You can slow the absorption of alcohol by eating when you drink. Drinking very large quantities of alcohol may cause confusion and loss of memory, loss of consciousness, coma, or, in extreme cases, death.

Some Asian people have a gene that causes an immediate adverse reaction to alcohol. Affected people have reactions such as nausea and facial flushing.

LONG-TERM EFFECTS Drinking alcohol within safe limits (opposite page) may protect against coronary heart disease (p.405) and stroke (p.532). Men over the age of 40 and postmenopausal women are most likely to benefit. However, when safe limits are exceeded, the risks outweigh the benefits. Since alcohol has a high calorie content, regular drinkers often put on weight (*see* CONTROLLING YOUR WEIGHT, p.53). Alcohol damages most body systems and is a major cause of liver disease (*see* ALCOHOL-RELATED LIVER DISEASE, p.646). In the brain, cells that control learning and memory may be damaged (*see* WERNICKE–KORSAKOFF SYNDROME, p.538). Drinking more than the safe alcohol limit increases the risk of cardiovascular disorders such as dilated cardiomyopathy (p.427), stroke, and high blood pressure (*see* HYPERTENSION, p.403). Excessive consumption of alcohol increases the risk of several kinds of cancer, especially cancer of the nasopharynx (p.480), cancer of the larynx (p.481), mouth cancer (p.634), and cancer of the oesophagus (p.638). If you also smoke, cancer risk is even greater.

Drinking too much alcohol reduces fertility. Many women give up drinking alcohol completely during pregnancy. While occasional, small drinks are unlikely to harm the fetus, there are definite risks from higher consumption.

Excessive drinking on a regular basis can lead to alcohol dependence (p.564) and is a major cause of social problems. In the UK, 65 per cent of the offenders and victims involved in murder, and 65 per cent of suicide victims, have been drinking, and alcohol is associated with 4 in 10 incidents of domestic violence. Regular drinking can damage relationships and lead to considerable stress to a drinker's family and friends.

ASSESSMENT DO YOU DRINK TOO MUCH?

If you drink more than two alcoholic drinks a day on most days, you may be putting your health at risk. The questions below may help you to judge the degree to which drinking is affecting your lifestyle and whether you are at risk of letting drinking become an uncontrollable habit.

1 *Have you ever thought that you ought to cut down on your drinking?*
☐ YES ☐ NO

2 *Have other people ever annoyed you by criticizing your drinking?*
☐ YES ☐ NO

3 *Have you ever felt guilty about your drinking?*
☐ YES ☐ NO

4 *Have you ever had an "eye-opener" drink first thing in the morning?*
☐ YES ☐ NO

ANALYSIS

If you have answered yes to two or more of these questions, your drinking may be becoming a problem. You should think about how you can change your drinking habits and seek help from either your doctor or a support group.

ASSESSING YOUR CONSUMPTION

If you think you may be drinking too much, consult your doctor, who might ask you to keep a diary for several weeks to record each drink you have.

Some people drink to relieve stress or painful emotions. Stress-related consumption may lead to the development of a drinking problem. Warning signs include drinking more than you intended on any occasion, severe hangovers, and being involved in accidents or arguments after drinking. Try completing a test (*see* DO YOU DRINK TOO MUCH?, above) to see if you have a problem.

WHAT YOU CAN DO

To enjoy alcohol safely, limit your intake. At social events, eat first, alternate alcoholic and nonalcoholic drinks, and finish each drink before refilling so that you know how many units you have had. Never drive if you intend to drink; try to go with a designated driver who will not drink. If you have children, set a good example for them. In addition, discuss the effects of alcohol with them and reinforce the message of any alcohol awareness programmes run by their school. To relieve emotional problems, try approaches such as counselling.

(WWW) ONLINE SITES: p.1026

Tobacco and health

The effects of tobacco on health and reasons for avoiding its use

Tobacco is most commonly smoked in cigarettes but can be smoked in cigars and pipes, inhaled as snuff, or chewed. However it is used, tobacco is harmful to health. In the UK, smoking is one of the main causes of death in people under the age of 65, leading to about 120,000 deaths each year. It is known to be a major contributing factor to coronary heart disease (p.405) and primary lung cancer (p.503). Smoking also damages the health of "passive smokers", who inhale other people's smoke from the air around them. The only way to avoid the risks associated with tobacco smoking is to avoid smoking and those situations in which you come into contact with other people's smoke.

In affluent countries such as the UK, the number of smokers declined from about half of the population in the early 1970s to less than 1 in 3 in the 1990s. The decline is due to increasing numbers of older people who stop. However, almost 1 in 4 15-year-olds smokes regularly, and the proportion of smokers is highest among people aged 20–24. It has been found that most of those people who continue to smoke are unemployed or manual workers.

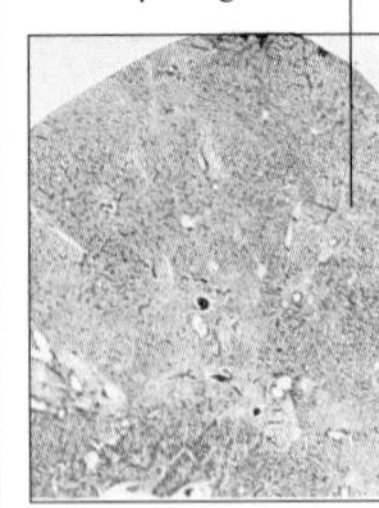

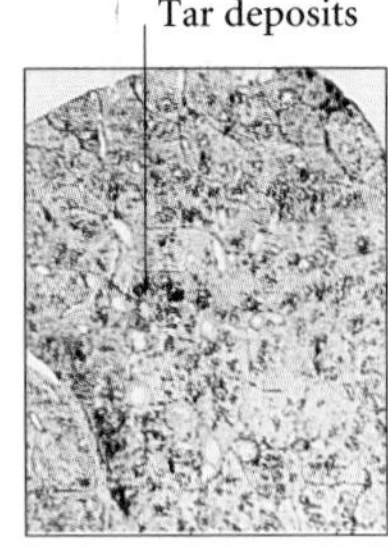

Effects of smoking on the lungs
Over time, the tar from cigarette smoke gradually builds up in the lungs, as these sections through the lungs of a long-term smoker and a nonsmoker show.

EFFECTS OF TOBACCO USE

Tobacco smoke contains many substances that are toxic or irritating to the body. The substances that have been studied most closely are tar, carbon monoxide, and nicotine. Tobacco smoke also contains carcinogenic (cancer-causing) substances that have toxic effects on the lungs and other organs.

Tar in tobacco smoke irritates and inflames the tissues of the lungs. Carbon monoxide attaches itself to red blood cells, reducing their capacity to carry oxygen. Nicotine acts as a tranquillizer, starting to take effect within 10 seconds of ingestion and producing a temporary feeling of well-being and relaxation. The substance is also known to increase the ability to concentrate. It stimulates the release of the hormone epinephrine (adrenaline) into the bloodstream, and this causes a rise in blood pressure. Nicotine is highly addictive, which is why most tobacco users find it hard to give up the habit. There are many damaging long-term effects of tobacco use, some of which are exacerbated by other aspects of a person's lifestyle, such as drinking excessive amounts of alcohol.

DAMAGE TO THE RESPIRATORY SYSTEM

Substances in cigarette smoke irritate the mucous membranes that line the air passages to the lungs, causing them to produce more mucus (sputum). These substances also paralyse the tiny hairs, called cilia, that help to expel sputum from the air passages. To clear their lungs, many smokers develop the characteristic "smoker's cough". Eventually, smoking may result in chronic obstructive pulmonary disease (p.487), which leads to severe shortness of breath.

Carcinogens in cigarette smoke cause over 8 in 10 of the deaths from lung cancer. In some countries, lung cancer has overtaken breast cancer as the leading cause of cancer-related deaths in women, a fact reflecting the large number of women who took up smoking during the second half of the 20th century. Smoking may also cause cancer of the nasopharynx (p.480) or cancer of the larynx (p.481). The risk of developing cancer of the larynx is even higher for cigar or pipe smokers and for people who both smoke and drink alcohol.

VASCULAR DAMAGE Smoking is known to cause permanent damage to the cardiovascular system and has been linked to about 1 in 4 deaths from cardiovascular disease. This damage is thought to be caused by the nicotine and carbon monoxide present in cigarette smoke, which may encourage the development of atherosclerosis (p.402), a condition in which the arteries become narrowed. Atherosclerosis in turn is known to increase the risk of stroke (p.532) and cardiovascular disorders such as coronary heart disease. In women over the age of 35, tobacco smoking increases the risk of developing disorders associated with the use of oral contraceptives (p.69), in particular deep vein thrombosis (p.437), stroke, and heart attacks (*see* MYOCARDIAL INFARCTION, p.410).

DAMAGE TO OTHER BODY SYSTEMS

Smokers are at increased risk of developing mouth cancer (p.634) and cancer of the oesophagus (p.638), particularly if they also drink alcohol. Carcinogenic chemicals from tobacco smoke that enter the bloodstream may also cause cancer in other parts of the body, such as the bladder (*see* BLADDER TUMOURS, p.715) and the cervix (*see* CANCER OF THE CERVIX, p.750).

The toxic effect of tobacco smoke may aggravate conditions such as peptic ulcers (p.640). Smoking may reduce fertility in men and women. If a pregnant woman smokes, her baby's birth weight is likely to be about 200 g (7 oz) lower than the average, and the baby is at greater risk of illness or death just after birth. The menopause may occur earlier in women who smoke. Smoking also affects the skin and accelerates skin changes, such as wrinkling, caused by aging and sunlight.

People who smoke cigars or pipes suffer less harm from smoke inhalation than those who smoke cigarettes. However, if you smoke cigars or a pipe you run a higher risk of developing mouth cancer and throat cancers. Snuff and chewing tobacco may also irritate the lining of the nose, mouth, and stomach.

RISKS OF PASSIVE SMOKING

Inhaling the smoke from other people's cigarettes is known as passive smoking. Secondhand smoke, also called environmental tobacco smoke (ETS), is a mixture of smoke from burning cigarettes and that exhaled by smokers.

In the short term, ETS irritates the eyes, nose, and throat and may cause headaches and nausea. The risk of developing lung cancer is up to one-third higher for nonsmokers who are regularly exposed to ETS than for those who are not exposed to it. The partners of smokers are at slightly greater risk of developing cardiovascular diseases than the partners of nonsmokers.

The children of smokers are particularly at risk from passive smoking. ETS aggravates respiratory disorders such as asthma (*see* ASTHMA IN CHILDREN, p.839). Children whose parents smoke are twice as likely to have asthma as those who have nonsmoking parents, and their asthma attacks may be more severe and more frequent. ETS can also provoke allergies, such as hay fever (*see* ALLERGIC RHINITIS, p.466).

Exposure to ETS raises children's susceptibility to infections such as sinusitis (p.475), acute bronchitis (p.486), colds, sore throats, and ear infections. Up to 1 in 3 cases of persistent ear infections (*see* CHRONIC SECRETORY OTITIS MEDIA, p.860), the most common cause of deafness in children, is linked to parental smoking. ETS is also a factor in sudden infant death syndrome (p.820).

WHAT YOU CAN DO

You can prevent disease by not smoking or by giving up smoking before you begin to develop heart or lung disease. However, no matter how long you have been smoking, you can prevent further damage to your health by giving it up (*see* HEALTH OF EX-SMOKERS, left). As soon as you give up smoking, you begin to reduce your risk of developing lung cancer and other respiratory disorders, cardiovascular disease, and stroke. You will also be less likely to suffer from a range of conditions that are associated with smoking, such as peptic ulcer. You are never too old to benefit from this reduction in risk; even elderly people who have been smoking for most of their adult lives can improve their health and life expectancy by stopping.

If you need help giving up smoking, consult your doctor. He or she may recommend an aid to stop cravings, such as nicotine gum or patches, or participation in a support group.

If you want to try on your own, plan in advance how you will stop. First, make a list of the reasons why you want to give up. Then work out the most common reasons why you smoke. You may crave cigarettes in certain situations or enjoy the ritual of smoking. Plan ways to cope with temptation and tell your family and friends so that they can offer support. Telephone helplines staffed by ex-smokers can provide help.

The next step is to choose a relatively stress-free day on which you will stop smoking completely. Dispose of all your cigarettes, lighters, and ashtrays, and distract yourself with enjoyable activities. Boost your willpower by looking at your list of reasons for giving up.

As soon as you give up, your body will start to repair the damage caused by smoking. You may feel withdrawal symptoms, such as irritability, and crave nicotine. If you relapse, work out why you felt the need to smoke, refer to your reasons for giving up, and try again.

Teach children about the health risks of smoking. Explain that people may enjoy smoking, but it makes them very ill. If your child's school runs an antismoking programme, try to reinforce its messages. Most smokers take up the habit in adolescence. If young people can be prevented from starting, they are more likely never to smoke. Teenagers may regard smoking as glamorous, and girls may think that it helps to control weight. Deter them by stressing the immediate drawbacks, such as bad breath.

(WWW) ONLINE SITES: p.1037

(HEALTH EFFECTS) HEALTH OF EX-SMOKERS

The body starts to repair damage caused by smoking as soon as the habit is stopped. The risk of developing lung cancer and other disorders such as cardiovascular disease and stroke lessens the longer smoking has been stopped; smokers who give up for 15 years or more reduce their risk of lung cancer by more than half.

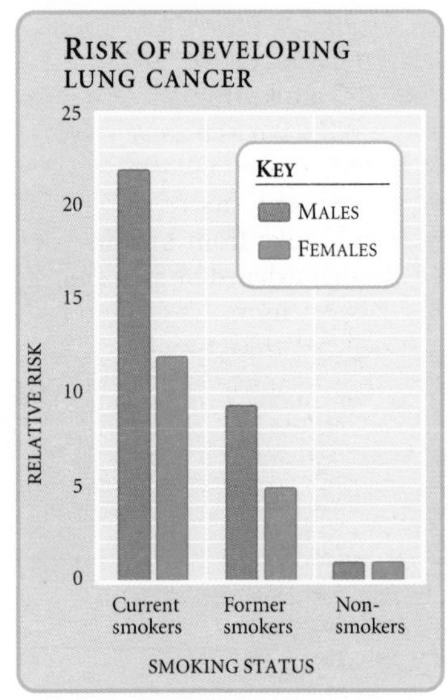

Smoking and lung cancer
This graph shows the risks for smokers and former smokers relative to the risk for nonsmokers. Statistics appear to show that women have a lower risk of lung cancer than men, but this may be due to different patterns of smoking.

Drugs and health

Health hazards associated with the recreational use of drugs

A drug is any chemical that alters the function of an organ or a process in the body. Drugs that have been developed to improve body functions or to treat disorders are known as medicines (*see* DRUG TREATMENT, pp.878–939). Some drugs, such as temazepam (*see* SLEEPING DRUGS, p.915), may be both used as medicines and abused for recreation. Other drugs, such as ecstasy, have no medicinal value and are used only for recreational purposes.

Recreational drug use can cause serious health problems, particularly if the user takes an overdose or becomes dependent on a drug (*see* DRUG DEPENDENCE, p.564). Since the sale or use of most recreational drugs is illegal, a user may be arrested and even face imprisonment. Alcohol and nicotine are also drugs that can be addictive and harmful (*see* ALCOHOL AND HEALTH, p.62, and TOBACCO AND HEALTH, p.63), as is caffeine, but they are viewed differently by society because they have been used for centuries and are sold legally.

"Hard" drugs, such as heroin and cocaine, are much less widely used than "soft" drugs, such as marijuana. For example, in 1994–5 almost 1 in 6 people in the UK who used recreational drugs daily used marijuana, but only 1 in 20 used heroin. However, hard drugs are more addictive than soft drugs, pose a much more serious threat to health, and may even carry a risk of death.

EFFECTS OF DRUG USE

Recreational drugs are usually used to alter mood. They are classified according to the predominant change that they cause but often have a mixture of effects. Stimulants, such as cocaine, cause increased physical and mental activity; relaxants, such as marijuana and heroin, produce a feeling of calm; intoxicants, such as glue, make users feel giggly and dreamy; and the main effect of hallucinogens, such as LSD, is to alter perception and cause the user to see or hear things that do not exist.

In addition, recreational drugs can affect functions such as breathing and temperature control. These effects can be damaging in both the short and the long term and some are potentially fatal. Some of the potential health risks, such as those of dependence or of an extreme reaction, apply to many or all drugs. Drugs that are injected carry additional risks associated with the use of needles. Each drug also carries a range of specific risks to the health of users (*see* RISKS OF SPECIFIC DRUGS, right). The health hazards associated with certain recently developed recreational drugs are not yet fully understood, although ecstasy use has been reported to lead to brain damage in the long term.

EXTREME REACTIONS Any recreational drug can be dangerous, even if not used regularly. One risk is an extreme reaction to a drug. The effects of any drug can vary among users, and a drug that has only mild effects on one person may severely affect another. In addition, a drug may be mixed with other substances, and the amount of active drug may vary considerably from dose to dose. Since the drugs are illegal, there is no control over the standards of drug purity. Many drugs, such as cocaine and LSD, can cause delusions, leading to abnormal or hazardous behaviour.

Uncertainty and recklessness about the strength of a drug may lead to overdose, which can be fatal. Alcohol and certain medicinal drugs, such as aspirin, interact with recreational drugs to produce intensified or unexpected effects.

DEPENDENCE Regular users of recreational drugs may face the problem of physical dependence. The body begins to crave the drug; the user feels ill if he or she does not take the drug regularly, and may come to need that substance simply in order to function normally. Physical dependence develops more rapidly if the drug is injected.

Even if a particular drug is not physically addictive, drug users may become psychologically dependent, coming to rely on the enjoyable effects of a drug or the rituals that surround its use. They may also risk psychological disturbance and malnutrition due to self-neglect or loss of appetite. Some users may also spend a lot of time taking or obtaining drugs and withdraw from ordinary life. Since illegal drugs are expensive, many users support their habit by crime.

HEALTH EFFECTS RISKS OF SPECIFIC DRUGS

People use drugs for recreation because they enjoy some of their effects, but there are also many short- and long-term effects that are unpleasant, harmful, or potentially fatal. It is important to be aware of the risks involved.

Hazardous effects

Short-term hazards may occur soon after taking a drug, possibly after only one dose. Long-term risks result from repeated use.

DRUG	SHORT-TERM HAZARDS	LONG-TERM HAZARDS
STIMULANTS		
Ecstasy	• Nausea • Tense muscles • Panic • Loss of temperature control and/or fluid retention, which can cause coma and death	• Sleep problems • Lethargy • Possible liver and kidney problems and brain damage
Amphetamines	• Tension • Anxiety • Overdose may be fatal • Effects include lethargy and depression	• Heart disorders • Severe psychological disorders
Cocaine	• Paranoia • Overdose can cause heart attack • Effects include lethargy and depression	• Damage to nose and lungs from sniffing drug • Anxiety • Paranoia • Heart disorders
Crack	• Loss of self-control • Violent or erratic behaviour • Burnt mouth and throat • Chest pain	• Heart disorders • Damage to lungs • Paranoia
RELAXANTS		
Marijuana (Cannabis)	• Decreased coordination and concentration • Impairment of skills, such as driving vehicles	• Apathy • Increased risk of lung cancer and other respiratory disorders
Heroin	• Overdose can cause coma and death • Infection with HIV or hepatitis if needles are shared	• Tremor • Apathy • Blood-vessel damage from repeated injections
INTOXICANTS		
Glue, petrol, aerosols	• Vomiting • Suffocation if inhaling from plastic bag • Loss of consciousness • Possibly fatal reaction upon inhalation	• Cough • Rash around nose and mouth • Damage to brain, liver, kidneys, and nervous system
HALLUCINOGENS		
Lysergic acid diethylamide (LSD)	• Extreme anxiety • Loss of self-control and increased risk of accidents	• Hallucinations that occur months or even years after use of drug
Phencyclidine, or phenocyclo-piperidine (PCP)	• Confusion • Vomiting • Sharp rise or fall in pulse rate and blood pressure • Seizures • Heart failure • Overdose may be fatal	• Loss of short-term memory and coordination • Paranoia • Speech difficulties • Violent behaviour • Depression

RISKS ASSOCIATED WITH INJECTION Users who inject drugs risk infection and damage to blood vessels, which can lead to tissue death (*see* GANGRENE, p.435) or septicaemia (p.299). If syringes and needles are shared, users also risk infection with HIV (*see* HIV INFECTION AND AIDS, p.297) and hepatitis B or C (*see* ACUTE HEPATITIS, p.644).

WHAT YOU CAN DO

If you or someone close to you abuses drugs, ask your doctor for information on health risks and advice on counselling and treatment. If you have children, tell them about the hazards of drug use. If their school has a drug awareness programme, reinforce its messages.

(WWW) ONLINE SITES: p.1030

SEX AND HEALTH

Human beings are unique among animals in having the capacity for sexual desire even when the female is not fertile and in retaining desire into old age, long after conception has ceased to be possible. The explanation may be that sex helps to maintain partnerships. Regular sex also seems to improve cardiovascular fitness and prolong life. People who are involved in stable sexual relationships live longer than those without sexual partners.

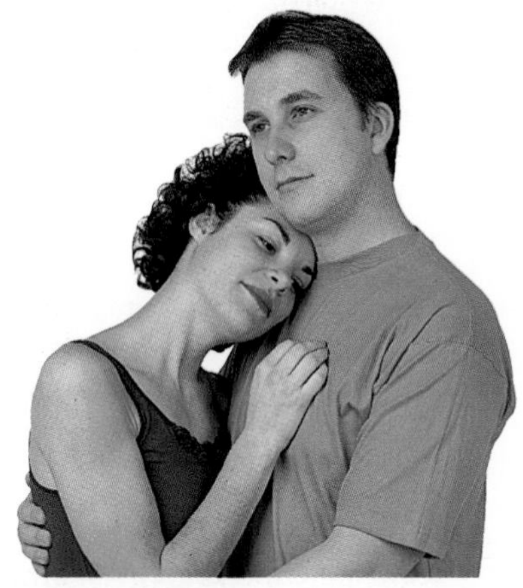

Enjoying intimacy
When two partners are establishing an intimate, sexual relationship, it is important for them to trust each other.

A satisfying sexual relationship is an important part of life but not always easy to achieve, and sexual contact may be risky. In particular, casual sex and sex with multiple partners carry the risks of unwanted pregnancy and sexually transmitted infections (STIs).

The first article in the section covers the basic elements of a healthy sexual relationship. The article on safe sex discusses ways to reduce your risk of exposure to sexually transmitted infections. The final article provides an overview of the advantages and disadvantages of different forms of contraception. Education about sex, pregnancy, and STIs is particularly important for teenagers, who often fail to make use of contraceptives and ignore advice about safe sex. In the UK, this has resulted in the highest rate of teenage conceptions in Western Europe.

Specific sexual problems and the symptoms and treatment of sexually transmitted infections are discussed in other sections of the book (*see* SEXUAL PROBLEMS, pp.769–773, and SEXUALLY TRANSMITTED INFECTIONS, pp.764–768), as are possible problems in conceiving (*see* INFERTILITY, pp.774–777).

Sexual relationships

The physical and emotional elements of satisfying sexual relationships

The physical maturity necessary for a sexual relationship is signalled by the onset of puberty, when the individual's body makes the transition from childhood to adulthood. The development of emotional maturity frequently takes much longer, and early sexual encounters, although sometimes exciting, may just as often be disappointing or cause anxiety. With age and experience, most people become better able to establish and fully enjoy sexual relationships.

A HEALTHY RELATIONSHIP

What constitutes a healthy sexual relationship varies widely from person to person. Sexual fulfilment depends on a blend of physical and psychological factors, and what is right for one couple may not suit another. You and your partner should both be happy with the frequency of sexual activity, and you should be able to discuss which sexual activities you find pleasant and which you find unappealing.

Anyone in a sexual relationship should be aware of the risks posed by sexually transmitted infections (STIs) and know how to minimize the risk of exposure to them (*see* SAFE SEX, p.68). In addition, to avoid an unwanted pregnancy, you should be familiar with the options for contraception (p.69), including emergency contraception. It is important that children approaching puberty are given education about STIs, safe sex, and contraception. Most schools provide sex-education programmes.

POTENTIAL PROBLEMS

It is normal to experience fluctuations in sex drive or occasional temporary loss of sexual desire, lack of sexual response, or inability to perform sexually. However, if sexual problems persist, they may be distressing and cause you anxiety, which further impairs your ability to enjoy sexual activity, and this creates a vicious circle.

Sexual problems may have a number of causes. Emotional difficulties in your current relationship will affect your sex life. External stress will also affect a relationship and may lead to problems. For example, ongoing problems at work or financial difficulties may cause anxiety, irritability, or lack of sleep, all of which may decrease your desire for sex. Past upsets of an emotional nature, such as the break-up of a former relationship, can affect your current situation even when the problem seems to have disappeared.

Decrease in sex drive or impaired sexual function may also be the result of complications of certain long-term physical conditions, such as diabetes mellitus (p.687); disabilities that cause pain and restrict movement; convalescence from surgery or severe illness; and the use of alcohol, recreational drugs, and certain medications.

WHAT YOU CAN DO

If there are matters that are bothering you, it is important to talk about them with your partner. If the problem is persistent, discuss it with your doctor, who can refer you for appropriate help. If you have a long-term illness or a disability that impairs your sex life, you may find it helpful to get in touch with an organization that has been established to help people with the problem.

(WWW) ONLINE SITES: p.1029, p.1036

Safe sex

Sexual practices that minimize your risk of contracting sexually transmitted infections

One of the hazards of sexual contact is exposure to certain infections. These range from uncomfortable but minor problems, such as pubic lice (p.768), to life-threatening disorders, such as HIV infection (*see* HIV INFECTION AND AIDS, p.297). Certain disorders, such as genital herpes (p.767), genital warts (p.768), and gonorrhoea (p.764), are almost always transmitted only by sexual contact and are known as sexually transmitted infections (STIs). Others, such as hepatitis B and C (*see* ACUTE HEPATITIS, p.644) and HIV infection, may be transmitted by other means as well as through sex. For example, people who inject drugs and share needles with others risk infection with HIV or hepatitis. In addition, some disorders, such as scabies (p.355), are transmitted by physical contact and are common among people living in overcrowded conditions and among schoolchildren. These disorders may also be transmitted during sexual intercourse.

Assessing the risks

It is important to assess your risk of exposure to STIs so that you can make informed choices about the level of risk that you find acceptable. To be able to do this, you need to understand how infection is spread and know which sexual activities carry the highest risks. If you think you are likely to be exposed to infection, or if you are not sure what your own risk might be, you should use a condom (see USING CONTRACEPTIVES, p.70) or avoid sex. It is essential that you and your partner do not have unprotected sex until your relationship is well established and monogamous and both of you are known to be free of disease.

HIGH-RISK ACTIVITIES Diseases such as hepatitis B and C and HIV infection may be spread through contact with semen, blood, or vaginal secretions. Other disorders, such as genital warts and genital herpes, are transmitted by contact with a wart or sore. The areas most vulnerable to infection are the skin of the genitals and mucous membranes such as the lining of the vagina, anus, mouth, and urethra (the tube that leads from the bladder to the outside of the body).

The sexual activities that pose the highest risks are those in which there is a chance that the mucous membranes will be damaged, allowing infectious agents from body fluids or body parts to enter the bloodstream. Vaginal, anal, and oral intercourse that involves penetration, and in which partners do not use a condom, are considered to be the activities carrying the highest risks. Anal penetration can be particularly hazardous because the lining of the anus and rectum is easily damaged.

SEXUAL HISTORY The risk of exposure to STIs increases with the more sexual partners that you have and the more times that you practise unsafe sex. A monogamous relationship with someone whom you know has been screened and found free of disease carries the lowest risk. You may be more vulnerable if your partner has had sex with someone else and has not told you, particularly if you do not use a condom with that partner. In addition, you or your partner may already have an STI and be infectious but have no symptoms. For example, chlamydial pelvic infections (p.765) affect both men and women but often cause no symptoms in women. In both sexes, infection with genital warts is followed by a latent period of about 9 months when you have no symptoms but are still infectious. Having casual sex without using a condom carries most risk because you are unlikely to know if your partner is infected.

Some STIs are particularly prevalent in certain groups of people. For example, HIV infection is more common among people living in some parts of Africa and Asia, prostitutes, people who inject recreational drugs and share needles, and people who have unprotected anal sex. You may run a higher than usual risk of infection if you have unsafe sex with a person from one of these groups.

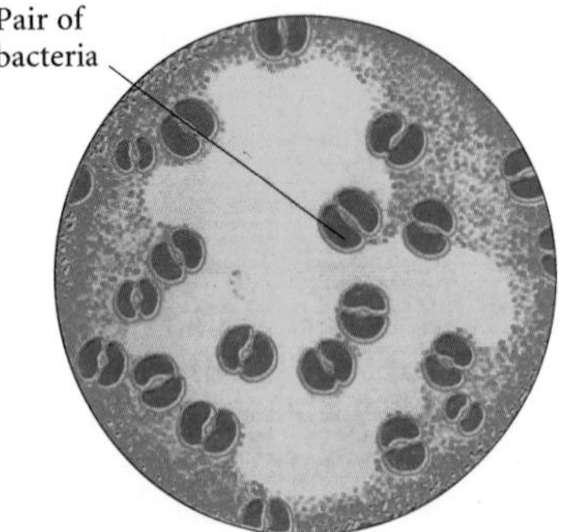

Gonorrhoea organisms
This highly magnified view shows the bacteria that cause gonorrhoea, Neisseria gonorrhoeae, *which may be found in genital, rectal, and throat secretions.*

What you can do

Condoms are able to protect you from infections that are transmitted during sexual intercourse. However, they do not protect you from contact with sores or warts on areas of the body that are not covered by the condom or from pubic lice or scabies.

If you choose not to use condoms, you should make sure that neither you nor your partner is carrying an infection. Discuss your past sexual contacts honestly, particularly if either of you is in a high-risk group. If you suspect that you have been exposed to infection, arrange to have a screening test at a clinic that specializes in treating STIs. With HIV infection, there is a latent period of at least 2–3 months between acquiring the infection and the time when the antibody to the virus can be detected in the test. For this reason, many clinics advise using condoms for the first 3 months of a new relationship before having an HIV test.

Once you and your partner are sure that you are free from STIs, the most effective way to protect yourselves is by remaining monogamous. If you do have sexual intercourse with other partners, make sure that you use condoms. If you are not using condoms and develop an STI, use condoms until you have been treated and are free of disease or abstain from penetrative sex. Both you and your partner should be treated at the same time to avoid the risk of reinfecting each other, and you should both be free of disease before you stop using condoms. Sexual activities that carry a relatively low risk of infection include kissing your partner's mouth (or body areas other than the genitals) and mutual masturbation by hand. The activities that have little or no risk are those that do not involve contact with your partner's genitals. These include intimate activities, such as cuddling, massage, and bathing together.

(WWW) ONLINE SITES: p.1031, p.1036

Contraception

Artificial and natural methods for controlling fertility

Contraception allows people to choose whether and when to have children. There are several types and each works differently (*see* USING CONTRACEPTIVES, p.70). Nearly all types, apart from the male condom and male sterilization, are designed for use by women.

Most contraceptives, apart from condoms, are supplied by your doctor, who considers your age, medical history, and sexual lifestyle. No contraceptive is entirely free from risk. Some types may not be suitable for you, while others have side effects that you must weigh against the benefits. In addition, you may need to change your contraceptive as you grow older, after having children, or if you alter your sexual lifestyle. It is important that you are happy with your contraceptive. Even if your doctor has recommended a particular type, do not accept it if you have doubts about it.

BARRIER METHODS

Barrier contraceptive methods include diaphragms, condoms, and cervical caps. They act by preventing sperm from entering the uterus and reaching the egg. Male condoms cover the penis, female condoms line the vagina, and caps and diaphragms cover the cervix. Barrier contraceptives do not disrupt normal body functions or affect fertility, but they are unreliable if not used correctly and can also affect the spontaneity of sex. Some people who use condoms may be allergic to the material from which the condoms are made.

When used correctly, condoms are an effective method of preventing unwanted pregnancy. Condoms are also thought to protect women from cancer of the cervix (p.750) by reducing the risk of infection with the human papilloma virus, some types of which have been linked with this type of cancer.

The male condom is the only contraceptive method that also protects users and their partners from sexually transmitted infections (*see* SAFE SEX, opposite page). Condoms may also be used for protection when one partner has a long-standing infection such as HIV (*see* HIV INFECTIONS AND AIDS, p.297).

HORMONAL METHODS

Hormonal contraceptives alter the hormone balance in a woman's body to prevent conception. They may be taken orally in the form of the combined pill or the progestogen-only pill. Hormones may also be injected into a muscle or implanted in a flexible rod under the skin. Hormonal methods are useful because they do not interrupt sexual activities, but they can cause side effects or health risks in some women. If you stop using them because you want to become pregnant, it may take a few months for your fertility to return. Oral contraceptives may not be reliable after a bout of vomiting or diarrhoea, and you should use alternative methods in this situation. Some antibiotics (p.885) may also reduce the effectiveness of oral contraceptives. For this reason, if you are taking an oral contraceptive, you should tell your doctor in case it interacts with other prescribed medication.

COMBINED PILL The combined contraceptive pill, containing both oestrogen and progestogen, is highly reliable. This is the most commonly used contraceptive among women under 35, who are in their most fertile period and need an effective method. There may be side effects, such as changes in weight and mood, but these usually disappear after the first few months of use.

The combined pill lowers the risk of cancer of the ovary (p.744) but increases the risk of some other disorders. It can cause a slight rise in blood pressure, so you may be advised not to use it if you have a family history of high blood pressure (*see* HYPERTENSION, p.403). It also causes blood to clot more readily, increasing your risk of stroke (p.532) and heart attacks (*see* MYOCARDIAL INFARCTION, p.410). The risk is substantially raised if you are over the age of 35 and smoke, but you should also avoid the combined pill if you are very overweight or have a family history of deep vein thrombosis (p.437), no matter what your age.

PROGESTOGEN-ONLY PILL This type of contraceptive pill contains only progestogen. It does not carry the health risks of the combined pill, but it is less effective and must be taken at the same time each day to be reliable. The progestogen-only pill often causes lighter periods but may also make your cycle irregular. However, its effect on menstruation does not alter its effectiveness as a contraceptive. There may be other side effects, such as acne and breast tenderness, but these should last only a few months. There is also a small risk of ovarian cysts (p.743) or of having an ectopic pregnancy (p.790) if you conceive while taking it.

INJECTIONS AND IMPLANTS Progestogen can be given as an injection or an implant – both provide reliable long-term contraception. They are useful if you do not want to have children for some years or at all or if you regularly forget to take pills. Initially, these may make your periods irregular or heavier. You may also gain 1–2 kg (2–4 lb). After the first period, most women stop menstruating with these methods.

MECHANICAL METHODS

Intrauterine devices (IUDs), also known as coils, are contraceptive devices that are inserted into the uterus by a doctor. They are made of plastic, and have threads that hang through the cervix so that the user can check that her device is still in place. Some IUDs contain copper; it is not known exactly how they work, but they are thought to cause an inflammatory reaction that kills sperm and prevents fertilized eggs from being implanted in the uterus. Other types contain progestogen, which thickens cervical mucus in order to repel sperm.

IUDs give immediate protection and last for several years. However, they may be difficult to insert in women who have never been pregnant and may be better for those who wish to defer future pregnancies or who have completed their families. The devices may increase your susceptibility to certain infections (*see* PELVIC INFLAMMATORY DISEASE, p.741) and may not be suitable if you have multiple short-term sexual contacts that increase your exposure to infections. There is a small risk that the IUD may be expelled from the uterus, or that it may pierce the uterus and cause a serious inflammation of the abdominal lining called peritonitis (p.665).

The IUD does not affect hormones or ovulation, but it may worsen heavy or painful periods, especially in the first few months after insertion (see MENORRHAGIA, p.735, and DYSMENORRHOEA, p.736). IUDs that contain progestogen usually make periods lighter and less painful after the first 3 months of use. For this reason, they can be useful for women with heavy periods or for those nearing the menopause. The devices may produce temporary side effects similar to those of the progestogen-only pill.

NATURAL METHODS

Natural birth control involves working out when you are fertile and avoiding intercourse at those times. It does not affect the body and has no side effects. If you wish, you can use it to determine when you can conceive. However, this method can disrupt the spontaneity of sex and should not be used without training. It also requires that you have a regular menstrual cycle. Natural birth control works best if you are in a long-term relationship and feel that you could accept an unplanned pregnancy.

SURGICAL METHODS

Surgical contraception, or sterilization, is an operation that makes you infertile. This surgery can be carried out on men (*see* VASECTOMY, p.721) or women (*see* FEMALE STERILIZATION, p.743). Since the operation is considered permanent, it is suitable only for those who are sure that they do not want children. The operations have low failure rates, of about 1 in 1,000 men and 7 in 1,000 women.

Male sterilization (vasectomy) is not immediately effective. The seminal vesicles (sacs that hold semen) still contain sperm after the operation, and a condom must be used until semen analysis (p.777) has shown that no sperm are left. Female sterilization is effective immediately after the operation, but it slightly increases the risk of ectopic pregnancy should it fail for any reason.

EMERGENCY METHODS

Emergency contraception is used to prevent pregnancy if you have had unprotected sex or if your contraception has failed. If it is less than 72 hours since unprotected sex, treatment is usually with two doses of progestogen. These pills can be obtained from your doctor or over the counter without a prescription. Alternatively, an IUD can prevent a pregnancy if it is inserted less than 5 days after unprotected sex.

(WWW) ONLINE SITES: p.1031

HEALTH OPTIONS USING CONTRACEPTIVES

Contraception provides a high degree of protection against unwanted pregnancy, although the effectiveness of different methods varies. For each method described here, effectiveness is defined as the number of women per hundred per year who do not become pregnant while using it and is expressed as a percentage. For most methods, apart from the IUD, your doctor will need to explain how to use them so that they are effective. It may take some time to learn how to use a diaphragm, a cap, or natural methods, and they are not suitable for times when you need contraception immediately. A condom is usually the best method in this situation.

BARRIER METHODS

Condoms, diaphragms, and caps form barriers between the penis and the uterus to prevent sperm from reaching the egg. They may be used with spermicide, a substance that kills sperm. Barrier methods are 92–98 per cent effective, and the male condom is the most effective. Most failures are due to incorrect use.

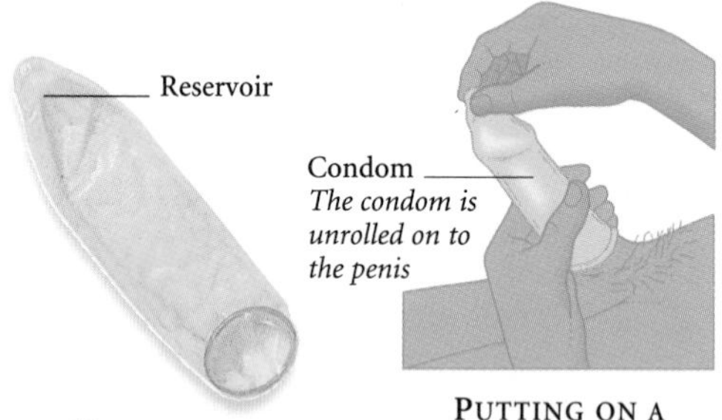

MALE CONDOM

PUTTING ON A MALE CONDOM

Male condom
Before a condom is unrolled on to the penis, the air must be squeezed out of the reservoir (end) so that the condom will not split. After intercourse, the penis must be withdrawn with the condom held on to prevent semen from leaking out.

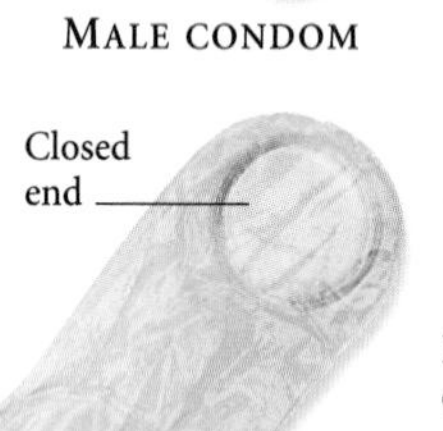

FEMALE CONDOM

Uterus
Cervix
Female condom
Vagina

INSERTING A FEMALE CONDOM

Female condom
The closed end of the condom is pushed up to the cervix. The open end extends just beyond the vaginal opening. Make sure that the penis goes inside the condom, not between the condom and the vaginal wall.

Cervical cap
The cap is partially filled with spermicide then pushed over the cervix. If intercourse does not occur within 3 hours of inserting it, extra spermicide must be added. To be effective, the cap must be left in place for at least 6 hours after intercourse.

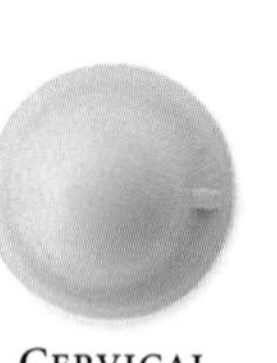

CERVICAL CAP

Uterus
Cervix
Cap
Vagina

IN POSITION

Diaphragm
The diaphragm is coated with spermicide on both surfaces. It is positioned so that the concave side covers the cervix. Like the cervical cap, it must be left in place for at least 6 hours after intercourse.

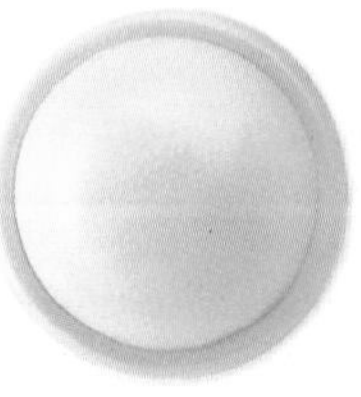

DIAPHRAGM

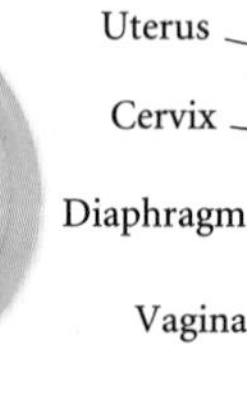

Uterus
Cervix
Diaphragm
Vagina

IN POSITION

Hormonal methods

Female hormones that prevent conception are prescribed as pills or injections. Some types of hormonal contraceptive contain only progestogen. This hormone thickens the cervical mucus so that sperm cannot pass through; it also suppresses ovulation and changes the receptivity of the lining of the uterus. The combined pill contains progestogen and oestrogen and prevents ovulation. Hormonal methods are over 99 per cent effective, but the instructions for taking pills must be followed exactly.

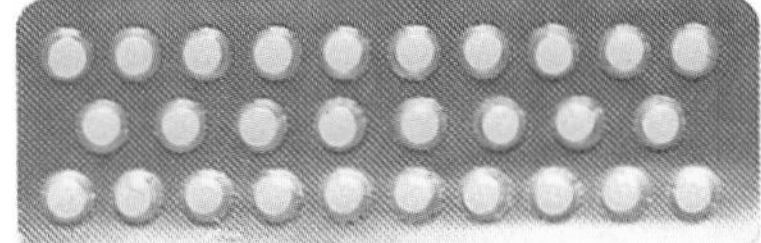

Progestogen-only pill
The progestogen-only pill must be taken at approximately the same time each day, for every day of the menstrual cycle.

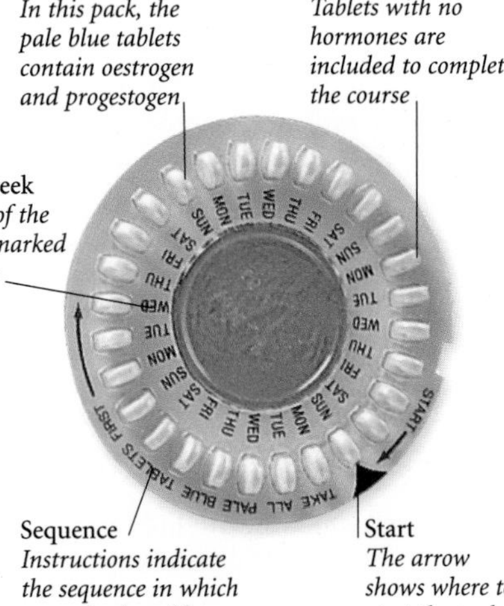

Combined oral contraceptive
The combined pill contains oestrogen and progestogen. There are various types. With some, you take pills for 21 days and then have 7 pill-free days. With others, you take 21 hormone pills and then 7 inactive pills. You must take the pills in the specified order.

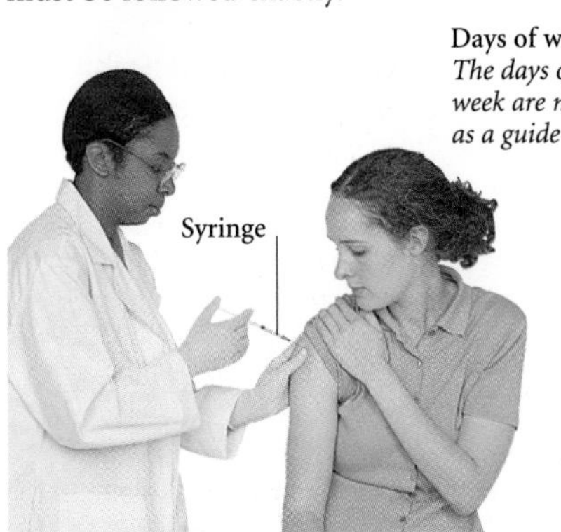

Contraceptive injection
Your doctor injects progestogen into a muscle in your arm or buttock, and it is released into your body over 8–12 weeks. Alternatively, an implant containing progestogen can be inserted under the skin of the upper arm and will remain effective for 3 years.

Mechanical methods

The intrauterine device (IUD) is fitted by a doctor and is left in place for 3–8 years, depending on the type. IUDs are thought to keep fertilized eggs from implanting in the uterus. Some also contain copper to kill sperm. Others contain progestogen, which thickens cervical mucus. IUDs are over 98 per cent effective.

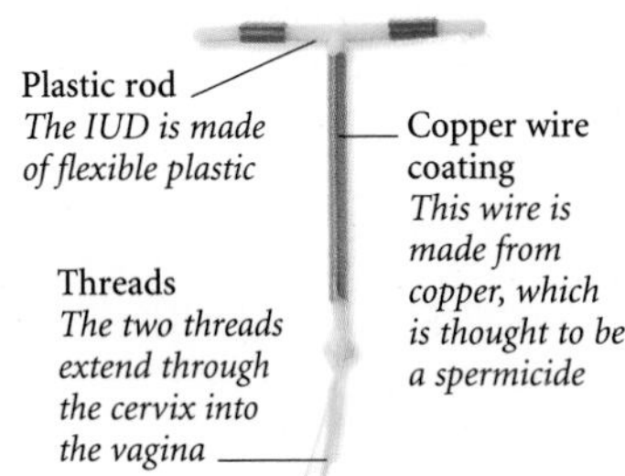

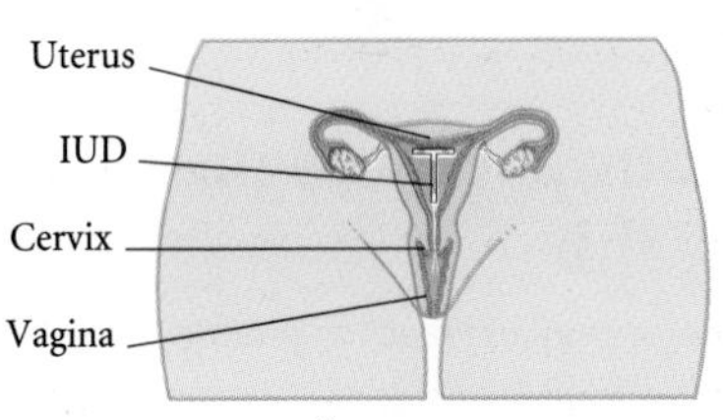

Intrauterine device (IUD)
An IUD has two threads that extend through the cervix. Once a month, the user should check that the threads are still there to make sure that the IUD has not been expelled during menstruation.

Natural methods

Natural methods of contraception are used to identify days in your menstrual cycle when you are fertile and times when you are less likely to conceive. Having identified these times, you can refrain from sex on your fertile days or use another form of contraception. The sympto-thermal method, which is only about 80 per cent effective, is the most commonly used natural method. It is based on two factors: body temperature rising just after ovulation (which occurs 12–16 days before each period) and staying high for at least 3 days; and increased amounts of mucus in the vagina around the time of ovulation. If you plan to use natural methods, seek advice from your doctor first.

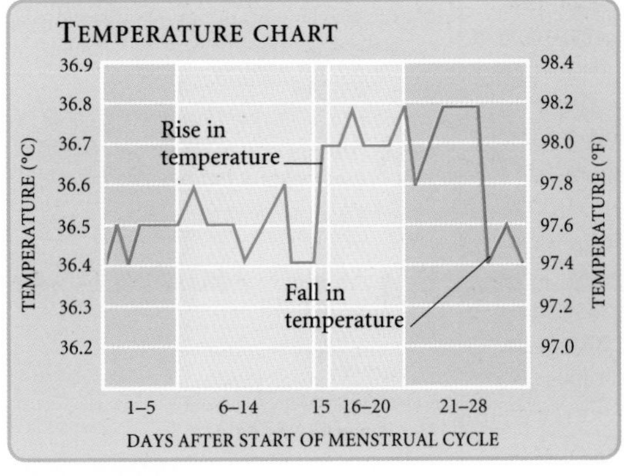

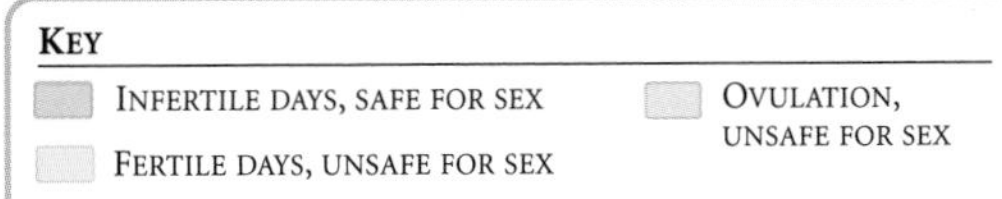

Using a temperature chart
You can monitor your fertility by recording your temperature on a chart like the one shown here. Take your temperature at the same time every day, immediately after waking and before getting up. Ovulation (on day 15 on this chart) is followed by a rise in temperature. When you have recorded higher temperatures for 3 days in a row, your fertile time is over. A time of infertility then follows, and this time continues until the last day of your next period.

PSYCHOLOGICAL HEALTH

Your physical and psychological health are closely linked. A long-term physical illness is likely to make you feel low, while a mental health disorder such as depression may cause physical symptoms. You can make changes in your lifestyle to improve your physical and psychological state so that you are better able to deal with the stresses and strains of daily life.

Some life events, such as a death in the family, inevitably cause stress. People's reactions to such stressful events depend in part on personality and in part on other current causes of stress, such as financial problems. The more stress you have to face, the greater your risk of developing a psychiatric disorder.

To help you to identify problems at an early stage, this section starts with a discussion of the difference between the normal range of well-being and a mental health disorder. The next two articles provide advice on how to develop good sleep habits and on ways to identify and minimize stress. The final article explains the process of grieving and suggests ways in which you might cope with your feelings.

Specific psychiatric disorders are covered elsewhere (*see* MENTAL HEALTH DISORDERS, pp.551–565).

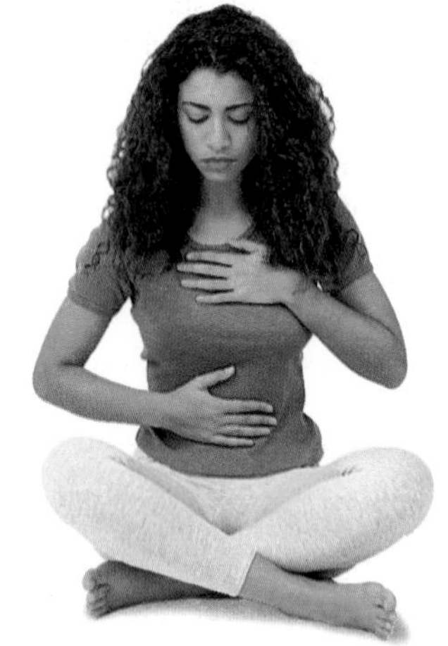

Maintaining psychological health
Learning how to relax by using techniques such as breathing exercises can be a key factor in maintaining psychological health.

Your psychological health

Your mental approach to dealing with everyday stress and life events

Growing up is a process of learning psychological responses to life events, both positive and negative. People vary in their ability to deal with these events, and everyone on occasion feels anger, frustration, sadness, mild depression, worry, loneliness, or uncertainty.

However, when these feelings prevent you from functioning normally for a sustained period, you may need to see your doctor. People have different personality traits and sometimes these can become sufficiently exaggerated to be classified as a disorder (*see* MENTAL HEALTH DISORDERS, pp.551–565).

Children and adults express their concerns differently. Recognizing early signs of problems enables action to be taken before they become serious.

RECOGNIZING PROBLEMS IN CHILDREN

Because children often cannot explain how they feel or what is upsetting them, they may express their feelings in unexpected ways, often as a change in behaviour. As a parent, it is important

ASSESSMENT HOW WELL DO YOU COPE?

How well you deal with the various aspects of your life depends mainly on your attitude and confidence. The eight questions below may be a guide to help you to judge how well you cope with the stresses of everyday life. Some surroundings are more stressful than others; for example, you may react differently depending on whether you are at home or at work.

1 *Do you live in a supportive environment and have friends or relatives nearby whom you can call on?*
☐ YES ☐ NO

2 *Are you able to cope with everyday stresses without resorting to alcohol, tobacco, or drugs (including caffeine)?*
☐ YES ☐ NO

3 *Are you able to express your positive and negative feelings clearly?*
☐ YES ☐ NO

4 *Do you fall asleep easily when you go to bed?*
☐ YES ☐ NO

5 *Are you able to adapt when faced with a difficult change or life event?*
☐ YES ☐ NO

6 *Are you assertive about what you need and want?*
☐ YES ☐ NO

7 *Are you good at organizing your time and being effective at work?*
☐ YES ☐ NO

8 *Can you deal with stress flexibly so that you don't suffer from stress-related complaints, such as headaches and upset stomach?*
☐ YES ☐ NO

ANALYSIS

If you answered a confident yes to all of the questions above, you clearly have a positive outlook. If you considered answering no or answered no to several of the questions, you may have a less confident disposition, and it may help to discuss your feelings with your doctor.

to be aware of warning signs. For example, your child may have a problem if he or she suddenly starts wetting the bed after a period of dryness or is unusually withdrawn, sad, or nervous. Children who are unhappy often complain of pain, typically stomach-ache. If your doctor cannot identify a physical cause, he or she may ask you about possible sources of stress.

RECOGNIZING PROBLEMS IN ADULTS

If you notice changes in your normal behaviour, such as increased moodiness, irritability, constant depression, anxiety attacks, trouble sleeping, poor concentration, or loss of appetite, you may be under some kind of emotional strain. If these feelings continue for a sustained period of time or grow more intense, they could signal a developing psychological problem. They may stem from a specific cause, such as the death of a relative (*see* LOSS AND BEREAVEMENT, p.76), but may develop for no apparent reason.

Your psychological health changes with age and may reflect your physical well-being. Physical and psychological problems often co-exist in older people, and if you become seriously ill or have a major operation you are more likely to suffer from psychological problems as a result (*see* MENTAL PROBLEMS DUE TO PHYSICAL ILLNESS, p.558).

If an aspect of your behaviour or personality is making you or someone close to you unhappy and you want to change but cannot, seek advice from your doctor or a therapist (*see* PSYCHOLOGICAL THERAPIES, pp.968–971).

(WWW) ONLINE SITES: p.1029, p.1034

Sleep

Understanding sleep and how it contributes to your health

Sleep is an important factor in maintaining good health. When you sleep well, you wake up feeling refreshed and alert; if you regularly sleep badly, every aspect of your life can suffer as a result. Occasional lack of sleep is a common experience. Usually, you should be able to overcome the problem by altering your lifestyle, but if you have persistent sleep problems you should consult your doctor (*see* INSOMNIA, p.554).

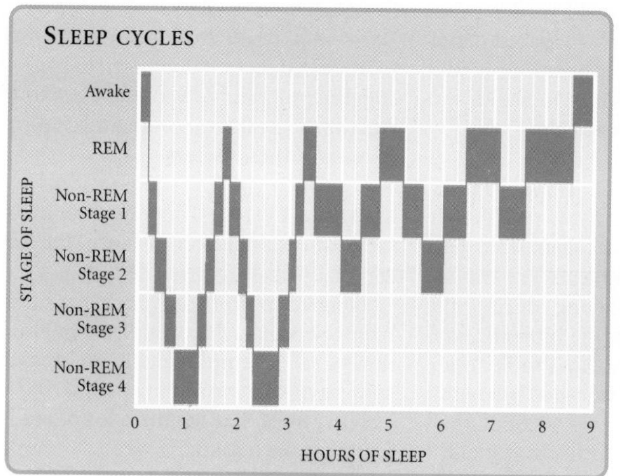

A typical night's sleep
The cycles in a night's sleep are made up of lengthening phases of REM sleep, when you dream, and four stages of non-REM sleep. In stages 1 and 2 you sleep lightly and wake easily; stages 3 and 4 are deep sleep, when you are difficult to wake.

WHY WE NEED TO SLEEP

Although scientists do not completely understand why people need to sleep, research shows that the body and mind require time to rest and recover from the day's activities. While you sleep, your body undergoes a series of repair processes and conserves energy.

There are two types of sleep: rapid eye movement (REM) sleep and non-REM sleep. During REM sleep, brain activity increases, dreaming occurs, and information is processed to reinforce memory and learning. Non-REM sleep consists of four stages: stage 1 is light sleep, in which you may wake spontaneously, and stage 4 is the deepest, in which you are very hard to wake. Each complete cycle of non-REM and REM sleep lasts about 90 minutes, starting with non-REM sleep. An average sleep cycle is made up of three-quarters non-REM sleep and one-quarter REM sleep.

SLEEP REQUIREMENTS

Sleep runs on a daily cycle regulated by an internal clock. Although people tend to sleep at night and are awake during the day, the cycle adapts to individual needs. The amount of sleep needed changes over a person's lifetime and depends on the individual. Newborn babies sleep up to 16 hours a day. Most people sleep an average of 7–8 hours a night, but generally the amount of sleep you need decreases as you grow older. Many people over 60 need only 6 hours sleep a night, although they may take a nap during the day.

Most people can cope with a couple of nights in which they have little or no sleep, without experiencing serious harmful effects on their health. At certain times, such as when you are ill or convalescing, you may find that you need more sleep than you usually have.

PROMOTING GOOD SLEEP

The most successful approach to getting a good night's sleep is to have a healthy lifestyle and to establish a regular routine before getting into bed.

A HEALTHY LIFESTYLE The key lifestyle factors that will help to ensure good sleep patterns are getting sufficient exercise, moderating your alcohol and caffeine intake, and not smoking.

Exercise promotes a sense of calm and well-being by increasing the production of endorphins in the brain (*see* THE BENEFITS OF EXERCISE, p.55). It also helps to tire you out physically.

Caffeine and nicotine are both central nervous system stimulants and may prevent you from falling asleep. Reduce your caffeine intake during the afternoon and evening. If you smoke, giving up may improve your sleep and also your general health (*see* TOBACCO AND HEALTH, p.63). Alcohol is a sedative (*see* ALCOHOL AND HEALTH, p.62), but you should not use it to help you to sleep because alcohol-induced sleep is not as refreshing as normal sleep.

BEDTIME ROUTINE By adopting a consistent bedtime routine, you may find it easier to relax and sleep normally. Your routine could include listening to the radio, reading, or practising relaxation exercises (p.75). Try soaking in a hot bath 2–4 hours before going to bed or having a warm drink made with milk at bedtime. Try to avoid working late into the evening. Make sure your bed is comfortable and your bedroom is well ventilated, not too hot or too cold, and sheltered from outdoor light.

Dealing with sleep problems

At some time in their lives, most people experience changes in their sleep patterns. Common problems are trouble getting to sleep, waking during the night or too early in the morning, and sleepiness during the day. Problems are often due to stress-associated behaviour such as drinking more alcohol than normal or working until late at night.

If you have a sleep problem, examine your lifestyle to see if a change in activity or behaviour could account for it. If you cannot sleep, get out of bed, walk around, read, or do some light household chores until you feel sleepy. Try to establish regular times for sleep and waking up. If you have a bad night, try not to sleep during the next day, but if you feel tired a nap of up to 20 minutes may improve your alertness.

If you continue to have difficulty sleeping, you should see your doctor. Your problem may be a symptom of an illness, such as depression (p.554), or a side effect of medication.

(WWW) ONLINE SITES: p.1036

Stress

How to identify signs of stress and find ways to manage it effectively

Stress is a physical or mental demand that provokes responses allowing us to meet challenges or escape from danger. The demand may be sudden, such as needing to avoid a speeding car, or long-term, such as pressures at work. Responses include both physical reactions, such as an increase in heart rate and sweating, and psychological reactions, such as an intense concentration on the source of stress.

A certain amount of stress can improve your performance in some sports and challenging physical activities, but excessive stress can be harmful to your health and interfere with your ability to cope with life. You can minimize harmful stress by identifying the types of situation that you find stressful and developing ways to avoid or limit them.

Sources of stress

Stress may result from external events or circumstances, your particular personality traits and how these affect your reaction to pressure, or a combination of both of these factors.

EXTERNAL EVENTS There are three main types of external circumstance that are especially likely to give rise to stress.

Long-term problems, such as an unhappy personal relationship, debilitating illness, or unemployment, are major sources of stress for many people.

Life events that require a lot of readjustment, such as marriage and moving house, can be highly stressful even if you consider the change a desirable one (*see* LIFE EVENTS AND STRESS, below).

An accumulation of minor everyday occurrences, such as being late for work or getting caught in a traffic jam, can cause you to reach a breaking point if you are already under a lot of strain.

ATTITUDES AND BEHAVIOUR Some patterns of behaviour may result in stress. For example, if you suffer from low self-esteem you may doubt your ability to cope with challenges that arise in your life. You may also feel that you are not entitled to receive help from other people when you are under excessive stress. Highly competitive people may find it difficult to relax and may have a higher than usual risk of developing stress-associated disorders. People who do not express anxiety or anger even when they are under stress may suffer from accumulated tension.

Recognizing stress

You may recognize that you have been stressed only when the source of the stress is removed. However, there are early warning symptoms of excessive stress that you can learn to recognize. If you experience any of the symptoms listed below, you may need to take action to reduce your stress level.

PHYSICAL SYMPTOMS Stress may affect your general health. You may feel tired, have problems such as tension headaches (p.518), mouth ulcers (p.632), or muscle pain, or be unusually susceptible to minor infections such as colds.

Excessive stress may also lead to or aggravate a range of disorders, such as high blood pressure (*see* HYPERTENSION, p.403), peptic ulcers (p.640), atopic eczema (p.334), irritable bowel syndrome (p.655), psoriasis (p.332), menstrual disorders (*see* MENSTRUAL, MENOPAUSAL, AND HORMONAL PROBLEMS, pp.734–740), and impotence (p.770).

PSYCHOLOGICAL SYMPTOMS If you feel very stressed, you may be anxious, tearful, or irritable. Even small problems may provoke an emotional response that is out of proportion to the cause.

(ASSESSMENT) Life events and stress

Major life events, such as divorce or retirement, are potential sources of stress. You are most likely to suffer from excessive stress if the event is unpleasant, if you view it as out of your control, or if several major events happen at once.

Assessing stress
Stress levels associated with major and minor life events are rated from very high to low.

Stress ratings of different life events

Very high	High	Moderate	Low
• Death of a spouse • Divorce or marital separation • Personal injury or illness • Loss of job • Moving house	• Retirement • Serious illness of family member • Pregnancy • Change of job • Death of close friend	• Large mortgage • Legal action over debt • Trouble with in-laws • Spouse begins or stops work • Trouble with boss	• Change in work conditions • Change in schools • Small mortgage or loan • Change in eating habits • Christmas or other holidays

HEALTH ACTION

RELAXATION EXERCISES

When you are under stress, your muscles tighten, your heart beats more rapidly, and your breathing becomes fast and shallow. A good way to relax both mind and body is to learn simple relaxation routines that slow down your body's stress responses. Two simple techniques are shown here. For further information, ask your doctor about relaxation classes.

BREATHING TECHNIQUES

Controlled breathing, which uses the diaphragm and the abdominal muscles, is the basis of all relaxation methods. To prepare for abdominal breathing exercises, you should wear loose clothing and try to find a quiet spot away from distractions. Sit or lie in a comfortable position.

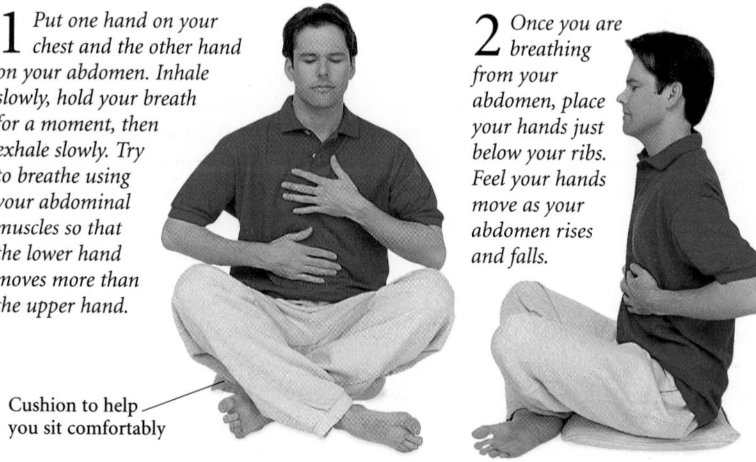

1 *Put one hand on your chest and the other hand on your abdomen. Inhale slowly, hold your breath for a moment, then exhale slowly. Try to breathe using your abdominal muscles so that the lower hand moves more than the upper hand.*

2 *Once you are breathing from your abdomen, place your hands just below your ribs. Feel your hands move as your abdomen rises and falls.*

MUSCLE RELAXATION

For muscle relaxation exercises, wear comfortable clothing and lie on a bed or on the floor. Put your arms by your sides and let your feet fall open. Tense and relax each part of your body in turn. During the exercise, keep your eyes closed. Breathe slowly using your abdominal muscles.

1 *Begin by taking one or two slow, deep breaths. Focus on your breathing. Starting with your feet, tense the muscles in each part of your body, hold for a count of three, then release the tension.*

Shoulders resting on floor

Head aligned with body

Pillow supporting head and neck

2 *When you have finished, lie still for a few moments, then roll onto your side. Support your body with your arms and knees. After a few minutes, open your eyes and get up slowly.*

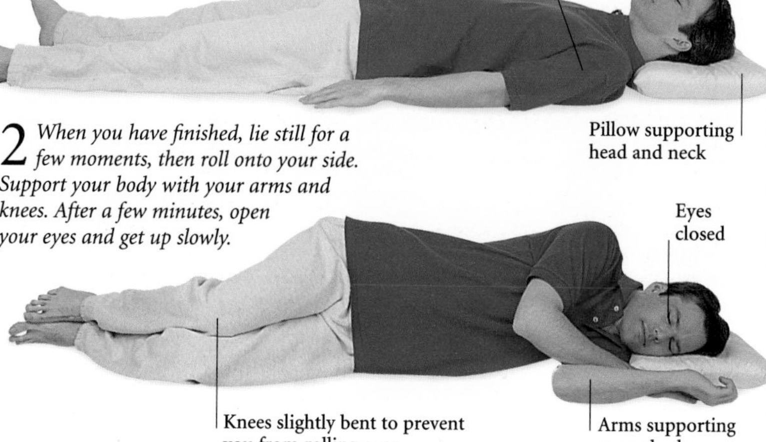

You may lack concentration and be unable to make decisions. Your sleep patterns may be disrupted. You may lose your appetite and find that you have less energy than you used to have. Relationships may suffer, especially if you become impatient or feel anxious when dealing with people. To distract yourself, you may begin to rely on alcohol, smoking, or drugs (*see* ALCOHOL, TOBACCO, AND DRUGS, pp.62–66), which may further affect your health.

MINIMIZING HARMFUL STRESS

To avoid excessive stress and maintain good health, you should learn to identify sources of stress and try to manage your life so that you can anticipate and prepare for problems or crises.

MAINTAINING GOOD HEALTH Attempt to improve your mental health and well-being by keeping up contact with your family, maintaining friendships, and pursuing leisure activities that give you pleasure without adding to your stresses. Exercising regularly can help to relieve physical tension (*see* THE BENEFITS OF EXERCISE, p.55), but you may also find it helpful to learn to relax your body consciously (*see* RELAXATION EXERCISES, left).

IDENTIFYING SOURCES OF STRESS A useful way to identify sources of stress is to keep a diary and record daily events and how you have responded to them. After a few weeks, look through your diary and identify events that you found stressful. Note whether the stress made you perform better or worse and try to identify activities that may have reduced your stress level.

ANTICIPATING PROBLEMS If you know that you will soon have to face a stressful event, prepare for it thoroughly so that you feel you have a good chance of managing it successfully. Break tasks or events down into smaller parts if they seem too big to cope with all at once. If you have several tasks to do in a limited time, list them and give the most important or urgent ones the highest priority. Limit the tasks that are not important or urgent in order to conserve your time and energy. If other people regularly make heavy demands on you, try to set limits.

Dealing with a crisis

Stress is a normal response to crises, and in most cases it need not be a cause for concern. However, if it leads to unmanageable symptoms, it has itself become a crisis. Seek help from your family and friends. Ask your doctor for help with the symptoms. He or she may refer you for counselling (p.971) if needed.

(WWW) ONLINE SITES: p.1036

Loss and bereavement

Understanding and coping with the feelings, emotions, and stress that characterize the grieving process

Many types of change may result in a sense of loss. Events that may provoke this feeling include the break-up of a relationship, children leaving home, job loss, or sudden disability. The loss felt after the death of a relative, a close friend, or a pet is called bereavement.

Loss provokes overwhelming physical and emotional reactions that can have a serious effect on your health. For example, bereaved people, especially widowed men, are at increased risk of dying from disease or suicide in the first year of bereavement, and their risk of developing depression (p.554) also increases. The process of gradual adjustment to loss, known as grieving, takes time. Understanding this process should help you to anticipate and handle your feelings and reduce the health risks associated with loss.

Normal reactions to loss

The grieving process has several elements, which may appear in a different order for different people and may overlap. You may not experience all of them. At any one time, you are likely to experience a mixture of emotions, some stronger than others. Throughout the grieving process, you may find that you oscillate between focusing on your loss and distracting yourself with work or plans for the future.

INITIAL REACTIONS At first, you may be overcome by shock or feel numb and detached. You may even act as though nothing has happened. These reactions are a natural psychological mechanism that shields you from the immediate impact of the loss. You are likely to experience signs of stress (p.74), such as loss of appetite, inability to sleep, and lack of energy. You may feel run down and become susceptible to minor illnesses.

PROTEST After the initial shock, you may feel overcome with intense emotions. The most common emotion is sadness. Other feelings may include anger, guilt, or fear. The emotional pain may be interrupted by periods in which feelings of emptiness predominate.

You may think about your loss constantly as your mind challenges the fact that the event has occurred. If a loved one has died, you may find yourself searching for him or her and may have hallucinations in which you are sure that you have seen or heard the person.

DISORGANIZATION As your mind accepts the reality of the loss, you may feel bleakness, apathy, and confusion and have no hope in the future. You may even feel suicidal.

REORGANIZATION As time passes, you accept the loss and achieve a new normality, even though your life may have changed forever. You may feel stronger as a result of coping with the loss. You can remember happy times and hope to be happy again without forgetting the loss or minimizing its impact.

How to cope with grief

If you know that you are going to suffer a loss – for example, if someone close to you has a terminal illness – find out about the grieving process in advance. By doing so, you may be able to cope more easily with your grief. Once the loss has occurred, it is important for you to acknowledge it in some way, such as by viewing the dead body of a loved person and attending the funeral service if you feel you can.

It is also important for you to recognize the difference between normal and abnormal responses to loss. The most common abnormal reactions are very intense emotions that last for a long time; inability to stop grieving, even after several years; and the inability to grieve at all. To cope with any of these reactions, it may be helpful to contact an organization that counsels bereaved people or allows grieving people to offer each other mutual support.

When supporting other people who have suffered a loss, take time to listen to them and acknowledge their painful feelings but try to avoid giving advice about how they should overcome their emotions. People who are grieving may also appreciate practical help, perhaps with shopping or child care, especially in the days immediately after a loss.

Very young children may not realize that death is permanent, but by about the age of 5 more than half of them fully understand. Be honest but gentle with a grieving child. Explain what has happened and avoid euphemisms for death. Allow time for the child to talk about the loss. He or she might like to make a scrapbook of pictures and writings to commemorate the deceased. You and the child may also find it helpful to have professional counselling (p.971).

(WWW) ONLINE SITES: p.1029

The grieving process

Grieving is like a loop in the course of normal life. You will eventually come to terms with your feelings and achieve a new form of normality.

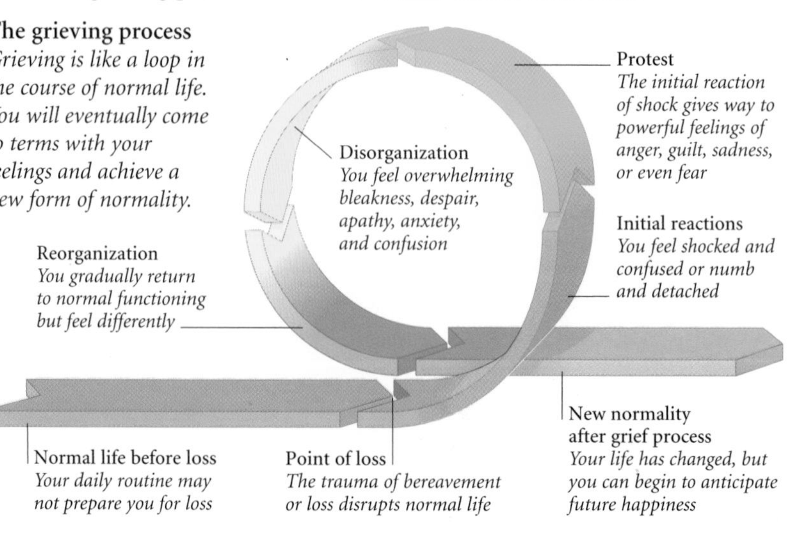

SAFETY AND HEALTH

Although most deaths and disabilities are the result of disease, a substantial number have other causes. About 1 in 50 deaths in the UK is caused by an accident. At home, on the road, at work, during recreational activities, and when travelling, accidents result in injuries to millions of people every year.

Accidents are the most significant single cause of death in children and young adults and are a major cause of death and disability in elderly people. They are also a major cause of serious injury in people of all ages. For example, in 1998 nearly 4,000 people were killed, and over 40,000 were seriously injured, in traffic accidents. These injuries have substantial social and economic costs and may also have psychological effects such as post-traumatic stress disorder.

The prevention of accidents has become a major concern for both medical and economic reasons. This section is designed to alert you to potentially dangerous circumstances in your everyday life, whether you are at work or at home. The first article addresses safety and health in your home and is followed by others on health and safety in the garden, in the sun, in and around water, with pets, at work, on the road, and when travelling.

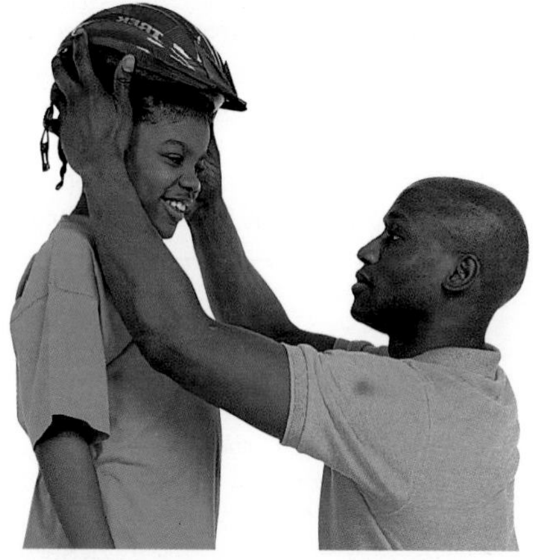

Family safety
When taking part in sports or travelling by road, make yourself aware of potential dangers and take action to minimize the risks to you and your family.

Home safety and health

How to prevent accidents and avoid health problems in the home

Almost half of all serious accidents take place in the home. Each year in the UK, more than 4,000 people are killed and almost 3 million have injuries needing medical treatment due to accidents in their homes. Many accidents are preventable, and with a few simple precautions you can make your home safer (*see* MAKING YOUR HOME SAFE, p.78).

Age is the major factor influencing people's risk of accidents. People over the age of 75 and children under the age of 5 have the highest rates of accidents in the home needing medical treatment. In older people, falls are one of the most common causes of accidents. In children, a significant cause is poisoning by substances such as drugs and chemicals used for household cleaning. Other causes of accidents in the home include fires, electrocution, drowning, and suffocation. A significant risk to health is posed by poor hygiene in the kitchen, which can cause digestive system upsets as a result of food poisoning (*see* FOOD HYGIENE, p.79).

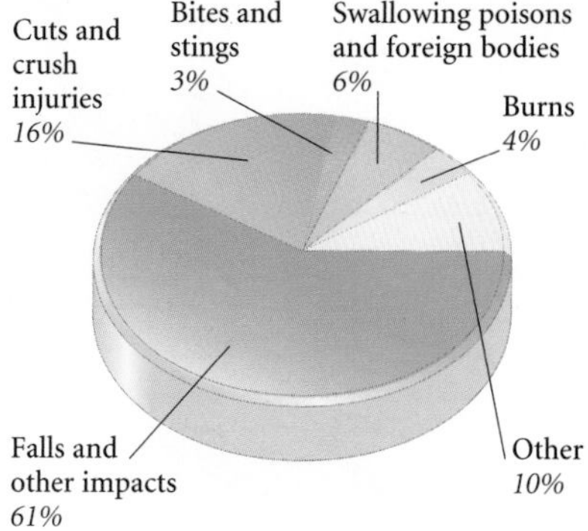

Accidental injuries in the home
In the UK in 1995, about 4 in 10 of all accidents serious enough to require medical attention occurred at home.

PREVENTING FALLS

About 4 in 10 of all injuries that occur in the home are the result of falls. Elderly people are especially vulnerable because they are often frail and less steady on their feet than people in younger age groups, and they may have attacks of fainting or dizziness. Elderly people are also more likely to have poor vision. To prevent falls in the home, make sure that the lighting in your house is adequate, that floor coverings are secure, that no objects are left on the stairs, and that safety rails are installed in the bathroom.

If you have a baby or a toddler, you can reduce the risk of falls by installing a stair gate, which restricts the child's access to stairways.

AVOIDING POISONING

Poisoning accounts for about 1 in 50 of all injuries that take place in the home. The poisons responsible include prescription and over-the-counter drugs, household cleaning materials, gases such as carbon monoxide, and lead. Since children are particularly at risk of poisoning, all drugs, cleaning materials, and other household chemicals should be kept out of their reach.

CARBON MONOXIDE Incomplete combustion of any fuel produces carbon monoxide, a colourless and odourless gas. If inhaled, this gas can be fatal because it reduces the ability of the blood to carry oxygen. To prevent the build-up of carbon monoxide, you should have chimneys and flues checked, and heating systems and gas appliances inspected, yearly. For extra protection you could also fit carbon monoxide alarms, available in DIY shops. The engines in cars, motorcycles, and some lawn mowers release carbon monoxide and should never be run in a closed garage.

LEAD Children are particularly vulnerable to the effects of lead, which can damage the brain, nerves, red blood cells, and digestive system. One common source of lead is drinking water supplied through lead pipes in older

HEALTH ACTION MAKING YOUR HOME SAFE

Accidents and injuries can occur in any part of the home. Roughly 1 in 10 of all accidents takes place in the living room/dining area and the same proportion occurs in the kitchen. About 1 in 14 accidents occurs on the stairs or in the bedroom, and about 1 in 40 happens in the bathroom.

Bathroom
The main hazards in the bathroom are slipping on wet surfaces, drowning, electrocution, and scalding yourself with hot water.

Shower
Always test the water temperature before getting into the shower

Safety rail
Install a firm handrail over the bath

Electrical outlet
Electrical outlets in the bathroom are for the use of shavers only

Nonslip mats
Use nonslip mats in the shower and bath

Living room
The living room is where people spend most of their waking time when they are at home. Many accidents in this area involve electrical appliances, falls, or fire.

Flexes
Do not let flexes trail across the floor or under the carpet

Electrical outlets
Do not overload outlets

Fire
Keep fire guards around the fire at all times

Toys
Put away children's toys after use

Furnishings
All furnishings should be flame-resistant

Rugs
Use nonslip mats under rugs

Bookcases
Secure bookcases and other items of heavy furniture to a wall to prevent them from falling over

Kitchen
Most accidents in the kitchen involve fires caused by hot cooking oil, scalds from hot liquids or solids, cuts from knives or broken glass, or electrocution from electrical appliances.

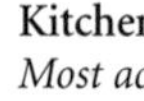

Cooker hood
Replace the filter at regular intervals

Saucepan handles
Turn pan handles away from the front of the stove

Fire extinguisher
Keep an extinguisher in the kitchen and make sure that you know how to use it

Knife block
Store knives safely in a knife block

Cooker
Use the back burners of cookers in preference to the front ones

Appliance flexes
Fit electrical appliances with coiled flexes and keep the appliances near the wall

Floor
Wipe up spilt liquid immediately and make sure that floors are dry before walking on them

houses. If there are lead pipes in your home, they should be replaced with copper or plastic pipes. Any lead-based paint in your house should be removed by professional contractors. If you have any children's toys made before 1980, make sure that the toys are not coated with lead-based paint.

Preventing fires

Fire is one of the greatest hazards in the home. If you have an open fire, put a fire guard in front of it to prevent burning embers from falling on the floor, and have both the fireplace and the chimney swept regularly. If you smoke, extinguish smoking materials carefully after use, and never leave lit materials unattended. When cooking, take care if using hot oil, and never leave frying pans or deep-fat fryers unattended. Keep a fire blanket or extinguisher in the kitchen. Teach children never to play with matches. To prevent electrical fires, take care not to overload sockets with adapters. Keep highly flammable materials, such as certain paints and paintbrush cleaners, locked away, ideally in a shed or a garage. In addition, have smoke detectors installed on every floor of your house in case a fire does break out.

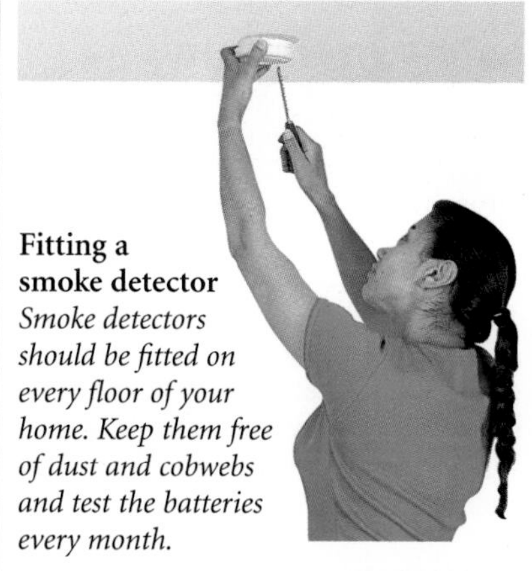

Fitting a smoke detector
Smoke detectors should be fitted on every floor of your home. Keep them free of dust and cobwebs and test the batteries every month.

Monitoring air pollution in and around the home

Air pollution may cause irritation of the respiratory tract and may trigger flare-ups of asthma (p.483). Causes of air pollution in the home include tobacco smoke and house dust. Outside the home, sources of air pollution include industrial plants, such as power stations and factories, and various types of vehicle, particularly cars, buses, and lorries. Your local authority is responsible for monitoring the air quality in your area. If you are concerned about a source of air pollution near your home, you should contact your local authority or the Department of the Environment, Transport and the Regions.

Pollutants from motor vehicles and industrial plants can cause a range of disorders. For example, nitrogen dioxide, sulphur dioxide, and ozone irritate the airways and aggravate the symptoms of respiratory diseases. The fine particles from diesel exhaust can also irritate the airways, and some types of particle have been found to cause cancer in laboratory animals.

Other sources of pollution include older refrigerators and freezers, and dry cleaning, which produce chlorofluorocarbons, and granite rock, which releases radon. Radon is an odourless, colourless, radioactive gas. It can damage the lungs if inhaled in large amounts, and can even cause lung cancer. If you live in an area where much of the underlying rock is granite, such as south-west England or the highlands of Scotland, seek advice from a specialist in radon protection. Although it is not possible to radon-proof your home, you can reduce the risk of exposure to radon by keeping your home well ventilated and sealing cracks in floors and walls.

(WWW) ONLINE SITES: p.1036

HEALTH ACTION Food hygiene

Food poisoning is usually caused by eating food contaminated by bacteria. The risk of poisoning is increased if food is left at room temperature because any bacteria present can multiply rapidly. Food is usually safe if stored in the refrigerator because the low temperature prevents bacteria from multiplying.

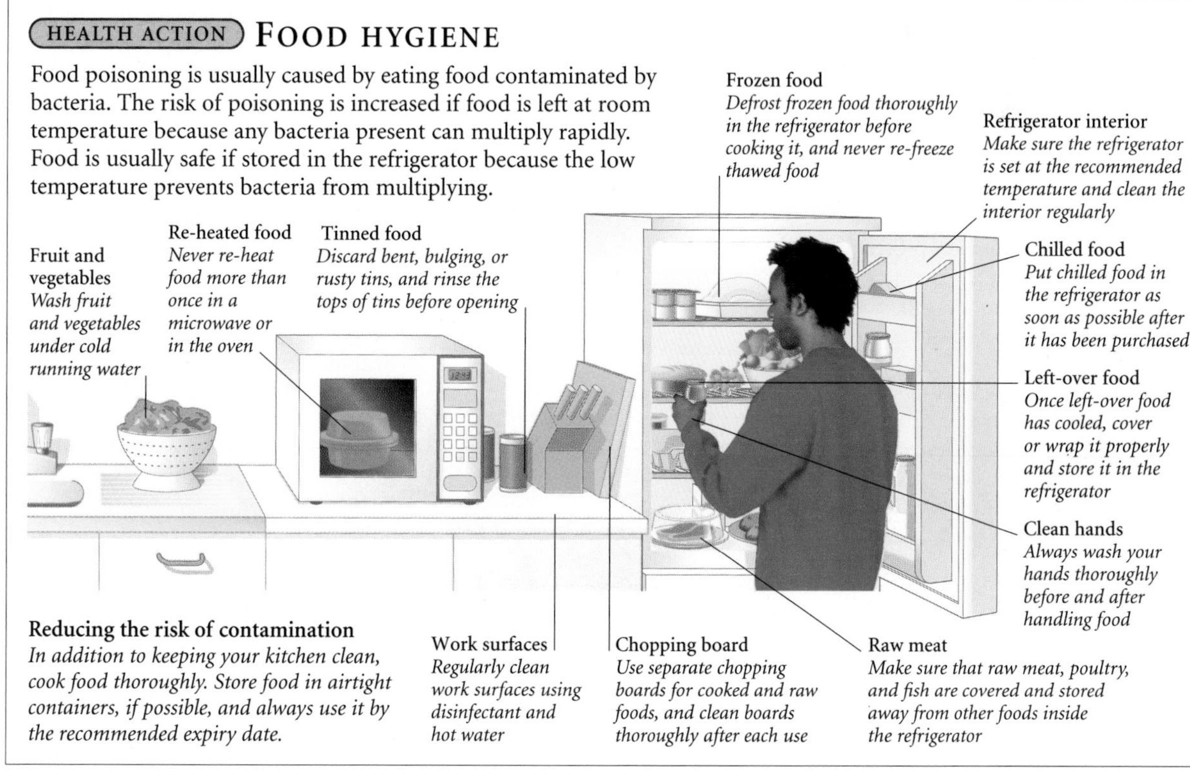

Reducing the risk of contamination
In addition to keeping your kitchen clean, cook food thoroughly. Store food in airtight containers, if possible, and always use it by the recommended expiry date.

Safety in the garden

Taking precautions to keep your garden safe for all age groups

Every year about 400,000 people in the UK have accidents in their gardens that need medical treatment. The greatest risk is from water in ponds or pools (*see* SAFETY IN AND AROUND WATER, p.81), although poisonous plants and chemicals, garden tools, barbecues, and play equipment also pose significant risks.

AVOIDING POISONOUS PLANTS

Some plants may cause irritation if they come into contact with the skin. Other plants, if swallowed, may cause symptoms ranging from irritation of the mouth, throat, and stomach to nausea and vomiting. A few plants may be lethal if eaten in sufficient quantities. Children should be taught that touching or eating plants may be dangerous. If a child does swallow anything poisonous, consult your doctor immediately, or take the child to the accident and emergency department of a hospital, taking a sample of the plant with you.

USING GARDEN CHEMICALS AND TOOLS SAFELY

Many chemicals for use in the garden are poisonous. Consider safe alternatives, such as removing weeds by hand or applying chemical-free pesticides. If you do use poisonous products, store them in a locked shed or cabinet and follow the manufacturer's instructions.

Sharp tools should not be left where children can find them. Wear protective clothing, such as goggles, ear protectors, gloves, long trousers, and boots, when using tools such as chainsaws.

USING BARBECUES SAFELY

Barbecues should always be supervised in case children wander too close to them. Avoid lighting barbecues in a high wind, do not wear loose clothing near flames, and never pour flammable liquids onto smoking charcoal. When using a gas-fired barbecue, check for gas leaks and make sure that the flame is blue. A yellow flame indicates incomplete combustion or the production of carbon monoxide. Keep an outdoor fire extinguisher on hand.

(WWW) ONLINE SITES: p.1036

Safety in the sun

Precautions and procedures to avoid skin damage and overexposure to heat

Overexposure to sunlight may lead to sunburn (p.357), premature aging, skin cancer (p.344), and damage to the eyes. Tanning, once fashionable, is now considered to be harmful. Too much sun can contribute to heat exhaustion and heatstroke. If you are outdoors in strong sunlight, protect yourself with suitable clothing, sunscreens, and sunglasses.

DAMAGING EFFECTS OF SUN

Exposure to strong sunlight without adequate protection can result in sunburn. Skin damage is caused by ultraviolet (UV) light, of which there are two main types: UVA light and UVB light. Overexposure to UVB light is known to cause skin cancer and cataracts (p.573). UVA light may also play a part in these conditions. In addition, repeated exposure to UV light can damage fibres called elastin in the skin, leading to premature aging.

UV light is partially filtered by haze or clouds in the atmosphere; the UV content of sunlight is greater at high altitudes, where the cloud cover is thinner. However, you can still burn on a cloudy day at lower altitudes because some UV light penetrates clouds. Snow and ice reflect up to three-quarters of UV light, and water may reflect almost all of it.

Certain drugs, such as tetracycline antibiotics (p.885), may make the skin more sensitive to sunlight (*see* PHOTOSENSITIVITY, p.338), and you will need to stay out of the sun if you are taking them.

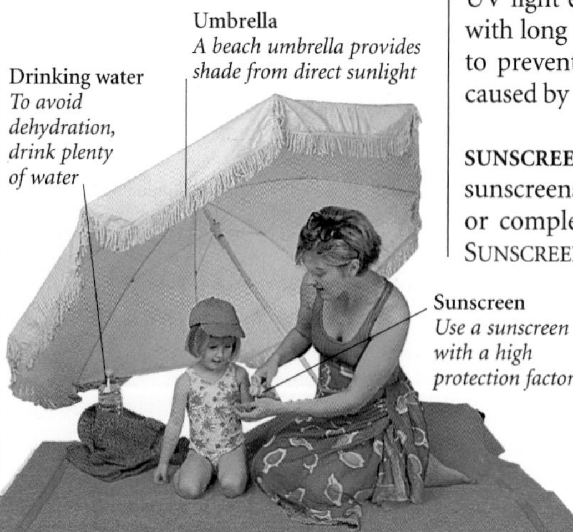

Protection at the beach
At the beach, you need to take extra care of your skin because sunlight is intensified when it is reflected by water, and sea breezes can keep you deceptively cool.

Oral contraceptives may cause areas of patchy skin pigmentation after exposure to the sun; if you are affected in this way, you may wish to use alternative contraception. Some perfumes and deodorants may cause skin discoloration in strong sunlight and should be avoided.

In the UK, skin cancer is the second most common form of cancer, with over 40,000 new cases each year. The most dangerous form is malignant melanoma (p.346), which causes about 1,500 deaths a year. The risk of skin cancer is greater if you had severe sunburn as a child. You are also at greater risk if you have red or blond hair and green or blue eyes because your skin contains a low level of melanin, a pigment that absorbs UVB light. Even if you have never had severe sunburn, exposure to the sun over many years can increase your risk of skin cancer. Whatever their skin type, babies and small children are more vulnerable to the sun than adults.

PROTECTION FROM THE SUN

You can minimize the risk of sun damage by staying out of the sun between 11 am and 3 pm. If you have to be in the sun, there are three main types of protection: clothing, sunscreens, and sunglasses.

CLOTHING Wear a wide-brimmed hat and tightly woven clothing that covers your shoulders and neck. Check that pale-coloured clothes do not become translucent when wet and thus offer little protection. Protective clothing is available for children, such as a "legionnaire's hat" to cover the back of the neck, and swimwear that protects the body from UV light even when wet. Loose clothes with long sleeves and trousers may help to prevent prickly heat (p.342), a rash caused by sweat trapped under the skin.

SUNSCREENS The chemicals included in sunscreens protect the skin by partially or completely absorbing UV rays (*see* SUNSCREENS AND SUNBLOCKS, p.893).

Opaque white or coloured sunblocks block sunlight completely and can be used to protect exposed skin, especially on vulnerable areas such as the nose and lips. Sunscreens are less effective than sunblocks because they only partially absorb UV rays, but because they are more transparent, they are more acceptable for all-over use.

The effectiveness of a sunscreen is rated by a sun protection factor (SPF). The higher the factor, the greater the protection, although the degree of protection also depends on your skin type. Sunscreens should be applied liberally 15–30 minutes before you go outside and re-applied every 2 hours. They are especially necessary if you are near water, snow, or ice or at high altitudes. Wear sunscreens even in the shade and on cloudy days. They are not suitable for babies under 6 months old, who should be kept out of direct sun.

SUNGLASSES Sunglasses should have British Standard mark BS2724 and give maximum protection from both UVA and UVB light. Never look at the sun directly, even when wearing sunglasses, or view it through a camera, since the light can damage your eyes.

(WWW) ONLINE SITES: p.1036

Safety in and around water

Avoiding accidents and injuries in and around water

Water can be a deadly hazard. Although fatalities from drowning declined in the UK during the late 1990s, 440 adults and children died in this way in 1997. Drowning is the third most common cause of accidental death in children under the age of 16. Water-borne infections may also be a danger to anyone who spends time in or near the water.

PREVENTING DROWNING AND NEAR-DROWNING

The situations that most often result in drowning or near-drowning are swimming in a strong current or very cold water and swimming or boating after drinking alcohol. In particular, children should be closely supervised when they are playing in or around water.

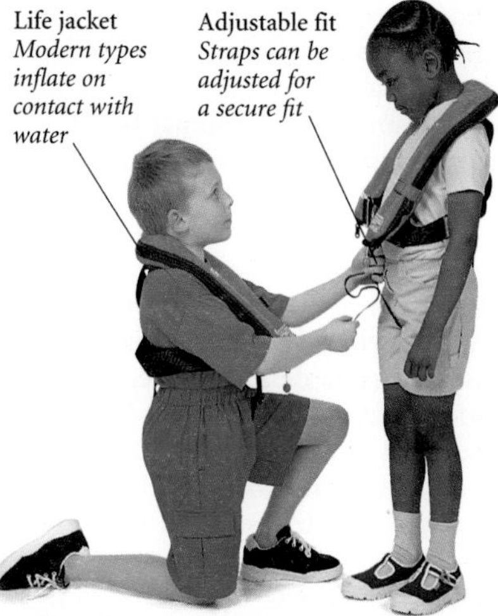

Life jackets
A life jacket should be worn for activities in which there is a risk of falling into water. It should fit comfortably, support the head, and allow the arms to move freely.

UNDERSTANDING WATER CONDITIONS
Many victims of drowning are strong swimmers who have been caught in currents or an undertow. Even confident swimmers should always heed advice about local swimming conditions.

Avoid swimming in very cold water because low water temperature may lead to drowning. A person immersed in water loses heat up to 27 times faster than a person in air at the same temperature. Water below 5°C (41°F) stiffens muscles and may cause cardiac arrest (*see* HYPOTHERMIA, p.323).

AVOIDING ALCOHOL More than one-third of victims of drowning accidents have a significant amount of alcohol in their blood (*see* ALCOHOL AND HEALTH, p.62). You should never drink alcohol before going swimming or boating since it will make you more likely to take risks. Alcohol will also make you less able to tackle difficulties that may arise and more susceptible to panic.

SUPERVISING CHILDREN Do not leave young children alone when they are swimming or in the bath because it is possible to drown in only a few centimetres of water. If you have a pond, well, or swimming pool in your garden, it should be fenced off or covered when not in use. Children should be taught how to swim as early as possible. In many countries there is now legislation that limits the age at which children may use public pools without adult supervision. If you leave older children or teenagers to swim without supervision, make sure that they swim in a safe place and that no child swims alone.

FIRST AID If someone has been submerged in cold water long enough to have stopped breathing, artificial respiration (pp.982–983) or cardiopulmonary resuscitation (pp.984–985) should be administered immediately. Even if a person appears to have drowned, he or she may be resuscitated when body temperature rises (*see* DROWNING AND NEAR-DROWNING, p.325).

AVOIDING HAZARDS IN WATER

Drowning is not the only hazard associated with water. Shallow water, hidden objects, marine and freshwater animals, and infections all present dangers.

SHALLOW WATER AND HIDDEN OBJECTS
Every year, thousands of people injure their spines by diving into water that is too shallow or that contains hidden objects. Many of these accidents result in permanent paralysis. Always check the depth of water before diving or jumping, and check for rocks, fallen trees, or glass below the surface.

ANIMAL LIFE AND INFECTIONS Marine and freshwater life can be a hazard in some areas. When on holiday, follow warnings about local dangers, such as sharks, and swim only in areas that have been designated as safe. Look out for animals that may sting or bite if you step on or touch them, such as jellyfish (*see* POISONOUS BITES AND STINGS, p.327). Coral can cause cuts and abrasions, which may become infected.

The sea near large coastal resorts and rivers downstream from cities may be polluted with sewage. Freshwater that is contaminated with rat or fox urine can cause a flu-like, potentially fatal infection called leptospirosis (p.302). In tropical countries, swimming or wading in lakes, rivers, or ponds is inadvisable due to the risk of contracting schistosomiasis (p.312). This infestation, also known as bilharzia, is caused by larvae that burrow through the skin, and may result in damage to the liver and urinary system.

(WWW) ONLINE SITES: p.1036

Pets and health

Minimizing health risks associated with domestic pets

Diseases contracted from pets are uncommon. However, animals can cause allergies, and infections and infestations with microorganisms, worms, or insects may spread to people. Pets such as dogs can bite; they should never be left alone with young children. Exotic pets may also pose health hazards. For example, tarantula hairs can cause eye damage.

Check cats and dogs regularly to look for ticks. If your pet scratches more than usual or develops bald patches, consult your veterinary surgeon in case your pet has a fungal infection, such as ringworm (p.352), that could infect you.

Cat and dog faeces contain a number of dangerous organisms, such as the eggs of the toxocara worm. If ingested, these worm eggs may cause toxocariasis (p.310), a potentially serious disease that may lead to blindness. Cat faeces may also contain toxoplasma protozoa. Pregnant women in particular should avoid contact with cat faeces, because toxoplasmosis (p.307) may cause serious harm to the developing fetus. Worm pets regularly and dispose of their faeces hygienically. Teach children to wash their hands after touching animals.

(WWW) ONLINE SITES: p.1036

Safety and health at work

Practical steps to promote safety and health in the workplace

There are well-established connections between conditions in the workplace and certain health problems. Some types of work carry especially high risks of specific disorders. As a result, measures have been developed to protect employees from a variety of occupational disorders.

Each year, despite preventive measures, 2.2 million people in the UK have illnesses caused or aggravated by their work; many of these disorders lead to absence from work. In addition, 1.6 million people suffer job-related injuries, and accidents at work cause about 350 deaths. If you develop symptoms of ill health or disease while you are at work and you suspect that your symptoms are due to conditions in your work environment, you should talk to your supervisor or occupational health department, or to your doctor.

Reducing risks in the office

Your office may be a surprising source of health hazards, particularly if you spend much of your day using a computer. If you work at a desk, you need to think carefully about the layout of your work area (*see* USING A WORK STATION, below). Over 1 million people are believed to develop disorders such as lower back pain (p.381) and repetitive strain injury (p.389) because of their work. Repetitive strain injury (RSI), which is caused by repeated movement of one part of the body, is a risk if you use a keyboard. You can reduce the risk by using a wrist rest or a specially designed keyboard.

Sick building syndrome is a group of symptoms sometimes reported by workers in offices. Symptoms include loss of energy, headaches, and sore throat. The cause is unknown but has been attributed to air-conditioning, lack of natural light, exposure to tobacco smoke, poor ventilation, and dust, solvents, and ozone emitted by printers and photocopiers.

Strained relationships with your colleagues or poor job satisfaction can be causes of stress. If this is the case, seek advice on managing stress (p.74).

Reducing risks in the industrial workplace

Some occupations are inherently dangerous. If your work involves contact with heavy machinery, organic solvents, loud noise, or extreme heat or cold, you should be aware of the dangers and be provided with protective equipment.

HEALTH ACTION — Using a work station

Your work area should be designed so that everything is easy to reach and use. Make sure that you have good lighting and ventilation. If you are working at a computer, take breaks from using the keyboard and monitor every 40 minutes. Focus on a distant object occasionally to relax your eye muscles and to prevent your eyes from getting tired.

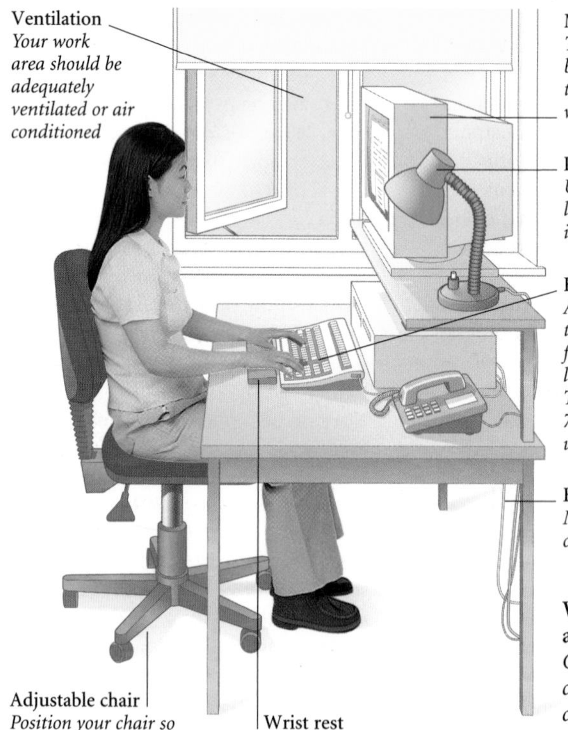

Working at a computer
Good posture and a correctly positioned chair and monitor may prevent problems such as back pain and repetitive strain injury.

Many substances in the workplace can cause occupational lung diseases (p.499). The most common of these conditions is asthma (p.483), which causes severe breathing problems if untreated. More than 200 substances, ranging from latex in gloves to the isocyanates used in paint spraying, are known to trigger the disorder. Your doctor can arrange for tests to identify asthma triggers. A number of other lung disorders are linked with the inhalation of specific particles. Occupations that carry particular risks include mining, farming, and any work involving contact with asbestos or silica (a constituent of sand and many types of rock).

Substances such as detergents may irritate your skin and cause disorders such as eczema (p.333) or contact dermatitis (p.355). To avoid these problems, you need to wear protective clothing and use barrier creams (*see* EMOLLIENTS AND BARRIER PREPARATIONS, p.890).

If your work involves lifting heavy loads or sitting for long periods with poor back support, you are vulnerable to back pain. Make sure that you have any necessary training, be aware of your posture, and try to lift heavy objects safely (*see* PREVENTING BACK PAIN, p.382).

TAKING RESPONSIBILITY FOR HEALTH AT WORK

In many countries, employers are required by law to meet safety standards, monitor employees' health, offer screening (p.42) if needed, and compensate workers who develop permanent health problems. Employees should be aware of the health hazards associated with their occupation and of legally required safety practices. In the UK, both employers and employees are responsible for maintaining a safe working environment.

(WWW) ONLINE SITES: p.1036

Safety on the road

Safety precautions for motorists, motorcyclists, cyclists, and pedestrians

Accidents involving motorists, motorcyclists, cyclists, and pedestrians are among the leading causes of accidental death in the developed world. In recent decades there have been improvements in vehicle safety (p.84) and in public compliance with speed limits and with drinking and driving laws, which have compensated for the risks associated with increased numbers of cars on the roads. However, in the UK, thousands of people still die or suffer serious injury each year in road accidents. In 1998, nearly 4,000 people died and more than 40,000 were injured.

Nearly all of the road traffic accidents that occur in the UK are due to human error; only about 1 in 20 accidents are associated with mechanical faults. Alcohol abuse is the greatest individual factor associated with deaths on the road: 1 in 6 deaths is due to drink–driving. Other significant causes of accidents include poor eyesight, tiredness, the use of illegal drugs, taking certain prescription drugs such as tranquillizers or antidepressants, or even taking over-the-counter drugs such as antihistamines and cough medicines. These factors can increase your reaction times, making it more difficult for you to avoid hazardous situations.

Serious medical conditions, such as heart attack (*see* MYOCARDIAL INFARCTION, p.410), diabetes mellitus (p.687), or epilepsy (p.524), can also affect your ability to drive safely. Before you learn to drive, or before resuming driving, you should ask your doctor about restrictions associated with medical conditions or contact the Driver and Vehicle Licensing Agency (DVLA) for information. In addition, even if you are a careful driver, bear in mind that other drivers may possibly involve you in accidents.

STAYING SAFE IN CARS

The most important vehicle safety device is the seat belt, which is believed to have prevented thousands of deaths and hundreds of thousands of injuries since its use first became compulsory. Airbags have also saved many lives. In addition to seat belts and airbags, modern cars and lorries have a variety of other built-in safety features, including headrests, specially designed seats for children of different ages (*see* CHILDREN'S CAR SEATS, p.29), anti-lock brakes, and tyres that are designed to run safely when deflated, even after a serious puncture. Although these devices reduce the risk of injury for the occupants of a vehicle, research shows that they do not make travelling safer for other road users. Take care not to drive less cautiously merely because you are reassured by the safety features on your own vehicle.

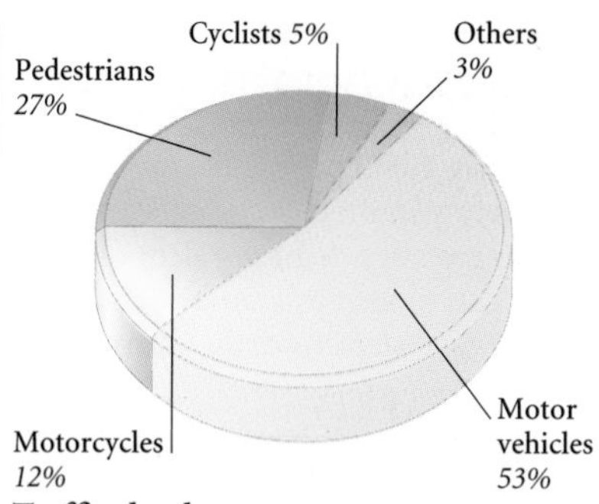

Traffic deaths
Occupants of motor vehicles accounted for just over half of all traffic deaths in the UK in 1997, mainly because the majority of people travel by car.

STAYING SAFE ON MOTORCYCLES AND BICYCLES

Although car occupants still account for most traffic fatalities, motorcyclists are more than 20 times as likely as car drivers to be killed or seriously injured. Motorcyclists need helmets and other special clothing to give them sufficient protection from the road surface, other vehicles, and the weather.

Cyclists account for about 1 in 20 of all those killed or injured on the roads, with the highest proportion of casualties among children aged 12–15 years. Cyclists are particularly at risk of head injuries, so wearing a cycling helmet is essential. It is important that a helmet fits you well. If you have an accident that damages your helmet, you should buy a new helmet. You should also have training in road safety and take extra care if cycling in wet or icy conditions, when braking ability is reduced.

STAYING SAFE AS A PEDESTRIAN

In the UK, more than 1 in 4 of the people killed and about 1 in 7 of those injured in traffic accidents are pedestrians. Nearly all injuries to pedestrians happen in urban areas. Children aged 5–14 years are most at risk of accidents.

If there is no pavement, you should walk on the same side of the road as the oncoming traffic. If you plan to go out walking or jogging at night, you should wear bright clothes and reflectors so that you can be seen by drivers. Teach children to be alert when out on busy streets and, wherever possible, to use pedestrian crossings, tunnels, or overpasses when they cross the road.

(WWW) ONLINE SITES: p.1036

HEALTH ACTION VEHICLE SAFETY

Nearly 4,000 people die on roads in the UK every year, and many more are severely injured. Accidents are more often the result of carelessness or driving after drinking alcohol than of mechanical failure. Whether travelling by car, motorcycle, or bicycle, you should maintain your vehicle properly and take steps to make yourself less vulnerable and to protect other drivers.

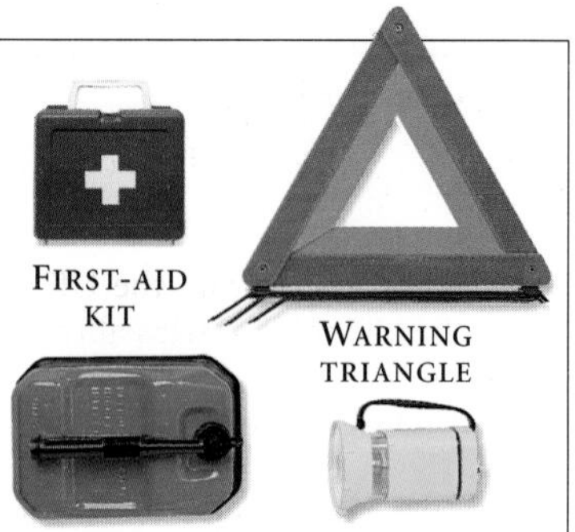

FIRST-AID KIT

WARNING TRIANGLE

EMPTY FUEL CAN

TORCH

Essential equipment
Carry a torch, an empty fuel can, a first-aid kit, and a hazard triangle in the boot of your car.

CAR SAFETY

Make sure that you use built-in safety features according to the manufacturer's guidelines. Children under the age of 12 should not travel in a seat that has front or side airbags, and small adults should not use side airbags.

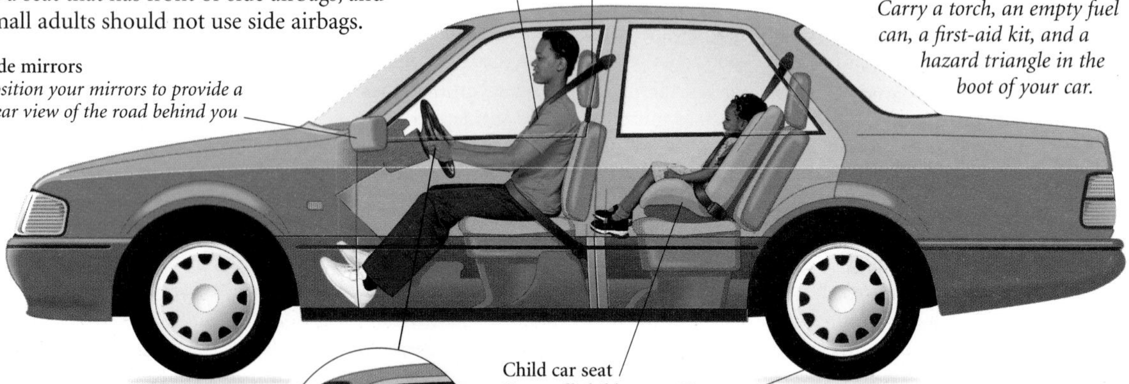

Seat belt
Every passenger should wear a seat belt

Headrest
A well-positioned headrest reduces neck injuries

Side mirrors
Position your mirrors to provide a clear view of the road behind you

Airbag
An airbag inflates on impact in a collision. A front airbag prevents your upper body from hitting the steering wheel or windscreen. A side airbag protects your body in the event of side-on collisions.

Child car seat
For small children, use approved child seats suitable for their weight (see CHILDREN'S CAR SEATS, p.29). Never put small children in seats with airbags.

Tyres
Inflate your tyres to the recommended pressure and check them regularly for signs of wear

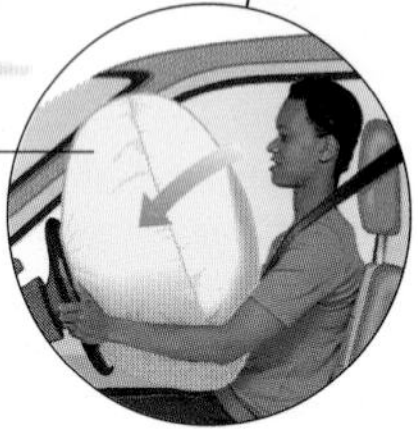

Safety features
All safety features in your car must be checked regularly and may need adjustment periodically. If you have children, take care to reassess their safety needs as they grow.

MOTORCYCLE SAFETY

Specialized motorcycle clothing helps to prevent or reduce injuries caused by a crash or fall and helps you to stay comfortable in all weather conditions. Additionally, modern motorcycles have several built-in safety features to help you to see and be seen.

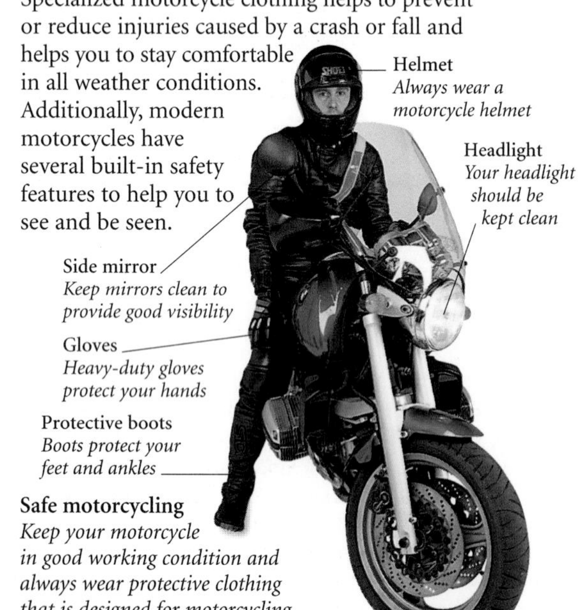

Safe motorcycling
Keep your motorcycle in good working condition and always wear protective clothing that is designed for motorcycling.

BICYCLE SAFETY

Lights, reflectors, and light-coloured or reflective clothing make cyclists more visible to drivers and pedestrians. You should protect your head with a cycling helmet whether you are cycling on or off the road.

Safe cycling
Keep your bicycle well maintained and be aware of drivers and pedestrians.

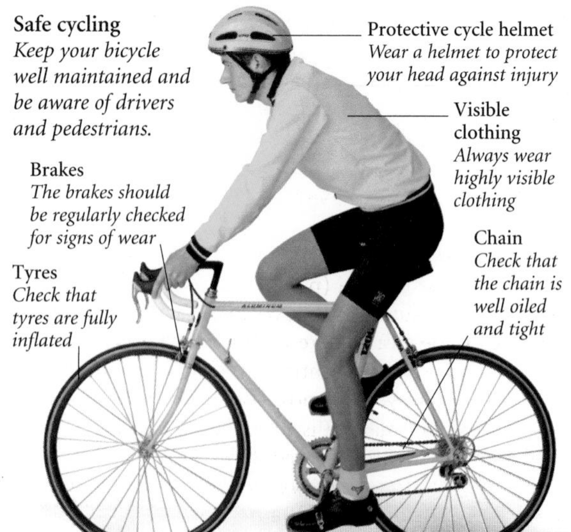

Travel health

Staying healthy and avoiding accidents when travelling abroad

Every year, people from the UK make more than 30 million trips abroad. Although most people complete their trips safely, going abroad still carries some health risks. The most common problems are digestive upsets, injuries in traffic accidents, and sexually transmitted infections. Tropical diseases are rare. You can minimize the risks by finding out about your destination, and about hotels and other facilities, before you travel, and by being prepared for both minor illnesses and emergencies.

Preparing to travel

Before visiting another country, contact your doctor, travel clinic, the country's embassy, or the Medical Advisory Service for Travellers Abroad (MASTA). These sources can advise you on immunizations, preventing disease, and local medical facilities. It is advisable to take out medical insurance before travelling. You may also need an application form for an E111, which entitles you to free or reduced-cost emergency care in EU countries and several other countries. The form is available from post offices.

IMMUNIZATIONS Immunization needs depend on your destination, state of health, current immune status, the duration and type of travel, and the time available before you travel. Seek advice on recommended immunizations at least 8 weeks before travelling because some immunizations require more than one dose to take effect (*see* TRAVEL IMMUNIZATIONS, p.86). Most countries do not require visitors to have specific immunizations, but a few ask for a certificate for yellow fever (p.296).

PREVENTING MALARIA You cannot be vaccinated against malaria (p.305), but you can take precautions to prevent it. Depending on the area you are visiting, your doctor may suggest antimalarial drugs (p.888). However, the most effective way to prevent malaria is to avoid mosquito bites. Pack long-sleeved shirts and long trousers, mosquito repellents containing the chemical DEET, a mosquito net to sleep under (*see* PREVENTING MALARIA, p.305), and mosquito pellets or coils to burn in the evening, when mosquitoes are most active. These precautions can also prevent dengue fever (p.296), another mosquito-borne disease. In addition, scratching insect bites can lead to infection. To relieve itching, pack bite treatment or antihistamine cream (*see* ANTIPRURITIC DRUGS, p.891).

MEDICATION If you are taking medication for an existing condition, take an extra supply in your hand luggage in case of delays. Keep medication in its original packaging and carry a doctor's letter describing your treatment.

EMERGENCY MEDICAL TRAVEL KIT The recommended contents of a medical travel kit depend on your destination. If you are travelling to a developed country, you may need only a mild painkiller (such as paracetamol), antihistamine cream to treat insect bites, and oral rehydration treatment for diarrhoea. If you visit a developing country, you should take sterile needles, 10-ml syringes (for blood tests), and materials for stitching wounds, for use by local medical personnel. These types of medical kit can be purchased at travel clinics and chemists.

Staying healthy in transit

If you are affected by motion sickness (p.604), avoid alcohol and eat only a small amount of food before travelling. Choose the most stable part of the vehicle, do not read, and stay close to a source of air. Your doctor or chemist can also advise you on drugs that prevent motion sickness (*see* ANTIHISTAMINES, p.906, and ANTIEMETIC DRUGS, p.922).

Flying across time zones may disrupt your cycle of sleeping and waking, a condition known as jet lag. To reduce its effects when flying east, go to bed about an hour earlier each night a few days before you fly. When flying west, go to bed about an hour later each night. Avoid heavy meals and salty or fatty food during the flight, and drink plenty of nonalcoholic fluids.

You should avoid air travel if you have had a recent heart attack (*see* MYOCARDIAL INFARCTION, p.410) or have severe lung disease, sinusitis (p.475), or an infection in the middle ear (*see* OTITIS MEDIA, p.597, and ACUTE OTITIS MEDIA IN CHILDREN, p.860). Seek your doctor's advice if you have recently had surgery or if you have been ill. Most airlines will not allow a woman who is more than 35 weeks pregnant to fly; women who are more than 28 weeks pregnant may need a doctor's certificate.

In countries in which people drive on the right, pay extra attention to traffic safety (*see* SAFETY ON THE ROAD, p.83). It is also advisable not to travel at night.

Staying healthy at your destination

Upsets of the digestive system and sexually transmitted infections are the most common problems associated with travelling abroad, but hot weather and local wildlife can also present hazards.

DIGESTIVE-SYSTEM PROBLEMS The most common travel illness is diarrhoea, which may result from a change in the bacteria normally present in the bowel or from water- or food-borne gastroenteritis (p.628), which is usually due to poor hygiene. To reduce the risk of gastroenteritis, wash your hands with soap and water before meals; avoid raw vegetables, salads, shellfish, and ice cream; and peel all fruit. If you are unsure whether the water is clean, use bottled water for drinking and brushing your teeth, or purify water using tablets or a filter. Avoid adding ice that may contain tap water to cold drinks.

Before you travel, ask your doctor about suitable drugs to treat traveller's diarrhoea. Such treatments include over-the-counter antidiarrhoeal drugs (p.924) and possibly a 3-day course of antibiotics (p.885), such as ciprofloxacin. If you develop diarrhoea, rest for at least a day, eat nothing, and drink plenty of fluids (preferably rehydration fluids that contain glucose and salt). If diarrhoea persists, seek medical help.

SEXUALLY TRANSMITTED INFECTIONS The best defence against sexually transmitted infections is abstinence from sex with new partners. You can also reduce the risk of infection by practising safe sex (p.68). Since good-quality condoms are not always available, take some with you.

HOT WEATHER Hot and humid climates result in nearly constant perspiration. Moist skin is an excellent growth medium for bacteria and fungi, especially

HEALTH ACTION

TRAVEL IMMUNIZATIONS

The immunizations that you will need before travelling depend on the area you intend to visit, although some diseases can be contracted almost anywhere. Wherever you are planning to go, make sure that you have been immunized against tetanus and polio (*see* ROUTINE IMMUNIZATIONS, p.45), and have had booster doses if necessary. Advice on other necessary immunizations may change from time to time. Before travelling, always ask your doctor or travel clinic for up-to-date information.

Immunization advice
The immunizations you need depend on your destination, the purpose of your visit, and your immunization history. Timings of the doses you receive may differ from those shown here.

DISEASE	NUMBER OF DOSES	WHEN EFFECTIVE	PERIOD OF PROTECTION	WHO SHOULD BE IMMUNIZED
Diphtheria (p.300)	1 injection	Immediately	10 years	People travelling to the countries of the former USSR and expatriates living in developing countries.
Hepatitis A (p.644)	1 injection (gamma globulin)	Immediately	3–6 months	People travelling to Mediterranean or developing countries on a single occasion.
	2 injections (active vaccine)	2–4 weeks after 1st dose	10 years	Frequent travellers to Mediterranean or developing countries.
Hepatitis B (p.644)	3 injections over 6 months, at least 4 weeks apart	Immediately after 2nd dose	3–5 years	People travelling to countries in which hepatitis B is prevalent; those who might need medical or dental treatment while travelling in a developing country; and people likely to have unprotected sex.
Japanese B encephalitis	2–3 injections 1–2 weeks apart	10–14 days after last dose	About 2 years	People staying for an extended period in rural areas of the Indian subcontinent, China, Southeast Asia, and the Far East.
Meningitis A and C (p.527)	1 injection	After 15 days	3–5 years	People travelling to Saudi Arabia and remote areas of Sub-saharan Africa, Nepal, and Brazil; immunization certificate needed if travelling to Mecca.
Rabies (p.296)	3 injections. 1 week between 1st and 2nd doses, 3 weeks between 2nd and 3rd doses	Immediately after 3rd dose	2–3 years	People travelling to areas where rabies is endemic and who are at high risk (veterinary surgeons, people working with animals, and those travelling into remote country).
Typhoid (p.301)	1 or 2 injections or 3 oral doses	10 days after last injection or dose	3 years	People travelling to areas with poor sanitation.
Yellow fever (p.296)	1 injection	After 10 days	10 years	People travelling to parts of South America and Africa.

in the skin folds under the breasts, the armpits, between the toes and fingers, the groin, and sometimes the scalp. However, most skin and fungal infections can be prevented by frequently showering and changing clothes, drying completely before dressing, wearing loose clothing preferably made from natural fibres, and taking precautions to avoid the harmful effects of strong sunlight (*see* SAFETY IN THE SUN, p.80).

BITES AND STINGS Mosquitoes are not the only biting pests that you may encounter when you travel. Other possible hazards may include poisonous spiders, scorpions or snakes. Even in the UK, parasites such as ticks can transmit diseases, such as Lyme disease (p.303).

Precautions against mosquitoes will help to prevent other stings and bites (*see* AVOIDING BITES AND STINGS, p.327). In addition, you should keep your bed away from the wall, shake clothes and shoes before you wear them, and put on shoes whenever you get out of bed.

Check your body regularly for bites. If you find you have an attached tick after walking in grass or woodland, remove it with tweezers taking care not to leave the head or mouthparts embedded (*see* TICK BITES, p.995).

STAYING HEALTHY AFTER RETURNING HOME

Some diseases contracted while travelling might not show up until you have returned home. For example, malaria can cause fever, severe headaches, shivering, and aching joints several weeks after your return. Consult a doctor and report the details of the places that you visited, including any stopovers. If you develop unusual or persistent symptoms, such as an unexplained rash or diarrhoea that lasts for 10 days or longer, seek medical advice so that the doctor can exclude infections due to travel.

(WWW) ONLINE SITES: p.1037

ASSESSING YOUR SYMPTOMS

This section describes and explains common or worrying symptoms using a series of question-and-answer charts. The charts help you to determine how serious the symptom is and suggest possible causes. They also help you to decide when you can treat the symptom yourself and when you should seek medical help. The section contains charts for everybody, in addition to charts specifically for men, women, and children up to the age of 12.

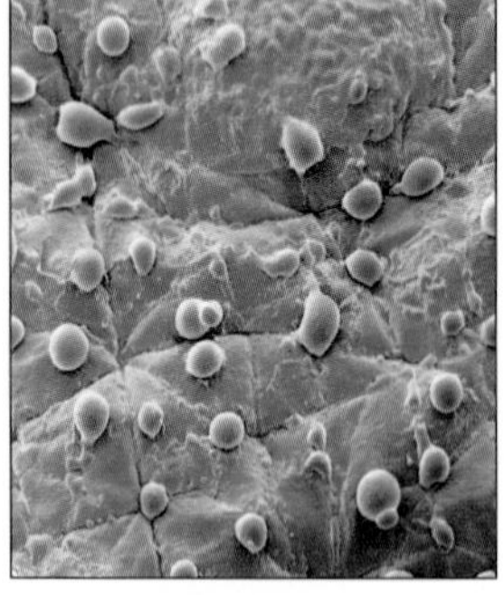

Droplets of sweat
The secretion of sweat helps to control body temperature. Excessive sweating is a common symptom of feverish illnesses.

INTRODUCTION

THE BODY FUNCTIONS RELIABLY most of the time, and we are not aware of the internal processes that keep us alive and enable us to carry out our everyday activities. However, sometimes we experience warning signals, called symptoms, that tell us something is wrong. Most of these symptoms are caused by minor illness or injury and clear up within a few days. However, it is important to be able to tell when a symptom may require medical attention, and it is the purpose of the question-and-answer symptom charts in this section to provide such guidance.

Symptoms take many forms. Some symptoms involve a new sensation, such as pain in the chest, that only you can perceive. Others involve a change in a normal body function, such as frequent passing of urine, or a change in appearance, such as the development of a rash. Such new sensations or changes in the way we look or function alert us to the possibility of illness and may prompt us to seek medical help. However, when investigating the cause of your problem, your doctor does not rely only on a description of your symptoms. He or she will also look for signs of illness. Signs are physical evidence of a disorder or illness that the doctor can detect during a physical examination but of which you may be unaware. For example, if you have a lung condition, shortness of breath might be one of the symptoms that you experience. When the doctor listens to your chest through a stethoscope, he or she may detect abnormal sounds with each breath; these are a sign of the disorder. The combination of symptoms and signs provides the doctor with a pattern that may suggest a diagnosis.

UNDERSTANDING SYMPTOMS

Doctors learn by experience to recognize patterns of symptoms and signs, and most of us learn to do the same for a particular illness if we have had similar symptoms on several occasions. For example, a person who has recurrent attacks of migraine is usually able to recognize the symptoms at an early stage and knows the best way to bring the attacks under control. Similarly, the symptoms of many common infectious illnesses have become general knowledge. Most people recognize aching muscles, runny nose, tiredness, and fever as the usual symptoms of flu. However, dealing with unfamiliar symptoms is not as easy. In these cases, you should make a note of your symptoms so that you can describe them accurately to your doctor or to another health professional. Information that may be helpful includes when the symptom started; which part of the body is affected; whether it came on suddenly or developed gradually; and whether it is

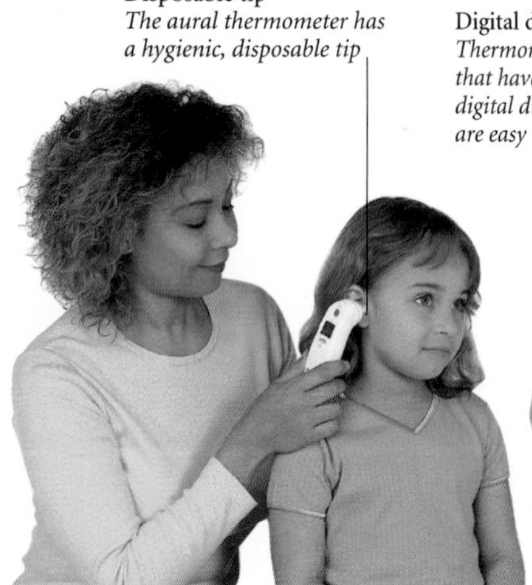

Disposable tip
The aural thermometer has a hygienic, disposable tip

AURAL METHOD

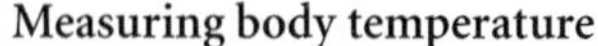

Digital display
Thermometers that have a digital display are easy to read

CONVENTIONAL METHOD

Measuring body temperature
A temperature above 37°C (98.6°F) is a common symptom of infectious illness. Temperature can be measured using a thermometer placed in the mouth or armpit. For children, using an aural thermometer, the tip of which is gently inserted into the ear, is a safer alternative. Modern thermometers have easy-to-read digital displays.

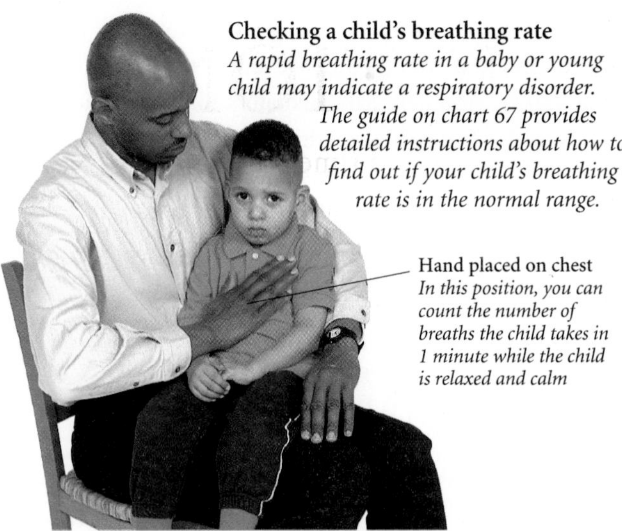

Checking a child's breathing rate
A rapid breathing rate in a baby or young child may indicate a respiratory disorder. The guide on chart 67 provides detailed instructions about how to find out if your child's breathing rate is in the normal range.

continuous or intermittent. If you have a pain, it may also be useful for you to determine how it feels, such as whether it is dull, sharp, burning, or throbbing.

Certain symptoms can be assessed very accurately because they can be measured. Probably the most familiar example is assessing whether or not a person has a fever and, if so, how high the fever is, by measuring body temperature using a thermometer. It is especially useful to be able to measure a symptom in young children because they may not be able to understand or tell you how they are feeling.

Most people are motivated to seek treatment for symptoms that they find troublesome, but it is not wise to assume that an apparently harmless symptom does not require treatment. For example, a rash may cause distress even though it is unlikely to have a serious cause, but a painless swelling may be the first sign of cancer and should not be ignored.

What the charts are for

The charts contained in this section guide you through a series of questions about your symptoms in order to suggest possible causes and the most appropriate course of action. The charts tell you whether you can safely treat your symptoms yourself or whether you need medical attention. They also say how urgently medical help should be sought if required.

Some symptoms, such as loss of consciousness or vomiting blood, are obvious emergencies. If a symptom could indicate a medical emergency in some circumstances, this point is clearly highlighted on the charts. Other symptoms, such as a sore throat or a runny nose, are often due to a minor infection and are likely to clear up whether or not they are treated. In these cases, the charts provide advice about self-help measures or first aid that may help to relieve discomfort in the meantime. If over-the-counter remedies would be appropriate, the charts will tell you. However, you should always consult your doctor if you are unsure whether a particular remedy is suitable for you and read the manufacturer's instructions before taking medication. The charts give you guidance on how long to continue treating yourself and when you need to see your doctor.

Although the charts can help you to decide on the best way to deal with your symptoms, they do not apply to all situations. For example, even apparently minor complaints should receive medical attention when they occur in people who are elderly or in those with reduced immunity, such as people having chemotherapy as part of cancer treatment.

Consulting your doctor

If you do need to see your doctor, he or she will assess your condition by asking you detailed questions about the nature of your symptoms. The questions on the charts should help you to think about your symptoms so that you will be able to describe them accurately to the doctor. The doctor will probably carry out a physical examination and will usually arrange tests to confirm whatever diagnosis is suggested by your symptoms and signs.

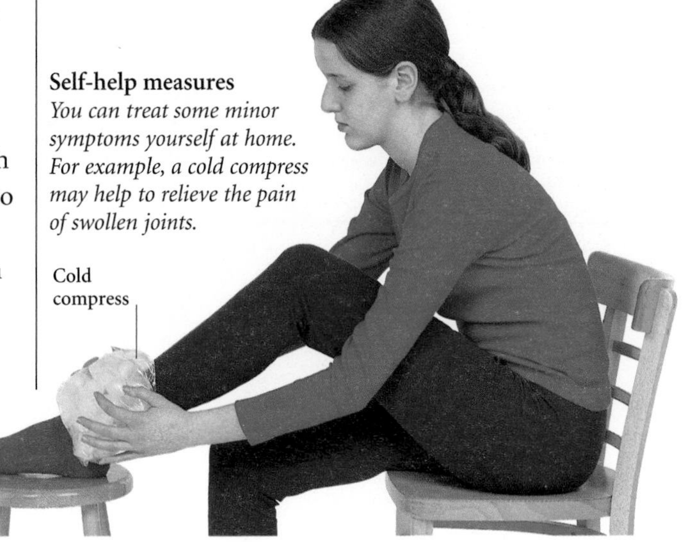

Self-help measures
You can treat some minor symptoms yourself at home. For example, a cold compress may help to relieve the pain of swollen joints.

How to use the charts

A complete list of the 70 symptom charts in this section can be found in the contents list at the beginning of this book. If you have more than one symptom, choose the chart that describes the main one. If the chart that you have selected contains a danger sign box, read that information first and, if you have any of the symptoms listed, call an ambulance immediately. Similarly, you should read warning boxes, which highlight advice that applies only in certain circumstances, before other

Special boxes
There are three different types of box. Danger sign boxes alert you to situations in which emergency medical help may save a life. Warning boxes highlight specific advice that applies in particular circumstances. Symptom assessment boxes tell you how to gather the information that you need to answer the questions in the chart

Introductory text
This text describes common causes of the symptom concerned and lists key information that you may need to know

Starting point
The starting point is always at the top left side of the chart. From here, arrow pathways guide you around the chart through each question to the possible cause or causes of your symptom

Question box
Each question is followed by two or more possible answers. Choose the one that is most applicable and follow the arrows to another location on the chart

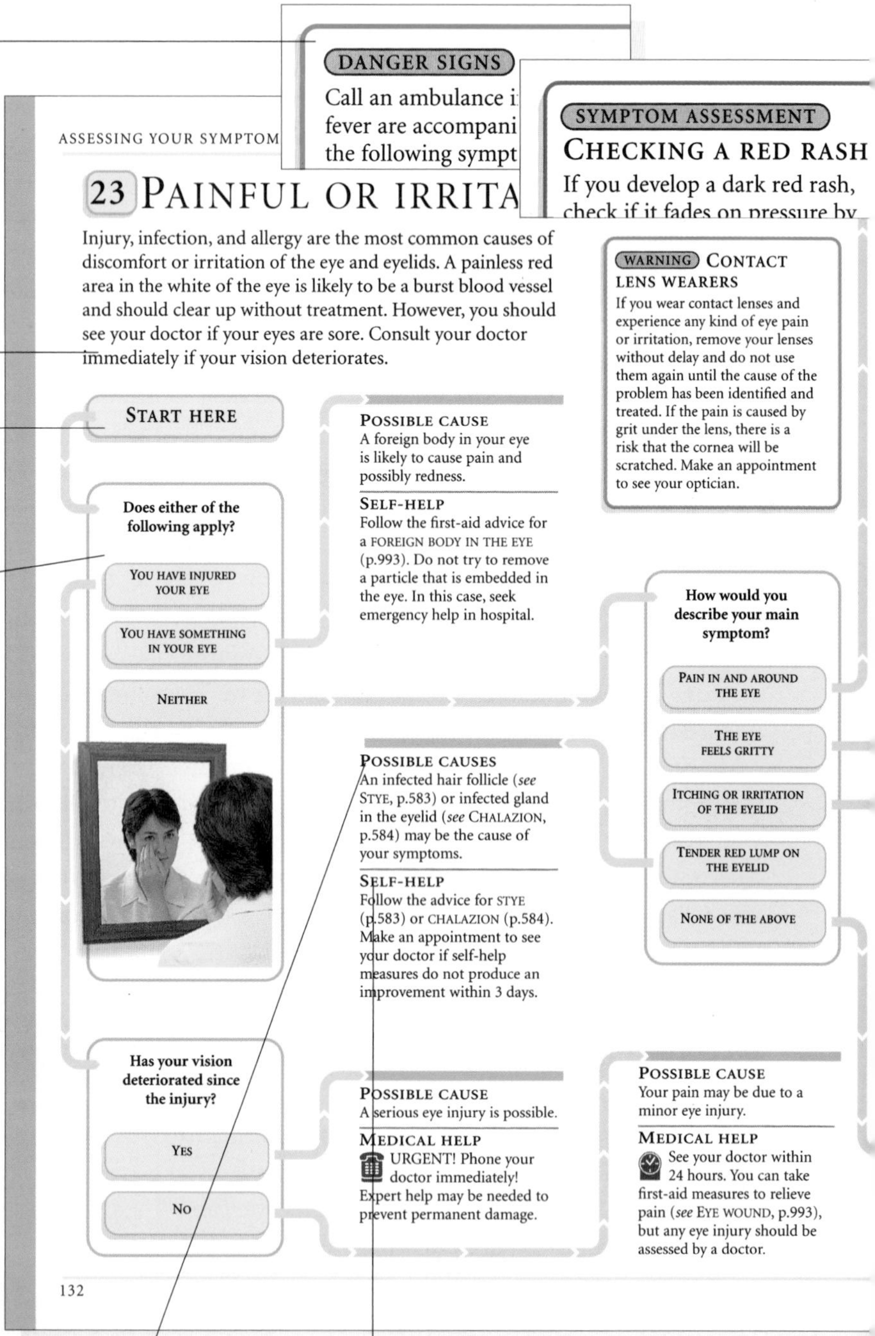
ASSESSING YOUR SYMPTOM

DANGER SIGNS
Call an ambulance i
fever are accompani
the following sympt

SYMPTOM ASSESSMENT
CHECKING A RED RASH
If you develop a dark red rash,
check if it fades on pressure by

23 PAINFUL OR IRRITA

Injury, infection, and allergy are the most common causes of discomfort or irritation of the eye and eyelids. A painless red area in the white of the eye is likely to be a burst blood vessel and should clear up without treatment. However, you should see your doctor if your eyes are sore. Consult your doctor immediately if your vision deteriorates.

WARNING CONTACT LENS WEARERS
If you wear contact lenses and experience any kind of eye pain or irritation, remove your lenses without delay and do not use them again until the cause of the problem has been identified and treated. If the pain is caused by grit under the lens, there is a risk that the cornea will be scratched. Make an appointment to see your optician.

START HERE

Does either of the following apply?
YOU HAVE INJURED YOUR EYE
YOU HAVE SOMETHING IN YOUR EYE
NEITHER

POSSIBLE CAUSE
A foreign body in your eye is likely to cause pain and possibly redness.
SELF-HELP
Follow the first-aid advice for a FOREIGN BODY IN THE EYE (p.993). Do not try to remove a particle that is embedded in the eye. In this case, seek emergency help in hospital.

How would you describe your main symptom?
PAIN IN AND AROUND THE EYE
THE EYE FEELS GRITTY
ITCHING OR IRRITATION OF THE EYELID
TENDER RED LUMP ON THE EYELID
NONE OF THE ABOVE

POSSIBLE CAUSES
An infected hair follicle (*see* STYE, p.583) or infected gland in the eyelid (*see* CHALAZION, p.584) may be the cause of your symptoms.
SELF-HELP
Follow the advice for STYE (p.583) or CHALAZION (p.584). Make an appointment to see your doctor if self-help measures do not produce an improvement within 3 days.

Has your vision deteriorated since the injury?
YES
NO

POSSIBLE CAUSE
A serious eye injury is possible.
MEDICAL HELP
URGENT! Phone your doctor immediately!
Expert help may be needed to prevent permanent damage.

POSSIBLE CAUSE
Your pain may be due to a minor eye injury.
MEDICAL HELP
See your doctor within 24 hours. You can take first-aid measures to relieve pain (*see* EYE WOUND, p.993), but any eye injury should be assessed by a doctor.

132

Possible causes
This text suggests what may have caused the symptom. Bear in mind that these are likely diagnoses only, and not all possibilities are covered

Self-help advice
This text describes what you can do to treat the symptom yourself at home and tells you how soon you need to contact a doctor if there is no improvement in your symptom

ORGANIZATION How this section is organized

There are four colour-coded groups of charts for symptoms appropriate to different groups of people.

GENERAL CHARTS p.92
These symptom charts apply to people of all ages. Some symptoms in children are also covered in a separate group of children's charts.

MEN'S CHARTS p.180
Symptoms that are experienced only by men, such as impotence, are dealt with in these charts.

WOMEN'S CHARTS p.184
This group of charts covers symptoms that are specific to women, such as menstrual problems.

CHILDREN'S CHARTS p.198
These charts feature certain important symptoms in children under the age of 12 for which special advice is needed.

parts of the chart. Otherwise, begin at the box that reads "Start here", follow the arrow to the first question, and choose the most appropriate answer. Follow the arrows and answer further questions until you reach an endpoint. If this point suggests a possible cause for the symptom, the chart will advise you on whether you need to seek medical help or whether you can safely treat the symptom yourself. Alternatively, you could consult NHS Direct, a telephone and internet information service staffed by nurses.

Cross-references
The charts feature cross-references that direct you to articles containing further information

Medical help
The icons and text indicate how urgently you should see a doctor

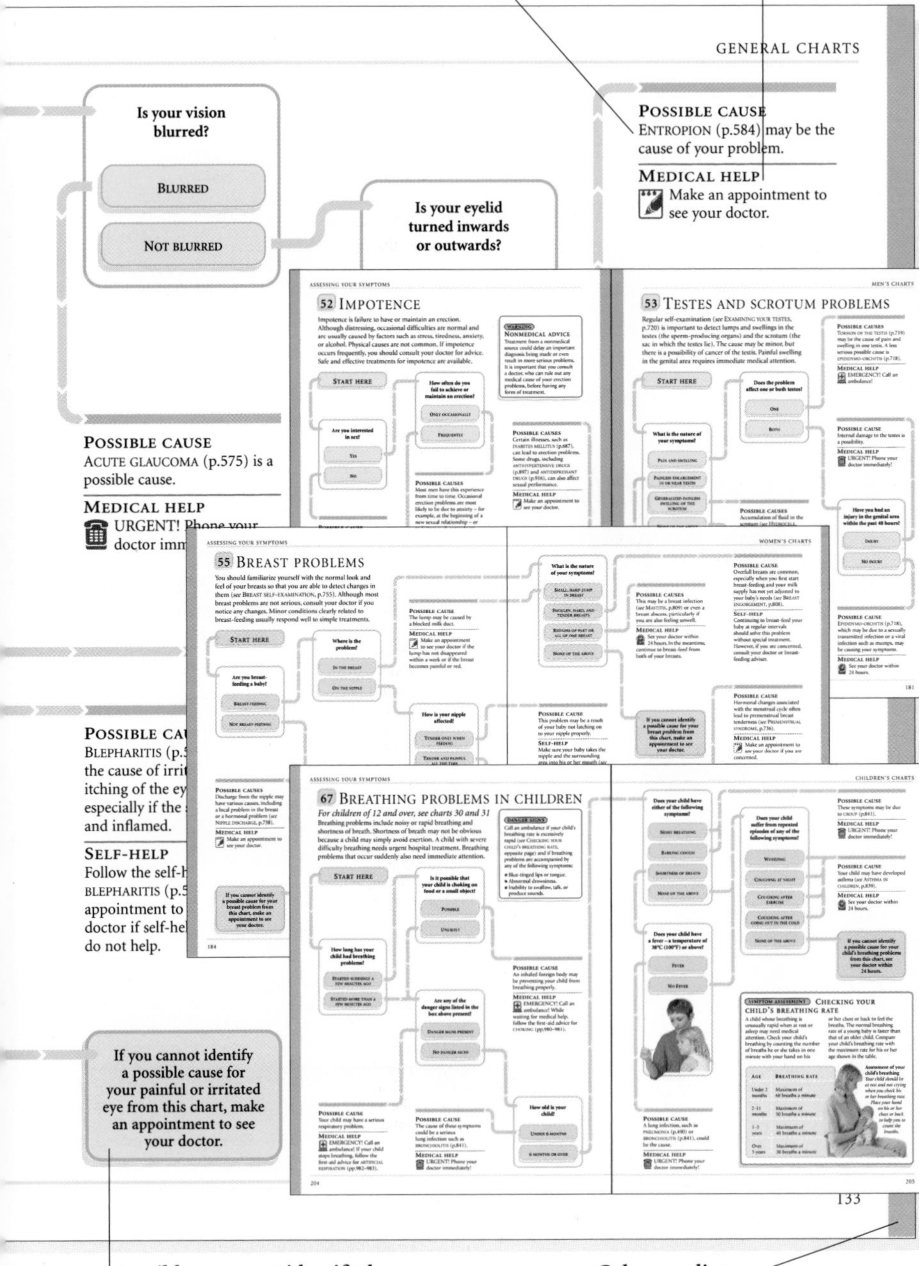

GENERAL CHARTS

Is your vision blurred?

BLURRED

NOT BLURRED

Is your eyelid turned inwards or outwards?

POSSIBLE CAUSE
ENTROPION (p.584) may be the cause of your problem.

MEDICAL HELP
Make an appointment to see your doctor.

POSSIBLE CAUSE
ACUTE GLAUCOMA (p.575) is a possible cause.

MEDICAL HELP
URGENT! Phone your doctor immediately!

52 IMPOTENCE

53 TESTES AND SCROTUM PROBLEMS

55 BREAST PROBLEMS

67 BREATHING PROBLEMS IN CHILDREN

If you cannot identify a possible cause for your painful or irritated eye from this chart, make an appointment to see your doctor.

Possible cause not identified
In some cases, your symptoms do not suggest a diagnosis. The chart then recommends that you should see your doctor, who will decide if the symptom needs further investigation

Colour-coding
The colour-coding at the edge of each page indicates whether the chart applies to everyone or specifically to men, women, or children

ACTION MEDICAL HELP

At the end of a pathway, medical help symbols with accompanying text tell you that you need to seek medical advice and indicate how soon you should contact a doctor. Four levels of medical urgency are indicated, which range from a life-threatening emergency to a situation that can be dealt with next time you see your doctor.

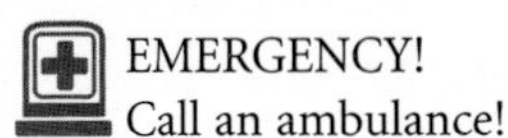

Your condition may be life-threatening unless treated quickly
Dial 999 for the emergency services because you may need trained care while you are in transit. If there is a delay in obtaining an ambulance, going by car may be the quickest way to get to hospital.

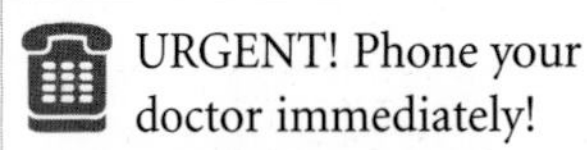

Your symptoms require immediate medical assessment
Contact the doctor, day or night, by telephone. Dial 999 if you fail to make contact within 1 hour. Admission to hospital may be necessary.

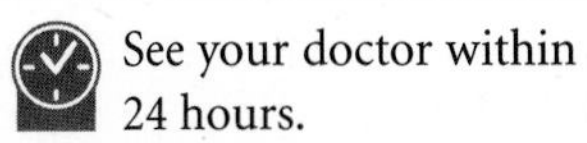

A short delay should not cause your condition to worsen
Symptoms should be assessed and, if necessary, treated by a doctor within 24 hours of their onset.

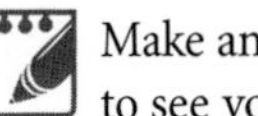

Make an appointment to see your doctor.

Your symptoms do not require urgent medical assessment
Your condition may require medical treatment, but a reasonable delay is unlikely to lead to problems.

1 FEELING UNWELL

There may be times when you feel unwell without being able to pinpoint a precise symptom. This feeling is commonly caused by the onset of a minor viral illness, psychological pressures, or just an unhealthy lifestyle. You should always consult your doctor if the feeling persists because there may be a more serious underlying problem.

START HERE

Do you have a fever – a temperature of 38°C (100°F) or above?

- FEVER
- NO FEVER

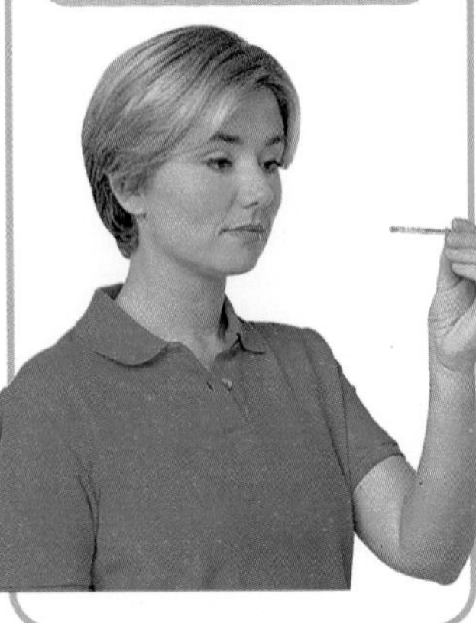

Have you lost more than 4 kg (9 lb) in weight over the past 10 weeks without a deliberate change in eating habits?

- LOST OVER 4 KG (9 LB)
- LOST UNDER 4 KG (9 LB) OR GAINED WEIGHT

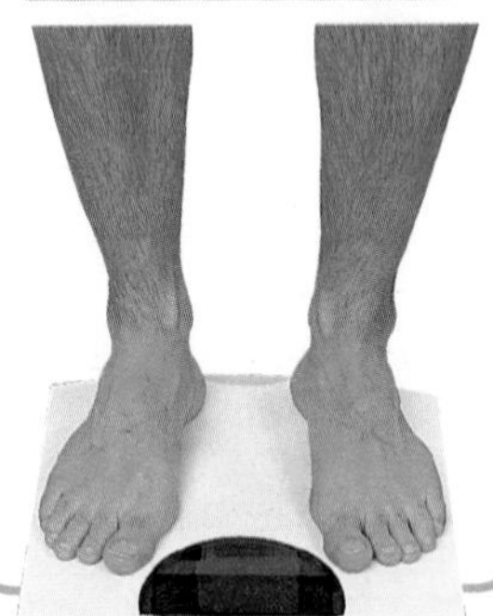

Go to chart 3 LOSS OF WEIGHT

Do you have any of the following symptoms?

- FEELING CONSTANTLY ON EDGE
- DIFFICULTY SLEEPING
- INABILITY TO CONCENTRATE OR TO MAKE DECISIONS
- NONE OF THE ABOVE

Are you currently taking any prescribed or over-the-counter medication?

- MEDICATION
- NO MEDICATION

POSSIBLE CAUSE

A mild fever is likely to make you feel unwell (*see* chart 6, FEVER if you are 12 or over or chart 66, FEVER IN CHILDREN for a child under 12).

POSSIBLE CAUSE

Your symptoms may be a side effect of the medication.

MEDICAL HELP

Make an appointment to see your doctor. Stop taking any over-the-counter medicines but continue to take prescribed medication unless advised to stop by your doctor.

POSSIBLE CAUSES
Your symptoms may be due to an ANXIETY DISORDER (p.551). DEPRESSION (p.554) can also cause some of these symptoms.

MEDICAL HELP
Make an appointment to see your doctor.

Might you be pregnant?

- POSSIBLY PREGNANT
- NOT PREGNANT

POSSIBLE CAUSE
Body changes that start to occur soon after conception can make you feel unwell (*see* COMMON COMPLAINTS OF NORMAL PREGNANCY, p.784).

SELF-HELP
If you are not sure whether you are pregnant, use a HOME PREGNANCY TEST (p.232) or consult your doctor.

Are you feeling more tired than usual?

- MORE TIRED
- NO CHANGE

Go to chart 2
TIREDNESS

Do you regularly drink more than the recommended limit of alcohol (*see* SAFE ALCOHOL LIMITS, p.62)?

- MORE THAN THE LIMIT
- WITHIN THE LIMIT

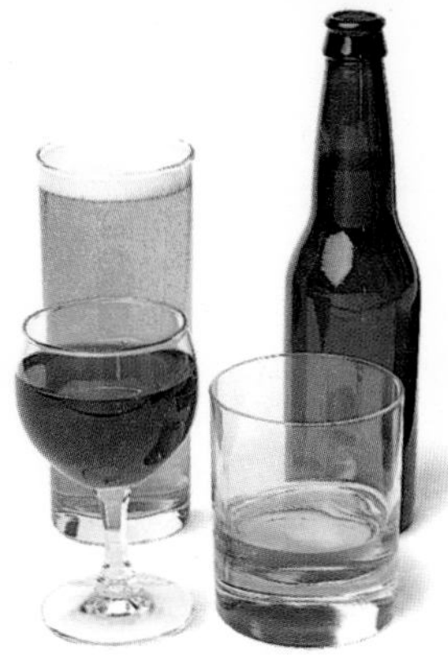

POSSIBLE CAUSE
Regularly drinking too much alcohol is likely to make you feel unwell (*see* ALCOHOL AND HEALTH, p.62).

MEDICAL HELP
Make an appointment to see your doctor for advice about reducing the amount of alcohol you drink.

Do you have any of the following symptoms?

- LOSS OF APPETITE
- NAUSEA
- DIARRHOEA
- NONE OF THE ABOVE

POSSIBLE CAUSE
You may have a mild digestive upset as a result of infection or having eaten something that disagrees with you (*see* GASTROENTERITIS, p.628).

SELF-HELP
Avoid rich or spicy foods and drink plenty of clear fluids. Consult your doctor if you do not feel better in 2 days or if other symptoms develop.

If you cannot identify a possible cause for feeling unwell from this chart, make an appointment to see your doctor.

2 TIREDNESS

For tiredness caused by poor sleep, see chart 5

It is normal to feel tired during the day if you have had difficulty sleeping or if you have been working hard or exercising. You should not be concerned unless your tiredness is persistent and severe. If you are uncertain about the cause of your tiredness, you should consult your doctor.

START HERE

Do you have any of the following symptoms?

- FEELING FAINT OR PASSING OUT
- SHORTNESS OF BREATH
- PALER SKIN THAN NORMAL
- NONE OF THE ABOVE

Have you lost more than 4 kg (9 lb) in weight over the past 10 weeks without a deliberate change in eating habits?

- LOST UNDER 4 KG (9 LB) OR GAINED WEIGHT
- LOST OVER 4 KG (9 LB)

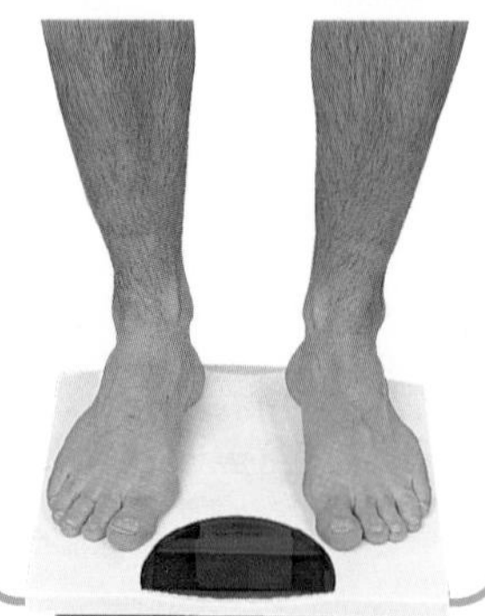

Do you have any of the following symptoms?

- INCREASED DRYNESS OR ROUGHNESS OF THE SKIN
- FEELING THE COLD MORE THAN YOU USED TO
- GENERALIZED HAIR THINNING
- NONE OF THE ABOVE

Have you been experiencing any of the following symptoms?

- INCREASED THIRST
- PASSING MORE URINE THAN NORMAL
- BLURRED VISION
- NONE OF THE ABOVE

POSSIBLE CAUSE

ANAEMIA (p.446) is a possible cause of your symptoms.

MEDICAL HELP

 See your doctor within 24 hours.

POSSIBLE CAUSE

DIABETES MELLITUS (p.687) may be a possibility.

MEDICAL HELP

 See your doctor within 24 hours.

Go to chart 3 LOSS OF WEIGHT

POSSIBLE CAUSE
HYPOTHYROIDISM (p.680) is a possible cause.

MEDICAL HELP
 Make an appointment to see your doctor.

POSSIBLE CAUSE
Regularly drinking too much alcohol can cause tiredness (*see* ALCOHOL AND HEALTH, p.62).

MEDICAL HELP
Make an appointment to see your doctor for advice about reducing the amount of alcohol you drink.

Go to chart 17
FEELING DEPRESSED

Are you currently taking any prescribed or over-the-counter medication?

- MEDICATION
- NO MEDICATION

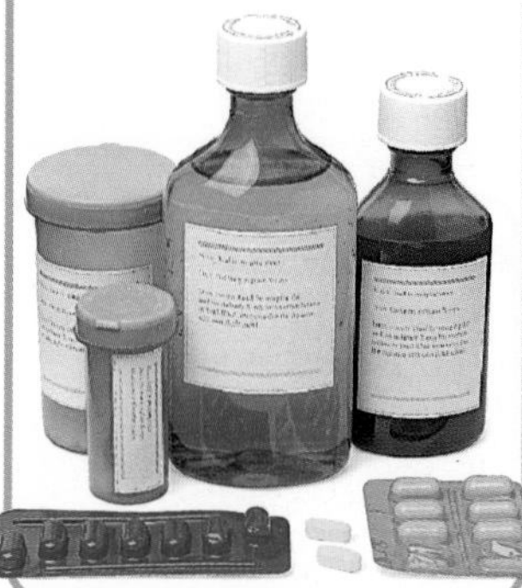

Do you regularly drink more than the recommended limit of alcohol (*see* SAFE ALCOHOL LIMITS, p.62)?

- MORE THAN THE LIMIT
- WITHIN THE LIMIT

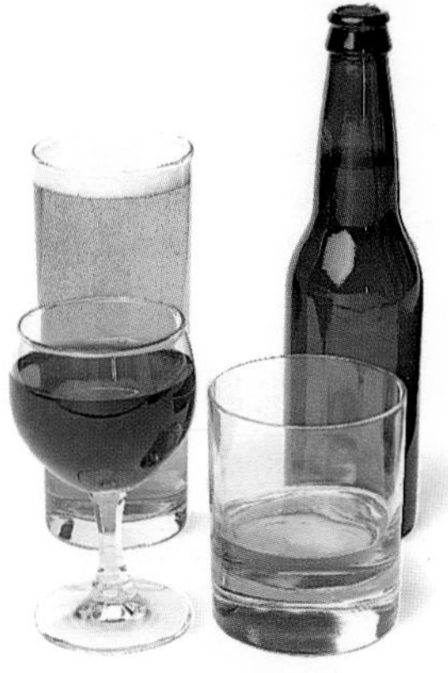

Do you have any of the following symptoms?

- LOW SELF-ESTEEM
- INABILITY TO CONCENTRATE OR TO MAKE DECISIONS
- LACK OF INTEREST IN SEX
- NONE OF THE ABOVE

Have you recently had a viral illness such as flu?

- RECENT ILLNESS
- NO RECENT ILLNESS

POSSIBLE CAUSE
Certain drugs, particularly some of those used to treat high blood pressure (*see* ANTIHYPERTENSIVE DRUGS, p.897), may cause tiredness.

MEDICAL HELP
Make an appointment to see your doctor. Stop taking over-the-counter medicines but continue any prescribed medication unless advised to stop by your doctor.

POSSIBLE CAUSE
It may take several weeks to recover from an illness, particularly from some viral infections, such as INFECTIOUS MONONUCLEOSIS (p.291).

MEDICAL HELP
Make an appointment to see your doctor if you are still feeling tired 1 month after any other symptoms you had have disappeared.

If you cannot identify a possible cause for your tiredness from this chart, make an appointment to see your doctor.

3 LOSS OF WEIGHT

For children under 12, see chart 70

Most people experience small fluctuations in their weight. However, weight loss is of concern if you lose more than 4 kg (9 lb) in 10 weeks or less without a deliberate change in diet and/or increased exercise. Consult your doctor if you have been losing weight without an obvious cause.

START HERE

How much weight have you lost in the past 10 weeks?

- 4 KG (9 LB) OR MORE
- LESS THAN 4 KG (9 LB)

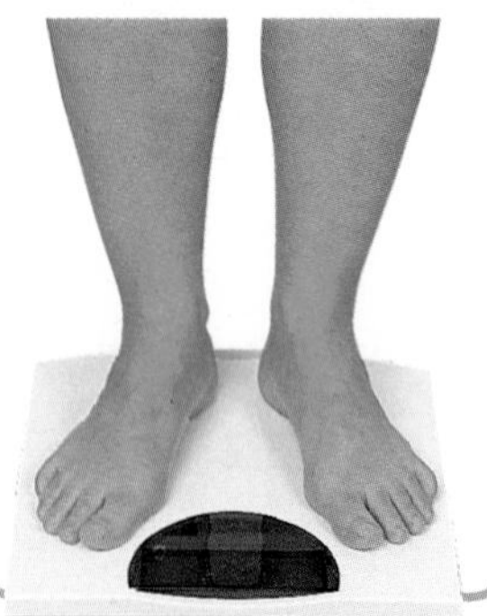

How has your appetite been lately?

- POOR
- NORMAL OR INCREASED

Have you been experiencing any of the following symptoms?

- RECURRENT FEVER
- PROFUSE SWEATING AT NIGHT
- PERSISTENT COUGH
- BLOODSTAINED SPUTUM
- NONE OF THE ABOVE

Have you been experiencing any of the following symptoms?

- INCREASED THIRST
- PASSING MORE URINE THAN USUAL
- BLURRED VISION
- NONE OF THE ABOVE

Do you have any of the following symptoms?

- FEELING CONSTANTLY ON EDGE
- INCREASED SWEATING
- BULGING EYES
- NONE OF THE ABOVE

POSSIBLE CAUSE

Your weight loss is unlikely to be a serious cause for concern unless you are below your ideal weight (*see* ARE YOU A HEALTHY WEIGHT?, p.53).

SELF-HELP

Increase the amount of food you eat (*see* CONTROLLING YOUR WEIGHT, p.53). Make an appointment to see your doctor if you continue to lose weight or have fallen below the ideal weight for your height.

POSSIBLE CAUSE

DIABETES MELLITUS (p.687) is a possible cause.

MEDICAL HELP

See your doctor within 24 hours.

POSSIBLE CAUSES

HYPERTHYROIDISM (p.679) is a possibility. However, ANXIETY DISORDERS (p.551) can cause some of these symptoms.

MEDICAL HELP

Make an appointment to see your doctor.

Possible causes
A chronic infection, such as TUBERCULOSIS (p.491) or an AIDS-related illness (*see* HIV INFECTION AND AIDS, p.297), could be the cause of your symptoms. An underlying CANCER (pp.274–283) is also a possible cause.

Medical help
 See your doctor within 24 hours.

Possible causes
An intestinal infection, such as GIARDIASIS (p.307), or a long-term bowel condition, such as ULCERATIVE COLITIS (p.659) or CROHN'S DISEASE (p.658), could be the cause of your symptoms. COLORECTAL CANCER (p.665) is also a possibility.

Medical help
 See your doctor within 24 hours.

Possible causes
DEPRESSION (p.554) could be the cause. However, ANXIETY DISORDERS (p.551) sometimes produce similar symptoms.

Medical help
 Make an appointment to see your doctor.

Have you noticed any of the following symptoms?

- Recurrent diarrhoea
- Recurrent constipation
- Recurrent abdominal pain
- Blood in faeces
- None of the above

Possible cause
You are probably eating less than you need to meet your energy requirements.

Medical help
Make an appointment to see your doctor to make sure that an underlying problem is not responsible for your weight loss.

Do you have any of the following symptoms?

- Difficulty sleeping
- Low self-esteem
- Lack of interest in sex
- Inability to concentrate or to make decisions
- Lack of energy
- None of the above

Have you recently increased the amount of exercise you do?

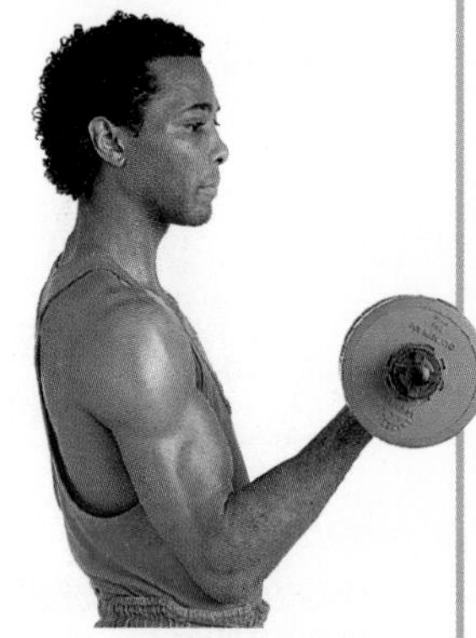

- No increase
- Increased exercise

Possible cause
Your increase in energy output is the most probable cause of your weight loss.

Self-help
Increase the amount of food you eat to make up for your increased energy needs (*see* CONTROLLING YOUR WEIGHT, p.53). Make an appointment to see your doctor if you continue to lose weight or are below the ideal weight for your height (*see* ARE YOU A HEALTHY WEIGHT?, p.53).

If you cannot identify a possible cause for your weight loss from this chart, call your doctor within 24 hours.

4 BEING OVERWEIGHT

For children under 12, see chart 70

You are overweight if you are heavier than the ideal weight for your height (*see* ARE YOU A HEALTHY WEIGHT?, p.53). Being overweight is most often due to eating more than you need and/or lack of exercise. If you are very overweight, you are at risk of various medical problems (*see* OBESITY, p.631).

START HERE

In the past, has your weight been consistently within ideal limits?

- PREVIOUSLY IDEAL WEIGHT
- PREVIOUSLY UNDERWEIGHT
- ALWAYS OVERWEIGHT

Do you have any of the following symptoms?

- TIREDNESS
- INCREASED DRYNESS OR ROUGHNESS OF THE SKIN
- FEELING THE COLD MORE THAN YOU USED TO
- GENERALIZED HAIR THINNING
- NONE OF THE ABOVE

POSSIBLE CAUSE
A hormone disorder, such as HYPOTHYROIDISM (p.680), is a possible cause.

MEDICAL HELP
 Make an appointment to see your doctor.

Are you currently taking any prescribed medication?

- MEDICATION
- NO MEDICATION

POSSIBLE CAUSE
Your weight gain may be a side effect of the medication.

MEDICAL HELP
Make an appointment to see your doctor. Continue to take your medication unless advised to stop by your doctor.

Are or were your parents overweight?

- OVERWEIGHT
- IDEAL WEIGHT OR UNDERWEIGHT

POSSIBLE CAUSE
A family tendency to being overweight may result from unhealthy family eating habits and/or a genetic predisposition to put on weight.

SELF-HELP
Adopt a sensible reducing diet (*see* CONTROLLING YOUR WEIGHT, p.53) and get more exercise. Make an appointment to see your doctor if you have not started to lose weight within 2 weeks.

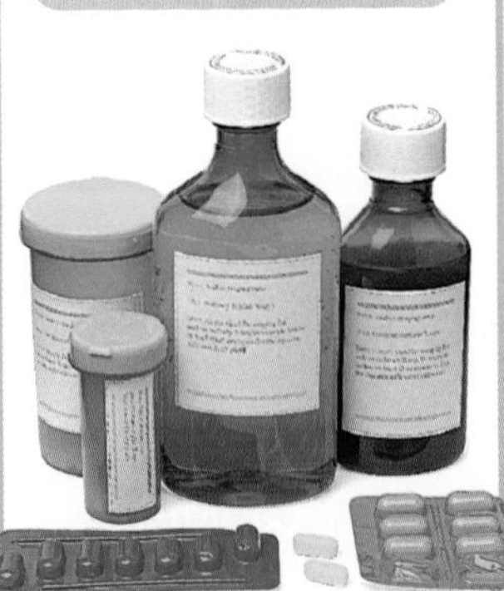

Do any of the following apply?

- You have recently had a baby
- You have recently given up smoking
- You have been suffering from depression or stress
- You have reduced your level of physical activity
- None of the above

Possible cause
Giving up smoking often leads to a temporary weight gain. However, the benefits to your health from giving up smoking far outweigh the much smaller risk from any excess weight.

Self-help
When you are sure that you have overcome your smoking habit, start a sensible reducing diet (*see* Controlling your weight, p.53).

Possible cause
During pregnancy, women often put on weight that they find hard to lose after the baby has been born.

Self-help
You will probably lose excess weight gradually over the next few months or so. If you are breast-feeding, it is not a good idea to reduce your calorie intake substantially. If you are still unhappy with your weight when you have finished breast-feeding, consult your doctor.

Possible cause
Reducing your level of physical activity without cutting down the amount of food that you eat will usually lead to weight gain (*see* Controlling your weight, p.53).

Self-help
Be sure to maintain a healthy level of exercise (*see* Taking regular exercise, p.57) and follow a sensible diet (*see* A healthy diet, p.48).

Possible causes
Both depression (p.554) and anxiety disorders (p.551) can cause weight gain.

Medical help
 Make an appointment to see your doctor.

How old are you?

- Under 40 years
- 40 years or over

Possible cause
Regularly eating more than you need is the most likely cause of your weight gain.

Self-help
Adopt a sensible reducing diet (*see* Controlling your weight, p.53) and get more exercise. Make an appointment to see your doctor if you have not started to lose weight within 2 weeks.

Possible cause
It is normal to gain a little weight as you become older.

Self-help
If you are above the ideal weight for your height, adopt a sensible reducing diet (*see* Controlling your weight, p.53) and get more exercise. Make an appointment to see your doctor if you have not lost any weight within 2 weeks.

If you cannot identify a possible cause for your weight problem from this chart, adopt a sensible reducing diet (*see* Controlling your weight, p.53). Make an appointment to see your doctor if you have not started to lose weight within 2 weeks.

5 DIFFICULTY SLEEPING

Most people are affected by difficulty sleeping on occasion. The causes include worry, drinking too much caffeine, or insufficient exercise. If you wake feeling unrested but are not aware of difficulty sleeping, the cause may be interruption of breathing during sleep (*see* SLEEP APNOEA, p.477). Consult your doctor if you have frequent sleeping problems.

START HERE

What kind of sleeping difficulty have you been experiencing?

- DIFFICULTY GETTING TO SLEEP
- DIFFICULTY STAYING ASLEEP

Are you awakened from sleep by attacks of shortness of breath?

- NO
- YES

Go to chart 30
SHORTNESS OF BREATH

Do you have any of the following symptoms?

- LACK OF ENERGY
- LOW SELF-ESTEEM
- INABILITY TO CONCENTRATE OR TO MAKE DECISIONS
- LACK OF INTEREST IN SEX
- NONE OF THE ABOVE

Go to chart 17
FEELING DEPRESSED

Do you take sleeping pills regularly or have you recently stopped taking them?

- TAKING SLEEPING PILLS
- RECENTLY STOPPED
- NEITHER

POSSIBLE CAUSE
The regular use of sleeping pills can lead to a gradual reduction in their effectiveness (*see* SLEEPING DRUGS, p.915).

MEDICAL HELP
Make an appointment to see your doctor.

POSSIBLE CAUSE
Withdrawal from sleeping pills can lead to difficulty sleeping as your body adapts (*see* SLEEPING DRUGS, p.915).

SELF-HELP
Follow the advice for getting a good night's sleep (*see* SLEEP, p.73). Make an appointment to see your doctor if difficulty sleeping continues.

POSSIBLE CAUSES
HYPERTHYROIDISM (p.679) is a possible cause. However, ANXIETY DISORDERS (p.551) can also cause these symptoms.

MEDICAL HELP

Make an appointment to see your doctor.

POSSIBLE CAUSE
Consumption of any of these can lead to difficulty sleeping.

SELF-HELP
Follow the advice for getting a good night's sleep (*see* SLEEP, p.73). Make an appointment to see your doctor if difficulty sleeping continues.

On nights that you have difficulty sleeping, have you consumed any of the following?

- LARGE AMOUNTS OF COFFEE, TEA, OR COLA
- LARGE AMOUNTS OF ALCOHOL
- A LATE, HEAVY MEAL
- NONE OF THE ABOVE

Do you have either of the following symptoms?

- FEELING CONSTANTLY ON EDGE
- INABILITY TO CONCENTRATE
- NEITHER

POSSIBLE CAUSE
Your symptoms may be a side effect of the medication.

MEDICAL HELP
Make an appointment to see your doctor. Stop taking over-the-counter medicines but continue any prescribed medication unless advised to stop by your doctor.

Are you currently taking any prescribed or over-the-counter medication?

- MEDICATION
- NO MEDICATION

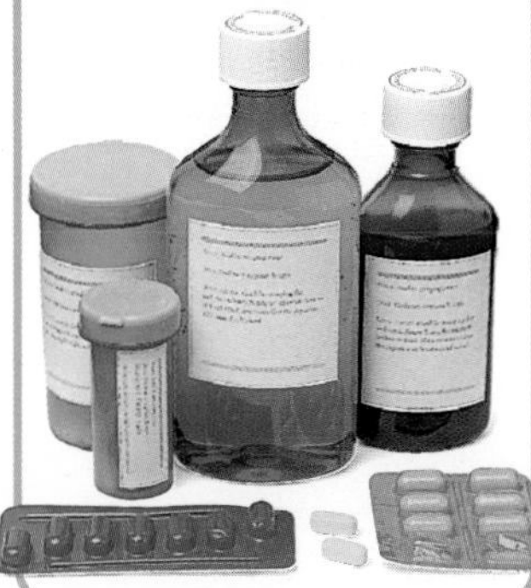

POSSIBLE CAUSE
Insufficient physical activity in the day can lead to sleeping problems at night.

SELF-HELP
Build more exercise into your daily routine (*see* TAKING REGULAR EXERCISE, p.57). Make an appointment to see your doctor if problems with sleeping persist.

POSSIBLE CAUSE
You may need less sleep than you think. It is possible that some of the sleep that you need has been taken as naps during the day.

SELF-HELP
Follow the advice for getting a good night's sleep (*see* SLEEP, p.73). Make an appointment to see your doctor if difficulty sleeping continues.

On nights that you have difficulty sleeping, have either of the following applied?

- YOU HAVE TAKEN A NAP DURING THE DAY
- YOU HAVE BEEN AWAKE FOR FEWER THAN 18 HOURS
- NEITHER

How physically active is your usual daily routine?

- MAINLY SEDENTARY
- PHYSICALLY ACTIVE

If you cannot identify a possible cause for your difficulty sleeping from this chart, make an appointment to see your doctor.

6 FEVER

For children under 12, see chart 66

Normal temperature varies from one person to another, but if your temperature is 38°C (100°F) or above, you have a fever. Most fevers are due to infection, but heat exposure or certain drugs can also raise body temperature. In all cases, follow the self-help advice for BRINGING DOWN A FEVER (p.289).

WARNING HIGH TEMPERATURE

If you are feeling unwell, you should take your temperature every 4 hours. Call your doctor immediately if your temperature rises to 39°C (102°F) or above, and take steps to lower the fever without delay (*see* BRINGING DOWN A FEVER, p.289).

START HERE

Do you have a rash?

RASH

NO RASH

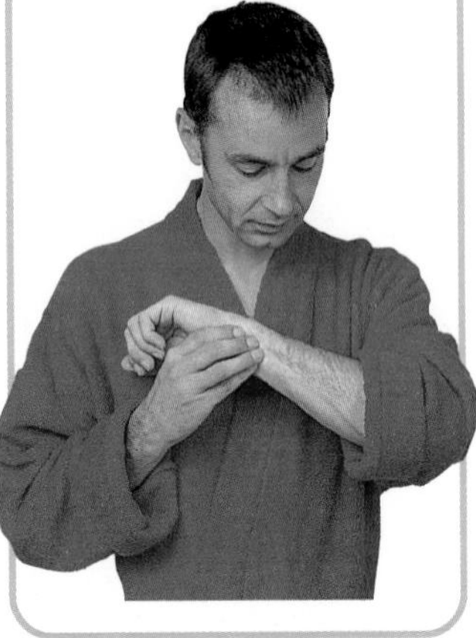

Go to chart 21 RASH WITH FEVER

Do you have a headache?

SEVERE HEADACHE

MILD HEADACHE

NO HEADACHE

Do you have any of the following symptoms?

DROWSINESS OR CONFUSION

DISLIKE OF BRIGHT LIGHT

NECK PAIN ON BENDING THE HEAD FORWARDS

NONE OF THE ABOVE

POSSIBLE CAUSE

There is a possibility that you have MENINGITIS (p.527).

MEDICAL HELP

EMERGENCY! Call an ambulance!

Are you having problems breathing?

YOU ARE SHORT OF BREATH

BREATHING IS PAINFUL

BREATHING IS NORMAL

Do you have a cough?

COUGH

NO COUGH

POSSIBLE CAUSES

CYSTITIS (p.709) is the most likely cause of your symptoms, but PYELONEPHRITIS (p.698) is also possible, especially if you have back pain.

MEDICAL HELP

 See your doctor within 24 hours.

Possible cause
A chest infection, such as PNEUMONIA (p.490), is a possible cause.

Medical help
URGENT! Phone your doctor immediately!

Possible cause
A chest infection, such as ACUTE BRONCHITIS (p.486), may cause your symptoms.

Self-help
Follow the self-help advice for ACUTE BRONCHITIS (p.486). Consult your doctor if your symptoms worsen or if you are no better in 2 days.

Have you been coughing up sputum?

- Sputum
- No sputum

Do you have either of the following symptoms?

- Generalized aches and pains
- Runny nose
- Neither

Possible causes
A viral illness, such as a severe cold (*see* COMMON COLD, p.288) or INFLUENZA (p.289), is the most probable cause of your symptoms.

Self-help
Follow the self-help advice for BRINGING DOWN A FEVER (p.289). Consult your doctor if your symptoms worsen, if you are no better in 2 days, or if other symptoms develop.

Have you had several bouts of fever over the past few weeks?

- Recurrent fever
- No other recent fever

Possible causes
A long-term infection, such as INFECTIVE ENDOCARDITIS (p.426) or an AIDS-related illness (*see* HIV INFECTION AND AIDS, p.297), may cause recurrent fever. An underlying cancer, such as LYMPHOMA (p.459), is also possible.

Medical help

See your doctor within 24 hours.

Do you have a sore throat?

- Sore throat
- No sore throat

Do you have any urinary problems?

- Pain on passing urine
- Passing urine too frequently
- Neither

Go to chart 27
SORE THROAT

If you cannot identify a possible cause for your fever from this chart, see your doctor within 24 hours.

7 EXCESSIVE SWEATING

Sweating is one of the body's cooling mechanisms. It is a normal response to heat, exercise, and stress or fear. Some people naturally sweat more than others. Wearing natural fibres, such as cotton, and using an antiperspirant often help to reduce sweating. You should consult your doctor if you sweat excessively and are unsure of the cause.

START HERE

Do you have a fever – a temperature of 38°C (100°F) or above?

- FEVER
- NO FEVER

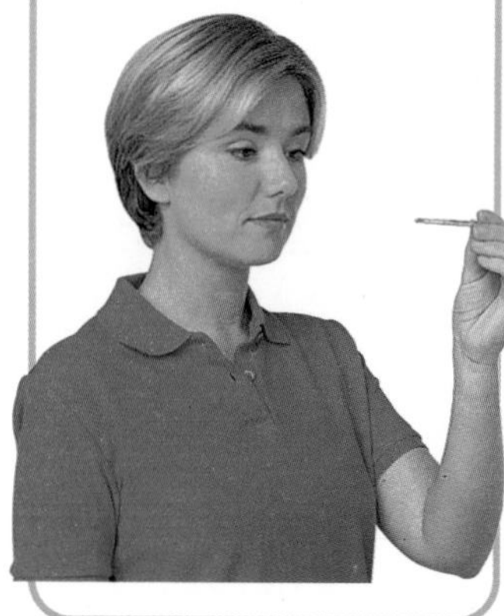

POSSIBLE CAUSE
A fever will generally cause increased sweating. Go to chart 6, FEVER if you are 12 or over or chart 66, FEVER IN CHILDREN for a child under 12.

When does the sweating occur?

- MAINLY AT NIGHT
- AT OTHER TIMES

Do you feel otherwise well?

- WELL
- UNWELL

POSSIBLE CAUSES
A chronic infection, such as TUBERCULOSIS (p.491), or an AIDS-related illness (*see* HIV INFECTION AND AIDS, p.297) may cause your symptoms. A cancer such as LYMPHOMA (p.459) is also a possibility.

MEDICAL HELP
 See your doctor within 24 hours.

Do you have any of the following symptoms?

- WEIGHT LOSS WITH INCREASED APPETITE
- FEELING CONSTANTLY ON EDGE
- BULGING EYES
- NONE OF THE ABOVE

POSSIBLE CAUSES
HYPERTHYROIDISM (p.679) is a possibility. However, ANXIETY DISORDERS (p.551) can cause some of these symptoms.

MEDICAL HELP
 Make an appointment to see your doctor.

Does either of the following apply?

- SWEATING OCCURS WITH MENSTRUAL PERIODS
- MENSTRUAL PERIODS HAVE BECOME IRREGULAR
- NEITHER

POSSIBLE CAUSE
Hormonal changes associated with the menstrual cycle or the menopause (*see* HEALTH AT THE MENOPAUSE, p.36) may cause excessive sweating.

MEDICAL HELP
 Make an appointment to see your doctor.

Is your weight within ideal limits (*see* ARE YOU A HEALTHY WEIGHT?, p.53)?

- OVERWEIGHT
- IDEAL WEIGHT
- UNDERWEIGHT

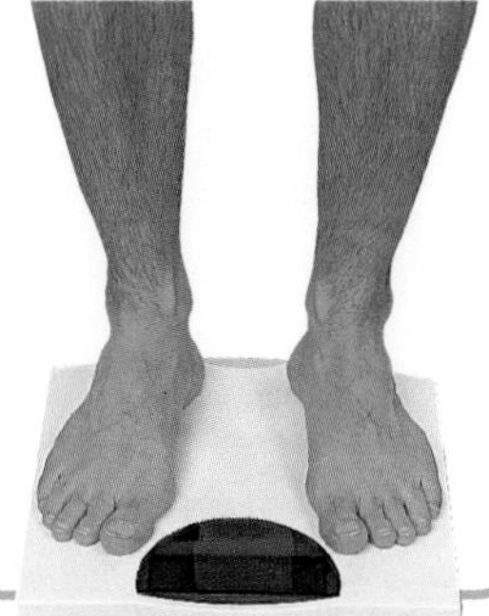

POSSIBLE CAUSE
Being overweight can lead to excessive sweating, particularly after physical exertion.

MEDICAL HELP
Make an appointment to see your doctor. Adopt a sensible reducing diet (*see* CONTROLLING YOUR WEIGHT, p.53) and follow the advice for HYPERHIDROSIS (p.342).

Do you regularly drink more than the recommended limit of alcohol (*see* SAFE ALCOHOL LIMITS, p.62)?

- MORE THAN THE LIMIT
- WITHIN THE LIMIT

POSSIBLE CAUSE
Drinking excessive amounts of alcohol can lead to increased sweating (*see* ALCOHOL AND HEALTH, p.62).

MEDICAL HELP
Make an appointment to see your doctor for advice about reducing the amount of alcohol you drink.

Are you currently taking any prescribed or over-the-counter medication?

- MEDICATION
- NO MEDICATION

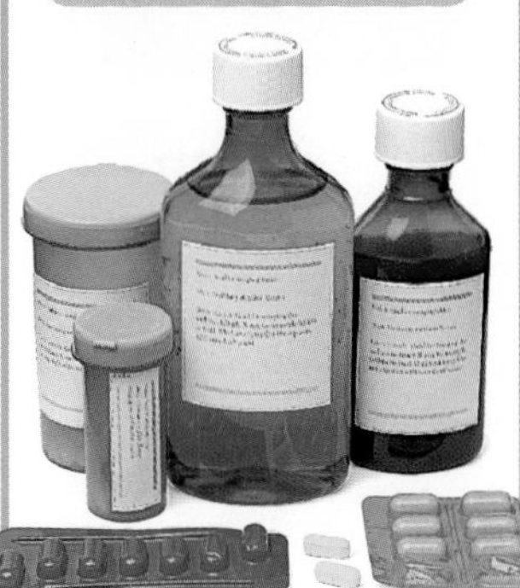

POSSIBLE CAUSE
Your symptoms may be a side effect of the medication.

MEDICAL HELP
Make an appointment to see your doctor. Stop taking any over-the-counter medicines but continue to take prescribed medication unless advised to stop by your doctor.

Is the excessive sweating limited to certain parts of the body?

- MAINLY HANDS
- MAINLY FEET
- OTHER PARTS AFFECTED

POSSIBLE CAUSE
Excessive sweating that chiefly affects the hands and feet is a fairly common problem.

SELF-HELP
Try self-help measures (*see* HYPERHIDROSIS, p.342). Make an appointment to see your doctor if your symptoms do not improve.

If you cannot identify a possible cause for your excessive sweating from this chart, see your doctor within 24 hours.

8 LUMPS AND SWELLINGS

Lumps and swellings under the skin, particularly in the neck, under the arms, or in the groin, are often enlarged lymph nodes (glands). These glands usually become swollen due to an infection. The swelling subsides shortly after the infection clears up. If the lumps are painful or if they are persistent but painless, you should consult your doctor.

WARNING PAINLESS LUMPS OR SWELLINGS
Any painless lump or swelling that does not disappear within 2 weeks should be seen by a doctor.

START HERE

What are the characteristics of the lump or swelling?

- RED AND PAINFUL
- OTHER

Are the lumps or swellings in more than one area?

- ONE AREA ONLY
- SEVERAL AREAS

Do you have a rash?

- RASH
- NO RASH

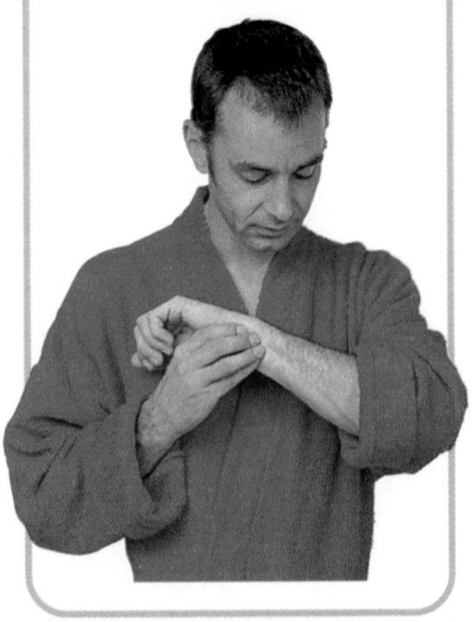

POSSIBLE CAUSE
An abscess or a BOIL (p.351) may be the cause of a painful, inflamed swelling.

MEDICAL HELP
 See your doctor within 24 hours.

Do you have a fever – a temperature of 38°C (100°F) or above?

- FEVER
- NO FEVER

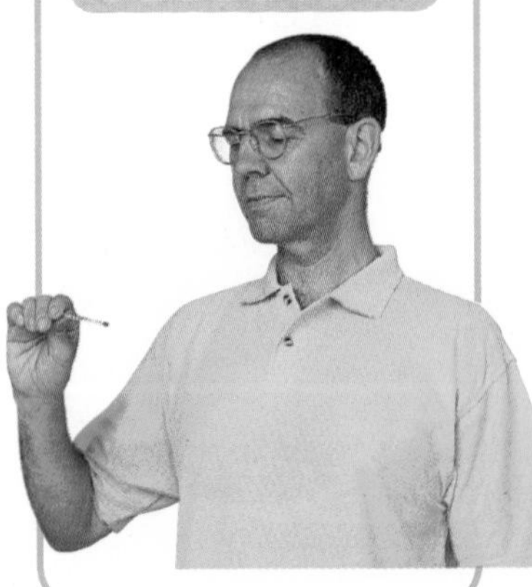

POSSIBLE CAUSE
INFECTIOUS MONONUCLEOSIS (p.291) is a possible cause of swelling of the lymph nodes in several areas, especially if you feel generally unwell.

MEDICAL HELP
 See your doctor within 24 hours.

POSSIBLE CAUSES
A viral infection is the most likely cause. There is also a possibility of a cancer of the lymphatic system (*see* LYMPHOMA, p.459) or an AIDS-related illness (*see* HIV INFECTION AND AIDS, p.297).

MEDICAL HELP
 See your doctor within 24 hours.

Where is the lump or swelling?

- TESTIS
- GROIN
- BREAST
- SIDES OR BACK OF NECK
- OTHER

Go to chart 53
TESTES AND SCROTUM PROBLEMS

What happens to the swelling if you press on it or if you lie down?

- IT DISAPPEARS
- IT REDUCES IN SIZE
- NO CHANGE

POSSIBLE CAUSE
You may have an inguinal hernia (*see* HERNIAS, p.661).

MEDICAL HELP

Make an appointment to see your doctor.

POSSIBLE CAUSE
Lymph nodes in the groin often become swollen in response to an infection.

MEDICAL HELP
Make an appointment to see your doctor.

Go to chart 55
BREAST PROBLEMS

POSSIBLE CAUSES
A number of viral illnesses can cause swollen glands and a rash. LYME DISEASE (p.303) is another possibility, particularly if you think you may have been bitten by a tick recently.

MEDICAL HELP

See your doctor within 24 hours.

Do you have a sore throat?

- SORE THROAT
- NO SORE THROAT

Go to chart 27
SORE THROAT

Do you have a recent injury near the site of the swelling?

- INJURY
- NO INJURY

POSSIBLE CAUSES
An injury is likely to cause some swelling as a result of damage to the tissues. An infected wound or a localized rash can also cause nearby lymph nodes to swell (*see* LYMPHADENOPATHY, p.458).

SELF-HELP
Make sure the wound is clean and protect it with an adhesive bandage or light dressing. Consult your doctor if there is any pain, redness, or pus around the wound, or if the swelling persists after the wound has healed.

If you cannot identify a possible cause for your lumps or swellings from this chart, make an appointment to see your doctor.

9 FEELING FAINT AND PASSING OUT

Feeling faint is a sensation of dizziness or light-headedness. It may be followed by passing out (loss of consciousness). The cause is usually lack of food or a reduction in blood flow to the brain. A brief episode of feeling faint without other symptoms is not a cause for alarm, but you should consult your doctor if such episodes recur or if you have passed out.

WARNING

UNCONSCIOUSNESS

If someone remains unconscious for more than a minute or so, whatever the suspected cause, you should get emergency medical help. If you need to leave the person to call for help, first lay him or her in the recovery position (p.979). Do not move the person if you suspect spinal injury.

START HERE

Have you had any of the following symptoms?

- DISTURBED VISION
- NUMBNESS, TINGLING, OR WEAKNESS IN ANY PART OF THE BODY
- CONFUSION
- DIFFICULTY IN SPEAKING
- NONE OF THE ABOVE

Are any of your symptoms still present?

- SYMPTOMS PRESENT
- SYMPTOMS NO LONGER PRESENT

POSSIBLE CAUSE

It is possible that you have had a STROKE (p.532).

MEDICAL HELP

 EMERGENCY! Call an ambulance!

POSSIBLE CAUSE

A TRANSIENT ISCHAEMIC ATTACK (p.531) is a possibility.

MEDICAL HELP

 URGENT! Phone your doctor immediately!

Have you noticed any of the following?

- BLOODSTAINED VOMIT
- RED BLOOD IN THE FAECES
- BLACK, TARRY FAECES
- NONE OF THE ABOVE

POSSIBLE CAUSE

You may have bleeding in the digestive tract, perhaps from a PEPTIC ULCER (p.640).

MEDICAL HELP

EMERGENCY! Call an ambulance!

Did any of the following occur when you passed out?

- YOU TWITCHED UNCONTROLLABLY
- YOU BIT YOUR TONGUE
- YOU PASSED URINE
- NONE OF THE ABOVE

POSSIBLE CAUSE

You may have had a seizure, which could be due to EPILEPSY (p.524).

MEDICAL HELP

EMERGENCY! Call an ambulance if this is your first attack. Otherwise, make an appointment to see your doctor as soon as possible. For first-aid advice on what to do, see MAJOR SEIZURES (p.989).

Did you feel faint or pass out immediately after either of the following?

- GETTING UP SUDDENLY
- EMOTIONAL SHOCK
- NEITHER

POSSIBLE CAUSE
Sudden psychological shock can result in feeling faint or passing out.

SELF-HELP
Rest and ask someone to stay with you until you feel better. If it happens again, make an appointment to see your doctor.

POSSIBLE CAUSE
The most likely explanation is a temporary drop in blood pressure due to a change in position; it is usually not a cause for concern (*see* HYPOTENSION, p.414).

MEDICAL HELP
See your doctor within 24 hours if you passed out. Make an appointment to see your doctor in the next few days even if you did not pass out.

Does either of the following apply?

- YOU HAVE DIABETES
- YOU HAD NOT EATEN FOR SEVERAL HOURS BEFORE PASSING OUT
- NEITHER

POSSIBLE CAUSE
Low blood sugar levels are a possible cause of feeling faint or passing out, often with sweating, anxiety, and nausea (*see* DIABETES MELLITUS, p.687, and HYPOGLYCAEMIA, p.691).

MEDICAL HELP

URGENT! Phone your doctor immediately! Eat or drink something sweet.

Do you have any of the following symptoms?

- SHORTNESS OF BREATH
- PALER SKIN THAN NORMAL
- UNDUE TIREDNESS
- NONE OF THE ABOVE

POSSIBLE CAUSE
ANAEMIA (p.446) is a possible cause of your symptoms.

MEDICAL HELP
See your doctor within 24 hours.

Might you be pregnant?

- POSSIBLY PREGNANT
- NOT PREGNANT

POSSIBLE CAUSE
Changes in blood flow during pregnancy can cause faintness.

MEDICAL HELP
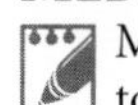
Make an appointment to see your doctor. If you are unsure whether or not you are pregnant, do a HOME PREGNANCY TEST (p.232).

Does either of the following apply?

- YOU HAVE HAD CHEST PAIN OR YOU HAVE A HEART CONDITION
- YOU HAVE HAD PALPITATIONS
- NEITHER

POSSIBLE CAUSES
You may have low blood pressure (*see* HYPOTENSION, p.414) due to worsening of a pre-existing heart condition or an irregular heartbeat (*see* ARRHYTHMIAS, p.415).

MEDICAL HELP

URGENT! Phone your doctor immediately!

If you cannot identify a possible cause for passing out from this chart, phone your doctor immediately. If you cannot identify a possible cause for feeling faint, see your doctor within 24 hours.

10 HEADACHE

Tension in head and neck muscles and fever are common causes of headache. Too much alcohol, caffeine, or nicotine may also cause a headache. Most headaches do not last for more than a few hours. If your headache lasts for more than 24 hours, is not improved by over-the-counter painkillers, or recurs several times in a week, consult your doctor.

DANGER SIGNS

Call an ambulance if a headache is accompanied by any of the following symptoms:

- Drowsiness or confusion.
- Weakness of a limb.
- Blurred vision.
- Dislike of bright light.
- Temporary unconsciousness.

START HERE

Have you hit your head within the past 24 hours?

- HEAD INJURY
- NO HEAD INJURY

Do you have a fever – a temperature of 38°C (100°F) or above?

- FEVER
- NO FEVER

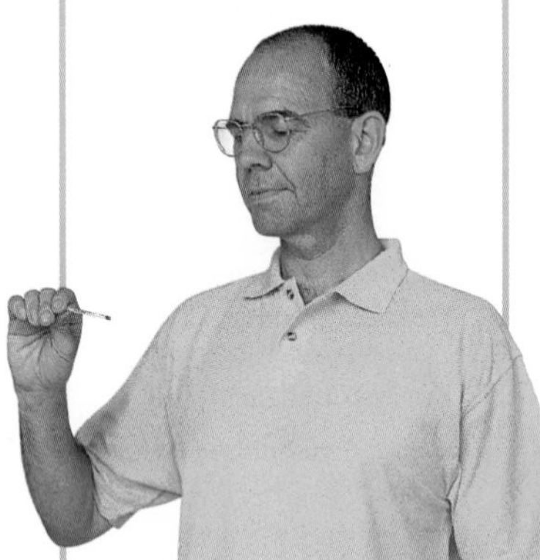

POSSIBLE CAUSES

Many minor illnesses associated with fever are accompanied by a headache. However, a serious illness such as MENINGITIS (p.527) may also be the cause. Go to chart 6, FEVER if you are 12 or over or chart 66, FEVER IN CHILDREN for a child under 12.

Are any of the danger signs listed in the box (above right) present, or have you vomited?

- DANGER SIGNS PRESENT
- VOMITED AFTER HEAD INJURY
- NO DANGER SIGNS OR VOMITING

Have you experienced nausea and/or vomiting with your headache?

- YES
- NO

POSSIBLE CAUSE

There may be damage to the tissues that surround the brain (*see* HEAD INJURIES, p.521).

MEDICAL HELP

EMERGENCY! Call an ambulance!

POSSIBLE CAUSE

A mild headache is common following a minor head injury (*see* HEAD INJURIES, p.521).

SELF-HELP

Take a painkiller (not aspirin). If your headache lasts for more than 2 hours or if you develop other symptoms, phone your doctor immediately.

POSSIBLE CAUSE

SINUSITIS (p.475) is the likely cause of your headache.

SELF-HELP

Try STEAM INHALATION (p.475). Get medical advice if you feel no better in 2 days.

How is your vision?

- BLURRED VISION
- DISTURBED IN OTHER WAYS
- UNCHANGED

POSSIBLE CAUSE
ACUTE GLAUCOMA (p.575) is a possibility, particularly if the pain is around your eye.

MEDICAL HELP
URGENT! Phone your doctor immediately!

POSSIBLE CAUSE
Your symptoms may be a side effect of the medication.

MEDICAL HELP
Make an appointment to see your doctor. Stop taking any over-the-counter medicines but continue to take prescribed medication unless advised to stop by your doctor.

Where is the pain?

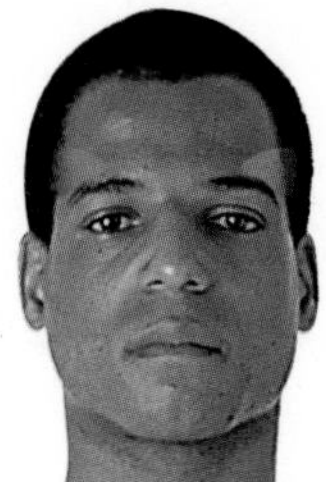

SITES OF PAIN

- OVER ONE OR BOTH TEMPLES AS SHOWN
- ELSEWHERE

POSSIBLE CAUSES
MIGRAINE (p.518) is the most likely cause of your headache, particularly if any visual problems occurred before the headache started. However, the possibility of another disorder, such as a STROKE (p.532), needs to be ruled out.

MEDICAL HELP
URGENT! Phone your doctor immediately if this is your first attack. Although the condition is probably not dangerous, your doctor should confirm the diagnosis.

Are you currently taking any prescribed or over-the-counter medication?

- MEDICATION
- NO MEDICATION

Have you had this type of headache before?

- YES
- NO

Does either of the following apply?

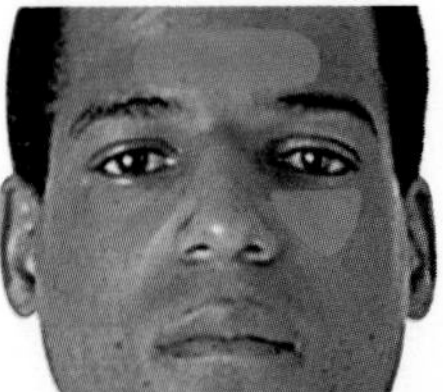

SITES OF PAIN

- THE PAIN IS FELT CHIEFLY IN THE AREAS SHOWN
- YOU HAVE RECENTLY HAD A RUNNY OR STUFFY NOSE
- NEITHER

POSSIBLE CAUSE
TEMPORAL ARTERITIS (p.464) is a possibility, particularly if you are over the age of 50 and have been feeling unwell.

MEDICAL HELP

URGENT! Phone your doctor immediately!

If you cannot identify a possible cause for your headache from this chart, make an appointment to see your doctor.

POSSIBLE CAUSE
A recurrent HEADACHE (p.518) for which there is no obvious cause, such as drinking too much alcohol, should always be investigated by your doctor.

MEDICAL HELP

Make an appointment to see your doctor.

11 VERTIGO

Vertigo is the sensation that your surroundings are moving around you. It can be very unpleasant and is often associated with nausea and vomiting. Healthy people may experience vertigo temporarily after a ride at an amusement park or after drinking too much alcohol. You should consult your doctor if you develop vertigo for no obvious reason.

WARNING **RECURRING ATTACKS OF VERTIGO**

If you have been experiencing attacks of vertigo, it is very important to avoid certain potentially hazardous activities. You should not climb ladders, operate machinery, or drive until the cause of your symptoms has been diagnosed and treated.

START HERE

Have you had any of the following symptoms?

- DISTURBED VISION
- NUMBNESS, TINGLING, OR WEAKNESS IN ANY PART OF THE BODY
- CONFUSION
- DIFFICULTY SPEAKING
- NONE OF THE ABOVE

Are any of these symptoms still present?

- SYMPTOMS PRESENT
- SYMPTOMS NO LONGER PRESENT

Have you noticed either of the following?

- HEARING LOSS
- RINGING IN THE EARS
- NEITHER

Have you experienced either of the following?

- NAUSEA OR VOMITING
- DIFFICULTY KEEPING YOUR BALANCE
- NEITHER

POSSIBLE CAUSE

There is a possibility that you have had a STROKE (p.532).

MEDICAL HELP

EMERGENCY! Call an ambulance!

POSSIBLE CAUSE

A TRANSIENT ISCHAEMIC ATTACK (p.531) is a possible cause of your symptoms.

MEDICAL HELP

URGENT! Phone your doctor immediately!

POSSIBLE CAUSE

An infection of the inner ear (see LABYRINTHITIS, p.604) is a likely cause of your symptoms.

MEDICAL HELP

See your doctor within 24 hours. In the meantime, minimize symptoms by lying down or by trying to move around as little as possible.

POSSIBLE CAUSES
MÉNIÈRE'S DISEASE (p.604) may be the cause of your symptoms. ACOUSTIC NEUROMA (p.605) is another, although less likely, possibility.

MEDICAL HELP

See your doctor within 24 hours.

Are you currently taking any prescribed medication?

- MEDICATION
- NO MEDICATION

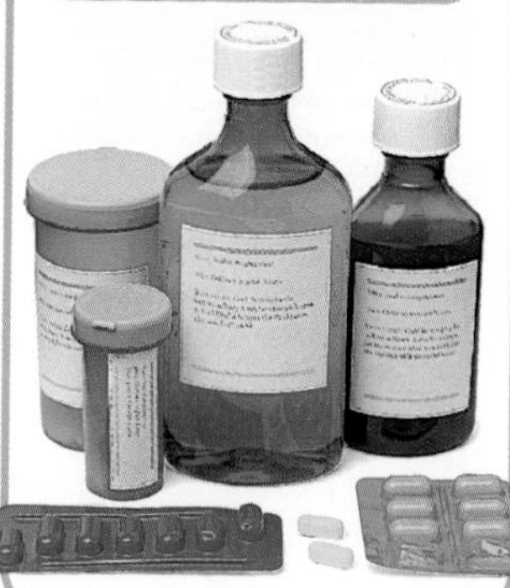

POSSIBLE CAUSE
Your symptoms may be a side effect of your medication.

MEDICAL HELP
URGENT! Phone your doctor immediately! He or she may advise you to stop taking a particular drug.

Have you been drinking alcohol?

- YES
- NO

POSSIBLE CAUSE
Your symptoms are most likely to be caused by drinking more alcohol than usual or drinking on an empty stomach (*see* ALCOHOL AND HEALTH, p.62).

SELF-HELP
The effects of alcohol should wear off within a few hours. Meanwhile, drink plenty of water. Consult your doctor if the sensation persists for longer than 12 hours.

How old are you?

- 50 OR OVER
- UNDER 50

Does turning or raising your head bring on vertigo?

- BRINGS ON VERTIGO
- NO NOTICEABLE EFFECT

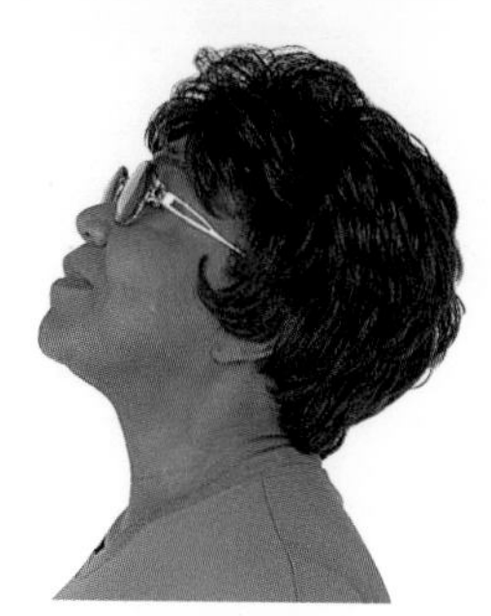

POSSIBLE CAUSE
A possible cause of your vertigo is arthritis in the neck (*see* CERVICAL SPONDYLOSIS, p.376). This disorder can result in pressure on arteries supplying areas of the brain that influence balance.

MEDICAL HELP
Make an appointment to see your doctor.

If you cannot identify a possible cause for your vertigo from this chart, see your doctor within 24 hours.

12 NUMBNESS AND/OR TINGLING

Almost everyone has experienced numbness, the loss of sensation in a part of the body, after sitting or lying in an awkward position for a while. Tingling, a prickly feeling, often occurs as sensation returns to a numb area. You should consult this chart if you experience numbness and/or tingling for which there is no obvious cause.

DANGER SIGNS

Call an ambulance if the numbness and/or tingling is accompanied by any of the following:

- Feeling faint or passing out.
- Disturbed vision.
- Confusion.
- Difficulty speaking.
- Weakness in a limb.

START HERE

Did the numbness and/or tingling occur in either of the following circumstances?

- AFTER SITTING IN ONE POSITION FOR A LONG TIME
- ON WAKING FROM A DEEP SLEEP
- NEITHER

POSSIBLE CAUSE

Pressure on nerves or on the blood vessels that supply them is the most likely cause of the numbness and tingling.

SELF-HELP

Sensation should return to normal within a few minutes of changing position. Consult your doctor if numbness or tingling persists for longer than 1 hour.

Where is the numbness and/or tingling?

- HAND OR ARM
- ELSEWHERE

Have you noticed any stiffness in your neck?

- NO STIFF NECK
- STIFF NECK

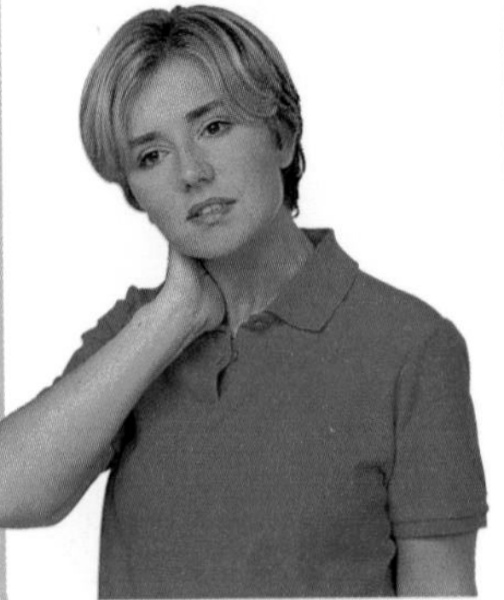

Does either of the following apply?

- NUMBNESS AND/OR TINGLING IS WORSE AT NIGHT
- PAIN SHOOTS INTO PALM OF HAND
- NEITHER

POSSIBLE CAUSE

CERVICAL SPONDYLOSIS (p.376) is a possible cause of this combination of symptoms.

MEDICAL HELP

 Make an appointment to see your doctor.

Possible cause
Carpal tunnel syndrome (p.547) is probably the cause of your symptoms.

Medical help
Make an appointment to see your doctor.

Are the affected areas on only one side of the body?
- One side only
- Both sides

Have you had any of the following symptoms?
- Feeling faint or passing out
- Disturbed vision
- Confusion
- Difficulty speaking
- Weakness in a limb
- None of the above

Possible cause
There is a possibility that you have had a stroke (p.532).

Medical help
EMERGENCY! Call an ambulance!

Are any of these symptoms still present?
- Symptoms present
- Symptoms no longer present

Do your fingers become numb and white or blue in either of the following circumstances?
- In cold weather
- When using vibrating machinery
- Neither

Possible cause
A transient ischaemic attack (p.531) is a possible cause of your symptoms.

Medical help
URGENT! Phone your doctor immediately!

Possible cause
This type of numbness is most likely to be caused by hand–arm syndrome (p.436), which is associated with long-term use of vibrating machinery.

Medical help
Make an appointment to see your doctor.

If you cannot identify a possible cause for your numbness and/or tingling from this chart, make an appointment to see your doctor.

Possible causes
Raynaud's phenomenon and Raynaud's disease (p.436) are two possible causes.

Medical help

Make an appointment to see your doctor.

13 TWITCHING AND TREMOR

Twitching (intermittent, isolated movements) and tremor (persistent trembling) are movements that cannot be controlled. Involuntary movements affect most people during times of anxiety or excitement or when falling asleep. You should consult your doctor, however, if you develop twitching or tremor at any other time.

START HERE

Was the twitching and/or tremor accompanied by either of the following?

- LOSS OF CONSCIOUSNESS
- LOSS OF CONCENTRATION OR AWARENESS
- NEITHER

POSSIBLE CAUSE

You may have had a seizure, a possible cause of which is EPILEPSY (p.524).

MEDICAL HELP

EMERGENCY! Call an ambulance if this is the first attack. Otherwise, make an appointment to see your doctor as soon as possible. For first-aid advice on what to do, see MAJOR SEIZURES (p.989).

Before the onset of tremor had you done any of the following?

- CONSUMED LARGE AMOUNTS OF COFFEE, TEA, OR COLA
- STOPPED DRINKING ALCOHOL AFTER A PERIOD OF HEAVY DRINKING
- STOPPED TAKING SLEEPING PILLS OR TRANQUILLIZERS
- NONE OF THE ABOVE

POSSIBLE CAUSES

Tremor following alcohol withdrawal indicates that you may have become dangerously dependent (*see* ALCOHOL DEPENDENCE, p.564). Stopping sleeping pills or tranquillizers after a long period of regular use can sometimes produce similar symptoms.

MEDICAL HELP

Call your doctor within 24 hours.

What kind of involuntary movement have you been experiencing?

- TREMOR (TREMBLING) OF THE HANDS
- TWITCHING OF A SMALL PART OF THE BODY SUCH AS AN EYELID
- OTHER

POSSIBLE CAUSE

NERVOUS TICS (p.550) are very common, and they are unlikely to be a sign that you have an underlying condition.

MEDICAL HELP

Make an appointment to see your doctor if you are worried about the twitching.

POSSIBLE CAUSE
Excessive caffeine intake is most likely to be the cause of your tremor.

SELF-HELP
Abstain from all products that contain caffeine for at least 24 hours. If the tremor persists, make an appointment to see your doctor.

POSSIBLE CAUSES
HYPERTHYROIDISM (p.679) is a possibility. However, ANXIETY DISORDERS (p.551) can cause some of these symptoms.

MEDICAL HELP
Make an appointment to see your doctor.

POSSIBLE CAUSE
Your symptoms may be a side effect of the medication.

MEDICAL HELP
Call your doctor within 24 hours. Stop taking over-the-counter medicines but continue to take any prescribed medication unless advised to stop by your doctor.

Do you have any of the following symptoms?

- WEIGHT LOSS WITH INCREASED APPETITE
- FEELING CONSTANTLY ON EDGE
- INCREASED SWEATING
- BULGING EYES
- NONE OF THE ABOVE

POSSIBLE CAUSE
PARKINSON'S DISEASE (p.539) could be the cause.

MEDICAL HELP

Make an appointment to see your doctor.

Are you currently taking any prescribed or over-the-counter medication?

- MEDICATION
- NO MEDICATION

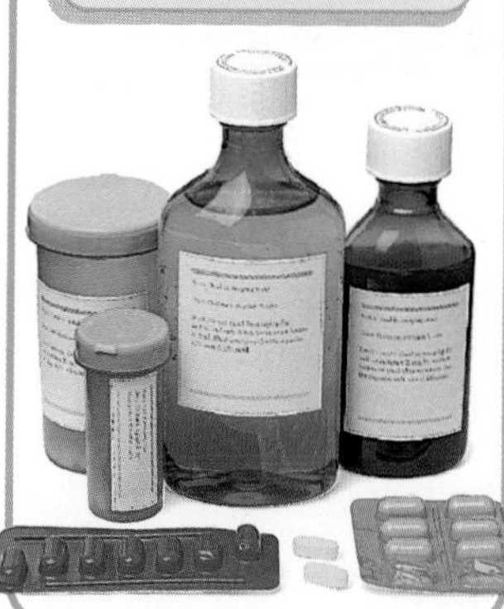

How old are you?

- 55 OR OVER
- UNDER 55

Do any of the following apply?

- SYMPTOMS ARE WORSE WHEN THE AFFECTED PART IS AT REST
- YOUR FACE HAS BECOME EXPRESSIONLESS
- YOU HAVE DIFFICULTY INITIATING ANY MOVEMENT
- NONE OF THE ABOVE

If you cannot identify a possible cause for your twitching or tremor from this chart, make an appointment to see your doctor.

14 FACIAL PAIN

Pain in the face may be sharp and stabbing or dull and throbbing. Inflammation of structures in the face, such as the sinuses or teeth, is the most common cause of facial pain. Facial pain is usually short-lived, but some types, such as neuralgia, may persist. Consult your doctor if the pain is persistent, unexplained, or not relieved by taking painkillers.

START HERE

Where is the pain?

- OVER ONE OR BOTH TEMPLES
- IN OR AROUND THE EYE
- ELSEWHERE

Do any of the following apply?

- YOUR SCALP IS SENSITIVE TO TOUCH
- YOU HAVE BEEN FEELING UNWELL
- PAIN COMES ON WHEN CHEWING
- NONE OF THE ABOVE

Go to chart 23 PAINFUL OR IRRITATED EYE

POSSIBLE CAUSE

TEMPORAL ARTERITIS (p.464) is a possibility, especially if you are over the age of 50.

MEDICAL HELP

 URGENT! Phone your doctor immediately!

Which of the following describes your pain?

- STABBING PAIN THAT OCCURS WHEN TOUCHING THE FACE OR CHEWING
- ACHING PAIN ON CHEWING AND/OR YAWNING
- DULL ACHING AROUND ONE OR BOTH CHEEKBONES
- NONE OF THE ABOVE

POSSIBLE CAUSE

TRIGEMINAL NEURALGIA (p.546) is a possible cause of this type of pain.

MEDICAL HELP

 Make an appointment to see your doctor.

POSSIBLE CAUSE

TEMPOROMANDIBULAR JOINT DISORDER (p.616) is a possible cause of this type of pain.

MEDICAL HELP

 Make an appointment to see your doctor or dentist.

POSSIBLE CAUSES

SINUSITIS (p.475) is the likely cause of your symptoms, especially if you have recently had a cold and both sides of your face are affected. If only one side is affected, a dental problem is more likely (*see* DENTAL ABSCESS, p.611).

SELF-HELP

Try STEAM INHALATION (p.475) if you think you may have sinusitis. Get advice from your doctor or dentist if you do not feel better within 2 days.

If you cannot identify a possible cause for your facial pain from this chart, make an appointment to see your doctor.

15 DIFFICULTY SPEAKING

Difficulty speaking includes the recent development of slurred or unclear speech and the inability to find or use words. These symptoms may have an obvious cause, such as drinking too much alcohol, or a more serious condition affecting the brain's speech centres may be to blame. If your speech suddenly deteriorates, consult your doctor urgently.

START HERE

Have you had any of the following symptoms?

- DISTURBED VISION
- NUMBNESS, TINGLING, OR WEAKNESS IN ANY PART OF THE BODY
- FEELING FAINT OR PASSING OUT
- CONFUSION
- INABILITY TO MOVE THE MUSCLES ON ONE SIDE OF THE FACE
- NONE OF THE ABOVE

Are any of your symptoms still present?

- SYMPTOMS PRESENT
- SYMPTOMS NO LONGER PRESENT

POSSIBLE CAUSE
A STROKE (p.532) is a possible cause of your symptoms.

MEDICAL HELP
EMERGENCY! Call an ambulance!

POSSIBLE CAUSE
It is possible that you have had a TRANSIENT ISCHAEMIC ATTACK (p.531).

MEDICAL HELP
URGENT! Phone your doctor immediately!

POSSIBLE CAUSES
A type of FACIAL PALSY (p.548), such as Bell's palsy, is a possible cause of your symptoms.

MEDICAL HELP
URGENT! Phone your doctor immediately!

Do any of the following apply?

- YOU HAVE A SORE MOUTH OR TONGUE
- YOU HAVE BEEN DRINKING ALCOHOL
- YOU HAVE BEEN TAKING MEDICATION OR DRUGS OF ANY KIND
- NONE OF THE ABOVE

POSSIBLE CAUSE
Pain or soreness of the mouth or tongue from a condition such as GLOSSITIS (p.633) can impair speech.

MEDICAL HELP

Make an appointment to see your doctor.

POSSIBLE CAUSE
Drinking even a moderate amount of alcohol can cause slurred speech.

MEDICAL HELP

If you regularly drink enough alcohol to cause slurred speech, you should make an appointment to see your doctor for advice about reducing your alcohol intake.

POSSIBLE CAUSE
Your symptoms may be a side effect of medication or drugs.

MEDICAL HELP
See your doctor within 24 hours. He or she may advise you to stop taking a particular medication.

If you cannot identify a possible cause for your speech difficulty from this chart, see your doctor within 24 hours.

16 FORGETFULNESS AND/OR CONFUSION

Most people are forgetful sometimes, especially if they are very busy. Absent-mindedness is also a natural part of the aging process. Confusion is the inability to think clearly and may include forgetfulness. You should consult your doctor if episodes of forgetfulness and/or confusion occur frequently or are severe enough to disrupt everyday life.

WARNING SUDDEN ONSET OF CONFUSION
Phone a doctor immediately if a person suddenly becomes very confused or disoriented about time or place or if someone seems to be seeing or hearing things that are not there.

START HERE

Has the forgetfulness and/or confusion come on since a head injury?

- HEAD INJURY
- NO HEAD INJURY

POSSIBLE CAUSE
Damage to the brain may cause such symptoms (*see* HEAD INJURIES, p.521).

MEDICAL HELP

URGENT! Phone your doctor immediately!

Have you had any of the following symptoms?

- DISTURBED VISION
- NUMBNESS, TINGLING, OR WEAKNESS IN ANY PART OF THE BODY
- VERTIGO OR LOSS OF CONSCIOUSNESS
- DIFFICULTY SPEAKING
- NONE OF THE ABOVE

Are any of these symptoms still present?

- SYMPTOMS PRESENT
- SYMPTOMS NO LONGER PRESENT

POSSIBLE CAUSE
A TRANSIENT ISCHAEMIC ATTACK (p.531) is a possible cause of your symptoms.

MEDICAL HELP

URGENT! Phone your doctor immediately!

POSSIBLE CAUSE
There is a possibility that you have had a STROKE (p.532).

MEDICAL HELP

EMERGENCY! Call an ambulance!

Do you have a fever – a temperature of 38°C (100°F) or above?

- FEVER
- NO FEVER

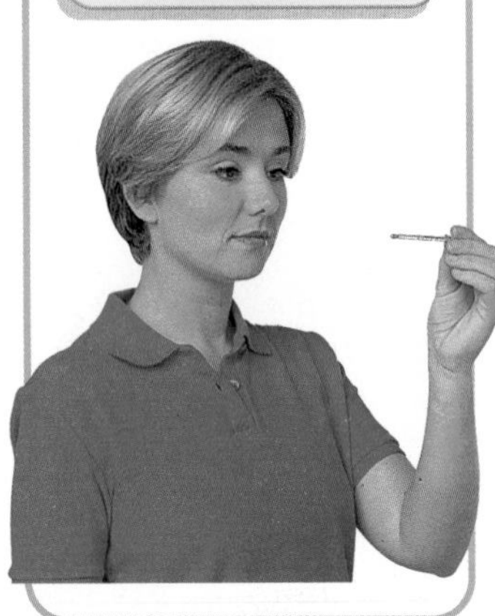

POSSIBLE CAUSES
Fever, especially a temperature that is over 39°C (102°F), may itself be a cause of confusion. However, confusion may be due to a number of serious diseases, such as PNEUMONIA (p.490), that also cause fever.

MEDICAL HELP
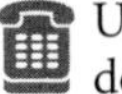
URGENT! Phone your doctor immediately!

Do you suffer from any of the following?

- HEART DISEASE
- LUNG DISEASE
- DIABETES MELLITUS
- NONE OF THE ABOVE

POSSIBLE CAUSES
Lack of oxygen to the brain caused by a worsening of your underlying condition may cause confusion (*see* CHRONIC OBSTRUCTIVE PULMONARY DISEASE, p.487, and CHRONIC HEART FAILURE, p.413).

MEDICAL HELP
URGENT! Phone your doctor immediately!

POSSIBLE CAUSE
Confusion may indicate low or very high blood sugar levels in someone with diabetes (*see* HYPOGLYCAEMIA, p.691, and DIABETES MELLITUS, p.687).

MEDICAL HELP
URGENT! Phone your doctor immediately! You should also eat or drink something sweet at once.

Are you currently taking any prescribed or over-the-counter medication?

- MEDICATION
- NO MEDICATION

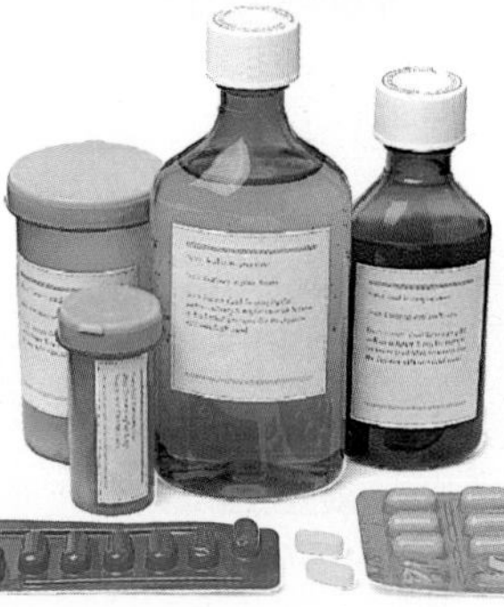

POSSIBLE CAUSE
Your symptoms may be a side effect of the medication.

MEDICAL HELP
See your doctor within 24 hours. Stop taking over-the-counter medicines but continue to take any prescribed medication unless advised to stop by your doctor.

Have you been drinking alcohol within the past few hours?

- YES
- NO

POSSIBLE CAUSE
Drinking too much alcohol can cause confusion and, more seriously, can also lead to loss of memory (*see* ALCOHOL AND HEALTH, p.62).

MEDICAL HELP
Make an appointment to see your doctor for advice about reducing the amount of alcohol you drink.

Is gradually increasing forgetfulness and confusion in an elderly person accompanied by any of the following?

- PERSONALITY CHANGE
- REDUCED ATTENTION TO PERSONAL HYGIENE
- INABILITY TO MANAGE EVERYDAY PROBLEMS
- NONE OF THE ABOVE

POSSIBLE CAUSES
These symptoms may indicate a decline in brain function (*see* DEMENTIA, p.535). However, DEPRESSION (p.554) may cause similar symptoms.

MEDICAL HELP

Make an appointment to see your doctor.

If you cannot identify a possible cause for forgetfulness and/or confusion from this chart, make an appointment to see your doctor.

17 FEELING DEPRESSED

Feeling depressed may include a lack of energy, sadness, and low self-esteem. It is normal to feel down from time to time, especially after disappointments. More severe feelings of depression are also natural after major upsets, such as the death of someone close. You should consult your doctor if depression is severe or if it persists for more than 2 weeks.

WARNING HAVING SUICIDAL THOUGHTS

Anyone who considers suicide is in need of urgent medical help. If you cannot persuade the person to contact a doctor, try to encourage him or her to seek other professional help or to call a suicide prevention hotline such as the Samaritans, who counsel people in despair and are available day and night.

START HERE

Do you have any of the following symptoms?

- LACK OF ENERGY
- DIFFICULTY SLEEPING
- LOW SELF-ESTEEM
- INABILITY TO CONCENTRATE OR TO MAKE DECISIONS
- LACK OF INTEREST IN SEX
- NONE OF THE ABOVE

POSSIBLE CAUSE
You are unlikely to be suffering from serious depression. Your low spirits are probably the result of a temporary stress or disappointment.

MEDICAL HELP
Make an appointment to see your doctor if your feelings of depression last for more than 2 weeks, if your depression gets worse, or if you develop other symptoms.

Did your depression develop after any of the following?

- BEREAVEMENT
- DIVORCE
- JOB LOSS
- OTHER DISTRESSING LIFE EVENT
- NONE OF THE ABOVE

POSSIBLE CAUSE
Grief and depression are normal following the loss of someone close (*see* LOSS AND BEREAVEMENT, p.76).

MEDICAL HELP
Make an appointment to see your doctor, who may provide support while you come to terms with your loss.

POSSIBLE CAUSE
Some life events can be devastating and a period of DEPRESSION (p.554) is natural.

MEDICAL HELP

Make an appointment to see your doctor.

Do any of the following apply?

- YOU HAVE RECENTLY HAD A BABY
- YOU HAVE RECENTLY HAD A VIRAL ILLNESS
- YOU ARE RECUPERATING FROM MAJOR SURGERY OR A SERIOUS ILLNESS
- NONE OF THE ABOVE

POSSIBLE CAUSE
Major hormonal changes after childbirth sometimes lead to depression (*see* DEPRESSION AFTER CHILDBIRTH, p.807).

MEDICAL HELP
Make an appointment to see your doctor.

POSSIBLE CAUSE
A serious accident, major surgical operation, or serious illness can be followed by DEPRESSION (p.554).

MEDICAL HELP
Make an appointment to see your doctor.

POSSIBLE CAUSE
Viral illnesses may sometimes be followed by a period of mild DEPRESSION (p.554).

SELF-HELP
Follow a healthy diet and get plenty of sleep to rebuild your strength. If your depression continues longer than 2 weeks after the viral symptoms have gone, make an appointment to see your doctor.

POSSIBLE CAUSE
Regularly drinking too much alcohol leads to depression in some people (*see* ALCOHOL DEPENDENCE, p.564).

MEDICAL HELP
Make an appointment to see your doctor for advice about cutting down your alcohol intake.

Do you regularly drink more than the recommended limit of alcohol (*see* SAFE ALCOHOL LIMITS, p.62)?

- MORE THAN THE LIMIT
- WITHIN THE LIMIT

POSSIBLE CAUSE
STRESS (p.74) is a common cause of depression.

SELF-HELP
Try to reduce the impact of stress in your life (*see* STRESS, p.74). Make an appointment to see your doctor if you have severe depression or if it is interfering with your normal everyday activities.

Have you been suffering from particular stress at home or at work?

- YES
- NO

Are you male or female?

- MALE
- FEMALE

Do you feel depressed only in the days before your period is due?

- YES
- NO

POSSIBLE CAUSE
Your depression may be related to your monthly hormonal changes (*see* PREMENSTRUAL SYNDROME, p.736).

MEDICAL HELP
Make an appointment to see your doctor.

POSSIBLE CAUSE
Your symptoms may be a side effect of the medication.

MEDICAL HELP
Make an appointment to see your doctor. Continue to take the medication unless advised to stop by your doctor.

Are you currently taking any prescribed medication or recreational drugs?

- MEDICATION
- RECREATIONAL DRUGS
- NEITHER

POSSIBLE CAUSE
Recreational drugs can cause psychological disturbances, including depression (*see* DRUGS AND HEALTH, p.65).

MEDICAL HELP

See your doctor within 24 hours.

If you cannot identify a possible cause for your depression from this chart, make an appointment to see your doctor.

18 ANXIETY

A feeling of unease or agitation, anxiety is a normal response to stress. A new job or problem in a relationship may result in anxiety. It may also occur as an effect of caffeine or certain drugs. Often, there is no obvious cause. Anxiety can cause palpitations and sweating, and it may interfere with sleep. If anxiety disrupts your daily activities, consult your doctor.

START HERE

Do you feel anxious in either of the following situations?

- WHEN FACED WITH CERTAIN ANIMALS, OBJECTS, OR SITUATIONS
- WHEN YOUR USUAL WAY OF DOING THINGS IS DISRUPTED
- NEITHER OR BOTH OF THE ABOVE

POSSIBLE CAUSES
Anxiety when faced with social situations such as public speaking is a normal reaction. Unfounded anxiety related to animals, objects, or situations is termed a PHOBIA (p.552).

MEDICAL HELP
Make an appointment to see your doctor if anxiety is interfering with normal everyday activities.

POSSIBLE CAUSE
You may have an OBSESSIVE–COMPULSIVE DISORDER (p.553).

MEDICAL HELP
Make an appointment to see your doctor if anxiety is interfering with normal everyday activities.

Have you been feeling anxious since stopping addictive behaviour, such as smoking, drinking alcohol, taking drugs, or gambling?

- NO
- YES

POSSIBLE CAUSES
Withdrawal from an addictive behaviour, such as gambling, or from an addictive substance, including alcohol or some prescribed drugs, is likely to cause strong feelings of anxiety.

MEDICAL HELP
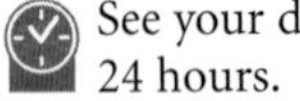
See your doctor within 24 hours.

Do you have any of the following symptoms?

- LACK OF ENERGY
- LOW SELF-ESTEEM
- LACK OF INTEREST IN SEX
- NONE OF THE ABOVE

POSSIBLE CAUSE
You may be suffering from DEPRESSION (p.554) as well as an ANXIETY DISORDER (p.551).

MEDICAL HELP

Make an appointment to see your doctor.

Do you have either of the following symptoms?

- WEIGHT LOSS DESPITE GOOD APPETITE
- BULGING EYES
- NEITHER

POSSIBLE CAUSE
HYPERTHYROIDISM (p.679) is a possible cause.

MEDICAL HELP

Make an appointment to see your doctor

If you cannot identify a possible cause for your anxiety from this chart, make an appointment to see your doctor.

19 ITCHING

Itching – irritation of the skin that leads to an intense desire to scratch – has many possible causes, including allergy and infection. Itchiness can affect the whole body or may be confined to a small area. It may be accompanied by skin changes, sometimes due to scratching, but may also occur with no noticeable change in the appearance of the skin.

START HERE

Is the itching confined to any of the following areas?

- SCALP → *Go to chart 22* HAIR AND SCALP PROBLEMS
- GENITAL AREA (WOMEN) → *Go to chart 62* GENITAL IRRITATION IN WOMEN
- GENITAL AREA (MEN) → see below
- ANUS → *Go to chart 38* ANAL AND RECTAL PROBLEMS
- NONE OF THE ABOVE

POSSIBLE CAUSES
Itching of the genital area in men may be due to a fungal infection (*see* RINGWORM, p.352) or PUBIC LICE (p.768).

MEDICAL HELP
Make an appointment to see your doctor.

Is there a rash in the itchy area?

- RASH
- NO RASH

Are you currently taking any prescribed or over-the-counter medication?

- MEDICATION
- NO MEDICATION → *Go to chart 20* GENERAL SKIN PROBLEMS

POSSIBLE CAUSE
Your symptoms may be a side effect of the medication.

MEDICAL HELP
Make an appointment to see your doctor. Stop taking any over-the-counter medicines but continue to take prescribed medication unless advised to stop by your doctor.

Do you have either of the following symptoms?

- YELLOW SKIN AND YELLOW WHITES OF EYES
- VERY DRY, SCALY SKIN
- NEITHER

POSSIBLE CAUSE
JAUNDICE (p.643) sometimes causes itching.

MEDICAL HELP

See your doctor within 24 hours.

POSSIBLE CAUSE
Dry skin is often itchy.

SELF-HELP
Apply moisturizing cream daily. If this does not relieve itching, make an appointment to see your doctor.

If you cannot identify a possible cause for your itching from this chart, make an appointment to see your doctor.

20 GENERAL SKIN PROBLEMS

Skin problems are often caused by localized infection, allergy, or irritation. They are not usually serious, although widespread skin problems may be distressing. You should consult your doctor if a skin problem lasts more than a month or causes severe discomfort; a new lump appears, especially if it is dark-coloured; or a sore fails to heal.

START HERE

What type of skin problem do you have?

- RASH
- OTHER SKIN PROBLEM

Do you have a fever – a temperature of 38°C (100°F) or above?

- FEVER
- NO FEVER

Go to chart 21 RASH WITH FEVER

Is the affected skin itchy?

- ITCHY
- NOT ITCHY

Have you noticed any of the following?

- RED, TENDER, AND HOT AREA OF SKIN
- NEW MOLE OR A CHANGE IN AN EXISTING MOLE
- AN OPEN SORE THAT HAS NOT HEALED AFTER 3 WEEKS
- HARD, SKIN-COLOURED LUMP ON HAND OR SOLE
- NONE OF THE ABOVE

POSSIBLE CAUSE
CELLULITIS (p.352) may be the cause of your symptoms.

MEDICAL HELP

URGENT! Phone your doctor immediately!

POSSIBLE CAUSE
SKIN CANCER (p.344) is a possible cause.

MEDICAL HELP

Make an appointment to see your doctor.

POSSIBLE CAUSES
This is likely to be a wart or verruca (*see* WARTS, p.354), or a callus (*see* CALLUSES AND CORNS, p.349).

MEDICAL HELP
Make an appointment to see your doctor if you are uncertain about the diagnosis.

POSSIBLE CAUSE
PSORIASIS (p.332) can produce this type of rash.

MEDICAL HELP

Make an appointment to see your doctor.

Does your skin problem fit any of the following descriptions?

- A PAINFUL, BLISTERY RASH IN ONLY ONE AREA ON ONE SIDE OF THE BODY
- REDDENED PATCHES COVERED WITH SILVERY SCALES
- BLISTERY, OOZING RASH ON OR AROUND THE LIPS
- A PAINFUL RED LUMP WITH A YELLOW CENTRE
- NONE OF THE ABOVE

POSSIBLE CAUSE
This may be a BOIL (p.351).

SELF-HELP
Follow the self-help measures for a BOIL (p.351). Phone your doctor if the condition has not improved in 24 hours.

What does the affected skin look like?

- AREAS OF INFLAMED SKIN WITH A SCALY SURFACE
- ONE OR MORE RED BUMPS WITH A CENTRAL DARK SPOT
- ONE OR MORE RED RAISED AREAS (WEALS) THAT COME AND GO
- NONE OF THE ABOVE

POSSIBLE CAUSE

URTICARIA (p.468) is possible.

SELF-HELP

Soothe the irritation with cold compresses or calamine lotion. Over-the-counter antihistamine tablets may help. Get medical advice at once if breathing difficulties develop.

POSSIBLE CAUSE

Shingles (*see* HERPES ZOSTER, p.290) is a possible cause of this type of rash.

MEDICAL HELP

 See your doctor within 24 hours.

POSSIBLE CAUSES

You may have IMPETIGO (p.351). However, if this is a recurring problem, a COLD SORE (p.354) is more likely.

MEDICAL HELP

See your doctor within 24 hours if the diagnosis is not clear. For COLD SORES (p.354), use self-help measures.

What do the edges of the rash look like?

- MERGE INTO SURROUNDING SKIN
- CLEARLY DEFINED MARGINS

POSSIBLE CAUSE

RINGWORM (p.352) may be the cause of your rash.

MEDICAL HELP

 Make an appointment to see your doctor.

POSSIBLE CAUSE

Insect bites, possibly from fleas or mosquitoes, may be the cause of such itchy bumps.

SELF-HELP

The first-aid advice for INSECT STINGS (p.995) may help to relieve symptoms.

Does either of the following apply?

- YOU HAVE A RASH THAT SPREADS OUT FROM A CENTRAL RED SPOT
- YOU HAVE BEEN BITTEN BY A TICK
- NEITHER

POSSIBLE CAUSE

There is a possibility that you have LYME DISEASE (p.303).

MEDICAL HELP

 See your doctor within 24 hours.

POSSIBLE CAUSES

SEBORRHOEIC DERMATITIS (p.335) or ECZEMA (p.333) may be causing your rash.

SELF-HELP

Avoid using harsh soaps or detergents on the skin. A mild emollient cream should help to soothe the rash. Make an appointment to see your doctor if your rash does not improve within 1 week or if other symptoms develop.

POSSIBLE CAUSE

Your symptoms may be a side effect of the medication.

MEDICAL HELP

URGENT! Phone your doctor immediately! He or she may advise you to stop taking a particular medication.

Are you currently taking any prescribed or over-the-counter medication?

- MEDICATION
- NO MEDICATION

If you cannot identify a possible cause for your skin problem from this chart, make an appointment to see your doctor.

21 RASH WITH FEVER

If you have a rash without fever, see chart 20

If you or your child has a temperature of 38°C (100°F) or above, you should check whether a rash is also present. A rash with fever is usually caused by a viral infection. Most viral infections are not serious. However, a rash may alert you to the possibility of potentially life-threatening meningitis.

DANGER SIGNS

Call an ambulance if a rash and fever are accompanied by any of the following symptoms:

- Abnormal drowsiness.
- Seizures.
- Temperature of 39°C (102°F) or above.
- Abnormally rapid breathing (*see* CHECKING YOUR CHILD'S BREATHING RATE, p.205).
- Noisy or difficult breathing.
- Severe headache.

START HERE

What are the features of the rash?

- WIDESPREAD ITCHY, BLISTERY RASH
- A RASH THAT SPREADS OUT FROM A CENTRAL RED SPOT
- FLAT, DARK RED SPOTS THAT DO NOT FADE WHEN PRESSED
- DULL RED SPOTS OR BLOTCHES THAT FADE WHEN PRESSED
- BRIGHT RED RASH, PARTICULARLY AFFECTING THE CHEEKS
- LIGHT RED OR PINK RASH MAINLY ON THE TRUNK AND/OR FACE
- NONE OF THE ABOVE

POSSIBLE CAUSE

CHICKENPOX (p.290) is a possible cause of this type of rash with fever.

MEDICAL HELP

See your doctor within 24 hours. Meanwhile, follow the advice for BRINGING DOWN A FEVER (p.289).

POSSIBLE CAUSE

There is a possibility that you have LYME DISEASE (p.303).

MEDICAL HELP

See your doctor within 24 hours. Meanwhile, follow the advice for BRINGING DOWN A FEVER (p.289).

POSSIBLE CAUSES

RUBELLA (p.294), also known as German measles, may be the cause of these symptoms. ROSEOLA INFANTUM (p.830), which mainly affects infants under 4 years, is another possibility, particularly if the rash was preceded by fever.

MEDICAL HELP

See your doctor within 24 hours to confirm the diagnosis. Meanwhile, follow the advice for BRINGING DOWN A FEVER (p.289).

POSSIBLE CAUSE

A PARVOVIRUS INFECTION (p.294) may be the cause of such a rash and other symptoms in a young child.

MEDICAL HELP

See your doctor within 24 hours. Meanwhile, follow the advice for BRINGING DOWN A FEVER (p.289).

If you cannot identify a possible cause for your rash and fever from this chart, see your doctor within 24 hours.

Do you have any of the following symptoms?

- Severe headache
- Drowsiness or confusion
- Dislike of bright light
- Neck pain on bending the head forwards
- Nausea or vomiting
- None of the above

Possible cause

Meningitis (p.527) could be a cause of your symptoms.

Medical help

 EMERGENCY! Call an ambulance!

Possible causes

This type of rash may be due to a severe allergic reaction, such as a reaction to penicillin (*see* Drug allergy, p.467). It may also be the result of a blood disorder, such as thrombocytopenia (p.453) or, in children, Henoch–Schönlein purpura (p.838).

Medical help

 URGENT! Phone your doctor immediately!

SYMPTOM ASSESSMENT

Checking a red rash

If you develop a dark red rash, check if it fades on pressure by pressing the side of a drinking glass on to it. If the rash is visible through the glass, it may be a form of purpura (p.339), a rash caused by bleeding from tiny blood vessels in the skin. Purpura can be caused by one of several serious disorders and needs prompt medical attention. You should call an ambulance if you have a high fever, severe headache, or any other danger sign (opposite).

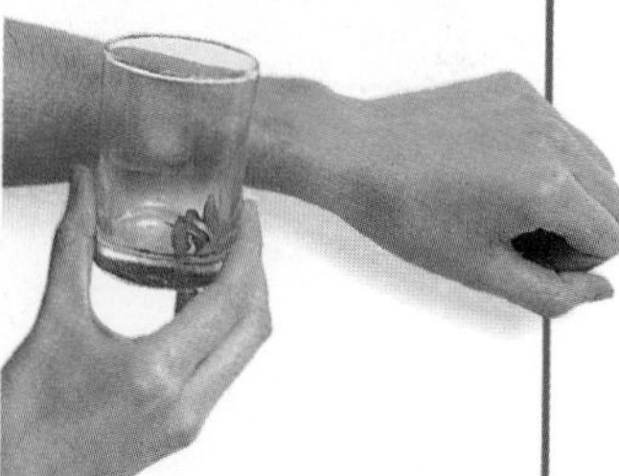

Checking a rash
In this example, the rash has faded under the glass – a sign that the rash is not serious.

Have you noticed any of the following symptoms in the past few days?

- Runny nose
- Cough
- Red eyes
- None of the above

Possible cause

Measles (p.293) is a possible cause of your symptoms.

Medical help

See your doctor within 24 hours. Meanwhile, follow the advice for bringing down a fever (p.289).

Do you have a severe sore throat?

- Yes → *Go to chart 27* Sore throat
- No → **If you cannot identify a possible cause for your rash and fever from this chart, see your doctor within 24 hours.**

22 HAIR AND SCALP PROBLEMS

The condition and appearance of your hair can be affected by your general state of health. Hair is also susceptible to damage and usually becomes thinner with age, especially in men. The scalp may be affected by the same skin problems as other areas of the body. You should consult your doctor if you are particularly worried about a hair or scalp problem.

START HERE

Have you noticed either of the following?

- GENERALIZED HAIR THINNING
- HAIR LOSS FROM LOCALIZED AREAS
- NEITHER

Have any of the following occurred in the past 2–3 months?

- YOU HAVE HAD A PROLONGED OR SERIOUS ILLNESS
- YOU HAVE HAD A BABY
- YOU HAVE STOPPED TAKING ORAL CONTRACEPTIVES
- NONE OF THE ABOVE

POSSIBLE CAUSE
Any of these events can cause temporary hair thinning.

MEDICAL HELP
Make an appointment to see your doctor if hair growth does not start to return to normal within a few weeks.

Do you have any of the following symptoms?

- TIREDNESS
- INCREASED DRYNESS OR ROUGHNESS OF THE SKIN
- FEELING THE COLD MORE THAN YOU USED TO
- UNEXPLAINED WEIGHT GAIN
- NONE OF THE ABOVE

Do you have either of the following problems affecting the scalp?

- FLAKING WITH OR WITHOUT ITCHING
- ITCHING
- NEITHER

POSSIBLE CAUSE
An itchy scalp may indicate HEAD LICE (p.831), especially in children.

SELF-HELP
Follow the advice for TREATING HEAD LICE (p.831). See your doctor if you are uncertain about the diagnosis.

POSSIBLE CAUSES
DANDRUFF (p.358) is the most common cause of a flaky scalp. However, PSORIASIS (p.332) is also a possibility.

SELF-HELP
Use an antidandruff shampoo. Make an appointment to see your doctor if this self-help measure does not bring about an improvement in your symptoms within a month.

POSSIBLE CAUSE
HYPOTHYROIDISM (p.680) may be a possibility.

MEDICAL HELP
Make an appointment to see your doctor.

POSSIBLE CAUSE
Your hair loss may be a side effect of the medication.

MEDICAL HELP
Make an appointment to see your doctor. Continue to take the medication unless advised to stop by your doctor.

POSSIBLE CAUSE
Any of these forms of styling can damage the hair, leading to overall hair thinning.

SELF-HELP
Your hair should recover if you do not use heat and harsh chemicals and avoid braiding your hair. If your hair has been severely damaged, it may help to have it cut short.

Are you currently taking any prescribed medication?

- MEDICATION
- NO MEDICATION

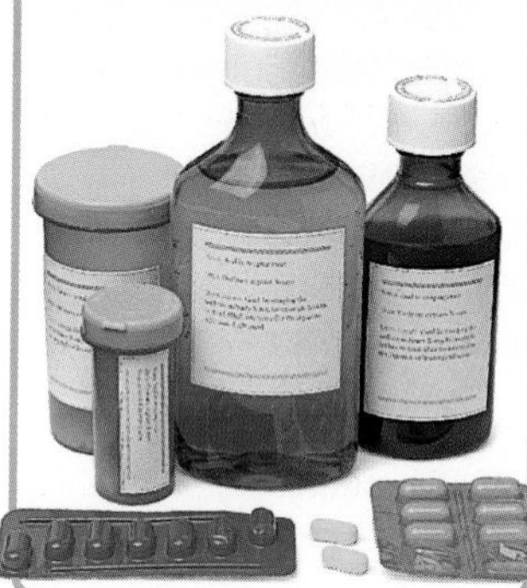

POSSIBLE CAUSE
MALE-PATTERN BALDNESS (p.359) typically causes this type of hair loss in adult men. It may also occur in women with a hormone imbalance.

MEDICAL HELP
Make an appointment to see your doctor if you are concerned about hair loss.

Have you used any of the following hair-styling methods?

- TIGHT BRAIDING
- HEATED ROLLERS OR TONGS
- BLEACHING, PERMING, OR DYEING
- NONE OF THE ABOVE

What type of hair loss have you noticed?

- THINNING HAIR FROM THE FOREHEAD OR CROWN
- BALD PATCHES SURROUNDED BY NORMAL HAIR GROWTH
- NONE OF THE ABOVE

POSSIBLE CAUSES
Patchy hair loss may be the result of RINGWORM (p.352) of the scalp or ALOPECIA (p.358).

MEDICAL HELP

Make an appointment to see your doctor.

If you cannot identify a possible cause for your hair or scalp problem from this chart, make an appointment to see your doctor.

23 PAINFUL OR IRRITATED EYE

Injury, infection, and allergy are the most common causes of discomfort or irritation of the eye and eyelids. A painless red area in the white of the eye is likely to be a burst blood vessel and should clear up without treatment. However, you should see your doctor if your eyes are sore. Consult your doctor immediately if your vision deteriorates.

WARNING CONTACT LENS WEARERS

If you wear contact lenses and experience any kind of eye pain or irritation, remove your lenses without delay and do not use them again until the cause of the problem has been identified and treated. If the pain is caused by grit under the lens, there is a risk that the cornea will be scratched. Make an appointment to see your optician.

START HERE

Does either of the following apply?

- YOU HAVE INJURED YOUR EYE
- YOU HAVE SOMETHING IN YOUR EYE
- NEITHER

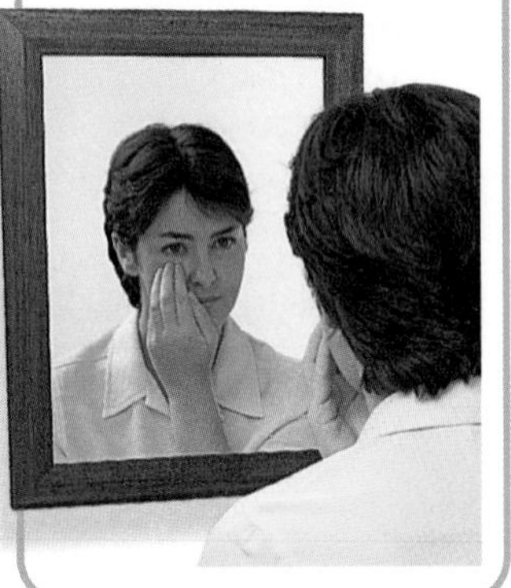

POSSIBLE CAUSE

A foreign body in your eye is likely to cause pain and possibly redness.

SELF-HELP

Follow the first-aid advice for a FOREIGN BODY IN THE EYE (p.993). Do not try to remove a particle that is embedded in the eye. In this case, seek emergency help in hospital.

How would you describe your main symptom?

- PAIN IN AND AROUND THE EYE
- THE EYE FEELS GRITTY
- ITCHING OR IRRITATION OF THE EYELID
- TENDER RED LUMP ON THE EYELID
- NONE OF THE ABOVE

POSSIBLE CAUSES

An infected hair follicle (*see* STYE, p.583) or infected gland in the eyelid (*see* CHALAZION, p.584) may be the cause of your symptoms.

SELF-HELP

Follow the advice for STYE (p.583) or CHALAZION (p.584). Make an appointment to see your doctor if self-help measures do not produce an improvement within 3 days.

Has your vision deteriorated since the injury?

- YES
- NO

POSSIBLE CAUSE

A serious eye injury is possible.

MEDICAL HELP

URGENT! Phone your doctor immediately! Expert help may be needed to prevent permanent damage.

POSSIBLE CAUSE

Your pain may be due to a minor eye injury.

MEDICAL HELP

See your doctor within 24 hours. You can take first-aid measures to relieve pain (*see* EYE WOUND, p.993), but any eye injury should be assessed by a doctor.

Is your vision blurred?

- BLURRED
- NOT BLURRED

POSSIBLE CAUSES
ACUTE GLAUCOMA (p.575) or UVEITIS (p.574) are possible causes.

MEDICAL HELP
 URGENT! Phone your doctor immediately!

Is your eyelid turned inwards or outwards?

- EYELID TURNED INWARDS
- EYELID TURNED OUTWARDS
- APPEARS NORMAL

POSSIBLE CAUSE
ENTROPION (p.584) may be the cause of your problem.

MEDICAL HELP
 Make an appointment to see your doctor.

POSSIBLE CAUSE
ECTROPION (p.584) may be the cause of your problem.

MEDICAL HELP
 Make an appointment to see your doctor.

POSSIBLE CAUSE
CLUSTER HEADACHES (p.519) are a possible cause, especially if the eye is red and/or watery.

MEDICAL HELP
 See your doctor within 24 hours.

POSSIBLE CAUSE
BLEPHARITIS (p.583) may be the cause of irritation or itching of the eyelids, especially if the skin is scaly and inflamed.

SELF-HELP
Follow the self-help advice for BLEPHARITIS (p.583). Make an appointment to see your doctor if self-help measures do not help.

Is there any discharge from the eye?

- WATERY DISCHARGE
- STICKY DISCHARGE
- NO DISCHARGE

POSSIBLE CAUSE
CONJUNCTIVITIS (p.570), which can occur as a result of allergy or infection, is the likely explanation.

MEDICAL HELP
 Make an appointment to see your doctor.

POSSIBLE CAUSE
KERATOCONJUNCTIVITIS SICCA (p.585), in which the eye fails to produce enough tears, can lead to discomfort.

MEDICAL HELP
 Make an appointment to see your doctor.

If you cannot identify a possible cause for your painful or irritated eye from this chart, make an appointment to see your doctor.

24 DISTURBED OR IMPAIRED VISION

Disturbed or impaired vision might include blurred vision or seeing double. You may also see flashing lights or floating spots. Visual disturbances may be caused by a problem in one or both eyes or by damage to the areas in the brain that process visual information. If your vision deteriorates suddenly, you should consult your doctor immediately.

START HERE

Do you have pain in the affected eye?

- PAIN → *Go to chart 23* PAINFUL OR IRRITATED EYE
- NO PAIN → How long has your vision been disturbed or impaired?

How long has your vision been disturbed or impaired?

- LESS THAN 24 HOURS → Have you injured your head in the past 48 hours?
- 24 HOURS OR LONGER → Do you have diabetes?

Have you injured your head in the past 48 hours?

- RECENT HEAD INJURY
- NO HEAD INJURY

POSSIBLE CAUSE
You may have damaged the part of the brain that is responsible for vision (*see* HEAD INJURIES, p.521).

MEDICAL HELP
EMERGENCY! Call an ambulance, or go to hospital immediately.

Do you have diabetes?

- YES
- NO → How old are you?

POSSIBLE CAUSES
DIABETIC RETINOPATHY (p.579) or a high blood sugar level can lead to blurred vision.

MEDICAL HELP

See your doctor within 24 hours.

How old are you?

- 50 OR OVER → What kind of visual disturbance or impairment have you been experiencing?
- UNDER 50

What kind of visual disturbance or impairment have you been experiencing?

- BLURRED VISION
- INCREASING DIFFICULTY IN FOCUSING ON NEARBY OBJECTS
- OTHER DISTURBANCE

What is the nature of your disturbed or impaired vision?

- SUDDEN LOSS OF ALL OR PART OF THE VISION IN ONE OR BOTH EYES
- BLURRED VISION
- SEEING FLASHING LIGHTS OR FLOATING SPOTS
- DOUBLE VISION
- NONE OF THE ABOVE

POSSIBLE CAUSES
Blockage of a blood vessel that supplies the brain or eye or a serious eye condition such as RETINAL DETACHMENT (p.578) are possible causes.

MEDICAL HELP
EMERGENCY! Call an ambulance, or go to hospital immediately.

POSSIBLE CAUSE
MIGRAINE (p.518) is a possible cause, but urgent medical assessment is needed to rule out a more serious condition.

MEDICAL HELP
URGENT! Phone your doctor immediately if this is a first attack. Otherwise, make an appointment to see your doctor.

POSSIBLE CAUSES
This may be due to bleeding inside the brain (*see* STROKE, p.532, and SUBARACHNOID HAEMORRHAGE, p.534). It may also be due to an abnormality in the muscles moving the eyes (*see* DOUBLE VISION, p.589).

MEDICAL HELP
EMERGENCY! Call an ambulance!

If you cannot identify a possible cause for your disturbed or impaired vision from this chart, phone your doctor immediately.

Are you currently taking any prescribed or over-the-counter medication?

- MEDICATION
- NO MEDICATION

POSSIBLE CAUSE
A CATARACT (p.573) can cause blurred vision in older people.

MEDICAL HELP
Make an appointment to see your doctor.

POSSIBLE CAUSE
Your symptoms may be a side effect of the medication.

MEDICAL HELP
See your doctor within 24 hours. Stop taking over-the-counter medicines but continue to take any prescribed medication unless advised to stop by your doctor.

POSSIBLE CAUSE
You may be developing PRESBYOPIA (p.589) as part of the normal aging process.

MEDICAL HELP
Make an appointment to see your optician.

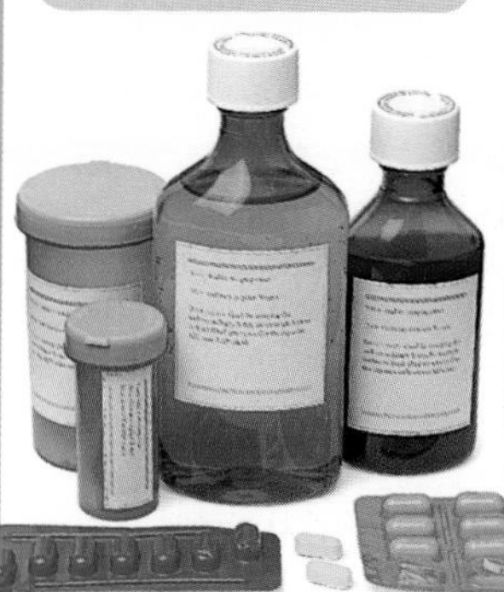

If you cannot identify a possible cause for your disturbed or impaired vision from this chart, see your doctor within 24 hours.

25 HEARING LOSS

Hearing loss is a sudden or gradual reduction in the ability to hear clearly in one or both ears. Total, permanent hearing loss is rare. Wax blockage or an ear infection may cause temporary hearing loss. The normal aging process may result in partial, permanent hearing loss, which can sometimes be treated with surgery or with a hearing aid.

START HERE

Do you have earache?

- EARACHE → *Go to chart 26* EARACHE
- NO EARACHE

Have you noticed any discharge from the ear?

- DISCHARGE
- NO DISCHARGE

Do any of the following apply?

- YOUR EAR FEELS BLOCKED
- YOU HAVE BEEN FEELING DIZZY
- YOU HAVE RINGING IN THE EAR
- NONE OF THE ABOVE

Do you have either of the following symptoms?

- RUNNY OR STUFFY NOSE
- SORE THROAT
- NEITHER

POSSIBLE CAUSE
An infection of the outer ear is a possible cause (*see* OTITIS EXTERNA, p.596).

MEDICAL HELP
Make an appointment to see your doctor.

POSSIBLE CAUSES
You could have MÉNIÈRE'S DISEASE (p.604). ACOUSTIC NEUROMA (p.605) or another problem of the nervous system are also possibilities.

MEDICAL HELP
Make an appointment to see your doctor.

POSSIBLE CAUSE
It is likely that the tube linking your middle ear and throat has become blocked as a result of a COMMON COLD (p.288).

SELF-HELP
STEAM INHALATION (p.475) can help. Make an appointment to see your doctor if your hearing has not returned to normal 1–2 days after the other cold symptoms have disappeared or if new symptoms develop.

POSSIBLE CAUSE
Your symptoms may be a side effect of the medication.

MEDICAL HELP
Make an appointment to see your doctor. Stop taking any over-the-counter medicines but continue to take prescribed medication unless advised to stop by your doctor.

Have you recently had any of the following illnesses?

- MENINGITIS
- ENCEPHALITIS
- NONE OF THE ABOVE

POSSIBLE CAUSE
These infections sometimes cause damage to hearing, which may not become obvious until later.

MEDICAL HELP
 Make an appointment to see your doctor.

Has hearing loss developed since you started any medication?

- MEDICATION
- NO MEDICATION

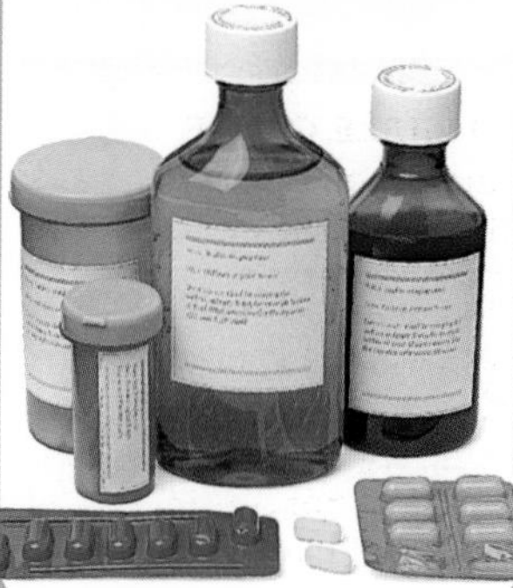

Does either of the following apply?

- YOU REGULARLY LISTEN TO LOUD MUSIC
- YOU ARE EXPOSED TO LOUD NOISE AT WORK
- NEITHER

POSSIBLE CAUSE
Exposure to loud noise can result in damage to your hearing (*see* NOISE-INDUCED HEARING LOSS, p.601).

MEDICAL HELP
 Make an appointment to see your doctor.

Have other family members suffered from increasing hearing loss that started before the age of 50?

- NO FAMILY HISTORY OF HEARING LOSS
- FAMILY HISTORY OF HEARING LOSS

POSSIBLE CAUSES
OTOSCLEROSIS (p.598) or one of a group of rare inherited disorders that affect hearing are possibilities.

MEDICAL HELP
 Make an appointment to see your doctor.

How old are you?

- 50 OR OVER
- UNDER 50

POSSIBLE CAUSES
Gradual loss of hearing that develops in later life may be due to PRESBYACUSIS (p.601). WAX BLOCKAGE (p.597) can also cause hearing loss.

MEDICAL HELP
 Make an appointment to see your doctor.

If you cannot identify a possible cause for your hearing loss from this chart, make an appointment to see your doctor.

26 EARACHE

Pain in one or both ears is a distressing symptom, especially for children. Earache is usually caused by an infection in the outer or middle ear. Mild discomfort, however, may be due to wax blockage. Consult your doctor if you have earache, particularly if it is persistent. A severe or recurrent middle-ear infection may damage hearing.

START HERE

Does pulling the ear lobe make the pain worse?

- INCREASES PAIN
- PAIN IS NO WORSE

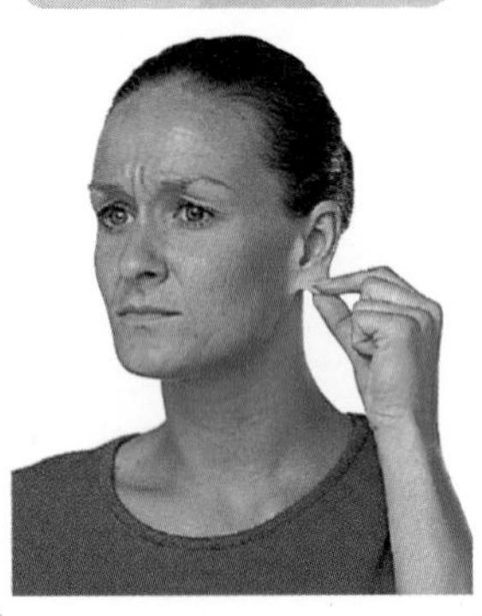

INCREASES PAIN →

POSSIBLE CAUSES

Your earache is probably due to an infection of the outer ear (*see* OTITIS EXTERNA, p.596) or a BOIL (p.351) in the ear canal.

MEDICAL HELP

Make an appointment to see your doctor.

PAIN IS NO WORSE →

Is there a discharge from the affected ear?

- DISCHARGE
- NO DISCHARGE

DISCHARGE →

POSSIBLE CAUSES

You may have a middle-ear infection (*see* OTITIS MEDIA, p.597) with a perforated eardrum; an outer-ear infection (*see* OTITIS EXTERNA, p.596) is another possibility.

MEDICAL HELP

See your doctor within 24 hours.

NO DISCHARGE →

Do you have a runny or stuffy nose?

- YES
- NO

YES →

POSSIBLE CAUSES

A cold (*see* COMMON COLD, p.288) is often accompanied by mild earache. Persistent or severe earache is likely to be due to a middle-ear infection (*see* OTITIS MEDIA, p.597).

SELF-HELP

Take decongestants to relieve stuffiness and painkillers to relieve discomfort. Make an appointment to see your doctor if pain is severe or persists for longer than 2 days.

NO →

Did the pain start during or immediately after an aeroplane flight?

- DURING OR IMMEDIATELY AFTER AN AEROPLANE FLIGHT
- UNRELATED TO AIR TRAVEL

DURING OR IMMEDIATELY AFTER AN AEROPLANE FLIGHT →

POSSIBLE CAUSE

BAROTRAUMA (p.598) may be the cause of your pain.

MEDICAL HELP

Make an appointment to see your doctor if the discomfort persists for longer than 24 hours.

UNRELATED TO AIR TRAVEL →

If you cannot identify a possible cause for your earache from this chart, see your doctor within 24 hours.

27 SORE THROAT

A raw or rough feeling in the throat is a symptom that most people have from time to time. A sore throat is often the first sign of a common cold and is also a feature of other viral infections. You can treat a sore throat yourself at home unless you also have other, more serious symptoms. However, if your sore throat persists or is severe, consult your doctor.

START HERE

Do you have a fever – a temperature of 38°C (100°F) or above?

- FEVER
- NO FEVER

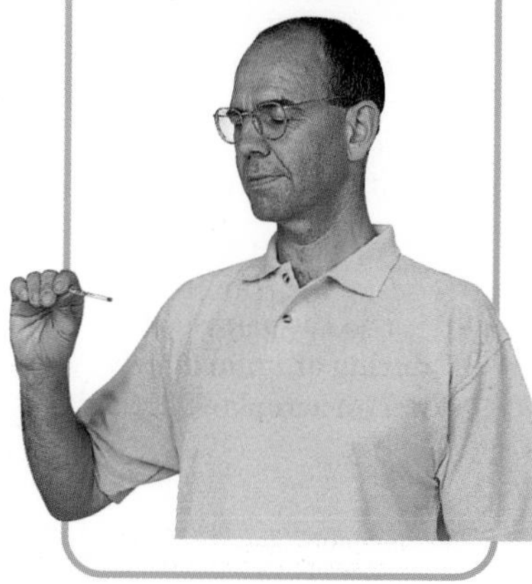

Do you have swelling in your groin and/or armpits ?

- YES
- NO

POSSIBLE CAUSE
INFECTIOUS MONONUCLEOSIS (p.291) can cause a sore throat and swollen lymph nodes.

MEDICAL HELP
 Make an appointment to see your doctor.

Do you have any of the following symptoms?

- GENERALIZED ACHES AND PAINS
- RUNNY NOSE
- HEADACHE
- COUGH
- NONE OF THE ABOVE

POSSIBLE CAUSE
A throat infection is a possible cause (*see* PHARYNGITIS AND TONSILLITIS, p.479).

MEDICAL HELP
Make an appointment to see your doctor. Follow the advice for SOOTHING A SORE THROAT (p.479) to help relieve your symptoms.

POSSIBLE CAUSE
A viral illness, such as a severe cold (*see* COMMON COLD, p.288) or INFLUENZA (p.289), is the most probable cause.

SELF-HELP
Follow the advice for BRINGING DOWN A FEVER (p.289). If your symptoms worsen, change, or are no better after 2 days, consult your doctor.

Before the onset of your sore throat had you been doing any of the following?

- SMOKING HEAVILY OR BREATHING SMOKE
- SHOUTING OR SINGING LOUDLY
- NONE OF THE ABOVE

POSSIBLE CAUSE
These activities are likely to result in inflammation of the throat (*see* PHARYNGITIS AND TONSILLITIS, p.479).

SELF-HELP
Follow the advice for SOOTHING A SORE THROAT (p.479). If your symptoms worsen, change, or are no better in 2 days, consult your doctor.

You may be developing a cold. Follow the advice for SOOTHING A SORE THROAT (p.479). Make an appointment to see your doctor if you are no better in 2 days.

28 HOARSENESS AND/OR VOICE LOSS

The sudden onset of hoarseness or huskiness of the voice is a common symptom of upper respiratory tract infections that involve the larynx or vocal cords. Such infections are almost always caused by viruses. Hoarseness and loss of voice that develop gradually are most commonly caused by overuse of the voice, smoking, or, rarely, cancer of the larynx.

WARNING PERSISTENT CHANGE IN THE VOICE

It is important to seek medical advice if you develop hoarseness or any other voice change that lasts for more than 2 weeks because the slight possibility of CANCER OF THE LARYNX (p.481) needs to be ruled out.

START HERE

How long ago did the hoarseness or loss of voice develop?

- OVER A WEEK AGO
- WITHIN THE PAST WEEK

Do you use your voice a lot; for example, are you a singer, actor, or teacher?

- NORMAL VOICE USE
- REGULAR LOUD VOICE USE

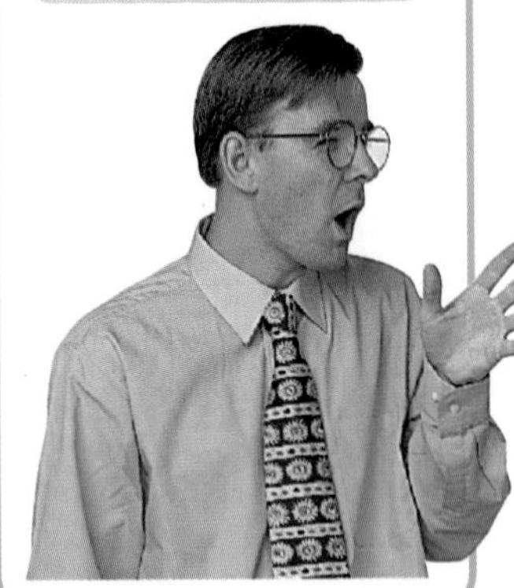

POSSIBLE CAUSES

Regular overuse of your voice can lead to inflammation of the vocal cords (*see* VOCAL CORD NODULES, p.480, and LARYNGITIS, p.479).

MEDICAL HELP

Make an appointment to see your doctor.

Have you had any of the following symptoms in the past week?

- RUNNY NOSE AND/OR SNEEZING
- COUGH
- SORE THROAT
- NONE OF THE ABOVE

POSSIBLE CAUSE

A viral throat infection has probably affected your vocal cords (*see* LARYNGITIS, p.479).

SELF-HELP

STEAM INHALATION (p.475) may help to relieve symptoms. Make an appointment to see your doctor if you do not feel better in 2 days or if other symptoms develop.

Before the onset of hoarseness, had you been shouting, singing, or using your voice more than usual?

- MORE VOICE USE THAN USUAL
- NORMAL VOICE USE

Do you smoke, or have you smoked in the past?

- YES
- NO

POSSIBLE CAUSES

Smoking, particularly smoking heavily over a long period of time, can result in chronic inflammation of the vocal cords (*see* LARYNGITIS, p.479). Another possibility is CANCER OF THE LARYNX (p.481), which is more common in people who smoke regularly.

MEDICAL HELP

 Make an appointment to see your doctor.

POSSIBLE CAUSE

HYPOTHYROIDISM (p.680) can cause increasing huskiness.

MEDICAL HELP

 Make an appointment to see your doctor.

Do you have any of the following symptoms?

- TIREDNESS
- INCREASED SKIN DRYNESS OR ROUGHNESS
- FEELING THE COLD MORE THAN YOU USED TO
- UNEXPLAINED WEIGHT GAIN
- GENERALIZED HAIR THINNING
- NONE OF THE ABOVE

POSSIBLE CAUSE

Excessive use of the voice can inflame the vocal cords (*see* LARYNGITIS, p.479).

SELF-HELP

STEAM INHALATION (p.475) may help. You should also rest your voice as much as possible. Make an appointment to see your doctor if your voice is no better in 2 days or if you develop other symptoms.

POSSIBLE CAUSE

Breathing in dust, fumes, or smoke can severely inflame the respiratory tract.

MEDICAL HELP

 URGENT! Phone your doctor immediately!

Did either of the following apply before the onset of hoarseness?

- YOU HAD INHALED DUST, CHEMICAL FUMES, OR SMOKE FROM A FIRE
- YOU HAD SPENT TIME IN A SMOKY ATMOSPHERE
- NEITHER

POSSIBLE CAUSE

Being in a smoky atmosphere can inflame the vocal cords (*see* LARYNGITIS, p.479).

SELF-HELP

STEAM INHALATION (p.475) may be helpful. Rest your voice as much as possible and avoid smoky environments. Make an appointment to see your doctor if your voice is no better in 2 days or if you develop other symptoms.

If you cannot identify a possible cause for your hoarseness or loss of voice from this chart, make an appointment to see your doctor.

29 COUGHING

For children under 12, see chart 68

Coughing is the body's defence mechanism for clearing the airways of inhaled particles or secretions. Persistent coughing may be due to infection or inflammation in the lungs or to the effects of irritants such as tobacco smoke. Persistent coughing should be investigated by your doctor.

WARNING COUGHING UP BLOOD

If you cough up sputum that contains streaks of blood on one occasion only, the most likely cause is a small tear in the lining of the windpipe; if you feel well, you need not be concerned. However, if you have more than one such episode, there may be a more serious cause; you should see a doctor without delay.

START HERE

How long have you had a cough?

LESS THAN 48 HOURS

OVER 48 HOURS

Do you have a fever – a temperature of 38°C (100°F) or above?

FEVER

NO FEVER

Are you coughing up sputum?

SPUTUM

NO SPUTUM

Are you currently taking any prescribed medication?

MEDICATION

NO MEDICATION

POSSIBLE CAUSE

Your symptoms may be a side effect of the medication.

MEDICAL HELP

Make an appointment to see your doctor. Continue to take the medication unless advised to stop by your doctor.

POSSIBLE CAUSES

A persistent dry cough may be due to ASTHMA (p.483), GASTRO-OESOPHAGEAL REFLUX (p.636), or exposure to irritants in your workplace (*see* OCCUPATIONAL LUNG DISEASES, p.499). However, the slight possibility of PRIMARY LUNG CANCER (p.503) needs to be excluded.

MEDICAL HELP

Make an appointment to see your doctor.

POSSIBLE CAUSE

Being in a smoky atmosphere can irritate the lungs.

SELF-HELP

Move into a well-ventilated area. See your doctor if you become breathless or develop other symptoms.

Are you a smoker?

SMOKER

NONSMOKER

If you cannot identify a possible cause for your cough from this chart, make an appointment to see your doctor.

Are you having either of the following problems with breathing?

- BREATHING IS PAINFUL
- YOU ARE SHORT OF BREATH
- NEITHER

POSSIBLE CAUSE
PNEUMONIA (p.490) may be the cause of these symptoms.

MEDICAL HELP
 URGENT! Phone your doctor immediately!

Have you coughed up sputum?

- SPUTUM
- NO SPUTUM

POSSIBLE CAUSE
ACUTE BRONCHITIS (p.486) is a possibility.

SELF-HELP
Follow the self-help advice for ACUTE BRONCHITIS (p.486). Consult your doctor if your symptoms worsen or if you are no better in 2 days.

POSSIBLE CAUSE
A viral illness such as a severe cold (*see* COMMON COLD, p.288) or INFLUENZA (p.289) is a likely cause of your cough.

SELF-HELP
Follow the self-help advice for BRINGING DOWN A FEVER (p.289). Consult your doctor if you are no better in 2 days or if other symptoms develop.

POSSIBLE CAUSE
Coughing is the body's natural response to a foreign body that has lodged in the lungs.

MEDICAL HELP
 Call your doctor if coughing has not subsided within 1 hour.

Have you inhaled any of the following in the last few hours?

- PARTICLE OF FOOD
- TOBACCO SMOKE
- DUST, FUMES, OR SMOKE FROM A FIRE
- NONE OF THE ABOVE

POSSIBLE CAUSE
Severe inflammation of the respiratory tract can occur as a result of breathing in any of these substances.

MEDICAL HELP
 URGENT! Phone your doctor immediately!

Do you have either of the following symptoms?

- RUNNY NOSE
- SORE THROAT
- NEITHER

POSSIBLE CAUSE
A cold (*see* COMMON COLD, p.288) is the probable cause of your cough.

SELF-HELP
STEAM INHALATION (p.475) may help. Consult your doctor if your breathing becomes painful or you start to wheeze, if you are no better in 2 days, or if other symptoms develop.

POSSIBLE CAUSES
A persistent smoker's cough that produces sputum may be due to CHRONIC OBSTRUCTIVE PULMONARY DISEASE (p.487) or, in rare cases, to PRIMARY LUNG CANCER (p.503).

MEDICAL HELP
 Make an appointment to see your doctor.

POSSIBLE CAUSES
A cough without any other symptoms may be caused by ASTHMA (p.483). CHRONIC HEART FAILURE (p.413) is a less likely possibility.

MEDICAL HELP
 Make an appointment to see your doctor.

30 SHORTNESS OF BREATH

For children under 12, see chart 67

Shortness of breath can be expected after strenuous exercise. Breathing should return to normal after resting. If you are short of breath at rest or after normal activities, such as getting dressed, you should consult your doctor because your symptom may be due to a serious heart or lung disorder.

DANGER SIGNS

Call an ambulance if either you or someone you are with has one of the following symptoms:

- Sudden, severe shortness of breath.
- Blue-tinged lips.

While waiting for medical help, loosen any tight clothing and help the person to sit upright.

START HERE

Is breathing painful?

- PAINFUL → *Go to chart 41* CHEST PAIN
- NOT PAINFUL

Have you been wheezing?

- WHEEZING → *Go to chart 31* WHEEZING
- NO WHEEZING

How quickly did the shortness of breath start?

- GRADUALLY OVER A FEW DAYS OR LONGER
- SUDDENLY WITHIN THE PAST 48 HOURS

Do you have either of the following symptoms?

- SWOLLEN ANKLES
- COUGH WITH SPUTUM ON MOST DAYS
- NEITHER

Do any of the following apply?

- YOU HAVE RECENTLY HAD A SURGICAL OPERATION
- YOU HAVE RECENTLY BEEN IMMOBILE BECAUSE OF INJURY OR ILLNESS
- YOU HAVE HAD A BABY WITHIN THE PAST 2 WEEKS
- NONE OF THE ABOVE

POSSIBLE CAUSE

It is possible that you have a blood clot in the lung (*see* PULMONARY EMBOLISM, p.495).

MEDICAL HELP

EMERGENCY! Call an ambulance!

Do you have any of the following symptoms?

- TEMPERATURE OF 38°C (100°F) OR ABOVE
- FROTHY PINK OR WHITE SPUTUM
- WAKING AT NIGHT FEELING BREATHLESS
- NONE OF THE ABOVE

POSSIBLE CAUSE
A possible cause of your symptoms is CHRONIC HEART FAILURE (p.413).

MEDICAL HELP
 See your doctor within 24 hours.

POSSIBLE CAUSES
One possible cause is CHRONIC OBSTRUCTIVE PULMONARY DISEASE (p.487). This is particularly likely if you have been a smoker for several years.

MEDICAL HELP
 Make an appointment to see your doctor.

POSSIBLE CAUSE
Your symptoms may be due to PNEUMONIA (p.490); this is particularly likely if you also have a cough.

MEDICAL HELP
 URGENT! Phone your doctor immediately!

POSSIBLE CAUSE
Your symptoms may be caused by fluid on the lungs (*see* ACUTE HEART FAILURE, p.412).

MEDICAL HELP
 URGENT! Phone your doctor immediately!

POSSIBLE CAUSE
Your symptoms may be the result of an OCCUPATIONAL LUNG DISEASE (p.499).

MEDICAL HELP
 Make an appointment to see your doctor.

Do you have, or have you ever had, regular exposure to or contact with the following?

- DUST OR FUMES
- GRAIN CROPS, CAGED BIRDS, OR ANIMALS
- NEITHER

POSSIBLE CAUSE
You may have had a panic attack brought on by stress (*see* ANXIETY DISORDERS, p.551).

MEDICAL HELP
 URGENT! Phone your doctor immediately if this is a first attack. Otherwise, follow the advice for COPING WITH A PANIC ATTACK (p.552).

Did the shortness of breath start immediately after a stressful event?

- YES
- NO

POSSIBLE CAUSE
Your shortness of breath may be the result of an allergic reaction (*see* EXTRINSIC ALLERGIC ALVEOLITIS, p.502).

MEDICAL HELP
 Make an appointment to see your doctor.

POSSIBLE CAUSE
ANAEMIA (p.446) is a possible cause of your symptoms.

MEDICAL HELP
 See your doctor within 24 hours.

Do you have any of the following symptoms?

- FAINTNESS OR FAINTING
- PALER SKIN THAN NORMAL
- UNDUE TIREDNESS
- NONE OF THE ABOVE

If you cannot identify a possible cause for your shortness of breath from this chart, see your doctor within 24 hours.

31 WHEEZING

For children under 12, see chart 67

Wheezing, a whistling or rasping sound on exhaling, occurs when the air passages become narrowed. Narrowing may be caused by inflammation due to infection, asthma, or inhaled dust, or, in rare cases, may be due to a tumour. If you have persistent wheezing, you should see your doctor.

START HERE

Has the wheezing come on suddenly within the past few hours or gradually over days or weeks?

- SUDDEN ONSET → **Do you have either of the following symptoms?**
  - FROTHY PINK OR WHITE SPUTUM
  - WAKING AT NIGHT FEELING BREATHLESS
  - NEITHER → **Are you short of breath?**
- GRADUAL ONSET → **Do you have a fever – a temperature of 38°C (100°F) or above?**
  - FEVER
  - NO FEVER → **Do you cough up sputum?**
    - MOST DAYS
    - SELDOM OR NEVER

Are you short of breath?

- SHORT OF BREATH
- NOT SHORT OF BREATH

(Short of breath)

POSSIBLE CAUSE
You could be having an attack of ASTHMA (p.483).

MEDICAL HELP
 URGENT! Phone your doctor immediately!

(Frothy pink or white sputum / Waking at night feeling breathless)

POSSIBLE CAUSE
There is a possibility of fluid on the lungs (*see* ACUTE HEART FAILURE, p.412).

MEDICAL HELP
URGENT! Phone your doctor immediately!

(Not short of breath)

POSSIBLE CAUSE
A mild asthma attack (*see* ASTHMA, p.483) is the most likely cause of wheezing without shortness of breath.

MEDICAL HELP
 See your doctor within 24 hours.

(Fever)

POSSIBLE CAUSE
ACUTE BRONCHITIS (p.486) is a possible cause.

SELF-HELP
Follow the self-help advice for ACUTE BRONCHITIS (p.486). If you are no better within 2 days, consult your doctor.

(Most days)

POSSIBLE CAUSE
Your symptoms may be caused by CHRONIC OBSTRUCTIVE PULMONARY DISEASE (p.487), especially if you are a smoker.

MEDICAL HELP
 Make an appointment to see your doctor.

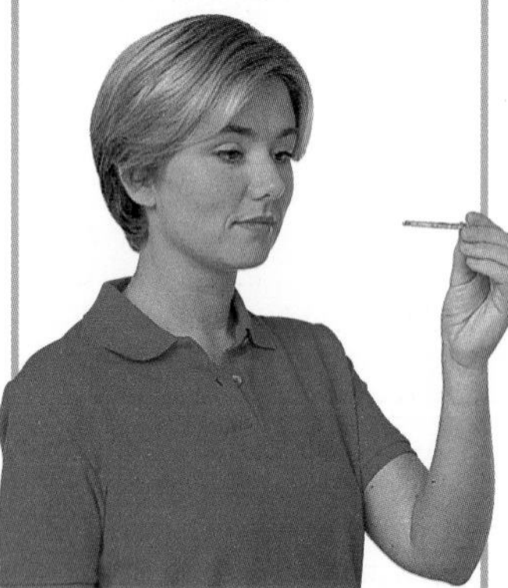

(Seldom or never)

If you cannot identify a possible cause for your wheezing from this chart, see your doctor within 24 hours.

32 DIFFICULTY SWALLOWING

Difficulty swallowing is most commonly the result of a sore throat due to infection. Self-treatment should ease the soreness and allow normal swallowing. However, persistent difficulty with swallowing may be due to a disorder of the stomach or oesophagus, the tube connecting the throat to the stomach, and should be investigated by your doctor.

START HERE

Is your throat sore?

- SORE
- NOT SORE

Is it possible that you have swallowed something sharp, such as a fish bone?

- POSSIBLE
- UNLIKELY

POSSIBLE CAUSE

Something may have either scratched your throat or become lodged in it.

MEDICAL HELP

URGENT! Phone your doctor immediately!

Which of the following applies?

- FOOD SEEMS TO STICK HIGH UP IN THE CHEST
- YOU HAVE A FEELING OF SOMETHING BEING STUCK IN THE THROAT
- NEITHER

POSSIBLE CAUSE

ANXIETY DISORDERS (p.551) may be a cause of this type of difficulty with swallowing.

MEDICAL HELP

Make an appointment to see your doctor.

Go to chart 27
SORE THROAT

If you cannot identify a possible cause for your difficulty swallowing from this chart, make an appointment to see your doctor.

Do you often get a burning pain in the centre of the chest in either of the following situations?

- WHEN YOU BEND FORWARD
- WHEN YOU LIE DOWN
- NEITHER

POSSIBLE CAUSE

GASTRO-OESOPHAGEAL REFLUX (p.636) is a likely cause.

MEDICAL HELP

Make an appointment to see your doctor.

Does either of the following apply?

- THE SWALLOWING DIFFICULTY IS GETTING WORSE
- YOU HAVE LOST WEIGHT
- NEITHER

POSSIBLE CAUSES

These symptoms may be due to a narrowed oesophagus, which could be caused by GASTRO-OESOPHAGEAL REFLUX (p.636) or rarely CANCER OF THE OESOPHAGUS (p.638).

MEDICAL HELP

See your doctor within 24 hours.

33 VOMITING

For children under 12, see chart 64

Vomiting is most often caused by irritation or inflammation of the digestive tract. It may also be triggered by conditions affecting the brain or by an inner-ear disorder, or it can be a side effect of medication. If you have been vomiting for longer than a day, consult chart 34, RECURRENT VOMITING (p.150).

DANGER SIGNS

Call an ambulance if your vomit contains blood, which may appear as any of the following:

- Bright red streaks.
- Black material that resembles coffee grounds.
- Blood clots.

START HERE

Have you vomited repeatedly in the past week?

- ON 2 OR MORE DAYS
- TODAY ONLY

Go to chart 34
RECURRENT VOMITING

Do you have pain in the abdomen?

- SEVERE PAIN
- MILD PAIN
- NO PAIN

Do you have pain in or around an eye?

- EYE PAIN
- NO EYE PAIN

POSSIBLE CAUSE
ACUTE GLAUCOMA (p.575) is a possibility, especially if your vision is also blurred.

MEDICAL HELP
URGENT! Phone your doctor immediately!

Do you have a headache?

- HEADACHE
- NO HEADACHE

Do you have any of the following symptoms?

- TEMPERATURE OF 38°C (100°F) OR ABOVE
- DIARRHOEA
- DIZZINESS
- NONE OF THE ABOVE

POSSIBLE CAUSE
You could have a serious abdominal condition, such as APPENDICITIS (p.664).

MEDICAL HELP

URGENT! Phone your doctor immediately!

POSSIBLE CAUSE
LABYRINTHITIS (p.604) is a possible cause of these symptoms.

MEDICAL HELP
See your doctor within 24 hours. In the meantime, minimize symptoms by lying down or by trying to move around as little as possible.

WARNING

Vomiting and medications

If you are taking any oral medication, including oral contraceptives, an episode of vomiting may reduce the effectiveness of the drug because your body cannot absorb the active ingredients. If you use oral contraceptives, continue taking the pills as usual, but take extra contraceptive precautions as well. You should continue using these precautions for a further 7 days after the vomiting has stopped. If you have not been able to take your contraceptive pills because of vomiting, consult your doctor for advice on how to restart them. You should also see your doctor if you are taking any other prescribed medicine and have been vomiting.

Go to chart 10 HEADACHE

Possible cause

Your symptoms may be the result of infection (*see* GASTROENTERITIS, p.628).

Self-help

Follow the self-help advice for PREVENTING DEHYDRATION (p.627). Consult your doctor if you are no better in 2 days or if other symptoms develop.

Have you eaten or drunk any of the following?

- An unusually large or rich meal
- A large amount of alcohol
- Food that may have been contaminated
- None of the above

Possible cause

You may be suffering from FOOD POISONING (p.629).

Self-help

Follow the self-help advice for PREVENTING DEHYDRATION (p.627). Consult your doctor if you are no better in 2 days or if other symptoms develop.

Possible cause

Your symptoms may be a side effect of the medication.

Medical help

See your doctor within 24 hours. Stop taking over-the-counter medicines but continue to take any prescribed medication unless advised to stop by your doctor.

Possible cause

The lining of your stomach has probably become inflamed (*see* GASTRITIS, p.640).

Self-help

Follow the self-help measures for GASTRITIS (p.640). Consult your doctor if you are no better in 2 days or if other symptoms develop.

Are you currently taking any prescribed or over-the-counter medication?

- Medication
- No medication

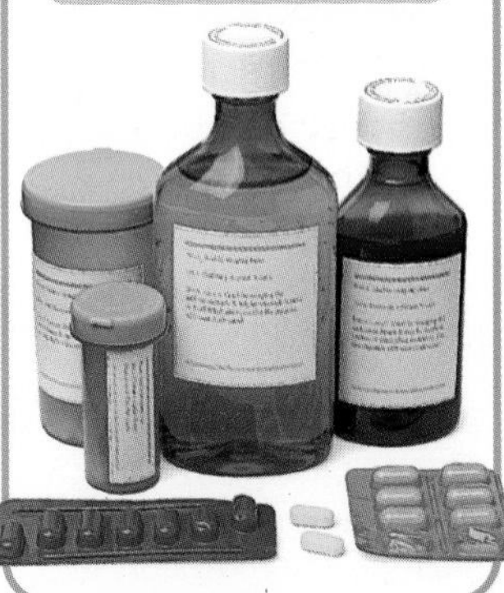

If you cannot identify a possible cause for your vomiting from this chart, see your doctor within 24 hours.

34 RECURRENT VOMITING

For children under 12, see chart 64

Consult this chart if you have been vomiting repeatedly over a number of days or weeks. Recurrent vomiting may be caused by a digestive tract disorder but is also common in early pregnancy. You should consult your doctor if you have persistent or recurrent vomiting.

START HERE

Could you be pregnant?

- POSSIBLY PREGNANT
- NOT PREGNANT

POSSIBLE CAUSE (Possibly pregnant)

Nausea and/or vomiting are often the first indicators of pregnancy (*see* COMMON COMPLAINTS OF NORMAL PREGNANCY, p.784).

MEDICAL HELP

Make an appointment to see your doctor if vomiting is preventing you from keeping down fluids. If you are not sure whether you are pregnant, do a HOME PREGNANCY TEST (p.232).

Have you experienced any of the following kinds of recurrent pain? (Not pregnant)

- BURNING CENTRAL CHEST PAIN IF YOU BEND OR LIE DOWN
- PAIN IN THE UPPER RIGHT ABDOMEN THAT MAY SPREAD TO THE BACK
- PAIN IN THE CENTRE OF THE UPPER ABDOMEN THAT IS RELATED TO EATING
- NONE OF THE ABOVE

POSSIBLE CAUSES (Burning central chest pain)

GASTRO-OESOPHAGEAL REFLUX (p.636) and NONULCER DYSPEPSIA (p.626) are possible causes of your symptoms.

MEDICAL HELP

Make an appointment to see your doctor.

POSSIBLE CAUSE (Pain in the upper right abdomen)

GALLSTONES (p.651) could be the cause of your symptoms.

MEDICAL HELP

See your doctor within 24 hours.

POSSIBLE CAUSE (Pain in the centre of the upper abdomen)

Your symptoms may be due to a PEPTIC ULCER (p.640).

MEDICAL HELP

Make an appointment to see your doctor.

Have you noticed either of the following symptoms? (None of the above)

- YELLOWING OF THE SKIN
- YELLOWING OF THE WHITES OF THE EYES
- NEITHER

POSSIBLE CAUSE (Yellowing)

Yellowing of the skin and the whites of the eyes, known as JAUNDICE (p.643), is often accompanied by vomiting. Jaundice has many possible causes but in most cases is due to liver disease such as hepatitis (*see* ACUTE HEPATITIS, p.644).

MEDICAL HELP

See your doctor within 24 hours.

POSSIBLE CAUSES
Your symptoms may be the result of a PEPTIC ULCER (p.640), but there is also a possibility of STOMACH CANCER (p.642).

MEDICAL HELP

Make an appointment to see your doctor.

Have you noticed changes in your weight or appetite since you began vomiting?

- LOSS OF OVER 4 KG (9 LB) IN WEIGHT
- LOSS OF APPETITE
- NEITHER

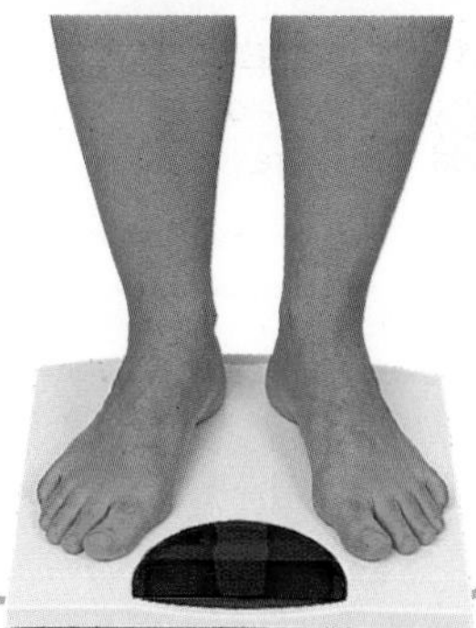

POSSIBLE CAUSES
Recurrent headaches with vomiting but no nausea may, in rare cases, indicate pressure on the brain due to bleeding or a tumour (*see* SUBDURAL HAEMORRHAGE, p.535, and BRAIN TUMOURS, p.530).

MEDICAL HELP

See your doctor within 24 hours.

Do you regularly drink more than the recommended limit of alcohol (*see* SAFE ALCOHOL LIMITS, p.62)?

- MORE THAN THE LIMIT
- WITHIN THE LIMIT

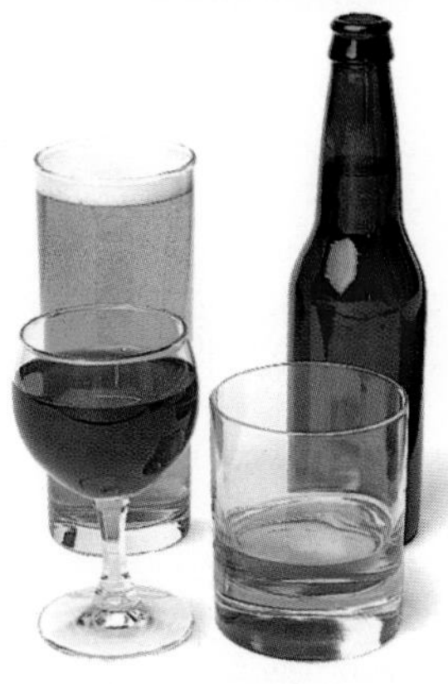

Have you been suffering from recurrent headaches?

- HEADACHES WITH VOMITING BUT NO NAUSEA
- HEADACHES WITH VOMITING AND NAUSEA
- NO HEADACHES

POSSIBLE CAUSE
You may be suffering from MIGRAINE (p.518).

MEDICAL HELP

Make an appointment to see your doctor, who can review your diagnosis. He or she may recommend that you take a preventive medication in future.

POSSIBLE CAUSE
Excessive consumption of alcohol over a prolonged period can cause long-term inflammation of the stomach lining (*see* GASTRITIS, p.640).

MEDICAL HELP

Make an appointment to see your doctor.

POSSIBLE CAUSE
Your symptoms may be a side effect of the medication.

MEDICAL HELP
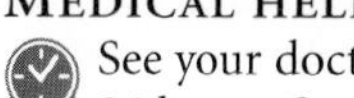
See your doctor within 24 hours. Stop taking over-the-counter medicines but continue to take any prescribed medication unless advised to stop by your doctor.

Are you currently taking any prescribed or over-the-counter medication?

- MEDICATION
- NO MEDICATION

If you cannot identify a possible cause for your recurrent vomiting from this chart, make an appointment to see your doctor.

35 ABDOMINAL PAIN

For children under 12, see chart 69

Mild abdominal pain is often due to a stomach or bowel upset that will clear up without treatment. However, severe or persistent abdominal pain, especially if it is accompanied by other symptoms, may indicate a more serious problem that your doctor should investigate.

DANGER SIGNS

Call an ambulance if you have severe abdominal pain that lasts for longer than 4 hours and is associated with any of the following additional symptoms:

- Vomiting.
- Fever.
- Swollen or tender abdomen.
- Feeling faint, drowsy, or confused.
- Blood in the urine or faeces.

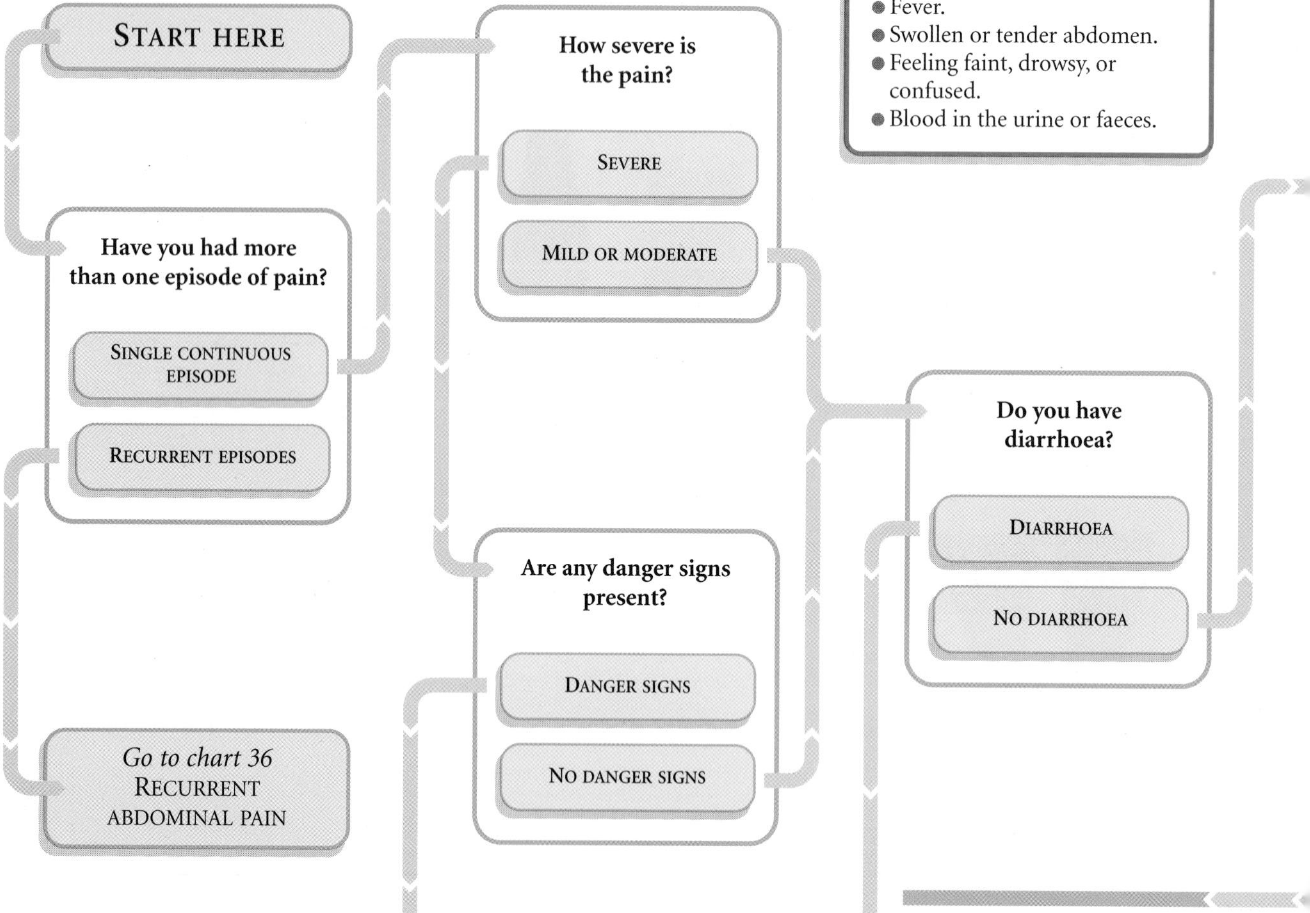

START HERE

Have you had more than one episode of pain?

SINGLE CONTINUOUS EPISODE

RECURRENT EPISODES

Go to chart 36 RECURRENT ABDOMINAL PAIN

How severe is the pain?

SEVERE

MILD OR MODERATE

Are any danger signs present?

DANGER SIGNS

NO DANGER SIGNS

Do you have diarrhoea?

DIARRHOEA

NO DIARRHOEA

POSSIBLE CAUSE

Severe abdominal pain may be an indication of a serious abdominal condition, such as APPENDICITIS (p.664).

MEDICAL HELP

EMERGENCY! Call an ambulance!

POSSIBLE CAUSE

Your pain may be the result of GASTROENTERITIS (p.628).

SELF-HELP

Maintain fluid intake (*see* PREVENTING DEHYDRATION, p.627). Consult your doctor if you are no better in 2 days or if other symptoms develop.

POSSIBLE CAUSE

GALLSTONES (p.651) are a possibility, especially if you have vomited.

MEDICAL HELP

See your doctor within 24 hours.

POSSIBLE CAUSE
You may have KIDNEY STONES (p.701), especially if you have been vomiting.

MEDICAL HELP
 URGENT! Phone your doctor immediately!

Do any of the following apply?

- PAIN IS RELATED TO EATING
- PAIN IS RELIEVED BY ANTACIDS
- PAIN COMES ON WHEN LYING OR BENDING OVER
- NONE OF THE ABOVE

POSSIBLE CAUSES
Your abdominal pain may be caused by NONULCER DYSPEPSIA (p.626) or GASTRO-OESOPHAGEAL REFLUX (p.636).

MEDICAL HELP
Make an appointment to see your doctor. In the meantime, follow the self-help measures for PREVENTING INDIGESTION (p.627).

Go to chart 41 CHEST PAIN

What kind of pain have you been experiencing?

- PAIN THAT STARTS IN THE BACK AND MAY MOVE TO THE GROIN
- PAIN IN THE CENTRE OF THE UPPER ABDOMEN
- PAIN IN THE UPPER RIGHT ABDOMEN THAT MAY SPREAD TO THE BACK
- PAIN MAINLY BELOW THE WAIST
- NONE OF THE ABOVE

Do you have either of the following symptoms?

- PAIN ON PASSING URINE
- PASSING URINE MORE OFTEN THAN USUAL
- NEITHER

POSSIBLE CAUSE
You may have a urinary tract infection (*see* PYELONEPHRITIS, p.698, and CYSTITIS, p.709).

MEDICAL HELP
 See your doctor within 24 hours.

Are you female or male?

- FEMALE
- MALE

Go to chart 60 LOWER ABDOMINAL PAIN IN WOMEN

If you cannot identify a possible cause for your abdominal pain from this chart, see your doctor within 24 hours

36 RECURRENT ABDOMINAL PAIN

For children under 12, see chart 69

Abdominal discomfort that has occurred on more than one day in the past month may be a symptom of a digestive tract disorder or, less commonly, of a urinary tract problem. It is important to consult your doctor if you experience recurrent attacks of abdominal pain even if they are short-lived.

START HERE

Where is the pain mainly felt?

- BELOW THE WAIST
- ABOVE THE WAIST

Is pain accompanied by bouts of diarrhoea and/or constipation?

- DIARRHOEA AND/OR CONSTIPATION
- NO CHANGE IN BOWEL HABIT

POSSIBLE CAUSE
GASTRO-OESOPHAGEAL REFLUX (p.636) is the most likely cause of this type of upper abdominal pain.

MEDICAL HELP
 Make an appointment to see your doctor.

Do you have either of the following symptoms?

- SWELLING IN THE GROIN
- DISCOMFORT IN THE GROIN MADE WORSE BY LIFTING OR COUGHING
- NEITHER

What kind of pain have you been experiencing?

- BURNING CENTRAL CHEST PAIN WHEN YOU BEND OR LIE DOWN
- PAIN THAT IS RELATED TO MEALS
- PAIN IN THE UPPER RIGHT ABDOMEN THAT MAY SPREAD TO THE BACK
- NONE OF THE ABOVE

POSSIBLE CAUSES
Your symptoms may be due to a PEPTIC ULCER (p.640). STOMACH CANCER (p.642) is also a remote possibility.

MEDICAL HELP
Make an appointment to see your doctor.

Do you have any of these symptoms?

- BLOOD IN THE URINE
- PAIN ON PASSING URINE
- PASSING URINE MORE OFTEN THAN USUAL
- NONE OF THE ABOVE

POSSIBLE CAUSE
GALLSTONES (p.651) are a possible cause.

MEDICAL HELP
Make an appointment to see your doctor.

Do you have any of the following symptoms?

- BLOOD IN THE FAECES
- LOST OVER 4 KG (9 LB) IN THE LAST 10 WEEKS
- NEITHER

POSSIBLE CAUSES

Recurrent abdominal pain in association with weight loss or blood in the faeces may be the result of a long-term intestinal condition, for example DIVERTICULAR DISEASE (p.663), CROHN'S DISEASE (p.658), or ULCERATIVE COLITIS (p.659). However, the possibility of COLORECTAL CANCER (p.665) needs to be excluded.

MEDICAL HELP

 Make an appointment to see your doctor.

POSSIBLE CAUSES

It is possible that you have a long-term intestinal condition such as IRRITABLE BOWEL SYNDROME (p.655). However, the possibility of COLORECTAL CANCER (p.665) also needs to be ruled out.

MEDICAL HELP

 Make an appointment to see your doctor.

POSSIBLE CAUSE

Such symptoms suggest the possibility of a HERNIA (p.661).

MEDICAL HELP

 Make an appointment to see your doctor.

POSSIBLE CAUSES

You may have a urinary tract infection, such as CYSTITIS (p.709) or PYELONEPHRITIS (p.698). However, there is also the slight possibility of a BLADDER TUMOUR (p.715) or KIDNEY CANCER (p.704).

MEDICAL HELP

 See your doctor within 24 hours.

POSSIBLE CAUSE

Your symptoms may be a side effect of the medication.

MEDICAL HELP

Make an appointment to see your doctor. Stop taking any over-the-counter medicines but continue to take prescribed medication unless advised to stop by your doctor.

Go to chart 60
LOWER ABDOMINAL PAIN IN WOMEN

Are you currently taking any prescribed or over-the-counter medication?

- MEDICATION
- NO MEDICATION

Are you female or male?

- FEMALE
- MALE

If you cannot identify a possible cause for your recurrent abdominal pain from this chart, make an appointment to see your doctor.

37 SWOLLEN ABDOMEN

Enlargement of the abdomen is usually due to weight gain or poor muscle tone from lack of exercise. A swollen abdomen may also result from a disorder of either the digestive system or the urinary system. If you have abdominal swelling that has come on rapidly, you should consult your doctor irrespective of any other symptoms you may have.

START HERE

How long has your abdomen been swollen?

- LESS THAN 24 HOURS
- LONGER THAN 24 HOURS

Do you have abdominal pain?

- SEVERE PAIN
- MILD PAIN
- NO PAIN

Go to chart 35
ABDOMINAL PAIN

POSSIBLE CAUSES
You may be suffering from excessive intestinal gas or CONSTIPATION (p.628). Either of these symptoms may suggest you have IRRITABLE BOWEL SYNDROME (p.655).

MEDICAL HELP
Make an appointment to see your doctor.

Is pain relieved by passing wind or having a bowel movement?

- RELIEVED
- UNRELIEVED

POSSIBLE CAUSE
The swelling could be due to an abnormally full bladder (*see* URINARY RETENTION, p.713).

MEDICAL HELP
 See your doctor within 24 hours.

Do any of the following apply?

- YOUR ANKLES ARE SWOLLEN
- YOU COULD BE PREGNANT
- YOU HAVE DIFFICULTY PASSING URINE
- YOU PASS ONLY SMALL VOLUMES OF URINE
- NONE OF THE ABOVE

Go to chart 51
SWOLLEN ANKLES

POSSIBLE CAUSE
A swollen abdomen may be the the first sign of an unsuspected pregnancy, especially if you have been using contraception or if your periods tend to be irregular.

SELF-HELP
If you think that you might be pregnant, carry out a HOME PREGNANCY TEST (p.232).

If you cannot identify a possible cause for your swollen abdomen from this chart, make an appointment to see your doctor.

38 ANAL AND RECTAL PROBLEMS

The anus is the opening of the lower large intestine (rectum) to the outside. Discomfort during bowel movements may be due to a disorder of the rectum, the anus, or the skin around the anus. Rectal or anal bleeding is often due to haemorrhoids but can also be an early symptom of cancer. Consult your doctor if you have any bleeding or persistent discomfort.

START HERE

Have you noticed bleeding from the anus?

- BLEEDING → Possible causes (haemorrhoids)
- NO BLEEDING → Do you have either of the following?

POSSIBLE CAUSES
HAEMORRHOIDS (p.668) may be responsible. Bowel movements following CONSTIPATION (p.628) may also cause this symptom. However, COLORECTAL CANCER (p.665) or ANAL CANCER (p.669) is also a possibility.

MEDICAL HELP
 See your doctor within 24 hours.

Do you have either of the following?

- PAIN IN OR AROUND THE ANUS OR RECTUM → Possible causes (haemorrhoids)
- SORE AREA IN THE CREASE ABOVE THE ANUS → Possible cause (pilonidal sinus)
- NEITHER → Do you have itching around the anus?

POSSIBLE CAUSE
You may have a PILONIDAL SINUS (p.360).

MEDICAL HELP
 See your doctor within 24 hours.

Do you have itching around the anus?

- ITCHING → Does either of the following apply?
- NO ITCHING → Do you have small, irregular, fleshy lumps around the anus?

Does either of the following apply?

- YOU HAVE NOTICED WHITE "THREADS" IN YOUR FAECES → Possible cause (threadworm)
- ITCHING IS WORSE WHEN YOU ARE IN BED → Possible cause (threadworm)
- NEITHER → Possible causes (haemorrhoids / anal itching)

POSSIBLE CAUSE
A THREADWORM INFESTATION (p.310) is a possibility.

MEDICAL HELP
 Make an appointment to see your doctor.

POSSIBLE CAUSES
HAEMORRHOIDS (p.668) are a possible cause, but ANAL ITCHING (p.669) can also occur for no obvious reason.

MEDICAL HELP
Make an appointment to see your doctor if anal itching continues for longer than 3 days.

Do you have small, irregular, fleshy lumps around the anus?

- YES → Possible cause (genital warts)
- NO → If you cannot identify a possible cause...

POSSIBLE CAUSE
It is possible that you have GENITAL WARTS (p.768).

MEDICAL HELP
 Make an appointment to see your doctor.

If you cannot identify a possible cause for your anal problem from this chart, make an appointment to see your doctor.

39 DIARRHOEA

For children under 12 years, see chart 65

Diarrhoea, which is the frequent passing of abnormally loose or watery faeces, is usually a result of infection. However, persistent diarrhoea may be caused by a serious gastrointestinal disorder. Consult your doctor if diarrhoea continues for more than 2 days or if it recurs.

WARNING

DEHYDRATION

A person with severe diarrhoea can become dehydrated if fluids are not replaced quickly enough. The symptoms of dehydration include drowsiness or confusion, a dry mouth, loss of elasticity in the skin, and failure to pass urine for several hours. Elderly people are particularly at risk. Seek urgent medical help if a person has symptoms of dehydration.

START HERE

Have you noticed blood in your faeces?

- BLOOD
- NO BLOOD

POSSIBLE CAUSES

You may be suffering from an intestinal infection, such as AMOEBIASIS (p.306), or an inflammatory condition of the intestines, such as ULCERATIVE COLITIS (p.659). However, there is a slight possibility of COLORECTAL CANCER (p.665).

MEDICAL HELP

See your doctor within 24 hours.

Have you suffered from repeated bouts of diarrhoea over the past few weeks?

- RECURRENT DIARRHOEA
- FIRST ATTACK

Has the diarrhoea been alternating with bouts of constipation?

- CONSTIPATION AND DIARRHOEA
- DIARRHOEA ALONE

POSSIBLE CAUSES

IRRITABLE BOWEL SYNDROME (p.655) is the most likely cause of your symptoms. In rare cases, these symptoms may be an indication of COLORECTAL CANCER (p.665).

MEDICAL HELP

Make an appointment to see your doctor.

Have you recently consumed either of the following?

- FOOD THAT MAY HAVE BEEN CONTAMINATED
- WATER THAT MAY HAVE BEEN CONTAMINATED
- NEITHER

POSSIBLE CAUSE

Your symptoms may be due to FOOD POISONING (p.629).

SELF-HELP

Maintain your fluid intake (*see* PREVENTING DEHYDRATION, p.627). Consult your doctor if you are no better within 2 days or if any other symptoms develop.

Do you have either of the following symptoms?

- NAUSEA OR VOMITING
- TEMPERATURE OF 38°C (100°F) OR ABOVE
- NEITHER

Have the attacks of diarrhoea occurred since a visit abroad?

FOREIGN TRAVEL

NO FOREIGN TRAVEL

POSSIBLE CAUSE
You may have picked up an intestinal infection, such as GIARDIASIS (p.307), during your foreign visit.

MEDICAL HELP

See your doctor within 24 hours.

POSSIBLE CAUSES
There is a possibility that you have a FOOD ALLERGY (p.467) or FOOD INTOLERANCE (p.657).

MEDICAL HELP

Make an appointment to see your doctor.

Do you have recurrent pain in the lower abdomen?

YES

NO

Is your diarrhoea associated with either of the following?

EATING PARTICULAR FOODS

PERIOD OF STRESS

NEITHER

POSSIBLE CAUSE
ANXIETY DISORDERS (p.551) can be a cause of diarrhoea.

MEDICAL HELP

Make an appointment to see your doctor.

Go to chart 36
RECURRENT ABDOMINAL PAIN

Are you currently taking any prescribed or over-the-counter medication?

MEDICATION

NO MEDICATION

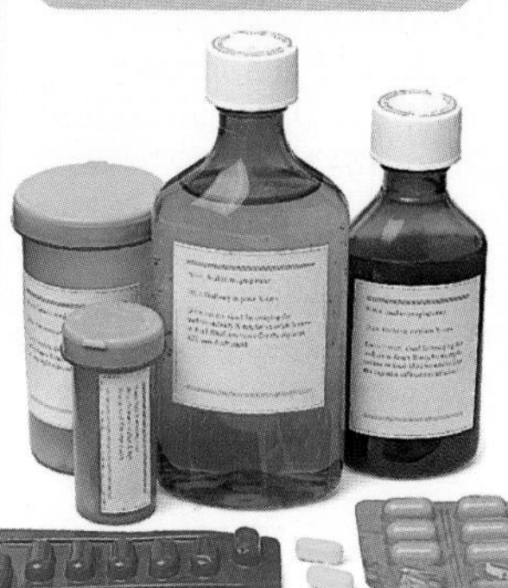

POSSIBLE CAUSE
Your symptoms may be a side effect of the medication.

MEDICAL HELP
Make an appointment to see your doctor. Stop taking any over-the-counter medicines but continue to take prescribed medication unless advised to stop by your doctor.

POSSIBLE CAUSES
GASTROENTERITIS (p.628) or FOOD POISONING (p.629) are the most likely possibilities.

SELF-HELP
Maintain your fluid intake (*see* PREVENTING DEHYDRATION, p.627). Consult your doctor if you are no better within 2 days or if other symptoms develop.

If you cannot identify a possible cause for your diarrhoea from this chart, make an appointment to see your doctor.

40 CONSTIPATION

Some people have a bowel movement once or twice a day; others do so less frequently. If you have fewer bowel movements than is usual for you or if your faeces are small and hard, you are constipated. The cause is often a lack of fluid or fibre-rich foods in the diet. If constipation occurs suddenly or persists despite a change in your diet, consult your doctor.

WARNING **BLOOD IN THE FAECES**

Blood can appear in the faeces as red streaks or in larger amounts. It can also make the stools look black. Small amounts of blood in the faeces are usually caused by minor anal problems, such as HAEMORRHOIDS (p.668), but you should always consult your doctor if you notice blood in the faeces because it is vital that other causes, such as COLORECTAL CANCER (p.665), are ruled out.

START HERE

How long have you suffered from constipation?

- FOR A FEW WEEKS OR LESS
- FOR SEVERAL MONTHS OR YEARS

Do you have pain in your rectum or anus when you move your bowels?

- PAIN
- NO PAIN

Do you have intermittent bouts of cramping pain in the lower abdomen?

- CRAMPING PAIN
- NO CRAMPING PAIN

POSSIBLE CAUSE

Your bowel reflexes may have become sluggish as a result of being constantly resisted.

SELF-HELP

Try following the advice for PREVENTING CONSTIPATION (p.628). Consult your doctor if your symptoms have not improved within 2 weeks.

POSSIBLE CAUSES

Pain on defaecation can cause or worsen constipation. HAEMORRHOIDS (p.668) or ANAL FISSURE (p.669) may be the cause of your symptoms.

MEDICAL HELP

Make an appointment to see your doctor.

Does either of the following apply?

- YOU REGULARLY IGNORE THE URGE TO MOVE YOUR BOWELS
- YOU REGULARLY USE STIMULANT LAXATIVES
- NEITHER

POSSIBLE CAUSE

Regular use of stimulant laxatives (p.924) can seriously disrupt the normal functioning of the bowels.

MEDICAL HELP

Make an appointment to see your doctor.

POSSIBLE CAUSES

Your constipation is probably due to a lack of fibre or fluid in your diet. Lack of exercise may also be a factor if you are not physically active (*see* CONSTIPATION, p.628).

SELF-HELP

Try following the advice for PREVENTING CONSTIPATION (p.628). Consult your doctor if your symptoms have not improved within 2 weeks.

POSSIBLE CAUSES
IRRITABLE BOWEL SYNDROME (p.655) is a possible cause, especially if your constipation alternates with bouts of diarrhoea. However, other causes, such as COLORECTAL CANCER (p.665), may need to be ruled out.

MEDICAL HELP
Make an appointment to see your doctor.

Are you currently taking any prescribed or over-the-counter medication?

- MEDICATION
- NO MEDICATION

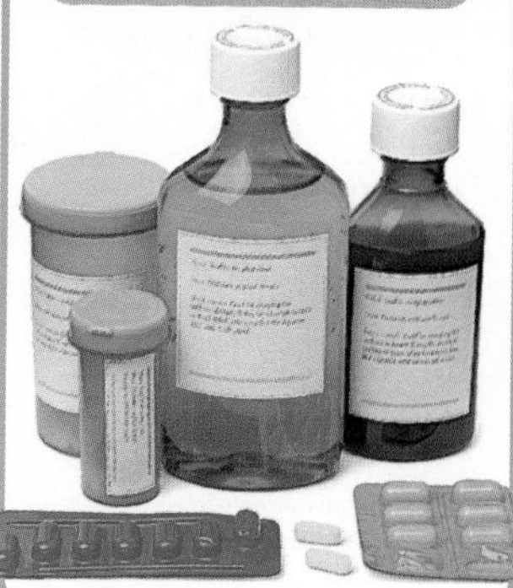

POSSIBLE CAUSE
Your symptoms may be a side effect of the medication.

MEDICAL HELP
Make an appointment to see your doctor. Stop taking any over-the-counter medicines but continue to take prescribed medication unless advised to stop by your doctor.

POSSIBLE CAUSE
A change in your regular diet, especially if you are travelling, can make you constipated.

SELF-HELP
Try following the advice for PREVENTING CONSTIPATION (p.628). Consult your doctor if your symptoms have not improved within 2 weeks.

POSSIBLE CAUSE
HYPOTHYROIDISM (p.680) is a possible cause.

MEDICAL HELP

Make an appointment to see your doctor.

Do you have any of the following symptoms?

- TIREDNESS
- INCREASED DRYNESS OR ROUGHNESS OF THE SKIN
- FEELING THE COLD MORE THAN YOU USED TO
- UNEXPLAINED WEIGHT GAIN
- GENERALIZED HAIR THINNING
- NONE OF THE ABOVE

Do any of the following apply?

- YOU ARE PREGNANT
- YOU HAVE BEEN DRINKING LESS FLUID THAN USUAL
- YOU HAVE CHANGED YOUR DIET
- NONE OF THE ABOVE

POSSIBLE CAUSE
Constipation is common in pregnancy (*see* COMMON COMPLAINTS OF NORMAL PREGNANCY, p.784).

SELF-HELP
Try following the advice for PREVENTING CONSTIPATION (p.628). Consult your doctor if your symptoms have not improved within 2 weeks.

POSSIBLE CAUSE
Lack of fluid in the bowel as a result of an inadequate fluid intake or excessive fluid loss can lead to constipation.

SELF-HELP
Be sure to drink plenty of fluids, especially if the weather is hot. Consult your doctor if your symptoms have not improved within 2 weeks.

If you cannot identify a possible cause for your constipation from this chart, make an appointment to see your doctor.

41 CHEST PAIN

Chest pain includes any discomfort felt in the front or back of the ribcage. Most chest pain is due to minor disorders such as muscle strain or indigestion. However, you should call an ambulance if you have a crushing pain in the centre or left side of your chest, if you are also short of breath or feel faint, or if the pain is unlike any pain you have had before.

START HERE

What kind of pain are you experiencing?

- CRUSHING
- SPREADING FROM THE CENTRE OF THE CHEST TO THE NECK, ARMS, OR JAW
- NEITHER OF THE ABOVE

Are you short of breath?

- SHORT OF BREATH
- NOT SHORT OF BREATH

Do any of the following apply?

- YOU HAVE RECENTLY HAD A SURGICAL OPERATION
- YOU HAVE RECENTLY BEEN IMMOBILE DUE TO INJURY OR ILLNESS
- YOU HAVE HAD A BABY WITHIN THE PAST 2 WEEKS
- NONE OF THE ABOVE

Is pain related to breathing?

- NOT RELATED TO BREATHING
- RELATED TO BREATHING

Does the pain subside after you rest for a few minutes?

- PAIN SUBSIDES
- PAIN PERSISTS

POSSIBLE CAUSE
Recurrent chest pain could be an indication of ANGINA (p.407), especially if pain in the chest occurs with exertion and disappears with rest.

MEDICAL HELP
URGENT! Phone your doctor immediately!

Does the pain have any of the following features?

- RELATED TO EATING OR TO PARTICULAR FOODS
- RELIEVED BY ANTACIDS
- BROUGHT ON BY BENDING OR LYING DOWN
- NONE OF THE ABOVE

Have you had this kind of pain before?

- PREVIOUS EPISODES OF THIS KIND OF PAIN
- NEVER BEFORE

POSSIBLE CAUSE
You may be having a heart attack (*see* MYOCARDIAL INFARCTION, p.410).

MEDICAL HELP
EMERGENCY! Call an ambulance! While waiting, chew half an aspirin unless you are allergic to it.

Possible cause
You may have a blood clot in the lung (*see* PULMONARY EMBOLISM, p.495).

Medical help
 EMERGENCY! Call an ambulance!

Do you have a fever – a temperature of 38°C (100°F) or above?

- FEVER
- NO FEVER

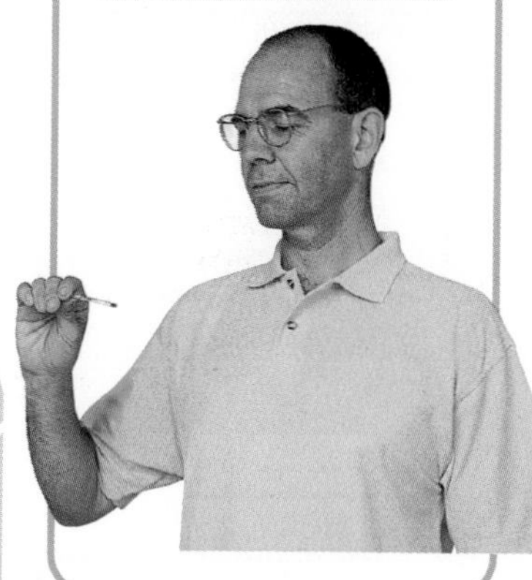

Possible cause
It is possible that you have a chest infection, such as PNEUMONIA (p.490).

Medical help
 URGENT! Phone your doctor immediately!

Possible cause
There is a possibility that you have a partially collapsed lung (*see* PNEUMOTHORAX, p.496).

Medical help
 URGENT! Phone your doctor immediately!

Is the chest sore to touch?

- SORE TO TOUCH
- NOT SORE TO TOUCH

Possible cause
Muscle strain and/or bruising is the most likely cause of your symptoms.

Self-help
Take a painkiller and rest for 24 hours. If the pain has not improved after this time, make an appointment to see your doctor.

Does either of the following apply?

- YOU HAVE HAD A CHEST INJURY
- YOU HAVE BEEN EXERCISING
- NEITHER

Possible cause
You may have PLEURISY (p.493), particularly if you have a cough and/or fever.

Medical help
 See your doctor within 24 hours.

Possible cause
This type of chest pain may be due to NONULCER DYSPEPSIA (p.626) or GASTRO-OESOPHAGEAL REFLUX (p.636).

Medical help
 Make an appointment to see your doctor.

Possible cause
You may be having a heart attack (*see* MYOCARDIAL INFARCTION, p.410).

Medical help
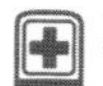 EMERGENCY! Call an ambulance! While waiting, chew half an aspirin unless you are allergic to it.

If you cannot identify a possible cause for your chest pain from this chart, make an appointment to see your doctor.

42 PALPITATIONS

Palpitations are an awareness of abnormally fast or irregular heartbeats. They are most often caused by stimulants, such as caffeine and nicotine, or by anxiety. Palpitations may also occur as a side effect of medication or because of a heart disorder. Call your doctor immediately if palpitations are frequent or persistent or if you have other symptoms.

START HERE

Do you have any of the following symptoms?

- SHORTNESS OF BREATH
- CHEST DISCOMFORT
- FEELING FAINT OR PASSING OUT
- NONE OF THE ABOVE

POSSIBLE CAUSE
You may have a serious arrhythmia (p.415) due to an underlying heart disorder.

MEDICAL HELP

EMERGENCY! Call an ambulance!

Do you have any of the following symptoms?

- WEIGHT LOSS WITH INCREASED APPETITE
- FEELING CONSTANTLY ON EDGE
- INCREASED SWEATING
- BULGING EYES
- NONE OF THE ABOVE

POSSIBLE CAUSES
HYPERTHYROIDISM (p.679) is a possibility. However, ANXIETY DISORDERS (p.551) can cause some of these symptoms.

MEDICAL HELP

Make an appointment to see your doctor.

Do any of the following apply?

- YOU HAVE BEEN DRINKING A LOT OF COFFEE, TEA, OR COLA
- YOU HAVE BEEN SMOKING MORE THAN USUAL FOR YOU
- YOU ARE TAKING MEDICATIONS
- NONE OF THE ABOVE

POSSIBLE CAUSE
Caffeine (in coffee, tea, and cola) and nicotine (in tobacco) are stimulants that can disturb heart rhythm.

SELF-HELP
Avoid all stimulants. Consult your doctor if your symptoms have not disappeared within 24 hours or if other symptoms also develop.

POSSIBLE CAUSE
Your symptoms may be a side effect of the medication.

MEDICAL HELP

See your doctor within 24 hours. Stop taking over-the-counter medicines but continue to take any prescribed medication unless advised to stop by your doctor.

Have you been feeling tense or under stress?

- FEELING UNDER STRESS
- NO STRESS

Go to chart 18 ANXIETY

If you cannot identify a possible cause for your palpitations from this chart, make an appointment to see your doctor.

43 POOR BLADDER CONTROL

If passing urine is painful, see chart 45

Inability to control the passage of urine may result in leakage of urine or difficulty urinating. These symptoms may be due to a bladder, nerve, or muscle disorder. In men, an enlarged prostate gland is a common cause. Urinary tract infections can also cause leakage of urine, especially in elderly people.

WARNING INABILITY TO PASS URINE

Inability to pass urine, even though the bladder is full, is a serious symptom. It may be the result of an obstruction or damage to nerves supplying the bladder, or it may be a side effect of certain drugs. You should phone your doctor immediately.

START HERE

Are you female or male?

- FEMALE
- MALE

Have you been experiencing either of the following symptoms?

- A STRONG URGE TO URINATE WITH LITTLE URINE PASSED
- LEAKAGE OF URINE WHEN YOU COUGH, SNEEZE, LAUGH, OR RUN
- NEITHER

POSSIBLE CAUSE

You may be suffering from an irritable bladder (*see* URGE INCONTINENCE, p.712).

MEDICAL HELP

Make an appointment to see your doctor.

POSSIBLE CAUSE

STRESS INCONTINENCE (p.711) is the most likely cause.

SELF-HELP

Try PELVIC FLOOR EXERCISES (p.712). Consult your doctor if there is no improvement within 1 month.

Do you have either of the following symptoms?

- DIFFICULTY STARTING TO PASS URINE
- WEAK URINARY STREAM
- NEITHER

POSSIBLE CAUSES

You may have an ENLARGED PROSTATE GLAND (p.725), especially if you are over 55, or a URETHRAL STRICTURE (p.714).

MEDICAL HELP

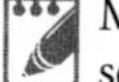
Make an appointment to see your doctor.

Are you currently taking any prescribed or over-the-counter medication?

- MEDICATION
- NO MEDICATION

POSSIBLE CAUSE

Some drugs, particularly those that act on urine production or the nervous system, can affect bladder control.

MEDICAL HELP

Make an appointment to see your doctor. Stop taking any over-the-counter medicines but continue to take prescribed medication unless advised to stop by your doctor.

If you cannot identify a possible cause for your poor bladder control from this chart, make an appointment to see your doctor.

44 FREQUENT URINATION

If passing urine is painful, see chart 45

How often you pass urine depends largely on how much you drink and how much your bladder can hold before you feel the need to empty it. If your urine looks abnormal, the appearance may give a clue to the cause of the problem (*see* CHECKING THE APPEARANCE OF YOUR URINE, p.169).

START HERE

How much urine do you pass each time you go to the toilet?

- LESS THAN USUAL
- AS MUCH OR MORE THAN USUAL

Have you been feeling more thirsty than usual?

- MORE THIRSTY
- NO INCREASED THIRST

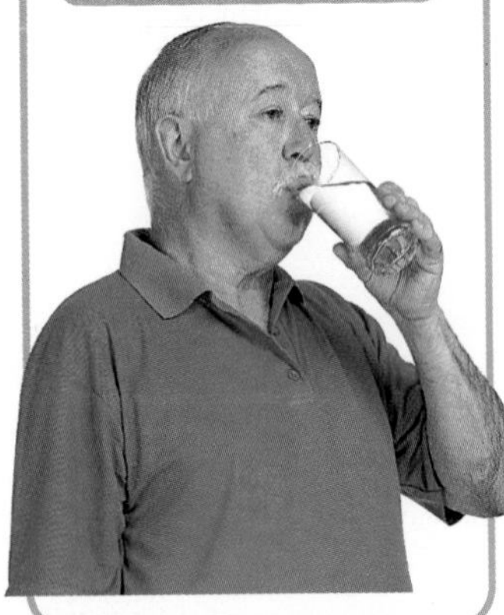

Are you female or male?

- FEMALE
- MALE

Have you been experiencing either of the following?

- UNEXPLAINED WEIGHT LOSS
- BLURRED VISION
- NEITHER

POSSIBLE CAUSE
DIABETES MELLITUS (p.687) is a possible cause of your symptoms.

MEDICAL HELP
 See your doctor within 24 hours.

Have you been drinking large amounts of the following?

- COFFEE OR TEA
- ALCOHOL
- NEITHER

POSSIBLE CAUSE
Substances in these drinks may increase the need to pass urine.

SELF-HELP
Reduce your consumption of such drinks. If you continue to be troubled by passing urine too frequently, consult your doctor.

POSSIBLE CAUSES
A kidney disorder, such as GLOMERULONEPHRITIS (p.699), or a hormonal disorder, such as DIABETES INSIPIDUS (p.678), are possible causes.

MEDICAL HELP
 Make an appointment to see your doctor.

Could you be pregnant?

- NOT PREGNANT
- POSSIBLY PREGNANT

POSSIBLE CAUSE
An increase in the frequency of passing urine is common in early, as well as later, pregnancy (*see* COMMON COMPLAINTS OF NORMAL PREGNANCY, p.784).

SELF-HELP
Carry out a HOME PREGNANCY TEST (p.232) if you are not sure whether you are pregnant.

Have you been experiencing either of the following ?

- A STRONG URGE TO PASS URINE WITH LITTLE URINE PASSED
- DIFFICULTY CONTROLLING URINATION
- NEITHER

POSSIBLE CAUSES
Your symptoms may be due to an irritable bladder (*see* URGE INCONTINENCE, p.712) or to a urinary tract infection, such as CYSTITIS (p.709).

MEDICAL HELP

Make an appointment to see your doctor.

Are you currently taking any prescribed or over-the-counter medication?

- MEDICATION
- NO MEDICATION

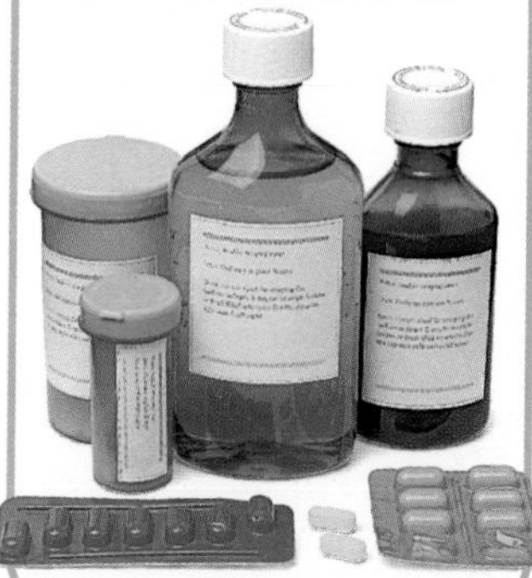

POSSIBLE CAUSE
Your symptoms may be a side effect of the medication.

MEDICAL HELP
Make an appointment to see your doctor. Stop taking any over-the-counter medicines but continue to take prescribed medication unless advised to stop by your doctor.

Do you feel the need to pass urine frequently when you are anxious?

- RELATED TO ANXIETY
- NOT RELATED TO ANXIETY

POSSIBLE CAUSE
ANXIETY DISORDERS (p.551) commonly cause an urge to pass urine frequently, even when the bladder is not full.

MEDICAL HELP
Make an appointment to see your doctor to discuss the causes of your anxiety.

If you cannot identify a possible cause for your frequent urination from this chart, make an appointment to see your doctor.

Do you have either of the following symptoms?

- DIFFICULTY STARTING TO PASS URINE
- WEAK URINARY STREAM
- NEITHER

POSSIBLE CAUSE
You may have an ENLARGED PROSTATE GLAND (p.725), especially if you are over 55.

MEDICAL HELP
Make an appointment to see your doctor.

45 PAINFUL URINATION

Pain or discomfort while passing urine is usually caused by inflammation of the urinary tract, often due to infection. In women, pain when passing urine may be due to vaginal infection. Discoloured urine sometimes accompanies this type of pain but can occur in the absence of disease (*see* CHECKING THE APPEARANCE OF YOUR URINE, opposite page).

START HERE

Do you have either of the following symptoms?

- PAIN IN THE BACK JUST ABOVE THE WAIST
- A TEMPERATURE OF 38°C (100°F) OR ABOVE
- NEITHER

POSSIBLE CAUSE

A kidney infection is a possible cause of your symptoms (*see* PYELONEPHRITIS, p.698).

MEDICAL HELP

URGENT! Phone your doctor immediately!

Have you felt the need to pass urine more frequently than usual?

- INCREASED FREQUENCY
- NO INCREASED FREQUENCY

Do you have any of the following symptoms?

- LOWER ABDOMINAL PAIN
- BLOOD IN THE URINE
- CLOUDY URINE
- NONE OF THE ABOVE

POSSIBLE CAUSE

A urinary tract infection, such as CYSTITIS (p.709), is possible.

MEDICAL HELP

See your doctor within 24 hours. Meanwhile, follow the self-help advice for CYSTITIS (p.709).

Are you female or male?

- FEMALE
- MALE

Do you have an unusual discharge from your penis?

- DISCHARGE
- NO DISCHARGE

Have you noticed soreness or itching in the genital area?

- SORENESS
- ITCHING
- NEITHER

POSSIBLE CAUSE
A vaginal yeast infection is the most likely possibility (*see* VAGINAL THRUSH, p.752).

MEDICAL HELP
Make an appointment to see your doctor if this is the first time you have had these symptoms. Otherwise, try using an over-the-counter antifungal preparation recommended by your pharmacist.

POSSIBLE CAUSE
A urinary tract infection, such as CYSTITIS (p.709), is possible.

MEDICAL HELP
See your doctor within 24 hours. Meanwhile, follow the self-help advice for CYSTITIS (p.709).

Do you have an unusual vaginal discharge?

- THICK, WHITE DISCHARGE
- YELLOWISH-GREEN DISCHARGE
- NO UNUSUAL DISCHARGE

POSSIBLE CAUSE
A sexually transmitted infection, such as GONORRHOEA (p.764) or NONGONOCOCCAL URETHRITIS (p.765), may be causing your symptoms.

MEDICAL HELP
See your doctor within 24 hours, or go to a clinic specializing in sexually transmitted infections.

POSSIBLE CAUSES
The most likely cause is either a vaginal infection, such as TRICHOMONIASIS (p.767), or a sexually transmitted infection, such as GONORRHOEA (p.764).

MEDICAL HELP

See your doctor within 24 hours.

If you cannot identify a possible cause for your symptoms from this chart, make an appointment to see your doctor.

SYMPTOM ASSESSMENT

CHECKING THE APPEARANCE OF YOUR URINE

The appearance of urine varies considerably. For example, urine is often darker in the morning than later in the day. Some drugs and foods may also cause a temporary colour change in the urine. Beetroot, for example, may turn the urine red.

A change in your urine can indicate a disorder. Very dark urine may be a sign of liver disease (*see* ACUTE HEPATITIS, p.644); red or cloudy urine may be due to bleeding or infection in the kidney or bladder.

If you are not sure about the cause of a change in the appearance of your urine, consult your doctor.

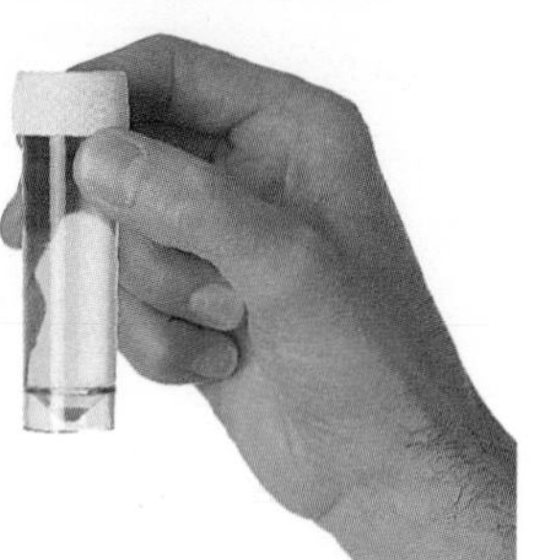

Normal appearance of urine
Normally, urine is clear, pale, and straw-coloured but may be cloudy at first in the morning.

If you cannot identify a possible cause for your symptoms from this chart, make an appointment to see your doctor.

46 BACK PAIN

Mild back pain is usually caused by poor posture, sudden movements, or lifting heavy objects, all of which may strain the back. Back pain is also common in pregnancy. Persistent or severe back pain may be the result of a more serious problem. You should consult your doctor if pain is severe or does not start to improve after 48 hours.

DANGER SIGNS

Call an ambulance if you have back pain that is associated with one of the following symptoms:

- Difficulty in controlling your bladder.
- Difficulty in controlling your bowels.

START HERE

Did the pain in your back come on after either of the following?

- AN INJURY OR FALL
- A SUDDEN, AWKWARD MOVEMENT
- NEITHER

Do you have either of the following?

- PAIN IN THE BACK JUST ABOVE THE WAIST
- A TEMPERATURE OF 38°C (100°F) OR ABOVE
- NEITHER

POSSIBLE CAUSE

PYELONEPHRITIS (p.698) is a likely cause of your symptoms.

MEDICAL HELP

URGENT! Phone your doctor immediately!

Did the pain occur after any of the following?

- LIFTING A HEAVY WEIGHT
- A FIT OF COUGHING
- STRENUOUS OR UNACCUSTOMED PHYSICAL ACTIVITY
- NONE OF THE ABOVE

Have you noticed any of the following symptoms?

- DIFFICULTY IN MOVING A LEG
- NUMBNESS OR TINGLING IN A LEG
- LOSS OF BLADDER CONTROL
- NONE OF THE ABOVE

POSSIBLE CAUSE

Your symptoms indicate that there may be spinal damage (*see* SPINAL INJURIES, p.524).

MEDICAL HELP

URGENT! Phone your doctor immediately!

POSSIBLE CAUSE

Your back is probably strained and/or bruised (*see* MUSCLE STRAINS AND TEARS, p.395).

SELF-HELP

Take a painkiller and rest. A covered hot-water bottle or a heat pad placed against your back may give you additional pain relief. Consult your doctor if you are no better within 24 hours.

Does either of the following apply?

- PAIN MAKES ANY MOVEMENT DIFFICULT
- PAIN SHOOTS FROM THE BACK DOWN THE BACK OF THE LEG
- NEITHER

POSSIBLE CAUSE

You have probably strained some of the muscles in your back or sprained some of the ligaments (*see* LOWER BACK PAIN, p.381).

SELF-HELP

See the advice for LOWER BACK PAIN (p.381). Consult your doctor if you do not feel any better in 2 or 3 days or if other symptoms develop.

Have you been suffering from increasing pain and stiffness over several months or longer?

- YES
- NO

POSSIBLE CAUSE

Fracture of a vertebra as a result of thinning of the bones is a possible cause (*see* OSTEOPOROSIS, p.368).

MEDICAL HELP

See your doctor within 24 hours.

POSSIBLE CAUSES

You may have a fractured vertebra (*see* OSTEOPOROSIS, p.368) or SCIATICA (p.546), caused by a PROLAPSED OR HERNIATED DISK (p.384).

MEDICAL HELP

See your doctor within 24 hours.

How old are you?

- 45 OR OVER
- UNDER 45

POSSIBLE CAUSE

ANKYLOSING SPONDYLITIS (p.378) is a possible cause of your symptoms, especially if you are male.

MEDICAL HELP

Make an appointment to see your doctor.

Does either of the following apply?

- YOU HAVE RECENTLY BEEN IMMOBILE DUE TO ILLNESS OR INJURY
- YOU ARE OVER 60
- NEITHER

POSSIBLE CAUSE

OSTEOARTHRITIS (p.374) in the back is the most likely cause of your symptoms.

MEDICAL HELP

Make an appointment to see your doctor.

POSSIBLE CAUSE

New back pain or a worsening of existing back pain may indicate the start of labour.

MEDICAL HELP

URGENT! Phone your doctor or midwife immediately if you think that you may be going into labour.

Are you in the last 3 months of pregnancy?

- PREGNANT
- NOT PREGNANT

If you cannot identify a possible cause for your back pain from this chart, make an appointment to see your doctor.

47 NECK PAIN OR STIFFNESS

Pain and/or stiffness in the neck is usually due to a minor problem, such as muscle strain or ligament sprain, that does not require treatment. However, if the pain occurs with fever, meningitis is a possibility. Neck pain or stiffness becomes more common as a person gets older and may then be due to a disorder of the bones and joints of the neck.

DANGER SIGNS

Call an ambulance if you have neck pain associated with either of the following symptoms:

- Difficulty in controlling your bladder.
- Difficulty in controlling your bowels.

START HERE

How long have you had pain and/or stiffness in the neck?

- LESS THAN 24 HOURS
- 24 HOURS OR LONGER

Have you jolted or injured your neck, for example in a car accident or fall?

- NECK INJURY
- NO NECK INJURY

Have you noticed any of the following symptoms?

- DIFFICULTY MOVING AN ARM OR LEG
- PAIN, NUMBNESS, OR TINGLING IN AN ARM OR LEG
- LOSS OF BLADDER CONTROL
- NONE OF THE ABOVE

POSSIBLE CAUSE
Your symptoms indicate that there may be spinal damage (*see* SPINAL INJURIES, p.524).

MEDICAL HELP
EMERGENCY! Call an ambulance!

POSSIBLE CAUSE
Your neck is probably strained and/or bruised (*see* MUSCLE STRAINS AND TEARS, p.395).

SELF-HELP
Take a PAINKILLER (p.912) and rest lying down. A heat pad placed against your neck may give you additional pain relief. Consult your doctor if you are no better in 24 hours.

Which of the following describes your symptoms?

- GRADUALLY WORSENING PAIN AND STIFFNESS OVER MANY MONTHS
- NECK PAIN WITH NUMBNESS OR PAIN IN THE ARM AND/OR HAND
- NEITHER

Do you have any of the following symptoms?

- TEMPERATURE OF 38°C (100°F) OR ABOVE
- SEVERE HEADACHE
- ABNORMAL DROWSINESS OR CONFUSION
- DISLIKE OF BRIGHT LIGHT
- NAUSEA OR VOMITING
- NONE OF THE ABOVE

Does either of the following apply?

- PAIN IS SEVERE ENOUGH TO PREVENT MOVEMENT
- PAIN SHOOTS DOWN ONE ARM FROM THE NECK
- NEITHER

POSSIBLE CAUSES
Your neck pain may be due to pressure on a nerve as a result of a PROLAPSED OR HERNIATED DISK (p.384) or CERVICAL SPONDYLOSIS (p.376).

MEDICAL HELP

See your doctor within 24 hours.

POSSIBLE CAUSES
You may have neck strain (*see* MUSCLE STRAINS AND TEARS, p.395) or TORTICOLLIS (p.388).

SELF-HELP
Rest your neck as much as possible by lying down and take a NONSTEROIDAL ANTI-INFLAMMATORY DRUG (p.894) to ease the pain. Keeping your neck warm with a heat pad may also help. Consult your doctor if you are no better in 3 days.

POSSIBLE CAUSE
MENINGITIS (p.527) could be the cause of these symptoms.

MEDICAL HELP
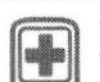
EMERGENCY! Call an ambulance!

Can you feel any tenderness or swelling at the sides or the back of the neck?

- YES
- NO

Go to chart 8
LUMPS AND SWELLINGS

Did either of the following apply in the 24 hours before the onset of pain?

- YOU EXERCISED UNUSUALLY STRENUOUSLY
- YOU SAT OR SLEPT IN AN AWKWARD POSITION
- NEITHER

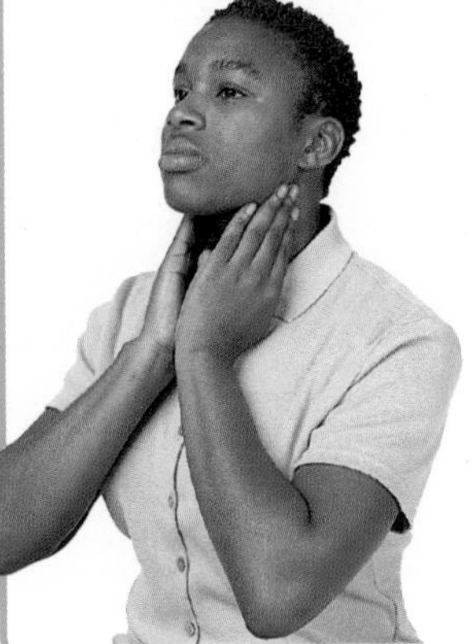

POSSIBLE CAUSE
The cause of your symptoms may be CERVICAL SPONDYLOSIS (p.376), especially if you are over the age of 45.

MEDICAL HELP

Make an appointment to see your doctor.

If you cannot identify a possible cause for your neck pain or stiffness from this chart, make an appointment to see your doctor.

48 PAINFUL ARM OR HAND

If you have painful joints, see chart 50

Pain in the arm or hand is often caused by injury or a problem in the neck or shoulder. Rarely, pain in the arm is due to a heart attack or a serious neck disorder. Consult your doctor if the pain is severe, recurrent, or persistent.

START HERE

Did the pain start during or soon after either of the following?

- AN INJURY OR FALL
- REPETITIVE MOVEMENTS OF THE AFFECTED ARM OR HAND
- NEITHER

POSSIBLE CAUSES
A serious injury is possible (*see* MUSCLE STRAINS AND TEARS, p.395, and FRACTURES, p.392).

MEDICAL HELP
URGENT! Phone your doctor immediately if you are in severe pain. Otherwise, use first-aid measures (*see* SPRAINS AND STRAINS, p.991), but make an appointment to see your doctor if the pain is no better after 48 hours or if other symptoms develop.

POSSIBLE CAUSE
REPETITIVE STRAIN INJURY (p.389) is a possible explanation for your symptoms.

MEDICAL HELP

Make an appointment to see your doctor.

Is the pain associated with any of the following symptoms?

- CHEST TIGHTNESS
- SHORTNESS OF BREATH
- NAUSEA, SWEATING, OR FEELING FAINT
- NONE OF THE ABOVE

POSSIBLE CAUSE
You may be having a heart attack (*see* MYOCARDIAL INFARCTION, p.410).

MEDICAL HELP
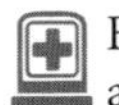
EMERGENCY! Call an ambulance! While waiting, chew half an aspirin unless you are allergic to it.

What are the features of the pain?

- LOCALIZED IN UPPER ARM OR SHOULDER
- SHOOTS DOWN THE LENGTH OF THE ARM
- EXTENDS FROM THE WRIST INTO THE PALM AND LOWER ARM
- NONE OF THE ABOVE

POSSIBLE CAUSES
Inflammation around the shoulder may be the cause (*see* POLYMYALGIA RHEUMATICA, p.464, and TENDINITIS AND TENOSYNOVITIS, p.390).

MEDICAL HELP

Make an appointment to see your doctor.

POSSIBLE CAUSES
You may have a pinched nerve in your neck, particularly if you also have neck pain (*see* PROLAPSED OR HERNIATED DISK, p.384, and CERVICAL SPONDYLOSIS, p.376).

MEDICAL HELP

See your doctor within 24 hours.

POSSIBLE CAUSE
You may have CARPAL TUNNEL SYNDROME (p.547), particularly if you also have numbness or tingling in your fingers.

MEDICAL HELP
Make an appointment to see your doctor.

If you cannot identify a possible cause for your painful arm or hand from this chart, make an appointment to see your doctor.

49 PAINFUL LEG

If you have painful joints, see chart 50

Leg pain due to a pulled muscle or torn ligament usually goes away without treatment. Pain may also result from a problem in the lower back or in the blood vessels in the leg. If your leg is also swollen, hot, or red, see your doctor at once.

START HERE

Did the pain start during or soon after either of the following?

- AN INJURY OR FALL → see *Possible causes* (serious injury)
- UNACCUSTOMED EXERCISE → see *Possible cause* (strained muscle)
- NEITHER → **What are the features of the pain?**

POSSIBLE CAUSES
A serious injury is possible (*see* MUSCLE STRAINS AND TEARS, p.395, and FRACTURES, p.392).

MEDICAL HELP
URGENT! Phone your doctor immediately if you are in severe pain. Otherwise, use first-aid measures (*see* SPRAINS AND STRAINS, p.991), but make an appointment to see your doctor if the pain is no better after 48 hours or if other symptoms develop.

POSSIBLE CAUSE
You may have strained a muscle (*see* MUSCLE STRAINS AND TEARS, p.395).

SELF-HELP
Try first-aid measures (*see* SPRAINS AND STRAINS, p.991).

What are the features of the pain?

- AFFECTS A SMALL AREA THAT IS ALSO RED AND HOT
- SUDDEN TIGHTENING OF THE MUSCLES IN THE CALF
- CONSTANT PAIN IN THE CALF, WHICH MAY BE SWOLLEN
- SHOOTING PAIN DOWN THE BACK OF THE LEG
- HEAVY, ACHING LEGS
- NONE OF THE ABOVE

POSSIBLE CAUSES
Your symptoms may be caused by an infection under the skin (*see* CELLULITIS, p.352) or an inflamed vein (*see* SUPERFICIAL THROMBOPHLEBITIS, p.439).

MEDICAL HELP

See your doctor within 24 hours.

POSSIBLE CAUSES
You may have MUSCLE CRAMP (p.388), but, if the pain occurs with exercise and disappears with rest, you may have narrowing of the blood vessels in the leg (*see* LOWER LIMB ISCHAEMIA, p.434).

MEDICAL HELP

Make an appointment to see your doctor.

POSSIBLE CAUSE
You may have a blood clot in a vein in your leg (*see* DEEP VEIN THROMBOSIS, p.437).

MEDICAL HELP

URGENT! Phone your doctor immediately!

POSSIBLE CAUSE
SCIATICA (p.546) is a likely cause of your symptoms.

MEDICAL HELP

Make an appointment to see your doctor.

Does sitting down with your feet up relieve the pain?

- YES
- NO

POSSIBLE CAUSE
VARICOSE VEINS (p.438) are a possible cause.

MEDICAL HELP

Make an appointment to see your doctor.

If you cannot identify a possible cause for your painful leg from this chart, make an appointment to see your doctor.

50 PAINFUL JOINTS

If you have a painless swollen ankle, see chart 51

Pain in a joint may be caused by injury or strain and often gets better without a cause being found. Gout or a joint infection can cause a joint to become red, hot, and swollen. Joint pain may be due to arthritis or a reaction to an infection. Consult your doctor if pain is severe or persistent.

START HERE

Have you injured the joint?

- INJURY
- NO INJURY

Does either of the following apply?

- YOU ARE UNABLE TO MOVE THE JOINT
- THE JOINT APPEARS MISSHAPEN OR SWOLLEN
- NEITHER

POSSIBLE CAUSE
A ligament around the joint is probably sprained.

SELF-HELP
Try the first-aid measures for SPRAINS AND STRAINS (p.991). Consult your doctor if the joint is no better in 24 hours.

Do you have either of the following?

- HOT JOINT(S)
- RED JOINT(S)
- NEITHER

POSSIBLE CAUSES
A severe injury is possible (*see* FRACTURES, p.392; MUSCLE STRAINS AND TEARS, p.395; and LIGAMENT INJURIES, p.394).

MEDICAL HELP
URGENT! Phone your doctor immediately! You should also follow the first-aid advice for FRACTURES (p.992).

POSSIBLE CAUSE
OSTEOARTHRITIS (p.374) is the most likely cause of pain and stiffness in the joints.

MEDICAL HELP
Make an appointment to see your doctor.

How many joints are affected?

- ONE JOINT
- MORE THAN ONE

POSSIBLE CAUSES
SEPTIC ARTHRITIS (p.381), GOUT (p.380), or PSEUDOGOUT (p.381), can all cause a single joint to become red, hot, and painful.

MEDICAL HELP

See your doctor within 24 hours.

Does moving the joint affect the pain?

- CONSIDERABLY WORSENS IT
- SLIGHTLY WORSENS IT OR NO CHANGE

Did the pain come on gradually over months or years?

- YES
- NO

Have you recently had either of the following?

- AN INFECTION WITH A RASH
- AN INFECTION WITHOUT A RASH
- NEITHER

POSSIBLE CAUSES
Some viral illnesses, such as RUBELLA (p.294), can cause joint pain, but LYME DISEASE (p.303) is also a possibility, particularly if you have been bitten by a tick.

MEDICAL HELP

See your doctor within 24 hours.

POSSIBLE CAUSES
Certain bacterial infections of the intestines and genital tract may cause a reaction that leads to painful joints (*see* REACTIVE ARTHRITIS, p.379).

MEDICAL HELP

See your doctor within 24 hours.

POSSIBLE CAUSES
RHEUMATOID ARTHRITIS (p.377) is a possible cause of your symptoms.

MEDICAL HELP

See your doctor within 24 hours.

Is the problem in a child under the age of 12 or in someone aged 12 or over?

- UNDER 12
- 12 OR OVER

POSSIBLE CAUSE
A FROZEN SHOULDER (p.385) could be the cause.

MEDICAL HELP

Make an appointment to see your doctor.

Which joint or joints are affected?

- HIP
- SHOULDER
- NECK
- OTHER JOINT(S)

POSSIBLE CAUSES
Most childhood hip problems are not serious, but a SLIPPED FEMORAL EPIPHYSIS (p.834) or PERTHES' DISEASE (p.833) are rare possibilities.

MEDICAL HELP
See your doctor within 24 hours.

POSSIBLE CAUSES
Your symptoms are probably a result of overuse of a joint, for example as a result of excessive exercise. A recent minor viral illness may also be the cause of such symptoms.

MEDICAL HELP

Make an appointment to see your doctor if there is no improvement in 48 hours.

Go to chart 47
NECK PAIN OR STIFFNESS

If you cannot identify a possible cause for your painful joints from this chart, make an appointment to see your doctor.

51 SWOLLEN ANKLES

If you have painful swollen ankles, see chart 50

Slight, painless swelling of the ankles is most often caused by fluid accumulating in the tissues after long periods of sitting or standing still, but it may be due to heart, liver, or kidney disorders. It is common in pregnancy. If swelling persists or if you have other symptoms, consult your doctor.

START HERE

Are both ankles affected?

- BOTH ANKLES
- ONE ANKLE

Have you been suffering from increasing shortness of breath?

- SHORTNESS OF BREATH
- NO SHORTNESS OF BREATH

POSSIBLE CAUSES

Swelling of the ankles (due to fluid retention) and shortness of breath may be a result of CHRONIC HEART FAILURE (p.413). Other possible causes of these symptoms are liver problems (*see* CIRRHOSIS, p.647) or kidney problems (*see* NEPHROTIC SYNDROME, p.700).

MEDICAL HELP

See your doctor within 24 hours.

Are you pregnant?

- PREGNANT
- NOT PREGNANT

POSSIBLE CAUSE

Swelling can persist or recur for several weeks following an injury. This is unlikely to be a cause for concern.

SELF-HELP

If the injury occurred within the past 48 hours, follow the first-aid advice for SPRAINS AND STRAINS (p.991). For a less recent injury, try resting the limb. Make an appointment to see your doctor if swelling persists despite rest or if the ankle is painful, tender, or inflamed.

POSSIBLE CAUSE

You may have a blood clot in a vein in your leg (*see* DEEP VEIN THROMBOSIS, p.437).

MEDICAL HELP

URGENT! Phone your doctor immediately!

Is the calf of the affected leg either of the following?

- SWOLLEN
- TENDER
- NEITHER

Have you injured your ankle within the past few weeks?

- RECENT INJURY
- NO RECENT INJURY

POSSIBLE CAUSE

Several hours of inactivity can lead to accumulation of fluid in the ankles due to less efficient circulation. The decreased cabin pressure in a plane increases this tendency.

SELF-HELP

Encourage the circulation by getting up and walking around at regular intervals during any long journey. When seated, keep your legs raised and take a brisk walk when you reach your destination.

Does either of the following apply?

- YOUR FACE OR FINGERS ARE SWOLLEN
- YOU HAVE GAINED OVER 2 KG (4.5 LB) IN THE PAST WEEK
- NEITHER

POSSIBLE CAUSE
Retaining excessive amounts of fluid may be a sign of pre-eclampsia (*see* PRE-ECLAMPSIA AND ECLAMPSIA, p.794).

MEDICAL HELP
URGENT! Phone your doctor or midwife immediately!

POSSIBLE CAUSE
You may have VARICOSE VEINS (p.438), which can cause fluid to accumulate in the ankles.

SELF-HELP
Avoid standing still for long periods. Walk as much as possible, and when sitting down try to keep your feet raised. Make an appointment to see your doctor if the swelling worsens or if other symptoms develop.

POSSIBLE CAUSE
Fluid retention, leading to swollen ankles, is common in pregnancy (*see* COMMON COMPLAINTS OF NORMAL PREGNANCY, p.784).

SELF-HELP
Avoid standing still for long periods and put your feet up whenever possible to reduce swelling. Consult your doctor if your face and/or fingers become swollen or if you start to put on weight rapidly.

POSSIBLE CAUSE
Your symptom may be a side effect of the drug.

MEDICAL HELP
Make an appointment to see your doctor. Stop taking any over-the-counter medicines but continue to take prescribed medication unless advised to stop by your doctor.

Do you have prominent veins in the leg or legs affected by swelling?

- PROMINENT VEINS
- NO PROMINENT VEINS

Are you currently taking any prescribed or over-the-counter medication?

- MEDICATION
- NO MEDICATION

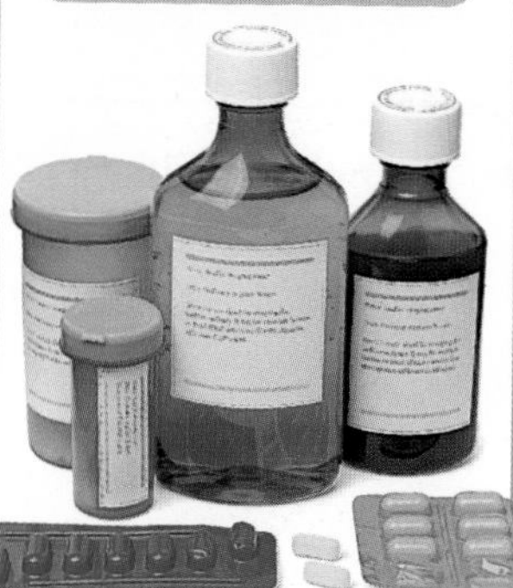

Did your ankles become swollen after either of the following?

- A LONG TRIP BY CAR OR TRAIN
- AN AEROPLANE FLIGHT
- NEITHER

If you cannot identify a possible cause for your swollen ankles from this chart, make an appointment to see your doctor.

52 IMPOTENCE

Impotence is failure to have or maintain an erection. Although distressing, occasional difficulties are normal and are usually caused by factors such as stress, tiredness, anxiety, or alcohol. Physical causes are not common. If impotence occurs frequently, you should consult your doctor for advice. Safe and effective treatments for impotence are available.

WARNING

NONMEDICAL ADVICE

Treatment from a nonmedical source could delay an important diagnosis being made or even result in more serious problems. It is important that you consult a doctor, who can rule out any medical cause of your erection problems, before having any form of treatment.

START HERE

Are you interested in sex?

- YES
- NO

POSSIBLE CAUSE

Lack of interest in sex is likely to reduce your ability to achieve an erection (*see* DECREASED SEX DRIVE, p.769).

MEDICAL HELP

Make an appointment to see your doctor.

How often do you fail to achieve or maintain an erection?

- ONLY OCCASIONALLY
- FREQUENTLY

POSSIBLE CAUSES

Most men have this experience from time to time. Occasional erection problems are most likely to be due to anxiety – for example, at the beginning of a new sexual relationship – or to factors such as tiredness or having too much alcohol to drink (*see* IMPOTENCE, p.770).

MEDICAL HELP

Make an appointment to see your doctor if you are concerned about problems with your sexual performance.

Do you wake with an erection?

- SOMETIMES
- NEVER

POSSIBLE CAUSE

Anxiety about your sexual performance is the most likely explanation for your problem (*see* IMPOTENCE, p.770). A physical cause is unlikely.

MEDICAL HELP

Make an appointment to see your doctor.

Are you currently receiving treatment for an illness?

- TREATMENT
- NO TREATMENT

POSSIBLE CAUSES

Certain illnesses, such as DIABETES MELLITUS (p.687), can lead to erection problems. Some drugs, including ANTIHYPERTENSIVE DRUGS (p.897) and ANTIDEPRESSANT DRUGS (p.916), can also affect sexual performance.

MEDICAL HELP

Make an appointment to see your doctor.

If you cannot identify a possible cause for your erection problem from this chart, make an appointment to see your doctor.

53 TESTES AND SCROTUM PROBLEMS

Regular self-examination (*see* EXAMINING YOUR TESTES, p.720) is important to detect lumps and swellings in the testes (the sperm-producing organs) and the scrotum (the sac in which the testes lie). The cause may be minor, but there is a possibility of cancer of the testis. Painful swelling in the genital area requires immediate medical attention.

START HERE

What is the nature of your symptoms?

- PAIN AND SWELLING → Does the problem affect one or both testes?
- PAINLESS ENLARGEMENT IN OR NEAR TESTIS → Possible causes: epididymal cyst
- GENERALIZED PAINLESS SWELLING OF THE SCROTUM → Possible causes: accumulation of fluid
- NONE OF THE ABOVE → If you cannot identify a possible cause

Does the problem affect one or both testes?

- ONE → Possible causes: torsion of the testis
- BOTH → Have you had an injury in the genital area within the past 48 hours?

Have you had an injury in the genital area within the past 48 hours?

- INJURY → Possible cause: internal damage
- NO INJURY → Possible cause: epididymo-orchitis

POSSIBLE CAUSES

TORSION OF THE TESTIS (p.719) may be the cause of pain and swelling in one testis. A less serious possible cause is EPIDIDYMO-ORCHITIS (p.718).

MEDICAL HELP

 EMERGENCY! Call an ambulance!

POSSIBLE CAUSE

Internal damage to the testes is a possibility.

MEDICAL HELP

 URGENT! Phone your doctor immediately!

POSSIBLE CAUSES

Accumulation of fluid in the scrotum (*see* HYDROCELE, p.721), varicose veins in the scrotum (*see* VARICOCELE, p.720), or an inguinal hernia (*see* HERNIAS, p.661) are the most likely causes of your symptoms. However, there is a possibility that you may have CANCER OF THE TESTIS (p.719).

MEDICAL HELP

 Make an appointment to see your doctor.

POSSIBLE CAUSES

An EPIDIDYMAL CYST (p.718) is the probable cause of your symptoms. However, there is a possibility that you have CANCER OF THE TESTIS (p.719).

MEDICAL HELP

 Make an appointment to see your doctor.

If you cannot identify a possible cause for your testes or scrotum problem from this chart, make an appointment to see your doctor.

POSSIBLE CAUSE

EPIDIDYMO-ORCHITIS (p.718), which may be due to a sexually transmitted infection or a viral infection such as mumps, may be causing your symptoms.

MEDICAL HELP

 See your doctor within 24 hours.

54 PROBLEMS WITH THE PENIS

If you are impotent, see chart 52

Pain or soreness of the penis that is not related to injury is often due to infection in the urinary tract or of the skin of the penis. Inflammation may be caused by friction during sexual intercourse. You should consult your doctor if there is any change in the appearance of the skin of the penis.

WARNING BLOOD IN THE SEMEN

Blood-streaked semen is usually caused by leakage from small blood vessels in the testes or epididymis. A single episode is unlikely to be a cause for concern, but, if it recurs, you should consult your doctor. It is also important to consult your doctor if you notice a blood-stained discharge that is not related to ejaculation or if you notice blood in your urine.

START HERE

What kind of problem are you experiencing?

- PAINFUL OR SORE PENIS
- DISCHARGE FROM PENIS
- FORESKIN PROBLEM
- CHANGE IN APPEARANCE OF ERECT PENIS
- NONE OF THE ABOVE

When does the pain occur?

- ONLY WITH AN ERECTION
- ONLY WHEN PASSING URINE
- AT OTHER TIMES

Go to chart 45
PAINFUL URINATION

How is the foreskin affected?

- HAS BEEN RETRACTED BUT CANNOT BE REPLACED
- AFTER CHILDHOOD, CANNOT BE FULLY RETRACTED
- BALLOONS WHEN PASSING URINE
- NONE OF THE ABOVE

POSSIBLE CAUSE

Inability to replace a retracted foreskin is called paraphimosis (*see* PHIMOSIS, p.721).

MEDICAL HELP

EMERGENCY! Call an ambulance! While waiting for help, surround the affected area with an ice pack.

POSSIBLE CAUSE

You may have a sexually transmitted infection, such as GONORRHOEA (p.764).

MEDICAL HELP

See your doctor within 24 hours or go to a clinic specializing in sexually transmitted infections.

POSSIBLE CAUSE

Your problem may be caused by PEYRONIE'S DISEASE (p.723).

MEDICAL HELP

Make an appointment to see your doctor.

POSSIBLE CAUSE

An abnormally tight foreskin (*see* PHIMOSIS, p.721) may cause these problems.

MEDICAL HELP

Make an appointment to see your doctor.

Has the painful erection now subsided?

- SUBSIDED
- STILL PRESENT

POSSIBLE CAUSE
PRIAPISM (p.723), in which there is an obstruction to the flow of blood leaving the penis, could be the cause of your symptoms.

MEDICAL HELP

URGENT! Phone your doctor immediately!

POSSIBLE CAUSE
If you are not circumcised, the cause may be an abnormally tight foreskin (*see* PHIMOSIS, p.721).

MEDICAL HELP

Make an appointment to see your doctor.

Has your penis become inflamed?

- ONLY TIP INFLAMED
- WHOLE PENIS INFLAMED
- NEITHER

POSSIBLE CAUSE
This may be BALANITIS (p.722).

MEDICAL HELP

Make an appointment to see your doctor.

POSSIBLE CAUSE
An allergic reaction, such as to the latex in condoms or to a contraceptive cream, may cause inflammation of this type (*see* ECZEMA, p.333, and CONTACT DERMATITIS, p.335).

MEDICAL HELP

Make an appointment to see your doctor.

Do you have any of the following on the skin of your penis?

- ULCERS
- SORE AREAS
- BLISTERS
- NONE OF THE ABOVE

POSSIBLE CAUSE
Any of these skin symptoms may be the result of a sexually transmitted infection, such as GENITAL HERPES (p.767).

MEDICAL HELP
Make an appointment to see your doctor or go to a clinic specializing in sexually transmitted infections.

Have you noticed either of the following on your penis?

- FLAT, PAINLESS SORE
- SMALL, FLESHY LUMPS
- NEITHER

POSSIBLE CAUSES
This may be a chancre (*see* SYPHILIS, p.766) or CANCER OF THE PENIS (p.723).

MEDICAL HELP
Make an appointment to see your doctor or go to a clinic for sexually transmitted infections.

POSSIBLE CAUSE
You probably have GENITAL WARTS (p.768).

MEDICAL HELP
Make an appointment to see your doctor or go to a clinic specializing in sexually transmitted infections.

If you cannot identify a possible cause for your problem from this chart, make an appointment to see your doctor.

55 BREAST PROBLEMS

You should familiarize yourself with the normal look and feel of your breasts so that you are able to detect changes in them (*see* BREAST SELF-EXAMINATION, p.755). Although most breast problems are not serious, consult your doctor if you notice any changes. Minor conditions clearly related to breast-feeding usually respond well to simple treatments.

START HERE

Are you breast-feeding a baby?

- BREAST-FEEDING
- NOT BREAST-FEEDING

Where is the problem?

- IN THE BREAST
- ON THE NIPPLE

POSSIBLE CAUSE
The lump may be caused by a blocked milk duct.

MEDICAL HELP
Make an appointment to see your doctor if the lump has not disappeared within a week or if the breast becomes painful or red.

How is your nipple affected?

- TENDER ONLY WHEN FEEDING
- TENDER AND PAINFUL ALL THE TIME

What is the nature of your breast problem?

- SINGLE LUMP IN THE BREAST
- A NIPPLE HAS CHANGED IN APPEARANCE
- DISCHARGE FROM THE NIPPLE
- BREASTS FEEL TENDER
- BREASTS FEEL LUMPY AND HARD
- NONE OF THE ABOVE

POSSIBLE CAUSES
Discharge from the nipple may have various causes, including a local problem in the breast or a hormonal problem (*see* NIPPLE DISCHARGE, p.758).

MEDICAL HELP
Make an appointment to see your doctor.

POSSIBLE CAUSES
These symptoms may not have a serious cause (*see* BREAST LUMPS, p.754, and ABNORMAL NIPPLES, p.757). However, such changes must be investigated promptly to rule out the possibility of BREAST CANCER (p.759).

MEDICAL HELP
Make an appointment to see your doctor.

If you cannot identify a possible cause for your breast problem from this chart, make an appointment to see your doctor.

What is the nature of your symptoms?

- SMALL, HARD LUMP IN BREAST
- SWOLLEN, HARD, AND TENDER BREASTS
- REDNESS OF PART OR ALL OF ONE BREAST
- NONE OF THE ABOVE

POSSIBLE CAUSE
Overfull breasts are common, especially when you first start breast-feeding and your milk supply has not yet adjusted to your baby's needs (*see* BREAST ENGORGEMENT, p.808).

SELF-HELP
Continuing to breast-feed your baby at regular intervals should solve this problem without special treatment. However, if you are concerned, consult your doctor or breast-feeding adviser.

POSSIBLE CAUSES
This may be a breast infection (*see* MASTITIS, p.809) or even a breast abscess, particularly if you are also feeling unwell.

MEDICAL HELP
See your doctor within 24 hours. In the meantime, continue to breast-feed from both of your breasts.

If you cannot identify a possible cause for your breast problem from this chart, make an appointment to see your doctor.

POSSIBLE CAUSE
This problem may be a result of your baby not latching on to your nipple properly.

SELF-HELP
Make sure your baby takes the nipple and the surrounding area into his or her mouth (*see* AVOIDING CRACKED NIPPLES, p.809). If you are still having problems when you use the correct feeding technique, consult your doctor or breast-feeding adviser.

POSSIBLE CAUSE
Hormonal changes associated with the menstrual cycle often lead to premenstrual breast tenderness (*see* PREMENSTRUAL SYNDROME, p.736).

MEDICAL HELP
Make an appointment to see your doctor if you are concerned.

Does either of the following apply?

- MENSTRUATION IS DUE TO START WITHIN 10 DAYS
- YOU MIGHT BE PREGNANT
- NEITHER

POSSIBLE CAUSE
Breast tenderness is common in pregnancy (*see* COMMON COMPLAINTS OF NORMAL PREGNANCY, p.784).

SELF-HELP
If you are not sure whether you are pregnant, do a HOME PREGNANCY TEST (p.232).

POSSIBLE CAUSE
Your symptoms may be due to CRACKED NIPPLES (p.808).

SELF-HELP
Keep your nipples dry between feeds and use moisturizing cream. If the problem persists or makes breast-feeding difficult, consult your doctor or breast-feeding adviser.

If you cannot identify a possible cause for your breast problem from this chart, make an appointment to see your doctor.

56 ABSENT PERIODS

The menstrual cycle varies from one woman to the next, but, once a pattern is established, periods usually occur regularly every 3–5 weeks. Pregnancy or the menopause are the most common causes of absent periods. Stress or loss of weight may also cause menstruation to stop or occur less often. Consult your doctor if your periods stop unexpectedly.

START HERE

Have you ever had a period?

PREVIOUS PERIODS

NEVER HAD A PERIOD

Could you be pregnant?

NOT PREGNANT

POSSIBLY PREGNANT

WARNING **POSSIBLE PREGNANCY**

Any sexually active woman who misses a period should consider the possibility that she might be pregnant, even if she has taken contraceptive measures during sexual intercourse.

In the years leading up to the menopause, periods become erratic. However, ovulation may still occur until menstruation has stopped completely for at least 6 months. It is, therefore, possible for a woman to become pregnant while she is going through the menopause.

If you think that you might be pregnant, check using a HOME PREGNANCY TEST (p.232).

POSSIBLE CAUSE

A missed period is a key indicator of pregnancy.

SELF-HELP

If you are not sure whether you are pregnant, do a HOME PREGNANCY TEST (p.232).

Have you had a baby within the past 6 months?

NO

YES

POSSIBLE CAUSE

Some girls, especially those who are small and slim, may develop late but, provided there are no other symptoms of ill health, there is unlikely to be a cause for concern.

MEDICAL HELP

Make an appointment to see your doctor if you are underweight (*see* ARE YOU A HEALTHY WEIGHT?, p.53) or if you have other symptoms.

How old are you?

UNDER 14

14 OR OVER

POSSIBLE CAUSES

Late puberty may be the result of hormonal imbalance, low weight, or regular strenuous exercise (*see* ABNORMAL PUBERTY IN FEMALES, p.739).

MEDICAL HELP

Make an appointment to see your doctor.

Do any of the following apply?

- YOU HAVE RECENTLY LOST OVER 4 KG (10 LB) IN WEIGHT
- YOU HAVE RECENTLY BEGUN A PROGRAMME OF STRENUOUS EXERCISE
- YOU HAVE RECENTLY STOPPED TAKING ORAL CONTRACEPTIVES
- NONE OF THE ABOVE

POSSIBLE CAUSES

Sudden weight loss, whatever the cause, and/or rigorous physical training can cause menstruation to stop (*see* AMENORRHOEA, p.735).

MEDICAL HELP

Make an appointment to see your doctor.

POSSIBLE CAUSE

It may take several weeks for normal menstruation to begin again after stopping oral contraceptives.

MEDICAL HELP

Make an appointment to see your doctor if you have not had a period within 3 months of stopping.

Are you under particular stress at home, school, or work?

- YES
- NO

POSSIBLE CAUSE

Emotional stress can disrupt the menstrual cycle (*see* AMENORRHOEA, p.735).

SELF-HELP

Try RELAXATION EXERCISES (p.75) to relieve stress. If your symptoms continue, consult your doctor.

How old are you?

- OVER 40
- 40 OR UNDER

POSSIBLE CAUSE

It is not unusual to miss a period around the time of the menopause (*see* HEALTH AT THE MENOPAUSE, p.36).

MEDICAL HELP

Make an appointment to see your doctor. In addition, you should keep a record showing when your periods occur so that the doctor can confirm the diagnosis.

If you cannot identify a possible cause for your absence of periods from this chart, make an appointment to see your doctor.

POSSIBLE CAUSE

It can take several months for menstruation to become reestablished after childbirth. This delay is likely to be extended if you are breast-feeding your baby frequently (*see* AMENORRHOEA, p.735).

MEDICAL HELP

Make an appointment to see your doctor if your periods have not restarted within 1 month of stopping breast-feeding. If you have not breast-fed, see your doctor if your periods have not restarted within 3 months of the birth.

57 PAINFUL PERIODS

Many women experience mild cramping pain in the lower abdomen during menstruation. This pain is considered normal unless it interferes with everyday activities; it can usually be relieved with painkillers. If you regularly have severe pain or if your periods become more painful than usual, you should consult your doctor.

START HERE

How does the pain you are currently experiencing compare with that of previous periods?

- NO WORSE THAN USUAL
- WORSE THAN USUAL

POSSIBLE CAUSE
Some menstrual pain is quite normal; it is known as primary DYSMENORRHOEA (p.736).

SELF-HELP
Take a painkiller. Make an appointment to see your doctor if pain interferes with normal activities.

Have you had an unusual vaginal discharge between periods?

- NO DISCHARGE
- DISCHARGE

POSSIBLE CAUSE
You could have an infection (*see* PELVIC INFLAMMATORY DISEASE, p.741).

MEDICAL HELP
 See your doctor within 24 hours.

Have you had any of the following symptoms?

- LOWER ABDOMINAL PAIN BETWEEN PERIODS
- LOW BACK PAIN BETWEEN PERIODS
- FEVER
- NONE OF THE ABOVE

Do you have an intrauterine contraceptive device (IUD)?

- IUD
- NO IUD

POSSIBLE CAUSE
An increase in menstrual pain is often a side effect of IUDs (*see* CONTRACEPTION, p.69).

MEDICAL HELP
 Make an appointment to see your doctor.

Have your periods become heavier or longer as well as more painful?

- HEAVIER
- LONGER
- NEITHER

POSSIBLE CAUSES
You may possibly have a gynaecological disorder such as FIBROIDS (p.745) or ENDOMETRIOSIS (p.742).

MEDICAL HELP
 Make an appointment to see your doctor.

If you cannot identify a possible cause for your painful periods from this chart, make an appointment to see your doctor.

58 HEAVY PERIODS

If you bleed between periods, see chart 59

Some women lose more blood than others during their periods. If normal sanitary protection is not sufficient, clots are passed, or bleeding lasts longer than 5 days, the bleeding is probably excessive. If you are concerned about heavy periods, consult your doctor.

START HERE

How does the bleeding of your most recent period compare with that of your usual periods?

- ABOUT THE SAME
- HEAVIER OR LONGER

Do you have an intrauterine contraceptive device (IUD)?

- IUD
- NO IUD

POSSIBLE CAUSE
Some IUDs can cause heavier periods than normal (*see* CONTRACEPTION, p.69).

MEDICAL HELP
Make an appointment to see your doctor.

Have you had a single heavy period that was also later than usual?

- YES
- NO

POSSIBLE CAUSES
Heavy, painful periods may be an indication that you have FIBROIDS (p.745) or ENDOMETRIOSIS (p.742).

MEDICAL HELP

Make an appointment to see your doctor.

Are your periods more painful than they used to be?

- MORE PAINFUL
- THE SAME OR LESS PAINFUL

POSSIBLE CAUSE
Some women regularly have heavy periods (*see* MENORRHAGIA, p.735).

MEDICAL HELP
Make an appointment to see your doctor. You could be susceptible to IRON-DEFICIENCY ANAEMIA (p.447).

POSSIBLE CAUSES
Late periods may be heavier than usual. However, if you are sexually active there is a possibility that you have had an early MISCARRIAGE (p.791).

MEDICAL HELP
Make an appointment to see your doctor if you are concerned about the cause of your late period.

If you cannot identify a possible cause for your heavy periods from this chart, make an appointment to see your doctor.

59 ABNORMAL VAGINAL BLEEDING

Vaginal bleeding is considered abnormal if it occurs outside the normal menstrual cycle, during pregnancy, or after the menopause. Although there is often a simple explanation, you should always see your doctor if you have any abnormal vaginal bleeding. If you are pregnant and you are bleeding, you should consult your doctor or midwife at once.

WARNING BLEEDING IN PREGNANCY

If you have any vaginal bleeding during pregnancy, you should contact your doctor or midwife urgently. If the bleeding is heavy, call an ambulance. Although most causes of bleeding are not serious, it is important to rule out MISCARRIAGE (p.791) or a problem such as a low-lying placenta (*see* PLACENTA PRAEVIA, p.798) or partial separation of the placenta from the wall of the uterus (*see* PLACENTAL ABRUPTION, p.799).

START HERE

Are you pregnant?

- MORE THAN 14 WEEKS PREGNANT
- LESS THAN 14 WEEKS PREGNANT
- NOT PREGNANT

POSSIBLE CAUSE

Bleeding at this stage of pregnancy could be due to a problem with the placenta (*see* VAGINAL BLEEDING IN PREGNANCY, p.791).

MEDICAL HELP

URGENT! Phone your doctor or midwife immediately! Rest in bed until you receive medical advice.

Do you have unaccustomed pain in the lower back or abdomen?

- LOWER BACK PAIN
- ABDOMINAL PAIN
- NEITHER

POSSIBLE CAUSES

You may be having a MISCARRIAGE (p.791) or you may have an ECTOPIC PREGNANCY (p.790).

MEDICAL HELP

URGENT! Phone your doctor or midwife immediately! Rest in bed until you receive medical advice.

POSSIBLE CAUSE

Bleeding at this stage of pregnancy could be the first sign of a threatened MISCARRIAGE (p.791).

MEDICAL HELP

URGENT! Phone your doctor or midwife immediately! Rest in bed until you receive medical advice.

Is the bleeding similar to that of a normal period?

- LIKE A PERIOD
- DIFFERENT

How long has it been since your last period?

- LESS THAN 6 MONTHS
- MORE THAN 6 MONTHS

Does either of the following apply?

- YOU HAVE ONLY RECENTLY STARTED HAVING PERIODS
- YOU ARE OVER 40
- NEITHER

POSSIBLE CAUSE
Irregular periods are fairly common in the first year or so of menstruation.

MEDICAL HELP

Make an appointment to see your doctor if you are concerned.

POSSIBLE CAUSE
Your periods may become irregular as you approach the menopause (*see* HEALTH AT THE MENOPAUSE, p.36).

MEDICAL HELP
Make an appointment to see your doctor if you are concerned.

POSSIBLE CAUSE
Having an occasional irregular period is unlikely to indicate that you have a serious problem if the period was normal in all other respects.

MEDICAL HELP
Make an appointment to see your doctor if you are concerned or if your pattern has not returned to normal within three menstrual cycles.

WARNING HORMONAL CONTRACEPTIVES
In the first few menstrual cycles after either starting hormonal contraception or changing to a different type of contraceptive pill, spotting is fairly common (*see* CONTRACEPTION, p.69). If abnormal bleeding persists or develops when there have previously been no problems, you should consult your doctor. He or she may examine you and change the dosage or type of hormonal contraceptive that has been prescribed.

Have you had sexual intercourse in the past 3 months?

- INTERCOURSE
- NO INTERCOURSE

Have you noticed bleeding within a few hours of intercourse?

- BLEEDING AFTER INTERCOURSE
- BLEEDING UNRELATED TO INTERCOURSE

POSSIBLE CAUSES
You may have an abnormality of the cervix (*see* CERVICAL DYSPLASIA, p.749; CERVICAL EROSION, p.749; and CANCER OF THE CERVIX, p.750).

MEDICAL HELP

Make an appointment to see your doctor.

POSSIBLE CAUSES
Bleeding, especially if it is accompanied by pain in the lower abdomen, may be the first sign of an ECTOPIC PREGNANCY (p.790) or of an impending MISCARRIAGE (p.791), even if you were not aware of being pregnant.

MEDICAL HELP

URGENT! Phone your doctor immediately!

POSSIBLE CAUSES
Bleeding after the menopause may be due to a minor problem affecting the vagina or cervix, such as CERVICAL EROSION (p.749), but the possibility of CANCER OF THE UTERUS (p.748) needs to be ruled out.

MEDICAL HELP

Make an appointment to see your doctor.

If you cannot identify a possible cause for your abnormal bleeding from this chart, make an appointment to see your doctor.

60 LOWER ABDOMINAL PAIN IN WOMEN

First refer to chart 35, ABDOMINAL PAIN

Several disorders specific to women can cause discomfort or pain in the lower abdomen. Many of these conditions are related to the reproductive tract (ovaries, uterus, or fallopian tubes) or to pregnancy. Abdominal pain that occurs during pregnancy should always be taken seriously.

WARNING ABDOMINAL PAIN IN PREGNANCY

Intermittent, mild abdominal pains are common throughout pregnancy due to stretching of the muscles and ligaments of the abdomen. Abdominal pain that occurs in early pregnancy can be due to complications, such as MISCARRIAGE (p.791) or an ECTOPIC PREGNANCY (p.790). In later pregnancy, pain is most commonly caused by the onset of labour. Rarely, partial separation of the placenta from the uterine wall may occur (*see* PLACENTAL ABRUPTION, p.799). If you develop severe pain, phone your doctor immediately.

START HERE

Do you have pain when you pass urine?

YES → POSSIBLE CAUSE

NO → Are you pregnant?

POSSIBLE CAUSE

You may have CYSTITIS (p.709).

MEDICAL HELP

See your doctor within 24 hours. Meanwhile, drink plenty of water and take a painkiller.

Are you pregnant?

MORE THAN 14 WEEKS PREGNANT → POSSIBLE CAUSES (late miscarriage)

LESS THAN 14 WEEKS PREGNANT → POSSIBLE CAUSES (threatened miscarriage)

DO NOT THINK SO → Have you had sexual intercourse in the past 3 months?

Have you had sexual intercourse in the past 3 months?

YES → Did your last period occur at the time you expected?

NO → continued

Did your last period occur at the time you expected?

ON TIME → continued

MISSED OR LATE → continued

POSSIBLE CAUSES

You could be having a late MISCARRIAGE (p.791) or the placenta may have partly separated from the wall of the uterus (*see* PLACENTAL ABRUPTION, p.799).

MEDICAL HELP

URGENT! Phone your doctor immediately! Rest in bed until you receive medical advice.

POSSIBLE CAUSES

Pain at this stage of pregnancy may indicate a threatened MISCARRIAGE (p.791) or an ECTOPIC PREGNANCY (p.790).

MEDICAL HELP

URGENT! Phone your doctor immediately! Rest in bed until you receive medical advice.

Do you have any of the following symptoms?

- Abnormal vaginal discharge
- Fever
- Pain during intercourse
- None of the above

Possible cause
Pelvic inflammatory disease (p.741) is a possible cause of these symptoms.

Medical help

See your doctor within 24 hours.

Have you been through the menopause?

- Premenopausal
- Postmenopausal

Is the pain related to your menstrual cycle?

- Occurs just before and/or during a period
- Occurs briefly in midcycle
- Unrelated

Do you have an intrauterine contraceptive device (IUD)?

- IUD
- No IUD

Possible cause
This form of contraception (p.69) often causes increased period pain, particularly for the first few cycles after it has been inserted.

Medical help

Make an appointment to see your doctor.

Possible cause
Some women regularly have pain associated with ovulation.

Medical help

Make an appointment to see your doctor to rule out other possible causes.

Possible cause
There is a possibility of an ectopic pregnancy (p.790).

Medical help

URGENT! Phone your doctor immediately!

If you cannot identify a possible cause for your lower abdominal pain from this chart, make an appointment to see your doctor.

Go to chart 57
Painful periods

61 ABNORMAL VAGINAL DISCHARGE

If the discharge contains blood, see chart 59

A thin, clear or whitish discharge from the vagina is normal. This discharge varies in consistency and quantity with the stage of the menstrual cycle, during sexual arousal, and during pregnancy. An abnormal discharge is usually caused by infection and should be investigated by your doctor.

START HERE

What are the characteristics of your discharge?

- THICK AND WHITE
- NORMAL APPEARANCE BUT HEAVIER THAN USUAL
- GREENISH YELLOW
- NONE OF THE ABOVE

POSSIBLE CAUSE
A vaginal yeast infection is a likely cause of your discharge, particularly if it is associated with genital irritation (*see* VAGINAL THRUSH, p.752).

MEDICAL HELP
Make an appointment to see your doctor if this is the first time you have had this symptom. Otherwise, try using an over-the-counter product recommended by a pharmacist.

Do any of the following apply?

- YOU ARE TAKING ORAL CONTRACEPTIVES
- YOU HAVE AN IUD
- YOU ARE PREGNANT
- NONE OF THE ABOVE

POSSIBLE CAUSE
These forms of contraception may cause an increase in normal vaginal secretions.

MEDICAL HELP
Make an appointment to see your doctor if you are concerned or if you develop genital irritation.

POSSIBLE CAUSE
Increased vaginal secretion is normal in pregnancy.

MEDICAL HELP
Make an appointment to see your doctor if you are concerned or if you develop genital irritation.

Do you have either of the following symptoms?

- FEVER
- LOWER ABDOMINAL PAIN
- NEITHER

POSSIBLE CAUSE
You could have an infection (*see* PELVIC INFLAMMATORY DISEASE, p.741).

MEDICAL HELP

See your doctor within 24 hours.

POSSIBLE CAUSE
A vaginal infection such as TRICHOMONIASIS (p.767) is a possible cause.

MEDICAL HELP
Make an appointment to see your doctor or go to a clinic specializing in sexually transmitted infections.

POSSIBLE CAUSE
CERVICAL EROSION (p.749) may be the cause of your increased discharge.

MEDICAL HELP

Make an appointment to see your doctor.

If you cannot identify a possible cause for your discharge from this chart, make an appointment to see your doctor.

62 GENITAL IRRITATION IN WOMEN

Genital irritation, which may include itching and/or soreness in the genital area, is most often caused by chemicals in toiletries or detergents. Avoiding these products should prevent irritation from occurring. Genital irritation may also be due to infection, but often the symptom has no obvious cause. If the irritation is persistent, consult your doctor.

START HERE

Have you noticed an unusual vaginal discharge?

- UNUSUAL DISCHARGE
- NORMAL DISCHARGE

Go to chart 61 ABNORMAL VAGINAL DISCHARGE

Have you noticed any change in the appearance of the skin in the genital area?

- SKIN CHANGES
- NO SKIN CHANGES

POSSIBLE CAUSE
You may have a skin condition, such as ECZEMA (p.333), that affects the genital area.

MEDICAL HELP
 Make an appointment to see your doctor.

Have you been using a new soap, bath product, or other toiletry item, or have you switched to a new washing powder?

- YES
- NO

POSSIBLE CAUSE
You may be sensitive to one of the ingredients contained in the new product you are using (*see* VULVOVAGINITIS, p.752).

SELF-HELP
Discontinue use of the new product and use only plain water to wash your genital area. Make an appointment to see your doctor if the irritation has not cleared up in 3–4 days.

Does either of the following apply?

- YOU ARE OVER 45
- YOUR PERIODS ARE IRREGULAR OR HAVE STOPPED
- NEITHER

Go to chart 44 FREQUENT URINATION

Have you been passing urine more frequently than usual?

- INCREASED FREQUENCY
- NO INCREASED FREQUENCY

POSSIBLE CAUSES
PUBIC LICE (p.768) are a possible cause. However, the symptom sometimes occurs for no obvious reason (*see* VULVOVAGINITIS, p.752).

MEDICAL HELP
Make an appointment to see your doctor.

POSSIBLE CAUSE
A change in hormone levels may be the cause of your symptoms (*see* MENOPAUSAL PROBLEMS, p.737).

MEDICAL HELP
 Make an appointment to see your doctor.

63 PAINFUL INTERCOURSE IN WOMEN

Pain or discomfort during sexual intercourse may be due to anxiety or lack of arousal, particularly if there is stress within the relationship. Pain may also be caused by an infection or a disorder affecting the organs in the pelvis. Consult your doctor if intercourse is often painful because this may have a harmful effect on your relationship.

START HERE

Have you had a baby within the past 6 weeks?

YES

NO

Have you noticed an abnormal vaginal discharge?

NO ABNORMAL DISCHARGE

ABNORMAL DISCHARGE

Is penetration difficult and painful because your vagina feels tight and dry?

YES

NO

Does pain during intercourse occur only occasionally or only when in particular positions?

OCCASIONAL PAIN

ASSOCIATED WITH PARTICULAR POSITIONS

ALWAYS PAINFUL

Go to chart 61 ABNORMAL VAGINAL DISCHARGE

Does either of the following apply?

YOU ARE OVER 45

YOUR PERIODS ARE IRREGULAR OR HAVE STOPPED

NEITHER

Have your menstrual periods become more painful recently?

NO CHANGE

MORE PAINFUL

POSSIBLE CAUSE

Soreness around the vagina or in the abdomen is normal following the birth of a baby (*see* PAINFUL INTERCOURSE IN WOMEN, p.772).

SELF-HELP

Avoid sexual intercourse while you are still sore. Make an appointment to see your doctor if intercourse is still painful 6 weeks or more after the birth.

POSSIBLE CAUSE

ENDOMETRIOSIS (p.742) is a possible cause.

MEDICAL HELP

Make an appointment to see your doctor.

POSSIBLE CAUSE
Low hormone levels can lead to dryness of the vagina and consequent discomfort during intercourse (*see* MENOPAUSAL PROBLEMS, p.737).

SELF-HELP
Try using lubricating jelly to moisten your vagina. Make an appointment to see your doctor if the problem persists.

Do you have any general or specific anxieties?

- YOU ARE UNDER STRESS AT HOME AND/OR AT WORK
- YOU HAVE BEEN FEELING DEPRESSED RECENTLY
- YOU ARE WORRIED THAT YOU MIGHT BECOME PREGNANT
- YOU OR YOUR PARTNER HAVE ANXIETIES ABOUT SEXUAL PERFORMANCE
- NONE OF THE ABOVE

POSSIBLE CAUSE
Fear of pregnancy can make sexual arousal difficult and cause pain during intercourse (*see* VAGINISMUS, p.773).

MEDICAL HELP

Make an appointment to see your doctor.

POSSIBLE CAUSE
Tension that may arise out of such anxieties is likely to reduce vaginal lubrication and cause painful intercourse (*see* VAGINISMUS, p.773).

MEDICAL HELP
Make an appointment to see your doctor if the problem persists.

POSSIBLE CAUSES
Pressure on an ovary during intercourse may be the cause of such pain. However, an OVARIAN CYST (p.743) is also a possible cause.

MEDICAL HELP
Make an appointment to see your doctor.

POSSIBLE CAUSES
STRESS (p.74) and DEPRESSION (p.554) can both reduce sexual desire, which in turn may lead to painful intercourse.

MEDICAL HELP
Make an appointment to see your doctor. Meanwhile, try to reduce your stress level (*see* STRESS, p.74).

POSSIBLE CAUSE
Dryness of the vagina in a woman who has not reached the menopause is usually due to lack of sexual arousal (*see* PAINFUL INTERCOURSE IN WOMEN, p.772).

SELF-HELP
Try using lubricating jelly to moisten your vagina. Make an appointment to see your doctor if the problem persists.

Have you just started your first or a new sexual relationship?

- FIRST SEXUAL RELATIONSHIP
- NEW SEXUAL RELATIONSHIP
- NEITHER

POSSIBLE CAUSE
Bruising and/or soreness of the vagina may follow the start of a new sexual relationship (*see* PAINFUL INTERCOURSE IN WOMEN, p.772).

SELF-HELP
Abstaining from intercourse for a few days should allow any soreness or bruising to heal.

If you cannot identify a possible cause for your pain during intercourse from this chart, make an appointment to see your doctor.

64 VOMITING IN CHILDREN

For children of 12 and over, see chart 33

Children vomit as a result of many illnesses, including ear infections and urinary and digestive tract disorders. Anxiety or excitement may also cause vomiting. Rarely, vomiting may be due to an infection or injury to the brain. If vomiting is persistent, you should consult your doctor urgently.

DANGER SIGNS

Call an ambulance if your child's vomiting is accompanied by any of the following symptoms:

- Greenish-yellow vomit.
- Abdominal pain for 4 hours.
- Flat, dark-red or purple spots that do not fade when pressed.
- Refusal to drink or feed (in babies) for over 6 hours.
- Abnormal drowsiness.
- Sunken eyes.
- Dry tongue.
- Passing no urine during the day for 3 hours (if child is under 1 year old) or 6 hours (in an older child).
- Black or bloodstained faeces.

START HERE

Has your child had a recent head injury?

- HEAD INJURY
- NO HEAD INJURY

POSSIBLE CAUSE

Concussion (*see* HEAD INJURIES, p.521) is a possibility.

MEDICAL HELP

EMERGENCY! Call an ambulance! Do not allow your child to eat or drink.

Does your child have any of the following symptoms?

- SEVERE HEADACHE
- ABNORMAL DROWSINESS OR CONFUSION
- DISLIKE OF BRIGHT LIGHT
- NECK PAIN ON BENDING THE HEAD FORWARDS
- NONE OF THE ABOVE

POSSIBLE CAUSE

Meningitis (*see* MENINGITIS IN CHILDREN, p.848) is possible.

MEDICAL HELP

EMERGENCY! Call an ambulance!

How old is your child?

- UNDER 3 MONTHS
- 3 MONTHS OR OVER

Apart from the vomiting, does your baby seem generally unwell – for example, is he or she feverish or drowsy?

- UNWELL
- WELL

POSSIBLE CAUSES

There may be many possible causes for these symptoms. However, any young baby who seems unwell and vomits needs prompt medical attention.

MEDICAL HELP

URGENT! Phone your doctor immediately!

Does your child seem to have abdominal pain?

- YES
- NO

POSSIBLE CAUSE

These symptoms may indicate a serious abdominal condition, such as APPENDICITIS (p.664).

MEDICAL HELP

URGENT! Phone your doctor immediately!

What are the characteristics of the vomiting?

- FREQUENT AND EFFORTLESS VOMITING AFTER FEEDS
- FORCEFUL VOMITING AFTER SEVERAL FEEDS
- OCCASIONAL VOMITING NOT NECESSARILY ASSOCIATED WITH FEEDING

POSSIBLE CAUSES
This type of regurgitation is rarely serious and has several possible causes (*see* FEEDING PROBLEMS IN BABIES, p.819).

SELF-HELP
Make sure you "wind" your baby after feeding. Consult your doctor if your baby seems unwell or fails to gain weight (*see* GROWTH CHARTS FOR BABIES, pp.40–41).

POSSIBLE CAUSE
This type of vomiting may be the result of a digestive tract problem, such as PYLORIC STENOSIS IN INFANTS (p.863).

MEDICAL HELP

See your doctor within 24 hours.

POSSIBLE CAUSE
Babies often vomit for no particular reason, and this is no cause for concern if your baby seems generally well and is gaining weight (*see* FEEDING PROBLEMS IN BABIES, p.819).

SELF-HELP
Be sure to "wind" your baby after each feed. Consult your doctor if your baby seems unwell or vomits frequently.

Did vomiting follow a violent bout of coughing?

- FOLLOWED COUGHING
- NO COUGHING

POSSIBLE CAUSES
Your child may have PERTUSSIS (p.492). An infection that causes severe coughing, such as BRONCHIOLITIS (p.841) or PNEUMONIA (p.490), can also cause vomiting.

MEDICAL HELP

URGENT! Phone your doctor immediately!

Does your child have diarrhoea?

- DIARRHOEA
- NO DIARRHOEA

POSSIBLE CAUSE
This could be a digestive tract infection (*see* VOMITING AND DIARRHOEA, p.864).

MEDICAL HELP
URGENT! Phone your doctor immediately if your child is under 6 months old. For older children, follow the self-help measures for VOMITING AND DIARRHOEA (p.864) and consult your doctor if there is no improvement in 24 hours or if other symptoms develop.

Does your child have any of the following symptoms?

- PAIN ON PASSING URINE
- RENEWED BEDWETTING OR DAYTIME "ACCIDENTS"
- TEMPERATURE OF 38°C (100°F) OR ABOVE
- NONE OF THE ABOVE

POSSIBLE CAUSE
Your child may have a URINARY TRACT INFECTION (p.871).

MEDICAL HELP

See your doctor within 24 hours.

POSSIBLE CAUSES
Illnesses with fever, such as ACUTE HEPATITIS (p.644), ACUTE OTITIS MEDIA (p.860), or a URINARY TRACT INFECTION (p.871), often cause vomiting.

MEDICAL HELP

See your doctor within 24 hours.

If you cannot identify a possible cause for your child's vomiting from this chart, see your doctor within 24 hours.

65 DIARRHOEA IN CHILDREN

For children of 12 and over, see chart 39

Diarrhoea is the passage of loose or watery faeces more often than normal. Breast-fed babies may pass loose faeces several times a day, and this is normal. If your child has diarrhoea, he or she should drink plenty of clear fluids to avoid dehydration. If symptoms do not improve, consult your doctor.

DANGER SIGNS

Call an ambulance if your child's diarrhoea is accompanied by any of the following symptoms:

- Abnormal drowsiness.
- Severe abdominal pain or abdominal pain that lasts for 4 hours or more.
- No urine passed during the day for 3 hours (if under 1 year) or 6 hours (in an older child).
- Refusal to drink or feed (in babies) for over 6 hours.
- Blood in the faeces.

START HERE

How long has your child had diarrhoea?

- LESS THAN 3 DAYS
- 3 DAYS OR MORE

Does your child have any of the following symptoms?

- ABDOMINAL PAIN
- TEMPERATURE OF 38°C (100°F) OR ABOVE
- VOMITING
- NONE OF THE ABOVE

Is your child taking prescribed or over-the-counter drugs?

- YES
- NO

POSSIBLE CAUSE

Your child may have GASTROENTERITIS (p.628).

MEDICAL HELP

URGENT! Phone your doctor immediately if your child is under 6 months old. If your child is older, follow the self-help advice for PREVENTING DEHYDRATION (p.627), and consult your doctor if your child is no better in 24 hours.

POSSIBLE CAUSE

Persistent constipation can lead to faeces trickling from the anus (*see* CONSTIPATION IN CHILDREN, p.865). This may be mistaken for diarrhoea.

MEDICAL HELP

Make an appointment to see your doctor.

Was your child constipated before the onset of diarrhoea?

- CONSTIPATED
- NOT CONSTIPATED

What is the appearance of your child's faeces?

- UNIFORMLY RUNNY
- CONTAINS RECOGNIZABLE PIECES OF FOOD

Is your child gaining weight and growing normally (*see* GROWTH CHARTS, pp.40–43)?

- YES
- NO

Possible cause
Your child's symptoms may be a side effect of the drug.

Medical help
See your doctor within 24 hours. Stop giving over-the-counter medicines but continue to give any prescribed medication unless advised to stop by your doctor.

Possible cause
Young children often fail to chew and digest food properly, which can lead to toddler's diarrhoea (*see* VOMITING AND DIARRHOEA, p.864).

Self-help
No special action is needed provided that your child is well. Consult your doctor if your child develops other symptoms.

Possible cause
Foods that are new to your baby may be the cause of digestive upsets.

Self-help
Withhold the food that seems to be causing the trouble for at least 1 week. Consult your doctor if your baby is no better in 24 hours or develops other symptoms.

How old is your child?

- Under 12 months
- 12 months – 3 years
- Over 3 years

Is your child experiencing unusual stress, anxiety, or excitement?

- Stress or anxiety
- Excitement
- Neither

Was your baby given any of the following before the onset of diarrhoea?

- Unfamiliar foods
- Sugary foods or sweetened drinks
- None of the above

If you cannot identify a possible cause for your child's diarrhoea from this chart, see your doctor within 24 hours.

Possible causes
It is possible that your child has a condition affecting the digestive tract, such as FOOD INTOLERANCE (p.657) or COELIAC DISEASE (p.658).

Medical help
Make an appointment to see your doctor.

Possible cause
Psychological stress or unusual excitement can cause diarrhoea.

Self-help
The diarrhoea should stop as soon as the cause has disappeared. Consult your doctor if there is a long-term cause of anxiety in your child's life or if your child develops other symptoms.

Possible cause
Sugar in food and drink can cause diarrhoea in babies.

Self-help
Avoid giving your baby sweetened foods and drinks. Consult your doctor if your baby is no better in 24 hours or develops other symptoms.

66 FEVER IN CHILDREN

For children of 12 and over, see chart 6

A fever is a temperature of 38°C (100°F) or above. If your child is unwell, you should take his or her temperature because a high fever may need urgent treatment. If a feverish child becomes unresponsive, call an ambulance. In all cases, follow the advice for BRINGING DOWN A FEVER (p.289).

DANGER SIGNS

Call an ambulance if your child's temperature rises above 39°C (102°F) and he or she has any of the following symptoms:

- Abnormally rapid breathing (*see* CHECKING YOUR CHILD'S BREATHING RATE, p.205).
- Abnormal drowsiness.
- Severe headache.
- Dislike of bright light.
- Refusal to drink for more than 6 hours.

START HERE

How old is your child?

- UNDER 6 MONTHS
- 6 MONTHS OR OVER

POSSIBLE CAUSE
Fever in young babies is unusual unless it occurs within 48 hours of immunization; it may indicate a serious illness.

MEDICAL HELP
URGENT! Phone your doctor immediately!

Does your child have a rash?

- RASH
- NO RASH

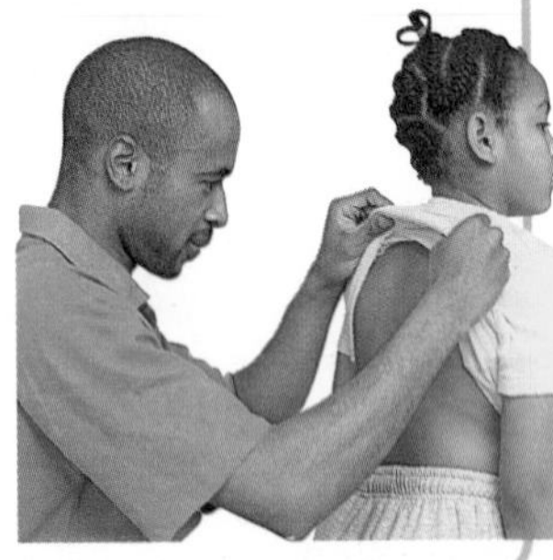

Go to chart 21
RASH WITH FEVER

Does your child have any of the following symptoms?

- SEVERE HEADACHE
- ABNORMAL DROWSINESS, IRRITABILITY, OR CONFUSION
- DISLIKE OF BRIGHT LIGHT
- NECK PAIN ON BENDING THE HEAD FORWARDS
- NONE OF THE ABOVE

POSSIBLE CAUSE
Meningitis (*see* MENINGITIS IN CHILDREN, p.848) is a possible cause of these symptoms.

MEDICAL HELP
EMERGENCY! Call an ambulance!

Is your child reluctant to move an arm or leg?

- YES
- NO

POSSIBLE CAUSE
Your child could have an infection in a bone or joint (*see* OSTEOMYELITIS, p.372, and SEPTIC ARTHRITIS, p.381).

MEDICAL HELP
URGENT! Phone your doctor immediately!

POSSIBLE CAUSE
Your child may have an infection of the middle ear (*see* ACUTE OTITIS MEDIA IN CHILDREN, p.860).

MEDICAL HELP
 See your doctor within 24 hours.

Possible cause
Your child could have a respiratory infection, such as PNEUMONIA (p.490).

Medical help
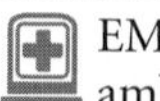
EMERGENCY! Call an ambulance!

Is your child's breathing abnormally noisy or rapid (*see* CHECKING YOUR CHILD'S BREATHING RATE, p.205)?

- Abnormally rapid
- Noisy
- Neither

Possible cause
This may be a severe episode of CROUP (p.841).

Medical help
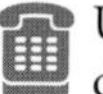
URGENT! Phone your doctor immediately.

Does either of the following apply?

- Your child has been pulling at one ear
- Your child has complained of earache
- Neither

Does your child have either of the following symptoms?

- Cough
- Runny nose
- Neither

Does your child have a sore throat?

- Sore throat
- No sore throat

Does your child have either of the following symptoms?

- Pain on passing urine
- Diarrhoea with or without vomiting
- Neither

If you cannot identify a possible cause for your child's fever from this chart, see your doctor within 24 hours.

Possible cause
A viral illness, such as a severe cold (*see* COMMON COLD, p.288) or INFLUENZA (p.289), is the most likely cause of your child's symptoms.

Self-help
See the advice for BRINGING DOWN A FEVER (p.289). Consult your doctor if your child's symptoms worsen, if your child is no better in 2 days, or if he or she develops other symptoms.

Possible cause
Your child could be suffering from a throat infection, such as TONSILLITIS (p.843).

Self-help
See the advice for BRINGING DOWN A FEVER (p.289). If your child is no better in 24 hours or if other symptoms develop, make an appointment to see your doctor.

Possible cause
A URINARY TRACT INFECTION (p.871) is a possibility.

Medical help

See your doctor within 24 hours.

Possible cause
It is possible that your child has a digestive tract infection (*see* GASTROENTERITIS, p.628).

Medical help
URGENT! Phone your doctor immediately if your child is under 6 months old. For older children, follow the self-help measures for VOMITING AND DIARRHOEA (p.864), and consult your doctor if your child is no better in 24 hours or if he or she develops other symptoms.

67 BREATHING PROBLEMS IN CHILDREN

For children of 12 and over, see charts 30 and 31

Breathing problems include noisy or rapid breathing and shortness of breath. Shortness of breath may not be obvious because a child may simply avoid exertion. A child with severe difficulty breathing needs urgent hospital treatment. Breathing problems that occur suddenly also need immediate attention.

DANGER SIGNS

Call an ambulance if your child's breathing rate is excessively rapid (*see* CHECKING YOUR CHILD'S BREATHING RATE, opposite page) and if breathing problems are accompanied by any of the following symptoms:

- Blue-tinged lips or tongue.
- Abnormal drowsiness.
- Inability to swallow, talk, or produce sounds.

START HERE

How long has your child had breathing problems?

STARTED SUDDENLY A FEW MINUTES AGO

STARTED MORE THAN A FEW MINUTES AGO

Is it possible that your child is choking on food or a small object?

POSSIBLE

UNLIKELY

POSSIBLE CAUSE
An inhaled foreign body may be preventing your child from breathing properly.

MEDICAL HELP
EMERGENCY! Call an ambulance! While waiting for medical help, follow the first-aid advice for CHOKING (pp.980–981).

Are any of the danger signs listed in the box above present?

DANGER SIGNS PRESENT

NO DANGER SIGNS

POSSIBLE CAUSE
Your child may have a serious respiratory problem.

MEDICAL HELP
EMERGENCY! Call an ambulance! If your child stops breathing, follow the first-aid advice for ARTIFICIAL RESPIRATION (pp.982–983).

How old is your child?

UNDER 6 MONTHS

6 MONTHS OR OVER

POSSIBLE CAUSE
The cause of these symptoms could be a serious lung infection such as BRONCHIOLITIS (p.841).

MEDICAL HELP
URGENT! Phone your doctor immediately!

Does your child have either of the following symptoms?

- NOISY BREATHING
- BARKING COUGH
- SHORTNESS OF BREATH
- NONE OF THE ABOVE

POSSIBLE CAUSE
These symptoms may be due to CROUP (p.841).

MEDICAL HELP

URGENT! Phone your doctor immediately!

Does your child suffer from repeated episodes of any of the following symptoms?

- WHEEZING
- COUGHING AT NIGHT
- COUGHING AFTER EXERCISE
- COUGHING AFTER GOING OUT IN THE COLD
- NONE OF THE ABOVE

POSSIBLE CAUSE
Your child may have developed asthma (*see* ASTHMA IN CHILDREN, p.839).

MEDICAL HELP

See your doctor within 24 hours.

If you cannot identify a possible cause for your child's breathing problems from this chart, see your doctor within 24 hours.

Does your child have a fever – a temperature of 38°C (100°F) or above?

- FEVER
- NO FEVER

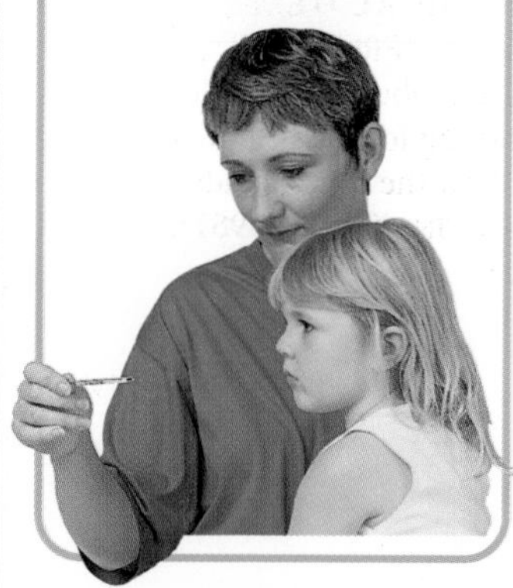

POSSIBLE CAUSE
A lung infection, such as PNEUMONIA (p.490) or BRONCHIOLITIS (p.841), could be the cause.

MEDICAL HELP
URGENT! Phone your doctor immediately!

SYMPTOM ASSESSMENT

CHECKING YOUR CHILD'S BREATHING RATE

A child whose breathing is unusually rapid when at rest or asleep may need medical attention. Check your child's breathing by counting the number of breaths he or she takes in one minute with your hand on his or her chest or back to feel the breaths. The normal breathing rate of a young baby is faster than that of an older child. Compare your child's breathing rate with the maximum rate for his or her age shown in the table.

AGE	BREATHING RATE
Under 2 months	Maximum of 60 breaths a minute
2–11 months	Maximum of 50 breaths a minute
1–5 years	Maximum of 40 breaths a minute
Over 5 years	Maximum of 30 breaths a minute

Assessment of your child's breathing
Your child should be at rest and not crying when you check his or her breathing rate. Place your hand on his or her chest or back to help you to count the breaths.

68 COUGHING IN CHILDREN

For children of 12 and over, see chart 29

Coughing is a normal reaction to irritation in the throat or lungs. Most coughs are due to minor infections of the nose and/or throat, but the sudden onset of coughing may be caused by choking. Coughing is unusual in babies under 6 months old and may indicate a serious lung infection.

DANGER SIGNS

Call an ambulance if your child is coughing and has any of the following symptoms:

- Blue-tinged lips or tongue.
- Abnormal drowsiness.
- Inability to talk or produce sounds.
- Inability to drink.

START HERE

How long has your child been coughing?

- STARTED SUDDENLY A FEW MINUTES AGO
- STARTED MORE THAN A FEW MINUTES AGO

Is is possible that your child is choking on food or a small object?

- POSSIBLE
- UNLIKELY

POSSIBLE CAUSE
An inhaled foreign body may be the cause of the coughing.

MEDICAL HELP
EMERGENCY! Call an ambulance! While waiting for medical help, follow the first-aid advice for CHOKING (pp.980–981).

How old is your child?

- 6 MONTHS OR OVER
- UNDER 6 MONTHS

POSSIBLE CAUSE
There is a possibility that your baby may be suffering from a serious lung infection (*see* BRONCHIOLITIS, p.841).

MEDICAL HELP
URGENT! Phone your doctor immediately!

Is your child's breathing abnormally rapid (*see* CHECKING YOUR CHILD'S BREATHING RATE, p.205) or noisy?

- ABNORMALLY RAPID
- NOISY
- NEITHER

Go to chart 67
BREATHING PROBLEMS IN CHILDREN

Does the cough have either of these characteristics?

- COMES IN FITS ENDING WITH A WHOOP
- IS ACCOMPANIED BY VOMITING
- NEITHER

POSSIBLE CAUSE
PERTUSSIS (p.492) may be the cause of your child's cough.

MEDICAL HELP

See your doctor within 24 hours.

Does your child have a runny nose?

- MOST OF THE TIME OR VERY OFTEN
- HAS DEVELOPED A RUNNY NOSE WITHIN THE PAST FEW DAYS
- NO RUNNY NOSE

POSSIBLE CAUSES
Your child may have an allergy (*see* ALLERGIC RHINITIS, p.466) or ENLARGED ADENOIDS (p.842), both of which may cause these symptoms.

MEDICAL HELP

Make an appointment to see your doctor.

POSSIBLE CAUSE
A viral illness, such as a COMMON COLD (p.288) or INFLUENZA (p.289), is the most likely cause of your child's symptoms.

SELF-HELP
See the advice for BRINGING DOWN A FEVER (p.289). Consult your doctor if symptoms get worse, if your child is no better in 2 days, or if other symptoms develop.

Does your child have a fever – a temperature of 38°C (100°F) or above?

- FEVER
- NO FEVER

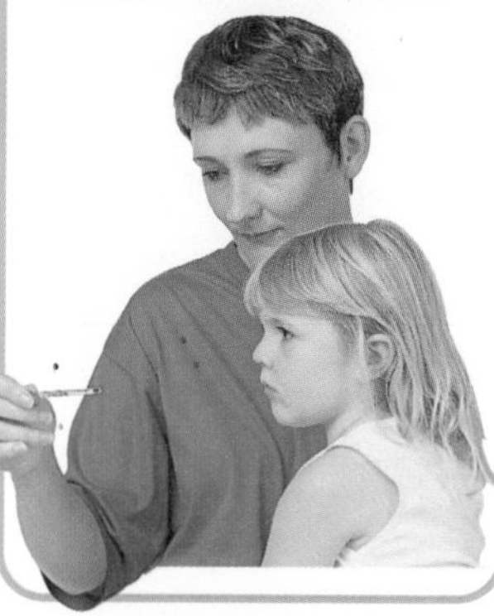

POSSIBLE CAUSE
Your child probably has a COMMON COLD (p.288).

SELF-HELP
STEAM INHALATION (p.475) may help to relieve the cough. Consult your doctor if symptoms get worse, if your child is no better in 2 days, or if other symptoms develop.

When does the coughing occur?

- MAINLY AT NIGHT
- AFTER EXERCISE
- WHEN OUT IN THE COLD
- NONE OF THE ABOVE

POSSIBLE CAUSE
Your child's cough may be a response to being in a smoky atmosphere or to smoking.

SELF-HELP
Make sure that no one smokes in the house and avoid taking your child into a smoky atmosphere. If you suspect that your child may be smoking, encourage him or her to stop.

Are there smokers in the home or might your child have been smoking?

- SMOKERS IN THE HOME
- CHILD MIGHT SMOKE
- NEITHER

POSSIBLE CAUSE
There is a possibility that your child has asthma (*see* ASTHMA IN CHILDREN, p.839).

MEDICAL HELP

See your doctor within 24 hours.

If you cannot identify a possible cause for your child's cough from this chart, see your doctor within 24 hours.

69 ABDOMINAL PAIN IN CHILDREN

For children of 12 and over, see chart 35

Many children suffer from abdominal pain at some time, and some children have recurrent episodes. Usually, the cause is not serious, and the pain subsides in a few hours without treatment. In rare cases, abdominal pain is a symptom of a serious disorder that requires prompt medical attention.

DANGER SIGNS

Call an ambulance if your child's abdominal pain is accompanied by any of the following symptoms:

- Greenish-yellow vomit.
- Pain in the groin or scrotum.
- Blood in the faeces.
- Pain has been continuous for more than 4 hours.

START HERE

Does your child have severe pain in either of the following places?

- GROIN
- SCROTUM
- NEITHER

POSSIBLE CAUSES
A strangulated inguinal hernia (*see* HERNIAS, p.661) or TORSION OF THE TESTIS (p.719) is possible.

MEDICAL HELP
EMERGENCY! Call an ambulance! Do not allow your child to eat or drink.

Does your child have any of the following symptoms?

- CONTINUOUS PAIN FOR MORE THAN 4 HOURS
- BLOOD IN THE FAECES
- GREENISH-YELLOW VOMIT
- NONE OF THE ABOVE

POSSIBLE CAUSE
Continuous abdominal pain for this length of time could be an indication of a serious abdominal condition, such as APPENDICITIS (p.664).

MEDICAL HELP
EMERGENCY! Call an ambulance! While waiting, do not allow your child to eat or drink.

POSSIBLE CAUSES
Abdominal pain accompanied by blood in the faeces could indicate INTUSSUSCEPTION (p.864) in a young child. In older children, the cause of these symptoms may be an intestinal infection due to FOOD POISONING (p.629).

MEDICAL HELP
EMERGENCY! Call an ambulance! Do not allow your child to eat or drink.

POSSIBLE CAUSE
An INTESTINAL OBSTRUCTION (p.663) is possible.

MEDICAL HELP
EMERGENCY! Call an ambulance! Do not allow your child to eat or drink.

Does your child have diarrhoea?

- NO DIARRHOEA
- DIARRHOEA

Has pain been relieved by either of the following?

- VOMITING
- PASSING WIND OR FAECES
- NEITHER

Does your child have any of the following symptoms?

- SORE THROAT
- COUGH
- RUNNY NOSE
- NONE OF THE ABOVE

POSSIBLE CAUSE

Young children often have abdominal pain in association with an upper respiratory tract infection, such as a COMMON COLD (p.288).

SELF-HELP

STEAM INHALATION (p.475) may help. Call an ambulance if your child develops danger signs (opposite page).

POSSIBLE CAUSE

Your child could have a digestive tract infection (*see* GASTROENTERITIS, p.628).

MEDICAL HELP

URGENT! Phone your doctor immediately if your child is under 6 months old. For older children, follow the advice on PREVENTING DEHYDRATION (p.627) and consult your doctor if your child is no better in 24 hours or if other symptoms develop.

Does your child have any of the following symptoms?

- PAIN ON PASSING URINE
- TEMPERATURE OF 38°C (100°F) OR ABOVE
- RENEWED BEDWETTING OR DAYTIME "ACCIDENTS"
- NONE OF THE ABOVE

POSSIBLE CAUSE

Your child may have a URINARY TRACT INFECTION (p.871).

MEDICAL HELP

See your doctor within 24 hours.

POSSIBLE CAUSE

Recurrent abdominal pain in children can sometimes be related to anxiety.

MEDICAL HELP

Make an appointment to see your doctor.

Has your child suffered from similar bouts of abdominal pain over the past few weeks?

- PREVIOUS ABDOMINAL PAIN
- NO PREVIOUS PAIN

If you cannot identify a possible cause for your child's abdominal pain from this chart, see your doctor within 24 hours.

70 WEIGHT PROBLEMS IN CHILDREN

For children of 12 and over, see charts 3 or 4

Check your child is within healthy limits by regularly measuring his or her weight and height (*see* GROWTH CHARTS FOR CHILDREN, pp.42–43). An abnormality in a child's weight may be due to disease. A long-term weight problem may increase your child's risk of future health problems.

WARNING

SPECIAL DIETS

The dietary needs of children differ from those of adults. An unbalanced diet can adversely affect growth and development. You should not put your child on a reducing diet or restrict specific food groups except on the advice of your doctor.

START HERE

What is your concern about your child's weight?

- OVERWEIGHT FOR HEIGHT
- UNDERWEIGHT FOR HEIGHT

POSSIBLE CAUSES

Your child may be eating more than is needed for the amount of exercise he or she is getting. Rarely, weight gain is due to a hormonal disorder or to prescribed drugs such as CORTICOSTEROIDS (p.930).

MEDICAL HELP

Make an appointment to see your doctor.

Has your child been underweight for long?

- YES
- NO

POSSIBLE CAUSE

It is likely that your child's thinness is constitutional, particularly if either parent is thin.

MEDICAL HELP

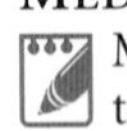
Make an appointment to see your doctor to confirm that there is no additional medical cause.

How is your child's appetite?

- GOOD
- POOR

Does your child have either of the following symptoms?

- DIARRHOEA
- INCREASED THIRST AND NEED TO PASS URINE
- NEITHER OF THE ABOVE

POSSIBLE CAUSES

Your child may be unable to absorb food properly due to a condition such as LACTOSE INTOLERANCE (p.657) or COELIAC DISEASE (p.658).

MEDICAL HELP

Make an appointment to see your doctor.

POSSIBLE CAUSE

Your child could have the metabolic disorder DIABETES MELLITUS (p.687), particularly if he or she has also had recurrent infections and been generally unwell.

MEDICAL HELP

URGENT! Phone your doctor immediately!

If you cannot identify a possible cause for your child's loss or gain in weight, make an appointment to see your doctor.

Looking for Disease

There are numerous medical tests available that are routinely used for investigating disease. This section describes the most common screening and diagnostic procedures and explains why and when they are used. It begins with what to expect when visiting your doctor and what kind of test sample may be taken. The section then examines how the most common imaging and viewing techniques work and explains how they are used.

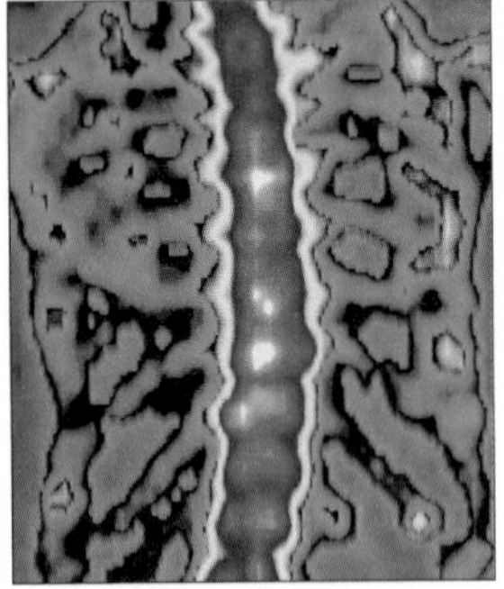

Bone scan of the chest
Radionuclide scanning is often used to detect cancer that has spread to the bones, visible here as light areas along the spine.

INTRODUCTION

THE DIAGNOSTIC METHOD IS THE PROCESS by which a doctor identifies the disease or disorder that is causing symptoms. The doctor may use various tests to confirm or eliminate a particular diagnosis or to help to decide between several possible diagnoses. The process may include finding an underlying agent, such as a virus or bacteria. Screening tests are used to detect early signs of disease in large groups of people or are used individually to look for risk factors that predispose a person to an illness, such as cancer, in the future.

There are a number of reasons for why you might visit a doctor. You may have a pain or other sensation that worries you, have noticed a change in your body's appearance, or simply be anxious about your general physical or mental state. At other times, you may need to see your doctor for a health checkup in connection with your work, or because an insurance company requires you to have a full medical examination.

If you have a particular health problem, your doctor will base his or her diagnosis on your symptoms, medical history, a physical examination, and possibly tests. If you are having a health check, you will have a physical examination, which typically includes measurement of your weight, temperature, respiratory and pulse rates, and blood pressure. Your doctor will also examine you to look for signs of a disorder, such as enlargement of the liver or abnormal sounds in the heart or lungs. You may also be asked to have screening tests appropriate to your age, gender, and lifestyle.

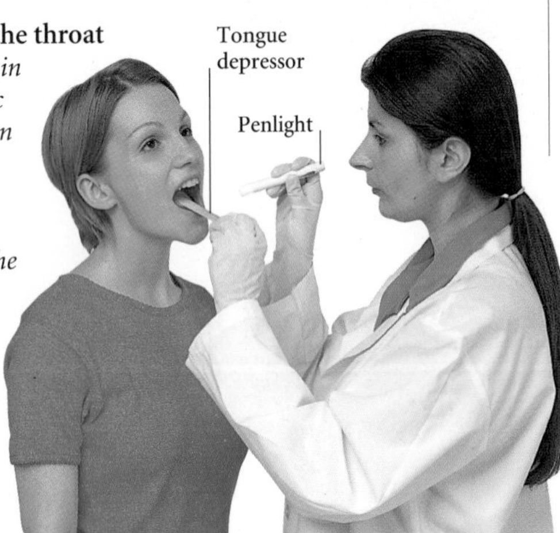

Examining the throat
The first step in the diagnostic process is often a physical examination. If you have a sore throat, the doctor will inspect it for signs of infection

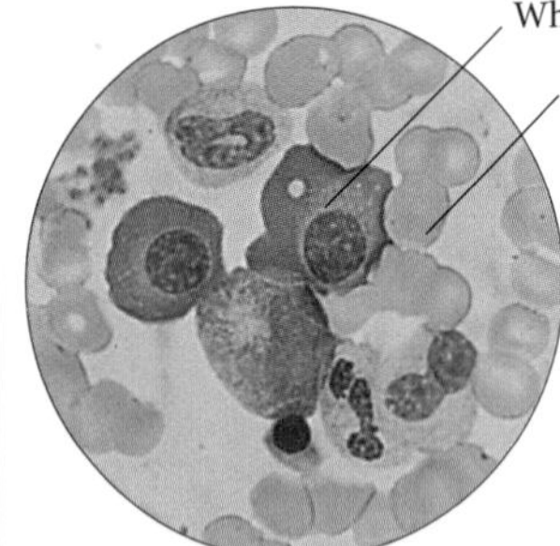

Blood smear
Examination of a blood sample under a microscope can help the doctor to make a diagnosis. On this smear, there are more white blood cells than normal, suggesting that the body is responding to an infection.

WHY TESTS ARE DONE

When you visit your doctor with a health problem, he or she begins the diagnostic process by asking you questions about your general health and any specific symptoms you may have. The next step is to take a complete medical history. This may involve asking you questions about past illnesses, family history of disease, lifestyle, personal relationships, and occupation. You will also have a physical examination. If you have symptoms or signs characteristic of a common disease or disorder, your doctor may be able to arrive at an immediate diagnosis. If he or she is unable to do this, you may be asked to have some tests.

At particular stages of you life, you may be advised to have a screening test. Screening uses one or more of the same tests as diagnosis, but, because the aim is to detect diseases before symptoms develop, not all tests are appropriate. People having tests because they are ill are usually prepared to tolerate a degree of discomfort or an element of risk. However, a person being screened who has no current concerns about his or her health might not tolerate tests that are risky, painful, or generally uncomfortable.

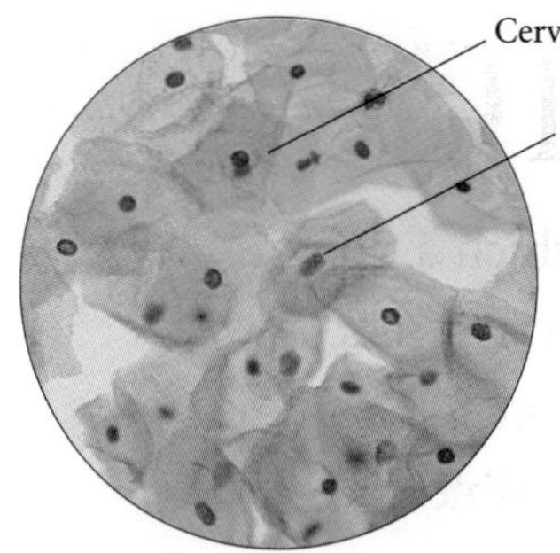

Cervical smear test result
A smear test is used to detect abnormal cervical cells that might become cancerous. This common screening test enables treatment to be given at an early stage. The cells shown here are healthy.

Types of test

Medical tests can be simple enough to be carried out in your doctor's surgery or more complex, requiring sophisticated equipment in a hospital or laboratory. Tests may be performed on body fluids, such as urine or blood, or on tissue, such as cells from the cervix. Viewing tests involve the use of instruments such as endoscopes, viewing tubes through which a doctor can look directly into the body, usually through a natural opening such as the mouth or nose. Imaging tests, such as MRI, CT scanning, and ultrasound, use complex equipment to create images of internal body structures to detect abnormalities. Certain tests, such as mammography (X-rays of the breasts), can be used for both diagnosis and screening.

Your doctor will choose an appropriate medical test to answer a specific diagnostic question or to screen for a particular disorder. You and your doctor will balance the medical value and reliability of the test against any health risks and discomfort.

Reliability

Some tests, such as diagnostic tests on tissue samples, are extremely accurate, but most are less reliable. There may be inaccuracies in the test equipment, the procedure, or in the interpretation of results. These and other human errors can lead to false results. A false positive result indicates the presence of disease in a person who is in fact healthy. A false negative result indicates that a person is free of the disease when he or she actually has it. False positive results cause anxiety and necessitate further tests to confirm or reject the diagnosis. A false negative result may delay diagnosis until symptoms develop, at which stage treatment may be less effective. Good tests give only a small proportion of false positive and false negative results. Since most tests are not totally reliable, results must be carefully assessed and always considered in the context of a person's medical history and examination.

COMPARISON Imaging techniques

Many imaging techniques use radiation, which may be from an outside source, as in plain and contrast X-rays, or injected into the body, as in PET scanning and other types of radionuclide scanning. Some techniques, such as MRI and ultrasound scanning, use no radiation and so avoid the risks that are associated with it. The particular technique a doctor chooses depends on what he or she is looking for. Although MRI produces highly detailed information about internal tissues, fractures are better detected by a simple X-ray. The images here show how different types of information about structures in the head can be obtained using different imaging techniques.

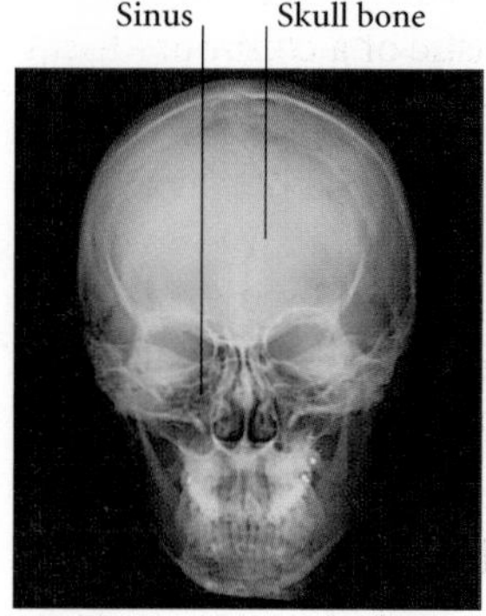

X-ray
Plain X-rays can produce clear images of dense structures, such as bones, and air-filled cavities, such as the sinuses in the skull.

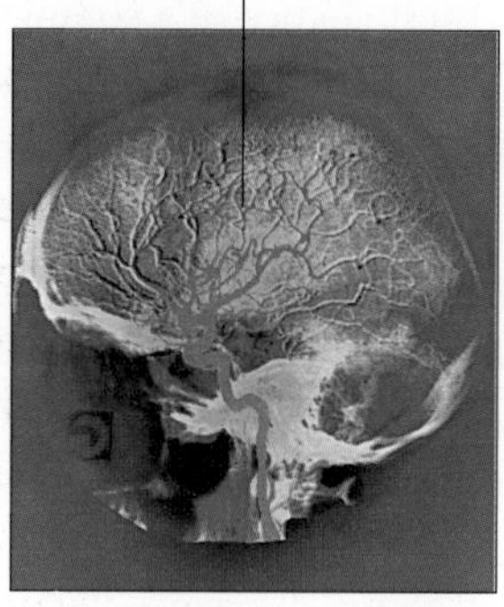

Contrast X-ray
Structures not normally visible on X-rays, such as blood vessels, can be seen after introducing a contrast medium into them.

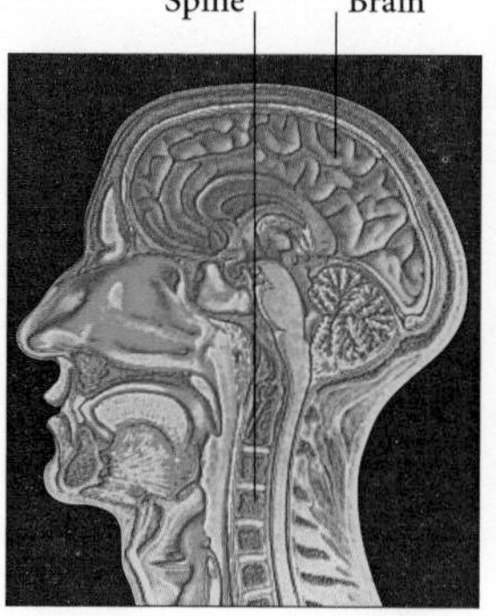

MRI scan
Magnetic resonance imaging (MRI) uses magnetic fields to give detailed structural images without using radiation.

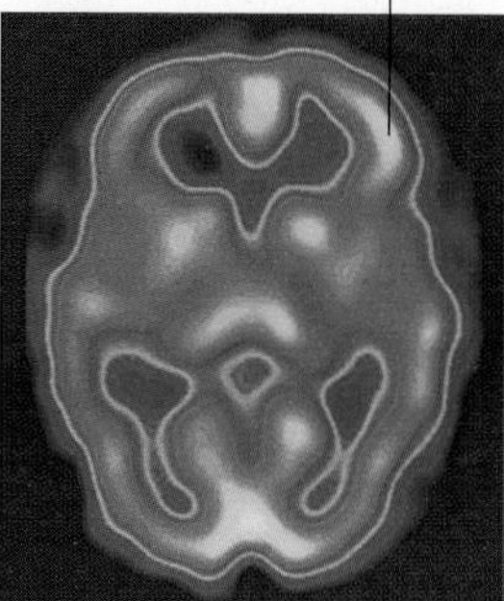

PET scan
Positron emission tomography (PET) uses injected radioactive substances, which are taken up and reflect the activity in tissues.

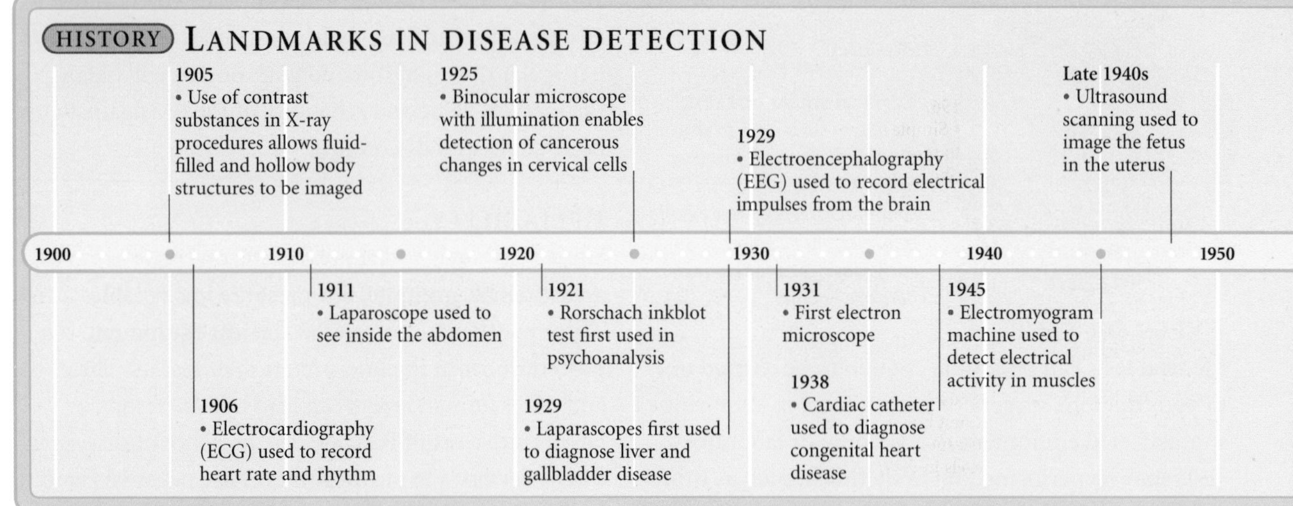

Trends in disease detection during the 20th century
Diagnostic and screening tests are now safer, more accurate, and less invasive because of the growth of computer technology. The mortality rates of some diseases, such as cervical cancer, have been greatly reduced as a result of efficient screening programmes.

Costs, risks, and acceptability

In addition to the cost of the test itself, having a test may involve less obvious expenses. For example, the results of a diagnostic test may affect your life insurance status. Some tests also carry health risks. For example, coronary angiography, which is used to view blood vessels to diagnose coronary artery disease, carries a very small risk of causing a stroke or heart attack. In addition to these costs and risks, the degree of discomfort or pain that the test causes must also be considered. However, the drawbacks of a test need to be weighed against the potential usefulness of the test result. A risky or painful test may still be justified medically and be acceptable to the person having it if it yields information that could be lifesaving.

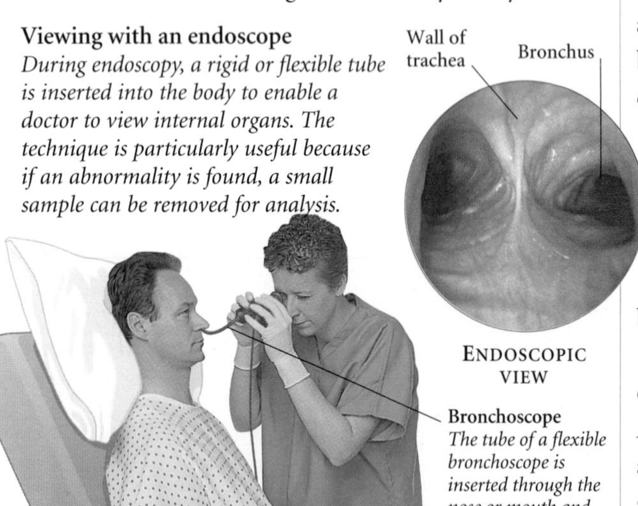

Viewing with an endoscope
During endoscopy, a rigid or flexible tube is inserted into the body to enable a doctor to view internal organs. The technique is particularly useful because if an abnormality is found, a small sample can be removed for analysis.

Bronchoscope
The tube of a flexible bronchoscope is inserted through the nose or mouth and extends to the lungs

Screening

Screening tests can have one of three basic aims. Many are used to identify people who already have a disease but who have not yet developed symptoms. This type of test is used only if there is a treatment available for an early stage of the disease that can improve the outcome. For example, breast cancer screening is a routine procedure because early detection gives the best chance of a complete cure. On the other hand, screening for Alzheimer's disease is not routine because no effective treatment is currently available.

A second type of screening test looks for risk factors or a genetic predisposition to developing a disease. A typical test might look for high blood cholesterol, associated with coronary artery disease, or for the genes associated with breast cancer. Screening may also be used to detect healthy carriers of abnormal genes, which may be passed on to children. These tests may be offered to couples who are planning to have children and pregnant women who have a family history of a genetic disorder.

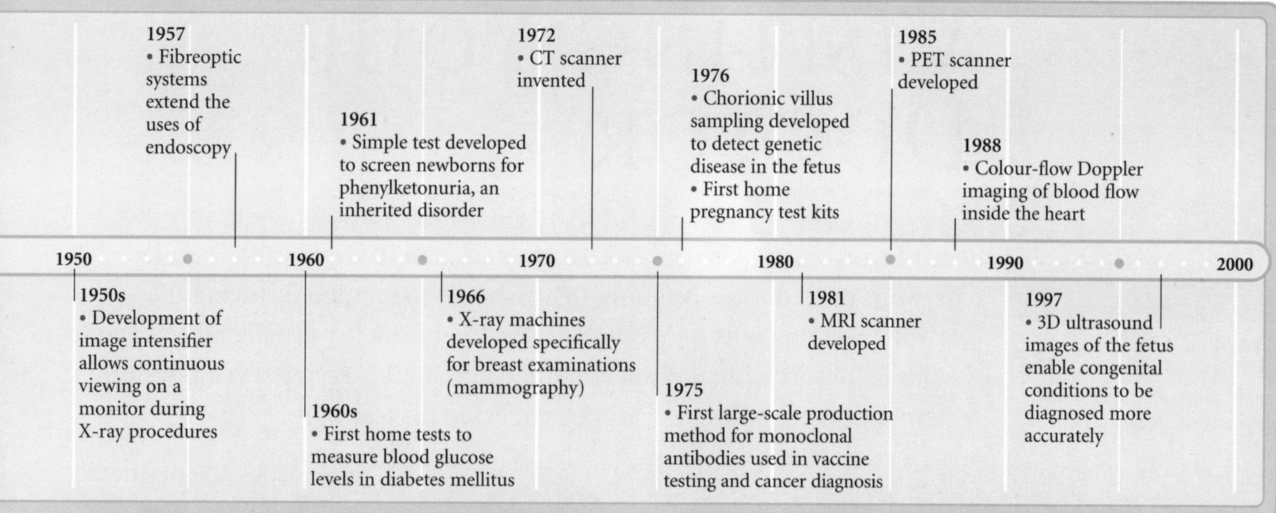

Successful screening relies on careful selection of the population to be tested. If the disorder is rare, the proportion of false positive test results tends to be high, even if the test is relatively precise. There is also little point in testing many people at great expense when few are likely to have the disease. To be reliable and cost-effective, screening programmes must be targeted at groups at increased risk. For example, breast cancer screening usually starts after the age of 50, when the disease becomes more common, and screening for sickle-cell disease can be limited to black people, a group that has a high incidence of the disease.

Trends in disease detection

Technological advances, such as endoscopy and increasingly sophisticated imaging tests, are making diagnosis safer and less invasive. In addition, the use of computers is making the analysis, storage, and retrieval of test results quicker and more reliable.

There are a number of reliable home tests now available, such as tests for blood sugar (necessary in diabetes) and blood pressure monitors. Used under the supervision of a doctor, these tests can help you to take responsibility for your own health and monitor long-term illnesses and the effects of treatments.

ORGANIZATION How this part of the book is organized

This part of the book tells you what happens when you visit the doctor with a problem, including the consultation, physical examination, and taking of samples for testing. Laboratory testing of samples and the technology and uses of imaging tests are then described. Tests specific to a body system or organ are described with the relevant system.

Visiting your doctor p.216
Explains the process by which your doctor arrives at a diagnosis; describes the doctor's surgery and the equipment he or she uses.

Medical history and examination p.218
Questions your doctor asks you and why; practicalities of the physical examination.

Obtaining samples for testing p.221
What is involved when samples of body fluids or tissues are taken for tests.

Testing samples p.224
Description of the medical laboratory and what happens to specimens.

Tests on blood structure and function p.226
Tests on the cellular components of blood; blood grouping; blood clotting tests.

Chemical tests p.229
Tests that can be carried out on samples of blood and urine, including cholesterol and pregnancy tests; tests on faecal samples.

Tests for microorganisms p.234
Various tests to identify microorganisms; testing bacteria for sensitivity to drugs.

Cell and tissue tests p.236
Tests in which cell and tissue samples are examined visually under a microscope.

Genetic tests p.238
How genetic tests are performed and what they can reveal about your future health.

Visualizing internal organs p.242
An overview of the techniques used for viewing and imaging body tissues.

Imaging techniques p.244
Details of imaging technologies, including X-rays, MRI, and ultrasound scanning.

Viewing techniques p.254
Looking inside the body using simple viewing instruments and endoscopes.

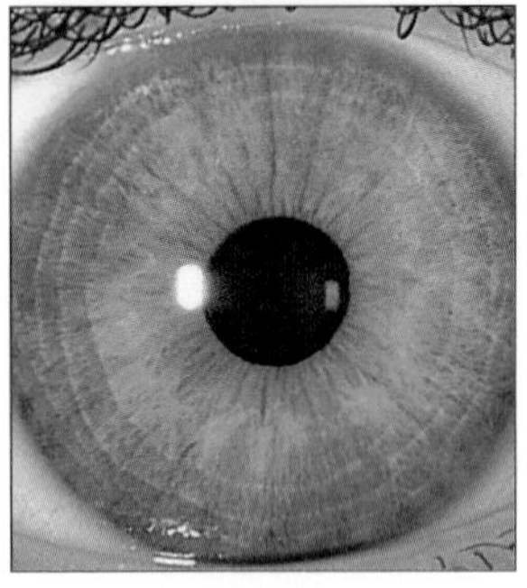

View of the eye
Your doctor may examine your eyes when you have a routine physical examination.

Visiting Your Doctor

You may need to visit your doctor for advice about symptoms or other health issues, or your doctor may ask you to come in for regular checkups or to discuss ongoing treatment. What happens during the consultation depends on its purpose, but your doctor usually assesses your health by observation, asking you questions, and carrying out a physical examination. Samples may also be collected for testing.

You may decide to visit your doctor because you feel ill or because you are concerned about a physical change, such as a swelling or stiffness in a joint. You may need advice about a lifestyle change, such as losing weight or giving up smoking. If you have a long-term condition, such as diabetes mellitus, you will need regular checkups. Even if you are healthy, you may be asked to attend the surgery for screening procedures, such as blood pressure measurement and cervical smear tests.

Preparing for a visit

Whatever your reason for visiting your doctor, you may find it helpful to decide on the issues that you want to discuss before you have the appointment. For example, if you have specific symptoms, you should think about how often they occur and whether certain activities bring the symptoms on or relieve them. Your doctor also needs to know about medications or supplements that you are taking, allergies that you have to particular treatments, and any alternative therapies that you are currently using.

The consultation

There are many ways in which your doctor can assess your health. First of all, he or she will note your general appearance, such as your weight, and look for signs of anxiety or depression. Your doctor will then ask you a series of questions, known as taking your medical history, before he or she performs a physical examination. The questions that you are asked and the extent of the physical examination depend on the purpose of the consultation.

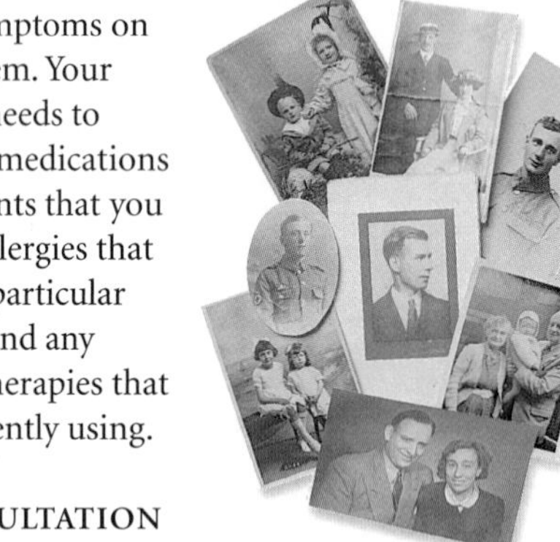

Family history
Some disorders may run in your family. Your doctor needs to know about these to help make a diagnosis.

If you are visiting a doctor for the first time, he or she may take a full medical history, including details of diseases that run in your family, illnesses that you have had in the past, and lifestyle factors such as your diet. If the doctor already has your medical record, he or she may refer to it. If you have specific symptoms, the doctor will concentrate on them in order to make a diagnosis.

A full physical examination is usually given only as part of a general checkup, such as for a new insurance policy. If you have symptoms, the doctor usually checks only relevant areas of your body. Even if you are not given a full examination, your doctor may inspect certain areas, such as your skin and nails, to assess your general health.

Your doctor may need to collect a sample, such as blood or urine. Samples are tested to confirm a diagnosis or to monitor a disease. Simple tests may be performed in the doctor's surgery, but more complex procedures are usually carried out in a laboratory. The doctor may ask you to telephone the surgery for the test results or to make another appointment to discuss the results and their implications for your health.

(Equipment) The doctor's basic equipment

Your doctor may use one or more basic pieces of equipment when performing a physical examination. Each has a specific function. Some instruments enable your doctor to examine certain parts of the body more closely. Others are used to listen for abnormal sounds or to check the reflexes.

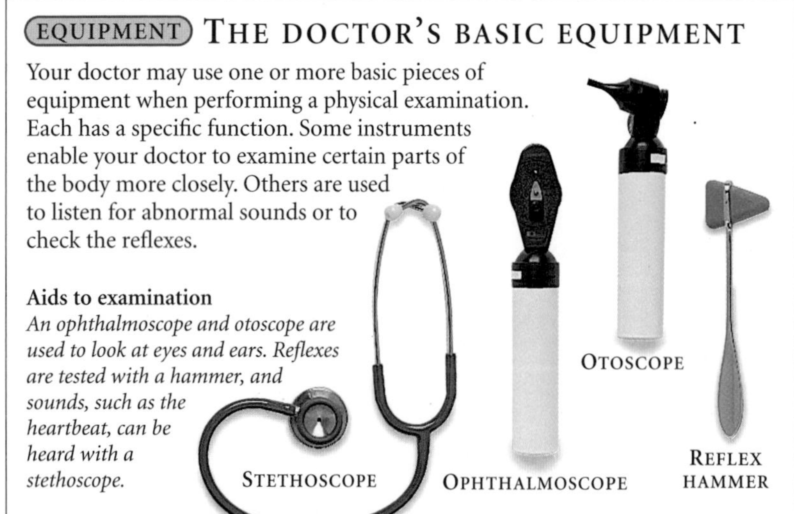

Aids to examination
An ophthalmoscope and otoscope are used to look at eyes and ears. Reflexes are tested with a hammer, and sounds, such as the heartbeat, can be heard with a stethoscope.

SETTING THE DOCTOR'S SURGERY

The doctor's surgery is designed to make the visit as efficient and comfortable as possible and to provide privacy so that you can talk freely to the doctor during the consultation. The surgery may contain various charts and measures that enable the doctor or nurse to collect basic information, such as your height and weight. The physical examination is often carried out in a special partitioned area of the surgery that contains all the necessary equipment.

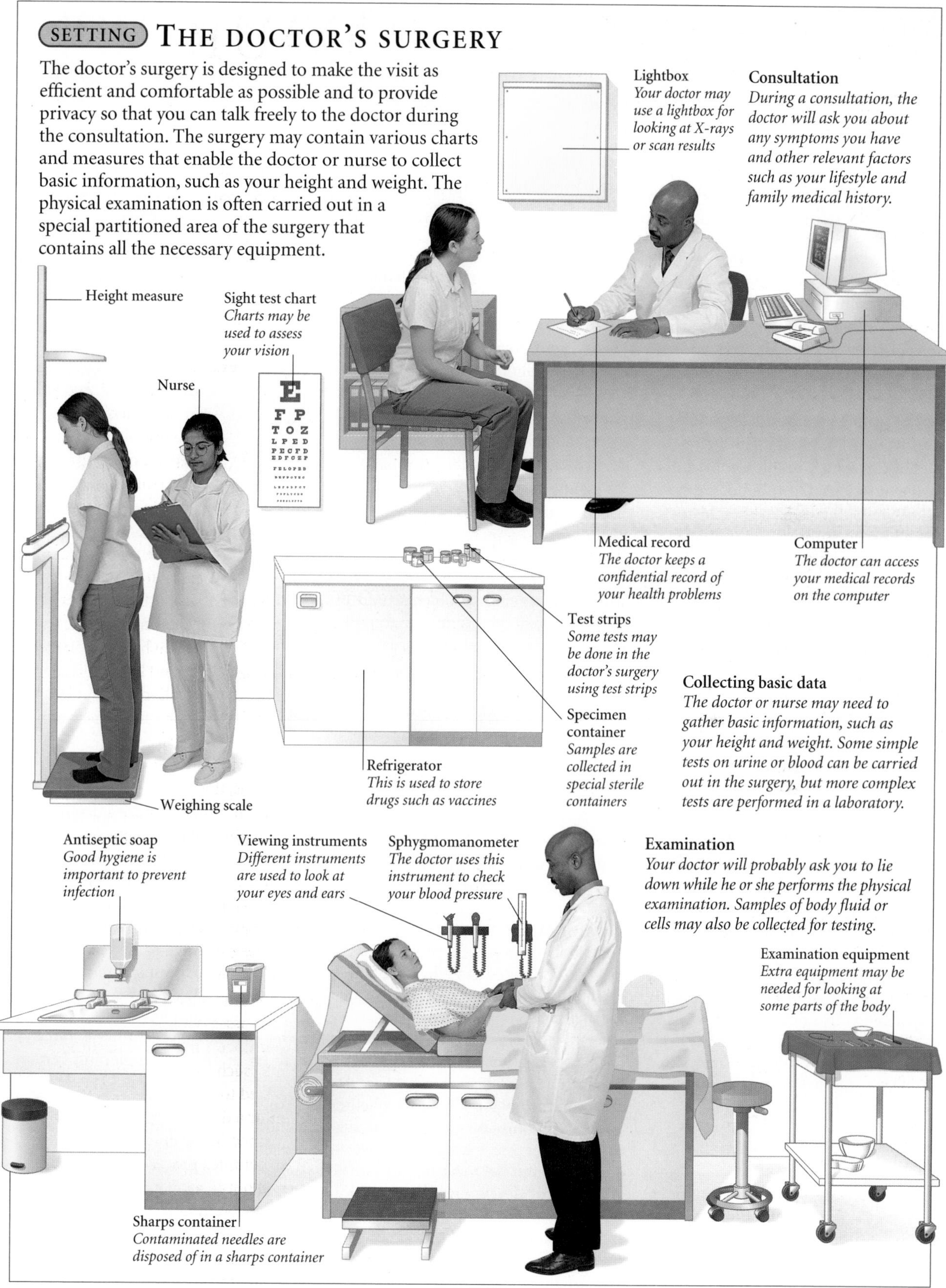

MEDICAL HISTORY AND EXAMINATION

You may visit your doctor for a checkup or if you are feeling ill. If you have symptoms, your doctor will ask various questions and carry out an examination to take the first steps towards a diagnosis. Occasionally, this may be all that is needed for your doctor to decide what is causing your illness and what action is needed. In other cases, tests are used to gather more information.

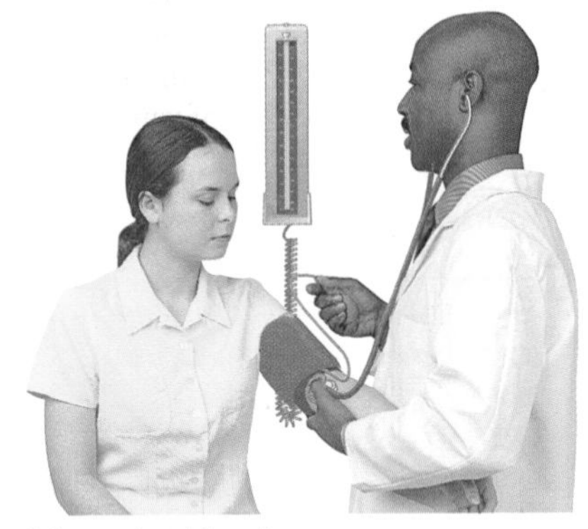

Measuring blood pressure
A physical examination may include measuring your blood pressure. High blood pressure increases the risk of stroke.

From the moment that you walk into the surgery, your doctor starts to gather information about you from your appearance. This information may provide clues to your general health and state of mind. The doctor obtains further information about your health from a medical history and by performing a physical examination.

The first article in this section looks at the questions that your doctor may ask when taking your medical history. Such questions are an important way of gathering information about past illnesses, disorders that run in your family, and your lifestyle.

Once he or she has taken your history, your doctor may examine you to look for abnormalities or confirm a suspected diagnosis. Some common physical examination procedures are described in the second article.

If you need a medical examination for insurance purposes, your doctor will look for early signs of disease or for factors that may increase your risk of developing disease. Routine checkups in childhood, during pregnancy, and for the elderly are discussed elsewhere (*see* HEALTH CHECKUPS, p.40).

Medical history

A medical record of a person's past and present health

A medical history is compiled from a series of questions that your doctor asks to help him or her to diagnose a disorder or assess your risk of developing a disease. The questions may centre on your current symptoms, but you may also be asked about past illnesses, medications or treatments you are taking, your family medical history, or your lifestyle.

If you visit your doctor with symptoms, your medical history will help him or her to reach a diagnosis and decide what action to take. You may visit your doctor for a checkup if you have recently registered with a new practice or if you are elderly. At the checkup, you are likely to be asked about lifestyle factors that influence your health, such as your diet (*see* HEALTH CHECKUPS, p.40).

PAST MEDICAL HISTORY AND MEDICATIONS

Since some health problems recur or affect more than one part of the body, it is important that your doctor is aware of disorders and operations that you have had. This may help him or her to decide whether a previous problem could be causing current symptoms. For example, if you have had the joint disorder arthritis (p.374), it may recur in the same joint or in one or more different joints.

Symptoms may be a side effect of or an allergic reaction to a treatment, so it is important to tell your doctor if you are taking any medications or supplements. You should also tell him or her if you are having or using any alternative therapies. Your doctor needs to ensure that new medication will not react with anything that you are already taking.

FAMILY HISTORY

Your doctor may ask you about illnesses or causes of death in close family members because many disorders, such as hypertension (p.403), coronary artery disease (p.405), and diabetes mellitus (p.687), sometimes run in families. If you have a family history of a particular disorder, the doctor will check whether your symptoms are due to that disorder. He or she may also be able to suggest preventive measures to reduce your risk of developing the condition in the future. For example, if you have a family history of heart disease, your doctor is likely to advise you to restrict your intake of high-fat foods.

LIFESTYLE

Although you may not think that questions about your lifestyle are relevant, what you eat, what you do, and where you live can all influence your health.

DIET, ALCOHOL, AND TOBACCO Your doctor may ask you whether you have a balanced diet and take exercise regularly. You may also be asked how much alcohol you drink, if you smoke, and if you use recreational drugs.

WORK, HOME LIFE, AND TRAVEL Your doctor may ask you questions about your job, because your work may have an effect on your health. Past occupations may also be important because some work-related diseases take years to appear. For example, people who work or have worked in the mining industry may be at risk of developing certain occupational lung diseases (p.499).

Your personal relationships, living conditions, and financial circumstances can also influence your health, particularly your psychological wellbeing.

If you have travelled abroad recently, you should tell your doctor which country or countries you have visited as there is a possibility that your symptoms may be due to an unusual infectious disease.

TECHNIQUE **INSPECTION**

Before your doctor starts to examine you, he or she has already gained important clues about your health from certain aspects of your overall appearance. For example, the condition of your skin reflects your general state of health and can indicate hormonal imbalances within the body.

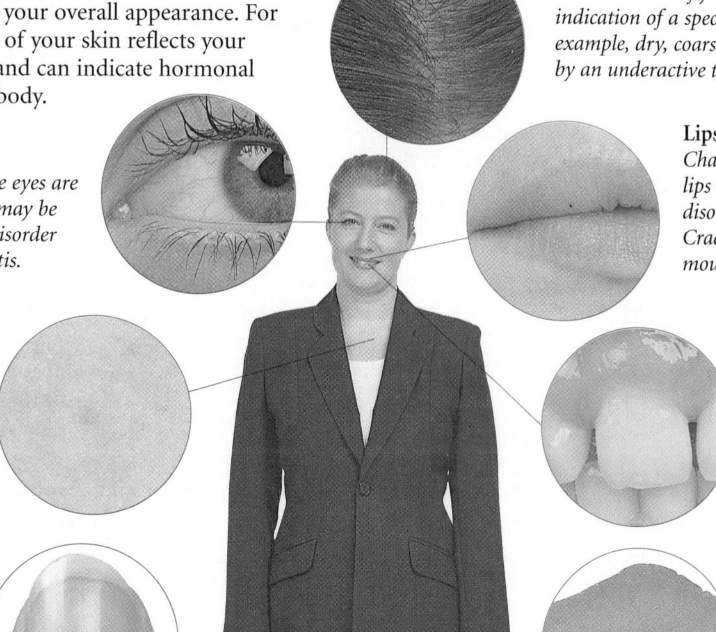

Hair
The condition of your hair may be an indication of a specific disorder. For example, dry, coarse hair may be caused by an underactive thyroid gland.

Eyes
Normally, the whites of the eyes are clear. A yellow coloration may be one of the first signs of a disorder of the liver, such as hepatitis.

Lips and mouth
Changes in the colour of your lips may reflect a blood disorder, such as anaemia. Cracks at the corners of the mouth suggest iron deficiency.

Skin
Obvious rashes may be due to skin disorders, such as eczema. The appearance of your skin may also be an indicator of disorders elsewhere in the body.

Gums
Inflamed or bleeding gums indicate gum disease, usually due to poor dental hygiene. Receding gums may also be caused by poor hygiene.

Nails
The appearance of the nails varies from person to person, but a change in nail shape or colour may indicate an underlying problem.

Joints
A red, swollen, or inflamed joint could be a sign of a joint disorder, such as arthritis, or the result of a joint injury.

Physical examination

An examination by a doctor to check the condition or health of various body systems and organs

A physical examination is often an essential part of the diagnostic process. You may also have a physical examination if you are visiting your doctor for a general checkup (p.40).

If you have symptoms, your doctor will concentrate on the areas of your body related to your symptoms or in which abnormalities can be detected. Even if you think that your symptoms are restricted to a certain part of your body, your doctor may want to check other areas. For example, the doctor may examine your ankles if you have symptoms of heart disease, such as shortness of breath, because heart disease is associated with swelling of the ankles.

Your doctor uses several basic techniques to carry out an examination (*see* INSPECTION, above, and BASIC EXAMINATION TECHNIQUES, p.220).

SKIN, HAIR, AND NAILS

Obvious skin problems include rashes, discoloration, and very rough or thin skin. These problems are usually symptoms of a skin disorder, but some may indicate a more widespread problem such as systemic lupus erythematosus (p.461), a disease that can cause inflammation of connective tissue.

The condition of your hair and nails can also be affected by certain disorders. For example, generalized thinning of your hair may be caused by a hormonal disorder, and a change in the shape or colour of your nails may indicate iron-deficiency anaemia (p.447).

HEART AND CIRCULATION

Your doctor may check the strength and rate of your pulse, usually at the wrist or the side of the neck. A rapid or uneven pulse suggests a heart problem. Pulses at other points, such as in the groin, may provide more information about your circulation. For example, weak pulses in one leg may indicate poor circulation in that leg.

Your doctor will use a stethoscope to listen to your heart. Valves in the heart make distinctive sounds as they open and close. Additional sounds, known as heart murmurs, may indicate heart valve damage. Blood pressure measurement (p.404) is a routine part of most physical examinations. High blood pressure (*see* HYPERTENSION, p.403) may increase your risk of stroke (p.532), heart disease, or kidney failure (p.705).

LUNGS

Your doctor will have noticed if you have difficulty in breathing. He or she may listen to your chest and back with a stethoscope while you breathe deeply. Abnormal sounds, such as wheezing, may indicate narrowed airways. The doctor may also tap the surface of your chest to check for fluid in the lungs.

ABDOMEN AND RECTUM

The abdomen contains major organs including the stomach, liver, kidneys, and intestines. By feeling and tapping your abdomen, your doctor can detect

TECHNIQUE BASIC EXAMINATION TECHNIQUES

Once your doctor has looked for obvious signs of disease (*see* INSPECTION, p.219), he or she may use any of three basic techniques to examine you. An examination may include auscultation, in which a stethoscope is used to listen to your chest or other parts of your body; palpation, in which an area is felt with the hands; and percussion, which involves listening to sounds made by tapping certain areas.

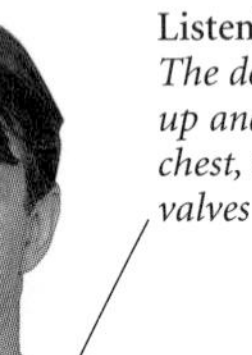

Listening to the chest
The doctor uses a stethoscope to pick up and amplify sounds within the chest, such as sounds made by heart valves as they open and close

Auscultation
A stethoscope can be used to listen not only to the chest but also to sounds made by the intestines or by blood passing through blood vessels. The doctor interprets these sounds to determine whether or not they are normal.

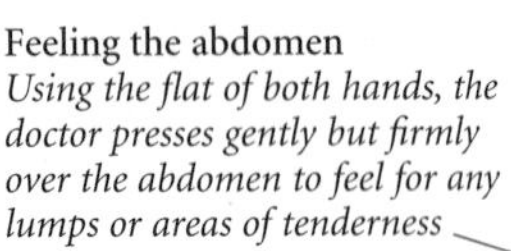

Feeling the abdomen
Using the flat of both hands, the doctor presses gently but firmly over the abdomen to feel for any lumps or areas of tenderness

Palpation
The doctor applies pressure with one or two hands and slowly feels over the entire abdomen. He or she will be able to detect enlarged or tender internal organs or abnormal swellings.

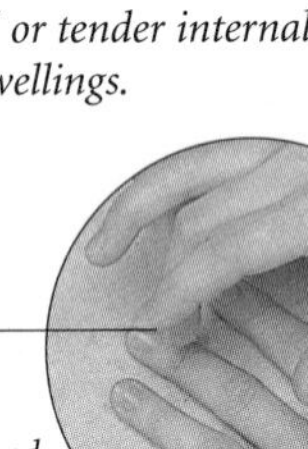

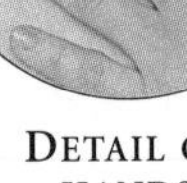

Percussing the chest
A finger of one hand is pressed on to the chest and tapped by a finger of the other hand to produce a sound

DETAIL OF HANDS

Percussion
By tapping different parts of the chest and abdomen and listening to the sounds that are produced, the doctor can distinguish solid tissue and fluids from gas-filled areas.

abnormal swellings. Listening to the intestines with a stethoscope may help to confirm the presence of a blockage.

Your doctor may decide to perform a rectal examination if you have certain symptoms, such as constipation. A rectal examination may also be carried out to look for colorectal cancer (p.665), especially in people over 50. In men, a rectal examination may also be performed to check for an enlarged prostate gland (p.725) or prostate cancer (p.726). Your doctor will ask you to lie on your left side while he or she inserts a gloved, lubricated finger into the rectum to feel for lumps or areas of tenderness.

REPRODUCTIVE ORGANS

In men, the scrotum and testes may be routinely examined to detect lumps or swellings. The penis may also be examined for signs of infection. Boys may be checked to make sure that both of their testes have descended properly.

In women, internal pelvic examinations may be used to look for disorders of the female reproductive organs. Your doctor inserts two gloved fingers inside the vagina before pressing down on the lower abdomen with the other hand. By using both hands, he or she can feel the size and shape of the uterus, the ovaries, and the fallopian tubes, in addition to any areas of tenderness. A cervical smear test (p.749) should be performed every 3–5 years in sexually active women to screen for early signs of cancer of the cervix (p.750). Your doctor may inspect your breasts for nipple abnormalities or unusual puckering of the skin and may feel your breasts for any unusual lumps or swellings.

BONES, JOINTS, AND MUSCLES

Your doctor may want to examine a joint for swelling or tenderness, either of which could indicate a joint disorder such as arthritis (p.374). He or she may also check the range of pain-free movement that you have in a joint and check that the ligaments and muscles around the joint are working normally.

NERVOUS SYSTEM

A full examination of the nervous system is a complex procedure and usually involves testing a range of functions, such as strength and sensation.

Your doctor may ask you to do tests to check your strength, coordination, and balance. For example, you may be asked to touch the end of your nose several times. Your doctor may also test your response to different sensations, such as a light touch, and check other senses, such as sight and smell. By testing reflexes, such as a knee jerk, your doctor will be able to assess the function of some of your nerves. He or she may also ask you questions to check mental functions, such as memory.

Occasionally, your doctor may ask you additional questions to assess your mental state. For example, if you have not been sleeping properly, he or she may ask if you are feeling depressed.

OBTAINING SAMPLES FOR TESTING

Almost any body fluid or tissue can be collected for testing. The procedures involved in obtaining most types of sample are straightforward and painless and may be carried out by a doctor or nurse as part of a visit to the surgery or by yourself at home. More complex sampling procedures are performed in hospital. Samples are usually sent to a laboratory for testing.

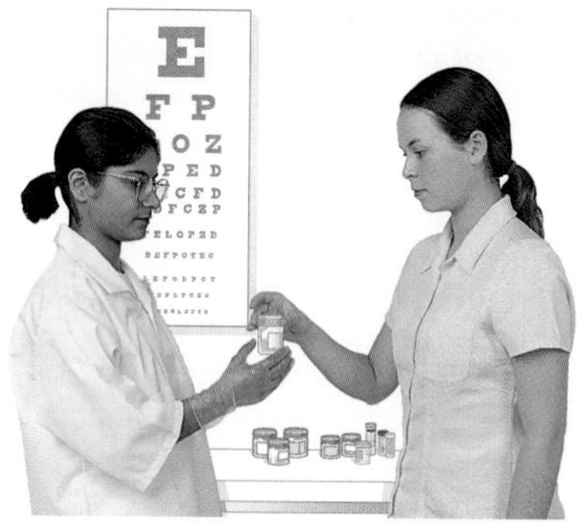

Providing a sample
When you visit the doctor, he or she may ask you to provide a specimen of your urine in a sterile container for testing.

Laboratory analysis of fluid or tissue samples can often provide useful medical information. It is one of the most important ways of confirming the cause of an illness or checking the condition of a body system or organ.

If the tests are to provide accurate information, the manner in which a sample is taken must be carefully controlled. The sample must be fresh and should not be contaminated with any other substances. For example, faecal samples should not contain urine. If your doctor has asked you to collect a sample at home, you should follow his or her instructions carefully. All samples should be stored in a sealed container that has been labelled and dated. The samples must be delivered to the doctor or laboratory as soon as possible. If samples are kept overnight, they need to be refrigerated.

The general principles of collecting samples are discussed in this section. In the first three articles, methods for collecting blood, urine, and faecal samples are described. Such samples are easy to collect and are often used in initial investigations or to monitor a chronic (long-term) disease, such as diabetes mellitus. Other fluids, cells, or tissues are collected only in certain circumstances, such as for cancer diagnosis. The principles of collecting these samples are covered in the final two articles. If a special procedure is used to collect a sample from a specific site, the technique is described with the relevant body system. For example, lumbar puncture (p.527), in which a sample of fluid is taken from around the spinal cord, is covered in disorders of the nervous system.

Blood samples

Small volumes of blood that can be collected and used to screen for or diagnose a wide range of disorders

Having a blood sample taken is a common medical procedure and is often performed by a doctor as part of a health checkup (p.40). Blood tests can help the doctor to assess your state of health and look for risk factors associated with certain diseases. For example, blood may be taken in order to check your blood cholesterol level (*see* BLOOD CHOLESTEROL TESTS, p.231), which is one indicator of your risk of developing coronary artery disease (p.405).

If you visit your doctor with specific symptoms, a blood test may help to diagnose the cause of your illness. Having a blood sample taken is also often a routine procedure when you are admitted to hospital. If you have a long-term illness, you may have regular blood tests to monitor your response to treatment or the progress of your condition.

HOW ARE SAMPLES OBTAINED?

Blood can be taken from various blood vessels, including the veins, the capillaries (small blood vessels), and, under some circumstances, the arteries. The choice of site depends on how much blood is needed and the purpose of the test. Blood samples are usually taken by a doctor, a nurse, or a phlebotomist, a technician who specializes in collecting blood. In some circumstances, you may need to collect small amounts of blood yourself. For example, people who have diabetes mellitus (p.687) learn to take blood samples at home in order to monitor their blood sugar levels.

VENOUS BLOOD The vast majority of blood samples are taken from a vein using a hollow needle attached to a vacuum bottle or syringe. The vein on the inside of the elbow is the most commonly used site (*see* HAVING A BLOOD SAMPLE TAKEN, p.222), although in children blood is often taken from a vein on the back of the hand or the foot. A topical anaesthetic spray can be applied beforehand to make the procedure less painful. Most tests require only a few millilitres of blood to be taken; even less is needed for children and babies.

CAPILLARY BLOOD If only a drop or two of blood is needed, a sterile instrument called a lancet is used to pierce the skin on a fingertip or, in a newborn or infant, on the heel. A drop of blood can then be squeezed out and collected.

ARTERIAL BLOOD If the blood levels of oxygen and carbon dioxide need to be measured, usually to assess the severity of lung disease, a sample is taken from an artery in the wrist or groin (*see* MEASURING BLOOD GASES, p.501). This procedure is usually performed by a doctor. A local anaesthetic may be used.

WHAT ARE SAMPLES USED FOR?

Blood samples may be used for a wide variety of tests. Some simple tests, such as tests for blood glucose levels, may be done in the doctor's surgery. More complex tests are usually performed in a

PROCEDURE HAVING A BLOOD SAMPLE TAKEN

Blood samples can be used to screen for or diagnose a variety of different disorders. In adults, blood is usually taken from a vein on the inside of the elbow. The blood is drawn up through a needle and collected into one or more bottles, depending on the tests needed. Usually, the blood is then sent to a laboratory to be tested. Once blood has been taken, pressure is applied to the wound to prevent the vein from leaking, which may cause a bruise to develop.

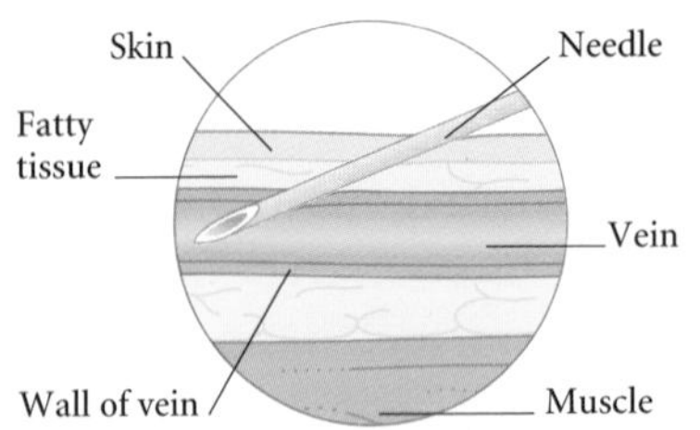

POSITION OF NEEDLE IN VEIN

During the procedure
The skin around the vein is cleaned. A hollow needle attached to a syringe is inserted into the vein and blood is taken.

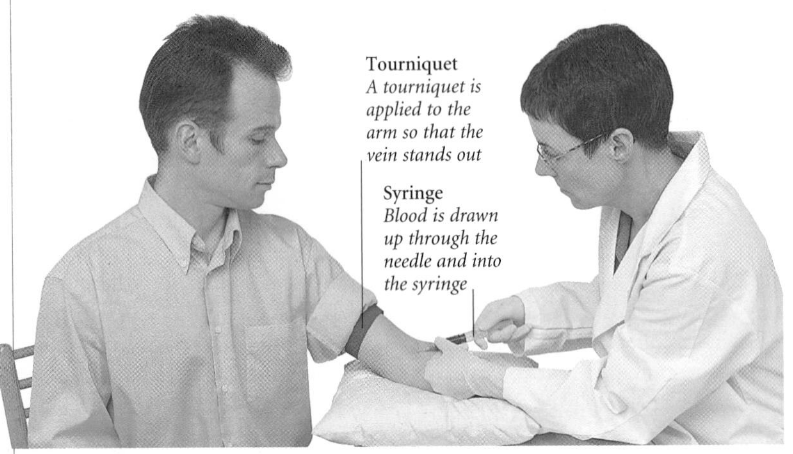

laboratory. These may include tests for microorganisms (pp.234–235), chemical tests (pp.229–233), and genetic tests (pp.238–241), as well as tests designed to look at the different types and numbers of blood cell and their function (*see* TESTS ON BLOOD STRUCTURE AND FUNCTION, pp.226–228).

Urine samples

Quantities of urine collected to investigate the function of different body systems, particularly the kidneys and urinary tract

You may be asked to provide a urine sample when you visit the doctor for a health checkup (p.40) or if you have symptoms, such as frequent urination, that need investigation. Urine tests can provide information about the condition of the urinary tract to help your doctor to confirm a diagnosis. The urine also reflects changes in blood chemistry associated with disorders of other systems, such as diabetes mellitus (p.687).

HOW ARE SAMPLES OBTAINED?

When you arrive at the doctor's surgery, the nurse may give you a container in which to collect a small sample of urine. Alternatively, you may be provided with a sterile container and asked to collect a urine sample at home.

Before collecting a urine sample, you should clean your genital area thoroughly with soap and water. You should then pass a small amount of urine into the toilet and stop urinating. When you start to pass urine again, collect some of the urine in the sterile container. The first few drops of urine passed are not collected in the container because they can become contaminated with bacteria as they pass from the normally sterile bladder through the urethra to the outside of the body. For some tests, you may need to collect all the urine that you pass during a 24-hour period.

If you need to collect a urine sample from a baby or a small child, your doctor may give you an adhesive bag and a sterile container. You should wash your child's genital area, dry it thoroughly, and attach the bag around his or her genitals. As soon as your child has passed urine, you should transfer the urine to the sterile container. Alternatively, the doctor may use a catheter to take a urine sample. The catheter is passed through the urethra and up into the child's bladder. The catheter is removed when enough urine has been collected.

Your doctor may make a preliminary assessment of your urine in the surgery by carrying out simple tests to detect evidence of infection or traces of protein or blood (*see* DIPSTICK TESTING OF URINE, p.231). However, in many cases, the sample has to be sent to the laboratory for further analysis (*see* ROUTINE URINE CHEMISTRY, p.230, and TESTS FOR MICROORGANISMS, pp.234–235).

Faecal samples

Small amounts of faeces that are collected to screen for or diagnose disorders affecting the digestive system

Your doctor may ask you to provide a faecal sample if you have symptoms, such as diarrhoea, that suggest a digestive disorder, especially if they are likely to have been caused by an infection. In adults over the age of 50, a faecal sample may be required for a screening test designed to detect early signs of colorectal cancer (p.665).

In order to provide a faecal sample, you should defaecate into a clean, wide-mouthed receptacle and then transfer a small sample to a container. Your doctor may give you a special container that has a spoon fixed to the inside of the lid to make this process easier. Try not to contaminate the sample with urine and avoid putting toilet paper in the container. If you pass liquid faeces, you should collect both solid and liquid material together. If you need to collect a faecal sample from a baby, do not use the contents of a nappy because liquid faeces will have been absorbed.

Some samples can be tested by the doctor in the surgery, but most samples are sent to a laboratory. Tests are most commonly performed to look for microscopic amounts of blood in the faeces (*see* FAECAL OCCULT BLOOD TEST, p.233) or for evidence of infection (*see* TESTS FOR MICROORGANISMS, pp.234–235).

Samples of body fluids

Secretions and other body fluids obtained to diagnose a wide range of disorders

Some body fluids have a protective role, such as the mucus lining the respiratory tract and the fluid that surrounds the spinal cord. Other body fluids, such as pus from a wound or fluid surrounding a lung, form or increase in volume as a result of disease.

Most body fluids are collected to look for evidence of infection or for cancer. However, certain body fluids may be collected for other purposes. For example, the amniotic fluid that surrounds and protects a fetus in the uterus contains shed fetal skin cells that can be used for genetic tests (*see* ANTENATAL GENETIC TESTS, p.787), and semen can be analysed to assess a man's fertility (*see* SEMEN ANALYSIS, p.777).

HOW ARE SAMPLES OBTAINED?

You can collect some samples yourself, including sputum, saliva, and semen. Your doctor may provide you with a sterile container for the sample. Other fluids, particularly those within body cavities or discharges from a wound, are usually collected by a nurse or doctor.

Fluids or secretions from the skin surface or from mucous membranes, such as those lining the throat or the vagina, are usually collected on sterile cotton swabs (*see* HAVING A THROAT SWAB, below). In order to collect fluids from body cavities or internal organs, the doctor uses a hollow needle and a syringe. In some cases, local anaesthesia is needed for this procedure. Techniques for collecting specific body fluids are covered in the section on your body and disease with the information on the relevant body system. For example, joint aspiration (p.380), in which a small sample of fluid is taken from a swollen joint to determine the cause of swelling, is covered in the section on joint disorders.

Fluid samples are usually sent to a laboratory for analysis. They may be examined for infection (*see* TESTS FOR MICROORGANISMS, pp.234–235), or the cells in the fluid may be separated and examined to detect other abnormalities (*see* CELL TESTS, p.236).

Cell and tissue samples

Individual cells or pieces of tissue obtained for screening or diagnostic tests

Cell and tissue samples are often used to diagnose disorders such as cancer. Collecting cell samples is a safe and usually painless procedure performed by a doctor or nurse. However, taking a tissue sample can sometimes involve a small risk of bleeding or damage to the surrounding organs and is often performed in hospital. Removal of a sample of tissue for examination is known as a biopsy. Tissue samples are usually taken only when other tests have failed to confirm a diagnosis or when a serious disease, such as cancer, is thought to have developed in a particular organ.

HOW ARE SAMPLES OBTAINED?

Samples of cells can sometimes be extracted from urine or other body fluids. For example, a urine sample may be spun at high speed in a machine called a centrifuge to separate the cells present in urine from the liquid. Cells may also be scraped painlessly from the tissue surfaces of a body cavity, such as the mouth or vagina. The cervical smear test (p.749), which screens for early signs of cervical cancer, analyses cells scraped from the surface of the cervix and is the most common procedure using this technique. Cells can also be taken from a solid structure, such as a lump in the breast, with a needle and syringe (*see* ASPIRATION OF A BREAST LUMP, p.756).

In some circumstances, a larger piece of tissue is required. Tissue samples may be taken from almost anywhere in the body, and the procedure used depends on the site. For example, samples of skin tissue are removed using a scalpel (*see* SKIN BIOPSY, p.344), and cores of tissue the size of a match may be removed from internal organs by using a biopsy needle. For example, if the liver disorder cirrhosis (p.647) is suspected, a sample of liver tissue is taken and analysed to confirm the diagnosis and determine the severity of the disease (*see* LIVER BIOPSY, p.647). Tissue samples may also be obtained when tissue is removed for the treatment of a disorder.

Cell and tissue samples are examined under a microscope in a laboratory to look for abnormal cells (*see* CELL AND TISSUE TESTS, pp.236–237).

PROCEDURE HAVING A THROAT SWAB

If you have a sore throat, you may need to have a throat swab taken to see if you have a bacterial infection. The doctor or nurse holds your tongue down with a depressor and uses a plastic stick with a sterile cotton end (swab) to collect a fluid sample from your throat. The swab is then sent to a laboratory. The procedure can be carried out quickly in the doctor's surgery and is not painful. However, you may gag briefly when the swab touches your throat.

Swab

Tongue depressor

Tongue depressor

Back of throat

Palate

Tonsil

Swab

VIEW OF THROAT

During the procedure

The doctor holds your tongue down with a depressor and wipes a swab over your tonsils and the back of your throat.

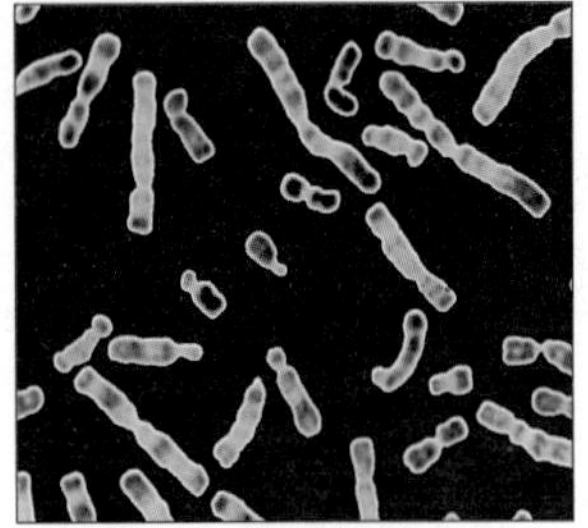

Magnified chromosomes
Chromosomes can be isolated from blood or cell samples to detect genetic disorders.

TESTING SAMPLES

TESTS CAN BE CARRIED OUT on almost any body fluid or tissue. Samples such as blood and urine are easy to obtain and are used for a wide range of tests, including some that you can carry out at home. Other samples, such as tissue, are more difficult to collect and are usually taken only if other tests cannot provide enough information. Test results may be used to confirm a diagnosis, assess the extent of a disorder, screen for disease, or monitor a chronic (long-term) condition or the effects of treatment.

Tests on samples are often the simplest and the quickest way for your doctor to confirm a suspected diagnosis or to assess your health. Having taken your medical history and examined you, your doctor may be left with certain questions. For example, he or she may want to know if particular organs have been affected by an illness.

The sample needed and the types of tests to be carried out depend on the information that is required. Blood and urine tests can check the function of various organs. Tests on faeces may identify disorders of the digestive tract. Sputum or other body fluids, cells, or tissues may be tested to look for various diseases, such as cancer.

Sometimes, several tests are needed. For example, if a kidney or a liver disorder is suspected, a blood test may be arranged. If the result is abnormal and scans or other noninvasive techniques are inconclusive, a tissue sample may be taken. Often, just one type of test is used to monitor a long-term condition, such as diabetes mellitus, or to screen for disease, but it may be repeated at periodic intervals.

COMPARISON DIFFERENT TESTS AND SAMPLES

The test and sample chosen depend on the information that your doctor needs. Some samples, such as blood or urine, can be used for many tests. For example, blood can be tested to assess levels of chemicals, search for infection, and assess numbers and types of blood cells. Other samples, such as tissue, are used for only a few tests, such as to look for cancer.

CHEMICAL TESTS

GENETIC TESTS

FAECES

URINE

BLOOD

BODY FLUIDS

CELLS AND TISSUES

BLOOD STRUCTURE AND FUNCTION TESTS

MICROORGANISM TESTS

CELL AND TISSUE TESTS

How samples are tested
One type of sample is often tested in several different ways. The types of test that may be carried out on samples are shown here.

TYPES OF TEST

Many test results are measurements, such as the amount of a chemical in a sample. These measurements are often produced by automated machines that process precise data rapidly. Such machines usually measure several substances in one sample and often process many samples at once.

Other tests rely on observations made by a technician. These tests may include the identification of abnormal cells or of a microorganism. Such tests require the samples to be carefully prepared before they are interpreted. Mostly, obtaining results takes several days, but it can take up to 6 weeks.

A few tests, such as monitoring blood sugar levels in diabetes mellitus, can be carried out yourself at home.

INTERPRETING RESULTS

When the test results are returned to your doctor, he or she assesses them to see if the tests have answered his or her questions. Occasionally, additional tests on samples may be needed. In other cases, further investigations, such as imaging tests, may be required. However, results of tests on samples often provide enough information to enable your doctor to make a diagnosis, assess the severity of a disorder, or decide on the best form of treatment.

SETTING THE MEDICAL LABORATORY

Laboratories contain a wide range of equipment, but they often specialize in one area of testing. For example, some laboratories contain automated machines that analyse blood and urine. Other laboratories may be used to examine tissue samples or to grow microorganisms from samples and examine them under the microscope. Three different types of laboratory are shown here.

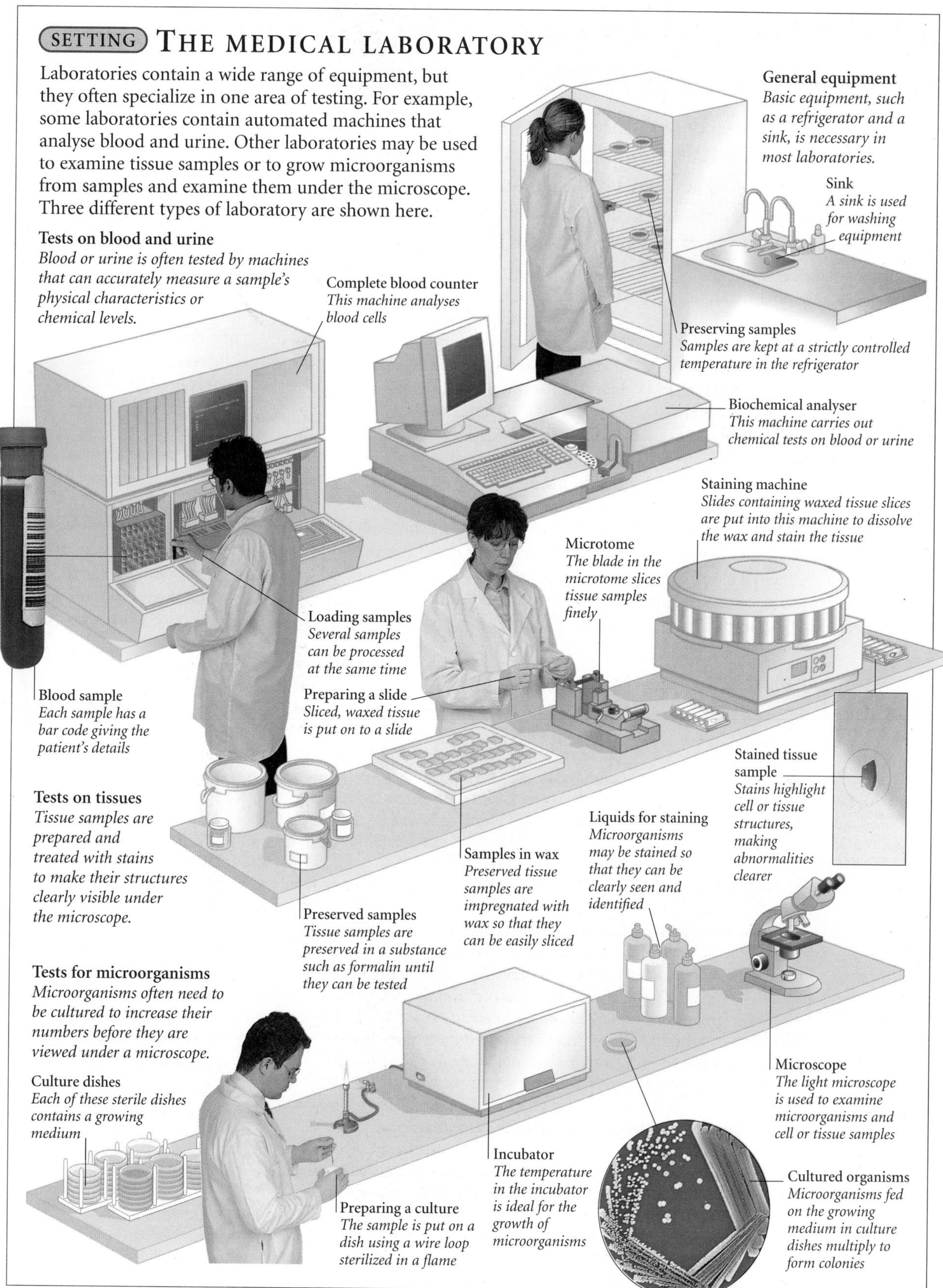

TESTS ON BLOOD STRUCTURE AND FUNCTION

Tests on the composition of blood are some of the most common methods used to look for disease and may also be done routinely to assess general health. They may be carried out on any blood component: red blood cells, white blood cells, tiny cells called platelets, and proteins, all of which are carried in liquid plasma.

This section describes the tests most commonly performed on a blood sample to measure the amounts of the various blood components and investigate their structures. Tests that measure the chemicals carried in the blood are discussed elsewhere (*see* CHEMICAL TESTS, pp.229–233).

The first article discusses tests that measure the number of the different types of cell in the blood and look at their structure to help to diagnose a wide range of diseases and disorders.

Proteins attached to red blood cells determine a person's blood group, and these proteins can be identified by using blood typing tests, which are discussed next. Blood typing is carried out on donated blood and on people before surgical procedures to ensure that if a blood transfusion is needed, blood of the correct group is given.

Blood clotting tests, which are used to diagnose disorders in which blood either does not clot properly or clots too readily, are also covered. These tests assess the time it takes for blood to clot. They also measure the levels of proteins in the blood called clotting factors and levels of platelets, both of which are necessary for blood clotting. Finally, immune function tests, which assess the immune system's strength and identify immune disorders, are discussed. These tests measure blood components that fight infection, such as antibodies and white blood cells.

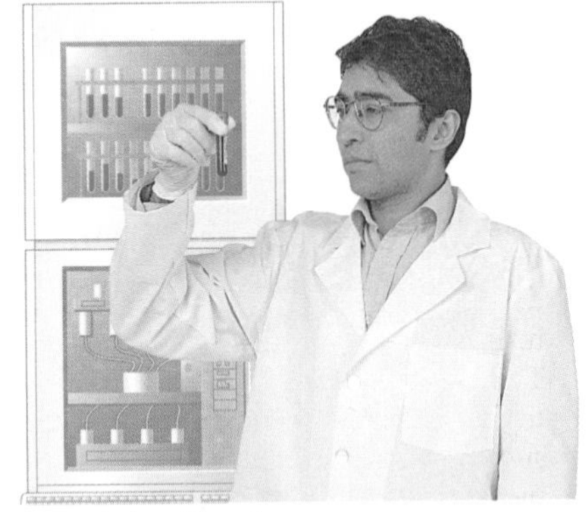

Examining blood
In a laboratory, scientists use automated machines to perform tests on blood to assess health and diagnose disease.

Blood cell tests

Studies to detect abnormalities in the numbers or structure of blood cells

Blood contains three main cell types: red blood cells, which contain haemoglobin (an oxygen-carrying pigment); white blood cells, which help to protect the body against disease; and platelets, tiny cells that play a role in blood clotting. Blood cell tests can help doctors to diagnose diseases of the blood or of the bone marrow (where the blood cells are made). The tests may also be used to look for evidence of infection or inflammation because both involve an immune reaction that increases the number of white blood cells in the circulation.

WHAT MIGHT BE STUDIED?

The different types of cell in a known volume of blood may be counted by an automated machine to give a full blood count. The structure of the blood cells may also be examined by smearing a drop of blood on to a glass slide and looking at it under a microscope.

FULL BLOOD COUNT In this test, a machine counts the numbers of red and white blood cells and platelets in a cubic millilitre of blood. A full blood count also measures the sizes of the cells, the proportion of the blood that is made up of red blood cells (the haematocrit), and the level of haemoglobin in the red blood cells.

If a lower than normal number of red blood cells or a low level of haemoglobin is found, a diagnosis of anaemia (p.446) may be made. The average size of the red blood cells may give a clue to the cause of the anaemia. For example, if the red blood cells are small and pale, there may be a deficiency in iron, which is needed to make haemoglobin. Red blood cells that are larger than normal may indicate that vitamin deficiency is a more likely cause of the anaemia.

A much higher than normal number of white blood cells may be caused by the bone marrow disorder leukaemia (p.453). However, a moderately raised number of white blood cells is usually due to infection or inflammation. There are many different types of white blood cell, and an increase in one type may indicate the cause of the infection or inflammation. For example, an increase in the number of white blood cells known as neutrophils may be a sign of a bacterial infection, and an increase in the number of cells called eosinophils may be a sign of an allergy.

If the total number of white blood cells is lower than normal, the immune system may be weakened. This may be

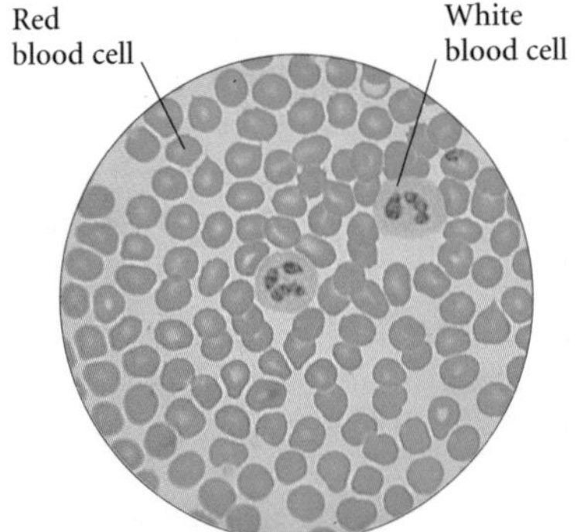

Cells in a blood smear
This highly magnified view of a drop of blood smeared on a slide shows normal red and white blood cells.

the result of malnutrition, HIV infection (*see* HIV INFECTION AND AIDS, p.297), or treatment with anticancer drugs (p.907).

Platelets play an important part in preventing bleeding by helping blood clots to form. A lower than normal number of platelets present in the blood is a condition known as thrombocytopenia (p.453), which can lead to excessive bruising or internal bleeding.

BLOOD SMEAR If information about the structure of blood cells is required, a drop of blood is smeared on to a slide to form a thin film called a blood smear. The blood is stained with special dyes to make the cells more visible, and the slide is examined under a microscope by a trained technician. A blood smear may be used to detect parasites in the blood, such as those that cause malaria (p.305). A blood smear can also identify cells with abnormal shapes that cannot be detected in an automated cell count, such as sickle-shaped red blood cells, which are a characteristic feature of sickle-cell disease (p.448).

WILL I NEED FURTHER TESTS?

If blood cell tests indicate anaemia, you may have chemical tests to measure the levels of vitamins and minerals in your blood that are needed for the production of red blood cells. If there is an abnormal number of white blood cells, your doctor may arrange for immune function tests (p.228) that assess the immune system's strength or tests for microorganisms (pp.234–235) to identify possible infections. You may also have tests that examine the bone marrow to see if blood cell production is impaired (*see* BONE MARROW ASPIRATION AND BIOPSY, p.451).

Blood typing

Identifying proteins on red blood cells to establish a person's blood group

Blood typing is a method of identifying your blood group, which is determined by proteins, called antigens, on the surfaces of the red blood cells (*see* BLOOD GROUPS, p.441). The fluid part of the blood (the plasma) contains antibodies that will react with antigens of a different blood group, causing the red blood cells to stick together. The clumps of red cells are then attacked by the immune system, and this immune response may lead to haemolytic anaemia (p.450) or internal bleeding. Blood typing is therefore essential for safe blood transfusions and is carried out before an operation in case a blood transfusion (p.447) is required during surgery. If you donate blood, your blood group is identified through blood typing so that your blood can be used in someone of the correct blood group. Blood typing may also be used to help to determine paternity.

WHAT MIGHT BE STUDIED?

There are at least 20 ways of classifying blood. The major blood types, which are the ones tested for most often, are ABO and Rh (Rhesus). Testing blood for minor blood types is not normally necessary. However, if you have regular blood transfusions, you may develop antibodies to one of the minor blood group antigens, and your blood may need to be tested for these antigens.

ABO TYPES This blood typing system consists of four blood groups: A, B, AB, and O. Type O is the most common in the UK (found in about 47 per cent of people), followed by type A (42 per cent), type B (8 per cent), and type AB (3 per cent). These proportions vary among different ethnic groups. For example, type B blood group is more common among Asian people.

RH TYPES Blood is classified as either Rh positive or Rh negative, although in reality the system is more complex. About 3 in 20 people in the UK are Rh negative. The Rh system is tested for during pregnancy because, if the mother is Rh negative and the fetus is Rh positive, the mother may produce antibodies against Rh factor in the fetal blood (*see* RHESUS INCOMPATIBILITY, p.795).

HOW IS IT DONE?

There are many different blood typing tests, but they are all based on the reaction between antibodies and antigens. Antibodies against the different blood groups are added to a blood sample. The blood group can be determined by seeing if the cells then form visible clumps or not. For example, if a blood sample forms clumps only when it is mixed with antibodies against type A blood, the blood group is A. If clumps form when the blood sample is mixed with antibodies against both type A and B blood, the blood group is AB.

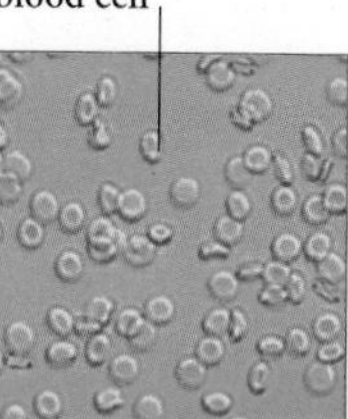

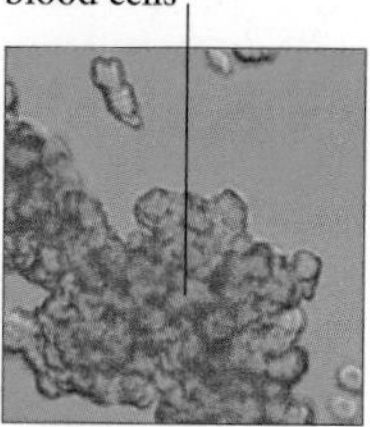

Identifying blood groups
Blood groups are identified by mixing samples of blood with antibodies against known blood groups and watching for a reaction that makes the red blood cells stick together to form a clump.

WILL I NEED FURTHER TESTS?

If a transfusion is needed during an operation, a small amount of the blood that is to be transfused is mixed with a sample of your own blood. This test is called cross-matching and is used to exclude the small possibility that the transfused blood is incompatible with yours because of a reaction between antibodies and antigens of one of the minor blood groups.

Blood clotting tests

Tests that are used to identify and assess abnormalities in the blood clotting process

When blood vessels are damaged, blood clots normally form to stop bleeding. Blood clots start to form when platelets (very small blood cells) clump together and stick to the lining of the damaged blood vessel. These clumped platelets release chemicals that act on dissolved proteins in the blood known as clotting factors. This process leads to the formation of a clot that seals the vessel and prevents further bleeding. Other substances in blood, known as anticlotting factors, prevent the blood from clotting spontaneously in undamaged vessels. Blood clotting tests will be performed if you have symptoms that suggest your blood is clotting either more slowly than is usual (*see* BLEEDING DISORDERS, p.451) or more readily than is usual (*see* HYPERCOAGULABILITY, p.453).

WHY AM I HAVING THE TESTS?

Your doctor may arrange for blood clotting tests if you have had an episode of severe or prolonged bleeding or if you bruise very easily. There are several inherited bleeding disorders that can be diagnosed with blood clotting tests. For example, if your doctor suspects that you have the disorder haemophilia (*see* HAEMOPHILIA AND CHRISTMAS DISEASE, p.452), you will have clotting tests to measure a type of blood clotting factor called factor VIII. In haemophilia, this clotting factor is found in a much lower concentration than is usual.

Blood clotting tests are performed routinely if you have a liver disease, such as acute hepatitis (p.644), because clotting factors are made by the liver. You will also have regular tests if your doctor has prescribed drugs that prevent blood clotting (p.904), such as warfarin. The tests ensure that the drug is working and that the prescribed dose will not cause internal bleeding.

Some disorders, such as deep vein thrombosis (p.437) or stroke (p.532), are due to blood clots forming in uninjured blood vessels. If you have one of these disorders, you may have tests to determine whether your blood is clotting too readily. For example, tests may show the presence of factor V Leiden, which is an abnormal form of clotting factor V that makes clots form easily.

HOW ARE THEY DONE?

Blood clotting tests measure the time it takes for a sample of blood to clot in the laboratory. If the results of these tests are abnormal, a further test may be carried out to measure the blood levels of clotting factors and anticlotting factors in order to see if the cause of the abnormal clotting can be identified.

To measure clotting times, a sample of blood is collected in a bottle containing chemicals that prevent blood from clotting. In the laboratory, substances are added to encourage the blood to clot. The time taken for a clot to form is measured under a range of conditions and compared with the normal time that it takes for blood to clot under the same conditions. The results show if there is a possible bleeding disorder or if the blood clots too easily.

If clotting times are abnormal, an automated machine measures the levels of different clotting factors and anticlotting factors in the blood. There may be an abnormality in just one specific clotting factor, as in haemophilia, or in many factors, as in liver disease.

WILL I NEED FURTHER TESTS?

Since some bleeding disorders are due to low numbers of platelets, you may also have a full blood count (*see* BLOOD CELL TESTS, p.226) to help to confirm the diagnosis. You may also have blood chemistry tests to look for vitamin or mineral deficiencies that could be the cause of a low clotting factor concentration in the blood. The tests may need to be repeated to monitor treatment.

Immune function tests

Measuring numbers of white blood cells, antibodies, and autoantibodies in the blood to identify immune system disorders

The immune system protects the body against infections and cancer. Immune function tests assess the function of the immune system by measuring the levels of its main elements, which are lymphocytes (a type of white blood cell) and antibodies (proteins that are produced by lymphocytes in response to infection). Some drugs or disorders may make the responses of the immune system either weaker than usual or overactive. A weak immune system is less capable of fighting infections. An overactive immune system may produce antibodies against a normally harmless substance, causing an allergy to that substance.

Autoimmune disorders occur when the immune system functions abnormally and makes autoantibodies, which are antibodies against the body's own cells that cause damage to body tissues.

WHY AM I HAVING THE TESTS?

Your doctor may suggest that you have immune function tests if you are particularly susceptible to infections. The tests can show if you have an immune deficiency and, if so, its type and severity. You may also be advised to have the tests if your symptoms suggest that you have an allergy, such as hay fever (*see* ALLERGIC RHINITIS, p.466). In addition, immune function tests may show if you have an autoimmune disorder, such as rheumatoid arthritis (p.377).

WHAT MIGHT BE STUDIED?

Immune function tests involve measuring the blood levels of lymphocytes and antibodies and the numbers of the different types of lymphocyte. The tests can also detect autoantibodies if they are present in blood. The tests may be carried out with an automated machine.

LYMPHOCYTES Tests can measure the total number of lymphocytes as well as the numbers of the different types. An increase in the total number may indicate an immune response to an infection or to an organ transplant. A drop in lymphocytes may be due to treatment with certain drugs, such as immunosuppressant drugs (p.906) or corticosteroids (p.930). Some infections cause lowered numbers of lymphocytes. A decrease in just one type of lymphocyte may indicate the type of infection. For example, HIV infection (*see* HIV INFECTION AND AIDS, p.297) affects lymphocytes called CD4 cells.

ANTIBODIES If immune function tests detect high levels of antibodies, this may indicate infection or an allergy. However, raised antibody levels may also be caused by multiple myeloma (p.456), a cancer of the bone marrow in which white blood cells that produce antibodies multiply uncontrollably. A very low level of one or more antibodies may be a sign of immunodeficiency (*see* ACQUIRED IMMUNODEFICIENCY, p.460).

AUTOANTIBODIES Tests may look for autoantibodies that damage just one organ in the body, such as the thyroid gland (*see* HYPOTHYROIDISM, p.680), or for autoantibodies that attack many organs in the body, as occurs in the autoimmune disorder systemic lupus erythematosus (p.461). If you have one autoimmune disorder, it is possible that you also have another. For example, if autoantibodies to the thyroid gland are found, you may have tests to detect autoantibodies that attack the adrenal glands (*see* ADDISON'S DISEASE, p.686).

WILL I NEED FURTHER TESTS?

Immune function tests may be repeated during the course of certain illnesses, such as HIV infection, to monitor the progress of disease and assess the effectiveness of treatment.

CHEMICAL TESTS

Most healthy tissues contain chemicals that may be released into body fluids, including blood and urine. A disorder can lead to abnormal levels of these chemicals in the blood or urine, which can be detected by chemical tests. These tests help your doctor to make a diagnosis or screen for a disease. In some cases, they may be repeated to monitor the progress of an existing disorder.

This section begins by looking at common analyses that are carried out on blood and urine samples. These routine tests for abnormal levels of chemicals can detect a wide range of disorders, including kidney and liver problems, diabetes mellitus, bone and muscle diseases, and heart attacks.

The next articles discuss specialized tests performed on blood and urine samples. These include tests to screen for high blood cholesterol levels, which identify people at increased risk of heart attacks and stroke, and tests for hormonal disorders, such as thyroid disorders. Other specialized tests include those for inflammation, which are often the first tests to be carried out when a diagnosis is not immediately obvious, and testing for blood in faecal samples, a common screening test for colorectal cancer.

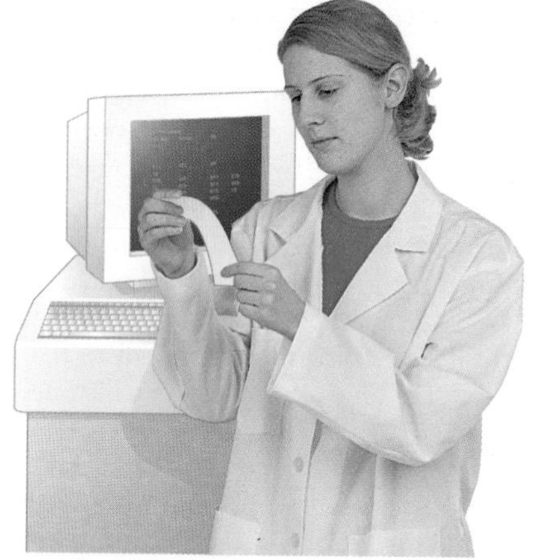

Obtaining results
Chemical tests are often performed by automated machines that can measure many chemicals at the same time. The results are printed out by a computer.

Routine blood chemistry

Measurement of a wide range of chemicals in a blood sample to assess the functioning of certain organs or body systems

Waste products and many other chemicals constantly move between the cells in the body tissues and blood in the circulation. Blood levels of these chemicals may become abnormal when cells and organs are not functioning adequately. Routine blood chemistry tests can detect abnormal levels by analysing the chemicals in a blood sample and are a simple way of finding out which cells and tissues are not functioning normally. The tests are carried out in a laboratory by an automated machine (*see* ANALYSIS OF BLOOD OR URINE, p.230).

WHY AM I HAVING THE TESTS?

Blood chemistry tests are sometimes performed routinely as part of a general health assessment or may be carried out to investigate specific symptoms. These tests can be used to identify disorders that produce abnormal levels of chemicals, and they may be used to confirm a diagnosis or to monitor the levels of particular chemicals in the blood during a course of treatment.

WHAT ARE THE TYPES?

There are many chemicals present in blood, but the ones that are tested for most often are those that change in level as a result of disorders of the kidneys, liver, or muscles. Standard diagnostic procedures include tests to detect proteins, salts, and enzymes. Tests may also be used to identify disorders that affect levels of bone minerals such as calcium.

TESTS FOR KIDNEY DAMAGE The principal function of the kidneys is to filter excess water, salts, and waste products from the blood and excrete them as urine. The kidneys also keep the fluid balance in the body constant by adjusting the quantities of water and salts that are excreted. Blood tests that look for kidney damage measure the levels of certain waste products and dissolved salts in the blood. If the levels of these substances are outside the normal range, a kidney disorder may be indicated.

The waste products urea and creatinine are two of the most frequently measured chemicals. Urea is produced when proteins in the body are broken down and is normally excreted by the kidneys in the urine. High levels of urea in the blood may therefore indicate that the kidneys are not performing their normal function. However, since urea comes mainly from protein in the diet, the level of urea in the blood varies depending on the amount of protein in the diet. The results of a urea test may be misleading in someone who is not eating properly or who is dehydrated.

Creatinine is a waste product that is produced by muscles and excreted in urine by the kidneys. The ability of the kidneys to filter blood efficiently can be assessed by measuring the blood level of creatinine. This may then be compared to the amount of creatinine that is excreted in urine over 24 hours (*see* ROUTINE URINE CHEMISTRY, p.230).

Tests to look for kidney damage also measure the blood levels of dissolved salts, which are known as electrolytes, such as potassium, sodium, bicarbonate, and chloride. The kidneys usually regulate the blood levels of these salts by excreting certain amounts in the urine. Measuring the level of potassium in the blood is especially important because an abnormal level of potassium can lead to irregularities in the heartbeat.

TESTS FOR LIVER DAMAGE High levels of enzymes may appear in the blood if liver cells have been damaged, which can occur as a result of infection with a virus, such as hepatitis A, B, or C, or by excessive alcohol consumption. Tests for enzymes are among the most common measures of liver function. The enzyme gamma glutamyl transferase is often used as a measure of liver damage due to alcohol (*see* ALCOHOL-RELATED LIVER DISEASE, p.646).

Other blood tests to look for liver damage measure the levels of chemicals that are usually excreted by the liver in bile, or proteins produced by the liver. One test measures bilirubin, which is formed when red blood cells break down. A high blood level of bilirubin (*see* JAUNDICE, p.643) may indicate that the liver is not working properly or that there are blockages, such as gallstones (p.651), in the bile ducts. The blood level of albumin, a protein that is made in the liver, is commonly measured as it can fall in a wide range of conditions, including heart failure, kidney disease, and cirrhosis (p.647).

TESTS FOR MUSCLE DAMAGE These tests can detect chemicals that are released when skeletal or heart muscle is damaged. When muscle is damaged, an enzyme called creatine kinase leaks into the blood. Raised blood levels may indicate damage due to many different disorders that affect skeletal muscle, ranging from muscle tears to muscular dystrophy (p.826). The tests are therefore of limited use in making a definite diagnosis. However, a particular type of creatine kinase occurs only in the heart muscle, and measurements can indicate if a heart attack (*see* MYOCARDIAL INFARCTION, p.410) has occurred. Levels of this chemical peak about 24 hours after a heart attack and remain high for about 3 days following the attack.

Another substance that can be measured is troponin, a protein that occurs exclusively in heart muscle and enters the blood only when the heart muscle is damaged. Since troponin is released into the blood within a few hours of a heart attack, its presence often provides the earliest chemical confirmation that a heart attack has occurred. The amount of troponin detected provides a measure of the amount of damage caused to the heart muscle by a heart attack.

TESTS FOR BONE MINERALS Most of the calcium and phosphate in the body is found in the bones, with a tiny amount in the blood. These minerals constantly move between the bones and the blood, and this movement is regulated by parathyroid hormone and vitamin D.

Tests for bone minerals help to diagnose disorders resulting in higher than normal levels of minerals being released from the bones, such as bone tumours and overactivity of the parathyroid gland (*see* HYPERPARATHYROIDISM, p.682). One test measures blood levels of the enzyme alkaline phosphatase because high levels are associated with conditions in which bone is broken down and built up again at an increased rate, such as Paget's disease of the bone (p.370).

WILL I NEED FURTHER TESTS?

If the results of routine blood tests are abnormal, you may need to have further tests before a diagnosis can be made. For example, X-rays (p.244) or ultrasound scanning (p.250) may be carried out to image the organ thought to be affected. A tissue sample may be taken for examination under a microscope. If a heart attack is suspected, you may be given an ECG (p.406), a procedure in which the electrical activity of the heart is recorded. Following a heart attack, blood tests may be repeated at regular intervals to monitor your progress.

TECHNIQUE ANALYSIS OF BLOOD OR URINE

Most chemical tests on blood or urine are carried out by a machine called a biochemical analyser, which can measure a range of substances. Tests on blood are carried out on the liquid part (the plasma) after all the cells have been removed. The sample is mixed with a chemical that changes colour according to how much of a substance is present in the sample. The machine measures the intensity of colour with a light beam.

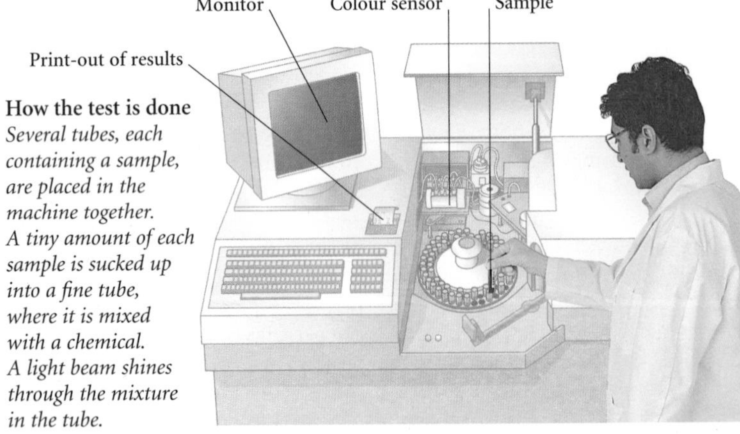

How the test is done
Several tubes, each containing a sample, are placed in the machine together. A tiny amount of each sample is sucked up into a fine tube, where it is mixed with a chemical. A light beam shines through the mixture in the tube.

Routine urine chemistry

Measurement of chemicals in urine that may reflect the health of certain body systems, particularly the urinary tract

Urine consists of waste products that are filtered from the blood by the kidneys in a mixture with water, salts, and other chemicals. Abnormal levels of chemicals or salts in the urine, or the presence of substances not normally found in urine, may indicate a problem with the filtering ability of the kidneys. In addition, certain hormonal disorders alter body chemistry and may affect the composition of the urine. Urine tests can be used to help in making a diagnosis or in monitoring such disorders.

Many urine tests are quick to perform, simply requiring a urine sample and the appropriate dipstick test (*see* DIPSTICK TESTING OF URINE, opposite page). They can be done in the doctor's surgery and are usually the first tests to be performed if a urinary tract disorder is suspected. More detailed urine testing (*see* ANALYSIS OF BLOOD OR URINE, left) may be helpful in the assessment of certain hormonal and kidney disorders. Your doctor may wish to monitor a kidney problem by measuring the amount of a substance, such as protein, excreted in the urine over a period of 24 hours.

TECHNIQUE DIPSTICK TESTING OF URINE

By using a special test dipstick, a sample of urine can quickly be tested in the doctor's surgery for a range of substances, including glucose, blood, enzymes, and protein. Nitrites from bacteria can also be detected. Squares of chemically impregnated paper along a stick change colour when they react with one of the test substances. The intensity of the colour change shows the amount of substance that is present in the urine.

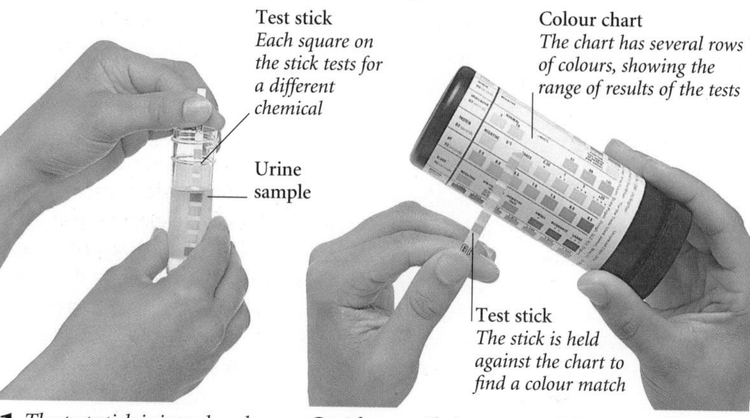

1 *The test stick is introduced into the urine. Chemicals in the squares along the stick react and cause a colour change.*

2 *After specified amounts of time, the colours of the squares on the stick are compared to the chart. The colours on the stick indicate the concentration of different substances in the urine.*

WHAT MIGHT BE STUDIED?

Substances that are commonly measured in urine are glucose, proteins, calcium, and creatinine. In addition to chemical tests, a urine sample may also be examined under the microscope to look for microorganisms (*see* MICROSCOPY FOR INFECTIOUS AGENTS, p.234), blood cells, and other elements that can provide evidence of underlying disease.

GLUCOSE Although glucose is not usually found in urine, some may appear if the glucose level in blood is abnormally high. The presence of glucose in urine may indicate diabetes mellitus (p.687), although the appearance of glucose in urine can be normal during pregnancy.

PROTEINS Healthy people do not usually excrete proteins in urine because they are too large to be filtered from the blood by the kidneys. Proteins may be found in the urine if there is a problem with the filtering units of the kidneys, as in glomerulonephritis (p.699).

CALCIUM To maintain the correct balance of calcium in the body, small amounts are normally excreted in urine. Hormone disorders, such as hyperparathyroidism (p.682), disturb this balance and cause high levels of calcium in the blood, which often result in an increased level of calcium in the urine.

CREATININE Tests for creatinine levels in the urine can show if the kidneys are filtering this waste product out of the blood effectively. If the kidneys are not functioning normally, there will be a low level of creatinine in the urine and a high level in the blood. The creatinine clearance test compares the level of creatinine in a blood sample (*see* ROUTINE BLOOD CHEMISTRY, p.229) with the level in urine collected over 24 hours.

WILL I NEED FURTHER TESTS?

If the results of urine tests are abnormal, other tests, such as blood tests, will probably be needed in order to confirm a diagnosis or to monitor treatment. If protein is detected in the urine, further tests may be needed to determine how much protein is excreted and to diagnose the underlying disorder.

If urine tests suggest a problem with your kidneys, you may need to undergo imaging procedures, such as ultrasound scanning (p.250) or MRI (p.248), to look for kidney abnormalities.

Blood cholesterol tests

Measurement of the levels of cholesterol and other lipids (fatty substances), such as triglycerides, in the blood

Blood cholesterol tests measure levels of the lipids (fatty substances) cholesterol and triglycerides in the blood. Although lipids are necessary for the normal functioning of the body, a high level of these substances in the blood increases the risk that they will form fatty deposits in arteries (*see* ATHEROSCLEROSIS, p.402). These fatty deposits narrow the arteries, restricting blood flow, and may result in coronary artery disease (p.405) and stroke (p.532).

Some medical organizations recommend that everyone over the age of 20 should have a blood cholesterol test at least every 5 years (*see* SCREENING, p.42). Having a cholesterol test is particularly important if you are already at increased risk of heart disease or stroke because you are overweight, smoke, have diabetes mellitus (p.687), or have a family history of heart disease or raised lipid levels (*see* INHERITED HYPERLIPIDAEMIAS, p.692).

WHAT MIGHT BE STUDIED?

Blood cholesterol tests measure the total level of cholesterol, other lipids such as triglycerides, and the amounts of two types of cholesterol in the blood, known as HDL (high-density lipoprotein) and LDL (low-density lipoprotein). HDL seems to have a protective effect against atherosclerosis, but a high blood level of LDL is a risk factor (*see* HYPERCHOLESTEROLAEMIA, p.691).

If your blood cholesterol level is high, the test will be repeated after an overnight fast to make sure that the high cholesterol level was not partly due to a recent meal. If you are found to have an unexpectedly high cholesterol level, your doctor may carry out other blood tests in order to exclude the possibility that an underlying disorder such as diabetes mellitus or hypothyroidism (p.680) is the cause of the condition.

HOW ARE THE RESULTS INTERPRETED?

Your doctor will take into account other risk factors for coronary artery disease that may be present when discussing the results of the cholesterol tests with you.

If your total blood cholesterol is more than 200 mg/dL (5.2 mmol/L), your doctor will probably order further tests to measure the amounts of HDL and LDL cholesterol and triglycerides in the blood. Depending on the results, your doctor may advise you about making changes to your diet or may prescribe lipid-lowering drugs (p.935) or both.

Hormone tests

Measurement of chemicals produced by the endocrine glands

Hormones are a group of chemicals that are mainly secreted by glands of the endocrine system, particularly the pituitary gland, thyroid gland, adrenal glands, ovaries, and testes. Hormone tests measure the levels of these chemicals to determine whether a gland is producing abnormal amounts of hormones. The tests may be performed if you have symptoms, such as tiredness, a change in weight, or menstrual problems, that could be the result of a hormonal disorder. Hormone tests may also be carried out to investigate the cause of infertility, abnormal growth in children, or early or delayed puberty. A common reason for having a hormone test is to confirm a pregnancy.

Most hormone tests are carried out on blood samples. However, in some cases, tests measure the amount of a hormone excreted in the urine over 24 hours or the level of a specific hormone in the urine. The amount of a hormone in a sample is usually measured automatically by a machine in the laboratory (*see* ANALYSIS OF BLOOD OR URINE, p.230). However, pregnancy tests can be done at home using an over-the-counter test kit (*see* HOME PREGNANCY TEST, below).

WHAT ARE THE TYPES?

In some cases, a diagnosis can be made by using a basic test, in which the level of hormones produced by a gland is measured. If basic tests are insufficient to make a diagnosis, you may need hormone stimulation tests, which establish whether a disorder is caused by faulty control of a gland rather than by an abnormality in the gland itself.

BASIC HORMONE TESTS Sometimes, a diagnosis can be made by detecting or measuring the level of one hormone only. For example, the placental hormone human chorionic gonadotropin (HCG) is normally produced only during pregnancy, and its presence is usually regarded as an accurate indication of pregnancy. However, some tests are more complicated because the level of hormones produced by one gland is often controlled by hormones produced by the pituitary gland or hypothalamus in the brain. Tests that measure the level of the controlling hormone may also be necessary. For example, tests for suspected thyroid disorders routinely estimate the level of thyroxine, which is produced by the thyroid gland. In addition, the level of thyroid-stimulating hormone (TSH), the pituitary hormone that stimulates the thyroid gland to produce thyroxine, may be measured. Analysis of TSH levels provides information about the underlying cause of a thyroid hormone imbalance that helps the doctor to choose the most appropriate treatment.

HORMONE STIMULATION TESTS These tests are used to make a diagnosis when it is known that there is a fault in hormone production, but the underlying cause needs to be identified. For example, if low levels of both thyroid hormones and TSH have been found, the pituitary gland may be responsible. To establish whether the fault is with the pituitary gland, you may be given a drug that should stimulate a healthy pituitary gland to produce TSH. If the gland fails to produce TSH in response to the drug, your doctor will know that a pituitary gland disorder is responsible for the hormonal imbalance.

TECHNIQUE HOME PREGNANCY TEST

Pregnancy testing kits are available from pharmacies and allow pregnancy testing to be carried out at home. All of the kits test for the hormone human chorionic gonadotropin (HCG) in a sample of urine. This hormone is normally produced only by a developing placenta, and therefore the tests are extremely accurate, even early in pregnancy. Details for using a test vary with different brands.

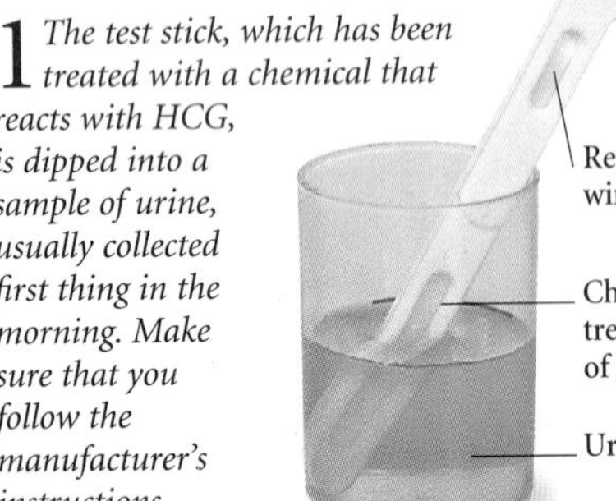

1 The test stick, which has been treated with a chemical that reacts with HCG, is dipped into a sample of urine, usually collected first thing in the morning. Make sure that you follow the manufacturer's instructions.

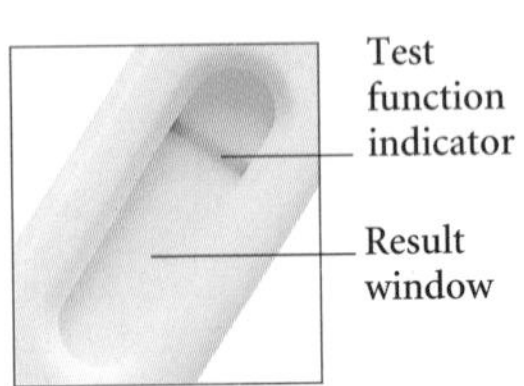

NEGATIVE RESULT

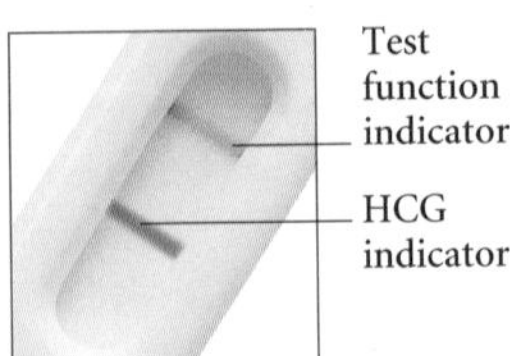

POSITIVE RESULT

2 The result is obtained a few minutes later. In the test shown here, the first line that becomes visible in the result window shows that the test has worked. A second line appears if HCG is present.

Tests for inflammation

Measurement of chemicals in blood that change in response to inflammation

The body responds to inflammation as a result of damage or infection by producing higher than normal amounts of particular proteins, the inflammatory proteins. The common tests for inflammation are based on assessment of the levels of these proteins in the blood.

Tests for inflammation are often the first tests that are carried out when you see your doctor with unexplained symptoms. The tests are used to detect inflammation in the body that would otherwise not be apparent, such as that caused by an infection. The tests may also be used to monitor the progression of certain inflammatory disorders, such as rheumatoid arthritis (p.377), and to assess their response to treatment.

What are the types?

One of the most specific indicators of inflammation is the inflammatory protein C-reactive protein. Measuring the level of this protein in the blood is therefore an important means of finding out whether inflammation is present and of assessing its severity. C-reactive protein levels in a sample of blood may be measured directly by a machine (*see* ANALYSIS OF BLOOD OR URINE, p.230). Alternatively, since inflammatory proteins increase the tendency of the red blood cells (erythrocytes) to clump together, this effect can be observed as an indirect means of measuring levels of these proteins.

C-reactive protein measurements

The level of C-reactive protein in the blood rises and falls rapidly in association with the severity of inflammation. Therefore, testing for C-reactive protein is useful for assessing response to treatment because the levels of the protein may fall following an effective treatment even before any symptoms of inflammation have started to subside.

Erythrocyte sedimentation test

This test measures the rate at which red blood cells settle to the bottom of a sample of blood, leaving the liquid part at the top. If inflammation is present, the red blood cells clump together and settle more rapidly than usual. The speed at which red blood cells settle, called the erythrocyte sedimentation rate (ESR), is related to the severity of inflammation.

Will I need further tests?

Tests for inflammation may indicate the severity of the inflammation, but they do not diagnose the cause or identify the site. If the result of a test for inflammation is positive, a variety of different disorders could be the cause, including infections due to bacteria or viruses, an autoimmune condition, or widespread cancer. Before a diagnosis can be made, you may need to provide a further blood sample or a urine sample to be tested for infection (*see* TESTS FOR MICROORGANISMS, p.234) or an autoimmune disease, such as rheumatoid arthritis (*see* IMMUNE FUNCTION TESTS, p.228). Imaging tests, such as X-rays (p.244), MRI (p.248), or radionuclide scanning (p.251), may also be needed to find a tumour or detect the site of inflammation, such as an abscess.

Tumour marker tests

Measurements of blood proteins that are produced by cells in tumours

A few cancerous tumours produce substances, such as proteins or hormones, that can be detected in blood and, in some cases, in urine. These substances are known as tumour markers. Tumour marker tests are used to detect the levels of these substances in a person with cancer or who is suspected of having cancer because of his or her symptoms or the results of other diagnostic tests.

Tumour marker measurements are usually carried out automatically by a machine in the laboratory (*see* ANALYSIS OF BLOOD OR URINE, p.230).

Why am I having the tests?

Tumour marker tests are usually used to assess the response of a tumour to treatment such as chemotherapy (p.280) or surgery. The level of a marker can indicate whether the tumour has been completely removed or eradicated or if cancer had spread to other areas of the body before treatment. Repeated measurements of marker levels may be used to monitor how well the cancer is responding to treatment. A sudden rise in the marker levels may indicate a recurrence of the tumour.

What might be studied?

Some of the tumour markers most commonly tested for are present in small amounts in healthy people. For example, although prostate cancer (p.726) is often associated with a rise in the blood level of prostate specific antigen (PSA), this protein is found at low levels in the blood of all men. The hormone human chorionic gonadotropin (HCG) is normally produced by the placenta during pregnancy. However, HCG is also associated with cancer of the testis (p.719) and choriocarcinoma (p.748), which is a cancer of the uterus.

Will I need further tests?

In most cases, tumour marker tests are repeated at intervals in order to monitor the effects of treatment. Blood tests and imaging tests, such as MRI (p.248), CT scanning (p.247), or radionuclide scanning (p.251), may be used to detect the spread of the cancer.

Faecal occult blood test

A test on a sample of faeces to detect small amounts of blood that are not visible to the naked eye

A faecal occult blood test detects small amounts of blood invisible to the naked eye that may be contained in a sample of faeces. Nonvisible (occult) blood may be due to a disorder that causes bleeding in the digestive tract, such as polyps in the colon (p.660), gastritis (p.640), or colorectal cancer (p.665).

Why am I having the test?

Testing for faecal occult blood to screen for colorectal cancer in anyone over the age of 50 is becoming standard practice (*see* SCREENING, p.42). The test should be repeated annually. You may also have the test if you have symptoms, such as abdominal pain, or have anaemia (p.446) due to unrecognized blood loss. There are various causes of this kind of anaemia, and a faecal occult blood test can show whether the blood is being lost from your digestive system. However, the test cannot identify which part of the digestive tract is bleeding.

How is it done?

The test is performed by smearing a sample of faeces on to a piece of paper or stool card and adding a chemical to the sample. If a colour change occurs, occult blood is present. The doctor may carry out the test in his or her surgery or send the sample to be tested in a laboratory, or you may be asked to apply stool samples to indicator cards yourself and then bring them to the doctor. Over-the-counter tests that work in a similar way to laboratory tests are available from pharmacies for home use.

Will I need further tests?

The test is usually repeated three times over several days because blood may not be present in every sample. If blood is detected, further tests will be carried out to look for the cause. An endoscope (viewing tube) may be used to examine the digestive tract and identify the cause of the bleeding (*see* ENDOSCOPY, p.255). Alternatively, contrast X-rays (p.245) are sometimes used to look for disorders of the digestive tract, such as tumours or ulcers, that may cause bleeding.

TESTS FOR MICROORGANISMS

Although many diseases due to microorganisms can be prevented by immunization or effectively treated by drugs, infectious diseases are still a major cause of illness and death worldwide. Identifying microorganisms responsible for disease is an essential step in the diagnosis and treatment of infectious illnesses.

Tests to identify microorganisms that cause infections play an increasingly important role in medicine today. Tests for bacteria may also play a part in diagnosing noninfectious diseases. For example, one specific species of bacterium, *Helicobacter pylori*, is a key cause of peptic ulcers.

This section begins by discussing traditional tests to identify organisms, such as cultures and microscopy. Some organisms are becoming resistant to the drugs used to treat them, especially antibiotics, and tests to detect drug sensitivity are also covered.

More modern techniques identify microorganisms by using proteins on the surface of the organism, known as antigens, or specific antibodies made by the body in response to infection. Other tests use the organism's genetic material. These tests are covered last and can identify an infectious organism within hours or even minutes.

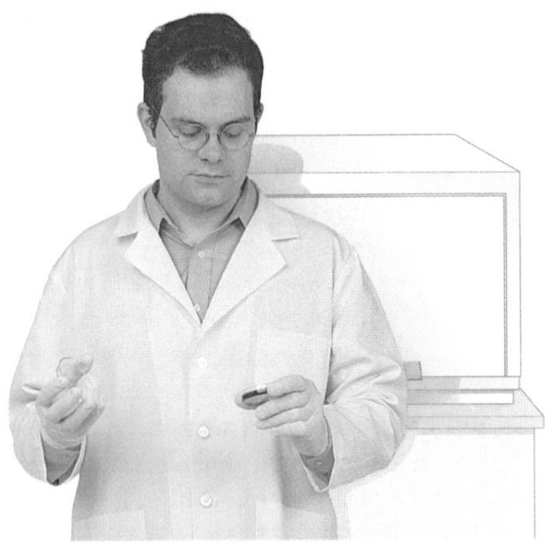

Examining a culture
Laboratories use special culture plates containing nutrients to grow large numbers of organisms from a sample. The organisms can then be identified.

Microscopy for infectious agents

Microscopic examination to detect or identify harmful microorganisms

Individual microorganisms, such as viruses, bacteria, and fungi, are too small to see without using a microscope. In microscopy, highly magnified images of microorganisms are produced so that they can be seen and identified. Microscopy can be performed on any type of sample from the body, such as blood, urine, or other body fluids.

Sometimes, a test sample is examined immediately in the doctor's surgery or in a laboratory. For example, a sample of urine may be examined under a microscope to identify bacteria. However, a sample often contains so few organisms that they cannot be detected easily. In these cases, the microorganisms may be grown (cultured) to increase their numbers before microscopy or other tests are performed (*see* CULTURE AND TESTS FOR DRUG SENSITIVITY, right).

HOW IS IT DONE?

Different microscopes are used to identify different organisms. Bacteria are usually identified with a light microscope. Viruses, which are much smaller than bacteria, are examined with a more powerful electron microscope.

Most samples are treated with stains before viewing to aid the detection and identification of any microorganisms they contain. The Gram stain is one of the most commonly used stains for differentiating between the different types of bacterium. Samples to be examined using an electron microscope have to be set in wax, thinly sliced, and coated with metals beforehand.

When the samples have been prepared, any microorganisms present are studied under a microscope. Different types of microorganism can be recognized by their size, their shape, and how they react with the stains.

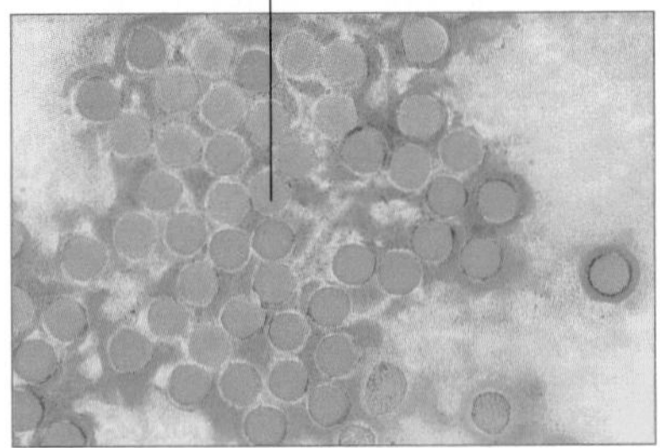

Highly magnified viruses
Tiny organisms, such as viruses, can be seen only with an electron microscope. This image shows a highly magnified cluster of hepatitis A viruses.

Culture and tests for drug sensitivity

Methods of increasing the numbers of microorganisms to aid their identification and test for sensitivity to antibiotics

Many tests require large numbers of microorganisms and, to obtain these, the organisms are cultured. Culturing encourages the organisms to reproduce. Most double in number every 20–30 minutes. The organisms generally form clusters, known as colonies. Although it usually takes up to 18 hours to obtain a result, some organisms, such as the bacterium that causes tuberculosis, may take up to 6 weeks to grow sufficient numbers to be easily identified. After they have been cultured, bacteria may be tested to determine which antibiotics are most effective against them.

HOW ARE THEY DONE?

Viruses and some other organisms can be grown only in cultures of living cells, but most microorganisms are grown in a sterile plastic dish containing a nutrient gel on which they feed. The sample to be cultured is spread on to the gel. If a particular organism is thought to be present, the culture is set up specifically to encourage that microorganism while

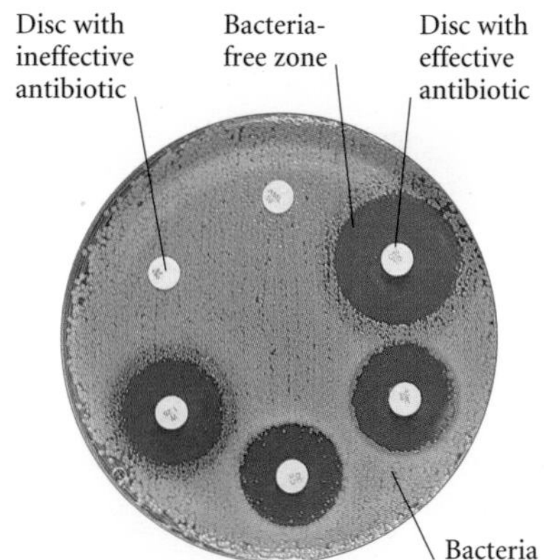

Antibiotic sensitivity test
Paper discs containing different antibiotics have been placed on this culture dish to see which drug can halt bacterial growth.

suppressing others. The culture dish is kept at a suitable temperature until colonies of microorganisms have grown, and it is then examined. Some microorganisms have specific features that may identify them. For example, the bacterium *Staphylococcus aureus* forms small, golden yellow colonies when cultured.

After culturing, a small portion of the colony may be carefully removed from the dish, stained, and examined under a microscope to identify the organisms present. Other chemical tests may be performed to help in identification.

When bacteria have been identified, drug sensitivity tests may be performed. Paper discs containing different types and amounts of antibiotics are added to the bacterial culture. After 24 hours, the culture is examined to see which antibiotics have been the most effective in destroying the bacteria.

Tests for antigens and antibodies

Tests on samples of body fluids to detect antigens and antibodies in the body

Every microorganism that enters the body has proteins on its surface, called antigens, that the immune system recognizes as foreign. When white blood cells of the immune system detect a foreign antigen, they produce antibodies that exactly fit on to that antigen and help to destroy the organism. Since every microorganism has unique antigens, and one antibody will lock on to only one particular antigen, tests for antigens and antibodies can identify microorganisms quickly and accurately.

Antibody tests are usually performed on samples of blood because antibodies are made by white blood cells. Antigen tests may be performed on any type of body fluid, such as urine or saliva.

Why are they done?

Antigen tests are useful when a rapid diagnosis is needed or when there are not enough microorganisms in a sample to be visible under a microscope. For example, finding the antigen of the bacterium that causes bacterial meningitis (p.527) in a sample of the fluid that surrounds the brain can provide a diagnosis in minutes.

Testing for antibodies is useful for diagnosing a persistent infection, such as HIV infection (*see* HIV INFECTION AND AIDS, p.297), or for confirming your immunity from a previous infection, such as rubella (p.294). Antibody tests are not useful for diagnosing recent infections because the immune system takes about 10 days to make an antibody against a new microorganism.

How are they done?

Antigens and antibodies cannot be seen separately, but when they join together they form a large clump that can be seen by the naked eye. In antigen tests, small beads or red blood cells may be coated with an antibody that reacts with the antigens on one particular microorganism. The sample that is to be tested is then added to the antibody-coated beads. If the suspected organism is present in the sample, its antigens will become attached to the antibody beads and make them clump together.

In antibody tests, antigens from a known microorganism may be coated on to small beads. A sample of body fluid is then added to the beads. If the immune system has produced antibodies against the organism, the antibodies will attach to the antigen beads, producing visible clumping.

Although the clumps of antigen and antibody may be seen without a microscope, the test can be made more sensitive by attaching a fluorescent or radioactive marker to either the antigens or the antibodies before they are added to the test sample.

Gene tests for microorganisms

Identifying infectious microorganisms by using their genetic material

Gene tests are relatively new techniques for identifying microorganisms. These tests can be carried out on samples of body fluid, such as blood or urine, and give a diagnosis within a few hours.

Gene tests can give a positive diagnosis even when there are few organisms in a sample. This allows a diagnosis to be made very early in the course of a disease, which is important in people who cannot fight infections because their immune system is damaged, such as people with HIV infection (*see* HIV INFECTION AND AIDS, p.297).

How are they done?

Microorganisms can be identified using gene probes or genetic fingerprinting. The basis of these tests is that each microorganism has a different sequence of chemicals in its genetic material, which can be DNA (deoxyribonucleic acid) or, rarely, RNA (ribonucleic acid).

A gene probe is a strand of DNA with a sequence of chemicals that will join to the DNA of just one type of microorganism. The test sample is treated to extract a small amount of DNA or RNA from the microorganisms. The probe is added to this genetic material and will join to it only if it is an exact match. The probe is radioactively labelled so that it can be detected after joining to the DNA. This test shows if a suspected organism is present in the sample.

In genetic fingerprinting, DNA from the microorganisms in the sample is cut into different-sized pieces by enzymes. DNA from a known organism is treated in the same way. The two sets of DNA are placed in a gel through which an electric current is passed. The current causes the cut pieces of DNA to separate into patterns. If the patterns match, the two organisms are the same.

Although gene tests can be performed with a small number of organisms, the amount of DNA can be increased using a process called polymerase chain reaction. This process takes about 5 hours and makes millions of copies of the microorganism's DNA or RNA.

CELL AND TISSUE TESTS

Microscopic studies of individual cells (cytology) or of a larger sample of tissue containing a variety of different cells (histology) are among the most important and definitive tests carried out. Other tests, such as blood tests or imaging tests, may suggest an abnormality, but in many cases the diagnosis is determined definitively by direct examination of the cells or tissues involved.

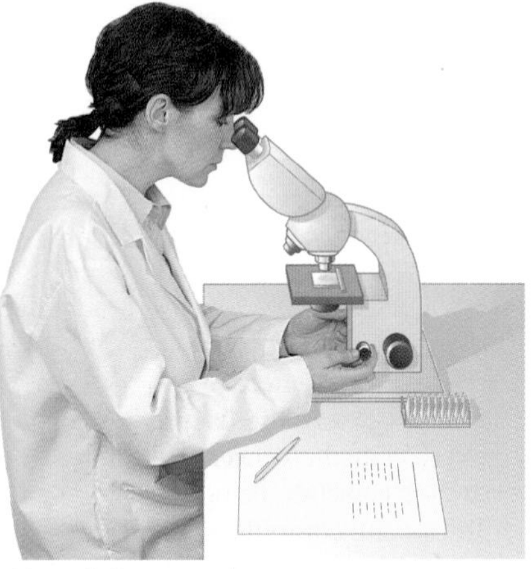

Examining samples
Highly trained technicians and doctors can obtain detailed information about the structure of cells or tissues by using powerful microscopes in the laboratory.

Each type of tissue in the body is made up of different cells, all of which have characteristic differences that enable them to be identified when they are examined under a microscope. Many disorders, such as cancer, can cause individual cells to look abnormal. In other diseases, the tissues may contain cells that would not normally be there. For example, infected or damaged tissues may contain inflammatory cells that are not normally present.

In this section, tests on cells are discussed first. These tests are often used at an earlier stage than other tests because they are easy to perform and the samples can be collected easily.

Some cell tests, such as the cervical smear test (p.749), are used for routine screening to detect precancerous cells or cancer cells at an early stage. If such cells are found, treatment can be given early, when it is most effective.

The second article covers tissue tests. Tissue tests are not carried out as often as cell tests because the samples are not as easy to obtain and require more preparation before being examined. However, a tissue test may provide more information than a cell test alone, because a tissue sample can show the proportion of abnormal cells within the tissue and therefore the extent of the disease.

Other cell tests are covered elsewhere. These include tests on blood structure and function (pp.226–228) and tests for genetic diseases (*see* GENETIC TESTS, pp.238–241).

Cell tests

Examination of cells under a microscope to detect abnormal changes

The study of cells under a microscope is known as cytology. Samples of cells can be examined to detect abnormalities in the appearance of individual cells or to detect cells that are not normally present in healthy tissue.

WHY AM I HAVING THE TESTS?

Cell tests are commonly used to screen for cancer. Such tests detect precancerous or cancerous cells before symptoms develop and are therefore used to detect certain cancers at an early stage. For example, cells taken during a cervical smear test (p.749) are examined under the microscope to look for abnormal cells in the cervix (*see* CANCER OF THE CERVIX, p.750). If abnormal cells are found, treatment can be started early, when it is most likely to be successful.

Your doctor may also arrange for you to have a cell test if symptoms develop that could be caused by cancer. For example, a small sample of cells may be taken from a swelling in your breast (*see* ASPIRATION OF A BREAST LUMP, p.756). These cells will then be analysed in a laboratory to determine whether or not the breast lump is cancerous.

HOW ARE THEY DONE?

Samples of cells may be obtained by scraping cells off tissue surfaces such as the lining of the cervix or by washing them off surfaces such as the lining of the lungs (*see* BRONCHOSCOPY, p.504). Individual cells can also be taken from solid tissue using a needle and syringe. In other cases, samples of cells may be obtained from certain body fluids, such as urine or sputum.

Individual cells taken from the surface of a tissue or obtained from solid tissue are usually transferred to a glass slide immediately. However, cells contained in a fluid sample, such as urine, need to be separated from the fluid. By spinning the fluid sample at high speed in a special machine called a centrifuge, the cells in the sample are pushed to the bottom of the liquid, which can then be drained off. The separated cells are then placed on a glass slide.

Before being examined, the cells are treated with preservative. They are then stained with a dye to make them easier to see. The cells are viewed under a high-powered light microscope.

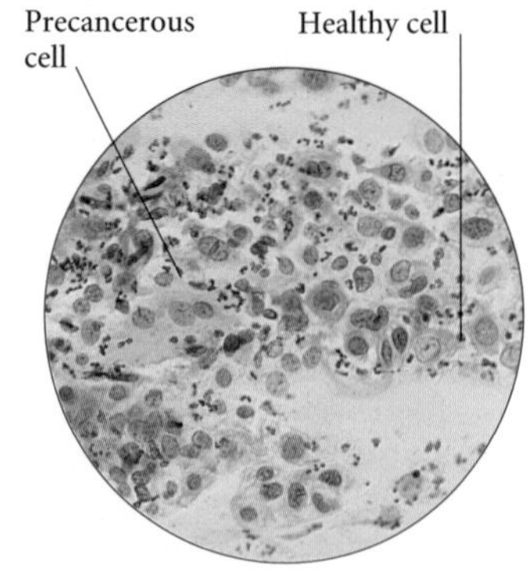

Cells from a cervical smear test
In this view through a microscope, both normal and abnormal (precancerous) cells that have been taken from the surface of the cervix are clearly visible.

How are the results interpreted?

The cells are studied by a cytologist, a technician or doctor trained to analyse cell structures, who looks for abnormal changes suggesting cancer. He or she may also look for other signs of disease, such as inflammatory cells.

If abnormal cells are found in a sample, the cytologist assesses the extent to which they differ from healthy cells to determine whether they are cancerous or likely to become cancerous. Training and experience are needed to make an accurate diagnosis and to predict the likelihood that the cancer will spread. Research is currently being carried out on the use of computers to perform preliminary surveys on the cells before the cytologist makes a detailed analysis.

Will I need further tests?

Cell tests cannot show the proportion of abnormal cells in a tissue or how widely the affected cells are distributed. Therefore, if abnormal cells are found, you may need a tissue test (below) to determine the extent of the disease.

Tissue tests

Examination of tissue samples under a microscope to diagnose or assess the severity of a condition

Some disorders disrupt the proportion of different types of cells within an organ or cause the individual cells to look abnormal. These changes can be detected by tissue tests, in which small samples of tissue are examined under a microscope. Such tests may enable doctors to make a diagnosis or to assess the severity of a disorder.

Why am I having the tests?

Your doctor may arrange for a tissue test if other tests have not established a diagnosis. Tissue tests are often used to distinguish between certain disorders that have similar symptoms, such as the inflammatory bowel conditions ulcerative colitis (p.659) and Crohn's disease (p.658). Tests on a small sample of the inflamed colon may be able to distinguish between the two conditions.

In addition to confirming a diagnosis, tissue tests may also be used to look for a cause. For example, a tissue test on a sample of liver tissue may confirm a diagnosis of cirrhosis (p.647), in which fibrous tissue develops, and suggest a cause from the distribution of the cells.

A tissue test may also be performed to determine the extent of a disease once a diagnosis has been made. For example, if you have had an area of skin removed to treat a cancerous tumour, a tissue test may show whether the edges of the removed skin are free of abnormal cells, indicating that the entire tumour has been removed, or if cancerous cells have reached the edges of the removed tissue, suggesting that the tumour has spread beyond the margins of the sample.

Finally, tissue tests may help your doctor to decide on the most appropriate treatment. For example, if a tissue test shows that cancer has spread from the original site of the tumour, more extensive treatment may be needed.

How are they done?

Samples of tissue are often obtained by a biopsy. During this procedure, a small piece of tissue is removed specifically to make a diagnosis. In other cases, a tissue sample may have been removed as part of the treatment for a particular disorder. For example, a section of the colon may be removed during treatment for colorectal cancer (p.665).

The tissue sample is immersed in a preservative substance such as formalin. The sample is then thinly sliced and stained to highlight the different structures in the tissue. Preparation of the tissue may take several days.

Tissue samples are usually examined under a light microscope, but certain changes may be seen only using a more powerful electron microscope. For example, a sample of kidney tissue taken from a person with nephrotic syndrome (p.700) may appear normal when viewed under a light microscope, but an electron microscope may reveal abnormalities.

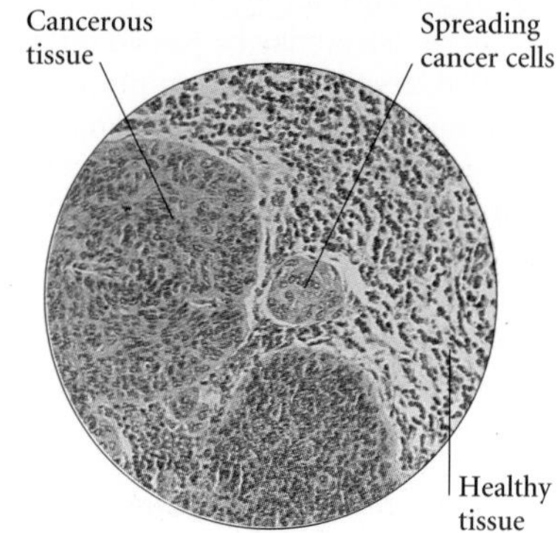

Tissue sample from the cervix
Cancerous cells can be seen spreading into healthy tissue in this highly magnified view of a tissue sample taken from the cervix.

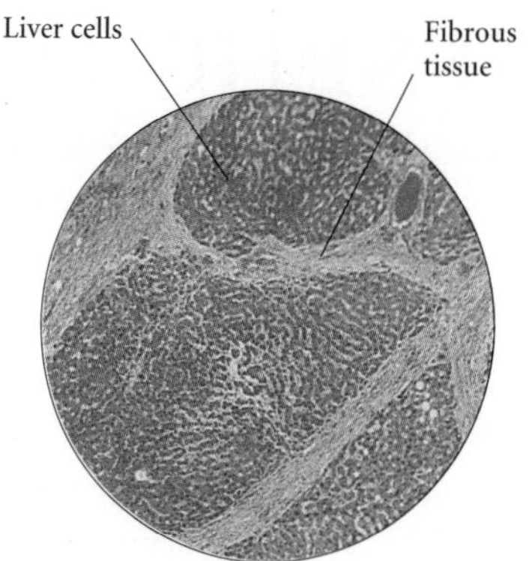

Liver tissue sample
This highly magnified view of a tissue sample from the liver shows excess fibrous tissue compressing the liver cells. This condition is known as cirrhosis.

How are the results interpreted?

A pathologist, a doctor who is specially trained to analyse tissue samples, usually examines several slides prepared from a single biopsy sample or from different areas of a surgically removed piece of tissue. He or she looks for the presence of abnormal cells or an abnormal balance of cells. The extent to which the tissue is different from healthy tissue indicates the severity of the disease. The slides are usually retained in case they need to be reviewed later.

Will I need further tests?

Tissue tests provide a definitive diagnosis for many conditions in which tissue is damaged. However, further tests may be necessary to determine whether other areas of the body are affected. For example, if tissue tests have confirmed that a growth in your intestine is cancerous, you may have CT scanning (p.247) or MRI (p.248) of your liver to look for evidence that the cancer has spread from the intestine to the liver.

Occasionally, you may need to have repeated tissue tests to monitor disease progression or response to treatment. For example, repeated tissue samples may be taken from an organ transplant to detect early signs of rejection.

GENETIC TESTS

Although genetic tests are less frequently performed than other types of test, the results may have profound effects on your life. Knowledge of your genetic make-up gives you the information you need to make decisions about your lifestyle. If you know that you carry a faulty gene that could be passed on, you may want to take this into consideration before starting a family.

Genes are sets of instructions in chemical form that control the way cells in the body function. They are located in the nucleus of body cells in structures called chromosomes (*see* GENES AND INHERITANCE, pp.264–269). Occasionally, genes or chromosomes are faulty, resulting in a disorder or increased susceptibility to a disorder. With the development of more sophisticated tests, an increasingly wide range of genetic abnormalities can now be identified.

Tests for genetic abnormalities may look directly for faulty chromosomes or genes or for the chemical effects that these produce within body cells. This section starts by describing tests that look for abnormalities in chromosome number or structure and tests to detect abnormal genes. Tests designed to look at the effects that certain abnormal chromosomes and genes have on body chemistry are then discussed.

You may be offered genetic tests if you develop symptoms of a genetic disorder, members of your family have a genetic disorder (*see* YOUR FAMILY MEDICAL HISTORY, p.24), or you are at increased risk of a particular disorder.

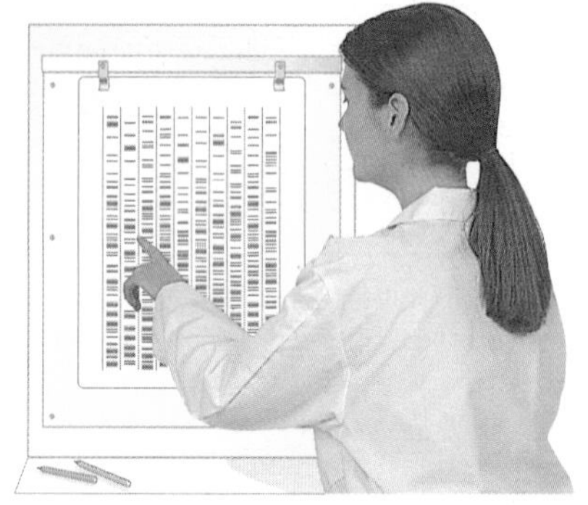

Looking for abnormal genes
Scientists now use techniques that enable small amounts of genetic material to be replicated and studied to look for abnormal genes.

Tests may be carried out antenatally if there is a higher than average risk of a disorder such as Down's syndrome. You should discuss the results with a professional counsellor (*see* GENETIC COUNSELLING, p.272).

Tests for chromosomal abnormalities

Studies of chromosomes to detect abnormalities in number or structure

Chromosomes are thread-like structures found within the nucleus of cells in the body that carry genetic information. Abnormalities can occur in the number of chromosomes or in the structure of individual chromosomes, resulting in a variety of disorders.

Normally, the cells of the body contain 22 pairs of chromosomes called autosomes and two sex chromosomes, which determine whether a person is male or female. This complete set of chromosomes in the body cells is known as a karyotype. In chromosome tests, the karyotype is analysed to determine whether abnormalities are present. Differences in the number of chromosomes are the most common types of chromosomal abnormality. Less commonly, part of a chromosome may be in the wrong place or may be missing.

Chromosomal abnormalities are usually due to a fault in the way that the chromosomes are divided during the formation of egg and sperm cells, but occasionally abnormalities arise during the early stages of cell division following the fertilization of an egg cell (*see* CHROMOSOME DISORDERS, p.270).

In many cases, chromosomal abnormalities result in miscarriage (p.791). If a fetus survives, there may be multiple physical abnormalities or generalized learning disabilities (p.854). Some alterations in the structure of a chromosome may not cause any obvious abnormalities in an affected individual, but the structural defect may be passed on in a way that results in symptoms in the next generation. However, abnormalities in chromosome number are not likely to recur in the same family.

WHY ARE THEY DONE?

Chromosome tests or karyotype analysis may be done to determine whether a condition could be caused by a chromosomal abnormality. For example, tests may be performed on a baby who has been born with abnormal physical characteristics that suggest a chromosome disorder, such as those seen in some cases of Turner's syndrome (p.823). Slow development or learning difficulties in a child may also lead the doctor to recommend these tests.

Chromosome tests may be performed during pregnancy. For example, they are usually offered to pregnant women identified by ultrasound scanning (*see* ULTRASOUND SCANNING IN PREGNANCY, p.793) and blood tests as being at increased risk of having a baby affected by Down's syndrome (p.821). Tests may

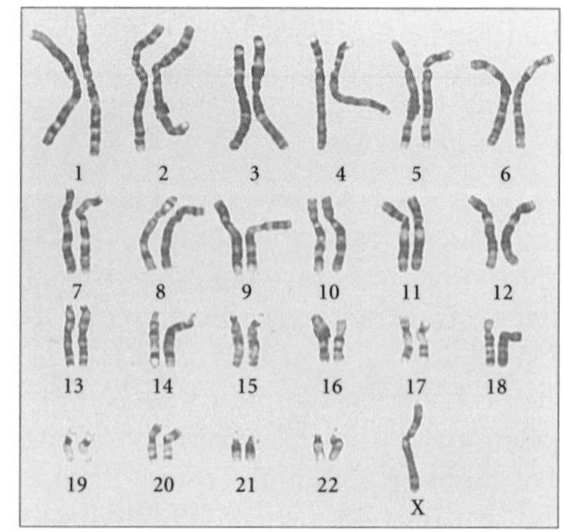

Karyotype
This set of chromosomes (karyotype) from a female with Turner's syndrome shows only one X chromosome rather than the two that are normal for a female.

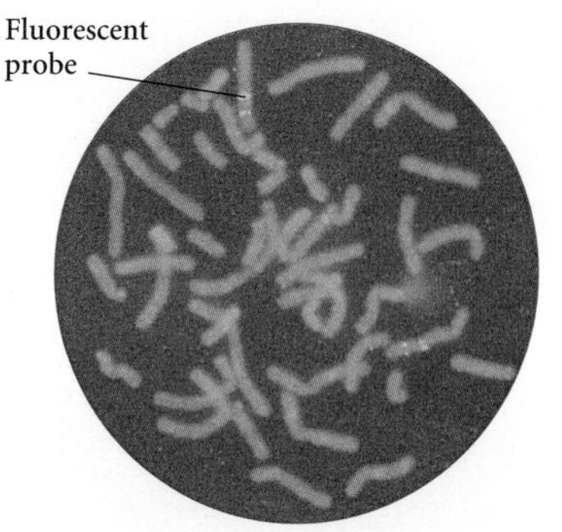

Fluorescently labelled chromosomes
Fluorescent probes may be used to detect chromosomal abnormalities. This normal result shows a fluorescent spot on each of the matching chromosomes of a pair.

also be carried out if routine ultrasound scanning during the pregnancy has suggested that a fetus has a physical defect that could be the result of a chromosomal abnormality. Karyotype analysis may also be carried out on the parents of a child with a chromosomal abnormality to predict the chance that any subsequent children they have will also be affected by the disorder.

HOW ARE THEY DONE?

Karyotype analysis on a fetus uses fetal skin cells taken from the fluid that surrounds the fetus in the uterus or fetal cells taken from the placenta (*see* ANTENATAL GENETIC TESTS, p.787). For adults and children, the test is commonly performed on white blood cells taken from a routine blood sample.

To examine chromosomes, the cells are placed in a nutrient liquid, where they start to divide. When the chromosomes can be seen easily, the cells are treated with a chemical to stop them dividing. The chromosomes can then be examined in several ways.

In one technique, the chromosomes are stained so that they can be identified under the microscope. All of the chromosomes from a cell are identified to find out whether there are any extra or missing chromosomes or if part of a chromosome is missing or misplaced. The complete set of the cell's chromosomes, which is known as the karyotype, can then be photographed in order to form a permanent record.

Another technique enables chromosomal abnormalities to be detected by using fluorescent probes that attach themselves to specific areas of chromosomes. This test enables scientists to see entire chromosomes or to label abnormalities that are too small to be seen by using other techniques.

HOW ARE THE RESULTS INTERPRETED?

If a fetus or a child is found to have a chromosomal abnormality, the results of the tests may help doctors to predict how severe a disability will be and the course that the disorder may take. If a fetus has a chromosomal abnormality that could cause considerable disability, parents may wish to discuss with their doctor whether or not to continue with the pregnancy. Parents may also wish to have genetic counselling (p.272) to discuss the chance of the disorder being passed on to any future children.

Tests for abnormal genes

Tests used to find abnormal genes known to cause a disease or to increase a person's susceptibility to a disease

Within every cell are many thousands of genes that control the cell's structure and functions. If a gene is abnormal, the structure of the cell or the way that it carries out its chemical processes may be altered. The result may be a genetic disorder or increased susceptibility to a disorder. Tests can identify abnormal genes that are known to cause disorders or that are associated with a greater than average susceptibility to a disorder.

Genes are located on 23 pairs of structures called chromosomes that are found in the nucleus of a cell. Each gene consists of a length of DNA (deoxyribonucleic acid) made up of chemicals called nucleotide bases linked together in a specific sequence. Abnormal changes to the sequence of DNA within a gene can occur, and these are known as mutations. Most mutations consist of a missing segment of DNA or a change in the sequence of the nucleotide bases (*see* GENES AND INHERITANCE, pp.264–269).

For certain genetic conditions, such as cystic fibrosis (p.824) and the blood disorder sickle-cell disease (p.448), the normal DNA sequence and the way in which the abnormal genes are inherited are known (*see* GENE DISORDERS, p.271). For many other genetic disorders, the precise gene abnormality is not known, but the position of the relevant gene on a chromosome has been established. This information can be used to help to predict a person's chance of inheriting the genetic disorder.

WHY ARE THEY DONE?

Tests for mutated genes may be performed to confirm a suspected diagnosis of a genetic disorder. Tests may also be offered to the relatives of a person with a disorder, who may want to find out if they have the abnormal gene and are at risk of passing it on to their children. Many genetic disorders occur only if both parents are carriers of an abnormal gene. Carriers do not have symptoms of the disorder themselves. However, if two carriers have children, some of their children may be expected to inherit an abnormal gene from each parent and develop the disorder. In these circumstances, genetic tests may be performed on couples before they have children or on the fetus in early pregnancy.

HOW ARE THEY DONE?

Genetic tests for an adult or a child are usually carried out on white blood cells that are taken from a blood sample or on cells collected by scraping the inside of the cheek. Tests on a fetus either use fetal cells from the placenta or fetal skin cells taken from the amniotic fluid that surrounds the fetus in the uterus (*see* ANTENATAL GENETIC TESTS, p.787).

A cell sample usually contains only a small amount of DNA. A technique called PCR (polymerase chain reaction) can provide enough DNA for a test by making millions of copies of the DNA in a sample. If the precise chemical sequence of a gene has been established, direct identification of mutations may be possible but, for other genetic disorders, an indirect method of testing for the mutated gene may be needed.

DIRECT TESTS These tests are used to look for an abnormal gene when the nucleotide sequence of the normal gene is known. In one technique, the DNA in the sample is cut into fragments, and the fragments are separated according to their size. Abnormal genes produce differently sized fragments from those

PROCEDURE LOOKING FOR ABNORMAL GENES

Genes control every cell in the body, and a defect in the structure of a gene can cause disease. Tests look for abnormalities in the sequence of chemicals called nucleotide bases, which make up the genes in DNA. There are many different methods for detecting abnormal genes. The order of nucleotide bases in the gene can be determined directly by sequencing the DNA. Some tests use a reaction in which the section of DNA containing the normal or abnormal gene is copied many times (amplified). Other tests (as shown below) detect a difference in how the abnormal and normal genes are cut by chemicals. The DNA fragment containing the gene can be visualized using a radioactive probe.

1 Cells are taken from a sample of blood or scraped from the lining of the mouth. For antenatal tests, cells come from the placenta or from the fluid surrounding the fetus.

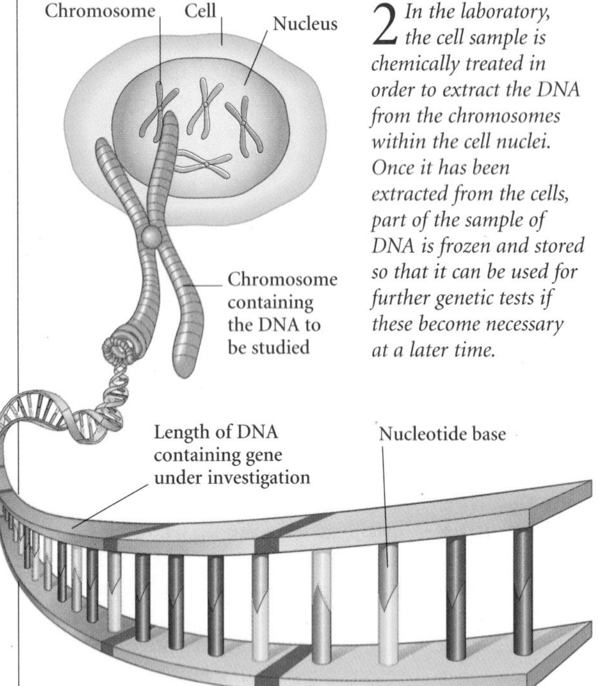

2 In the laboratory, the cell sample is chemically treated in order to extract the DNA from the chromosomes within the cell nuclei. Once it has been extracted from the cells, part of the sample of DNA is frozen and stored so that it can be used for further genetic tests if these become necessary at a later time.

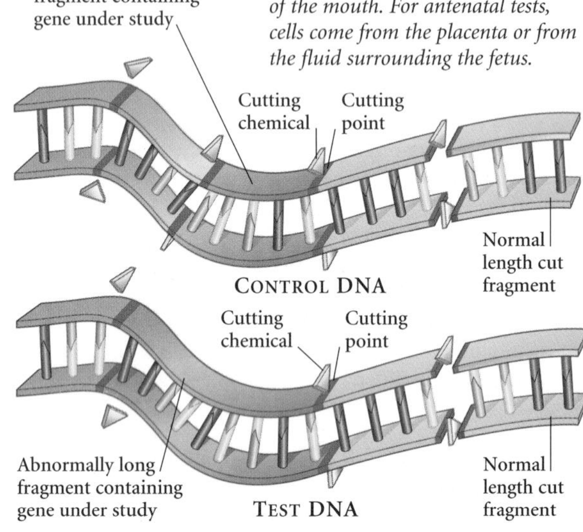

3 A chemical that cuts the DNA at specific places is added to the sample and also to a control (normal) sample. If the nucleotide sequence of the DNA in a gene is abnormal, it will be cut in different places from that of the control DNA, creating abnormally long or short fragments of DNA.

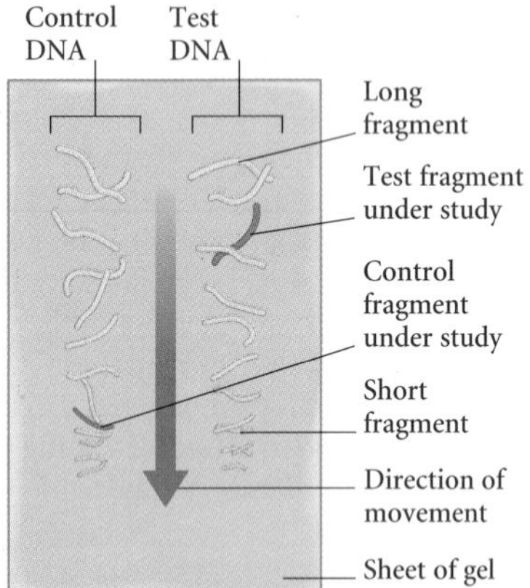

4 The DNA fragments are placed on the surface of a sheet of gel. An electric current is passed through the gel, causing the fragments of DNA to separate according to size. Short fragments move farther along the gel than long ones.

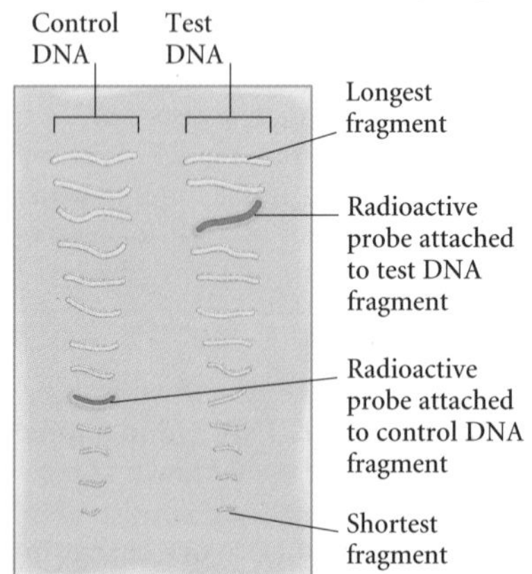

5 After separation, the DNA of the gene under study is located by adding DNA probes, which are pieces of DNA that match the nucleotide sequence of the gene and bind to it. A radioactive label is then attached to the probe so that it can be identified.

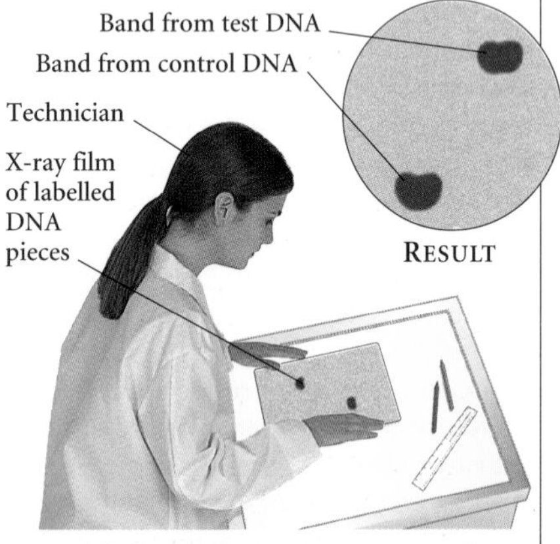

6 The radioactive probes are exposed to X-ray film and produce visible bands on the film. If the bands from the two samples are in the same positions, the gene is normal. If the positions are different, the gene is abnormal.

of normal genes. These fragments can be detected either by staining the DNA with chemicals to make it visible or by using a radioactive DNA probe that is specially designed to stick to a specific abnormal gene (*see* LOOKING FOR ABNORMAL GENES, opposite page).

INDIRECT TESTS When the exact gene abnormality that causes a disorder has not been identified, tests known as linkage analysis are used instead. These tests depend on the use of markers (distinctive sequences of DNA) that are almost always inherited with an abnormal gene because they are close to it on the same chromosome. These indirect tests are designed to identify the marker rather than the abnormal gene itself.

To find a suitable marker for a genetic disorder, relatives with the disorder and unaffected relatives are asked to provide samples from which DNA can be extracted. The DNA is analysed to detect a marker known to be closely linked to (found very near) the abnormal gene that occurs only in affected relatives. A tested person with this marker is likely to have inherited the abnormal gene.

HOW ARE THE RESULTS INTERPRETED?

Direct testing shows definitely whether an abnormal gene is present or not. If indirect tests indicate a linked genetic marker, the likelihood that an abnormal gene is present depends on how closely linked the marker and the gene are. The closer the marker and the abnormal gene are on the chromosome, the more likely that both have been inherited.

People shown to have an abnormal gene may have a disorder; they may be at risk of developing one; or they may be carriers, who have no symptoms but can pass the abnormal gene on to the next generation. The effects of an abnormal gene vary according to whether the gene is dominant or recessive. Mutated genes inherited in a dominant fashion cause a disorder in all the people with the abnormal gene, and there is a 1 in 2 chance of this gene being passed on to children. Mutations in recessive genes usually cause no symptoms in carriers. However, the children of two carriers of a recessive gene are at risk of inheriting two copies of the abnormal gene and having symptoms of the disorder.

Tests for gene products or biochemical markers

Identifying an abnormal gene by analysing its effects on body chemistry

A gene is a length of DNA (deoxyribonucleic acid). The chemical sequence of DNA in each gene contains the necessary instructions to make a protein that controls a specific cell function. If a gene is faulty, a cell may not function properly, leading to a genetic disorder.

The protein coded for by a gene is known as the gene product. In some genetic disorders, it may be possible to measure the gene product directly. In others, direct measurement of the gene product is not possible or is very difficult. However, the abnormality is likely to affect chemical processes in the cell, leading to abnormal amounts of other substances in the body. Sometimes, it is possible to measure the levels of these substances, which are called biochemical markers, as an indirect means of detecting genetic disorders.

WHY ARE THEY DONE?

The tests may be performed to confirm a diagnosis if you have symptoms that indicate a genetic disorder. In some cases, tests may be used to look for carriers of an abnormal gene. Carriers do not have symptoms of a disorder but can pass the gene on to their children, who may develop the disorder.

Since tests for biochemical markers are often easier and cheaper than tests for gene products, they are often used to screen large groups of people. For example, newborn babies are routinely screened for phenylketonuria (p.867), a disorder that can cause brain damage if not detected early. Routine screening may also be recommended for certain ethnic groups with a higher than normal risk of inheriting a disorder.

WHAT MIGHT BE STUDIED?

The levels of a gene product or a biochemical marker are usually measured by analysing a sample of blood or urine. Often, only a small amount of the sample is needed for testing. The tests are performed in a laboratory, usually by an automated machine (*see* ANALYSIS OF BLOOD OR URINE, p.230).

GENE PRODUCTS Chemicals that may be present in abnormal amounts as a result of a genetic disorder include hormones, blood proteins, and enzymes. For example, in the disorder haemophilia (*see* HAEMOPHILIA AND CHRISTMAS DISEASE, p.452), an abnormal gene results in a reduced amount of a protein necessary for normal blood clotting. The level of this protein, called Factor VIII, can be measured directly in a sample of blood. Another condition that can be diagnosed by measuring levels of a gene product is alpha$_1$-antitrypsin deficiency (p.489). Affected people have a low level of the enzyme alpha$_1$-antitrypsin, which may cause lung and liver damage.

BIOCHEMICAL MARKERS The way that a cell's chemical processes are disrupted determines the type of substance that can be used as a biochemical marker. For example, in the disorder phenylketonuria, phenylalanine (a chemical that is found naturally in many foods) accumulates because the enzyme that normally breaks it down is missing. Chemical tests can detect high levels of phenylalanine in the blood of babies born with this condition.

Some genetic abnormalities result in damage to body tissues, causing them to release substances into the blood that may be used as biochemical markers. For example, muscles damaged as a result of the inherited disorder muscular dystrophy (p.826) release an enzyme called creatine kinase. High levels of creatine kinase are found in the blood of people with muscular dystrophy.

HOW ARE THE RESULTS INTERPRETED?

Gene products are unique to a particular illness, and test results therefore provide a definite diagnosis. However, a test for a biochemical marker may sometimes only suggest the presence of an abnormality. For example, the blood level of creatine kinase is raised in people with muscular dystrophy, but the level is also high in people with other conditions causing muscle damage. In these cases, it may be necessary to measure the gene product itself, if possible. Family medical history may also need to be taken into account to assess an individual's risk of having or developing a particular disease.

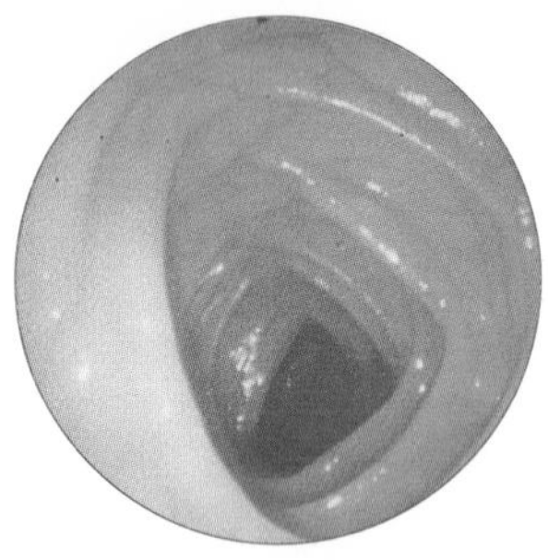

Endoscopic view of the colon
Body cavities and hollow organs such as the colon (above) can be viewed using an instrument called an endoscope.

VISUALIZING INTERNAL ORGANS

MODERN TECHNOLOGICAL ADVANCES have changed the way in which we investigate the human body, and today a wide variety of visualizing techniques is available. Imaging creates pictures, usually on film or a computer, of internal organs and structures. Viewing techniques use specialized devices, including endoscopes, to allow hollow structures in parts of the body such as the digestive tract to be looked at directly.

Imaging and viewing techniques are often used to confirm a diagnosis or to make one if other tests are not conclusive. These techniques may also be used to screen for some disorders and to monitor the progress of a disease or treatment. Most imaging techniques, and some complex viewing techniques, are carried out in hospital. Other techniques, such as simple X-rays and basic viewing, may be performed in the doctor's surgery or an outpatient clinic.

IMAGING TECHNIQUES

Imaging uses modern technology to create a picture of internal organs or body structures. The oldest form of imaging, which is still in use today, consists of "shadow pictures", mainly of the skeleton, cast by X-ray radiation on to photographic film.

Since the 1940s, there have been major advances in the field of medical imaging. Today, advanced techniques such as CT scanning use X-rays to produce detailed images of soft tissues and structures other than the skeleton. Liquids called contrast media can also be introduced into structures, such as blood vessels, enabling hollow areas or fluid-filled structures to be seen using X-rays. Radionuclide scanning detects the radiation emitted by radioactive substances that are introduced into the body, allowing doctors to assess cell activity in body tissues.

Other modern techniques include MRI, which uses radio waves and magnets to produce clear, detailed images, and ultrasound scanning, which uses sound waves. Both of these techniques do not use radiation.

Some scanning techniques, such as spiral CT scanning, are so advanced that a computer can create a video image that gives an impression of travelling through parts of the body.

VIEWING TECHNIQUES

Depending on the problem, a direct view of part of the body sometimes provides more useful information than an artificial picture created by an imaging technique. Structures near the surface of the body, such as the eardrum, can be viewed directly using simple instruments. Endoscopes are used to look deeper inside the body.

Endoscopy was first used more than 100 years ago, when short, rigid devices were used to look inside the bladder and the colon. Today, rigid endoscopes are still used to view some body cavities and to carry out certain types of surgery. However, advances in technology have also led to the development of a range of flexible endoscopes. These endoscopes are used to examine the internal walls of hollow structures that can be reached through natural body openings. For example, the upper digestive tract may be viewed through the mouth.

COMPARISON IMAGING AND VIEWING

The type of visualizing test that is used depends on the part of the body and the problem being investigated. Imaging creates an artificial picture built up from information about the nature of a tissue, such as its density or the activity of its cells. Viewing, such as endoscopy, provides a direct view of body cavities and the internal walls of hollow organs.

Brain
Nasal cavity
PLANE OF SCAN

Image produced by MRI scanning
An MRI scan shows all the structures, tissues, and cavities within the area being scanned. In this MRI, the nasal cavity and brain tissues are normal.

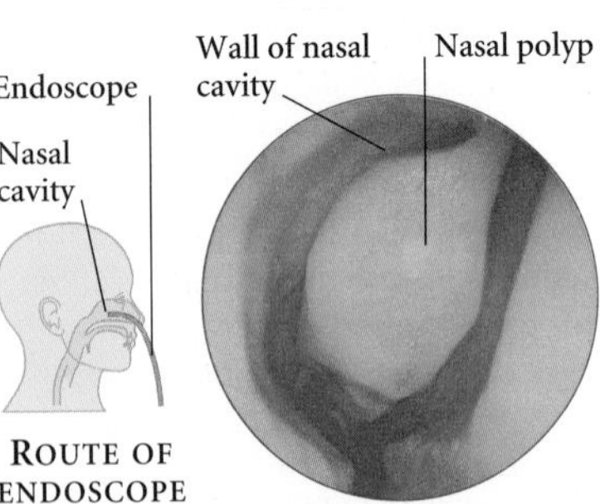

View down an endoscope
One use of endoscopy is to investigate and view abnormalities within body cavities. This view through an endoscope shows a polyp inside the nasal cavity.

COMPARISON IMAGING USING DIFFERENT TECHNIQUES

The imaging technique that your doctor uses depends on the part of the body being studied and the type of information needed. X-rays show dense tissue, such as bone, most clearly, whereas contrast X-rays provide a clear image of hollow or fluid-filled parts of the body. MRI and CT scanning can provide information about many types of tissue in great detail. An ultrasound scan can assess function by detecting movement, such as blood flow, and radionuclide scanning, such as SPECT, gives detailed information about organ function.

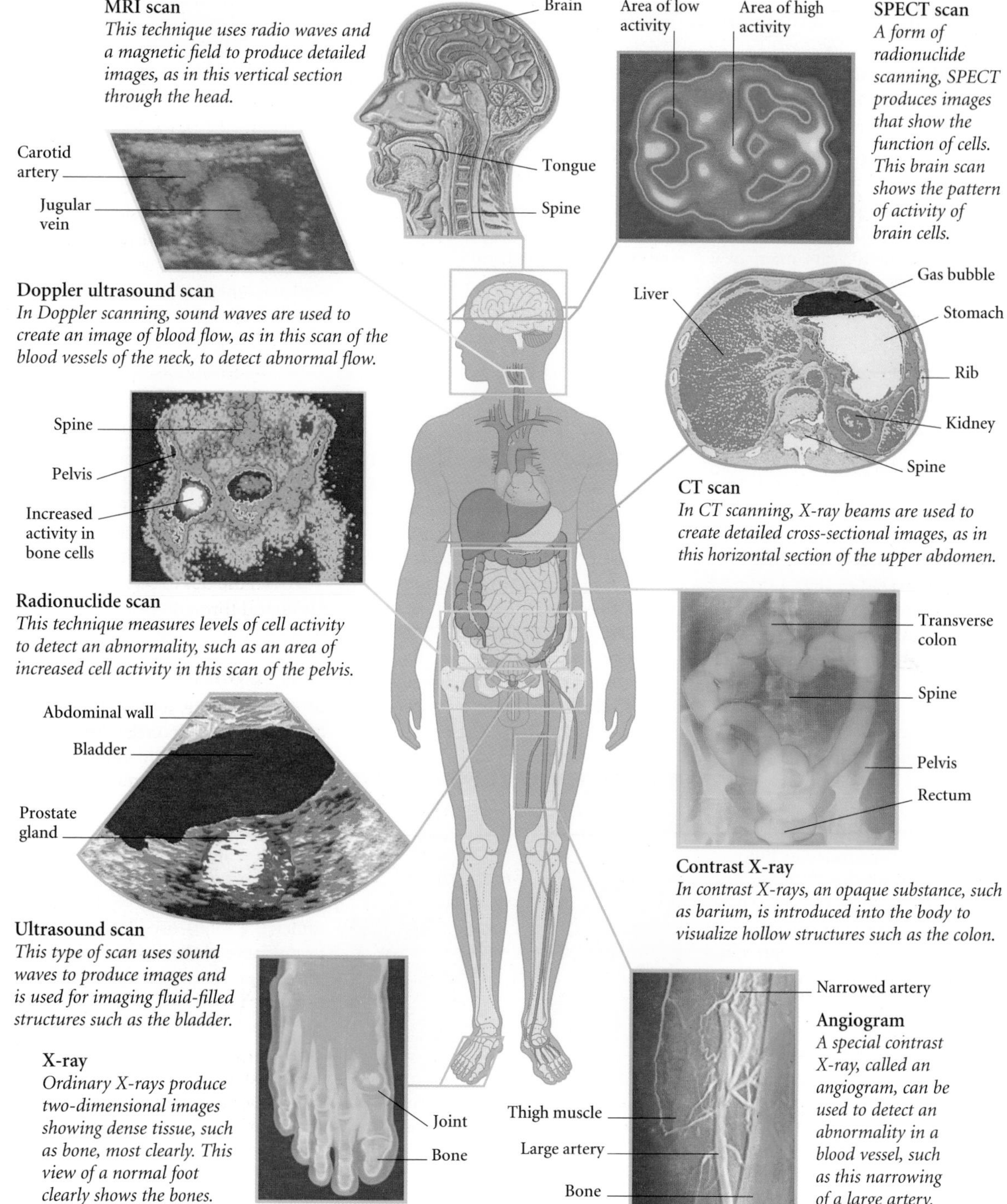

MRI scan
This technique uses radio waves and a magnetic field to produce detailed images, as in this vertical section through the head.

SPECT scan
A form of radionuclide scanning, SPECT produces images that show the function of cells. This brain scan shows the pattern of activity of brain cells.

Doppler ultrasound scan
In Doppler scanning, sound waves are used to create an image of blood flow, as in this scan of the blood vessels of the neck, to detect abnormal flow.

CT scan
In CT scanning, X-ray beams are used to create detailed cross-sectional images, as in this horizontal section of the upper abdomen.

Radionuclide scan
This technique measures levels of cell activity to detect an abnormality, such as an area of increased cell activity in this scan of the pelvis.

Contrast X-ray
In contrast X-rays, an opaque substance, such as barium, is introduced into the body to visualize hollow structures such as the colon.

Ultrasound scan
This type of scan uses sound waves to produce images and is used for imaging fluid-filled structures such as the bladder.

X-ray
Ordinary X-rays produce two-dimensional images showing dense tissue, such as bone, most clearly. This view of a normal foot clearly shows the bones.

Angiogram
A special contrast X-ray, called an angiogram, can be used to detect an abnormality in a blood vessel, such as this narrowing of a large artery.

IMAGING TECHNIQUES

The aim of imaging is to provide detailed and reliable pictorial information about structures within the body with the minimum risk and discomfort. Most imaging is now highly computerized and has largely replaced exploratory surgery in establishing the presence and extent of disease. Recent techniques are also able to indicate how well a tissue or an organ is functioning.

The first techniques used for imaging the body were based on X-rays, a form of high-energy radiation that is able to pass through body tissues. Some X-rays require particular substances, called contrast media, to improve the visibility of certain structures.

Over the last 30–40 years, many new techniques have been introduced, most of which involve the use of computers that control the imaging equipment and are able to create images of the body in three dimensions.

This section begins by explaining the basic imaging methods that use X-rays, which include ordinary and contrast X-rays and CT scanning. Other imaging techniques are then covered, such as MRI and ultrasound scanning, which do not involve the use of radiation, and different types of radionuclide scanning.

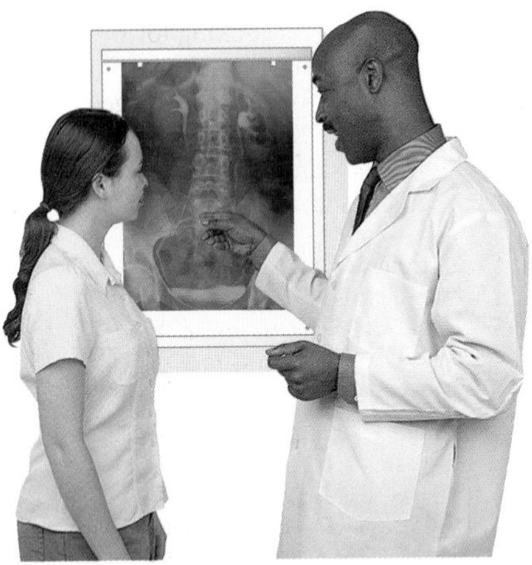

Looking at imaging results
Your doctor may show you your X-ray or scan and explain the results by pointing out the various structures that are visible along with any areas of abnormality.

X-rays

Images produced using high-energy radiation; especially suitable for looking at bone and some soft tissues

X-rays have been used in imaging since they were discovered in 1895. Ordinary X-rays, called plain X-rays, are mainly used for imaging bones and certain soft tissues, such as the breasts. Structures that are hollow or fluid-filled, such as the digestive tract or blood vessels, do not show up well on ordinary X-rays and are more successfully imaged using contrast X-rays (opposite page).

Ordinary X-rays are still commonly used in imaging, despite the development of more sophisticated techniques, such as CT scanning (p.247) and MRI (p.248). This is because X-rays are inexpensive, quick, simple to perform, and usually provide the doctor with sufficient information to make a diagnosis.

HOW DO THEY WORK?

X-rays are a form of radiation similar to light waves but with a higher energy. This high energy enables X-rays to pass through body tissues. The ability of X-rays to penetrate structures depends on the tissue's density. X-rays easily penetrate soft tissues but pass less readily through dense tissue, such as bone. X-rays blacken photographic film. If a single beam of X-rays is focused on to the body, the parts that allow X-rays through, such as air in the lungs, appear black on the film. Soft tissues, such as skin, fat, and muscle, appear as varying shades of grey. Dense substances, such as bone, are seen as white. As a result of these differences, the final image of the body created by the X-rays on the film looks like a photographic negative.

X-rays only create two-dimensional images, which means that occasionally two or more X-rays must be taken from different angles to pinpoint a condition. For example, to determine the position of a tumour in the lung, X-rays would be taken of the body from the front and from the side or at a slanting angle.

Rib
Spine
Breast
Heart
Lung

Chest X-ray
In this X-ray of a healthy woman's chest, bones appear white, soft tissue appears as shades of grey, and air appears black.

WHAT ARE THEY USED FOR?

Ordinary X-rays produce clear images of bone and are often used to look for fractures (*see* HAVING AN X-RAY, opposite page). Chest X-rays (p.490) may be performed to look for an enlarged heart or damaged lung tissue in a person with symptoms, such as chest pain, that may be due to heart or lung disease.

At lower doses, X-rays are useful for examining soft tissues, such as those of the breast, in detail, and they are widely used to screen for breast cancer (*see* MAMMOGRAPHY, p.759). Bone densitometry (p.369) uses low-dose X-rays to measure bone density. This technique is used to screen for and diagnose osteoporosis (p.368), a common condition in postmenopausal women.

WHAT ARE THE RISKS?

There are no immediate risks from having ordinary X-rays, but there is some risk that radiation may cause damage to body cells, possibly leading to cancer later in life. This risk increases if you are repeatedly exposed to X-ray radiation

PROCEDURE HAVING AN X-RAY

X-rays are ideal for looking for fractures in bone and imaging certain soft tissues. You are positioned on or against a special table or surface so that the part of your body to be imaged lies between a drawer containing a film cassette and the X-ray source. After positioning the X-ray machine, the radiographer stands behind a screen. You are exposed to X-rays for a fraction of a second, and the whole procedure takes only a few minutes.

During the procedure
The source of the X-rays is positioned directly above the area being examined. You have to keep still so that the X-ray image is clear. In some cases, a second X-ray may be taken from a different angle to give more information.

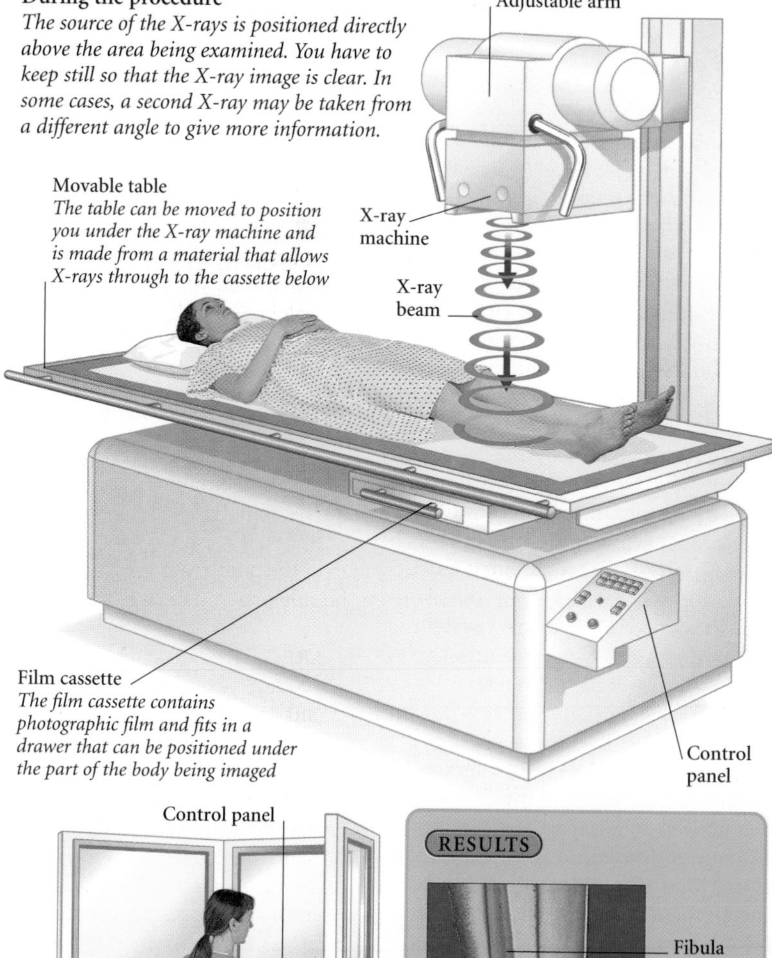

Movable table
The table can be moved to position you under the X-ray machine and is made from a material that allows X-rays through to the cassette below

Film cassette
The film cassette contains photographic film and fits in a drawer that can be positioned under the part of the body being imaged

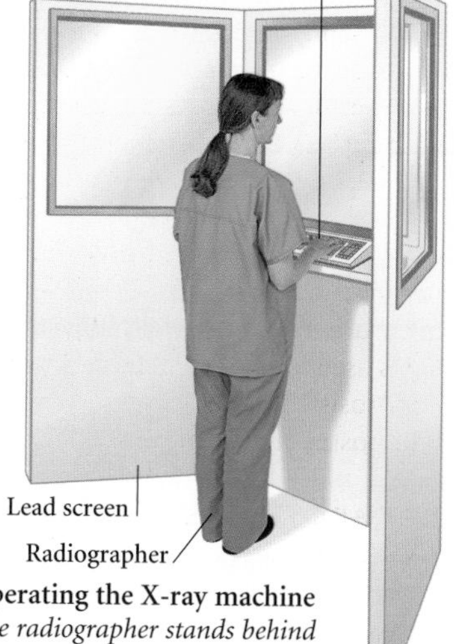

Operating the X-ray machine
The radiographer stands behind a protective screen to minimize his or her exposure to X-rays.

RESULTS

Fibula
Fracture
Tibia

X-ray image
This X-ray clearly shows the two bones of the lower leg, the tibia and the fibula. The main bone, the tibia, has an obvious fracture.

(*see* RADIATION DOSES, p.246). The earlier in life you are exposed to radiation, the greater the risk. Radiographers always try to use the minimum amount of radiation when taking X-rays, and modern equipment makes it possible to produce good-quality images with lower doses of radiation than in the past.

During X-ray procedures, areas that are not being imaged may be shielded. For example, when X-raying the pelvis, special care is often taken to shield the reproductive organs to avoid damage to sperm or eggs. Women are always asked if they may be pregnant before having an X-ray because radiation may cause fetal abnormalities in early pregnancy. Radiographers are always protected by a lead apron or screen to avoid repeated exposure to radiation.

Contrast X-rays

Images produced using radiation and a substance that makes hollow or fluid-filled structures visible

Hollow or fluid-filled body structures, such as the intestines or blood vessels, do not show up well on an ordinary X-ray image (*see* X-RAYS, opposite page). A substance called a contrast medium can be introduced into these structures to make them visible. Contrast media are opaque to radiation in the same way as dense body tissues, such as bone. X-rays cannot pass through the media, and areas containing these substances will appear white on an X-ray image.

The contrast medium is injected into the body or introduced orally or rectally, depending on the structure to be imaged. This procedure is generally straightforward, but it may cause discomfort and involve some risks, such as an adverse reaction to the dye. Contrast X-ray procedures are increasingly being replaced by other techniques, in particular CT scanning (p.247), MRI (p.248), and ultrasound scanning (p.250), all of which cause less discomfort and involve fewer risks to health.

WHAT ARE THEY USED FOR?

Contrast X-rays can produce images of various hollow or fluid-filled structures that do not show up well on ordinary X-rays. Contrast X-rays are often used to image the blood vessels, urinary system, and digestive tract. Different types of contrast media that may be used include iodine (which is soluble in water) and barium sulphate (which is insoluble).

BLOOD VESSELS Water-soluble iodine dyes can be carried around the body in the bloodstream. For this reason, and because they show up well on X-rays, these dyes are used to check whether blood is flowing normally in the blood vessels. Imaging of blood vessels by using X-rays is known as angiography. In this technique, the dye is injected through a catheter that has been introduced into a blood vessel and guided until its tip is near the vessel to be studied. The dye flows into the appropriate vessels, making abnormalities, such as blockages, visible on X-rays.

Angiography is often used to look at arteries that have become narrowed or blocked due to fatty deposits in the vessel walls (*see* ATHEROSCLEROSIS, p.402). Coronary angiography (p.408) images the blood vessels supplying the heart, and femoral angiography (p.433) is used to image blood vessels in the leg. Better-quality images may be produced using a computer to remove unwanted background information, a procedure called digital subtraction angiography.

URINARY SYSTEM When injected into a vein, dye circulates in the bloodstream and becomes concentrated in the kidneys before it is excreted in urine. The dye can therefore be used to image various structures in the urinary system. As

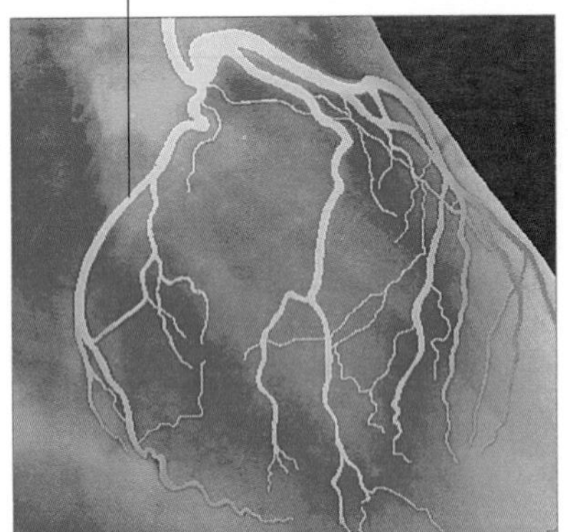

Contrast X-ray of blood vessels
These normal blood vessels supplying the heart muscle contain a water-soluble iodine dye, making them stand out on this colour-enhanced contrast X-ray image.

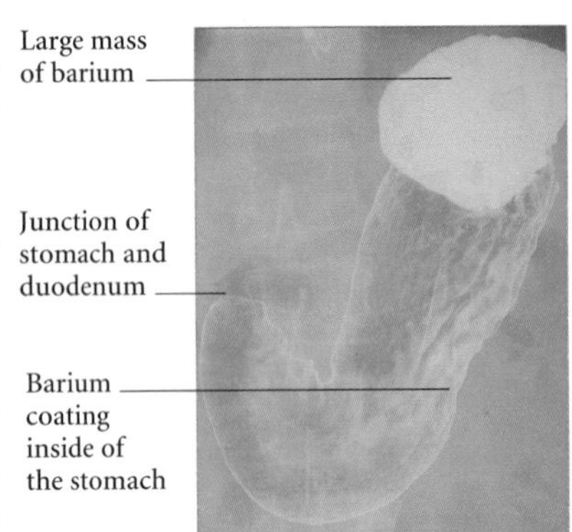

Barium contrast X-ray
A swallowed barium solution makes this normal stomach visible on an X-ray image. The barium is at the top of the stomach because the person is lying head down.

the dye passes through the urinary tract, it outlines the ureter (the tube linking the kidneys and the bladder) and the bladder. If the bladder and urethra (the tube that takes urine from the bladder to the outside of the body) alone are to be imaged by the X-rays, the contrast medium may be introduced directly into the bladder through a catheter that is passed up through the urethra. Contrast X-rays are often used to look for suspected kidney disease and obstructions in the urinary system due to kidney stones or tumours (*see* INTRAVENOUS UROGRAPHY, p.699).

DIGESTIVE TRACT Barium sulphate is a thick, insoluble, chalky liquid that does not allow X-rays to pass through it and shows up well on X-ray images. Barium liquid moves slowly through the digestive tract and is not absorbed by the body. All these qualities make barium a good contrast medium for examining the digestive tract. Barium X-ray examinations can also be useful for studying function, such as swallowing. However, endoscopy (p.255), in which tube-like instruments are used to look at internal organs, may sometimes be more appropriate than barium investigations.

Barium sulphate is drunk if the upper digestive tract from the oesophagus to the duodenum (the first part of the small intestine) is to be examined. This procedure is known as a barium swallow (p.637) or a barium meal. Barium meals can be used to investigate most problems of the upper digestive tract, including swallowing difficulties and indigestion (*see* NONULCER DYSPEPSIA, p.626). The progression of the barium through the digestive tract after it has left the duodenum can be followed by taking a number of X-rays at intervals or recording moving images on video.

Barium sulphate is also used to image the colon. It is given as an enema after a laxative has been taken to empty the bowel. Barium enemas can be used to detect abnormal growths in the colon lining, such as polyps (*see* POLYPS IN THE COLON, p.660).

In double-contrast radiography, air is introduced into the digestive tract after the barium. The air replaces the

COMPARISON

RADIATION DOSES

Radiation can potentially damage body cells, which may increase the long-term risk of cancer. Low levels of background radiation are always present in the environment, but higher radiation levels are used in imaging. Different radiation doses are received from different imaging procedures. The greater the dose, the longer the exposure, and the earlier in life exposure occurs, the higher the related risk.

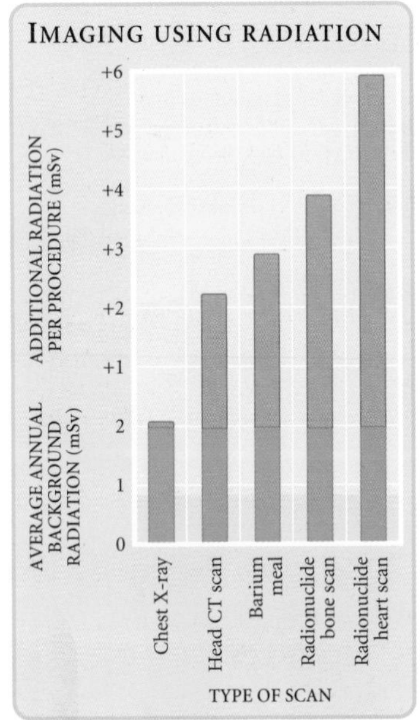

Measuring the potential for harm
This graph shows the radiation doses received from different types of imaging in millisieverts (mSv). The doses shown include average background radiation.

PROCEDURE HAVING A CT SCAN

A CT scanner uses a series of X-ray beams to build up images of the body in "slices". Several individual scans may be carried out to create detailed images of the area that is being investigated. CT scanning can detect hundreds of levels of density and is used to produce pictures of many different parts of the body. The radiographer positions you on a motorized bed and moves you into the scanner. If you feel anxious, you may be given a sedative.

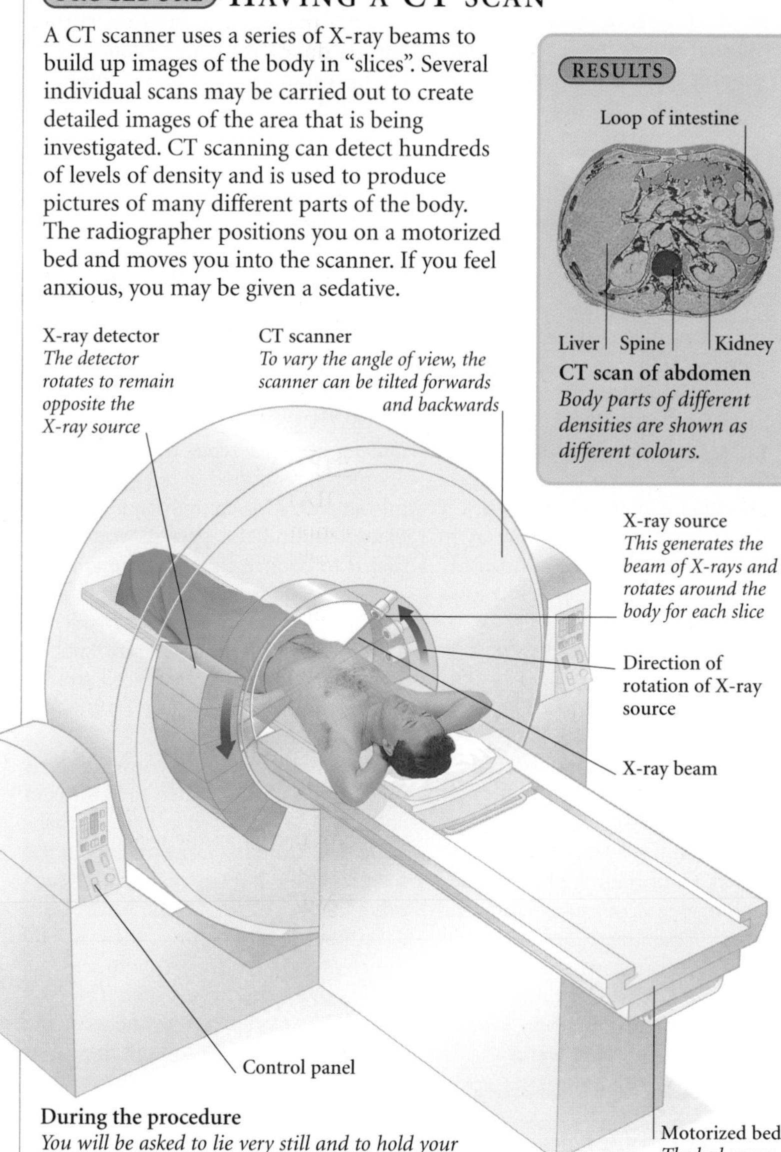

CT scan of abdomen
Body parts of different densities are shown as different colours.

During the procedure
You will be asked to lie very still and to hold your breath while each scan is taken, to avoid blurring the image. Several scans may be carried out, and the whole procedure may take about 30 minutes.

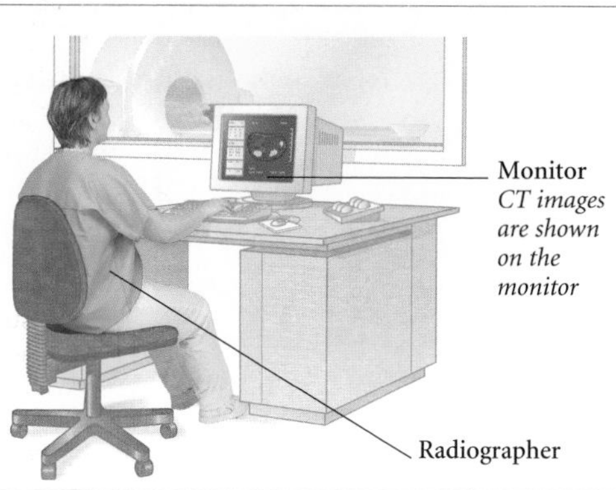

Operating the CT scanner
The radiographer moves to an adjacent room to operate the scanner by using a computer. A microphone allows him or her to communicate with you. Being in a separate room protects the radiographer from radiation. A doctor may oversee a scan or control the scanner.

barium, which remains only on the lining of the digestive tract. This technique gives a detailed image of the lining and is useful for detecting changes due to conditions such as Crohn's disease (p.658).

WHAT ARE THE RISKS?

Radiation can cause damage to body cells, which may rarely lead to cancer later in life. Contrast X-rays expose you to a relatively large quantity of radiation because they require many X-rays (*see* RADIATION DOSES, opposite page).

Injecting contrast media carries a minor risk of serious complications such as anaphylaxis (p.469). People who have asthma triggered by an allergy or who have a known sensitivity to iodine are advised not to have contrast X-rays or are pretreated with certain drugs, such as antihistamines (p.906) and corticosteroids (p.930), or other contrast media may be used. Most people experience a flushing sensation as dye is injected.

Barium sulphate can cause constipation, and your doctor may prescribe a laxative after a barium X-ray.

CT scanning

Computer-assisted imaging using a succession of X-ray beams to produce cross-sectional images through the body

Computerized tomography (CT) scanning uses X-rays (p.244) in conjunction with a computer. A series of X-rays is passed through the body at slightly different angles to produce highly detailed cross-sectional images ("slices") of the body, called tomograms. CT scanning makes it possible to gather detailed information about organs painlessly and with minimal exposure to radiation.

HOW DOES IT WORK?

The CT scanner consists of an X-ray source and an X-ray detector, both of which rotate during the procedure so that they remain opposite each other. CT scanning uses X-rays in a different way from an ordinary X-ray machine to give a higher-quality image. The film used in ordinary X-rays can show only a few levels of density, such as dense tissues, soft tissues, and air. The detector within a CT scanner can see hundreds of different levels of density. For this reason, a CT scan is able to show details

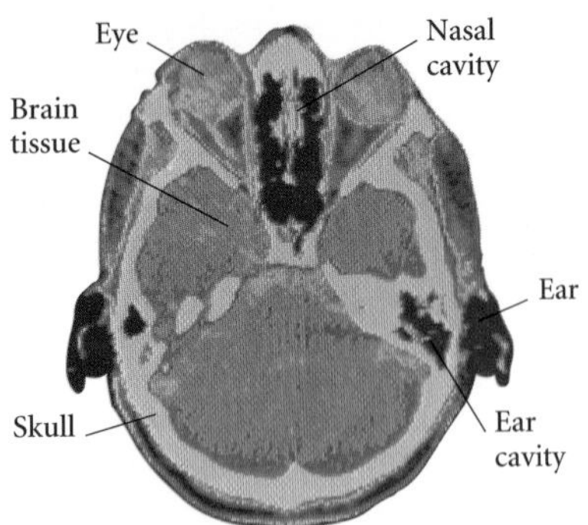

CT scan of the head
This normal CT scan of the head viewed from above clearly shows the different structures and cavities within the skull.

that are impossible to see using ordinary X-rays, including fibrous tissue in solid organs such as the liver. Instead of sending one beam of radiation through your body, the X-ray source inside a CT scanner emits a succession of narrow beams as it moves through an arc. The X-ray detector then picks up the radiation after it has passed through various body tissues (*see* HAVING A CT SCAN, p.247). After each arc is completed, the bed is moved forwards a small distance.

The information from the detector is then sent to the computer, which builds up cross-sectional images of the body and displays them on a monitor. These resulting images can be stored either as computer files or on conventional X-ray film. More sophisticated computers can produce three-dimensional images from standard CT data.

Newer CT scanners use the spiral (or helical) technique, in which the scanner rotates around you as the bed moves forwards slowly so that the X-ray beams follow a spiral course. This type of CT scanning produces three-dimensional images and reduces the time taken for the scans to be completed.

WHAT IS IT USED FOR?

The CT scans performed most often are those of the head and the abdomen. CT scanning of the head is a valuable technique that is commonly used to investigate the brain following a stroke (p.532) or if a brain tumour (p.530) is suspected. Abdominal CT scans are frequently used to detect tumours and to diagnose disorders in which organs are enlarged or inflamed, such as polycystic kidney disease (p.704). CT scans can also be used to investigate the lungs and to guide biopsy procedures, in which cells or tissue are taken from internal organs for examination.

CT scanning is able to produce much more clear images of bone than MRI (below). Blood vessels can also be imaged. These images may be enhanced by using a contrast medium (a substance that makes a fluid-filled or hollow structure visible on the image).

WHAT ARE THE RISKS?

Imaging techniques that use radiation may damage body cells, which may increase the risk of cancer in the long term (*see* RADIATION DOSES, p.246). The dose for a CT procedure depends on the number of cross sections imaged. Scanning time is reduced for spiral CT scans, but the dose is the same as in a normal CT scan. Radiation exposure during CT scans is generally quite low.

MRI

A radiation-free, computer-assisted imaging technique that uses a strong magnetic field and radio waves

The technique of magnetic resonance imaging (MRI) has been used since the early 1980s to provide highly detailed sectional images of internal organs and structures. These images are created by a computer using information received from a scanner. MRI does not involve potentially harmful radiation; instead, it uses magnets and radio waves.

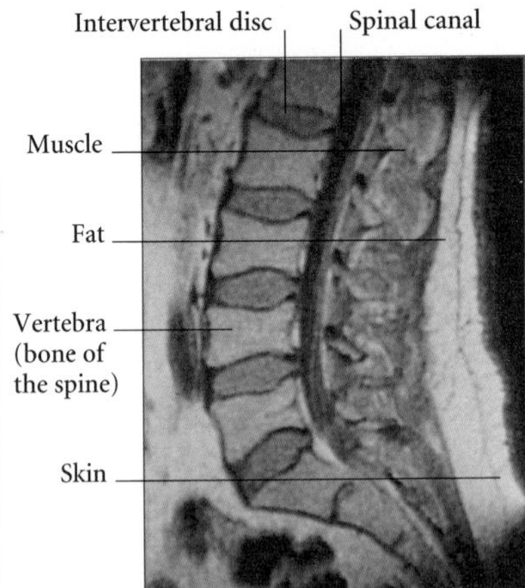

MRI of the lower spine
This MRI scan of a healthy person's lower spine clearly shows the different structures, including muscle, skin, and bone.

Although MRI is a relatively expensive procedure and MRI scans tend to take longer than other techniques, it does have several advantages. Images from MRI are similar to those produced by CT scanning (p.247), but MRI can distinguish abnormal tissue, such as a tumour, from normal tissue much more clearly. MRI scans can also be taken at a greater range of planes through the body than is possible with CT scanning and therefore can be used to image any part of the body. MRI is radiation-free and is considered to be one of the safest imaging techniques available.

HOW DOES IT WORK?

During an MRI scan, you lie inside a scanner surrounded by a large, powerful magnet. A receiving magnet is then placed around the part of your body that is to be investigated. If large areas, such as the abdomen, are to be imaged, the receiving magnet is fitted inside the MRI scanner; for smaller areas, such as a joint, a magnet may be placed around the part to be scanned (*see* HAVING AN MRI SCAN, opposite page).

Your body, like everything else, is made up of atoms. When the atoms in your body are exposed to a strong magnetic field from the large magnet in the scanner, they line up parallel to each other. Short pulses of radio waves from a radiofrequency source then briefly knock the atoms out of alignment. As they realign, the atoms emit tiny signals, which are detected by the receiving magnet. Information about these signals is then passed on to a computer, which builds up an image based on the signals' strength and location.

MRI images can be enhanced by the use of a contrast medium to highlight particular structures in the body, such as tumours and blood vessels.

WHAT IS IT USED FOR?

MRI can provide clear images of any part of the body. This type of scanning is especially useful for looking at the brain and for detecting brain tumours (p.530). MRI is also valuable for looking at the spinal cord and may be used to investigate lower back pain (p.381). Sports injuries (p.391), especially in the knee (*see* TORN KNEE CARTILAGE, p.395), are increasingly being examined using MRI. In a small number of cases, MRI

PROCEDURE Having an MRI scan

MRI scanning is most commonly used to investigate the brain but is also used for looking at the spine and, increasingly, for sports injuries. You are positioned on a motorized bed and a receiving magnet is placed around the part of your body to be examined. You are then moved into the tunnel of the scanner. Several individual scans will be taken. You will have to lie within the scanner for up to an hour, and therefore it is important that you are as comfortable as possible. You may be given earplugs or headphones because the scanner can be noisy. Your doctor may give you a sedative if you are anxious or claustrophobic.

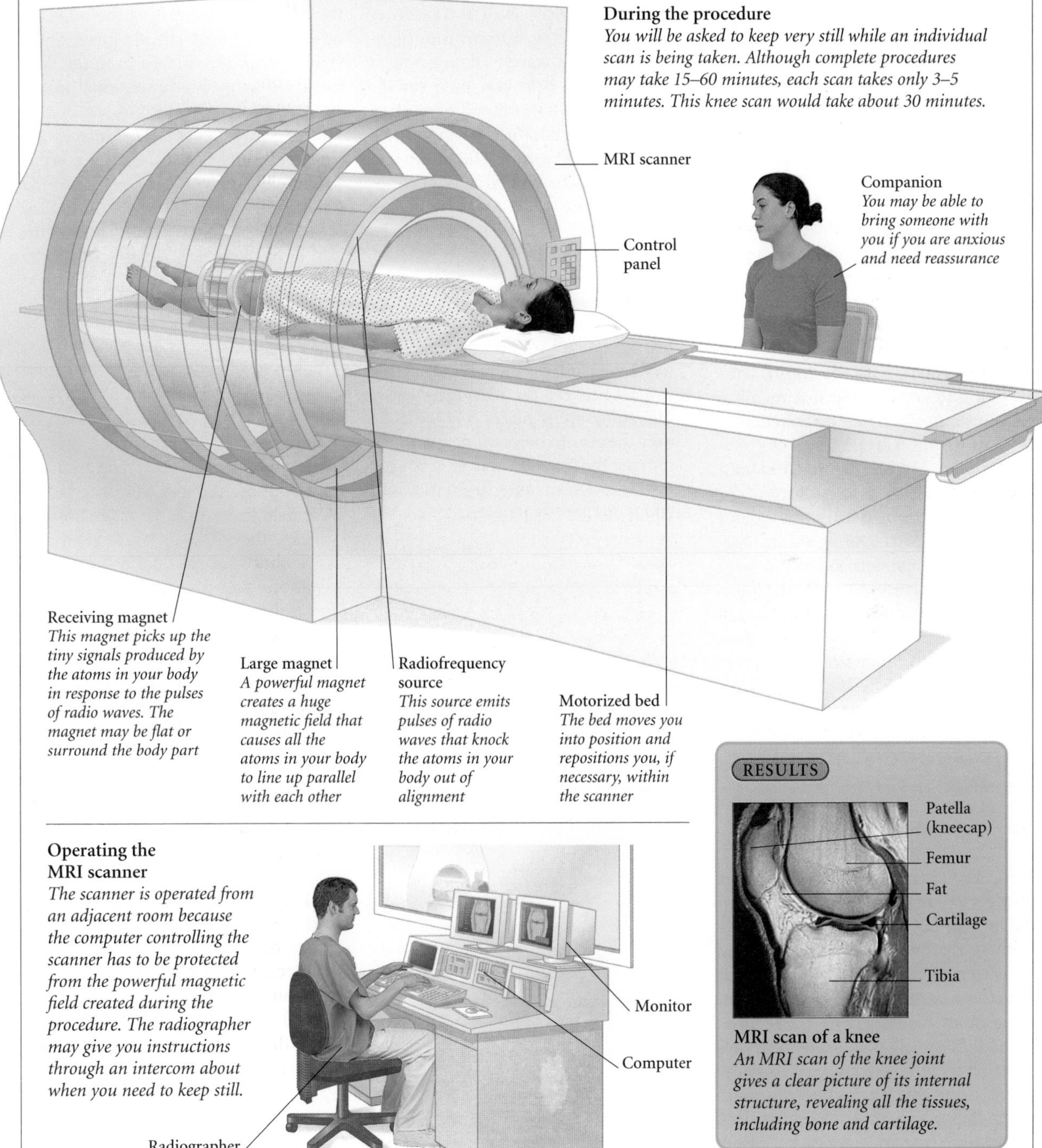

During the procedure
You will be asked to keep very still while an individual scan is being taken. Although complete procedures may take 15–60 minutes, each scan takes only 3–5 minutes. This knee scan would take about 30 minutes.

Companion
You may be able to bring someone with you if you are anxious and need reassurance

Receiving magnet
This magnet picks up the tiny signals produced by the atoms in your body in response to the pulses of radio waves. The magnet may be flat or surround the body part

Large magnet
A powerful magnet creates a huge magnetic field that causes all the atoms in your body to line up parallel with each other

Radiofrequency source
This source emits pulses of radio waves that knock the atoms in your body out of alignment

Motorized bed
The bed moves you into position and repositions you, if necessary, within the scanner

Operating the MRI scanner
The scanner is operated from an adjacent room because the computer controlling the scanner has to be protected from the powerful magnetic field created during the procedure. The radiographer may give you instructions through an intercom about when you need to keep still.

MRI scan of a knee
An MRI scan of the knee joint gives a clear picture of its internal structure, revealing all the tissues, including bone and cartilage.

has been used to examine the breasts. MRI scans show the location of tumours within the breast tissue more accurately than plain two-dimensional X-rays (*see* MAMMOGRAPHY, p.759). In addition, since MRI does not use radiation, MRI scans can be repeated often, allowing doctors to monitor a condition safely.

A particular type of MRI, called magnetic resonance angiography (MRA), enables doctors to look at blood flow by comparing the signals received from stationary tissue with those from flowing blood. MRA can be performed without a contrast medium and is therefore safer and causes less discomfort than angiography using contrast X-rays (p.245).

WHAT ARE THE RISKS?

The long-term effects of magnetization are not yet known, although many people have undergone repeated scans with no ill effects. Doctors recommend that women in early pregnancy avoid having an MRI scan if possible, since the risks (if any) to the developing fetus are not known. The contrast medium gadolinium, which may be used during MRI, causes no side effects.

If you could have any metal in your body, such as a surgical implant or shrapnel, you should tell your doctor before having MRI. During a scan, magnetic metal fragments lodged in your body will move around under the influence of the magnetic field and could cause serious damage. Before an MRI scan, your doctor may request X-rays to look for metal in your body.

Ultrasound scanning

A technique that uses high-frequency sound waves to image internal structures or a fetus in the uterus

Ultrasound scanning uses sound waves of a very high frequency, inaudible to the human ear. The sound waves travel through the body and their echoes are processed to create images of internal structures or of a fetus in the uterus. Ultrasound scanning is a versatile technique that can show movement as well as structure, and the range of examinations using this method is constantly expanding. For example, organs situated deep within body cavities, such as those in the pelvis, which were previously difficult to image, can now be examined using ultrasound scanning. Since ultrasound does not involve radiation, it is thought to be completely safe.

HOW DOES IT WORK?

The principle of ultrasound scanning is similar to that used in naval sonar, in which sound waves are bounced off objects deep in the ocean. In ultrasound scanning, a device called a transducer converts an electric current into high-frequency sound waves. The transducer is usually hand-held and used on the skin surface, but it is sometimes inserted on a probe into a natural opening such as the vagina or rectum. The transducer may also be incorporated into an endoscope, a viewing tube, to image deeper inside the body. Sound waves emitted by the transducer are focused in a narrow beam that passes through different parts of the body as the transducer is moved back and forth. Sound waves pass readily through soft tissue and fluid and are reflected at a point where different densities meet, such as where fluid in the bladder meets the bladder wall.

In addition to sending out the sound waves, the ultrasound transducer acts as the receiver by converting the reflected echoes back into electrical signals. These signals are processed by a computer and displayed as a two-dimensional image on a monitor (*see* HAVING AN ULTRASOUND SCAN, below). The images are updated continuously, enabling scans to show movement, such as that of the fetus in the uterus (*see* ULTRASOUND SCANNING IN PREGNANCY, p.793) or

PROCEDURE HAVING AN ULTRASOUND SCAN

In ultrasound scanning, a device called a transducer emits high-frequency sound waves and receives their echoes to produce images on a monitor. To ensure good contact between the transducer and the body, the radiographer places gel on the skin over the area to be examined before moving the transducer over it. An ultrasound scan takes 10–30 minutes and is completely painless.

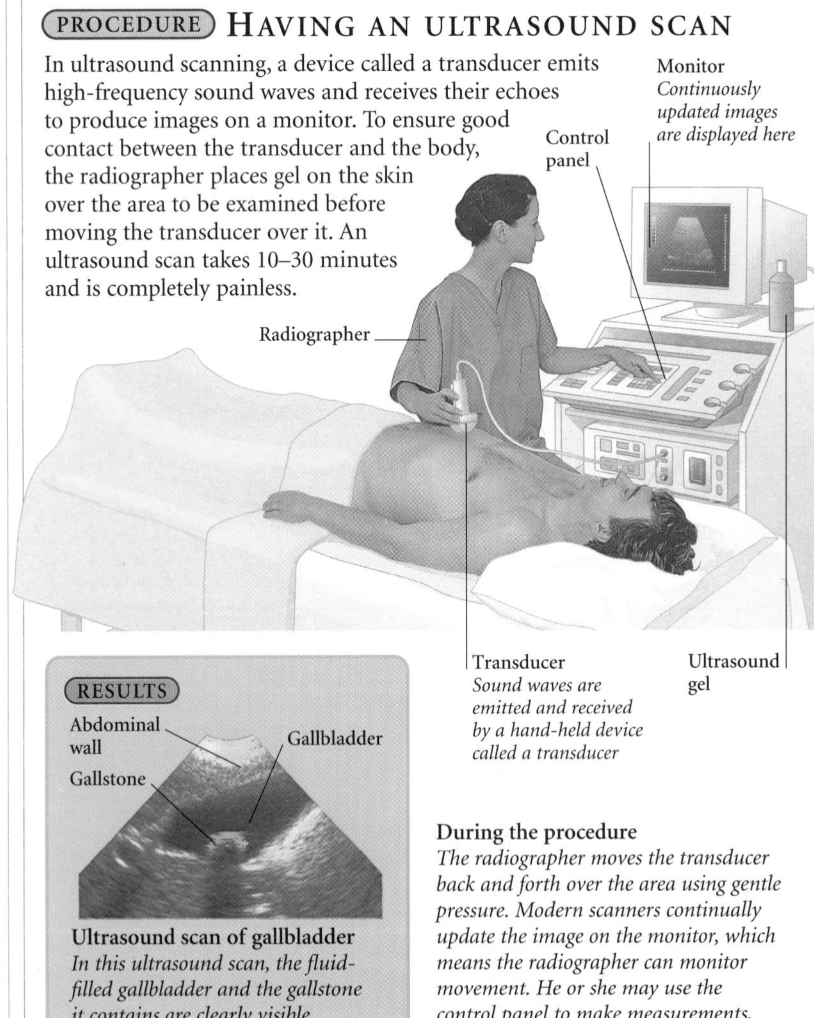

Ultrasound scan of gallbladder
In this ultrasound scan, the fluid-filled gallbladder and the gallstone it contains are clearly visible.

During the procedure
The radiographer moves the transducer back and forth over the area using gentle pressure. Modern scanners continually update the image on the monitor, which means the radiographer can monitor movement. He or she may use the control panel to make measurements, such as the diameter of a gallstone.

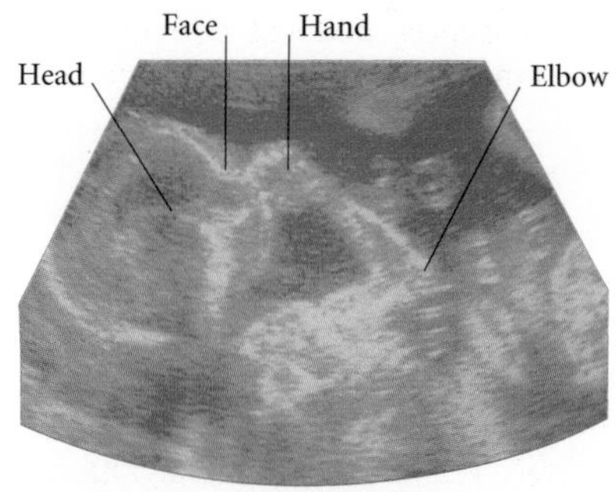

Ultrasound scan of a fetus
Imaging using ultrasound is a useful technique for looking at the movement of a fetus and monitoring fetal growth. There is no known risk to the health of the fetus.

valves opening and closing within the heart (*see* ECHOCARDIOGRAPHY, p.425). A specific type of ultrasound known as Doppler ultrasound scanning (p.432) uses short pulses of ultrasound to look at the direction and the speed of blood flow. Blood that is flowing away from the Doppler probe appears blue on the scan, while blood that is flowing towards it appears red. A mixture of colours indicates turbulence. The speed of blood flow is measured by a computer.

WHAT IS IT USED FOR?

Most pregnant women will have at least one ultrasound scan to examine the growing fetus. Ultrasound can also be used to image the brain of a newborn baby through the fontanelles (the soft spots in a baby's head between the bones of the skull). Using ultrasound in this way can identify bleeding into the brain from the surrounding blood vessels, a potential problem in premature babies.

Ultrasound scanning is commonly used to investigate internal organs because it produces good images of soft tissue, such as the liver, and fluid-filled structures, such as the gallbladder. It can also be used to examine the structure of the heart and its movement. Used endoscopically through the oesophagus, ultrasound can provide more detailed information on the heart or investigate organs deep within the body, such as the stomach and pancreas. The transducer can also be inserted into the vagina on a probe to examine the female reproductive organs. Ultrasound can be used on the eye to locate foreign bodies or to investigate disorders, such as retinal detachment (p.578). It can also be used to guide tissue sampling by pinpointing an abnormal area, such as in a prostate gland biopsy (p.726).

Doppler ultrasound scans are routinely used to investigate blood vessels in which blood flow may be reduced. For example, Doppler scans are often used to detect blood clots in the veins (*see* DEEP VEIN THROMBOSIS, p.437) and to detect thickened artery walls, particularly in the arteries in the neck (*see* CAROTID DOPPLER SCANNING, p.531). In pregnant women with high blood pressure, Doppler ultrasound may be used to investigate the uterine artery, which carries blood to the uterus.

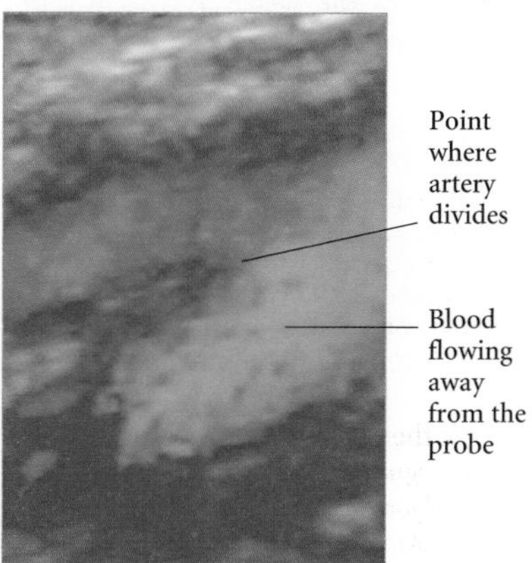

Doppler ultrasound scan of an artery
The colour of the blood on a Doppler ultrasound scan indicates direction of flow. The blue in the scan above indicates blood that is flowing away from the probe.

WHAT ARE THE RISKS?

Ultrasound scanning is not thought to cause any adverse effects and can be repeated as often as necessary. It is the only imaging technique considered safe for routine screening of a fetus.

Radionuclide scanning

A technique in which a radioactive substance is introduced into the body to assess structure and function of tissues

The technique of radionuclide scanning produces images using radiation emitted from a substance within the body. The radioactive substance, called a radionuclide, is introduced into the body and taken up by the organ or tissue to be imaged. A counter positioned outside the body detects the radiation that is emitted by the radionuclide and transmits this information to a computer. The computer then converts the information into images. Radionuclide scanning is used both to image the structure of many internal organs and to provide a measure of their function. SPECT scanning (p.253) and PET scanning (p.253) are two specialized forms of radionuclide scanning.

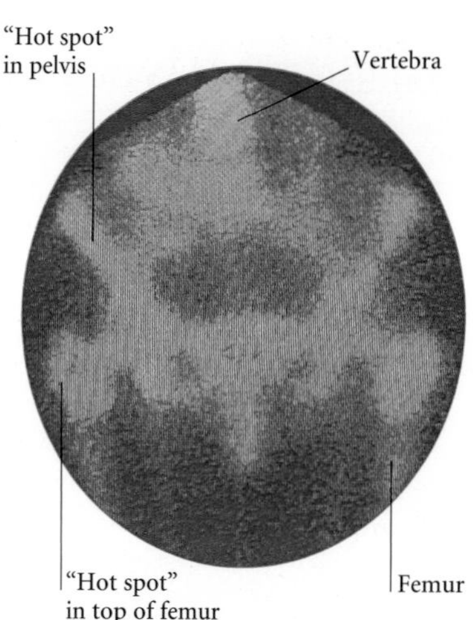

Radionuclide bone scan
This radionuclide scan of the pelvis shows "hot spots" where there is increased uptake of radioactive substance by the bone tissue. In this case, they are cancerous deposits.

HOW DOES IT WORK?

Radionuclides are normally introduced into the body by a single intravenous injection and are then carried in the bloodstream to the tissues (*see* HAVING A RADIONUCLIDE SCAN, p.252). Xenon gas, one particular type of radionuclide used during a lung scan, is inhaled (*see* RADIONUCLIDE LUNG SCANNING, p.494).

Different tissues take up different radionuclides. A specific radionuclide is chosen because it will accumulate in the particular tissues to be investigated. For example, iodine is taken up by the thyroid gland, and radioactive iodine is therefore injected intravenously to produce a radionuclide scan of the gland.

A radionuclide emits radiation in the form of gamma rays, which are similar to X-rays. The gamma rays are detected outside the body by a device called a gamma camera. Within the camera are detectors that pick up the radiation and convert information about its quantity and location into a form that can be analysed by a computer. The computer

PROCEDURE HAVING A RADIONUCLIDE SCAN

Radionuclide scanning is used both to image structures and to assess their function. In most cases, an injection of a radioactive substance (radionuclide) is given before the scan, but you may be asked to inhale radioactive gas if your lungs are being scanned (*see* RADIONUCLIDE LUNG SCANNING, p.494). The choice of radionuclide depends on the structure being imaged. During the scan, you lie still on a motorized bed and the radiographer moves you and a camera into position. The camera detects radiation emitted by the radionuclide, and a computer builds up an image.

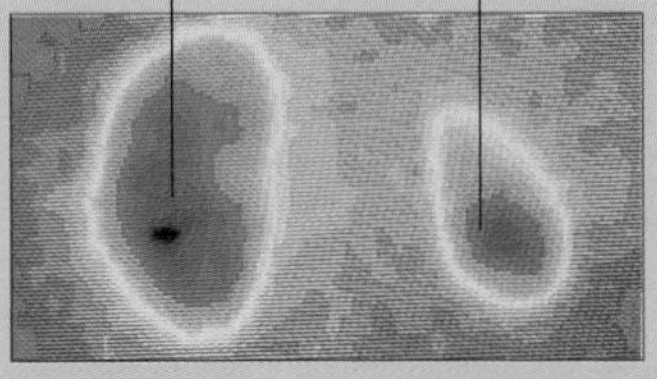

Radionuclide scan of kidneys
The kidney seen on the right emits less radiation because it is damaged and takes up less of the radionuclide.

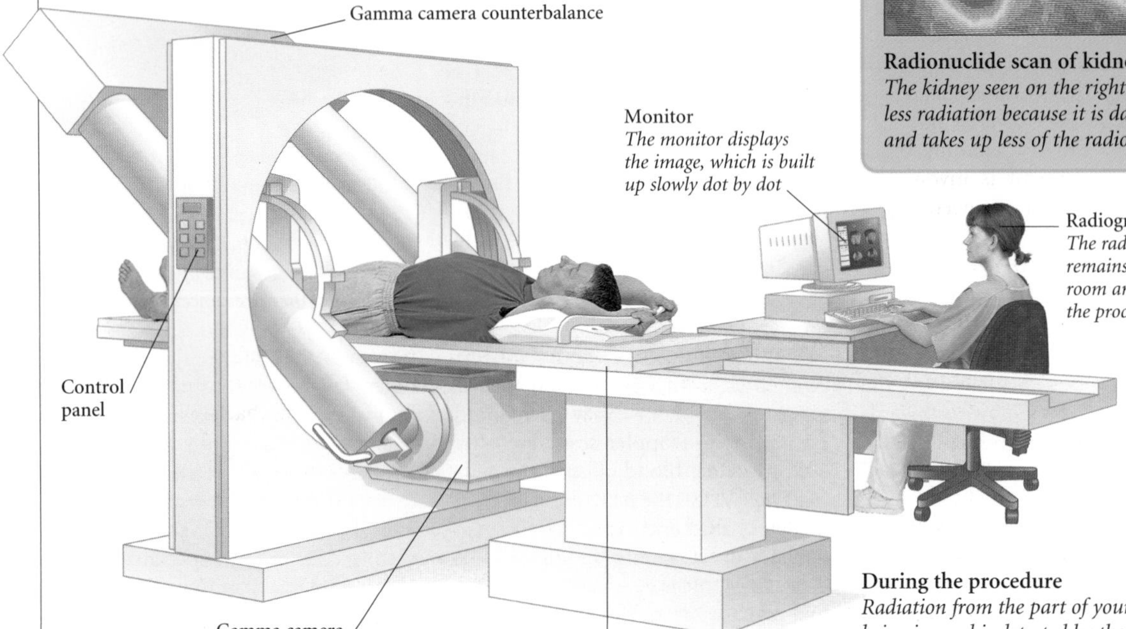

During the procedure
Radiation from the part of your body being imaged is detected by the gamma camera, and the information is sent to a computer. Most scans last 30–60 minutes.

then builds up an image and displays it on a monitor. The image is built up dot by dot, with each dot representing a certain amount of radiation.

Radionuclide scans show parts of the body as areas of colour of varying intensity. Areas of intense colour are called hot spots; these are areas where there is a high uptake of radionuclide. Areas of less intense colour, called cold spots, are areas where the radionuclide uptake is low. The greater the amount of tissue activity, the greater the uptake.

WHAT IS IT USED FOR?

An important feature of radionuclide scanning is that it can produce a "map" of an organ based on the activity of its tissues, therefore providing information about how that organ or tissue is functioning. This imaging technique may be used to detect abnormal levels of activity in organs such as the thyroid gland and kidneys, and it is useful for detecting some tumours of these organs. A radionuclide scan of bone will indicate areas that have increased activity, which might be due to problems such as Paget's disease of the bone (p.370) or cancer. Changes in the function of a tissue or an organ often develop before structural changes occur, and radionuclide scanning can detect some diseases at a significantly earlier stage than most other imaging techniques. For example, a radionuclide scan of bone can detect infection of bone tissue (*see* OSTEOMYELITIS, p.372) weeks before it would become apparent on an ordinary X-ray.

Radionuclide scans are particularly useful for assessing how well a treatment has worked. Scans may be done before and after a particular treatment to compare the function of an organ.

Two particular types of radionuclide scanning may be used to look at the function of the heart. Thallium scanning reveals areas of the heart muscle with a poor blood supply and is used to look at the activity of the heart muscle during exercise (*see* EXERCISE TESTING, p.407). MUGA (multiple-gated acquisition scanning) is a technique in which the blood flow into and out of the heart is measured to assess how efficiently the heart pumps blood around the body.

WHAT ARE THE RISKS?

Radionuclide scanning has no immediate risks, but radiation-based imaging may damage the body cells, leading to an increased risk of cancer in later life (*see* RADIATION DOSES, p.246). However, radionuclides are always administered in very small amounts, and they break down quickly in the body.

SPECT scanning

A type of radionuclide scanning that produces images of blood flow to tissues

First used in the 1970s for research, single-photon-emission computerized tomography (SPECT) scanning is now used for imaging. This technique is a specialized type of radionuclide scanning (p.251) and provides information on blood flow to various body tissues.

SPECT scanning is extremely sensitive and can target certain organs more easily than ordinary radionuclide scanning procedures. However, only a few centres offer SPECT scanning because expensive equipment is involved and specialist technicians are needed.

How does it work?

Before a SPECT scan, a radioactive substance (radionuclide) is intravenously injected. Radionuclides are distributed in the blood and are taken up by specific tissues. The more blood flowing through the tissues, the more radionuclide is taken up. The radionuclide emits radiation in the form of particles called photons. Photons are detected outside the body by a rotating camera, which can move through 360°. A computer converts the information from the camera into cross-sectional images, on which the different tissues or organs can be coloured to assist identification. SPECT scanning can be used to produce both vertical and horizontal cross sections through the body, and the data can also be manipulated by a computer to produce three-dimensional images.

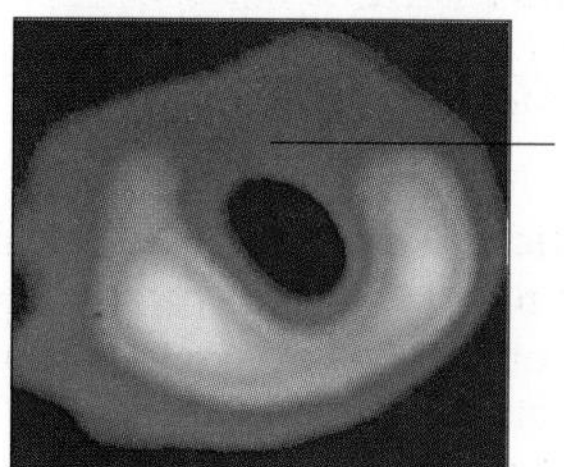

BEFORE SURGERY

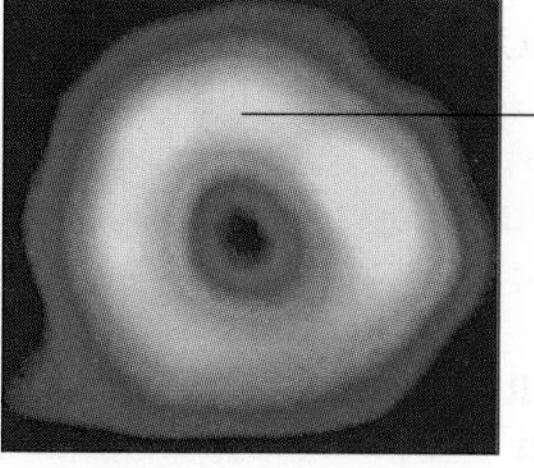

AFTER SURGERY

SPECT scans of heart muscle

These SPECT scans show horizontal cross sections through the heart. Before surgery, the absence of radionuclide in part of the heart indicates there is no blood flow in that area. Surgery restores the blood flow.

What is it used for?

SPECT scanning is mainly used to find out how well an organ is functioning by looking at the supply of blood to its tissues. SPECT scanning is particularly useful for assessing the function of the brain, heart, liver, and lungs.

What are the risks?

SPECT scanning presents no immediate risks to health, but it does involve radioactive substances and therefore has the potential to damage the body cells, which may increase the risk of cancer in later life (*see* RADIATION DOSES, p.246). However, SPECT scanning uses only small amounts of radionuclides, which break down quickly in the body.

PET scanning

A type of radionuclide scanning that creates an image based on the function of individual cells within an organ or tissue

Positron emission tomography (PET) scanning is a special form of radionuclide scanning (p.251). The technique was originally used as a research tool in the 1970s, and until recently its use was often restricted to research and teaching because the equipment it involves is expensive. However, PET scanning is now increasingly being used for imaging. Unlike certain other techniques, such as CT scanning (p.247), PET does not produce good structural images; instead, it gives information about the chemical activity of tissues or organs. It can also be used to assess blood flow.

How does it work?

By measuring the uptake by a tissue or organ of certain molecules, such as glucose or oxygen, doctors can assess how well an organ is functioning. The molecules that are to be taken up by the tissue or organ are labelled with a radioactive substance (radionuclide) before being introduced into the body.

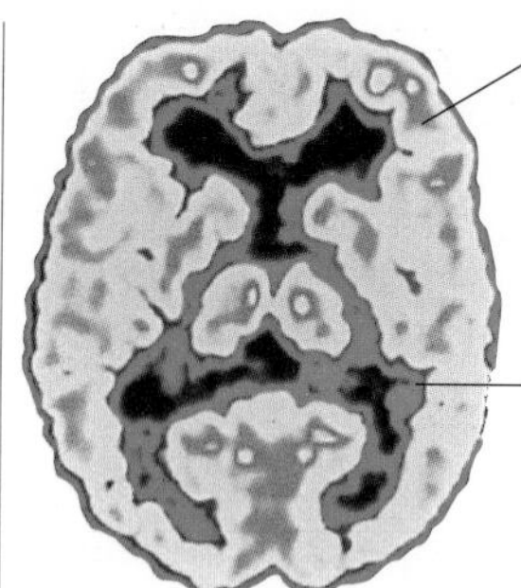

PET scan of brain

This normal PET scan shows high activity on the outside of the brain, the grey matter, and lower activity deeper inside.

PET uses radionuclides that emit particles called positrons. The radiation that these particles generate is detected by a PET scanner. The number of positrons emitted by an area of tissue or an organ indicates how much radionuclide it has taken up and therefore how chemically active that region is. A PET scanner is a doughnut-shaped machine incorporating detectors that pick up radiation all around the patient. The technique produces cross-sectional images that can be colour coded according to the concentration of radioactivity.

What is it used for?

PET is mainly used to study the brain and the heart. The radionuclides used in PET can label the molecules related to blood flow as well as those involved in chemical activity. Consequently, PET can show areas of decreased blood flow while also establishing whether the cells in the area being studied are still chemically active and capable of recovery or whether they are dead. PET scanning is used to locate the origin of epileptic activity (*see* EPILEPSY, p.524) in the brain and investigate brain function in certain mental health problems, such as depression (p.554). PET is also used to detect tumours because the level of chemical activity in abnormal tissue is higher than that in healthy tissue.

What are the risks?

Like in other radiation-based imaging techniques, PET scanning carries a risk of cell damage that may lead to cancer later in life (*see* RADIATION DOSES, p.246). However, radionuclides are used in small amounts and rapidly break down into harmless elements.

VIEWING TECHNIQUES

Viewing structures or organs in the body is often important for screening, diagnosis, or monitoring disease. Structures that are easily accessible, such as the ears, may be viewed directly using basic viewing instruments; those deeper inside the body are usually viewed indirectly, using complex optical instruments called endoscopes to transmit images on to a monitor screen.

Some viewing techniques may be used as part of a routine examination. For example, your doctor can look at your ears, eyes, and throat simply and quickly in his or her surgery. Each of the instruments used is designed to view a particular part of the body. For example, an otoscope is used to look at the ears and an ophthalmoscope to look at the eyes. The first article covers these basic viewing techniques.

To view other organs deeper within the body, your doctor may arrange for an endoscopic investigation. Endoscopy is discussed in the second article. An endoscope is a tube-like viewing device through which body cavities or hollow internal organs can be inspected. Endoscopes may be flexible or rigid and vary in length and diameter. Each type of endoscope is designed to view a particular part of the body.

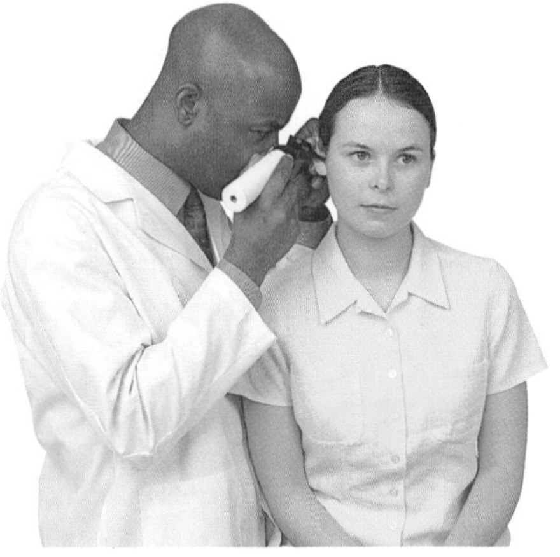

Inspecting the ear
During a routine checkup, your doctor may use a special viewing device called an otoscope to look inside the ear and examine the ear canal and eardrum.

Basic viewing techniques

The use of simple instruments to look at tissues near the surface of the body

Instruments that can be used to view body structures and organs directly have been developed and improved considerably over the past 100 years. Some of these instruments have been replaced by endoscopes (*see* ENDOSCOPY, opposite page). However, some basic viewing instruments are still frequently used in a doctor's surgery as part of a routine examination because they are simple to use and cause minimal discomfort.

HOW DO THEY WORK?

In order to examine the interior of a natural opening, such as the ear canal, your doctor will usually need a source of light that can be focused on the area to be examined and some form of magnification. These two elements are often incorporated into a single viewing instrument, such as an otoscope, which is used for inspecting the ear.

For other natural openings, such as the vagina or nose, your doctor may need to use an additional instrument, called a speculum, to hold the passage open and keep other structures out of the way during viewing. In some cases, a speculum may also be used to make access easier and to enable the doctor to take samples of tissue.

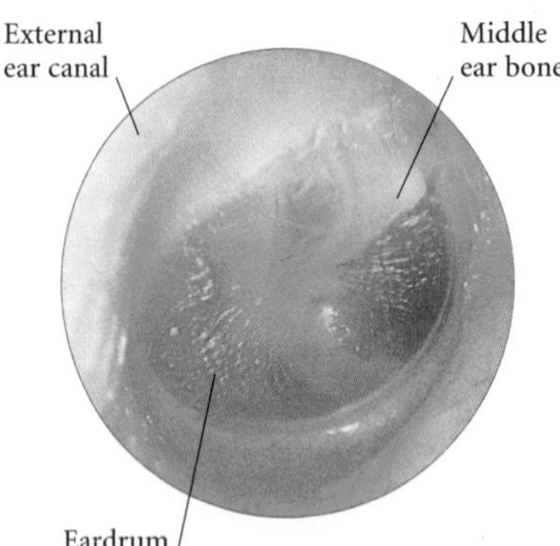

View through an otoscope
This view shows a healthy eardrum and ear canal as a doctor would see it through an otoscope. One of the bones of the middle ear is visible through the eardrum.

The light-sensitive retina at the back of the eye can be viewed from the outside through the pupil. The instrument used to do this, called an ophthalmoscope, incorporates magnifying lenses and a source of light.

WHAT ARE THEY USED FOR?

Your doctor may perform basic viewing techniques as part of a routine physical examination to assess a particular area of the body or to investigate symptoms in that area. For example, if you have earache, your doctor may examine your ear (*see* OTOSCOPY, p.597), and to investigate hoarseness, your doctor may look at your larynx (voice box) by using a procedure known as mirror laryngoscopy (p.481). Basic viewing techniques can also be part of screening procedures. For example, if you have a long-term disorder such as diabetes mellitus (p.687), which is associated with retinal damage, your doctor may examine your eyes by means of ophthalmoscopy (p.578) and slit-lamp examination (p.574) so that he or she can detect damage at an early stage. In addition, some types of tissue sample, such as tissue from the cervix, can be taken with the help of a viewing instrument (*see* COLPOSCOPY, p.750).

In some cases, it is possible to take photographs through basic viewing instruments, such as an ophthalmoscope. Photographs taken at different times can be compared to monitor a condition.

WHAT ARE THE RISKS?

An examination using basic viewing techniques is completely safe and may be repeated as often as necessary to monitor or screen for a disorder. Most examinations cause little or no discomfort, and anaesthesia is not usually necessary. However, when viewing the larynx and throat, a local anaesthetic spray may be used to numb the throat.

PROCEDURE FLEXIBLE ENDOSCOPY

Flexible endoscopy uses a specially designed viewing instrument to investigate organs and structures inside the body. Before you undergo an endoscopic examination, you may be given an anaesthetic or sedative. The endoscope is inserted through a natural opening, such as the mouth, and is guided to the appropriate area by the specialist. A tiny camera at the tip of the endoscope sends views back to the eyepiece and monitor. Very fine surgical instruments may be passed down the endoscope, allowing minor procedures, such as the removal of tissue samples, to be carried out.

During the procedure
For an investigation of the stomach and duodenum, you will be asked to lie on your side. You may be sedated or have local anaesthetic sprayed on the back of your throat. A flexible endoscope is then passed into your digestive tract through your mouth.

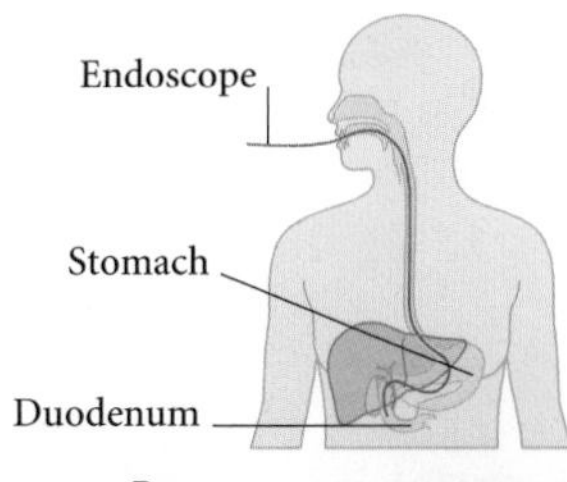

ROUTE OF ENDOSCOPE

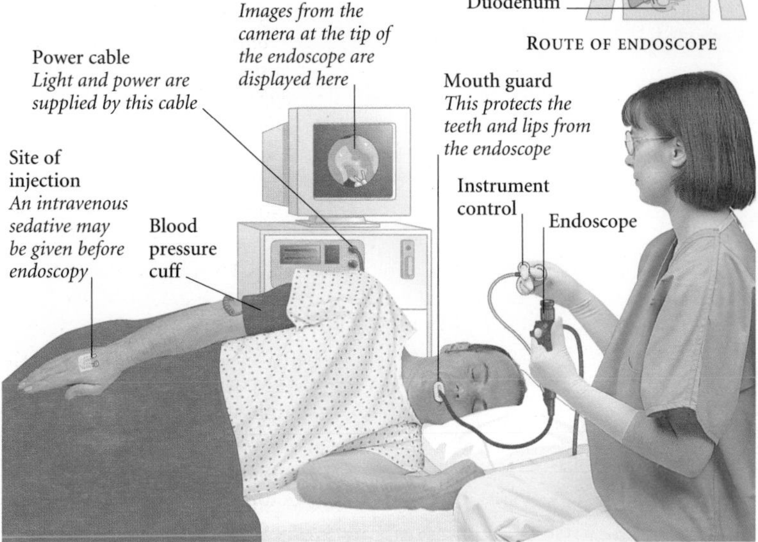

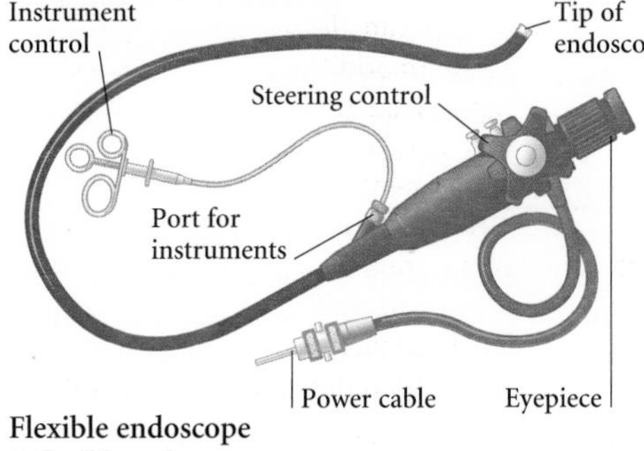

Flexible endoscope
A flexible endoscope contains separate channels to carry water, air, a camera lens, instruments, and optical fibres. A steering control guides the tip around bends in the structure to be viewed.

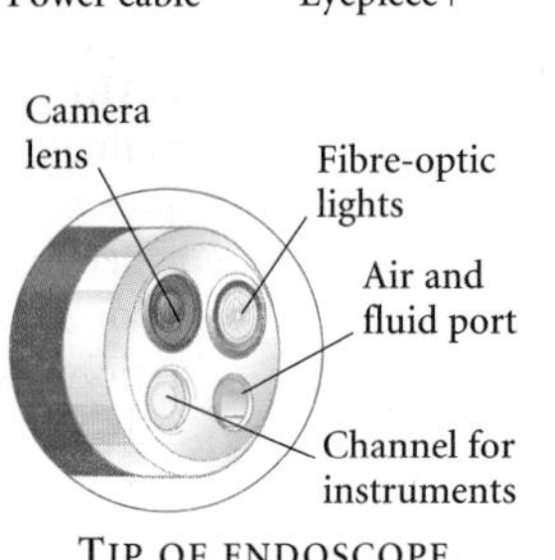

TIP OF ENDOSCOPE

VIEW

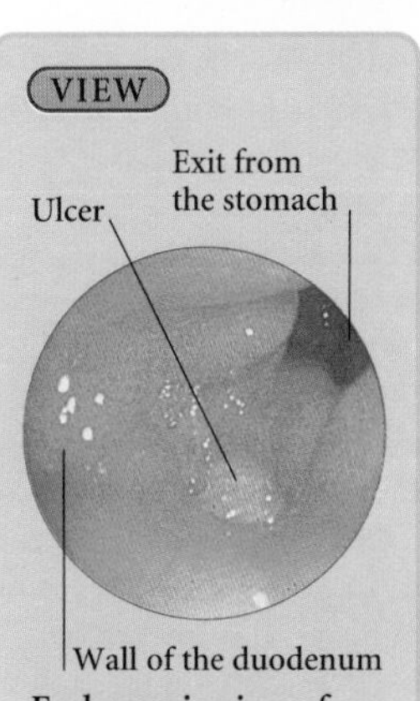

Endoscopic view of the duodenum
This endoscopic view shows the inside of the duodenum. An ulcer is visible on the wall.

Endoscopy

The use of tube-like instruments to look at organs or structures deep within the body

During endoscopy, a tube-like optical instrument known as an endoscope is introduced deep into the body so that internal structures can be examined visually. Access into the body is usually through a natural opening, such as the mouth or anus, although some endoscopes are introduced through small incisions made in the skin.

The first endoscopes were rigid, but various flexible instruments have been developed since the 1960s. Although most endoscopes now in routine use are flexible, rigid types are preferred in certain cases, including investigations in which there is a short distance from the skin to the structure being viewed, such as in an examination of the knee joint.

HOW DO THEY WORK?

There are many types of endoscope, each specifically designed to investigate a particular part of the body. Flexible and rigid endoscopes differ in appearance, but they share many of the same features and operate in a similar way. For example, both forms of endoscope use light, reflection, and magnification to show body structures clearly.

FLEXIBLE ENDOSCOPES The development of flexible endoscopes has been made possible by the invention of fibre-optics. Fibre-optics use thin, flexible fibres of glass or plastic (optical fibres) that transmit light along their length by internal reflections. The main part of a flexible endoscope consists of a long, thin tube containing several channels that run along its length. Some channels in the endoscope carry optical fibres to provide light or transmit the image back up to the eyepiece. Other channels contain wires to control the direction of the endoscope. Channels may also be used to pump or suck air or fluid into or out of the area being examined. Other channels may be used to pass down various instruments, such as biopsy forceps or scissors.

Most flexible endoscopes now have a miniature camera built into their tip, and the view recorded by the camera is displayed on a monitor. This facility

PROCEDURE RIGID ENDOSCOPY

Rigid endoscopes can be used to examine various internal organs and structures, especially joints and the external surfaces of organs within the abdominal cavity, such as the ovaries. The most frequently investigated joint is the knee, primarily because damage to it is common. Investigations using rigid endoscopes are often carried out under general anaesthesia. The endoscope is inserted through a small incision made in the skin. Further small incisions may be made for other instruments, such as forceps. The internal structures may be viewed on a monitor or through an eyepiece.

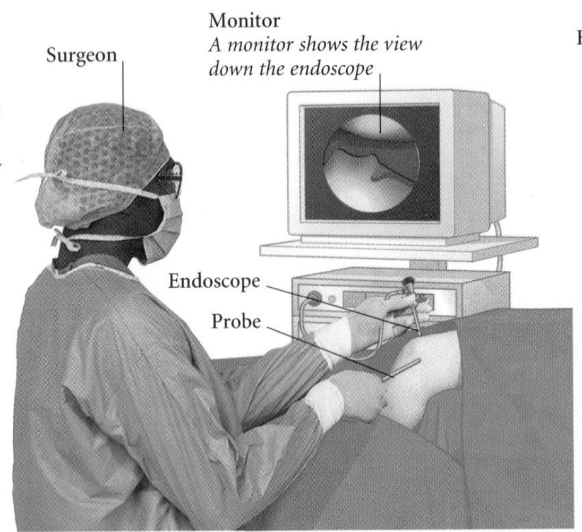

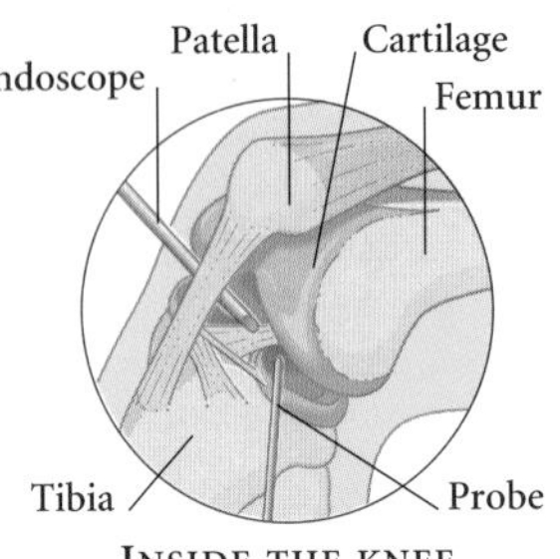

INSIDE THE KNEE

During the procedure
For endoscopy of the knee joint, you will be given a general anaesthetic. Small incisions are made on either side of the knee through which the endoscope and other instruments are passed.

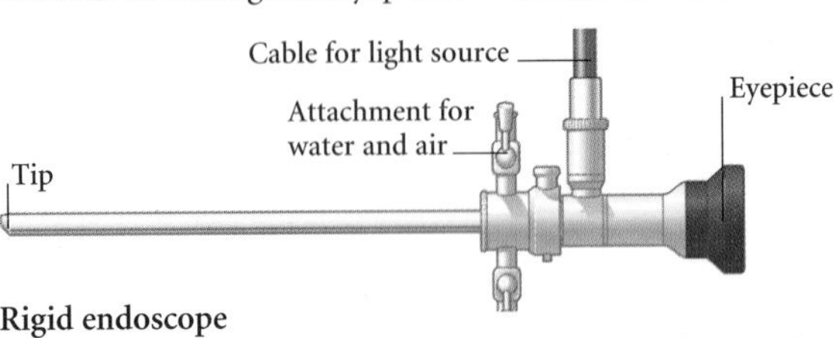

Rigid endoscope
A rigid endoscope is a straight, narrow metal tube with an eyepiece at one end to which a camera can be attached if necessary. A light source is connected to the endoscope and illuminates the structure or organ. Water and air can be pumped down the tube if necessary.

VIEW

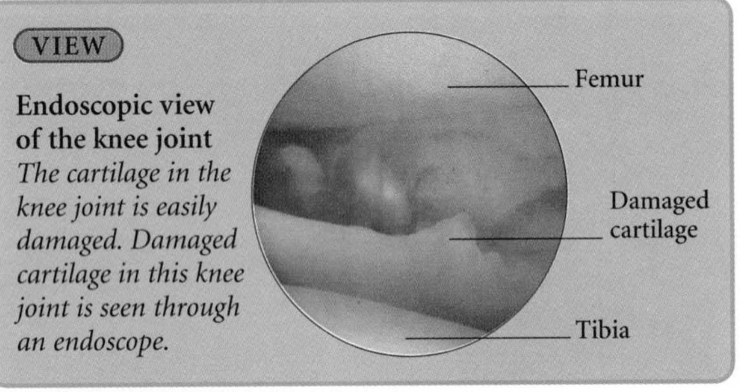

Endoscopic view of the knee joint
The cartilage in the knee joint is easily damaged. Damaged cartilage in this knee joint is seen through an endoscope.

allows the doctor and his or her colleagues, and sometimes the patient, to observe an investigation together and makes it possible for a videotaped record to be kept for reference.

RIGID ENDOSCOPES These endoscopes are normally much shorter than flexible endoscopes and are usually inserted through an incision in the skin. Like flexible endoscopes, rigid endoscopes use a fibre-optic light source. However, other instruments, such as those used to hold tissues out of the way or to perform a surgical procedure, are passed through a separate incision rather than down the endoscope.

To allow the surfaces of the different organs or structures to be seen clearly, investigations using rigid endoscopes often involve expanding the organ or body cavity with gas or fluid to separate tissue surfaces. For example, air may be pumped into the abdomen during a laparoscopy (p.742) so that the abdominal organs can be examined.

WHAT ARE THEY USED FOR?

Flexible endoscopes are particularly useful for looking at the digestive and respiratory tracts, which bend in places (*see* FLEXIBLE ENDOSCOPY, p.255). For example, nasendoscopes are very thin, short, flexible endoscopes that are used to inspect the nasal cavity and the surrounding sinuses (*see* ENDOSCOPY OF THE NOSE AND THROAT, p.476). Rigid endoscopes are used to investigate the abdominal cavity and joints (*see* RIGID ENDOSCOPY, above), where the structure to be viewed is near the skin surface.

If an abnormality is discovered during endoscopy, samples can be taken and, in some cases, treatment can be administered immediately. Instruments may be passed either down the channels of an endoscope or through small incisions in the skin in order to enable the doctor to carry out certain procedures such as taking tissue samples or removing foreign bodies. An endoscope can also be used to introduce a contrast medium into a particular site so that detailed images can then be produced on X-rays (*see* ERCP, p.653).

Some surgical procedures, such as removal of the gallbladder, that used to require a lengthy operation and a large incision can now be carried out far more quickly and easily using instruments together with a rigid endoscope (*see* ENDOSCOPIC SURGERY, p.948).

WHAT ARE THE RISKS?

Endoscopy is generally very safe, but, in rare cases, the endoscope may perforate an organ's wall. For example, if the endoscope is in the stomach, it may pierce the digestive tract. Immediate surgery will then be needed to repair the damage. If a tissue sample is taken, there may be some bleeding from the site.

For some endoscopic investigations, general anaesthesia or sedation may be required (*see* HAVING A GENERAL ANAESTHETIC, p.944), and these carry risks of their own. Your doctor will therefore make sure that you are in sufficiently good health to undergo the procedure.

Your Body and Disease

This section covers a comprehensive range of diseases and disorders arranged mainly by body system. The normal anatomy and functioning of each body system is explained first, followed by articles on the disorders that affect that body system. Each article investigates the causes, symptoms, diagnosis, treatment options, and prognosis of the disorder concerned. Most of the articles direct you to online sites where further information can be found.

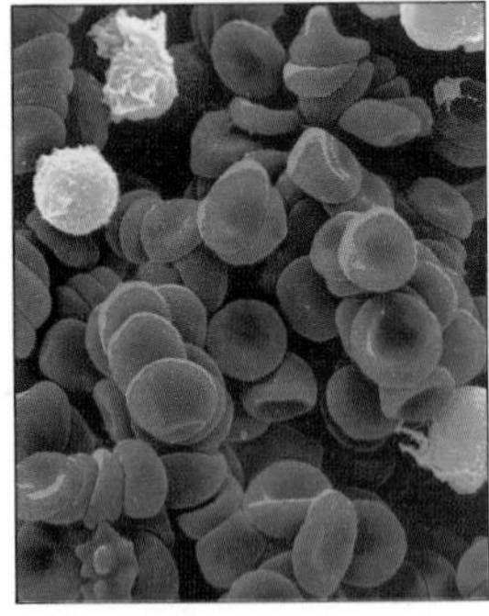

Blood cells
Two components of blood that are essential to health are white blood cells to fight disease and red blood cells to carry oxygen.

INTRODUCTION

HUMAN BEINGS ARE ROBUST AND ADAPTABLE, able to survive in a wide range of environments and to endure physical and psychological stress. The body's design incorporates systems that renew and repair it continuously and others that protect it from harm. Many trivial injuries or potential illnesses heal themselves or are controlled before we are even aware of them. However, throughout a lifetime, we are exposed to a relentless stream of minor and more serious diseases and injuries with a wide variety of effects on the body.

You become ill when something disrupts the normal healthy working of your body. Why you become ill at any particular time is a question with multiple answers, many of which focus on your genes. Some rare diseases are caused by an inherited faulty gene, but genes are also a contributing factor in many other illnesses. In particular, they predict to some extent your chance of developing some of the major diseases of adult life, such as cancer and stroke. Genes also help to determine your susceptibility to many mental health problems. However, genes are only part of the story. Your age, your environment, and the way you live are all factors that affect your chance of falling ill.

One hundred years ago, people were most at risk from infectious diseases. New drugs, immunizations, and advances in hygiene and public sanitation have dramatically reduced mortality from infectious diseases in the developed world, although they remain a major threat to health in the developing world. Today, the major causes of death in the UK are heart disease, cancer, stroke, and accidents. These causes are strongly associated with lifestyle, and the risk of each one can be reduced by changes in behaviour. As a result, the emphasis in medicine has changed, and doctors now recognize that prevention is as important as treatment.

When you are ill
Recovery from most minor illnesses is usually quick, but at some time in life you may have a more serious disease that needs hospital treatment.

UNDERSTANDING THE BODY

When you become ill, you want to know what has caused the problem, how it will affect you, and how it can be treated. Understanding disease is easier if you already have some appreciation of the normal structure and function of your body and the way in which its various components are organized.

The body can be divided into a number of major systems that carry out vital functions. For example, the respiratory system enables you to breathe, and the immune system protects you from infection and some diseases. The bones, muscles, nerves, skin, blood, and other tissues that make up body systems are made of billions of connected cells. Each cell is a specialized, fully functioning unit, and all its activities are controlled by the genetic code contained in the DNA (deoxyribonucleic acid) in its nucleus.

In this book, diseases and disorders are mainly grouped in sections under the body system that they affect. Each section begins with a description of the normal anatomy and physiology of a body system to help you to understand the disorders that follow.

STRUCTURE AND FUNCTION THE HUMAN BODY

The body consists of various systems that interact with each other. Making up these systems are organs and tissues that work together to carry out a specific body function, such as digestion. The different types of tissue that make up organs and other body parts are highly specialized. For example, the stomach has muscular walls for churning food and a mucosa lining that secretes gastric juices and protective mucus. The interconnected cells that make up these tissues each contain genes that programme cell activities.

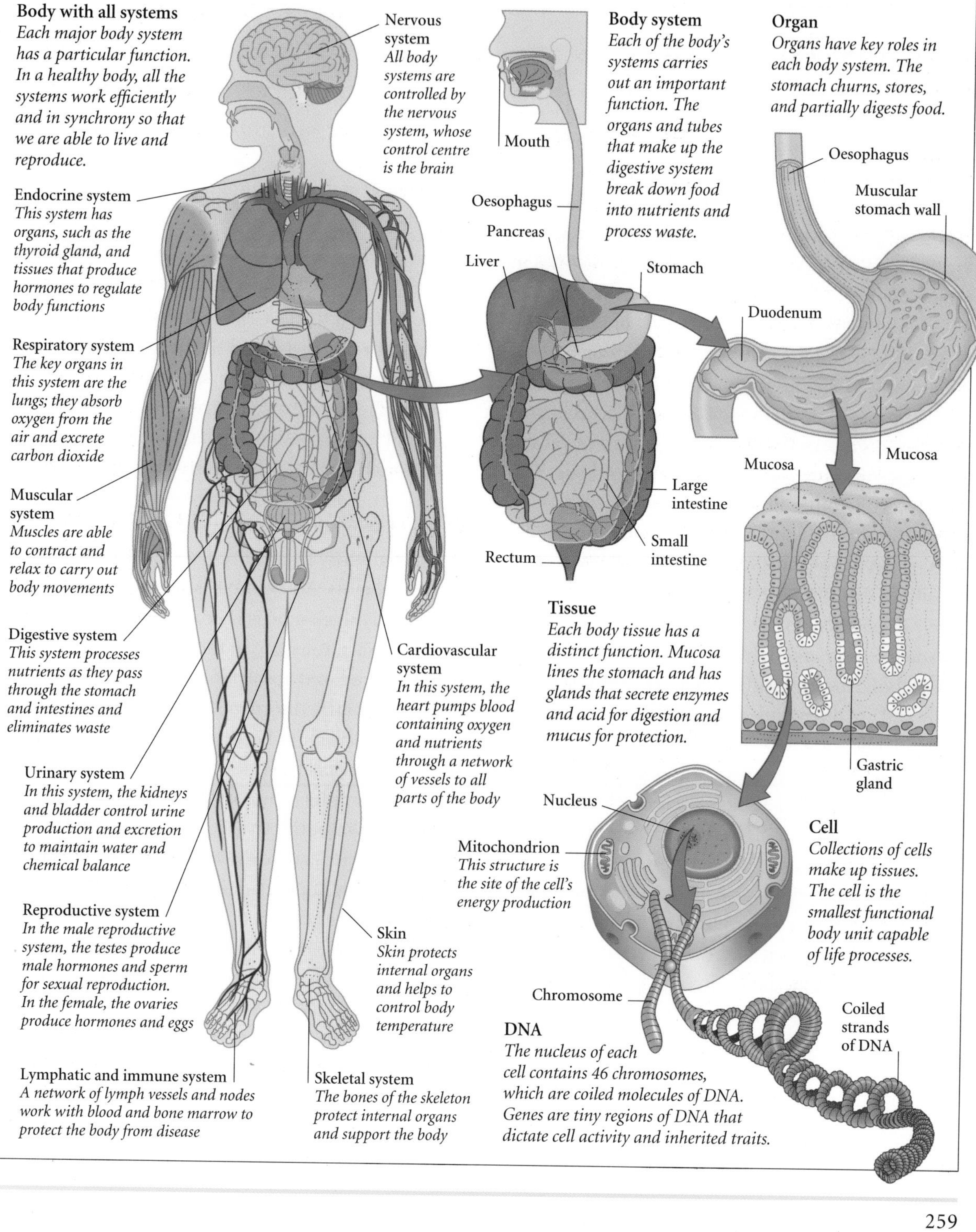

Body with all systems
Each major body system has a particular function. In a healthy body, all the systems work efficiently and in synchrony so that we are able to live and reproduce.

Endocrine system
This system has organs, such as the thyroid gland, and tissues that produce hormones to regulate body functions

Respiratory system
The key organs in this system are the lungs; they absorb oxygen from the air and excrete carbon dioxide

Muscular system
Muscles are able to contract and relax to carry out body movements

Digestive system
This system processes nutrients as they pass through the stomach and intestines and eliminates waste

Urinary system
In this system, the kidneys and bladder control urine production and excretion to maintain water and chemical balance

Reproductive system
In the male reproductive system, the testes produce male hormones and sperm for sexual reproduction. In the female, the ovaries produce hormones and eggs

Lymphatic and immune system
A network of lymph vessels and nodes work with blood and bone marrow to protect the body from disease

Nervous system
All body systems are controlled by the nervous system, whose control centre is the brain

Cardiovascular system
In this system, the heart pumps blood containing oxygen and nutrients through a network of vessels to all parts of the body

Skin
Skin protects internal organs and helps to control body temperature

Skeletal system
The bones of the skeleton protect internal organs and support the body

Body system
Each of the body's systems carries out an important function. The organs and tubes that make up the digestive system break down food into nutrients and process waste.

Mouth
Oesophagus
Pancreas
Liver
Stomach
Large intestine
Small intestine
Rectum

Organ
Organs have key roles in each body system. The stomach churns, stores, and partially digests food.

Oesophagus
Muscular stomach wall
Duodenum
Mucosa
Mucosa

Tissue
Each body tissue has a distinct function. Mucosa lines the stomach and has glands that secrete enzymes and acid for digestion and mucus for protection.

Gastric gland

Cell
Collections of cells make up tissues. The cell is the smallest functional body unit capable of life processes.

Nucleus

Mitochondrion
This structure is the site of the cell's energy production

Chromosome

Coiled strands of DNA

DNA
The nucleus of each cell contains 46 chromosomes, which are coiled molecules of DNA. Genes are tiny regions of DNA that dictate cell activity and inherited traits.

When you have a problem, you may be referred to a doctor who specializes in disorders that affect a particular body system or organ. For example, you may see a gastroenterologist for digestive system disorders or a dermatologist for skin disorders. However, diseases can also be categorized according to the mechanisms by which they damage the body.

How disease affects the body

The different ways in which diseases damage the body are called disease processes. Several body systems may be damaged by the same process. For example, the major cause of disability and death in the UK, coronary artery disease, comes under the heading of ischaemic disease. This term applies to all diseases in which there are changes in blood vessels, such as a build-up of fatty deposits, that restrict blood flow and starve organs and tissues of oxygen-carrying blood.

Similarly, cancerous tumours, which are the second leading cause of death in the UK, can affect many different organs and tissues, but all consist of cells that reproduce uncontrollably, invade healthy tissue, and may spread to other sites in the body.

Infections form another category and range from minor skin complaints, such as boils, to major infectious diseases, such as meningitis. Infections occur when microscopic organisms, such as bacteria, invade the body, multiply, and disrupt cell function.

Metabolic disorders affect chemical processes in the body and are often caused by a failure to produce a particular enzyme or by malfunction of a hormone-producing gland. For example, in one type of diabetes mellitus, normal blood sugar levels cannot be maintained because cells in the pancreas produce insufficient amounts of the hormone insulin.

A number of neurological illnesses and mental health problems are caused by disorders of brain chemistry. Diseases such as Alzheimer's disease and depression are associated with imbalances in the levels of neurotransmitters, chemicals that transmit nerve signals. However, no chemical or structural factor has been found for many other mental health problems.

Autoimmune disorders are a group of complicated diseases in which the immune system, which helps to protect the body from infections and cancer, attacks the body's own tissue. Cells or tissues are slowly damaged or destroyed, and the function of an organ or gland may be affected. For example, in rheumatoid arthritis, the immune system attacks and damages the linings of joints, causing pain and sometimes disability.

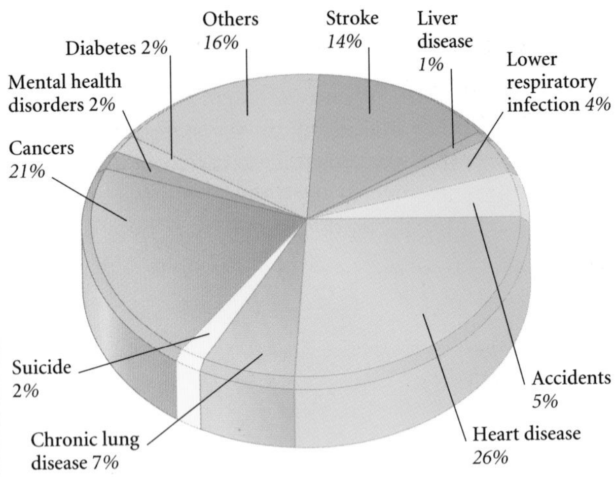

Major causes of death in Europe
Heart disease is the major cause of death in Europe, followed by cancers, stroke, and chronic lung disease. Incidence of these diseases is high because they occur later in life, and people are living longer, and because of lifestyle factors, such as smoking.

Although inheritance is increasingly being found to play a part in many major diseases, there is a distinct group of several thousand rare genetic disorders that are caused solely by a faulty gene inherited from one or both parents. An example is cystic fibrosis, in which abnormally thick mucus is produced in the lungs and digestive tract, resulting in the destruction of lung tissue and reduced absorption of food.

In degenerative disorders, the structure and function of tissues and organs become gradually impaired by the loss of specialized cells or tissues. One of the most familiar examples is osteoarthritis, a gradual wearing away of the smooth cartilage that covers the surfaces of joints. Degenerative diseases have been traditionally associated with aging, but a growing number of diseases, such as cataract (a loss of transparency in the lens of the eye), are being found to have other causes, such as exposure to strong sunlight, toxins, radiation, and prolonged use of certain drugs.

Injury is a category that covers all types of deliberate and accidental damage to the body. Every year in the UK, there are about 16,000 fatal injuries. The major cause of these injuries is traffic accidents, followed by falls, fires, homicides, and drowning.

Your susceptibility to disease

Some of the factors that contribute to your chance of becoming ill are your genes, ethnicity, age, and social and geographical environment. However, against this largely unalterable background, you can reduce your risk of illness by following the guidelines for healthy living described in another section of this book (*see* TAKING CONTROL OF YOUR HEALTH, pp.15–86).

Many illnesses can occur at any age. For example, at any time in life people may find themselves under the kind of pressures that can lead to psychological disorders. However, there are particular age groups that are vulnerable to certain types of illness or behave in a way that makes them susceptible to injury.

Babies are susceptible to infectious disease because their immune system is not fully developed and they have not had previous exposure to infections, and young children tend to have frequent accidents while their physical skills are still developing.

In their teens and in early adulthood, people have a relatively small chance of developing a serious illness

(PROCESS) Categories of disease

Many disorders have features in common and can be grouped into clear categories, according to the effect they have on the body. For example, all cancers are growths of faulty cells and all infections are caused by microorganisms invading the body. The other main groups of diseases are ischaemic, degenerative, genetic, metabolic, and autoimmune. Injury is a category that covers a wide variety of damage to the body.

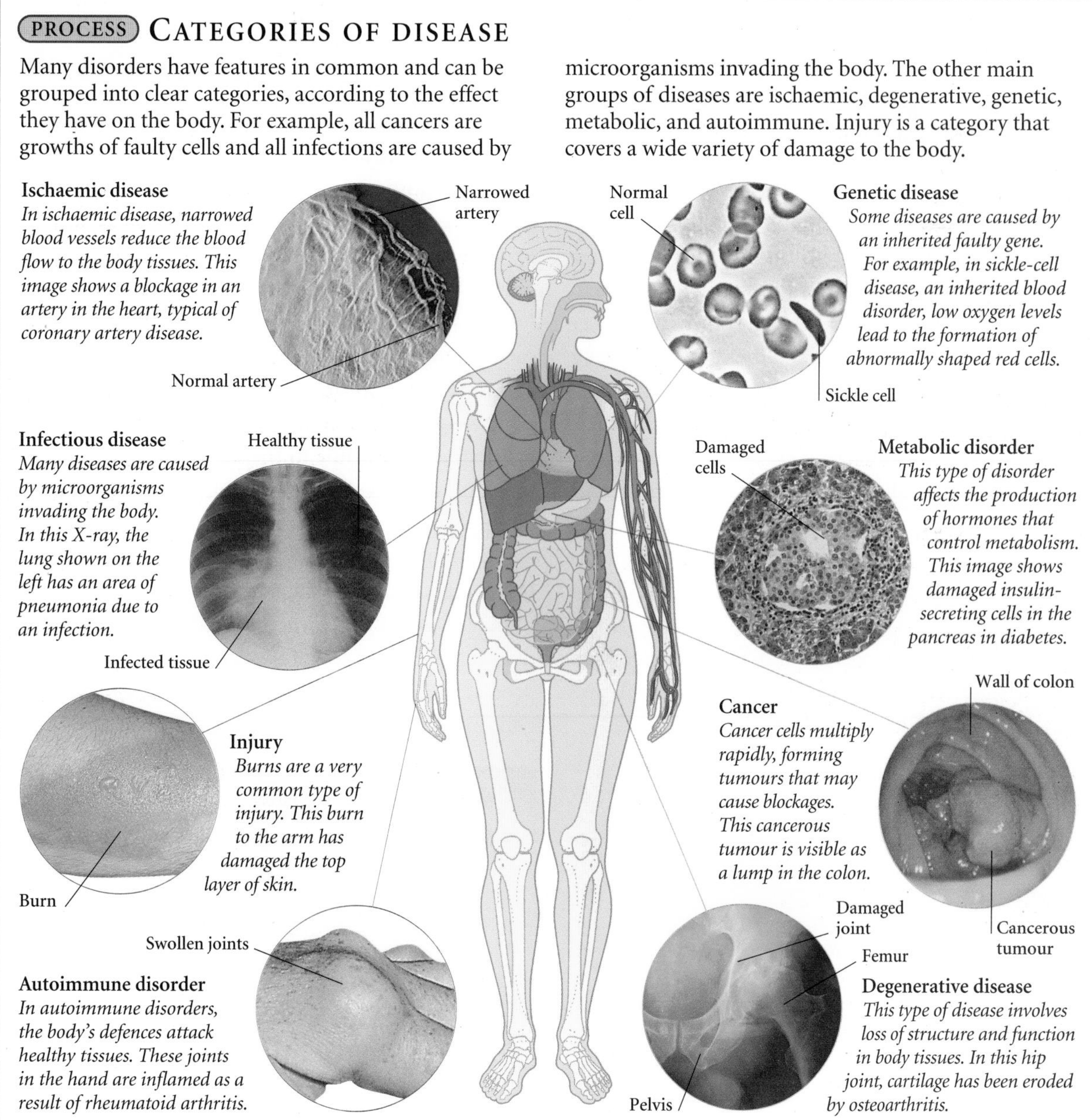

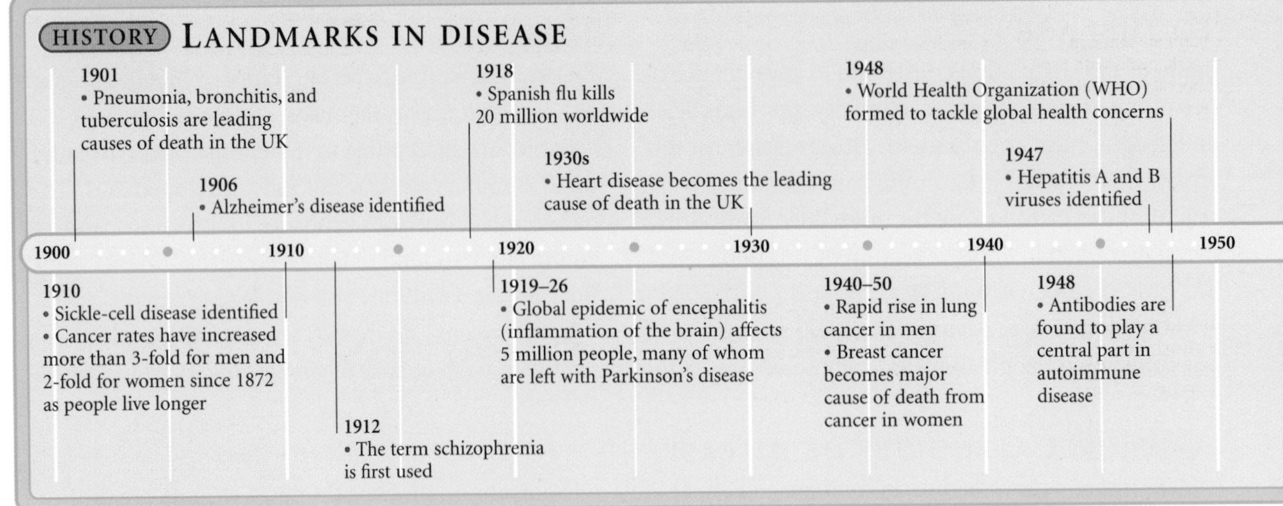

The rise and fall of disease
The decline, control, and, in some cases, eradication of infectious diseases during the past 100 years was countered by a steady rise in heart disease, cancers, and stroke. These major causes of death in the developed world are now becoming global health problems.

such as cancer but are more likely to injure themselves. For example, most disability and death in young men is associated with risk-taking behaviour involving vehicles and weapons. Adolescents are prone to eating disorders, depression, and substance abuse. A feeling of invulnerability in young people leads many to eat unhealthily, take insufficient exercise, smoke, and drink too much alcohol. These lifestyle factors mean trouble for the future because they contribute to many of the major diseases, such as heart disease, cancer, and stroke, that are increasingly common from middle age onwards. As people age, the incidence of long-term illness and disability increases, and, for some people, poor physical health leads to mental health problems.

Susceptibility to disease is closely linked to social factors. Some of the patterns of ill health seen in poorer countries are repeated in people with incomes below the poverty line. In the UK, rates of heart disease are three times higher in poor families than in those with a reasonable standard of living.

Changing patterns of disease

During the past 50 years, many major infectious diseases have been brought under control in the developed world, and smallpox, one of the oldest diseases of humanity, has been eradicated globally. However, AIDS, a deadly new disease caused by HIV infection, has emerged and is now a leading cause of death. In addition, tuberculosis (TB) has become harder to control, both because some strains have become resistant to antibiotics and because of the reduced immunity to disease in HIV-infected people.

For most of the 20th century, cardiovascular disease, cancer, and stroke have been major causes of death in developed parts of the world. They are also becoming increasingly common in developing societies, where factors that contribute to them, such as a high-fat diet, smoking, and a sedentary lifestyle, are seen as an integral part of a more affluent way of life.

The high incidence of these diseases is due in part to the increasing age of the population. As the number of people over the age of 65 is predicted to double by the year 2025, and the proportion of younger people is predicted to fall, these long-term diseases are likely to continue to be major global threats to health.

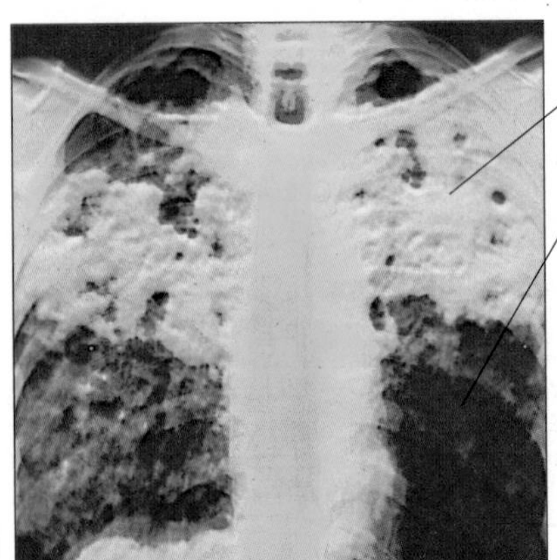

Lungs damaged by tuberculosis
This colour-enhanced chest X-ray shows areas of infected tissue at the top of the lungs due to tuberculosis.

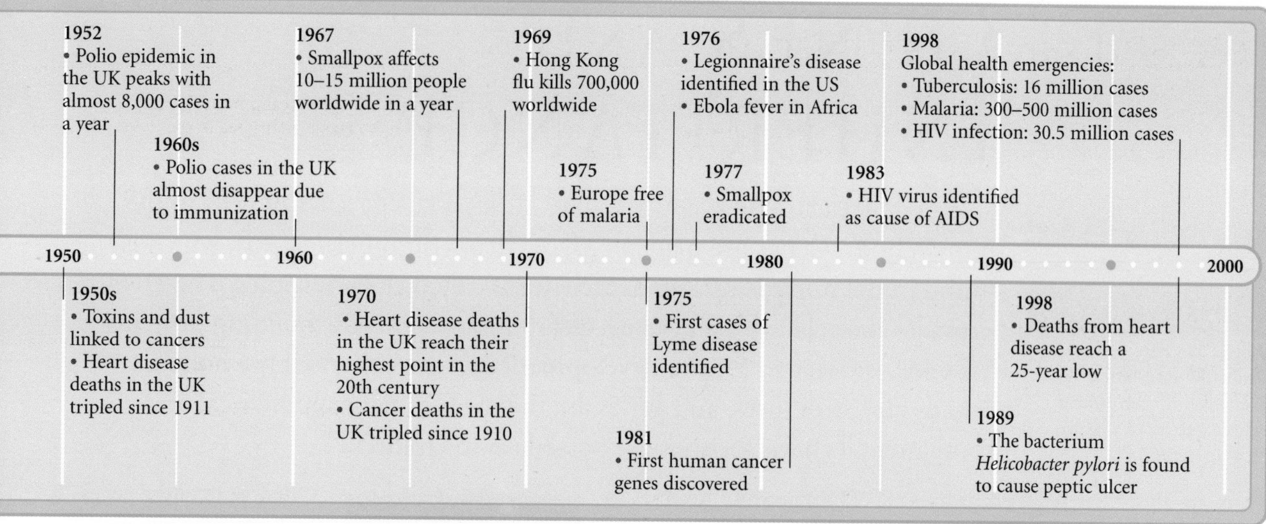

ORGANIZATION HOW THIS PART OF THE BOOK IS ORGANIZED

Most of this part of the book is organized into major body systems. Each of these sections begins with an illustrated guide to the structure and function of the system and its organs, followed by articles on the diseases affecting that system. There are separate sections on infections, which can affect any body system, serious multi-system injuries, and the principles of cancer. Disorders related to sex and reproduction and pregnancy and childbirth have their own sections, as do problems that exclusively affect children or problems that have different effects in children.

GENES AND INHERITANCE p.264
Introduction to disorders caused by chromosomal and genetic abnormalities.

CANCER p.274
The nature of cancer and the principles of its management. Specific cancers are covered with the relevant body system.

INFECTIONS AND INFESTATIONS p.284
Diseases resulting from infections and infestations. Some infections are covered with the body system they affect.

SERIOUS INJURIES AND ENVIRONMENTAL DISORDERS p.314
Major types of injury and their effects on the body; the effects of poisoning and adverse environmental factors.

SKIN, HAIR, AND NAILS p.328
Widespread and localized skin conditions; minor injuries; hair and nail disorders.

MUSCULOSKELETAL SYSTEM p.362
Diseases and injuries affecting joints, ligaments, bones, muscles, and tendons.

CARDIOVASCULAR SYSTEM p.396
Major diseases of the heart plus disorders affecting heart rate and rhythm; diseases of the major arteries and veins.

BLOOD AND THE LYMPHATIC AND IMMUNE SYSTEMS p.440
Disorders affecting blood and bone marrow and the vessels in the lymphatic system; immune disorders and allergies.

RESPIRATORY SYSTEM p.470
Nose and throat disorders, followed by diseases affecting the lungs.

NERVOUS SYSTEM AND MENTAL FUNCTION p.508
Diseases and disorders of the brain, spinal cord, and nerves; mental health problems.

EYES AND VISION p.566
Diseases, abnormalities, and injuries of the eyes, including vision disorders.

EARS, HEARING, AND BALANCE p.592
Ear disorders, including those affecting hearing and the balance mechanism.

TEETH AND GUMS p.606
Teeth and gum disorders, routine dental care, dental and orthodontic treatments.

DIGESTIVE SYSTEM p.620
Problems and disorders affecting the organs involved in digestion, including the stomach, intestines, liver, pancreas, and gallbladder; nutritional disorders.

HORMONES AND METABOLISM p.670
Diseases of endocrine glands and tissues that affect hormone production and the body's chemical processes (metabolism).

URINARY SYSTEM p.694
Disorders of the kidneys, bladder, and the urethra, the urine outlet from the bladder.

MALE REPRODUCTIVE SYSTEM p.716
Disorders of the male reproductive organs, the testes, scrotum, penis, and prostate gland; male hormonal disorders.

FEMALE REPRODUCTIVE SYSTEM p.730
Disorders of the female reproductive organs; menstrual, menopausal, and hormonal problems; breast disorders.

SEX AND REPRODUCTION p.762
Infertility; sexually transmitted infections; problems with sexual function.

PREGNANCY AND CHILDBIRTH p.778
Problems and complications that may occur during pregnancy, labour, childbirth, and following delivery.

INFANCY AND CHILDHOOD p.810
Problems in babies; genetic disorders first apparent in childhood; diseases affecting children exclusively or in a different way.

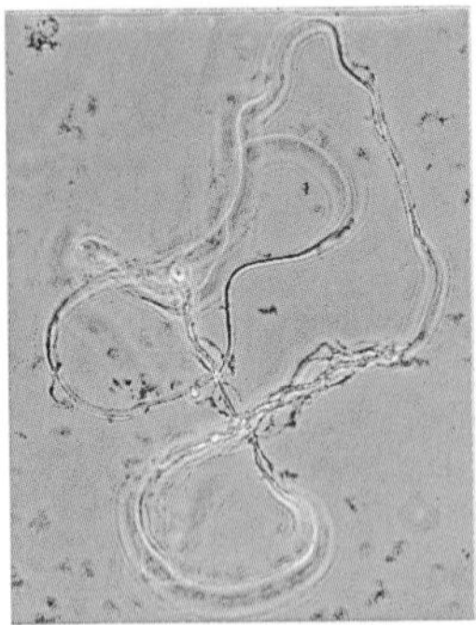

DNA
Genes are made of DNA, a double-stranded helical molecule that is found in the nucleus of cells.

GENES AND INHERITANCE

GENES CONTROL THE GROWTH, REPAIR, AND FUNCTIONS of cells in the human body. Genes are made of DNA (deoxyribonucleic acid), which is found in the nucleus of cells as structures called chromosomes. The DNA provides the cells with all the necessary instructions for building proteins. Proteins are needed for the development and growth of all the body's organs and structures, and genes are the means by which physical and some mental characteristics are passed on to children.

There are about five billion cells in the adult human body, and all of them, except red blood cells, have a set of genes made of DNA. This chemical has a double helix shape and is made of two strands of molecules joined together in the centre by a series of nucleotide bases. The DNA is coiled into structures called chromosomes that are stored in the nucleus of cells.

GENE ORGANIZATION

Human genes are arranged on 22 pairs of matching chromosomes, plus two sex chromosomes. One chromosome in each pair is inherited from each parent. Therefore, body cells contain two copies of genes, with the genes for the same characteristic carried on the matching chromosomes in a pair. Egg and sperm cells, called sex cells, have 23 single chromosomes so that a paired set of genes is created when a sperm cell fertilizes an egg.

There are about 35,000 pairs of genes in a human body cell. Every gene has one function, which is to provide the cell with the information that allows it to make one protein when needed. The order of nucleotide bases along the DNA provides this information. Each body cell contains the same genes, but each tissue or organ needs to make different proteins. For this reason, many genes in an individual body cell are permanently switched off, and a system exists to turn on genes only when they are required.

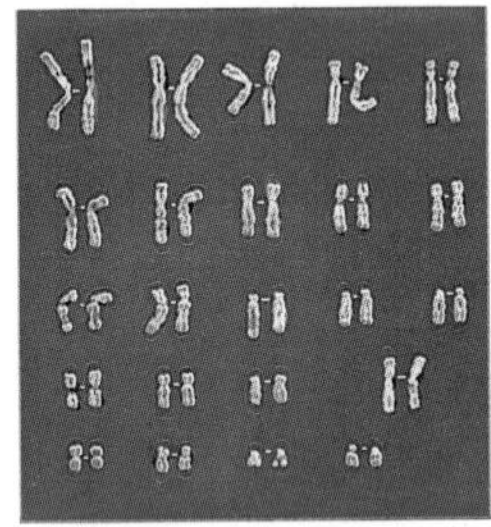

Human chromosomes
Human body cells contain 46 chromosomes, which are organized in 23 pairs.

Often, both of the genes in a matching pair are identical. However, some matching genes occur in slightly different forms called alleles. Some genes may have two to several hundred different alleles. These different forms account for differences between individuals, such as shade of hair colour or length of nose. Differences in just 0.1 per cent of our DNA create all our unique features.

Most of the differences that occur between genes do not affect function. For example, blue eyes work as well as brown ones. However, some genetic differences have important effects. For example, inherited diseases, such as cystic fibrosis and sickle-cell disease, are caused by different forms of abnormal genes. Genes also play a part in disorders such as coronary artery disease and some common cancers, such as colorectal and breast cancer.

COPYING GENES

Every time a cell divides into two during growth or repair, its genes are duplicated so that each new cell has a full set. When sperm and egg cells are made, the chromosomes join together and exchange genes between each other before the cell divides. This exchange ensures that when an egg and a sperm fuse, the new child is different both from its parents and from its siblings.

(STRUCTURE) THE HUMAN GENOME

The human genome contains about 35,000 pairs of genes. In 1990, an international research programme called the Human Genome Project was set up to identify each gene, its function, and its sequence of nucleotide bases (the building blocks of DNA). The information gained from this project will give a better understanding of how disorders are passed from parent to child and may aid the development of treatments. Some genes for disorders, including many on the X chromosome, have already been identified.

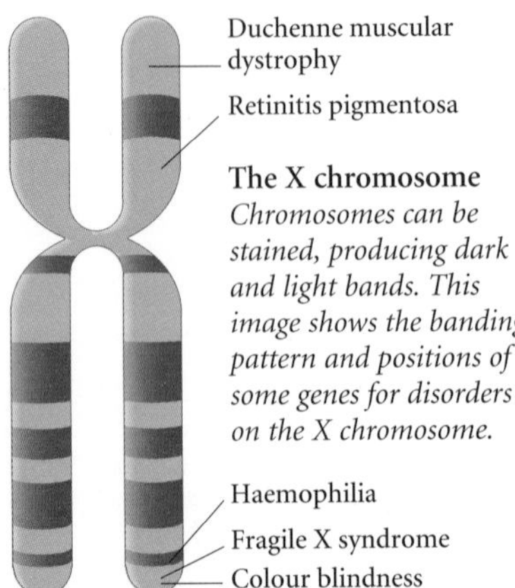

The X chromosome
Chromosomes can be stained, producing dark and light bands. This image shows the banding pattern and positions of some genes for disorders on the X chromosome.

STRUCTURE Structure of genetic material

Genes are made up of DNA, which is shaped like a twisted ladder with rungs made of molecules called nucleotide bases linked together in specific pairs. The arrangement of these bases along the DNA provides the cell with instructions on making proteins. DNA is tightly coiled into rod-shaped structures called chromosomes, which are stored in the nucleus of the cell. There are 22 pairs of chromosomes in each body cell plus two sex chromosomes.

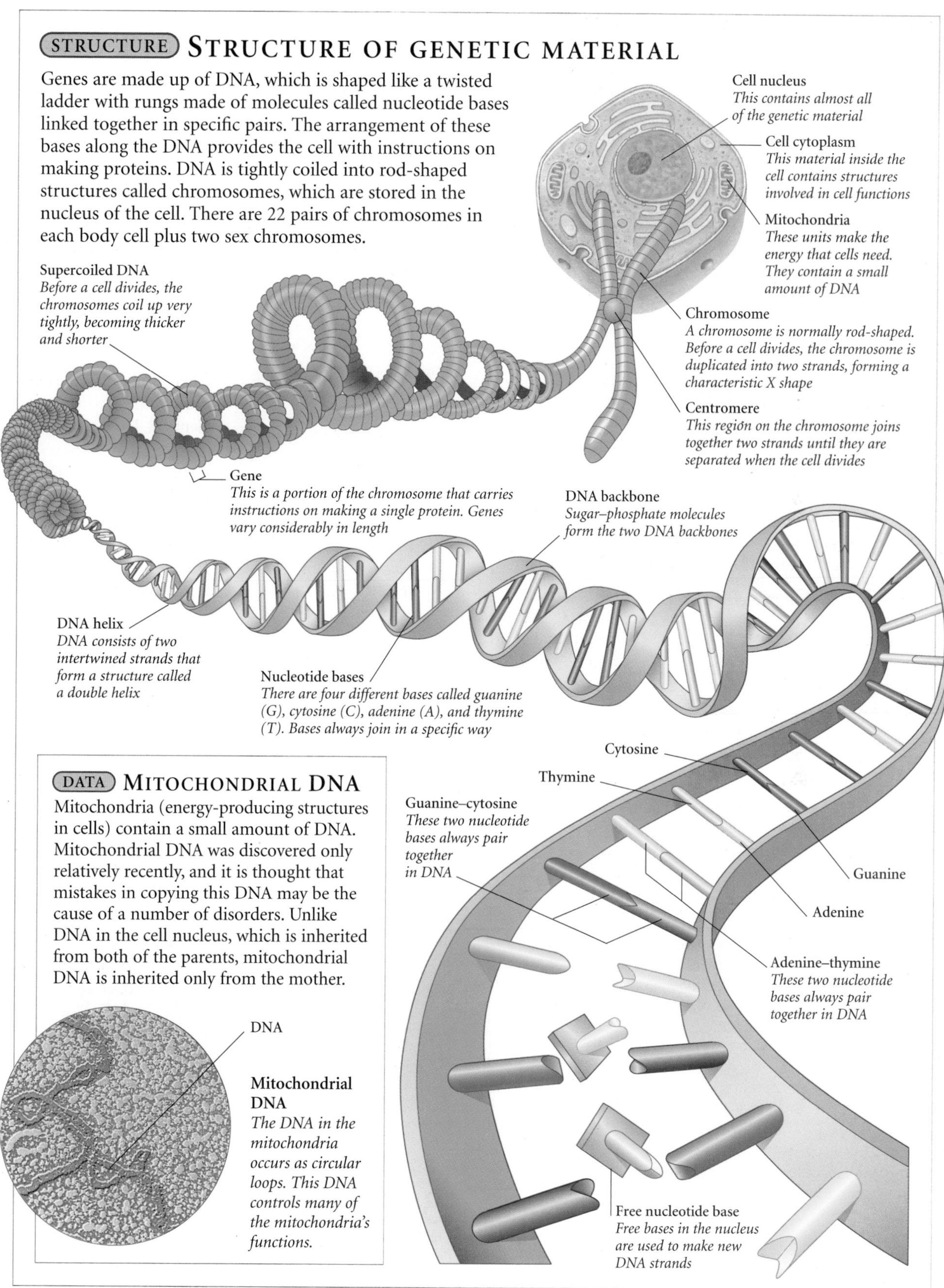

DATA Mitochondrial DNA

Mitochondria (energy-producing structures in cells) contain a small amount of DNA. Mitochondrial DNA was discovered only relatively recently, and it is thought that mistakes in copying this DNA may be the cause of a number of disorders. Unlike DNA in the cell nucleus, which is inherited from both of the parents, mitochondrial DNA is inherited only from the mother.

FUNCTION THE ROLE OF DNA

DNA contains instructions for making proteins, which have many roles in the body. Some make up body structures, such as skin and hair; others are hormones or enzymes that control cell activities. Proteins are made from amino acids, of which there are 20 types, according to instructions relayed by messenger RNA (mRNA). An mRNA strand is a copy of a gene, which is a particular section of DNA. mRNA has four bases; three are the same as those of DNA, one is unique to mRNA.

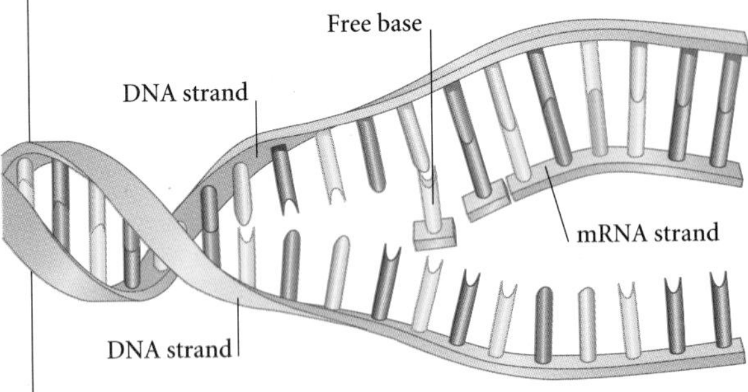

1 *Strands of DNA separate along a stretch of the molecule. Free bases attach to corresponding bases on one DNA strand to make mRNA. The newly formed mRNA carries the instructions for making a protein and moves into the cytoplasm.*

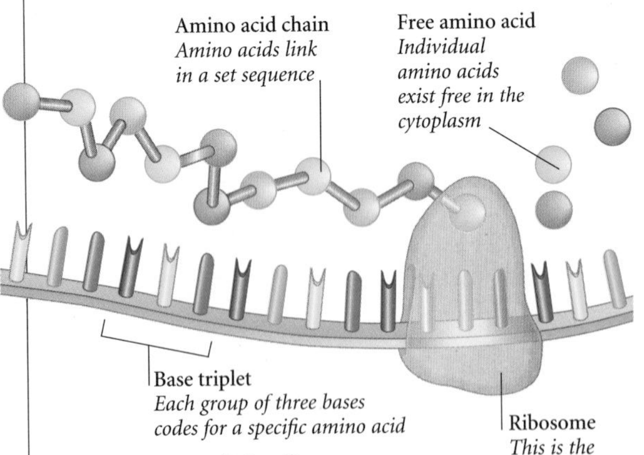

2 *A structure called a ribosome moves along the strand of mRNA three bases at a time. The ribosome brings specific amino acids into place according to the sequence of bases in the mRNA triplets.*

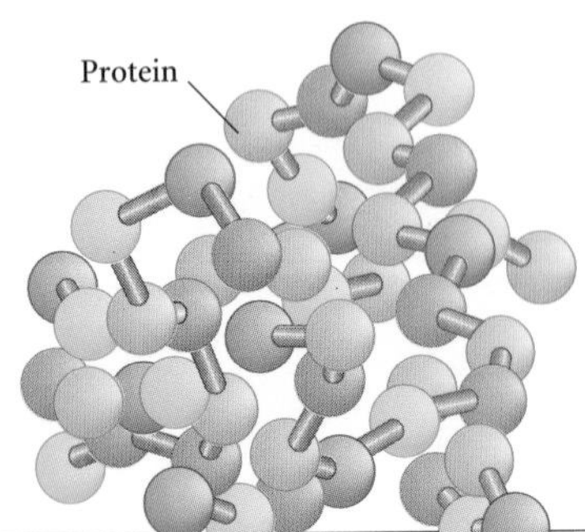

3 *When the ribosome reaches the end of the mRNA strand, it detaches itself from the assembled chain of amino acids. The chain then folds up to form the newly completed protein.*

PROCESS CELL DIVISION

The process of growth requires body cells to divide and multiply constantly. Cells also divide to replace those that have become worn out. When a cell divides, its genetic material is copied. This type of cell division is called mitosis. A slightly different process of cell division, called meiosis, results in the production of egg and sperm cells. In this process, the resulting cells have only half the amount of DNA and the genes are rearranged to create a mix of genetic information.

REPLICATION OF DNA

Before a cell can divide to make new body cells or egg and sperm cells, the DNA in the cell must be copied. Each of the two strands in the original DNA acts as a template against which two new strands are built.

1 *The original DNA double helix splits open at several points along its length. This process produces areas where there are two separate single strands.*

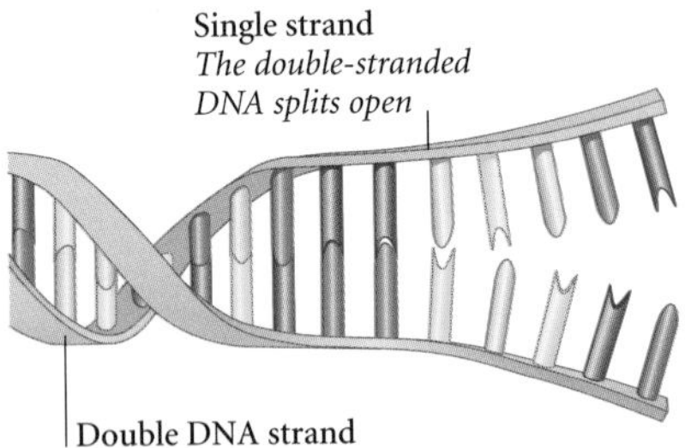

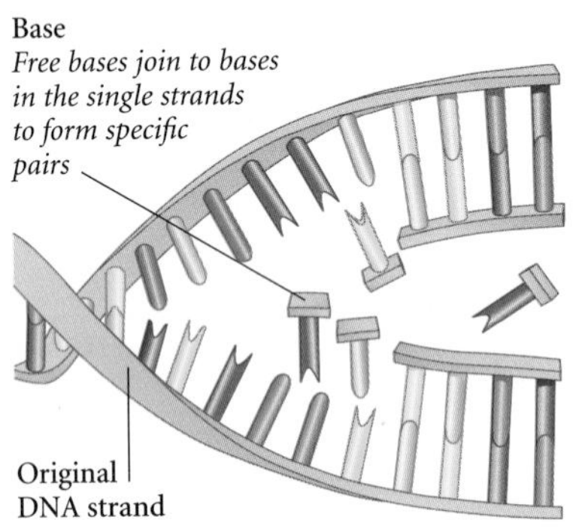

2 *New free bases (units of DNA) are attached to both of the single strands of DNA. The order in which free bases join to the single DNA strands is determined by the DNA bases that are already present on the single strand.*

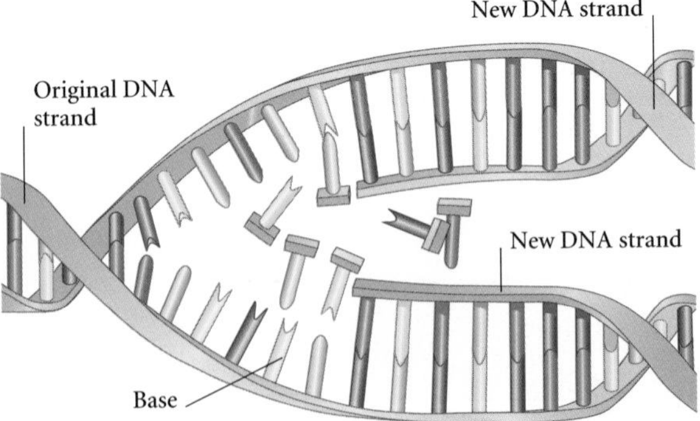

3 *While the bases attach to the strand, each of the two newly formed double strands starts to twist. The process continues along the whole length of the DNA, eventually producing two identical double DNA strands.*

Mitosis

When body cells divide, their genetic material has to be duplicated so that each new cell has a complete set of genes. This process of division is called mitosis and results in cells identical to the original cell. In the diagram below, only four chromosomes are shown for simplicity.

1 *The DNA in the chromosomes is copied to form two identical strands joined in the centre by a structure called the centromere.*

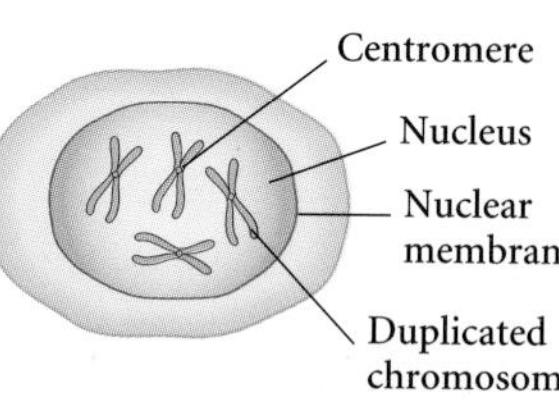

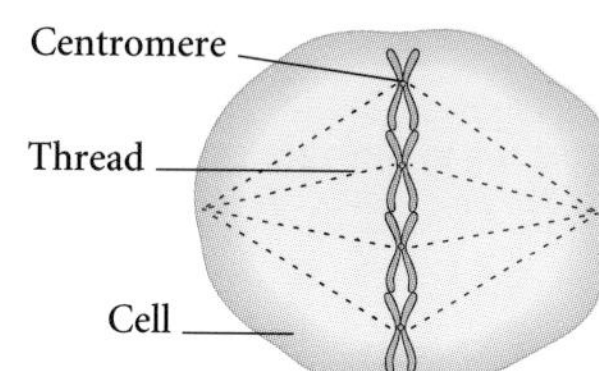

2 *The membrane around the nucleus breaks down and threads form across the cell. The chromosomes line up on the threads.*

3 *The duplicated chromosomes are pulled apart by the threads. The single chromosomes move to opposite sides of the cell.*

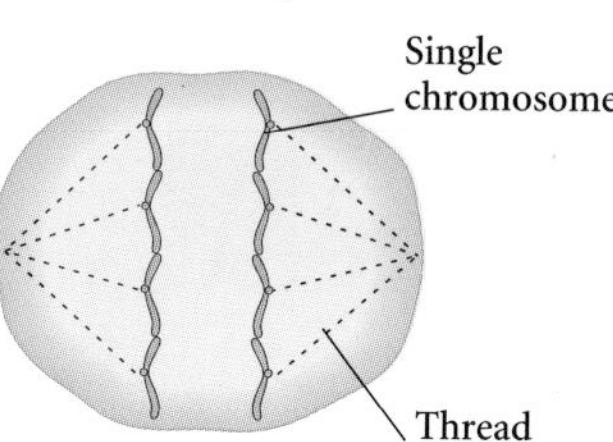

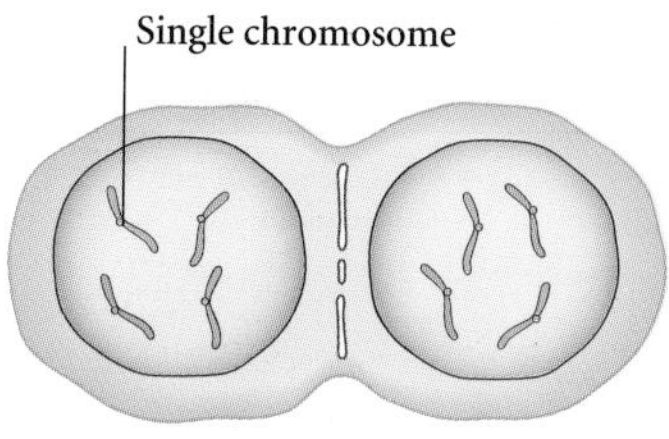

4 *A nuclear membrane forms around each set of single chromosomes. The cell begins to divide into two new cells.*

5 *Two new cells form. Each cell has a central nucleus containing an identical set of chromosomes.*

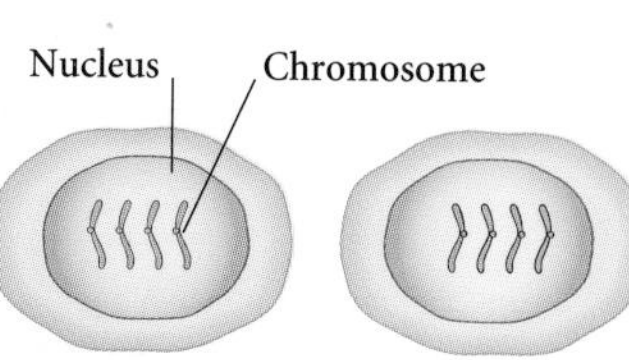

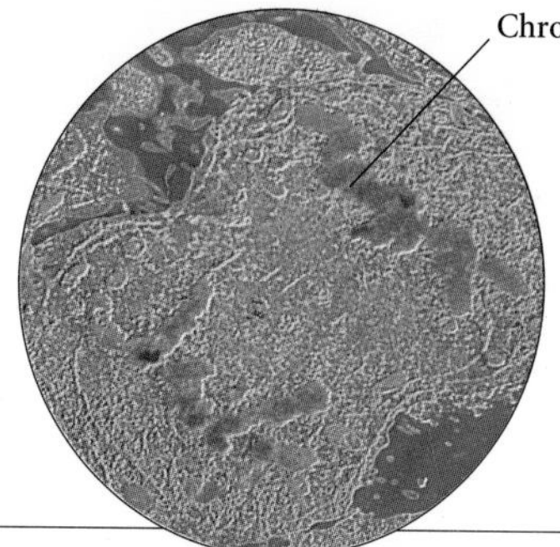

Dividing cell
This highly magnified image shows a body cell dividing by mitosis. Separated chromosomes can be seen in the middle of each of the new cells.

Meiosis

Sperm cells in males and egg cells in females are produced by a form of cell division called meiosis. In this process, the amount of genetic material in the new cells is halved during two stages of cell division. This process ensures that a complete set of genes is obtained when an egg and sperm fuse. During meiosis, matching pairs of chromosomes exchange genetic material randomly. Each of the resulting sperm or egg cells then has a slightly different mixture of genes from each other.

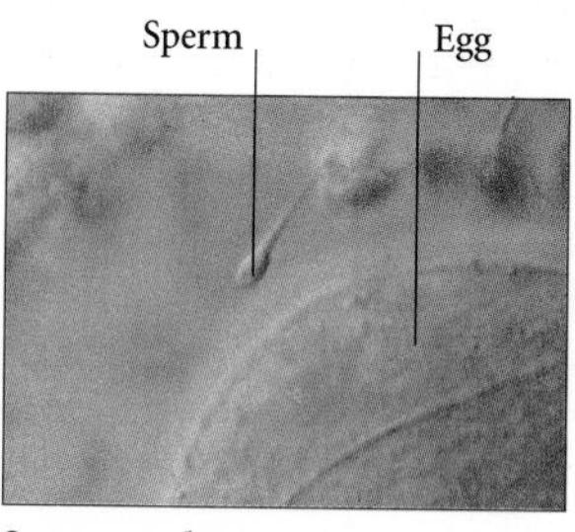

Sperm and egg
This magnified view shows an egg and sperm just before fertilization. Each of these sex cells is made by a process of division called meiosis.

1 *DNA in the chromosomes is duplicated to form X-shaped double chromosomes. Each of these is joined in the centre by a structure called a centromere.*

Duplicated chromosome
Nucleus

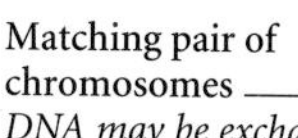

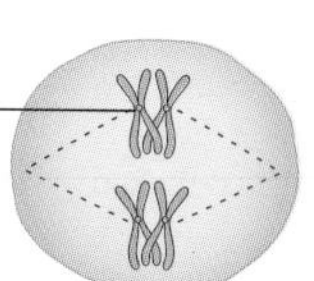

2 *The membrane around the nucleus disappears. Matching chromosomes touch in random places and may exchange genetic material.*

3 *Each of the duplicated chromosomes has a mixture of genetic material. Threads form in the cell to pull the pairs of chromosomes apart.*

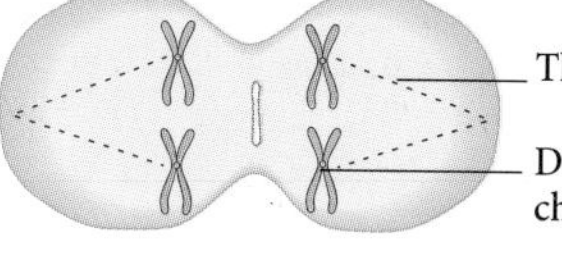

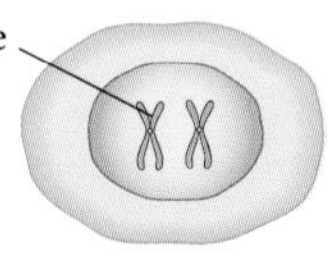

4 *The cell divides to produce two new cells. Each new cell has a full set of 23 duplicated chromosomes from the original cell.*

5 *The duplicated chromosomes line up. More threads attach to each chromosome. Each duplicated chromosome is pulled apart to form two single chromosomes.*

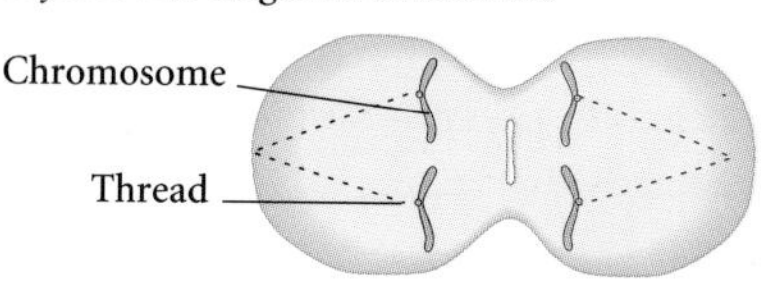

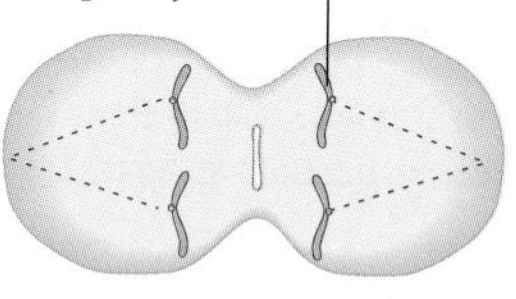

6 *The two cells divide to produce four cells from the original single cell, each with half the amount of genetic material. Each cell has a slightly different mixture of genes.*

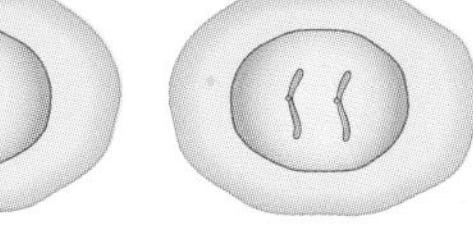

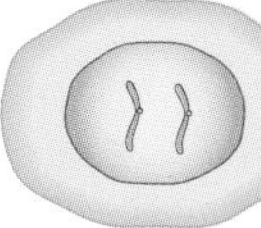

STRUCTURE AND FUNCTION INHERITANCE

Physical characteristics, many disorders, and some aspects of behaviour are at least partly determined by genes passed from parents to children. Genes for each characteristic are always found at the same place on the same chromosome. At fertilization, each of the 23 single chromosomes in an egg cell and a sperm cell matches up into pairs, making a full set of 46 chromosomes that contains two copies of each gene.

HOW GENES ARE INHERITED

Half of a child's genes are inherited from its mother and half from its father. In turn, the child's parents inherited half of their genes from each of their own parents. Therefore, approximately one-quarter of a child's genes has been inherited from each of its grandparents.

GRANDPARENTS

Maternal grandmother | Maternal grandfather | Paternal grandmother | Paternal grandfather

PARENTS

Mother | Father

Genes from maternal grandmother | Genes from paternal grandfather

Genes from maternal grandfather | CHILD | Genes from paternal grandmother

Child's genetic make-up
A child's genes are a mix of genes from his or her parents and grandparents. About one-quarter of each child's genes are inherited from each grandparent.

HOW GENDER IS DETERMINED

There are two sex chromosomes, X and Y, that determine gender. Females have two X chromosomes and males have an X and a Y chromosome, in addition to the 22 other chromosomes. Therefore, all eggs have an X chromosome, while sperm may contain an X or a Y chromosome. The gender of a child depends on whether the sex chromosome in the sperm that fertilizes the egg is X or Y.

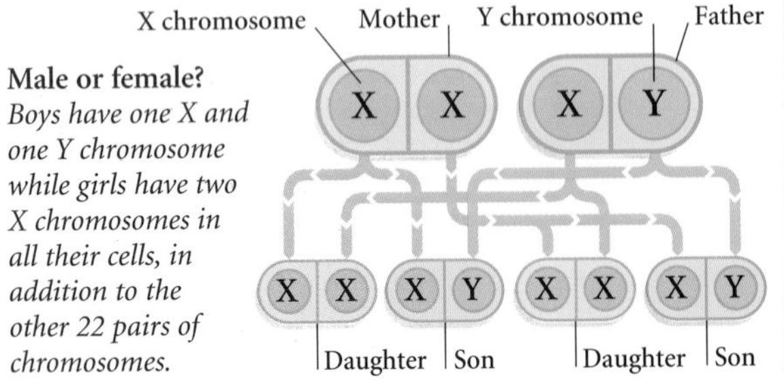

Male or female?
Boys have one X and one Y chromosome while girls have two X chromosomes in all their cells, in addition to the other 22 pairs of chromosomes.

DOMINANT AND RECESSIVE INHERITANCE

Many characteristics are determined by a single pair of genes. Each gene in a pair may have a dominant or recessive effect. A dominant gene overrides the effect of a recessive gene, with the result that one dominant gene produces the dominant characteristic and a recessive characteristic occurs only if no dominant genes are present. For example, blue eye colour is recessive and brown eye colour is dominant as shown below.

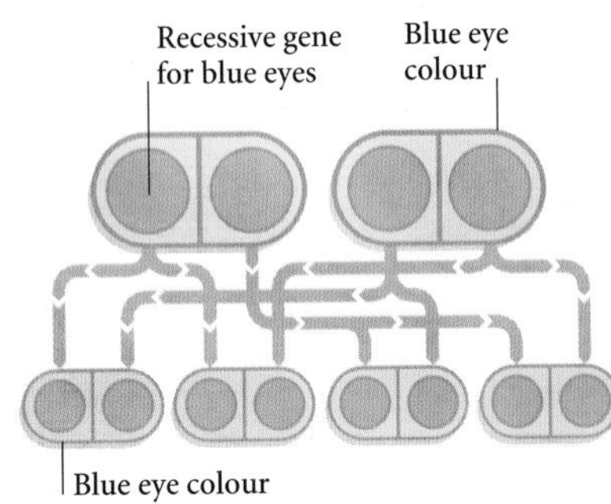

Recessive and recessive
Each child inherits two recessive genes for blue eyes, one from each parent. Since there are no dominant genes to override the effect of the recessive gene, all of the children have blue eyes.

Recessive gene for blue eyes | Blue eye colour | Brown eye colour | Dominant gene for brown eyes

Blue eye colour | Brown eye colour

Recessive and mixed
Each child inherits a recessive gene from one parent, and either a recessive or a dominant gene from the other parent. Each child therefore has a 1 in 2 chance of having brown eyes.

Mixed and mixed
Each child has a 3 in 4 chance of inheriting at least one dominant gene from a parent and having brown eyes. Each child has a 1 in 4 chance of inheriting two recessive genes and having blue eyes.

Recessive gene for blue eyes | Dominant gene for brown eyes

Blue eye colour | Brown eye colour | Brown eye colour

Recessive gene for blue eyes | Dominant gene for brown eyes

Brown eye colour

Dominant and recessive
Each child inherits a recessive gene from one parent and a dominant gene from the other parent. Since the recessive gene is overridden in each child, all of the children will have brown eyes.

SEX-LINKED INHERITANCE

Sex-linked traits and disorders are usually due to recessive genes on the X chromosome. These characteristics and conditions therefore have different patterns of inheritance in females and males. Females with one abnormal gene are carriers if the gene is recessive but affected if the gene is dominant. In males, an abnormal recessive gene behaves as if it is dominant since there is only one X chromosome. One example of an X-linked disorder is colour blindness. Its inheritance is illustrated in the diagram below.

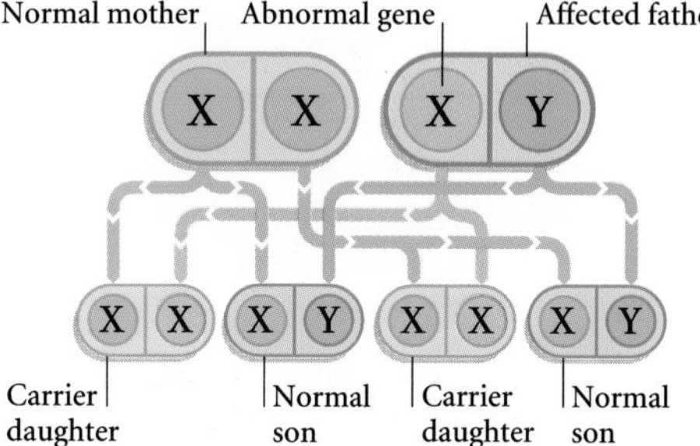

Colour-blind father and normal mother
A colour-blind father passes the abnormal gene on his X chromosome to all his daughters. These daughters are not colour blind, although they can pass the gene on to the next generation. Sons inherit the X chromosome from their mother and are normal.

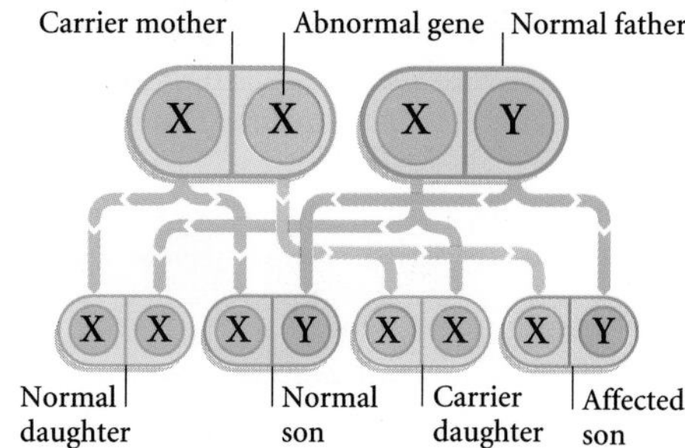

Carrier mother and unaffected father
Each child of a carrier mother has a 1 in 2 chance of inheriting the abnormal gene. Sons inheriting the gene are colour blind as they have no other X chromosome. Daughters who inherit the gene are carriers.

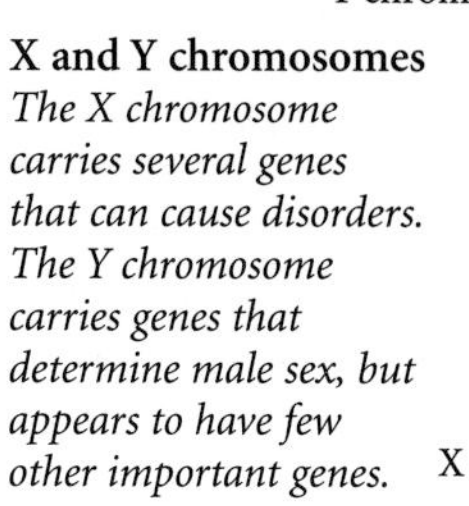
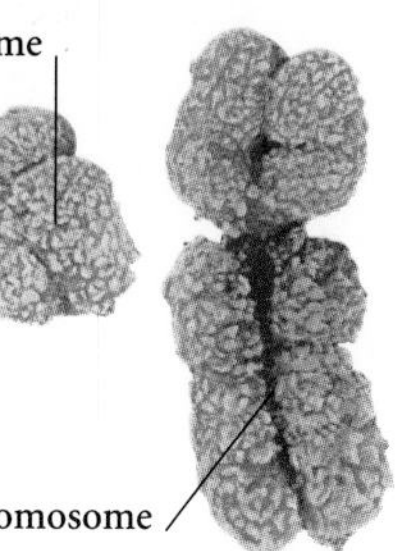

X and Y chromosomes
The X chromosome carries several genes that can cause disorders. The Y chromosome carries genes that determine male sex, but appears to have few other important genes.

PROCESS MUTATIONS

When DNA is duplicated, errors may occur that result in a change in a gene. These changes are called mutations and they may have a dramatic effect on the way a cell functions. Mutations may occur either in egg or sperm cells or in body cells but can only be passed on to a child when they occur in eggs or sperm. Mutations are important for three reasons: they form the basis of evolution by providing a species with a better chance of survival if the mutation is beneficial; they account for a fraction of certain inherited disorders, such as haemophilia; and some mutations cause cells to become cancerous.

HOW MUTATIONS OCCUR

Most mutations involve a change in just one base (unit of DNA). Mutations may occur spontaneously as random errors in copying or may be caused by exposure to UV light, such as that present in sunlight, certain chemicals (mutagens), and radiation.

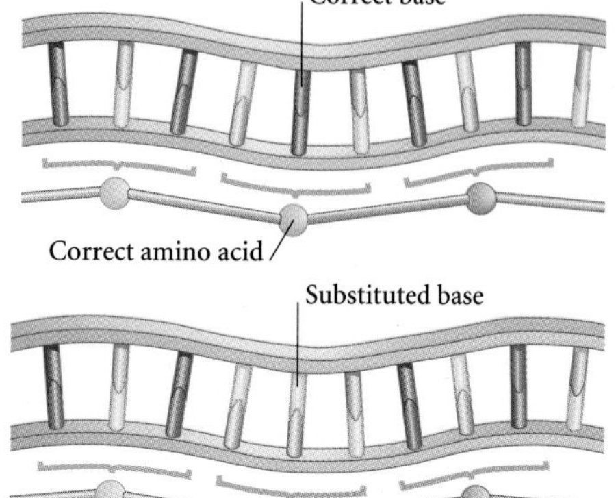

Normal gene
The sequence of bases in a gene provides the cell with the correct sequence of amino acids that are needed to make a functioning protein.

Mutated gene
If a base in a gene is incorrect, the wrong amino acid sequence may be used to make the new protein. The resulting protein may function poorly or not at all.

MUTATIONS IN EGGS AND SPERM

A mutation in an egg or sperm cell is transmitted to a child at fertilization, and it then exists in every cell in the child's body. Some of these inherited mutations are harmless, but some may cause severe abnormalities in the child.

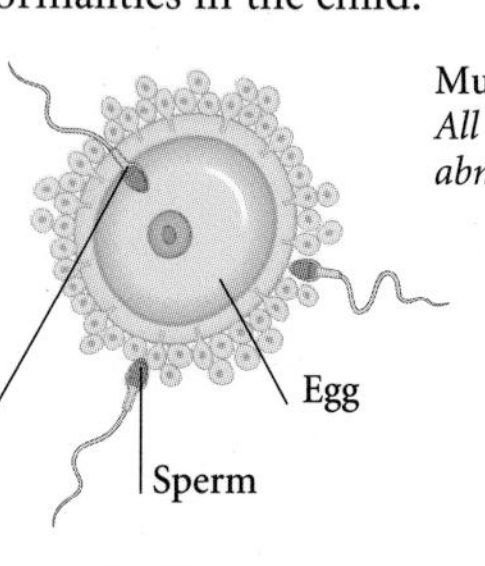

1 *An abnormal sperm that contains a gene carrying a genetic mutation fertilizes a normal egg cell.*

2 *The mutated gene from the abnormal sperm is copied into every new cell as the fertilized egg begins to divide.*

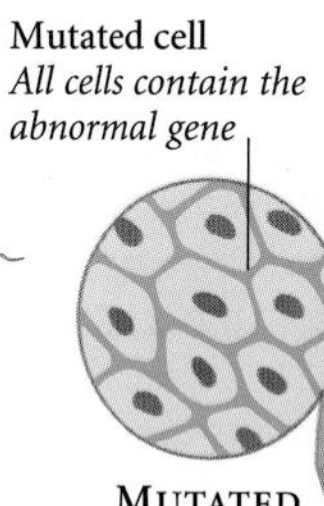

3 *The child has the abnormal gene in every cell in his or her body. The presence of this gene may result in a genetic disorder.*

GENETIC DISORDERS

Genes play a part in the cause of many common diseases, such as asthma and diabetes mellitus. In these diseases, a number of genes interact with factors in the environment. However, some other rarer disorders are caused solely by defective genes or abnormal chromosomes and may be passed on from parent to child.

This section discusses the principles of chromosome and gene disorders and explains how these disorders may be inherited. The specific details of individual disorders are covered more fully in other parts of the book.

The first article discusses the way in which chromosomal abnormalities cause disease. The most common and well-known abnormality is Down's syndrome, in which a child has one extra chromosome in every cell. Since the same chromosomes occur in every cell, abnormalities often cause problems affecting many systems of the body. The second article describes single gene disorders, which may be passed on through a family or may occur without a family history as the result of a gene mutation. People who have a family history of a gene disorder may find genetic counselling useful. Information about genetic testing is given elsewhere (*see* GENETIC TESTS, pp.238–241).

KEY ANATOMY

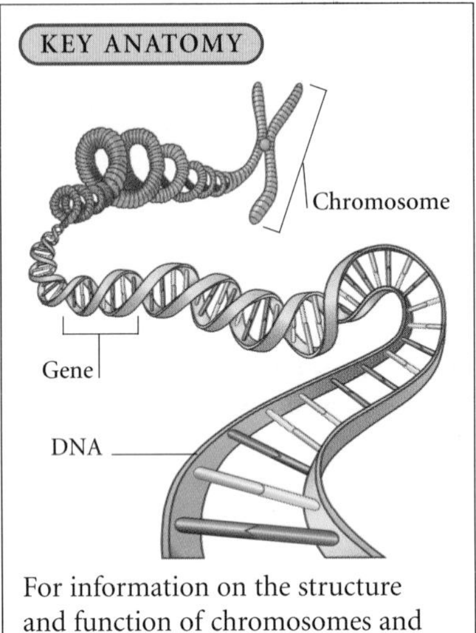

For information on the structure and function of chromosomes and genes, *see* pp.264–269.

Chromosome disorders

Disorders that result from inheriting an incorrect number of or structurally altered chromosomes

 AGE Always present at birth but effects may not become apparent until later

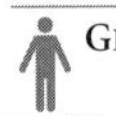 GENDER Risk factors depend on the type

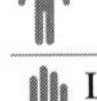 LIFESTYLE Not a significant factor

About 1 in 150–200 babies is born with a chromosomal abnormality. Some of these abnormalities do not affect health, but most may cause multiple problems, including physical abnormalities and learning difficulties. About 50–60 per cent of all miscarriages are the result of chromosome disorders. However, there are many chromosome disorders, such as Turner's syndrome (p.823), Klinefelter's syndrome (p.822), and Down's syndrome (p.821), that are not fatal.

Every cell in the body, apart from eggs and sperm, carries 46 chromosomes arranged in 22 pairs plus the 2 sex chromosomes. One of each pair is inherited from each parent. The sex chromosomes determine an individual's gender. Females have two X chromosomes; males have one X and one Y chromosome. The other 22 pairs are known as autosomes. Each cell is estimated to contain about 35,000 pairs of genes on these chromosomes, providing instructions for making proteins involved in the growth, multiplication, and function of the body's cells.

Chromosomal abnormalities are usually due to a fault in the division of chromosomes that occurs when eggs and sperm are formed. This process, called meiosis, involves a halving of the number of chromosomes in normal body cells. This process results in each sex cell having only 23 chromosomes. Occasionally, a chromosomal abnormality can arise early in the division of the fertilized egg. Chromosomal abnormalities usually have major physical and/or mental effects on the individual.

Several factors increase the likelihood of a couple having a child with a chromosomal abnormality, such as already having a child with a chromosome disorder or a maternal age of over 35 years.

WHAT ARE THE TYPES?

A chromosomal abnormality involves either an incorrect number of chromosomes or a defect in the structure of a chromosome. These abnormalities can affect any one of the 44 autosomal chromosomes or one of the sex chromosomes. Disorders that are caused by autosomal chromosome abnormalities are usually more severe.

NUMERICAL ABNORMALITIES Mistakes occasionally occur in the way chromosome pairs are divided between the new egg or sperm cells during meiosis, with one cell having too many chromosomes while the other has too few. If an egg containing an extra chromosome is fertilized by a normal sperm, the embryo will have an extra chromosome in every cell in its body. Alternatively, if a sperm with a missing chromosome fertilizes a normal egg, the fetus will have one less chromosome in each of its cells. About two-thirds of all chromosome disorders are caused by cells that contain the wrong number of chromosomes.

Extra or missing autosomal chromosomes usually result in miscarriage of the embryo. One exception to this is the inheritance of an extra chromosome 21, known as trisomy 21. Although fetuses with this extra chromosome are often miscarried, a number survive, and they have the condition Down's syndrome. Abnormalities in the number of sex chromosomes tend to have a less severe effect on the embryo and, in some cases, there are no obvious signs of a disorder. About 1 in 500 babies is born with an extra X or Y chromosome. An extra X chromosome in a girl or Y chromosome in a boy may have little or no physical effect. However, boys who are born with an extra X chromosome

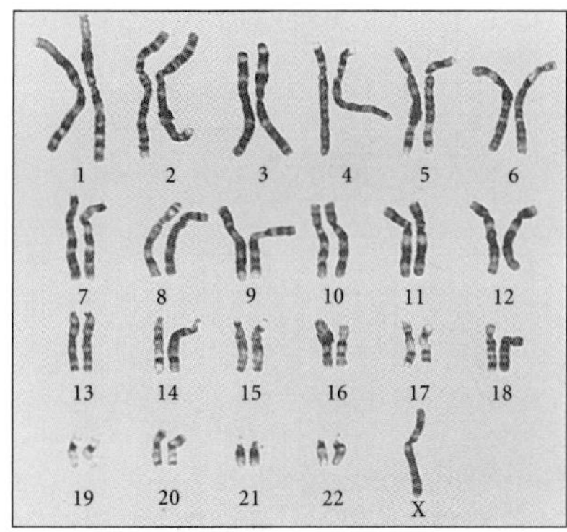

Chromosomes in Turner's syndrome
This set of chromosomes (karyotype) from a female with Turner's syndrome shows only one X chromosome rather than the two that are normal for a female.

(XXY) have a disorder known as Klinefelter's syndrome, which may prevent normal male secondary sexual characteristics developing. About 1 in 2,500 girls is born with only one X chromosome instead of the usual two, a condition known as Turner's syndrome. Girls with this condition have a short stature and, if they do not receive treatment, fail to develop normal secondary sexual characteristics at puberty. Girls with Turner's syndrome are infertile.

STRUCTURAL ABNORMALITIES There is a natural exchange of genetic material between pairs of chromosomes during meiosis. This mixing ensures that the genetic make-up of each egg and sperm is slightly different. Occasionally, faults occur during this process, resulting in a structural chromosomal abnormality. A small section of chromosome may be deleted, duplicated, or inserted the wrong way around (inverted). These types of structural abnormalities in the chromosome may result in miscarriage or birth defects, ranging from mild to extremely severe. The effect on the fetus depends on the amount and type of genetic material that is altered. Material may also be exchanged between two different chromosomes following breaks in each one. This process is known as translocation. If no genetic material is gained or lost during this process, it is known as a balanced translocation. Balanced translocations are carried by about 1 in 500 people. A translocation rarely causes health problems in the affected person. However, when a person with a translocation has a child of his or her own, serious chromosomal abnormalities may occur in the child as a result of inheriting too much or too little chromosomal material.

MOSAICISM In this condition, a person has some body cells that contain a normal set of chromosomes and other cells that contain an abnormal number of chromosomes. Mosaicism occurs when there is a fault in cell division in the embryo soon after fertilization, creating some cells that have an incorrect number of chromosomes. These cells can usually be detected by analysis of a blood sample. The effects of mosaicism depend on the proportion of cells containing abnormal chromosomes.

HOW ARE THEY DIAGNOSED?

Many chromosome disorders are obvious either at birth or once symptoms appear. The diagnosis can be confirmed by a blood test (*see* TESTS FOR CHROMOSOMAL ABNORMALITIES, p.238).

If a fetus dies in the womb, is stillborn, or is miscarried, it can usually be tested to look for chromosomal defects. During a pregnancy, chromosomal abnormalities can be detected by taking a sample of fetal cells and analysing the chromosomes (*see* ANTENATAL GENETIC TESTS, p.787). Antenatal genetic tests may be offered to women at increased risk of having an affected baby due to advanced maternal age or when Down's syndrome in a relative is known to be caused by an inherited chromosomal abnormality. Certain routine antenatal blood tests carried out in early pregnancy may also indicate an increased risk. In such cases, women may be offered specific antenatal tests, such as amniocentesis or chorionic villus sampling, which can confirm the diagnosis of Down's syndrome in a fetus.

WHAT IS THE TREATMENT?

There is no cure for disorders caused by chromosomal abnormalities. However, surgery in infancy may rectify physical abnormalities, such as intestinal abnormalities or heart defects, and some people with sex chromosome disorders may be treated with hormone replacement. For example, girls with Turner's syndrome can be given hormones to induce puberty and increase height.

When there is a history of chromosomal abnormality within the family or if recurrent miscarriages have occurred, prospective parents may wish to consider genetic counselling (p.272) so that they can assess the risk of a child developing a chromosome disorder before deciding to begin a pregnancy.

(WWW) ONLINE SITES: p.1032

Gene disorders

Disorders that result from inheriting a faulty gene or genes

 AGE Always present at birth but effects may not become apparent until later

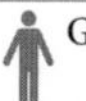 GENDER Risk factors depend on the type

 LIFESTYLE Not a significant factor

Genes provide instructions to the cells to make enzymes and other proteins that the body needs to grow and function. A defective gene may have mild, moderate, or potentially fatal consequences or no effect at all, depending on the role of the protein for which the gene codes. The development of many common disorders, such as diabetes mellitus (p.687) and asthma (p.483), is linked with genetic factors but is also influenced by environment and lifestyle.

Several thousand disorders are the result of abnormalities in single genes, but the majority of these conditions are extremely rare. Some of the most common single gene disorders include haemophilia (*see* HAEMOPHILIA AND CHRISTMAS DISEASE, p.452), cystic fibrosis (p.824), sickle-cell disease (p.448), and thalassaemia (p.449). About 1 in 100 babies is born with a disorder that is caused by a single faulty gene.

Some communities have particularly high frequencies of abnormal genes for certain disorders. For example, the abnormal gene that produces Tay–Sachs disease (p.868) is more common among Ashkenazi Jews, and the gene for thalassaemia is more common in people from Mediterranean countries and Asia.

Some gene disorders are obvious soon after birth or in the first few months of life. Other disorders caused by a single abnormal gene, such as Huntington's disease (p.538), do not become apparent until adult life when the symptoms first appear.

WHAT ARE THE CAUSES?

In most gene disorders, an individual has the defective gene or genes in all cells of the body from the first stages in the development of the embryo. There are two possible reasons for the presence of the abnormal gene. First, the defective gene may have been passed on from parent to child. Second, a normal gene may have become faulty (mutated) during meiosis, the process of division by which eggs and sperm form. In this way, certain gene disorders can occur without a previous family history.

WHAT ARE THE TYPES?

Genes occur in pairs; one of each pair is inherited from the mother, the other from the father. The genes may be dominant or recessive. Dominant genes override the effects of genes that are recessive. Genes are found on the 22 pairs of chromosomes known as autosomes and also on the X and Y sex chromosomes (predominantly on the X chromosome). Single gene disorders are classified by their pattern of inheritance: autosomal dominant, autosomal recessive, or X-linked. In addition, many common disorders are the result of an interaction between genes, the environment, and lifestyle. These are known as multifactorial disorders.

AUTOSOMAL DOMINANT DISORDERS In these disorders, an abnormal gene needs to be inherited from only one parent to lead to a disorder. A normal gene inherited from the other parent does not mask the effect of a dominant gene mutation. If a person has an autosomal dominant disorder, each of his or her children has a 1 in 2 chance of inheriting the abnormal gene and developing the disorder. Familial hypercholesterolaemia is one of the most common conditions to follow this particular pattern of inheritance (*see* INHERITED HYPERLIPIDAEMIAS, p.692). In this disorder, there are high levels of blood cholesterol, leading to an increased risk of early coronary artery disease (p.405). About 1 in 500 people of European descent has this gene and is affected by the disorder.

AFFECTED PARENT

UNAFFECTED PARENT

Abnormal gene

Normal gene

AFFECTED CHILDREN

UNAFFECTED CHILDREN

Autosomal dominant disorder

In this example, one of the parents has the abnormal gene and the other parent is unaffected. Each child has a 1 in 2 chance of inheriting the faulty gene and therefore developing the disorder.

AUTOSOMAL RECESSIVE DISORDERS A person must inherit two copies of a faulty gene, one from each parent, to develop an autosomal recessive disorder. If a person inherits one copy of the faulty gene but the gene from the other parent is normal, the person is a carrier. A carrier does not develop the disease but may pass the gene on to his or her children. Since two genes, one from each parent, are necessary to produce the disease, autosomal recessive disorders are rare. Cystic fibrosis, a disease that affects certain glands, is the most common autosomal recessive disorder in white Europeans. About 1 in 20 people is a carrier of the disease. The chance of one cystic fibrosis carrier having children with another carrier is about 1 in 400, and, since there is a 1 in 4 risk of a child inheriting two faulty genes, cystic fibrosis affects 1 in 1,600 people. The most common autosomal recessive disorder among black people is sickle-cell disease, for which 1 in 10 people is a carrier and about 1 in 400 has the disorder.

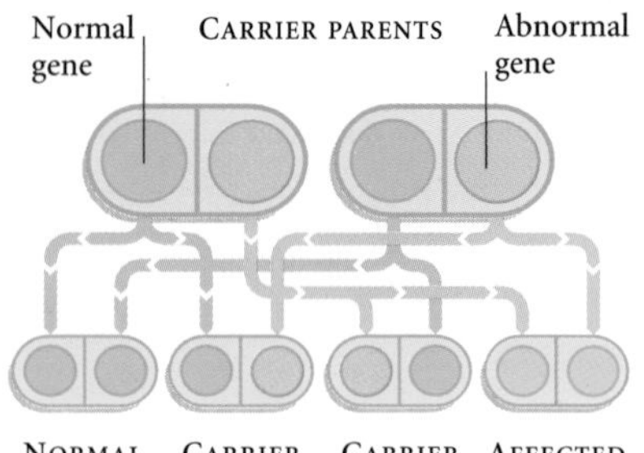

Autosomal recessive inheritance

In this example, both parents carry the abnormal gene but do not have the disease. Their children may be unaffected (1 in 4 chance), may be carriers of the faulty gene (1 in 2), or may have the disease (1 in 4).

X-LINKED RECESSIVE DISORDERS In a disorder of this type, such as haemophilia, the faulty gene is carried on the X chromosome. Women who have just one faulty gene are unaffected carriers because they have a second X chromosome that almost always carries a normal gene and can mask the effect of the abnormal one. However, they may pass on the abnormal gene to their children. Since each child inherits one X chromosome from the mother, each child of a carrier has a 1 in 2 chance of inheriting the abnormal gene. If a boy inherits the abnormal gene, he will definitely develop the disorder because he cannot inherit a second X chromosome. The girls are carriers because the X chromosome inherited from their father masks the abnormal gene. An affected man will pass on the faulty gene to his daughters but not to his sons.

(TEST) GENETIC COUNSELLING

Genetic counselling can help people to plan their families if there is a history of an inherited disease. Counsellors use the most up-to-date information and test results to estimate the chance that a given single gene disorder will recur in the same family. They may discuss the options available for reducing the risk of a child being born with the particular disorder.

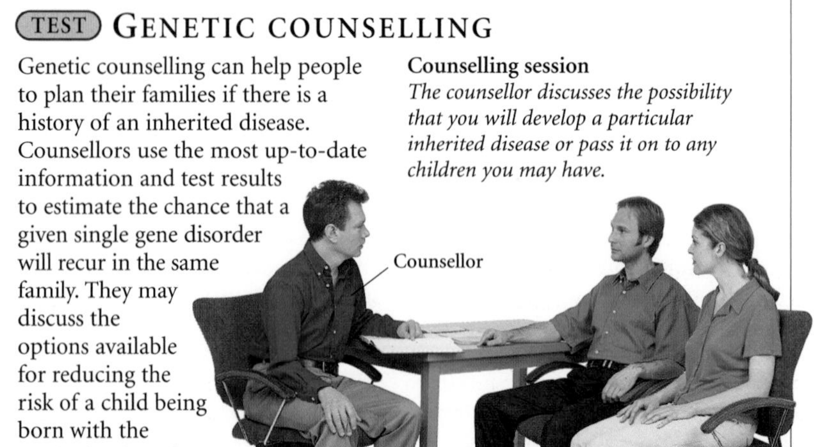

Counselling session

The counsellor discusses the possibility that you will develop a particular inherited disease or pass it on to any children you may have.

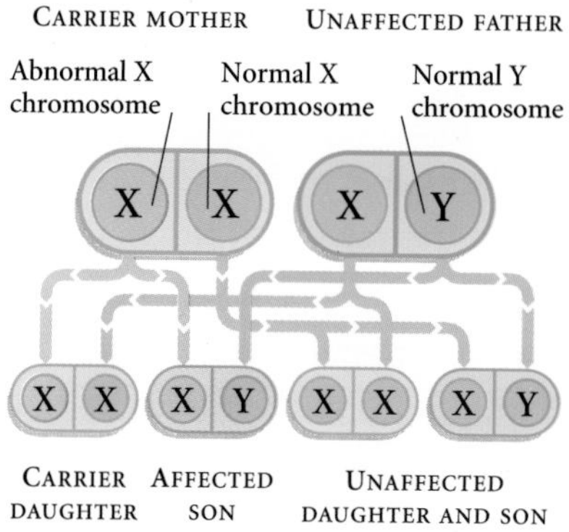

CARRIER MOTHER
UNAFFECTED FATHER
Abnormal X chromosome
Normal X chromosome
Normal Y chromosome
X X X Y
X X X Y X X X Y
CARRIER DAUGHTER
AFFECTED SON
UNAFFECTED DAUGHTER AND SON

X-linked recessive inheritance
In this example, a mother carries the abnormal gene on the X chromosome but is unaffected. The sons have a 1 in 2 chance of inheriting the disease; the daughters have a 1 in 2 chance of being carriers but will not have the disease.

MULTIFACTORIAL DISORDERS There are many common disorders, including asthma, that run in families but for which no single gene appears to be responsible. In these disorders, it is likely that several different genes interact to cause the disease and that lifestyle and environmental factors also play a role. Certain disorders are known to be associated with a group of proteins called HLAs. These proteins form part of the body's immune system and determine a person's tissue type. HLAs are inherited, and each individual has a unique combination of them. In some people, particular HLAs increase susceptibility to certain disorders, such as ankylosing spondylitis (p.378) and systemic lupus erythematosus (p.461).

WHAT MIGHT BE DONE?

The underlying cause of single gene disorders cannot be treated, although gene therapy, in which abnormal genes are replaced by normal genes, is currently an area of intense research. The symptoms of many gene disorders can be treated successfully. For example, people who have haemophilia and are unable to produce an important protein involved in blood clotting, called factor VIII, are treated with regular injections of the missing protein (*see* DRUGS THAT PROMOTE BLOOD CLOTTING, p.903). Similarly, over the past 20 years, improved treatment for people with cystic fibrosis, including physiotherapy (p.961) and antibiotics (p.885), has increased life expectancy. However, some disorders due to a single gene, such as Huntington's disease, are not easily treated and are eventually fatal.

CAN THEY BE PREVENTED?

People who have a blood relative with an inherited disorder may be able to have screening to determine whether they have the faulty gene (*see* GENETIC TESTS, pp.238–241). Screening is available only for certain disorders, such as cystic fibrosis and sickle-cell disease, in which the faulty gene has been identified. Screening may be offered to whole communities in which there is a high incidence of a faulty gene. For example, Ashkenazi Jews may be screened for Tay–Sachs disease, which is common in this group. A couple with a family history of a gene disorder may opt for genetic counselling (opposite page) before conceiving or have antenatal genetic tests (p.787) for fetal abnormalities.

(WWW) ONLINE SITES: p.1032

GENE DISORDERS

AUTOSOMAL DOMINANT DISORDERS

Achondroplasia p.833
A disorder of bone growth, resulting in short stature and abnormal proportions

Huntington's disease p.538
A brain disorder that causes abnormal movements and dementia in adulthood

Inherited hyperlipidaemias p.692
Excessive levels of lipids in the blood, of which the most common form is familial hypercholesterolaemia

Marfan's syndrome p.824
A rare disorder that mainly affects the skeleton, heart, and eyes

Neurofibromatosis p.827
A disorder in which numerous swellings develop on the covering of nerves

Polycystic kidney disease (in adults) p.704
A disorder in which fluid-filled cysts replace normal kidney tissue

Porphyria p.693
A disorder in which chemicals called porphyrins build up in the body, causing psychological and physical symptoms

Von Willebrand disease p.452
A bleeding disorder due to a deficiency of a substance needed for blood clotting

AUTOSOMAL RECESSIVE DISORDERS

Albinism p.868
A lack of the pigment melanin, which gives colour to the skin, hair, and eyes

Cystic fibrosis p.824
Abnormally thick secretions, leading to digestive and respiratory problems

Galactosaemia p.868
Inability to break down a form of sugar, leading to its accumulation in the blood

Haemochromatosis p.692
A condition in which too much iron is deposited in various organs

Phenylketonuria p.867
Deficiency of an enzyme needed to digest a component of protein-containing foods

Polycystic kidneys (in children) p.704
A disorder in which fluid-filled cysts replace normal kidney tissue, usually apparent at birth

Retinitis pigmentosa p.581
Progressive degeneration in the retina, the light-sensitive membrane at the back of the eye, leading to loss of vision

Sickle-cell disease p.448
A blood disorder in which red blood cells become an abnormal shape and blood flow through vessels is impeded

Tay–Sachs disease p.868
A severe disorder in which harmful substances build up in the brain

Thalassaemia p.449
A blood disorder in which production of haemoglobin, the oxygen-carrying component of red blood cells, is abnormal

X-LINKED DISORDERS

Colour blindness p.591
Impaired ability to distinguish between certain colours

Fragile X syndrome p.822
A disorder that produces severe learning disabilities and a characteristic appearance

Haemophilia and Christmas disease p.452
Disorders in which the blood does not clot normally due to a clotting factor deficiency

Muscular dystrophy p.826
A disorder causing progressive weakness and wasting of muscles

Inheritance of single gene disorders
This table lists the major single gene disorders that are covered in this book. Some disorders exist in more than one form, with different inheritance patterns. The most common pattern is indicated.

CANCER

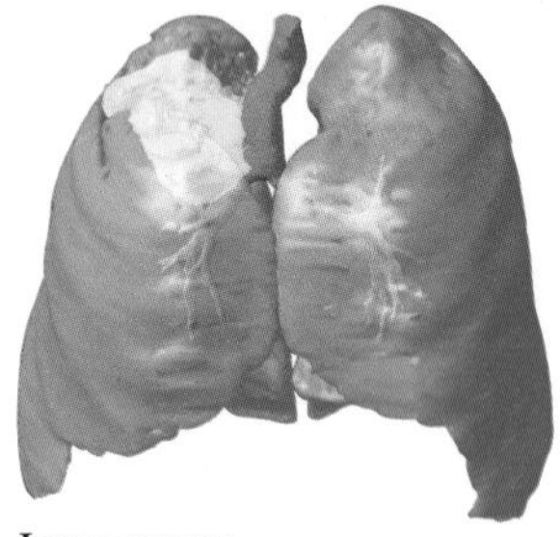

Lung cancer
The yellow and white area in this colour-enhanced CT scan of the lungs is a cancerous tumour, probably caused by smoking.

CANCER IS A DISEASE in which body cells grow uncontrollably because their normal regulatory mechanisms have been damaged. Of the many types of cancer, the majority form solid tumours in a specific part of the body, commonly the skin, breast, lung, bowel, or prostate gland. The disease may then spread through the blood and lymphatic systems. As our understanding of cancer has advanced during the past 20 years, changes in lifestyle, efficient screening programmes, and new types of therapy have improved prevention and treatment of the disease.

The term "cancer" comes from the Greek word for crab. The ancient Greek physician Hippocrates likened a spreading cancerous tumour to the shape of a crab's claw. Although our understanding of the disease has advanced dramatically since then, the description is still apt. An important feature of a cancerous tumour is its ability to spread within the body.

GENETIC BASIS OF CANCER

The discovery in the late 1970s that damage to genetic material underlies cancer was one of the most important breakthroughs in cancer research. Every cell contains genetic information in the form of about 35,000 pairs of genes that control the activities of cells. A cell may become cancerous when certain genes that control vital processes such as cell division become damaged. These faulty genes may be inherited or caused by carcinogens (cancer-causing agents), such as sunlight and tobacco smoke. Cells are continually exposed to carcinogens, but they rarely become cancerous for several reasons: cells can usually repair their damaged genes; more than one gene must be damaged before cancer develops; and the body's immune system often destroys any abnormal cells before they are able to multiply enough to form a cancerous tumour.

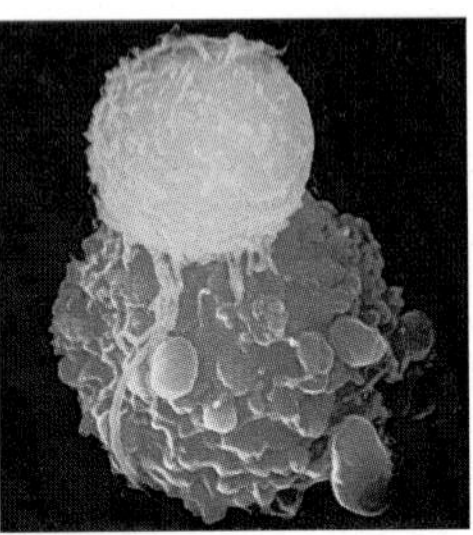

Destroying cancer cells
In this highly magnified image, a white blood cell is chemically destroying the larger cancerous cell.

AGING AND CANCER

Cancer is most common among older people, largely because their cells have had more time to accumulate genetic damage, but also because the body's defences against cancer, particularly the cells and proteins of the immune system, gradually become less efficient with age. In addition, a cancer that began earlier in life may not be diagnosed until old age because it often takes many years for some types of tumour to grow large enough to produce noticeable symptoms. Since life expectancy increased significantly in developed countries during the second half of the 20th century, cancer has now become one of the most common causes of death in the UK, second only to coronary artery disease.

TREATING CANCER

For 2,000 years, doctors have attempted to cure cancer by surgically removing visible tumours. For some localized cancers, radiotherapy can be effective; this treatment is often combined with surgery with the aim of achieving a cure. Treatment with anticancer drugs, known as chemotherapy, may be used instead of or in combination with surgery to destroy cancers that have spread around the body.

New therapies for the treatment of cancer that are currently being assessed include inactivating damaged genes and boosting the immune system's ability to destroy cancerous cells. However, as with many other diseases, the most effective ways to lower the number of deaths are currently prevention through a healthy lifestyle and screening to detect cancer early.

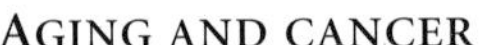

DATA CAUSES OF CANCER

Although most cancers appear to be caused by several factors, including inherited ones, a main environmental cause can often be identified for a particular cancer. The most common carcinogens (cancer-causing agents), such as tobacco smoke, are avoidable. Smoking has caused a major lung cancer epidemic throughout the world in the 20th century.

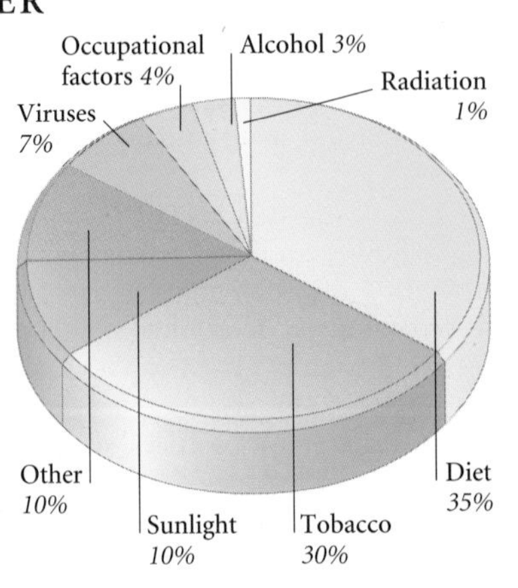

Carcinogens in the environment
Although radiation other than sunlight is commonly cited as a cause of cancer, its contribution is actually very small.

STRUCTURE CANCEROUS TUMOURS

A cancerous (malignant) tumour is a collection of many abnormal cells, most of which divide uncontrollably. Cancerous tumours infiltrate neighbouring tissues by forcing their way between normal cells and can spread to distant body parts through blood or lymph vessels. Cancerous cells are extremely irregular in shape and size and often bear little resemblance to the cells from which they arose. This characteristic irregular appearance of cancerous cells is often used to help diagnose cancer.

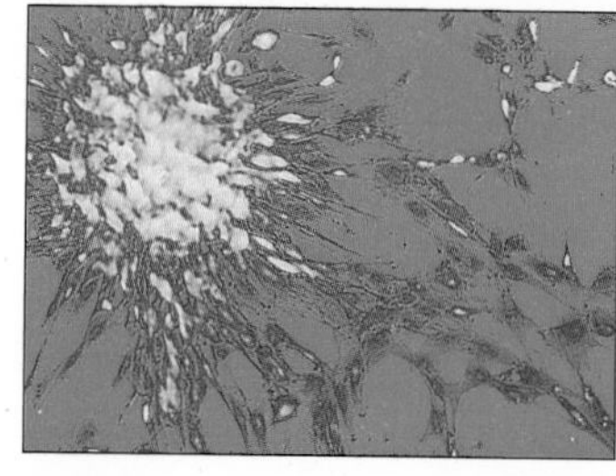

Migration of cancerous cells
In this magnified image, cancerous cells are migrating after separating from a tumour. Some of these cells will settle at new sites and divide to form tumours.

Normal cell
Bands of normal cells remain between the spreading cancerous cells

Dividing cell
Cancerous cells often divide more frequently than normal cells

Cancerous cell
Cancerous cells have large nuclei and tend not to resemble the cells from which they originated

Epithelial layer
Tumours often form in epithelial tissue, which covers the body and lines body cavities and organs

Ulcerated area
The tumour may erode the epithelial layer completely

Bleeding
Inside the tumour, bleeding often occurs because fast-growing cancer cells breach blood vessel walls

Nerve fibre
Involvement of nerve fibres in a cancerous tumour may cause pain

Dead tissue
Inside the tumour, cancerous cells may die if the tumour has outgrown its blood supply

Calcium deposits
Calcium deposits build up in some tumours and may be visible on X-rays

Blood vessel
Involvement of blood vessels in a tumour provides a route for distant spread of cancer

Lymph vessel
Involvement of lymph vessels in a tumour provides a route for the spread of cancer to nearby lymph nodes

Tumour outgrowth
The tumour cells form outgrowths that spread into surrounding tissue

STRUCTURE NONCANCEROUS TUMOURS

Noncancerous (benign) tumours are common and include lipomas, which are fatty lumps beneath the skin, and many other skin lesions. These types of tumour do not invade tissue, but they may compress nearby structures as they grow. Noncancerous tumours do not spread around the body.

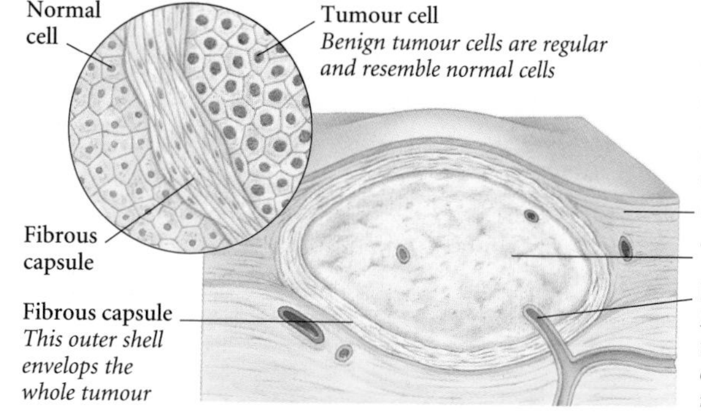

Structure of a noncancerous tumour
A noncancerous tumour has an outer fibrous capsule that separates it from the surrounding normal tissue.

PROCESS HOW CANCER STARTS

Cells are continually bombarded by carcinogens (cancer-causing agents such as sunlight and certain viruses). Carcinogens damage specific genes (sections of DNA that control specific cell functions), known as oncogenes, that regulate vital processes such as cell division. Most damaged genes are repaired, but this process occasionally fails. Progressive damage to oncogenes may cause the cell to function abnormally and eventually become cancerous.

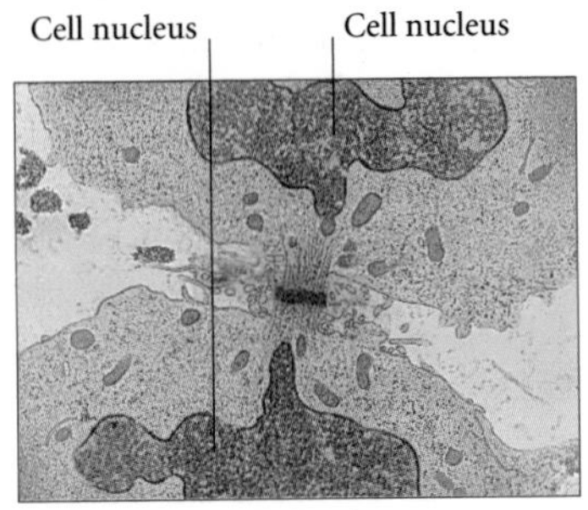

A cancerous cell dividing
In this magnified image, a cancerous cell is dividing to form two cells that contain damaged genetic material.

GENETIC DAMAGE

Oncogenes regulate the rate at which a cell divides. They also repair damaged genes and programme faulty cells to self-destruct. In time, carcinogens may cause irreparable damage to a cell's oncogenes. As damage accumulates, the oncogenes may start to function abnormally, causing the cell to become cancerous. If a faulty oncogene is inherited, a cell may become cancerous much more quickly.

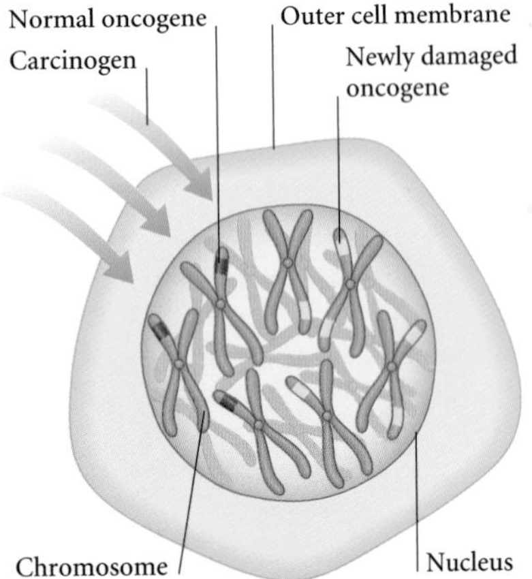

1 *Carcinogens penetrate the cell and cause repeated damage to oncogenes on the chromosomes. Most newly damaged oncogenes are repaired.*

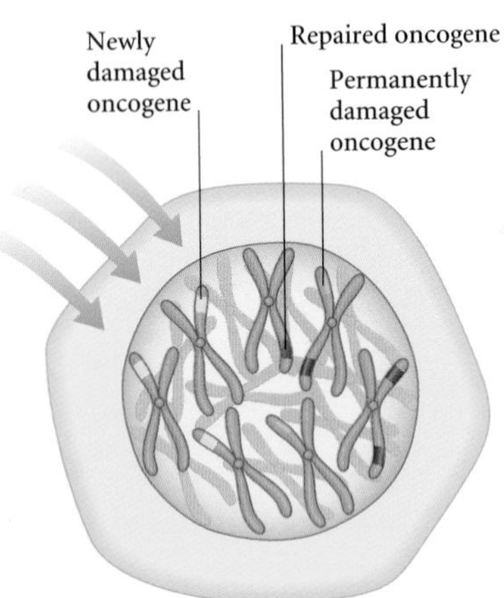

2 *The damage and repair of oncogenes continues. With time, some of the oncogenes in the cell become permanently damaged and cannot be repaired.*

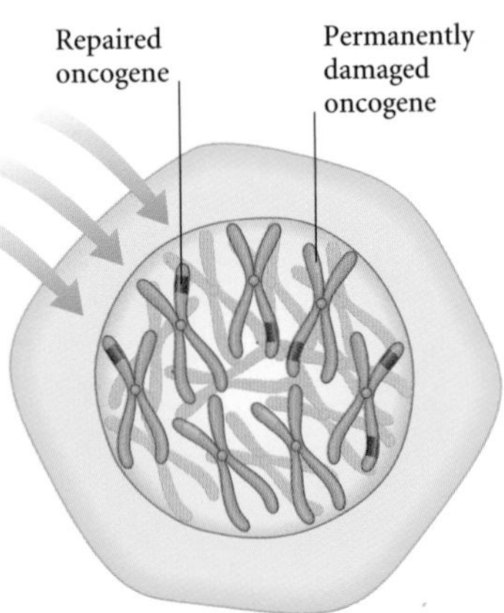

3 *If a number of oncogenes controlling key cell functions are permanently damaged, the cell no longer functions normally and becomes cancerous.*

FORMATION OF A TUMOUR

A cancerous tumour begins as a single cell. If the cell is not destroyed by the body's immune system, it will multiply uncontrollably, dividing to form two cells, which in turn divide to form four, and so on. Tumour growth rates are measured by the time taken for the number of cells in a tumour to double (the "doubling time"). The doubling time of a tumour generally varies from about 1 month to 2 years.

Doubling time
A solid tumour can usually be detected after 25–30 doublings. At this stage in its growth, a tumour contains about a billion cells and has a diameter of about 13 mm (½ in).

Tumour growth
After only four cell divisions, a cancerous tumour contains 16 cells. The cells double in number regularly, causing the tumour to grow larger.

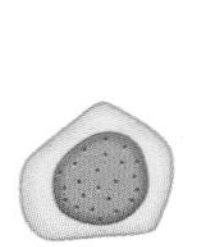

CANCEROUS CELL

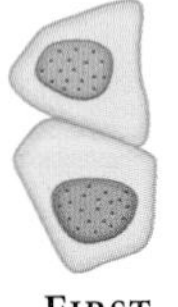

FIRST DOUBLING

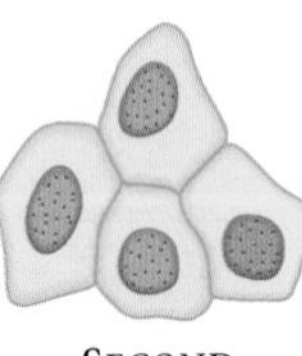

SECOND DOUBLING

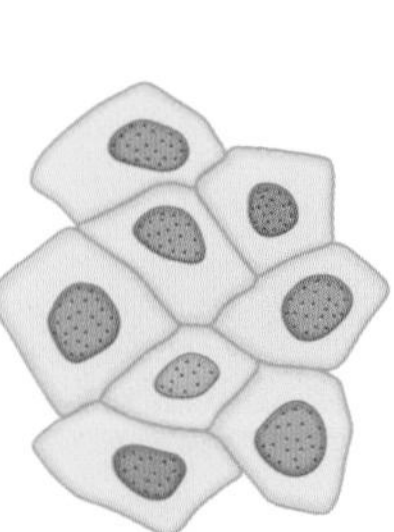

THIRD DOUBLING

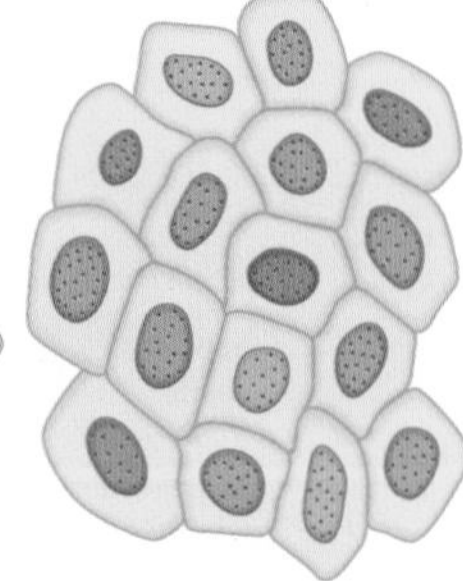

FOURTH DOUBLING

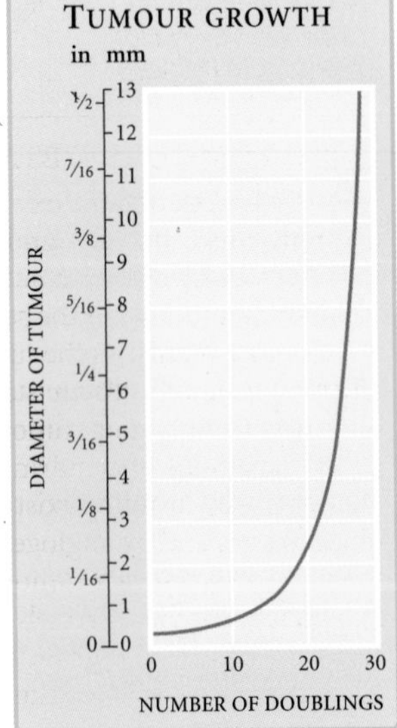

PROCESS HOW CANCER SPREADS

The defining feature of a cancerous tumour is its ability to spread not only locally but also to distant sites in the body by a process called metastasis. In metastasis, a cancerous cell detaches from a tumour and travels in the blood or lymph to a new location. The cell must overcome many obstacles if it is to settle in a new site and form a secondary tumour, also known as a metastasis. It must survive attacks from the immune system and stimulate the growth of blood vessels (angiogenesis) to provide oxygen and nutrients.

SPREAD IN THE LYMPH FLUID

Cancerous cells may spread into the lymphatic system, which is a network of vessels that drains lymph fluid to nearby lymph nodes, where the fluid is filtered. A cell may become trapped in a lymph node and multiply to form a tumour. Immune cells in the lymph node attack the tumour and may halt the progression of the cancer.

1 As a tumour grows, it invades surrounding tissues and can enter nearby lymph vessels. If some of the cancerous cells from the tumour detach themselves in the lymph vessel, they may be carried along the vessel until they reach and settle in a lymph node.

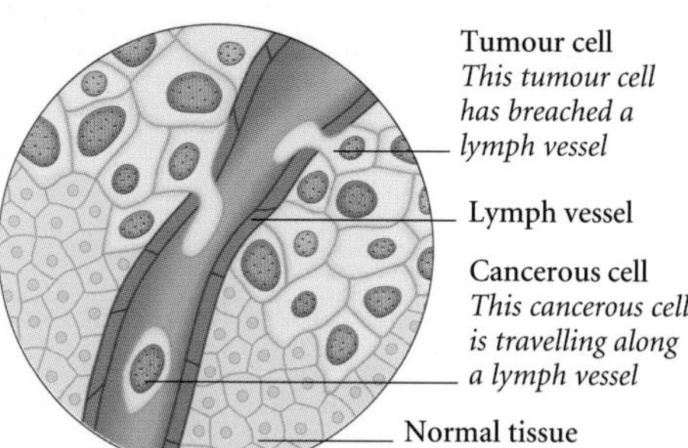

2 A cancerous cell enters a local lymph node, where it begins dividing to form a tumour. The tumour usually remains within the node, and the cells of the immune system may temporarily stop it from spreading to other parts of the body.

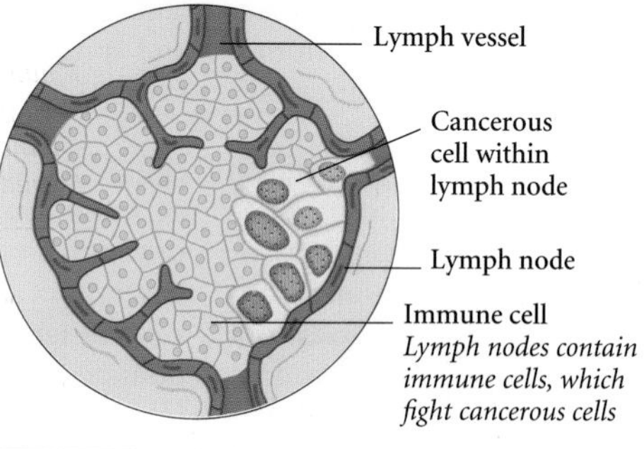

SPREAD IN THE BLOOD

Cancer often spreads to sites in the body that have a good blood supply, such as the liver, lungs, bone, and brain. The liver is a particularly common site since it receives blood from the heart and intestines. When cancerous cells reach very small blood vessels, they pass through the walls to invade tissues.

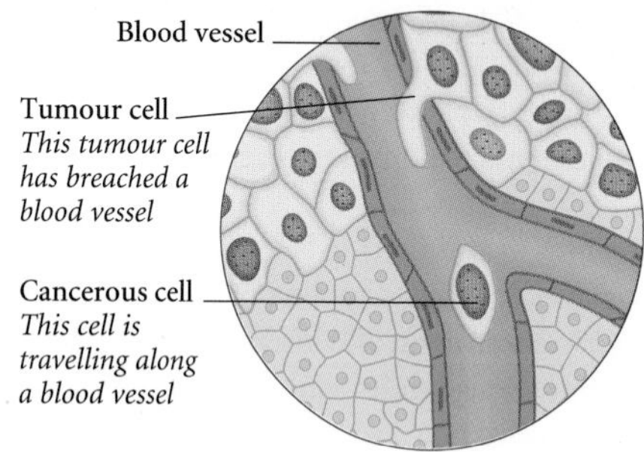

1 The growing tumour ruptures the walls of nearby blood vessels. Some cancerous cells detach from the tumour and pass through blood vessel walls into the blood circulation.

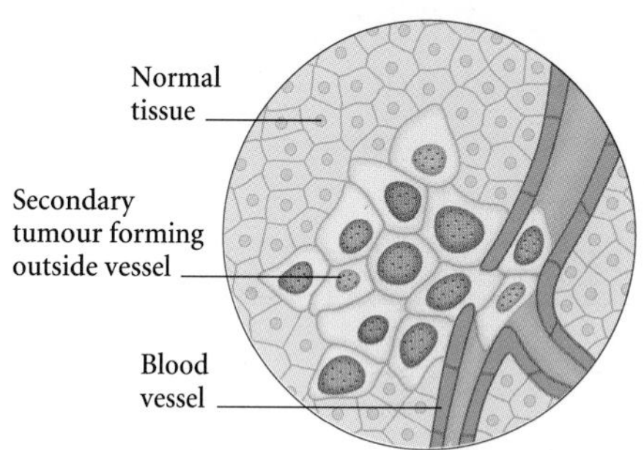

2 A cancerous cell travels in the bloodstream until it becomes lodged in a capillary (tiny blood vessel) at a distant site. The cell then starts dividing to form a secondary tumour.

HOW TUMOURS OBTAIN NUTRIENTS

A cancerous cell obtains oxygen and nutrients from surrounding blood vessels by diffusion across its outer membrane, in the same way as normal cells. As the tumour enlarges, its inner cells are starved of nutrients. Enlarging tumours use two methods of acquiring nutrients – by invading existing blood vessels and by angiogenesis, the process by which a tumour stimulates new blood vessels to form. To survive and grow, a tumour must be able to stimulate angiogenesis successfully.

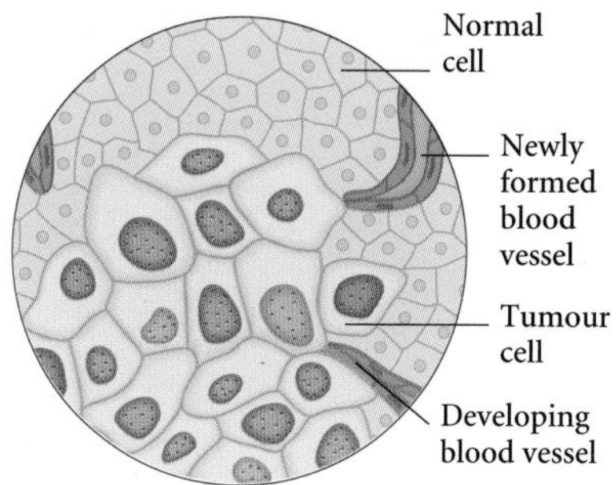

Angiogenesis
In angiogenesis, tumour cells produce chemicals that stimulate the growth of blood vessels towards the tumour.

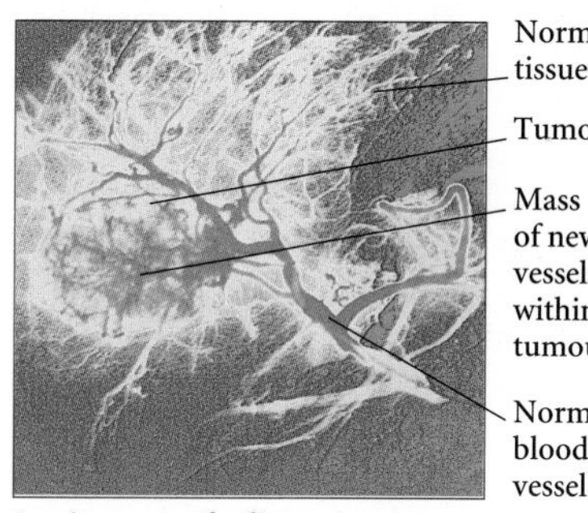

Angiogram of a liver tumour
This contrast X-ray of a tumour within the liver shows a large number of new blood vessels in the area of the tumour.

LIVING WITH CANCER

In recent years, improved techniques in the early diagnosis and treatment of cancer have led to more cures than ever before. However, cancer is primarily a disease of old age, and, as life expectancy increases, so does the proportion of people who will eventually develop some form of cancer in later life.

Cancer is not a single disease. Tumours arising in different tissues behave in different ways and respond differently to treatment. However, all cancers have some elements in common, such as their invasive growth.

The aim of this section is to look at the general principles applied to the diagnosis, treatment, and aftercare of all cancers. Research is being carried out to produce new treatments and cures. Some modern cancer treatments are still experimental but will probably eventually increase the proportion of people who survive. Even if a cancer cannot be cured, many treatments are available to relieve symptoms and improve quality of life.

Cancers that arise in a specific part of the body are covered in the relevant body system section. For example, lung cancer (p.503) is covered in the section on lung disorders, and breast cancer (p.759) in the breast disorders section.

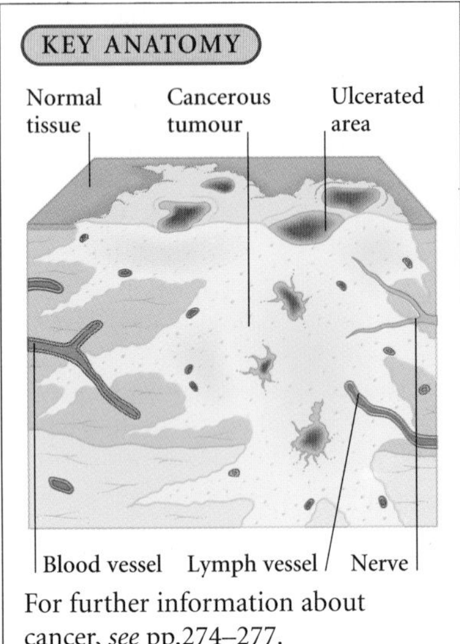

For further information about cancer, *see* pp.274–277.

Cancer and its management

The different causes of cancer and its management

AGE GENDER GENETICS LIFESTYLE
Risk factors depend on the type

Cancer is the second most common cause of death after heart disease in most western countries. In some countries, it is the leading cause of death. Although about 1 in 3 people develops cancer at some stage in life, many people can be cured because of advances in diagnosis and treatment.

Many types of cancer produce a solid tumour that forms in an organ, such as the breast, intestine, or bladder. If not detected and treated, these cancers may spread to other body tissues. Other cancers are often widespread from early on, such as cancer of the lymph nodes (*see* LYMPHOMA, p.459) and cancer of blood-forming cells in the bone marrow (*see* LEUKAEMIA, p.453).

WHAT ARE THE CAUSES?

Cancer occurs when cells divide and grow in an uncontrolled manner. Cell division and cell functioning are controlled by genes, and defects in some of these genes can lead to a cell becoming cancerous. In both children and adults, these defects (mutations) in the genes may be caused by environmental factors such as chemicals (especially from smoking), viruses, ultraviolet light, or other types of radiation. In some cases, an abnormal gene is inherited from a parent. The main causes of cancer vary in different age groups.

Children and adults with reduced immunity, such as those with AIDS (*see* HIV INFECTION AND AIDS, p.297) or people who are taking immunosuppressants (p.906), have an increased risk of developing certain types of cancer. In such people, agents such as viruses are more likely to cause cancer.

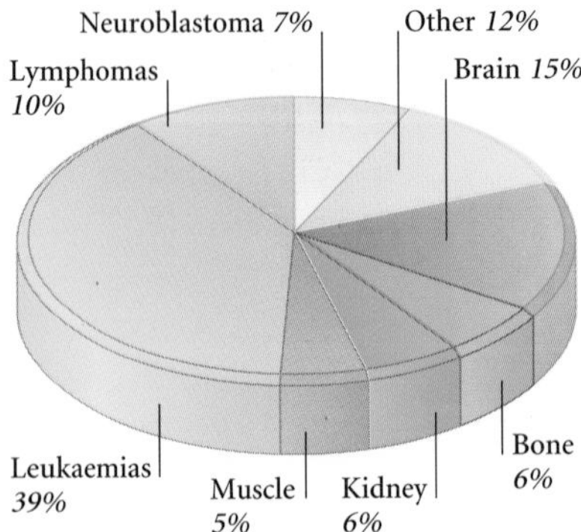

Cancer in children

The various types of leukaemia (cancer of the bone marrow) are by far the most common cancers affecting children.

CANCER IN CHILDREN Cancers in children are rare, affecting about 1 in 600 children in the UK, but they are still a major cause of death in infancy. The most common childhood cancers are leukaemia and tumours of the brain and spinal cord (*see* BRAIN AND SPINAL CORD TUMOURS IN CHILDREN, p.850).

The cause of most types of cancer in children is not known. Some cancers, such as a neuroblastoma (p.850), occur primarily in children. A neuroblastoma develops in an adrenal gland or the nervous system from tissue that normally disappears during fetal development. Cancers of this type are most common during infancy. Other types of childhood cancer, such as primary bone cancer (p.373), affect older children.

Occasionally, cancer is due to abnormal genes that may be inherited. About half of all cases of the eye cancer retinoblastoma (p.858) are mainly genetic in origin, and kidney cancer (*see* WILMS' TUMOUR, p.872) sometimes runs in families. In such cases, one or more family members may have the same cancer.

The risk of cancer is increased in some genetic disorders. For example, children with Down's syndrome (p.821) are 10–20 times more likely than other children to develop leukaemia.

Some cancers in children may be caused by environmental factors. For example, certain viruses, such as the Epstein–Barr virus, are known to cause some types of cancer, including one type of childhood lymphoma.

CANCER IN ADULTS Cancer occurs much more commonly in adults than in children. In the UK, about 1 in 3 people develops cancer at some time in adult life. The most common types of cancer that occur in adults are lung cancer (p.503), skin cancer (p.344), breast cancer (p.759), colorectal cancer (p.665), and prostate cancer (p.726).

Many cancers in adults under the age of 40 have a significant inherited factor. Up to 1 in 10 cases of cancer of the ovary (p.744), breast cancer, prostate cancer, and colorectal cancer are due in part to inheritance of abnormal genes. In older people, a combination of several factors eventually leads to cancer. The most common factors are carcinogens (cancer-causing agents), which include certain chemicals (particularly those found in tobacco smoke), dietary factors, some viruses, and specific types of radiation, including the ultraviolet light in natural sunlight.

In adults over the age of 50, the total number of newly diagnosed cancer cases roughly doubles each decade. Therefore, an 80-year-old person is eight times more likely to have cancer than a 50-year-old person. Some cancers, such as certain types of skin cancer and prostate cancer, are very common in old age, but these cancers may often be present without causing serious problems.

What are the symptoms?

Sometimes, a cancer is detected before it causes symptoms, often during a routine screening test. However, cancer is more often discovered when symptoms gradually develop and become noticeable over a period of weeks or months, prompting a person to visit a doctor. The symptoms of cancer may include:

- A lump, which is often firm and painless, in or beneath the skin.
- Changes in the appearance of a mole.
- A nonhealing wound.
- Blood in the urine or sputum.
- Changes in bowel habits.
- A discharge containing blood from the bowel or vagina.
- Persistent abdominal pain.
- Hoarseness or changes in the voice.
- Difficulty with swallowing.
- Severe, recurrent headaches.

Many cancers also produce more general symptoms, which may include:

- Weight loss.
- Unexplained tiredness.
- Loss of appetite and nausea.

If you experience one or more of these symptoms, you should consult your doctor as soon as possible.

How is it diagnosed?

Routine screening (p.42) is constantly improving the early diagnosis of cancer. Screening aims to detect disease before symptoms are present. An example is examination of the large intestine, such as a colonoscopy (p.661) or a rectal examination, to look for colorectal cancer. Other screening tests that are commonly used include mammography (p.759) to check for breast cancer

TEST Staging cancer

If you are diagnosed with cancer, your doctor will need to know if the cancer has spread from its primary site to nearby lymph nodes or to other parts of the body. This assessment of the spread of a cancer is known as staging and may involve surgery and imaging tests. Staging allows doctors to plan the best treatment and to determine the prognosis.

Size and local spread

The first part of staging involves measuring the size of the tumour and assessing the extent of its invasion into nearby tissues. A biopsy may be performed, in which a sample of tissue is taken from the tumour and examined, or the whole tumour may be removed for examination.

Biopsy sample of a tumour
This biopsy sample taken from an abnormal area of the colon confirms the presence of cancerous tissue. The junction between normal and cancerous tissue is clearly visible.

Normal tissue

Cancerous tissue

Lymph node involvement

If a cancer spreads, it often first affects nearby lymph nodes, causing them to enlarge. Cancer in lymph nodes can be detected by examination under a microscope after surgical removal or by imaging techniques such as CT scanning (p.247).

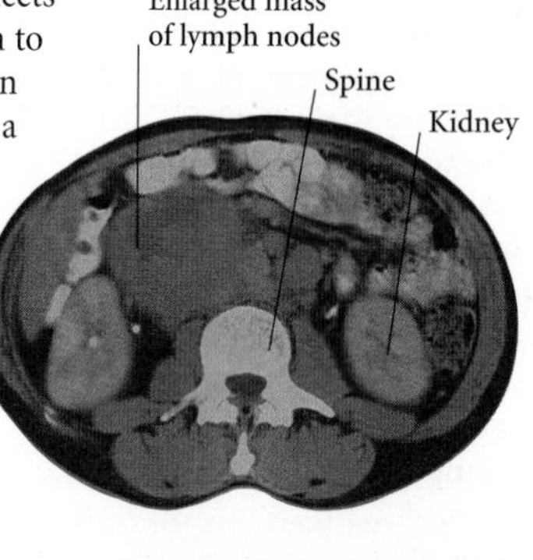

Cancer in the lymph nodes
This CT scan of the abdominal cavity shows an enlarged mass of cancerous lymph nodes. In this case, the cancer has spread from a testis.

Distant spread

If cancer cells enter the bloodstream, metastases (secondary tumours) may develop in other parts of the body. Imaging of the most common sites of metastases, such as the liver, lungs, and bones, may therefore be performed after a primary tumour is diagnosed.

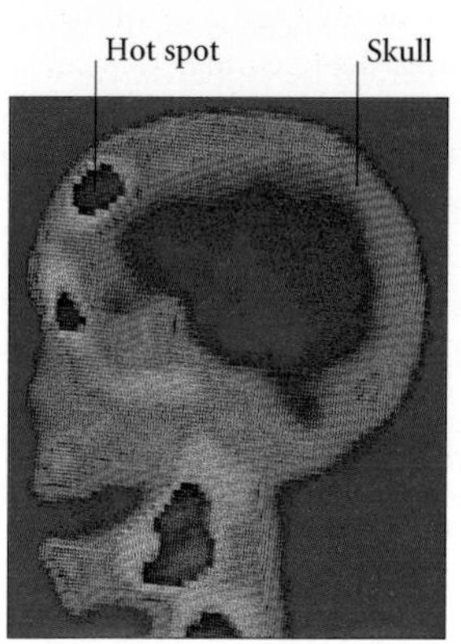

Bone metastases
In this radionuclide scan of the skull, "hot spots" show areas of increased cell activity. Such areas indicate the presence of cancer that has spread from elsewhere in the body.

and the cervical smear test (p.749) to look for precancerous cells that may lead to cancer of the cervix (p.750).

Alternatively, cancer may be diagnosed as a result of tests to investigate symptoms. Such tests may include imaging tests, such as X-rays (p.244), ultrasound scanning (p.250), CT scanning (p.247), or MRI (p.248). In a few cases, blood tests may be performed. For example, one test looks for proteins that indicate a particular type of tumour (*see* TUMOUR MARKER TESTS, p.233). To confirm a diagnosis, it is usually necessary to have a biopsy, in which a sample of abnormal tissue is removed and tested to find out if cancer is present (*see* CELL AND TISSUE TESTS, p.236). If cancer is present, further tests will identify the type of cell in the tissue that has become cancerous, which can give an indication of how fast the tumour is likely to grow and the best way to treat it. Once a diagnosis of cancer has been made, you will probably have tests to investigate how far the cancer has spread from its original site (*see* STAGING CANCER, p.279).

WHAT ARE THE TREATMENTS?

Although cancer can develop at many different sites around the body, the general principles of treatment are the same. The chances of a cancer being curable are highest if it is detected by screening at a sufficiently early stage before it causes symptoms.

The three main techniques used to treat cancer are surgery, chemotherapy (right), and radiotherapy (opposite page). Other treatments include biological and hormonal therapies.

Depending on the type and the stage of cancer, treatment may be intended to cure the cancer, slow the growth of the cancer, or be palliative (in which treatment is intended to help a person live as comfortably as possible rather than attempt to cure the cancer).

In most cases, curative treatment involves the surgical removal of a tumour. In addition to surgery, nonsurgical treatments, such as chemotherapy and radiotherapy, are often given with the aim of destroying any cancer cells that have spread beyond the obvious solid tumour. Nonsurgical treatments may also be used if a cure is not possible with the aim of slowing the growth of certain types of cancer rather than curing them. Palliative care can control the symptoms of cancer, maximize quality of life, and provide psychological help for you and your family as you come to terms with the process of dying.

Treatment is tailored to the type and the extent of the cancer, your age, your general health, and your wishes after discussing the outlook and options with doctors and family. For example, attempts to cure a cancer may not be appropriate in extreme old age because of the adverse effects of the treatment. Instead, treatment may be offered to relieve symptoms and to improve quality of life for the time left (*see* CARING FOR A TERMINALLY ILL PERSON, p.965).

SURGERY Surgical removal of a tumour is the main treatment for most common solid tumours at an early stage. During surgery, it is usual to remove some normal tissue surrounding the tumour to maximize the chances that all cancerous cells are removed from the body. Sometimes, the lymph nodes near the tumour are also removed because cancer often spreads to these nodes first. Less commonly, surgery aims to remove tumours that have spread to more distant sites in the body.

Surgery may not be appropriate if a tumour is inaccessible. For example, surgery to remove a tumour deep inside the brain may cause great damage to healthy brain tissue. Surgery may also not be the best treatment if the cancer has already spread to other parts of the body. In such cases, other treatments, including chemotherapy or radiotherapy, may be appropriate.

Surgery may be used as a palliative treatment for certain types of cancer (*see* PALLIATIVE SURGERY FOR CANCER, p.282). For example, surgery may be carried out to remove a tumour that is blocking the bowel or bile duct or to treat fractures of bones that have been weakened by cancer.

TREATMENT WITH ANTICANCER DRUGS
In chemotherapy (below), anticancer drugs (p.907) are used to kill cancerous cells. This is the principal treatment for leukaemias and other cancers that are widespread in the body. It may also be used for solid tumours that have spread to other parts of the body or to reduce the risk of further spread. Like surgery, chemotherapy may be used to cure cancer or as a palliative treatment. The side effects vary with the type of drug, but can include nausea and vomiting, temporary hair loss (*see* ALOPECIA, p.358), constipation, diarrhoea, tiredness, and rarely kidney damage or anaemia (p.446). You may be offered treatments for some of these side effects, such as antiemetic drugs (p.922) for nausea and vomiting or blood transfusions (p.447) for anaemia. The duration of treatment varies depending on the type of cancer and the aim of the treatment.

TREATMENT CHEMOTHERAPY

Treatment of cancer with anticancer drugs (p.907) is known as chemotherapy. The drugs may be taken orally but are more often given directly into the bloodstream by injection into a vein. You may need to take the drugs daily, weekly, or monthly. Treatment by injection will usually be given in hospital.

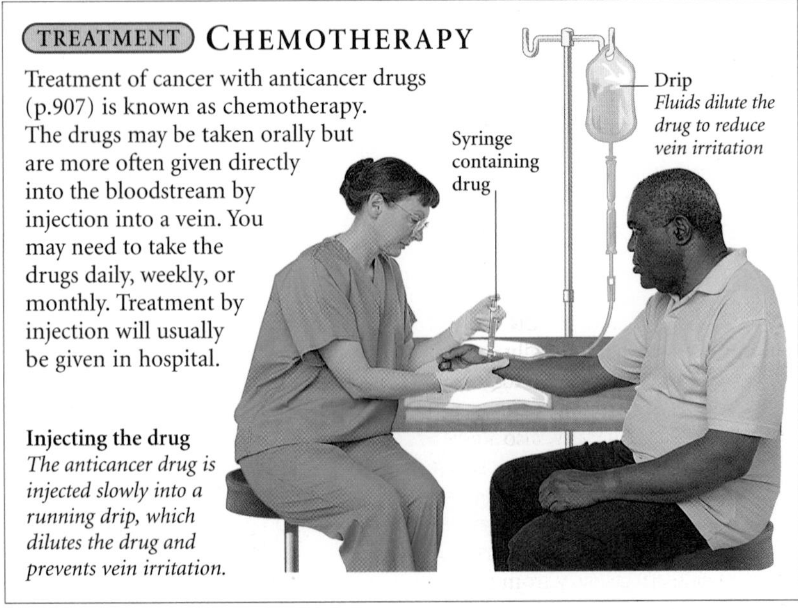

Injecting the drug
The anticancer drug is injected slowly into a running drip, which dilutes the drug and prevents vein irritation.

TREATMENT RADIOTHERAPY

During radiotherapy, cancer cells are destroyed by using high-intensity radiation. Treatment can be either external or internal depending on the site of the tumour. The dose and position of the radiation is carefully calculated so that normal cells receive as little radiation as possible, allowing them to recover with little or no long-term damage. The treatment is painless at the time, but side effects such as nausea may develop as treatment continues. Radiotherapy may be used alone or with other cancer treatments.

EXTERNAL RADIATION

External radiation is often carried out using a linear accelerator, which produces X-rays, gamma rays, or electron beams. The type of radiation used depends on the type of cancer. The skin is usually marked with ink to outline the area to be treated. Treatment may be given once, several times a week, or several times a day, depending on the cancer and type of radiation used.

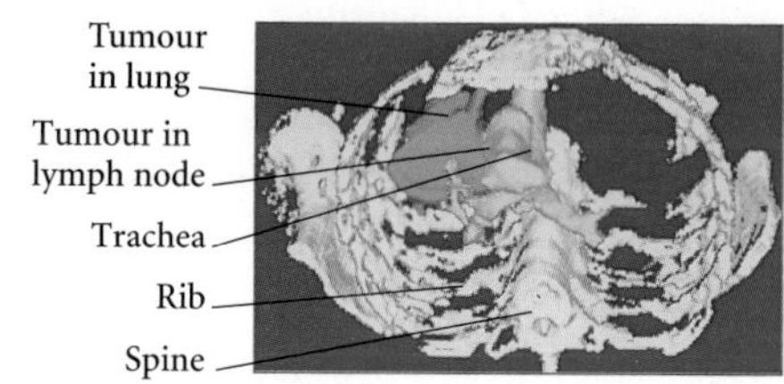

Lung tumour
Multiple CT scans are taken at different angles and used to construct a 3-D computer map of the tumours in a lung and a nearby lymph node. Such maps are used as an accurate plan of the area that will receive radiation.

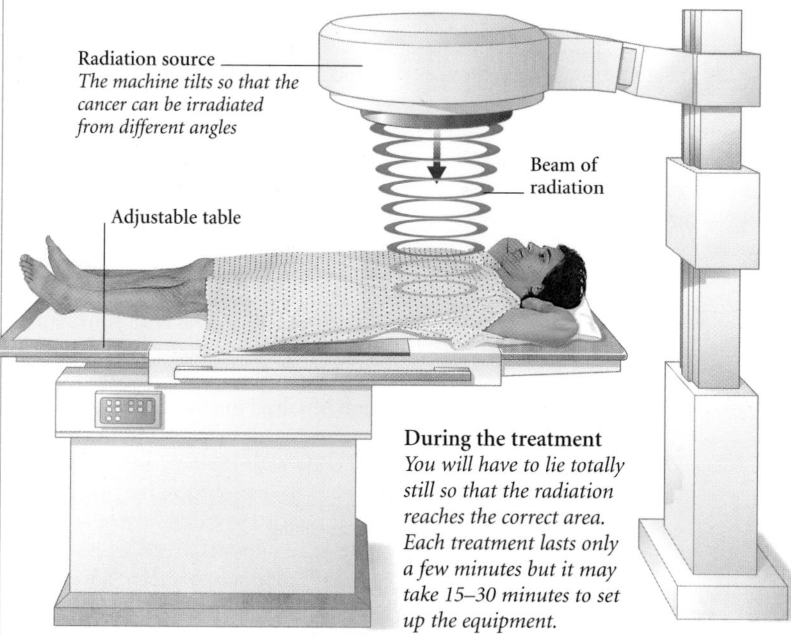

During the treatment
You will have to lie totally still so that the radiation reaches the correct area. Each treatment lasts only a few minutes but it may take 15–30 minutes to set up the equipment.

INTERNAL RADIATION

During this procedure, radioactive materials are placed directly into or around the cancer. For example, temporary radioactive implants may be placed within hollow organs, such as the uterus or vagina. Occasionally, a radioactive substance may be taken orally or injected into a body cavity. In some instances, small radioactive seeds may be placed directly into the affected organ and left in place while they gradually release radiation.

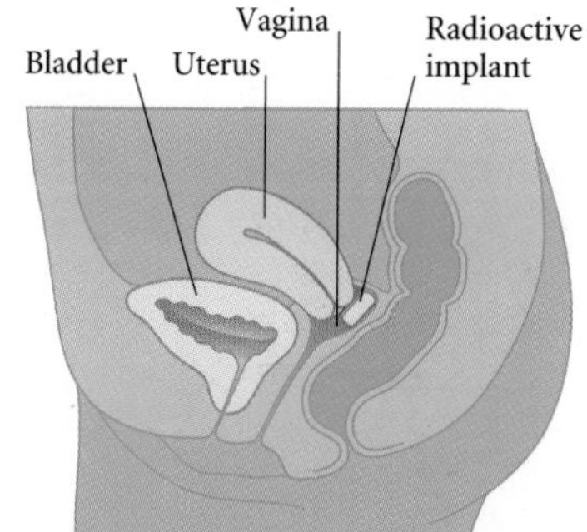

Radioactive implants in the vagina
Implants containing radioactive substances are sometimes used to treat cancers of the uterus, the cervix, and the vagina.

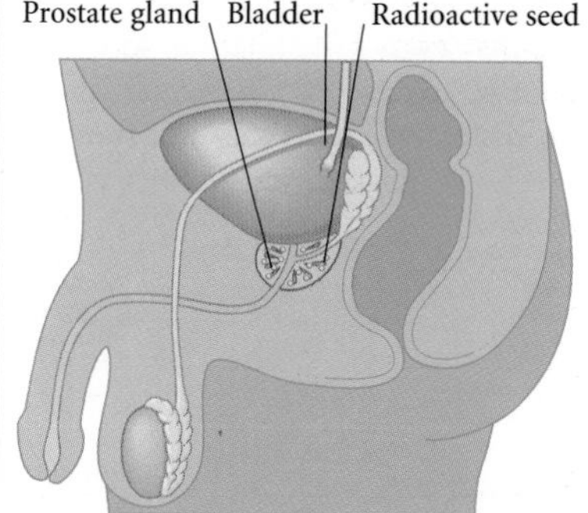

Radioactive seeds in the prostate
Prostate cancer may be treated by the insertion of radioactive seeds. The seeds emit radiation for several months.

TREATMENT WITH RADIATION In this technique, radiation is carefully focused on an area of cancerous tissue to destroy it or to slow its growth (*see* RADIOTHERAPY, above). Radiotherapy, also known as radiation therapy, can have severe side effects. However, your doctor will recommend radiotherapy if he or she believes that it will be worthwhile. Common side effects vary from person to person and may include reddened or painful skin at the site of treatment, loss of appetite, nausea and vomiting, and tiredness. If you have radiotherapy to the head or neck, you may temporarily lose your hair (*see* ALOPECIA, p.358) and experience pain in the throat and a permanently dry mouth. Radiotherapy to the large bowel may cause inflammation and persistent diarrhoea. Many of these side effects can be relieved using drugs and clear up when treatment has been completed. Radiotherapy can be used either curatively or palliatively.

HORMONAL THERAPIES Certain types of hormone affect the cell growth and replication of some cancers. For example, the female sex hormone oestrogen is known to stimulate the growth of

TREATMENT PALLIATIVE SURGERY FOR CANCER

The aim of palliative surgery is to relieve the symptoms or to prevent complications rather than to cure the cancer. Palliative surgery may be performed to remove an unsightly growth; to relieve or remove an obstruction that is due to a tumour, particularly within the digestive or respiratory tract; to cut nerves that transmit pain signals; or to prevent fractures of bones that are weakened by cancerous deposits. Two common examples of palliative surgery for cancer are described below.

RELIEVING AN OBSTRUCTION

If narrowing of an airway or of the intestine is causing symptoms, a rigid incompressible tube, known as a stent, can help to keep the passage unblocked. Under general anaesthesia, the stent is pushed through the obstruction to open up or widen the affected passage.

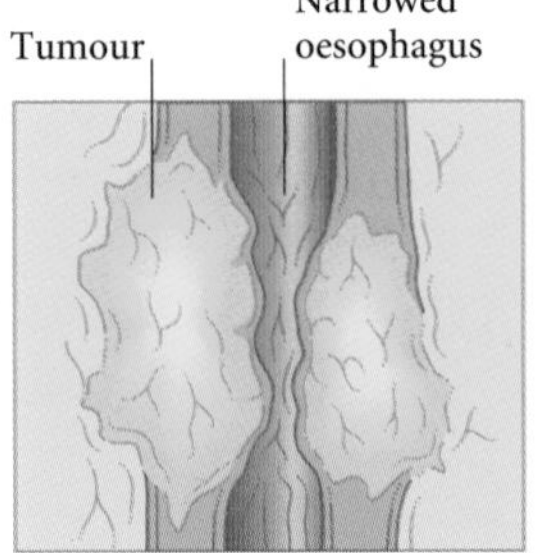

BEFORE SURGERY

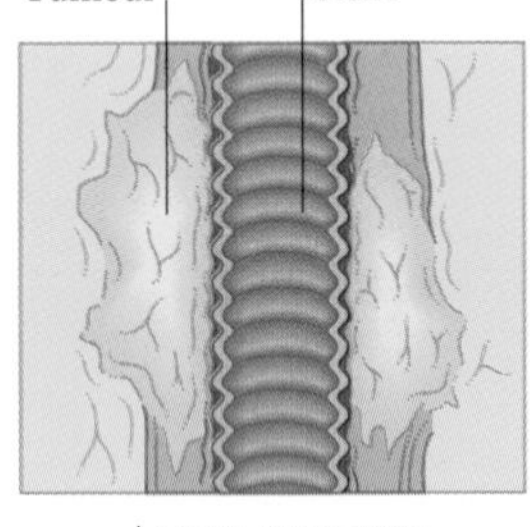

AFTER SURGERY

LOCATION

Oesophageal stent
The oesophagus has become narrowed by a tumour, which makes swallowing difficult. A rigid plastic tube (stent) inserted to widen the oesophagus makes swallowing easier.

PREVENTING FRACTURES

If cancer spreads from elsewhere in the body to an area of the bone, the affected bone becomes weak and thin and may eventually fracture. To help to prevent fractures from occurring and allow a person to remain as active as possible, the bone may be pinned using a metal rod.

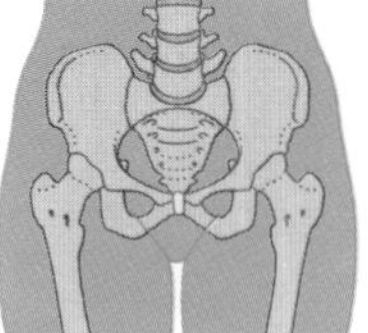
LOCATION

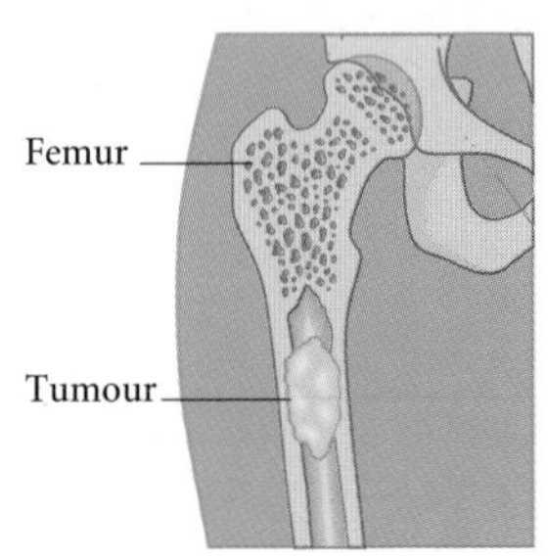

BEFORE SURGERY

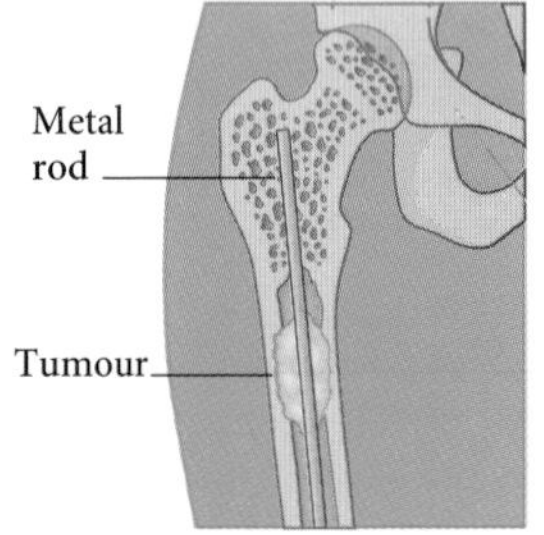

AFTER SURGERY

Pinning the femur
Cancer has spread to the femur from elsewhere in the body. The metal rod supports the affected area of bone to prevent a fracture.

most breast cancers and also suppress the growth of prostate cancer. Treatment with sex hormones plays an important part in the management of these types of cancer (*see* SEX HORMONES AND RELATED DRUGS, p.933).

BIOLOGICAL THERAPIES These newer types of treatment are currently under investigation and are not yet used for most cancers. Biological therapies may involve taking drugs known as "cancer vaccines" to stimulate the immune system, which is the body's natural defence mechanism. For example, substances such as interferons, which trigger some types of white blood cell to attack abnormal cells, can be manufactured synthetically and given as interferon drugs (p.907). You may also be given synthetically created antibodies (proteins that recognize and attack foreign cells or particles in the body) that deliver a radioactive substance or anticancer drug directly to a cancer.

Two promising experimental biological therapies are gene therapy and angiogenesis inhibition. Gene therapy involves introducing a gene into the genetic material of cancerous cells by using a virus. The new gene is responsible for producing a natural substance that can help destroy the cancerous cells. Experiments using animals have shown that this approach can shrink small tumours. In angiogenesis inhibition, drugs are given to halt the growth of new blood vessels that allow a tumour to continue to grow. When starved of an adequate supply of nutrients and oxygen, the tumour shrinks.

Biological therapies have now been used successfully to treat kidney cancer (p.704), malignant melanoma (p.346), and certain types of lymphomas and leukaemias. These treatments may cause side effects such as fever, muscle aches, vomiting, and fatigue.

SUPPORTIVE CARE A diagnosis of cancer and its treatment can be stressful and frightening. The aim of supportive care is to make life continue as normally as possible. You will be offered relief for the symptoms of cancer, such as pain (*see* PAIN RELIEF FOR CANCER, opposite page). Side effects due to cancer treatments, such as vomiting, will also be treated. You and your family will probably be offered psychological support and advice from the medical team involved in your treatment. These specialists will help you to understand and cope with the diagnosis and treatment of the cancer. You may wish to see a counsellor to obtain advice and psychological support (*see* COUNSELLING, p.971). Such support can boost your emotional well-being and self-esteem, which may be particularly affected if treatment has caused obvious physical changes, such as removal of a breast or hair loss. Research appears to show that people with a positive mental attitude survive longer than those who simply resign themselves to the disease.

Sharing problems with people who have had similar personal experiences can be reassuring, and it may be possible to join a support group for people with cancer and their families.

WHAT IS THE PROGNOSIS?

The earlier a cancer is diagnosed, the more likely it is that treatment will be successful and the cancer can be cured. The prognosis is usually expressed in terms of a 5-year survival rate (the percentage of people alive 5 years after the diagnosis of cancer is made). For most types of cancers, the outlook has been greatly improved during the last few decades, especially in children.

These days, as many as 7 in 10 children and 1 in 2 adults diagnosed with cancer are alive 5 years later (*see* SURVIVING CANCER, below). Even in cases where the cancer cannot be cured, there is still a good chance of long-term survival with a fairly good quality of life, often for many years after the diagnosis.

(WWW) ONLINE SITES: p.1028, p.1035

Surviving cancer

An overview of the features of life after successful treatment for cancer

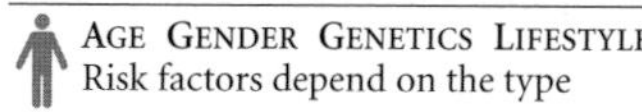

Cure rates may be higher than 9 in 10 for some types of cancers and lower than 1 in 10 for others. The chances of a cure depend on various factors, including the age and general health of the affected person, the type of cancer and the stage it has reached, and the effectiveness of treatment (*see* CANCER AND ITS MANAGEMENT, p.278). Full remission occurs when all the symptoms disappear and there is no evidence of any cancerous cells in the body. If cancer does not recur for 5 years, there is a good chance that it has been cured. A relapse may be indicated by the return of symptoms or by evidence of cancer in follow-up tests.

Sometimes, treatment may damage the immune system (*see* ACQUIRED IMMUNODEFICIENCY, p.460). Radiotherapy (p.281) and chemotherapy (p.280) may increase the risk of a second type of cancer developing in previously normal tissue. For example, chemotherapy may increase the risk that leukaemia (p.453) or lymphoma (p.459) will develop.

ARE THERE COMPLICATIONS?

Cancer treatment often causes physical changes that may be psychologically difficult to deal with. For example, a breast may have been removed because of breast cancer (p.759). Mental abilities may also be affected, especially after treatment for brain and spinal cord tumours in children (p.850).

Emotional problems after treatment may understandably include a fear that the cancer is going to recur. You may also become depressed as a reaction to the physical changes caused by the treatment (*see* DEPRESSION, p.554).

You may encounter discrimination at work. Some employers may be reluctant to employ or promote you if you have been treated for cancer. They may be unwilling to invest money in you and assume that you are going to die soon or that you will claim large amounts of money from pension and health insurance plans. Employers may also have an unfounded belief that survivors of cancer are unproductive workers and may fear that you will need a long time off work. However, there are organizations that can offer emotional support and legal advice if you face discrimination.

WHAT MIGHT THE DOCTOR DO?

You will be advised to visit the doctor for follow-up evaluations once the cancer has gone into remission. Follow-up involves routine checkups at intervals after treatment. These checkups may involve having imaging tests, such as X-rays (p.244) or CT scanning (p.247), endoscopy (p.255), or blood tests (*see* TUMOUR MARKER TESTS, p.233). Some cancers can be successfully treated if a recurrence is detected early enough.

WHAT CAN I DO?

You should attend any recommended follow-up appointments and try not to feel too anxious or fearful about these checkups. They will be scheduled less frequently over time and are often required only annually after 5 years. Follow-up is carried out to maximize the chances of diagnosing and successfully treating any recurrence of cancer early.

Once your cancer has been cured, you may feel the need to improve the quality of your life by making a change in your priorities. Many cancer survivors decide to leave or change their jobs in order to fulfill lifelong ambitions or to spend more time with their families. You and your family may also wish to join a self-help organization, usually run by cancer survivors, which can offer support and advice to other survivors and their families.

If you develop cancer before the age of 50, it may have a genetic cause. If this genetic cause has been inherited then other family members may also be at increased risk of developing the same cancer. For example, a small proportion of cases of colorectal cancer (p.665), breast cancer (p.759), cancer of the ovary (p.744), and prostate cancer (p.726) have an inherited genetic cause.

If your family has a higher than normal incidence of a particular type of cancer, it is important for relatives at risk to be regularly screened for that cancer (*see* SCREENING, p.42).

(WWW) ONLINE SITES: p.1028

(TREATMENT) PAIN RELIEF FOR CANCER

It should be possible to control pain due to cancer by using drugs. Painkillers (p.912) of increasing strength can be prescribed and most are taken orally as pills or liquids, or applied as skin patches. If pain is severe and not controlled by these types of drugs, morphine or other powerful painkillers may be injected continuously at home using a portable syringe driver, which allows a person to pursue normal activities.

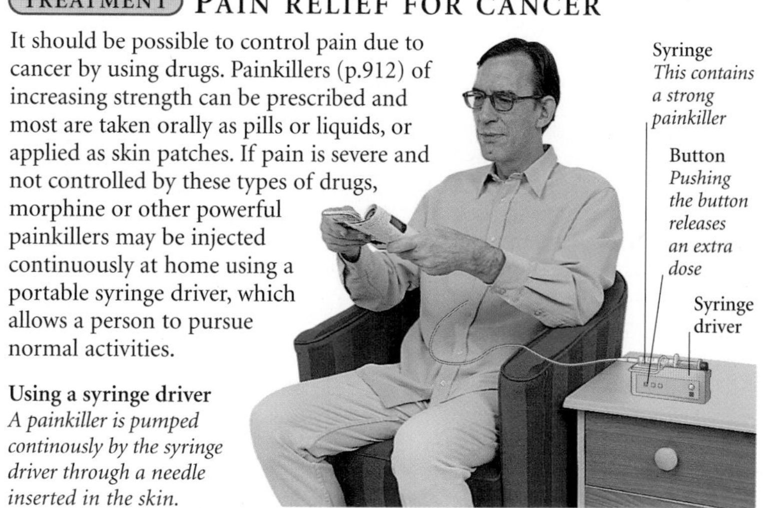

Using a syringe driver
A painkiller is pumped continously by the syringe driver through a needle inserted in the skin.

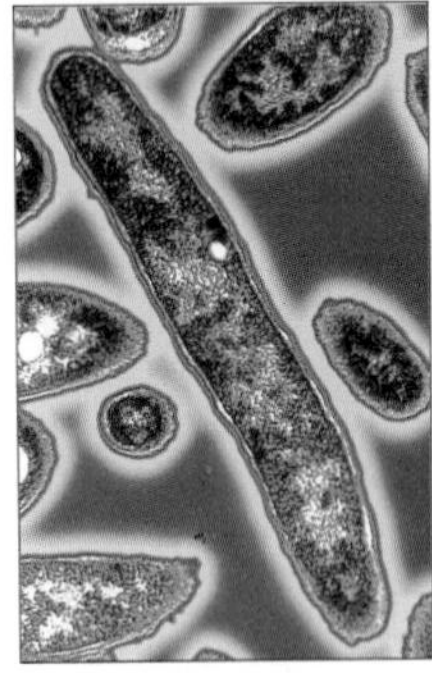

Legionella bacteria
These bacteria, which can cause pneumonia, are sometimes found in air conditioners.

INFECTIONS AND INFESTATIONS

THE MOST COMMON CAUSE OF DISEASE is infection by microorganisms that find their way into internal body tissues, where they multiply and disrupt normal cell function. These organisms, which are commonly known as germs, take a wide range of forms and contain the groups classified broadly as viruses, bacteria, protozoa, and fungi. Disease can also be caused by larger, more complex organisms, such as parasitic worms and their larvae, which may infest various parts of the body, especially the intestine.

The likelihood of serious illness from infectious disease is largely influenced by the environment. In the developed world, most infections can be treated effectively or prevented. However, in the developing world, where children are often malnourished, many of the common infections, such as measles, can be fatal. People living in temperate regions are rarely affected by cholera, malaria, or parasitic worms, but in the tropics such disorders are frequent causes of ill health and death.

Sometimes, an infectious disease spreads rapidly worldwide. Influenza, for example, tends to occur in annual outbreaks in all countries. Future global health threats include several newly emerged diseases, such as AIDS, and long-established diseases, such as tuberculosis, in which organisms have become resistant to common drugs.

HOW INFECTIONS ARE TRANSMITTED

The organisms that cause disease enter the body in a variety of ways. Some are breathed in or swallowed in food and water; others may gain entry through a break in the skin or be transmitted during sexual contact. An infection may spread throughout the body, affecting several organs at once. However, certain infectious organisms target and damage only one particular organ or part of the body, such as the liver, respiratory tract, or intestine.

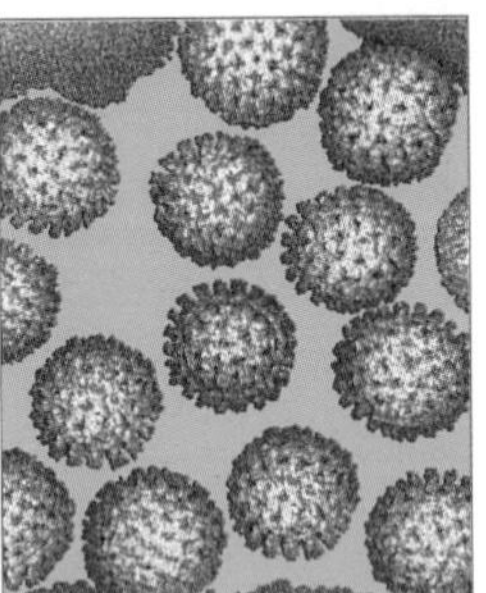

Rotaviruses
These wheel-shaped viruses are a common cause of gastrointestinal infections.

Infections are more likely to develop if the number of infecting organisms is large or if a person's resistance to disease is reduced. Reduced resistance may be due to factors such as extremes of age, poor nutrition, or an immune system already weakened by disease.

CONTROLLING INFECTION

Over the last 100 years, great advances have been made in the control of infections, largely due to improvements in diet, housing, and hygiene. In addition, the increasing availability of routine immunizations and drugs such as antibiotics have made it possible to cure or even wipe out many infectious diseases. International programmes to monitor the occurrence of infections have also helped to check the spread of many often fatal diseases.

COMPARISON SIZES OF ORGANISMS

There are vast differences in size between the various infectious organisms. However, an organism's size does not determine the severity of the disease it causes. A microscopic virus can lead to a life-threatening illness, and a tapeworm 6 m (20 ft) long may cause only mild symptoms.

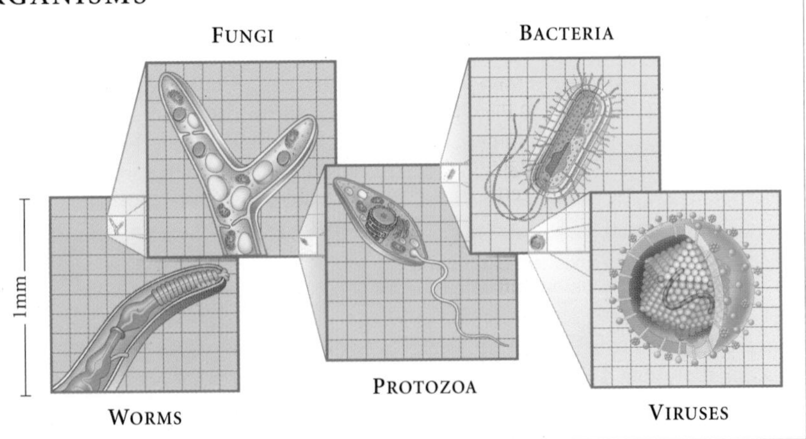

Relative dimensions of organisms
Worms are the largest disease-causing organisms. In this diagram, each successive picture after worms represents a 100-fold magnification. The smallest disease-causing organisms are the viruses.

STRUCTURE AND FUNCTION VIRUSES

Viruses are the smallest infectious organisms, and they are so tiny that millions of them could fit inside a single human cell. Viruses are only capable of reproduction inside a living cell, called a host cell, that they invade. A virus consists of little more than a single or double strand of genetic material surrounded by a protein shell. However, some types of virus also have a protective outer envelope.

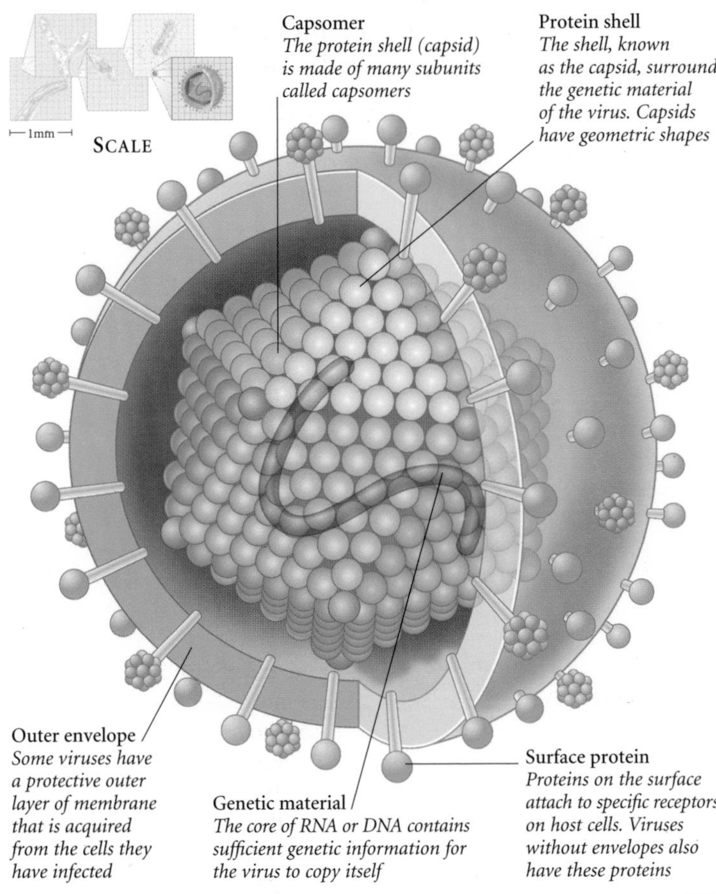

Capsomer
The protein shell (capsid) is made of many subunits called capsomers

Protein shell
The shell, known as the capsid, surrounds the genetic material of the virus. Capsids have geometric shapes

Outer envelope
Some viruses have a protective outer layer of membrane that is acquired from the cells they have infected

Genetic material
The core of RNA or DNA contains sufficient genetic information for the virus to copy itself

Surface protein
Proteins on the surface attach to specific receptors on host cells. Viruses without envelopes also have these proteins

CHANGES IN VIRUSES

The immune system recognizes viruses by the proteins that are on their surfaces (antigens). When viruses reproduce, the antigens on the new viruses may become slightly different to prevent the immune system from recognizing the virus. This is known as antigenic drift. Much larger changes (antigenic shifts) may result in epidemics.

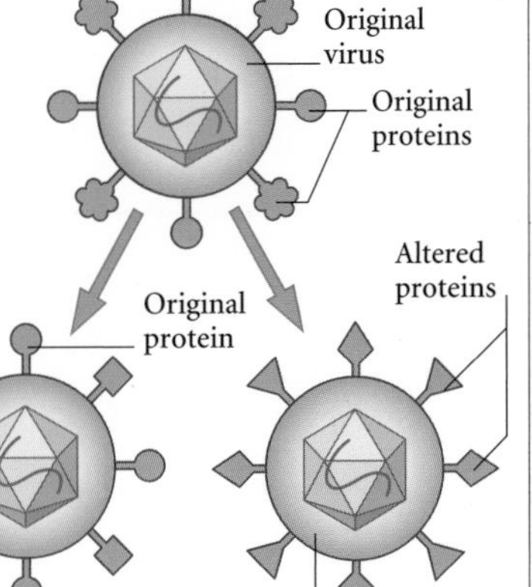

Antigenic drift and shift
A minor change to a virus is known as antigenic drift; a larger change is known as an antigenic shift.

HOW VIRUSES REPRODUCE

To survive, viruses must reproduce inside living cells. The genetic material from an infecting virus takes over the functions of the host cell to make millions of new virus particles.The new viruses leave the host cell by bursting out of the cell or by budding out from the cell surface.

1 *Proteins on the virus attach to specific receptors on the surface of a host cell. The virus may enter the cell by being engulfed by the cell membrane or by fusing into the cell membrane.*

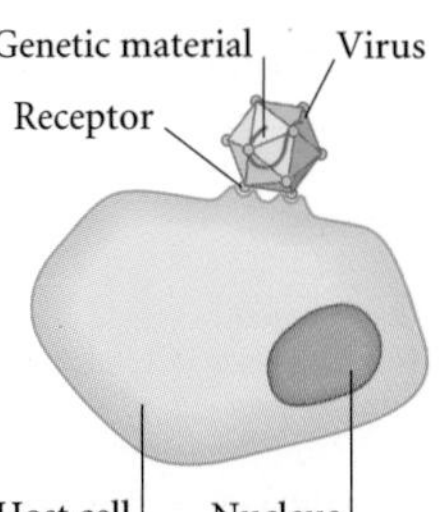

2 *When inside the cell, the virus sheds its protein shell. The genetic material of the virus reproduces, using substances from inside the cell.*

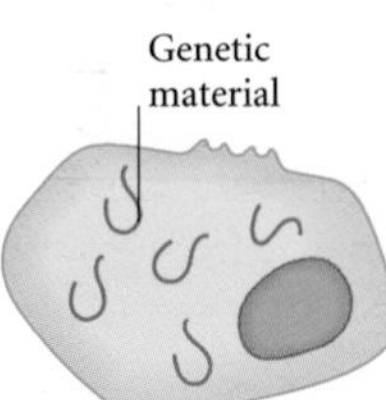

3 *Each copy of the genetic material programmes the formation of a new protein shell. Once the shells have formed, the new viruses are complete.*

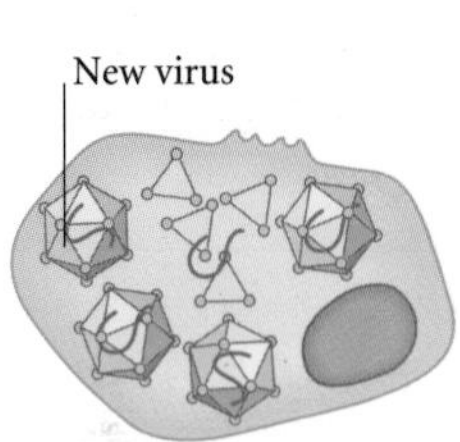

4 *The viruses leave the cell either by suddenly rupturing the cell membrane, which destroys the host cell, or by slowly budding out from the surface of the cell membrane.*

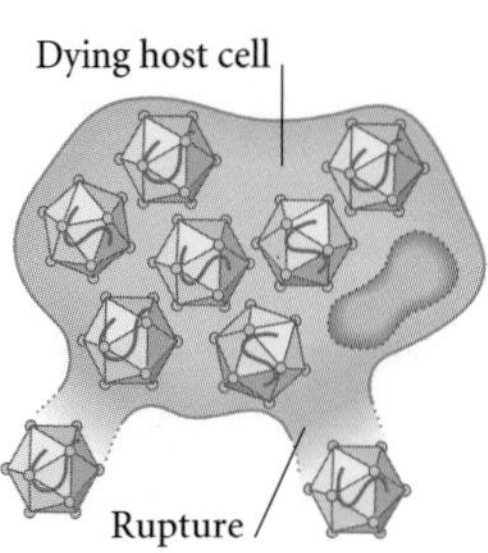

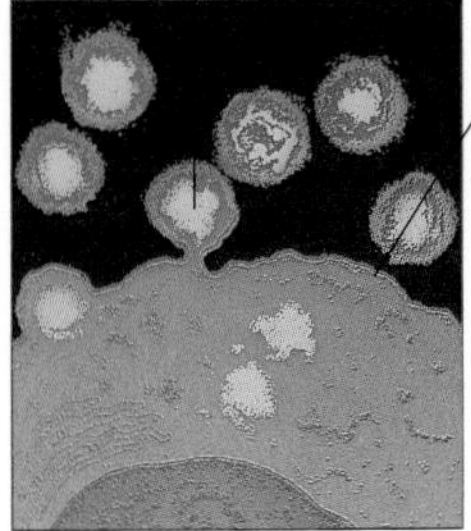

Budding viruses
When certain viruses bud out from their host cell, they envelop themselves in host cell surface membrane.

STRUCTURE AND FUNCTION BACTERIA

Bacteria are microscopic single-celled organisms that are found in every environment. Some bacteria live in or on our bodies without causing disease. There are thousands of different types of bacterium, but relatively few of these cause disease in humans. Bacteria have a variety of shapes that are broadly classified as cocci (spheres), bacilli (rods), and spirochetes and spirilla (curved forms).

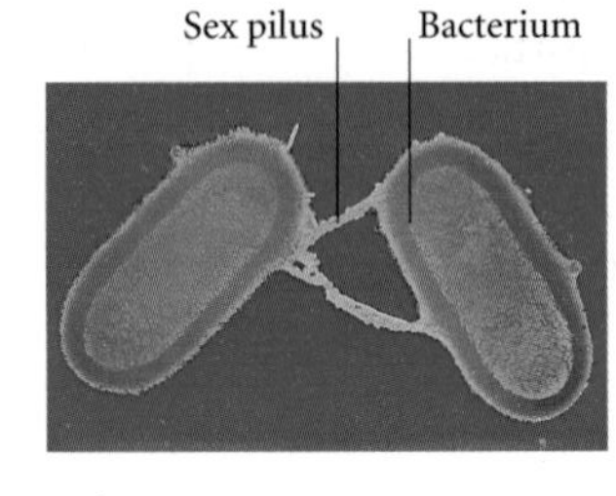

Conjugation
Bacteria may exchange genes in a process called conjugation. Plasmids, which may contain genes that give the bacteria resistance to antibiotics, are passed through tubes called sex pili.

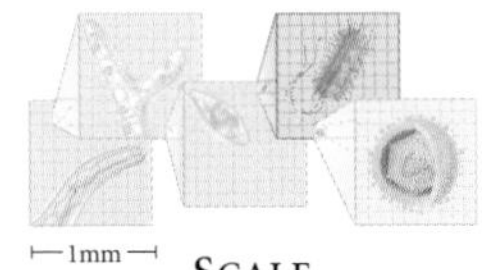

SCALE

Cell wall
Most bacteria have rigid cell walls made of complex sugars and amino acids

Capsule
Some bacteria are encased in a capsule that provides extra protection from the host's immune system

Cytoplasm
All metabolic processes necessary for life occur in this fluid

Plasma membrane
This layer controls the entrance and exit of chemicals, water, and waste from the cell

Nucleoid
This area contains the cell's DNA (genetic material)

Plasmid
This circle of DNA contains some extra beneficial genes

Mesosome
This infolding of plasma membrane may have a role in cell division

BACILLUS

Flagellum
This hair-like projection is used in movement

Pilus
The delicate but rigid pili anchor the bacteria to other cells

Ribosome
This structure is involved in the manufacture of proteins

Ribosome

Nucleoid

Capsule

COCCUS

Capsule

Ribosome

Flagellum
This spirillum has flagella coiled within its cell wall

SPIROCHETE

EFFECTS OF TOXINS

Some bacteria cause disease by producing poisonous chemicals known as toxins. These chemicals may destroy specific body cells or enter cells and alter their chemical processes. Some toxins are released from bacteria when they die and may cause shock and fever.

1 *The toxin is released into the body by the bacterium. The toxin attaches to a body cell and is absorbed into the fluid cytoplasm.*

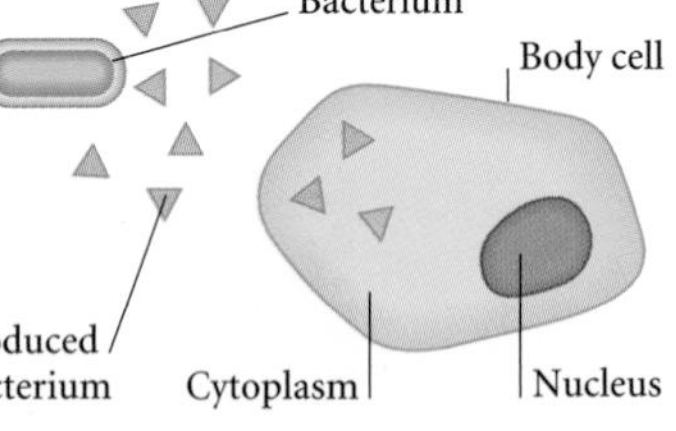

2 *The toxin disrupts normal chemical reactions inside the cell, so that the cell is unable to function and dies.*

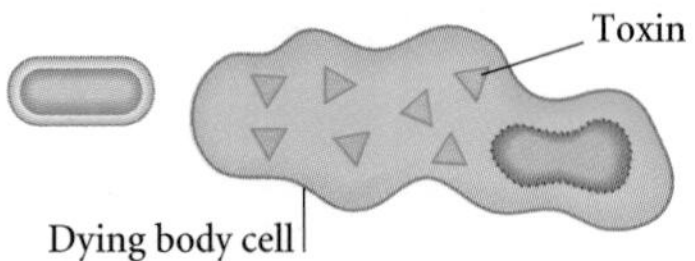

BACTERIAL INVASION OF A CELL

A few bacteria damage tissues in the human body not by secreting toxins but by directly invading the cells. Once inside body cells, the bacteria reproduce and eventually burst out, rupturing the cell membrane.

1 *Different bacteria are specifically attracted to certain body cells. Bacteria enter the cell through the membrane and use the cell nutrients.*

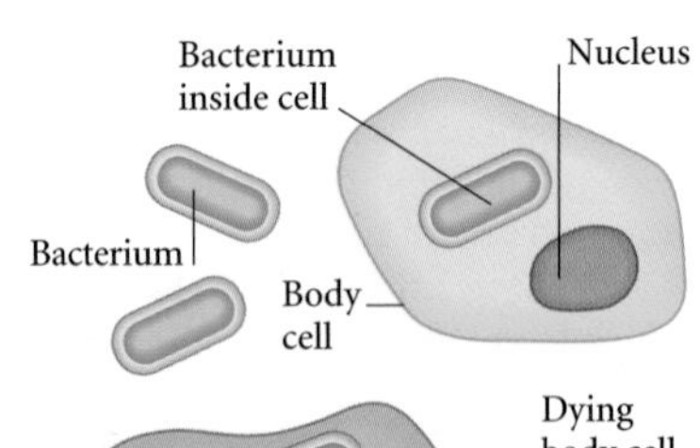

2 *The bacteria multiply rapidly in the cell. They kill the cell by breaking its membrane then spread to other areas of the body.*

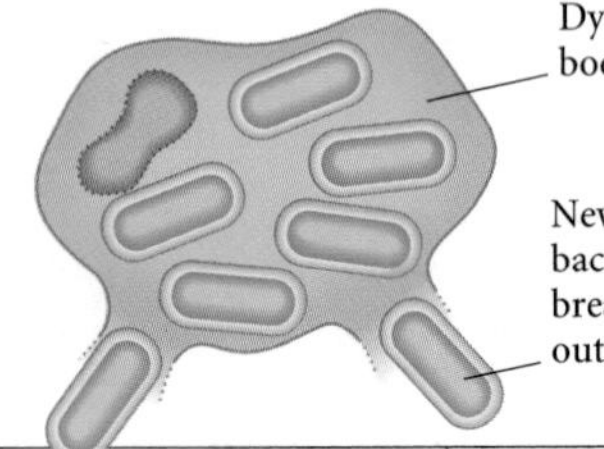

STRUCTURE PROTOZOA

Protozoa are single-celled organisms that feed by scavenging for particles and other microorganisms, such as bacteria, or by absorbing nutrients from their environment. Many types of protozoa live in moist places, such as soil, water, or sewage, and some of these may infect humans and other animals, causing disease. Other types of disease-causing protozoa depend on bloodsucking insects, such as mosquitoes, to spread them among human hosts. Most cases of protozoal infection occur in the tropical regions of the world.

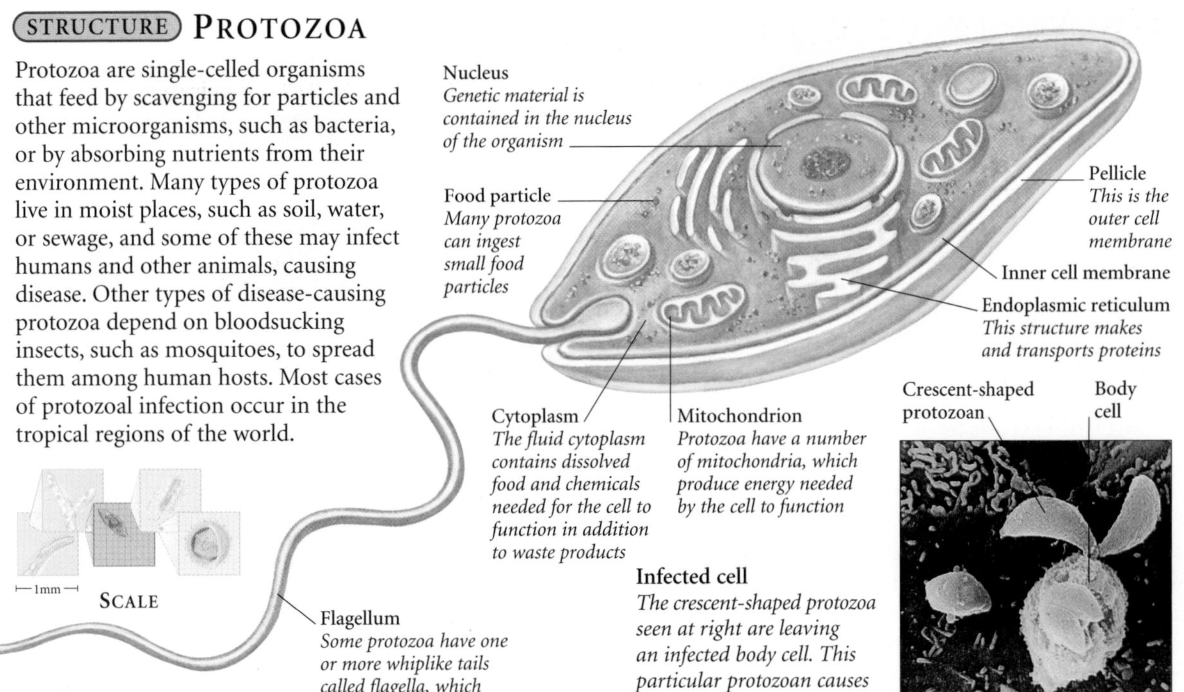

Infected cell
The crescent-shaped protozoa seen at right are leaving an infected body cell. This particular protozoan causes the disease toxoplasmosis.

STRUCTURE FUNGI

Disease-causing fungi can be divided into two broad groups: the filamentous fungi, which grow as branching threads called hyphae; and the single-celled yeasts. Some fungi have features of both groups. Fungi may form spores that remain dormant for years before causing disease.

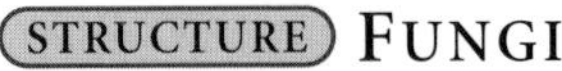

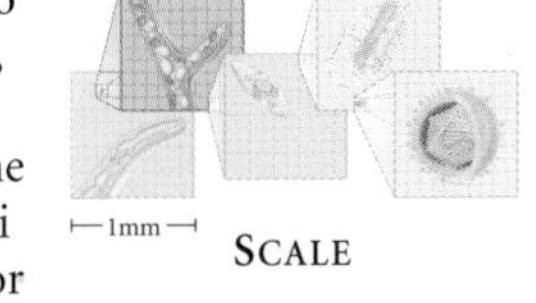

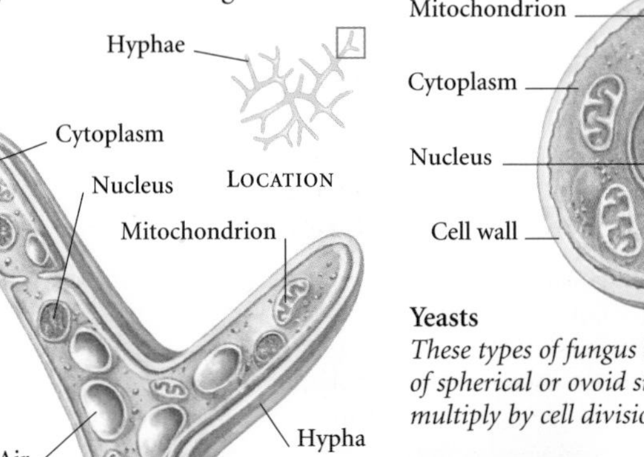

Filamentous fungi
These fungi form long tubular branches known as hyphae that may be divided into segments by cross walls called septa.

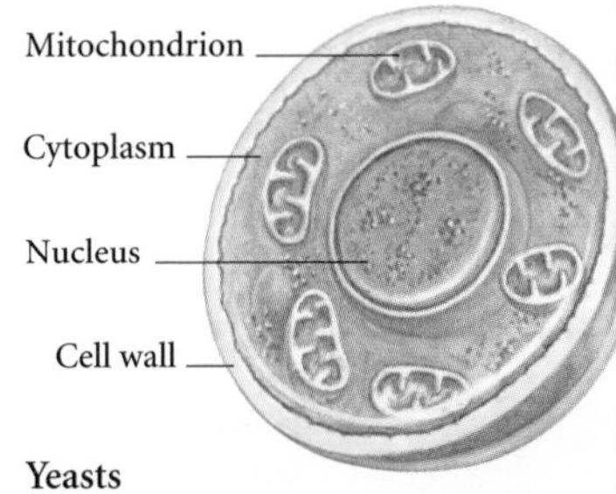

Yeasts
These types of fungus live in colonies of spherical or ovoid single cells. They multiply by cell division and budding.

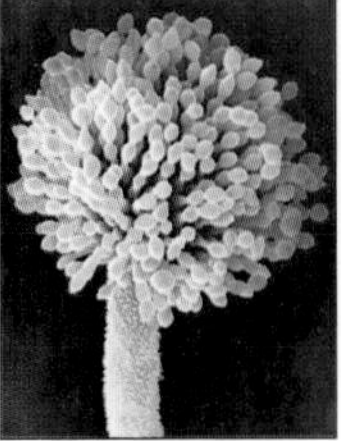

Fungal spores
Various types of fungus, including aspergillus fungi (left), produce dormant forms called spores that may cause illness if inhaled.

STRUCTURE WORMS

Worms are complex organisms that range in size from microscopic to several metres long. There are two types, flatworms and roundworms, that are adapted to infest humans. Adult worms or immature larvae infest various parts of the body, including the intestines and blood vessels.

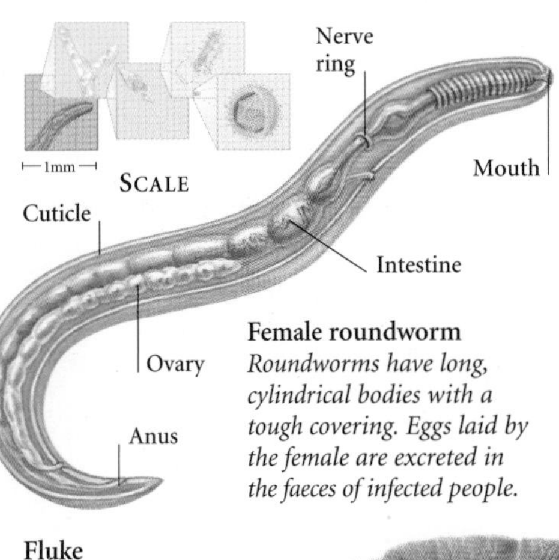

Female roundworm
Roundworms have long, cylindrical bodies with a tough covering. Eggs laid by the female are excreted in the faeces of infected people.

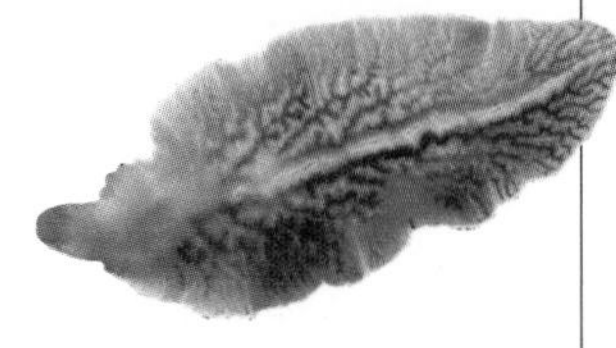

Fluke
Most common in the tropics, flukes are flat and leaf-shaped or elongated parasitic flatworms.

VIRAL INFECTIONS

Some of the most familiar minor illnesses, such as coughs, sore throats, and attacks of diarrhoea and vomiting, are often caused by viral infections. However, viruses are responsible not only for minor infections but also for potentially fatal diseases, such as rabies and HIV infection and AIDS.

The first articles discuss frequently occurring viral infections such as the common cold and influenza, the related infections chickenpox and herpes zoster, and herpes simplex infections. The next articles describe the once-common viral infections of childhood, measles, mumps, and rubella. Until the second half of the 20th century, almost all children experienced these illnesses. Routine immunization has now made such diseases rare in developed countries. However, some of these viruses can still affect adults who have not been immunized, producing symptoms that are often severe. Articles follow on a number of viral diseases, including yellow fever and dengue fever, that may be encountered in the developing world. The section ends with an article on HIV infection and AIDS.

Viral infections that affect only one body system are covered elsewhere in the book. For example, acute hepatitis (p.644) and chronic hepatitis (p.645) are covered in liver and gallbladder disorders, and genital herpes (p.767) and genital warts (p.768) are covered in sexually transmitted infections.

KEY STRUCTURES

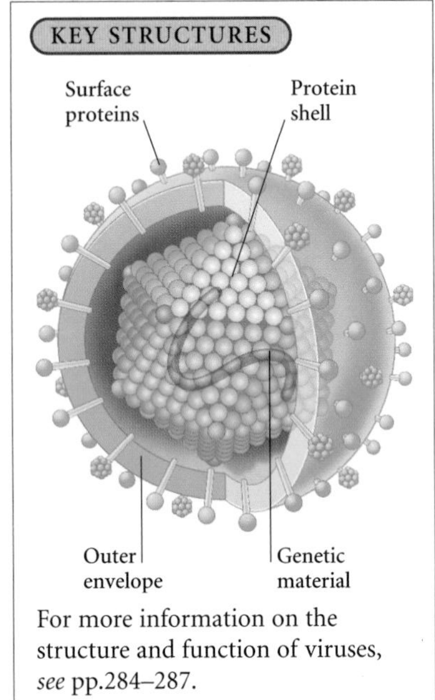

For more information on the structure and function of viruses, *see* pp.284–287.

Common cold

An infection of the nose and throat that can be caused by many different viruses

 AGE More common in children

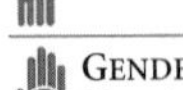 GENDER GENETICS LIFESTYLE Not significant factors

There are at least 200 highly contagious viruses that are known to cause the common cold. These viruses are easily transmitted in the minute airborne droplets sprayed from the coughs or sneezes of infected people. In many cases, the viruses are also spread to the nose and throat by way of hand-to-hand contact with an infected person or by way of objects that have become contaminated with the virus.

Colds can occur at any time of the year, although infections are more frequent in the autumn and winter. About half of the population of Europe and the US develops at least one cold each year. Children are more susceptible to colds than adults because they have not yet developed immunity to the most common viruses and also because viruses usually spread very quickly in communities such as nurseries and schools.

WHAT ARE THE SYMPTOMS?

The initial symptoms of a cold usually develop between 12 hours and 3 days after infection. Symptoms usually intensify over 24–48 hours, unlike those of influenza (opposite page), which worsen rapidly over a few hours. If you have a cold, symptoms may include:

- Frequent sneezing.
- Runny nose with a clear watery discharge that later becomes thick and green coloured.
- Mild fever and headache.
- Sore throat and, sometimes, a cough.

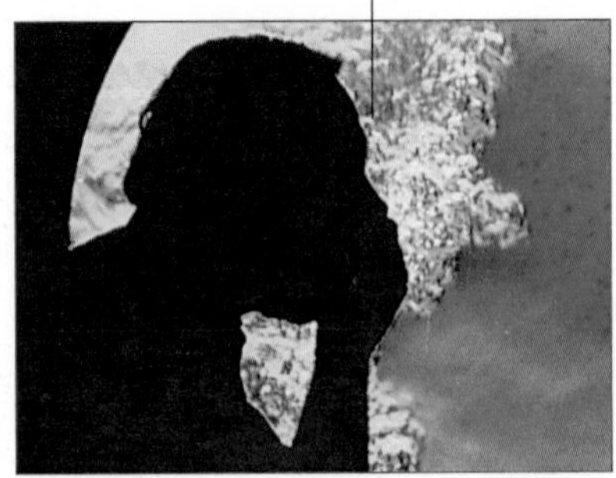

Spreading the cold virus
Cold viruses are easily spread by coughs and sneezes. This specialized photograph shows how far droplets are sprayed by a sneeze, even when a handkerchief is used.

In some people, a common cold may be complicated by a bacterial infection such as an infection of the chest (*see* ACUTE BRONCHITIS, p.486) or of the sinuses (*see* SINUSITIS, p.475). Bacterial ear infections, which may cause earache, are a common complication of colds (*see* OTITIS MEDIA, p.597, and ACUTE OTITIS MEDIA IN CHILDREN, p.860).

WHAT CAN I DO?

Most people recognize their symptoms as those of a common cold and do not seek medical advice.

Despite a great deal of scientific research, there is no cure for the common cold, but over-the-counter drugs (*see* COLD AND FLU REMEDIES, p.910) can help to relieve the symptoms. These drugs include painkillers (p.912) to relieve a headache and reduce a fever, decongestants (p.909) to clear a stuffy nose, and cough remedies (p.909) to soothe a tickling throat. It is important to drink plenty of cool fluids, particularly if you have a fever (*see* BRINGING DOWN A FEVER, opposite page). Many people take large quantities of vitamin C to prevent infection and treat the common cold, but any benefit from this popular remedy is unproved.

If your symptoms do not improve in a week or your child is no better in 2 days, you should consult a doctor. If you have a bacterial infection, your doctor may prescribe antibiotics (p.885), although they are ineffective against viruses.

The common cold usually clears up without treatment within 2 weeks, but a cough may last longer.

(WWW) ONLINE SITES: p.1033

Influenza

An infection of the upper respiratory tract (airways), commonly known as flu

AGE GENDER GENETICS LIFESTYLE
Not significant factors

Influenza, also known as flu, is a highly contagious viral disease that tends to occur in epidemics during the winter. The infection mainly affects the upper respiratory tract (airways) and can be transmitted easily in airborne droplets from the coughs and sneezes of infected people. Influenza viruses can also be transmitted from person to person through direct contact.

Many different viral infections can result in mild flu-like symptoms, but true influenza is caused by two principal types of influenza virus: A and B. The type A virus, in particular, often changes its structure (mutates) and produces new strains to which very few people have immunity.

The number of influenza cases varies from year to year, but particularly virulent strains can spread worldwide and cause millions of deaths in major outbreaks, known as pandemics. Twentieth century pandemics include Spanish flu in 1918, Asian flu in 1957, Hong Kong flu in 1968, and Russian flu in 1977.

WHAT ARE THE SYMPTOMS?

The symptoms of influenza develop 24–48 hours following infection. Many people believe that they have influenza when they have only a common cold (opposite page), but the symptoms of influenza are far more severe than those of a cold. The first symptom may be slight chills. Other symptoms, which develop later and worsen rapidly in just a few hours, may include the following:

- High fever, sweating, and shivering.
- Aching muscles, especially in the back.
- Severe exhaustion.
- Frequent sneezing, stuffy or runny nose, sore throat, and cough.

Following an attack of flu, tiredness and depression are often experienced after other symptoms have disappeared.

The most common complications are bacterial infections of the airways (*see* ACUTE BRONCHITIS, p.486) and lungs (*see* PNEUMONIA, p.490). Such infections can be life-threatening to people in high-risk groups. These include babies, elderly people, those with long-term heart or lung disease, and people with reduced immunity, such as those with AIDS (*see* HIV INFECTION AND AIDS, p.297) or diabetes mellitus (p.687).

WHAT MIGHT BE DONE?

For most normally healthy people, the best way to relieve the symptoms of influenza is to rest in bed, drink plenty of cool fluids, and follow the advice for bringing down a fever (below). Painkillers (p.912), such as paracetamol, and other over-the-counter remedies may help to ease aching muscles and other symptoms (*see* COLD AND FLU REMEDIES, p.910). If self-help measures do not provide relief, your doctor may prescribe antiviral drugs (p.886), such as amantadine, which usually have a rapid effect against influenza viruses provided that they are given within 24 hours of the onset of symptoms.

You should see your doctor immediately if you have difficulty in breathing or if your fever lasts for longer than 2 days. He or she may arrange for you to have a chest X-ray (p.490) to rule out a chest infection such as pneumonia. If a bacterial infection is found, your doctor will prescribe antibiotics (p.885). However, these drugs have no effect on the influenza virus itself.

A doctor should be consulted immediately when flu symptoms first appear in people in high-risk groups who are at increased risk of complications.

WHAT IS THE PROGNOSIS?

If there are no complications, most of the symptoms of influenza usually disappear after 6–7 days, although a cough may persist for over 2 weeks. Tiredness and depression may last for even longer. However, for anyone in one of the high-risk groups, the complications of influenza may be life-threatening, and, in epidemics, deaths from associated pneumonia are very common.

(SELF-HELP) BRINGING DOWN A FEVER

A fever is a body temperature that is above 38°C (100°F). If you or your child develops a fever, look at the symptom charts on p.102 and p.202 to check whether medical help is required. Anyone who has a fever should drink plenty of cool fluids and relieve discomfort with an over-the-counter painkiller. Babies over 3 months of age and children under 12 years may be given liquid paracetamol but should not be given aspirin. They may be cooled by a facecloth moistened with tepid water and sometimes by fanning. Young children are susceptible to febrile convulsions if they have a high fever and should be watched closely.

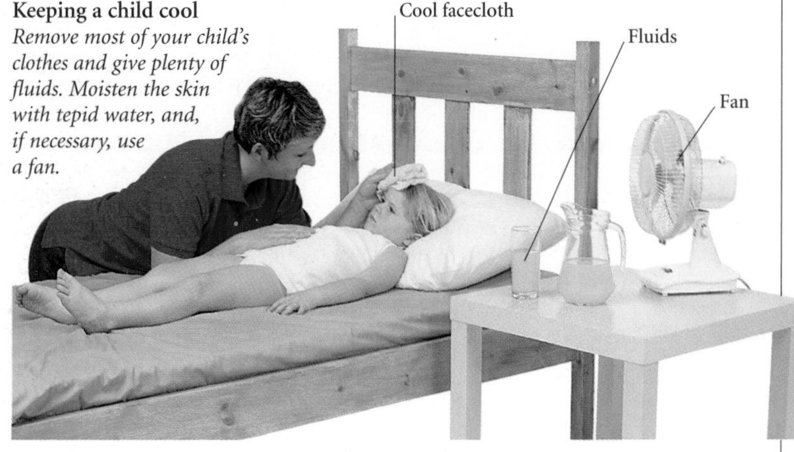

Keeping a child cool
Remove most of your child's clothes and give plenty of fluids. Moisten the skin with tepid water, and, if necessary, use a fan.

Immunization can give effective protection. It is especially recommended for people in high-risk groups (excluding babies) and people who are particularly likely to be exposed to the influenza virus, such as health workers or carers of elderly people.

Immunization prevents infection in about two-thirds of people who are vaccinated annually. However, the vaccine can never be completely effective because the viruses frequently mutate, and different strains are responsible for outbreaks each year. The World Health Organization recommends which types of vaccine are issued each autumn, depending on which strains of virus are expected to be prevalent in particular regions. However, if a virus mutates substantially, protection from the vaccine will be minimal, and there is a greater risk of epidemics occurring.

(WWW) ONLINE SITES: p.1033

Chickenpox

A childhood infection that causes a fever and widespread crops of blisters

 AGE Mainly affects unimmunized children between the ages of 2 and 10

 GENDER GENETICS LIFESTYLE Not significant factors

Chickenpox, sometimes called varicella, is a common viral infection that mostly affects young children. The infection, with its characteristic rash of blisters, is caused by the varicella zoster virus, which also causes herpes zoster (right). The virus is easily transmitted in airborne droplets from the coughs and sneezes of infected people or by direct contact with the blisters. You can catch chickenpox from someone who has either chickenpox or herpes zoster if you are not immune.

The illness is usually mild in children, but symptoms are more severe in young babies, older adolescents, and adults. Chickenpox can also be more serious in people with reduced immunity, such as those with AIDS (*see* HIV INFECTION AND AIDS, p.297).

WHAT ARE THE SYMPTOMS?

The symptoms of chickenpox appear 1–3 weeks after infection. In children, the illness often starts with a mild fever or headache; in adults, there may be

Chickenpox rash
Itchy, fluid-filled blisters are usually widespread all over the head and body in chickenpox. The blisters, seen here on the abdomen, form scabs within 24 hours.

more pronounced flu-like symptoms (*see* INFLUENZA, p.289). As infection with the virus progresses, the following symptoms usually become apparent:

- Rash in the form of crops of tiny, red spots that rapidly turn into itchy, fluid-filled blisters. Within 24 hours the blisters dry out, forming scabs. Successive crops occur for 1–6 days. The rash may be widespread or consist of only a few spots, and it can occur anywhere on the head or body.
- Sometimes, discomfort during eating caused by spots in the mouth that have developed into ulcers.

A person is contagious from about 2 days before the rash first appears until it fully crusts over in about 10–14 days.

The most common complication of chickenpox is bacterial infection of the blisters due to scratching. Other complications include pneumonia (p.490), which is more common in adults, and, rarely, inflammation of the brain (*see* VIRAL ENCEPHALITIS, p.528). Newborn babies and people with reduced immunity are at higher risk of complications. Rarely, if a woman develops chickenpox in early pregnancy, the infection may result in fetal abnormalities.

WHAT MIGHT BE DONE?

Chickenpox can usually be diagnosed from the appearance of the rash. Children with mild infections do not need to see a doctor; rest and simple measures to reduce fever (*see* BRINGING DOWN A FEVER, p.289) are all that are needed for a full recovery. Calamine lotion (*see* ANTIPRURITIC DRUGS, p.891) may help to relieve the itchiness of the rash. To prevent skin infections, especially in children, keep fingernails short and avoid scratching. People who are at risk of severe attacks, such as babies, older adolescents, adults, and people with reduced immunity, should be seen by their doctor immediately. An antiviral drug (p.886) may be given to limit the effects of the infection, but it must be taken in the early stages of the illness in order to be effective.

Children who are otherwise healthy usually recover within 10–14 days from the onset of the rash, but they may be left with permanent scars where the blisters have been scratched and then developed a bacterial infection. Adolescents, adults, and people who have reduced immunity take longer to recover from chickenpox.

CAN IT BE PREVENTED?

One attack of chickenpox gives lifelong immunity to the disease. However, the varicella zoster virus remains dormant within nerve cells and may reactivate years later, causing herpes zoster. Immunization against chickenpox is not recommended for healthy children in the UK, but in some other countries it has been introduced as a routine measure for babies aged 12–18 months.

(WWW) ONLINE SITES: p.1028, p.1033

Herpes zoster

An infection, also known as shingles, that causes a painful rash of blisters along the path of a nerve

 AGE Most common between the ages of 50 and 70

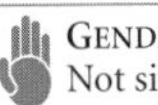 GENDER GENETICS LIFESTYLE Not significant factors

Herpes zoster, often known as shingles, is characterized by a painful crop of blisters that erupts along the path of a nerve. The rash commonly occurs on only one side of the body and usually affects the skin on the chest, abdomen, or face. In older people, discomfort may continue for months after the rash has disappeared. This prolonged pain is called postherpetic neuralgia.

Herpes zoster infection is caused by the varicella zoster virus. This virus initially causes chickenpox (left) but then remains dormant in nerve cells. If the virus is reactivated later in life, it causes herpes zoster. The reason for reactivation is unknown, but herpes zoster often occurs at times of stress or ill health. The disorder most commonly occurs in people aged 50–70 years. People with reduced immunity, such as those with AIDS (*see* HIV INFECTION AND AIDS, p.297) or those undergoing chemotherapy (p.280), are more susceptible to herpes zoster. People with AIDS are particularly likely to have severe outbreaks of herpes zoster.

The varicella zoster virus is easily spread by direct contact with a blister and will cause chickenpox in a person who is not immune to the disease.

WHAT ARE THE SYMPTOMS?

Initially, you may experience tingling, itching, and a sharp pain in an area of skin. After a few days, the following symptoms may also develop:

- Painful rash of red spots that turn into fluid-filled blisters.
- Fever.
- Headache
- Tiredness.

Within 3–4 days, the blisters form scabs. These scabs heal and drop off within 10 days but may leave scars in some people. If a nerve that supplies the eye is affected, it may cause a potentially serious inflammation of the cornea (*see* CORNEAL ULCER, p.571). Rarely, infection of a facial nerve causes weakness or paralysis on one side of the face (*see* FACIAL PALSY, p.548).

WHAT MIGHT BE DONE?

Herpes zoster can be difficult to diagnose until the rash appears, and severe pain around the ribs can be mistaken for the chest pain of angina (p.407). Your doctor may prescribe antiviral drugs (p.886) to reduce the severity of the symptoms and the risk of postherpetic neuralgia. If your eyes are affected or if you have reduced immunity, you will need immediate treatment with antiviral drugs. Painkillers (p.912) may help to relieve discomfort, and carbamazepine (*see* ANTICONVULSANT DRUGS, p.914) may help to relieve the prolonged pain of postherpetic neuralgia. Most people who develop herpes zoster recover within 2–6 weeks, but up to half of all affected people over the age of 50 develop postherpetic neuralgia.

A single attack of herpes zoster does not provide immunity to the disease, and the infection may recur.

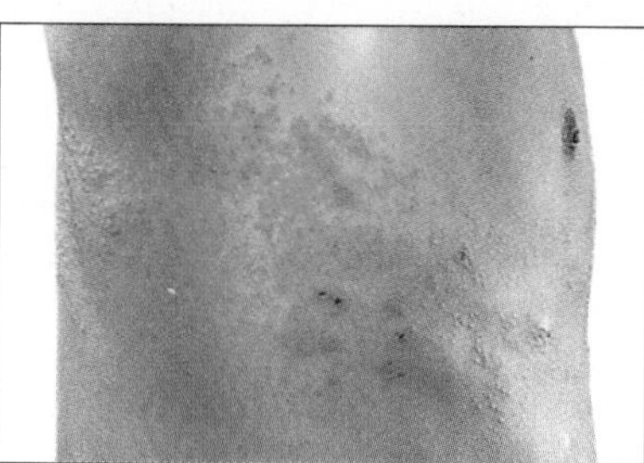

Herpes zoster rash
A rash of blisters develops along the path of a nerve in herpes zoster. The blisters often occur on the skin over the ribs on only one side of the body, as shown here.

(WWW) ONLINE SITES: p.1033

Herpes simplex infections

Infections that can cause painful blisters on or around the lips or genitals

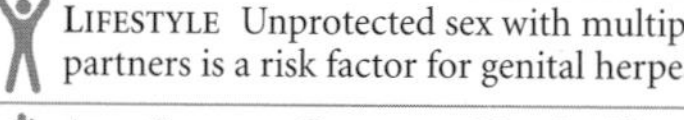

LIFESTYLE Unprotected sex with multiple partners is a risk factor for genital herpes

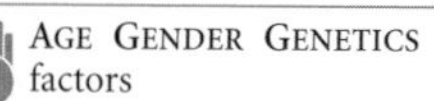

AGE GENDER GENETICS Not significant factors

The highly contagious herpes simplex viruses cause a number of different disorders characterized by small, painful blisters on the skin and mucous membranes, most commonly on or around the lips (*see* COLD SORE, p.354) or genital area (*see* GENITAL HERPES, p.767). Herpes simplex virus (HSV) infection is transmitted by contact with a blister.

Infection with HSV does not give immunity against future attacks. The viruses remain dormant in the nerves and may be reactivated at times of stress or illness. Like many viral infections, outbreaks are more frequent and more severe in people with reduced immunity, such as those with AIDS (*see* HIV INFECTION AND AIDS, p.297).

WHAT ARE THE TYPES?

There are two types of HSV: HSV1 usually causes infections of the lips, mouth, and face; and HSV2 typically causes infections of the genitals.

Most people have been infected with HSV1 by the time they are adults. In most cases, initial infection produces no symptoms. However, some children may develop blisters on the inside of the mouth (*see* STOMATITIS, p.632), and children with the skin disorder eczema may develop eczema herpeticum (*see* ECZEMA IN CHILDREN, p.829). After the initial infection, the virus becomes dormant but may reactivate periodically later in life, causing cold sores.

HSV2 is usually sexually transmitted and causes genital herpes. This condition, like cold sores, tends to recur. HSV2 can also be responsible for a life-threatening infection in a newborn baby if the baby comes into contact with the mother's genital blisters during birth (*see* CONGENITAL INFECTIONS, p.817).

Both HSV1 and HSV2 can affect the eyes, causing inflammation and a discharge (*see* CONJUNCTIVITIS, p.570). In rare cases, infection with HSV results in severe inflammation of the brain (*see* VIRAL ENCEPHALITIS, p.528).

WHAT MIGHT BE DONE?

HSV infection can be diagnosed from the appearance and site of the blisters. Mild cold sores can usually be treated with over-the-counter topical antiviral drugs (p.886). However, if you have genital herpes or severe or repeated attacks of cold sores, you may be treated with oral antiviral drugs.

(WWW) ONLINE SITES: p.1033

Infectious mononucleosis

An infection causing swollen lymph nodes and a sore throat that is common in adolescence and early adulthood

AGE Most common between the ages of 12 and 20

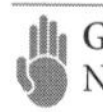

GENDER GENETICS LIFESTYLE Not significant factors

Infectious mononucleosis is known as the "kissing disease" of adolescence and early adulthood because it is mainly transmitted in saliva. Another name is glandular fever because the symptoms include swollen lymph nodes (glands) and a high temperature. The illness is usually characterized by tonsillitis (*see* PHARYNGITIS AND TONSILLITIS, p.479), which may be severe.

WHAT IS THE CAUSE?

Infectious mononucleosis is caused by the Epstein–Barr virus (EBV), which attacks lymphocytes, the white blood cells that are responsible for fighting infection. EBV infection is very common; about 9 in 10 people have been infected by the age of 50. More than half of all infected people do not develop symptoms and, consequently, are unaware that they have been infected.

What are the symptoms?

If symptoms of infectious mononucleosis develop, they usually do so 4–6 weeks after infection and appear over several days. Symptoms may include:

- High fever and sweating.
- Extremely sore throat, causing difficulty in swallowing.
- Swollen tonsils, often covered with a thick, greyish-white coating.
- Enlarged, tender lymph nodes in the neck, armpits, and groin.
- Tender abdomen as the result of an enlarged spleen.

These symptoms are often accompanied by poor appetite, weight loss, headache, and tiredness; sometimes, there may be a rash on the trunk and face. In some people, the sore throat and fever clear up quickly, and the other symptoms last less than a month. Other people may be ill for longer and feel lethargic for months after the infection.

What might be done?

Your doctor will probably diagnose the infection from your enlarged lymph nodes, sore throat, and fever. A blood test may be carried out to look for antibodies against EBV. A throat swab may also be taken to exclude bacterial infection, which would need to be treated with antibiotics (p.885).

There is no specific treatment for infectious mononucleosis, but simple measures may help to relieve symptoms.

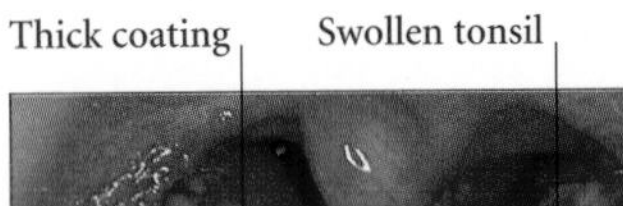

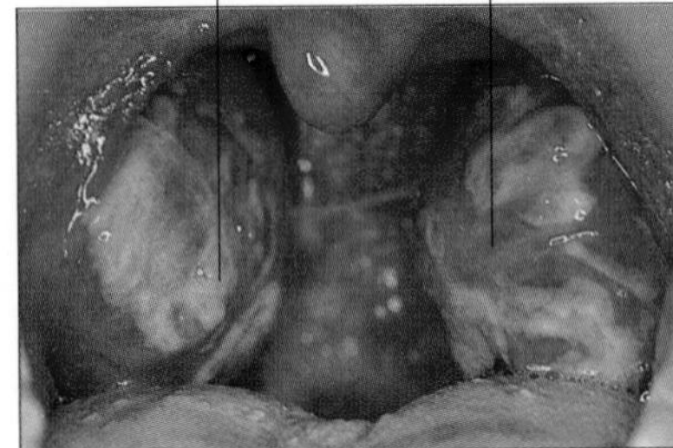

Swollen tonsils

In infectious mononucleosis, the tonsils become swollen, causing a very sore throat. They may also become covered with a thick, greyish-white coating.

Drinking plenty of cool fluids and taking over-the-counter painkillers (p.912), such as paracetamol, may help to control the fever and pain. Contact sports should be avoided while the spleen is enlarged because of the risk of rupture, which causes severe internal bleeding and can be life-threatening.

What is the prognosis?

Almost everyone who has infectious mononucleosis makes a full recovery eventually. However, in some people, recovery may be slow, and tiredness may last for weeks or even months after the symptoms first appear. One attack of the disease, with or without symptoms, provides lifelong protection.

(WWW) ONLINE SITES: p.1033

Cytomegalovirus infection

An infection that usually produces no symptoms but can cause fatal illness in people with reduced immunity

Gender More common in males

Age Genetics Lifestyle Not significant factors

Infection with cytomegalovirus (CMV) is very common and affects most adults at some time in their lives. However, most people do not develop symptoms and are not aware that they have been infected with the virus, although they will carry CMV for life in an inactive form. CMV is a type of herpesvirus.

People with reduced immunity, such as those who have AIDS (*see* HIV INFECTION AND AIDS, p.297), are at risk of serious illness from a first infection, and CMV can also be reactivated in this group. In addition, the virus can seriously affect a fetus if a woman is infected during pregnancy (*see* CONGENITAL INFECTIONS, p.817).

The virus can be passed in saliva, in minute droplets from the coughs or sneezes of infected people; during sexual intercourse; through a blood transfusion; during an organ transplant; and across the placenta to a fetus if the mother becomes infected during pregnancy. In developed countries, blood that is used for transfusion to high-risk groups is screened for CMV.

What are the symptoms?

CMV infection can produce widely differing symptoms, depending on the age and general health of the person affected. Most people have no symptoms from a first infection with the virus. If symptoms are present, they are often vague and may include:

- Tiredness.
- Fever.
- Sore throat.
- Nausea, vomiting, and diarrhoea.

In teenagers and young adults, symptoms may resemble those of infectious mononucleosis (p.291).

The symptoms of CMV infection are more severe in people with reduced immunity. In such cases, first infection or reactivation of the virus can result in a fever lasting for 2–3 weeks, a nonitchy rash, and inflammation of the liver (*see* ACUTE HEPATITIS, p.644), which causes yellowing of the skin and whites of the eyes (*see* JAUNDICE, p.643). In addition, the virus can cause inflammation of the brain (*see* VIRAL ENCEPHALITIS, p.528) and the lungs (*see* PNEUMONIA, p.490). In people with reduced immunity, CMV can also cause retinitis, inflammation of the light-sensitive cells at the back of the eye, which may result in blindness.

If a woman is infected with the virus during the first 24 weeks of pregnancy, there is a 1 in 7 risk that the baby will develop abnormalities, such as deafness. The baby may also be seriously ill at birth with jaundice, liver enlargement, and certain blood disorders.

What might be done?

In a person who is otherwise healthy, CMV infection usually goes unnoticed, causes no problems, and is not treated. If your symptoms are severe and your doctor suspects CMV infection, he or she may arrange for a blood test to look for antibodies against the virus. The symptoms are often relieved by early treatment with antiviral drugs (p.886).

For people with reduced immunity, complications can be life-threatening. These people may be given antiviral drugs to protect against infection or, if a blood test shows that the virus is already present, to prevent symptoms from developing. Drugs may also be given to a pregnant woman who has the infection in order to protect the fetus.

(WWW) ONLINE SITES: p.1032, p.1033

Measles

A childhood illness that causes fever and a widespread nonitchy rash

AGE Mainly affects unimmunized children between the ages of 1 and 5

GENDER GENETICS LIFESTYLE Not significant factors

Measles is a highly contagious viral illness that causes a distinctive rash and fever and mainly affects young children. Rare in the developed world because of routine immunization, the disease kills up to 1 million unimmunized children in the developing world each year.

The measles virus is easily transmitted in minute airborne droplets from the coughs and sneezes of infected people. A child who has measles may feel very ill, and there is a small risk of complications, especially if the child has reduced immunity or is severely malnourished. Measles is contagious for 1–2 days before the rash appears and for about 5 days afterwards.

WHAT ARE THE SYMPTOMS?

Symptoms of measles usually develop 10 days after infection and may include:

- Fever.
- Tiny white spots with a red base, known as Koplik spots, on the insides of the cheeks.
- After 3–4 days, a red, nonitchy rash that starts on the head and spreads downwards. At first, the rash consists of separate flat spots. The spots then merge to give a blotchy appearance.
- Painful, red, watery eyes (*see* CONJUNCTIVITIS, p.570).
- Stuffy or runny nose.
- Hacking cough.

The most common complications of measles are bacterial infections of the middle ear (*see* ACUTE OTITIS MEDIA IN CHILDREN, p.860) and the lungs (*see* PNEUMONIA, p.490). In about 1 in 1,000 cases, the brain is affected (*see* VIRAL ENCEPHALITIS, p.528), a serious complication that starts 7–10 days after the appearance of the rash.

WHAT MIGHT BE DONE?

Your doctor will probably be able to diagnose measles from the combination of symptoms. In most children, rest and simple measures to reduce a fever (*see* BRINGING DOWN A FEVER, p.289) are all that are needed for a full recovery. If there are no complications, symptoms usually disappear in 7 days. Antibiotics (p.885) may be prescribed if a bacterial infection develops.

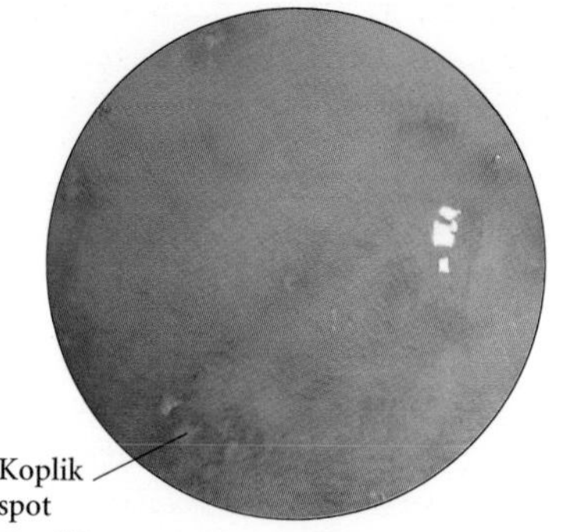

Koplik spots in measles
These tiny white spots may appear on the insides of the cheeks when the symptoms of measles first develop, shortly before the onset of the rash on the head and body.

CAN IT BE PREVENTED?

Babies are immunized against measles with a measles, mumps, and rubella (MMR) vaccine, given at 12–15 months and again between 3 and 5 years (*see* ROUTINE IMMUNIZATIONS, p.45). Immunization or an attack of measles gives lifelong immunity to the disease.

WWW ONLINE SITES: p.1028, p.1033

Mumps

An illness causing swelling of the salivary glands on one or both sides of the jaw

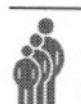
AGE Mainly affects unimmunized schoolchildren and young adults

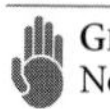
GENDER GENETICS LIFESTYLE Not significant factors

Mumps is a mild viral infection that was common among schoolchildren until routine immunization was introduced. The mumps virus is spread in saliva and in minute airborne droplets from the coughs and sneezes of infected people. The virus causes swelling and inflammation of one or both of the parotid salivary glands, which are situated below and just in front of the ears. If both glands are affected, the child's face may have a hamster-like appearance. In adolescent boys and men, the virus may affect the testes; rarely, this effect may result in problems with fertility (*see* MALE INFERTILITY, p.777).

WHAT ARE THE SYMPTOMS?

Up to half of all people with mumps develop no symptoms, and in most other people the symptoms are mild. The main symptoms appear 2–3 weeks after infection and may include:

- Pain and swelling on one or both sides of the face, below and just in front of the ear, lasting about 3 days.
- Pain when swallowing.

A person who is infected with the mumps virus may also have a sore throat and fever, and the salivary glands under the chin may become painful. He or she is contagious for up to 7 days before symptoms first appear and for about 10 days afterwards.

About 1 in 4 adolescent boys or adult men with mumps also develops painful inflammation of one or both testes (*see* EPIDIDYMO-ORCHITIS, p.718). Rarely, the inflammation may result in infertility. A few people who develop mumps also develop viral meningitis (p.527), in which the membranes that surround the brain and spinal cord become inflamed. Inflammation of the pancreas (*see* ACUTE PANCREATITIS, p.652) is a rare complication of mumps.

WHAT MIGHT BE DONE?

Your doctor will probably diagnose the disorder from the distinctive swelling of the parotid glands. There is no specific treatment, but drinking plenty of cool fluids and taking over-the-counter painkillers (p.912), such as paracetamol, may relieve discomfort. Most people recover without further treatment, but adolescent boys and men who have severe inflammation of the testes may be prescribed a stronger painkiller. If complications develop, other types of treatment may be recommended.

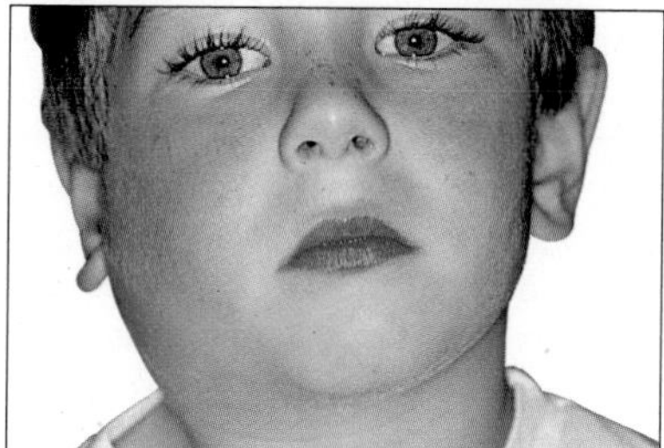

Inflamed parotid gland
The parotid glands are situated below and just in front of each ear. In the viral infection mumps, one (as shown above) or both parotid glands may become swollen.

Can it be prevented?

Babies are immunized against mumps as part of the measles, mumps, and rubella (MMR) immunization given at 12–15 months and then between 3 and 5 years (*see* ROUTINE IMMUNIZATIONS, p.45). Immunization or an attack of mumps give lifelong immunity.

(WWW) ONLINE SITES: p.1028, p.1033

Rubella

An illness, also known as German measles, that is usually mild but can severely damage a developing fetus

AGE GENDER GENETICS LIFESTYLE
Not significant factors

Rubella, also called German measles, usually causes little more than a mild rash. However, because it can cause serious birth defects in a fetus if the mother contracts the illness during early pregnancy, unimmunized pregnant women should avoid contact with an infected person. The disease is caused by the highly contagious rubella virus, which is transmitted through airborne droplets from the coughs and sneezes of infected people. Rubella has become less common in the developed world because of routine childhood immunization.

What are the symptoms?

The symptoms of rubella appear from 2–3 weeks after infection and may include all or some of the following:

- Swollen lymph nodes at the back of the neck and behind the ears. In some cases, lymph nodes throughout the body are swollen, including those in the armpits and groin.
- After 2–3 days, a pink, nonitchy rash, first on the face and then the body, that usually disappears within 3 days.

Children may have mild fever, but adolescents and adults can develop high fever and headache. Rarely, several joints may become inflamed for a short time (*see* REACTIVE ARTHRITIS, p.379). A person who has rubella is highly infectious from up to 10 days before the pink rash appears to about 10 days afterwards.

Are there complications?

If you contract rubella in early pregnancy, your baby is at serious risk of being born with abnormalities, such as congenital deafness (p.859), congenital heart disease (p.836), clouding of the lens in the eye (*see* CATARACT, p.573), and the nervous system disorder cerebral palsy (p.846). The greatest risk is during the first 4 months of pregnancy, and the earlier rubella occurs, the more likely the baby will be seriously affected.

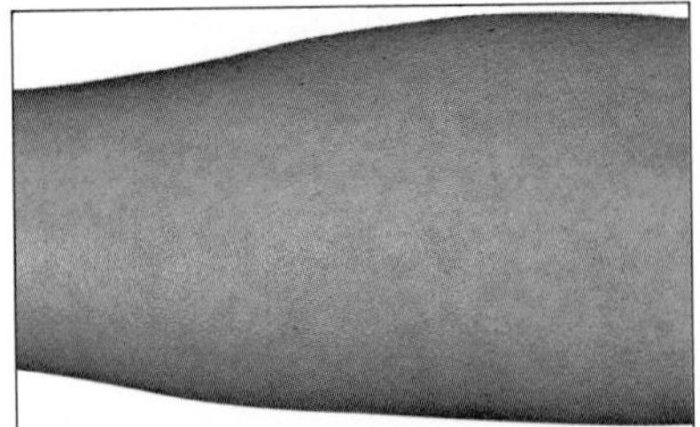

Rubella rash
The light pink rash of rubella is shown here on an arm. The rash usually first develops on the face and gradually spreads to the trunk and then to the limbs.

What might be done?

Your doctor may suspect rubella from the symptoms, but the rash is not distinctive and other viral infections can produce similar symptoms. He or she may arrange for a blood test to confirm the diagnosis. There is no specific treatment, but drinking plenty of cool fluids and taking over-the-counter painkillers (p.912), such as paracetamol, may help to reduce fever and ease discomfort. Most affected people recover in about 10 days, and one attack gives lifelong immunity against the virus.

If you are pregnant and have rubella or have been in contact with someone with the disease, you may wish to discuss with your doctor the risk to the fetus and how best to proceed.

Can it be prevented?

Babies are routinely immunized against rubella as part of the standard measles, mumps, and rubella (MMR) immunization that is given at 12–15 months and then again between 3 and 5 years (*see* ROUTINE IMMUNIZATIONS, p.45). Immunization or an attack of rubella provides lifelong immunity. Ideally, all unimmunized women who are planning a pregnancy should be tested for antibodies against rubella and should receive advice about immunization (*see* HEALTH IN PREGNANCY AND AFTER CHILDBIRTH, p.33).

(WWW) ONLINE SITES: p.1028, p.1033

Parvovirus infection

An infection that causes a rash and inflammation of the joints

AGE GENDER GENETICS LIFESTYLE
Not significant factors

In children, parvovirus infection is a mild illness with a fever that often goes unnoticed. It is also known as fifth disease or slapped cheek disease. The virus occurs only rarely in adults, when it may cause severe joint pain. Parvovirus is transmitted in airborne droplets from the coughs and sneezes of infected people; it is occasionally transmitted by a blood transfusion. Infection causes a brief halt in the production of red blood cells by the bone marrow, and, for this reason, can have serious consequences in people with anaemia (p.446).

What are the symptoms?

Many children do not develop symptoms; in others, these symptoms may appear within 7–14 days of infection:

- Bright red rash on the cheeks that may spread to the trunk and limbs.
- Mild fever.
- In rare cases, mild inflammation of the joints (*see* ARTHRITIS, p.374).

Adults are likely to develop more severe symptoms that may include:

- Rash on the palms and soles.
- Severe inflammation and pain in the joints of the knees, wrists, and hands.

Some women develop a serious form of arthritis that can last for up to 2 years.

In people with reduced immunity, such as those taking immunosuppressant drugs (p.906) or those with AIDS (*see* HIV INFECTION AND AIDS, p.297), the infection may become long-term and can cause anaemia. In people who already have anaemia, parvovirus infection may exacerbate the condition. If a pregnant woman becomes infected during the first 6 months of pregnancy, there is a risk of miscarriage (p.791).

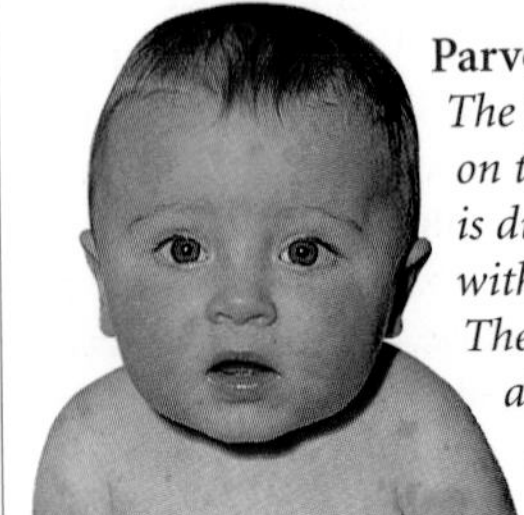

Parvovirus rash
The bright red rash on this baby's face is due to infection with parvovirus. The condition is also known as slapped cheek disease.

What might be done?

Your doctor may be able to diagnose parvovirus infection from your symptoms. If the diagnosis is not clear, he or she may arrange for a blood test to detect antibodies against the virus. If you have painful joints, your doctor may arrange for further blood tests and for X-rays (p.244) of the joints to exclude other causes of arthritis. In most people, the infection clears up within 2 weeks without treatment. However, people at risk of severe anaemia may need hospital treatment. One attack of parvovirus infection provides lifelong immunity.

(WWW) ONLINE SITES: p.1033

Poliomyelitis

A rare infection, commonly known as polio, that can affect the nervous system

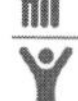
AGE Mainly affects unimmunized children but can affect unimmunized adults

LIFESTYLE Travel in some parts of Asia and Africa is a risk factor

GENDER GENETICS Not significant factors

Poliomyelitis is a highly infectious disease that varies in severity from a mild condition with few or no symptoms to a severe disorder affecting the nervous system. In a few instances, the disease can lead to paralysis. Poliomyelitis is caused by infection with the polio virus, which is transmitted by contact with the faeces of an infected person, through contaminated food and drinking water, or in contaminated swimming pools.

Since routine immunization began in the 1950s, polio has become rare in developed countries. However, in some parts of Africa and Asia, the disease remains a serious risk for travellers who do not have up-to-date immunization.

What are the symptoms?

For most infected people, polio produces no symptoms or results in a mild illness with a slight fever and sore throat that develops 3–21 days after infection. In about 1 in 500 infected people, the brain and spinal cord become inflamed, and symptoms include a high fever, severe headache, backache, and a stiff neck. In a few cases, one or more limbs may be paralysed, and in addition the muscles of the respiratory system may be affected, causing breathing problems.

What might be done?

In most cases, polio is undiagnosed and untreated. If the disease is suspected from the symptoms, the diagnosis can be confirmed by tests to look for the presence of the virus in faeces. There is no specific treatment for polio, but mild symptoms can usually be relieved with painkillers (p.912) and bed rest. People who have severe symptoms are admitted to hospital, and mechanical ventilation may be given if the respiratory muscles are paralysed.

Most people make a full recovery from milder forms of the disease. Of those who become paralysed, many improve within 6 months. Physiotherapy (p.961) can help people to recover the use of weakened limbs, but in some people affected muscles may become permanently weakened and affected limbs may eventually become wasted. In other people, muscle pain and weakness may recur many years after the illness. This recurrence is known as postpolio syndrome.

Can it be prevented?

Polio vaccine provides complete protection against the virus. In the UK, immunization against the disease is routine in early childhood (*see* ROUTINE IMMUNIZATIONS, p.45). Before travelling to parts of the world where infection with polio is still a risk, adults should have a booster dose of vaccine (*see* TRAVEL IMMUNIZATIONS, p.86).

(WWW) ONLINE SITES: p.1033, p.1037

Viral haemorrhagic fevers

A group of infections that cause abnormal bleeding and may be fatal

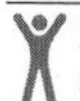
LIFESTYLE Travel in some parts of Africa is a risk factor for some infections

AGE GENDER GENETICS Not significant factors

Viral haemorrhagic fevers, which cause severe abnormal bleeding, occur predominantly in Africa and rarely reach the developed world. Hantavirus infection is the only one of these fevers that is native to some parts of Europe and the US. The other fevers, which include Marburg fever, Ebola fever, and Lassa fever, occur only in localized outbreaks in Africa. African haemorrhagic fevers have made international news headlines in recent years because there is a slight risk that travellers may be infected with these potentially fatal diseases and spread them to the developed world.

Hantavirus and Lassa fever virus are carried by rodents, such as rats, and are transmitted to people through contact with the animals' urine, faeces, or saliva. Marburg fever virus is carried by monkeys, but the animal carrier of Ebola fever virus is unknown. All of these viruses can be transmitted in body secretions and are highly contagious.

What are the symptoms?

The symptoms of viral haemorrhagic fevers develop slowly from 1 to 3 weeks after infection and may include:

- Flu-like symptoms, including headache, fever, sore throat, and tiredness.
- Rash, which causes peeling skin in Ebola fever.
- Abnormal bleeding from the skin and mucous membranes.

The symptoms of hantavirus infection vary from mild to severe. Lassa fever may produce no symptoms at all. Ebola and Marburg fevers produce severe symptoms. The complications of Ebola and Marburg fevers include acute kidney failure (p.706), serious breathing difficulties, and shock (p.414).

What might be done?

Viral haemorrhagic fevers are diagnosed from the symptoms and a blood test to look for antibodies against the virus. There are no specific treatments for Hantavirus infection, Marburg fever, or Ebola fever. However, Lassa fever may respond to antiviral drugs (p.886) if the treatment is given in the first week. Most people with these infections are admitted to hospital for treatment and to limit the spread of the virus. Dialysis (p.707) may be necessary if kidney function is impaired, and mechanical ventilation will be required for serious breathing difficulties.

The outlook depends on the type of virus and the medical care available. Lassa fever is fatal in up to 1 in 50 cases; Hantavirus infection has a death rate of up to 1 in 10; Marburg fever is fatal in about 1 in 4; and Ebola fever has a death rate of up to 9 in 10 cases.

(WWW) ONLINE SITES: p.1033, p.1037

Yellow fever

An infection, mainly confined to Africa, that is transmitted by mosquitoes

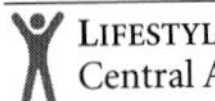
LIFESTYLE Travel to Africa and South and Central America is a risk factor

AGE GENDER GENETICS Not significant factors

The tropical viral infection yellow fever was given its name because it can cause severe jaundice (p.643), in which the skin turns bright yellow. The virus is transmitted by mosquitoes from monkeys to humans and then by mosquitoes from person to person. More than 9 in 10 cases occur in Africa; the remainder occur mainly in South and Central America. The disease has become less common with routine immunization, but epidemics still occur in Africa.

The symptoms of yellow fever appear suddenly, 3–6 days after a bite from an infected mosquito. In some cases, there may be a mild flu-like illness. However, in other cases there may be abnormal bleeding, liver failure (p.650), or kidney failure (p.705). Severe bleeding may lead to shock (p.414). Rarely, the infection leads to convulsions and coma (p.522).

Diagnosis is based on the symptoms and confirmed by a blood test to look for antibodies against the virus. There is no specific treatment for yellow fever, and the disease is fatal in 2–5 out of 10 people. An attack provides lifelong immunity. Immunization gives protection for 10 years and is recommended for people travelling to high-risk areas (*see* TRAVEL IMMUNIZATIONS, p.86).

(WWW) ONLINE SITES: p.1033, p.1037

Dengue fever

An infection, also known as breakbone fever, that is spread by mosquitoes

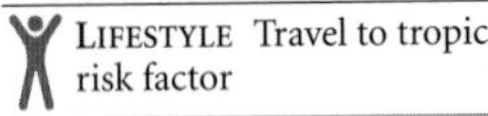
LIFESTYLE Travel to tropical countries is a risk factor

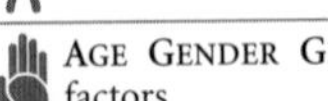
AGE GENDER GENETICS Not significant factors

Dengue fever occurs in many tropical areas of the world, and an estimated 40–80 million people, including many travellers, become infected each year. The dengue fever virus is carried and transmitted by the mosquito *Aedes aegypti*, which is found in suburban and rural areas and usually bites during the daytime. Since the disease causes severe pain in the muscles and joints, it is also known as "breakbone fever".

The symptoms of dengue fever appear 4–8 days after a bite from an infected mosquito. They include a high temperature, headache, severe backache, muscle pain and weakness, and joint pain. Small red spots may also develop on the skin during the first few days of the illness. The fever often subsides for 3–4 days but then recurs before subsiding again. In severe cases, abnormal bleeding may occur from areas such as the gums and nose and from injection sites.

WHAT MIGHT BE DONE?

Dengue fever can usually be diagnosed from the symptoms. There is no specific treatment, but it is important to rest and drink plenty of cool fluids. Over-the-counter painkillers (p.912), such as paracetamol, may help to relieve symptoms and reduce fever. Severely affected people may need observation and treatment in hospital, but life-threatening complications are uncommon. Recovery usually takes several weeks.

An attack of dengue fever gives immunity for only about a year, and there is no vaccine against the virus. Travellers to areas where it is common should use mosquito repellents and wear clothing that completely covers the arms and legs (*see* TRAVEL HEALTH, p.85).

(WWW) ONLINE SITES: p.1033, p.1037

Rabies

A serious infection of the nervous system, usually transmitted in saliva from a bite by an infected animal

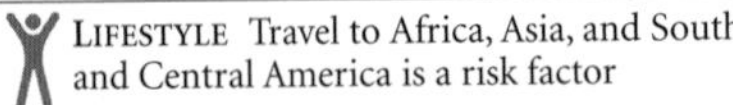
LIFESTYLE Travel to Africa, Asia, and South and Central America is a risk factor

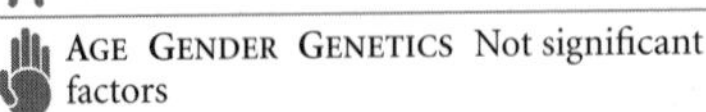
AGE GENDER GENETICS Not significant factors

The rabies virus mainly affects animals but can be passed to humans by an animal bite or a lick over a break in the skin. After entering the wound, the virus can travel along nerves to the brain and cause potentially fatal inflammation. Immunization against the virus and prompt medical treatment give complete protection against the disease, but, if left untreated, about half of all people bitten by a rabid animal develop rabies and almost inevitably die.

Rabies is very rare in developed countries, although only a few, including the UK, Japan, and Australia, are completely free from the disease. Africa and many parts of Asia are high-risk areas. In developed countries, most cases are due to bites from bats, and worldwide most cases result from bites by dogs that have been infected by wild animals. Some animals infected with the rabies virus act aggressively and salivate excessively.

WHAT ARE THE SYMPTOMS?

An infected person may develop symptoms within 10 days to 2 months of a bite, although, rarely, the virus can lie dormant for several years. Rabies usually starts with flu-like symptoms (*see* INFLUENZA, p.289) that last for about 2–7 days, followed by:

- Paralysis of face and throat muscles.
- Extreme thirst.
- Painful throat spasms leading to an inability to drink and a fear of water.
- Disorientation and agitation.
- Loss of consciousness.
- Paralysis of limbs.

Once symptoms have developed, the condition is usually fatal.

WHAT MIGHT BE DONE?

Wash all suspect animal bites immediately with soap and water. Seek medical advice without delay because treatment must be started at once to be effective. Treatment consists of injections of antibodies against the rabies virus, followed by a rabies vaccination to stimulate production of more antibodies. If possible, the animal that inflicted the bite should be captured and observed for 10 days. If the animal remains free from symptoms, treatment can stop; if it is rabid, treatment is continued and the animal is destroyed. Alternatively, it may be destroyed immediately and then examined for evidence of the virus.

There is no cure once the symptoms have developed. Diagnosis may not be obvious from the symptoms, and blood and saliva tests are usually arranged to confirm the presence of the virus.

Rabies can be prevented by a vaccine, which is recommended for people working with animals in high-risk areas (*see* TRAVEL IMMUNIZATIONS, p.86). All travellers in these areas should avoid contact with stray animals.

(WWW) ONLINE SITES: p.1033

HIV infection and AIDS

A long-term infection that, left untreated, results in reduced immunity to other infections

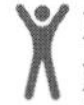
LIFESTYLE Unprotected sex with multiple partners and intravenous drug use are risk factors

AGE GENDER GENETICS Not significant factors

Infection with the human immunodeficiency virus (HIV), which can lead to acquired immunodeficiency syndrome (AIDS) if left untreated, has been the most written about and most researched disease of the past 20 years. Despite the development of effective drugs to limit the progression of the infection, there is still no vaccine against the virus, and the number of people with HIV infection continues to rise, especially in developing countries.

HIV is believed to have originated in Africa, where a similar virus is carried by some species of primate. The virus is thought to have spread from monkeys to humans through saliva in bites, then around the world from person to person by sexual contact or through other exchange of body fluids. The first recognized cases of AIDS occurred in 1981, when there was an outbreak of unusual cases of pneumonia and skin cancer in young homosexual men in Los Angeles. Two years later, the virus was isolated and identified as HIV.

HIV infects and gradually destroys cells in the immune system, weakening the response to infections and cancers. People infected with HIV may have no symptoms for many years, or they may experience frequent or prolonged mild infections. When the immune system becomes severely weakened, people are susceptible to serious infections caused by organisms that are usually harmless, and they are also susceptible to certain types of cancer. The development of some specific diseases or cancers leads to a diagnosis of AIDS.

WHO IS AFFECTED?

By the end of 1998, about 22,000 people in the UK were infected with HIV, with about 2,000 new cases every year. Worldwide, over 33 million people were thought to be infected, 9 in 10 of whom were unaware that they had the condition. As a result of developments in drug treatment, deaths due to AIDS have fallen dramatically in the developed world since 1995. In the UK, the total number of deaths in known HIV-positive individuals fell from 1,667 in 1995 to 444 in 1998. The problem of AIDS is much greater in developing countries, where most people with HIV infection live and where the new drugs are unavailable or unaffordable.

HOW IS HIV TRANSMITTED?

HIV is carried in body fluids, including blood, semen, vaginal secretions, saliva, and breast milk. It is most commonly transmitted sexually, by anal, oral, or vaginal intercourse. People are at higher risk of HIV infection and more likely to transmit the virus if they have another sexually transmitted infection.

People who use intravenous drugs and share or reuse needles contaminated with the virus are at high risk of infection. Medical workers are also at risk from accidental skin punctures with contaminated needles (*see* NEEDLESTICK INJURY, p.356), but the risk is low.

HIV infection can be passed from an infected woman to the fetus or to the baby at birth (*see* CONGENITAL INFECTIONS, p.817) or by breast-feeding. The virus can also be transmitted through organ transplants or blood transfusions. However, in developed countries, screening of blood, organs, and tissues for HIV is routine, making the risk of infection by this route extremely low.

HIV infection cannot be transmitted by everyday human contact, such as shaking hands, or by coughs or sneezes, and there is no risk to your health from working or living with someone who is infected with the virus.

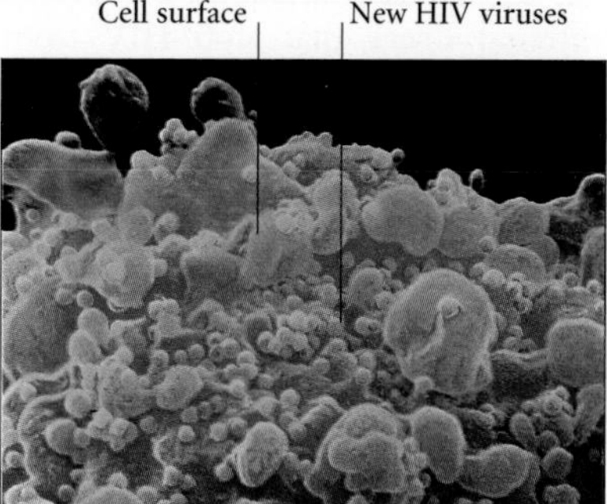

Human immunodeficiency virus
This highly magnified view of a white blood cell known as a CD4 lymphocyte shows tiny, newly formed HIV viruses budding out of the cell's uneven surface.

WHAT IS THE CAUSE?

HIV enters the bloodstream and infects cells with a special structure called the CD4 receptor on their surfaces. These cells include a type of white blood cell known as a CD4 lymphocyte, which is responsible for fighting infection. The virus reproduces rapidly within the cells and destroys them in the process.

At first, the immune system is able to function normally despite the infection, and symptoms may not develop for years. However, the number of CD4 lymphocytes eventually begins to fall, especially if the infection is untreated, causing increased susceptibility to other infections and some types of cancer.

WHAT ARE THE SYMPTOMS?

The first symptoms of HIV infection can appear within 6 weeks of the virus entering the body. Some people experience a flu-like illness that may include some or all of the following symptoms:

- Swollen lymph nodes (*see* LYMPHADENOPATHY, p.458).
- Fever.
- Tiredness and aching muscles.
- Rash.
- Sore throat.

These symptoms usually clear up after a few weeks, and many people with HIV infection feel completely healthy. However, in some people, any of the following minor disorders may develop:

- Persistent, swollen lymph nodes.
- Mouth infections such as thrush (*see* CANDIDIASIS, p.309).
- Furred white patches in the mouth (*see* ORAL LEUKOPLAKIA, p.634).
- Gum disease (*see* GINGIVITIS, p.617).
- Persistent herpes simplex infections (p.291), such as cold sores (p.354).
- Extensive genital warts (p.768).
- Itchy, flaky skin (*see* SEBORRHOEIC DERMATITIS, p.335).
- Weight loss.

The time between infection with HIV and the onset of AIDS varies and can be between 1 and 14 years. Often, people are unaware for years that they are infected with HIV until they develop one or more serious infections or cancers known as AIDS-defining illnesses.

ARE THERE COMPLICATIONS?

The single complication of HIV infection is the development of AIDS. A person infected with HIV is said to have AIDS if he or she has developed a particular AIDS-defining illness. These illnesses include opportunistic infections (infections that occur only in people with reduced immunity), certain cancers, and nervous system disorders that may result in dementia (p.535), confusion, and memory loss.

OPPORTUNISTIC INFECTIONS These infections may be caused by protozoa, fungi, viruses, or bacteria, and they can often be life-threatening.

One of the most common illnesses in people with AIDS is a severe infection of the lungs by the parasite *Pneumocystis carinii* (*see* PNEUMOCYSTIS INFECTION, p.308). Other common diseases are the protozoal infections cryptosporidiosis (p.307), which may result in prolonged diarrhoea, and toxoplasmosis (p.307), which can affect the brain.

Candida albicans is a fungus that can cause mild superficial infections in healthy people but may produce much more serious infections in people who have developed AIDS (*see* CANDIDIASIS, p.309). The cryptococcus fungus (*see* CRYPTOCOCCOSIS, p.308) may cause fever, headaches, and lung infections.

People with AIDS suffer from severe bacterial and viral infections. Bacterial infections include tuberculosis (p.491) and listeriosis (p.301), which may lead to blood poisoning (*see* SEPTICAEMIA, p.299). Viral infections include those caused by the herpesviruses. Herpes simplex infections can affect the brain, causing meningitis and viral encephalitis (p.528). Cytomegalovirus infection (p.292) may cause a number of severe conditions, including pneumonia, viral encephalitis, and a type of eye inflammation that can result in blindness. However, people who have AIDS are not more susceptible to common infections such as colds.

CANCERS The most common type of cancer that affects people with AIDS is Kaposi's sarcoma (p.346), a type of skin cancer that can also affect the inside of the mouth and internal organs, including the lungs. Other types of cancer that commonly develop in people with AIDS include lymphomas (p.459), such as non-Hodgkin's lymphoma. Cancer of the cervix (p.750) is an AIDS-defining illness in women infected with HIV.

HOW IS IT DIAGNOSED?

If you suspect that you may have been exposed to HIV infection, you should have a blood test to check for antibodies against the virus. You may also have this blood test if you have symptoms that suggest HIV infection, and it is often offered as part of antenatal care. Consent is always obtained before the test, and counselling is given both before and afterwards to discuss the implications of a positive result.

If your HIV test result is negative, you may be advised to have another test in 3 months because antibodies take time to develop. HIV infection can also be difficult to diagnose in the baby of an infected woman because the mother's antibodies may remain in the baby's blood for up to 18 months.

AIDS is diagnosed when an AIDS-defining illness, such as pneumocystis infection, develops or when a blood test shows that the CD4 lymphocyte count has dropped below a certain level.

WHAT IS THE TREATMENT?

If your HIV test result is positive, you will probably be referred to a special centre where you will receive monitoring, treatment, and advice from a team of health-care professionals.

Drug treatment may be started when you are diagnosed with HIV infection, or when blood tests show that virus levels are increasing or that the CD4 lymphocyte level is falling. Advances in the use of combinations of specific antiviral drugs that stop HIV from replicating have made it possible to prevent progression of HIV infection to AIDS and to suppress the viral infection to undetectable levels in some people (*see* DRUGS FOR HIV INFECTION AND AIDS, p.887).

Once AIDS has developed, opportunistic infections are dealt with as they occur. In some cases, there may also be long-term preventive treatment against the most common infections. Emotional support and practical advice can be obtained from the many groups and charitable organizations that help people with HIV infection and AIDS.

WHAT IS THE PROGNOSIS?

There is no cure for HIV infection, but the drug treatments available in the developed world have made it possible to regard the condition as a long-term illness rather than a rapidly fatal one. Since the introduction of antiviral drug combination therapies, deaths from AIDS in the developed world have been reduced dramatically. However, for most of the people with HIV who live in the developing world, the outlook is bleak. Few of them will have access to up-to-date treatment, and, left untreated, half of all people infected with the virus develop AIDS within 10 years and die.

CAN IT BE PREVENTED?

HIV infection can be prevented by teaching at an early age about the risks of infection. The two main precautions that everyone can take to avoid sexual transmission are to use a condom during sexual intercourse and to avoid sex with multiple partners (*see* SEX AND HEALTH, p.67). It is also recommended that both partners have an HIV test before having unprotected sex in a new relationship. Specific groups also need to take special precautions. For example, people who inject drugs intravenously must use a clean needle every time.

People who are HIV positive need to take special care to prevent others from coming into contact with their blood or body fluids and should always inform dental or medical staff that they have HIV infection. Women who are HIV positive and pregnant may be given antiviral drugs to reduce the risk of transmission to the fetus, and they may also be advised to have a caesarean section (p.802) and avoid breast-feeding to reduce the risk of transmitting the virus to their babies.

Medical professionals take many steps to prevent transmission of HIV, including screening all blood products and tissues for transplant and using disposable or carefully sterilized equipment.

Extensive research is being carried out both to develop a vaccine against HIV and to prevent the development of AIDS. However, although researchers are optimistic they will succeed, there will inevitably be millions more deaths worldwide before an affordable cure is found and made available to everyone.

(WWW) ONLINE SITES: p.1032, p.1033

BACTERIAL INFECTIONS

A large group of diseases is caused by bacteria entering the body and multiplying too fast to be destroyed by the immune system. Some types of bacteria also release powerful poisons, known as toxins, that rapidly damage tissues. In the past, bacterial diseases were a major cause of death; today, most serious infections can be treated effectively with antibiotics.

Each of the bacterial infections covered in this section affects many areas of the body simultaneously. The most serious of these infections is septicaemia, described in the first article, which can be due to almost any bacterium. The diseases in the following articles are caused only by particular bacteria. They include both relatively recently identified infections, such as toxic shock syndrome, and those that have long been recognized, such as diphtheria and plague. The final articles describe illnesses caused by the rickettsiae bacteria, some of which may be transmitted to humans through insect bites.

Many other bacterial infections, such as pneumonia (p.490), tuberculosis (p.491), and meningitis (p.527), cause damage to certain organs, and for this reason they are covered in the sections on specific body systems.

Bacterial skin infections, such as boils, are discussed in skin infections and infestations (pp.351–355).

KEY STRUCTURES

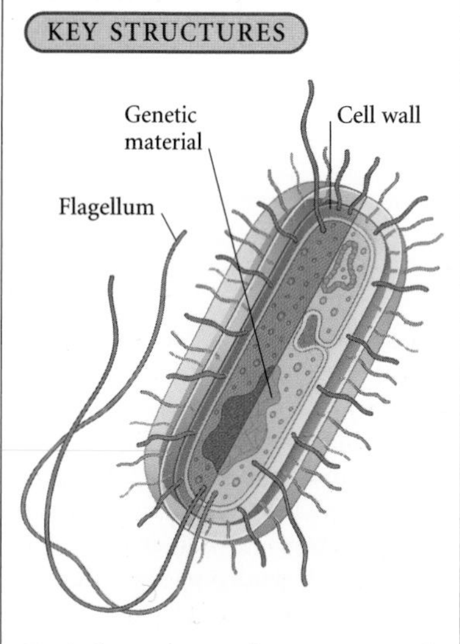

For information on the structure and function of bacteria, *see* pp. 284–287.

Septicaemia

An infection, also known as blood poisoning, in which bacteria multiply in the bloodstream

 AGE More common in children and elderly people

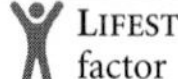 LIFESTYLE Intravenous drug use is a risk factor

 GENDER GENETICS Not significant factors

Septicaemia, also known as blood poisoning, is a potentially fatal condition in which bacteria multiply rapidly in the bloodstream. It is common for bacteria to enter the bloodstream in small numbers through sites such as a breach in the skin or through the mouth when the teeth are brushed. The bacteria are usually destroyed by the immune system and cause no symptoms. However, if bacteria enter the bloodstream in large numbers from a major source of infection, such as a kidney infection (*see* PYELONEPHRITIS, p.698), blood poisoning can result. Septicaemia can develop as a complication of almost all types of serious infectious diseases.

The infection is more likely to occur in people with reduced immunity due to disorders such as diabetes mellitus (p.687) or HIV infection (*see* HIV INFECTION AND AIDS, p.297) or due to treatment with chemotherapy (p.280) or immunosuppressant drugs (p.906). Young children and elderly people are also more susceptible. Others at increased risk are intravenous drug users, who may introduce bacteria into their blood from contaminated needles.

WHAT ARE THE SYMPTOMS?

The symptoms of septicaemia develop suddenly and include:

- High fever.
- Chills and violent shivering.

If septicaemia is left untreated, the bacteria may produce toxins that damage blood vessels, causing a drop in blood pressure and widespread tissue damage. In this dangerous condition, called septic shock, symptoms may include:

- Faintness.
- Cold, pale hands and feet.
- Restlessness and irritability.
- Rapid, shallow breathing.
- In many cases, delirium and eventual loss of consciousness.

In some people, bacteria may lodge on the heart valves, especially if the heart has previously been damaged by disease. This serious condition is called infective endocarditis (p.426). In rare cases, septicaemia may result in a lack of the blood cells involved in blood clotting (*see* THROMBOCYTOPENIA, p.453), which increases the risk of excessive bleeding.

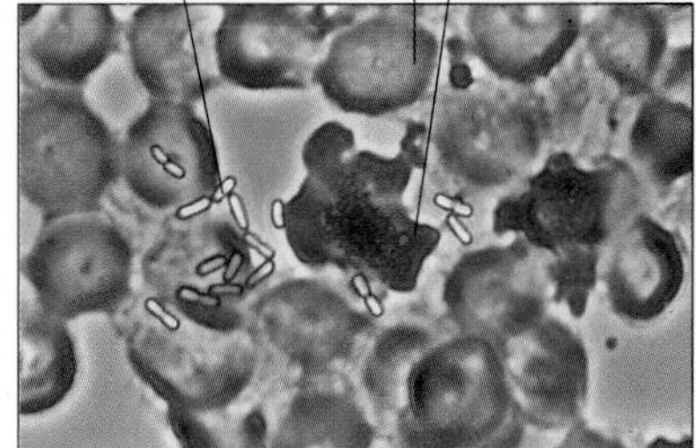

Bacteria in blood
This magnified blood sample from a person with septicaemia shows small, rod-shaped bacteria among the blood cells.

WHAT MIGHT BE DONE?

If your doctor suspects that you have septicaemia, you will be admitted to hospital for immediate treatment. Intravenous antibiotics (p.885) are given first, and then blood tests are performed to identify the bacterium causing the infection. Once the bacterium has been identified, specific antibiotics are given. With prompt treatment, most people make a complete recovery.

(WWW) ONLINE SITES: p.1033

Toxic shock syndrome

A rare but serious condition caused by staphylococcal or streptococcal toxins

 AGE Most common between the ages of 15 and 20

 GENDER More common in females

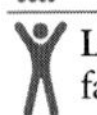 LIFESTYLE Using tampons may be a risk factor

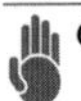 GENETICS Not a significant factor

First recognized in the late 1970s, toxic shock syndrome is an uncommon but potentially fatal infection. The condition is caused by a toxin produced by *Staphylococcus aureus* and some streptococcal bacteria, which enter the bloodstream from a localized site of infection.

Toxic shock syndrome mainly affects young adults, and about half of all cases occur in menstruating women. The infection may be linked to the use of tampons, which can provide a site for bacterial growth in the vagina, particularly if a tampon is left in place longer than the recommended time.

The symptoms start suddenly and may include fever, vomiting, diarrhoea, and severe muscular aches and pains. A widespread red, sunburn-like rash may appear, and confusion may occur. More serious complications can also develop, such as acute kidney failure (p.706).

Toxic shock syndrome requires immediate treatment in hospital with intravenous antibiotics (p.885). Treated promptly, 9 in 10 people recover fully.

(WWW) ONLINE SITES: p.1033, p.1037

Scarlet fever

A rare streptococcal infection causing a red rash and a sore throat

 AGE Most common between the ages of 6 and 12

 GENDER GENETICS LIFESTYLE Not significant factors

Once a common and dangerous childhood disease, scarlet fever has become rare in developed countries since the introduction of antibiotics (p.885). This infection is caused by the bacterium *Streptococcus pyogenes*, transmitted in microscopic droplets from coughs and sneezes. A prominent feature of the condition is a widespread scarlet rash.

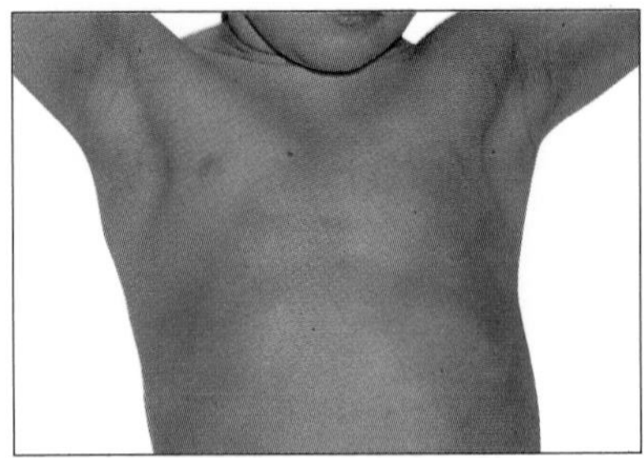

Scarlet fever
The characteristic red rash of scarlet fever begins on the trunk and is often most obvious in the armpits.

WHAT ARE THE SYMPTOMS?

About 1–3 days after infection, the following symptoms may develop:

- Sore throat and headache.
- Fever and vomiting.
- Raised, red rash, spreading rapidly on the neck, trunk, armpits, and groin.

A thick, white coating may develop on the tongue, disappearing in a few days to leave the tongue bright red with a pimpled "strawberry" appearance.

WHAT MIGHT BE DONE?

Scarlet fever is usually diagnosed from the symptoms. To confirm the diagnosis, a throat swab may be taken.

The infection is treated with antibiotics, and the symptoms usually begin to improve within 24–48 hours. Most people recover within a week.

(WWW) ONLINE SITES: p.1028, p.1033

Diphtheria

A rare throat infection that can cause breathing difficulties

 AGE More common in children

 GENDER GENETICS LIFESTYLE Not significant factors

Now rare in developed countries, diphtheria was a common cause of death in children until immunization became routine. In this disease, the bacterium *Corynebacterium diphtheriae* multiplies in the throat and may release toxins into the blood. The infection is usually transmitted through airborne droplets from coughs or sneezes of infected people.

Diphtheria bacteria may also infect the skin. This form of the disease, known as cutaneous diphtheria, is more common in tropical countries but it can affect people elsewhere, especially if their standards of hygiene are poor. Outbreaks of diphtheria tend to occur among overcrowded communities.

WHAT ARE THE SYMPTOMS?

The symptoms of diphtheria develop 1–4 days after infection and include:

- Sore throat.
- Fever.
- Swollen lymph nodes in the neck.
- In many cases, a grey membrane that grows across the throat, causing difficulty in breathing.

In the cutaneous form of the disorder, deep sores may develop. If diphtheria is not treated, bacterial toxins may spread in the blood and cause potentially fatal complications such as acute heart failure (p.412) and paralysis.

WHAT MIGHT BE DONE?

Diphtheria may be diagnosed from the symptoms, but a throat swab is taken for confirmation. Most people recover fully if treated immediately with antibiotics (p.885) and antitoxin injections in hospital. Routine immunization (p.45) in children and boosters in adults provide protection against the disease.

(WWW) ONLINE SITES: p.1033

Brucellosis

A rare infection, contracted from farm animals and dairy products, that may cause recurrent illness

 LIFESTYLE Working with farm animals is a risk factor

 AGE GENDER GENETICS Not significant factors

Brucellosis is caused by various types of brucella bacteria, which can be transmitted to humans through contact with infected farm animals and in unpasteurized milk and other dairy products. The disease rarely occurs in developed countries, where domestic animals are normally free of the infection.

The symptoms of brucellosis vary considerably from person to person. In some cases, depression and weight loss are the only signs of infection, although many people develop fever with night sweats, tiredness, headache, and pain in the joints. Left untreated, the illness can become persistent, recurring at intervals over months or sometimes years.

WHAT MIGHT BE DONE?

A lack of specific symptoms makes brucellosis difficult to diagnose, although the bacteria can be identified by a blood test. It is usually treated with antibiotics (p.885), which are sometimes given with corticosteroids (p.930). With treatment, most people recover within 2–3 weeks.

(WWW) ONLINE SITES: p.1033

Listeriosis

An uncommon infection transmitted through contaminated food

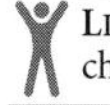
LIFESTYLE Eating certain foods, such as soft cheeses and meat pâté, is a risk factor

AGE GENDER GENETICS Not significant factors

The bacterium that causes listeriosis, *Listeria monocytogenes*, is widespread in the soil and is present in most animal species. It can pass to humans through food products, particularly soft cheeses, milk, meat pâtés, and prepackaged salads. The risk of listeriosis is increased by incorrect storage of these foods. The bacteria multiply in the intestines and may spread in the blood (*see* SEPTICAEMIA, p.299) and affect other organs.

The symptoms of listeriosis vary from one person to another. The infection often goes unnoticed in healthy adults, although some people may develop flu-like symptoms such as fever, sore throat, headache, and aching muscles.

In elderly people and people with reduced immunity, such as those with HIV infection (*see* HIV INFECTION AND AIDS, p.297) or those taking immunosuppressant drugs (p.906), listeriosis can lead to meningitis (p.527), a potentially fatal inflammation of the membranes covering the brain. In pregnant women, infection can pass to the fetus, causing miscarriage (p.791) or stillbirth (p.805).

WHAT MIGHT BE DONE?

Listeriosis is usually diagnosed from a blood test. In otherwise healthy people, mild listeriosis clears up without treatment in a few days. People with serious infection, especially during pregnancy, need urgent treatment in hospital with intravenous antibiotics (p.885).

Hygienic handling and storage of food reduces the risk of listeriosis (*see* HOME SAFETY AND HEALTH, p.77).

(WWW) ONLINE SITES: p.1030, p.1033, p.1035

Typhoid and paratyphoid

Infections caused by salmonella bacteria that result in high fever followed by a rash

LIFESTYLE Visiting or living in areas where the disease occurs is a risk factor

AGE GENDER GENETICS Not significant factors

Typhoid and paratyphoid are almost identical diseases that are caused by the bacteria *Salmonella typhi* and *S. paratyphi*, respectively. The bacteria multiply in the intestines and spread to the blood and to other organs, such as the spleen, gallbladder, and liver. The diseases are transmitted through infected faeces and most commonly occur in areas where hygiene and sanitation are poor. Infection is commonly due to food or water contaminated by unwashed hands.

WHAT ARE THE SYMPTOMS?

Symptoms of both diseases appear 7–14 days after infection and may include:

- Headache and high fever.
- Dry cough.
- Abdominal pain and constipation, usually followed by diarrhoea.
- Rash of rose-coloured spots appearing on the chest, abdomen, and back.

Both infections can lead to serious complications, such as intestinal bleeding and perforation of the intestines.

WHAT MIGHT BE DONE?

Typhoid and paratyphoid can be diagnosed by testing blood or faecal samples for the bacteria. The diseases are usually treated with antibiotics (p.885) in hospital. Symptoms normally subside 2–3 days after treatment is begun, and most people recover fully in a month.

Even with treatment, the bacteria are excreted for about 3 months after the symptoms have disappeared. Some people who do not have treatment may become lifelong carriers of the bacteria and transmit the infection to others, although they appear to be healthy.

Good hygiene is the best protection against infection (*see* TRAVEL HEALTH, p.85). Several vaccines are available, and, if you intend to travel to a developing country, immunization may be advisable (*see* TRAVEL IMMUNIZATIONS, p.86).

(WWW) ONLINE SITES: p.1033, p.1037

Cholera

An intestinal infection that causes profuse, watery diarrhoea

LIFESTYLE Visiting or living in areas where the disease occurs is a risk factor

AGE GENDER GENETICS Not significant factors

Cholera typically occurs in epidemics and has caused millions of deaths over the centuries. It is due to infection of the small intestine by the bacterium *Vibrio cholerae*. Usually associated with areas of poor sanitation, cholera can be spread through contaminated water or food.

The illness starts suddenly, 1–5 days after infection, with vomiting and profuse, watery diarrhoea. In some cases, fatal dehydration develops.

WHAT MIGHT BE DONE?

Cholera is usually diagnosed from the characteristic "rice water" appearance of the diarrhoea. To confirm the diagnosis, a faecal sample may be checked for the presence of the bacteria.

Urgent hospital treatment is needed to replace lost fluids and minerals, which are given orally or intravenously. Antibiotics (p.885) may be given to reduce the risk of passing the infection to others. If treated without delay, most people make a complete recovery.

Cholera vaccines are relatively ineffective. In regions where cholera may occur, good hygiene is the best protection (*see* TRAVEL HEALTH, p.85).

(WWW) ONLINE SITES: p.1033, p.1037

Botulism

A rare, life-threatening form of poisoning in which a bacterial toxin in food damages the nervous system, causing paralysis

LIFESTYLE Eating home-preserved food is a risk factor

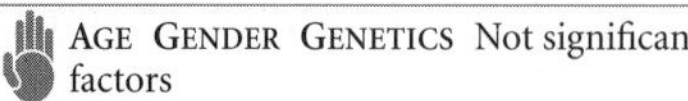
AGE GENDER GENETICS Not significant factors

The toxin that causes botulism is one of the most dangerous poisons known to humanity. This toxin is produced by the bacterium *Clostridium botulinum*, which can multiply rapidly in canned or preserved foods. If a contaminated food is eaten, absorption of even minute amounts of toxin can cause severe damage to the nervous system.

Strict controls on commercial canning have made botulism caused by shop-bought products rare. The foods most commonly affected are home-preserved vegetables, fish, and fruit. Babies, who are especially susceptible to the effects of the toxin, may develop botulism after being given contaminated honey.

What are the symptoms?

The symptoms of botulism appear very suddenly, 8–36 hours after eating contaminated food. In the initial stages, the symptoms usually include:

- Nausea and constipation.
- Dry mouth.

Within 24 hours, these symptoms are followed by muscle weakness that starts in the eyes, causing blurred vision, and then progresses down the body. Without treatment, the respiratory muscles may become paralysed, causing suffocation.

What might be done?

Botulism needs immediate treatment in hospital with antitoxin drugs. For people whose breathing is affected, mechanical ventilation may be necessary. If given treatment without delay, 9 in 10 people make a full recovery.

To reduce the risk of poisoning, you should pressure-cook home-preserved food for at least 30 minutes at 120°C (250°F) and ensure that all containers are sterilized. Babies under the age of 12 months should not be given honey.

(WWW) ONLINE SITES: p.1030, p.1033

Tetanus

A wound infection, caused by a bacterial toxin, that produces severe muscle spasms

AGE GENDER GENETICS LIFESTYLE Not significant factors

Tetanus is caused by a toxin produced by the bacterium *Clostridium tetani*, which lives in soil and in the intestines of humans and other animals. If the bacteria enter a wound, they multiply, and an infection may develop that acts on the nerves controlling muscle activity. The condition, also called lockjaw, is rare in developed countries because most people have been immunized.

The symptoms of tetanus usually appear 5–10 days after infection. Fever, headache, and muscle stiffness in the jaw, arms, neck, and back are typical. As the condition progresses, painful muscle spasms may develop. In some people, the muscles of the throat or chest wall are affected, leading to breathing difficulties and possible suffocation.

What might be done?

Diagnosis of tetanus is based on details of the injury and on the symptoms. The disease needs immediate treatment in hospital with antitoxin injections, antibiotics (p.885), and sedatives (*see* ANTIANXIETY DRUGS, p.916) to relieve muscle spasm. Mechanical ventilation may be necessary to aid breathing. If given prompt treatment, most people make a complete recovery. If treatment is delayed, tetanus is usually fatal.

To reduce the risk of tetanus, you should thoroughly clean wounds, especially those contaminated with soil, and treat them with antiseptic. Deep puncture wounds, which are especially likely to become infected, should be seen by your doctor, who may give you antibiotics to prevent infection.

Vaccination against tetanus, usually given in early childhood (*see* ROUTINE IMMUNIZATIONS, p.45), is highly effective. Boosters should be given every 10 years to maintain protection.

(WWW) ONLINE SITES: p.1033

Hansen's disease

An infection, also known as leprosy, that affects nerves and skin, causing numbness and disfigurement

AGE GENDER GENETICS LIFESTYLE Not significant factors

Hansen's disease, commonly known as leprosy, is a long-term infection caused by the bacterium *Mycobacterium leprae*, which damages the skin and nerves. The limbs and face, in particular, may be affected. Infection is thought to be transmitted in airborne droplets produced when an infected person coughs or sneezes and through skin contact. Contrary to popular belief, the disease is not easily transmitted from person to person. Only people who live in prolonged, close contact with an infected person are at risk of infection, and most people are naturally resistant to the bacteria. The disease is rare in developed countries and is most common in Asia, Africa, and South America.

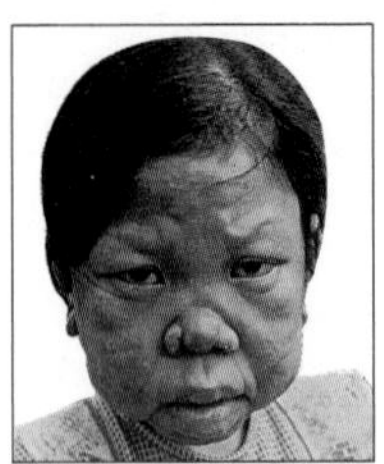
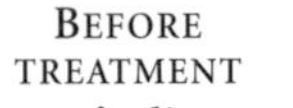
BEFORE TREATMENT

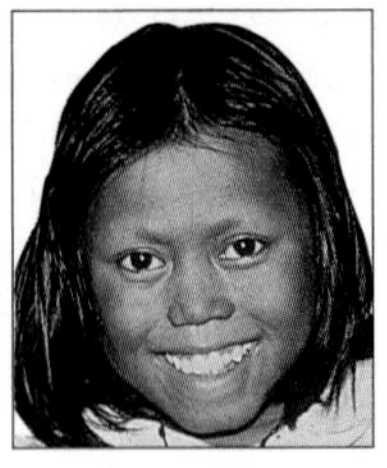
AFTER TREATMENT

Hansen's disease
At the age of 7, this girl had thickened facial skin due to Hansen's disease. After 2 years of treatment with antibiotics, her appearance had improved dramatically.

Hansen's disease develops very slowly, the first symptoms appearing 3–5 years after infection. Initially, nerve damage causes numbness of the skin on the face, hands, and feet. The affected skin may also become thickened and discoloured. Hansen's disease is infectious only while these early symptoms are developing. Lack of sensation may lead to injury or even loss of fingers and toes.

Diagnosis is based on the symptoms and examination of a sample of skin tissue to identify the bacterium. Treatment with antibiotics (p.885), for up to 2 years, prevents further nerve damage and reduces areas of thickened skin. However, nerve damage that has already occurred is irreversible.

(WWW) ONLINE SITES: p.1033

Leptospirosis

A group of infections transmitted to humans by rats and other animals

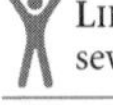
LIFESTYLE Working on farms or with sewage is a risk factor

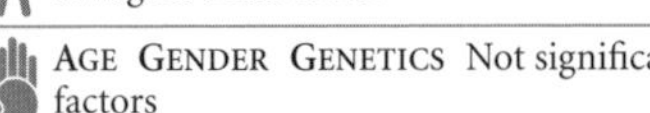
AGE GENDER GENETICS Not significant factors

Infections caused by different types of *Leptospira* bacteria are known generally as leptospirosis. The bacteria are carried by animals such as rats or foxes and excreted in their urine. Infection is usually transmitted to humans by contact with contaminated water or soil. In most cases the infection causes a flu-like illness. However, in its most severe form, which is known as Weil's disease, leptospirosis may be life-threatening.

Leptospirosis most commonly occurs in farmers and sewage workers, but the disease can affect anyone who comes into contact with contaminated water, such as swimmers or those taking part in watersports. In the UK, about 8 cases of leptospirosis are reported each year.

What are the symptoms?

The symptoms of leptospirosis usually appear abruptly 2–20 days after infection. They may include:

- Fever.
- Intense headache and muscle pain.
- Flat, red rash.
- Inflammation of the eyes and eyelids (*see* CONJUNCTIVITIS, p.570).

The symptoms tend to disappear after a few days but may recur if immediate treatment is not given. If the disease goes untreated, it frequently causes a potentially dangerous inflammation of the membranes covering the brain (*see* MENINGITIS, p.527).

About 1 in 10 infected people develops Weil's disease. This disorder leads to widespread internal bleeding, damage to the kidneys and liver, and jaundice (p.643), which causes the skin and the whites of the eyes to turn yellow.

What might be done?

To diagnose leptospirosis, your doctor may arrange for blood and urine tests to check for the presence of bacteria. If treated with antibiotics (p.885) at an early stage, most people recover fully.

As a preventive measure, workers at particular risk of infection are usually given antibiotics after minor injuries such as cuts and scrapes.

(WWW) ONLINE SITES: p.1033

Lyme disease

An infection transmitted by ticks that causes a rash and flu-like symptoms

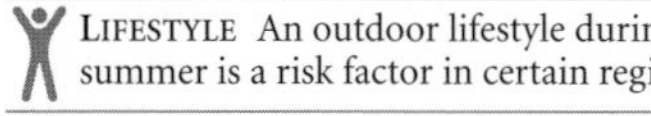 LIFESTYLE An outdoor lifestyle during summer is a risk factor in certain regions

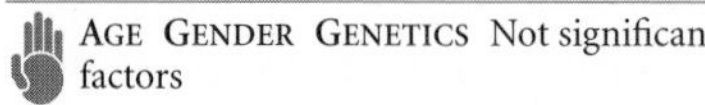 AGE GENDER GENETICS Not significant factors

Named after Old Lyme, the North American town where the disease was first recognized, Lyme disease is caused by a bacterium called *Borrelia burgdorferi.* The infection is transmitted to humans by ticks that usually live on deer. If a person is bitten by an infected tick that remains attached to his or her skin, bacteria can enter the bloodstream and may then spread throughout the body. A tick may be infected with more than one type of bacterium, and as a result a single bite may cause other, similar infections at the same time.

Although Lyme disease is most widely reported in the US, the infection is now becoming recognized as a problem in the UK, particularly in areas of woodland or parkland where there are deer. People who go camping or walking in such areas during the summer months are most at risk of being bitten by a tick carrying Lyme disease bacteria.

What are the symptoms?

A bite from an infected tick usually produces a red lump with a scab on the skin, although some people who have been bitten may not notice this initial sign. Within 2 days to 4 weeks after the bite, the following symptoms may develop:

- Spreading circular rash at the site of the bite that may clear in the centre.
- Tiredness.
- Flu-like chills and fever.
- Headache and joint pains.

If the infection is left untreated, these symptoms may persist for several weeks. In some people who have Lyme disease, dangerous complications may develop up to 2 years later that may affect the heart, nervous system, and joints.

What might be done?

Your doctor may suspect from your symptoms that you have Lyme disease and may also arrange for a blood test to confirm the diagnosis.

If they are given prompt treatment with antibiotics (p.885), most people make a complete recovery. Nonsteroidal anti-inflammatory drugs (p.894) can help to relieve joint pain. Complications are extremely rare. For people at particular risk, vaccines are now available that offer 70 per cent protection against Lyme disease. Vaccination needs to be repeated every 2 years.

In regions known to be tick-infested, you should cover your arms and legs to reduce the risk of being bitten (*see* PREVENTING TICK BITES, above) and immediately remove any ticks that you find attached to your skin (*see* FIRST AID: TICK BITES, p.995).

(WWW) ONLINE SITES: p.1033

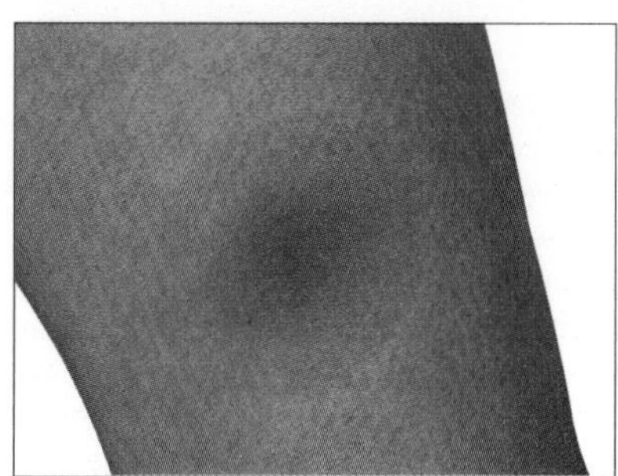

Lyme disease
A bite from a tick infected with the bacterium that causes Lyme disease typically produces an expanding circular red rash, as seen here on the thigh.

(SELF-HELP) Preventing tick bites

Ticks are tiny, spider-like parasites that are difficult to see, and their bites often go unnoticed. If you are walking or camping in tick-infested areas you should take the following precautions to minimize the risk of being bitten:

- Wear light-coloured clothes, so that ticks can be seen more easily.
- Keep your skin covered by wearing long sleeves and tucking trousers into socks.
- Where there is vegetation, do not sit directly on the ground.
- Whenever possible, keep to well-trodden trails and pathways, and avoid walking through overgrown vegetation.
- While out walking, stop to make occasional checks for ticks, especially on children and dogs.
- Before going to bed at night, carefully examine your own and your children's skin and clothing for ticks.

Plague

A serious infection carried by rodents and transmitted to humans by flea bites

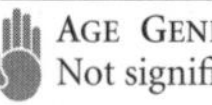 AGE GENDER GENETICS LIFESTYLE Not significant factors

Plague is the result of infection by the bacterium *Yersinia pestis,* which usually affects rodents but can be transmitted to humans through flea bites. During the Middle Ages, the disease caused pandemics (widespread epidemics), one of the largest of which was the so-called Black Death of the 14th century, which killed over 25 million people in Europe. Today, small outbreaks occur in Asia, Africa, and South America, and there are a few cases each year in the US, but plague is unknown in Europe.

There are two main forms of plague: bubonic plague, which affects the lymph nodes, and pneumonic plague, which occurs if the infection spreads to the lungs. The symptoms of both forms develop rapidly and include a high fever and chills. In bubonic plague, painful swellings known as buboes develop in the lymph nodes, usually in the groin and armpits. Pneumonic plague causes a severe cough, shortness of breath, and chest pain. Once the lungs are infected, plague can be transmitted from person to person through airborne droplets from coughs and sneezes.

Plague is diagnosed from the symptoms and by a blood test. People given immediate treatment with antibiotics (p.885) usually make a complete recovery. However, if treatment is delayed, the disease is frequently fatal.

(WWW) ONLINE SITES: p.1033

Rocky Mountain spotted fever

A rickettsial infection, transmitted to humans by animal ticks, that causes fever and a spotted rash

LIFESTYLE An outdoor lifestyle during summer is a risk factor in certain regions

AGE GENDER GENETICS Not significant factors

Despite its name, Rocky Mountain spotted fever occurs not only in the Rocky Mountain states of the US but also in eastern US states and South America. The disease is caused by the bacterium *Rickettsia rickettsii*, which is transmitted to humans through bites from infected animal ticks. Although the disease does not occur in Europe, visitors to the US who go camping or walking in woodland areas may be at risk, especially during spring and summer.

The initial symptoms appear suddenly about a week after infection and may include severe headache, muscle pains, chills, and fever. Within a few days, a rash of tiny pink spots develops, usually appearing first on the limbs and then spreading rapidly over the rest of

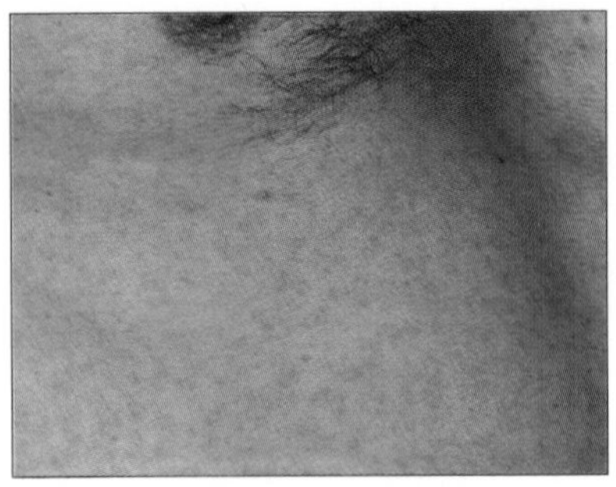

Rocky Mountain spotted fever
The rash of Rocky Mountain spotted fever often begins on the limbs and spreads over the body, as seen here on the chest.

the body. This rash gradually becomes darker. If the condition is left untreated, potentially fatal complications, such as gangrene (p.435) and kidney failure (p.706), may develop.

Rocky Mountain spotted fever is usually diagnosed from the appearance of the rash, but blood or tissue tests may be carried out. If given prompt treatment with antibiotics (p.885), most infected people make a rapid recovery.

In regions known to be infested with ticks, you should keep your arms and legs covered to reduce the risk of being bitten (*see* PREVENTING TICK BITES, p.303) and promptly remove any ticks that attach themselves to your skin (*see* FIRST AID: TICK BITES, p.995).

(WWW) ONLINE SITES: p.1033

Q fever

A rickettsial infection transmitted to humans by contact with farm animals

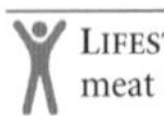
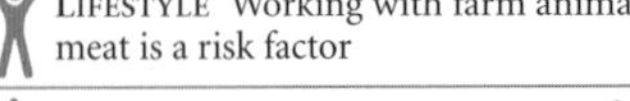
LIFESTYLE Working with farm animals or meat is a risk factor

AGE GENDER GENETICS Not significant factors

Labelled Q for "query" before the source of the infection was identified, Q fever is caused by the rickettsial bacterium *Coxiella burnetti*. The bacteria are carried by livestock such as cows, sheep, and goats and can be transmitted through urine, faeces, and milk, or inhaled in dust contaminated with particles of tissue from infected animals.

Within 2–3 weeks of infection, a high fever, severe headache, muscle pain, and cough may suddenly occur. The symptoms usually disappear in 1–2 weeks, but, in some people, infection spreads and damages the heart valves (*see* INFECTIVE ENDOCARDITIS, p.426) and the liver (*see* ACUTE HEPATITIS, p.644).

Q fever is diagnosed by a blood test and is usually treated successfully with antibiotics (p.885). Vaccines give some protection against the infection for several years and are available for people who are at high risk, such as farmers and slaughterhouse workers.

(WWW) ONLINE SITES: p.1033

Typhus

A serious rickettsial infection transmitted to humans by lice, fleas, or mites

LIFESTYLE Living in overcrowded, unhygienic conditions is a risk factor

AGE GENDER GENETICS Not significant factors

There are three main forms of typhus, all of which are caused by different types of rickettsial bacteria.

Epidemic typhus is transmitted by body lice, usually in overcrowded conditions, and has resulted in hundreds of thousands of deaths in times of war or famine. Today, the disease is rare except in some areas of tropical Africa and South America. Endemic typhus, which is also known as murine typhus, is a rare disease that can be transmitted from rats to humans by fleas; a few cases occur each year in North and Central America. Scrub typhus, which is transmitted by mites, has been reported in India and Southeast Asia.

The first sign of infection with scrub typhus is a black scab over the site of the bite. In all types of typhus, flu-like symptoms may develop in 1–3 weeks of infection, followed a few days later by a widespread, blotchy pink rash. In severe cases of typhus, delirium and coma (p.522) occur. If the disease is not treated, dangerous complications such as pneumonia (p.490) or kidney failure (p.705) are also likely to develop.

WHAT MIGHT BE DONE?

Typhus is often diagnosed from the symptoms, but a blood test may be carried out. Treatment with antibiotics (p.885) is usually effective. Without treatment, the bacteria can lie dormant in the body for years before being reactivated and causing the disease to recur.

(WWW) ONLINE SITES: p.1033

Protozoal and Fungal Infections

Protozoa and fungi are simple organisms, capable of living in many different habitats. Some protozoa and fungi are parasites of humans. They acquire all their food from our bodies and often cause disease. One protozoal infection, malaria, affects hundreds of millions of people worldwide each year and is often fatal.

Protozoal infections are discussed first, starting with malaria, the most important health hazard for visitors to the tropics. Further articles deal with other protozoal infections, including diseases that are common causes of diarrhoea, such as amoebiasis and cryptosporidiosis. The protozoal infection trichomoniasis, which is transmitted sexually, is covered with other such sexually transmitted diseases (*see* TRICHOMONIASIS, p.767).

Fungal infections are discussed next. Like most protozoal infections, fungal infections may be serious in people with reduced immunity, such as those who have AIDS. The types of fungi described in this section can spread around the body from the initial site of infection, sometimes causing long-term illness. Common fungal infections that affect particular areas of the body, such as the skin and vagina, are covered in the sections on specific body systems.

KEY STRUCTURES

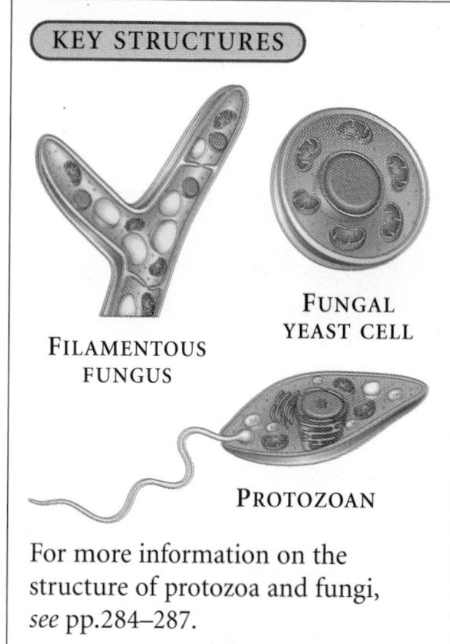

For more information on the structure of protozoa and fungi, *see* pp.284–287.

Malaria

A parasitic infection of red blood cells spread by mosquitoes

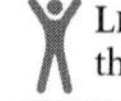
LIFESTYLE Visiting or living in areas where the disease occurs are risk factors

AGE GENDER GENETICS Not significant factors

Malaria, a parasitic infection that leads to the destruction of red blood cells, is one of the greatest public health problems in the world. In tropical countries, where the infection is most likely to be contracted, about 10 million new cases of malaria and 2 million deaths due to the disease occur every year. Most of those who die of malaria are children. The disease is the most serious health threat to travellers and holidaymakers who visit the tropics.

The World Health Organization has been trying to control malaria for many years but with only intermittent success. Malarial parasites are transmitted to humans by mosquitoes of the anopheles group, which have now become resistant to a number of insecticides. In many areas, the malarial parasite itself has now also become resistant to the common antimalarial drugs (p.888). Currently, no effective vaccine has been developed to protect against infection with the malarial parasite.

If you live in a region where malaria is common, you may have several mild episodes of infection that increase your resistance, making you less likely to develop a serious infection. However, this protection is lost within a year if you move to a malaria-free region. Therefore, if you emigrate from a malaria-affected area and later return for a holiday, you will need to take preventive measures (*see* PREVENTING MALARIA, right). If you become ill after a visit to the tropics, you should tell your doctor where you have been and when you went there.

What are the types?

The characteristics of malaria have been known for over 2,000 years. However, the cause of the disease was only identified in 1880. Four species of protozoal parasites from the plasmodium group cause malaria in humans, each species causing a different type of malaria. The most dangerous type of malaria is falciparum malaria, caused by *Plasmodium falciparum*. This type of malaria results in the most deaths and is often fatal within 48 hours of the first symptoms if it is left untreated. The other three types of malaria, caused by *Plasmodium malariae, Plasmodium ovale,* and *Plasmodium vivax*, are less severe.

All types of malarial parasite are transmitted to humans by a bite from an infected mosquito. Initially, the parasites multiply in the liver and are then released into the bloodstream, where they penetrate red blood cells. After 48–72 hours, depending on the species of parasite, the infected cells rupture, releasing parasites that invade other red blood cells. If a noninfected mosquito bites the infected person, the insect itself

SELF-HELP Preventing Malaria

If you plan to visit an area where malaria occurs, your doctor will be able to give you up-to-date advice about antimalarial drugs (p.888) for that area. You may need to start taking the drugs several days before you leave and continue taking them during and after your visit. To protect yourself against mosquito bites, you should:

- Keep your body covered as much as possible.
- Sleep under a mosquito net that is impregnated with insecticide.
- Use insect repellent on clothes and exposed skin.

These measures against mosquito bites are especially important between dusk and dawn, when malaria-carrying mosquitoes bite.

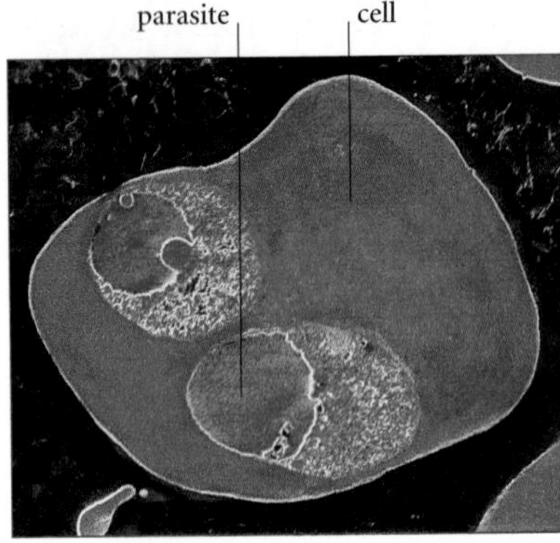

Infected red blood cell
The protozoa that cause malaria infect red blood cells. Attacks of the disease occur when the protozoa burst out of the cells.

becomes infected and can then spread the disease to other people. In all types of malaria, the disease can pass from an infected pregnant woman to her fetus.

WHAT ARE THE SYMPTOMS?

The symptoms of malaria usually begin between 10 days and 6 weeks after being bitten by an infected mosquito. However, in some cases, symptoms may not develop for months or years, especially if preventive drugs were being taken at the time of infection.

If not treated, malaria due to *P. vivax*, *P. ovale*, and *P. malariae* causes recurrent attacks of symptoms with each episode of red blood cell destruction by the parasites. Each attack usually lasts for 4–8 hours and may occur at intervals of 2 or 3 days, depending on the species of parasite. Symptoms of an attack include:

- High fever.
- Shivering and chills.
- Heavy sweating.
- Confusion.
- Tiredness, headache, and muscle pain.

Between each attack, extreme tiredness may be the only symptom.

Falciparum malaria causes a continuous fever that may be mistaken for influenza (p.289). It is more severe than the other types, and attacks may lead to loss of consciousness and kidney failure (p.705) and may be fatal.

WHAT MIGHT BE DONE?

Your doctor may suspect malaria if you have an unexplained fever within a year after a trip to a region where the infection occurs. Diagnosis is confirmed by identifying the malarial parasite in a blood smear under a microscope.

If you are diagnosed with malaria, you should be given antimalarial drugs (p.888) as early as possible to avoid complications. Treatment depends on the type of malaria, how resistant the parasite is to drugs, and the severity of the symptoms. If you have falciparum malaria, you may be treated in hospital with oral or intravenous antimalarial drugs. Treatment may also involve a blood transfusion (p.447) to replace destroyed red blood cells or kidney dialysis (p.707) if kidney function is impaired. Other types of malaria are usually treated on an outpatient basis with oral antimalarial drugs.

If treated early, the outlook is usually good, and most people make a full recovery. However, malaria caused by *P. vivax* and *P. ovale* may recur after treatment.

Preventive measures, including using antimalarial drugs, should be taken to reduce the risk of infection when visiting areas where malaria occurs.

(WWW) ONLINE SITES: p.1033, p.1037

Amoebiasis

An intestinal infection that causes diarrhoea and may spread to the liver

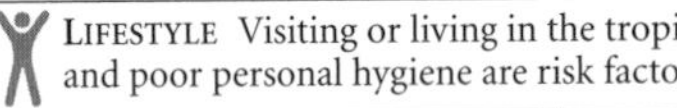
LIFESTYLE Visiting or living in the tropics and poor personal hygiene are risk factors

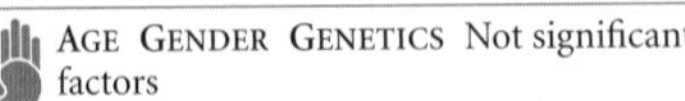
AGE GENDER GENETICS Not significant factors

The intestinal infection amoebiasis is caused by the protozoan parasite *Entamoeba histolytica.* Worldwide, the disease is very common, affecting about 500 million people. It is mostly contracted in developing countries in the tropics. Usually, infection results from drinking water or eating food contaminated with the parasite, which is excreted in the faeces of infected people. In severe cases, ulcers develop in the walls of the intestine, and the condition is then known as amoebic dysentery.

WHAT ARE THE SYMPTOMS?

Most infected people do not develop symptoms or have only mild, intermittent symptoms, which may include:

- Diarrhoea.
- Mild abdominal pain.

If you develop amoebic dysentery, the symptoms usually first appear between 5 days and several weeks after the initial infection. Symptoms may include:

- Watery, bloody diarrhoea.
- Severe abdominal pain.
- Fever.

In some cases, dehydration and anaemia (p.446) may develop. In addition, there is a risk of infection spreading through the bloodstream to the liver, causing high fever, painful liver abscesses, extreme tiredness, and loss of appetite.

WHAT MIGHT BE DONE?

Diagnosis of amoebiasis is usually made from examination of a sample of faeces under a microscope to look for the parasite. Your doctor may also arrange for you to have a blood test to look for antibodies that are produced by the body in response to the parasite. If your doctor suspects that you have liver abscesses, he or she will arrange for you to have imaging tests, such as CT scanning (p.247) or ultrasound scanning (p.250). Amoebiasis can be successfully treated with antibiotics (p.885), which usually kill the parasite within a few days. With drug treatment, most affected people make a full recovery from the infection within a few weeks.

CAN IT BE PREVENTED?

There are several preventive measures you can take against amoebiasis if you visit a region where the disease is common. You should drink only bottled or thoroughly boiled water to be certain that it is safe (*see* TRAVEL HEALTH, p.85). You should also avoid eating raw vegetables, salads, or fruits with skins that cannot be peeled because their skins may be contaminated with the parasite.

(WWW) ONLINE SITES: p.1033, p.1037

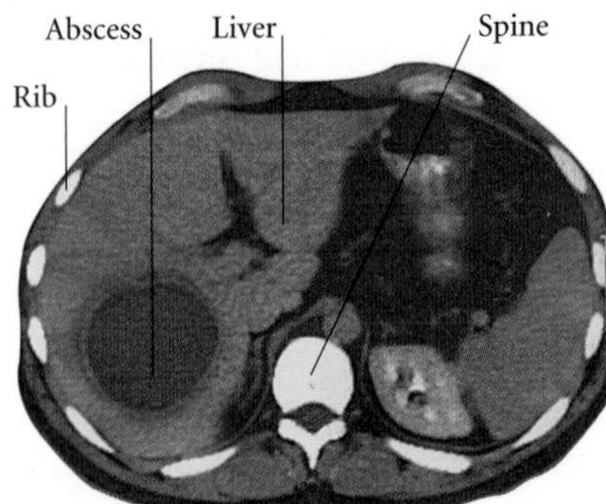

Liver abscess due to amoebiasis
In some people with amoebiasis, infection spreads to the liver and forms an abscess, as seen in the CT scan above.

Giardiasis

An intestinal infection with a protozoal parasite, often leading to diarrhoea

 AGE More common in early childhood

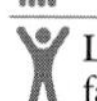 LIFESTYLE Poor personal hygiene is a risk factor

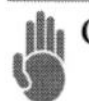 GENDER GENETICS Not significant factors

Giardiasis is caused by a minute parasite known as *Giardia lamblia,* which infects the small intestine. Cysts (the dormant stages) of the parasite are excreted in the faeces of infected people and animals. The disease occurs mainly as a result of drinking water contaminated with cysts. The infection may also spread as a result of poor personal hygiene.

Infections are more serious in people with reduced immunity due to disorders such as HIV infection and AIDS (p.297) or treatment with immunosuppressant drugs (p.906).

Giardiasis occurs mainly in developing countries. In developed countries, the infection usually affects children, walkers who drink from contaminated streams, and people who have returned from travelling in developing countries.

WHAT ARE THE SYMPTOMS?

Some people may not have symptoms, but, if symptoms do develop, they usually appear within 2 weeks of infection with the parasite and may include:

- Diarrhoea.
- Excessive flatulence and belching.
- Bloating and abdominal pain.
- Nausea.

If the symptoms last longer than a week, the infection may damage the lining of the small intestine, preventing the absorption of food and vitamins (*see* MALABSORPTION, p.655). This may result in weight loss and, in some cases, the blood disorder anaemia (p.446).

WHAT MIGHT BE DONE?

If your doctor suspects that you have giardiasis, you will probably be asked to provide a sample of faeces, which will be examined for the parasite cysts. If no parasites are found but your doctor still suspects you have the disease from your symptoms, he or she may recommend that you undergo upper digestive tract endoscopy (p.641) to examine the

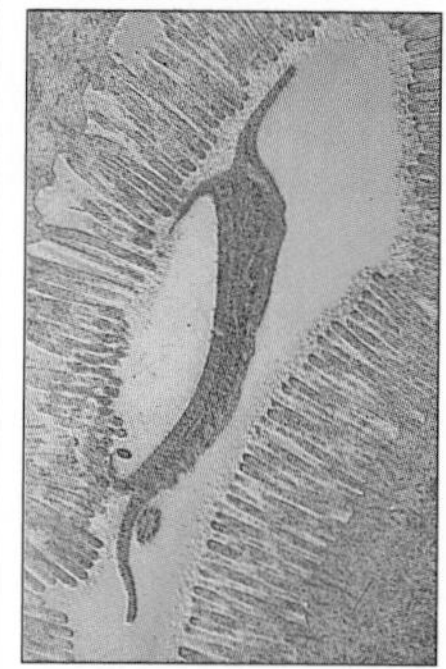

Parasite in body tissue *This highly magnified image shows the parasite* Giardia lamblia *in a sample of tissue taken from the small intestine of a person with giardiasis.*

inside of the small intestine. A sample of tissue or contents from the intestine may be removed during the procedure and examined under the microscope for evidence of infection. If giardiasis is diagnosed, your doctor will prescribe antibiotics (p.885), which usually kill the parasite in a few days. However, the infection may recur.

CAN IT BE PREVENTED?

If you are visiting a region where giardiasis occurs, you can prevent infection by boiling your drinking water for at least 10 minutes to kill the cysts. You should also follow strict standards of personal hygiene. Washing hands thoroughly after bowel movements and before preparing food should help to prevent the spread of the infection.

(WWW) ONLINE SITES: p.1033, p.1037

Cryptosporidiosis

An intestinal infection caused by a protozoal parasite, often leading to watery diarrhoea and fever

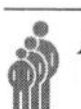 AGE More common in children

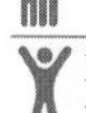 LIFESTYLE Poor personal hygiene is a risk factor

 GENDER GENETICS Not significant factors

Cryptosporidiosis is caused by a protozoal parasite known as *Cryptosporidium parvum.* It is an intestinal infection that is spread through contact with infected people or animals or by eating food or drinking water contaminated with the parasite. The disease occurs worldwide, but it is more common in developing countries because poor hygiene helps to spread infection. In developed countries, outbreaks may be due to contamination of reservoirs. Cryptosporidiosis is often severe in people with reduced immunity, such as those with AIDS (*see* HIV INFECTION AND AIDS, p.297). In the 1990s, the number of cases of diarrhoea caused by cryptosporidiosis increased, especially in children.

In some cases, there are no symptoms. In others, watery diarrhoea, abdominal pain, fever, nausea, and vomiting may develop a week after infection. The symptoms usually last 7–10 days. People with reduced immunity may have persistent symptoms and develop severe malnutrition and dehydration, which can be fatal.

WHAT MIGHT BE DONE?

Cryptosporidiosis is usually diagnosed by examining a sample of faeces under a microscope for the parasite. There is no effective treatment to cure this infection, but, if your symptoms are severe, you may need hospital treatment with intravenous fluids and antidiarrhoeal drugs (p.924). If a local outbreak of the disease occurs, you should boil all your drinking water to kill the parasite.

(WWW) ONLINE SITES: p.1033

Toxoplasmosis

A protozoal infection that can seriously affect fetuses and people who have reduced immunity

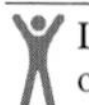 LIFESTYLE Contact with cats and eating raw or undercooked meat are risk factors

 AGE GENDER GENETICS Not significant factors

The protozoal infection toxoplasmosis is caused by *Toxoplasma gondii.* Cysts (dormant stages) of the parasite are excreted in the faeces of infected cats and can be passed to people by direct contact with cats or by handling cat litter. Another source of infection is the raw or undercooked meat of animals that have eaten food contaminated with cysts from the faeces of infected cats.

In most people, the infection does not cause symptoms because the cysts are dormant. However, people with reduced immunity, such as those with AIDS (*see* HIV INFECTION AND AIDS, p.297), may become seriously ill either from an initial infection or if dormant cysts are reactivated. If a woman develops toxoplasmosis while pregnant, the parasites may infect the fetus and cause abnormalities (*see* CONGENITAL INFECTIONS, p.817).

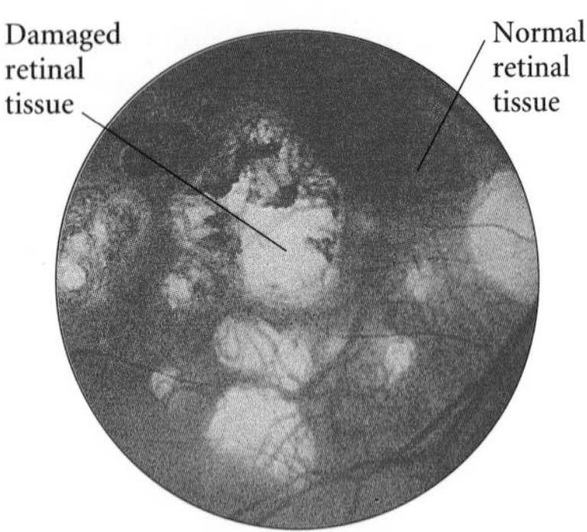

Toxoplasmosis affecting the retina
Areas of damage, caused by the protozoan Toxoplasma gondii, *are visible in this view of the retina as seen through an ophthalmoscope (a viewing instrument).*

WHAT ARE THE SYMPTOMS?

Most otherwise healthy people do not develop symptoms. However, in some, mild symptoms appear 1–3 weeks after the initial infection and include:

- Painless, enlarged lymph nodes, usually in the neck.
- Tiredness.
- Fever and headache.

The heart, muscles, skin, and eyes may become damaged by the infection, and, in people with reduced immunity, it may affect the brain. In such cases, the symptoms may develop suddenly or over several weeks and include:

- Fever and headache.
- Paralysis affecting a limb or one side of the body.
- Partial loss of vision.
- Confusion.
- Lethargy.

In some people with reduced immunity, toxoplasmosis causes seizures. If a fetus is infected, toxoplasmosis may damage the eyes and cause blindness.

WHAT MIGHT BE DONE?

Toxoplasmosis is diagnosed by microscopic examination of affected tissue or by blood tests. Usually, no treatment is necessary, although pyrimethamine (*see* ANTIMALARIAL DRUGS, p.888) and antibiotics (p.885) may be prescribed for people whose immunity is reduced or pregnant women. People with reduced immunity may need to take the drugs for life to prevent reactivation of cysts.

Infection can be prevented by avoiding contact with cats and by not eating undercooked or raw meat.

(WWW) ONLINE SITES: p.1033, p.1035

Pneumocystis infection

A parasitic infection that is a common cause of pneumonia in people with reduced immunity

 AGE GENDER GENETICS LIFESTYLE
Not significant factors

People with reduced immunity, such as those who have AIDS (*see* HIV INFECTION AND AIDS, p.297) or those receiving chemotherapy (p.280), may develop a form of pneumonia called pneumocystis infection, caused by inhaling the *Pneumocystis carinii* parasite. In people who have a healthy immune system, the parasite does not cause pneumonia. In developing countries, children who are malnourished often have the infection.

WHAT ARE THE SYMPTOMS?

The symptoms of pneumocystis infection generally develop gradually over weeks, but, in some people, they may develop quickly. Symptoms include:

- Tiredness.
- Feeling unwell.
- Fever.
- Dry cough.
- Shortness of breath on mild exertion.

As the infection progresses, shortness of breath may develop even at rest.

HOW IS IT DIAGNOSED?

Pneumocystis infection is diagnosed by a physical examination, a chest X-ray (p.490), or by examining a sample of sputum for the parasite. Sometimes, the parasite is hard to isolate. In such cases, a bronchoscopy (p.504) may be performed. In this procedure, secretions from the bronchi (the main airways of the lungs) and/or a piece of lung tissue are removed and examined for evidence of pneumocystis infection.

WHAT IS THE TREATMENT?

Pneumocystis pneumonia is treated with antibiotics (p.885), initially administered intravenously and then orally, for at least 3 weeks. Your doctor may also prescribe corticosteroids (p.930).

Once the infection has cleared up, you may need to continue taking low doses of antibiotics, depending on the cause of reduced immunity. People with AIDS may remain on antibiotics for life. Those receiving chemotherapy may need antibiotics until the therapy is finished.

WHAT IS THE PROGNOSIS?

Fewer than 1 in 10 cases of initial pneumocystis infection are fatal. However, without treatment with preventive antibiotics, the infection may recur. In the developed world, many people with HIV infection or AIDS are now treated for pneumocystis infection before their immunity is seriously impaired.

(WWW) ONLINE SITES: p.1033

Cryptococcosis

A rare fungal infection that most commonly affects the brain or lungs

 AGE GENDER GENETICS LIFESTYLE
Not significant factors

Cryptococcosis is caused by the fungus *Cryptococcus neoformans*, which occurs in soil contaminated by bird droppings. If the fungal spores are inhaled, infection may develop in the lungs and/or the fungus may be absorbed into the blood, spreading to other parts of the body, most commonly the brain, skin, and bones.

People whose immunity is reduced, such as those who have AIDS (*see* HIV INFECTION AND AIDS, p.297) or who are undergoing chemotherapy (p.280), are most at risk from cryptococcosis. The fungus rarely causes serious illness in people who are otherwise healthy.

In its most dangerous form, cryptococcosis can cause inflammation of the membranes covering the brain and spinal cord (*see* MENINGITIS, p.527). Symptoms may include fever, severe headache, and a stiff neck. Lung infections may result in chest pain, coughing, and shortness of breath. Infection of the skin may cause ulcers to develop. Affected bones may be painful.

WHAT MIGHT BE DONE?

A diagnosis of cryptococcosis is based on the presence of the fungus in blood, sputum, or body tissues. If meningitis is suspected, samples of fluid from the spine will be tested (*see* LUMBAR PUNCTURE, p.527). If the lungs have been affected, the levels of oxygen and other gases in the blood may be measured to assess lung function (*see* MEASURING BLOOD GASES, p.501).

For severe cryptococcal infections, antifungal drugs (p.889) are given and in some cases need to be administered intravenously. In people with AIDS, it can be difficult to eradicate the fungus from the body, although the symptoms can often be well controlled. A mild lung infection in a person whose general health is normally good should clear up without treatment.

(WWW) ONLINE SITES: p.1033

Aspergillosis

A fungal infection that can affect the lungs and spread to other organs

AGE GENDER GENETICS LIFESTYLE Not significant factors

Aspergillosis is caused by spores of the aspergillus fungus, which occur in dust, soil, and decaying plants. The spores are harmless if a healthy person inhales them. However, the fungus can cause lung disease and other serious illnesses in people who are vulnerable to infection because of particular sensitivity, pre-existing lung damage, or reduced function of the immune system.

WHAT ARE THE TYPES?

There are three forms of aspergillosis. In some people, a sensitivity to the fungus eventually develops into a disorder known as allergic bronchopulmonary aspergillosis, the symptoms of which are similar to those of asthma (p.483).

In people who already have damaged lungs as a result of a long-term disease, such as tuberculosis (p.491) or bronchiectasis (p.496), the fungi spores may become lodged in cavities in the lung tissue caused by the disease. Eventually, the spores grow into masses known as "fungus balls". This condition usually causes a cough that may be accompanied by bloody sputum.

The fungus can also cause a serious infection of the lungs in people whose immune systems are suppressed, such as those with AIDS (*see* HIV INFECTION AND AIDS, p.297) or those receiving chemotherapy (p.280). The result of this infection is a pneumonia-like illness. In severe cases, the infection may spread to other body organs, including the heart, brain, and kidneys.

WHAT MIGHT BE DONE?

Aspergillosis is diagnosed by examining a sample of sputum under a microscope to look for the fungus or by a blood test for antibodies. A chest X-ray

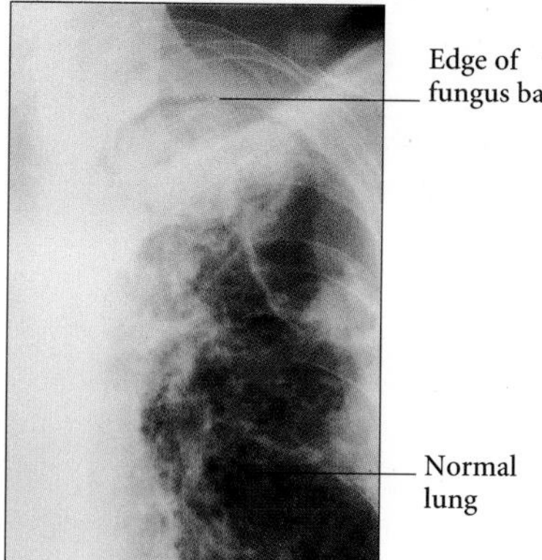

Aspergillosis in the lungs
In this X-ray, an aspergillus fungus ball can be seen. The fungus ball has formed in a cavity in the top of the lung.

(p.490) may also be carried out. Treatment usually involves antifungal drugs (p.889). It may be necessary to remove a fungus ball surgically. Aspergillosis is sometimes fatal in people who have impaired immunity.

(WWW) ONLINE SITES: p.1033, p.1034, p.1036

Sporotrichosis

A fungal infection that usually affects only the skin but sometimes spreads to other parts of the body

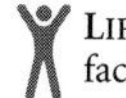
LIFESTYLE Working with plants is a risk factor

AGE GENDER GENETICS Not significant factors

The fungus that causes sporotrichosis, *Sporothrix schenkii*, normally grows on plants, especially moss and tree bark. Florists and gardeners are at particular risk of infection, which usually occurs when the fungus enters the skin, for example through injury with a thorn.

If a wound has become infected with the fungus, a reddened, painless lump usually develops 1–3 months later. The infection may spread, producing small lumps beneath the skin around the wound. In people with reduced immunity, such as those with AIDS (*see* HIV INFECTION AND AIDS, p.297) or people who are taking immunosuppressant drugs (p.906), the fungus may spread to other parts of the body, including the lungs and joints.

Diagnosis is usually obvious from the appearance of lumps below the skin and can be confirmed by a skin biopsy (p.344), in which a small sample of affected skin is removed for examination. In some cases, the infection clears up spontaneously. In otherwise healthy people, sporotrichosis is usually treated with antifungal drugs (p.889). If the infection is widespread in people with reduced immunity, long-term treatment with antifungal drugs may be necessary. In such cases, the disease can be difficult to eradicate.

(WWW) ONLINE SITES: p.1033

Candidiasis

A fungal yeast infection that usually affects only one part of the body but can be serious if it spreads around the body

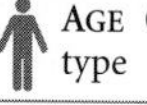
LIFESTYLE Using intravenous drugs is a risk factor

AGE GENDER Risk factors depend on the type

GENETICS Not a significant factor

In healthy people, the yeast *Candida albicans* normally exists on the surface of certain moist areas of the body, including the mouth, throat, and vagina. Sometimes, the fungus overgrows in localized areas, causing minor forms of candidiasis such as oral thrush (p.862) and vaginal thrush (p.752). However, in people who have reduced immunity, such as those with AIDS (*see* HIV INFECTION AND AIDS, p.297) or diabetes mellitus (p.687), the fungus sometimes spreads into the blood and other tissues. Infection that spreads throughout the body may also occur in people who have long-term urinary catheters or intravenous catheters, or people who have had prolonged courses of antibiotics or use intravenous drugs.

Widespread candidiasis can be diagnosed by culturing the fungus from a sample of blood or other body fluid or tissue specimens. A chest X-ray (p.490) may also be carried out to look for signs of infection in the lungs. Treatment consists of antifungal drugs (p.889), which may be given either orally or intravenously, depending on the severity of the infection. Untreated, candidiasis can spread throughout the body and may eventually be fatal. The outlook depends on the extent of infection and on the person's general health.

(WWW) ONLINE SITES: p.1033, p.1037

WORM INFESTATIONS

Most animals, including humans, can be infested with parasitic worms that derive all their nutrients from their hosts. Most of these worms live in the intestines for at least part of their life cycle. In many cases, worm infestations are long-term diseases that produce few symptoms in their early stages.

Various types of the family of worms known as roundworms can infest humans. Most affect only people in the developing world. However, some roundworms, such as threadworm, commonly affect people in developed countries. The first five articles in this section describe several types of roundworm infestation: threadworm infestation, toxocariasis, ascariasis, hookworm infestation, and tropical worm infestations, such as filariasis.

Infestations in humans that are caused by other types of worms known as flatworms, which include tapeworms and flukes, are covered in the last three articles on schistosomiasis, tapeworm infestation, and hydatid disease.

It is possible to acquire a tropical worm infestation abroad but not to experience symptoms until some months later. If you become ill after visiting the tropics, you should visit a doctor familiar with tropical diseases.

KEY ANATOMY

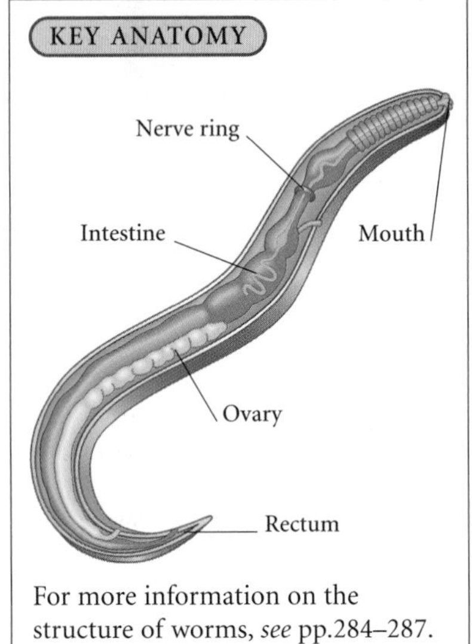

For more information on the structure of worms, *see* pp.284–287.

Threadworm infestation

An infestation of thin worms that lay eggs around the anus, causing intense itching

 AGE More common in children

 LIFESTYLE Poor sanitation and inadequate personal hygiene are risk factors

 GENDER GENETICS Not significant factors

Threadworm infestation is caused by the roundworm *Enterobius vermicularis* and is the most common parasitic worm infestation affecting humans in the UK. Usually, infestation occurs by ingesting worm eggs in contaminated food, on fingers, or in house dust. If they are swallowed, the eggs develop into adult threadworms in the intestine. At night, female threadworms crawl out of the anus to lay eggs around the anal region, causing intense itching. Threadworm infestation mainly affects children.

WHAT ARE THE SYMPTOMS?

In most cases, the symptoms of threadworm infestation include:

- Intense itching in the anal region at night when the worms lay eggs.
- Inflammation of the anus as a result of constant scratching.
- In some cases, mild abdominal pain.

Sometimes, tiny, white threadworms can be seen wriggling in the faeces after a bowel movement. In rare cases, infestation causes appendicitis (p.664).

WHAT MIGHT BE DONE?

The diagnosis can be confirmed by identification of threadworm eggs in a swab taken from the anal region. Your doctor will probably prescribe a single dose of an anthelmintic drug (p.889) to kill the worms effectively and speed recovery. Usually, the entire household is treated, and treatment is repeated after 2 weeks. Reinfection is common because the eggs can be picked up under the fingernails when scratching and accidentally swallowed. The cycle of infestation then begins again. Underwear, nightwear, and bedlinen may also be contaminated.

Threadworm infestation is usually easy to control. The risk of reinfection is reduced by scrupulous attention to personal hygiene: washing hands after going to the toilet, avoiding scratching the anal area, and washing clothes and bedlinen regularly.

(WWW) ONLINE SITES: p.1028, p.1033

Threadworm egg Larva inside egg

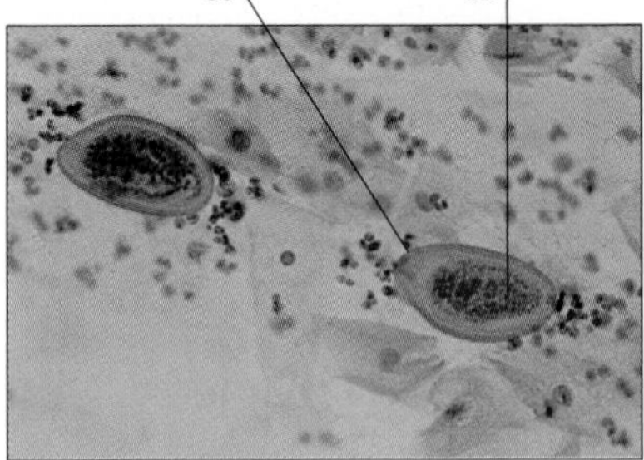

Threadworm eggs
Threadworms infest the intestine and emerge from the anus at night to lay eggs in the anal region, causing itching. Larvae can be seen inside the magnified eggs above.

Toxocariasis

The infestation of various organs with roundworm larvae, which may cause fever

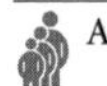 AGE More common in children

 LIFESTYLE Owning pet dogs or cats may be a risk factor

 GENDER GENETICS Not significant factors

The adult forms of the roundworms *Toxocara canis* and *Toxocara cati* normally infest dogs and cats, which excrete faeces containing worm eggs. However, the larvae (immature forms) of the worms can infest humans, usually as a result of ingestion of soil contaminated with worm eggs. Children are particularly susceptible because they are more likely to play in soil and then put their fingers in their mouths.

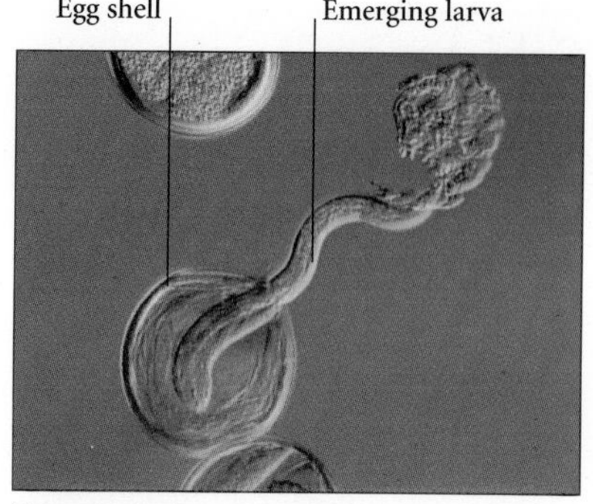

Toxocariasis
A larva (immature form) of the worm that causes the disease toxocariasis can be seen in this highly magnified image. The larva has just hatched from the egg.

Once the eggs have been swallowed, they hatch in the intestine into tiny larvae, which may then migrate to other parts of the body, including the lungs and liver. In rare cases, the larvae can migrate to the eyes and the brain.

What are the symptoms?

In most cases of toxocariasis, symptoms do not develop. However, in some cases, symptoms may include:

- Mild fever.
- Feeling unwell.

A heavy infestation of the larvae in the lungs may cause wheezing and a dry cough. If larvae reach the brain, they may cause epilepsy (p.524), and infestation of the eyes may damage the retina (the light-sensitive membrane at the back of the eye), causing blindness that is likely to be permanent (p.591).

What might be done?

If your doctor suspects that you or your child has toxocariasis, he or she may arrange for a blood test to confirm the diagnosis. Most people recover completely from the infestation without needing treatment. However, your doctor may prescribe an anthelmintic drug (p.889) to kill the worms. In severe cases in which the brain is affected, anticonvulsant drugs (p.914) will probably be given. Brain or eye damage due to toxocariasis is usually permanent.

It is important to deworm pets regulary to prevent toxocariasis, and dogs or cats should be prevented from defaecating in places where children are likely to play, such as in a sandpit.

(WWW) ONLINE SITES: p.1033

Ascariasis

An intestinal roundworm infestation that may cause diarrhoea and abdominal pain

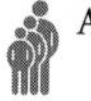 AGE More common in children

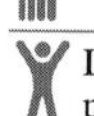 LIFESTYLE Poor sanitation and inadequate personal hygiene are risk factors

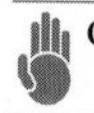 GENDER GENETICS Not significant factors

The roundworm *Ascaris lumbricoides* is responsible for ascariasis, one of the most common parasitic infestations of humans. About 1 in 4 people in the world has ascariasis at some time in his or her life. The disease is most common in tropical and subtropical areas, and children are affected more often than adults. Ascariasis is rare in developed countries such as the UK.

People usually become infested with roundworms by eating food or drinking water contaminated with the worm eggs. Poor sanitation, the use of human excrement as fertilizer and inadequate personal hygiene all contribute to the spread of ascariasis among humans. Once swallowed, the worm eggs hatch into larvae in the intestine. The larvae then travel in the blood to the lungs and later return to the intestine, where they develop into adults, breed, and lay eggs.

What are the symptoms?

In most cases, ascariasis does not cause symptoms. However, in large numbers, the roundworms may cause:

- Diarrhoea.
- Abdominal pain.

Worm larvae in the lungs may cause wheezing and coughing. A large number of worms in the intestine may cause appendicitis (p.664) or a blockage (*see* INTESTINAL OBSTRUCTION, p.663).

What might be done?

Ascariasis is usually diagnosed by identification of the worm eggs in a sample of faeces or of the worm itself, which is pale pink and has a long cylindrical body approximately 20–30 cm (8–12 in) in length. In most people, treatment consists of taking a single dose of an anthelmintic drug (p.889) to kill the worms. However, the infestation will recur if roundworm eggs are swallowed again after treatment.

(WWW) ONLINE SITES: p.1033

Hookworm infestation

An infestation of small, blood-sucking roundworms that may cause abdominal pain, cough, and fever

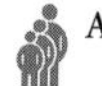 AGE More common in children

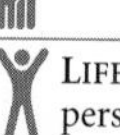 LIFESTYLE Poor sanitation and inadequate personal hygiene are risk factors

 GENDER GENETICS Not significant factors

The two main species of hookworms that can infest humans are *Ancylostoma duodenale* and *Necator americanus*. People are usually infested by direct contact with hookworm larvae (immature forms of the worm), which live in soil and can penetrate human skin. The larvae travel in the blood to the lungs and trachea (windpipe) and then to the intestines, where they develop into adult worms that can reach up to 1 cm (½ in) in length. The adults attach to the intestinal wall with hook-like teeth and feed by sucking blood from the wall. The female worms lay eggs, which pass out in the faeces of an affected person and develop into larvae in the soil.

Poor sanitation, inadequate personal hygiene, and the use of human faeces as fertilizer may increase the spread of the disorder. Hookworm is very common in tropical areas, affecting up to 1 in 2 people, especially children, at any one time. In the UK, people with hookworm have almost always acquired the infestation abroad through walking barefoot in water contaminated by sewage.

What are the symptoms?

In the early stages of hookworm infestation, the only symptom may be an itchy rash at the site where the larvae have pierced the skin. As the infestation progresses, symptoms may include:

- Dry cough and mild fever due to the presence of larvae in the lungs.

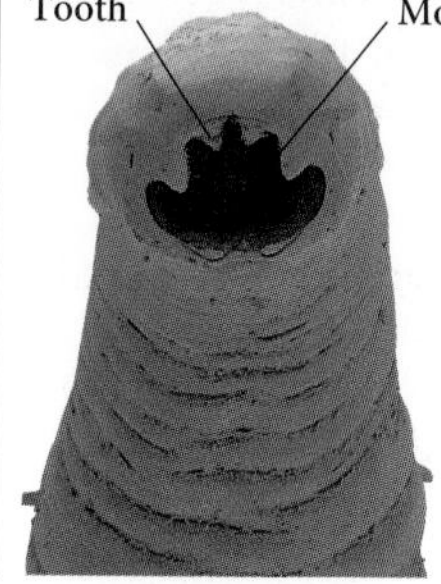

Hookworm
This magnified image shows the mouth of a hookworm. The "teeth" attach the worm to the wall of the intestine.

- Abdominal pain due to the presence of worms in the intestines.

Left untreated, large numbers of worms in the intestines may cause gradual, heavy blood loss, which may lead to iron-deficiency anaemia (p.447). If the anaemia is severe, it may cause chronic heart failure (p.413).

WHAT MIGHT BE DONE?

Your doctor will arrange for a sample of faeces to be examined for worm eggs if he or she suspects hookworm infestation. You will be given anthelmintic drugs (p.889) to kill the worms and, if anaemia has developed, iron supplements. Rarely, if the anaemia is severe, a blood transfusion (p.447) is necessary.

In order to prevent hookworm infestation when travelling in tropical and subtropical regions, you should wear waterproof shoes in villages and other populated areas if the ground is wet.

(WWW) ONLINE SITES: p.1033

Tropical worm infestations

Diseases caused by parasitic roundworms that are widespread in tropical regions

LIFESTYLE Poor sanitation and inadequate personal hygiene are risk factors

AGE Risk factors depend on the type

GENDER GENETICS Not significant factors

Parasitic worms that infest humans are most common in tropical and subtropical regions. Both poor sanitation and poor personal hygiene contribute to the spread of parasites among people, especially children. In the UK, tropical worm infestations are very rare and usually occur only in people who have visited or lived in the tropics.

WHAT ARE THE TYPES?

There are four main types of roundworm infestation that normally affect only people in tropical and subtropical regions, such as Central and South America, Africa, and Southeast Asia.

TRICHINOSIS This disease is caused by a tiny worm called *Trichinella spiralis*. People usually become infested by eating undercooked pork containing cysts (larval stages of the worm). In severe cases, symptoms may include vomiting, diarrhoea, abdominal and muscle pains, and fever. In some cases, trichinosis can cause acute heart failure (p.412) or an illness similar to meningitis (p.527).

STRONGYLOIDIASIS The minute worm *Strongyloides stercoralis* causes this condition. Infestation is usually a result of walking barefoot on soil contaminated with larvae. If severe, infestation may result in abdominal pain and diarrhoea between periods of constipation and weight loss. Infestations may be present for years without causing symptoms, but symptoms will appear if immunity becomes reduced due to conditions such as HIV infection (*see* HIV INFECTION AND AIDS, p.297).

FILARIASIS Various types of worm or their larvae cause filariasis. The parasites are transmitted to people by certain bloodsucking insects. Different parts of the body are affected, depending on the type of worm. A severe infestation with some types may lead to a massive, painful, disfiguring swelling in the limbs or in the scrotum known as elephantiasis. Infestation with a type of worm known as *Onchocerca volvulus* sometimes results in blindness.

TRICHURIASIS This infestation is due to *Trichuris trichuria*, also known as whipworm, and it is most common in children. People become infested when they ingest worm eggs. Adult worms live in the intestines, and a severe case of trichuriasis may cause bloody diarrhoea, abdominal pain, and weight loss.

WHAT MIGHT BE DONE?

The diagnosis depends on the type of worm but is usually confirmed when eggs, larvae, or adult worms are found in a sample of faeces, blood, or tissue. Treatment also varies with the infestation, but anthelmintic drugs (p.889) are commonly prescribed. Most people make a full recovery if treated early, but reinfection is common in tropical countries. Preventive measures include not walking barefoot on soil, not eating undercooked meat or other foods that may be contaminated, and using insect repellents and mosquito nets.

(WWW) ONLINE SITES: p.1033

Schistosomiasis

An infestation of flukes that can damage the liver and bladder

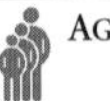
AGE More common in children

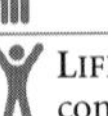
LIFESTYLE Swimming in fresh water containing infested snails is a risk factor

GENDER GENETICS Not significant factors

People who bathe in lakes, canals, or unchlorinated freshwater pools in the tropics are at risk of schistosomiasis, also known as bilharzia. The disease is caused by any of five species of fluke (types of flatworm) of the schistosoma group. Freshwater snails release larvae (immature forms) of the parasite, which can penetrate the skin of bathers. Once inside the body, the parasites mature into adults, and the females lay eggs, which may cause inflammation. Schistosomiasis affects about 200 million people worldwide, mainly in developing countries. People in the UK become infested only when visiting tropical regions.

WHAT ARE THE SYMPTOMS?

The symptoms of schistosomiasis vary depending on the species of fluke. Most people experience itching (known as "swimmer's itch") at the site where the parasite has entered the skin. The itching usually occurs within a day of exposure to the parasite. Some people may have no further symptoms, whereas others may develop them within 4–6 weeks. Symptoms may include:

- Fever.
- Muscle pains.
- Diarrhoea.
- Coughing and vomiting.
- Passing urine more frequently, with a burning sensation.

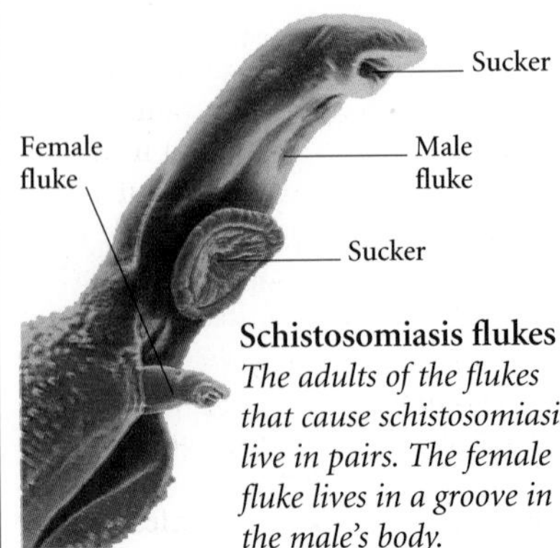

Schistosomiasis flukes
The adults of the flukes that cause schistosomiasis live in pairs. The female fluke lives in a groove in the male's body.

- Blood in the urine, especially at the end of the stream.

Without treatment, schistosomiasis may damage the liver or the urinary system. In many cases, this damage is life-threatening. A long-standing, untreated infestation may cause colorectal cancer (p.665) and bladder tumours (p.715).

WHAT MIGHT BE DONE?

Schistosomiasis is usually diagnosed by finding fluke eggs in a sample of either urine or faeces. Sometimes, the condition is diagnosed by a rectal biopsy, in which a sample of tissue is taken from the rectum and examined under a microscope for eggs. The biopsy is usually accompanied by a blood test to look for antibodies that the body produces against the parasite. In nearly all cases, the infestation is treated with an anthelmintic drug (p.889), which is usually effective in killing the worms. Schistosomiasis can be prevented by not swimming or wading in fresh water in the regions of the world where the infestation is known to occur.

(WWW) ONLINE SITES: p.1033

Tapeworm infestation

An intestinal infestation of ribbon-shaped parasitic flatworms that may cause abdominal pain and diarrhoea

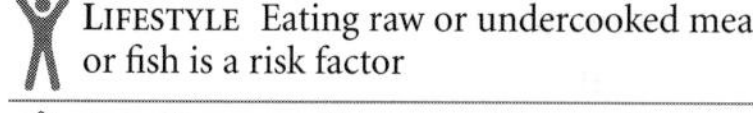
LIFESTYLE Eating raw or undercooked meat or fish is a risk factor

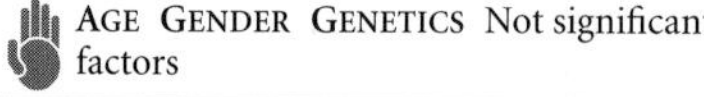
AGE GENDER GENETICS Not significant factors

Three types of large, adult tapeworms infest humans. These worms are the pork tapeworm (*Taenia solium*), the beef tapeworm (*Taenia saginata*), and the fish tapeworm (*Diphyllobothrium latum*). Infestation usually occurs by eating raw or undercooked meat or fish that contains larvae (immature stages of the worms). Once in the intestines, the worms mature into adults, which may reach 6–9 m (20–30 ft) in length. Tapeworm eggs are passed out in the faeces and, in the case of pork tapeworm, may cause reinfection. Certain other species of tapeworm may live as slow-growing larval cysts in humans (*see* HYDATID DISEASE, right).

Pork and beef tapeworm infestations occur most commonly in developing countries. Fish tapeworm infestation is most common in regions where raw fish dishes, such as sushi, are popular. These regions include Eastern Europe, Scandinavia, and Japan.

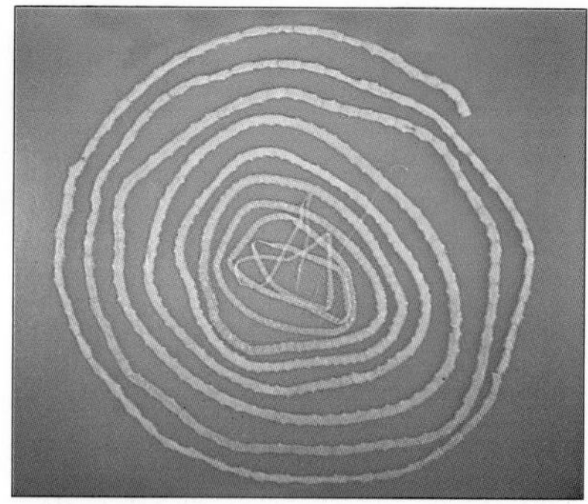

Tapeworm
This coiled beef tapeworm was removed from a human intestine, where it had grown to several metres in length.

WHAT ARE THE SYMPTOMS?

In many people, a tapeworm infestation does not produce any symptoms. However, you may experience:

- Mild abdominal pain.
- Diarrhoea.
- In beef and pork tapeworm infestations, an increase in appetite.

If you are infested with beef tapeworm, you may feel segments of the worm wriggling out of your anus. Rarely, fish tapeworms may cause the blood disorder megaloblastic anaemia (p.448).

A disorder called cysticercosis may develop if pork tapeworm eggs enter the stomach, either in food contaminated with eggs or if an adult worm in the intestine lays eggs that then travel to the stomach. Larvae hatch from the eggs and migrate to the intestine. They burrow through the intestinal wall and travel around the body in the blood. Epilepsy (p.524) may result if larvae reach the brain, and, if they infest the eyes, they may cause blindness (p.591).

WHAT MIGHT BE DONE?

A diagnosis is made if tapeworm segments or eggs are present in the faeces. To kill the worms, a single dose of an anthelmintic drug (p.889) is prescribed. Tapeworm infestation can be prevented by freezing or cooking meat and fish thoroughly. To prevent reinfection and cysticercosis, wash your hands carefully after a bowel movement.

(WWW) ONLINE SITES: p.1033

Hydatid disease

A rare infestation of tapeworm cysts that may affect the liver, lungs, or bones

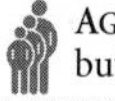
AGE Infestation usually occurs in children but normally becomes apparent in adults

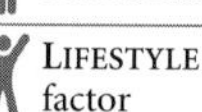
LIFESTYLE Owning pet dogs may be a risk factor

GENDER GENETICS Not significant factors

Infestation with cysts that contain the larvae (immature stages) of the tapeworm *Echinococcus granulosus* is called hydatid disease. The cyst stage of the worm normally affects livestock such as sheep. If a dog eats raw offal containing a cyst, the larvae mature into egg-laying adults in the dog's intestines. Worm eggs pass out in the dog's faeces and can be transmitted to humans who eat food that is contaminated with eggs. The eggs hatch into larvae when they reach the human intestine. The larvae then move to the liver, lungs, or bones, where they develop into slow-growing cysts up to 20 cm (8 in) in diameter.

Hydatid disease occurs most commonly in sheep-farming regions where sheepdogs are used, such as Australia, New Zealand, and, to a lesser extent, the UK. The infestation also occurs in Middle Eastern countries.

WHAT ARE THE SYMPTOMS?

Infestation mainly occurs in childhood, but symptoms may not develop until adulthood because the hydatid cysts are so slow-growing. In many cases, there are no symptoms. However, a hydatid cyst in the liver may cause:

- Pain.
- Nausea.
- Yellowing of the skin and whites of the eyes (*see* JAUNDICE, p.643).

A cyst in the lungs may lead to chest pain and coughing, and a cyst in bone may cause pain and fractures (p.392) in the long bones of the limbs.

WHAT MIGHT BE DONE?

Diagnosis is made from the symptoms and by ultrasound scanning (p.250) or X-rays (p.244). The larvae can be killed by an anthelmintic drug (p.889), but cysts must be surgically removed. The spread of hydatid disease can be stopped by controlling and deworming dogs.

(WWW) ONLINE SITES: p.1033

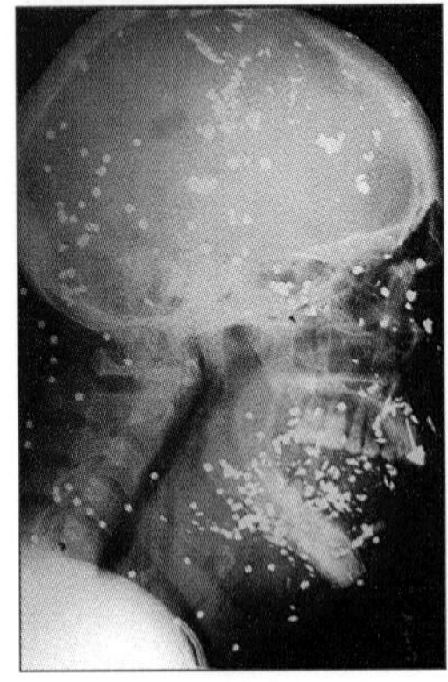

Shotgun injuries
This X-ray of a skull and neck shows multiple injuries that have been caused by the pellets from a shotgun.

Serious Injuries and Environmental Disorders

Most people know somebody who has experienced a potentially fatal injury or accident, even if they have not been involved in one themselves. Susceptibility to injury is linked to lifestyle, environment, and gender, with more than twice as many men as women sustaining a life-threatening injury. Age is also an important factor, and statistics show that most injuries and accidents tend to happen in adolescence and early adulthood.

By the end of 1990s, there were about 16,000 deaths each year due to injury or poisoning in the UK, at least 10,000 of which were accidental.

One of the most common causes of fatal serious injuries is road traffic accidents. In 1998, almost 4,000 people in the UK were killed on the roads and a further 45,000 were seriously injured.

Poisoning, either due to a deliberate drug overdose or accidental ingestion, is the cause of about 2,000 deaths each year in the UK. About 50,000 people are treated in hospital as a result of poisoning. In adults, poisoning is most often due to a drug overdose. However, most nonfatal accidental poisonings occur in children under the age of 5. Burns cause about 250 deaths in the UK each year and 130,000 people need treatment in hospital. The very young and the elderly are most likely to be seriously injured as a result of burns.

Illness and injury that result from environmental factors, such as altitude and low temperatures, are becoming more common, particularly in young adults. Disorders such as frostbite, hypothermia, and altitude sickness can occur when young people take risks on holidays in remote areas with extreme climates. Hypothermia is a particular threat to elderly people, even at home. This is because the body's ability to regulate body temperature becomes less effective with old age. However, the most common cause of fatal injury in elderly people is a fall, which often results in one or more bone fractures. More than 1,700 elderly people die each year in England and Wales as the result of falls.

Some accident statistics indicate improving trends. For example, vehicle safety features are improving survival rates for traffic accidents. The medical management of serious injuries has also improved. Paramedics can now provide resuscitation at the scene of accidents, patients are taken to hospital more quickly, accident departments are better staffed, and intensive care units have more effective procedures for dealing with multiple injuries and shock. In addition, trauma centres have been established that specialize in treating patients who are seriously ill.

DATA Accidental Deaths at Different Ages

In England and Wales, most accidental deaths occur between late adolescence and middle age. In most age groups except the elderly, accidents are a more frequent cause of death in males than in females. However, over the age of 75 there are many more women in the population than men, and this accounts for the greater number of accidental deaths in elderly women.

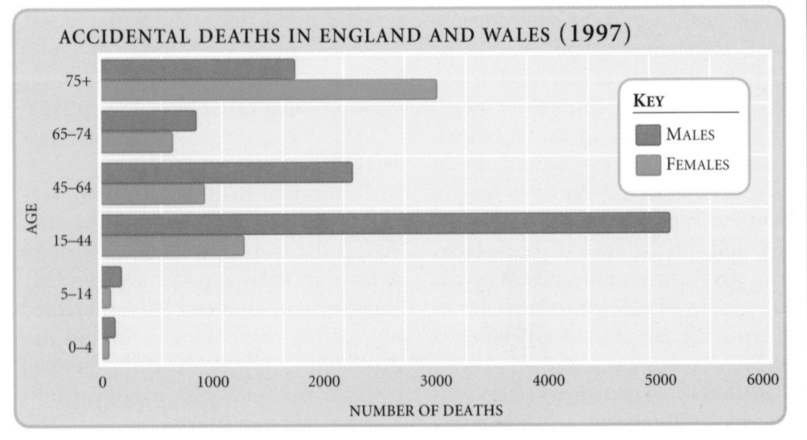

Accidental deaths in men and women
Most deaths due to accidents occur between the ages of 15 and 44. In 1997 more than 5,000 men and 1,000 women in this age range died as a result of accidents.

DATA SERIOUS INJURIES TO THE BODY

The nature and location of an injury determines its severity. For example, crush injuries to the torso tend to be more serious than those to the limbs because they may damage internal organs. The severity of gunshot and stab injuries depends on the precise location of the wounds and whether major organs or blood vessels are involved. Poisoning and drowning usually affect entire systems and may damage several vital organs.

Blood clot

Distorted brain tissue

Bullet

Bleeding inside the skull
A single gunshot to the head has caused a blood clot to form just inside the skull, as shown on this CT scan. The brain tissue is swollen and distorted.

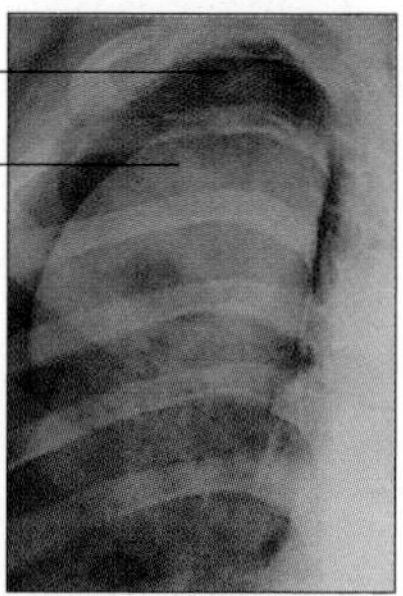

Collapsed lung
This X-ray shows air between the lung and the chest wall following an injury. The lung has collapsed.

Brain
The brain may be damaged when a blow to the head causes internal bleeding and swelling

Skull
The skull is susceptible to fractures. Bone fragments may damage the brain beneath

Trachea (windpipe)
If the trachea is crushed or obstructed by a foreign body, asphyxia (a potentially fatal lack of oxygen) may result

Lung
A lung may collapse following a penetrating wound or become inflamed by inhaled gases or smoke in an accident or fire

Heart
The heart may be directly damaged by physical injuries, such as a stab wound, or its function may be impaired by toxic substances in a drug overdose

Spleen
The spleen may rupture when crushed or following a severe blow to the abdomen, resulting in severe internal bleeding

Liver
When the liver is injured by a cut or a blow, a large amount of blood may be lost. Drug overdoses may also damage the liver

Spine
If the spine is injured, the vertebrae may be fractured or displaced and damage the spinal cord, causing paralysis or death

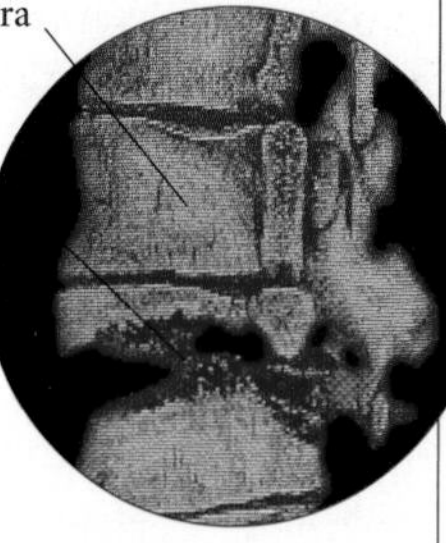

Fractured vertebra
This 3D CT scan shows a fractured vertebra in side view. Part of the bone is displaced.

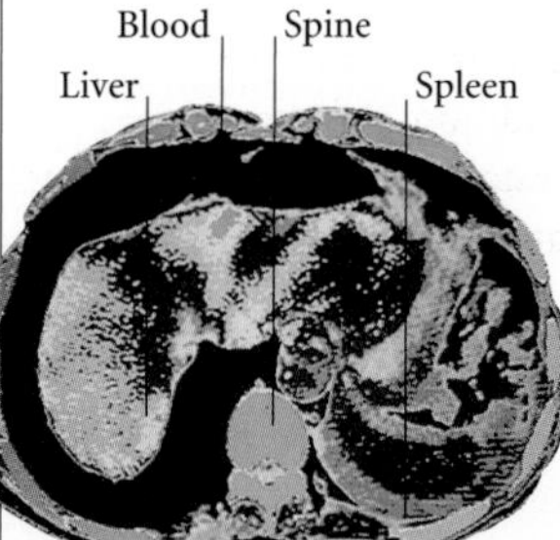

Ruptured spleen
The spleen and liver on this CT scan are surrounded by blood. The bleeding is from the spleen, which has been ruptured by a severe blow.

Hand
The hands are vulnerable to injury. In an accident, fingers may be severed, or the skin and tendons may be damaged

Kidney
A lacerated kidney may leak urine into the surrounding tissue, which causes inflammation. An injury that tears the kidney from its blood supply causes profuse bleeding

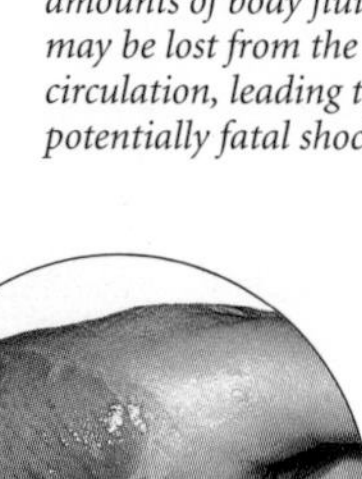

Skin
The skin's protective layer may be damaged by a burn. Large amounts of body fluid may be lost from the circulation, leading to potentially fatal shock

Intestines
If the intestinal wall is damaged, the contents may leak into the abdomen, causing serious infection

Artery
Bleeding from a severed artery is profuse and life-threatening

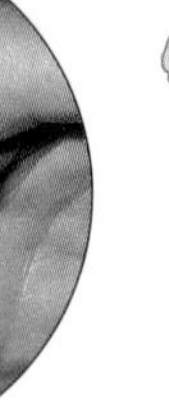

Toes
Toes may be crushed or severed by heavy objects. Severe frostbite of the toes may lead to gangrene

Severe burn
Here, the inside of the wrist has been badly burned. The overlying skin has been lost, leaving a red, raw area.

Neck of femur

Hip joint

Fracture in pelvis

Fractured pelvis
A pelvic fracture can be clearly seen in the X-ray. This type of injury may be caused by a fall.

SERIOUS INJURIES

Injuries can affect any part of the body, but they are most often serious if they affect the head, chest, or abdomen. Such injuries may be the result of an accident or a deliberate act of violence by another person. In addition to their physical impact, serious injuries may have long-term psychological and emotional effects.

The first half of this section covers serious injuries that usually have an accidental cause. Crush injuries, which are the most common form of serious injury, often result from a road traffic accident. The number of deaths from traffic accidents has fallen in recent years, mainly as a result of improved design of cars and other factors such as drink–drive laws. However, every day 10 people are killed on the roads in the UK. The next two articles discuss burns and electrical injuries. Burns are extremely common and may result from a wide variety of accidents. Most burns are due to minor accidents and occur around the home. Severe burns often occur in industrial environments and may result in permanent scarring or even death. Electrical injuries are a specific form of burn injury, often causing damage to internal tissues that may not be initially apparent. Such injuries may occur in the home but are often a result of an accident in the electrical or construction industries.

The next two articles cover injuries that are usually associated with crime: stab and gunshot injuries. In the UK, the number of injuries due to the use of guns has risen in recent years, but these are still relatively uncommon. The final article discusses sexual assault, which is regarded as one of the most complex serious injuries. Sexual assault may involve severe physical injuries, and it may take a victim many years to recover from the emotional trauma.

Injuries that are specific to one area of the body are covered elsewhere (*see* HEAD INJURIES, p.521, SPINAL INJURIES, p.524, MUSCULOSKELETAL INJURIES, pp.391–395, and EYE INJURIES, p.582).

Crush injuries

Injury to any part of the body caused by compression, most frequently as a result of a road traffic accident

 GENDER More common in males

 LIFESTYLE Risk factors depend on the cause

 AGE GENETICS Not significant factors

Crush injuries are most often caused by road traffic accidents, which account for nearly 4,000 deaths in the UK each year. Accidents that occur in the construction industry and explosions can also cause crush injuries to any part of the body. This type of injury may range in severity from simple bruising to life-threatening damage to internal organs and tissues. Men are at greater risk of sustaining crush injuries because they are more likely to work in the construction industry and engage in high-risk activities.

WHAT ARE THE TYPES?

Most damage sustained by crushing is internal, and often the only obvious external evidence is bruising. Fractures (p.392) are common, especially to the limbs, and, if the chest is crushed, one or more ribs are likely to be broken and may puncture the lungs. Multiple rib fractures may result in a flail chest, in which breathing may become sufficiently impaired to cause respiratory failure (p.507) and shock (p.414). Crush injuries may lead to a pneumothorax (p.496), in which air is trapped between the two-layered membrane covering the lungs. Damage to the heart can also occur.

If the abdomen has been crushed, the intestines, liver, spleen, or kidneys may be damaged. The contents of a ruptured intestine may leak out into the abdominal cavity and cause an infection (*see* PERITONITIS, p.665). If the spleen or the liver is ruptured, massive internal bleeding may occur.

In addition to specific injuries, more general complications may develop. For example, if a large proportion of the body's tissues is compressed, chemicals released from the damaged tissue may impair kidney function (*see* KIDNEY FAILURE, p.705), which may be fatal.

WHAT MIGHT BE DONE?

Anyone with a suspected crush injury should be freed as soon as possible and receive emergency first aid (*see* FIRST AID: ABC OF RESUSCITATION, p.978). If possible, call an ambulance while first aid is being performed. Once the person reaches hospital, treatment depends on the injuries sustained. General measures include emergency resuscitation and giving oxygen and intravenous fluids. Painkillers (p.912) are given as needed. If bleeding is excessive, a blood transfusion (p.447) may be necessary.

After emergency measures have been carried out, internal damage is assessed using imaging techniques, such as chest X-rays (p.490), CT scanning (p.247), and MRI (p.248). Treatment is then directed at specific injuries. Fractures are treated by resetting the broken bones in their correct position and immobilizing the affected part if needed (*see* FRACTURE TREATMENTS, p.393). If limbs have been crushed, surgery may be done to repair blood vessels and nerves (*see* MICROSURGERY, p.950). Amputation may be necessary if limb damage is irreparable. A person with rib fractures may need

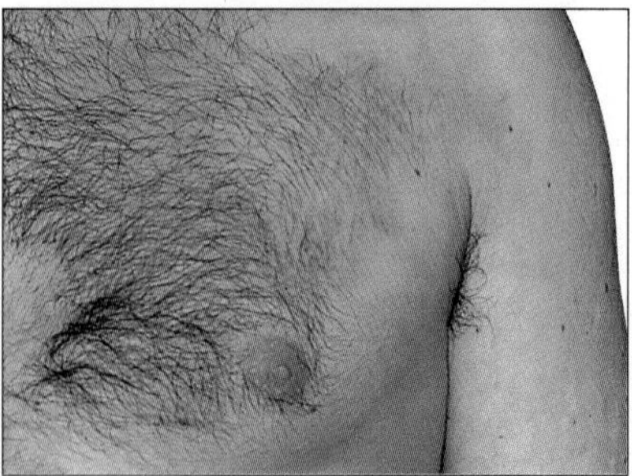

Crush injury
Skin bruising may be the only visible sign of a crush injury. This bruise is due to a seat belt pressing across the chest.

mechanical ventilation to assist breathing (*see* INTENSIVE CARE UNIT, p.958).

If internal bleeding into the abdominal cavity is suspected, a procedure called peritoneal lavage may be carried out, in which a small tube is inserted into the abdominal cavity, and sterile fluid is introduced into the abdomen. This fluid is then withdrawn, and, if it contains blood, surgery is performed to look for and repair the source of bleeding (*see* ENDOSCOPIC SURGERY, p.948).

Antibiotics (p.885) are prescribed to treat peritonitis and other infections. Additional complications, such as kidney failure, are treated as they arise.

The outlook depends on the type of crush injury, the length of time that the person was crushed, and the speed with which treatment was initiated.

(WWW) ONLINE SITES: p.1036

Burns

Areas of damage to tissue, usually skin, caused by heat, chemicals, or electricity

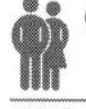

GENDER More common in males

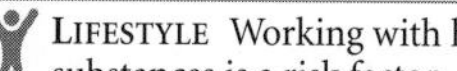

LIFESTYLE Working with hot or caustic substances is a risk factor

AGE GENETICS Not significant factors

Each year as many as 130,000 people in the UK require treatment for burns and scalds and around 250 die as a result of their injuries. Elderly people and young children are particularly vulnerable to the effects of burns.

Most burns are minor and are caused by accidents in the home, such as scalding with hot water. Although almost all minor burns heal quickly, more severe burns often require hospital treatment and can be life-threatening. The degree of severity depends on how deep the burn extends into tissue and the size of the area affected. Burns to sensitive areas, such as the face, hands, feet, or genitals, can be particularly serious.

Burns are usually due to heat, such as fire, hot fluids, or sunlight. However, caustic chemicals, such as certain paint strippers, and electricity (*see* ELECTRICAL INJURIES, p.318) can also cause burns. These burns tend to be more common in men because they are more likely to work in chemical or electrical industries. Burns usually involve the skin, but caustic substances can produce burns in the oesophagus and stomach if they are swallowed. Hot smoke can burn the windpipe and airways.

WHAT ARE THE TYPES?

The skin is made up of two layers: the surface layer, called the epidermis, and the more sensitive dermis underneath. Burns are categorized as first-degree, second-degree, or third-degree, according to the depth of tissue damage.

FIRST-DEGREE BURNS Burns that affect only the epidermis are known as first-degree burns and are the least severe type of burn. The burned area may be red, slightly swollen, and sensitive to the touch, but blisters do not form. Within a few days, the skin heals and the damaged layer of skin may peel off. Sunburn (p.357) is one of the most common causes of first-degree burns.

SECOND-DEGREE BURNS Once the epidermis has been destroyed, the more sensitive lower dermis layer is vulnerable to damage. Damage to both of these two layers is known as a second-degree burn and is usually very painful. The skin becomes red and covered with large blisters filled with clear fluid. After about 3 days, the pain usually decreases, and most second-degree burns should be fully healed within 14 days.

THIRD-DEGREE BURNS The most serious and deepest type of burn is known as a third-degree burn. In this type, the epidermis, dermis, and the underlying fat are destroyed. Sometimes, this damage may extend into the muscle tissue. The area becomes numb, thickened, and discoloured. Healing is very slow since the damaged dermis cannot regenerate itself, and new skin can grow only from the edges of the damaged area.

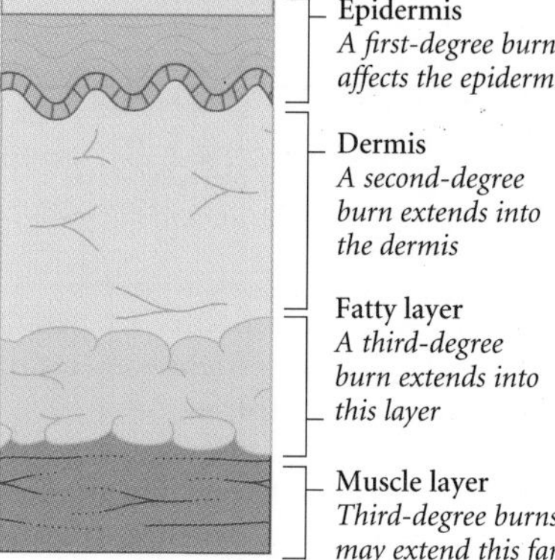

Degrees of severity of burns

Burns are categorized depending on the extent of damage to the different layers of tissue. The more severe the burn, the more layers of tissue are affected.

ARE THERE COMPLICATIONS?

In large second-degree and third-degree burns, fluid is lost from the damaged areas, which may lead to shock (p.414) and damage to the kidneys (*see* KIDNEY FAILURE, p.705). Breathing difficulties may arise if the lungs have been damaged by smoke (*see* ASPHYXIATION, p.326).

Burns are particularly susceptible to infection because the damaged skin can no longer act as a barrier against infection. Infection with bacteria is most common after third-degree burns and may delay healing. If bacteria enter the bloodstream, they may multiply and cause septicaemia (p.299).

WHAT CAN I DO?

Immediately after a burn or scald, the damaged skin should be cooled with large amounts of cold water and first-aid should be started (*see* FIRST AID: MINOR BURNS AND SCALDS, p.988, and FIRST AID: SEVERE BURNS, p.988). Do not put creams on a burn because this may make the burn worse.

Seek medical assistance for anything but minor burns. Large second-degree and all third-degree burns require specialized hospital care, ideally in a burns unit. You should seek medical advice if you have any doubt about the severity of a burn. Anyone with burns on the face or lips needs to be admitted to hospital immediately in case swelling of the affected tissues causes the airways to close up and makes breathing difficult. Hospital admission is also necessary if you have inhaled smoke.

WHAT MIGHT THE DOCTOR DO?

Minor burns are cleaned and dressed. Dressings are usually changed several times a day. An antibacterial cream (*see* PREPARATIONS FOR SKIN INFECTIONS AND INFESTATIONS, p.892) may be applied to help to prevent infection. If an infection does develop, it is usually treated with intravenous antibiotics (p.885).

If the burns are extensive, intravenous fluids, painkillers (p.912), and oxygen may be given. Mechanical ventilation (*see* INTENSIVE CARE UNIT, p.958) may be needed if breathing problems develop due to smoke inhalation.

Anyone with severe burns will be monitored to make sure that his or her fluid levels are maintained and that kidney function is not affected. Skin grafting (right) will be considered to aid healing for most severe second-degree burns and for all third-degree burns.

Scar tissue, which is fragile and sensitive, often develops following severe second-degree and third-degree burns. Scarred areas should be protected from the sun with clothing or sunscreen (*see* SUNSCREENS AND SUNBLOCKS, p.893). Scars may cause itching, which can be relieved with antipruritic drugs (p.891). Scarred areas may also become taut and inflexible, restricting movement if skin over a joint is affected, and skin grafting may be required. Physiotherapy (p.961) sometimes helps to improve movement.

WHAT IS THE PROGNOSIS?

With correct treatment, minor burns usually heal within a few days; more severe burns may take several weeks. Third-degree burns may take months to heal even if skin grafts are used, and some scarring may be permanent.

(WWW) ONLINE SITES: p.1036

TREATMENT SKIN GRAFTING

Skin grafting involves using a section of normal skin from one part of the body (the donor site) to cover another site where the skin has been lost as a result of an injury, such as a burn, or a disorder, such as an ulcer. There are several different methods of skin grafting. The two examples shown here use small donor sites to cover large areas of missing skin.

MESHED GRAFT

A meshed graft is used when a very large area of missing skin needs to be covered and donor sites are limited. The donor skin is removed and made into a mesh using angled cuts. The meshed graft can then be stretched to cover the large area of missing skin.

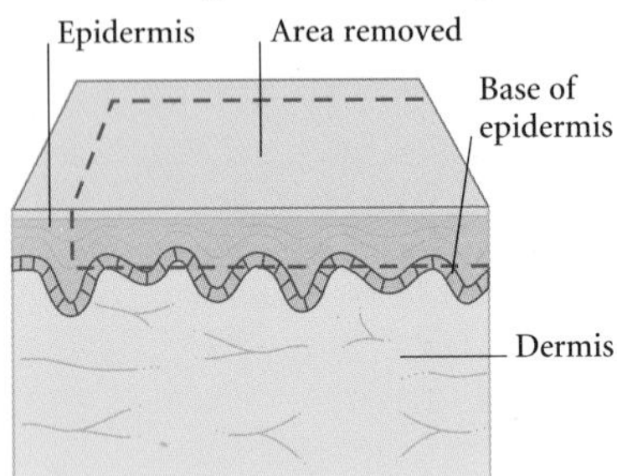

Taking the donor skin
A very thin slice of skin is shaved off the donor site. A sufficient number of cells are left at the base of the epidermis to allow the skin to regrow over the wound.

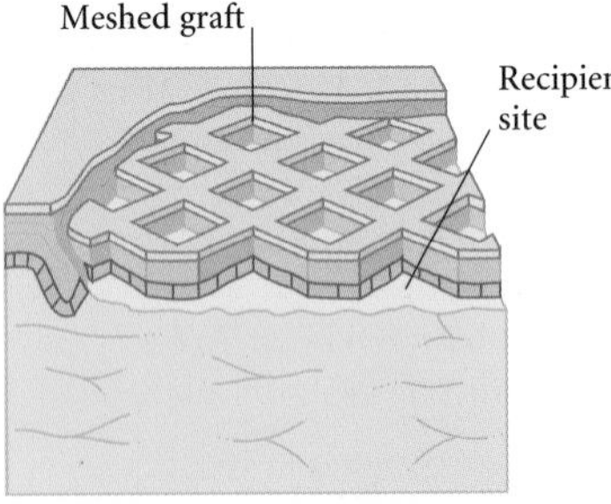

Positioning the meshed graft
The donor skin is cut and stretched to form a mesh that fits in the larger recipient site. Once in place, new skin grows to fill the spaces around the mesh.

PINCH GRAFTS

Pinch grafts are very small pieces of skin that are often used to help skin ulcers to heal. Multiple small grafts are pinched up and removed from the donor site. The pinch grafts are then placed over the larger area of missing skin and grow to cover the area.

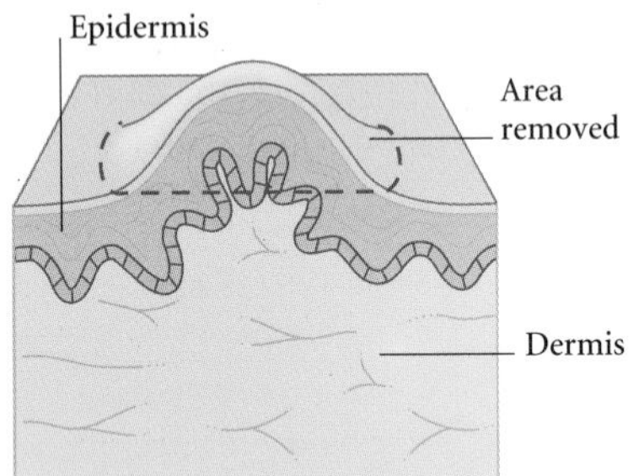

Taking the pinch grafts
Small sections of skin are pinched up at the donor site and cut using scissors or a scalpel. The donor site can heal because the removed sections are small.

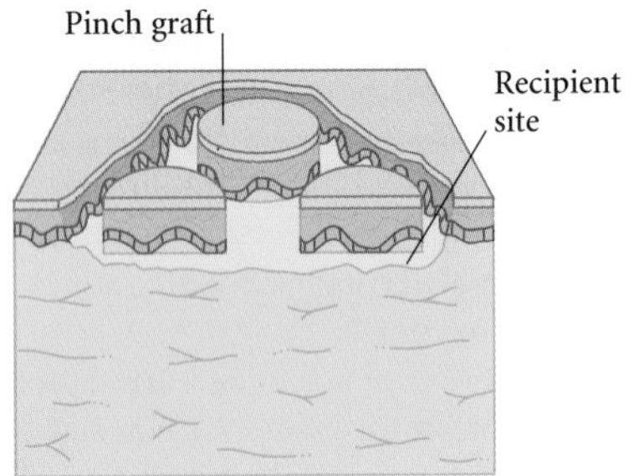

Positioning the pinch grafts
Multiple small pinch grafts are placed on the recipient site. The grafts will gradually grow outwards to form a new sheet of healthy skin in about 10–14 days.

Electrical injuries

Damage to body tissues caused by the passage of an electric current through the body

 GENDER More common in males

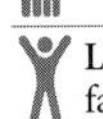 LIFESTYLE Working with electricity is a risk factor

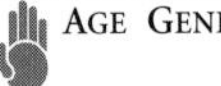 AGE GENETICS Not significant factors

An electrical current passing through the body can generate intense heat and burn the tissues. Although burns may occur internally, they are often most obvious on the skin (*see* BURNS, p.317). The current may also disrupt the normal functioning of the heart or brain and may be immediately fatal.

Each year in the UK there are about 3,000–4,000 electricity-related injuries and 40–50 resulting deaths. Causes of electrical injuries include accidents in the home and lightening strikes. This type of injury also occurs in people who work in the electricity-generating or construction industries.

The majority of electrical injuries occur as a result of touching exposed electrical wires, faulty switches, or water that is electrified by a wire or device. The danger of receiving an electrical injury is greatly increased in the presence of water because water acts as an excellent conductor of electricity.

Men are at greater risk than women of sustaining an electrical injury because they are more likely to work in industries involving electricity.

WHAT ARE THE SYMPTOMS?

General symptoms that are common to many electrical injuries include:

- Loss of consciousness, which may be short-lived.
- Dazed, confused behaviour.

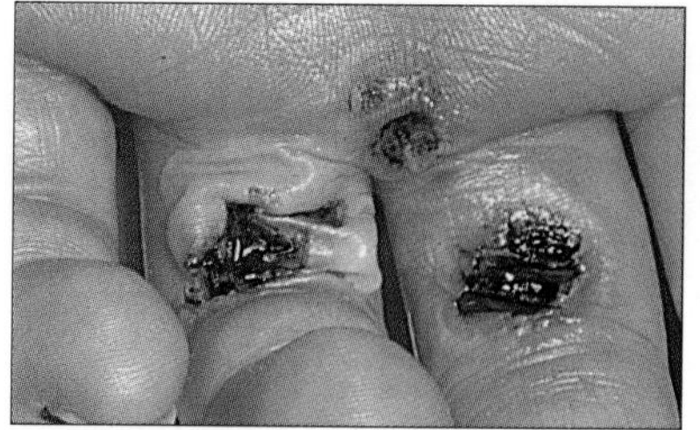

Electrical burns
These two fingers have sustained deep burns as a result of direct contact with an uninsulated electrical cable.

- Burns on the skin.
- Rapid, shallow breathing.

The severity of these symptoms depends on the voltage of the electricity and the duration of contact with the electrical current. In addition, the muscles may become rigid, preventing a person from breaking contact with the electrical current. Severe muscle spasms may lead to bone fractures (p.392).

Specific symptoms vary depending on the route taken by the electrical current through the body. For example, if the current passes through the heart, it may disrupt the rhythm of the heartbeat (*see* ARRHYTHMIAS, p.415) and occasionally lead to cardiac arrest (p.419). If the current passes through the brainstem, which controls automatic body functions such as breathing, the shock may be fatal (*see* BRAIN DEATH, p.523). If the person survives such a shock, irreversible brain damage may have occurred.

WHAT CAN I DO?

You should call for medical assistance for anything more than a minor electric shock. If you find someone who has had an electric shock, make sure that the electricity is turned off before you attempt to touch him or her. Check his or her breathing and pulse rate and initiate resuscitation measures if necessary (*see* FIRST AID: ABC OF RESUSCITATION, p.978). Continue these measures until medical help arrives. You should also carry out these procedures if you come across someone who has an injury as a result of being struck by lightning.

Never attempt to rescue a person injured by high-voltage electricity (over 1,000 volts) because the electricity may jump from the victim to you. Keep at least 18 m (60 ft) from the person and call for medical assistance immediately.

WHAT MIGHT THE DOCTOR DO?

Once the person has been admitted to hospital, a full physical examination will be carried out and tissue damage will be assessed. The heartbeat may be monitored to detect an abnormal rhythm. Oxygen may be given and mechanical ventilation (*see* INTENSIVE CARE UNIT, p.958) may be required. An irregular heart rhythm will probably be treated with an antiarrhythmic drug (p.898). Most people recover if they receive first-aid and medical treatment promptly.

(WWW) ONLINE SITES: p.1036

Stab injuries

Injuries to any part of the body inflicted by a sharp object

 AGE More common in young adults

 GENDER More common in males

 LIFESTYLE Living in urban areas is a risk factor

 GENETICS Not a significant factor

Stab injuries are the cause of about 200 deaths every year in the UK, mostly in young men living in urban areas. Stab wounds vary in severity, depending on the site and depth of the wound. Chest or abdominal wounds are particularly likely to cause internal bleeding, which can be life-threatening.

Medical attention is always essential after a stab injury because visible bleeding is often minor in relation to the severity of the internal injuries.

WHAT ARE THE TYPES?

Shallow wounds may damage skin and muscle only. However, deeper wounds can cause significant internal bleeding, which may lead to loss of consciousness and shock (p.414).

Stab injuries may also cause damage to specific body organs. For example, a stab wound to the chest may result in a pneumothorax (p.496), in which air enters the space between the two-layered membrane that surrounds the lungs, causing breathing difficulties. If the abdomen is wounded in a stab injury, there is a risk of the intestines being punctured and the contents leaking into the abdominal cavity, which can result in infection (*see* PERITONITIS, p.665).

WHAT CAN I DO?

Make sure that the person is breathing and has a pulse (*see* FIRST AID: ABC OF RESUSCITATION, p.978) and then call for medical help. Try to stop external bleeding by applying pressure (*see* FIRST AID: SEVERE BLEEDING, p.986). If the weapon is still in the body, it should be left in place until doctors can remove it safely.

WHAT MIGHT THE DOCTOR DO?

Shallow wounds may only need stitching. An injection to prevent tetanus (*see* VACCINES AND IMMUNOGLOBULINS, p.883) and antibiotics (p.885) to prevent infection may be given.

Deeper stab injuries require a full assessment to check for internal damage. Emergency measures may include giving oxygen and intravenous fluids. A blood transfusion (p.447) may also be needed. CT scanning (p.247) and MRI (p.248) may be done to look for internal bleeding, and exploratory surgery may be carried out to locate and repair the site of internal bleeding. If a chest X-ray (p.490) shows a pneumothorax, a tube is inserted to allow the air to escape (*see* CHEST DRAIN, p.497).

The outlook depends on the type of stab injury. Counselling (p.971) may be offered to help to reduce the risk of post-traumatic stress disorder (p.553).

(WWW) ONLINE SITES: p.1036

Gunshot injuries

Injuries to any part of the body inflicted by a bullet or shotgun pellets

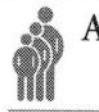 AGE More common in young adults

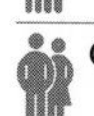 GENDER More common in males

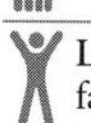 LIFESTYLE Living in urban areas is a risk factor

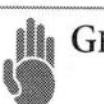 GENETICS Not a significant factor

The effects of a gunshot injury depend on the site of the injury, the type of weapon and bullets used, and the range from which the weapon was fired. In addition to tissue damage, there is a high risk of infection. Wounds to the head or trunk are often life-threatening. In the UK, injury due to the use of guns is not common. However, when such injuries do occur, the victims are usually young men living in urban areas.

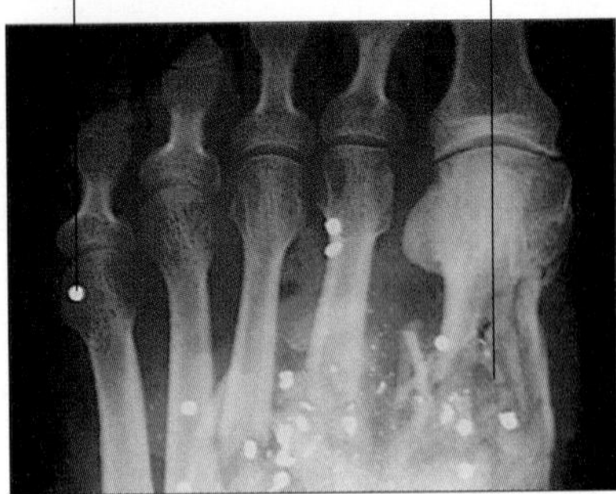

Gunshot injury
Multiple shotgun pellets can be seen in and between the bones of the toes and foot in this X-ray. The bone at the base of the big toe is also shattered.

What are the types?

A gunshot injury to a limb may damage muscle only or cause a fracture (p.392). Such limb injuries are often not serious. However, damage to vital organs may be life-threatening. For example, a gunshot injury to the chest will probably cause breathing difficulties and may result in a pneumothorax (p.496), in which air enters the space between the two-layered membrane that surrounds the lungs. If the spleen or the liver is damaged, life-threatening bleeding may occur, leading to loss of consciousness and shock (p.414). A gunshot injury to the intestines may cause their contents to leak into the abdominal cavity, which can cause infection (*see* PERITONITIS, p.665). Gunshot injuries to the heart or the brain are often fatal.

What can I do?

If you are with someone who has been shot, check his or her breathing and pulse (*see* FIRST AID: ABC OF RESUSCITATION, p.978) and call an ambulance. Try to stop external bleeding by applying pressure to the affected area (*see* FIRST AID: SEVERE BLEEDING, p.986). If shock develops, initiate first-aid measures (*see* FIRST AID: SHOCK, p.987).

What might the doctor do?

Anyone with a gunshot injury needs to be taken to hospital, where initial measures may include controlling blood loss and administering oxygen and intravenous fluids. If a lot of blood has been lost, a blood transfusion (p.447) may be needed. An injection to prevent tetanus (*see* VACCINES AND IMMUNOGLOBULINS, p.883) and antibiotics (p.885) to prevent infection are given if necessary.

Following initial measures, the extent of internal tissue damage is investigated using imaging techniques, such as chest X-rays (p.490), CT scanning (p.247), and MRI (p.248). Almost all gunshot injuries require surgery to repair damaged organs and remove fragments of the bullet, shreds of clothing, and other debris in the wound. Once the wound has been cleaned and bleeding has been stopped, the wound is covered with sterile gauze for 4–5 days to help to prevent infection. The wound is then closed.

Certain injuries may need additional treatment. For example, if a pneumothorax develops, a chest drain (p.497) is inserted into the space between the two membranes to allow the air to escape. If breathing difficulties occur, mechanical ventilation may be necessary (*see* INTENSIVE CARE UNIT, p.958).

With prompt treatment, many gunshot injuries do not lead to long-term physical damage. If vital internal organs are affected, the injury may be fatal.

(WWW) ONLINE SITES: p.1036

Sexual assault

Physical and psychological damage resulting from rape or attempted rape

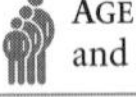 AGE Most common between the ages of 16 and 24

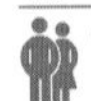 GENDER More common in females

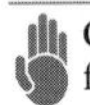 GENETICS LIFESTYLE Not significant factors

The number of cases of sexual assault recorded by the police, which includes both rape and attempted rape, has risen dramatically in recent years. In the UK, more than 6,000 rapes and a further 20,000 indecent assaults were reported to the police in 1997. However, sexual assault is known to be one of the most under-reported crimes, so that the true figure is likely to be much higher.

Many people are unwilling to report a sexual assault, especially if they know the perpetrator. However, help should always be sought. Calling the police or doctor without delay makes treatment for any infection more effective and the gathering of forensic evidence easier. It is best if forensic samples are collected as soon as possible after the assault.

Are there complications?

Hepatitis B and C (*see* ACUTE HEPATITIS, p.644) and other sexually transmitted diseases, such as HIV infection (*see* HIV INFECTION AND AIDS, p.297), syphilis (p.766), or gonorrhoea (p.764), may be contracted. A victim of sexual assault is likely to experience severe psychological trauma, and anxiety disorders (p.551), depression (p.554), or post-traumatic stress disorder (p.553) may develop.

What might be done?

If you report that you have been sexually assaulted, you will receive treatment for injuries and possible infections. You will also be offered support to help you to recover from the experience.

The doctor will examine you, noting bruises or other injuries. Swabs are taken and tested for infections and the presence of semen or other body fluids that may provide forensic evidence against the attacker. After you have received counselling, blood samples are taken to check for HIV infection. Other samples, such as clothes and nail clippings, may be retained for analysis. All examinations and collecting of material for forensic tests are carried out in a supportive environment and only after the doctor has explained what needs to be done and you have agreed.

You will be offered emergency contraception (p.69) if there is a possibility of pregnancy. Antibiotics (p.885) are given in order to prevent sexually transmitted diseases such as gonorrhoea and chlamydial infection (p.765). If there is a risk of developing HIV infection, a course of antiviral drugs may be prescribed to reduce this risk (*see* DRUGS FOR HIV AND AIDS, p.887).

Follow-up care may be offered about 7–10 days after the assault. Subsequent visits may be arranged at 6 weeks for syphilis and gonorrhoea tests and at 3 and 6 months for repeat HIV and hepatitis B and C testing.

Counselling (p.971) will usually be recommended following the attack, and you may also find it helpful to contact self-help organizations that can provide emotional support and practical advice for the victims of sexual assault. You may find that you need support for an extended time. Being able to talk about your feelings is likely to speed recovery.

(WWW) ONLINE SITES: p.1036

POISONING AND ENVIRONMENTAL DISORDERS

The natural environment can be hazardous, and, with increased travel and leisure, people today are more likely than ever to be exposed to potentially life-threatening conditions. Although the human body can adjust to some extent, it cannot cope with poisons or prolonged exposure to extremes of environment.

The first article in this section covers deliberate or accidental drug overdose and poisoning. In adults, many drug overdoses are intentional, whereas in children poisoning usually occurs as a result of the accidental ingestion of common household substances.

Disorders caused by extremes of temperature are described next. Heat exhaustion and heatstroke are almost inevitable consequences of spending too long in very high temperatures. In hypothermia, the body's temperature falls to life-threatening levels as a result of excessive cold. If the body tissues are cold enough, they may freeze. This condition is known as frostbite and is particularly likely to affect extremities that are inadequately protected.

Illness can also result from exposure to extremes of elevation, and this is described next. Altitude sickness not only affects mountaineers but may also occur in people travelling to cities at high altitudes. Decompression sickness, more commonly known as "the bends", usually results from a rapid decrease in pressure when a person surfaces too rapidly after a deep dive underwater.

The next articles in this section deal with environmental injuries that affect oxygen supply to the brain. Drowning and near-drowning are both caused by water preventing normal breathing. The more general term of asphyxiation is used to describe oxygen deprivation that results from a wider variety of causes, such as an object in the throat or carbon monoxide poisoning.

The final articles covered here deal with poisoning from snake and spider bites and scorpion stings. Such injuries are painful but rarely serious. Most of these environmental disorders can be easily prevented by simple measures.

Drug overdose and accidental ingestion

Deliberate or unintentional consumption of potentially harmful substances

AGE Accidental ingestion more common in young children

GENDER Drug overdose more common in females

LIFESTYLE Alcohol and drug abuse are risk factors

GENETICS Not a significant factor

In the UK, an estimated 50,000 people are treated for poisoning each year. Most accidental poisonings occur in children under the age of 5, and many are preventable (see HOME SAFETY AND HEALTH, p.77). However, poisoning in adults is most commonly the result of a deliberate overdose (see ATTEMPTED SUICIDE AND SUICIDE, p.556). Women are more likely than men to take a drug overdose.

Some substances, such as household bleach, are harmful regardless of how much is ingested. Prescribed drugs, such as sleeping drugs (p.915), usually cause harm only if the recommended dose is exceeded. Illegal substances, such as heroin, can have unpredictable effects, depending partly on the amount taken and on the person's susceptibility to the drug (see DRUGS AND HEALTH, p.65).

WHAT ARE THE SYMPTOMS?

The symptoms vary from mild to severe. They may develop immediately or over a number of days. Some common general symptoms include:

- Nausea and vomiting.
- Abdominal pain.
- Diarrhoea.
- Rapid heartbeat.
- Chest pain.
- Shortness of breath.
- Confusion.
- Seizures.
- Eventually, loss of consciousness.

There may also be local symptoms, such as burns in the mouth after swallowing caustic substances.

An overdose of certain drugs, such as tricyclic antidepressants (see ANTIDEPRESSANT DRUGS, p.916), can disturb the action of the heart and result in an irregular heart rhythm (see ARRHYTHMIAS, p.415) and sometimes a feeling of faintness. In some cases, an arrhythmia may even lead to cardiac arrest (p.419). Overdose of an opium-based drug, such as heroin, causes a reduction in breathing rate, which may be life-threatening. An overdose of certain substances may also damage the liver and kidneys. For example, liver failure (p.650) may result from an overdose of paracetamol (see PAINKILLERS, p.912). Rarely, ingestion of certain poisons can cause a severe allergic reaction (see ANAPHYLAXIS, p.469).

WHAT CAN I DO?

If the affected person is unconscious, check his or her breathing and pulse rate and call an ambulance (see FIRST AID: ABC OF RESUSCITATION, p.978). Continue first aid until help arrives (see FIRST AID: SWALLOWED POISONS, p.994).

Even if there are no symptoms and the quantity of poison ingested is small, you should always consult your doctor or poison centre for advice. Collect as much information as possible, including bottles or containers and remains of the substance that has been taken. If vomiting has occurred, you should collect a sample for analysis by the doctor. If the person is unconscious or reluctant to talk, you may be needed to provide vital information. Do not give the person anything to drink or try to induce vomiting unless instructed to do so.

What might the doctor do?

The doctor needs to know what has been taken and when. He or she will examine the person and, if a drug overdose has been taken, will arrange for blood tests to measure drug levels in the circulation. Other body fluids, such as vomit, may be analysed.

In some cases, admission to an intensive care unit (p.958) for monitoring and treatment may be required. If tricyclic antidepressants have been taken, the heart rhythm is monitored to detect any abnormalities. After a paracetamol overdose, blood tests are carried out to look for signs of liver damage.

Various methods may be used to try to eliminate the ingested substance from the digestive tract and to prevent it from being absorbed into the circulation. If the person is conscious and has ingested a noncaustic substance, syrup of ipecac may be given to induce vomiting. If he or she does not vomit, a tube may be passed through the mouth into the stomach to wash out the stomach with sterile water or a saline solution. If the person is unconscious, a tube may be passed into the windpipe to prevent liquid from entering the lungs as the stomach is emptied.

Alternatively, activated charcoal may be given orally. The toxic substance binds to the charcoal in the digestive tract and is then passed out in the faeces. If very high levels of a toxic substance are present in the circulation, elimination can be increased by filtering the blood (*see* DIALYSIS, p.707). Some substances can be inactivated by giving a specific antidote. For example, naloxone may be given for an opium-based overdose.

Complications are usually treated as they arise. For example, antiarrhythmic drugs (p.898) can be prescribed for an irregular heartbeat. If breathing difficulties are severe, mechanical ventilation may eventually be required.

If an overdose was taken deliberately, a psychiatric assessment will be carried out when the person is stable.

What is the prognosis?

Although poisoning may be fatal, most cases are treated successfully. However, in some cases, there may be permanent damage, such as liver damage following an overdose of paracetamol.

(WWW) ONLINE SITES: p.1026, p.1030, p.1032

Heat exhaustion and heatstroke

Conditions resulting from exposure to excessive heat, in which there is loss of fluids and a rise in body temperature

AGE May occur at any age but most common in babies and elderly people

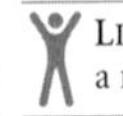
LIFESTYLE Exertion in a hot environment is a risk factor

GENDER GENETICS Not significant factors

In a hot environment, the body loses heat by diverting blood to the skin and by sweating. Profuse sweating may lead to an excessive loss of fluids and salts, resulting in heat exhaustion. This condition is rarely serious, but, if exposure to heat continues, heatstroke may occur as the body's normal cooling mechanisms break down and the temperature of the body rises. Heatstroke is a life-threatening medical emergency.

Heat exhaustion and heatstroke most commonly occur above 40°C (104°F). High humidity levels increase the risk of heatstroke because sweating is ineffective and heat loss is decreased.

EFFECT OF HUMIDITY ON THE RISK OF HEATSTROKE

KEY: EXTREME RISK; HIGH RISK; MODERATE RISK; LOW RISK

RELATIVE HUMIDITY (%): 100, 90, 80, 70, 60, 50, 40, 30, 20

AIR TEMPERATURE: 25, 30, 35, 40, 45, 50, 55 °C; 80, 90, 100, 110, 120, 130 °F

The risk of heatstroke

As the moisture in the atmosphere (the humidity) rises, it becomes more difficult to lose heat by sweating, and heatstroke may occur at lower temperatures.

Who is at risk?

Heat exhaustion and heatstroke may affect otherwise healthy people, particularly after physical exertion in a hot climate. People who come from temperate climates and travel to the tropics need time to acclimatize to the heat before they can safely exert themselves.

The body's cooling mechanisms are less efficient in infants and in elderly people, making them more susceptible to heat exhaustion and heatstroke. Diabetes mellitus (p.687), obesity (p.631), alcohol dependence (p.564), and chronic heart failure (p.413) all reduce the body's ability to lose heat. Diarrhoea (p.627) may contribute to dehydration and increase the risk of developing heat exhaustion and heatstroke.

What are the symptoms?

After prolonged exposure to hot conditions, the following symptoms of heat exhaustion may develop:

- Profuse sweating.
- Tiredness.
- Muscle cramps.
- Nausea and vomiting.
- Faintness and unsteadiness.
- Headache.

If exposure to heat continues, the body temperature rises and heatstroke may develop, causing symptoms such as:

- Fast, shallow breathing.
- Confusion and disorientation.
- Seizures.

Left untreated, heatstroke may progress to coma (p.522) in minutes. Death may be due to kidney failure (p.705), acute heart failure (p.412), or direct heat-induced damage to the brain.

What can I do?

Heat exhaustion can be treated easily. The affected person should rest in a cool place (ideally in an air-conditioned building) and sip cool, salty drinks until he or she feels comfortable. If heatstroke is suspected, he or she should be admitted to hospital as soon as possible.

What might the doctor do?

Once in hospital, the person is examined, and blood tests are carried out to assess the level of salts in the blood.

Treatment for heatstroke is usually carried out in an intensive care unit (p.958). Body temperature is lowered by sponging the body with tepid water or loosely wrapping the person in a wet sheet and placing him or her near a fan. Intravenous fluids are given. Once the body temperature has been reduced to 38°C (100°F), these cooling procedures are stopped to prevent the development of hypothermia. Monitoring is carried out continuously to make sure that the body temperature is returning to normal levels and that vital organs are functioning normally. In some severe cases, mechanical ventilation may be required to assist breathing.

Most people with heat exhaustion recover in a few hours if they are moved to a cooler place and fluids are gradually replaced. If heatstroke is treated promptly, most people recover after a few days of bed rest, although their body temperature may fluctuate for several weeks afterwards.

Can they be prevented?

Heat-related disorders can be largely prevented by avoiding strenuous exertion in the heat of the day, spending as much time as possible in the shade, consuming large quantities of liquids, and avoiding alcoholic drinks.

(WWW) ONLINE SITES: p.1036, p.1037

Hypothermia

A fall in body temperature to a dangerously low level

AGE May occur at any age but most common in babies and elderly people

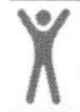
LIFESTYLE Homelessness and outdoor activities in cold climates are risk factors

GENDER GENETICS Not significant factors

Hypothermia is a condition that occurs when the body's temperature, normally about 37°C (98.6°F) falls below 35°C (95°F). The body normally has various warming mechanisms, including shivering, that replace lost heat. However, if the environment is too cold or if the body's warming mechanisms fail, hypothermia develops. Hypothermia may be associated with frostbite (p.324) and, if it is extreme, can be life-threatening.

Who is at risk?

Hypothermia is particularly common in climbers and walkers who are inadequately dressed for cold weather. People who are homeless in cold weather are also vulnerable. In addition, people who have reduced awareness of low temperatures due to alcohol or drug abuse may not realize they need to protect themselves and may develop hypothermia.

Certain disorders increase the risk of developing hypothermia. For example, hypothyroidism (p.680) slows down the body's functions and reduces the body temperature. People whose mobility is reduced following a stroke (p.532) or because of a disorder such as arthritis (p.374) generate little body heat and are also more susceptible to hypothermia.

Elderly people are particularly at risk of developing hypothermia. As the body ages, it becomes less able to maintain its normal body temperature in cold conditions. Elderly people may also be less aware of the cold and do not always notice if their body temperature drops. In some cases, dementia (p.535) may reduce an elderly person's awareness of temperature changes.

Babies are susceptible to hypothermia because they lose heat rapidly and, like elderly people, cannot easily maintain their body temperature.

In all cases, the rate of heat loss and therefore the risk of hypothermia is increased in high winds or wet conditions, and hypothermia may develop particularly quickly when a person is immersed in cold water.

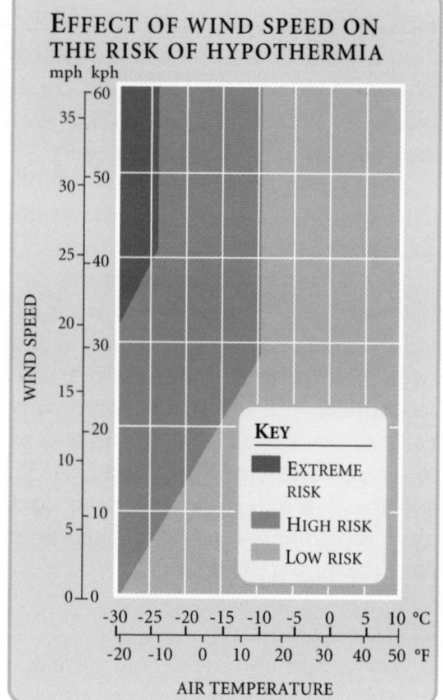

The risk of hypothermia
As the wind speed increases, heat is lost more rapidly from the body, making hypothermia more likely to occur at warmer temperatures.

What are the symptoms?

The symptoms of hypothermia usually develop gradually over hours or days but may develop in minutes in someone immersed in cold water or exposed to high winds. The person may not feel cold. Symptoms may include:

- Tiredness.
- Slow, clumsy movements.
- Confusion, impaired judgment, and slow reactions.
- Blue, cold hands and feet.

As the body temperature drops further, these symptoms become more obvious. In addition, the lips may turn blue, delirium or loss of consciousness may develop, and the heart may develop an abnormal rhythm (*see* ARRHYTHMIAS, p.415) or, eventually, even stop beating (*see* CARDIAC ARREST, p.419).

(SELF-HELP) Avoiding hypothermia in elderly people

Elderly people are particularly susceptible to hypothermia. If you are elderly, you should take care to protect yourself against the cold. The following measures may help:

- Keep all your windows closed in cold weather.
- Install an easy-to-read wall thermometer. The temperature in the room where you spend most of your time should be at least 20°C (68°F).
- Make sure that your home is warm before getting out of bed in the morning.
- Have at least one hot meal and several hot drinks each day.
- Try to move around at least hourly to create your own heat.
- Wear several layers of clothing if possible to trap warm air.
- Wear a hat to prevent loss of body heat through the scalp.
- If your clothes get wet, change into dry clothes as soon as possible to prevent the moisture in the clothes from conducting heat away from the body.

WHAT CAN I DO?

If you are with someone who has mild hypothermia, move him or her to a warm, sheltered place. If necessary, help remove damp clothes and replace them with warm, dry clothing, including a hat. Wrap the person in a warm blanket, and, if he or she is fully conscious, give him or her a warm, nonalcoholic drink. Do not give alcohol because it can exacerbate the condition. If hypothermia is more severe, call for medical help as soon as possible.

If you are stranded in a remote place with a person with severe hypothermia, you should follow as many of the above measures as possible until help arrives. If possible, get into a survival or sleeping bag together. Your body heat will help to warm the person up. If he or she becomes unconscious, carry out first-aid measures if necessary (*see* FIRST AID: ABC OF RESUSCITATION, p.978).

WHAT MIGHT THE DOCTOR DO?

The doctor will assess the degree of hypothermia using a rectal thermometer that can record low temperatures. People with severe hypothermia need slow rewarming in hospital, usually in an intensive care unit (p.958). Most people with mild to moderate hypothermia recover fully. The outlook is best for young, otherwise healthy people.

In most cases, hypothermia can be prevented by self-help measures, such as dressing warmly and keeping moving in cold weather.

(WWW) ONLINE SITES: p.1026, p.1036

Frostbite

Damage to the body tissues caused by exposure to extreme cold

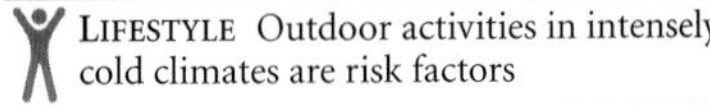
LIFESTYLE Outdoor activities in intensely cold climates are risk factors

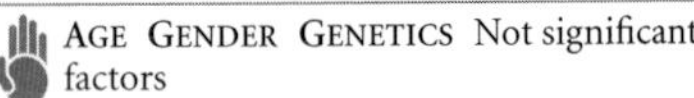
AGE GENDER GENETICS Not significant factors

Exposure to extreme cold can freeze the body tissues and damage them, a condition that is known as frostbite. If not treated, frostbite may result in tissue death and permanent damage to the affected area. Frostbite can develop at any temperature below 0°C (32°F). The lower the temperature, the more rapidly frostbite develops. The risk of frostbite is increased by windy conditions.

People who have impaired circulation, such as those with diabetic vascular disease (p.432), are at increased risk of frostbite. Certain drugs affecting circulation (*see* BETA-BLOCKER DRUGS, p.898) may also make frostbite more likely.

The extremities are most susceptible to frostbite and are affected first. White, cold patches of skin appear, accompanied by tingling. These symptoms are followed by numbness. When warmed, mildly affected tissues become red and swollen. If frostbite is more severe, blisters appear, and the area becomes very painful. Prolonged frostbite may lead to tissue death (*see* GANGRENE, p.435), and the skin may appear black or dark blue. Frostbite is often associated with hypothermia (p.323).

WHAT CAN I DO?

If you or someone with you develops frostbite, you should warm the affected areas only as long as there is no possibility of refreezing. Rewarming should be carried out slowly by immersing the affected areas in warm water that is not too hot to touch. Remove the affected areas from the water as they return to a normal colour. Do not rub frostbitten areas. You should not warm the skin with direct heat, such as a fire, because the skin may be burned before sensation returns. Place gauze between the frostbitten fingers and toes, and bandage the affected areas loosely.

WHAT MIGHT THE DOCTOR DO?

If the affected area does not completely recover with warming, go to hospital as soon as possible. In hospital, rewarming will be completed, and sterile dressings applied to reduce the risk of infection. Physiotherapy (p.961) may also be required to promote circulation to the affected areas. In very severe cases, and after all other means have been tried, amputation of dead areas may be necessary to preserve nearby healthy tissue.

Frostbite damage usually heals within 6 months, but lasting sensitivity to low temperatures is common. If frostbite is severe, stiffness, pain, and numbness may persist indefinitely.

Frostbite can be prevented by dressing warmly when going outside in very cold weather, paying particular attention to the extremities.

(WWW) ONLINE SITES: p.1036, p.1037

Altitude sickness

A condition experienced at high altitudes resulting from oxygen deficiency in the blood and tissues

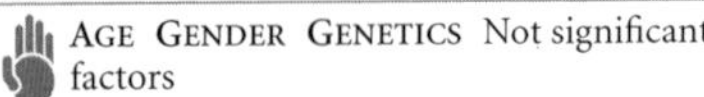
LIFESTYLE Rapidly ascending to high altitudes is a risk factor

AGE GENDER GENETICS Not significant factors

At high altitudes, the amount of oxygen in the air is reduced. The resulting low levels of oxygen in the blood and tissues cause symptoms such as tiredness, unsteadiness, headache, and nausea. This condition is known as altitude sickness. Altitude sickness usually affects mountaineers, but people flying from sea level to a high-altitude location may experience some mild altitude sickness upon arrival. The severity of the illness depends on how high and fast a person ascends, but altitude sickness does not normally occur below 2,400 m (8,000 ft).

WHAT ARE THE SYMPTOMS?

Symptoms may begin to develop about 6 hours after arriving at high altitude. Symptoms may include:

- Headache.
- Tiredness and weakness.
- Unsteadiness.
- Nausea.

These symptoms are usually mild and disappear within 1–2 days if you do not ascend further. In some people, more severe symptoms, including shortness of breath and vomiting, may develop within 36 hours. In rare cases, fluid may build up in the lungs and result in a cough with frothy sputum. The brain may swell, initially causing difficulty in walking and clumsy movements. If altitude sickness is left untreated, further symptoms may develop, including confusion, seizures, and even coma (p.522).

WHAT CAN I DO?

If you have mild altitude sickness, rest, painkillers (p.912), plenty of fluids, and a light diet should enable you to acclimatize to the altitude. A further ascent should not be attempted until all your symptoms have subsided.

In severe cases, a rapid descent to a lower altitude may be essential. Even descending only 300 m (1,000 ft) may lead to an improvement. If symptoms persist, hospital admission is necessary.

What might the doctor do?

In severe cases, immediate oxygen therapy is necessary. If the lungs and brain are affected, a delay in treatment may lead to permanent brain damage and possibly death. Bed rest will be recommended, and the drug dexamethasone (*see* Corticosteroids, p.930) may be given to relieve the symptoms.

Most people treated for altitude sickness recover fully within 1–3 days. Even if the lungs and brain are affected, a full recovery is likely, although in this case treatment may be needed over a longer period of several days or weeks.

Can it be prevented?

Good physical preparation and a high level of fitness are essential prerequisites for climbing at high altitudes. Ascents to high altitudes should be staged and gradual and should include intervals of a few days spent at intermediate altitudes before climbing higher.

Plenty of fluids should be taken on climbs. Occasionally, the drug acetazolamide may be prescribed beforehand to reduce susceptibility to altitude sickness. An oxygen supply should be part of the equipment for people climbing above 3,700 m (12,000 ft) because it may be necessary for treating unforeseen cases of altitude sickness.

(WWW) ONLINE SITES: p.1036, p.1037

Decompression sickness

A condition resulting from the formation of gas bubbles in the blood and tissues following a rapid decrease in pressure

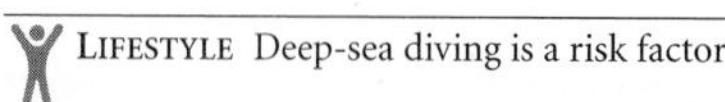
Lifestyle Deep-sea diving is a risk factor

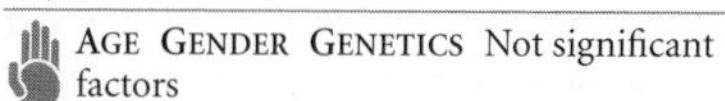
Age Gender Genetics Not significant factors

Decompression sickness, also known as "the bends", usually occurs when a person surfaces too quickly after a deep dive underwater. The condition may also result from working in pressurized tunnels, being exposed to sudden aircraft decompression at high altitude, or flying too soon after scuba diving.

At normal atmospheric pressure, a certain amount of gas is dissolved in the blood and other tissues. More gas accumulates in the tissues of divers due to the high-pressure gas mixture they breathe while underwater. If, during a slow ascent to the water's surface, the surrounding pressure is lowered gradually, excess gas is carried to the lungs by the blood and is exhaled. If the reduction in pressure during ascent is too rapid, gas cannot be carried away gradually and bubbles form in the blood and tissues, causing decompression sickness. Decompression sickness in people other than divers is also due to the formation of gas bubbles in blood and tissues.

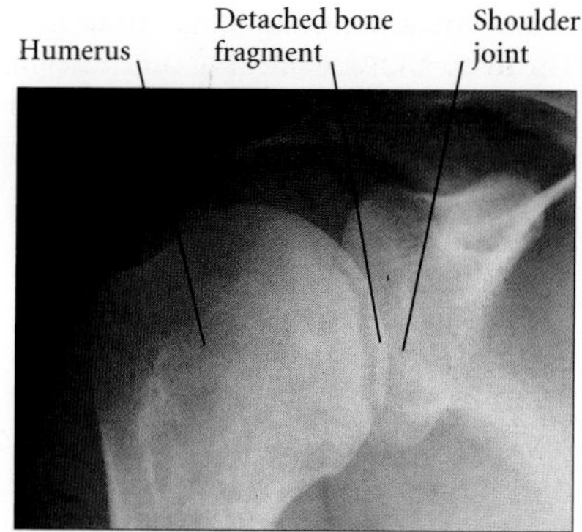

Effect of decompression sickness
A rapid reduction in atmospheric pressure may cause decompression sickness, resulting in bone damage, often near large joints.

What are the symptoms?

Symptoms usually occur within a few hours of the pressure being reduced but may take up to 24 hours to develop. They often include:

- Itching.
- Mottling of the skin.
- Severe pains in the larger joints, particularly the shoulders and knees.
- Headache.

Gas bubbles may lodge in the blood vessels that supply the heart or lungs, causing a tight pain across the chest. If bubbles lodge in the brain or spinal cord, weakness in the legs or problems with vision and balance may occur.

What might be done?

If you have symptoms of decompression sickness, you should be taken to a recompression chamber immediately. Once you are in the sealed chamber, air is pumped in to increase the pressure (recompression). The increased pressure forces the gas bubbles to redissolve into the tissues, thereby relieving the symptoms. Decompression can then be carried out slowly over several hours to prevent bubbles from forming again.

Prompt treatment usually leads to a full recovery. Serious, untreated cases may cause long-term paralysis. People who have repeated episodes of decompression sickness and recompressions may develop progressive degeneration of their bones and joints.

(WWW) ONLINE SITES: p.1036

Drowning and near-drowning

Suffocation after submersion in water, often leading to unconsciousness and even death

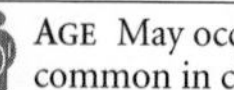
Age May occur at any age but most common in children and adolescents

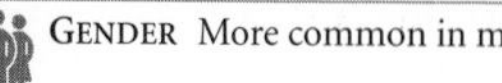
Gender More common in males

Lifestyle Access to unfenced water is a risk factor

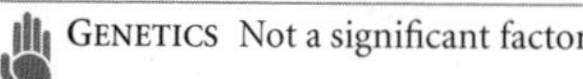
Genetics Not a significant factor

Drowning causes about 500 deaths each year in the UK and is a common cause of accidental death, particularly in children and adolescents. An even greater number have a near-drowning experience. The majority of cases of drowning are the result of water activities in a strong current or after drinking alcohol. However, young children who drown often do so in swimming pools or ponds at home. The risk of drowning can be greatly reduced by taking care around water and particularly by supervising children when they are swimming or playing in water (*see* Safety in and around water, p.81).

When a submerged person starts to choke, the larynx (voice box) goes into spasm, preventing water from entering the lungs but blocking normal breathing. Eventually, lack of oxygen causes loss of consciousness, and the larynx usually relaxes. If the face is submerged, water may then enter the lungs. In 1 out of 10 cases, the larynx stays closed and no water enters the lungs. This condition is known as dry drowning.

People who are drowning can often be revived by first aid. However, life-threatening complications may develop, and hospital treatment is still needed even if they have apparently recovered.

ARE THERE COMPLICATIONS?

Lack of oxygen can lead to brain damage and death. Even if breathing is restored, water may cause inflammation of the lining of the lungs, leading to acute respiratory distress syndrome (p.506). Debris in the lungs may cause infection and lung damage, impairing the ability of the lungs to function normally.

Inhaled water may alter blood chemistry. If fresh water is inhaled, it passes from the lungs to the bloodstream and destroys the red blood cells. If salt water is inhaled, the salt causes blood to enter the tissues of the lungs.

A drowning person can survive for longer in cold water because the body's processes slow down. As a result, many people who have been resuscitated after a near-drowning experience may also have hypothermia (p.323).

WHAT CAN I DO?

Only attempt to rescue a drowning person if you are sure that you can do so without putting yourself at risk.

If the person is conscious and close to you, throw him or her an object that will float, ideally with a rope attached. Alternatively, use a stick, pole, or even an item of clothing. If the person cannot reach the object, swim out only if it is safe. Otherwise, note the position of the person and call for assistance.

If you swim out to the person, basic resuscitation measures will be difficult or impossible to perform while you are in deep water. However, once you can stand, artificial respiration (pp.982–983) may be started. When you reach land, start to carry out full first-aid resuscitation measures as necessary (*see* FIRST AID: ABC OF RESUSCITATION, p.978).

If the person has fallen into cold water, wrap him or her in warm, dry clothing or blankets to try to reduce the risk of hypothermia. Continue resuscitating a person who is cold because nearly drowned people can survive far longer if they have hypothermia.

Even if the person seems well, medical attention should be sought to make sure that there are no complications.

WHAT MIGHT THE DOCTOR DO?

Even if the person is conscious when first seen in hospital, he or she is likely to be admitted for observation because problems can develop in the first 24–48 hours. Treatment may range from giving oxygen to monitoring and care in an intensive care unit (p.958). In some cases, mechanical ventilation may be needed to ease breathing difficulties. Additional treatment depends on complications. For example, corticosteroids (p.930) may be given to reduce inflammation in the lungs, and antibiotics (p.885) may be administered to counter possible lung infections.

If hypothermia has developed, the person is rewarmed slowly. Body temperature needs to be slowly returned to normal before an assessment for brain damage can be carried out.

WHAT IS THE PROGNOSIS?

The outlook is improved if the water is cold, the period of submersion is short, and the person is young and otherwise healthy. About 1 in 20 people who are resuscitated later die of a complication. Those who survive may have sustained some permanent brain damage.

(WWW) ONLINE SITES: p.1032, p.1036

Asphyxiation

Failure of oxygen to reach the brain for a variety of reasons

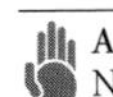
AGE GENDER GENETICS LIFESTYLE
Not significant factors

Asphyxiation is the term that is given to a potentially fatal condition in which oxygen is prevented from reaching the brain. If it is not treated within a few minutes, asphyxiation leads to loss of consciousness, irreversible brain damage, and, subsequently, to death.

WHAT ARE THE CAUSES?

Asphyxiation may be the result of an inability to breathe or insufficient oxygen in the inhaled air.

An inability to breathe can be due to a variety of factors. One of the most common causes is a foreign object that is lodged in the throat. Something held over the face may also block the airway, as may the person's tongue if he or she is unconscious. A severe head injury (p.521) or a drug overdose (*see* DRUG OVERDOSE AND ACCIDENTAL INGESTION, p.321) may slow down breathing or even stop it completely. Severe damage to the wall of the chest (*see* CRUSH INJURIES, p.316) may prevent the lungs from inflating, particularly if one or more of the ribs has been fractured. The neck may be compressed by accidental or deliberate strangulation.

Lack of oxygen in the air can occur as a result of carbon monoxide from a car exhaust. Smoke from a fire reduces the level of oxygen in the air, or oxygen may become depleted if a person is enclosed in an airtight space.

WHAT ARE THE SYMPTOMS?

Asphyxiation usually develops rapidly over a few minutes but can occur over several hours, depending on the cause. Most cases of asphyxiation lead to similar symptoms, including:

- Agitation.
- Confusion.
- Eventually, loss of consciousness.

In most cases, the skin, particularly the lips, turns blue. However, when carbon monoxide poisoning is the cause, the skin may turn a bright cherry red.

WHAT CAN I DO?

Only go to the aid of a person who is being asphyxiated if you are in no danger from smoke or other gases yourself. Check for an obstruction to breathing (*see* FIRST AID: CHOKING, pp.980–981) and carry out emergency resuscitation measures until help arrives (*see* FIRST AID: ABC OF RESUSCITATION, p.978).

WHAT MIGHT THE DOCTOR DO?

Once in hospital, medical treatment is directed at reversing the cause of the asphyxiation. For example, if the condition is due to a foreign body lodged in the throat, the object will be removed. If the object cannot be removed quickly, an incision may be made in the trachea (the windpipe) and a tube inserted to restore breathing until the airway can be cleared. Fractured ribs will be treated and painkillers (p.912) given. Drug overdoses are treated by eliminating as much of the ingested toxic substance as possible. In some severe cases in which the underlying cause of the asphyxiation cannot be treated rapidly, mechanical ventilation (*see* INTENSIVE CARE UNIT, p.958) may be required.

The shorter the period of oxygen deprivation, the better the prognosis. Following prolonged asphyxiation, there may be permanent brain damage.

(WWW) ONLINE SITES: p.1032, p.1036

Poisonous bites and stings

Penetrating injuries from snakes, scorpions, insects, or marine life that are followed by an injection of venom

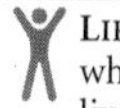
LIFESTYLE Walking or swimming in areas where venomous biting or stinging animals live is a risk factor

AGE GENDER GENETICS Not significant factors

The risk of receiving a poisonous bite or sting varies considerably in different parts of the world. The animals most commonly responsible for venomous bites and stings include snakes, spiders, scorpions, and marine animals such as jellyfish. If you are travelling abroad, it is important to seek advice about the risk of encountering venomous animals, especially if you intend to go camping, hiking, or swimming. You should also take appropriate precautions to prevent being bitten or stung (*see* AVOIDING BITES AND STINGS, right).

What are the causes?

Worldwide, there are many species of venomous snake, but only one of these, the adder, occurs naturally in the UK. Poisonous spiders are found in parts of America and Australia. For example, black widow and brown recluse spiders occur in North America, while Australia is home to the redback and funnel back spider. Venomous scorpions are found in several parts of the world, including North Africa, South America, and India.

Poisonous marine animals, including jellyfish and sea anemones, can be found around the shores of Britain. Poisonous fish, such as stingrays and scorpion fish, are found only in tropical waters.

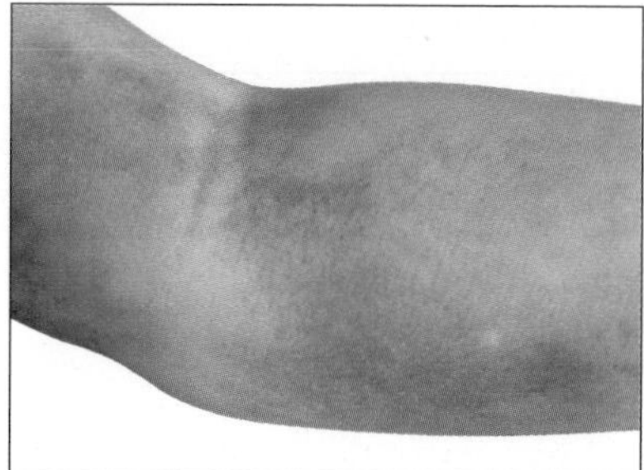

Effect of a snake bite
A bite by a poisonous snake may cause swelling and discoloration of surrounding tissues, obscuring the bite marks.

What are the symptoms?

If you are bitten by a snake and there are no fang marks, no venom has been injected and there will be no symptoms. If there is venom in the wound, symptoms may appear immediately or over the next few hours. Initial symptoms occur around the bite and may include:

- Swelling and discoloration.
- Pain and a burning sensation.

Later, symptoms of widespread poisoning may begin to appear, including:

- Pale skin and sweating.
- Confusion.
- Eventual loss of consciousness.

Blood pressure may fall, causing shock (p.414). Major organs may be affected, possibly resulting in respiratory failure (p.507) and acute heart failure (p.412).

Most scorpion stings are extremely painful but otherwise harmless. However, a sting from a bark scorpion, which is found in parts of America, may cause further symptoms, including sweating, restlessness, vomiting, diarrhoea, an irregular heartbeat, and muscle spasms.

The bite of a venomous spider, such as the black widow spider, usually causes generalized muscle pain, sweating, and headache and may lead to shock.

Stings by marine creatures may produce pain and swelling. Raised, red, itchy areas of skin may appear at the point of contact with a jellyfish or sea anemone. Rarely, stings from marine animals may result in symptoms such as diarrhoea, vomiting, and an irregular heartbeat.

What can I do?

If you, or someone with you, is bitten by a snake or poisonous spider, remove any clothing or jewellery that may cause constriction should the area around the bite start to swell. The affected person should move as little as possible and first aid carried out (*see* FIRST AID: POISONOUS BITES AND STINGS, p.994). If you have been bitten by a snake, note its appearance so that when you reach hospital the doctor can decide whether antivenom is required.

Most scorpion stings need only application of a cold compress to the wound and painkillers (p.912) for pain.

If you have been stung by a jellyfish or other marine animal, wipe off any stingers or tentacles with a towel or sand and wash the area with sea water before seeking medical attention.

SELF-HELP Avoiding bites and stings

The chance of being bitten or stung when hiking can be reduced by taking the following steps:

- Apply insect repellent before setting out on a hike.
- Wear a long-sleeved shirt tucked into your waistband and long trousers tucked into socks.
- Put a rubber band where trousers and socks meet to prevent insects from getting under clothing.
- Wear strong walking boots to protect the entire foot and ankle.
- Stay in the middle of paths when you are hiking and avoid areas of dense undergrowth.
- Make noise as you walk through areas where there may be snakes.
- If you come across a snake, retrace your steps because there may be others in the vicinity.

If you are swimming, the following measures will help you to avoid being stung by a marine animal:

- Look out for signs warning of the presence of jellyfish or other hazardous marine life.
- Do not touch unfamiliar marine creatures.
- Swim near a lifeguard.

What might the doctor do?

Hospital treatment for a snake bite may include resuscitation and intravenous fluids. You may also be given antivenom, and antianxiety drugs (p.916) may be helpful if you are panicking. Once your condition has stabilized, the affected area will be elevated and immobilized until the swelling subsides.

Treatment for a spider bite, or for a sting by a scorpion or marine animal, depends on the symptoms. Oxygen may be given for breathing difficulties. If the symptoms are severe, antivenom may be given to counteract the effects of the poison. Antivenoms are available for some scorpion stings and for the more dangerous species of poisonous marine animal. Pain can be relieved by applying a local anaesthetic (p.914) to the skin.

With the appropriate treatment, most symptoms improve within a few days and there are no long-lasting effects.

WWW ONLINE SITES: p.1032, p.1036

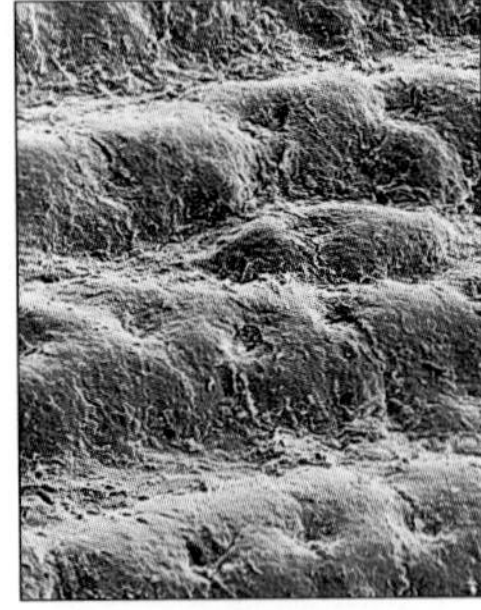

Surface of the skin
This magnified view of the hairless skin of the palm shows sweat pores arranged along ridges. The ridges help us to hold on to objects.

SKIN, HAIR, AND NAILS

WITH AN AVERAGE SURFACE AREA of about 2 sq. m ($2^1/_2$ sq. yd), the skin is one of the largest organs of the body. The skin forms a protective barrier between the harsh environment of the outside world and the body's muscles, internal organs, blood vessels, and nerves. Hair and nails grow from the skin and provide extra protection. The appearance of the skin varies widely, not only changing with factors such as increasing age but also acting as a barometer of our fluctuating emotions and general health.

The skin is a living organ. The topmost layer of the epidermis, which forms the surface of the skin, is made up of dead cells, and a person sheds about 30,000 of these cells every minute. However, live skin cells are continually produced in the lower part of the epidermis to replace them. Below the epidermis lies the dermis, which contains blood vessels, nerve endings, and glands. A layer of fat lies under the dermis and acts as an insulator, shock absorber, and energy store.

PROTECTING AND SENSING

Even though most parts of it are less than 6 mm ($^1/_4$ in) thick, the skin is still a robust protective layer. The main component of its surface is a tough, fibrous protein called keratin. This substance can also be found in hair, which provides protection and warmth, and in nails, which cover the delicate ends of the fingers and toes.

The skin forms a highly effective barrier against microorganisms and harmful substances, but it is most effective when the surface remains intact. Wounds may become infected and allow bacteria, some of which live on the skin's surface, to enter the bloodstream. Sebum, an oily fluid formed in the sebaceous glands in the dermis, helps to keep the skin supple and repels water. It is because skin is waterproof that we do not soak up water like a sponge when we bathe.

Our sense of touch comes from receptors in the skin's dermis that respond to pressure, vibrations, heat, cold, and pain. Every second, billions of signals from stimuli received all over the body are sent to the brain, where they are processed to create a sensory "image" and to warn of dangers, such as a hot cooker. Some sensory areas, such as the fingertips, have a high density of receptors.

The skin also plays a major part in regulating body temperature and, when exposed to sunlight, produces vitamin D, which is essential for strong bones.

A RESPONSIVE LAYER

Our skin responds to the life we lead. For example, the skin of a gardener's hands becomes thickened, giving extra protection. The aging process, during which the skin becomes wrinkled and less elastic, can be accelerated by smoking or excessive exposure to sun. Skin can also change colour. In direct sunlight, the epidermis and dermis produce extra melanin, a pigment that filters harmful ultraviolet rays and causes the skin to darken. People originating in areas that have strong sunlight tend to have darker skin, which does not burn as easily as lighter skin. The skin of people with fair complexions has less melanin and is more susceptible to sunburn.

STRUCTURE PARTS OF A NAIL

Protective plates called nails cover the ends of the fingers and toes. They consist mainly of keratin, the tough protein in hair and skin. Nails grow from the matrix, which lies below a fold of skin called the cuticle, and from the lunula, the crescent-shaped area at the base of the nail.

Nail structures
The most obvious part of a nail is the nail plate. This structure lies on the nail bed, an area rich in blood vessels.

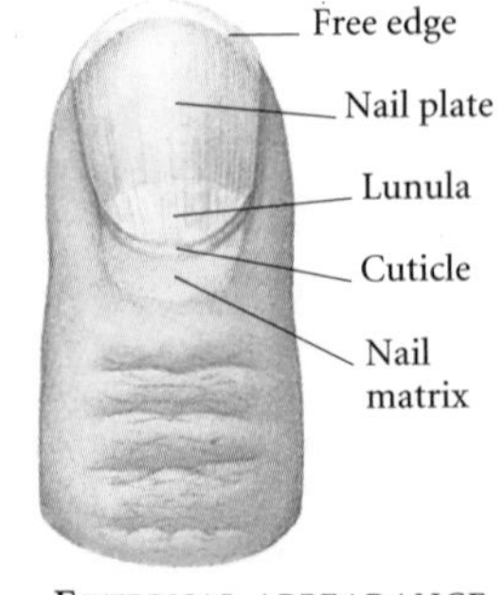

EXTERNAL APPEARANCE

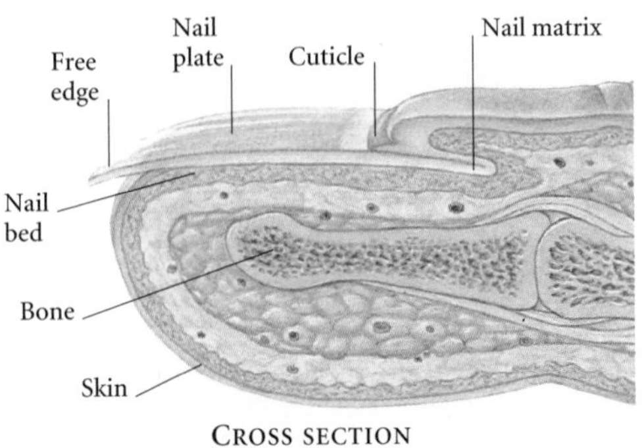

CROSS SECTION

STRUCTURE SKIN AND HAIR

The skin consists of two basic layers: the epidermis, which is the thin outer layer, and the dermis, which is the thick inner layer. The epidermis consists of sheets of tough, flat cells. Hair grows from hair follicles, which are modified regions of epidermis that reach into the dermis. New hair cells, made in the follicle, eventually die to form the scaly hair shaft. The dermis is made of strong, elastic tissue and contains blood vessels, glands, and nerve endings, which respond to stimuli such as heat, pressure, and pain.

Epidermal cell
Sweat pore

Pore surrounded by epidermal cells
Sweat from glands in the dermis reaches the skin's surface through pores such as this one. The large, upright flakes around the pore are dead epidermal cells.

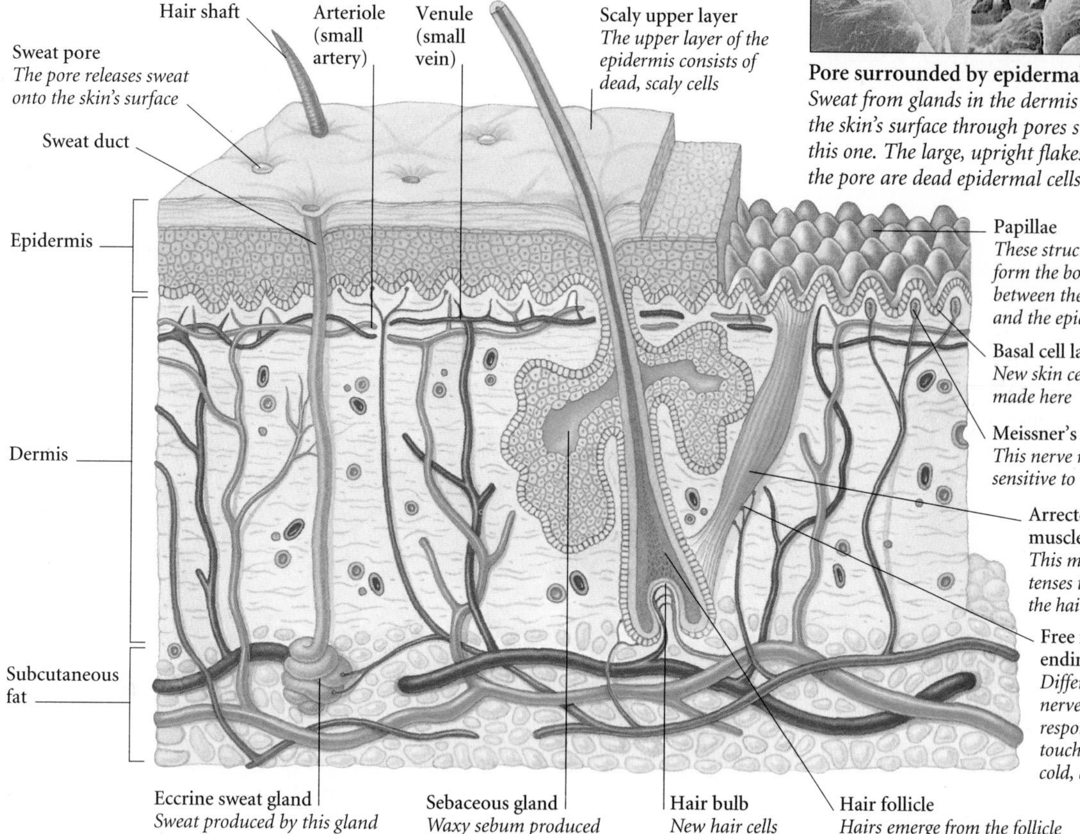

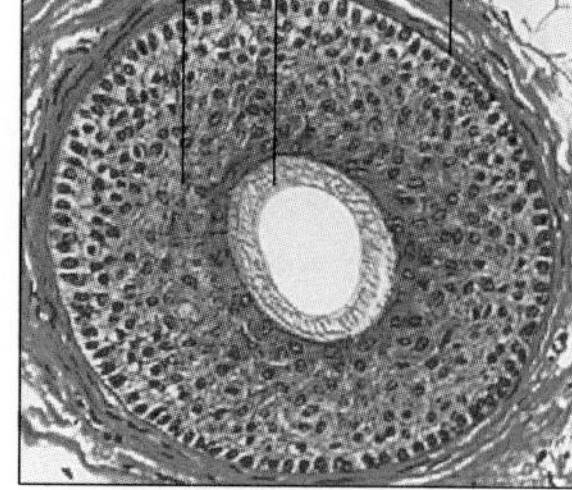

Magnified section of hair
Hair has three layers: the inner medulla (which is usually hollow), a thick pigmented cortex, and an outer cuticle.

STRUCTURE MUCOUS MEMBRANES

Mucous membranes are sheets of cells that protect body areas that must not dry out. These membranes line the mouth and nose; the insides of the eyelids; and the genital, digestive, and respiratory tracts. Special cells in the membranes, called goblet cells, secrete mucus, a sticky protein that lubricates and cleans. At the opening of body cavities, mucous membranes are continuous with the skin.

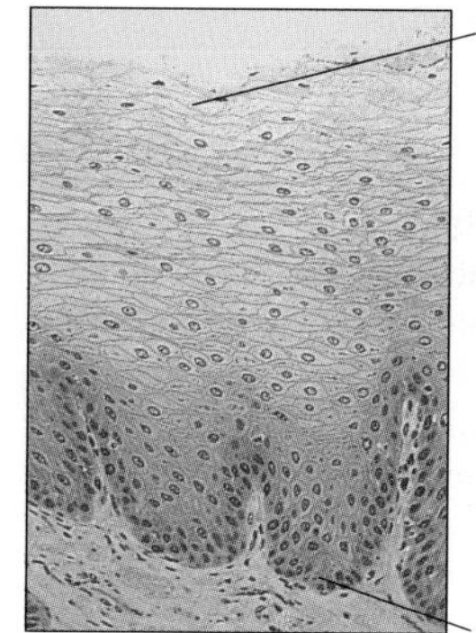

Membrane layers
The structure of mucous membranes – rapidly dividing cells in the basal layer below the layer of flat cells – is similar to that of the skin's epidermis, but lacks a thick, distinctive outer edge.

(FUNCTION) GROWTH AND REPAIR

The skin constantly renews itself by shedding dead cells from the surface and generating new cells below. As a result, surface cells that are lost through wear, damage, or disease are quickly replaced. New cells are made in the epidermis, the skin's upper layer, which serves as a tough, protective covering.

SKIN GROWTH

In most areas of the body, the epidermis has four layers. In the lowest, the basal layer, new cells are produced. As new cells move to the surface, they change to form intermediate layers of prickle cells and granular cells. The cells reach the surface in 1–2 months. The layer at the surface consists of dead, flat cells, which are continually shed.

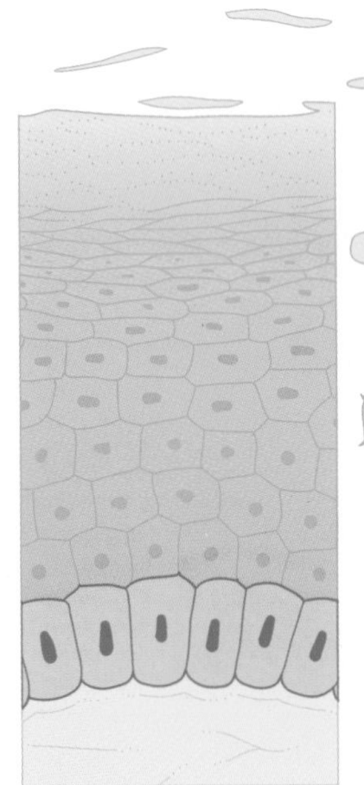

Surface layer cell
The dead, flat cells on the skin surface form a tough protective coating; the cells are constantly replaced as they wear away

Granular cell
The cells in the granular layer are flatter than the prickle cells, and their cellular structure has begun to break down

Prickle cell
Cells in the prickle cell layer have spiny projections that anchor them together, giving strength to the skin

Basal cell
The basal layer of cells adjoins the dermis. This area is where skin cells are continually dividing to make new cells, which then move up the layers

SKIN REPAIR

When the skin is injured, it responds by repairing the damaged tissue and replacing lost tissue with new cells. During the process of repair, dead or damaged tissue is initially supplanted by scar tissue and eventually by healthy new cells. In some cases, a scar remains. Skin repair takes place over a series of stages, shown below.

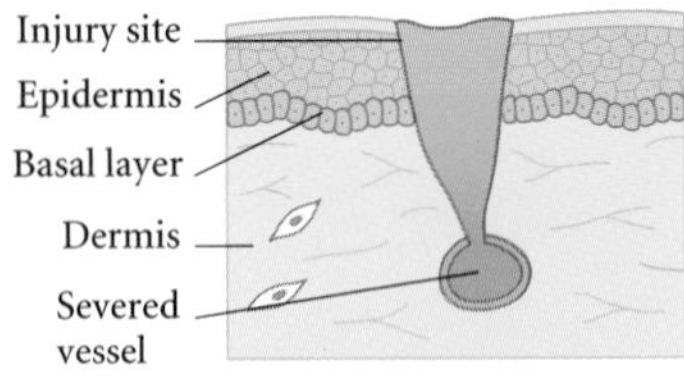

1 *Any injury in which the skin is broken, no matter how superficial the injury, may damage the blood vessels in the dermis and cause bleeding.*

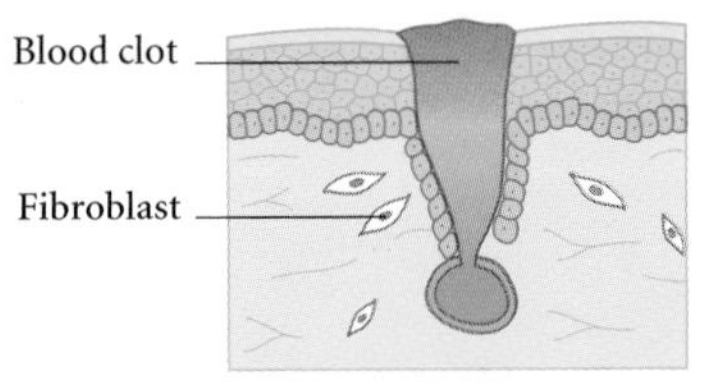

2 *Blood seeps from the blood vessels and forms a clot. Fibroblasts and other specialized repair cells multiply and migrate to the damaged area.*

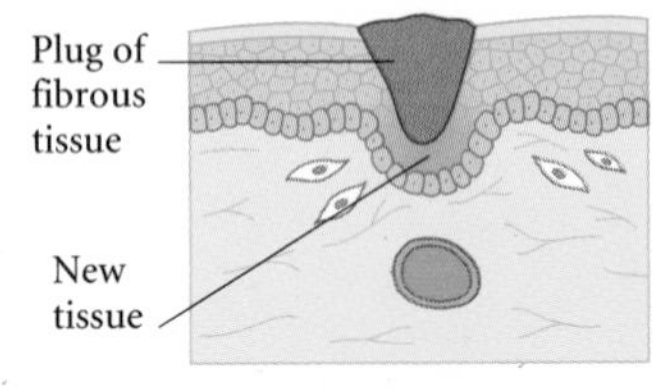

3 *Fibroblasts produce a plug of fibrous tissue within the clot. As strands of fibrin in the plug contract, the plug shrinks. New skin tissue forms beneath.*

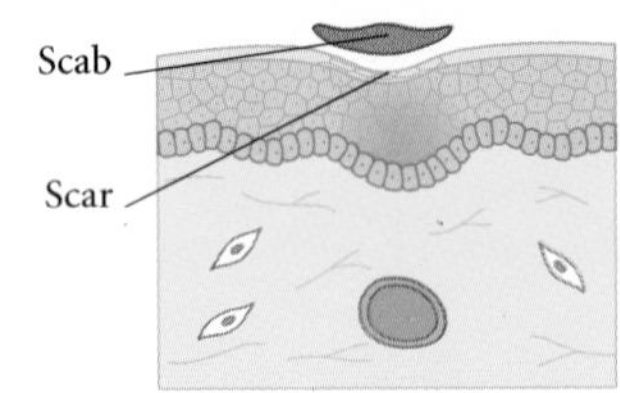

4 *The fibrous plug hardens to become a scab on the skin's surface, which falls off when new skin growth is complete. However, a scar may remain.*

HAIR GROWTH

Hair grows from a follicle, a specialized area of epidermis that grows down into the dermis. A hair is generated from rapidly dividing cells in the bulb at the base of the follicle. The papilla under the bulb contains blood vessels that carry nutrients. Each follicle has growth periods followed by rest phases. However, the phases of different follicles are not synchronized. Every day some hairs are growing while others are shed. A single hair grows between 6 mm (¼ in) and 8 mm (⅓ in) a month.

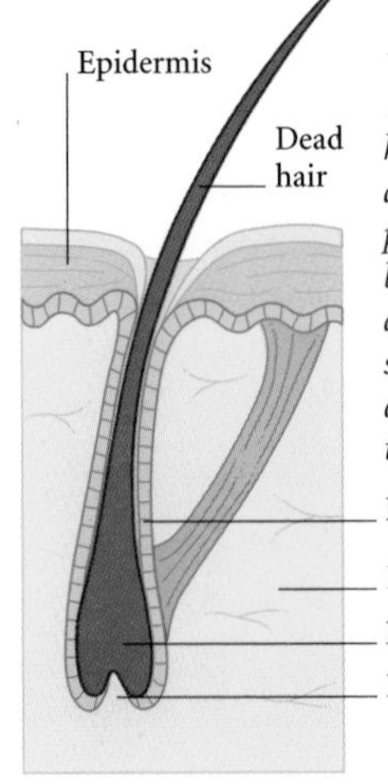

1 *During the rest phase of a hair follicle, cell activity in the papilla and hair bulb slows down and eventually stops. When cell activity stops, the hair dies.*

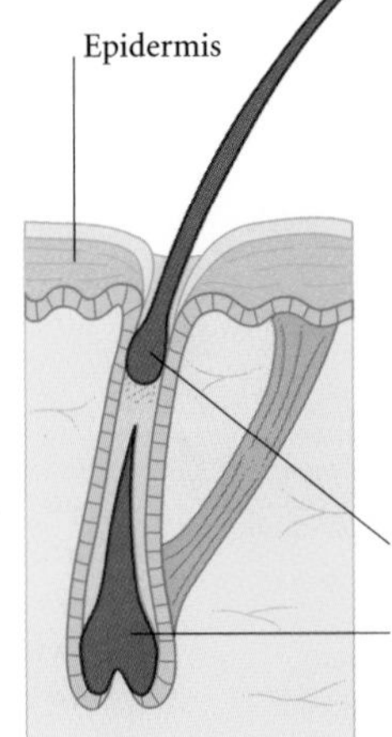

2 *During the growth phase, cells divide rapidly in the bulb and initiate the growth of a new hair. The new growing hair slowly pushes the dead hair out of the hair follicle.*

FUNCTION ROLES OF THE SKIN, HAIR, AND NAILS

All over the body, the skin carries out the same basic functions to protect us from injury and infection. The skin is important in thermoregulation (temperature control), which is controlled by the hypothalamus in the brain, and in responding to different stimuli. The pigment melanin gives the skin some protection from the harmful ultraviolet rays of the sun.

PROTECTION

Although the basic structure of the skin is the same over the entire body, there are local variations linked to differences in function. For example, the skin on the palms and soles has no hair. Further differences occur in colour and texture, and in the density of hair follicles, glands, nerve endings, and blood vessels.

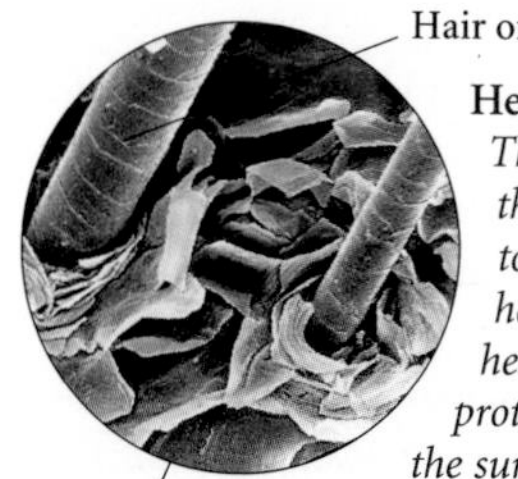

Head hair
Thick hair on the scalp helps to insulate the head against heat loss and protects it from the sun's effects.

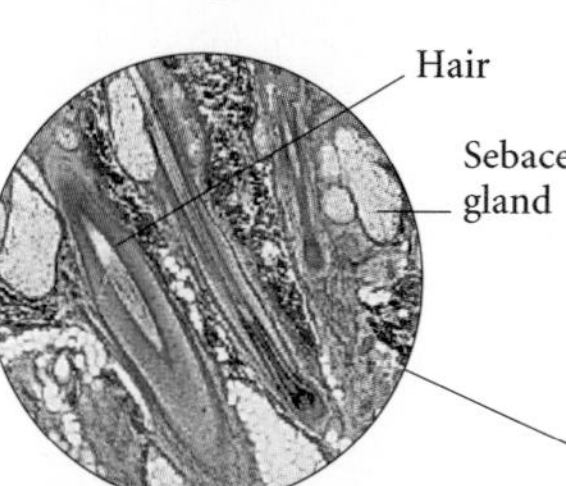

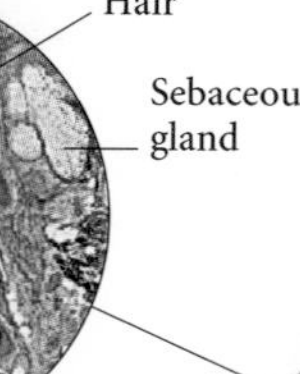

Sebaceous glands
These glands secrete sebum, which helps to waterproof and lubricate the skin.

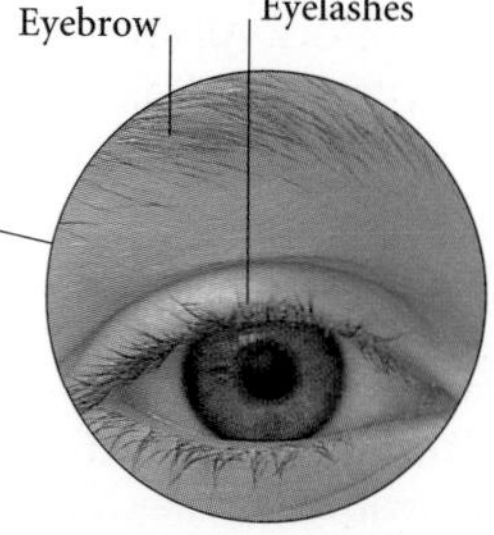

Eyelashes and eyebrows
Eyelashes protect the eye from foreign particles, and eyebrows direct sweat away from the eye.

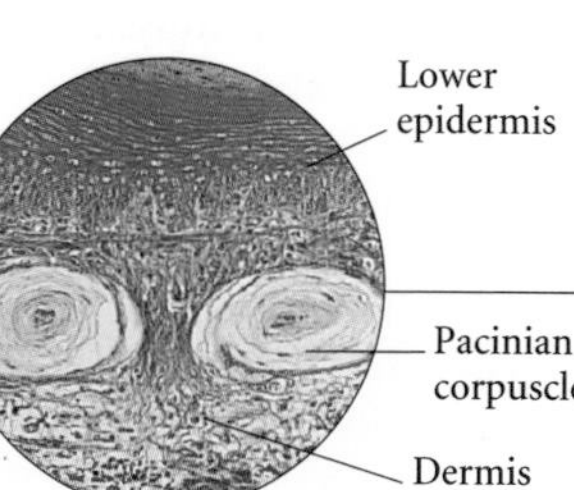

Pressure receptors
Pacinian corpuscles are receptors in the skin's dermis that warn of potentially damaging pressure.

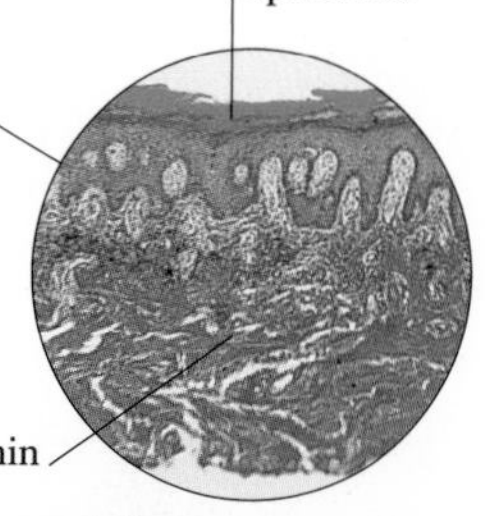

Pigmented skin
When exposed to sunlight, skin produces melanin, a pigment that filters out ultraviolet rays.

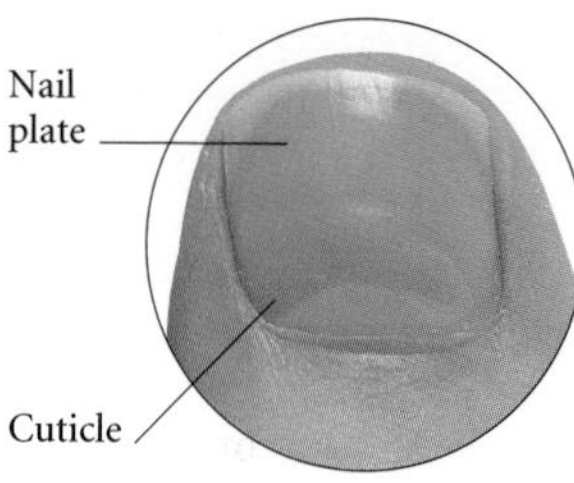

Nails
Tough plates made of keratin, a fibrous protein, cover the end of each digit to prevent injury.

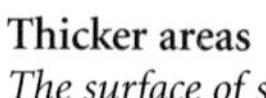

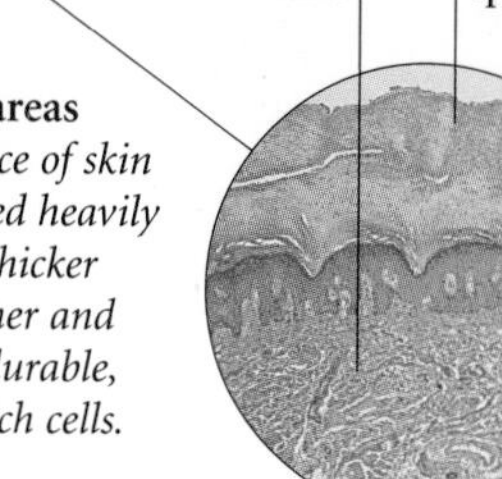

Thicker areas
The surface of skin that is used heavily becomes thicker and tougher and is full of durable, keratin-rich cells.

THERMOREGULATION

The skin plays a significant role in regulating body temperature. In contrast with some animals, humans do not possess a thick fur coat to provide warmth. Instead, we have a complex thermoregulation system that includes features such as special blood vessels in the skin that are concerned solely with conservation and loss of heat. A layer of fat under the skin provides extra insulation.

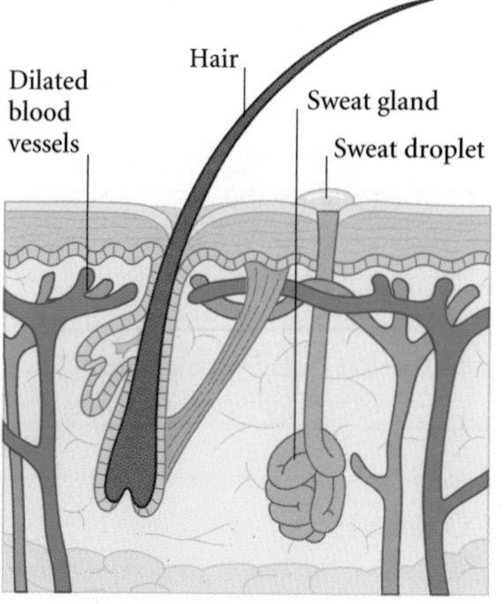

High body temperature
If the body is too hot, blood vessels dilate to let more blood reach the skin, where the blood cools. This causes the skin to look flushed. Sweat glands produce more sweat, which evaporates to cool the skin.

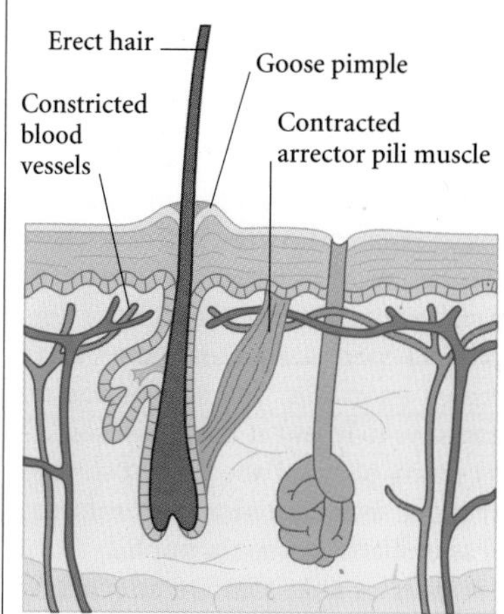

Low body temperature
If the body is too cold, the blood vessels narrow. The arrector pili muscles contract, lifting hairs and pulling on the skin to form goose pimples. The erect hairs trap an insulating layer of air next to the skin.

GENERALIZED SKIN CONDITIONS

Many skin disorders can affect several or all areas of the body surface at once. Some of these disorders have a strong inherited component, but often the cause of a particular condition is not known. Not all generalized skin problems are curable – some recur intermittently throughout life – but most can be controlled effectively with treatment and self-help measures.

Most generalized skin disorders do not pose a serious threat to health, but chronic conditions, such as psoriasis and eczema, can affect the quality of life and require long-term treatment. Other disorders cause only temporary discomfort and often clear up without treatment. Some conditions are the result of an allergy to substances such as drugs and disappear after the cause has been identified and eliminated.

The articles in this section discuss disorders that cause widespread rashes, itching, flaking, or blistering. Disorders that affect particular areas of skin are discussed elsewhere (*see* LOCALIZED SKIN CONDITIONS, pp.340–350, and SKIN INFECTIONS AND INFESTATIONS, pp.351–355). Disorders that affect the skin of children are discussed in a separate section (*see* INFANCY AND CHILDHOOD, pp.828–831). Rashes that affect the skin as part of an infectious disease, such as rubella or measles, are also found elsewhere (*see* INFECTIONS AND INFESTATIONS, pp.284–313).

KEY ANATOMY

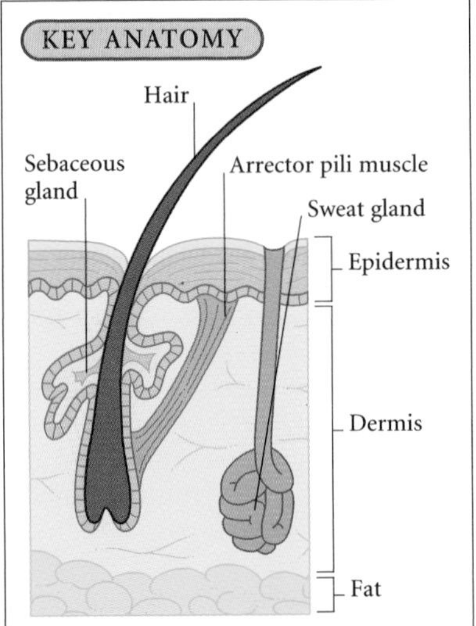

For further information on the structure and function of the skin, *see* pp.328–331.

Psoriasis

Patches of red, thickened, scaly skin, often affecting many areas of the body

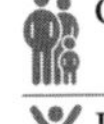 GENETICS Often runs in families

 LIFESTYLE May be aggravated by stress

 AGE Risk factor depends on the type

 GENDER Not a significant factor

Psoriasis is common in Western countries, Australia and South America, and parts of Asia and Africa. There are several types, most of which are difficult to control and flare up throughout life. Red, thickened, scaly skin occurs in all types of psoriasis. The scaly areas do not always itch, but if the condition affects many parts of the body, psoriasis may cause severe physical discomfort as well as embarrassment in public.

In areas of skin that are affected by psoriasis, new skin cells are produced at a much faster rate than dead cells are shed and the excess skin cells accumulate to form thick patches. The cause is not known, but an episode of psoriasis may be triggered or aggravated by infection, injury, or stress. The disorder often runs in families, which suggests that a genetic factor may be involved; approximately 1 in 3 people with psoriasis has a close relative who also has the condition. The use of certain drugs, such as antidepressants (p.916), antihypertensives (p.897), beta-blockers (p.898), and antimalarial drugs (p.888), can produce psoriasis in some people.

WHAT ARE THE TYPES?

There are four main types of psoriasis, each of which has a distinctive appearance. Some people may be affected by more than one type of the disorder.

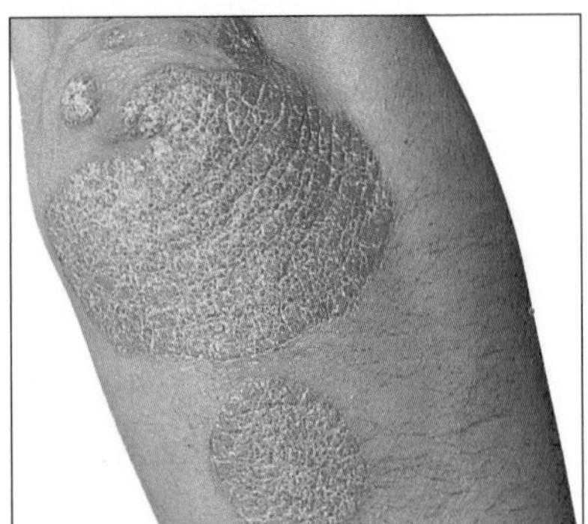

Plaque psoriasis on the elbow
The elbows are a common site for plaque psoriasis. The scaly surfaces of the patches are accumulations of dead skin cells.

PLAQUE PSORIASIS The most common form of psoriasis, plaque psoriasis is a lifelong disorder that may develop in people of any age. The condition may produce the following symptoms:

- Patches called plaques, consisting of thickened, red skin and scaly surfaces. They usually occur on the elbows, knees, lower back, and scalp; behind the ears; and at the hairline. In some cases, they develop on old scar tissue.
- Intermittent itching of affected areas.
- Discoloured nails that are covered with small pits. In severe cases, the nails lift away from the nail beds.

The symptoms of plaque psoriasis tend to continue for weeks or months and may recur intermittently.

GUTTATE PSORIASIS This form most commonly affects children and adolescents and often occurs after a bacterial throat infection. Typical symptoms are:

- Numerous coin-shaped, pink patches of scaly skin, each about 1 cm (3/8 in) across, mainly on the back and chest.
- Intermittent itching of the affected areas of skin.

These symptoms usually disappear in 4–6 months and do not recur, but more than half of those affected later develop another form of psoriasis.

Guttate psoriasis
The small, pink, scaly patches of guttate psoriasis are often spread over large areas. A typical site is the back, as shown above.

PUSTULAR PSORIASIS This is a rare but potentially life-threatening type of psoriasis that mainly affects adults. The condition may appear abruptly, with the following symptoms:

- Small blisters filled with pus that develop on the palms of the hands and the soles of the feet.
- Widespread areas of red, inflamed, and acutely tender skin.
- Some thickening and scaling of the inflamed areas.

In its most severe form, pustular psoriasis affects the entire body.

INVERSE PSORIASIS Elderly people are commonly affected by this type of psoriasis, in which large, moist, red areas develop in skin folds rather than over widespread body areas. The rash often affects the groin, the skin under the breasts, and sometimes the armpits. Inverse psoriasis usually clears up with treatment but may recur.

Are there complications?

About 1 in 10 people with psoriasis of any type develops a form of arthritis (p.374) that usually affects the fingers or knee joints. In pustular psoriasis, a massive loss of cells from the surface of the skin may lead to dehydration, kidney failure (p.705), infections, and high fever. If left untreated, the condition can be life-threatening.

What might be done?

Your doctor should be able to diagnose the type of psoriasis from its appearance. If you have only mild psoriasis that does not cause problems, you may decide not to treat the skin symptoms. Otherwise, you should follow the treatment that your doctor recommends.

TOPICAL TREATMENTS Psoriasis is commonly treated with emollients to soften the skin (*see* EMOLLIENTS AND BARRIER PREPARATIONS, p.890). Other common treatments are preparations containing coal tar or a substance called anthralin, which reduce inflammation and scaling. Coal tar and anthralin are effective but have an unpleasant smell and can stain clothing and bed linen. Anthralin should be applied to affected areas only because it can irritate healthy skin.

Alternatively, your doctor may prescribe a topical preparation containing the vitamin D derivative calcipotriol (*see* VITAMINS, p.927). The preparation is usually applied twice a day. It has no smell, does not stain skin or clothes, and is normally effective within about 4 weeks. You should follow the advice of your doctor because this treatment should not be used on the face or in the creases of the skin.

Topical corticosteroids (p.892) may also be prescribed. However, the drugs should be used sparingly because they may cause long-term side-effects, such as thinning of the skin.

GENERALIZED TREATMENTS For widespread psoriasis that does not respond to topical treatments, therapeutic exposure to ultraviolet (UV) light is often effective. UV therapy is usually given without oral medications. PUVA therapy involves using UV therapy together with psoralen, an oral drug that is taken before the ultraviolet light treatment and helps to make the skin more sensitive to the effects of light. This combined treatment slightly increases the risk of skin cancer and is given only under the supervision of a dermatologist.

Regular, short doses of sunlight often help to clear up psoriasis. Moderate exposure of affected areas to sunlight, if the weather is sufficiently warm, can be beneficial, but you should adopt sensible precautions to avoid sunburn (*see* SAFETY IN THE SUN, p.80).

In very severe cases of pustular psoriasis, for which topical preparations may not be effective, treatment with oral or intravenous drugs may be recommended. The drugs used for this treatment include retinoids (p.890), methotrexate (*see* ANTICANCER DRUGS, p.907), and cyclosporin (*see* IMMUNOSUPPRESSANTS, p.906). However, retinoid drugs and methotrexate can all cause abnormalities in a developing fetus. For this reason, you should not take any of these drugs if you are pregnant or planning to have a child.

What is the prognosis?

Although there is no cure for psoriasis, treatment can relieve the symptoms and help many people with the condition to lead a normal life. If psoriasis is a long-term problem, you may find it beneficial to join a self-help group.

(WWW) ONLINE SITES: p.1036

Eczema

Patches of red, blistering, itchy skin, also known as dermatitis

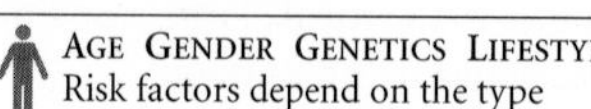

AGE GENDER GENETICS LIFESTYLE
Risk factors depend on the type

The main feature of eczema is red, inflamed, itchy skin that is often covered with small, fluid-filled blisters. In long-standing eczema, the affected skin may become thickened as a result of persistent scratching. Eczema tends to recur intermittently throughout life.

What are the types?

There are several different types of eczema. Some are triggered by particular factors, but others, such as nummular eczema, occur for no known reason.

ATOPIC ECZEMA This is the most common form of eczema. It usually appears first in infancy (*see* ECZEMA IN CHILDREN, p.829) and may continue to flare up during adolescence and adulthood (*see* ATOPIC ECZEMA, p.334). The cause of the condition is not known, but people who have an inherited tendency to allergies, including asthma (p.483), are more susceptible to it.

CONTACT DERMATITIS Direct contact with an irritant substance or an allergic reaction to a substance can result in a type of eczema known as contact dermatitis (p.335). It can occur at any age.

SEBORRHOEIC DERMATITIS This form of eczema affects infants and adults. The precise cause of seborrhoeic dermatitis (p.335) is unknown, although the condition is often associated with a yeast-like organism on the skin.

NUMMULAR ECZEMA Otherwise known as discoid eczema, this form of the condition is much more common in men than women. In nummular eczema, itchy, coin-shaped patches develop on the arms or legs, and the affected areas of skin may ooze and become scaly or blistered. The cause is not known.

ASTEATOTIC ECZEMA Most common in elderly people, this is caused by drying of the skin that occurs with aging. The scaly rash is random and cracked.

DYSHIDROTIC ECZEMA This type of eczema occurs where the skin is thickest, such as on the fingers, the palms of the hands, and the soles of the feet. Numerous itchy blisters develop, sometimes joining to form large, oozing areas. The cause is not known.

WHAT IS THE TREATMENT?

Try to keep your skin moist with emollients (*see* EMOLLIENTS AND BARRIER PREPARATIONS, p.890), take short, lukewarm showers or baths, and use mild soaps. Topical corticosteroids (p.892) help to reduce inflammation and itching. Avoid contact with substances that may irritate the skin. If contact dermatitis occurs, patch testing (opposite page) can be carried out to identify a trigger substance. Most forms of eczema can be controlled successfully.

(WWW) ONLINE SITES: p.1036

Atopic eczema

Itchy inflammation of the skin that appears in patches, usually in skin creases

AGE Usually first appears in infancy; sometimes persists into adulthood

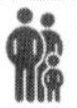
GENETICS Often runs in families

LIFESTYLE May be aggravated by extreme temperatures, certain foods, or stress

GENDER Not a significant factor

The intensely itchy rash that is typical of atopic eczema usually appears first in infancy and often disappears later in childhood (*see* ECZEMA IN CHILDREN, p.829). However, flare-ups of the rash can sometimes occur throughout adolescence and into adulthood. Atopic eczema often affects people with a family history of asthma (p.483) or other allergic disorders, such as hay fever (*see* ALLERGIC RHINITIS, p.466). Flare-ups in adulthood are sometimes linked to stress, temperature change, or an allergic reaction to certain foods. Often, there is no obvious reason for them.

WHAT ARE THE SYMPTOMS?

The rash usually appears in patches, typically on the hands, as well as in skin creases in areas such as the wrists, the backs of the knees, and the insides of the elbows. The symptoms may include:

- Redness and swelling of the skin.
- Small, fluid-filled blisters.
- Itching, especially at night.
- Dry, scaly, and cracked skin.
- Thickened skin as a result of continuous scratching.

Bacterial infection sometimes develops in the affected area, resulting in further swelling and discomfort.

WHAT MIGHT BE DONE?

Your doctor will probably be able to diagnose atopic eczema from the symptoms. He or she may suggest a topical corticosteroid (p.892) to reduce the inflammation. You should apply this sparingly and reduce the frequency of use when the rash begins to clear up. Avoid using topical corticosteroids on the face unless directed otherwise by your doctor. Oral antihistamines may help to relieve the itching (*see* ANTIPRURITIC DRUGS, p.891). If the rash is infected, you will be prescribed oral antibiotics (p.885) or topical antibiotics (*see* PREPARATIONS FOR SKIN INFECTIONS AND INFESTATIONS, p.892).

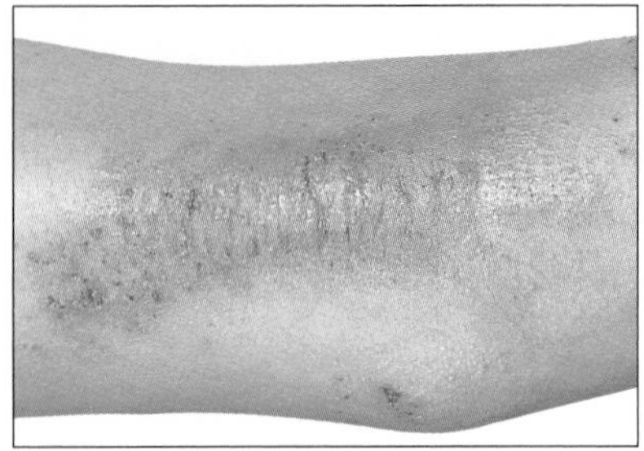

Atopic eczema
The itchy, dry, inflamed rash of atopic eczema typically develops in skin creases, such as the inside of the elbow.

You can relieve the symptoms by using emollients (*see* EMOLLIENTS AND BARRIER PREPARATIONS, p.890) and specially formulated bath oil that you can buy over the counter. Self-help measures can be used between flare-ups (*see* MANAGING HAND ECZEMA, below).

WHAT IS THE PROGNOSIS?

Atopic eczema can be controlled but not cured, and new patches of affected skin may appear at any time. However, the condition usually improves with age and is rare in elderly people.

(WWW) ONLINE SITES: p.1036

(SELF-HELP) MANAGING HAND ECZEMA

Eczema on the hands can be particularly persistent, painful, and unattractive. The following tips may help keep your eczema under control and reduce flare-ups:

- Avoid immersing your hands in water for long periods. If possible, wear cotton gloves inside rubber gloves for protection.
- Protect your hands with gloves or a barrier cream before cleaning, gardening, carrying out home repairs, or using irritant substances.
- Remove rings before using detergents or chemicals to prevent these irritant substances from becoming trapped against the skin.
- Apply emollient creams frequently to moisturize the skin, and wash with mild soaps.

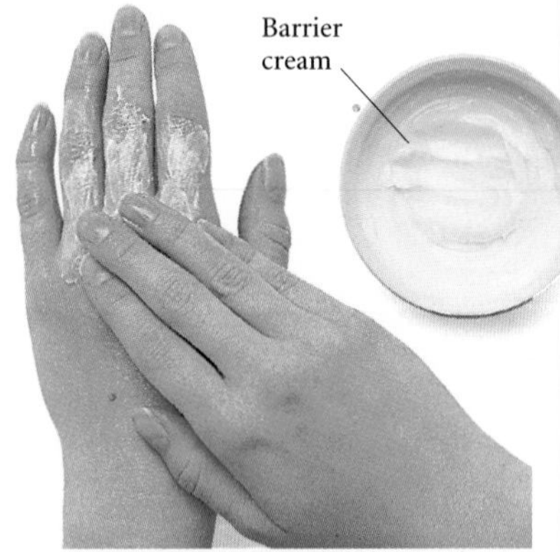

Applying barrier cream
You can help prevent irritants such as detergents from coming into contact with the skin by applying a barrier cream before carrying out chores. Emollient creams, which moisturize the skin, should be used after washing.

Contact dermatitis

Patches of red, itchy, and flaking skin caused by irritation or allergy

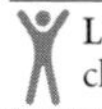
LIFESTYLE Work involving exposure to chemicals or detergents is a risk factor

AGE GENDER GENETICS Not significant factors

As its name implies, contact dermatitis is inflammation of the skin caused by contact with a specific substance. There are two types: irritant contact dermatitis, which is caused by primary irritants (substances, such as bleach, that harm anyone's skin); and allergic contact dermatitis, which occurs when a person comes into contact with a particular substance to which he or she has developed a sensitivity over time.

Substances that commonly trigger irritation or allergic reactions include some cosmetics; the nickel contained in jewellery, buttons, earrings for pierced ears, or watch straps; certain chemicals; drugs in some skin creams; and certain plants, such as ragweed.

WHAT ARE THE SYMPTOMS?

Contact dermatitis usually affects only the area that has been in direct contact with the substance that triggered the reaction. In irritant contact dermatitis, the skin inflammation develops soon after contact with the substance. The severity of the resulting rash depends both on the concentration of the irritant and on the duration of exposure.

Allergic contact dermatitis usually develops slowly over a period of time, and it is possible to have contact with a substance for several years without any skin inflammation occurring. However, once your skin has become sensitive to the substance, even a small amount of it or a short exposure time can trigger an allergic reaction.

In either form of contact dermatitis, the symptoms may include:

- Redness and swelling of the skin.
- Water- or pus-filled blisters that may ooze, drain, or become encrusted.
- Flaking skin, which may develop into raw patches.
- Persistent itching.

Consult your doctor if the cause of the contact dermatitis is not obvious or if the inflammation persists for a longer period of time than usual.

WHAT MIGHT BE DONE?

Your doctor will want to know when the skin inflammation developed and whether you have any known allergies. The site of the reaction is often a clue to its cause. For example, a patch of dermatitis on the wrist may be caused by an allergy to nickel in a watch or watch strap. People who handle chemicals at work often develop irritant or allergic contact dermatitis on their hands.

Your doctor may prescribe a topical corticosteroid (p.892) to relieve itching and inflammation. However, even with treatment, contact dermatitis may take a few weeks to clear up.

If you handle chemicals at work, it is particularly important to find the cause of your skin allergy. If the cause cannot easily be identified, you may need to have patch testing (below).

Once the trigger has been identified, try to avoid it as much as possible. If you cannot do so, you may need to cover your skin with creams (*see* EMOLLIENTS AND BARRIER PREPARATIONS, p.890), protective clothing, or gloves before you are exposed to the trigger.

(WWW) ONLINE SITES: p.1036

Seborrhoeic dermatitis

Patches of red, scaly, itchy skin that occur mainly on the scalp, face, and chest

LIFESTYLE Stress can trigger an attack

AGE GENDER GENETICS Not significant factors

Seborrhoeic dermatitis is a rash that commonly occurs in infants and adults. In infants, either the scalp or the nappy area may be affected by the rash (*see* CRADLE CAP, p.829, and NAPPY RASH, p.829). In adults, the rash tends to occur on the central part of the face, the eyebrows, and the scalp, where it often leads to flaking of the skin. Seborrhoeic dermatitis can also develop in the armpits, the groins, or the middle of the chest. In men, the condition sometimes develops in the beard area.

The cause is unknown, but seborrhoeic dermatitis is sometimes linked with the overgrowth of a yeast-like substance that is present naturally on the surface of the skin. The condition can recur and flare-ups may be triggered by a period of stress or illness.

(TEST) PATCH TESTING

Patch testing is carried out on people with contact dermatitis. The test is performed by a dermatologist to find out which substances provoke an allergic reaction. Possible allergens (substances that can cause an allergic reaction) are diluted and placed on small strips or discs. The test discs are then stuck to the skin using inert (nonallergenic) tape. After 48 hours, the discs are removed and the skin underneath them is examined. A red, inflamed patch indicates a positive reaction to an allergen. The tested area is examined again 2 days later to check for delayed reactions.

Inert tape

Disc of test substance

1 *Minute quantities of test substances are placed on small discs. The discs are stuck with inert tape to an inconspicuous area of the skin, usually on the back.*

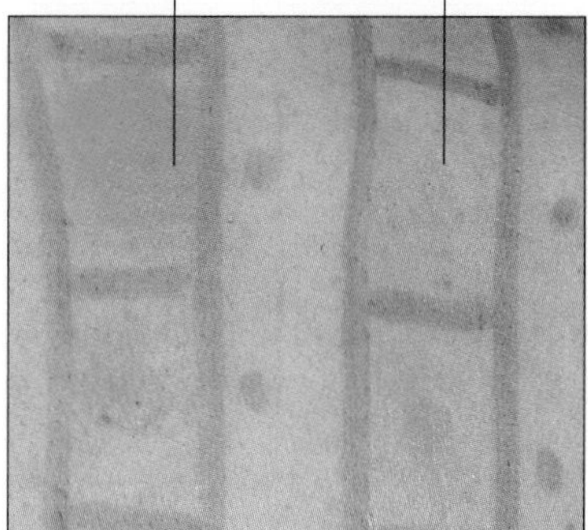

2 *When the discs are removed from the skin after 48 hours, positive reactions to allergens appear as red patches. In some cases, reactions may take longer to appear.*

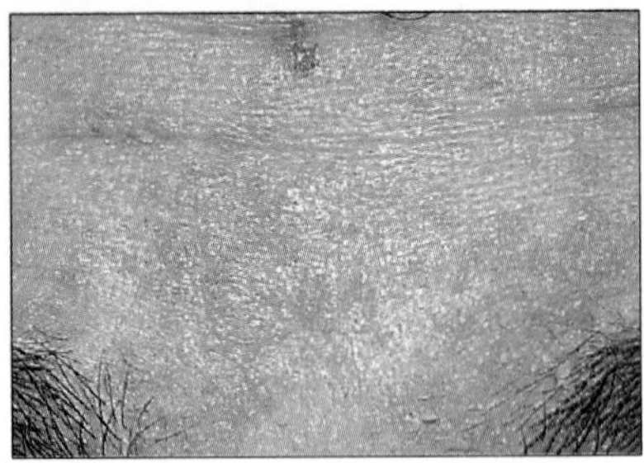

Seborrhoeic dermatitis on the forehead
The forehead and eyebrows are common sites for seborrhoeic dermatitis. Flakes of skin may become trapped in the eyebrows.

What are the symptoms?

The symptoms of seborrhoeic dermatitis may include the following:

- Scaly, red patches of inflamed skin, often with a yellow crust.
- Eyelids that are sore, red, and crusty (*see* BLEPHARITIS, p.583).
- Excessive dandruff (p.358).
- Occasional itching of affected areas.

The rash may flare up intermittently over a period of months or years.

What might be done?

If a yeast overgrowth is diagnosed, your doctor may prescribe a topical corticosteroid (p.892) or an antifungal drug (p.889). If your scalp is affected, he or she may prescribe an antifungal shampoo or recommend that you use a coal tar shampoo. Both should produce a rapid improvement in symptoms.

(WWW) ONLINE SITES: p.1036

Blistering diseases

Disorders of various types that cause eruptions of blisters

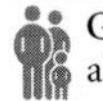
GENETICS Some types are due to an abnormal gene inherited from both parents

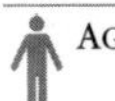
AGE Risk factor depends on the type

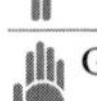
GENDER LIFESTYLE Not significant factors

There are several uncommon diseases that produce eruptions of blistering on the surface of the skin. These blistering diseases may either occur in particular sites or cover widespread areas of the body. In contrast to individual blisters (p.357), which are minor skin injuries, blistering diseases can be serious. Left untreated, these diseases may eventually become life-threatening.

What are the types?

Some rare types of blistering disease are present at birth and are caused by an abnormal gene inherited from both parents in an autosomal recessive manner (*see* GENE DISORDERS, p.271). These diseases cause the skin over the whole body to become very fragile and blister when touched. They may be fatal.

More commonly, blistering diseases are acquired in adulthood. There are three main types of these diseases; all of them are autoimmune disorders, in which the body produces antibodies that are damaging to the skin.

PEMPHIGOID The most common type of blistering disease is pemphigoid. The disorder affects people over the age of 60. It results in numerous tightly filled blisters, mainly on the legs and trunk, each measuring up to 3 cm (1¼ in) across. Initially, the blisters may itch.

PEMPHIGUS Less common than pemphigoid, pemphigus also usually affects people over the age of 60. In this condition, blisters may appear on any part of the body but often occur around the eyes and inside the mouth. The blisters are fragile and may rupture spontaneously, leaving patches of raw skin.

DERMATITIS HERPETIFORMIS This disorder is associated with an allergy to gluten, the protein in wheat (*see* COELIAC DISEASE, p.658). The condition results in itchy blisters, usually on the elbows, buttocks, and knees.

What might be done?

In all types of blistering disease, diagnosis is usually based on a skin biopsy (p.344). This procedure involves taking a sample of skin for examination.

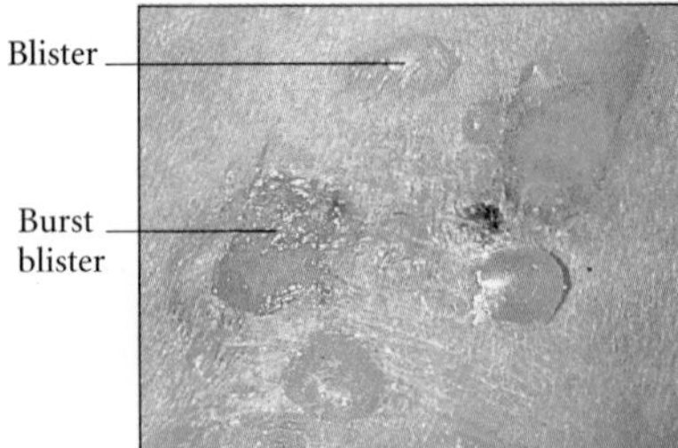

Blistering caused by pemphigoid
Severe blistering of the skin is the main symptom of pemphigoid, an autoimmune disorder usually affecting elderly people.

There is no effective treatment for inherited blistering diseases. Parents of babies who have these diseases may wish to seek genetic counselling (p.272) to discuss the likelihood of further children also being affected.

If you have either pemphigoid or pemphigus, your doctor will prescribe oral corticosteroids (p.930). Some people will also need immunosuppressants (p.906) for several weeks or months. If you have severe pemphigus, you may need immediate treatment in hospital with immunosuppressants.

In most cases, dermatitis herpetiformis disappears once the affected person has adopted a gluten-free diet, but the drug dapsone may also be needed to help clear up the blisters.

What is the prognosis?

The blistering diseases that affect adults can often be controlled with treatment, but very few cases can be permanently cured. Although pemphigoid may disappear spontaneously in 2–5 years, pemphigus often needs lifelong treatment with drugs. The allergic condition dermatitis herpetiformis may recur if gluten is reintroduced into the diet.

(WWW) ONLINE SITES: p.1033, p.1036

Lichen planus

An itchy rash consisting of small, raised, flat-topped lesions that are shiny and pink or purple in colour

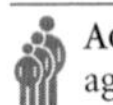
AGE More common in people over the age of 30

LIFESTYLE Stress may increase the risk

GENDER GENETICS Not significant factors

In lichen planus, small, shiny, itchy lesions appear in a dense cluster. Often, there is no obvious cause, but occasionally the rash may develop as a reaction to certain drugs, such as sulphonamide antibiotics (p.885) or gold-based antirheumatic drugs (p.895). Lichen planus may be associated with stress. It is more common in people over the age of 30.

What are the symptoms?

The rash can develop in patches on the lower back and on the inner surfaces of the wrists, forearms, and ankles. Lichen planus often appears suddenly and may

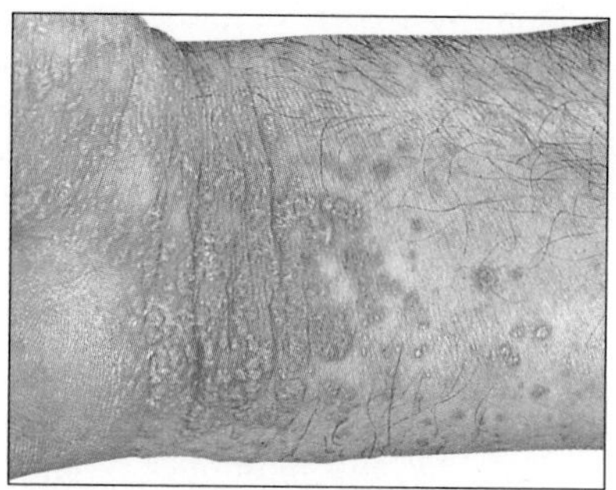

Lichen planus on the wrist
The inner surface of the wrist, shown above, is one of the areas where the itchy lesions of lichen planus may appear.

affect more than one area, but sometimes the rash spreads gradually over a period of a few months. The symptoms of lichen planus include:

- Groups of small, shiny, pink or purple, flat-topped lesions on the skin; the surface of some may be covered by a network of fine white lines.
- Intense itching, particularly at night.

The disorder can also affect the nails and scalp. If lichen planus develops in the nails, they become ridged along their length and, in some cases, fall off (*see* NAIL ABNORMALITIES, p.360).

If the scalp is affected, patchy hair loss with associated scarring of the scalp may occur. The lesions may also appear on the sites of skin injury such as scratches. Another form of lichen planus affects the mouth (*see* ORAL LICHEN PLANUS, p.634).

WHAT MIGHT BE DONE?

If the diagnosis is not obvious from the appearance of the rash, your doctor may arrange for a skin biopsy (p.344), in which a sample of skin is removed and examined under a microscope. To relieve the itching, the doctor may prescribe a strong topical corticosteroid (p.892). In addition, you can take an over-the-counter oral antihistamine (*see* ANTIPRURITIC DRUGS, p.891) for relief at night. If the rash is widespread and affects your nails or scalp, you may need oral corticosteroid drugs (p.930).

If a drug reaction is suspected, your doctor will advise you to stop taking the drug and may prescribe an alternative. Lichen planus usually persists for 12–18 months and may leave patches of darkened skin where it has healed.

WWW ONLINE SITES: p.1036

Erythema multiforme

A red rash usually forming concentric rings with purplish centres

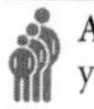
AGE Most common in children and young adults

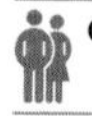
GENDER More common in males

GENETICS LIFESTYLE Not significant factors

Erythema multiforme develops rapidly and is characterized by distinctive red spots that grow bigger over a few days. The rash is widespread, and often includes the palms of the hands and the soles of the feet. It may affect the mucous membranes, such as the lining of the mouth and nose. The rash is most common in young people and affects more males than females. The disorder is not contagious and is usually mild, although a serious form sometimes occurs.

In most cases, the cause of erythema multiforme is unknown, but the rash can be triggered by infection with a virus such as herpes simplex, the virus that produces cold sores (p.354). Other factors that can trigger the rash include taking certain drugs, such as sulphonamide antibiotics (p.885), phenytoin (*see* ANTICONVULSANT DRUGS, p.914), or the vaccine for poliomyelitis (p.295). Erythema multiforme can also be caused by cancer or by radiotherapy (p.281).

WHAT ARE THE SYMPTOMS?

The symptoms, which develop suddenly, may include:

- Many small, red spots distributed symmetrically over the body. The spots usually enlarge to form red rings with purplish centres, called target lesions. The lesions may blister in the middle.

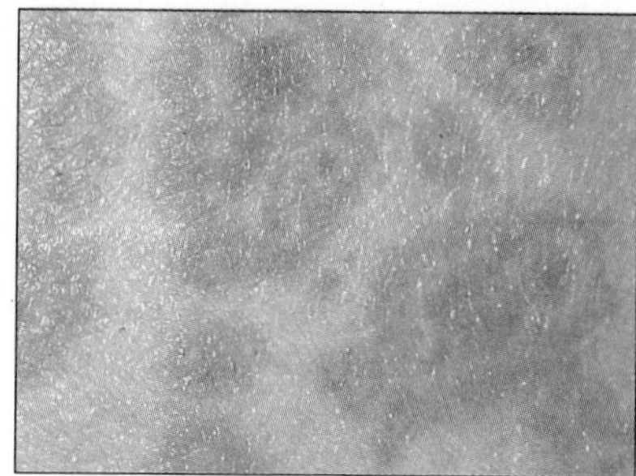

Erythema multiforme
The rash of erythema multiforme usually consists of concentric red rings, often with purplish centres (target lesions).

- Itching of the affected area.
- Painful, inflamed lesions within the mouth and nose.
- Fever, headache, and sore throat.
- Occasionally, diarrhoea.

In rare instances, most of the skin and mucous membranes throughout the body become severely inflamed and ulcerated. Such cases require emergency treatment because the condition may be life-threatening if it is left untreated.

WHAT MIGHT BE DONE?

Your doctor will probably make a diagnosis from the appearance of the rash. If the rash appeared shortly after you started taking a prescribed drug, the doctor may prescribe an alternative treatment. If itching is a problem, he or she may suggest an oral antihistamine (*see* ANTIPRURITIC DRUGS, p.891). In the case of severe erythema multiforme, particularly if the mouth is inflamed, you may need treatment in hospital; intravenous fluids, painkillers (p.912), and corticosteroids (p.930) may be given in an intensive care unit.

Erythema multiforme usually disappears over a few weeks. However, there is a possibility that it may recur. If a drug is thought to be the cause, you should avoid taking it in future.

WWW ONLINE SITES: p.1036

Pityriasis rosea

A rash of oval, pink, flat spots, most commonly affecting the trunk and limbs

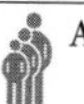
AGE Mainly affects young adults

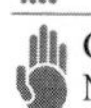
GENDER GENETICS LIFESTYLE Not significant factors

Pityriasis rosea produces a mild, pink rash. The condition most commonly occurs in young adults. It usually affects the trunk, arms, and upper thighs; more rarely, it affects the feet, hands, and scalp. The condition is thought to be caused by a viral infection.

WHAT ARE THE SYMPTOMS?

The symptoms change over time as the condition progresses. They usually develop in the following order:

- An oval patch, 2–6 cm (¾–2½ in) in diameter, known as a herald patch, appears. This patch resembles those that occur in ringworm (p.352).

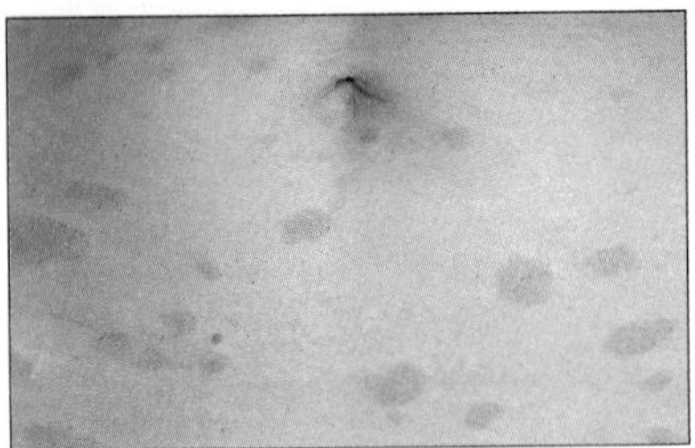

Pityriasis rosea
Oval, pink, flat spots, shown here on the abdomen, are typical of pityriasis rosea, which may affect several parts of the body.

- About 3–10 days later, a number of smaller oval, pink, flat spots, 1–2 cm (1/4–3/4 in) in diameter, appears. The rash begins on the trunk, spreading across the abdomen, along the thighs and upper arms, and up towards the neck. The spots on the back usually occur in sweeping lines, resembling the shape of a Christmas tree.
- A scaly margin may appear around the edges of the patches after a week.

Itching may occur and is occasionally troublesome. Although pityriasis rosea is not serious, it is important to consult your doctor to rule out conditions such as psoriasis (p.332) and eczema (p.333).

WHAT MIGHT BE DONE?

The distinctive rash makes the condition easy to diagnose. It usually clears up after about 6–8 weeks without treatment and is unlikely to reappear.

(WWW) ONLINE SITES: p.1036

Photosensitivity

Sensitivity of the skin to ultraviolet light, resulting in redness and discomfort

 AGE GENDER GENETICS LIFESTYLE
Not significant factors

Photosensitivity is defined as an abnormal reaction of the skin to the effects of ultraviolet rays in sunlight. The condition is sometimes present at birth and sometimes develops later in life.

Various substances may cause photosensitivity, including drugs such as tetracyclines (*see* ANTIBIOTICS, p.885), diuretics (p.902), and oral contraceptives. Photosensitivity may also result from the use of certain cosmetics. The condition sometimes occurs in people who have systemic lupus erythematosus (p.461), an autoimmune disorder in which the body attacks its own tissues. Sometimes there is no obvious cause. In these cases, the condition is referred to as primary photosensitivity.

WHAT ARE THE SYMPTOMS?

The reaction occurs in areas frequently exposed to sunlight, such as the face and hands. It usually develops shortly after exposure but may be delayed for 24–48 hours. The symptoms include:

- Red, often painful rash.
- Small, itchy blisters.
- Scaly skin.

At a later stage, the nails may lift from the nail beds. Sometimes, affected people also develop generalized redness on all exposed skin. In rare cases, people with severe photosensitivity are unable to go outdoors in daylight.

WHAT MIGHT BE DONE?

Your doctor will probably make a diagnosis from the appearance of the rash. If the reaction is thought to be caused by a drug, the doctor may prescribe an alternative. You may also need blood tests to check for underlying disorders.

To relieve the symptoms, you may need to take a topical corticosteroid (p.892) or oral antihistamine (*see* ANTIPRURITIC DRUGS, p.891). Severe cases are treated with controlled exposure to ultraviolet light, sometimes combined with drugs, to desensitize the skin.

You can help control the reaction by avoiding sunlight as much as possible. When outdoors, cover your skin, wear a hat, and use a high-factor sunblock (*see* SAFETY IN THE SUN, p.80).

(WWW) ONLINE SITES: p.1036

Drug-induced rashes

Many different kinds of rash that occur in some people during or after treatment with certain drugs

 AGE GENDER GENETICS LIFESTYLE
Not significant factors

Rashes are a common side-effect of drug treatment. The reaction is caused by an allergic response to the drug or to substances produced when the drug is broken down by the body.

Reactions to drugs can produce almost any type of rash, including some forms that mimic other disorders, such as lichen planus (p.336) or erythema multiforme (p.337). However, the majority of drug-induced rashes appear as raised areas of skin spread widely over the body. Drug-induced rashes may be accompanied by intense itching. Sometimes, even when a rash is mild, there may be other, more dramatic effects such as wheezing and collapse. Occasionally, people with severe reactions need hospital treatment.

The drugs that most often produce rashes are antibiotics (p.885), such as penicillin, but almost all drug treatments can cause an allergic reaction if a person becomes sensitive to them. Drug-induced rashes usually develop within the first few days of starting treatment but can also occur after a course of treatment has finished.

Sensitivity develops after at least one previous exposure to a drug. It is common for people to take a certain drug for the first time without experiencing any allergic reaction and then to develop a rash when the drug is taken in a subsequent course of treatment.

WHAT MIGHT BE DONE?

If you develop a rash while you are taking a drug, you should consult your doctor before the next dose is due. He or she may then stop the treatment or prescribe another drug.

If you have been taking several drugs and one of these could have caused the rash, you must tell your doctor about all the drugs you have taken recently, including over-the-counter treatments, drugs that have been prescribed in hospital, and medicines prescribed by another doctor. You should also tell the doctor about any recreational drugs that you may be taking.

Most drug-induced rashes disappear when the drug responsible is stopped. However, the symptoms may continue for weeks afterwards. If itching is a problem, your doctor may advise that you apply a topical corticosteroid (p.892) or take an oral antihistamine (*see* ANTIPRURITIC DRUGS, p.891); both types of drug are available over the counter and by prescription.

Once you know you are allergic to a drug, you should make sure you notify any doctor who treats you in future. If you have had a severe reaction to a particular drug, you should consider wearing a medical alert tag.

Itching

An irritating sensation in the skin, either localized or widespread

AGE GENDER GENETICS LIFESTYLE
Risk factors depend on the cause

Itching, also known as pruritus, is a very common symptom and is associated with many skin disorders. The irritation may be either restricted to a small area or widespread over the body. Continual scratching, which often damages the skin, aggravates the problem.

WHAT ARE THE CAUSES?

Localized itching can often be the result of an insect bite. Itching may also be associated with a rash. An itchy rash is the main symptom of conditions such as urticaria (p.468), eczema (p.333), lichen planus (p.336), and parasitic skin infestations such as scabies (p.355).

Widespread itching may develop as a result of dry skin, an irritant reaction to particular bath products or detergents, or an allergic reaction to certain drugs (*see* DRUG ALLERGY, p.467). It can also occur as a symptom of a serious underlying disorder, such as liver disease or chronic kidney failure (p.706).

Persistent patches of itchy skin may develop as a result of emotional stress. The itching typically affects the limbs and neck but can also involve other areas of the body. Frequent scratching, often unconsciously, causes the skin to thicken and can increase the itching, leading to a further cycle of scratching and itching. This condition, known as lichen simplex or neurodermatitis, is more common in females.

WHAT CAN I DO?

There are several measures that you can take to relieve itching and stop scratching. Emollients (*see* EMOLLIENTS AND BARRIER PREPARATIONS, p.890) will help to moisturize dry and itchy skin, particularly if you apply them after washing or bathing. To relieve severe itching, you may find that using over-the-counter oral antihistamines (*see* ANTIPRURITIC DRUGS, p.891), topical corticosteroids (p.892), or calamine is helpful.

As far as possible, you should avoid substances that are likely to irritate the skin, such as scented bath products, detergents, or woollen garments. You may benefit from wearing loose-fitting clothing made of fabric that does not irritate the skin and from keeping your fingernails cut short so that you cannot damage your skin when scratching.

You should contact your doctor if you have persistent itching for which there is no obvious cause.

WWW ONLINE SITES: p.1036

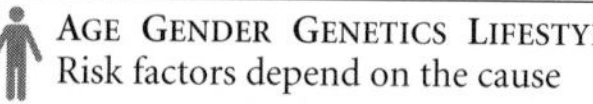

Purpura

A group of disorders in which reddish-purple spots appear on the skin

AGE GENDER GENETICS LIFESTYLE
Risk factors depend on the cause

In the conditions known as purpura, reddish-purple spots or bruise-like discolorations develop on the skin. The spots or bruises, called purpuric spots, result from small areas of bleeding under the skin and may be caused by damaged blood vessels or by an abnormality in the blood. The appearance of the spots varies, and they can range from the size of a pinhead to about 2.5 cm (1 in) in diameter. Unlike many other red rashes, purpuric spots do not fade when they are pressed.

The spots themselves are harmless, but purpura is sometimes a sign of a potentially serious underlying disorder.

WHAT ARE THE TYPES?

The most common type of purpura is senile purpura, which occurs mainly in elderly people. The condition gives rise to dark bruises, typically on the backs of the hands and forearms and on the thighs. Senile purpura is due to weakening of the tissues that support the blood vessels under the skin; these weakened blood vessels become susceptible to damage and bleed easily.

Very small purpuric spots, known as petechiae, often result from a reduction in the number of platelets (cells in the body that help the blood to clot). Platelet deficiency can be associated with many bone marrow disorders, such as leukaemia (p.453), or with autoimmune disorders (p.461). The condition may also occur as a side-effect of treatment with some drugs, such as diuretic drugs (p.902) or antibiotics (p.885).

Purpuric spots of variable size may be a sign of a serious bacterial infection of the blood (*see* SEPTICAEMIA, p.299). In some people, the infection may be due to a type of bacterium called meningococcus, which can result in potentially life-threatening meningitis (p.527). If purpura appears in conjunction with a fever, you should seek emergency medical advice.

Henoch-Schönlein purpura (p.838) is an uncommon type of purpura occurring in childhood and caused by inflammation of small blood vessels. The spots that appear in this condition are unlike those in other forms of purpura and resemble small, raised lumps.

WHAT MIGHT BE DONE?

Senile purpura is usually diagnosed from the bruise-like appearance of the spots. The condition is harmless, and no treatment is needed. The spots fade gradually but are likely to recur.

Any obvious underlying disorder, such as meningitis, will be treated. If the cause of the purpura is not obvious, your doctor may arrange for blood tests to find out if the platelet levels in the blood and the ability of the blood to clot are normal.

If blood tests show an abnormality, your doctor may refer you to a specialist for further investigations. If you are found to have a very low platelet count, you may be given platelet transfusions to prevent serious internal bleeding from occurring, especially in the brain, until the underlying disorder can be diagnosed and treated. The purpura should disappear once the cause has been successfully treated. If the condition is the result of an autoimmune disorder, your doctor may prescribe corticosteroid drugs (*see* IMMUNOSUPPRESSANTS, p.906) to clear it up.

WWW ONLINE SITES: p.1026, p.1033, p.1036

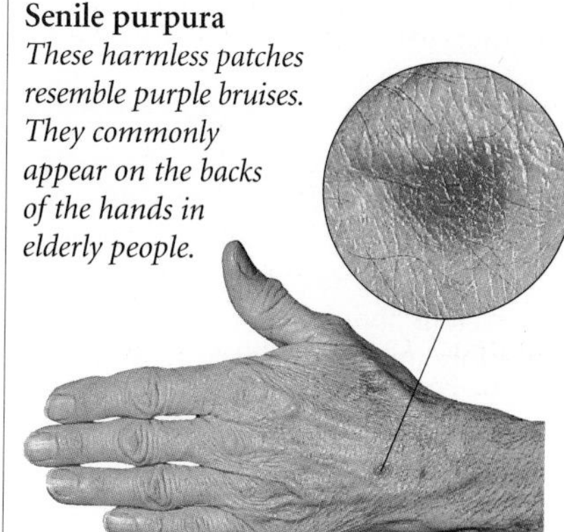

Senile purpura
These harmless patches resemble purple bruises. They commonly appear on the backs of the hands in elderly people.

LOCALIZED SKIN CONDITIONS

Localized skin conditions are those that affect the skin on only one part of the body or on a small area. Many of these conditions are related to specific sites because they are associated with structures such as particular glands in the skin, or because of the localized effects of factors such as pressure or exposure to sunlight.

Acne and rosacea, two types of rash that are usually confined to the face, are described first in this section. The next articles cover conditions that are associated with sweat glands or with under- or overproduction of melanin, the pigment that gives skin its colour.

Skin cancers, which are increasingly common, are given extensive coverage. It is important to be able to recognize the signs of cancerous changes in the skin, and the various types of skin cancer are described in detail to help you to identify them. Subsequent articles describe several noncancerous forms of swelling and growth. The final articles cover localized skin defects caused by factors such as friction or poor blood circulation.

Localized disorders due to infection are described in another section (*see* SKIN INFECTIONS AND INFESTATIONS, pp.351–355). Skin problems specific to babies are discussed elsewhere in the book (*see* INFANCY AND CHILDHOOD, pp.828–831), as are minor injuries such as sunburn (*see* MINOR SKIN INJURIES, pp.356–357).

KEY ANATOMY

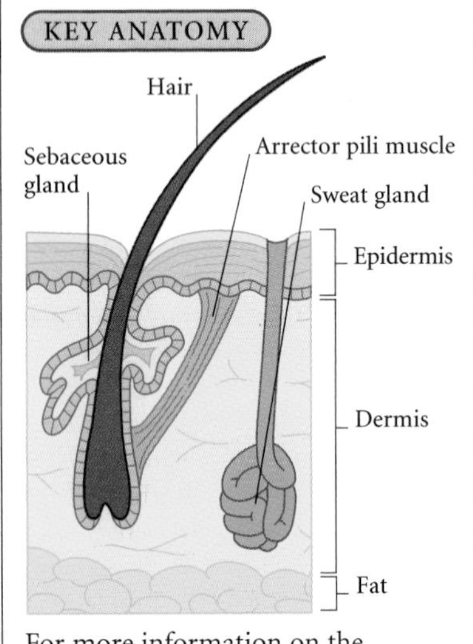

For more information on the structure and function of the skin, *see* pp.328–331.

Acne

A rash, usually on the face, due to blockage and inflammation of glands in the skin

 AGE Most common in adolescents

 GENDER More common in males

 GENETICS Sometimes runs in families

 LIFESTYLE Risk factors depend on the type

There are various types of acne. The most common form is acne vulgaris, which is the familiar rash that affects many teenagers. Acne vulgaris is more common and tends to be more severe in males. The condition is triggered by hormonal changes at puberty and may appear as early as the age of 10. The rash usually subsides after adolescence but may persist after the age of 30. Acne can cause great psychological distress, and teenagers may feel especially self-conscious about their appearance.

More unusual forms of acne include occupational acne, which results from exposure to certain types of industrial oil, and drug-induced acne, which is caused by some prescribed drugs, such as corticosteroids (p.930).

WHAT ARE THE CAUSES?

Acne vulgaris is caused by the overproduction of sebum, an oily substance secreted by the sebaceous glands in the skin. Normally, the sebum drains into hair follicles and flows out through the follicle openings on the skin's surface, thereby keeping the skin lubricated and supple. However, when the glands produce excess sebum, the follicles become blocked. If the sebum remains clogged in the follicle openings, it hardens and becomes dark, forming plugs called blackheads. In some cases, follicles are sealed by an excess of keratin, the tough, fibrous protein produced by the skin cells. When this happens, the trapped sebum hardens into white lumps, called whiteheads, under the surface of the skin. In both types of blockage, bacteria multiply in the sebum, causing inflammation of the surrounding tissues.

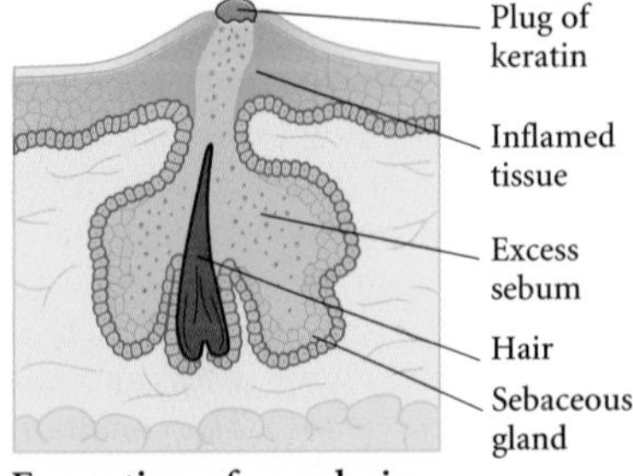

Formation of acne lesions
Acne develops when excess sebum, and in some cases the protein keratin, blocks hair follicles. Bacteria multiply in the trapped sebum, infecting the surrounding tissues and causing various types of lesion.

Acne starting at puberty is thought to result from increased sensitivity to androgens (male sex hormones), which are present in both boys and girls and levels of which are raised during puberty. Androgens cause the sebaceous glands to increase their output of sebum. There may be a genetic factor since acne can run in families. The use of anabolic steroids to improve performance in sports may also raise androgen levels. Other causes of acne vulgaris include hormonal disorders such as Cushing's syndrome (p.684), which is due to an excess of corticosteroid hormones.

Acne may become worse in times of stress. In girls, outbreaks may be affected by the hormonal fluctuations that occur during the menstrual cycle. The condition may also be exacerbated by the use of oil-based cosmetics.

Poor hygiene does not cause acne, although a build-up of oil and dead cells on the skin surface may increase the risk of blocked follicles and allow bacteria to multiply. There is no evidence that fatty foods, sweets, or chocolate either cause or aggravate acne.

Occupational acne is usually caused by long-term contact between the skin and oily clothes. The reasons for drug-induced acne are not known.

WHAT ARE THE SYMPTOMS?

Acne vulgaris occurs in areas of skin that have a high density of sebaceous glands. At puberty, the hair, face, and upper trunk normally become greasy due to increased production of sebum. However, in people with acne, oiliness is excessive. Acne tends to appear on the face, but other areas such as the upper back, centre of the chest, shoulders, and neck are also commonly affected. The disorder is usually more severe in winter and tends to improve in summer with increased exposure to sunlight. Lesions that are caused by occupational acne may appear on parts of the body that come into close contact with oily clothes, such as the thighs. All forms of acne may produce some or all of the following types of lesion:

- Tiny blackheads.
- Small, firm whiteheads.
- Red pimples, often with yellow pus-filled tips.
- Painful, large, firm, red lumps.
- Tender lumps beneath the skin without obvious heads (cysts).

All of the types of lesion listed above may develop at any one time, but the severity of acne varies greatly from person to person. Deep-seated lesions may leave scars after they have healed.

WHAT IS THE TREATMENT?

Self-help measures may help to clear up mild acne and prevent recurrence (*see* CONTROLLING ACNE, left). Your doctor may also recommend a topical drug treatment, such as benzoyl peroxide or retinoid cream (*see* RETINOID DRUGS, p.890) to loosen keratin that is sealing the hair follicles. The doctor may also prescribe topical antibiotics (*see* PREPARATIONS FOR SKIN INFECTIONS AND INFESTATIONS, p.892). Moderate acne is often successfully treated with a low-dose oral antibiotic (p.885), such as tetracycline or erythromycin.

If these treatments fail, you may be referred to a dermatologist. He or she may prescribe isotretinoin, an oral retinoid that acts to loosen keratin and reduce sebum secretion. However, the use of isotretinoin during pregnancy is known to result in fetal abnormalities. For this reason, sexually active women should take the drug only if they are using a reliable contraceptive. Some women may be prescribed the combined pill, which may relieve acne by counteracting the action of androgens.

There is no immediate cure for acne. However, scarring may be prevented if treatment is started at an early stage. Individual acne cysts may be treated with corticosteroid injections. If acne has already left noticeable scars, you may wish to consult a cosmetic surgeon and discuss techniques such as dermabrasion. In this procedure, the top layer of skin is removed under a general anaesthetic. The raw areas then heal to leave a more even layer of skin.

(WWW) ONLINE SITES: p.1036

SELF-HELP

CONTROLLING ACNE

Following these simple self-help measures may help clear up acne and prevent further episodes:

- Wash your skin twice a day with warm, but not hot, water and a mild cleanser. Do not scrub your skin too vigorously.
- Do not pick at pimples because this may make the condition worse and result in scarring.
- Apply a benzoyl peroxide cream daily to the affected areas.
- If you have occupational acne, keep work clothes clean to avoid prolonged contact with oils.

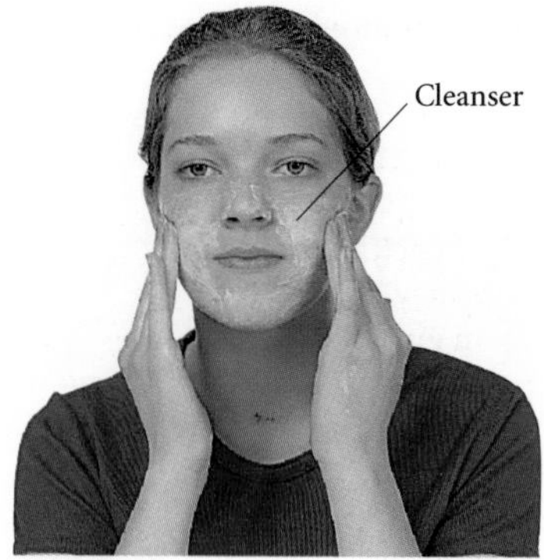

Cleansing your face
Wash your face with warm water and a mild cleanser. Scrubbing hard or using hot water can make the acne worse.

Rosacea

Long-term, possibly permanent, redness and pimples on the cheeks and forehead

 AGE Most common between the ages of 30 and 55

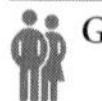 GENDER More common in females

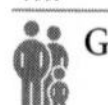 GENETICS Often runs in families

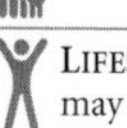 LIFESTYLE Alcohol, coffee, and spicy foods may trigger attacks

In rosacea, a rash develops on the central area of the face and often results in burning or itching. The cause of the disorder is unknown, but there may be a genetic factor because rosacea often runs in families. Women between the ages of 30 and 55 are most commonly affected. The rash may be triggered by eating a spicy meal, drinking alcohol or coffee, or entering a hot room.

WHAT ARE THE SYMPTOMS?

In most cases, the first symptom is red flushing, which often appears spontaneously on the cheeks and forehead after exposure to one of the trigger factors. Later, a rash develops, which is intermittent at first but may become permanent. Other symptoms include:

- Red, puffy skin.
- White- or yellow-headed pimples.
- Visible tiny blood vessels.
- Stinging, burning, or itching sensation in the affected area.

If the skin of the nose is affected, it may eventually thicken, swell, and become purplish red. This condition, which is known as rhinophyma, most commonly occurs in elderly men. About 1 in 4 people who has rosacea also develops irritation of the eyes.

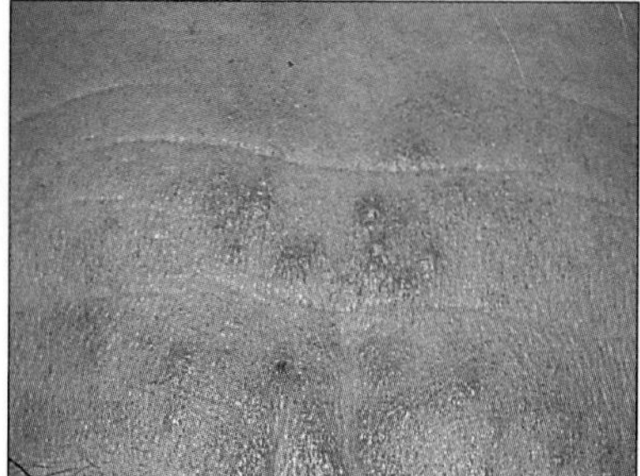

Rosacea pimples on the forehead
The white- and yellow-headed pimples associated with rosacea resemble acne lesions and often appear on the forehead.

WHAT MIGHT BE DONE?

You should avoid anything that triggers flushing, such as spicy food, alcohol, or coffee. In addition, avoid sunlight and the use of topical corticosteroids (p.892), both of which tend to aggravate rosacea.

To treat the condition, your doctor may prescribe metronidazole gel, a topical antibiotic (*see* PREPARATIONS FOR SKIN INFECTIONS AND INFESTATIONS, p.892), which is usually effective. However, if the rosacea does not improve, you may be prescribed the antibiotic tetracycline (*see* ANTIBIOTICS, p.885) or an oral retinoid drug (p.890). You may need several weeks of treatment before the rash eventually clears up.

If rhinophyma develops, the area of thickened skin on the nose can be pared away under general anaesthesia. Normal skin tissue will then form to cover the treated surface of the nose.

Rosacea usually comes and goes over a period of 5–10 years before finally disappearing. Occasionally, the condition may be lifelong, especially in men.

(WWW) ONLINE SITES: p.1036

Prickly heat

Multiple small, raised, itchy spots that appear on the skin in hot conditions

AGE Most common in infants and children

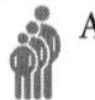
LIFESTYLE Being overweight and being in a hot, humid climate are risk factors

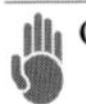
GENDER GENETICS Not significant factors

Prickly heat is an intensely itchy rash that most commonly occurs in hot weather. It develops when sweat glands are blocked by bacteria and dead skin cells. Sweat trapped in the glands then causes mild inflammation. The rash consists of tiny, red, itchy spots or blisters accompanied by a prickling or burning feeling. The most common sites are the hands, feet, armpits, and chest. Prickly heat is more likely to affect overweight people because they tend to become overheated and sweat easily. Infants and children are more likely than adults to have the condition, in which case the rash develops in the nappy area or on the face, chest, or back.

The rash often disappears on its own in a few days. You can help this process by wearing loose clothing made from natural fibres and, in babies, by leaving nappies off as much as possible. If the rash persists, your doctor may suggest using a mild topical corticosteroid (p.892), but this should not be used on the face. Consult a doctor before using a topical corticosteroid on a baby and always follow the doctor's instructions.

(WWW) ONLINE SITES: p.1036

Hyperhidrosis

Excessive sweating in specific areas or over the whole body

AGE Most common between the ages of 15 and 30

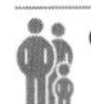
GENETICS Sometimes runs in families

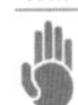
GENDER LIFESTYLE Not significant factors

Frequent and excessively heavy sweating is called hyperhidrosis. The condition usually first appears at puberty and disappears by the age of 30. In many cases, no cause can be found, but about half of all affected people have a family history of the condition, which suggests a genetic factor. Hyperhidrosis can be an indication of an underlying problem, such as an overactive thyroid gland (*see* HYPERTHYROIDISM, p.679) or diabetes mellitus (p.687). It may also occur in menopausal women. In some people, stress triggers sweating attacks.

Hyperhidrosis may occur in many areas of the body, particularly the feet, armpits, hands, and face. It is often accompanied by an unpleasant odour.

WHAT CAN I DO?

Wash away sweat regularly, and wear comfortable, loose clothing made from natural fibres that absorb sweat. Antiperspirant may help to reduce underarm sweating. If anxiety makes the problem worse, relaxation exercises (p.75) may help. If these methods do not provide relief, consult your doctor.

Your doctor may prescribe a topical treatment containing aluminium chloride to reduce the activity of the sweat glands. If you have hyperhidrosis in the armpits and other treatments have failed, he or she may suggest a minor operation to destroy the nerve centres that control sweating, thus ending the problem permanently.

(WWW) ONLINE SITES: p.1036

Vitiligo

Loss of normal pigment from patches of skin, most commonly occurring on the face and hands

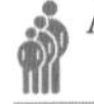
AGE More common in young adults

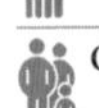
GENETICS Sometimes runs in families

GENDER LIFESTYLE Not significant factors

People who have vitiligo have irregular patches of pale skin caused by the loss of melanin, the pigment that gives the skin its colour. The disorder is more obvious in people with dark skin.

In about half of all cases, vitiligo develops before the age of 20. It does not cause physical discomfort, but some people become distressed by the discoloured appearance of their skin.

WHAT IS THE CAUSE?

It is thought that vitiligo is an autoimmune disorder in which the antibodies produced by the body react against its own tissues. In this condition, antibodies destroy the cells in the skin that produce melanin. About 1 in 3 people with vitiligo has a family history of the condition. About the same proportion also have another type of autoimmune disorder, such as pernicious anaemia (*see* MEGALOBLASTIC ANAEMIA, p.448).

WHAT ARE THE SYMPTOMS?

The loss of skin colour is gradual, occurring over several months or even years. The symptoms include:

- Depigmented skin patches that may occur on any part of the body but most commonly the face and hands.

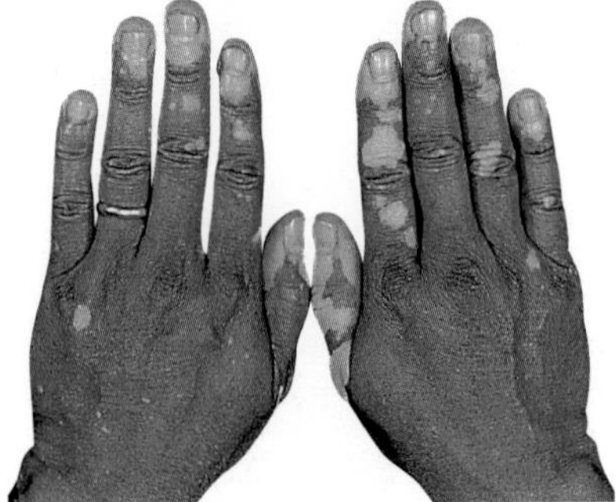

Vitiligo
The pale patches on these hands are due to vitiligo, a condition that causes a gradual loss of the skin pigment melanin.

- In some cases, white hair on affected areas of skin due to loss of pigment from the hair follicles.

In most people with vitiligo, the depigmented patches of skin are distributed symmetrically over the body.

WHAT MIGHT BE DONE?

The diagnosis is usually obvious, but your doctor may arrange for a skin test to exclude pityriasis versicolor (p.353), a fungal infection that may produce discoloured patches of skin. Blood tests may be done to make sure you do not have another autoimmune disorder.

In mild vitiligo, the discoloured areas can be hidden with cosmetics. No other treatment is needed. The affected areas cannot tan so you should avoid exposure to the sun and use a sunblock in direct sunlight (*see* SAFETY IN THE SUN, p.80). Phototherapy using ultraviolet light can help but takes several months to work. Before treatment, you may be given psoralen, a drug to increase the skin's sensitivity to light.

Occasionally, people may lose the pigment from extensive areas of skin. In these cases, the rest of the skin may be bleached so that the overall colour of the skin appears more even.

There is no cure for vitiligo, and often the depigmented patches continue to enlarge slowly. However, about 3 in 10 affected people regain their natural skin colour spontaneously.

(WWW) ONLINE SITES: p.1036

Freckles

Multiple small, brown-coloured spots on the skin that are usually harmless

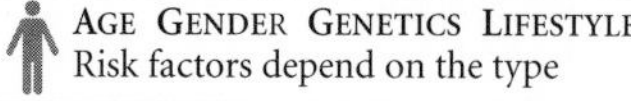

AGE GENDER GENETICS LIFESTYLE Risk factors depend on the type

Freckles result from an overproduction of melanin, the pigment that gives the skin its colour. There are two common types of freckle: the small, brown spots that appear on areas of skin frequently exposed to the sun; and the flat, lighter brown patches that can appear anywhere on the skin and affect most people with increasing age.

The tendency to develop freckles on exposure to the sun is usually inherited. It is more common in people with fair skin, particularly those with red hair. The patches are harmless and tend to fade during the winter, but fair, freckled skin is a sign of sensitivity to sunlight and of increased susceptibility to skin cancer (p.344). You should use suntan lotion daily to help protect you against sunburn (*see* SAFETY IN THE SUN, p.80).

The type of patch that develops with age is called an age spot, lentigo, or liver spot. These spots most commonly affect people over the age of 40. They can appear on covered and exposed parts of the body and do not fade in winter.

A lentigo is usually harmless, but some may eventually develop into malignant melanomas (p.346), particularly if they are on the face. A variation in colour may be a warning sign. If raised, brown lumps appear on a lentigo, consult your doctor as soon as possible so that he or she can analyse the spot and detect any cancerous changes in the cells.

Moles

Flat or raised growths on the skin that are rough or smooth and vary in colour from light to dark brown

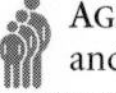

AGE Increasingly common in childhood and adolescence

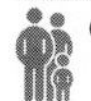

GENETICS Sometimes run in families

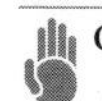

GENDER LIFESTYLE Not significant factors

Moles are caused by an overproduction of pigmented skin cells called melanocytes. They can form anywhere on the body, and there are several types. Moles may appear soon after birth (*see* BIRTHMARKS, p.828) or may appear during childhood and early adolescence; nearly all adults have 10–20 moles by the age of 30. Most moles are noncancerous, but in rare cases a mole may undergo changes that make it cancerous (*see* MALIGNANT MELANOMA, p.346). Alterations in the shape, colour, or size of moles are not always a sign of cancer, and changes during puberty or pregnancy are usually normal. However, changes should always be evaluated by a doctor.

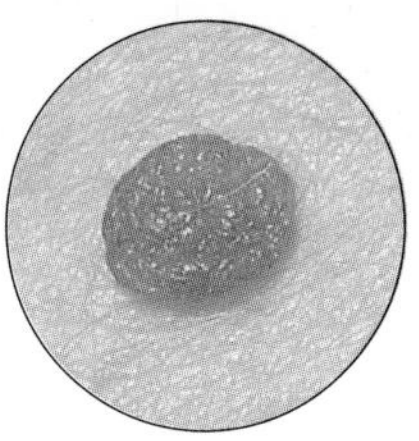

Raised mole
This noncancerous mole appears as a raised, brown spot; the pigmented area may extend deep into the skin.

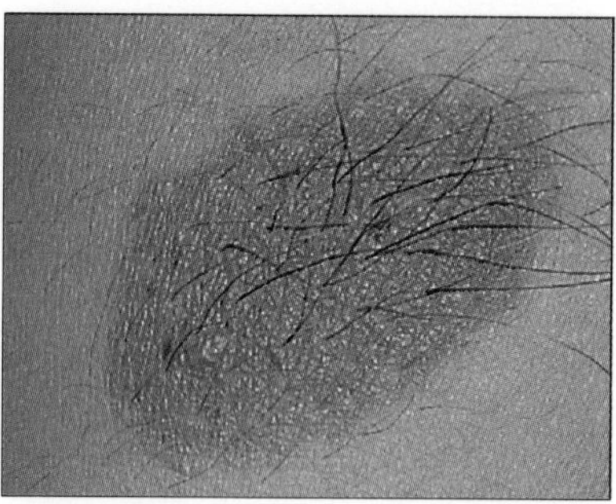

Hairy mole
Moles that are covered in hair, such as the one shown here, or moles with just a few hairs rarely become cancerous.

WHAT ARE THE TYPES?

Usually, moles are flat or raised growths that vary in colour from light to dark brown and measure less than 1 cm (3/8 in) in diameter. They may be rough or smooth, hairy or hairless.

One type of mole, known as a dysplastic naevus, is larger than usual and unevenly coloured. This type may appear in childhood or old age and may develop from a smaller mole. Dysplastic naevi sometimes run in families. Any type of mole may become cancerous, but dysplastic naevi are more likely to undergo cancerous changes than other moles. The risk of such changes is higher in people who have a family history of malignant melanoma or if the mole is frequently exposed to sunlight.

Blue naevi, moles that have a bluish-black colour, occur most commonly on the face, arms and legs, and buttocks.

A halo naevus is a mole from which pigment is disappearing, leaving a ring of paler skin around a shrinking central dark spot. Eventually, the mole may disappear completely.

WHAT MIGHT BE DONE?

You should consult a doctor immediately if you have a mole that is more than 1 cm (3/8 in) in diameter and is growing rapidly, that changes shade or colour, that becomes itchy or inflamed, or that starts bleeding.

If your doctor suspects that a mole is cancerous, he or she may recommend that you have it removed and examined for cancerous cells (*see* SKIN BIOPSY, p.344). Noncancerous moles can also be removed, either for cosmetic reasons or if they are being chafed by clothing.

(WWW) ONLINE SITES: p.1036

Skin cancer

Several types of cancer that originate in the skin, most of which are associated with prolonged exposure to sunlight

 GENETICS Fair-skinned people are most at risk

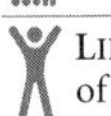 LIFESTYLE Exposure to the sun and the use of sunbeds are risk factors

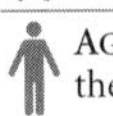 AGE GENDER Risk factors depend on the type

Skin cancer is the second most common form of cancer in the UK after lung cancer. In recent years, the global incidence has escalated, and the condition now affects millions of people.

The usual cause of skin cancer is prolonged exposure to the harmful ultraviolet radiation in sunlight. The risk is higher if you live or take holidays in areas with intense sun. The closer you are to the equator, the greater the risk. The recent depletion of the ozone layer is thought to play a part in increasing the incidence of skin cancer because the ozone layer acts as a shield against harmful ultraviolet light. In addition, sunbeds, which use ultraviolet light, may cause skin cancer.

If you work outdoors or have been sunburned (particularly in childhood), you could be vulnerable to skin cancer. People who have fair skin are especially susceptible because they have low levels of melanin, the pigment that gives the skin its colour and helps to protect it from the sun's harmful ultraviolet rays.

To reduce the risk of developing skin cancer, try to avoid exposure to the sun and protect your skin when outdoors (*see* SAFETY IN THE SUN, p.80). Examine your skin regularly, and ask someone else to check your back and scalp.

WHAT ARE THE TYPES?

There are three main types of skin cancer associated with overexposure to the sun. The most common type is basal cell carcinoma (right), which can be easily treated and rarely spreads. The next type is squamous cell carcinoma (opposite page). It may spread and be fatal but can be cured if detected early. Basal cell carcinoma and squamous cell carcinoma together account for 36,500 cases of skin cancer every year in the UK. The third type is malignant melanoma (p.346). This form of skin cancer is rare, although its incidence is increasing; about 6,000 cases are diagnosed each year. It can spread rapidly to other parts of the body and causes more deaths than other skin cancers.

An uncommon skin cancer known as Kaposi's sarcoma (p.346) usually occurs only in people with AIDS (*see* HIV INFECTION AND AIDS, p.297).

WHAT MIGHT BE DONE?

Skin cancer can usually be cured if it is diagnosed early. You should consult your doctor promptly if you notice any changes in your skin, such as enlarging lumps or sores that do not heal. You may need to have a skin biopsy (left). During this procedure, a small area of skin is removed and examined under a microscope for abnormal cells.

The type of skin cancer and spread of the disease determine the treatment and outlook. Sometimes, only the affected area of skin needs to be treated.

Most skin cancers can be removed surgically, but skin grafting (p.319) may be necessary if a cancer has invaded large areas of surrounding skin tissue. If the cancer spreads to other parts of the body, radiotherapy (p.281) or chemotherapy (p.280) may be needed.

(WWW) ONLINE SITES: p.1028, p.1036

(TEST) SKIN BIOPSY

A skin biopsy is a technique used to diagnose skin diseases, such as cancer. In this procedure, a sample of skin is removed from an anaesthetized site and sent to a laboratory to be examined under a microscope. A biopsy may be used to cut away a whole lesion from the skin, such as a mole, or to remove a small sample at the edge of a large patch of affected skin.

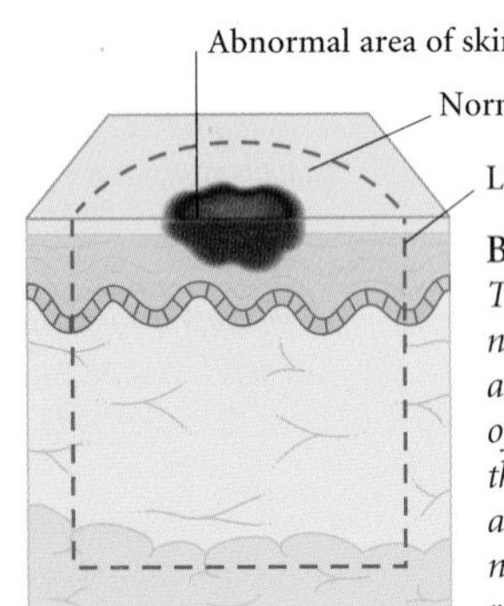

Biopsy site
The biopsy site is first numbed with a local anaesthetic. A section of tissue, including skin that looks abnormal and a surrounding area of normal skin, is then removed for analysis.

(RESULTS)

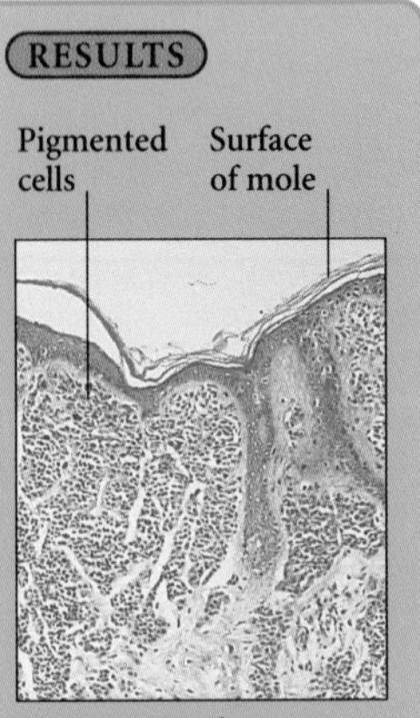

Biopsy sample
This magnified view shows part of a removed mole. The sample confirms that the mole has no cancerous cells.

Basal cell carcinoma

A skin cancer, usually affecting sun-exposed areas, that rarely spreads elsewhere in the body

 AGE Rare in people under the age of 40; increasingly common over 40

 GENDER More common in males

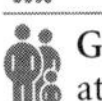 GENETICS Fair-skinned people are most at risk

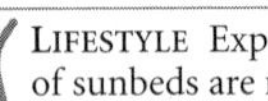 LIFESTYLE Exposure to the sun and the use of sunbeds are risk factors

The most common type of skin cancer, basal cell carcinoma is also the least dangerous because it usually remains localized and rarely spreads to other parts of the body. This cancer should not be left untreated because it can destroy bone and surrounding skin.

Basal cell carcinoma is characterized by pearly lesions that can occur on any part of the body but commonly appear on the face, often at the corner of an eye, near the ear, or on the nose.

The condition is usually caused by exposure to strong sunlight, which damages cells just below the surface of the skin. Fair-skinned people over the age of 40 are most susceptible.

You can minimize your risk of developing basal cell carcinoma by avoiding prolonged exposure to sunlight and by protecting your skin when you are outdoors (*see* SAFETY IN THE SUN, p.80).

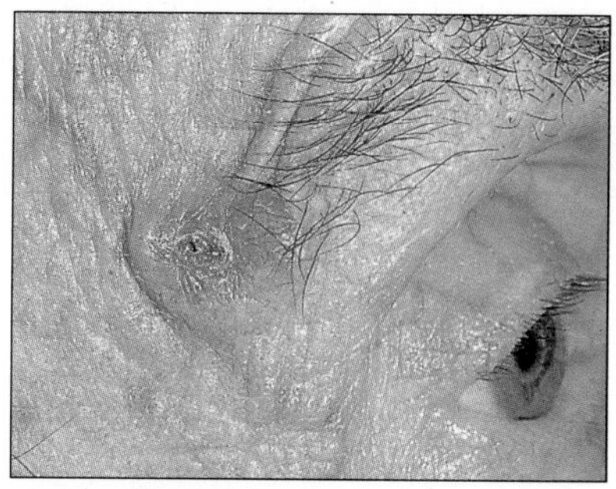

Basal cell carcinoma
This pink, shallow ulcer, with its waxy, rolled edge and central scab, is an example of an untreated basal cell carcinoma.

WHAT ARE THE SYMPTOMS?

Basal cell carcinoma grows slowly over months or even years. A typical lesion develops in the following way:

- A small, painless lump appears; it has a smooth surface with blood vessels, a pink to brownish-grey colour, and a waxy or pearl-like border.
- The lump gradually grows, usually spreading outwards and developing a central depression with rolled edges.

An untreated lump may form a shallow ulcer that may bleed intermittently and then form a scab but never fully heals.

If you notice an enlarging skin lump or a sore that fails to heal, you should consult your doctor promptly.

WHAT MIGHT BE DONE?

If your doctor suspects basal cell carcinoma, he or she will probably arrange for you to have a skin biopsy (opposite page) to confirm the diagnosis. During this procedure, a small lesion may be scraped away or frozen off. A large lesion may need to be removed surgically. If you have several lesions or if the affected area is difficult to treat surgically (for example, if it is near the eye), you may need to have radiotherapy (p.281). If the cancer has caused damage to underlying tissue, you may need plastic surgery (p.952).

WHAT IS THE PROGNOSIS?

About 9 in 10 people who develop basal cell carcinoma are successfully treated. There should be no further problems after treatment, but in a few cases the skin cancer may recur.

If you have already had an episode of basal cell carcinoma, you are more likely to develop further cancerous lesions on other parts of your body, usually within a period of 2–5 years. For this reason, you should continue to protect yourself against exposure to sunlight and inspect your skin regularly. Your doctor will probably recommend that you have periodic checkups in order to detect and treat any new lesions that develop while they are still small.

(WWW) ONLINE SITES: p.1028, p.1036

Squamous cell carcinoma

A skin cancer that usually affects the face but can spread to other parts of the body

 AGE Mainly affects people over the age of 60

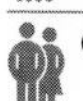 GENDER More common in males

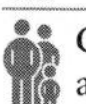 GENETICS Fair-skinned people are most at risk

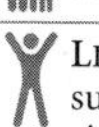 LIFESTYLE Exposure to the sun, the use of sunbeds, and working with oils and tars are risk factors

Squamous cell carcinoma is a common type of skin cancer that usually affects areas that have been exposed to sunlight but may also occur in other parts of the body, such as the genitals. This type of carcinoma is capable of spreading throughout the body, and for this reason early detection and treatment of the condition are essential.

WHAT ARE THE CAUSES?

Squamous cell carcinoma develops on areas of skin that have been constantly exposed to sunlight over many years. Sometimes, this form of skin cancer may develop from scaly growths known as solar keratoses (p.347). The condition is most common in fair-skinned men over the age of 60.

People who work with some industrial tars and oils are known to have a higher than normal risk of squamous cell carcinoma, but these people are normally protected by adequate health and safety measures.

Most squamous cell carcinomas can be prevented by avoiding prolonged exposure to sunlight. If this is not possible, you should take precautions to protect your skin, such as applying sunblock and wearing a hat, when you are outdoors (*see* SAFETY IN THE SUN, p.80).

WHAT ARE THE SYMPTOMS?

Squamous cell carcinoma begins as an area of thickened, scaly skin. The lesion then develops into:

- A hard, painless, gradually enlarging lump that has an irregular edge and is red to reddish brown in colour.
- Subsequently, a recurring ulcer that does not heal.

If you develop an enlarging skin lump or a sore that does not heal on any part of your body, you should consult your doctor as soon as possible.

WHAT MIGHT BE DONE?

If your doctor suspects squamous cell carcinoma, he or she may arrange for you to have a skin biopsy (opposite page), in which a small piece of tissue is removed under a local anaesthetic and examined under a microscope for the presence of cancerous cells.

Squamous cell carcinoma can usually be treated surgically if the lesions are detected at an early stage. Sometimes, radiotherapy (p.281) is used as an alternative to surgery. If you have several large lesions or if the cancer has spread into underlying tissues, chemotherapy (p.280) may also be necessary.

WHAT IS THE PROGNOSIS?

If the condition is detected early, about 9 in 10 people with squamous cell carcinoma are treated successfully. Lesions on the face respond particularly well to treatment. If the disease is detected late, the success of the treatment depends on how far the cancer has spread. Some lesions may recur, particularly larger ones, and your doctor will advise you to have regular checkups.

(WWW) ONLINE SITES: p.1028, p.1036

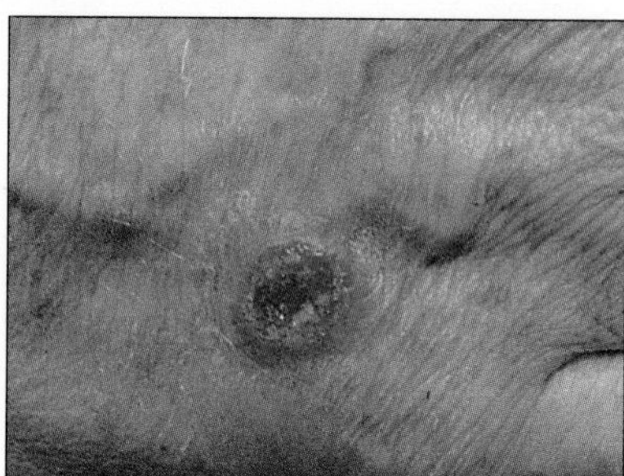

Squamous cell carcinoma
The face and hand are common sites for squamous cell carcinoma. Here, a lesion on the back of the hand has developed into an ulcer with a clearly defined edge.

Malignant melanoma

A skin cancer affecting the pigment-producing cells of the skin that can spread rapidly to other parts of the body

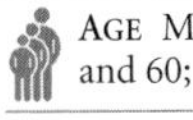

AGE Most common between the ages of 40 and 60; increasingly found in young adults

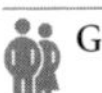

GENDER More common in females

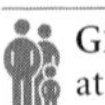

GENETICS Fair-skinned people are most at risk

LIFESTYLE Exposure to the sun and the use of sunbeds are risk factors

Malignant melanoma is a rare, serious form of skin cancer. A melanoma may begin as a new growth on normal skin or may develop from an existing mole. Left untreated, the cancer can spread to other parts of the body and may be fatal. As with most other skin cancers, the main cause is exposure to sunlight.

Worldwide, the number of cases of malignant melanoma, particularly in young adults, has increased dramatically over the past 10 years. This rise is probably due to the growing popularity of outdoor activities. The condition is most common in people aged 40–60 and in women. In the UK, there are about 6,000 new cases each year.

WHAT IS THE CAUSE?

Malignant melanoma is thought to result from damage to melanocytes (the skin cells that produce the pigment melanin) by sunlight. The cancer occurs more frequently in people with fair skin than in those with dark skin. People who are continually exposed to intense sunlight or who live in sunny climates have an increased risk of developing a malignant melanoma. In particular, severe sunburn (p.357) during childhood has been shown to double the chance of developing malignant melanoma in later life. Reducing exposure to the sun can help to decrease the risk of developing this type of cancer (*see* SAFETY IN THE SUN, p.80).

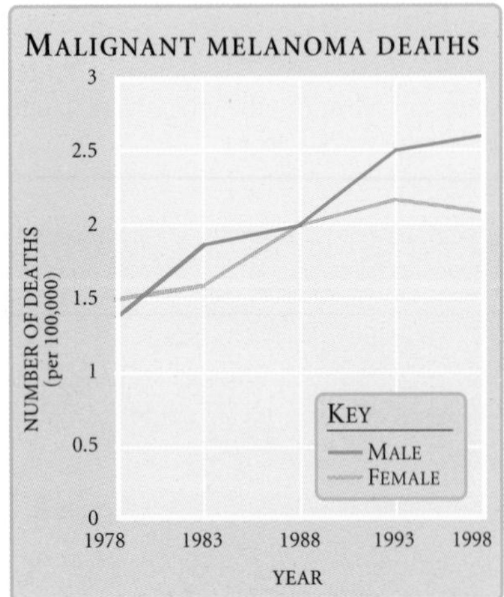

Increasing death rates
In the UK, deaths from malignant melanoma have increased since the 1970s. Although this cancer is more common in women, it is more often fatal in men.

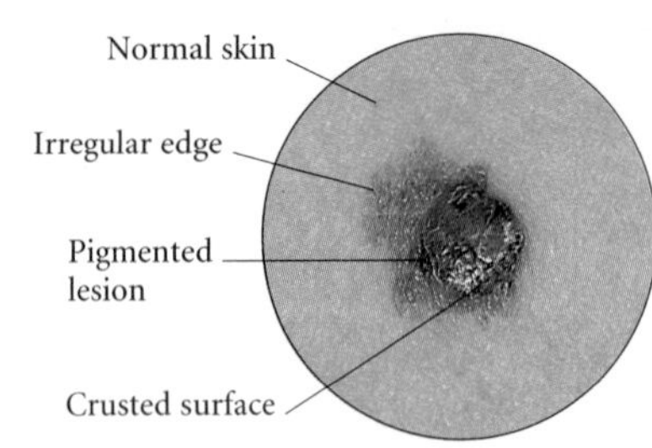

Malignant melanoma
The uneven colour, irregularly spreading edge, and crusted surface of this raised growth are characteristic features of a malignant melanoma.

WHAT ARE THE SYMPTOMS?

Malignant melanomas can develop on any part of the body but appear most commonly on sun-exposed areas. Some melanomas spread across the skin in irregular flat patches; others appear as fast-growing lumps. In older people, they may occur on the face as freckle-like spots, known as lentigo maligna, that grow slowly over many years. If they are not removed, all of these types of melanoma will grow down into the underlying layers of the skin.

You should suspect a malignant melanoma if a quickly growing, irregular, dark-coloured spot starts to develop on your skin or if you notice any of the following changes in an existing mole:

- Increasing size.
- Irregular and asymmetrical edges.
- Itching, inflammation, or redness.
- Thickening of the surface.
- Bleeding or crusting.
- Variation in shade or colour.

You should inspect your skin regularly and note the location and size of any moles. Ask another person to help you to examine your back and scalp. Changes in shade or colour in existing moles or the appearance of a new and enlarging spot, particularly one that is more than 6 mm (¼ in) in diameter or starts to vary in shade or colour, should be reported to your doctor.

WHAT MIGHT BE DONE?

If your doctor suspects that you have a malignant melanoma, he or she will arrange for the lesion and an area of surrounding skin to be removed to decrease the risk of malignant cells remaining. The tissue will be examined under a microscope (*see* SKIN BIOPSY, p.344). If the tissue is cancerous, a larger portion of skin may be removed, which may require a skin graft (p.319).

Samples may also be taken from the lymph nodes near the melanoma and examined for cancerous cells, the presence of which would indicate that the cancer has spread. If it has, you may have chemotherapy (p.280), radiotherapy (p.281), or biological therapies (*see* CANCER AND ITS MANAGEMENT, p.278).

WHAT IS THE PROGNOSIS?

Superficial melanomas that are treated early are usually cured, but melanomas are more often fatal in men, possibly because men do not always report symptoms to the doctor immediately. If melanomas are aggressive or penetrate deep into the skin, the outlook is less optimistic, and, if they spread to other areas of the body, they are often fatal.

(WWW) ONLINE SITES: p.1028, p.1036

Kaposi's sarcoma

A skin cancer, characterized by raised, pinkish-brown lesions, that is most often associated with AIDS

GENDER More common in males

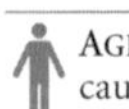

LIFESTYLE Unprotected sex with multiple partners and intravenous drug use are risk factors in AIDS-related cases

AGE GENETICS Risk factors depend on the cause

Kaposi's sarcoma used to be a very rare condition, appearing mainly in older men of Mediterranean or Jewish origin. It developed slowly and rarely spread. However, a more rapidly developing form now occurs increasingly in people with AIDS (*see* HIV INFECTION AND AIDS, p.297). In these cases, it is associated with infection by a herpes virus.

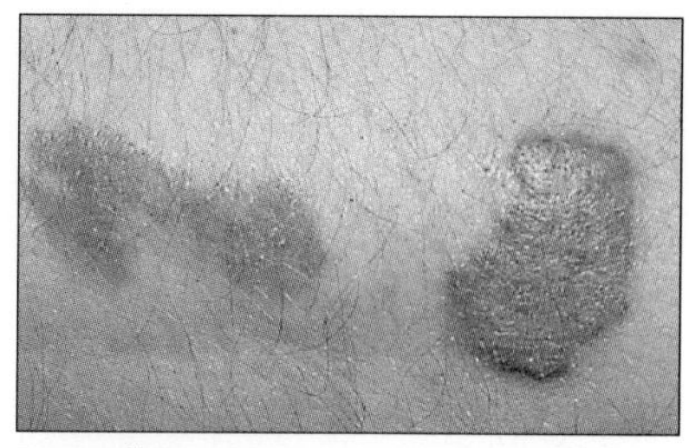

Kaposi's sarcoma
Sharply defined, pinkish-brown raised nodules and flat patches are the first signs of Kaposi's sarcoma. They may develop anywhere on the body.

The sharply defined lesions of Kaposi's sarcoma are pinkish brown and can occur anywhere on the skin. In AIDS-related cases, the lesions spread quickly; in severe cases, they may affect mucous membranes, especially of the palate and internal organs. Internal lesions can cause severe bleeding.

If detected early, localized Kaposi's sarcoma can be treated effectively with radiotherapy (p.281). If the cancer is more advanced, chemotherapy (p.280) may be needed. Kaposi's sarcoma is seldom the main cause of death in people with AIDS, although it may be fatal when the internal organs are affected.

(WWW) ONLINE SITES: p.1032, p.1036

Solar keratosis

A pinkish-red, scaly, rough-textured skin growth caused by prolonged exposure to sunlight; also called actinic keratosis

 **AGE** More common in people over the age of 40

 **GENDER** More common in males

 **GENETICS** Fair-skinned people are most at risk

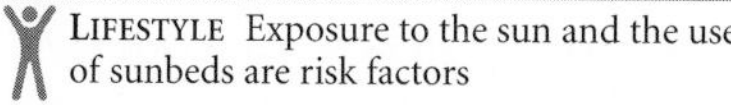 **LIFESTYLE** Exposure to the sun and the use of sunbeds are risk factors

Solar keratoses are small, scaly skin growths usually caused by years of exposure to sunlight. People under the age of 40 are not often affected by the condition, but the risk of solar keratoses increases after this age and is higher than normal in people (usually men) who work outdoors. The disorder is most common in fair-skinned people, who are often particularly sensitive to the sun.

The lesions are pinkish red and have a rough texture. They most commonly appear on uncovered areas of the skin, such as the face and the backs of the hands and on bald parts of the scalp. Usually, several lesions appear at the same time. Sometimes, a solar keratosis develops into squamous cell carcinoma (p.345), a type of skin cancer.

What might be done?

The lesions should always be removed; your doctor may freeze or scrape them off. If there are many growths in a large area, a cream containing the anticancer drug 5-fluorouracil (*see* ANTICANCER DRUGS, p.907) may be prescribed. The growths may recur after treatment.

To reduce the risk of developing this condition, protect your skin from exposure to the sun (*see* SAFETY IN THE SUN, p.80). People who are bald or have thin hair should wear a hat outdoors.

(WWW) ONLINE SITES: p.1036

Discoid lupus erythematosus

A disorder in which itchy, red, scaly patches develop, usually on the face and scalp and behind the ears

 **AGE** Most common between the ages of 25 and 45

 **GENDER** Much more common in females

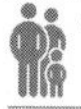 **GENETICS** Sometimes runs in families

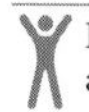 **LIFESTYLE** Strong sunlight triggers or aggravates the condition

Discoid lupus erythematosus (DLE) is an autoimmune disorder, in which the body attacks its own tissues. It causes a red, itchy, scaly rash to appear, particularly on the face and scalp, behind the ears, and on any parts of the body that are exposed to sunlight. The disorder most commonly occurs in women between the ages of 25 and 45. The cause is unknown, but a genetic factor may be involved because DLE tends to run in families. Exposure to sunlight tends to trigger the onset of the rash or to make an existing rash worse. Over a period of several years, DLE may subside and recur repeatedly with different degrees of severity.

In some cases, the rash disappears, but it can leave behind a scarred area in which the skin is thin and discoloured. If DLE occurs on the scalp, the damage to the skin can result in permanent loss of hair and patchy baldness of the scalp (*see* ALOPECIA, p.358).

What might the doctor do?

Your doctor will probably arrange for a small sample of skin to be removed from an affected area (*see* SKIN BIOPSY, p.344) to confirm the diagnosis. If you have DLE, your doctor may prescribe a topical corticosteroid (p.892), which you apply to the affected areas of skin two or three times a day.

If the skin has not healed after the corticosteroid treatment, your doctor may prescribe a course of chloroquine, an antimalarial drug (p.888) that often relieves the symptoms of DLE. The doctor will advise you to have regular eye examinations while you are on this drug because chloroquine may eventually cause damage to the eyes.

What can I do?

You can take steps to control the rash by staying out of the sun or by using a suntan lotion to protect your skin (*see* SAFETY IN THE SUN, p.80). Concealing creams may improve the appearance of skin that has become discoloured.

What is the prognosis?

Most cases of DLE can be successfully treated with corticosteroids, although scarring can occur. About 1 in 10 people with DLE goes on to develop a related, but frequently more serious, autoimmune disorder called systemic lupus erythematosus (p.461). This condition affects many parts of the body, including the lungs, kidneys, and joints.

(WWW) ONLINE SITES: p.1033, p.1036

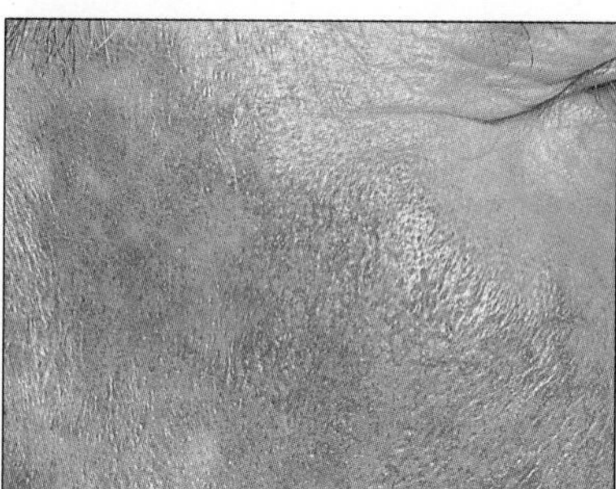

Rash of discoid lupus erythematosus
This red facial rash is characteristic of discoid lupus erythematosus. The distinct, discoloured patches are due to scarring from previous episodes of the disorder.

Erythema nodosum

Shiny, tender, red or purple swellings (nodules), usually on the shins

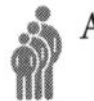 AGE Most common in young adults

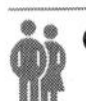 GENDER More common in females

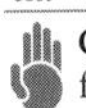 GENETICS LIFESTYLE Not significant factors

Many conditions may give rise to erythema nodosum, in which tender red or purple swellings known as nodules develop, usually on the shins.

Erythema nodosum is most common in young adults, and particularly in women. It may be linked with long-standing disorders such as tuberculosis (p.491) and the inflammatory disorder sarcoidosis (p.498). The condition may also be a reaction to drugs, in particular to some types of antibiotics (p.885). In children, it is often associated with a sore throat caused by a streptococcal infection. In some cases, there is no obvious cause for the condition.

WHAT ARE THE SYMPTOMS?

In many cases, erythema nodosum is accompanied by pains in the joints and muscles and fever. The nodules usually appear on the shins; less commonly, they develop on the forearms. They are:

- Shiny and bright red or purple.
- In general, between 1 cm (3/8 in) and 15 cm (6 in) in diameter.
- Very painful and tender.

The nodules fade over a few weeks and may begin to look like bruises.

WHAT MIGHT BE DONE?

A diagnosis is made from the symptoms and the appearance of the nodules. There is no specific treatment, but your doctor may advise you to rest in bed and keep your legs raised until the nodules have begun to subside. To reduce swelling, the doctor may also prescribe nonsteroidal anti-inflammatory drugs (p.894) and, occasionally, oral corticosteroids (p.930). In addition, he or she may arrange for blood tests and a chest X-ray (p.490) to be performed to check for an underlying disorder.

Most affected people recover over 4 to 8 weeks. However, in 1 in 5 people, erythema nodosum recurs.

(WWW) ONLINE SITES: p.1036

Skin tag

A small, harmless flap of skin, usually attached by a stalk to the neck, trunk, groin, or armpit

 AGE More common with increasing age

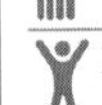 LIFESTYLE Being overweight is a risk factor

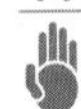 GENDER GENETICS Not significant factors

Tags are tiny flaps of skin, sometimes darker than the surrounding area, that are attached to the body by a stalk. They usually occur spontaneously but sometimes are the result of an imperfectly healed wound. Skin tags are found on any part of the body, typically on the neck and trunk, but they may also occur in the groin or armpit. While skin tags are harmless, they may bleed or become sore if they are rubbed by clothing. Elderly and overweight people are especially prone to skin tags.

Consult your doctor if you are unsure whether a growth is a skin tag or if a tag is irritated by your clothes. You may have the tag removed under a local anaesthetic by burning, scraping, or snipping with surgical scissors.

Seborrhoeic keratosis

A harmless, pigmented wart-like growth that most commonly occurs on the trunk

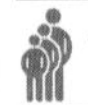 AGE More common with increasing age

 GENDER GENETICS LIFESTYLE Not significant factors

Seborrhoeic keratoses, also called seborrhoeic warts, are harmless skin growths, usually brown or black in colour. The growths occur on the trunk but may also affect the head, neck, and, less commonly, the backs of the hands and the forearms. They may appear singly or in groups. Seborrhoeic keratoses are common in elderly people.

WHAT ARE THE SYMPTOMS?

You may notice a seborrhoeic keratosis as a crusted patch that appears to be stuck on rather than in the skin. The growth is usually:

- Painless but occasionally itchy. You may find that scratching the growth causes soreness.

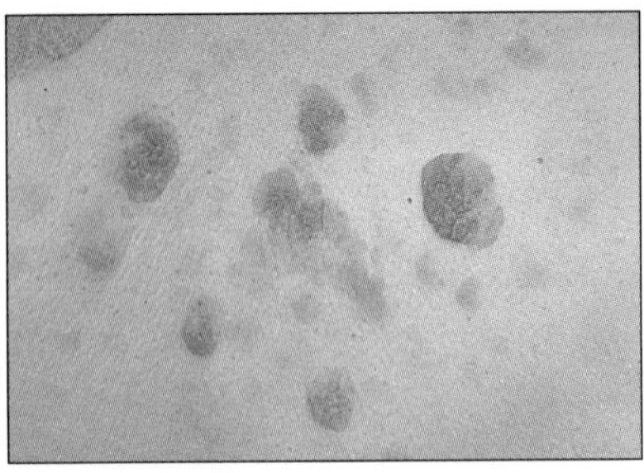

Seborrhoeic keratoses
Although they vary in colour and shape, seborrhoeic keratoses commonly take the form of rough, brown, raised patches.

- Up to 2 cm (3/4 in) in diameter.
- Greasy and rough on the surface.
- Brown or black in colour.
- Either raised or flat.

In rare cases, an individual may have hundreds of seborrhoeic keratoses.

WHAT MIGHT BE DONE?

If you have a pigmented patch, consult your doctor to check that it is not due to a serious condition. If it is a seborrhoeic keratosis, it may be removed by scraping or cutting it off or by freezing it. This will leave little or no scarring. The lesion is unlikely to recur, but in a person who is susceptible to seborrhoeic keratoses, new lesions may develop on other areas of the body.

(WWW) ONLINE SITES: p.1036

Sebaceous cyst

A harmless swelling under the skin that may become infected

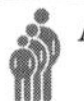 AGE More common in adults

 GENDER GENETICS LIFESTYLE Not significant factors

A sebaceous cyst, also called an epidermoid cyst, is a smooth lump that forms under the skin due to inflammation of a hair follicle. The sac is filled with dead skin cells and sebum, the oily secretion of the sebaceous glands. Some cysts have a dark central pore.

Sebaceous cysts commonly occur on the scalp, face, trunk, and genitals but may appear on any part of the body. Although harmless, the cysts occasionally grow large and become unsightly. A sebaceous cyst that is infected by bacteria may become inflamed and painful and eventually burst.

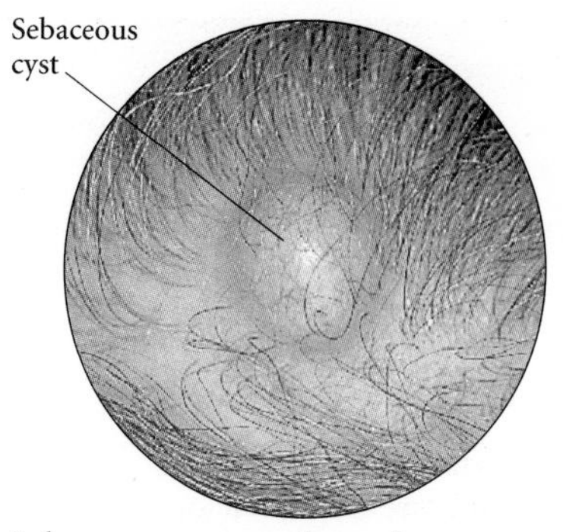

Sebaceous cyst on the scalp
The scalp is a typical site for a sebaceous cyst, which is a smooth, harmless lump that develops under the skin.

If a sebaceous cyst is not causing you any problems, it can safely be left untreated. However, if the cyst becomes very large or painful, it can be removed under a local anaesthetic. The cyst will usually be taken out intact because it can recur if the sac and its contents have not been completely removed. If it becomes infected, antibiotics (p.885) or incision and drainage may be required.

(WWW) ONLINE SITES: p.1036

Calluses and corns

Areas of thickened skin on the hands or feet caused by pressure or friction

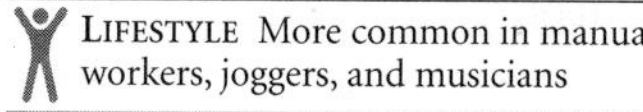
LIFESTYLE More common in manual workers, joggers, and musicians

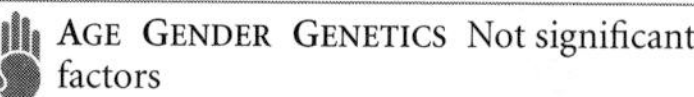
AGE GENDER GENETICS Not significant factors

If there is prolonged pressure or friction on a small area of the hand or foot, a patch of hard, thickened skin known as a callus may develop to protect the underlying tissues. Calluses are usually painless. They commonly occur on the hands of people such as musicians due to friction. The soles of the feet may become callused by the uneven pressure of body weight during walking.

Corns are patches of thickened skin that occur on the toes. They are usually due to wearing shoes that are too tight. The patches have a hard, clear centre and can be painful and persistent.

What is the treatment?

If you have a callus, you can remove some of the hardened skin by soaking the area in warm water for 10 minutes and then rubbing the callus gently with a pumice stone. Regular application of moisturizing cream may help to keep the skin soft. If possible, keep pressure off the area to aid recovery and to prevent recurrence of the callus. It is difficult to protect calluses that have developed on the sole of the foot, but well-fitting shoes may be of some help.

To relieve pressure on corns, wear shoes that do not press on the toes, and use corn pads (small rings of sponge that are available over the counter).

Your doctor or a chiropodist may reduce the size of a thickened area by paring it down with a scalpel, usually over several sessions. Once the source of pressure has been removed, calluses and corns should not recur.

Calluses or corns may become infected and ulcerated, especially in people with diabetes mellitus (p.687). If infection or ulceration occurs, do not try to treat the lesions yourself but get advice from a doctor or chiropodist.

(WWW) ONLINE SITES: p.1036

Keloid

A firm, raised, smooth overgrowth of scar tissue that develops after injury to the skin

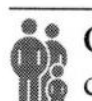
GENETICS May run in families; more common in black people

AGE GENDER LIFESTYLE Not significant factors

A keloid is an itchy, firm, irregularly shaped overgrowth of scar tissue. Keloids are smooth and shiny, appearing pinkish red on light skin and brown on dark skin. They usually form on the surface of a wound when a defective healing process causes overproduction of the skin protein collagen. Keloids are more common in black people, and susceptibility to them may run in families. If you are prone to the growths, you may find they appear after any kind of skin damage, including cuts, burns, acne, insect bites, tattoos, piercings for jewellery, and minor surgery. Rarely, they form spontaneously with no known cause. Keloids may develop almost anywhere on the body but usually occur on the chest, shoulders, and ear lobes. The growths are harmless, although large keloids may be unsightly.

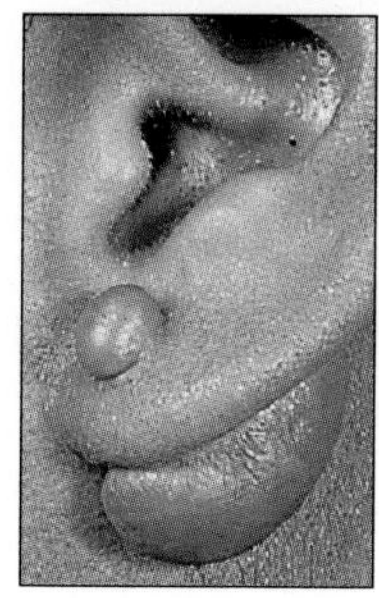

Keloid growth
An overgrowth of scar tissue called a keloid has formed on this ear lobe after ear-piercing. Susceptible people may develop keloids after even minor skin damage.

What is the treatment?

Your doctor may either inject a corticosteroid (p.930) into the scar tissue, or prescribe tape impregnated with a topical corticosteroid (p.892), which can be cut to size and placed over the keloid, causing the scar to shrink. Even with treatment, keloids often take up to a year to fade. Surgery and laser treatment are usually ineffective because the new scar tissue created forms another keloid.

(WWW) ONLINE SITES: p.1036

Stretch marks

Pink or purple lines on the skin, most commonly over the abdomen, buttocks, breasts, and thighs

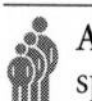
AGE Sometimes occur as a result of growth spurts at puberty

GENDER More common in females

LIFESTYLE More common in pregnant women and overweight people

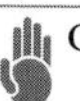
GENETICS Not a significant factor

Stretch marks, also called striae, occur when fibres of the skin protein collagen are broken due to rapid stretching of the skin or to hormonal changes that disrupt the fibres. The marks affect 3 in 5 pregnant women and are common in adolescent girls undergoing growth spurts. Overweight people may also develop them, especially if weight gain is rapid. They also occur in people with Cushing's syndrome (p.684) and in those using oral corticosteroids (p.930) or topical corticosteroids (p.892).

Stretch marks first appear as pink or purple raised lines on the abdomen, thighs, breasts, or buttocks. They vary in length and may be between 6 mm (1/4 in) and 12 mm (1/2 in) wide. Over a few months, they usually become pale and flatten, eventually becoming barely noticeable. There are no effective preventive measures or treatments.

(WWW) ONLINE SITES: p.1035, p.1036

Chilblains

Itchy, painful, reddish-purple swellings on the fingers or toes

AGE More common in children and elderly people

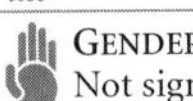

GENDER GENETICS LIFESTYLE Not significant factors

Chilblains result from excessive narrowing of blood vessels under the skin in cold weather. The reddish-purple swellings, which most commonly affect the fingers and toes, are painful when they are exposed to cold and are intensely itchy once the skin has become warm again.

Chilblains usually disappear without treatment but may recur. Children and elderly or inactive people in particular should wear sufficient clothing, including gloves, socks, and a hat, to keep warm and help to prevent chilblains from developing. If you are susceptible to chilblains and are exposed to cold weather, taking exercise may encourage blood flow to your hands and feet.

(WWW) ONLINE SITES: p.1036

Leg ulcer

A persistent open sore, usually on the lower part of the leg

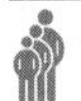

AGE More common in elderly people

LIFESTYLE People who are of limited mobility or bedridden are at risk

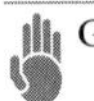

GENDER GENETICS Not significant factors

A leg ulcer occurs when an area of skin on the lower leg breaks down, usually as a result of poor blood circulation. An open sore may then develop, either spontaneously or following a minor injury, such as a scratch by a fingernail.

An ulcer appears as a shallow, pink area of broken skin; the surrounding skin may be swollen. Ulcers are slow to heal and often painful. They are most common in older people who have poor circulation or are not very mobile.

What are the types?

There are two main types of leg ulcer: venous ulcers and arterial ulcers. More than 9 in 10 of all leg ulcers are venous ulcers, which are caused by poor blood flow through the veins and therefore often occur in people with varicose veins (p.438). The ulcers usually form just above the ankle and may be surrounded by purplish-brown, scaly skin.

Arterial ulcers develop as a result of poor blood flow through the arteries supplying the limbs. People with diabetes mellitus (p.687) and those with sickle-cell disease (p.448) are especially susceptible to this type of ulcer. Arterial ulcers often form on the foot and are surrounded by pale, thin skin.

At the first sign of an ulcer, you should consult your doctor. Leg ulcers often become infected, and the infection may spread to the surrounding skin, causing cellulitis (p.352).

What might be done?

Your doctor may recommend Doppler ultrasound scanning (p.432) to assess blood flow in the affected leg. The ulcer should be dressed regularly and firmly bandaged to prevent infection, reduce swelling, and improve the blood circulation in that part of the leg. Wearing support stockings, exercising regularly, and keeping the leg raised when you are resting can also help to improve the circulation of the blood. If you have an arterial ulcer, you may need surgery.

What is the prognosis?

In susceptible people, leg ulcers may take several months to heal, and they often recur. In rare cases, skin grafting (p.319) may be necessary. If you are susceptible to leg ulcers, you should not neglect even minor wounds and you should consult your doctor at the first signs of soreness in a leg.

(WWW) ONLINE SITES: p.1036

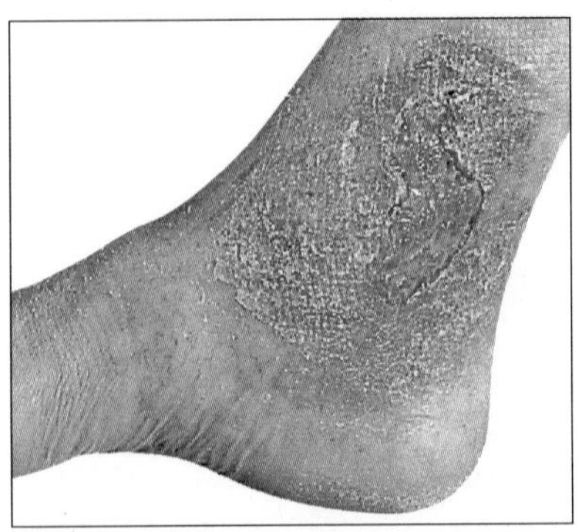

Leg ulcer on the ankle
A venous leg ulcer, such as the one shown here, consists of an open sore that is often surrounded by scaly, purplish-brown skin.

Pressure sores

Skin ulcers that develop in pressure spots, affecting people with limited mobility

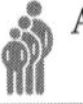

AGE Most common in elderly people

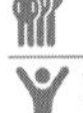

LIFESTYLE People who are of limited mobility or bedridden are at risk

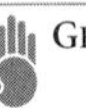

GENDER GENETICS Not significant factors

If people are paralysed or immobile, even for a few hours, small areas of their skin are subject to constant pressure from their own body weight. This pressure may restrict the normal supply of blood to the tissues. Sometimes, an area of tissue dies, leading to open sores, called pressure sores or bedsores. These usually affect elderly people, who are more likely to be immobile and have fragile skin. Urinary incontinence (p.710) may contribute to the development of pressure sores if it causes the skin to be continually damp.

What are the symptoms?

Common sites for pressure sores are the shoulders, hips, base of the spine, buttocks, heels, and ankles. The symptoms appear in the following stages:

- Affected areas of skin start to become red and tender.
- Painful areas become purple.
- The skin breaks down to form ulcers.

Left untreated, the sores become bigger and deeper and may become infected. Severe pressure sores may sometimes involve muscle, tendon, or bone under the damaged area of skin.

What might be done?

Bedridden people or those with limited mobility should have their skin checked regularly for signs of redness and tenderness. A bedridden person should have his or her position changed at least every 2 hours to relieve compression of the affected areas. It is important to keep the skin clean and dry. If a sore becomes infected, antibiotics (p.885) may be necessary. Usually, pressure sores gradually heal with treatment and good nutrition to improve the person's general health, but deep ulcers may take several months to clear up. If they are extensive, plastic surgery (p.952) may be necessary to promote healing.

(WWW) ONLINE SITES: p.1033, p.1036

SKIN INFECTIONS AND INFESTATIONS

The skin surface provides the body with protection from the environment and from infection, but the skin itself may become infected by bacteria, viruses, or fungi. Some of these organisms live naturally on the body and do not normally cause disease unless they breach the barrier of the skin's surface. Infestation of the skin by parasites, such as mites, may also occur.

Infectious organisms can enter the skin in various ways. Natural openings, such as a hair follicle or sweat gland, or broken skin at the site of an insect bite or a cut may provide a gateway for bacteria. Warm and moist areas, such as the skin between the toes, are more susceptible to fungal infections. Some common viral skin infections, such as warts, can be spread from one part of the body surface to another or may be passed from one person to another by direct skin contact.

In this section, bacterial skin infections are described first, followed by fungal and viral infections. The final article covers infestation by the scabies mite.

Diseases such as measles and rubella, in which a skin rash occurs due to an infection that also affects many other areas of the body, are covered elsewhere (*see* INFECTIONS AND INFESTATIONS, pp.284–313). The two common skin infestations head lice (p.831) and pubic lice (p.768) are also described in other sections of the book.

KEY ANATOMY

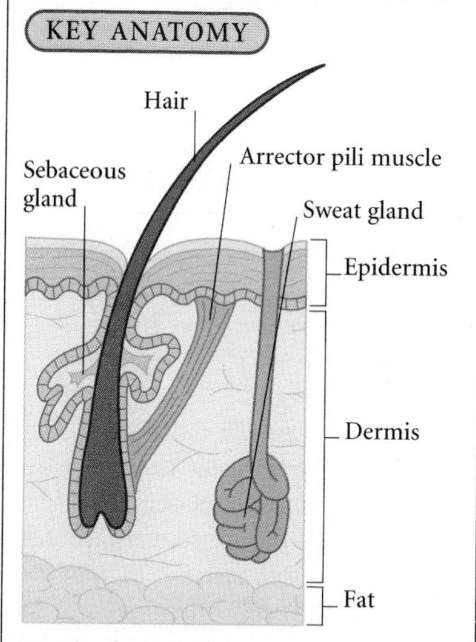

For further information on the structure and function of the skin, *see* pp.328–331.

Boil

A red, painful, pus-filled swelling of the skin caused by a bacterial infection

AGE GENDER GENETICS LIFESTYLE
Not significant factors

A boil develops when a hair follicle or sebaceous gland (which secretes sebum into the hair follicle) becomes infected. The infection then spreads and pus collects in surrounding tissues. Common sites for boils are moist areas, such as the groin, or areas where friction occurs, such as under a collar. Boils are usually due to infection with the bacterium *Staphylococcus aureus*, which some people normally carry on the skin or in the nose without symptoms. A cluster of connected boils is called a carbuncle.

Boils are most common in people whose resistance to infection is lowered by a disorder such as diabetes mellitus (p.687) or AIDS (*see* HIV INFECTION AND AIDS, p.297), but they can occur in those without immune problems.

WHAT ARE THE SYMPTOMS?

The symptoms develop gradually in the following order over several days:

- A small, red lump appears.
- The area becomes painful and tender.
- The lump and the tissues around it begin to swell as pus accumulates.
- A white or yellow head of pus appears at the centre of the boil.
- The affected area feels warm to the touch and throbs.

Boils often clear up without treatment. They may burst and release the pus or gradually subside and then disappear.

WHAT CAN I DO?

You can relieve pain and help the healing process by applying a cotton-wool ball or a clean cloth soaked in hot water to the area for about 30 minutes four times a day. Do not squeeze the boil because this may cause the infection to spread further. If a boil does not start to heal within a few days or it becomes large or painful, consult your doctor.

WHAT MIGHT THE DOCTOR DO?

Your doctor may drain the pus by making a small incision in the centre of the boil with a sterile needle. This procedure is usually painless. You may also be prescribed oral antibiotics (p.885) to treat the cause of the infection. Large boils may need to be lanced with a surgical knife under local anaesthesia.

If you develop recurrent boils, you may have blood and urine tests to look for an underlying disorder. Your doctor may also recommend that you use antiseptic soap or cream to kill the bacteria (*see* PREPARATIONS FOR SKIN INFECTIONS AND INFESTATIONS, p.892).

(WWW) ONLINE SITES: p.1033, p.1036

Impetigo

Blistering and crusting of the skin caused by a bacterial infection

AGE More common in children

GENDER GENETICS LIFESTYLE
Not significant factors

The blistering skin condition impetigo is caused by bacteria entering broken skin, typically where there is a cut, an area of eczema (p.333), or a cold sore (p.354). The condition is highly contagious and is spread by physical contact. It is more common in children.

WHAT ARE THE SYMPTOMS?

Impetigo can appear anywhere on the body but usually occurs on the face, especially around the nose and mouth. The following symptoms usually develop over a period of 1–2 days:

- Initially, the skin reddens and tiny, fluid-filled blisters appear.

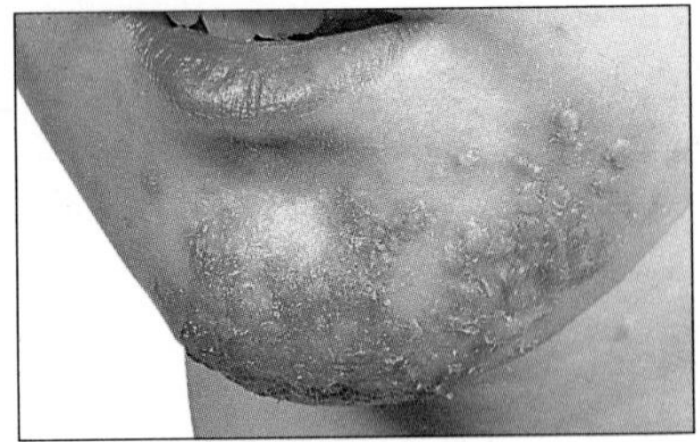

Impetigo on the face
The honey-coloured crust covering this child's chin has been formed by impetigo blisters that have burst and dried out.

- The blisters burst soon after they are formed, releasing a yellow fluid.
- The skin underneath the burst blisters becomes red and weeping.
- The blisters dry out to form an itchy, honey-coloured crust.

The blistered patch often spreads. Left untreated, it may become quite large.

WHAT IS THE TREATMENT?

Your doctor may prescribe topical antibiotics (*see* PREPARATIONS FOR SKIN INFECTIONS AND INFESTATIONS, p.892) or oral antibiotics (p.885). Soaking the crusts with warm salt water helps to remove them and relieve itching. With treatment, impetigo usually clears up in a few days. To avoid spreading the condition to others, wash your hands often and do not share face flannels. Keep an affected child home from school.

(WWW) ONLINE SITES: p.1026, p.1036

Folliculitis

Inflammation of the hair follicles that produces small, yellow, pus-filled pimples

 AGE More common in adults

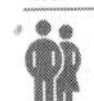 GENDER More common in males

LIFESTYLE Shaving and hair-plucking are risk factors

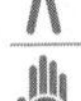 GENETICS Not a significant factor

Inflammation of the hair follicles due to bacterial infection is called folliculitis. The pus-filled pimples produced by this condition may develop on any part of the body but most commonly appear on the limbs and, in men, in the beard area. Shaving or plucking the hairs can increase the risk of inflammation. Folliculitis of the beard area is particularly common in black men, whose curly hairs often grow back into the skin and may cause an infection. The use of topical corticosteroids (p.892) may also cause folliculitis in some people.

Your doctor may prescribe topical antibiotics (*see* PREPARATIONS FOR SKIN INFECTIONS AND INFESTATIONS, p.892) to treat the infection or oral antibiotics (p.885) for acute, extensive folliculitis. To avoid spreading folliculitis, wash regularly with antibacterial soap and do not share razors or towels. Men may find that growing a beard helps to prevent folliculitis from developing on the face.

(WWW) ONLINE SITES: p.1036

Cellulitis

Bacterial infection of the skin and underlying tissues that causes redness and swelling

 AGE More common in elderly people

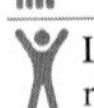 LIFESTYLE Intravenous drug use is a risk factor

 GENDER GENETICS Not significant factors

In cellulitis, an area of skin and the underlying tissues become infected by bacteria that enter through a small, possibly unnoticed, wound. The infection causes redness, pain, and swelling and most commonly affects the legs.

Elderly people are especially vulnerable to cellulitis because they are more likely to have poor circulation, which leads to oedema (fluid build-up in the tissues) or leg ulcers (p.350). These problems increase the risk of infection. Others who are at increased risk of cellulitis include intravenous drug users and people whose resistance to infection has been lowered by disorders such as diabetes mellitus (p.687) or AIDS (*see* HIV INFECTION AND AIDS, p.297).

WHAT ARE THE SYMPTOMS?

The symptoms appear gradually over several hours and include:

- Redness, swelling, and in some cases warmth in the affected area of skin.
- Pain and tenderness in the area.
- Occasionally, fever and chills.

If you develop these symptoms, consult your doctor without delay. Left untreated, cellulitis may cause septicaemia (p.299), a serious blood infection.

WHAT MIGHT BE DONE?

If you have an obvious wound, your doctor may take a swab from the area to identify the bacterium that is causing the infection. The doctor will probably prescribe oral antibiotics (p.885), which should take effect within 48 hours. In severe cases, you may need hospital treatment with intravenous antibiotics. If your leg is affected, you should keep it elevated to help to reduce the swelling. Cellulitis may recur if you have a persistent immune or circulatory problem.

(WWW) ONLINE SITES: p.1036

Ringworm

A fungal infection that produces itchy, red, circular patches on the scalp, groin, or elsewhere on the skin

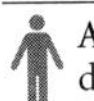 AGE GENDER LIFESTYLE Risk factors depend on the type

 GENETICS Not a significant factor

Despite the name, ringworm is caused not by worms but by fungi that infect the skin and cause itchy, red, ring-shaped patches. There are a number of common forms of the disorder, including scalp ringworm (tinea capitis), body ringworm (tinea corporis), and ringworm of the groin (tinea cruris).

Scalp ringworm, which is more common in children, can spread from one person to another or be acquired from cats and dogs. Ringworm of the groin mainly affects men, particularly those who have other fungal infections, such as athlete's foot (opposite page). All forms of ringworm are especially common in people with reduced immunity to infection due to disorders such as diabetes mellitus (p.687) or AIDS (*see* HIV INFECTION AND AIDS, p.297).

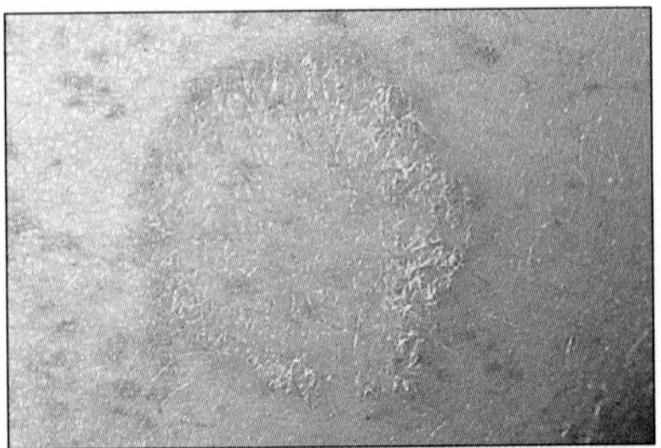

Ringworm on the body
The patch of ringworm shown here has already begun to spread, leaving a scaly, itchy, red ring surrounding normal skin.

WHAT ARE THE SYMPTOMS?

In all forms of ringworm, the following symptoms develop gradually over days or sometimes weeks:

- Initially, a small, round, scaly, itchy, red patch appears.
- After 1–2 weeks, more patches appear.
- Each patch grows larger and forms a scaly, red ring around a central area of normal skin.

In scalp ringworm, hairs may break off just above the surface of the skin, leading to irregular patches of stubble (*see* ALOPECIA, p.358). In ringworm of the groin, the rash occasionally spreads further to affect the skin on the inside of the thighs and the buttocks.

WHAT MIGHT BE DONE?

Your doctor will probably recognize ringworm from its appearance and may confirm the diagnosis by taking a skin scraping. The removed skin is examined under a microscope to confirm the presence of fungal infection.

Topical antifungal drugs may be obtained by prescription from your doctor or over the counter (*see* PREPARATIONS FOR SKIN INFECTIONS AND INFESTATIONS, p.892). If the ringworm affects your scalp or is widespread, you may be prescribed oral antifungal drugs (p.889), which you will need to take for several weeks to clear up the infection completely. If you have ringworm of the groin, you can help to prevent a recurrence by keeping the area clean and dry.

(WWW) ONLINE SITES: p.1026, p.1036

Athlete's foot

A fungal infection of the foot that produces cracked, sore, itchy skin between the toes

 AGE Most common in teenagers and young adults; rare in children

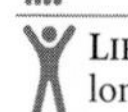 LIFESTYLE Wearing enclosed footwear for long periods is a risk factor

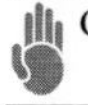 GENDER GENETICS Not significant factors

Athlete's foot, also called tinea pedis, is a common fungal infection of the feet that particularly affects the skin between the toes. The condition can be caused by several types of fungi that thrive in warm, humid conditions.

Athlete's foot often affects teenagers and young adults, who tend to sweat more and wear enclosed footwear, such as trainers, for long periods. It is rare in children. Athlete's foot can be picked up by walking barefoot in communal areas that are warm and humid, such as changing rooms and poolsides.

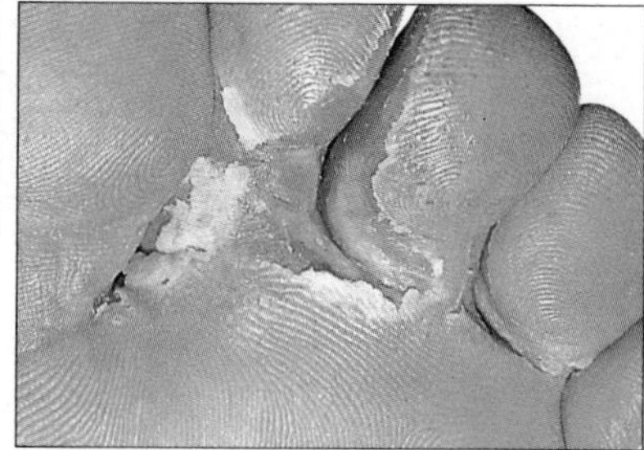

Athlete's foot
Toes affected by the fungal skin infection athlete's foot may become white and soggy, and the skin between and under them may peel away to leave painful raw areas.

WHAT ARE THE SYMPTOMS?

Athlete's foot most commonly occurs between the fourth and fifth toes and produces the following symptoms:

- Cracked, sore, and itchy areas of skin.
- Flaking, white, soggy skin.

Sometimes, the infection spreads on to the sole or the sides of the foot or affects the toenails, which then become yellowish, thickened, and brittle. People who have athlete's foot are more susceptible to ringworm (opposite page) of the groin, another fungal infection.

WHAT IS THE TREATMENT?

The affected area can be treated using an over-the-counter antifungal preparation, which should be applied at least twice a day (*see* PREPARATIONS FOR SKIN INFECTIONS AND INFESTATIONS, p.892). It is important that you continue to apply the preparation to affected areas for a few days after the symptoms have cleared up to make sure that the infection is eradicated. If over-the-counter preparations do not help or you are unsure of the diagnosis, consult your doctor, who can give you further advice about treatment or prescribe a stronger antifungal drug (p.889).

To prevent the infection from recurring, you should wash your feet at least once a day, more frequently if they become sweaty, and dry them thoroughly between the toes. At home, it may help to wear open-toed shoes or go barefoot.

(WWW) ONLINE SITES: p.1026, p.1036

Pityriasis versicolor

A fungal infection that produces patches of discoloured skin on the trunk

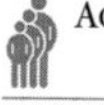 AGE More common under the age of 50

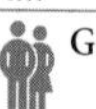 GENDER More common in males

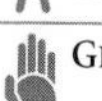 LIFESTYLE Hot and humid conditions are a risk factor

GENETICS Not a significant factor

Pityriasis versicolor, also called tinea versicolor, is a patchy skin condition caused by a fungus living in the hair follicles of the body. The fungus does not normally produce symptoms, but in hot and humid conditions, when the skin becomes moist, it grows and colonizes the outer layer of skin. If the skin is oily, the fungus is more likely to spread to the surface of the skin. The infection is more common in men, particularly those under the age of 50.

WHAT ARE THE SYMPTOMS?

The only symptom is the appearance of painless, discoloured patches on the skin. The upper trunk area, including the neck, chest, shoulders, and back, is usually affected. The patches are:

- Of variable size, round, and flat with clearly defined edges.
- Pinkish brown in colour on pale skin, becoming more noticeable if the surrounding skin tans. On dark skin, the patches are pale. In some people, affected areas are darkly pigmented.

Left untreated, the patches may become widespread and persist indefinitely.

WHAT MIGHT BE DONE?

Your doctor will probably be able to diagnose pityriasis versicolor from the appearance of the patches. Sometimes, skin scrapings may be taken to confirm the presence of the fungus. Treatment usually consists of washing the affected area regularly with an over-the-counter shampoo containing selenium sulphide, an antifungal drug (p.889). With thorough treatment, the infection usually clears up in 2–3 weeks, but it may take several more weeks for your skin to return to its normal colour. If you miss a patch of affected skin when applying the shampoo, the infection will recur.

(WWW) ONLINE SITES: p.1036

Cold sore

A painful cluster of tiny blisters, usually near the lips, caused by a viral infection

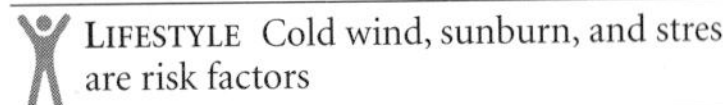

LIFESTYLE Cold wind, sunburn, and stress are risk factors

AGE GENDER GENETICS Not significant factors

Cold sores are painful clusters of blisters usually caused by herpes simplex virus type 1 (HSV-1). Most people have been infected with HSV-1 at least once by the time they reach adulthood. The initial infection often goes unnoticed but may cause blisters in the mouth. The virus then remains dormant in the nerve cells, but in some people it is reactivated and produces cold sores. Trigger factors include cold wind, sunburn, tiredness, stress, the common cold, menstruation, and fever. Some people have recurrent cold sores.

WHAT ARE THE SYMPTOMS?

Cold sores often develop on the skin around the lips. The symptoms usually appear in the following order:

- The affected site begins to tingle.
- One or more clusters of tiny, painful blisters develop, and the surrounding skin becomes inflamed.
- The blisters burst and become crusty.
- Usually, the blisters subside within 10–14 days.

If cold sores recur, the blisters usually reappear in the same areas on the face.

WHAT MIGHT BE DONE?

You may be able to prevent individual outbreaks by using an over-the-counter antiviral cream such as aciclovir (*see* PREPARATIONS FOR INFECTIONS AND INFESTATIONS, p.892), but you must apply the cream as soon as the first symptoms develop. In some cases, oral antiviral drugs (p.886) may be prescribed. Although prompt treatment can prevent individual outbreaks, the virus remains in the system and symptoms may recur. If you have recurrent cold sores, try to protect your skin from trigger factors such as sunburn or cold wind. To minimize the risk of spreading the virus, do not touch the blisters and avoid kissing. Sometimes, oral sex can transmit the virus from the mouth to the genitals (*see* GENITAL HERPES, p.767).

(WWW) ONLINE SITES: p.1033, p.1036

Warts

Firm, skin-coloured or darker growths on the skin caused by a viral infection

AGE Most common in children and young adults

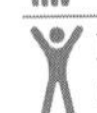

LIFESTYLE Warm, moist conditions are a risk factor

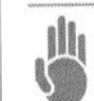

GENDER GENETICS Not significant factors

Warts, also called verrucas, are small growths caused by human papillomaviruses. The viruses invade skin cells and encourage them to multiply, thus creating thickened areas of skin. Warts usually occur on the hands or feet and are generally harmless. However, some types affect the genitals and are more serious (*see* GENITAL WARTS, p.768).

Warts are transferred by direct contact with an infected person or from virus particles on recently shed flakes of skin. The infection is commonly spread in warm, moist conditions.

Most people have at least one wart by the age of 20, but in some people warts recur. People with reduced immunity due to a disease such as AIDS (*see* HIV INFECTION AND AIDS, p.297) may develop large numbers of warts.

WHAT ARE THE TYPES?

There are three main types of wart. These types are classified according to their appearance and the different sites on the body on which they occur.

COMMON WARTS These warts most frequently occur on the hands. They are:

- Firm with a rough, raised surface.
- Usually round.
- Dotted with tiny black spots.

The black spots are small blood vessels. Common warts often grow in groups, which are known as crops.

PLANTAR WARTS These warts occur on the soles of the feet. Although plantar warts are the same as common warts, they grow into the skin because they are continually under pressure from the weight of the body. A group of plantar warts that have joined together is called a mosaic wart. Plantar warts are:

- Flattened into the sole of the foot.
- Firm, with a thickened surface.
- Usually painful to walk on.
- Dotted with tiny black spots.

The virus that causes plantar warts is usually picked up from walking barefoot in communal areas, such as changing rooms and swimming pools.

SELF-HELP TREATING A WART

You can treat common and plantar warts by using over-the-counter gels or lotions containing salicylic acid, which dissolves the thickened layer of skin. Apply the treatment daily for several weeks until the warts have disappeared. Keep equipment used for treating warts away from other bath items to avoid spreading the virus. Do not share bath items.

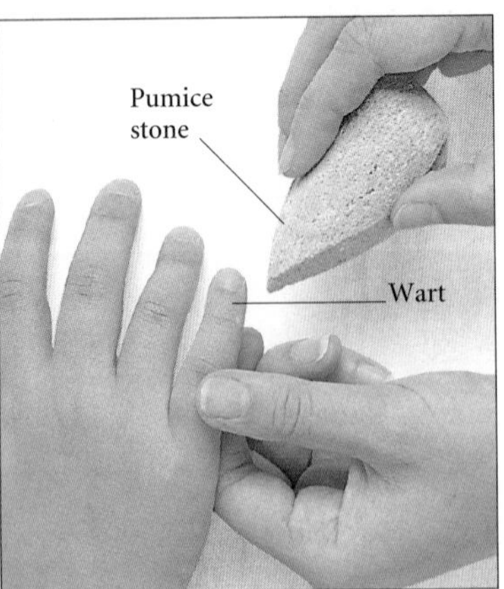

1 *Soak the wart in water to soften it. Then gently rub it with a pumice stone or an emery board to remove as much of the thickened skin as possible.*

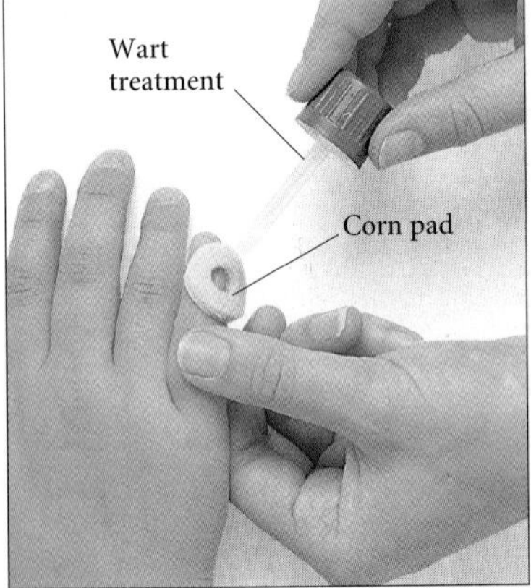

2 *Shield the surrounding skin with a corn pad or petroleum jelly. Carefully apply the wart treatment to the wart and cover the area with an adhesive bandage.*

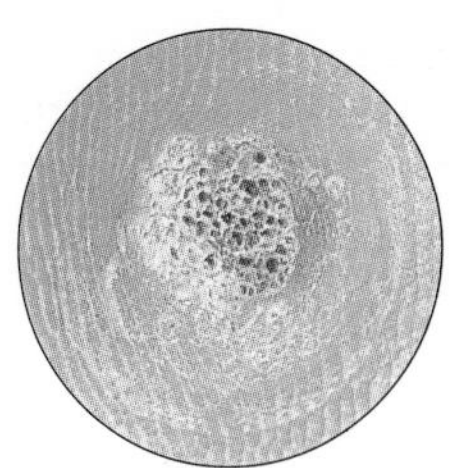

Plantar wart
This wart on the sole of the foot has been flattened by the body's weight and has developed a thickened surface.

FLAT WARTS Verruca plana, also known as flat warts, commonly occur on the wrists, backs of the hands, and face. Flat warts vary in size and are:

- Skin-coloured.
- Flat-topped and very slightly raised.
- Often itchy.

These warts often occur in lines where the virus has spread along a scratch.

WHAT MIGHT BE DONE?

Most warts disappear without treatment, but this can take months or years. Many over-the-counter wart treatments are available (*see* TREATING A WART, opposite page). If a wart persists despite self-help measures or if you are unsure whether a lesion is a wart, consult your doctor. You should tell your doctor if a wart is painful, appears on the face or genitals, or affects a child under the age of 5. The doctor may decide to remove a wart by freezing, scraping, or burning it off. In some cases, warts can recur.

(WWW) ONLINE SITES: p.1026, p.1036

Molluscum contagiosum

A viral infection producing multiple shiny, pearly-white pimples

AGE More common in children

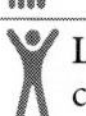

LIFESTYLE Close skin contact and, in some cases, sexual contact with an infected person are risk factors

GENDER GENETICS Not significant factors

Molluscum contagiosum is a viral skin infection in which pimples appear in clusters on the trunk and at the tops of the arms and legs. The condition is harmless but contagious and is spread by close skin contact. It is common in children, especially in those with atopic eczema, probably because they scratch their skin, and this allows the virus to enter (*see* ECZEMA IN CHILDREN, p.829). In adults, molluscum contagiosum is usually spread through sexual contact. In such cases, the pimples tend to occur on the lower abdomen, genitals, and thighs. The condition is more common and often more severe in people whose immune systems are weakened by disorders such as AIDS (*see* HIV INFECTION AND AIDS, p.297) or by treatment with immunosuppressants (p.906).

WHAT ARE THE SYMPTOMS?

The symptoms of molluscum contagiosum begin 2–8 weeks after infection. A single, itchy pimple appears, and the infection then spreads to form a cluster of pimples. The pimples are:

- Approximately 3–6 mm (1/8–1/4 in) in diameter.
- Smooth and pearly-white or pink.
- Dome-shaped with a tiny depression in the centre.

Molluscum contagiosum is not painful, but large pimples may bleed if they become caught on clothing.

WHAT MIGHT BE DONE?

Children with molluscum contagiosum are usually not treated because treatment may leave small scars and can be painful. The condition usually clears up by itself within 12 months. In adults, the pimples may be removed for cosmetic reasons. Your doctor may pierce them with a small probe, squeeze them with a pair of forceps, or scrape away a thin layer of skin under the pimples.

To prevent spread across the body, do not scratch the pimples. Avoid close physical contact and do not share towels or face flannels so that others are not infected. The condition can recur if you are re-exposed to infection or if your immune system becomes weakened.

(WWW) ONLINE SITES: p.1036

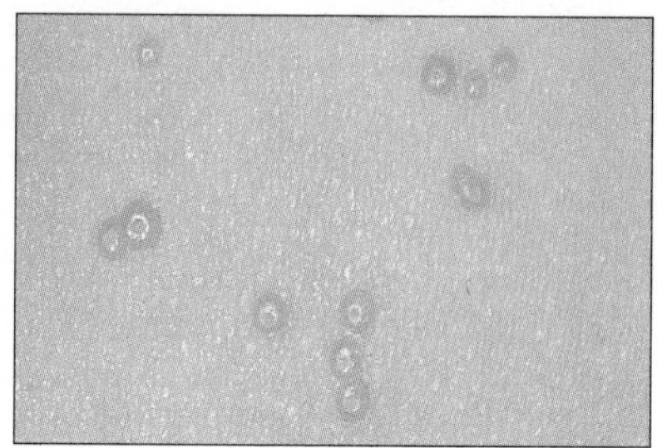

Molluscum contagiosum
These clusters of tiny, itchy, dome-shaped pimples are produced by the viral skin infection molluscum contagiosum.

Scabies

A mite infestation of the skin causing distinctive brown lines and an itchy rash

AGE Most common in children and young adults

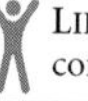

LIFESTYLE Living in overcrowded conditions is a risk factor

GENDER GENETICS Not significant factors

The skin infestation scabies is caused by a mite that burrows into the outer layer of skin to lay its eggs. For several weeks there are no symptoms, but as the larvae hatch and grow into mites the skin becomes sensitive to the faeces of the mites and intense itching develops.

Scabies can affect people of any age but is most common in children and young adults. It is highly contagious and is spread by close physical contact, especially in overcrowded living conditions. It can be passed on by sexual contact or by prolonged hand-holding.

WHAT ARE THE SYMPTOMS?

The symptoms of scabies appear within 4–6 weeks of infestation and include:

- A rash of raised, pinkish-red spots up to 1 cm (3/8 in) in diameter.
- Widespread itching, which is particularly severe at night.
- Light brown lines (burrows), which most often occur between the fingers and toes. In babies, they sometimes appear on the palms and soles.

The itching may occur before the rash appears, and it may persist for up to 3 weeks after the rash has disappeared.

WHAT MIGHT BE DONE?

Your doctor will probably be able to diagnose scabies from the appearance of the rash. To confirm the diagnosis, he or she may take a skin scraping from the area for examination under a microscope. Scabies is usually treated with an antiparasitic lotion applied to the body from the neck down and washed off 8–24 hours later (*see* PREPARATIONS FOR INFECTIONS AND INFESTATIONS, p.892). A topical corticosteroid (p.892) may also be prescribed to relieve itching. To prevent reinfection, people in close contact with you should be treated at the same time, and clothing and bedding should be washed thoroughly.

(WWW) ONLINE SITES: p.1036

MINOR SKIN INJURIES

The skin is remarkably resistant to the wear and tear of everyday life, but from time to time it may be affected by minor injury. Hands and feet are especially vulnerable to cuts, scrapes, and blisters. In a healthy person, superficial skin injuries normally heal rapidly, and most do not need attention from a doctor.

The most common types of skin injury are minor cuts and scrapes, in which the outer layer of the skin is broken. These types of wound are usually trivial, although they may be painful and there is a risk of infection entering the damaged site.

Sunburn is another common minor skin injury but one that is usually avoidable. Damage to the skin caused by overexposure to sunlight may not always appear serious, but, in the long term, sunburn increases the risk of potentially dangerous skin cancers.

Friction and burns can cause damage to tissues beneath the surface of the skin, which often remains unbroken. Leaking blood and other fluids from this damage are trapped under the skin and appear as bruises or blisters.

Simple self-help measures are often the only treatment needed for minor skin injuries. Emergency procedures for dealing with serious injuries are explained elsewhere (*see* FIRST AID, pp.976–998). Burns (p.317), which can be serious, are also discussed elsewhere in the book.

KEY ANATOMY

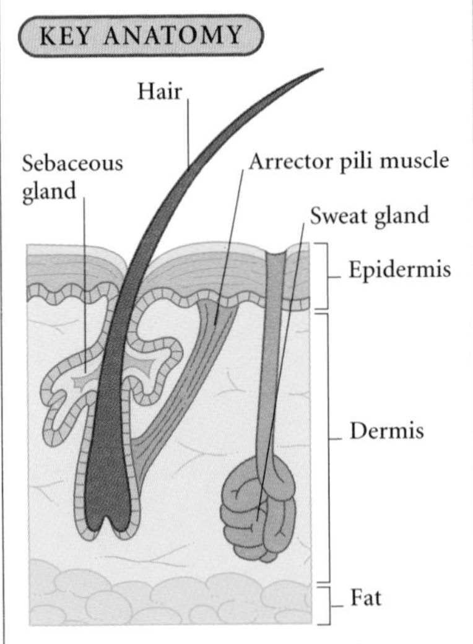

For further information on the structure and function of the skin, *see* pp.328–331.

Cuts and scrapes

Broken areas on the surface of the skin caused by minor injuries

AGE GENDER GENETICS LIFESTYLE Not significant factors

From time to time, the surface of the skin may be broken by small cuts and scrapes. Most of these minor injuries bleed to some extent, particularly those on the scalp or the palm of the hand.

A cut in the skin may be irregular or, if it results from injury caused by a sharp-edged implement such as a knife, clearly demarcated. Scrapes occur when the top layer of the skin rubs against a rough surface and is damaged. These superficial abrasions do not necessarily bleed but may ooze clear fluid.

WHAT CAN I DO?

Clean a cut or scrape as soon as you possibly can with soap and water and make sure that no dirt or foreign bodies are embedded in the wound. To control bleeding, press a clean gauze pad firmly over the area. Small injuries may heal more quickly if left uncovered, but, if dirt is likely to enter the wound, you should protect the area with an antiseptic cream and a sterile dressing.

WHAT MIGHT THE DOCTOR DO?

Minor injuries usually do not need medical attention. However, if a wound is slow to heal, becomes more swollen, red, and painful, or contains pus, it may be infected. You may need oral antibiotics (p.885) or topical antibiotics (*see* PREPARATIONS FOR SKIN INFECTIONS AND INFESTATIONS, p.892) from your doctor.

If a wound is deep or dirty, you may need an antitetanus injection, especially if you have not had one for more than 5 years (*see* ROUTINE IMMUNIZATIONS, p.45). Severe wounds may need stitches.

Needlestick injury

Accidental puncture of the skin by a used hypodermic needle

LIFESTYLE Working in health centres and visiting public leisure areas are risk factors

AGE GENDER GENETICS Not significant factors

Although a minor puncture of the skin with a used hypodermic needle may cause little pain or bleeding, a needlestick injury may have particularly serious implications for your health. Any needlestick injury needs to be investigated because of the risk that the needle carries organisms such as HIV, the virus that causes AIDS (*see* HIV INFECTION AND AIDS, p.297), or the hepatitis B virus (*see* ACUTE HEPATITIS, p.644).

Needlestick injuries may occasionally occur among hospital staff. People who frequently visit public areas, such as parks or beaches, may also be at risk from needles that have been discarded by intravenous drug abusers.

If you have a needlestick injury, you should wash the wound using soap and water and consult a doctor as soon as you can. If possible, take the needle with you because your doctor may be able to check for the presence of viruses in the blood remaining in the needle.

Depending on the circumstances of the injury, you may need to have blood tests to find out if you are already immune to hepatitis B or if you are HIV-positive. If a course of immunization is started immediately, hepatitis B can usually be prevented. Your doctor may also suggest treatment with antiviral drugs to reduce the chance of HIV infection (*see* DRUGS FOR HIV INFECTION AND AIDS, p.887). Blood tests are usually done again after 3 months, and may be repeated at 3-month intervals for up to 12 months. The tests will determine whether you are clear of infection.

(WWW) ONLINE SITES: p.1032, p.1036

Sunburn

Inflammation of the skin caused by overexposure to the sun

 GENETICS More common in fair-skinned people

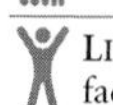 LIFESTYLE Outdoor activities are risk factors

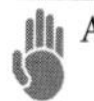 AGE GENDER Not significant factors

Sunburn occurs when the ultraviolet rays in sunlight damage cells in the outer layer of the skin, causing soreness, redness, and blistering. Damage is most likely to occur in the middle of the day when the sun is at its highest, but sunlight at any time of day can be harmful. It is possible for sunburn to occur even when the sky is overcast because ultraviolet rays can penetrate the cloud cover. Sunlight reflected off water or snow is especially damaging because its effects are intensified.

Fair-skinned people are more susceptible to sunburn because their skin produces only a small amount of the protective pigment melanin.

Sunburn or long-term exposure to the sun can cause the skin to age prematurely and increase the risk of developing skin cancer (p.344). To prevent sunburn, use sunscreens regularly (*see* SUNSCREEENS AND SUNBLOCKS, p.893) and avoid excessive exposure to the sun (*see* SAFETY IN THE SUN, p.80).

WHAT ARE THE SYMPTOMS?

Sunburn can occur after just 30 minutes of exposing the skin to the sun. The symptoms may take a few hours to develop and include:

- Sore, red, hot skin.
- Swelling of the affected area.
- In severe cases, blistering.

A few days after the initial sunburn, the skin may become dry and start to peel. Severe sunburn may be associated with heatstroke, which is a potentially fatal condition (*see* HEAT EXHAUSTION AND HEATSTROKE, p.322).

WHAT IS THE TREATMENT?

If you develop sunburn, stay in the shade and drink plenty of fluids. You may be able to relieve symptoms by applying aloe-based creams, calamine lotion, or sprays or lotions that contain the topical anaesthetic lidocaine to any affected areas (*see* LOCAL ANAESTHETICS, p.914). Cool baths and compresses may also help. Severe sunburn needs immediate medical attention, and you should consult your doctor as soon as possible. If you are severely burned and you also have heatstroke, you will need urgent treatment in hospital.

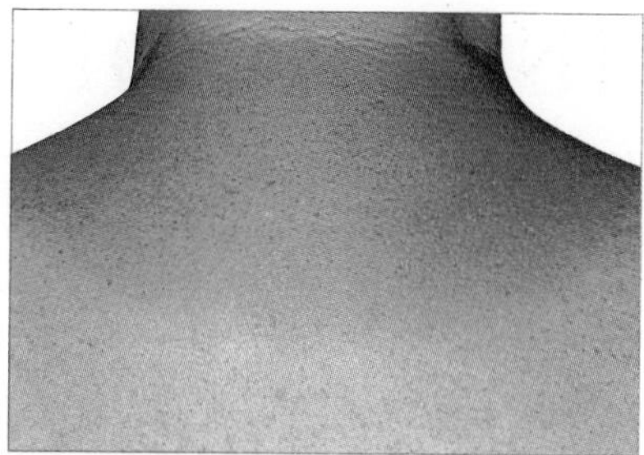

Sunburn
Even a short period of exposure to the sun can damage the surface of the skin, resulting in reddening and soreness.

(WWW) ONLINE SITES: p.1032, p.1036

Blister

A collection of fluid beneath the surface of the skin

 AGE GENDER GENETICS LIFESTYLE Not significant factors

A blister forms when fluid leaks from blood vessels in the skin, usually after minor injury, and collects to form a small, raised area just beneath the outer layer of skin. The most common causes of single blisters are friction, such as that caused by a badly fitting shoe, and burns, including sunburn (left). Widespread blistering may be caused by eczema (p.333), or it may occur in some viral infections, such as chickenpox (p.290) and shingles (*see* HERPES ZOSTER, p.290). The bacterial skin infection impetigo (p.351) may cause pus-filled blisters. There are also a number of much less common but potentially life-threatening conditions that result in blistering either on specific areas of skin or over the whole of the body (*see* BLISTERING DISEASES, p.336).

Blistering caused by minor damage usually heals rapidly without treatment. New skin develops beneath the blister, the fluid is gradually absorbed, and the top layer of skin dries and peels away. If the skin is broken, or if the blistered site is likely to be damaged further, you should protect the area with a dry, sterile dressing. Blistering due to disease or infection may need drug treatment.

You should not prick a blister to release the fluid because the skin acts as a barrier against infection. If the blisters are filled with pus or you notice spreading redness in the surrounding skin, consult your doctor.

Bruise

A discoloured area of skin caused by bleeding in underlying tissues

 AGE Most common in children and elderly people

 GENDER GENETICS LIFESTYLE Not significant factors

If the blood vessels beneath the skin are damaged by a blow or a fall, blood may leak into the surrounding tissues. This internal bleeding, even if it occurs deep in a muscle, will eventually show through the surface of the skin as black or blue patches called bruises. Over a period of a few days after the injury, the red cells in the leaked blood break down and the bruises gradually change colour, fading to green, light brown, or yellow. The discoloration normally disappears completely within a week.

After receiving an injury, you can reduce blood loss beneath the skin by applying firm pressure to the area with an ice pack. You should maintain the pressure for at least 5 minutes.

Children and elderly people bruise more easily than young and middle-aged adults. If severe bruising appears for no obvious reason at any age, you should consult your doctor because it may be a sign of a bleeding disorder such as von Willebrand's disease (p.452).

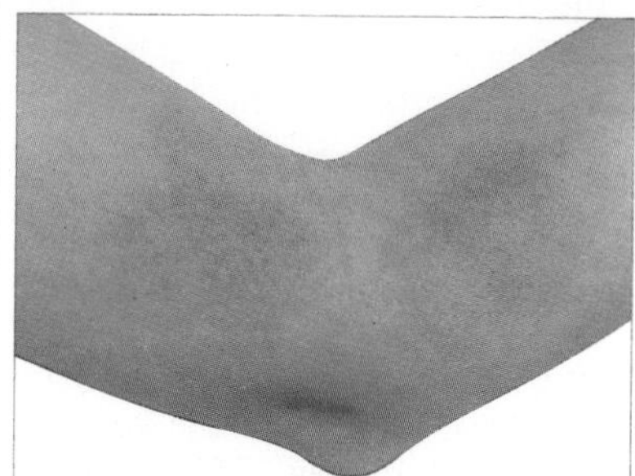

Bruising around the elbow
Prominent areas of the body, such as the elbow and knee, are vulnerable to injury and are common sites for bruises.

HAIR AND NAIL DISORDERS

Hair and nails, like the outer layers of skin, are made of dead cells that grow from a living base. The dead parts that show above the skin's surface can be cut or damaged without causing pain, but damage to the living roots is painful. The condition of the hair and nails often reflects general health. Changes in the nails, in particular, may indicate an underlying disease.

KEY ANATOMY

HAIR STRUCTURE

NAIL STRUCTURE

For more information on the structure and function of hair and nails, *see* pp.328–331.

Most hair and nail disorders are not a health threat but may be unsightly and cause embarrassment. However, some are caused by serious health problems. For example, excessive growth of body hair may be due to a hormonal imbalance, and spoon-shaped nails suggest iron deficiency. In these cases, treating the underlying disorder often improves the condition. Hair disorders may be due to factors such as drug treatments and localized skin diseases. Many nail abnormalities are due to minor injury or infection but can be difficult to treat. Topical preparations do not penetrate the nail, and oral drugs only affect its base. A damaged nail will not appear normal until it grows out, so the condition of the nails is sometimes an indication of past rather than present health.

This section begins by describing several disorders that affect scalp or body hair. The remaining articles describe abnormalities of the nails and the skin that surrounds them. Some common scalp problems are discussed elsewhere, including head lice (p.831) and seborrhoeic dermatitis (p.335).

Dandruff

Excessive shedding of flakes of skin from the scalp

AGE More common in young adults

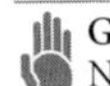
GENDER GENETICS LIFESTYLE Not significant factors

Dandruff is a harmless condition that involves an acceleration in the normal shedding of dead skin cells from the scalp. This dead skin accumulates as white flakes in the hair and sometimes causes itching. The condition is most common in young adults and may be a source of embarrassment.

Dandruff is most often caused by a yeast organism that grows in the scalp. Extensive dandruff is known as seborrhoeic dermatitis (p.335), a disorder that causes inflammation and scaling of the skin in other areas of the body, such as the face, chest, and back. Dandruff may be associated with inflammation of the eyelids (*see* BLEPHARITIS, p.583).

You can treat dandruff by washing your hair three to four times a week with a tar-based shampoo or a shampoo that contains an antiyeast agent, such as selenium sulphide or ketoconazole (*see* ANTIFUNGAL DRUGS, p.889).

If the dandruff persists despite treatment, you should consult your doctor because you may have developed a skin condition, such as eczema (p.333) or psoriasis (p.332), that also affects the scalp. These disorders may require specific treatment with prescription drugs.

(WWW) ONLINE SITES: p.1036

Alopecia

Loss of part or all of the hair, most commonly the hair on the scalp

AGE GENDER GENETICS LIFESTYLE Risk factors depend on the type

Alopecia, or hair loss, can occur in any body area but is particularly noticeable when it affects the scalp. The condition may be localized, in which hair is lost in patches, or generalized, in which there is thinning or total hair loss over the whole scalp. Hair loss can be temporary or permanent. Alopecia is not always associated with ill health, but it may cause embarrassment.

WHAT ARE THE CAUSES?

The most common cause of alopecia in men is oversensitivity to the hormone testosterone, producing a characteristic pattern of hair loss (*see* MALE-PATTERN BALDNESS, opposite page).

Patchy hair loss is usually due to alopecia areata, an autoimmune disorder that causes bald patches to appear on the scalp. These bald areas are surrounded by short, broken hairs. The hair usually regrows within 6 months, but in rare cases alopecia areata can cause permanent loss of all body hair.

Hairstyles that pull on the scalp are a common cause of patchy hair loss; if the pulling is continuous, hair loss may be permanent. Patchy hair loss may be the result of a rare psychological disorder in which the hair is compulsively pulled. Burns or skin disorders, such as ringworm (p.352), which scar the scalp may cause patchy hair loss.

Generalized hair loss is normal in elderly people. It may also occur temporarily after pregnancy and is a common side effect of chemotherapy (p.280). Other causes of thinning hair include acute illness, stress, and malnutrition.

WHAT IS THE TREATMENT?

Your doctor will probably be able to diagnose alopecia areata by the appearance of your scalp. This condition does not usually require treatment, but corticosteroids injected into the hairless patches may be effective in promoting regrowth. In most other cases of hair loss, the hair usually regrows once the underlying cause has been treated. Hair lost during pregnancy usually regrows about 3 months after childbirth.

If your scalp has patchy scarring, you may need a skin biopsy (p.344) to diagnose the underlying cause. Scarred areas may be treated with topical corticosteroids (p.892) or antifungal drugs (p.889), but if the damage is severe and has affected the hair follicles it is unlikely that new hair will grow.

(WWW) ONLINE SITES: p.1033, p.1036

Male-pattern baldness

Progressive loss of hair from the scalp, often in a characteristic pattern

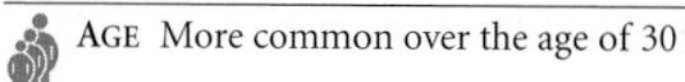

AGE More common over the age of 30

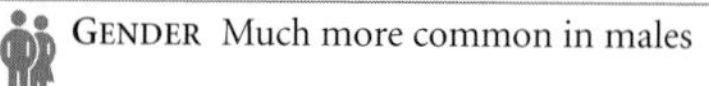

GENDER Much more common in males

GENETICS Often runs in families

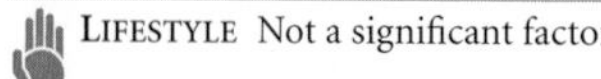

LIFESTYLE Not a significant factor

In male-pattern baldness, also called androgenic alopecia, hair is lost over several years, first from the temples and then from the crown, leaving a rim of hair around the scalp. The condition is very common in men over the age of 30 but may develop much earlier. In rare cases, it begins during puberty. This type of male-pattern baldness is often progressive and is thought to be caused by hypersensitivity of the follicles to the male sex hormone testosterone. There may be a family history of baldness in the male relatives on the mother's side.

Male-pattern baldness also occurs in women but is less common. Hair loss in women is usually due to hormonal disturbances, in particular those that take place after the menopause. In these cases, thinning is more generalized.

Your doctor may arrange for you to have tests to look for an underlying health problem (*see* ALOPECIA, opposite page). Over-the-counter solutions containing the substance minoxidil may stimulate regrowth temporarily, but new hair disappears when treatment is stopped. A more permanent way to replace hair in male-pattern baldness is by having a hair transplant (left).

(WWW) ONLINE SITES: p.1034, p.1036

(TREATMENT) HAIR TRANSPLANT

Baldness can be treated surgically by several different methods of hair transplantation. In the method shown here, a strip of skin and hair is taken from a donor site, usually at the back of your scalp or behind your ears. The removed hairs and their attached follicles are then inserted into the bald area on the scalp, which is called the recipient site. You will usually be given a mild sedative, and both the donor and recipient sites on the scalp are anaesthetized. The transplant process takes 1–1½ hours.

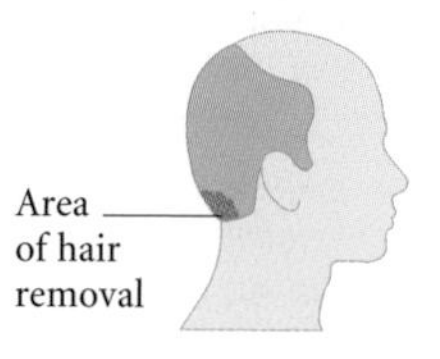

DONOR SITE

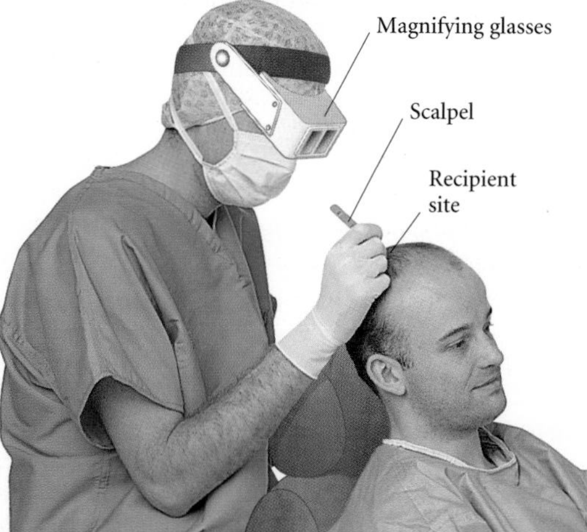

During the procedure
A strip of skin containing hairs with attached follicles is taken from the donor site, usually at the back of the scalp. The surgeon then makes numerous tiny incisions in the area that is to receive transplanted hair.

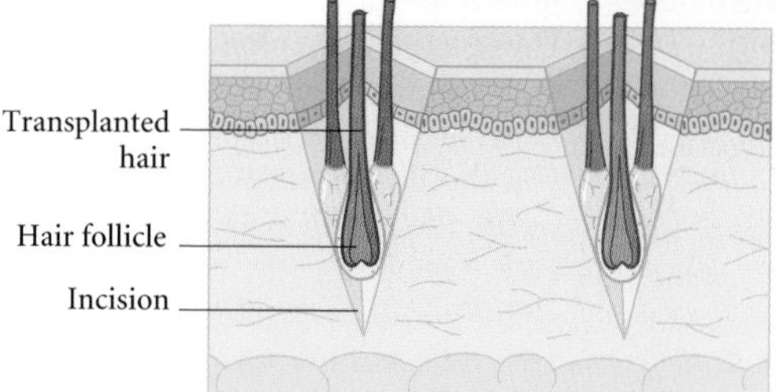

Transplanted hairs
The hairs from the donor site are inserted into the incisions using tweezers. The hairs themselves fall out shortly afterwards, but new hair starts to grow from the follicles 3 weeks to 3 months later. The donor site heals in about 5 days.

Excessive hair

Excessive growth of hair or hair growth in areas that would not normally have hair

AGE Occurs only after puberty; more common with increasing age

GENDER More common in females

GENETICS Sometimes runs in families

LIFESTYLE Not a significant factor

There are two types of excessive hair growth: hirsutism and hypertrichosis. Hirsutism affects women only. In this condition, excessive hair develops particularly on the face, trunk, and limbs. This type of excessive growth is more common in women over the age of 60, especially in those of Mediterranean, Asian, Hispanic, or Arab descent.

The second type of excessive hair growth, hypertrichosis, can affect both males and females. In this condition, hair grows all over the body, even in areas that do not normally have hair.

WHAT ARE THE CAUSES?

Mild hirsutism in women is often considered normal, especially following the menopause. In some cases, it may be a result of an increase in normally occurring male hormones in the female body (*see* VIRILIZATION, p.740), which may be caused by disorders such as polycystic ovary syndrome (p.744).

Hypertrichosis can occur with anorexia nervosa (p.562) or as a side effect of immunosuppressants (p.906) or antihypertensive drugs (p.897).

What might be done?

If you are a young woman with hirsutism, your doctor may arrange for a blood test to measure your male hormone levels. If these are high, you may be given a drug to block the hormones' effects and be treated for the underlying disorder. For example, polycystic ovary syndrome may be treated with hormones or surgery. If hypertrichosis is a side effect of a drug, stopping the treatment often reverses the condition.

You can deal with excessive hair yourself by bleaching it or by shaving, plucking, waxing, or using depilatory creams. The only way to remove hair permanently is by electrolysis, but it is a slow process and can be uncomfortable.

(WWW) ONLINE SITES: p.1033, p.1036

Pilonidal sinus

A pit, often containing hairs, at the top of the cleft between the buttocks

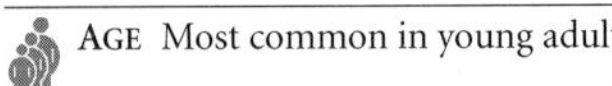
AGE Most common in young adults

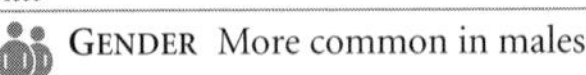
GENDER More common in males

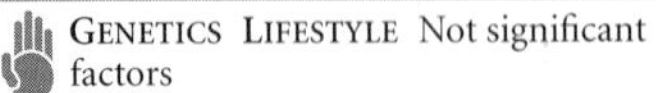
GENETICS LIFESTYLE Not significant factors

A pilonidal sinus is a small, enclosed pit beneath the skin at the top of the cleft between the buttocks. The condition occurs most commonly in men with a lot of body hair. The exact cause is unknown but may be a defect in the development of that area. Hair growth at the site tends to be directed inwards, which may cause infection in the sinus and result in a painful abscess.

Prompt action at the first signs of infection may prevent an abscess from forming. You should soak the area in warm water to relieve discomfort and consult your doctor as soon as possible. You may be prescribed oral antibiotics (p.885) to treat the infection. If pus has built up, the abscess will need to be drained under general anaesthesia and left open to heal. In most cases, the infection is unlikely to recur.

Nail abnormalities

Changes in the shape, colour, or texture of the nails, often due to injury, infection, or underlying disease

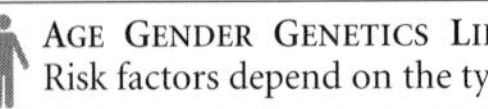
AGE GENDER GENETICS LIFESTYLE Risk factors depend on the type

The nails are particularly susceptible to damage. Injury is the most common cause of abnormalities in the shape, colour, or texture of the nails. Changes in general health and in the health of the skin at the nail bed may also lead to abnormalities. In addition, infection of the nail itself may alter its appearance.

What are the types?

Some forms of nail abnormality need treatment only if they are unsightly or painful; others may be signs of underlying health problems that may require medical investigation.

WHITE SPOTS Small white marks that appear on one or more nails occur naturally and are due to minor damage, such as from a knock or blow.

THICKENING Thickening of the nails, a condition known as onychogryphosis, may be due to neglect or a fungal infection or occur for no apparent reason. Distortion of the nail may result. The toenails are most likely to be affected.

RIDGES The occurrence of ridged lines running from the base of the nail to the tip is normal in people who are elderly. In younger people, these ridges may be a sign of rheumatoid arthritis (p.377) or of the skin conditions lichen planus (p.336) and eczema (p.333).

PITTING Multiple pits the size of a pinhead on the nail surface often indicate a general skin disorder, such as psoriasis or eczema (p.333). Pitting may also be associated with the hair disorder alopecia areata (*see* ALOPECIA, p.358).

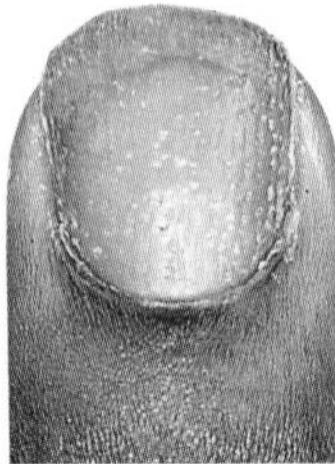

Pitted fingernail
Many small pits can be seen all over the surface of the fingernail. In this case, the pitting is caused by the skin disorder psoriasis.

NAIL SEPARATION If a nail is damaged through injury, it can lift away from the nail bed (a condition called onycholysis) and eventually fall off. Separation of the nail from the nail bed may also occur in some people who have psoriasis or lichen planus or in those with certain types of thyroid problem. Nail separation makes the nail bed susceptible to infection, which causes the lifted nail to appear green.

YELLOWING Yellow, crumbly nails may be due to a fungal infection (onychomycosis). Sometimes, heavy smoking causes discoloration of the nails.

CLUBBING Increased curvature of the nails and broadening of the fingertips is called clubbing. This condition often indicates a serious underlying disorder of the lungs, particularly cystic fibrosis (p.824), bronchiectasis (p.496), or lung cancer (p.503). Alternatively, clubbing of the nails may be a sign of liver disease, congenital heart disease (p.836), thyroid disease, or certain bowel disorders, such as Crohn's disease (p.658).

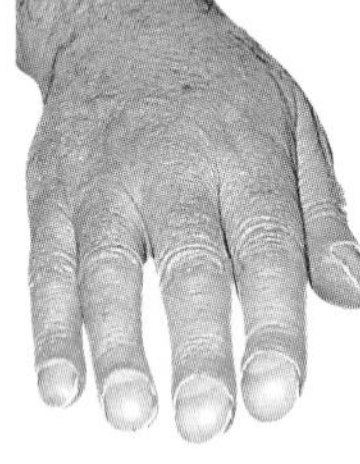

Clubbing of the fingernails
Increased curvature of the nails, known as clubbing, may result in loss of the normal indentation at the nail bed.

SPOON-SHAPED NAILS In this form of abnormality, known as koilonychia, the nails have a concave and spoon-shaped appearance. This condition is usually caused by a severe iron deficiency.

What might be done?

Minor nail abnormalities that are not associated with underlying disorders, such as white spots caused by minor injury, are unlikely to need treatment. However, if the colour, shape, or general condition of your nails changes when no obvious damage has occurred, you should consult your doctor to find out if the problem is caused by a disease. Clubbing that has existed from childhood is probably due to a hereditary defect. This form of clubbing is irreversible and need not be investigated. However, you should consult a doctor if you develop clubbing as an adult. Once the cause of an underlying disorder has been treated, the nails should begin growing normally again, and healthy nail will gradually replace the abnormal tissue. The process is slow; abnormal fingernails may take between 6 and 9 months to grow out, and toenails take even longer. In the meantime, the appearance of the damaged fingernails may be improved by having regular manicures, and a chiropodist may be able to treat distorted toenails.

Paronychia

Infection of the skin fold around a nail, causing a painful swelling

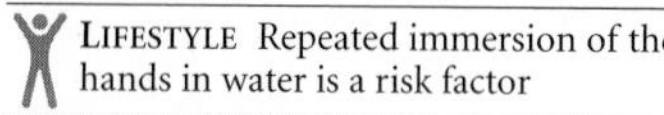
LIFESTYLE Repeated immersion of the hands in water is a risk factor

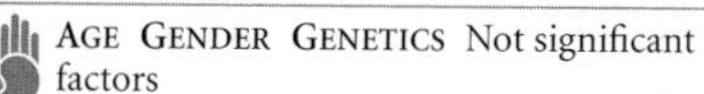
AGE GENDER GENETICS Not significant factors

Infection of the fold of skin surrounding a fingernail or toenail (nail fold) is called paronychia. The infection causes pain and swelling, which may develop either suddenly (acute paronychia) or gradually over several months (chronic paronychia), depending on the underlying cause. One or more nails may be affected by the condition.

What are the causes?

Acute paronychia is usually the result of a bacterial infection entering the nail fold through a cut or break in the skin. Chronic paronychia is common among people such as cooks who repeatedly immerse their hands in water. The skin around the nail separates from the nail, softens, and becomes infected, usually by a yeast organism. A secondary bacterial infection may then occur, resulting in acute paronychia. Some people with decreased resistance to infection, such as those with diabetes mellitus (p.687), are at increased risk of paronychia.

What are the symptoms?

Usually, the symptoms of acute paronychia become apparent about 24 hours after infection and include:

- Pain and swelling on one side of the nail fold.
- Build-up of pus around the nail.

If acute paronychia is left untreated, the nail may separate from the nail bed and eventually fall away. The symptoms of chronic paronychia develop over several months. The condition may cause some discomfort and swelling but does not usually produce a build-up of pus. Eventually, the affected nail thickens slightly and develops horizontal ridges and brownish discoloration.

What is the treatment?

Your doctor may prescribe oral antibiotics (p.885) for acute paronychia. In severe cases, pus may be drained under local anaesthesia. Chronic paronychia may be treated with an over-the-counter cream containing an antifungal drug (p.889), but if there is a secondary infection your doctor may prescribe stronger antifungals and oral antibiotics. Acute paronychia often clears up in a few days with treatment. Chronic paronychia may take several weeks.

To prevent chronic paronychia, you should dry your hands thoroughly after washing and wear cotton-lined rubber gloves when your hands are in water.

Ingrown toenail

Painful inward growth of the edges of a toenail into the surrounding skin

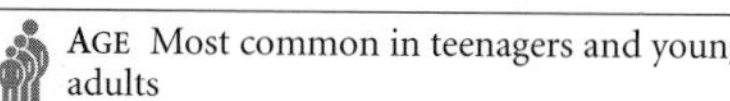
AGE Most common in teenagers and young adults

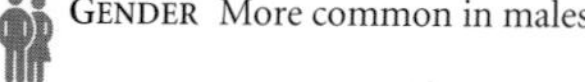
GENDER More common in males

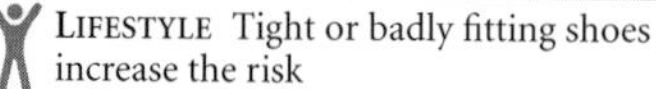
LIFESTYLE Tight or badly fitting shoes increase the risk

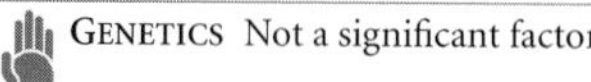
GENETICS Not a significant factor

An ingrown toenail curves under on one or both sides and cuts into the surrounding skin, causing inflammation and sometimes infection. The condition, which most commonly affects the big toe, is often due to ill-fitting shoes pressing on an incorrectly cut nail. In some cases, injury can cause the skin around the nail to overgrow and engulf part of the nail. Poor foot hygiene can also increase the risk of infection, leading to inflammation.

What are the symptoms?

The symptoms of an ingrown toenail may include the following:

- Pain, redness, and swelling around the toenail.
- Broken skin at the nail edge, which oozes clear fluid, pus, or blood.

You should consult your doctor as soon as you notice a toenail that has become ingrown because it is possible that your toe may be infected.

What is the treatment?

You can relieve the pain of an ingrown toenail by bathing your foot in warm salt water daily and taking painkillers (p.912). You should protect the affected toe by keeping it covered with a clean, dry gauze. If there is no improvement within a few days, you should consult your doctor. If your toenail is infected, he or she may prescribe oral antibiotics (p.885) or topical antibiotics (*see* PREPARATIONS FOR SKIN INFECTIONS AND INFESTATIONS, p.892).

To help to prevent an ingrown toenail from recurring, keep your feet clean and wear correctly fitting shoes. Your toenails should be cut straight across, rather than along a curve, to prevent them from growing into the skin. If the problem recurs, your doctor may suggest that you have part or all of the toenail removed to stop it growing into the toe (*see* REMOVAL OF AN INGROWN TOENAIL, below).

TREATMENT REMOVAL OF AN INGROWN TOENAIL

Minor surgery may be needed for an ingrown toenail. Your toe will be anaesthetized and cleaned with antiseptic, and a tourniquet will be applied to its base. The nail, or part of it, will be removed, and phenol will be applied to the exposed nail bed to kill it and prevent regrowth. You should be comfortable enough to walk within 24 hours of surgery, and the wound should heal within a week.

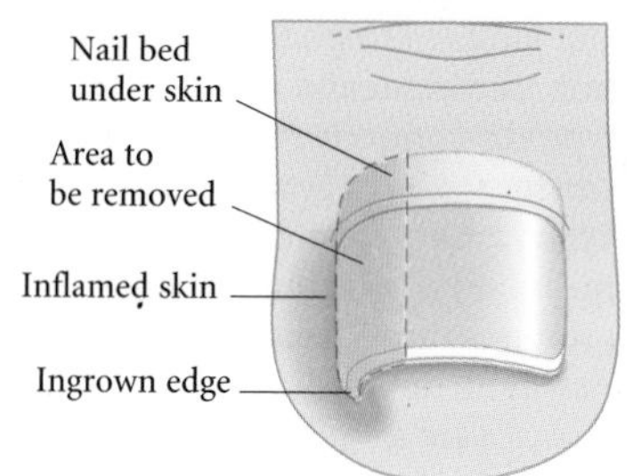

The operation
A vertical cut is made along the toenail. The ingrown part is removed and the nail bed treated to prevent regrowth.

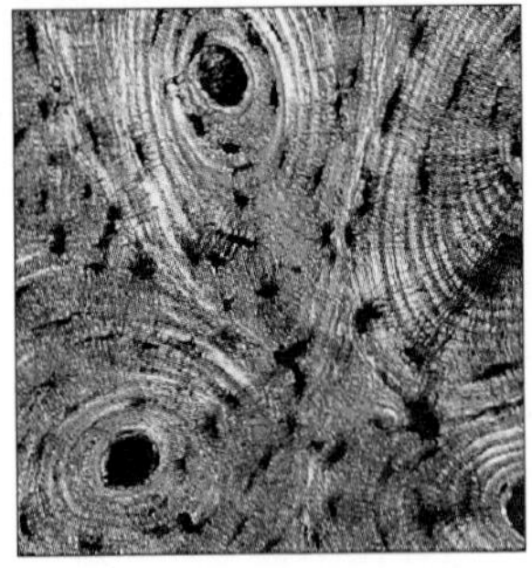

Structure of compact bone
The structural units of compact bone are called osteons (shown here in cross section). Osteons consist of rings of collagen (protein) around central canals.

MUSCULOSKELETAL SYSTEM

EVERY DAY WE USE OUR MUSCLES and joints to carry out voluntary movements. Many of these actions, such as walking, demand very little concentration, but complex tasks, such as playing the piano, require more conscious effort, supported by a subconscious system of coordination learned when the skill was first mastered. All movements are based on mechanical changes in the muscles, which contract or relax, making specific bones pivot, hinge, rotate, or glide at the joints.

Skeletal muscles move the body at its joints by contracting. In addition, they maintain a steady tension, or tone, that gives the body the support it needs to maintain its posture, such as keeping the head upright on the neck. This postural tone is automatic but does require alertness. Unlike horses, people cannot sleep standing up.

There are two other types of muscle in the body: cardiac muscle, found only in the heart; and smooth muscle, occurring in hollow organs such as the intestines. Most muscle of these types is not under conscious control.

TYPES OF BONE

Bones come in many shapes and sizes, ranging from the flat bones found in the skull to the long bones of the limbs. The outer layer of each bone is made of dense, heavy, compact bone. The inner layer consists of spongy bone that is made up of numerous trabeculae (struts) arranged in such a way that they provide maximum support without excessive weight.

Bone gives the body shape and supports the body's structure. It is a living tissue, which is constantly being renewed. Bone also serves as a reservoir for various minerals, such as calcium and phosphorus. Bone marrow, the soft, fatty substance that fills the cavities in bones, produces most of the body's blood cells (*see* FORMATION OF BLOOD CELLS, p.440).

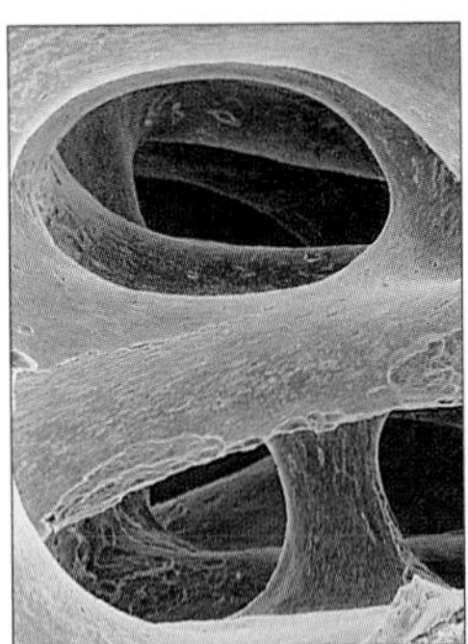

Struts in spongy bone
The trabeculae (struts) that form spongy bone make it light but strong.

MOVEMENT

Joints, which are formed where bones meet, are covered with lubricated cartilage that allows smooth movement. The range of movement of the joints is determined both by their structure and by the ligaments that stabilize and support them; the hip joint, for example, moves less freely than the shoulder. In contrast, the joints in the wrist, foot, and spine sacrifice mobility for stability; their bones are joined by strong, inflexible ligaments that allow little movement. Most of the skull bones fuse together and become immobile once growth has ceased.

FUNCTION HOW THE BODY MOVES

Movement of the body depends on the interaction of muscles, bones, and joints in response to signals from the brain and nerves. A muscle typically connects two bones and crosses the joint between them. When a muscle contracts, it pulls on the bones to which it is attached and produces movement. Muscles can only pull, not push. Therefore, many muscles are arranged in pairs, one on each side of a joint, so that they produce opposing movements. An example is the pairing of the triceps and biceps muscles in the upper arm.

Straightening the arm
The triceps and biceps muscles cross opposite sides of the elbow joint. While the triceps muscle contracts to pull down the bones of the forearm, the biceps relaxes.

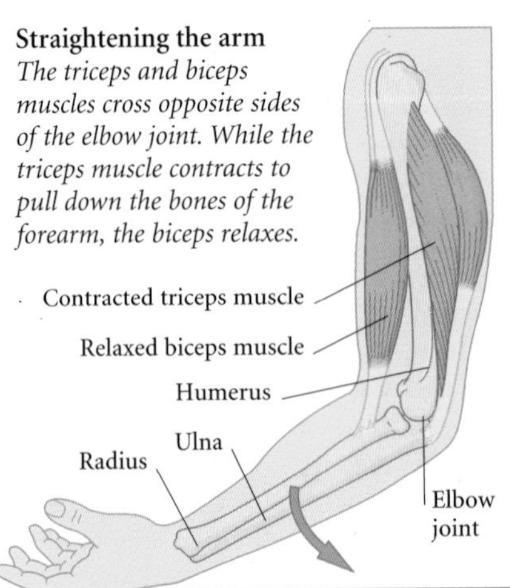

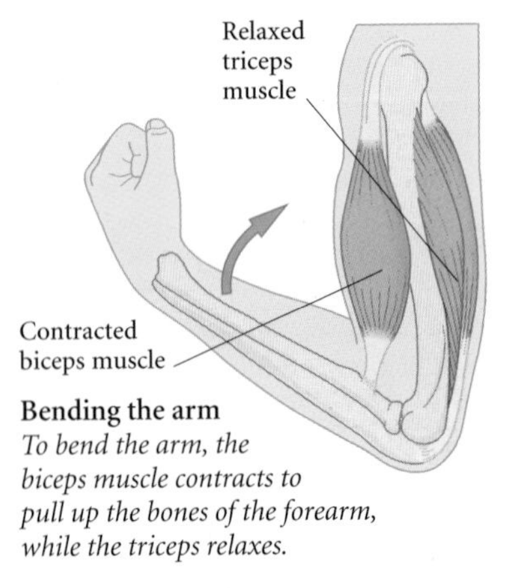

Bending the arm
To bend the arm, the biceps muscle contracts to pull up the bones of the forearm, while the triceps relaxes.

STRUCTURE THE BODY'S SKELETON

The adult human skeleton is a bony framework that supports the body and gives it shape. It also protects the internal organs and anchors the body's muscles. The skeleton is composed of 206 bones and is divided into two parts. The axial skeleton – the skull, spine, and rib cage – consists of 80 bones and protects the brain, spinal cord, heart, and lungs. The appendicular skeleton has 126 bones and consists of the bones of the limbs, the collarbones, the shoulder blades, and the bones of the pelvis.

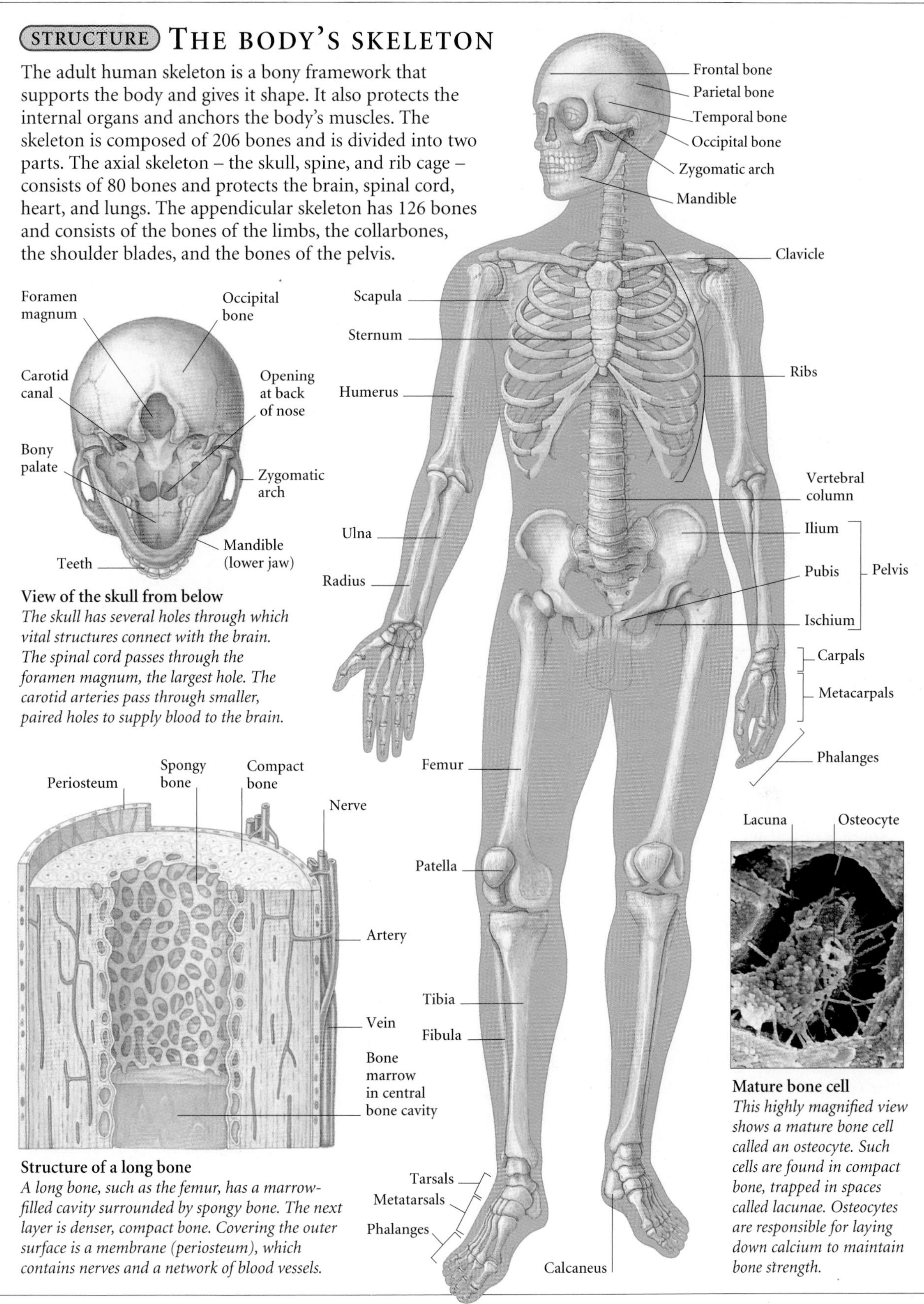

View of the skull from below
The skull has several holes through which vital structures connect with the brain. The spinal cord passes through the foramen magnum, the largest hole. The carotid arteries pass through smaller, paired holes to supply blood to the brain.

Structure of a long bone
A long bone, such as the femur, has a marrow-filled cavity surrounded by spongy bone. The next layer is denser, compact bone. Covering the outer surface is a membrane (periosteum), which contains nerves and a network of blood vessels.

Mature bone cell
This highly magnified view shows a mature bone cell called an osteocyte. Such cells are found in compact bone, trapped in spaces called lacunae. Osteocytes are responsible for laying down calcium to maintain bone strength.

STRUCTURE THE BACKBONE

The spine, also known as the vertebral column, holds the body upright, supports the head, and encircles the spinal cord. It consists of 33 bones called vertebrae. Joints and discs of fibrous tissue between most of the vertebrae make the spine flexible, while ligaments and muscles stabilize it and control movement.

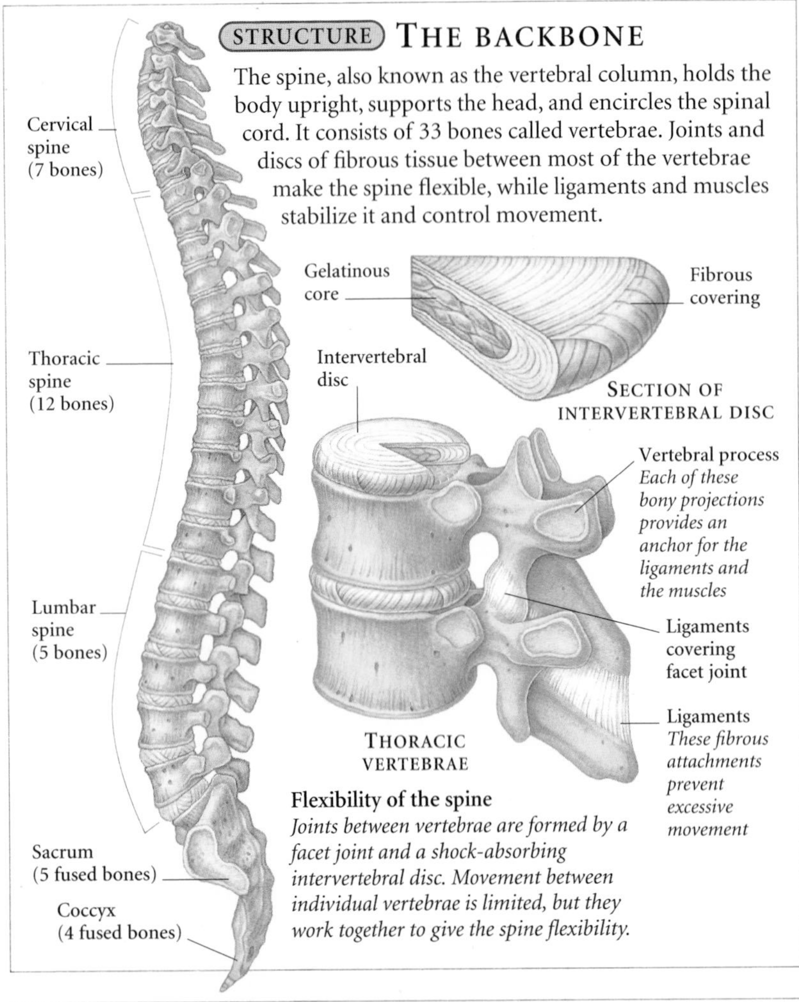

Flexibility of the spine
Joints between vertebrae are formed by a facet joint and a shock-absorbing intervertebral disc. Movement between individual vertebrae is limited, but they work together to give the spine flexibility.

FUNCTION HOW BONE REPAIRS ITSELF

A broken bone and any damaged blood vessels start to repair and heal themselves immediately. A fracture in a long bone, such as the collarbone, normally takes about 6 weeks to heal in an adult. However, some injured bones may not regain their full strength for several months, and healing may need to be aided by a plaster or resin cast or by mechanical fixation. In children, fractured bones usually heal more quickly.

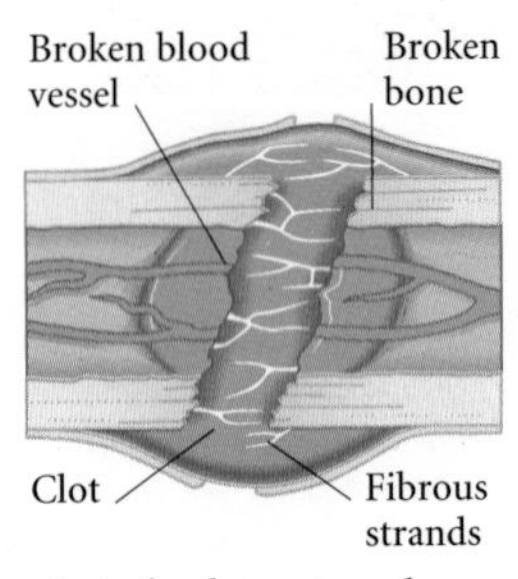

1 *A clot forms to seal broken blood vessels. Gradually, a mesh of fibrous tissue forms and starts to replace the clot.*

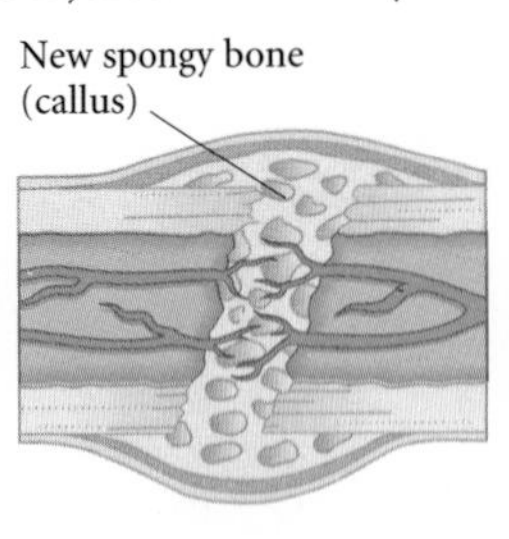

2 *New, soft, spongy bone called callus develops on the framework provided by the fibrous tissue, joining the broken ends.*

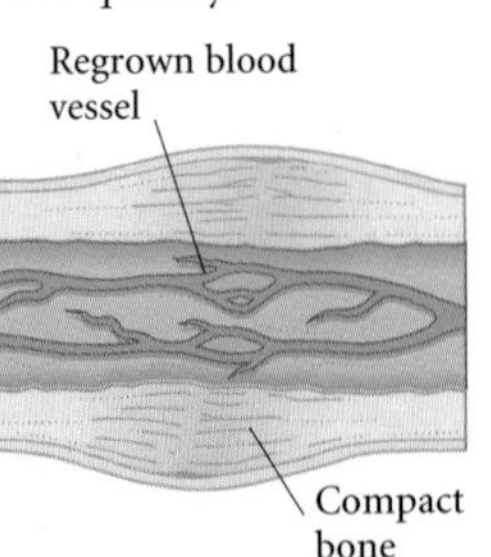

3 *Dense, compact bone gradually replaces the callus, and blood vessels regrow. Eventually, the bone regains its shape.*

STRUCTURE AND FUNCTION

THE JOINTS

Joints are formed where two or more bones meet. Most joints, including those of the limbs, move freely and are known as synovial joints. They are lubricated by synovial fluid secreted by the joint lining. In contrast, semi-movable joints, such as those in the pelvis and spine, are less flexible but give greater stability. A few joints, such as those of the skull, are fixed and allow no movement.

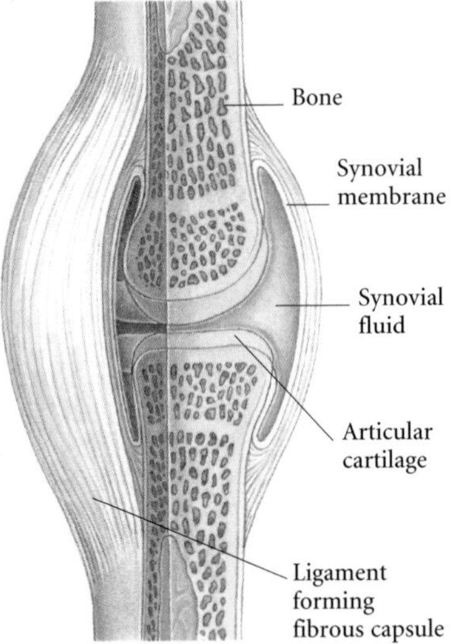

Structure of a synovial joint
The bones of synovial joints are held together by ligaments that form a fibrous capsule. The synovial membrane lining the capsule secretes a lubricating fluid, and articular cartilage on the bone ends provides a smooth surface for movement.

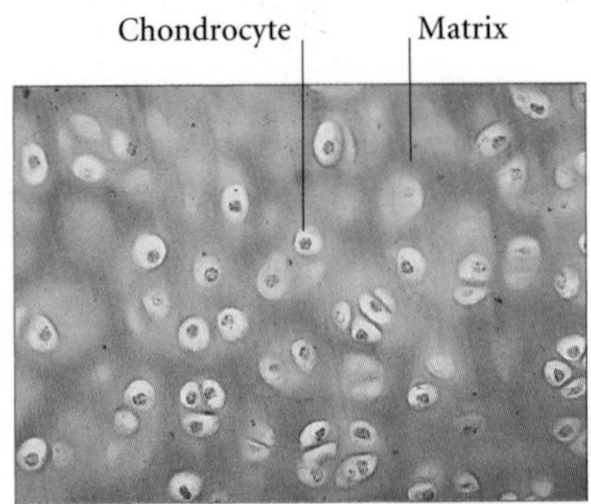

Composition of articular cartilage
Articular cartilage is composed of cells (chondrocytes) located in cavities in a tough matrix of collagen, forming a smooth, flexible surface.

TYPES OF JOINT

Illustrated here are six examples of synovial joints, each of a different type, and one fixed and one semi-movable joint. Synovial joints are classified according to how their articular surfaces (where bones meet) fit together and the movements each permits. The diagram accompanying each synovial joint illustrates its range of movement.

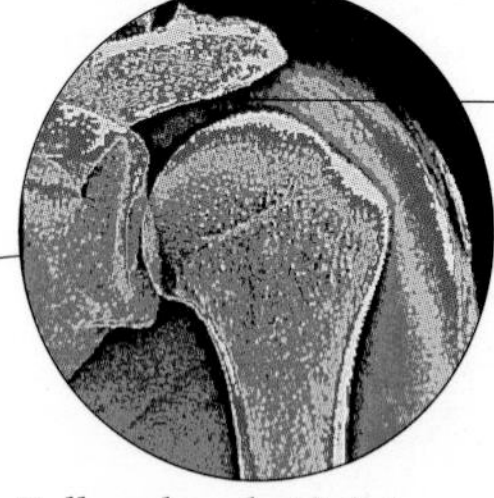

Fixed joint
In a fixed joint, the bones are bound together by fibrous tissue, allowing little or no movement. The fixed joints between the bones of the skull are called sutures.

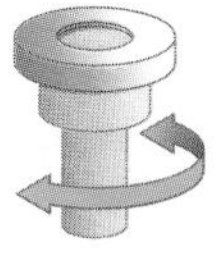

Pivot joint
In a pivot joint, one bone rotates within a collar formed by another. The pivot joint between the atlas and the axis, the uppermost bones of the neck, allows the head to turn to either side.

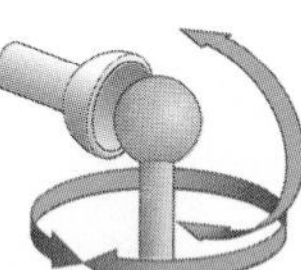

Ball-and-socket joint
In a ball-and-socket joint, the ball-shaped end of one bone fits into a cup-shaped cavity in another, allowing movement in all directions. The shoulder and hip are ball-and-socket joints.

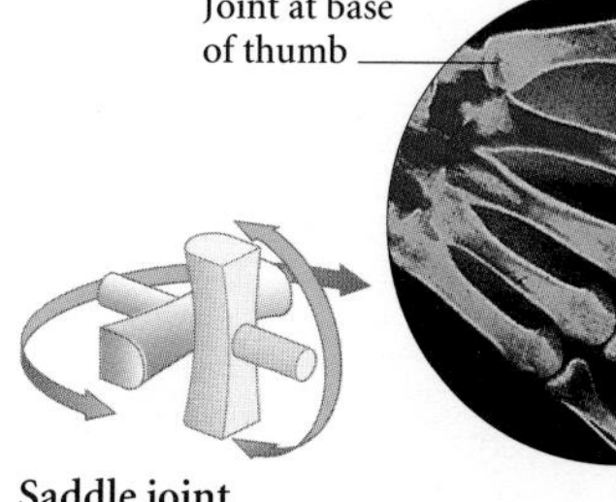

Saddle joint
Saddle-shaped bone ends that meet at right angles form a saddle joint. The bones can rotate a little and move sideways and back and forth. The body's only saddle joint is at the base of the thumb.

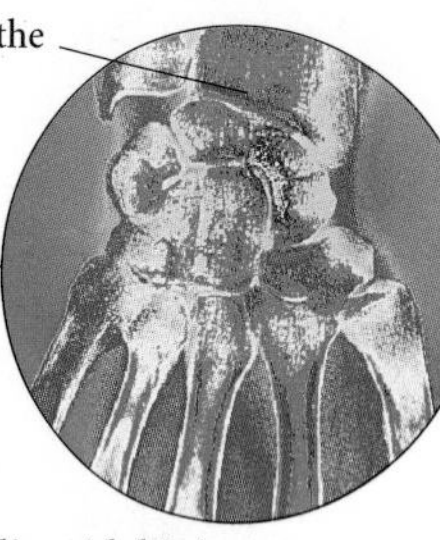

Ellipsoidal joint
The oval end of one bone fits into the oval cup of another in an ellipsoidal joint, allowing movement in most directions and limited rotation. The wrist is an ellipsoidal joint.

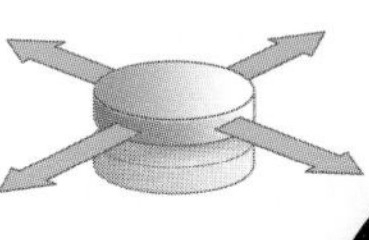

Plane joint
In a plane joint, surfaces that are almost flat slide over each other, back and forth and sideways. Some joints in the foot and wrist are plane joints.

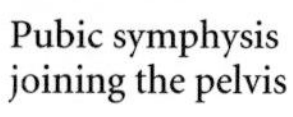
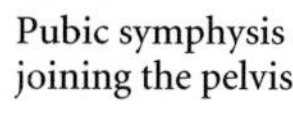

Hinge joint
The cylindrical surface of one bone fits into the groove of another to form a hinge joint. This type of joint either bends or straightens a limb. The knee, elbow, and finger joints are all examples of hinge joints.

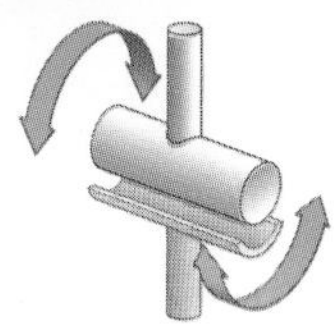

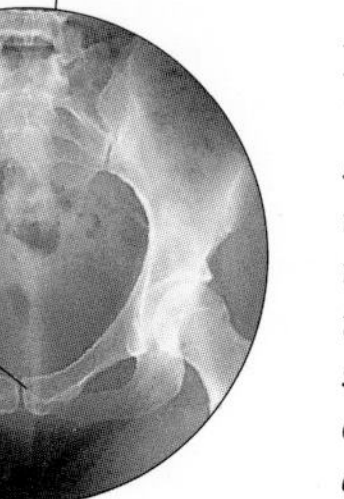

Semi-movable joint
In a semi-movable joint, the articular surfaces are fused to a tough pad of cartilage that allows only a little movement. Examples are the pubic symphysis, which joins the front halves of the pelvis, and the joints of the spine.

STRUCTURE THE BODY'S MUSCLES

Muscles consist of tissue that can contract powerfully to move the body, maintain its posture, and work the various internal organs, including the heart and blood vessels. These functions are performed by three different types of muscle (opposite page), of which skeletal muscle makes up the greatest bulk. (Many of the body's skeletal muscles are identified, right.) Usually each end of a skeletal muscle is attached to a bone by a tendon, a flexible cord of fibrous tissue. The skeletal muscles may be controlled consciously to produce movement.

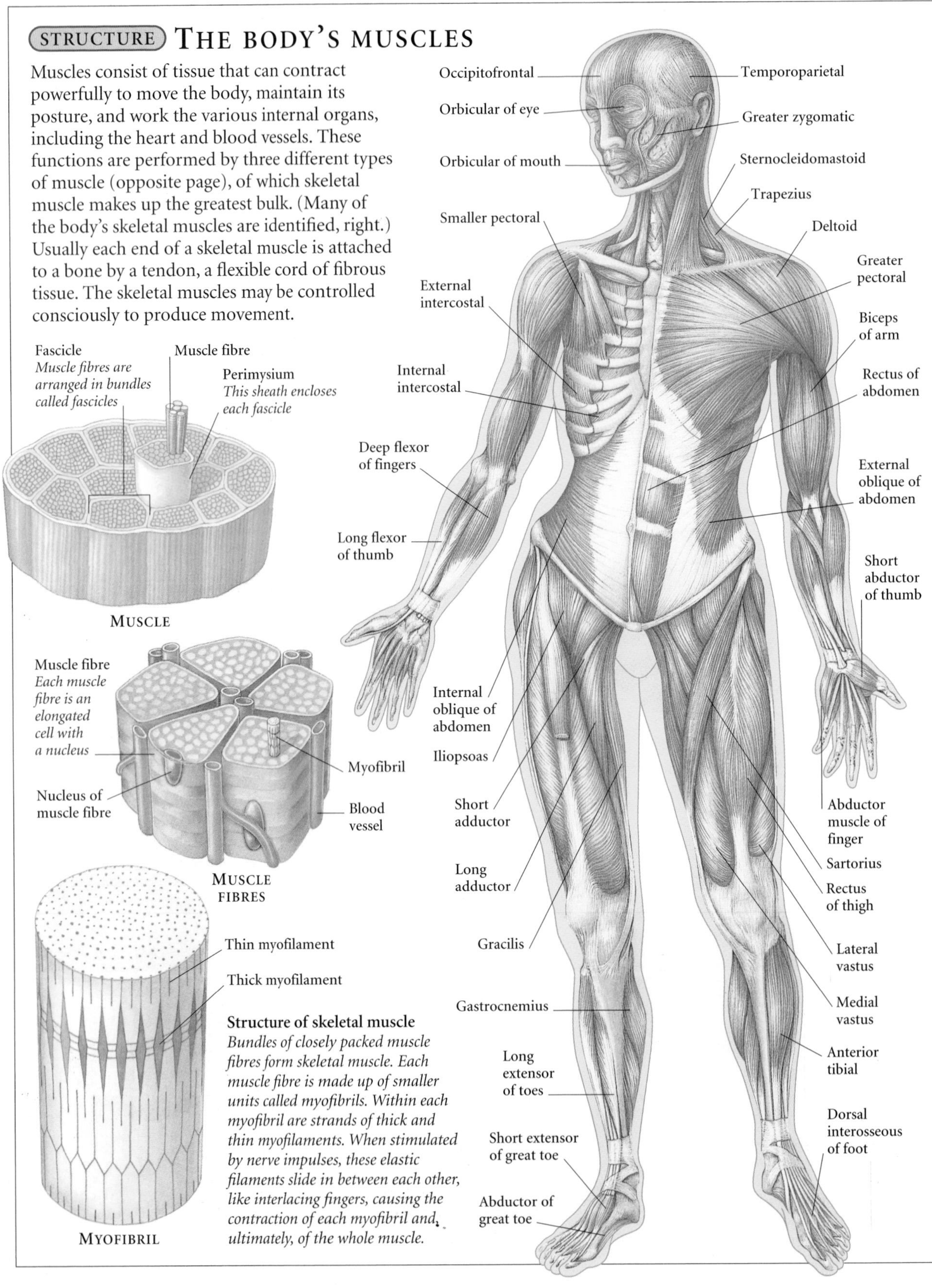

Structure of skeletal muscle
Bundles of closely packed muscle fibres form skeletal muscle. Each muscle fibre is made up of smaller units called myofibrils. Within each myofibril are strands of thick and thin myofilaments. When stimulated by nerve impulses, these elastic filaments slide in between each other, like interlacing fingers, causing the contraction of each myofibril and, ultimately, of the whole muscle.

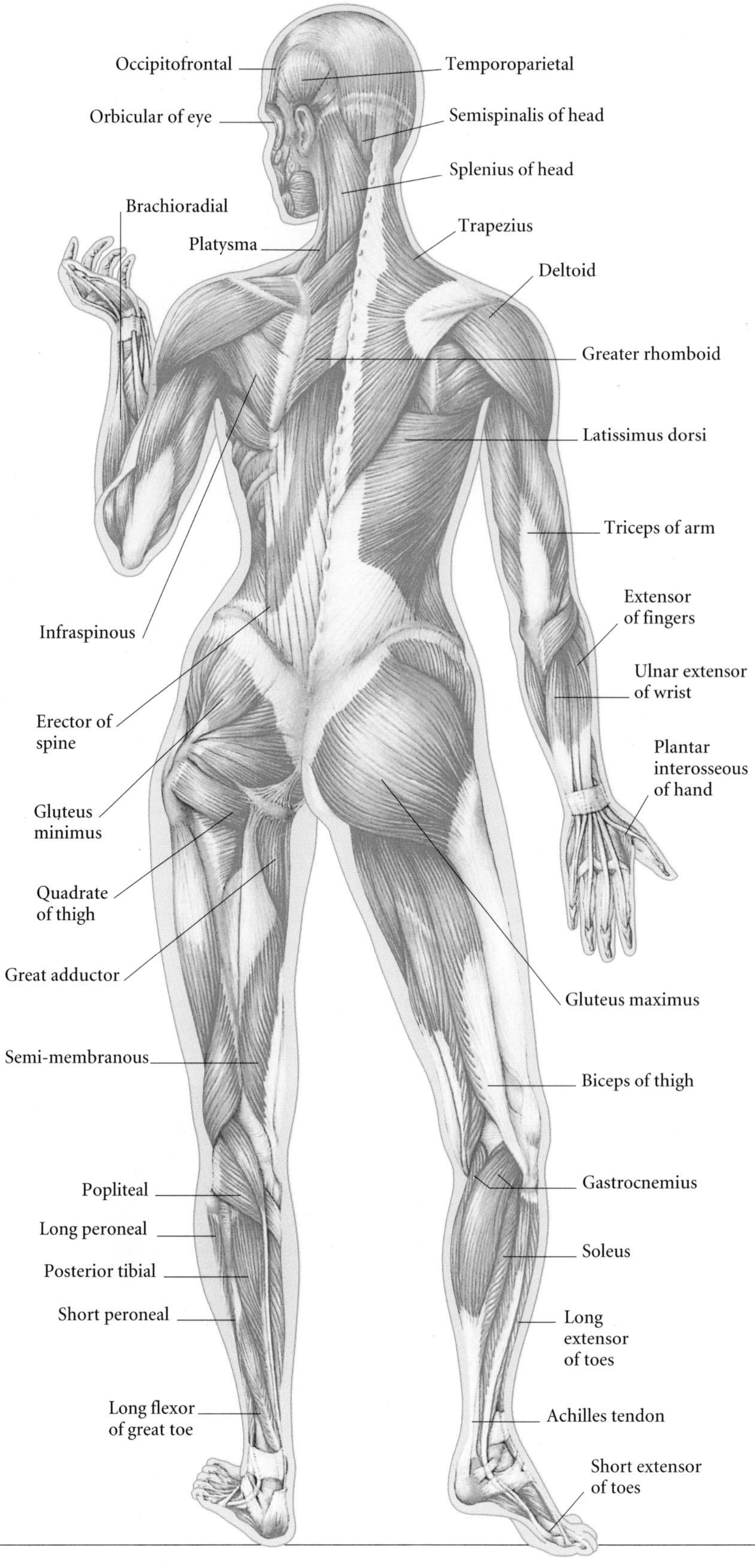

Occipitofrontal
Temporoparietal
Orbicular of eye
Semispinalis of head
Splenius of head
Brachioradial
Platysma
Trapezius
Deltoid
Greater rhomboid
Latissimus dorsi
Triceps of arm
Infraspinous
Extensor of fingers
Ulnar extensor of wrist
Erector of spine
Plantar interosseous of hand
Gluteus minimus
Quadrate of thigh
Great adductor
Gluteus maximus
Semi-membranous
Biceps of thigh
Popliteal
Gastrocnemius
Long peroneal
Soleus
Posterior tibial
Short peroneal
Long extensor of toes
Long flexor of great toe
Achilles tendon
Short extensor of toes

Types of muscle

The three types of muscle are skeletal muscle, which covers and moves the skeleton; cardiac (heart) muscle, which pumps blood around the body; and smooth muscle, which is found in the walls of the digestive tract, blood vessels, and the genital and urinary tracts. Smooth muscle performs the unconscious actions of the body, such as propelling food along the digestive tract.

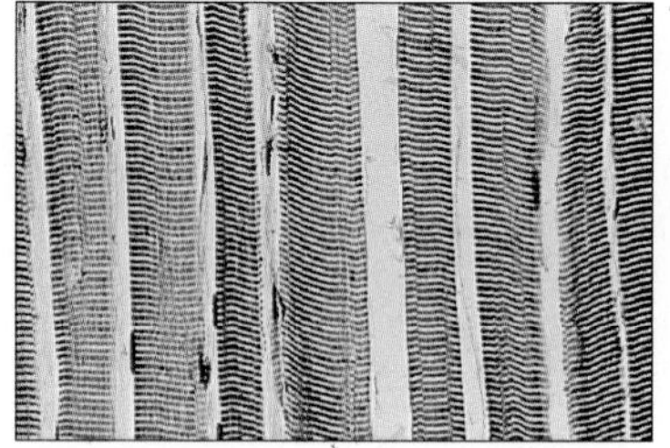

Skeletal muscle
This type of muscle is formed of long, strong, parallel fibres, which are able to contract quickly and powerfully, but can do so only for short periods of time.

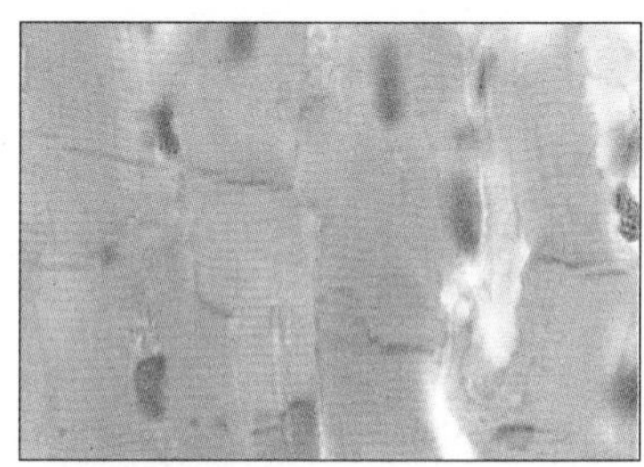

Cardiac muscle
Short, branching, interlinked fibres form a network within the wall of the heart. Cardiac muscle contracts rhythmically and continually without tiring.

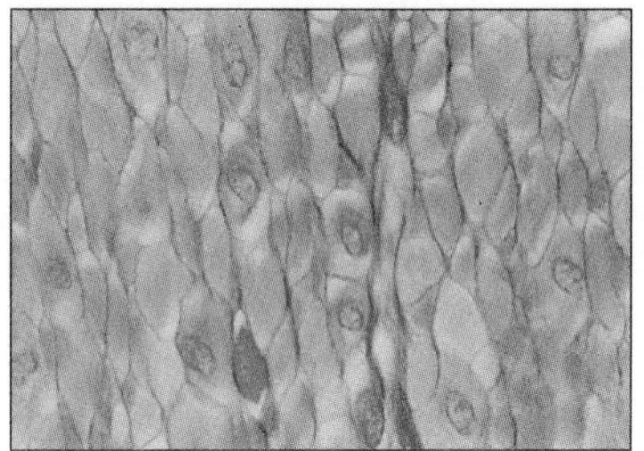

Smooth muscle
These fibres are short, spindle-shaped, and thinner than skeletal muscle fibres. Smooth muscle cells form sheets of muscle that can contract for prolonged periods.

BONE DISORDERS

Bone consists of a resilient protein framework strengthened by calcium and phosphate deposits. While people often think of bone as lifeless and unchanging, it is actually a living tissue, supplied with nerves and blood vessels, that is continually being broken down and rebuilt. Bone can be weakened by nutritional and hormonal factors and by certain long-term disorders.

This section starts by discussing the bone disorder osteoporosis, which is common in elderly people. This disorder affects the natural processes of bone breakdown and replacement, causing bones to become brittle and fracture more easily. The section also covers the other main disorders that affect bone formation, including osteomalacia and rickets, both of which are due to lack of vitamin D, and Paget's disease of the bone, the cause of which has yet to be established. Kyphosis, lordosis, and scoliosis, bone disorders that affect the curvature of the spine, are described next. Further articles discuss the bone infection osteomyelitis and noncancerous and cancerous tumours of the bones. Defects in the bone marrow are covered elsewhere in the book (*see* BLOOD DISORDERS, pp.446–457).

KEY ANATOMY

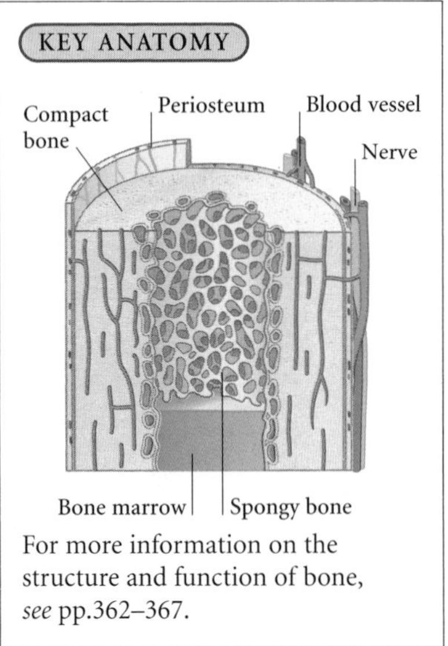

For more information on the structure and function of bone, *see* pp.362–367.

Osteoporosis

Loss of bone tissue, resulting in bones that are brittle and susceptible to fracture

 AGE Common over the age of 50

 GENDER More common in females

 GENETICS Sometimes runs in families; more common in white and Asian people

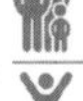 LIFESTYLE Poor diet, lack of exercise, smoking, and alcohol are risk factors

As people get older, their bones become thinner and lighter. By the age of 70, most people's skeletons are about a third lighter than they were at the age of 40. This loss of bone density, known as osteoporosis, is the result of an imbalance between the natural breakdown and replacement of bone. Eventually, all elderly people are affected by osteoporosis, but the severity of the condition varies from person to person. People who are thin, who do little exercise, and whose relatives have osteoporosis are likely to develop the condition to a greater degree than others.

Many people do not realize that they have osteoporosis until they fracture a wrist or hip as a result of a minor fall. In the UK, an estimated 60,000 fractures occur each year in people aged 65 or over. Osteoporosis is a major cause of these fractures, the hip being the most common site. In elderly people, hip fractures are often life-threatening or result in immobility.

WHAT ARE THE CAUSES?

Sex hormones are necessary for bone replacement. In both men and women, osteoporosis begins to develop as sex hormone production declines with age. Any condition that causes this decline to accelerate can increase the severity of age-related osteoporosis. In women, production of the sex hormone oestrogen declines rapidly at the menopause. Early menopause, which tends to occur in women who smoke, increases the risk of osteoporosis. In men, untreated hypogonadism (p.729) results in low levels of the sex hormone testosterone early in life and a low bone density.

Osteoporosis may occur as a result of long-term treatment with oral corticosteroids (p.930). People with rheumatoid arthritis (p.377), an overactive thyroid gland (*see* HYPERTHYROIDISM, p.679), or chronic kidney failure (p.706) are also at increased risk of osteoporosis.

Exercise is essential to maintain bone health. The density of bones declines rapidly in people who are confined to bed and in those whose daily activity is reduced by disorders such as arthritis (p.374) or multiple sclerosis (p.541).

Osteoporosis sometimes runs in families. Women who have a close relative with osteoporosis are more likely to develop the disorder themselves. White and Asian women, especially those who have a slight build, are at increased risk of developing the condition.

CAN IT BE PREVENTED?

Measures to prevent osteoporosis are most effective if started early in life. Teenagers and young adults should eat a balanced diet rich in calcium and vitamin D (*see* A HEALTHY DIET, p.48) and maintain it throughout life. Calcium is essential for bone strength, and vitamin

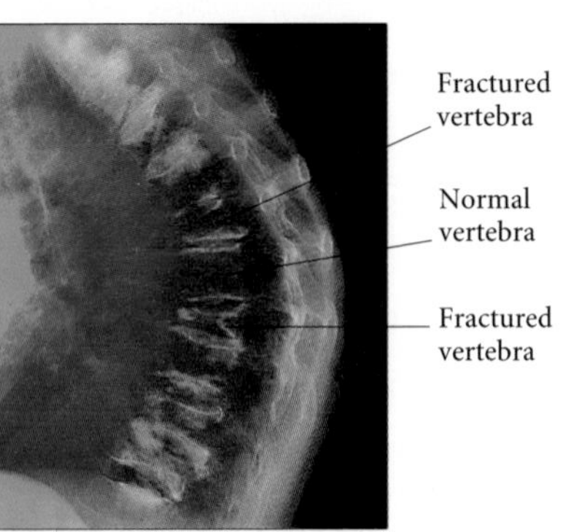

Spine affected by osteoporosis
This colour-enhanced X-ray shows severe curvature of the upper spine due to compression fractures of vertebrae that have been weakened by osteoporosis.

D aids calcium absorption in the body. Extra calcium is needed during pregnancy, while breast-feeding, and during and after the menopause; it may be advisable to take a supplement at such times (*see* VITAMIN AND MINERAL SUPPLEMENTS, p.927). Vitamin D is also produced in the skin in response to sunlight. People exposed to little sunlight may need vitamin D supplements.

Walking and other weight-bearing exercise help to increase bone density. Not smoking and limiting alcohol intake also reduce the risk of osteoporosis.

Women may be encouraged to use hormone replacement therapy (p.937) during and after the menopause, which may help to protect against osteoporosis, but there is no medical consensus on how long it should be continued.

Anyone thought to be at increased risk of osteoporosis, such as having a family history of the disorder, can have his or her bone density measured (*see* BONE DENSITOMETRY, below). Bone density testing is often used to assess a person's likelihood of having bone loss and also to monitor people who are taking preventive treatment.

WHAT ARE THE SYMPTOMS?

Some physical changes associated with aging are in fact due to osteoporosis. These include:

- Gradual loss of height.
- Rounding of the back.

For many people, the first evidence of osteoporosis is a painful fracture (p.392) of a bone after minor stress or injury. An example is sudden, severe back pain due to a compression fracture of the body of a vertebra (bone of the spine). In severe osteoporosis, a fracture may occur spontaneously.

WHAT MIGHT BE DONE?

The diagnosis will be made from your medical history and an examination. Bone densitometry, X-rays (p.244), and blood tests may also be performed to exclude other causes of the symptoms, such as osteomalacia (*see* OSTEOMALACIA AND RICKETS, p.370) and Paget's disease of the bone (p.370), and to look for various disorders that may cause osteoporosis, such as hyperthyroidism.

If you have back pain due to a fracture, your doctor may recommend that you take painkillers (p.912) or use a heat pad. Underlying disorders will be treated if possible. For example, you may be prescribed drugs to treat an overactive thyroid gland (*see* DRUGS FOR HYPERTHYROIDISM, p.932).

To slow the progression of osteoporosis, it is important to follow the advice given above for taking preventive measures. Most drugs simply slow the rate of bone loss (*see* DRUGS FOR BONE DISORDERS, p.896), although there is evidence that bisphosphonates reduce the risk of fractures. However, even if these measures are taken, some bone loss is inevitable in later life.

(WWW) ONLINE SITES: p.1035

(TEST) BONE DENSITOMETRY

This technique uses low-dose X-rays to measure the density of bone. The test is carried out to screen for and diagnose osteoporosis, a condition that is particularly common in postmenopausal women. The varying absorption of X-rays as they pass through the body is interpreted by a computer and displayed as an image. The computer calculates the average density of the bone and compares it with the normal range for the person's age and sex. The procedure takes about 10–20 minutes and is painless.

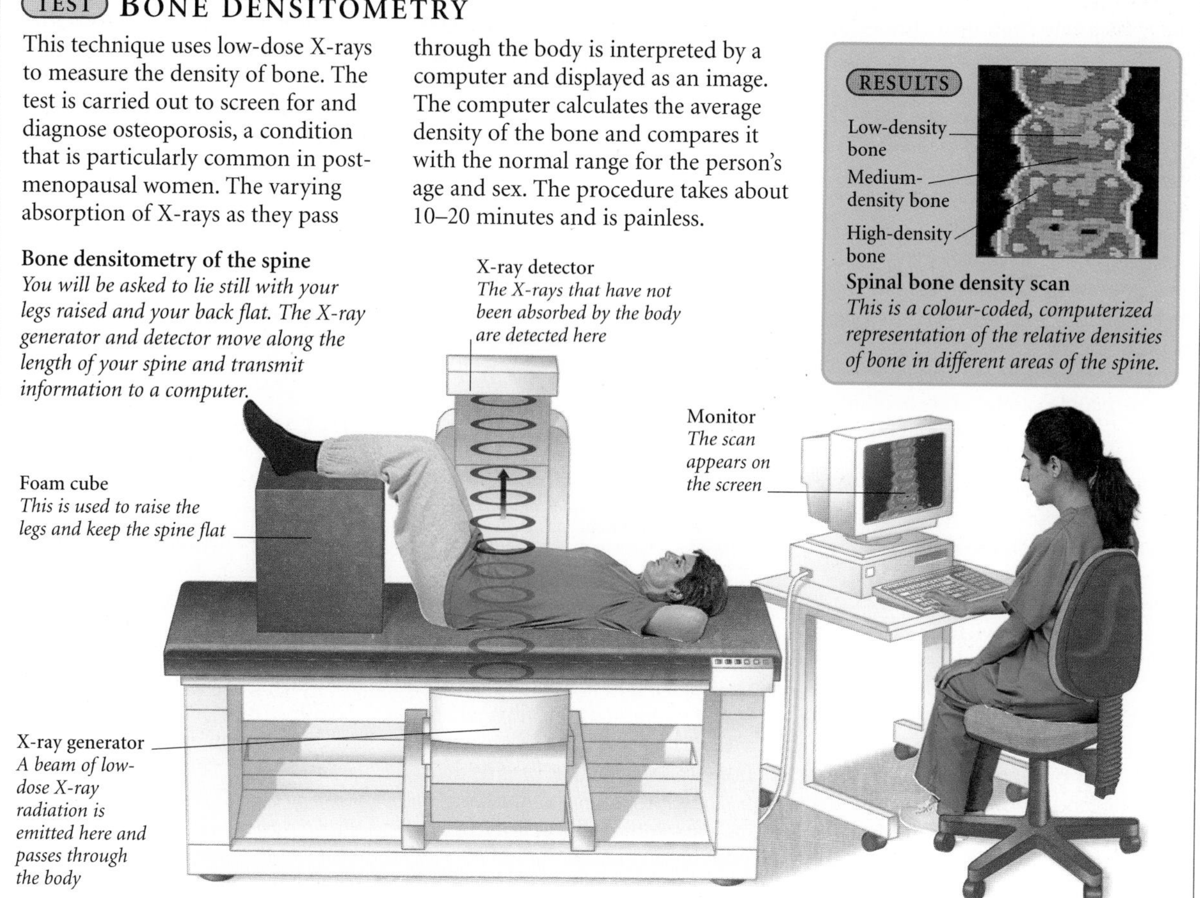

Bone densitometry of the spine
You will be asked to lie still with your legs raised and your back flat. The X-ray generator and detector move along the length of your spine and transmit information to a computer.

Spinal bone density scan
This is a colour-coded, computerized representation of the relative densities of bone in different areas of the spine.

Osteomalacia and rickets

Disorders due to a lack of vitamin D, resulting in weak, soft bones that become distorted or fracture easily

AGE Osteomalacia develops in adults; rickets develops in children

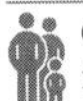
GENETICS In some cases, the cause is inherited

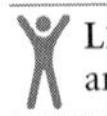
LIFESTYLE Minimal exposure to sunlight and vegan or fat-free diets are risk factors

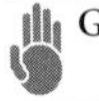
GENDER Not a significant factor

The minerals calcium and phosphate give bone its strength and density. A deficiency of vitamin D results in poor absorption of calcium from the diet, leading to weak and soft bones that are easily deformed or fractured. In adults, the condition is called osteomalacia; in children, it is known as rickets.

WHAT ARE THE CAUSES?

Healthy people obtain the vitamin D they need partly from their diet (from eggs, fish, green vegetables, fortified margarine, and milk) and partly from vitamin D production in the skin on exposure to sunlight. A deficiency of vitamin D, therefore, is most common in people who eat a restricted diet and receive little direct sunlight. In tropical countries, vitamin D deficiency is almost unknown, except in women who are required to cover their entire bodies. At higher latitudes, deficiency may occur in elderly, housebound people.

Some people cannot absorb vitamin D from food due to intestinal surgery or coeliac disease (p.658). Less commonly, osteomalacia and rickets may be caused by inherited disorders of vitamin D metabolism or chronic kidney failure (p.706). In rare cases, drugs used to treat epilepsy (*see* ANTICONVULSANT DRUGS, p.914) interfere with vitamin D metabolism and cause osteomalacia or rickets.

WHAT ARE THE SYMPTOMS?

The symptoms of osteomalacia develop over months or years and may include:

- Painful, tender bones, most often the ribs, hips, and bones of the legs.
- Difficulty in climbing stairs or in getting up from a squatting position.
- Bone fractures after a minor injury.

A child with rickets may experience similar symptoms, and may also have:

- Retarded growth.
- Swelling and tenderness at the growing ends of the bones.
- Prominence of the ribs where they join the breastbone.

Left untreated, bow legs or knock-knees may develop in affected children.

WHAT MIGHT BE DONE?

Your doctor may suspect osteomalacia or rickets from your symptoms and a physical examination. He or she may arrange for blood tests to check for low levels of calcium, phosphate, and vitamin D. A bone biopsy, in which a bone sample is taken for analysis, or X-rays (p.244) can confirm the diagnosis.

If you have a vitamin D deficiency, you should eat foods rich in vitamin D (*see* A HEALTHY DIET, p.48) and increase your exposure to sunlight. If you have a disorder that prevents absorption of the vitamin from food, you may need to have vitamin D injections (*see* VITAMINS, p.927). Calcium supplements (*see* MINERALS, p.929) may also be required.

After treatment, most people make a full recovery, although deformities that occur in childhood may be permanent.

(WWW) ONLINE SITES: p.1035

Paget's disease of the bone

A disorder of bone maintenance and repair, leading to weakened, distorted, and occasionally painful bones

AGE Rare under the age of 40; increasingly common over the age of 50

GENDER More common in males

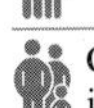
GENETICS Sometimes runs in families; rare in people of Asian or African origin

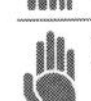
LIFESTYLE Not a significant factor

In a healthy person, bone is continually being broken down and replaced by new bone to maintain the normal bone structure. However, in Paget's disease of the bone (also known as osteitis deformans), the processes involved in the normal breakdown and replacement of bone tissue become disrupted in some parts of the skeleton. The condition may affect any bone in the body, but the pelvis, collarbone, vertebrae (bones of the spine), skull, and leg bones are those most commonly involved. The affected bones become larger and structurally abnormal, which progressively weakens them and makes them more liable to fracture.

Paget's disease usually develops after the age of 50 and affects 1 in 10 people over the age of 80. The disorder tends to run in families and affects more men than women. Paget's disease is most common in Europe, North America, and Australia. It is rare in people of Asian and African origin.

WHAT ARE THE SYMPTOMS?

Frequently, Paget's disease produces no symptoms and may be diagnosed only by chance when an X-ray has been taken for some other reason. If symptoms are present, they may include:

- Bone pain that is worse at night.
- Joint pain, especially in those joints near affected bones.
- Bone deformities, such as bow legs or enlargement of the skull.
- Fractures (p.392) that occur after a minor injury.

Long-standing Paget's disease may also lead to the following complications:

- Numbness, tingling, or weakness in the affected area if the bone presses on adjacent nerves.
- Hearing loss if abnormal growth of bone compresses nerves to the ear.

In rare cases, a further complication of Paget's disease is the development of a type of bone cancer (*see* PRIMARY BONE CANCER, p.373).

WHAT MIGHT BE DONE?

If your doctor suspects you have Paget's disease, he or she may arrange for you to have X-rays (p.244) to confirm the diagnosis. You may also have blood and urine tests to check for abnormal levels of substances involved in the formation and breakdown of bone. If your hearing is affected, you will probably have hearing tests (p.600).

Treatment is not necessary if you have no pain or other symptoms and are unlikely to be at risk of fractures. If you are in discomfort, your doctor will prescribe painkillers (p.912) or a nonsteroidal anti-inflammatory drug (p.894). If these drugs are inadequate then specific treatment may be needed.

The most common treatment is with bisphosphonates; less commonly, the hormone calcitonin may be prescribed (*see* DRUGS FOR BONE DISORDERS, p.896). Your response to these drugs may be monitored by blood tests.

Although drug treatment will not reverse any bone deformity that may have already developed, it will slow the progress of the disease.

WWW ONLINE SITES: p.1035

Kyphosis and lordosis

Excessive outward curvature at the top of the spine (kyphosis) or inward curvature in the lower back (lordosis)

LIFESTYLE Being overweight is a risk factor

AGE GENDER GENETICS Risk factors depend on the cause

Viewed from the side, a normal spine has two main curves along its length. If you have kyphosis or lordosis, these natural curves may become exaggerated. In kyphosis, there is an excessive outward curve at the top of the back, which results in a rounded back, or "hunchback". Lordosis affects the spine in the lower back, leading to an exaggerated "hollow back". Kyphosis and lordosis often occur together, resulting in excessive curvature both at the top and in the small of the back.

If kyphosis occurs in childhood, the cause is often not known. In adults, disorders that limit mobility, such as osteoarthritis (p.374), or that weaken the vertebrae (bones of the spine), such as osteoporosis (p.368), are the most common causes of kyphosis. Poor posture may also lead to kyphosis.

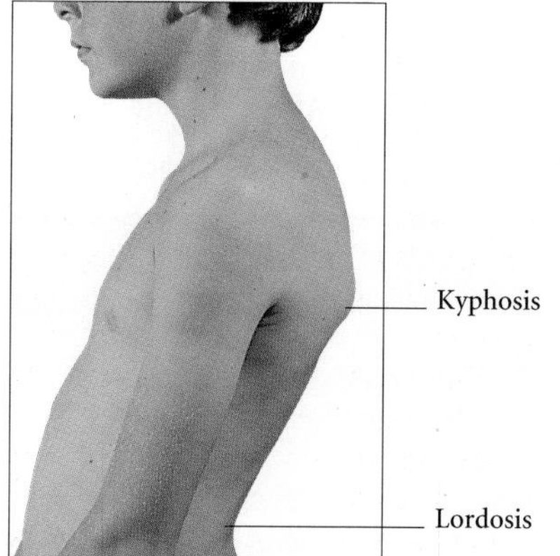

Kyphosis and lordosis
The child in this photograph has kyphosis, in which the back below the neck is curved out and rounded, and lordosis, in which the lower back is excessively hollow.

Kyphosis often leads to lordosis because the lower spine compensates for the imbalance of the curve at the top of the spine. Lordosis may also develop in people with weak abdominal muscles and poor posture. People who are very overweight are more likely to develop lordosis since they tend to lean backwards to improve their balance.

Your doctor may advise you on ways to improve your posture. He or she will probably recommend that you avoid strenuous activity and lose any excess weight. Posture can be improved by physiotherapy (p.961), which strengthens the muscles supporting the spine.

People with abnormal curvature of the spine have a predisposition to other spinal problems in later life, such as a prolapsed or herniated disc (p.384).

WWW ONLINE SITES: p.1035

Scoliosis

Abnormal curvature of the spine to the left or right

GENDER More common in females

GENETICS Sometimes runs in families

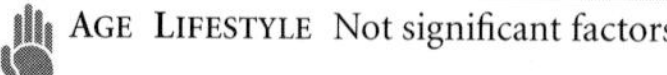

AGE LIFESTYLE Not significant factors

The spine normally forms a straight, vertical line when viewed from the back. Scoliosis is an abnormal sideways curvature of the spine, most commonly affecting the spine in the chest area and the lower back region. Scoliosis is more common in females. Early diagnosis is important because, if left untreated, the deformity can become worse.

WHAT ARE THE CAUSES?

In most cases, the cause of scoliosis is unknown. Genetic factors may be involved since the condition tends to run in families. In some cases, scoliosis is congenital (present from birth). Rarely, the curvature is the result of muscle weakness around the spine or due to a neuromuscular disease such as cerebral palsy (p.846) or poliomyelitis (p.295).

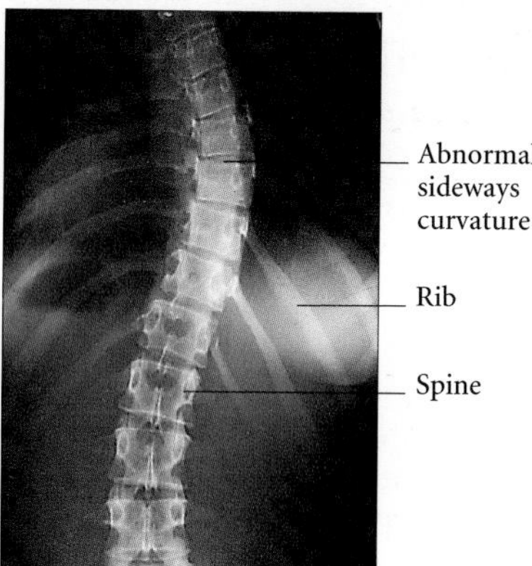

Scoliosis
In this X-ray, the upper spine curves to one side, a condition known as scoliosis. Left untreated, the curvature will increase.

Scoliosis may also be due to skeletal defects, such as unequal leg length. In rare cases, temporary scoliosis occurs as a result of muscle spasm following a spinal injury (p.524).

WHAT ARE THE SYMPTOMS?

Unless the condition is congenital or the result of a spinal injury, the symptoms develop gradually, usually during childhood or adolescence. The symptoms may include:

- Visible curving of the spine to one side, which is more obvious when bending forwards.
- Back pain.
- Abnormal gait.

If scoliosis is severe, the ribcage may become deformed, sometimes leading to heart and lung problems.

WHAT MIGHT BE DONE?

The doctor will probably diagnose scoliosis from a physical examination and X-rays (p.244). If possible, treatment is aimed at the underlying condition. For example, if your legs are of unequal length, your doctor may recommend wearing corrective shoes.

If there is no underlying cause and the spinal curvature is slight, you will probably only need regular checkups to monitor your condition. If scoliosis is severe or is progressing rapidly, it may be necessary for you to wear a spinal brace to limit further curvature. Surgery may be necessary to fuse the affected vertebrae or to straighten the spine with metal rods and wires.

WWW ONLINE SITES: p.1028, p.1035

Coccydynia

Severe, sharp pain in the coccyx, the small triangular bone at the base of the spine

LIFESTYLE Poor posture when sitting is a risk factor

AGE GENDER GENETICS Not significant factors

Pain in the coccyx, or coccydynia, may be due to injury, a baby pushing against the mother's coccyx during birth, or prolonged pressure due to poor posture while sitting. Often, no cause is found.

Before making a diagnosis, your doctor may carry out a rectal examination to rule out a tumour in the rectum. Women may also have a vaginal examination to look for a tumour in the uterus. Your doctor may also arrange for you to have an X-ray (p.244) of the lower spine to look for signs of injury.

Coccydynia may be relieved with a painkiller (p.912) or a nonsteroidal anti-inflammatory drug (p.894). You may also be able to ease the pain by applying heat to the area with a heat pad or cold with an ice pack. A local injection with a corticosteroid drug (*see* LOCALLY ACTING CORTICOSTEROIDS, p.895), often in combination with an anaesthetic, can sometimes provide relief. Usually no further treatment is necessary.

(WWW) ONLINE SITES: p.1035

Osteomyelitis

Infection of bone, causing pain and damage to surrounding tissue

AGE Most common in young children and elderly people but can occur at any age

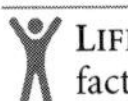
LIFESTYLE Use of intravenous drugs is a risk factor

GENDER GENETICS Not significant factors

Osteomyelitis is infection of bone, usually due to bacteria. The condition is most common in young children, but elderly people are also at risk. In other age groups, the condition is most common in people with reduced immunity, such as those with sickle-cell disease (p.448) or diabetes mellitus (p.687). In young children, the vertebrae (spinal bones) or one of the long bones of the limbs are usually affected. In adults, osteomyelitis most commonly affects the vertebrae or the pelvis.

What are the causes?

There are two forms of osteomyelitis: one that comes on suddenly (acute), and the other that develops more gradually and is long-term (chronic).

The acute form of osteomyelitis is usually a consequence of infection with *Staphylococcus aureus* bacteria. These bacteria normally live harmlessly on the skin but they can enter the bloodstream and result in osteomyelitis if they infect the bone tissue as a result of a wound, fracture (p.392), joint replacement (p.377), or intravenous injection with a contaminated needle.

The chronic form of osteomyelitis may be caused by tuberculosis (p.491) or, in rare cases, by a fungal infection. In some cases, acute osteomyelitis may develop into the chronic form.

What are the symptoms?

The symptoms of acute osteomyelitis develop suddenly and may include:

- Swelling of the skin and severe pain in the affected area.
- Fever.
- In young children, not wanting to move an affected arm or leg.

Chronic osteomyelitis develops more slowly. Its symptoms include:

- Weight loss.
- Mild fever.
- Persistent pain in the affected bone.

Pus may form in the bone and can make its way to the skin's surface, causing a discharging opening (a sinus).

How is it diagnosed?

If your doctor suspects that you have osteomyelitis, he or she may arrange for X-rays (p.244), radionuclide scanning (p.251), or MRI (p.248) to locate the infected area of bone. If pus is present, a sample may be aspirated (removed from the bone through a fine needle) for examination to identify the organism that is causing the disease.

What is the treatment?

Treatment with intravenous antibiotics (p.885) is usually begun in hospital and may continue after you return home. You may then need to continue taking antibiotics orally for a period of several months. When osteomyelitis is caused by tuberculosis, antituberculous drugs (p.886) may be prescribed for a period of 12–18 months.

In some cases, surgery may be necessary to remove infected bone. If a large area of bone is removed, you may need a bone graft, in which the infected bone is replaced by new bone taken from elsewhere in the body or from a donor. If the infection is associated with a joint replacement, the artificial joint will be removed, the infection treated, and a new joint put in its place.

The acute form of osteomyelitis is usually treated successfully, but the chronic form may take several months or years to clear up. In some cases, it may be necessary to take antibiotics indefinitely to suppress the infection.

(WWW) ONLINE SITES: p.1035

Noncancerous bone tumours

Noncancerous growths that may cause pain and deformity in a bone

AGE Most common in childhood or adolescence; rare over the age of 40

GENDER GENETICS LIFESTYLE Not significant factors

Noncancerous bone tumours may occur in any part of a bone. These tumours develop most commonly in the long bones of the limbs, such as the femur (thighbone). The bones of the hands are another common site. Noncancerous bone tumours most often develop during childhood or adolescence. They are rare in people over the age of 40.

Although the presence of a tumour normally causes no symptoms, sometimes there may be pain in the affected area, or the bone may become enlarged and deformed. Affected bone is more

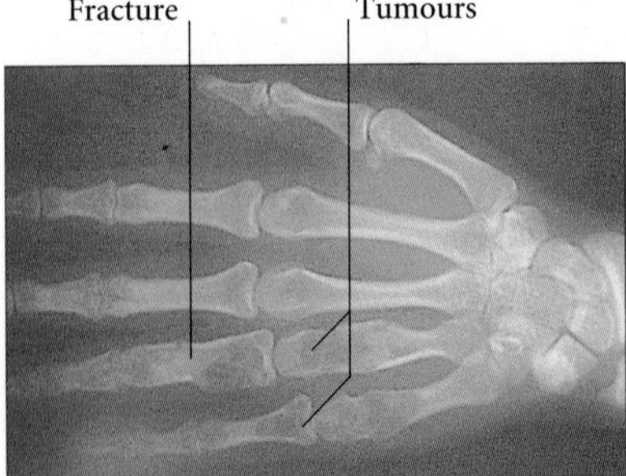

Noncancerous bone tumours
This X-ray shows several noncancerous tumours in the bones of the fingers. Some bones have become enlarged as a result of the tumours, and one has a fracture.

likely to fracture from even a minor injury. Occasionally, a tumour may press on nerves, causing a tingling sensation or numbness. In some cases, movement may be restricted, or pain may be felt on movement if the tumour presses on nearby tendons (fibrous bands that connect muscles to bones).

A bone tumour is usually diagnosed from X-rays (p.244), MRI (p.248), or radionuclide scanning (p.251). To confirm that the tumour is noncancerous, your doctor may arrange for a biopsy of the bone, in which a small piece of the affected bone is removed for analysis.

A tumour may be removed surgically if it is painful, causes deformity of the bone, or grows rapidly. You may subsequently need a bone graft, in which artificial bone or bone taken from elsewhere in your body or from a donor is used. Generally, surgery is successful in removing noncancerous tumours, although occasionally these recur and may require further surgery.

(WWW) ONLINE SITES: p.1035

Primary bone cancer

Cancerous tumours that originate within the bone tissue

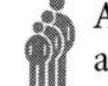 AGE Most common in childhood and adolescence

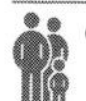 GENETICS Sometimes runs in families

 GENDER LIFESTYLE Not significant factors

Cancers originating in bone, known as primary bone cancers, are rare. They usually develop in children and teenagers. The causes are unknown, but some cases are associated with genetic factors. The most common site of primary bone cancer is the leg, either just above or just below the knee.

The first symptom is often painful, tender swelling of the affected area. If the cancer affects a bone in the leg, you may experience pain on standing or while you are at rest, and the pain may become worse at night. The diseased bone may fracture easily.

What might be done?

To confirm the diagnosis, your doctor will probably arrange for you to have X-rays (p.244) and possibly CT scanning (p.247) or MRI (p.248). He or she may also arrange for you to have chest X-rays (p.490) and radionuclide scanning (p.251) to check if the cancer has spread to other parts of the body.

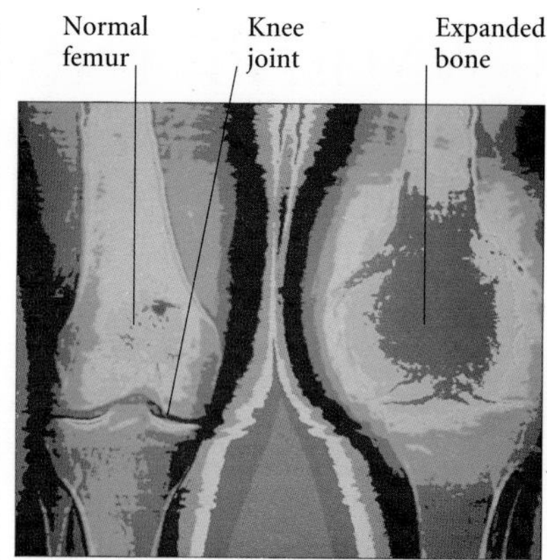

Primary bone cancer in the leg
This colour-coded CT scan of both legs reveals a primary bone cancer of one femur (thighbone) and associated swelling.

Radiotherapy (p.281) may reduce the size of the tumour. However, in most cases the tumour is removed surgically. Removed bone is replaced by artificial bone or by bone taken from elsewhere in the body or from a donor.

Following surgery, radiotherapy or chemotherapy (p.280) may be given to destroy any remaining cancerous cells. Amputation of a limb is rarely necessary. Most people treated for primary bone cancer have only a small chance of recurrence in the first 5 years. After this period, recurrence is unlikely.

(WWW) ONLINE SITES: p.1028, p.1035

Bone metastases

Cancerous tumours in bone that have spread from a cancer elsewhere in the body

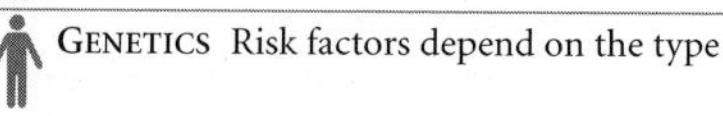 AGE More common in elderly people

GENETICS Risk factors depend on the type

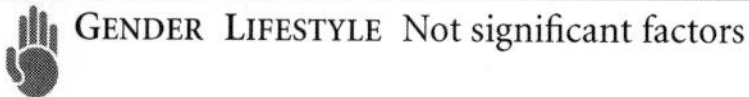 GENDER LIFESTYLE Not significant factors

Bone metastases, also known as secondary bone cancer, are tumours that have spread from another part of the body. Metastases most often develop in the ribs, pelvis, skull, or spine. The condition occurs much more commonly than primary bone cancer, especially in older people, who are more likely to have cancer elsewhere in their body. The cancers that most often spread to bone are those originating in the breast, the lung, the thyroid gland, the kidney, and the prostate gland.

What are the symptoms?

Bone metastases may cause the following symptoms in addition to those of the main cancer:

- Gnawing bone pain that may become worse at night.
- Swelling of the affected area.
- Tenderness over the affected area.

The affected bones fracture easily, often after minor injury.

What might be done?

If you already have a cancer somewhere else in your body, you may have X-rays (p.244) or radionuclide scanning (p.251) to check whether the cancer has spread to the bones. If the site of the primary cancer is unknown, you may need further tests to find out where the metastasis came from. For example, women may have a breast X-ray (*see* MAMMOGRAPHY, p.759) to look for evidence of breast cancer.

Your doctor will probably direct treatment at your original cancer. He or she may also make arrangements for you to have a course of chemotherapy (p.280), radiotherapy (p.281), or hormonal therapy to relieve bone pain.

The outlook for people with bone metastases usually depends on the site of the original cancer and how successfully it can be treated. However, the best that can usually be achieved after bone metastases is a period of remission.

(WWW) ONLINE SITES: p.1028, p.1035

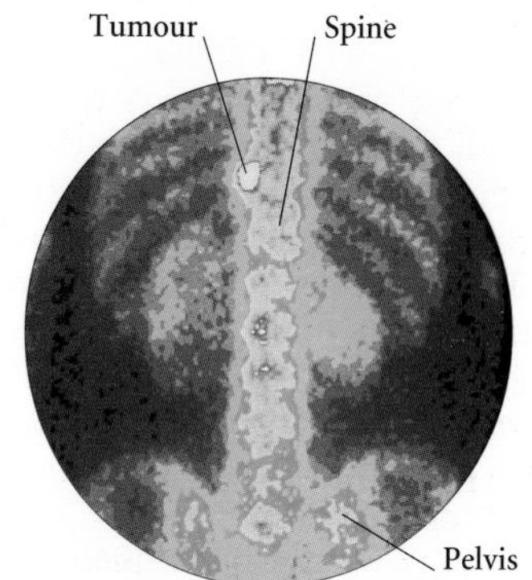

Bone metastases
This radionuclide scan gives a view of the trunk of a person with metastatic bone cancer. The scan reveals a cancerous tumour in a vertebra of the upper spine.

JOINT AND LIGAMENT DISORDERS

Joints occur where bones meet, and they allow our bodies to be flexible. Lubricated tissue called cartilage lines the ends of bones and prevents friction during movement, and fibrous ligaments surrounding the joint give strength and support. Joints may be damaged by arthritis, injury, infection, or degeneration of bone, cartilage, and ligaments caused by aging or disease.

Joint disorders are a major cause of disability and immobility, but the treatment of long-term joint disorders has greatly improved during the past 20 years, partly due to the availability of safe, reliable artificial joints.

The first article describes the many types of arthritis, a general term for disease of one or more joints. This is followed by separate articles on the most common types, including osteoarthritis, rheumatoid arthritis, gout, and reactive arthritis. Septic arthritis, which in the past was a major cause of crippling joint disease, is now usually curable with antibiotics. Next in this section is a detailed look at lower back pain together with self-help measures that can be taken to prevent back pain from occurring. The section ends with articles on nonarthritic conditions such as bursitis, in which the fluid-filled cushions around the joints become swollen and inflamed.

There is a similar but distinct form of rheumatoid arthritis that can develop in children (*see* JUVENILE CHRONIC ARTHRITIS, p.835).

KEY ANATOMY

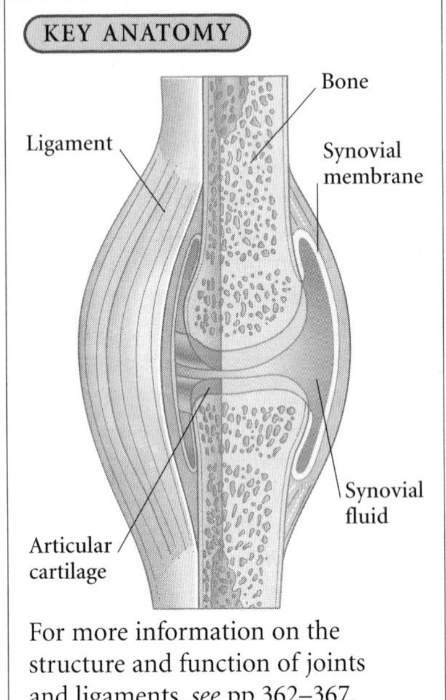

For more information on the structure and function of joints and ligaments, *see* pp.362–367.

Arthritis

Pain, inflammation, and stiffness in one or more joints

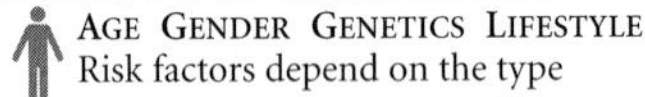

The term arthritis covers a group of inflammatory and degenerative conditions that cause stiffness, swelling, and pain in the joints. Arthritis may also be linked with disorders such as psoriasis (p.332) and Crohn's disease (p.658).

WHAT ARE THE TYPES?

There are several different types of arthritis, each having different characteristics. The most common form is osteoarthritis (right), which most often involves the knees, hips, and hands and usually affects middle-aged and older people. Cervical spondylosis (p.376) is a form of osteoarthritis that affects the joints in the neck.

Rheumatoid arthritis (p.377) is a damaging condition that causes inflammation in the joints and in other body tissues, such as the membranous heart covering, lungs, and eyes. The disorder has different effects in children (*see* JUVENILE CHRONIC ARTHRITIS, p.835).

Ankylosing spondylitis (p.378) is another persistent form of arthritis that initially affects the spine and the joints between the base of the spine and the pelvis. Other tissues, such as the eyes, may also be affected. The disorder may eventually cause the vertebrae (bones of the spine) to fuse together.

Reactive arthritis (p.379) typically develops in susceptible people after they have had an infection, most commonly of the genital tract or intestines. Reactive arthritis most often causes inflammation in an ankle or a knee.

Both gout (p.380) and pseudogout (p.381) are types of arthritis in which crystals are deposited in a joint, resulting in swelling and pain.

Septic arthritis (p.381) is a relatively rare condition that can develop when infection enters a joint either through a wound or from the bloodstream.

Treatment depends on the type of arthritis. Painkillers (p.912), such as paracetamol, and nonsteroidal anti-inflammatory drugs (p.894) may relieve symptoms. Physiotherapy (p.961) may keep joints mobile. Severely damaged joints may be replaced surgically (*see* JOINT REPLACEMENT, p.377).

(WWW) ONLINE SITES: p.1027

Osteoarthritis

Gradual degeneration of the cartilage covering the bone ends within joints

AGE Rare under the age of 45; increasingly common over the age of 60

GENDER Twice as common in females

GENETICS Sometimes runs in families

LIFESTYLE Past injuries and being overweight are risk factors

In a joint affected by osteoarthritis, the protective cartilage found at the ends of bones is worn away. As the condition develops, the bone around the affected joint thickens, and bony growths called osteophytes form. If the synovial tissue that lines the joint capsule becomes inflamed, fluid may accumulate within the joint. These changes cause pain, swelling, and stiffness of the joints, reducing their mobility.

Osteoarthritis is most common in weight-bearing joints, such as the knees and hips. However, the hands, feet, and shoulders may also be affected, as may the bones of the neck (*see* CERVICAL SPONDYLOSIS, p.376). Nearly everyone has developed a degree of osteoarthritis by the age of 70, but only some people have symptoms. Women are more commonly affected by osteoarthritis than men, and their symptoms are more severe. This form of arthritis sometimes develops in younger people, particularly in those who have had joint injuries.

What are the causes?

There is often no obvious cause for the onset of osteoarthritis, but there are known factors that may increase the risk of developing the disorder. Wear occurs most often in joints that have been damaged by repeated strenuous activity or by repeated minor injuries. For example, the pressure that ballet dancers exert on their feet makes them susceptible to developing osteoarthritis of the ankle. Osteoarthritis is also common in former athletes.

Damage to a joint early in life may lead to osteoarthritis later on. Excessive weight can also increase a person's risk of developing the condition because of the extra stress it places on the joints. Another risk factor is damage to cartilage caused by another joint disorder, such as septic arthritis (p.381). Finally, if a close member of your family has osteoarthritis, you are more likely to develop the condition yourself.

What are the symptoms?

Initially, the symptoms are mild, but they may slowly get worse. Often only one or two joints are badly affected, but sometimes osteoarthritis is more widespread. The symptoms may include:

- Pain and tenderness that worsen with activity and are relieved by rest.
- Swelling around the joint.
- Stiffness lasting a short time after a period of inactivity.
- Restricted joint movement.
- Enlarged, distorted finger joints if the hands are affected.
- Crackling noise (called crepitus) on moving the affected joint.

SELF-HELP Living with arthritis

If you have long-term arthritis, you may be able to manage your symptoms so that you can maintain an active lifestyle. Consult your doctor about pain relief and keeping joints mobile. Organizations concerned with arthritis can also provide you with valuable information and support.

Mobility

Gentle, regular exercise helps to relieve stiffness and improve mobility. Physical activity also helps to strengthen the muscles that support joints. However, if exercise causes swelling or pain, stop the activity and consult your doctor.

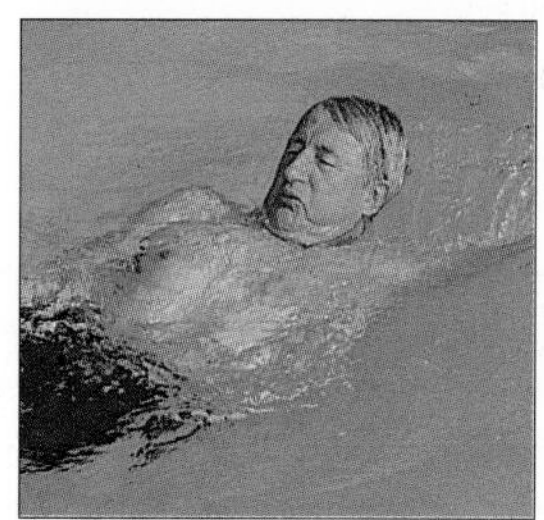

Exercising
Regular swimming is an ideal sport for maintaining your joint flexibility and stamina. Since the water supports your body, muscles can be exercised without straining your joints.

Pain relief

To relieve severe joint pain, apply heat or cold to the affected area. Heat increases blood flow, and cold helps to reduce swelling. Both decrease sensitivity to pain.

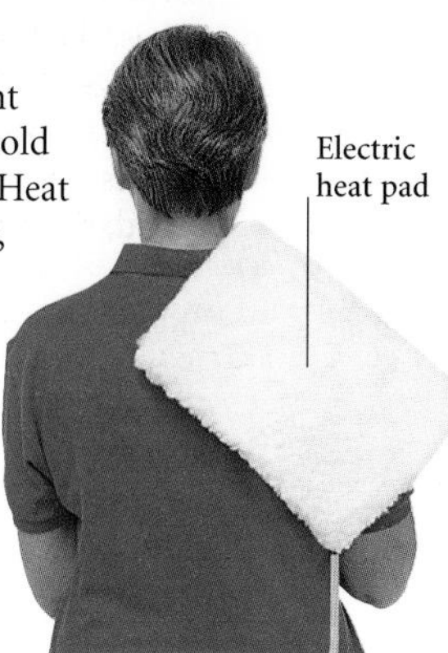

Using a heat pad
You can use a heat pad to provide a steady supply of heat to an aching joint.

Specialized equipment

Your doctor or a physiotherapist may be able to suggest specially adapted pieces of equipment to help you with household tasks. The equipment may have particular features, such as handles that are easy to grip or extending arms to help you reach objects without bending down.

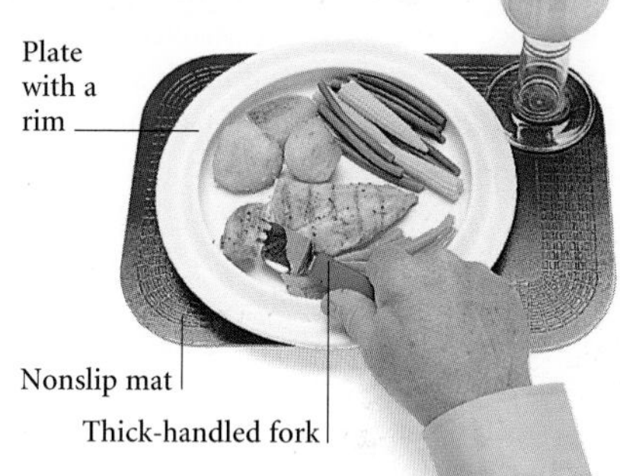

Eating and drinking
If arthritis restricts the movement in your hands, use cutlery with thick handles and glasses with wide stems that will be easier to grip. A plate with a rim may keep food from spilling, and a nonslip mat will help to hold your plate still during a meal.

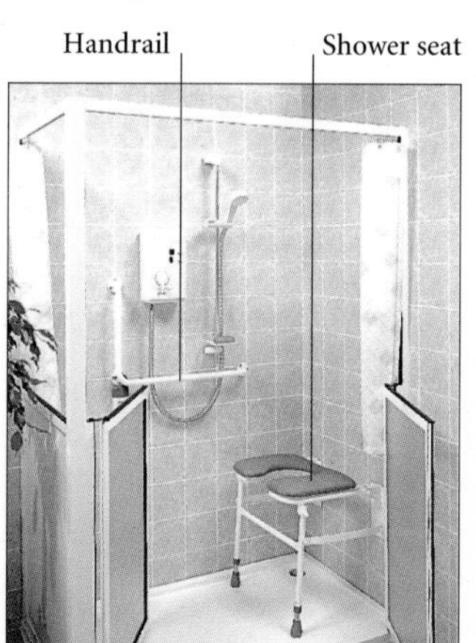

Taking a shower
A fixed seat in the shower cubicle allows you to sit down while you wash. Handrails and a nonslip floor surface reduce the risk of falls.

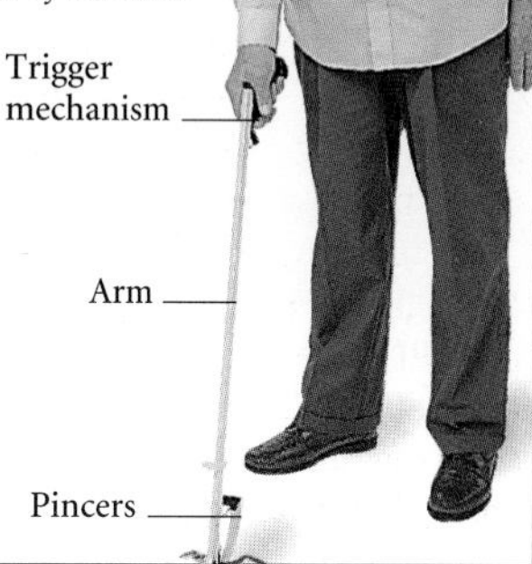

Picking up objects
Tongs enable you to pick up objects that are out of your reach without bending or stretching. Some types of tongs have a trigger mechanism that operates pincers at the end of the arm.

Referred pain, which is felt in areas remote from the site of damage but on the same nerve pathway as the affected joint, may develop. For example, an arthritic hip may cause referred pain in the knee. The pain may become worse towards the end of the day.

If movement is severely restricted, an affected person may be confined to the home. Lack of mobility may lead to weakness and wasting of muscles and sometimes to weight gain.

WHAT MIGHT THE DOCTOR DO?

Your doctor may suspect that you have osteoarthritis from your symptoms, a history of joint problems, and a physical examination. It is often possible to confirm a diagnosis of osteoarthritis, while at the same time ruling out other types of arthritis, by means of blood tests and X-rays (p.244).

Osteoarthritis cannot be cured, but with treatment most symptoms can be relieved. Your doctor may recommend that you take paracetamol (*see* PAINKILLERS, p.912) or a nonsteroidal anti-inflammatory drug (p.894). If you experience a severe flare-up of pain and inflammation in a single joint, your doctor may inject a corticosteroid drug directly into the affected joint to reduce swelling and relieve pain (*see* LOCALLY ACTING CORTICOSTEROIDS, p.895).

To improve muscle function around joints affected by osteoarthritis, your doctor may refer you for physiotherapy (p.961). If osteoarthritis is very severe, surgery may be necessary to repair or replace an affected joint (*see* JOINT REPLACEMENT, opposite page).

Healthy hip joint | Pelvis | Osteoarthritic hip joint | Femur

Osteoarthritis in a hip joint
In the hip joint seen on the right of this X-ray, the head of the femur (thighbone) has become worn where it fits into the pelvis, causing pain and stiffness.

WHAT CAN I DO?

If you have mild osteoarthritis, you may be able to participate in most everyday activities by adapting your lifestyle (*see* LIVING WITH ARTHRITIS, p.375). If you are overweight, ask your doctor for dietary advice to enable you to lose weight and reduce further wear on your joints. If possible, take gentle exercise to help to lose weight, maintain muscle tone, and delay the progression of the disease. Supportive shoes with rubber soles will absorb shock and reduce further wear. If you have a painful hip or knee, use a walking stick for support. Massage, warm baths, or a heat pad may ease joint pain and increase mobility.

(WWW) ONLINE SITES: p.1027, p.1035

Cervical spondylosis

A disease of bones and cartilage in the neck, which may lead to pain and stiffness

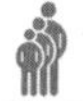
AGE Increasingly common over the age of 45

GENDER More common in males

GENETICS LIFESTYLE Not significant factors

Cervical spondylosis is osteoarthritis (p.374) affecting the upper spine. In this disorder, the vertebrae (bones of the spine) and the discs of cartilage between them begin to show signs of disease. The bones thicken, and bony outgrowths called osteophytes develop on the vertebrae. Inflamed joints and osteophytes may press on spinal nerves or compress blood vessels in the neck.

The condition is increasingly common over the age of 45 and affects more men than women. Rarely, it is triggered by injury and affects younger people.

WHAT ARE THE SYMPTOMS?

Many people do not have symptoms or may develop only very mild symptoms. When symptoms do become apparent, they may include:

- Restricted neck movement that may be painful.
- Pain at the back of the head.
- Aching or shooting pain that travels from the shoulders to the hands.
- Numbness, tingling, and muscle weakness in the hands and arms.

Sometimes, if the head is moved too quickly, the deformities in the upper spine may suddenly compress blood vessels that carry blood to the brain, resulting in dizziness, unsteadiness, or double vision (*see* VERTIGO, p.603).

In rare cases, joints that have severely degenerated may put prolonged pressure on the spinal cord, causing tingling and muscle weakness or paralysis in the legs or, sometimes, difficulty in controlling bladder or bowel function.

HOW IS IT DIAGNOSED?

Some people do not have symptoms and cervical spondylosis may be recognized only when an X-ray (p.244) is taken for another reason. However, if you experience neck pain or dizziness, consult your doctor, who may arrange for X-rays to look for signs of cervical spondylosis. If your doctor thinks that your symptoms may not be due solely to cervical spondylosis, he or she may arrange further tests to look for other causes, such as a prolapsed or herniated disc (p.384). You may also undergo nerve conduction studies and EMG (*see* NERVE AND MUSCLE ELECTRICAL TESTS, p.544) to assess nerve activity in your arms and hands. CT scanning (p.247) or MRI (p.248) may also be carried out to see whether there have been any changes affecting the bones of the spine, the discs of cartilage between them, or the tissues around them.

WHAT IS THE TREATMENT?

Changes in the spine are not inevitably progressive. There may be little deterioration for many years, and sometimes symptoms improve. To relieve symptoms in mild cases, your doctor may recommend painkillers (p.912) or prescribe nonsteroidal anti-inflammatory drugs (p.894). Once the initial pain has been relieved, the doctor may also suggest some simple exercises to maintain mobility and increase the strength of muscles in your neck.

If cervical spondylosis has damaged a nerve, surgery may be recommended to prevent the symptoms from getting worse. In this operation, the surgeon widens the natural opening between the vertebrae through which the nerve passes when it branches off the spinal cord. In a few rare cases, surgery may also be carried out to stabilize the spine by fusing together affected vertebrae.

(WWW) ONLINE SITES: p.1027, p.1035

Rheumatoid arthritis

A persistent disorder that can cause the joints to become painful, swollen, stiff, and deformed

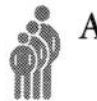
AGE Most common over the age of 40

GENDER Three times more common in females

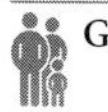
GENETICS May run in some families

LIFESTYLE Not a significant factor

In rheumatoid arthritis, the affected joints become stiff and swollen as a result of inflammation of the synovial membrane, which encloses each joint. If the inflammation persists, it may damage both the ends of the bones and the cartilage that covers them. Tendons and ligaments, which support the joints, may also become worn and slack, and deformity of the joints occurs.

In most cases, rheumatoid arthritis affects several joints. The disorder usually appears first in the small joints of the hands and feet but may develop in any joint. Rheumatoid arthritis usually tends to appear in similar areas on both sides of the body. Tissues in other parts of the body, such as the eyes, the lungs, the membranous sac around the heart, and blood vessels, may also be affected.

Rheumatoid arthritis is a long-term disease and usually recurs in episodes lasting for several weeks or months. Some people remain free of symptoms between episodes. The disorder affects about 1 in 100 people and is three times more common in women than in men. A similar but distinct arthritic disorder can develop in children (*see* JUVENILE CHRONIC ARTHRITIS, p.835).

Rheumatoid arthritis is an autoimmune disorder (p.461) in which the body produces antibodies that attack the synovial membrane and, in some cases, other body tissues. A genetic factor may be involved since the condition is common in some families.

WHAT ARE THE SYMPTOMS?

Rheumatoid arthritis usually develops slowly, although sometimes the onset of the inflammation can be abrupt. General symptoms associated with the condition may include tiredness, poor appetite, and loss of weight. Specific symptoms may include:

- Painful, swollen joints that are stiff on waking in the morning.
- Painless, small bumps (nodules) on areas of pressure, such as the elbows.

Since the condition can be both painful and debilitating, depression (p.554) is

TREATMENT JOINT REPLACEMENT

Joints that have been severely damaged by a disorder such as arthritis or by an injury may be surgically replaced with artificial joints made of metal, ceramic, or plastic. The joints in the body that are most commonly replaced are the hips, knees, and shoulders. During the operation, the ends of damaged bones are removed and the artificial components are fixed in place. The operation usually relieves pain and increases the range of movement in the affected joint.

HIP REPLACEMENT

The most commonly replaced joint in the body is the hip. During the operation, both the pelvic socket and the head of the femur (thighbone), which fits into the socket, are replaced. The operation is carried out under general anaesthesia and involves a short stay in hospital.

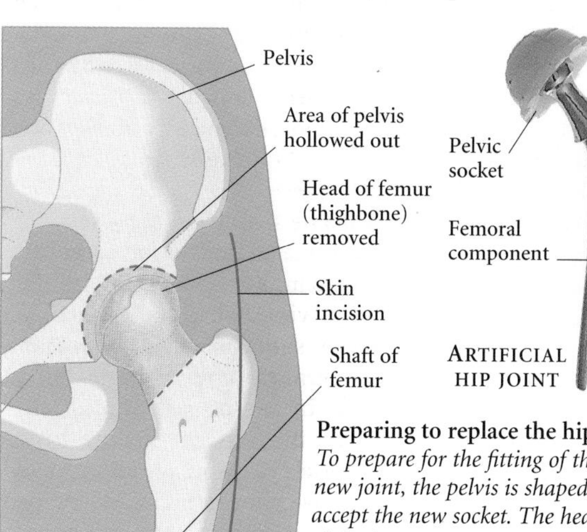

Preparing to replace the hip
To prepare for the fitting of the new joint, the pelvis is shaped to accept the new socket. The head of the femur is removed, and the centre of the bone is shaped to fit the femoral component.

Pelvic socket
Femoral component

Artificial hip in position
This X-ray shows an artificial hip joint in place, with the femoral component fitted into the femur (thighbone) and the socket fitted into the pelvis.

OTHER JOINTS

Many different types of joint in the body can be replaced, from tiny finger joints to large joints such as the knees.

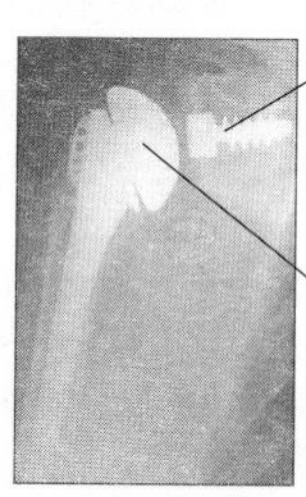

Artificial shoulder joint
This replacement shoulder joint has components fitted in the humerus and the scapula.

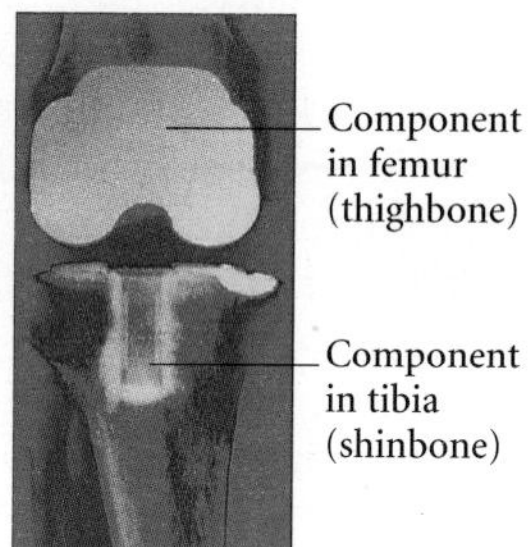

Artificial knee joint
This replacement knee joint has artificial components in the femur and the tibia.

common in people with rheumatoid arthritis. In women, the symptoms of rheumatoid arthritis may improve during pregnancy but may then flare up again after the baby is born.

ARE THERE COMPLICATIONS?

Over time, thinning of the bones (*see* OSTEOPOROSIS, p.368) and a greater susceptibility to fractures may develop in people with rheumatoid arthritis. This results partly from the disease itself and partly from reduced mobility.

The general symptoms of rheumatoid arthritis are partly due to anaemia (p.446), caused by a failure of the bone marrow to manufacture enough new red blood cells. Bursitis (p.387) may develop, in which one or more of the fluid-filled sacs around a joint become inflamed. Swelling that compresses the median nerve in the wrist may lead to a tingling feeling and pain in the fingers (*see* CARPAL TUNNEL SYNDROME, p.547). Spasm or narrowing of the walls of the arteries that supply the fingers and toes results in Raynaud's phenomenon (p.436), in which the digits become pale and painful on exposure to cold.

A less common complication is when the spleen and the lymph nodes enlarge (*see* LYMPHADENOPATHY, p.458). Inflammation may affect the membranous sac that surrounds the heart (*see* PERICARDITIS, p.428) and also the lungs (*see* FIBROSING ALVEOLITIS, p.497). In some cases, there may be inflammation of the white of the eye (*see* SCLERITIS, p.574), or the eyes may become very dry (*see* SJÖGREN'S SYNDROME, p.463).

HOW IS IT DIAGNOSED?

The diagnosis is usually based on your medical history and a physical examination. Your doctor may arrange for blood tests to check for the presence of an antibody known as rheumatoid factor, which is usually associated with rheumatoid arthritis. You may also have blood tests to measure the severity of the inflammation. X-rays (p.244) of the affected joints may be taken to assess the degree of damage.

WHAT IS THE TREATMENT?

There is no cure for rheumatoid arthritis. The aim of treatment is to control symptoms and reduce further joint damage by slowing the progression of the disease. Various types of drug are available, and your doctor's recommendation will depend on the severity and progression of the disease, your age, and your general health.

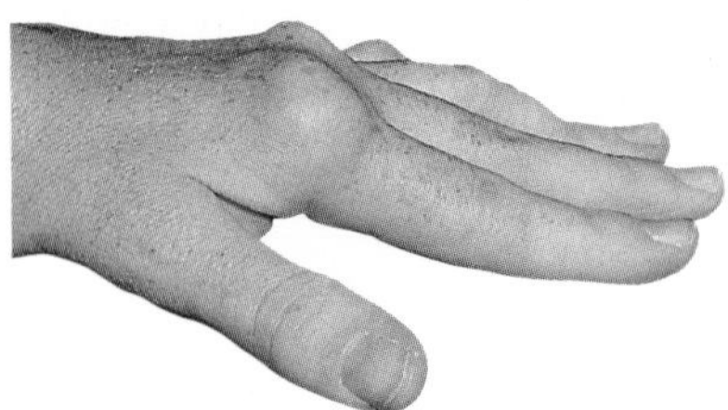

Swelling in rheumatoid arthritis
The swollen knuckles of this hand are caused by rheumatoid arthritis, a condition in which the joints become inflamed and may be damaged.

If your symptoms are usually mild, your doctor may simply prescribe a nonsteroidal anti-inflammatory drug (p.894). However, if your symptoms are severe, he or she may prescribe drugs that slow the progression of the disease (*see* ANTIRHEUMATIC DRUGS, p.895), which should limit permanent joint damage. These drugs may have to be taken for several months before the full benefits are felt. An antirheumatic such as sulfasalazine or hydroxychloroquine may be given first. If your symptoms persist, the doctor may prescribe a drug such as gold, penicillamine, methotrexate, or ciclosporin. Since these drugs can sometimes cause serious side effects, which include kidney damage and blood disorders, the doctor will closely monitor your condition.

Your doctor may recommend that you use a splint or brace to support a particularly painful joint and to slow down the development of deformities. Taking gentle, regular exercise may help to keep your joints flexible and prevent supporting muscles from weakening. Physiotherapy (p.961) may be given to improve your joint mobility and help to increase muscle strength. Hydrotherapy and heat or ice treatments may provide pain relief.

An intensely painful joint may be eased if your doctor injects it with a corticosteroid drug (*see* LOCALLY ACTING CORTICOSTEROIDS, p.895). If a joint is severely damaged, your doctor may suggest that you have surgery to replace the damaged joint with an artificial one (*see* JOINT REPLACEMENT, p.377).

WHAT IS THE PROGNOSIS?

Many people with rheumatoid arthritis are able to lead a normal life (*see* LIVING WITH ARTHRITIS, p.375), but lifelong drug treatment may be needed to control the symptoms. About 1 in 10 people becomes severely disabled as repeated attacks destroy the joints. To monitor progression of the disease and your response to treatment, regular blood tests will be needed. Sometimes, the attacks gradually cease, and the disease is said to have burned itself out, but some permanent disability may remain.

(WWW) ONLINE SITES: p.1027, p.1033

Ankylosing spondylitis

Persistent inflammation and stiffening of the joints, usually affecting the spine and pelvis

 AGE Usually begins in late adolescence or early adulthood; onset rare over the age of 45

 GENDER About four times more common in males

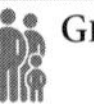 GENETICS Sometimes runs in families

 LIFESTYLE Not a significant factor

In ankylosing spondylitis, persistent joint inflammation affects the sacroiliac joints at the back of the pelvis and the vertebrae (bones of the spine) in particular. If the spine is severely diseased, new bone grows between the vertebrae, which eventually fuse together.

This form of arthritis is four times more common in men than in women. A variant of ankylosing spondylitis is associated, in some cases, with the persistent skin disorder psoriasis (p.332) or with inflammatory bowel disease, such as Crohn's disease (p.658).

WHAT ARE THE CAUSES?

The cause of ankylosing spondylitis is unknown, but about 9 in 10 affected people have a particular antigen (a substance that is capable of stimulating an immune response in the body) called HLA-B27 on the surface of most cells. This antigen is inherited, which helps to explain why ankylosing spondylitis runs in some families. Most people with HLA-B27 do not develop the condition, and a bacterial infection is thought to trigger ankylosing spondylitis in those who are predisposed.

WHAT ARE THE SYMPTOMS?

The symptoms of ankylosing spondylitis usually appear in late adolescence or early adulthood and develop gradually over a period of months or even years. Men are usually more severely affected. The main symptoms include:

- Lower back pain, which may spread down into the buttocks and thighs.
- Lower back stiffness that may be worse in the morning and improves with exercise.
- Pain in other joints, such as the hips, knees, and shoulders.
- Pain and tenderness in the heels.
- Tiredness, weight loss, and mild fever.

If left untreated, ankylosing spondylitis can distort the spine (*see* KYPHOSIS AND LORDOSIS, p.371), resulting in a stooped posture. If the joints between the spine and the ribs are affected, expansion of the chest becomes restricted. In some people, ankylosing spondylitis causes inflammation or damage to tissues in areas other than the joints, such as the eyes (*see* UVEITIS, p.574).

HOW IS IT DIAGNOSED?

Your doctor may suspect that you have ankylosing spondylitis from the pattern of your symptoms. He or she will perform a physical examination and may arrange for an X-ray (p.244) to look for evidence of fusion in the joints of the pelvis and the spine. Your doctor may also arrange for you to have blood tests to measure the level of inflammation and look for the HLA-B27 antigen.

WHAT IS THE TREATMENT?

Treatment of ankylosing spondylitis is aimed at relieving the symptoms and preventing the development of spinal deformity. Your doctor may prescribe a nonsteroidal anti-inflammatory drug (p.894) to control pain and inflammation. He or she may also refer you for physiotherapy (p.961), which may include breathing exercises and daily exercises to help to improve your posture, strengthen the back muscles, and prevent deformities of the spine (*see* PREVENTING BACK PAIN, p.382). You may also benefit from regular physical activity, such as swimming, which may help to relieve pain and stiffness. If a joint such as a hip is affected, you may eventually need to have it replaced surgically (*see* JOINT REPLACEMENT, p.377).

If your mobility is severely reduced, you may need occupational therapy (p.962). The therapist may suggest that you use specially designed equipment and furniture to make your life easier.

WHAT IS THE PROGNOSIS?

Although the condition is not curable, most people with ankylosing spondylitis are only mildly affected, causing minimum disruption of their everyday lives. In many cases, early treatment and regular exercise help to relieve pain and stiffness of the back and prevent deformity of the spine. However, about 1 in 20 people who develop ankylosing spondylitis may eventually become disabled and have difficulty in carrying out many routine activities. If disability is due to an affected joint, a replacement may be carried out.

(WWW) ONLINE SITES: p.1035

Reactive arthritis

Inflammation of joints as a result of an abnormal immune response to a recent infection elsewhere in the body

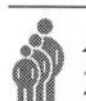
AGE Most common between the ages of 20 and 40

GENDER More common in males

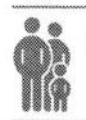
GENETICS Sometimes runs in families

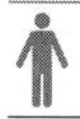
LIFESTYLE Risk factors depend on the cause

Reactive arthritis is usually a short-term disorder that develops after a bacterial infection of the genital tract, such as chlamydial infection (p.765) or nongonococcal urethritis (p.765), or the intestinal tract (*see* GASTROENTERITIS, p.628). Any of these infections may stimulate an abnormal immune response that causes tissues in the joints, usually the knee or ankle, to become inflamed. If inflammation also affects the eyes or the genital tract, the condition is known as Reiter's syndrome.

About 8 in 10 people who develop Reiter's syndrome have a particular antigen (a substance capable of stimulating an immune response in the body) known as HLA-B27. Although Reiter's syndrome is induced by infection, it usually develops in people who have a genetic predisposition to it. The disorder may therefore run in families.

WHAT ARE THE SYMPTOMS?

Depending on the infection that has triggered reactive arthritis or Reiter's syndrome, you may experience symptoms of a genital infection, such as pain on passing urine, or symptoms of gastroenteritis, such as diarrhoea. However, some people have no initial symptoms.

Both conditions develop 3–30 days after the initial infection has appeared. Symptoms may include:

- Painful, red, tender joints.
- Swelling around the joints.

Although the knees or ankles are most commonly affected, other joints may also be involved. If you have Reiter's syndrome, you may also notice:

- Sore, red eyes (*see* CONJUNCTIVITIS, p.570, and UVEITIS, p.574).
- Pain on passing urine and a discharge from the penis or vagina.

Less commonly, complications such as mouth ulcers (p.632), inflammation of the penis (*see* BALANITIS, p.722), lower back pain (p.381), and skin lesions on the hands and feet may develop.

WHAT MIGHT BE DONE?

Your doctor may diagnose reactive arthritis or Reiter's syndrome from your medical history and symptoms. He or she will probably take swabs from your urethra or cervix or collect a stool sample to try to establish the source of infection. Further tests may include a blood test to detect signs of inflammation and an X-ray (p.244) to look for evidence of joint damage.

If you are still affected by a genital or intestinal infection, your doctor may prescribe oral antibiotics (p.885). To relieve pain in your joints, he or she may recommend a nonsteroidal anti-inflammatory drug (p.894). If the pain is very severe and there is no infection present in the joint itself, you may be given a corticosteroid drug, injected directly into the joint (*see* LOCALLY ACTING CORTICOSTEROIDS, p.895).

WHAT IS THE PROGNOSIS?

The symptoms usually last for less than 6 months, and most people recover fully from reactive arthritis or Reiter's syndrome. People who are susceptible to Reiter's syndrome can reduce the risk of recurrence by taking care with personal hygiene and practising safe sex (p.68).

(WWW) ONLINE SITES: p.1027, p 1033

Gout

A type of arthritis in which crystalline deposits of uric acid form within joints, particularly at the base of the big toe

 **AGE** Most common between the ages of 30 and 60

 **GENDER** Twenty times more common in males

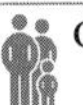 **GENETICS** Often runs in families

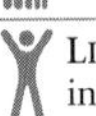 **LIFESTYLE** Being overweight and excessive intake of alcohol are risk factors

Gout causes sudden pain and inflammation, usually in a single joint. The base of the big toe is the most common site, but any joint may be affected. The disorder affects many more men than women. In women, gout rarely appears before the menopause.

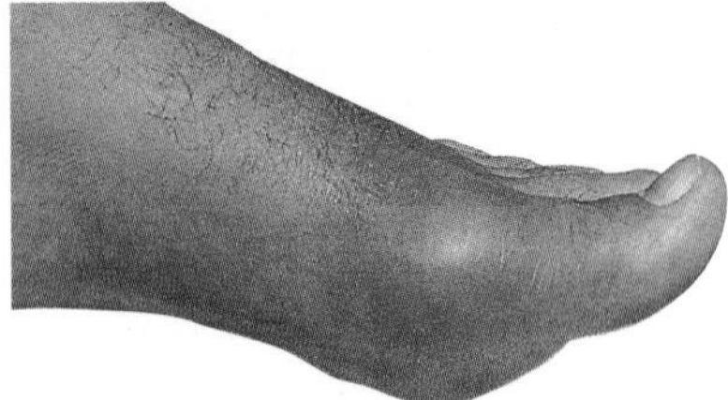

Swelling due to gout
As a result of an attack of gout, in which uric acid crystals form in a joint, the joint at the base of this big toe has become painful and swollen.

What are the causes?

An attack of gout is usually caused by raised blood levels of uric acid (a waste product of the breakdown of cells and proteins). An excess of uric acid may be caused by the overproduction and/or decreased excretion of uric acid and may lead to uric acid crystals being deposited in a joint. The underlying cause of gout is unknown, but the condition is often inherited. A few people with gout also develop kidney stones (p.701) formed from excess uric acid.

Gout may occur spontaneously or be triggered by surgery, being overweight, drinking alcohol, treatment with diuretics (p.902), or excess cell destruction associated with chemotherapy (p.280).

What are the symptoms?

The symptoms of gout usually flare up suddenly. They may include:

- Redness, tenderness, swelling, and warmth around the affected area.
- Pain, which may be severe, in the affected joint or joints.
- Mild fever.

In long-standing gout, deposits of uric acid crystals may collect in the earlobes and the soft tissues of the hands or feet, forming small lumps called tophi.

What might be done?

Your doctor may suspect that you have gout from your symptoms and arrange for blood tests to measure your uric acid levels. To confirm the diagnosis, he or she may arrange for you to have a joint aspiration (below), in which fluid is withdrawn from the affected joint and examined for uric acid crystals.

Gout may subside by itself after a few days. To reduce severe pain and inflammation, you may be treated with a nonsteroidal anti-inflammatory drug (p.894), the antigout drug colchicine, or with oral corticosteroids (p.930). If gout persists, your doctor may give you a corticosteroid injection directly into the affected joint (*see* LOCALLY ACTING CORTICOSTEROIDS, p.895).

If you have recurring gout, you may need lifelong treatment with preventive drugs such as allopurinol to reduce the production of uric acid or probenecid to increase the excretion of uric acid.

Your doctor may recommend that you reduce alcohol consumption and avoid foods such as liver. You may be able to reduce the frequency and severity of attacks by losing excess weight (*see* CONTROLLING YOUR WEIGHT, p.53).

What is the prognosis?

Gout is painful and can disrupt normal activities, but attacks can be controlled with drugs and changes in lifestyle. Repeated attacks may damage the joint.

(WWW) ONLINE SITES: p.1027, p.1036

TEST AND TREATMENT: Joint aspiration

During joint aspiration, fluid is withdrawn from a swollen joint with a needle and syringe, possibly under local anaesthesia. The fluid is then examined to find the cause of the swelling. Joint aspiration may also be carried out to relieve swelling due to excess fluid and to diagnose or treat disorders such as gout, pseudogout, and rheumatoid arthritis.

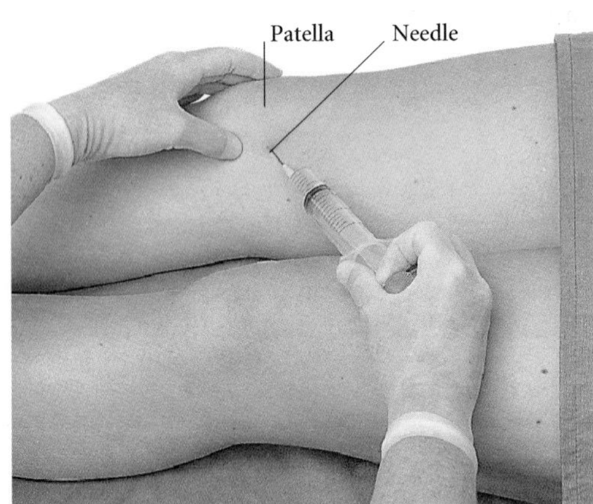

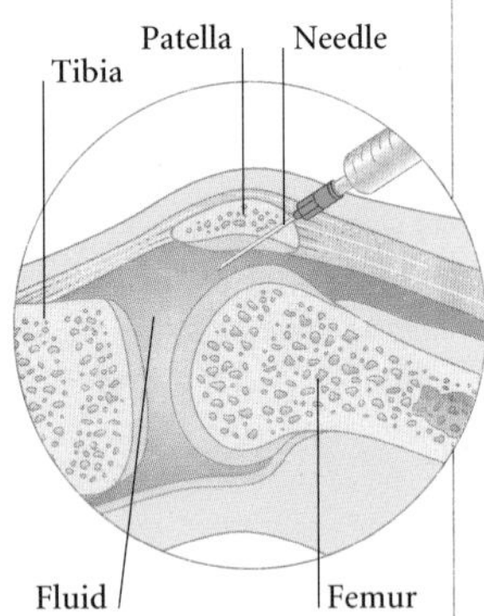

Knee joint aspiration
You will be asked to keep your knee relaxed so that the needle can be inserted easily. The patella is held still while the needle is passed into the space under the patella and fluid is withdrawn.

RESULTS

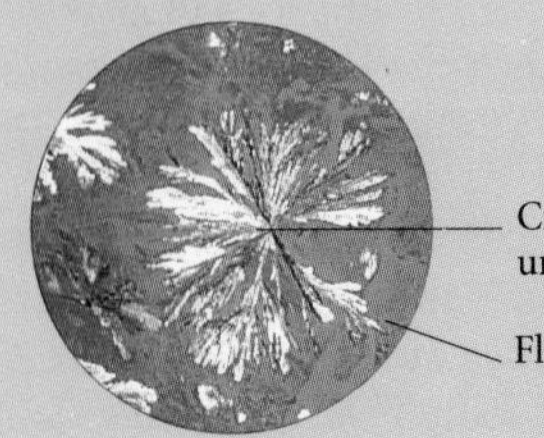

Fluid sample
A fluid sample withdrawn from a swollen joint is examined under a microscope. This magnified view of the fluid reveals the presence of uric acid crystals, which are indicative of gout.

Pseudogout

A type of arthritis in which crystals of calcium pyrophosphate or other chemicals are deposited in joints

 AGE Usually develops after the age of 60; more common with increasing age

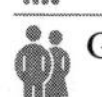 GENDER More common in females

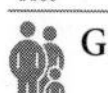 GENETICS Sometimes runs in families

 LIFESTYLE Not a significant factor

In pseudogout, crystals of calcium pyrophosphate or similar chemicals are deposited in joints, causing attacks of pain and stiffness. Usually, a single joint is affected. The most common sites are the knee and wrist, but crystals may be deposited in any joint. Although the process of formation and deposition of the crystals may start earlier, symptoms are less common before the age of 60.

In most people, the cause of pseudogout is unknown, although attacks may be triggered by surgery, infection, or injury. Pseudogout is often associated with other joint disorders, particularly osteoarthritis (p.374). Pseudogout may also be linked to hyperparathyroidism (p.682), a hormonal condition that leads to high blood levels of calcium, or haemochromatosis (p.692), a disorder in which the body is overloaded with iron. Pseudogout is more common in women and may run in families.

WHAT ARE THE SYMPTOMS?

Symptoms are similar to those of gout (opposite page). Attacks may cause:

- Severe pain, stiffness, swelling, and redness of the affected joint.
- Mild fever.

Some people have no pain between attacks, while others experience persistent pain and stiffness.

WHAT MIGHT BE DONE?

If your doctor suspects pseudogout, he or she may arrange for X-rays (p.244) of the affected joint. You may also need joint aspiration (opposite page), in which fluid is removed from a joint for analysis and to relieve swelling.

The symptoms of pseudogout may be relieved by simply removing fluid from the affected joint. In severe cases, a corticosteroid drug may be injected directly into the joint during the same procedure (*see* LOCALLY ACTING CORTICOSTEROIDS, p.895). You may also need nonsteroidal anti-inflammatory drugs (p.894). Once treatment starts, symptoms usually clear up within 48 hours.

There is no cure for pseudogout, but if the underlying cause is treated many people lead normal lives. Physiotherapy (p.961) can help to increase joint mobility and muscle strength.

(WWW) ONLINE SITES: p.1035

Septic arthritis

A type of arthritis resulting from infection of a joint

 AGE Most common in children and elderly people

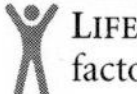 LIFESTYLE Intravenous drug use is a risk factor

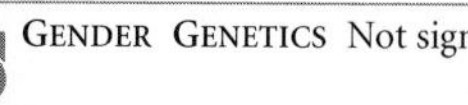 GENDER GENETICS Not significant factors

Septic arthritis is an infection in the synovial fluid or tissues of a joint, such as a hip or a knee. The condition is usually caused by bacteria that have entered the joint through a nearby open wound or have travelled through the bloodstream from an infection elsewhere in the body. For example, the bacteria that cause gonorrhoea (p.764) may spread from the genital tract through the bloodstream. The risk of developing septic arthritis is increased in people who have rheumatoid arthritis (p.377), who have been fitted with an artificial joint, or who use intravenous recreational drugs.

WHAT ARE THE SYMPTOMS?

The symptoms of septic arthritis usually appear suddenly and may include:

- Fever.
- Swelling, tenderness, redness, and warmth around the affected joint.
- Severe pain and restricted movement of the affected joint.

If pus builds up in an infected area, the joint may be damaged permanently. If you develop the above symptoms, consult your doctor immediately.

WHAT MIGHT BE DONE?

Your doctor may arrange for you to have a sample of fluid taken from the affected joint (*see* JOINT ASPIRATION, opposite page). The fluid is analysed to look for evidence of infection and to try to establish its cause.

Septic arthritis caused by bacteria is initially treated with intravenous antibiotics (p.885) for at least 4 weeks. Your doctor may then prescribe oral antibiotics for several weeks or months.

To help to relieve pain and inflammation, pus may be drained from the infected joint several times. Your doctor may also prescribe a nonsteroidal anti-inflammatory drug (p.894). You should rest the joint until the inflammation has completely subsided. Gentle movement is allowed and is important later on to prevent the joint becoming stiffened by shrinkage of the surrounding tissues. If the infected joint is an artificial joint, it may need to be replaced surgically with a new artificial joint to allow the infection to clear up.

WHAT IS THE PROGNOSIS?

If treatment is started early, the symptoms of septic arthritis should begin to subside within a few days, and eventually the inflammation may disappear completely. However, left untreated, the infection may be life-threatening and lead to irreversible joint damage.

(WWW) ONLINE SITES: p.1027, p.1033

Lower back pain

Pain in the back, below the waist, that may be sudden and sharp or persistent and dull

 AGE GENDER GENETICS LIFESTYLE Risk factors depend on the cause

Lower back pain affects about 6 in 10 adults during the course of a year. More working days are lost due to back pain than to any other medical condition. In most cases, the pain lasts for only a week or so, but many people find that their problem recurs. In a minority of people, persistent lower back pain causes long-term disability.

Lower back pain is usually caused by minor damage to the ligaments and muscles in the back. The lower back is vulnerable to these problems because it supports most of the body's weight and is under continual stress from movements such as bending and twisting. Less commonly, lower back pain may be a result of an underlying disorder such as a prolapsed or herniated disc (p.384) in the spine.

SELF-HELP PREVENTING BACK PAIN

Most people have experienced back pain at some time in their lives, but in many cases the problem could have been avoided. Back pain may be due to poor posture, weak abdominal or back muscles, or sudden muscle strain. You can improve your posture by wearing comfortable shoes, by standing or sitting with your spine properly aligned, and by choosing an appropriate mattress for your bed. Regular exercises strengthen abdominal and back muscles, and losing excess weight will relieve stress on joints and muscles. Learning how to perform physical tasks safely, including how to lift and carry objects, can help to prevent back strain. Ask your doctor or physiotherapist to give you advice on posture, exercises, and diet.

CORRECT BODY POSTURE

To break bad postural habits, you should be constantly aware of the way in which you stand, sit, move, and even sleep. The pictures on this page show how to carry out everyday activities comfortably, with minimal strain on your spine and back muscles.

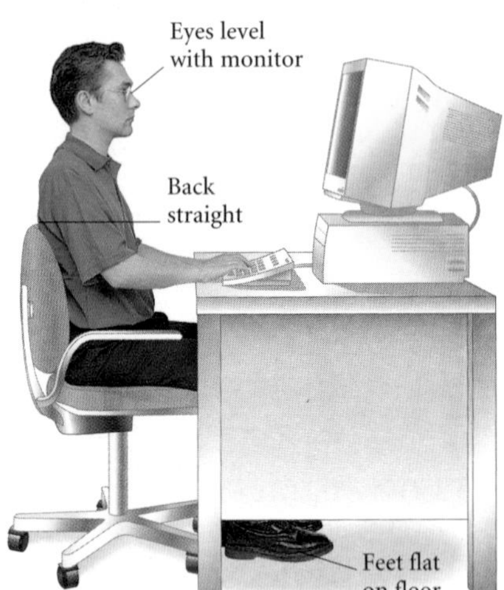

Sitting position
Sit with your back straight and both feet flat on the floor. Use a chair that supports the small of your back. When using a computer, position the monitor so that you can look straight at it.

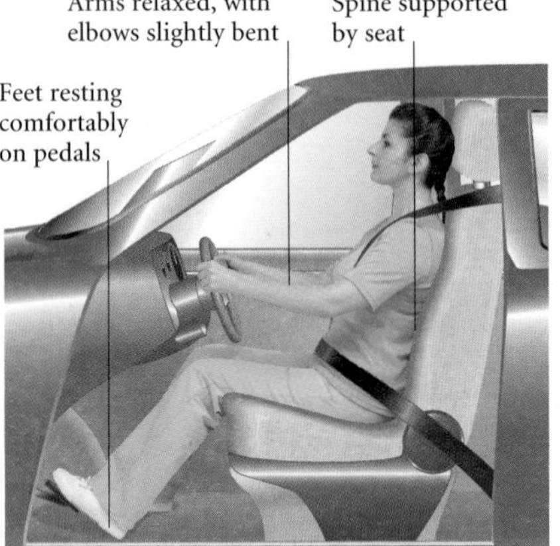

Driving position
Angle your seat backwards a little to support your spine, and position the seat so that you can reach the hand and foot controls easily.

Shoulders pulled back
Trunk held straight
Abdominal muscles tightened
Pelvis tilted slightly to align body

Standing position
Put your weight evenly on both feet. Hold your head up and shoulders back, allowing your spine to curve naturally. Balance your body over its centre of gravity, which is in the pelvis and lower spine.

LIFTING AN OBJECT

When lifting, pushing, or pulling a heavy object, keep the object close to you so that you can use your full strength to move it. To lift an object, hold the bottom edge so that you support the full weight of the object and keep your body balanced as you lift to avoid straining your spine.

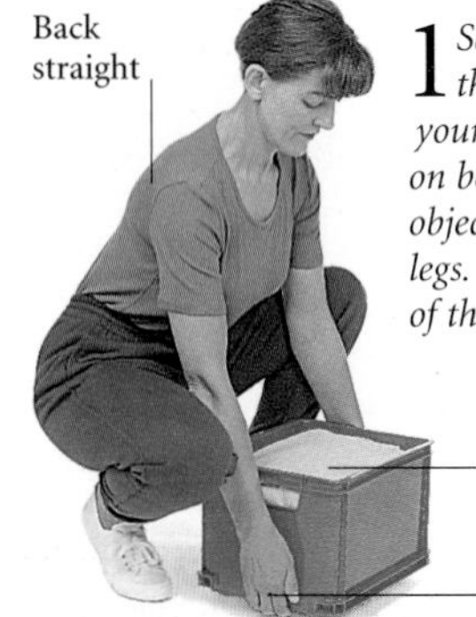

1 *Squat close to the object with your weight evenly on both feet and the object between your legs. Grasp the base of the object.*

2 *Keep your back straight and lean forwards slightly. Stand up in a single, smooth movement, pushing yourself up with your leg muscles and keeping the object close to you.*

Upper body straight
Weight of object balanced over thighs and feet
Legs pushing body straight upwards

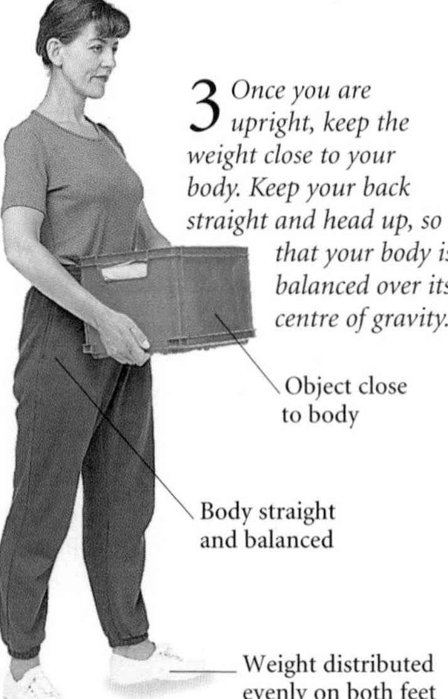

3 *Once you are upright, keep the weight close to your body. Keep your back straight and head up, so that your body is balanced over its centre of gravity.*

BACK-STRENGTHENING EXERCISES

You can help to prevent back pain by gently exercising the muscles in your back and abdomen. See a doctor or ask for a referral to a physiotherapist before starting a programme of exercise. You should not continue to do any exercise that causes you pain.

The movements shown below should make your back muscles stronger and your spine more flexible. Repeat each one 10 times if you can, and try to exercise daily. Do the exercises on a comfortable but firm, flat surface, such as a mat laid on the floor.

Lower back stretch

This stretch may relieve aching joints and muscles in the lower back. Lie on your back with your feet flat on the floor and with your knees bent. Lift your knees towards your body. With your hands, pull your knees into your chest. Hold for 7 seconds and breathe deeply. Keeping your knees bent, lower your feet to the floor one at a time.

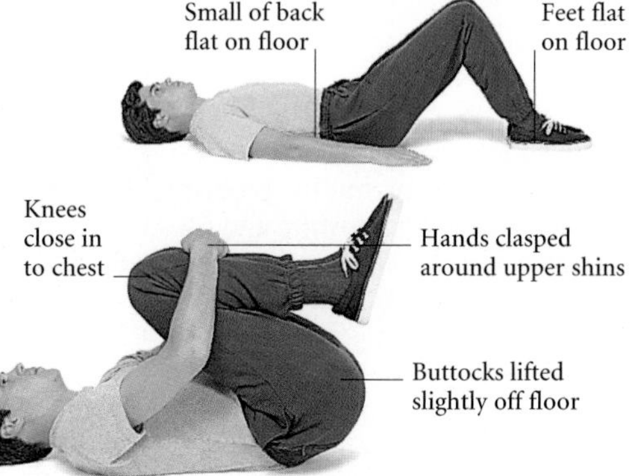

Pelvic tilt

This movement helps to stretch the muscles and ligaments of the lower back. Lie on your back with your knees bent and your feet flat on the floor. Press the small of your back into the floor. Tighten your abdominal and buttock muscles so that your pelvis tilts upwards and your buttocks rise slightly off the floor. Hold for 6 seconds and then relax.

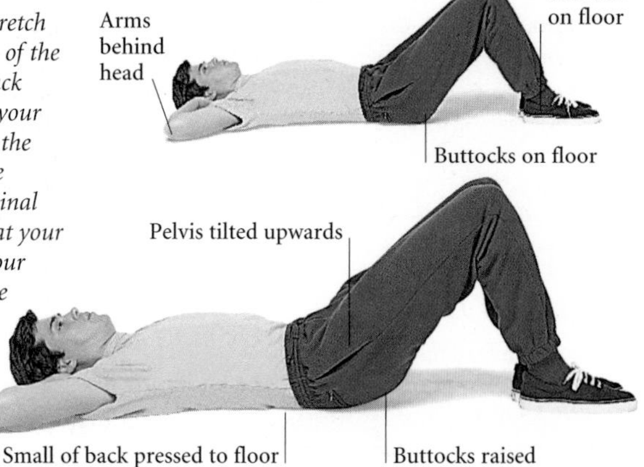

Hump and sag

The movements in this exercise should increase suppleness in the joints and muscles of the back. Support yourself on your hands and knees with your knees slightly apart. Tuck your chin into your chest, then gently arch your back. Hold for about 5 seconds. Look up, allowing your back to sag, and hold again for about another 5 seconds.

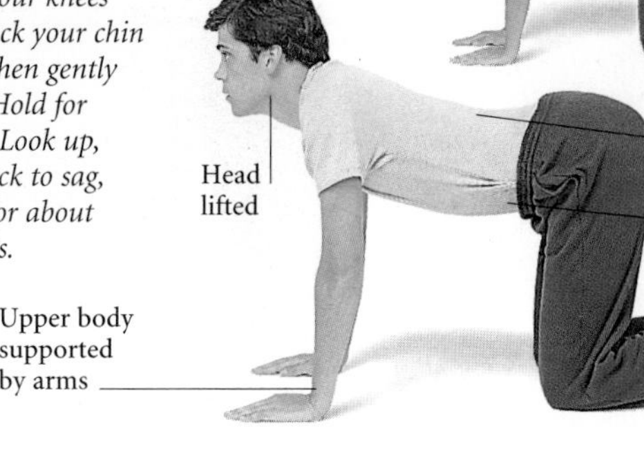

WHAT ARE THE CAUSES?

Lower back pain may come on suddenly (acute) or develop gradually over a period of weeks (chronic).

Acute back pain is often caused by a physical injury due to lifting heavy objects or to activities such as digging in the garden. The pain is commonly caused by a strained muscle or tendon. The injury may be aggravated by subsequent activity. In most cases, symptoms subside within 2–14 days.

Back pain that is more persistent may be improved by changing your posture, for example while sitting at a desk or driving a car. Pain may be aggravated by emotional stress and excessive muscle tension. Lower back pain may also occur during pregnancy, due both to changes in posture because of the extra weight of the baby and to softening of ligaments supporting the spine caused by hormonal changes.

Another cause of lower back pain is a prolapsed or herniated disc exerting pressure on a spinal nerve or the spinal cord. Back pain of this type may have a gradual or sudden onset and is accompanied by sciatica (p.546), in which severe shooting pain extends down the back of one or both legs.

Persistent lower back pain may be caused by joint disorders. In people over the age of 45, the most common joint problem is osteoarthritis (p.374), while in younger people the problem may be ankylosing spondylitis (p.378), which affects the joints of the spine. Less often, back pain results from bone disorders, such as Paget's disease of the bone (p.370), or cancer that has spread to bone from a tumour elsewhere in the body (*see* BONE METASTASES, p.373).

In some cases, disorders affecting internal organs can lead to pain in the lower back. Examples include certain disorders of the female reproductive system, such as pelvic inflammatory disease (p.741), and of the urinary system, such as prostatitis (p.724).

WHAT ARE THE SYMPTOMS?

Pain in the lower back can take various forms. You may experience:

- Sharp pain localized to a small area of the back.
- More general, aching pain in the back and buttocks, which is made worse by sitting and relieved by standing.

- Back stiffness and pain on bending.
- Pain in the back that radiates to the buttock and leg, sometimes accompanied by numbness or tingling.

Back pain that is associated with weight loss or difficulty in controlling your bowel or bladder may be due to a serious underlying disorder. You should consult your doctor immediately if you develop these symptoms.

WHAT CAN I DO?

In most cases, you should be able to treat lower back pain yourself by taking an over-the-counter painkiller (p.912). If the pain persists, additional relief may be provided by a heat pad or wrapped hot-water bottle and sometimes by ice placed against your back.

If the pain is severe, you may be more comfortable resting in bed, but you should not stay in bed for more than 2 days. Start moving around as soon as possible and gradually return to normal activities. If the pain worsens or is still too severe to allow you to move around after a few days, you should consult your doctor.

Once the pain has subsided, you can help to prevent recurrence if you pay attention to your posture, learn to lift correctly, and do regular exercises to strengthen the muscles of your back and make your spine more flexible (*see* PREVENTING BACK PAIN, p.382).

WHAT MIGHT THE DOCTOR DO?

If you need to consult your doctor because of severe or persistent lower back pain, he or she will probably carry out a full physical examination to assess your posture, the range of movement in your spine, and any areas of local tenderness. Your reflexes, the strength of different leg muscles, and the sensation in your legs may also be tested to look for evidence of pressure on spinal nerves or the spinal cord. A pelvic or rectal examination may be necessary if you have symptoms that are associated with the female reproductive organs or with the bowels.

You may have various blood tests and X-rays (p.244) to look for underlying causes of the pain, such as joint inflammation or bone cancer. If there is evidence of pressure on the spinal cord or spinal nerves, MRI (p.248) or CT scanning (p.247) may be carried out to detect abnormalities that require additional treatment, such as a prolapsed or herniated disc.

Unless there is a serious underlying cause for your back pain, your doctor will probably advise you to continue taking a painkilling drug. You may be given physiotherapy (p.961) to mobilize stiff and painful joints between the vertebrae. In some cases, an injection combining a local anaesthetic (p.914) with a corticosteroid (*see* LOCALLY ACTING CORTICOSTEROIDS, p.895) is given directly into areas of tenderness.

WHAT IS THE PROGNOSIS?

Most episodes of lower back pain clear up without treatment, but the problem may recur. Improving posture and lifting techniques reduces the risk.

In a small number of people, lower back pain may be a long-standing condition, severely disrupting their work and social life and sometimes leading to depression (p.554). Effective pain control is essential in these cases, and maintaining physical activity, despite some pain, reduces disability. People who become depressed because of their condition will benefit from treatment with antidepressants (p.916).

(WWW) ONLINE SITES: p.1035

Prolapsed or herniated disc

Protrusion of one of the shock-absorbing pads that lie between the vertebrae of the spine, also known as a "slipped disc"

AGE Most common between the ages of 25 and 45

GENDER Slightly more common in males

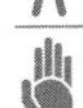
LIFESTYLE Being overweight and lifting objects incorrectly are risk factors

GENETICS Not a significant factor

The shock-absorbing discs between the vertebrae (bones of the spine) consist of a strong, fibrous outer coat and a soft, gelatinous core. A prolapsed disc occurs when the core pushes outwards, distorting the shape of the disc. If the outer coat ruptures, the condition is termed a herniated disc. When a disc prolapses or herniates, the surrounding tissues become inflamed and swollen. Then, together with the disc, the tissues may press on a spinal nerve or the spinal cord, causing pain.

Although discs in the lower back are most often affected, herniation of the discs in the neck and, rarely, the upper back can occur. People between the ages of 25 and 45 are most vulnerable to disc prolapse or herniation. The disorder is slightly more common in men.

WHAT ARE THE CAUSES?

With age, the discs begin to dry out. They also become more vulnerable to prolapse or herniation as a result of the normal stresses of daily life and minor injuries. Sometimes, a disc is damaged by bending forwards or a sharp twisting movement, or by lifting a heavy object incorrectly.

WHAT ARE THE SYMPTOMS?

Symptoms of a prolapsed or herniated disc may develop gradually over a period of weeks or may appear suddenly. They may include:

- Dull pain in the affected area.
- Muscle spasm and stiffness around the affected area that makes movement difficult.

If the disc presses on a spinal nerve, you may also have the following symptoms:

- Severe pain, tingling, or numbness in a leg (*see* SCIATICA, p.546) or, if the neck is affected, in an arm.
- Weakness or restricted movement in the leg or arm.

The pain is frequently relieved by rest but may be made worse by sitting, coughing, sneezing, bending, or bowel

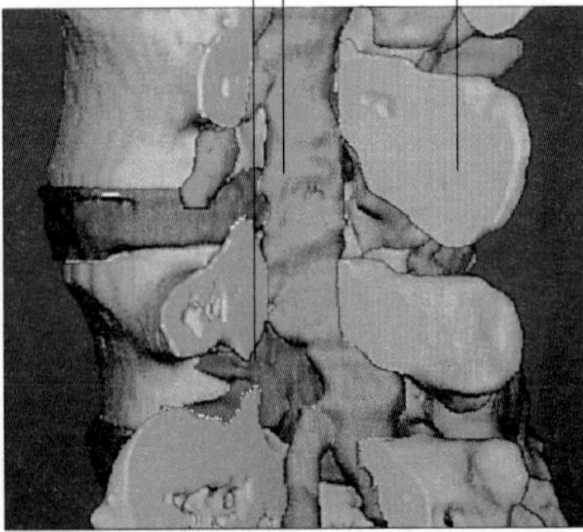

Herniated disc
This 3D CT scan shows a herniated disc in the spine. The soft core of the disc is protruding through the fibrous outer coat and pressing against the spinal cord.

TREATMENT MICRODISCECTOMY

Microdiscectomy is a surgical procedure used to treat a prolapsed or herniated disc pressing on a spinal nerve or the spinal cord. The protruding part of the disc is removed through an incision in the fibrous outer coat of the disc. The operation is performed under general anaesthesia and requires a brief stay in hospital.

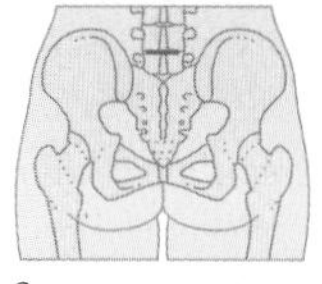

SITE OF INCISION

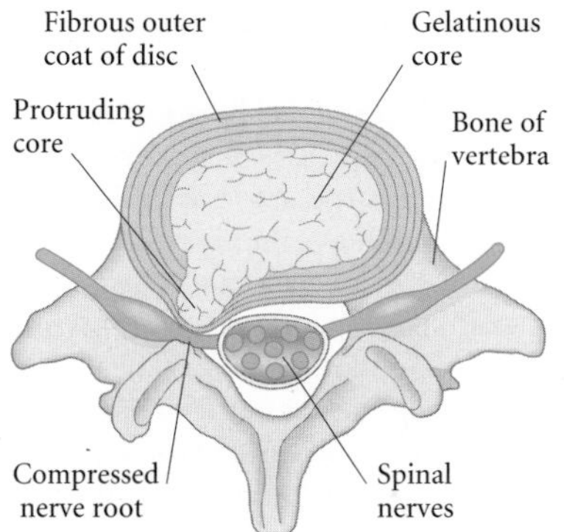

Before the operation
The soft core of the disc is pushed outwards, distorting (and sometimes rupturing) the outer coat. The protruding tissue presses on the spinal cord.

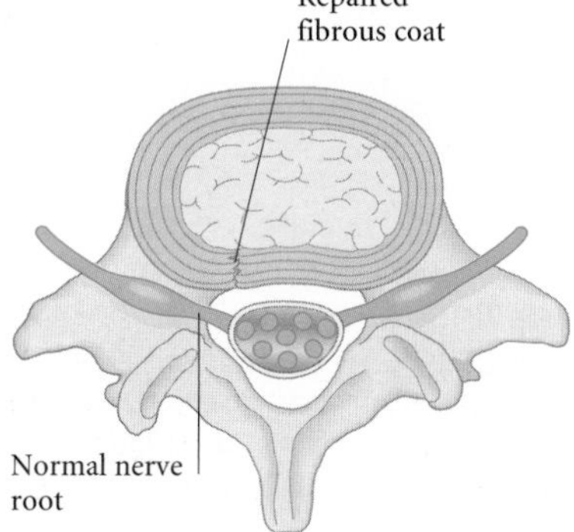

After the operation
The protruding tissue has been removed, and the incision in the outer coat of the disc has been closed up. The spinal cord is no longer compressed.

movements. Impaired bladder or bowel function may indicate pressure on the spinal cord, and you should consult a doctor urgently in such cases.

WHAT MIGHT BE DONE?

Diagnosis is usually made from your symptoms and a physical examination. Your doctor may also arrange for you to have an X-ray (p.244), to rule out other causes of back pain, and MRI (p.248) or CT scanning (p.247), which can locate the position of the prolapsed or herniated disc accurately.

Although the disc is permanently damaged, the pain usually improves over 6–8 weeks as the swelling subsides. Your doctor will probably suggest ways in which you can modify physical activities to avoid further stress on your back. He or she may also recommend painkillers (p.912) and refer you for physiotherapy (p.961), which can reduce muscle spasms and speed recovery.

Rarely, pain may be relieved with traction, in which the spine is gently stretched with weights to create more space around a nerve and reduce pressure on it. Some people benefit from an epidural injection (p.801) or a selective nerve root block, in which a local anaesthetic (p.914), sometimes used in combination with a corticosteroid drug (*see* LOCALLY ACTING CORTICOSTEROIDS, p.895), is injected around the compressed nerve to decrease swelling. If the damaged disc is in the neck, a supportive collar may be helpful.

In a few cases, if bladder or bowel function is impaired due to pressure on a nerve or the spinal cord or if there is severe pain or muscle weakness, urgent surgery on the disc may be required (*see* MICRODISCECTOMY, above).

(WWW) ONLINE SITES: p.1035

Spondylolisthesis

A disorder in which a vertebra (bone of the spine) slips forwards over one beneath it

AGE GENDER GENETICS LIFESTYLE Risk factors depend on the cause

In spondylolisthesis, a vertebra (bone of the spine) slides forwards to project over the vertebra below, distorting the spinal canal. Spondylolisthesis usually affects the vertebrae in the lower part of the back. The disorder may be caused by a deformity of the spine present from birth or a stress fracture due to overstretching, especially in people who take part in sports, such as cricketers and rowers. In elderly people, particularly women, spondylolisthesis may be the result of a joint disorder such as osteoarthritis (p.374). In rare cases, the condition is caused by a severe injury.

Many people with spondylolisthesis have no symptoms. However, sometimes pain and stiffness may be felt in the affected area of the spine. Pressure on the spinal roots of the sciatic nerve may lead to sciatica (p.546), a condition in which pain is felt in the lower back and travels down the leg.

A diagnosis of spondylolisthesis will need to be confirmed by X-rays (p.244). Procedures such as MRI (p.248) or CT scanning (p.247) may also be needed to exclude other possible causes of back pain such as a prolapsed or herniated disc (opposite page). Treatment may include wearing a support, such as a brace, and a course of physiotherapy (p.961), which helps to strengthen the muscles supporting the affected vertebrae (*see* PREVENTING BACK PAIN, p.382). Rarely, surgery may be needed to fuse the affected vertebrae together.

Normal activity can often be resumed about 6 months after treatment.

(WWW) ONLINE SITES: p.1035

Frozen shoulder

Pain and restriction of movement in the shoulder joint

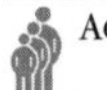

AGE More common over the age of 40

GENDER More common in females

GENETICS LIFESTYLE Not significant factors

Pain and stiffness in a shoulder joint, severely restricting its movement, is known as frozen shoulder. The condition may be due to inflammation resulting from an injury to the shoulder region. Frozen shoulder can also sometimes occur if the shoulder is kept immobilized for a long period of time, such as following a stroke (p.532). However, in many cases, frozen shoulder develops for no apparent reason. The condition occurs most frequently in people over the age of 40 and is more common in women. People who have diabetes mellitus (p.687) are more susceptible to the condition.

WHAT ARE THE SYMPTOMS?

The symptoms of frozen shoulder often begin gradually over a period of weeks or months. They may include:

- Pain in the shoulder, which is severe in the early stages of the condition and is often worse at night.
- With time, gradually decreasing pain but increasing stiffness and restricted joint movement.
- In severe cases, pain travelling down the arm to the elbow.

If you have pain in the shoulder that lasts for more than a few days, you should consult your doctor.

WHAT MIGHT BE DONE?

Your doctor will probably diagnose frozen shoulder from the symptoms and an examination of your shoulder. A painkiller (p.912) or a nonsteroidal anti-inflammatory drug (p.894) may be prescribed to relieve the discomfort and reduce inflammation.

If the pain persists or is severe, you may be given a corticosteroid drug by means of a direct injection into the shoulder joint (*see* LOCALLY ACTING CORTICOSTEROIDS, p.895). You may also be referred for physiotherapy (p.961). Despite these measures, your shoulder may remain stiff for up to 2 years.

Even when the stiffness has disappeared, recovery is usually slow and may take up to a further 6 months.

(WWW) ONLINE SITES: p.1035

Chondromalacia

Pain in the front of the knee due to an abnormality of the cartilage at the back of the kneecap

AGE Most common in teenagers and young adults

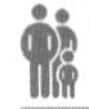
GENETICS Sometimes runs in families

LIFESTYLE Strenuous exercise can trigger symptoms

GENDER Not a significant factor

Chondromalacia, also referred to as patellofemoral pain syndrome, occurs when the cartilage surface of the back of the patella (kneecap) is damaged. The underlying cause of the condition is not known, but it can be triggered by strenuous exercise or repeated knee injuries. In teenagers, chondromalacia may be caused by increased weight-bearing on the knee joint during a growth spurt. The condition may also be associated with a misaligned or a recurrently dislocated patella or with muscle weakness in the upper leg.

WHAT ARE THE SYMPTOMS?

Symptoms vary in severity from person to person but may include:

- Pain in the knee when the leg is bent and straightened (such as when going up or down stairs).
- Stiffness after prolonged sitting.
- Crepitus (a crackling noise) during knee movement.

Chondromalacia usually occurs in only one knee, although the condition does sometimes develop in both knees.

WHAT MIGHT BE DONE?

Your doctor will examine your knee and press down on the patella to see if your symptoms worsen. He or she may arrange for X-rays (p.244) of the knee and back of the patella. In severe cases, arthroscopy (below) may be performed to examine the interior of the knee joint and remove damaged cartilage.

Your doctor may advise you to take a painkiller (p.912) or a nonsteroidal anti-inflammatory drug (p.894) and to apply ice packs for pain relief. He or she may also advise exercise to strengthen thigh and knee muscles and reduce stress on the knee joint. You may be advised to wear a knee support as a temporary measure. In rare cases, surgery is necessary to realign the patella.

WHAT IS THE PROGNOSIS?

Chondromalacia often improves over time and most people are not disabled, although they may have mild recurrences of pain in the knee. Regular exercise to strengthen the muscles of the thigh and the ligaments around the knee will reduce the risk of developing osteoarthritis (p.374) in later life.

(WWW) ONLINE SITES: p.1028, p.1035

(TEST AND TREATMENT) ARTHROSCOPY

In arthroscopy, the inside of a joint is inspected with a viewing instrument called an arthroscope. The procedure is most commonly used to inspect the inside of the knee joint and to treat disorders such as a damaged cartilage. It may be performed under general or local anaesthesia. The arthroscope is inserted into the joint through a small incision in the skin. Surgical instruments can then be passed down through the arthroscope or through other incisions. During the examination, the surgeon can remove or repair tissue, such as damaged cartilage, or shave the surface of the patella (kneecap).

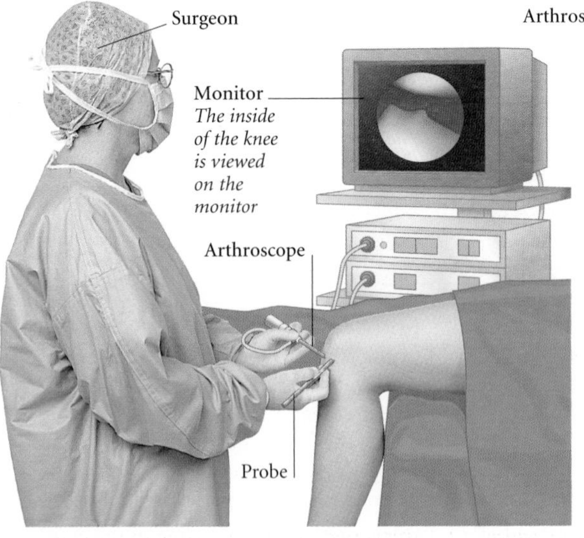

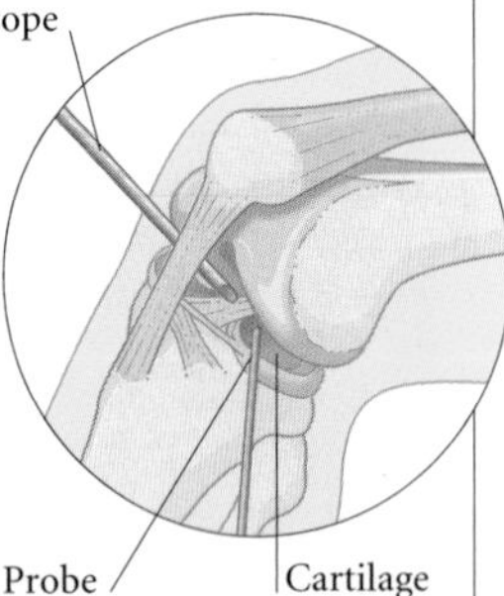

INSIDE THE KNEE

Surgical procedure
An arthroscope and a probe are inserted into the joint. The probe can be used to manipulate the cartilage and improve the view.

Bursitis

Inflammation of a bursa, one of the fluid-filled sacs located around joints

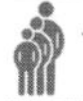
AGE More common in adults

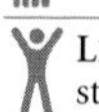
LIFESTYLE Occupations involving repeated stress on a joint are risk factors

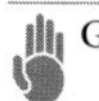
GENDER GENETICS Not significant factors

Bursae act as friction-reducing cushions around joints. Inflammation of a bursa, called bursitis, may occur if it is put under prolonged or repeated stress. The bursa becomes tender and swollen, and movement of the joint is restricted.

The knee is most commonly affected, especially as a result of frequent kneeling, but the elbow or other joints may also be affected. Bursitis may also follow injury or unaccustomed exercise. Certain joint diseases, such as rheumatoid arthritis (p.377) and gout (p.380), increase the risk of bursitis. Rarely, the condition is due to a bacterial infection.

Your doctor will probably diagnose bursitis from a physical examination. Treatment includes resting the affected joint. Your doctor may also recommend a nonsteroidal anti-inflammatory drug (p.894) and application of ice packs. However, if symptoms persist, he or she may drain the bursa and inject it with a corticosteroid drug (*see* LOCALLY ACTING CORTICOSTEROIDS, p.895) to reduce inflammation. If a bacterial infection is present, antibiotics (p.885) will be prescribed, in which case the symptoms usually subside within a few days. If bursitis is persistent or recurrent, surgical removal of the bursa may be necessary.

(WWW) ONLINE SITES: p.1035

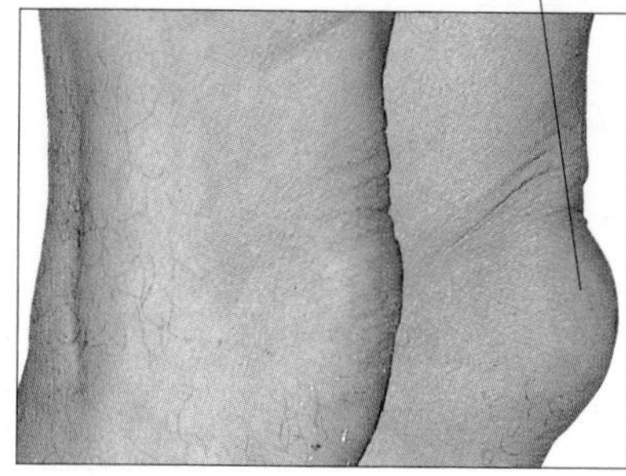

Bursitis in the knee
The knee seen on the right is swollen due to a fluid-filled, inflamed bursa, which can be caused by prolonged kneeling.

(TREATMENT) BUNION SURGERY

Surgery to treat a bunion is aimed at correcting the underlying bone deformity, known as hallux valgus. One common type of surgical procedure used to treat a bunion involves reshaping and realigning the deformed bone at the base of the big toe. The operation is performed under general anaesthesia and may require a brief stay in hospital. Normal activity can usually be resumed about 6 weeks after surgery.

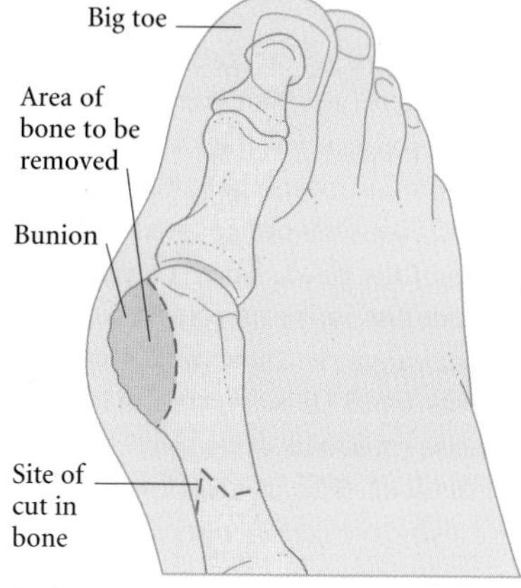

Before surgery
The big toe is turned towards the other toes. The bone has become obviously deformed, and the soft tissue around it has thickened, forming a painful bunion.

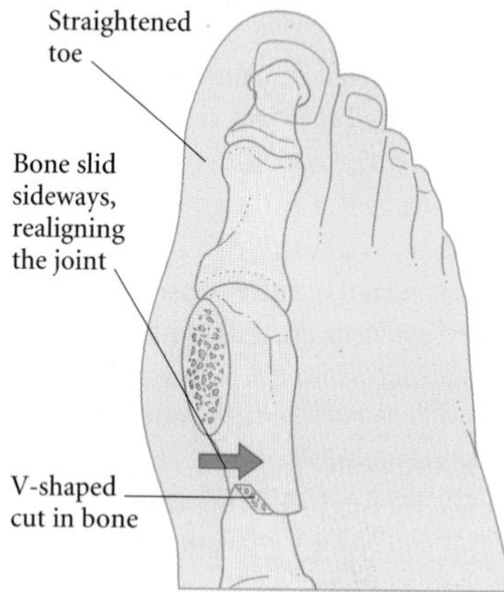

After surgery
The protruding part of the bone has been removed and a V-shaped cut made in the lower part of the bone. The big toe is straight due to realignment of the bone.

Bunion

Inflamed, thickened soft tissue and bony overgrowth at the base of the big toe

AGE Most common in young adults and older people

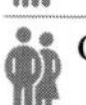
GENDER More common in females

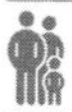
GENETICS Sometimes runs in families

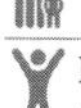
LIFESTYLE Wearing tight, pointed shoes, especially with high heels, is a risk factor

A bunion is a thickened lump at the base of the big toe. It often becomes inflamed and painful, making walking difficult. The underlying cause is usually a minor bone deformity, called hallux valgus, in which the joint at the base of the big toe develops an abnormal projection, which forces the tip of the toe to turn towards the other toes. The cause of hallux valgus itself is not known, but the condition runs in some families. As a result of pressure on the deformity, the surrounding tissues thicken. The term bunion refers to the thickened lump that is due to the combination of the bony deformity and thickening of the soft tissue around it. The condition is particularly common in young women who wear tight, pointed shoes with high heels.

In rare cases, the constant rubbing of tight shoes on the skin over a bunion may cause an abrasion, which then leads to a bacterial infection. People with diabetes mellitus (p.687) are particularly susceptible to infected bunions because the sensation in their feet may be reduced (*see* DIABETIC NEUROPATHY, p.545). In such people, damage to the skin tends to heal more slowly.

Without attention, a bunion may gradually worsen. Pain may be alleviated by wearing comfortable shoes and a special toe pad or corrective sock that straightens the big toe. However, if a bunion causes severe discomfort, your doctor may suggest that you have surgery to correct the underlying deformity by realigning the bone (*see* BUNION SURGERY, above). If the bunion becomes infected, your doctor will prescribe antibiotics (p.885). A bunion increases the chance of developing osteoarthritis (p.374) of the toe joint in later life.

(WWW) ONLINE SITES: p.1035

MUSCLE AND TENDON DISORDERS

Skeletal muscles contract and relax to move the body and are connected to bones by fibrous tissue known as tendons. Both muscles and tendons can be temporarily or permanently damaged by injury, overexertion, infection, or other disorders, causing pain, weakness, restricted movement, and tiredness.

Skeletal muscles account for half the weight of the body but are only rarely affected by disease. Injury to a muscle or tendon, either through strenuous exercise or as a result of a repetitive physical activity, is the cause of some of the disorders described in this section, including muscle cramps, torticollis, repetitive strain injury, and tennis and golfer's elbow. The next articles discuss inflammation of a tendon (tendinitis) or tendon sheath (tenosynovitis) and ganglia, which are fluid-filled cysts that commonly arise on the wrist or the back of the hand.

Some disorders that affect the skeletal muscles are covered in other parts of the book. These conditions include the immune system disorders polymyalgia rheumatica (p.464) and polymyositis (p.463) and the inherited disease muscular dystrophy (p.826). Musculoskeletal injuries (pp.391–395) are also covered elsewhere.

KEY ANATOMY

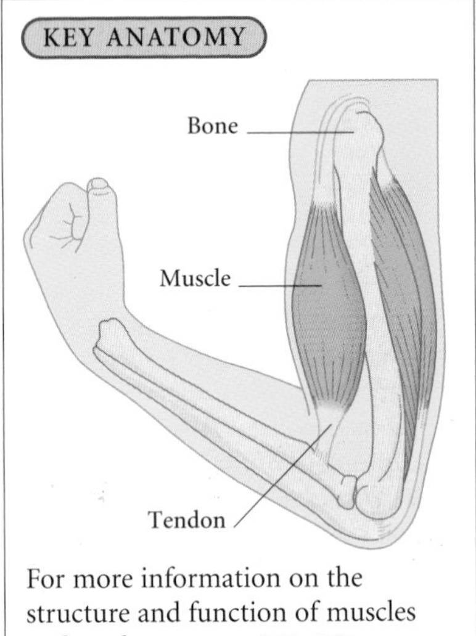

For more information on the structure and function of muscles and tendons, *see* pp.362–367.

Muscle cramps

Sudden painful spasms in a muscle or group of muscles

AGE GENDER GENETICS LIFESTYLE
Not significant factors

Muscle cramps affect almost everyone from time to time. Painful spasms, often lasting only a few minutes, make the affected muscle become hard and tender. Muscle cramps may occur in any muscle in the body but they are most common in leg muscles. When abdominal muscles are affected, the condition is also known as a "stitch".

Muscle cramps often develop during physical exercise, possibly as a result of reduction in the oxygen supply to the muscles or a build-up of chemical waste produced by muscles during exercise. Another possible cause is the loss of salt and water that occurs due to heavy sweating during hot weather or strenuous exercise. Muscle cramps may also develop if you have been sitting or lying in an awkward position for a long time. Sometimes, there is no obvious cause.

Cramps are not the only cause of attacks of muscle pain. If you develop recurrent muscle pain in your calves when walking, you should consult your doctor; the cause may be lower limb ischaemia (p.434), a disorder in which the arteries that supply blood to the leg muscles become narrowed.

The immediate self-help treatment for muscle cramps is to stretch and rub the affected area and to apply a heat pad. You should drink plenty of fluids and eat something salty. If you regularly have cramps at night, your doctor may prescribe a low dose of quinine, an antimalarial drug (p.888) that effectively relieves the symptoms.

(WWW) ONLINE SITES: p.1026

Torticollis

Muscle spasm in the neck causing twisting of the head; also known as wry neck

AGE GENDER GENETICS LIFESTYLE
Not significant factors

In torticollis, the muscles on one side of the neck contract and cause the head to be pulled over to one side. The condition is typically accompanied by pain and stiffness in the neck.

Torticollis may develop in babies after a difficult birth involving neck muscle damage. In children, the disorder may be a result of swollen glands in the neck caused by an infection. Torticollis in adults is often caused by physical injury to muscles or by sleeping in an awkward position. The disorder can also be a side effect of certain drugs, such as some tranquillizers (*see* ANTIPSYCHOTIC DRUGS, p.917). An uncommon cause of the condition is cervical spondylosis (p.376), a form of arthritis that affects the bones of the neck.

Your doctor may make the diagnosis from a physical examination. Torticollis in babies will gradually get better with physiotherapy (p.961). In adults and older children, painkillers (p.912), local heat, massage, and use of a neck collar may help to relieve the muscle spasm. Recovery usually takes only a few days but if torticollis persists, a local injection of botulinum toxin (*see* MUSCLE RELAXANTS, p.896) may be given. If the disorder is caused by a particular drug, it will improve once the drug is stopped.

(WWW) ONLINE SITES: p.1035, p.1036

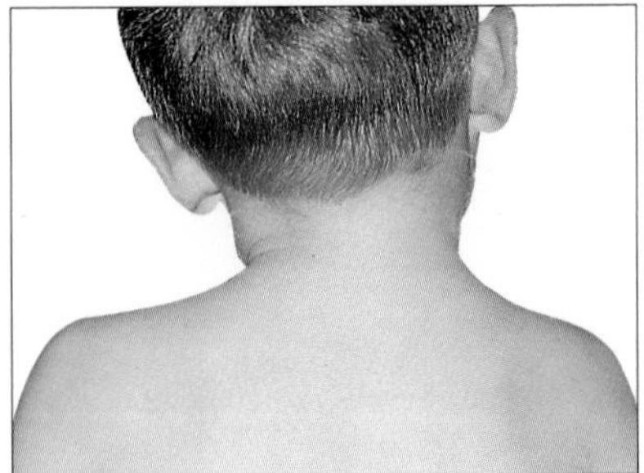

Torticollis
Muscle contraction on one side of the neck has caused this child's head to tip to the side. This condition is called torticollis.

Fibromyalgia

Pain, stiffness, and tiredness associated with muscle tenderness

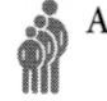
AGE Occurs mainly in adults

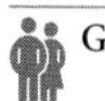
GENDER More common in females

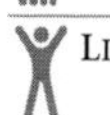
LIFESTYLE Stress may be a risk factor

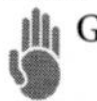
GENETICS Not a significant factor

Fibromyalgia is a disorder that causes widespread muscle pain and tenderness. The condition has no particular cause, and no visible abnormality has ever been identified in the muscle tissue. However, fibromyalgia commonly develops during periods of stress.

WHAT ARE THE SYMPTOMS?

The symptoms of fibromyalgia develop slowly over weeks and occur in a distinct pattern around the body. They may include the following:

- Muscle pain in the upper back, head, thighs, abdomen, and hips.
- Particularly tender areas of muscle, typically at the base of the skull and near the shoulder blades.

Fibromyalgia is commonly associated with headaches, tiredness, depression (p.554), anxiety disorders (p.551), and disturbed sleep patterns. Some people have irregular bowel movements (*see* IRRITABLE BOWEL SYNDROME, p.656). All of these symptoms usually become worse when levels of stress increase.

WHAT MIGHT BE DONE?

The diagnosis of fibromyalgia is often based on the symptoms and a physical examination, but your doctor may arrange for blood tests to rule out other disorders, such as rheumatoid arthritis (p.377). Although there is no specific treatment, the pain may be relieved by deep tissue massage and locally applied moist heat, ultrasound treatment, or an injection with a local anaesthetic. Your doctor may also prescribe a low dosage of amitriptyline (*see* ANTIDEPRESSANT DRUGS, p.916) to relieve pain. Regular exercise is also important. Many people make a full recovery or learn to manage their symptoms and maintain a normal lifestyle, but some may be disabled.

(WWW) ONLINE SITES: p.1035

Repetitive strain injury

Symptoms associated with repetitive physical activity

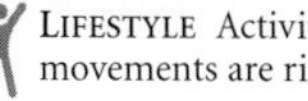
LIFESTYLE Activities that involve repeated movements are risk factors

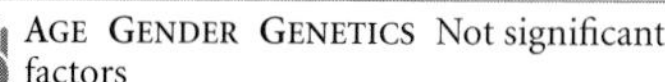
AGE GENDER GENETICS Not significant factors

Prolonged, repeated movements of one part of the body, particularly if the movements are rapid and forceful, can cause symptoms described as repetitive strain injury (RSI). Overuse injury and cumulative trauma disorder are other names for the same condition. RSI most commonly affects the muscles and tendons in the arms. The condition may be associated with stress in the workplace or the home.

People who often carry out repeated movements as part of their everyday work, such as those using a keyboard or working on a production line, are particularly at risk of RSI. Musicians and athletes are also susceptible. Other disorders that cause pain in the muscles and tendons, such as tendinitis and tenosynovitis (p.390) or carpal tunnel syndrome (p.547), can cause symptoms similar to those of RSI.

WHAT ARE THE SYMPTOMS?

The symptoms of RSI develop gradually and at first may occur only while performing the repetitive activity. The symptoms may include:

- Pain, aching, and tingling.
- Restricted movement in the affected part of the body.

In the early stages of RSI, the symptoms may disappear when the affected area is rested. Later, you may have symptoms at rest. If you develop RSI, you should consult your doctor without delay since the condition is more difficult to treat once it has become long-standing.

WHAT MIGHT THE DOCTOR DO?

Your doctor will ask about your lifestyle and any repetitive physical activities. Diagnosis is usually made after a physical examination. However, you may also have X-rays (p.244) and blood tests to rule out disorders such as rheumatoid arthritis (p.377). Your doctor may also recommend a painkiller (p.912) or nonsteroidal anti-inflammatory drug (p.894) to relieve discomfort.

WHAT CAN I DO?

If you believe the symptoms are related to your occupation, you should inform your employer and seek advice from an occupational doctor or nurse. He or she can give you advice about posture changes and special equipment, such as adjustable seating, that may help you to avoid unnecessary strain (*see* USING A WORK STATION, p.82). You should also make sure you take regular breaks from repetitive tasks. Rarely, a change in work or leisure activities may be advisable.

WHAT IS THE PROGNOSIS?

If RSI is recognized at an early stage and steps are taken to reduce stress at work, you should make a complete recovery. A physiotherapist will probably be able to give you advice on how to use your muscles and build up their strength (*see* PHYSIOTHERAPY, p. 961).

(WWW) ONLINE SITES: p.1036

Tennis elbow and golfer's elbow

Inflammation of a tendon at its attachment to the bone at the elbow

AGE More common over the age of 30

LIFESTYLE Common among recreational tennis players and golfers and among people carrying out repetitive activities

GENDER GENETICS Not significant factors

Tennis elbow and golfer's elbow both occur when the tendon attachment of the muscle to the bone at the elbow becomes damaged. In tennis elbow, the tendon on the outer side of the elbow is injured; in golfer's elbow, the tendon on the inner side of the elbow is affected.

Both conditions are caused by vigorous and repeated use of the forearm against resistance, which can occur when playing certain sports, such as tennis, or using a screwdriver. The tendon is repeatedly pulled at the point at which it is attached to the bone, which may cause small tears to develop. The resulting damage leads to tenderness and pain in the affected arm.

You should rest the affected painful arm as much as possible. Physiotherapy (p.961), ice packs, simple exercises to stretch and strengthen the muscles, and ultrasound treatment may help to relieve symptoms. You may also find that a nonsteroidal anti-inflammatory drug (p.894) helps. If the condition does not improve within 2–6 weeks, your doctor may inject a corticosteroid drug into the affected area (*see* LOCALLY ACTING CORTICOSTEROIDS, p.895). Once the symptoms have subsided, you should seek advice on ways to change your technique before resuming the sport or activity that gave rise to the condition.

(WWW) ONLINE SITES: p.1031, p.1035, p1036

Tendinitis and tenosynovitis

Painful inflammation of a tendon (tendinitis) or of a tendon sheath (tenosynovitis)

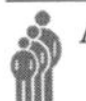 AGE More common in adults

 LIFESTYLE More common in athletes

 GENDER GENETICS Not significant factors

Tendinitis is inflammation of a tendon, the fibrous cord that attaches a muscle to a bone. Tenosynovitis is inflammation of the sheath of tissues that surrounds a tendon. These two conditions usually occur together. Tendons around the shoulder, elbow, wrist, fingers, thigh, knee, or back of the heel are most commonly affected.

Both conditions may be caused by injury of a particular tendon or, rarely, by an infection. Inflammation of the Achilles tendon between the heel and the calf may be the result of a sports injury (p.391) or of wearing ill-fitting shoes. Tenosynovitis may be associated with rheumatoid arthritis (p.377). In some cases, the cause is unknown.

WHAT ARE THE SYMPTOMS?

You may notice the following symptoms in the affected area, particularly during movement:

- Pain and/or mild swelling.
- Stiffness and restricted movement in the affected area.
- Warm, red skin over the tendon.
- A tender lump over the tendon.

Occasionally, you may feel a crackling sensation (known as crepitus) when the affected tendon moves.

WHAT MIGHT BE DONE?

Diagnosis is based on the symptoms and a physical examination. Your doctor will treat any underlying disorder. To reduce the pain and inflammation, he or she may recommend nonsteroidal anti-inflammatory drugs (p.894). You may also require an injection of a corticosteroid drug (*see* LOCALLY ACTING CORTICOSTEROIDS, p.895) into the tendon sheath. If the condition is due to an infection, a course of antibiotics (p.885) will be prescribed. In some cases, a tendon will heal more quickly if it is splinted. Tendinitis and tenosynovitis improve with treatment.

(WWW) ONLINE SITES: p.1031, p.1035

Dupuytren's contracture

Thickening and shortening of tissues in the palm of the hand, resulting in deformity of the fingers

 AGE More common over the age of 50

 GENDER Much more common in males

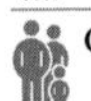 GENETICS Sometimes runs in families

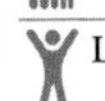 LIFESTYLE Alcohol abuse is a risk factor

In Dupuytren's contracture, the fibrous tissue in the palm of the hand becomes thickened and shortened. As a result, one or more fingers, often the fourth and fifth fingers, are pulled towards the palm into a bent position. Sometimes, painful lumps develop on the palm, and the overlying skin becomes puckered. In about half of all cases, both hands are involved. Rarely, the disorder affects the soles of the feet and the toes.

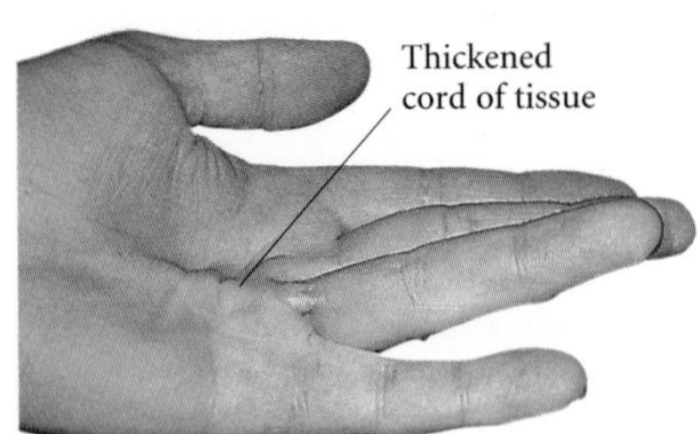

Dupuytren's contracture
The fourth finger of this hand is pulled towards the palm by fibrous tissue that has thickened and shortened. This is known as Dupuytren's contracture.

The tissue changes in Dupuytren's contracture develop slowly over months or years. The cause is unknown, but it occurs more commonly in men over the age of 50, in people with diabetes mellitus (p.687) or epilepsy (p.524), and in people who abuse alcohol. About 1 in 10 people with Dupuytren's contracture has a relative with the disorder.

WHAT MIGHT BE DONE?

In mild cases, no treatment may be needed. If your fingers are slightly bent, you may benefit from stretching exercises or short-term splinting. If you have painful lumps in your palm, a corticosteroid may be injected into the area (*see* LOCALLY ACTING CORTICOSTEROIDS, p.895). In severe cases, it may be necessary to surgically remove the thickened tissue in the palm to allow the fingers to straighten. The disorder can recur, especially in people who have a family history of Dupuytren's contracture and who are affected in both hands.

(WWW) ONLINE SITES: p.1035

Ganglion

A fluid-filled cyst that most commonly develops on the wrist or back of the hand and sometimes the foot

 AGE GENDER GENETICS LIFESTYLE Not significant factors

A ganglion is a cyst that develops under the skin near a joint and is filled with a jelly-like fluid. The ganglion is usually an outgrowth from the capsule surrounding a joint or from the sheath of a tendon, the fibrous cord that attaches muscle to bone. The fluid inside the ganglion is derived from the synovial fluid that lubricates tendons and joints.

Ganglia are extremely common and are usually painless. They most commonly occur on the wrist or the back of the hand but occasionally they develop on the foot. They vary in size from that of a small pea to that of a plum.

A ganglion may be felt as a lump under the skin and may be present for several years without causing a problem. However, some ganglia become very uncomfortable or even painful. A ganglion may disappear spontaneously, or it can be removed surgically under local anaesthesia. Ganglia sometimes recur.

(WWW) ONLINE SITES: p.1035

MUSCULOSKELETAL INJURIES

The bones, joints, muscles, and connective tissues of the body's musculoskeletal system are susceptible to injury from the stresses and strains placed on them during routine and leisure activities. The healing of minor injuries is usually rapid and complete, but major ones require expert treatment to avoid permanent damage.

Today, many people are aware of the health benefits of exercise and use part of their leisure time to pursue athletic activities. However, such pursuits may lead to musculoskeletal injuries if care is not taken. The first article in this section gives an overview of the main types of sports injury, the treatment of which has now become a specialized branch of medicine.

Injury may result in bone fractures of various types and these are covered next. The treatment of fractures has changed a great deal in the past 20 years as a result of various technical innovations, particularly for more complicated fractures in which the damaged bone is fragmented.

Injuries occurring in other parts of the musculoskeletal system, including joints, ligaments, muscles, and tendons, are also discussed. As with fractures, these injuries may cause long-term disability if not treated properly.

Damage to the musculoskeletal system may also occur as part of more widespread damage to the body following serious trauma, such as a motor vehicle accident (*see* SERIOUS INJURIES, pp.316–320).

KEY ANATOMY

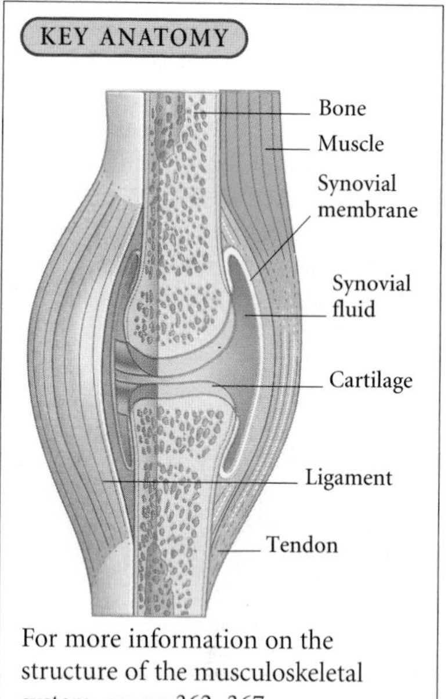

For more information on the structure of the musculoskeletal system, *see* pp.362–367.

Sports injuries

Damage to any part of the body as a result of athletic activity

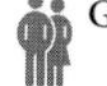 GENDER More common in males

 AGE Older participants may be more likely to be injured and injuries heal more slowly

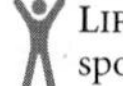 LIFESTYLE Playing sports, especially contact sports, is a risk factor

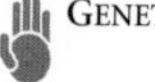 GENETICS Not a significant factor

Athletes and other people who exercise vigorously risk injury. Sports injuries often occur in people who are new to a sport, begin to exercise after prolonged inactivity, or do not warm up properly before exercise. Men are at greater risk because they play more contact sports.

WHAT ARE THE TYPES?

Any part of the musculoskeletal system may be injured while playing sports. In some sports, there is an increased risk of injury to a specific part of the body.

BONE INJURIES Many sports activities can cause damage to the bones, either through repetitive actions or as a result of an impact with another person, the ground, or equipment, such as a bat or a ball. Bones may be broken or cracked (*see* FRACTURES, p.392) during contact sports such as rugby. The repetitive jarring of bones of the lower limbs of runners may cause stress fractures.

JOINT INJURIES The bones that form a joint may partially or completely pull apart (*see* DISLOCATED JOINT, p.394) during sports that put them under great strain, such as javelin throwing. Dislocation is also a risk in all contact sports. A common injury among football players is damage to the cartilage pads in the knee joint (*see* TORN KNEE CARTILAGE, p.395).

LIGAMENT AND TENDON INJURIES The fibrous bands of tissue that hold the structures of the musculoskeletal system together are often injured during sports activities. Ligaments, which hold the bones together, may become damaged by a sudden twisting movement or during a fall (*see* LIGAMENT INJURIES, p.394). Tendons, which attach muscle to bone, may become torn during athletic activities, such as jumping, that involve a sudden muscle contraction (*see* RUPTURED TENDON, p.395).

MUSCLE INJURIES Most sports rely on strength and suppleness of the muscles, and damage to muscles is common in athletes (*see* MUSCLE STRAINS AND TEARS, p.395). For example, calf strain, overstretching of the muscles in the calf region, is a common injury in basketball players. Muscle injury is frequently caused by sudden, strenuous movements and lifting heavy objects.

CAN THEY BE PREVENTED?

Many sports injuries could be prevented by warming up correctly before starting exercise (*see* WARMING UP AND COOLING DOWN IN YOUR EXERCISE ROUTINE, p.60). Adequate preparation can increase flexibility and reduce stiffness in the muscles and joints. In sports such as running, you should start gently, gradually increasing your pace to prevent placing too much strain on your body. Wear clothes and footwear designed for your type of sport and use recommended safety equipment.

WHAT MIGHT BE DONE?

Many minor injuries to ligaments, tendons, and muscles can be treated using basic first-aid procedures (*see* FIRST AID: SPRAINS AND STRAINS, p.991) and nonsteroidal anti-inflammatory drugs (p.894). If a sports injury is causing intense or persistent pain, you should consult a doctor. He or she will examine you and may arrange for you to have an X-ray (p.244) to check whether you have sustained a fracture.

If you have a fracture, it may be necessary to immobilize the injured area by using a cast (*see* FRACTURE TREATMENTS, opposite page). Surgery may be required for some injuries, such as a ruptured tendon. You may also need physiotherapy (p.961) from a sports therapist. You should not participate in any sports until you are free of pain.

(WWW) ONLINE SITES: p.1031, p.1035, p.1036

Fractures

Breaks or cracks in bones anywhere in the body from a variety of causes

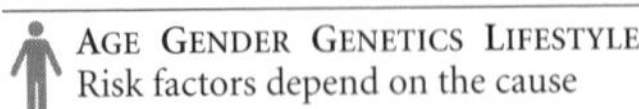

Any bone in the body can be fractured. Most fractures are caused by an injury such as a direct impact or a twisting movement, which may occur during an athletic activity or a fall.

Susceptibility to fractures increases with the bone disorder osteoporosis (p.368), which mainly affects women after the menopause and results in brittle bones. Fractures that occur in bones affected by tumours are called pathological fractures and may occur after minor injury or even spontaneously.

The most common sites of fracture in elderly people are the neck of the femur (thighbone) and the lower end of the radius bone of the forearm near the wrist. A fracture at the end of the radius, known as a Colles' fracture, may occur if a person trips and breaks his or her fall with an outstretched arm.

What are the types?

There are two main types of fracture: closed (simple), in which the broken bone does not break through the overlying skin; and open (compound), in which the bone pierces the skin and is exposed. Open fractures are more serious because of the risk of infection and an increased risk of damage to nerves and blood vessels. Open and closed fractures may be further subdivided according to their shape and pattern.

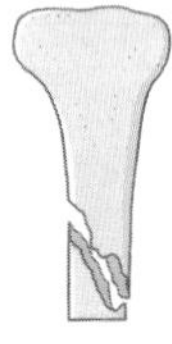

TRANSVERSE FRACTURE In a transverse fracture, there is a straight break across a bone. Transverse fractures, often in a long bone in the arm or leg, are usually due to a powerful blow, such as that sustained in a collision during a traffic accident.

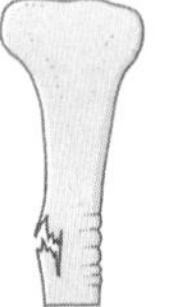

SPIRAL FRACTURE This type of fracture is also known as an oblique fracture. Spiral fractures are usually caused by sudden, violent, rotating movements, such as twisting the leg during a fall. Spiral fractures usually occur in arm and leg bones.

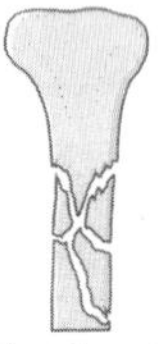

GREENSTICK FRACTURE If a long bone in the arm or leg bends, it may crack on one side only, producing a break called a "greenstick" fracture. This type of fracture occurs only in children, whose bones are still growing and flexible.

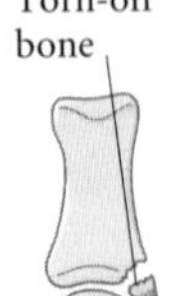

COMMINUTED FRACTURE In a comminuted fracture, the bone is broken into small fragments, which increases the likelihood of damage to soft tissues surrounding the broken bone. These fractures are usually caused by severe, direct forces.

AVULSION FRACTURE In this type of fracture, a piece of bone is pulled away from the main bone by a tendon, a fibrous band that attaches muscle to a bone. It usually results from a sudden violent twisting injury.

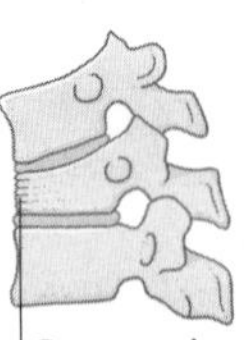

COMPRESSION FRACTURE A compression fracture occurs if spongy bone, like that in the vertebrae of the spine, is crushed. This type of fracture is often due to osteoporosis.

Fractures caused by repeated jarring of a bone are called stress fractures. They may occur in the feet or shinbones of long-distance runners. In the elderly, fractures may result from minor stress such as a cough, which can break a rib.

What are the symptoms?

The symptoms of a fracture depend on its type and may include:

- Pain and tenderness, which may limit movement of the affected area.
- Swelling and bruising.
- Deformity in the affected area.
- Crackling noise (crepitus) caused by grating of the ends of the bones on movement or pressure.
- In an open fracture, damage to skin, bleeding, and visible bone.

All fractures cause a certain amount of internal bleeding because of damage to blood vessels in the bone. The broken bone ends may cause further bleeding by damaging tissues and blood vessels in the injured area. In some fractures, blood loss may be severe and can occasionally lead to shock (p.414).

Various complications may be associated with a fracture. For example, if you fracture a rib, there is a risk that the broken rib may puncture a lung (*see* PNEUMOTHORAX, p.496). An open fracture may become infected.

Delay in treating a fracture properly may result in failure of the bone to heal and permanent deformity or disability. Consult a doctor immediately if you think that you have a fracture.

How is it diagnosed?

Your doctor will arrange for you to have X-rays (p.244) of the affected area to reveal the type and extent of the fracture. CT scanning (p.247) or MRI (p.248) may be needed to investigate complex fractures. If a fracture was not due to injury, your doctor may check for a possible underlying disorder that may have weakened your bones.

What is the treatment?

If the broken ends of the bone have been displaced, they will need to be returned to their original position to restore normal shape. This process is known as reduction. Depending on the location and severity of the fracture, a broken bone may be manipulated back into its correct position under a local or general anaesthetic, either without an incision (closed reduction) or through an incision in the skin (open reduction). The fractured bone may be held in place until it has healed fully by using one of several methods (*see* FRACTURE TREATMENTS, opposite page).

(TREATMENT) FRACTURE TREATMENTS

Although some broken bones do not need immobilization, most have to be returned to their correct position (reduction) and held in place so that the fractured ends are able to heal and join together properly. The method of immobilization chosen for a particular fracture depends on the type, location, and severity of the fracture.

IMMOBILIZATION IN A CAST

The simplest form of immobilization is a cast, a rigid casing that is applied to a limb and left in position for several weeks to hold the fractured bone ends together and prevent movement. Casts are usually made from plaster, plastic, or resin. They are removed using an electric saw, which cuts through the cast.

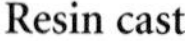

Resin cast
Resin casts are light, waterproof, and durable. The cast is applied as a bandage to fit the affected limb. It then sets and provides support without restricting the blood supply.

INTERNAL FIXATION

Bones that are severely fractured may need metal plates, screws, nails, wires, or rods to be inserted surgically to hold the broken bone ends together. A cast may not be required. Internal fixation is often used for fractures at the ends of bones.

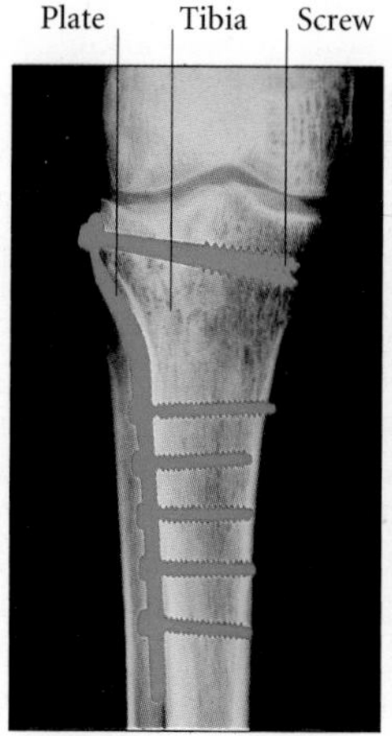

Plate and screws
A fracture in the tibia (shinbone) may be immobilized by a metal plate secured by screws.

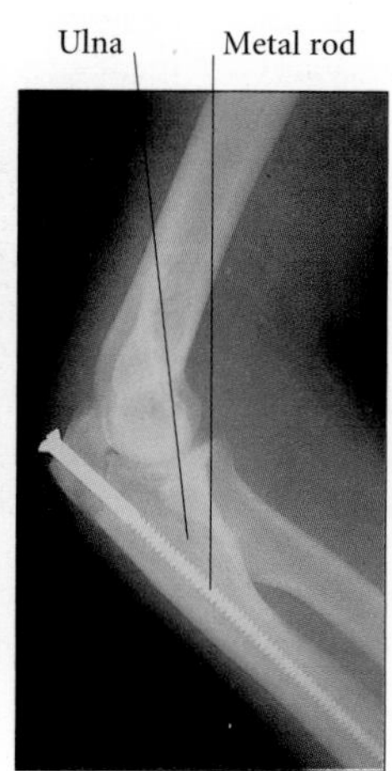

Inserted rod
A fractured ulna (lower arm bone) may be held together by a metal rod inserted into the bone.

EXTERNAL FIXATION

A specialized technique known as external fixation is often required to repair bones that are fractured in several places. In this technique, pins are inserted through the skin into the bone fragments. The pins are held in place by an external metal frame, which allows the affected limb to be used normally within a few days. The frame and pins are removed when the bone has healed.

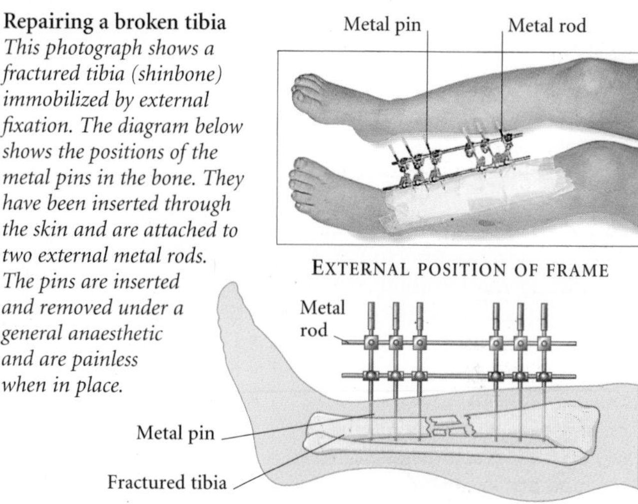

Repairing a broken tibia
This photograph shows a fractured tibia (shinbone) immobilized by external fixation. The diagram below shows the positions of the metal pins in the bone. They have been inserted through the skin and are attached to two external metal rods. The pins are inserted and removed under a general anaesthetic and are painless when in place.

TRACTION

Traction is used for the temporary immobilization of a fracture until further treatment of the injury can be carried out. The technique is often used for fractures in the shaft of the femur (thighbone). Weights are used to maintain alignment because the powerful muscles in the thigh would normally pull on the ends of the broken bone, forcing them out of alignment.

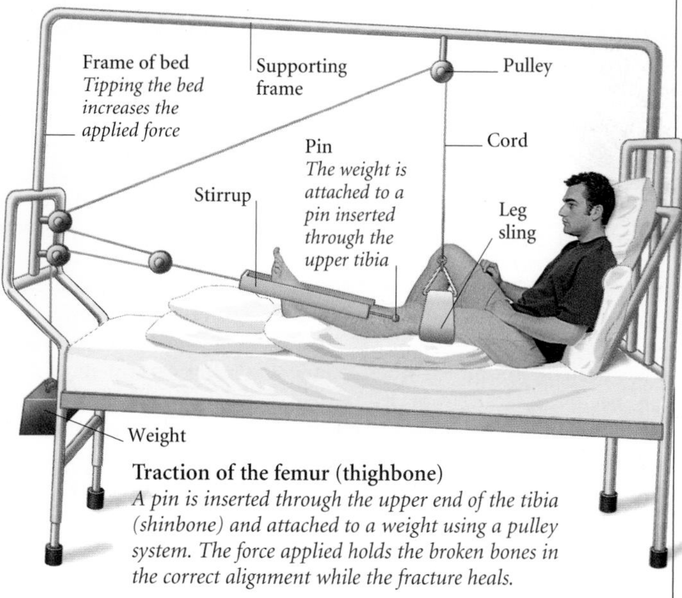

Traction of the femur (thighbone)
A pin is inserted through the upper end of the tibia (shinbone) and attached to a weight using a pulley system. The force applied holds the broken bones in the correct alignment while the fracture heals.

In some cases, it may not be appropriate to immobilize a broken bone. For example, a broken rib is generally not immobilized because the chest needs to to expand normally during breathing. This is important to reduce the risk of pneumonia (p.490), which can develop as a result of shallow breathing and an impaired ability to cough. As a preventive measure, you may be asked to take deep breaths regularly.

Occasionally, healing is slowed down because not enough blood can reach the fracture site or because the broken bone has not been immobilized effectively. In such cases, surgery may be needed; the splintered bone is removed and bone taken from a different part of the body is grafted in its place. A broken bone, such as a fracture in the femur close to the hip joint, may be replaced with an artificial substitute, in this case comprising either part of the femur or the entire hip joint (*see* JOINT REPLACEMENT, p.377).

You may need to have physiotherapy (p.961) after the fracture has healed to restore mobility to a nearby joint and strengthen the surrounding muscles.

WHAT IS THE PROGNOSIS?

In adults, most fractures take 6–8 weeks to heal. Fractures in children generally heal much more quickly. Fractures in babies may heal in a couple of weeks.

(WWW) ONLINE SITES: p.1035

Dislocated joint

Displacement of the bones in joints, usually as a result of injury

 GENDER More common in males

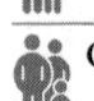 GENETICS Sometimes runs in families

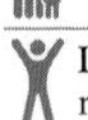 LIFESTYLE Playing contact sports, such as rugby, is a risk factor

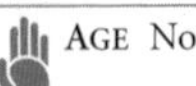 AGE Not a significant factor

A dislocated joint occurs when a bone has been displaced from its normal position. As a result of pain and the dislocation itself, movement of the joint is severely restricted. The ligaments that hold the bones in place are often torn during the process of dislocation (*see* LIGAMENT INJURIES, right), and the capsule that surrounds the joint may be damaged. Sometimes the bones within the joint also fracture (p.392). Shoulder and finger joints are particularly susceptible to dislocation.

WHAT ARE THE CAUSES?

Any powerful force acting against a joint may cause a dislocation. Contact sports, such as rugby, and heavy falls are common causes in men. Abnormally loose joints that are susceptible to dislocation may be an inherited condition. Dislocation may also be associated with a joint disorder, such as rheumatoid arthritis (p.377). Dislocation of the hip may be present from birth (*see* CONGENITAL HIP DYSPLASIA, p.832).

WHAT ARE THE SYMPTOMS?

If you dislocate a joint, the symptoms will appear suddenly and may include:

- Severe pain in the affected area.
- Deformity of the joint.
- Swelling around the joint.
- Bruising of the skin around the joint.

Displaced bones may cause damage to nearby nerves, tendons, and blood vessels, resulting in reduced circulation in tissues beyond the affected area.

If you think that you may have dislocated a joint, you should consult a doctor promptly. If a back injury causes dislocation of the vertebrae (bones of the spine), there may be damage to the spinal cord and consequent paralysis.

WHAT MIGHT BE DONE?

Diagnosis of a dislocated joint is usually obvious from the symptoms and a physical examination. However, you may have an X-ray (p.244) to confirm the dislocation and to check for a fracture. Dislocated joints can usually be manipulated back into position by a doctor. You may be given a painkiller (p.912) to relieve discomfort or, in some cases, a sedative to relieve muscle spasm while the joint is being manipulated. If manipulation is unsuccessful, you may need surgery to reposition the joint.

After treatment, the affected joint may be immobilized for 3–6 weeks and you may need physiotherapy (p.961) to help you start to use the joint again. There may be an increased risk that the joint will dislocate again. Joints that dislocate repeatedly may require surgical treatment to stabilize them.

(WWW) ONLINE SITES: p.1035

Ligament injuries

Damage to ligaments, the fibrous bands of tissue that hold bones together at a joint

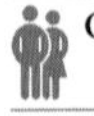 GENDER More common in males

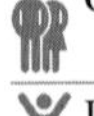 LIFESTYLE Playing sports is a risk factor

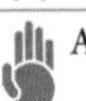 AGE GENETICS Not significant factors

Ligaments attach bones to each other within joints and help to keep joints stable. Ligaments are only slightly elastic and are easily damaged if they are overstretched. Possible injuries range from minor tears, also called sprains, to complete rupture. The most common cause of a ligament injury is a sudden twisting or wrenching movement due to a fall, playing sports, or exercising excessively. Such injuries occur more commonly in men because they exercise more vigorously. Failure to warm up properly before starting exercise is another cause of ligament injury. The ankle and knee are injured most often.

WHAT ARE THE SYMPTOMS?

Symptoms usually develop suddenly in the affected joint and may include:

- Pain, particularly on movement.
- Swelling and bruising.
- An abnormal range of movement at the joint.

If you are unable to use a joint after injuring it, you should consult your doctor promptly because tearing a ligament may lead to a dislocation of the bones within the affected joint (*see* DISLOCATED JOINT, left).

WHAT MIGHT BE DONE?

Most ligament injuries heal well within 8 weeks without treatment, but you can help speed up recovery of a mild sprain using first-aid measures (*see* FIRST AID: SPRAINS AND STRAINS, p.991). To relieve pain, you may be given nonsteroidal anti-inflammatory drugs (p.894). If the pain is severe, you may have an X-ray (p.244) to rule out a fracture (p.392). Physiotherapy (p.961) is often needed after severe injuries, and surgery may also be necessary. Sometimes, the ruptured ligament is beyond repair. In such cases, the ligament may be replaced with a nearby tendon or a donor graft.

(WWW) ONLINE SITES: p.1035

Torn knee cartilage

Damage to the cartilage pads (menisci) in the knee joints

 GENDER More common in males

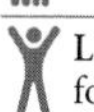 LIFESTYLE Playing contact sports, such as football, is a risk factor

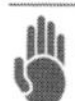 AGE GENETICS Not significant factors

Damage to cartilage commonly occurs in the knee joint, where two cartilage discs, known as menisci, act as shock absorbers between the femur (thighbone) and tibia (shinbone). These discs help to distribute body weight in the joint. A torn cartilage often occurs in football players and is therefore more common in men. The injury is usually caused by a sudden twisting of the leg, often with the knee bent and the foot on the ground. A cartilage can tear without sudden injury, and people whose occupation involves squatting down and placing strain on the knees are at risk.

If you do tear a cartilage abruptly, you will feel a sharp pain and may hear a noise at the time of the injury. Pain usually becomes worse on moving the joint, and swelling may develop immediately or several hours later. You will probably be unable to straighten the joint. A torn cartilage may prevent the leg from supporting your body weight.

WHAT MIGHT BE DONE?

Your doctor will examine your knee and probably arrange for an X-ray (p.244) to check for bone damage. The diagnosis may be confirmed by examining the knee using MRI (p.248) or arthroscopy (p.386). Sometimes, damaged knee cartilage is repaired surgically under a general anaesthetic, and most people are able to use the injured joint 2–3 weeks afterwards. Physiotherapy (p.961) may be needed to help to mobilize the affected joint. There is a risk that torn knee cartilage may lead to early development of osteoarthritis (p.374), a degenerative disorder of the joints.

(WWW) ONLINE SITES: p.1035

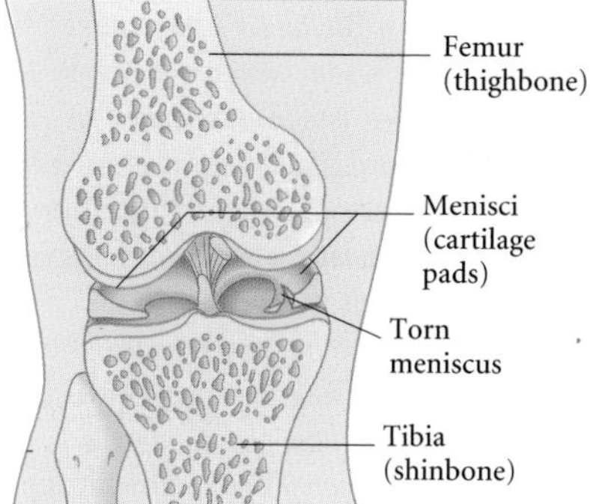

Cartilage in the knee

In the knee joint, two menisci (cartilage pads) act as cushions between the femur and tibia. The menisci are vulnerable to tearing, often as a result of acute injury.

Muscle strains and tears

Injuries of varying severity resulting from the overstretching of a muscle

 AGE More common with increasing age

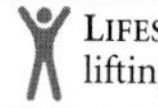 LIFESTYLE Intensive athletic training and lifting heavy weights are risk factors

 GENDER GENETICS Not significant factors

Muscle strain occurs when a muscle is overstretched, damaging some of its fibres. A tear occurs when the damage is severe and affects many muscle fibres. Both conditions are usually caused by sudden, strenuous movements and occur most often in people who play sports. Abdominal and back muscles may be injured by lifting heavy objects. Athletes are particularly susceptible to these injuries. Symptoms may include pain, swelling, and bruising.

Muscle strains and tears may be prevented by preparing adequately before sports activities (*see* WARMING UP AND COOLING DOWN IN YOUR EXERCISE ROUTINE, p.60). If you do strain or tear a muscle, follow first-aid procedures (*see* FIRST AID: SPRAINS AND STRAINS, p.991). When the pain and swelling subside, usually within 2 days, you can exercise the muscle gently. However, if the pain remains, consult your doctor.

Your doctor may suggest that you take a nonsteroidal anti-inflammatory drug (p.894). He or she may also advise you to rest the affected muscle and receive physiotherapy (p.961). If the injury is severe, you may have an X-ray (p.244) to rule out a fracture (p.392). Rarely, surgery may be needed to repair a muscle that has been badly torn.

(WWW) ONLINE SITES: p.1035

Ruptured tendon

A complete tear in one of the tough, fibrous bands that attach muscle to bone

LIFESTYLE Intensive sports training and lifting heavy weights are risk factors

AGE GENDER GENETICS Not significant factors

A tendon may rupture when the muscle to which it is attached contracts suddenly and powerfully, usually during vigorous physical activity such as playing sports or lifting a heavy object. Athletes tend to carry out these activities more often and are therefore more likely to sustain injury. A ruptured tendon may also result from a severe blow, deep cut, or fracture (p.392). In some cases, a ruptured tendon can occur spontaneously as a complication of long-term joint disease such as rheumatoid arthritis (p.377). The tendons in the limbs, particularly the Achilles tendon (which runs from the calf muscle to the heel bone) and those in the hands, are most susceptible to rupture.

You may feel a snapping sensation in the injured area at the time that the tendon ruptures. Other symptoms include pain, impaired movement, and swelling of the affected area.

WHAT MIGHT BE DONE?

Diagnosis is usually obvious from the symptoms and physical examination of the affected area. Your doctor may prescribe nonsteroidal anti-inflammatory drugs (p.894). In some cases of Achilles tendon rupture, surgery will be needed to join the torn ends of the tendon. Whether or not you have surgery for an Achilles tendon injury, the injured area will be immobilized by the successive application of different casts. The first cast holds the heel up and the toes down, to avoid stretching the tendon. Subsequent casts are used to flatten the foot gradually and return it to its normal position. You may also be advised to have physiotherapy (p.961) to help to strengthen the muscles in the injured area around the tendon.

The time taken for recovery varies, but motion is usually fully restored in 4–12 months. If an Achilles tendon was involved, you may be vulnerable to further injury on the opposite side.

(WWW) ONLINE SITES: p.1035

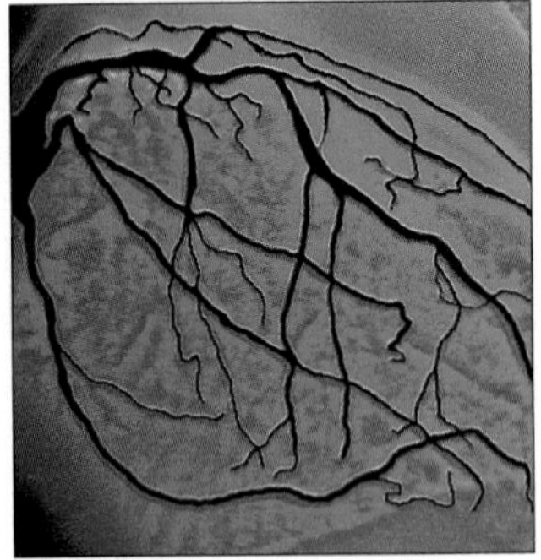

Blood supply to the heart
The extensive network of arteries that surround the heart and supply oxygenated blood to its muscle can be seen in this contrast X-ray.

CARDIOVASCULAR SYSTEM

THE CARDIOVASCULAR SYSTEM and the blood contained in its vessels are the body's transport system. The heart pumps blood around two circuits of blood vessels. The main (systemic) circuit carries blood that contains oxygen, vital nutrients, and hormones to every cell. The second (pulmonary) circuit takes blood to the lungs, where oxygen is absorbed and the waste product carbon dioxide is eliminated. Other waste products are taken to the liver for processing and finally eliminated by the kidneys.

The heart pumps the body's total volume of blood (about 5 litres or 9 pints) around the entire body about once a minute. In the systemic circulation, blood containing oxygen and vital nutrients is pumped to tissues and organs through blood vessels called arteries. Body cells absorb the oxygen and nutrients, while the blood absorbs waste products from the cells before returning to the heart through blood vessels called veins. The deoxygenated blood is then pumped to the lungs in the pulmonary circulation. After oxygen has been absorbed and carbon dioxide eliminated, the blood returns to the heart. During exercise, the rate of circulation may increase several times to meet the body's demand for oxygen. The blood supply to some muscles may increase twelvefold while that to the digestive system falls by a third.

THE HEART AND ITS CHAMBERS

About the size of a clenched fist, the heart is a muscular organ that lies in the centre of the chest, slightly to the left. It is divided into two halves, each of which contains an upper chamber (the atrium) and a lower chamber (the ventricle). The atria collect blood from various parts of the body, while the ventricles pump blood out of the heart. Each of the four chambers is joined to one or more blood vessels. The largest of these vessels, the aorta, is about the diameter of a garden hose. Forceful contractions of the ventricles pump blood out of the heart about 70 times per minute at rest. This pumping rate is called the heart rate and is measured in beats per minute. With each beat, a pressure wave travels along the arteries, causing their walls to expand. This wave, or pulse, can be felt where the arteries are close to the skin's surface. Between pulse waves, the elastic walls of the arteries rebound.

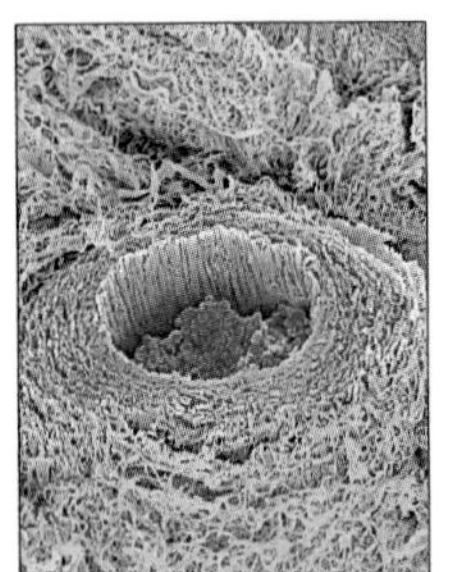

A small artery
The multi-layered wall of the artery seen in this highly magnified image contains muscle and elastic fibres. Individual red blood cells inside the artery are also visible.

Heart muscle (myocardium) must work continuously for 24 hours a day without rest. Therefore, myocardial cells contain more and larger energy-producing units (mitochondria) than other types of body cell.

HEART RATE AND BLOOD PRESSURE

Heart rate is regulated by electrical impulses from the heart's pacemaker, the sinoatrial node, which is a small area of nervous tissue in the wall of the right atrium. Each impulse causes a rapid sequence of contractions, first in the atria and then in the ventricles, that corresponds to one heartbeat.

Blood pressure depends on the rate and force of the heart's contractions, the volume of blood pumped out, and the resistance to blood flow in the blood vessels, which varies with their size. Heart rate and blood pressure are controlled by the nervous system in the short term and by hormones, which act over a longer period.

FUNCTION BLOOD FLOW THROUGH THE HEART

Blood flows through veins into the heart's upper chambers (atria) and is pumped into the arteries by the lower chambers (ventricles). Deoxygenated blood collects in the right atrium and flows into the right ventricle, which pumps it to the lungs. Oxygenated blood returns from the lungs to the left atrium. The left ventricle then pumps this blood around the body.

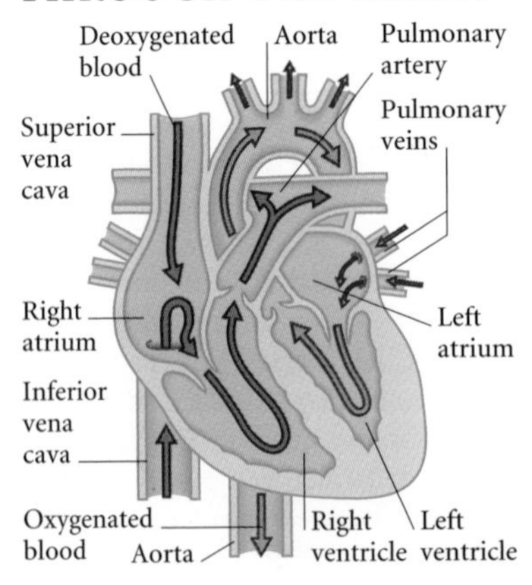

Two sides of the heart
The heart's right side pumps deoxygenated blood from the body to the lungs. The left side pumps oxygenated blood to the body.

STRUCTURE AND FUNCTION

THE BLOOD VESSELS

The cardiovascular system includes three types of blood vessel: arteries, veins, and capillaries. Placed end to end, they would circle the Earth nearly four times. The smallest vessels, the capillaries, make up 98 per cent of this length. The largest artery, the aorta, emerges from the heart and branches into a network of progressively smaller arteries that carry blood to every part of the body. The smallest arteries join capillaries, which in turn join a network of tiny veins that merge into larger veins as they return blood to the heart.

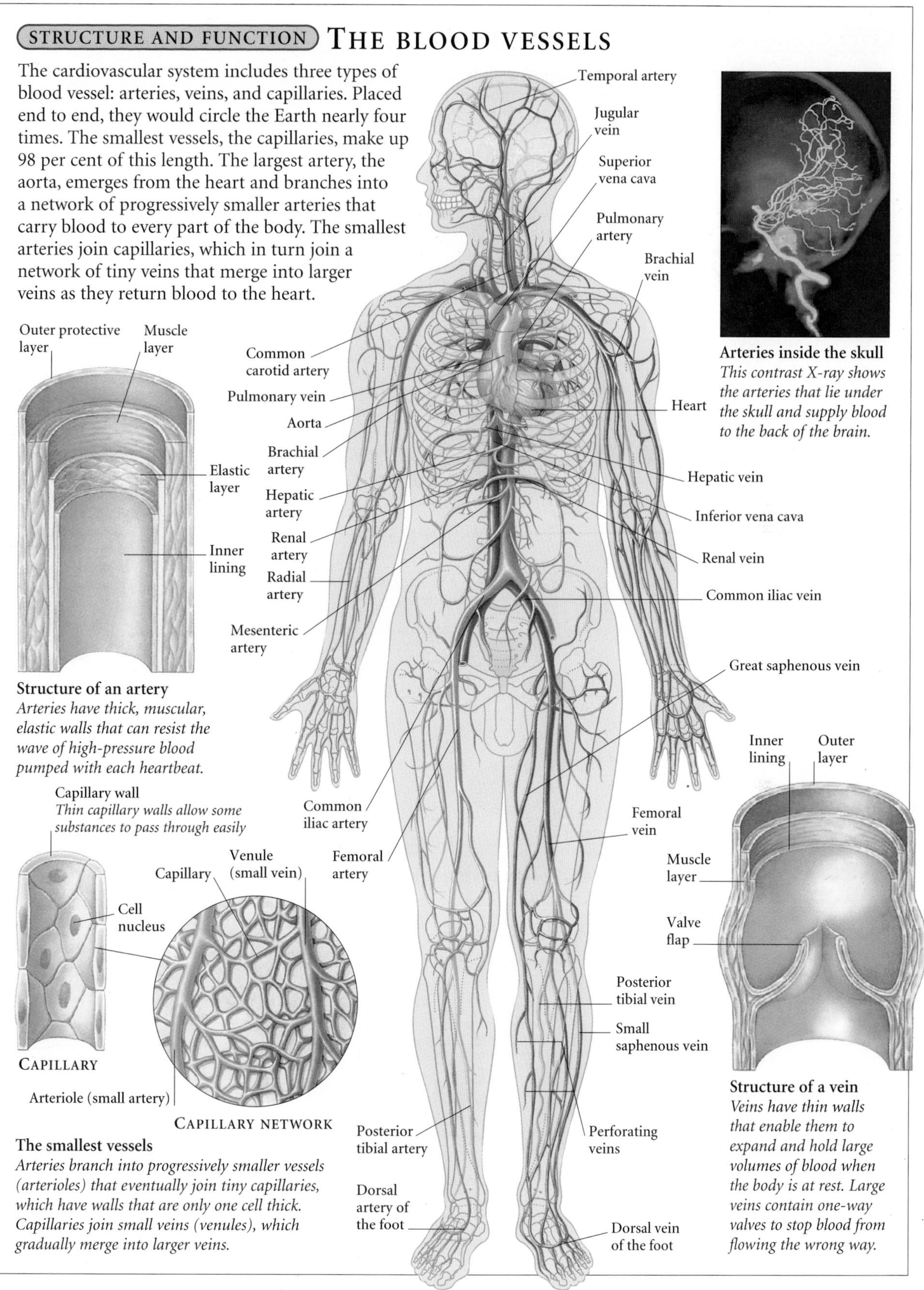

Arteries inside the skull
This contrast X-ray shows the arteries that lie under the skull and supply blood to the back of the brain.

Structure of an artery
Arteries have thick, muscular, elastic walls that can resist the wave of high-pressure blood pumped with each heartbeat.

The smallest vessels
Arteries branch into progressively smaller vessels (arterioles) that eventually join tiny capillaries, which have walls that are only one cell thick. Capillaries join small veins (venules), which gradually merge into larger veins.

Structure of a vein
Veins have thin walls that enable them to expand and hold large volumes of blood when the body is at rest. Large veins contain one-way valves to stop blood from flowing the wrong way.

STRUCTURE — STRUCTURE OF THE HEART

The heart is a hollow muscular pump consisting mainly of myocardium, a type of muscle that can work without resting. The interior of the heart is divided into two halves, each of which consists of an upper chamber and a lower chamber (the atrium and the ventricle). Each chamber connects to one or more blood vessels. Blood flow through these chambers is controlled by one-way valves.

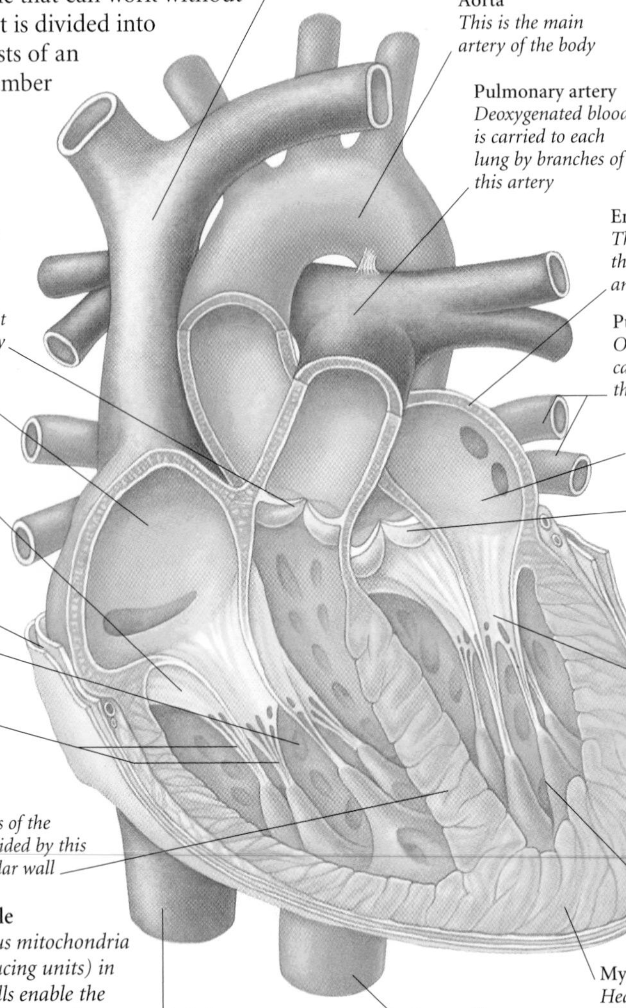

Superior vena cava

Aorta
This is the main artery of the body

Pulmonary artery
Deoxygenated blood is carried to each lung by branches of this artery

LOCATION

Endocardium
This smooth layer lines the interior of the heart and is one cell thick

Pulmonary veins
Oxygenated blood is carried from the lungs to the heart by these veins

Left atrium

Aortic valve
The three cusps (flaps) of the aortic valve allow one-way blood flow from the left ventricle into the aorta

Mitral valve
This valve has two cusps (flaps); it allows one-way blood flow from the left atrium into the left ventricle

Left ventricle

Myocardium
Heart muscle is three times thicker on the left side, which pumps blood to the body, than on the right

Pulmonary valve
This valve has three cusps (flaps); it allows blood to flow from the right ventricle into the pulmonary artery

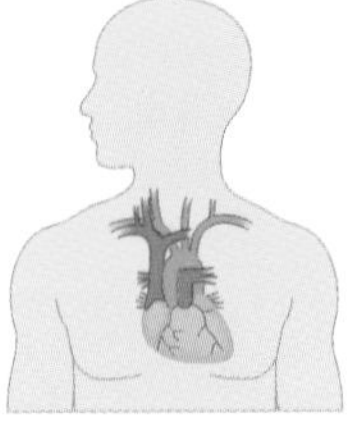

Right atrium

Tricuspid valve
The three cusps (flaps) of this valve allow one-way blood flow from the right atrium into the right ventricle

Pericardium
This double-layered membrane separates the heart from the lungs and chest wall

Right ventricle

Chordae tendineae
These fibrous strands attach the heart valve cusps (flaps) to the heart wall

Mitochondrion

Muscle cell

Septum
The two sides of the heart are divided by this thick, muscular wall

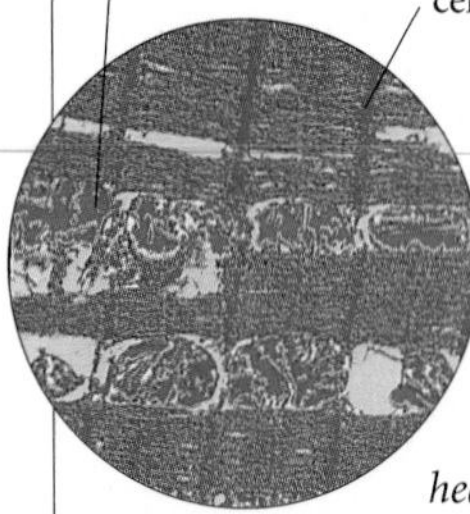

Heart muscle
The numerous mitochondria (energy-producing units) in heart muscle cells enable the heart to pump without resting.

Inferior vena cava

Descending aorta

FUNCTION — BLOOD SUPPLY TO THE HEART

The coronary arteries branch off the aorta and surround and penetrate heart muscle. Arterioles and capillaries branch off from the arteries to supply heart muscle with oxygen-rich blood. Deoxygenated blood drains into the coronary veins, which carry it back into the heart's right atrium.

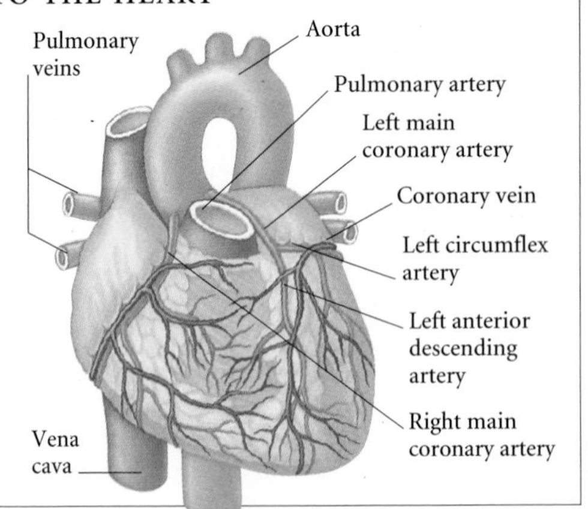

The coronary arteries
There are two main coronary arteries, the left and the right. The left one branches to form the left circumflex artery and the left anterior descending artery.

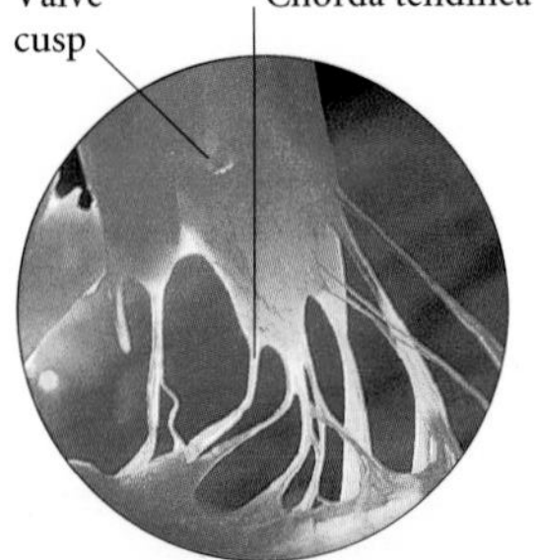

Anchoring the valves
String-like chordae tendineae anchor each valve cusp (flap) to the heart wall to prevent it from being turned inside out.

(FUNCTION) HOW THE HEART BEATS

A single pumping action of the heart is called a heartbeat. A healthy adult heart beats at a rate of 60–80 beats per minute at rest and at up to 200 beats per minute during strenuous exercise. One-way valves inside the heart prevent blood from being pumped in the wrong direction. The rhythmic "lub-dub" sound of the heart is due to the heart valves shutting tightly.

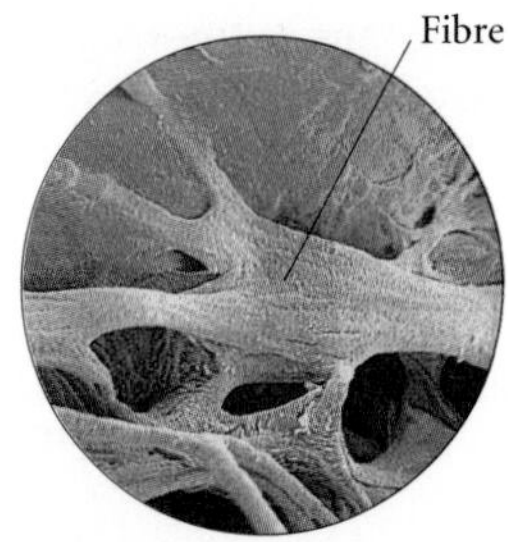

Conducting fibres
Specialized muscle fibres in the walls of the heart conduct electrical impulses that regulate the heartbeat.

THE HEART CYCLE

A heartbeat has three phases. In diastole, the heart relaxes. During atrial systole, the atria contract, and in ventricular systole, the ventricles contract. The sinoatrial node (the heart's pacemaker) regulates the timing of the phases by sending electrical impulses to the atria and ventricles.

Diastole
The heart muscle relaxes, and blood flows into the atria from the pulmonary veins and vena cava. Near the end of this phase, the sinoatrial node emits an electrical impulse.

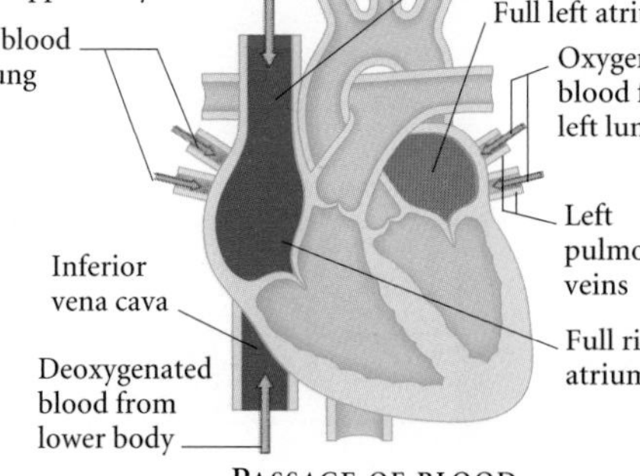

PASSAGE OF BLOOD

Sinoatrial node
Electrical impulse

ELECTRICAL ACTIVITY

Atrial systole
The electrical impulse spreads through both atria. The impulse causes their muscular walls to contract and push blood into the ventricles. By the end of atrial systole, the impulse reaches the atrioventricular node, which is in the right atrium.

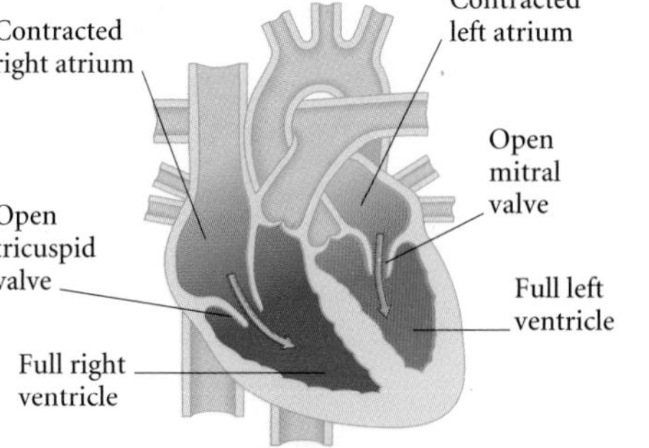

PASSAGE OF BLOOD

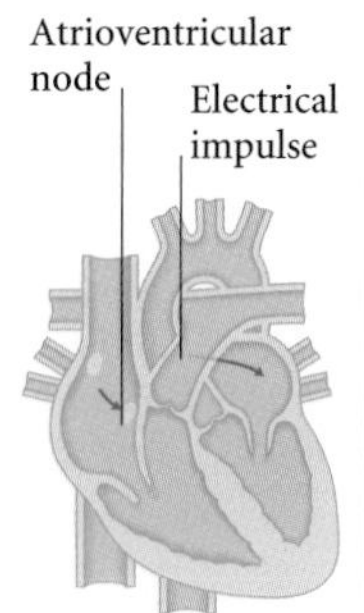

ELECTRICAL ACTIVITY

Ventricular systole
The impulse reaches the atrioventricular node, where it is momentarily delayed before it spreads throughout the walls of the ventricles. The impulse causes the ventricles to contract, pushing blood out into the aorta and the pulmonary arteries.

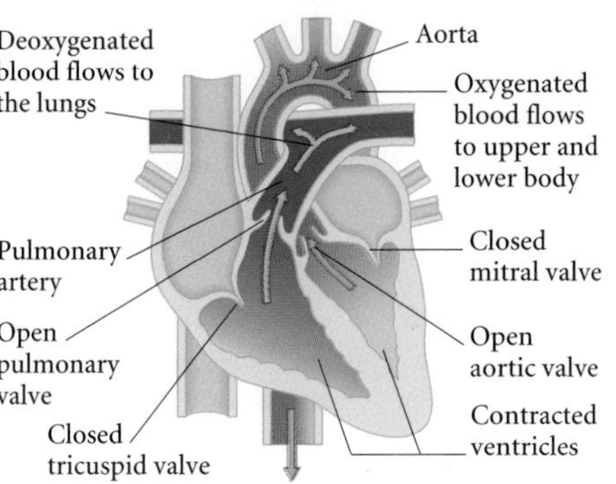

PASSAGE OF BLOOD

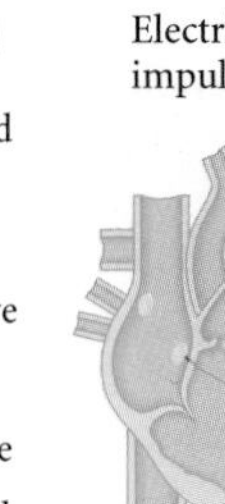

ELECTRICAL ACTIVITY

HEART VALVES

Heart valves consist of two or three cup-shaped cusps (flaps). The cusps consist mainly of collagen, a tough protein, and are covered in endocardium, a thin layer of tissue that lines the inside of the heart and joins the lining of the blood vessels.

Blood at low pressure
Flow of blood
Valve cusp (flap)
Blood at high pressure opens valve

Open heart valve
When a heart chamber contracts, the high pressure of the blood inside it pushes open the valve cusps, and blood flows through to the other side of the valve.

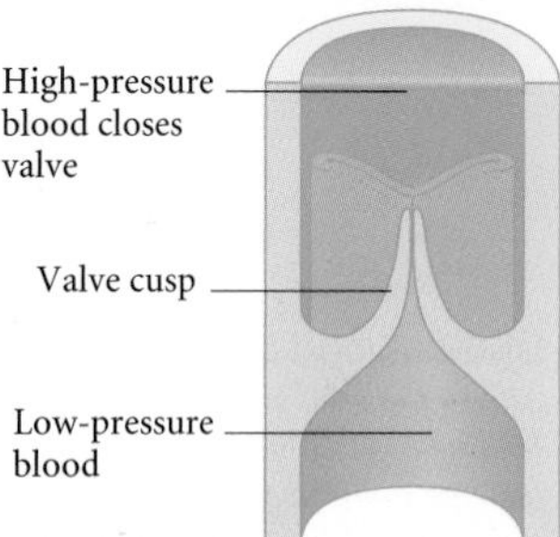

Closed heart valve
The pressure of blood on the other side of the valve rises and snaps shut the valve cusps. The closed valve prevents backflow.

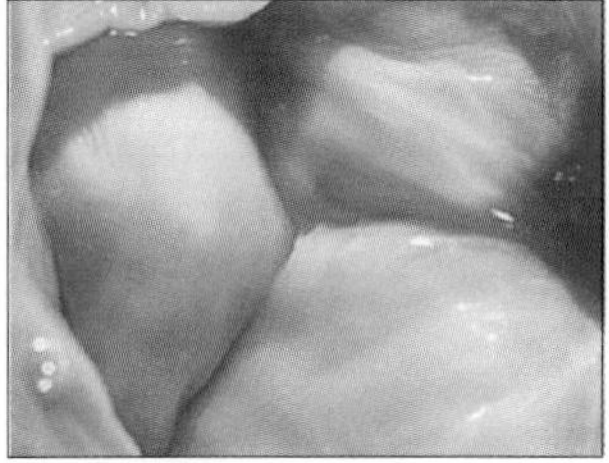

Closed pulmonary valve
The pulmonary valve has three cusps with rounded undersides that are attached to the inner wall of the pulmonary artery.

FUNCTION THE BLOOD CIRCULATION

Blood circulates in two linked circuits: the pulmonary, which carries blood to the lungs to be oxygenated, and the systemic, which supplies oxygenated blood to the body. Arteries carrying blood from the heart divide into smaller vessels called arterioles and then into capillaries, where nutrient and waste exchange occurs. Capillaries join up to form venules, which in turn join to form veins that carry blood back to the heart. The portal vein does not return blood to the heart but carries it to the liver.

A DOUBLE CIRCUIT

The heart powers the pulmonary and the systemic circulations. In the pulmonary circulation, deoxygenated blood (blue) travels to the lungs, where it absorbs oxygen before returning to the heart. This oxygenated blood (red) is pumped around the body in the systemic circulation. Body tissues absorb oxygen, and deoxygenated blood returns to the heart to be pumped to the lungs again.

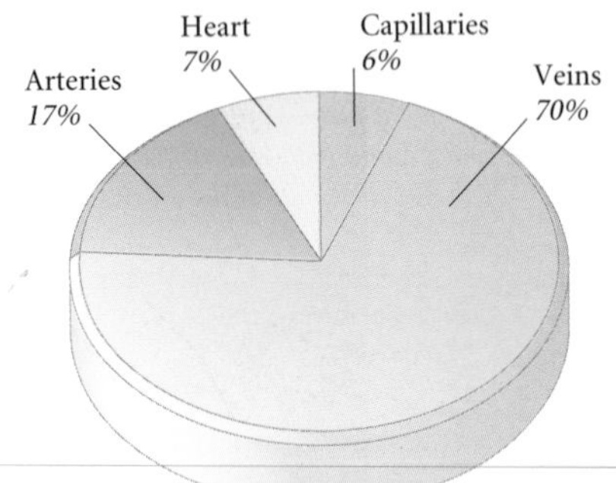

Distribution of blood in the circulation
At rest, the veins act as a reservoir for blood, holding most of the body's blood volume. If an increase in blood supply is needed, the veins constrict and return more blood to the heart.

Aorta
This major artery carries oxygenated blood to all parts of the body

Network of vessels in upper body

Pulmonary veins
Oxygenated blood is carried from the lungs back to the heart in these veins

Arteriole

Capillary

Venule

Network of vessels in right lung
Blood gives up carbon dioxide and absorbs oxygen in the capillaries

Network of vessels in left lung

Pulmonary artery
This takes deoxygenated blood to the lungs

Superior vena cava
This vein carries blood from the upper body to the heart

Portal vein
This vein carries blood rich in nutrients from the digestive system to the liver

Inferior vena cava
This vein carries blood from the lower body to the heart

Network of vessels in liver

Network of vessels in digestive system

Network of vessels in lower body

KEY
PULMONARY CIRCULATION
SYSTEMIC CIRCULATION

Blood supply
In both the pulmonary and systemic circulations, the exchange of oxygen, nutrients, and waste products occurs in the capillaries that join arterioles to venules.

VENOUS RETURN

The blood pressure in the veins is about a tenth of that in the arteries. Various physical mechanisms ensure that there is adequate venous return (blood flow back to the heart). Many deep veins lie within muscles. When the muscles contract, they squeeze the veins and force blood back to the heart. The action of inhalation during breathing also draws blood to the heart. In addition, venous return from the upper body is assisted by gravity.

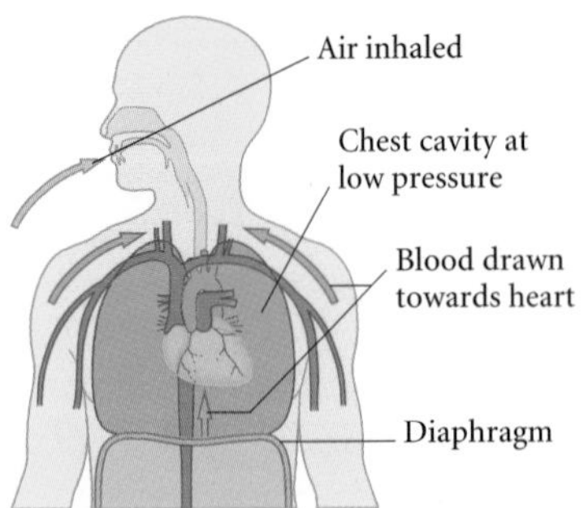

Respiratory pump during inhalation
While inhaling, the chest cavity expands, lowering the pressure in the chest. Higher pressure in the rest of the body pushes blood in the veins towards the heart.

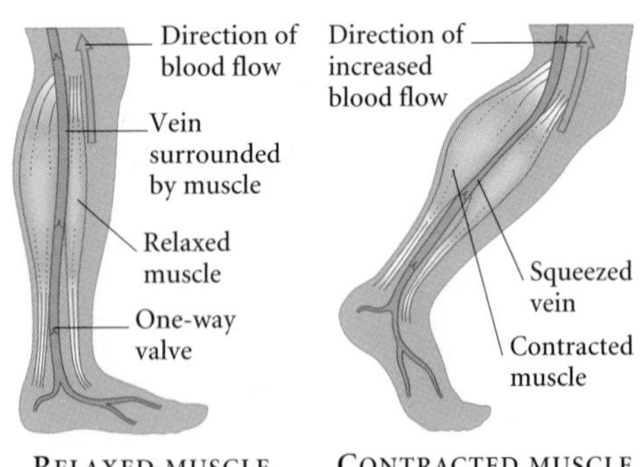

Muscular pump
Muscles contract and relax as we move, squeezing the veins that pass through them and pushing blood back to the heart. One-way valves prevent backflow.

FUNCTION CONTROL OF BLOOD PRESSURE

Blood pressure in the arteries must be regulated to ensure an adequate supply of blood, and hence oxygen, to the organs. If arterial blood pressure is too low, not enough blood reaches body tissues. If it is too high, it may damage blood vessels and organs. Rapid changes in blood pressure trigger compensatory responses from the nervous system within seconds. These autonomic nervous responses do not involve the conscious parts of the brain. Longer-term changes are largely regulated by hormones that affect the volume of fluid excreted by the kidneys. Hormonal responses work over several hours.

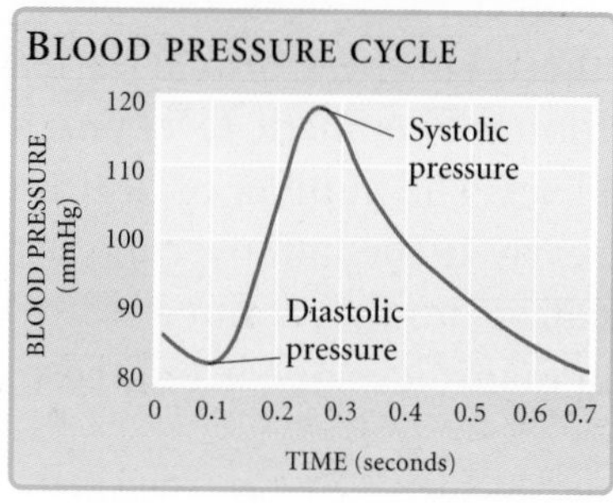

Systolic and diastolic pressure
Arterial pressure is low while the heart fills with blood (diastolic pressure) but rises as the heart pumps blood out (systolic pressure). The units of pressure are millimetres of mercury (mmHg).

SHORT-TERM CONTROL OF BLOOD PRESSURE

Heavy bleeding or a sudden change in posture may cause a rapid change in blood pressure, to which the nervous system immediately responds. Baroreceptors (stretch receptors in the walls of the major arteries) detect pressure changes and send signals along sensory nerves to the brain. An autonomic response adjusts the heart rate, volume of blood pumped, and arterial diameter to restore normal pressure.

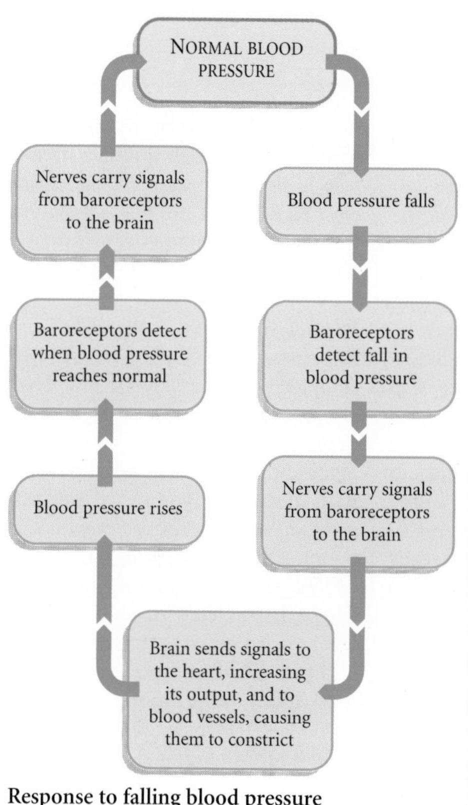

Response to falling blood pressure
Baroreceptors in the aorta and carotid arteries, which supply the head, detect a fall in blood pressure and send signals to the brain. The brain sends signals to the heart and blood vessels to restore normal pressure.

LONG-TERM CONTROL OF BLOOD PRESSURE

Blood pressure is controlled in the long term by the action of hormones. The kidneys respond to low blood pressure by secreting renin. This hormone is converted into angiotensin, which constricts arteries and raises blood pressure. The adrenal glands, hypothalamus, and heart also respond to high or low pressure by secreting aldosterone, vasopressin, and natriuretic hormone, respectively. These hormones alter the amount of fluid excreted by the kidneys, which affects the volume of blood in the body and hence the blood pressure.

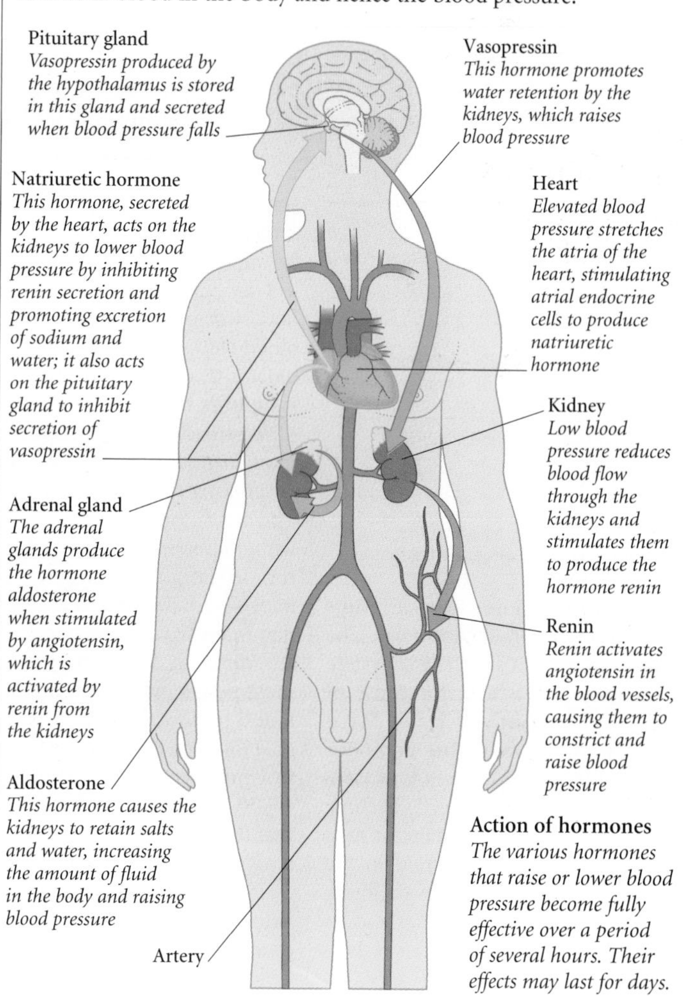

Action of hormones
The various hormones that raise or lower blood pressure become fully effective over a period of several hours. Their effects may last for days.

MAJOR CARDIOVASCULAR DISORDERS

By the middle of the 20th century, heart disease was the leading cause of death in northern Europe. Coronary artery disease was the primary cause, although rheumatic fever and high blood pressure also claimed lives. The number of deaths caused by heart disease peaked by the early 1980s, and over the last 20–30 years preventive treatments have brought about a steady decline in heart disease deaths in many developed countries.

This section covers the major disorders affecting the heart and the circulation. The first articles overlap to a certain extent because some cardiovascular disorders can lead to the development of others. Smoking, an unhealthy diet, being overweight, and lack of exercise are risk factors for the development of hypertension (high blood pressure) and atherosclerosis, in which the arteries are narrowed. Narrowing of the coronary arteries that supply the heart muscle can cause coronary artery disease, which itself is the major cause of angina and heart attacks. If the heart is damaged by coronary artery disease or a heart attack, it may be unable to pump blood efficiently around the rest of the body, resulting in heart failure. Heart failure can develop suddenly, or it may be a chronic disorder that develops over a number of years.

The last articles in the section cover hypotension, the medical term for low blood pressure, and shock. Shock is a medical emergency that requires immediate treatment in hospital.

KEY ANATOMY

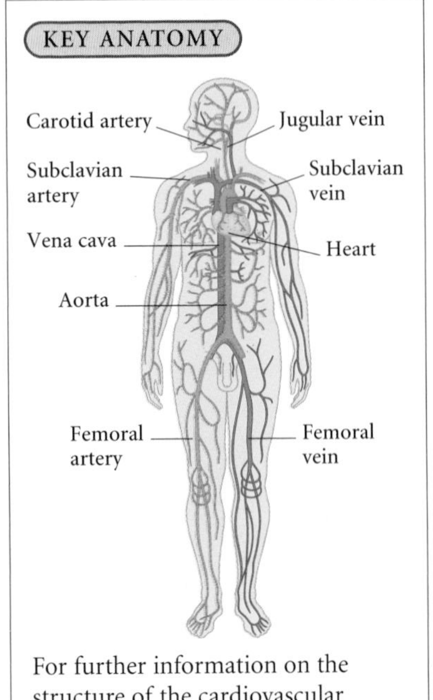

For further information on the structure of the cardiovascular system, *see* pp.396–401.

Atherosclerosis

Accumulation of cholesterol and other fatty substances in the walls of arteries, causing them to narrow

 AGE More common with increasing age

 GENDER More common in males until the age of 60, then equal incidence

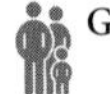 GENETICS Sometimes runs in families

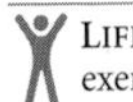 LIFESTYLE Smoking, a high-fat diet, lack of exercise, and excess weight are risk factors

Atherosclerosis is a disease that results in the arteries becoming narrowed. The condition can affect arteries in any area of the body and is a major cause of stroke (p.532), heart attack (*see* MYOCARDIAL INFARCTION, p.410), and poor circulation in the legs (*see* LOWER LIMB ISCHAEMIA, p.434). The arteries become narrowed when fatty substances, such as cholesterol, that are carried in the blood accumulate on the inside lining of the arteries and form yellow deposits called atheroma. These deposits restrict the blood flow through the arteries. In addition, the muscle layer of the artery wall becomes thickened, narrowing the artery even more. Platelets (tiny blood cells responsible for clotting) may collect in clumps on the surface of the deposits and initiate the formation of blood clots. A large clot may completely block the artery, resulting in the organ it supplies being deprived of oxygen.

Atherosclerosis is much more common in northern Europe than it is in developing countries in Africa and Asia. The condition becomes more common with increasing age and also tends to run in families. Autopsies on young men who have died in accidents reveal that many have already developed some atheroma in their large arteries, and most people who die in middle age are found to have a degree of atherosclerosis. However, it is rare for the condition to cause symptoms before the age of 45–50, and many people are unaware that they have atherosclerosis until they have a heart attack or a stroke.

The female sex hormone oestrogen helps protect against the development of atherosclerosis. As a result, the incidence of atherosclerosis is much lower in women before the menopause than in men. However, by the age of 60, a woman's risk of developing atherosclerosis is the same as a man's, although women who take hormone replacement therapy containing oestrogen may continue to be protected.

WHAT ARE THE CAUSES?

The risk of developing atherosclerosis is determined largely by the level of cholesterol in the bloodstream, which depends on dietary and genetic factors. Since cholesterol levels are closely linked with diet, atherosclerosis is most common in Western countries where most people eat a diet high in fat. Some disorders, such as diabetes mellitus (p.687), can be associated with a high cholesterol level regardless of diet. Certain inherited lipid disorders also result in a high level of fats in the blood (*see* INHERITED HYPERLIPIDAEMIAS, p.692).

In addition to high blood cholesterol levels, factors that make atherosclerosis more likely are smoking, lack of regular exercise, having high blood pressure (*see* HYPERTENSION, opposite page), and being overweight, especially if there is a concentration of fat around the waist.

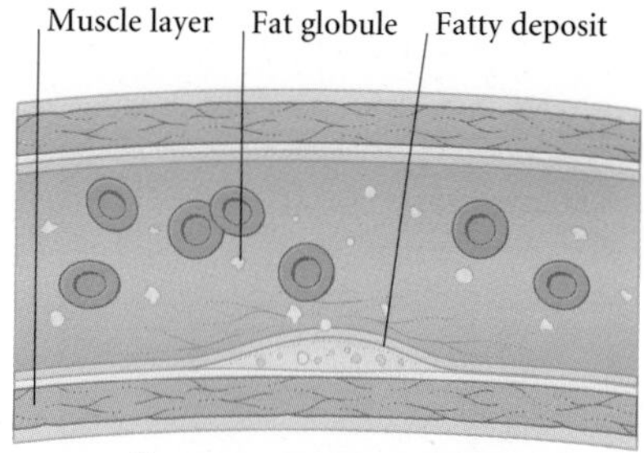

EARLY ATHEROSCLEROSIS

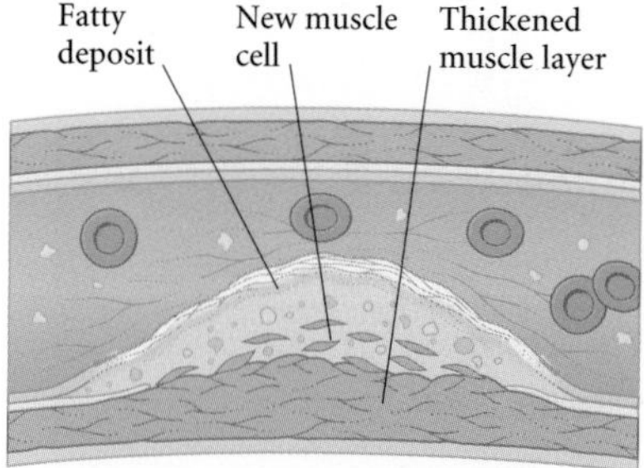

ADVANCED ATHEROSCLEROSIS

How atherosclerosis develops

Fatty substances gradually accumulate in the lining of the artery wall, and the muscle layer thickens as new muscle cells form in the fatty deposit. As a result, the artery becomes progressively narrowed.

WHAT ARE THE SYMPTOMS?

There are usually no symptoms in the early stages of atherosclerosis. Later, symptoms are caused by the reduced or total absence of a blood supply to the organs supplied by the affected arteries. If the coronary arteries, which supply the heart muscle, are partially blocked, symptoms may include the chest pain of angina (p.407). If there is a complete blockage in a coronary artery, there may be a sudden, often fatal, heart attack. Many strokes are a result of atherosclerosis in the arteries that supply blood to the brain. If atherosclerosis affects the arteries in the legs, the first symptom may be cramping pain when walking caused by poor blood flow to the leg muscles. If atherosclerosis is associated with an inherited lipid disorder, fatty deposits may develop on tendons or under the skin in visible lumps.

HOW IS IT DIAGNOSED?

Since atherosclerosis has no symptoms until blood flow has been restricted, it is important to screen for the disorder before it becomes advanced and damages organs. Routine medical checkups include screening for the major risk factors of atherosclerosis, particularly raised blood cholesterol levels, high blood pressure, and diabetes mellitus. One current recommendation is that all adults should have their cholesterol levels measured at intervals of 5 years at the least after the age of 20.

If you develop symptoms of atherosclerosis, your doctor may arrange tests to assess the damage both to the arteries and to the organs they supply. Blood flow in affected blood vessels can be imaged by Doppler ultrasound scanning (p.432) or coronary angiography (p.408). If your doctor thinks that the coronary arteries are affected, an ECG (p.406) may be carried out to monitor the electrical activity of the heart and imaging techniques, such as angiography and radionuclide scanning (p.251), may be used to look at the blood supply to the heart. Some of these tests may be done as you exercise to check how the heart functions when it is put under stress (*see* EXERCISE TESTING, p.407).

WHAT IS THE TREATMENT?

The best treatment is to prevent atherosclerosis from progressing. Preventive measures include following a healthy lifestyle by eating a low-fat diet, not smoking, exercising regularly, and maintaining the recommended weight for your height. These measures lead to a lower than average risk of developing significant atherosclerosis.

If have been found to have a high blood cholesterol level but are otherwise in a good state of health, you will be advised to adopt a low-fat diet. You may also be given drugs that decrease your blood cholesterol level (*see* LIPID-LOWERING DRUGS, p.935). For people who have had a heart attack, research has shown that there may be a benefit in lowering blood cholesterol levels, even if the cholesterol level is within the average range for healthy people.

If you have atherosclerosis and are experiencing symptoms of the condition, your doctor may prescribe a drug such as aspirin to reduce the risk of blood clots forming on the damaged artery lining (*see* DRUGS THAT PREVENT BLOOD CLOTTING, p.904).

If you are thought to be at high risk of severe complications, your doctor may recommend surgical treatment, such as coronary angioplasty (p.409), in which a balloon is inflated inside the artery to widen it and improve blood flow. If blood flow to the heart is severely obstructed (*see* CORONARY ARTERY DISEASE, p.405), you may have a bypass operation (*see* CORONARY ARTERY BYPASS GRAFT, p.411) to restore blood flow.

WHAT IS THE PROGNOSIS?

A healthy diet and lifestyle can slow the development of atherosclerosis in most people. If you do have a myocardial infarction or a stroke, you can reduce the risk of developing further complications by taking preventive measures (*see* LIFE AFTER A HEART ATTACK, p.412).

(WWW) ONLINE SITES: p.1032

Hypertension

Persistent high blood pressure that may damage the arteries and the heart

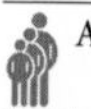 AGE More common with increasing age

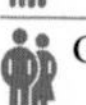 GENDER Slightly more common in males

 GENETICS Often runs in families; more common in black people

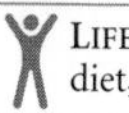 LIFESTYLE Stress, alcohol abuse, a high-salt diet, and excess weight are risk factors

In the UK, about 1 in 6 adults has persistent high blood pressure, also known as hypertension. The condition puts strain on the heart and arteries, resulting in damage to delicate tissues. If it is left untreated, hypertension may eventually affect the eyes and kidneys. The higher the blood pressure, the greater the risk that complications such as heart attacks (*see* MYOCARDIAL INFARCTION, p.410), coronary artery disease (p.405), and stroke (p.532) will develop.

Blood pressure varies naturally with activity, rising during exercise or stress and falling during rest. It also varies among individuals, gradually increasing with age and weight. Blood pressure is expressed as two values given in units of millimetres of mercury (mmHg). The blood pressure of a resting, healthy young adult should not be more than 120/80 mmHg. In general, a person is considered to have hypertension when his or her blood pressure is persistently higher than 140/90 mmHg, even at rest.

Hypertension does not usually cause symptoms, but, if your blood pressure is very high, you may have headaches,

TEST BLOOD PRESSURE MEASUREMENT

Blood pressure measurement is a routine part of having a physical examination. A measuring device called a sphygmomanometer gives a blood pressure reading as systolic pressure (the higher figure) when the heart contracts and diastolic pressure when the heart relaxes. A healthy young adult has a blood pressure of about 120/80 mmHg. Your blood pressure may be taken when you are sitting, standing, or lying down.

During the procedure
An inflatable cuff is wrapped around your upper arm and inflated using a bulb. The cuff is slowly deflated while the doctor listens to the blood flow through an artery in your arm using a stethoscope.

Sphygmomanometer

Inflatable cuff

Stethoscope

Bulb
The doctor uses the bulb to inflate and deflate the cuff

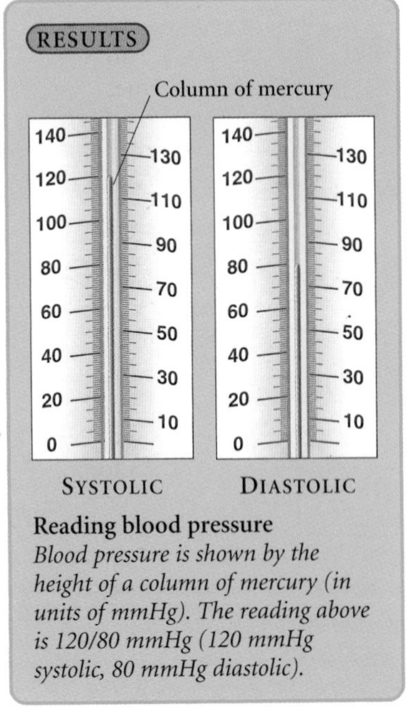

Reading blood pressure
Blood pressure is shown by the height of a column of mercury (in units of mmHg). The reading above is 120/80 mmHg (120 mmHg systolic, 80 mmHg diastolic).

dizziness, or blurred vision. However, usually the only symptoms that develop are those due to the damage caused by hypertension. By the time these arise and hypertension becomes evident, irreversible damage to arteries and organs has occurred. Hypertension is sometimes called the "silent killer" because individuals may have a fatal stroke or heart attack without warning.

In the last 20 years, health education and screening programmes have led to many more people being diagnosed with hypertension at an early stage before symptoms occur. Early diagnosis, together with improved treatments, have substantially reduced the incidence of heart attacks and strokes.

WHAT ARE THE CAUSES?

In about 9 in 10 people with hypertension, there is no obvious cause for the condition. However, both lifestyle and genetic factors may contribute. The condition is most common in middle-aged and elderly people because the arteries become more rigid with age. It is also marginally more common in men. People who are overweight or who drink excessive amounts of alcohol are more likely to develop hypertension, and a stressful lifestyle may aggravate the condition. Although hypertension occurs most often in developed countries, it is now a significant problem in the developing world too. The tendency to develop hypertension is thought to be inherited, and black people are more susceptible to the condition. The condition is rare in countries where people typically have a low-salt diet, suggesting that salt may be a contributing factor.

In a minority of cases, an underlying cause of the hypertension is identified, such as kidney disease or a hormonal disorder, such as hyperaldosteronism (p.685) or Cushing's syndrome (p.684). Some drugs, such as combined oral contraceptives and corticosteroids (p.930), can cause hypertension.

In pregnant women, hypertension can lead to the development of the potentially life-threatening conditions pre-eclampsia and eclampsia (p.794). The elevated blood pressure usually returns to normal after the birth.

ARE THERE COMPLICATIONS?

The risk of damage to the arteries, heart, and kidneys rises with the severity of hypertension and the length of time for which it is present. Arteries that have been damaged are at greater risk of becoming narrowed by atherosclerosis (p.402), in which fatty deposits build up in vessel walls, causing them to narrow and restricting blood flow.

Atherosclerosis is more likely in people who smoke or who have high blood cholesterol levels. Atherosclerosis of the coronary arteries may lead eventually to chest pain (*see* ANGINA, p.407) or to a heart attack. In other arteries in the body, atherosclerosis may result in disorders such as aortic aneurysm (p.430) or stroke. Hypertension puts strain on the heart that may eventually lead to chronic heart failure (p.413). Damage to the arteries in the kidneys may result in chronic kidney failure (p.706). The arteries supplying the retina in the eye may also be damaged by hypertension (*see* RETINOPATHY, p.579).

HOW IS IT DIAGNOSED?

It is important that you have your blood pressure measured routinely at least every 2 years after the age of 18 (*see* BLOOD PRESSURE MEASUREMENT, above). If your blood pressure is more than 140/90 mmHg, your doctor may ask you to return in a few weeks so that he or she can check it again. Some individuals become anxious when visiting their doctor, which may cause a temporary rise in blood pressure. Therefore, a diagnosis of hypertension is usually not made unless you have elevated blood pressure on three separate occasions. If your readings are variable, you may be offered a portable device to measure your blood pressure at home.

If you have hypertension, your doctor may arrange for tests that check for organ damage. Tests for heart damage include echocardiography (p.425) or electrocardiography (*see* ECG, p.406). Your eyes may be examined to look for damaged blood vessels. You may also have tests to look for other factors, such as a high blood cholesterol level, that may increase your risk of a heart attack.

If you are young or have severe hypertension, you may have tests to find the underlying cause. For example, you may have urine and blood tests and ultrasound scanning (p.250) to look for kidney disease or a hormonal disorder.

What is the treatment?

Hypertension cannot usually be cured but can be controlled with treatment. If you have mild hypertension, changing your lifestyle is often the most effective way of lowering your blood pressure. You should reduce your salt and alcohol consumption and try to keep your weight within the ideal range (*see* ARE YOU A HEALTHY WEIGHT?, p.53). If you smoke, you should give up.

If self-help measures are not effective in reducing your blood pressure, your doctor may prescribe antihypertensive drugs (p.897). These drugs work in different ways, and you may be prescribed just one type of drug or a combination of several. The type of drug and the dosage are tailored to the individual, and it may take some time to find the right combination and dosage. If you develop side effects, consult your doctor so that your medication can be adjusted. He or she may recommend that you measure your blood pressure regularly yourself to help to evaluate your treatment. You can now buy a small electronic blood pressure machine to use at home, but seek advice from your doctor first.

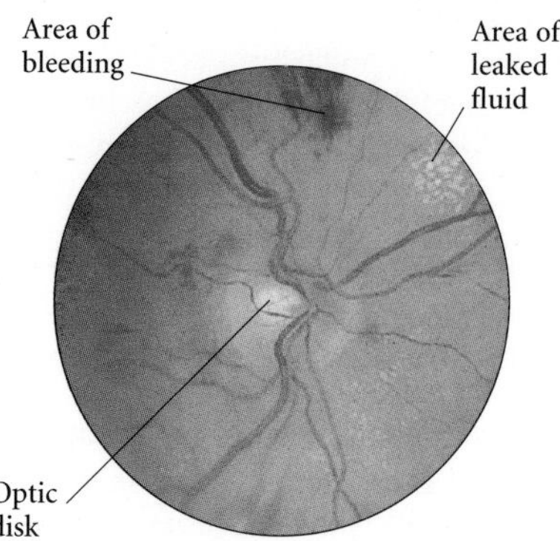

Retinal damage from hypertension
Damage to the small blood vessels in the retina at the back of the eye has resulted in blood and fluid leaking into the retina.

If your hypertension has an obvious underlying medical cause, such as a hormonal disorder, treatment of this disorder may result in your blood pressure returning to a normal level.

What is the prognosis?

The outlook depends on how high your blood pressure is and how long it has been high. For most people, lifestyle changes and drug treatment can control blood pressure and reduce the risk of complications. These measures usually need to be maintained for life. Long-standing, severe hypertension carries the greatest risk of complications.

(WWW) ONLINE SITES: p.1032

Coronary artery disease

Narrowing of the coronary arteries that supply the heart muscle with blood, leading to heart damage

AGE More common with increasing age

GENDER More common in males until the age of 60, then equal incidence

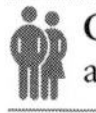
GENETICS Sometimes runs in families

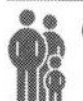
LIFESTYLE Smoking, a high-fat diet, lack of exercise, and excess weight are risk factors

The coronary arteries, which branch from the main artery in the body, the aorta, supply the heart muscle with oxygen-rich blood. In coronary artery disease (CAD), also known as coronary heart disease, one or more of the coronary arteries is narrowed. Blood flow through the arteries is restricted, leading to damage to the heart muscle. Heart disorders, including heart attacks (*see* MYOCARDIAL INFARCTION, p.410) and the chest pain of angina (p.407), are usually caused by CAD. The condition is therefore a leading cause of death in many developed countries. The number of deaths from CAD reached its peak in the UK in the early 1980s, with about 85 people per 100,000 dying each year. The death rate from CAD has since fallen by more than half as a result of health education about smoking and diet and the introduction of more effective treatments. However, in many parts of the world, including some developing countries, mortality from CAD is rising as a result of changing lifestyle factors.

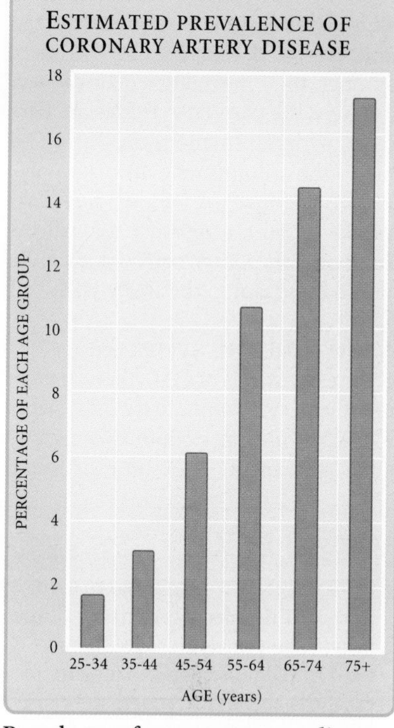

Prevalence of coronary artery disease
The percentage of people (the prevalence) affected by coronary artery disease, which causes restricted blood supply to the heart, steadily increases with age. More than 1 in 6 people over the age of 65 is affected.

What are the causes?

Coronary artery disease is usually due to atherosclerosis (p.402), a condition in which fatty deposits accumulate on the inside of the artery walls. These deposits narrow the arteries and restrict blood flow. If a blood clot forms or lodges in the narrowed area of an artery, the vessel can become completely blocked. CAD caused by atherosclerosis is more likely if your blood cholesterol level is high and you eat a high-fat diet. CAD is also linked to smoking, obesity, lack of exercise, diabetes mellitus (p.687), and high blood pressure (*see* HYPERTENSION, p.403).

In women, the hormone oestrogen may reduce the risk of developing CAD.

After the menopause, oestrogen levels fall, and by the age of 60 women have the same risk of developing CAD as men, although their mortality remains lower.

Rarely, the coronary arteries are narrowed by inflammation, which may be due to the autoimmune disorder polyarteritis nodosa (p.465) or Kawasaki disease (p.837), a disorder that affects children. Temporary narrowing can be caused by spasm in the artery wall.

What are the symptoms?

In the early stages of CAD, there are frequently no symptoms. In the later stages of CAD, the first symptom is usually either pain in the chest on exertion, a condition known as angina, or a heart attack. Some people with CAD develop an abnormality of the heart rhythm (*see* ARRHYTHMIAS, p.415), which may cause palpitations (awareness of heartbeats), light-headedness, and, sometimes, loss of consciousness. Some severe forms of arrhythmia can cause the heart to stop pumping completely (*see* CARDIAC ARREST, p.419), which accounts for most of the sudden deaths from CAD.

In elderly people, CAD may lead to a condition called chronic heart failure (p.413), in which the heart gradually becomes too weak to provide an adequate circulation of blood around the body. Chronic heart failure may then lead to the accumulation of excess fluid in the lungs and tissues, causing additional symptoms such as shortness of breath and swollen ankles.

How is it diagnosed?

CAD is usually diagnosed only when a person develops symptoms of the disease. Sometimes, a heart attack is the first sign. If you have symptoms that suggest CAD, such as chest pain, your doctor may arrange a series of tests to establish the severity of the problem. These tests include an ECG (left) to monitor the heart's electrical activity and radionuclide scanning (p.251) to show whether the blood supply to the heart muscle is adequate. You may have exercise testing (opposite page) to see how the heart performs under stress, as well as echocardiography (p.425), an ultrasound technique that images the heart muscle and valves. The imaging technique MRI (p.248) is increasingly used to detect heart abnormalities.

If these tests suggest that the blood supply to your heart is inadequate, you may be referred for coronary angiography (p.408), in which a dye is injected into the bloodstream to enable arteries to be seen on an X-ray. Angiography detects blocked or seriously narrowed sections of an artery and provides your doctor with the information he or she needs to decide whether or not surgical treatment is required.

What is the treatment?

Treatment for CAD falls into three categories: lifestyle changes to reduce the risk of CAD becoming worse, drug treatments to improve the function of the heart and help to relieve symptoms, and surgical procedures, such as coronary angioplasty (p.409), that improve the blood supply to the heart muscle.

If you are diagnosed as having CAD, you should adopt a healthier lifestyle, with a low-fat diet and regular exercise. If you smoke, you should stop.

The drugs used to treat CAD depend on your symptoms and their severity and on the cause of the disorder. If tests show that you have a high blood cholesterol level, you will be treated with lipid-lowering drugs (p.935). However, these may be prescribed even if you eat a diet low in fat and your cholesterol levels are within the acceptable range.

TEST ECG

ECG (electrocardiography) is used to record the electrical activity of the heart. The procedure is frequently used to diagnose abnormal heart rhythms and to investigate the cause of chest pain. Several electrodes are attached to the skin to transmit the electrical activity of the heart to an ECG machine. Several traces are produced at the same time. Each trace shows electrical activity in different areas of the heart. The test usually takes several minutes to complete and is safe and painless.

Technician

During the procedure
Small electrodes are attached to your chest, wrists, and ankles while you rest on a bed. Signals from the electrodes produce a trace.

Chest electrode

Trace

ECG machine

Ankle electrode

RESULTS

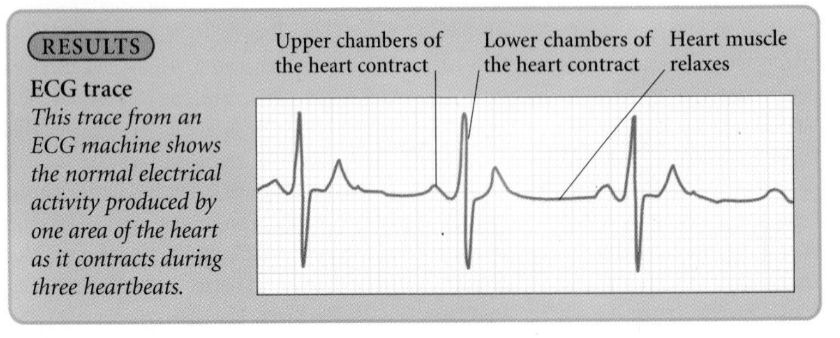

ECG trace
This trace from an ECG machine shows the normal electrical activity produced by one area of the heart as it contracts during three heartbeats.

TEST EXERCISE TESTING

Exercise testing is usually done when coronary artery disease is suspected. It is used to assess the function of the heart when it is put under stress. The test involves raising your heart rate by exercising, generally using a treadmill with an adjustable slope or an exercise bicycle, and monitoring the heart's function. The exercise is tailored to ensure that your heart is tested adequately without putting you at risk. Various monitoring methods may be used, including radionuclide scanning (p.251), which can image the heart's function, and ECG, which monitors the heart's electrical activity.

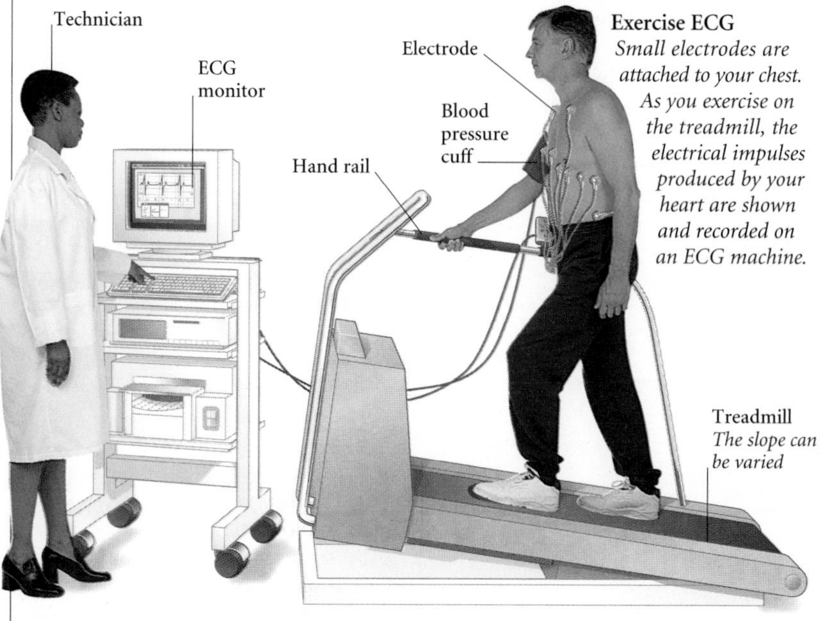

Exercise ECG
Small electrodes are attached to your chest. As you exercise on the treadmill, the electrical impulses produced by your heart are shown and recorded on an ECG machine.

RESULTS

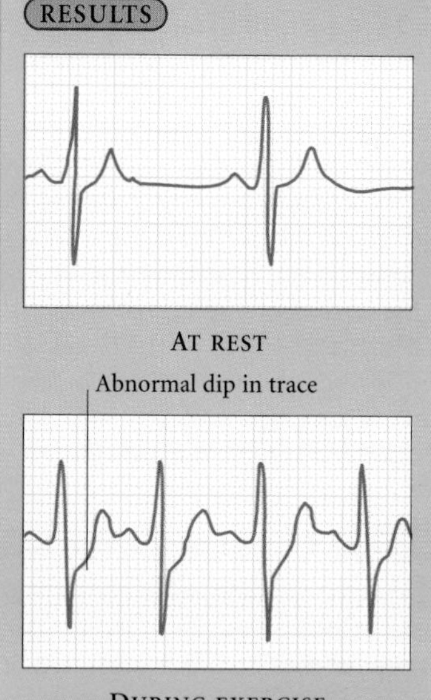

ECG tracing
These traces are from a person with coronary artery disease. At rest, the ECG trace is normal (top). During exercise, when the heart beats faster and requires more oxygen, the trace becomes abnormal (bottom), showing an exaggerated downward dip.

This is because treatment with lipid-lowering drugs slows the progression of CAD and, as a consequence, reduces the risk of a heart attack.

Angina may be treated with drugs, such as nitrate drugs (p.899) and beta-blocker drugs (p.898), that improve the blood flow through the arteries and help the heart to pump effectively. An abnormal heart rhythm is often treated using antiarrhythmic drugs (p.898).

If treatment fails to relieve the symptoms or if there is extensive narrowing of the arteries, your doctor will discuss several treatment options with you. If only small segments of the artery are affected, you may be offered coronary angioplasty, in which a balloon is inflated in the narrowed area of the affected blood vessel in order to widen it. During the procedure, a small hollow tube called a stent may be inserted into the affected artery to keep it open. Alternatively, your doctor may suggest a coronary artery bypass graft (p.411). In this procedure, blockages in one or more coronary arteries are bypassed using an artery on the inside of the chest wall or veins taken from a leg.

WHAT IS THE PROGNOSIS?

Coronary artery disease affects people in middle to old age and is more easily prevented than treated. The chance of developing the disease can be reduced by following a healthy lifestyle. More efficient methods of diagnosing CAD and screening for risk factors also make it possible to begin treatment early in the course of the disease. Effective drugs to prevent the progression of CAD and the success of both coronary angioplasty and bypass grafting have greatly improved the prognosis for CAD.

For an individual with CAD, the outlook depends on the number of blood vessels involved and how extensively the heart muscle is damaged when the condition is diagnosed.

WWW ONLINE SITES: p.1032

Angina

Pain in the chest, usually brought on by exertion and relieved by rest

 AGE More common with increasing age

 GENDER More common in males until the age of 60, then equal incidence

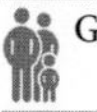 GENETICS Sometimes runs in families

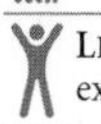 LIFESTYLE Smoking, a high-fat diet, lack of exercise, and excess weight are risk factors

Angina is chest pain that originates in the heart muscle during physical activity and is quickly relieved by rest. The pain is due to an inadequate supply of blood to the heart muscle. Angina affects both sexes but is less common in women under 60 because the hormone oestrogen protects against it. This protection gradually disappears when levels of oestrogen drop after the menopause.

Over the last 30 years, angina has become progressively less common in western Europe, mainly due to people adopting a healthy lifestyle. At the same time, treatment with drugs and surgery has improved the outlook for people who have the condition.

What are the causes?

The most common cause of angina is coronary artery disease (p.405), a narrowing of the arteries that supply the heart muscle. This narrowing is usually the result of fatty deposits building up on the inside of the artery walls (*see* ATHEROSCLEROSIS, p.402). The blood flow through the arteries may be sufficient for the heart while it is at rest but becomes inadequate during exertion. If the supply of oxygen-rich blood is insufficient, the heart muscle is starved of oxygen and toxic substances build up in the heart muscle, causing a constrictive, cramp-like pain. People who have a high blood cholesterol level (*see* HYPERCHOLESTEROLAEMIA, p.691), persistently high blood pressure (*see* HYPERTENSION, p.403), or diabetes mellitus (p.687) have an increased risk of developing atherosclerosis and angina. Having a close relative with the disorder also increases the risk of angina, as does smoking.

Angina can also be caused by temporary spasm of the coronary arteries, in which the arteries narrow for a short time, or by a damaged heart valve that causes a reduction in the blood flow to the heart muscle (*see* AORTIC STENOSIS, p.423). A rare cause of angina is anaemia, in which the ability of the blood to carry oxygen is impaired. This reduces the supply of oxygen to the heart.

What are the symptoms?

The chest pain of angina varies from mild to severe. It usually starts during exertion and is relieved after a short rest. The features of angina are:

- A dull, heavy, constricting sensation in the centre of the chest.
- A discomfort that spreads into the throat and down one or both arms, more often the left arm.

Angina usually occurs predictably at a particular level of exertion. For example, if you regularly walk uphill or climb stairs, the pain of angina will develop at about the same stage of the activity each time. Angina brought on by outdoor exertion often occurs more rapidly in cold or windy weather.

If you experience this type of chest pain for the first time or if your angina becomes more frequent or develops at rest, you should contact your doctor immediately. Worsening angina can be a warning that a blood clot has formed in the coronary artery, which may completely block it and cause a heart attack (*see* MYOCARDIAL INFARCTION, p.410). A prolonged and very severe attack of angina may be due to a heart attack.

How is it diagnosed?

Your doctor will usually make a diagnosis of angina from your symptoms. However, in some circumstances it may be difficult for your doctor to be certain that the pain is angina and is not caused by a gastrointestinal problem such as gastro-oesophageal reflux (p.636).

Your doctor will measure your blood pressure to see if you have hypertension (p.403). He or she may also arrange for you to have blood tests to check for anaemia or raised cholesterol levels. You will probably have an ECG (p.406) to monitor the electrical activity of the heart at rest and exercise testing (p.407) as a comparison. The ECG may show no abnormalities, but the exercise test will usually be abnormal if you have angina. The ECG may confirm that you have had a heart attack. If the tests confirm that there is a significant problem

TEST CORONARY ANGIOGRAPHY

Coronary angiography is used to image the arteries that supply the heart muscle with blood. Angiography can image narrowed or blocked coronary arteries, which are not visible on a normal X-ray. A local anaesthetic is injected, and a fine, flexible catheter is passed into the femoral artery, through the aorta, and into a coronary artery. Contrast dye is injected through the catheter, and a series of X-rays is taken. The procedure is painless, but you may feel a flushing sensation as the dye is injected.

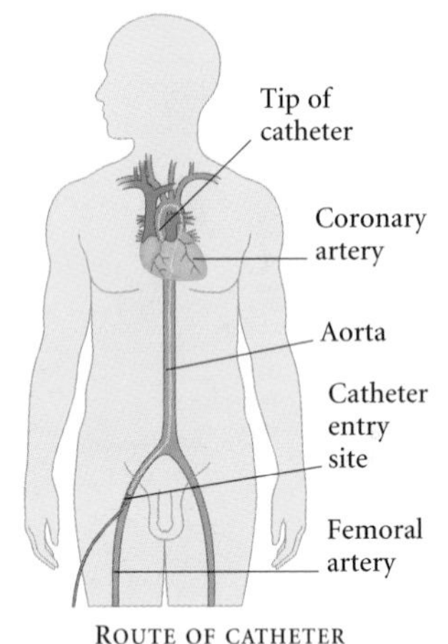

ROUTE OF CATHETER

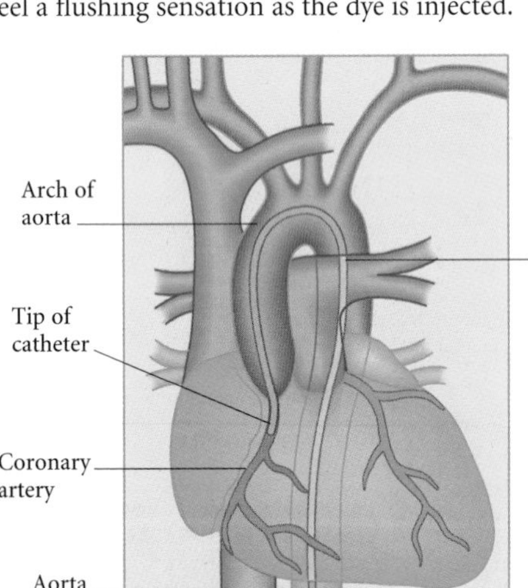

During the procedure
The catheter is positioned in the heart so that its tip rests in a coronary artery, and contrast dye is then injected. The artery and the small vessels leading from it are visualized by a series of X-rays. The catheter may be repositioned and the procedure repeated to check all the coronary arteries.

RESULTS

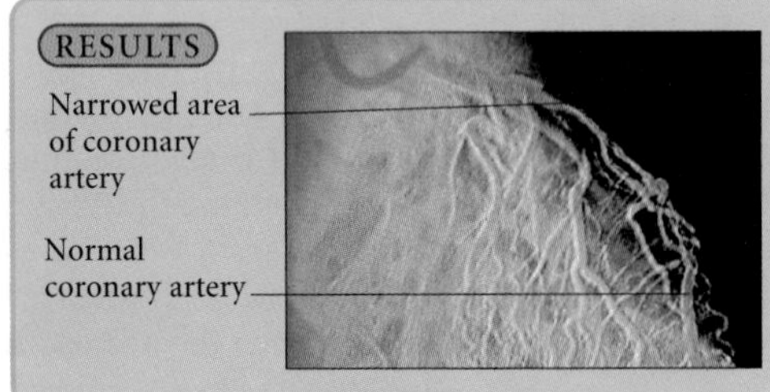

Coronary artery disease
This angiogram of the heart shows a section of coronary artery that has become narrowed by coronary artery disease, restricting blood flow.

(TREATMENT) CORONARY ANGIOPLASTY

Coronary angioplasty is used to widen coronary arteries that are narrowed or blocked by fatty deposits. The technique may be carried out at the same time as coronary angiography (opposite page). Under local anaesthesia, a guide wire is inserted through the femoral artery in the groin and up into the affected coronary artery. A balloon catheter is passed up the wire, and the balloon is inflated in the narrowed area to widen it. Sometimes, a metal tube called a stent is inserted afterwards to keep the artery open.

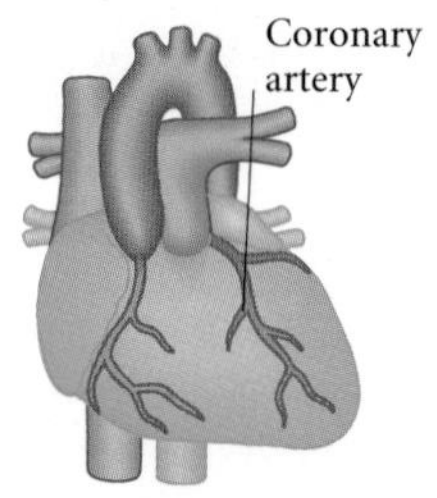

LOCATION

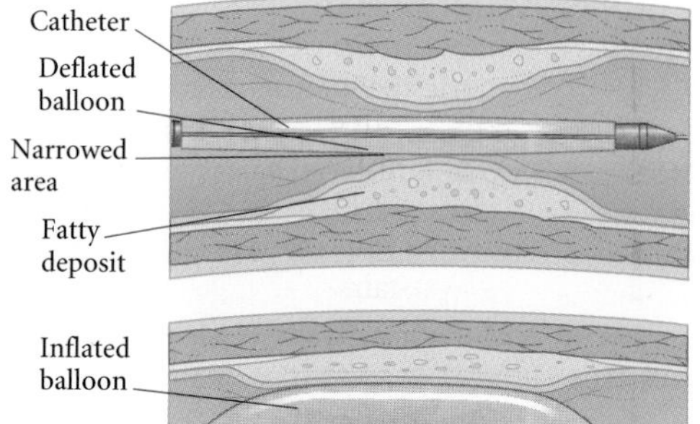

1 A catheter with a deflated balloon attached to its tip is threaded into the artery. The catheter is placed precisely so that the balloon is inside the narrowed area of the coronary artery.

Inflated balloon
Compressed fatty deposit

2 The balloon is inflated and deflated several times in order to compress the deposits and widen the narrowed area. The catheter is then withdrawn. A small tube (stent) may be inserted to keep the artery open.

(RESULTS)

Effect of treatment
X-rays using contrast dye are taken before and after coronary angioplasty. These images show that the blocked artery has been widened successfully and blood flow improved.

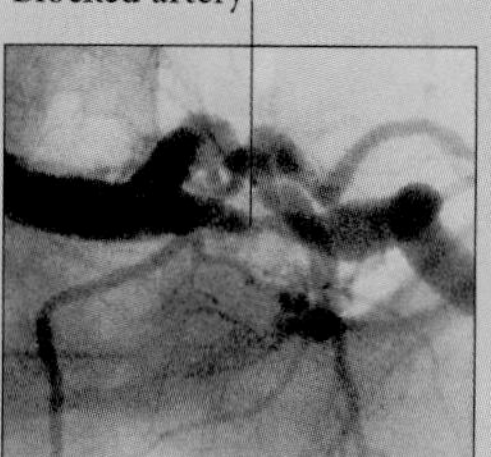

BEFORE TREATMENT

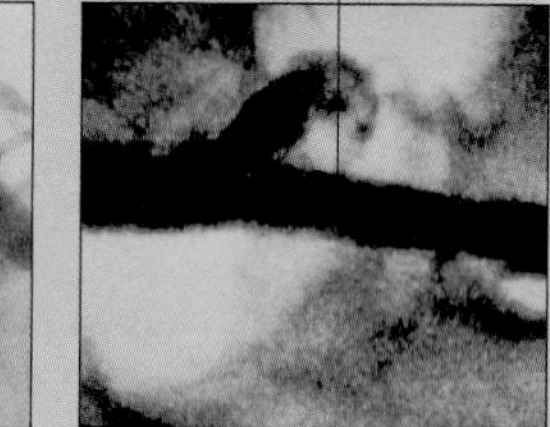

AFTER TREATMENT

with blood flow to the heart, you may need coronary angiography (opposite page), in which dye is injected into the coronary arteries so that narrowed areas can be detected on an X-ray.

WHAT IS THE TREATMENT?

The treatment of angina depends on its severity. Drugs are used to relieve acute episodes of pain and also to reduce the number and severity of attacks. Drug treatment of an acute attack of angina usually includes nitrate drugs (p.899) to widen the coronary arteries. Fast-acting nitrates can be administered in the form of a spray or soluble tablets. Longer-acting nitrates can be taken on a regular basis to prevent attacks from occurring. In addition, drugs may be used to reduce the heart's need for oxygen (*see* BETA-BLOCKERS, p.898). Doctors also advise that a daily low dose of aspirin be taken (*see* DRUGS THAT PREVENT BLOOD CLOTTING, p.904) because this makes the blood less sticky and reduces the risk of clots forming in an artery. If there is an underlying disorder contributing to the angina, such as aortic stenosis, hypertension, or diabetes mellitus, it will be treated.

Lifestyle changes can prevent worsening of angina and increase the level of exercise that you can achieve without experiencing pain. It is imperative that you stop smoking; cutting down is not sufficient. A diet that is low in saturated fat is important, and, if necessary, you should try to lose weight (*see* CONTROLLING YOUR WEIGHT, p.53). You may also be prescribed drugs to lower your blood cholesterol level (*see* LIPID-LOWERING DRUGS, p.935), even if it is within the normal range, because these drugs have been shown to slow down the progress of coronary artery disease. You should take as much regular exercise as you can within the limits prescribed by your doctor. Walking as little as 1.5–3 km (1–2 miles) every day can be enough to reduce the risk of a fatal heart attack.

If angina becomes more severe in spite of drug treatment, your doctor may advise you to consider surgery to either widen the arteries or improve the blood flow to the heart. You may have coronary angioplasty (left), in which a small balloon is placed within the narrowed area of artery and then inflated to widen it. Angioplasty is a straightforward procedure that normally requires only same-day or overnight admission to hospital. However, it is rarely suitable if several coronary arteries are narrowed, in which case you will probably be advised to have a coronary artery bypass graft (p.411), in which an artery inside the chest wall or a vein taken from a leg is used to bypass the diseased areas in the arteries. Coronary artery bypass grafting is a major surgical procedure that requires a brief stay in an intensive care unit (p.958) because it carries a small risk of complications. You will need 2–3 months of convalescence.

WHAT IS THE PROGNOSIS?

The outlook depends on the extent of coronary artery disease. If you have mild angina, the outlook is good provided that you make sensible changes to your lifestyle and follow treatment recommendations. People often have no further symptoms once treatment has started, and many are able to live a normal life apart from some restrictions on exercise. If you are otherwise in good health, you have a 1 in 2 chance of surviving for at least 10–12 years. If the arteries are badly damaged, the outlook is less favourable.

(WWW) ONLINE SITES: p.1032

Myocardial infarction

Loss of blood supply to part of the heart muscle due to a blockage in a coronary artery, commonly known as heart attack

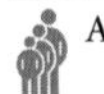 AGE More common with increasing age

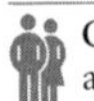 GENDER More common in males until the age of 60, then equal incidence

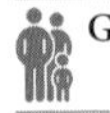 GENETICS Sometimes runs in families

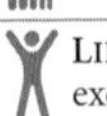 LIFESTYLE Smoking, a high-fat diet, lack of exercise, and excess weight are risk factors

Heart attack or "coronary" are common terms for the disorder myocardial infarction, which means, literally, death of part of the heart muscle following a blockage in its blood supply. Myocardial infarction is one of the major causes of death in developed countries such as the UK. However, the mortality rates have fallen significantly since the early 1980s due to recent improvements in treatment and an increasing awareness that following a healthier lifestyle helps to prevent heart attacks.

What are the causes?

Myocardial infarction is usually a result of coronary artery disease (p.405). In this condition, the coronary arteries that supply the heart muscle with fresh oxygenated blood become narrowed. This narrowing is usually due to atherosclerosis (p.402), in which droplets of fatty substances, such as cholesterol, build up on the inside of the artery wall. These substances form deposits called atheroma, which then become covered with a fibrous layer that may rupture or become roughened. Blood cells called platelets can stick to the rough or damaged area and trigger the formation of a blood clot. Once formed, the clot may completely block blood flow through the artery, leading to a heart attack.

If you have a family history of coronary artery disease (CAD), you are at increased risk of having a heart attack, especially if one or more members of your family developed CAD or had a heart attack under the age of 55. The risk is also increased if you have raised blood pressure (*see* HYPERTENSION, p.403) or cardiovascular problems as a result of diabetes mellitus (p.687).

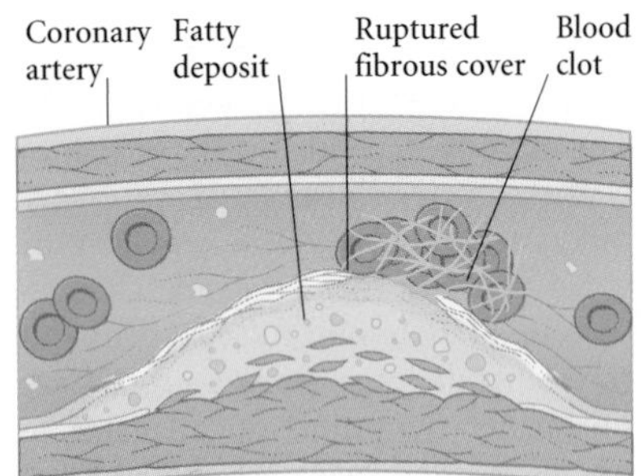

Cause of myocardial infarction

If a coronary artery is narrowed by a fatty deposit, the fibrous cover of the deposit may rupture, triggering the formation of a blood clot. If this clot blocks the artery, blood flow to an area of heart muscle stops, causing a myocardial infarction.

What are the symptoms?

The symptoms of a heart attack usually develop suddenly and may include:

- Severe, heavy, crushing pain in the centre of the chest that may spread up to the neck and into the arms, especially the left arm.
- Pallor and sweating.
- Shortness of breath.
- Nausea and, sometimes, vomiting.
- Anxiety, sometimes accompanied by a fear of dying.
- Restlessness.

If you develop these symptoms, you should always assume that you are having a heart attack and require urgent medical attention. Do not delay calling an ambulance to "see how things go" because this delay may be fatal. A well-equipped emergency ambulance is the most appropriate means of transportation to hospital because life-saving treatment may be required on the journey. While waiting for the ambulance, you should chew half an aspirin tablet if possible. Aspirin reduces the stickiness of the blood to prevent further clotting.

Sometimes, a myocardial infarction may cause a different pattern of symptoms. If you have been suffering from the chest pain of angina (p.407), your pain may have been getting steadily worse and may have been occurring at rest as well as on exertion. An episode of angina that does not respond to your usual treatment or one that lasts longer than 10 minutes may be a myocardial infarction and needs immediate emergency hospital treatment.

About 1 in 5 people does not have chest pain in a heart attack. However, there may be other symptoms, such as breathlessness, faintness, sweating, and pale skin. This pattern of symptoms is known as a "silent infarction". This type of heart attack is more common in elderly people and those with diabetes.

Are there complications?

In the first few hours and days after a heart attack, the main risks are the development of an irregular heartbeat, which may be life-threatening, or a cardiac arrest (p.419). Depending on the extent and site of the damaged muscle, other problems may develop. For example, in the weeks or months after the attack, the pumping action of the heart muscle may be too weak, leading to a condition called heart failure (*see* ACUTE HEART FAILURE, and CHRONIC HEART FAILURE, pp.412–413). Less common complications include damage to one of the heart valves (*see* MITRAL INCOMPETENCE, p.423) or inflammation of the membrane covering the heart's surface (*see* PERICARDITIS, p.428). Both these conditions may also lead to the development of heart failure.

How is it diagnosed?

In many cases, the diagnosis is obvious. An ECG (p.406), which is a tracing of the electrical activity of the heart, often shows changes that confirm myocardial infarction. The ECG can be valuable in assessing which part and how much of the heart muscle has been damaged and will establish whether the heart rhythm is still normal or is irregular. To confirm the diagnosis, blood samples may be taken to measure the levels of particular chemicals that leak into the blood from damaged heart muscle.

What is the treatment?

The immediate aims of treatment for myocardial infarction are to relieve pain and restore the blood supply to the heart muscle to minimize the amount of damage and prevent further complications. These aims are best achieved by immediate admission to an intensive care unit (p.958), where your heart rhythm and vital clinical signs can be monitored continuously. If you have severe chest pain, you will probably be given an injection of a powerful painkilling drug (p.912), such as morphine.

Within the first 6 hours of the attack, you may also be given a thrombolytic

TREATMENT CORONARY ARTERY BYPASS GRAFT

During this procedure, one or more narrowed coronary arteries are bypassed using blood vessels from the legs or chest. The operation takes about 2 hours. In most cases, the heart is stopped and a heart–lung machine is used to take over the function of the heart during surgery (*see* SURGERY USING A HEART–LUNG MACHINE, p.953). However, a less invasive technique using endoscopic surgery is being used increasingly. Afterwards, you will be monitored in an intensive care unit for several days.

MAMMARY ARTERY BYPASS GRAFT

If there is only one blockage in a coronary artery, one of the internal mammary arteries within the chest, usually the left artery, is used to create the bypass. Artery grafts are preferable to vein grafts because they are better able to take the pressure of the blood that normally flows through the coronary arteries and are less likely to become blocked over time.

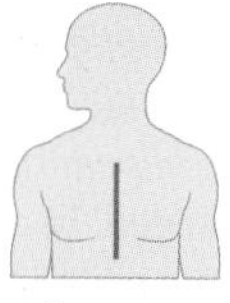

SITE OF INCISION

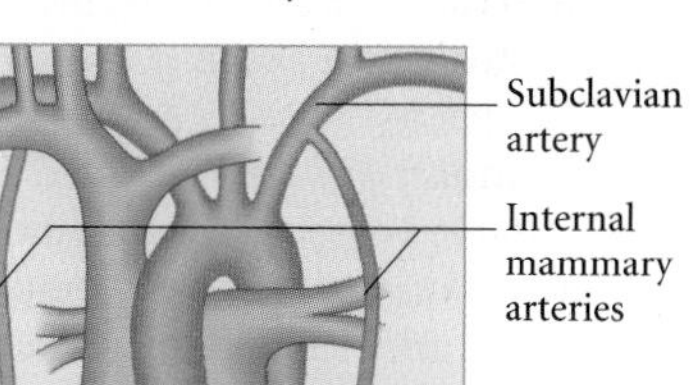

1 *The left internal mammary artery is cut where shown above. The upper end is left attached to the subclavian artery and the lower end is tied off.*

Blockage
Diverted artery joined to coronary artery
Tied end of mammary artery

2 *The free end of the mammary artery is connected to the coronary artery at a point beyond the blockage to supply blood to the heart muscle there.*

SAPHENOUS VEIN BYPASS GRAFT

If more than one blockage in a coronary artery needs to be bypassed or if the internal mammary artery is not suitable, sections of the saphenous vein (the vein that runs the length of the leg) are used after first being reversed. Sometimes, the vein is used in addition to the mammary artery, although vein grafts tend to become obstructed more quickly than arterial grafts.

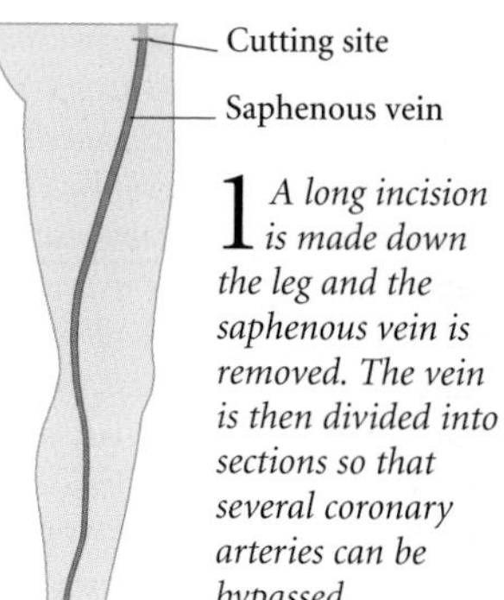

1 *A long incision is made down the leg and the saphenous vein is removed. The vein is then divided into sections so that several coronary arteries can be bypassed.*

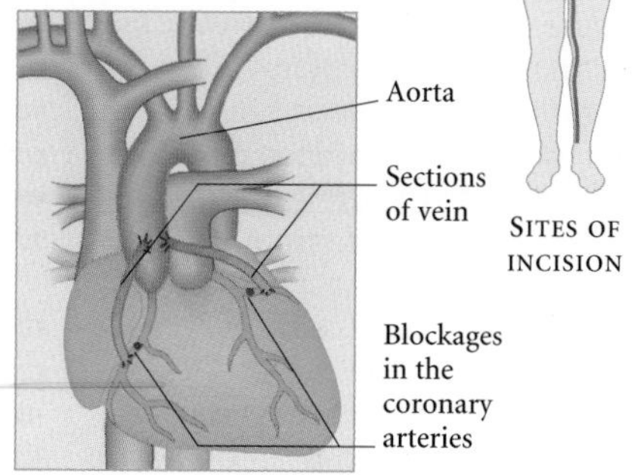

2 *Sections of the saphenous vein are used to bypass the blockages. One end of each section is attached to the aorta, and the other is attached to the coronary artery beyond a blockage.*

SITES OF INCISION

drug (p.904) to dissolve the blood clot that is blocking the coronary artery. Alternatively, you may have immediate coronary angioplasty (p.409) to widen the narrowed artery. If the blood flow to the damaged heart muscle can be restored within 6 hours, there is a greater likelihood of full recovery.

While you are in the coronary care unit, your heartbeat is monitored, and treatment is given if arrhythmias or symptoms of heart failure develop. If your progress is satisfactory, you will be allowed out of bed briefly after 24–48 hours. Soon afterwards, you can begin a rehabilitation programme, during which you are encouraged to spend gradually longer periods out of bed.

Once you have recovered from the attack, the condition of your coronary arteries and heart muscle is assessed. Tests such as echocardiography (p.425) and exercise electrocardiography (*see* EXERCISE TESTING, p.407) are used to help to decide on further treatment. For example, if the pumping action of the heart is impaired, you may be prescribed an ACE inhibitor (p.900) and/or a diuretic drug (p.902). If a coronary artery is blocked, you may need bypass surgery at a later stage (*see* CORONARY ARTERY BYPASS GRAFT, left). If tests reveal a persistent irregular heartbeat, you may need to have a pacemaker implanted in your chest (*see* CARDIAC PACEMAKER, p.419).

Certain drugs taken long-term can reduce the risk of another heart attack, and you may be prescribed a beta-blocker drug (p.898) and/or aspirin for this reason. You may also be advised to adopt a low-fat diet and to take lipid-lowering drugs (p.935) to lower your blood cholesterol level. These drugs are beneficial after a heart attack even if your cholesterol level is not elevated.

WHAT CAN I DO?

It is important to follow your doctor's advice about how soon to return to normal activities. It is natural to feel worried about your health, and many people experience some mild depression (p.554). It is important to avoid becoming disabled by the fear that you may have another heart attack. Many hospitals offer ongoing cardiac rehabilitation programmes after discharge from hospital to help people regain their confidence and share their experiences.

WHAT IS THE PROGNOSIS?

If you have not had a previous myocardial infarction, you are treated quickly, and there are no complications, the outlook is good. After 2 weeks, the risk of another heart attack is considerably reduced, and you have a good chance of living for another 10 years at least. The outlook is better if you stop smoking, reduce alcohol intake, exercise regularly, and follow a healthy diet.

If you have experienced a previous heart attack, the outlook depends on the amount of heart muscle that was damaged and whether you have additional complications. However, many people who have surgery or angioplasty live for 10 years or more.

(WWW) ONLINE SITES: p.1032

(SELF-HELP) LIFE AFTER A HEART ATTACK

Making changes in your lifestyle after a heart attack can help to speed your recovery and to reduce the risk of another attack:

- Stop smoking. This is the single most important factor in preventing a further attack.
- Eat a healthy diet and try to keep your weight within the ideal range for your height and build (*see* DIET AND HEALTH, p.48).
- If you drink alcohol, take only moderate amounts. You should have no more than 1–2 small glasses of wine or beer a day.
- Together with your doctor, agree on a programme of increasing exercise until you are able to engage in moderate exercise, such as swimming regularly, for 30 minutes or more at a time.

After a period of recovery, you can make a gradual return to your normal daily routine:

- You will probably be able to return to work within 8–12 weeks, or sooner if you have a desk job. You might consider working part-time at first.
- Try to avoid stressful situations.
- You should be able to drive a car within 4 weeks.
- You can resume having sexual intercourse about 4 weeks after a heart attack.

Acute heart failure

Sudden deterioration in the pumping action of the heart, usually leading to accumulation of fluid in the lungs

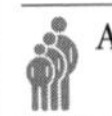 AGE More common over the age of 65

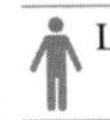 LIFESTYLE Risk factors depend on the cause

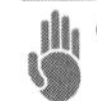 GENDER GENETICS Not significant factors

Heart failure is the term used when the heart's ability to pump efficiently is reduced. In acute heart failure, the condition develops suddenly, often due to a severe heart attack. In most cases, only the left side of the heart is affected by acute heart failure. This side of the heart receives blood rich in oxygen directly from the lungs and pumps it to the rest of the body. If acute heart failure develops, a back-up of blood occurs in the blood vessels leading from the lungs to the heart. Back pressure then causes fluid to accumulate in the lungs. This build-up of fluid is called pulmonary oedema, and, if it is not treated immediately, is life-threatening.

WHAT ARE THE CAUSES?

Acute heart failure may develop in people with complete heart block (p.418) or people with chronic heart failure (opposite page) if the weakened heart is put under strain. For example, a severe infection, such as pneumonia (p.490), may increase the workload on the heart and lead to acute heart failure. Another common cause of acute heart failure is a severe myocardial infarction (p.410) that damages a large area of heart muscle. The condition may also be caused by an acute infection of a heart valve (*see* INFECTIVE ENDOCARDITIS, p.426).

Right-sided acute heart failure is rare and is usually due to a blood clot blocking the pulmonary artery, which is the blood vessel that leads from the lungs to the right side of the heart (*see* PULMONARY EMBOLISM, p.495).

WHAT ARE THE SYMPTOMS?

The symptoms of acute heart failure usually develop rapidly and include:

- Severe shortness of breath.
- Wheezing.
- Cough with pink, frothy sputum.
- Pale skin and sweating.

Fluid in lung tissue

Heart

Normal area of lung

Lung oedema in acute heart failure
In acute heart failure, fluid accumulates rapidly in both lungs (a condition known as pulmonary oedema). This results in extreme shortness of breath.

If acute heart failure is caused by a heart attack, you may have additional symptoms such as intense, prolonged chest pain and feelings of anxiety. If heart failure is caused by a pulmonary embolism, you may cough up blood and have sharp chest pain that is worse when inhaling. If acute heart failure is not treated, it can cause dangerously low blood pressure (*see* SHOCK, p.414), and the condition may then be fatal.

WHAT MIGHT BE DONE?

Acute heart failure is a medical emergency and requires immediate hospital treatment. You will be treated sitting up and may be given oxygen through a face mask and diuretic drugs (p.902) intravenously to reduce fluid in the lungs. You may have electrocardiography (*see* ECG, p.406) and echocardiography (p.425) to assess your heart function and to look for the cause of heart failure, and a chest X-ray (p.490) to confirm the presence of fluid in the lungs. When your symptoms are under control, you may have coronary angiography (p.408) to look for blockages in the coronary arteries supplying the heart muscle.

Long-term treatments will focus on the underlying cause. When the cause cannot be treated, drugs such as ACE inhibitors (p.900) and digitalis drugs (p.901) may be given to help to prevent recurrence and slow deterioration in heart function. However, in spite of these treatments, the condition may be progressive and so be fatal.

(WWW) ONLINE SITES: p.1032

Chronic heart failure

Long-standing inefficient pumping action of the heart, leading to poor circulation of blood and accumulation of fluid in tissues

 AGE More common over the age of 65

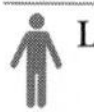 LIFESTYLE Risk factors depend on the cause

 GENDER GENETICS Not significant factors

In chronic heart failure, the heart is unable to pump blood around the body effectively, leading to a gradual build-up of fluid in the lungs and body tissues. Chronic heart failure is a common progressive condition that may be so mild at first that symptoms go unnoticed. It mostly affects people over 65. In most developed countries, the incidence is rising as the average lifespan increases.

Although the term chronic heart failure appears to imply a life-threatening disorder, it can often be treated, and people with mild chronic heart failure can live for many years. However, the condition may limit physical activity.

At first, one side of the heart may be predominantly affected, and, in these circumstances, the condition is termed right- or left-sided heart failure. Right heart failure leads to ankle swelling and accumulation of fluid throughout the body. Left heart failure causes fluid to accumulate in the lungs. Fluid in the lungs due to left-sided failure usually rapidly leads to right-sided failure, and the combination of the two, known as congestive heart failure, is the most common form of chronic heart failure.

WHAT ARE THE CAUSES?

Any condition that causes damage to the heart can lead to chronic heart failure. Whether the right or left side of the heart is first affected depends on the cause. In 8 out of 10 cases, chronic heart failure is caused by coronary artery disease (p.405), in which the blood supply to the heart muscle is reduced. Persistent high blood pressure (*see* HYPERTENSION, p.403) can lead to chronic heart failure because the heart works harder to pump blood through vessels in which pressure is abnormally high. These disorders initially produce left heart failure.

Failure of the right side of the heart is a common complication of chronic lung disease, particularly chronic obstructive pulmonary disease (p.487).

Other possible causes of chronic heart failure are heart valve disorders (p.421) and dilated cardiomyopathy (p.427). In rare cases, chronic heart failure may be due to anaemia (p.446), the hormone disorder hyperthyroidism (p.679), or extreme obesity (p.631). Some people who have diabetes mellitus (p.687) are at risk of developing the condition.

WHAT ARE THE SYMPTOMS?

The symptoms of chronic heart failure develop gradually, are often vague, and may include:

- Tiredness.
- Shortness of breath that is worse during exertion or when lying flat.
- Loss of appetite.
- Nausea.
- Swelling of the feet and ankles.
- In some cases, confusion.

People with chronic heart failure may also have sudden attacks of acute heart failure (opposite page), with symptoms of severe shortness of breath, wheezing, and sweating. These attacks usually occur during the night. Occasionally, acute heart failure develops if the heart is put under additional strain due to a heart attack or an infection. Acute heart failure needs immediate hospital treatment.

HOW IS IT DIAGNOSED?

If chronic heart failure is suspected, you may have electrocardiography (*see* ECG, p.406) to assess the electrical activity of your heart. You may also have echocardiography (p.425) to image the heart and check its function. A chest X-ray (p.490) may show signs of heart failure, such as an abnormally large heart or excess fluid in the lung tissue.

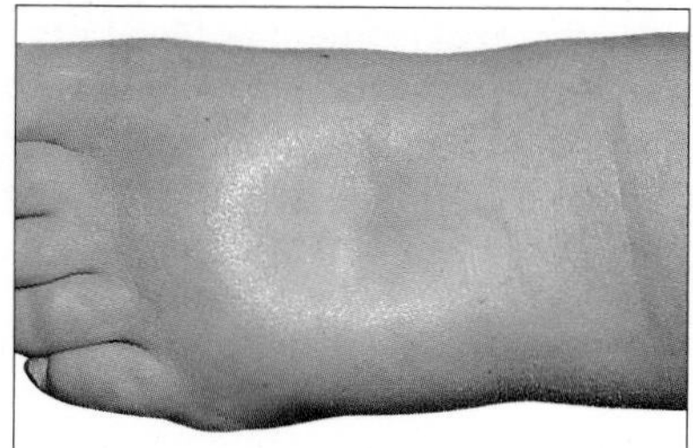

Fluid retention
In chronic heart failure, fluid collects in body tissues, most obviously in the feet. If the skin is pressed, an indentation remains at the site of pressure for a few minutes.

Your doctor may arrange for further tests to investigate the underlying cause of heart failure. For example, you may have coronary angiography (p.408) to diagnose narrowing of the coronary arteries or blood tests to check for anaemia or an overactive thyroid gland.

WHAT CAN I DO?

If you have chronic heart failure, you should avoid strenuous exercise and stressful situations. Regular gentle exercise, such as walking, may help if you have mild or moderate chronic heart failure. If you smoke, you should stop immediately. If necessary, you should try to lose excess weight to avoid putting unnecessary strain on your heart (*see* ARE YOU A HEALTHY WEIGHT?, p.53). You should also avoid salty foods, which can encourage your body to retain fluid.

HOW MIGHT THE DOCTOR TREAT IT?

Your doctor will probably prescribe diuretic drugs (p.902), which increase urine production, and ACE inhibitor drugs (p.900), which cause blood vessels to widen and reduce the workload on the heart. In addition, drugs that increase the efficiency of the heart, such as digoxin (*see* DIGITALIS DRUGS, p.901) or, in some cases, beta-blockers (p.898), may be given. You may also be treated to prevent progression of any underlying disorder. For example, if you have coronary artery disease, you may be advised to take a daily dose of aspirin, which reduces the risk of a heart attack (*see* DRUGS THAT PREVENT BLOOD CLOTTING, p.904). Your doctor will monitor your heart condition and adjust your drug treatment and dosage as needed.

In some cases, drug treatment may not be effective, and a heart transplant (p.427) may be considered if a person is otherwise in good health.

WHAT IS THE PROGNOSIS?

Treatment is usually initially successful in relieving symptoms and improving quality of life. However, in most cases, the underlying cause cannot be treated effectively. As a result, heart failure becomes progressively more severe, and symptoms are then difficult to control with drugs. In about half of these cases, the condition is fatal within 2 years.

(WWW) ONLINE SITES: p.1032

Hypotension

Lower than normal blood pressure due to a variety of causes

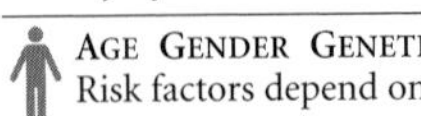

AGE GENDER GENETICS LIFESTYLE
Risk factors depend on the cause

Hypotension is the medical term for low blood pressure. The pressure with which the blood is pumped around the circulation varies between individuals and throughout the day. The normal range is that which is adequate to supply all of the organs and body tissues with blood. Blood pressure at the lower end of the normal range is not likely to produce symptoms. However, if the pressure in the circulation falls below the level needed to provide the brain with enough blood, light-headedness or fainting may occur.

A common type of hypotension is postural hypotension, in which suddenly standing or sitting up leads to light-headedness and fainting.

What are the causes?

In many people, low blood pressure occurs as a result of dehydration following loss of large amounts of fluid or salts from the body. For example, heavy sweating, loss of blood, or profuse diarrhoea may all cause hypotension.

Disorders that reduce the efficiency of the heart's pumping action are common causes of low blood pressure. These disorders include heart failure (*see* ACUTE HEART FAILURE, p.412, and CHRONIC HEART FAILURE, p.413), heart attack (*see* MYOCARDIAL INFARCTION, p.410), and an irregular heartbeat (*see* ARRHYTHMIAS, p.415).

Hypotension may also be caused by an abnormal widening of the blood vessels, which may occur as a result of an infection in the bloodstream (*see* SEPTICAEMIA, p.299) or a severe allergic reaction (*see* ANAPHYLAXIS, p.469).

Postural hypotension may be caused by disorders in which the nerve supply to the blood vessels is damaged, such as diabetic neuropathy (p.545) or peripheral neuropathies (p.543). Hypotension may also sometimes be the result of an adverse effect of certain drugs, particularly those used in the treatment of high blood pressure (*see* ANTIHYPERTENSIVE DRUGS, p.897) and certain types of antidepressant drugs (p.916).

What are the symptoms?

You may not have symptoms of hypotension unless your blood pressure is very low. Symptoms may include:

- Tiredness.
- General weakness.
- Light-headedness and fainting.
- Blurred vision.
- Nausea.

These symptoms are usually temporary, and blood pressure rises when the cause is treated. However, if blood pressure is too low to provide an adequate blood supply to vital organs, it can be fatal (*see* SHOCK, below).

What might be done?

Your blood pressure will be measured while you are lying down and then standing (*see* BLOOD PRESSURE MEASUREMENT, p.404). There may be an obvious reason for your low blood pressure. For example, you may be dehydrated and need treatment with intravenous fluids. If your doctor suspects an underlying disorder, such as a heart condition, you may be admitted to hospital for tests and treatment. If your medication is causing hypotension, your doctor will probably advise a change of drug or dosage.

(WWW) ONLINE SITES: p.1032

Shock

A severe reduction in blood pressure causing poor blood supply to major organs

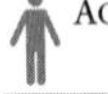

AGE Risk factor depends on the cause

GENDER GENETICS LIFESTYLE
Not significant factors

Shock is a potentially life-threatening condition that necessitates immediate medical attention. The medical term shock describes the cold, pale, collapsed state that results from low blood pressure due to serious injury or illness. Left untreated, the reduced blood supply deprives the vital organs and body tissues of oxygen and is eventually fatal.

The condition is unrelated to the psychological and emotional distress that may follow a traumatic experience.

What are the causes?

Shock may develop as a result of any situation in which the heart is unable to pump blood effectively or in which there is too little blood for the heart to pump. The heart is unable to function normally if it is damaged following a heart attack (*see* MYOCARDIAL INFARCTION, p.410) or if the heart rhythm is abnormal (*see* ARRHYTHMIAS, p.415).

Shock due to insufficient blood circulating around the body may be the result of major blood loss, such as bleeding from the digestive tract (p.630) or from a serious injury. The volume of blood circulating in the body may also be reduced by fluid loss due to severe burns or profuse diarrhoea.

Some conditions, such as severe allergic reactions (*see* ANAPHYLAXIS, p.469) or a blood infection (*see* SEPTICAEMIA, p.299), may cause the blood vessels in the body to widen, resulting in a significant drop in blood pressure and shock.

What are the symptoms?

Shock may not develop until hours after the injury or illness, but as soon as blood pressure falls, the symptoms develop suddenly. Symptoms may include:

- Confusion or agitation.
- Cold, clammy skin and sweating.
- Rapid, shallow breathing.
- Fast heartbeat.
- Loss of consciousness.

Symptoms of the underlying cause may also be present, such as prolonged chest pain due to a heart attack.

If shock is not treated immediately, the internal organs may be damaged, leading to various disorders including kidney failure (p.706) and acute respiratory distress syndrome (p.506).

What might be done?

A person in shock requires emergency admission to an intensive care unit for treatment and careful monitoring. The priority is to restore the blood and oxygen supply to the body's major organs regardless of the initial cause of shock. Immediate treatment usually includes oxygen therapy and intravenous fluids, blood or blood products, and drugs to increase blood pressure. Once the cause of shock has been established, specific treatment can be given. For example, antibiotics (p.885) may be prescribed to treat septicaemia. Surgery may be needed to stop bleeding. For treatment to be successful, the blood supply to the organs must be restored before permanent damage occurs.

(WWW) ONLINE SITES: p.1032

HEART RATE AND RHYTHM DISORDERS

Disorders of heart rate and rhythm are caused by disturbances in the heart's electrical system and are very common, particularly in elderly people. These disorders do not always cause symptoms and are sometimes detected only during routine health checkups. Treatment usually consists of drugs, although newer techniques that use carefully controlled electric currents are also used.

A healthy adult has a resting heart rate of 60–80 beats per minute, although this rate rises during exercise. Children have a higher resting heart rate, while that of very fit adults and the elderly may be as low as 50 beats per minute. Disorders that affect the pumping action of the heart may increase or decrease the heart rate, alter its rhythm, or, in cardiac arrest, stop the heart pumping altogether. Many of these disorders have coronary artery disease (p.405) as an underlying cause.

The first article in this section describes ectopic beats, which are extra, isolated heartbeats. This article is followed by an overview of arrhythmias, which are abnormal heart rates and rhythms, and a discussion of individual types of arrhythmias. The final article discusses cardiac arrest, which is the sudden and complete failure of the heart to pump blood caused by a disturbance in its electrical system. Cardiac arrest is a potentially fatal condition and requires emergency medical treatment.

KEY ANATOMY

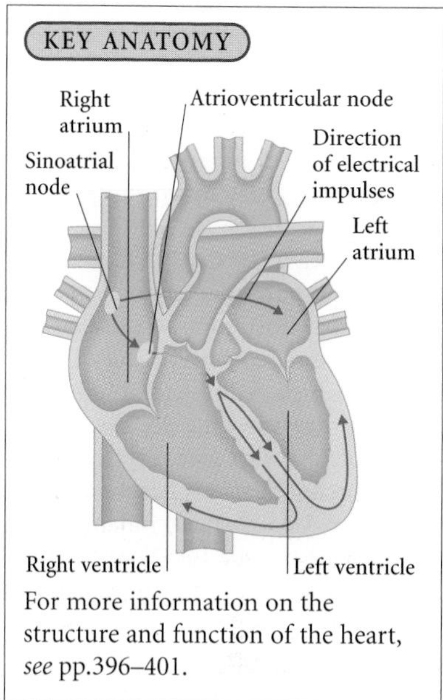

For more information on the structure and function of the heart, *see* pp.396–401.

Ectopic beats

Contractions of the heart that are out of the normal rhythmic pattern

AGE More common in young people and elderly people

LIFESTYLE Smoking and consumption of alcohol and caffeine are risk factors

GENDER GENETICS Not significant factors

An ectopic beat is an isolated, irregular heartbeat that rapidly follows a normal one. The interval between an ectopic beat and the next normal beat may be longer than usual. Most people experience ectopic beats at some time in their lives. Ectopic beats may originate either in the atria (the upper chambers of the heart) or in the ventricles (the lower chambers of the heart). Atrial ectopic beats are usually harmless. They typically occur in young people and are often associated with the use of nicotine and the consumption of caffeine and alcohol. Ventricular ectopic beats occur less frequently, usually in elderly people, and may indicate the presence of a more serious underlying disorder, such as coronary artery disease (p.405). They may also occur after a heart attack (*see* MYOCARDIAL INFARCTION, p.410).

Ectopic beats may be symptomless or may cause a thumping sensation in the chest as the heart briefly beats more strongly than usual.

WHAT MIGHT BE DONE?

Ectopic beats in young people are likely to be atrial and harmless. They may disappear if you stop smoking and reduce your intake of coffee and alcohol. If they persist, visit your doctor. Ectopic beats that are frequent or accompanied by light-headedness, shortness of breath, or chest pain, or that occur at an older age, are likely to be ventricular. They may have a serious underlying cause, requiring urgent medical attention.

Since ectopic beats are intermittent, your doctor may arrange for your heart to be monitored continuously over 24 hours or more (*see* AMBULATORY ECG, p.416). Tests may be carried out to look for an underlying cause of the ectopic beats, such as coronary artery disease.

The treatment of ventricular ectopic beats depends on the underlying cause. Antiarrhythmic drugs (p.898) reduce the frequency of the beats and are commonly prescribed. If the beats follow a heart attack, antiarrhythmic drugs lower the risk of cardiac arrest (p.419).

(WWW) ONLINE SITES: p.1032

Arrhythmias

Abnormal rates and/or rhythms of the heartbeat

AGE More common in elderly people

GENETICS LIFESTYLE Risk factors depend on the type

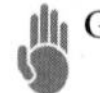
GENDER Not a significant factor

The normal resting adult heart rate is 60–80 beats per minute. Both heart rate and rhythm may be affected in arrhythmias, which may involve both the atria (upper heart chambers) and the ventricles (lower heart chambers). There are two types of arrhythmias: tachycardias, in which the heart rate is too high, and bradycardias, in which the rate is too low. Tachycardias may arise in the atria or the ventricles and can be regular or irregular. When tachycardias occur in the ventricles, they can deteriorate into ventricular fibrillation, a serious arrhythmia that may lead to cardiac arrest (p.419). Bradycardias include sick sinus syndrome (p.419) and complete heart block (p.418). Most arrhythmias are caused by disorders of the heart and its blood vessels. A heart rate outside the usual range is not always a cause for concern. An elevated heart rate is normal during exercise and pregnancy, and exceptionally fit people have a resting heart rate that is lower than normal.

Arrhythmias may reduce the pumping efficiency of the heart, causing too little blood to reach the brain. Although arrhythmias may cause alarming symptoms, such as a thumping heartbeat, the different types vary in seriousness.

WHAT ARE THE CAUSES?

Most arrhythmias are caused by heart disease, the most common underlying disorder being coronary artery disease (p.405), which reduces the blood supply to the heart and the electrical system that controls heart rate. Less common causes include various heart valve disorders (pp.421–429) and inflammation of the heart muscle (*see* MYOCARDITIS, p.426). Some types of arrhythmia present from birth are due to a defect of the heart, such as an abnormal electrical pathway between the atria and the ventricles. However, these arrhythmias only cause symptoms later in life.

Some arrhythmias occur in people with otherwise healthy hearts. Causes include an imbalance of thyroid hormones (*see* HYPERTHYROIDISM, p.679), or of blood chemistry, such as an excess of potassium. Some drugs, such as bronchodilators (p.910) and digitalis drugs (p.901) may cause arrhythmias, as may caffeine and tobacco, but sometimes their cause is unknown.

WHAT ARE THE SYMPTOMS?

Symptoms do not always develop, but, if they do, their onset is usually sudden. The symptoms may include:

- Palpitations (awareness of an irregular heartbeat).
- Light-headedness, sometimes leading to loss of consciousness.
- Shortness of breath.
- Pain in the chest or neck.

Complications include stroke (p.532), acute heart failure (p.412), and chronic heart failure (p.413).

WHAT MIGHT BE DONE?

Your doctor may suspect an arrhythmia from your symptoms and by checking your pulse. He or she may arrange for you to have electrocardiography (*see* ECG, p.406) to monitor electrical activity in the heart. Since some arrhythmias occur only intermittently, you may need to have a continuous ECG over 24 hours or be fitted with an event monitor (*see* AMBULATORY ECG, left). You may also have tests to detect abnormalities that affect electrical pathways of the heart (*see* CARDIAC ELECTROPHYSIOLOGICAL STUDIES, opposite page).

In some cases, antiarrhythmic drugs (p.898) can be used to treat arrhythmias. In other cases, electric shocks may be administered to restore a normal heartbeat (*see* CARDIOVERSION, p.420). Abnormal electrical pathways in the heart can be destroyed using a technique called radiofrequency ablation, which is carried out at the same time as electrophysiological studies. If the heart rate is too low, an artificial pacemaker may be inserted to stimulate the heart and restore a normal heartbeat (*see* CARDIAC PACEMAKER, p.419).

The outlook for an arrhythmia depends on the type. Supraventricular tachycardia usually is not serious and does not affect life expectancy, whereas ventricular fibrillation is a potentially fatal arrhythmia and requires emergency medical treatment.

(WWW) ONLINE SITES: p.1032

TEST AMBULATORY ECG

Ambulatory electrocardiography (ECG) is carried out using a wearable device called a Holter monitor that records the electrical activity of the heart using a number of electrodes attached to the chest. The device is usually worn for 24 hours and detects intermittent arrhythmias (abnormal heart rates and rhythms). An event monitor is a similar device that can be worn for longer periods but records only when it is activated by the user.

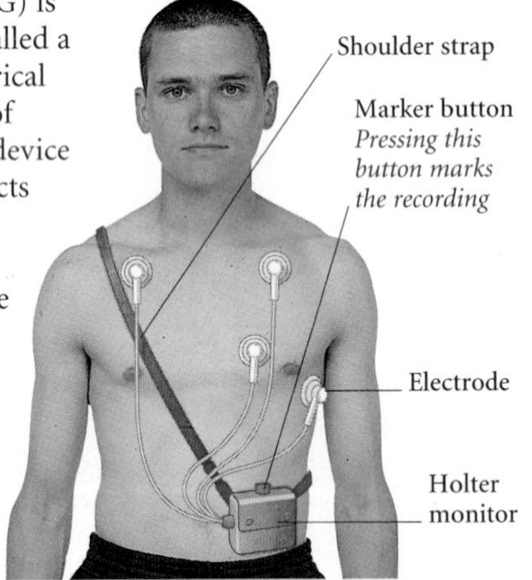

Using a Holter monitor
You press a button on the device to mark times when symptoms occur. A doctor can check if these markings coincide with periods of arrhythmia.

RESULT

Normal heartbeat
Early, abnormal heartbeat
Symptom marker
Delayed heartbeat

ECG trace
This trace shows normal heartbeats interrupted by an isolated abnormal beat, which coincides with a symptom marker.

Supraventricular tachycardia

Recurrent episodes of rapid heart rate arising in the upper chambers of the heart

- **AGE** Most common in children and young adults
- **GENETICS** Sometimes runs in families
- **LIFESTYLE** Exertion and consumption of alcohol and caffeine may trigger attacks
- **GENDER** Not a significant factor

Supraventricular tachycardia (SVT) is a type of arrhythmia caused by a fault in the electrical pathway that regulates the heart rate. During an episode of SVT, which may last up to several hours, the heartbeat is rapid but regular. The heart rate rises to 140–180 beats per minute and sometimes climbs even higher. In a heart that is working normally, each heartbeat is triggered by an electrical impulse from the sinoatrial node (the heart's pacemaker), located in the right atrium (one of the heart's upper chambers). The impulse passes to a second node, the atrioventricular node, which relays it to the ventricles. In SVT, the heartbeat is not controlled by the sinoatrial node. This may occur either because an abnormal pathway develops, causing an impulse to circulate continuously between the atrioventricular node and the ventricles, or because an extra area of cells develops and sends out pacemaking impulses.

SVT may first appear in childhood or adolescence, although it can occur at any age. In some cases, SVT is caused by an inherited abnormality in the heart's electrical pathways. Episodes generally occur for no apparent reason, but they may be triggered by exertion and by caffeine and alcohol.

What are the symptoms?

The symptoms of SVT usually develop suddenly. They last from a few seconds to several hours and include:

- Palpitations (awareness of an irregular or abnormally rapid heartbeat).
- Light-headedness.
- Pain in the chest or neck.

In rare cases, a prolonged episode of SVT may reduce blood pressure to a life-threatening level.

What might be done?

If your doctor suspects that you have SVT, you will probably have electrocardiography (*see* ECG, p.406) to record the electrical activity of your heart. This investigation may last 24 hours or more (*see* AMBULATORY ECG, opposite page) because SVT occurs only intermittently. You may have further tests to look for abnormalities in the heart's electrical pathways (*see* CARDIAC ELECTROPHYSIOLOGICAL STUDIES, above).

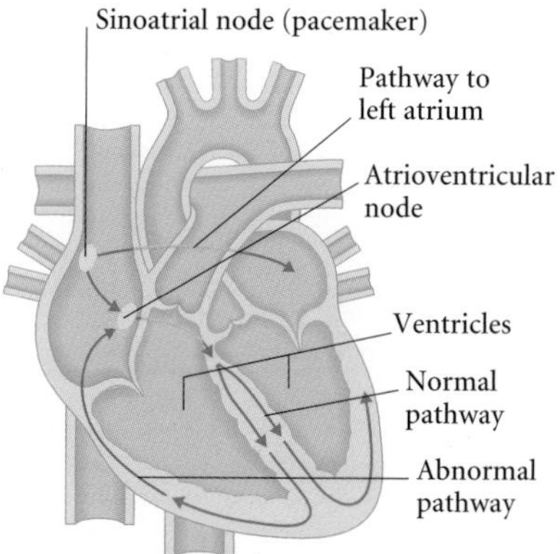

Supraventricular tachycardia (SVT)
Impulses from the sinoatrial node normally control heart rate. One cause of SVT is an abnormal electrical pathway, which allows an impulse to circulate continuously in the heart, taking over from the sinoatrial node.

TEST AND TREATMENT: Cardiac electrophysiological studies

Cardiac electrophysiological studies (EPS) are used to pinpoint abnormal pathways in the heart's electrical conducting system. A catheter that has electrodes at its tip is introduced into the heart and manipulated to record the electrical activity at different sites. Once an abnormal pathway is located, it can be destroyed by sending a current through the electrodes in a procedure known as radiofrequency ablation. Radiofrequency ablation can provide a permanent cure for some disorders in about 1 minute and has a high success rate.

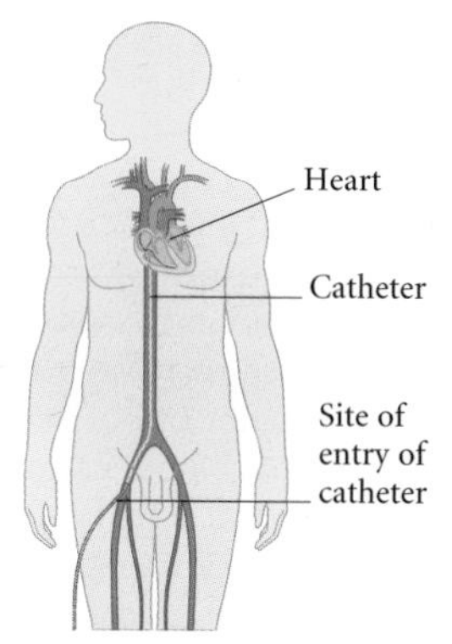

ROUTE OF CATHETER

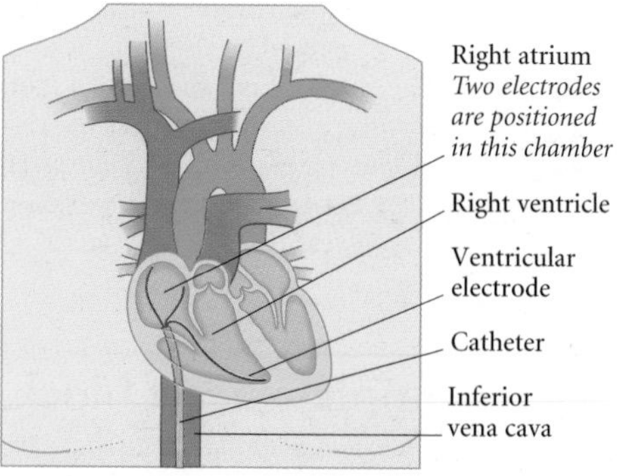

During EPS
A catheter is inserted into a vein in the groin under local anaesthesia and threaded into the heart. Electrodes at the tip of the catheter detect electrical activity and can be used to deliver a current to destroy abnormal pathways.

A prolonged and severe episode of SVT requires emergency hospital treatment. In hospital, you may be given oxygen and an intravenous injection of an antiarrhythmic drug (p.898). In some cases, an electric shock may be given to restore the heart to its normal rate (*see* CARDIOVERSION, p.420).

People who have occasional, brief episodes of SVT can control the symptoms by stimulating the vagus nerve, to slow the heart rate. One way to stimulate the nerve is to rub the area over the carotid artery in the neck, although this is not recommended in adults over the age of 50 because it may precipitate a stroke. Other techniques include plunging your face into ice-cold water or straining as if moving one's bowels. Your doctor can teach you these techniques.

Troublesome episodes of SVT may be treated with long-term antiarrhythmic drugs. SVT may be cured by radiofrequency ablation, a treatment carried out during cardiac electrophysiological studies. This treatment destroys abnormal electrical pathways but carries a small risk of causing complete heart block (p.418), in which the heart's electrical system fails. In most cases, SVT does not affect life expectancy.

(WWW) ONLINE SITES: p.1032

Atrial fibrillation

Rapid, uncoordinated contractions of the atria, the upper chambers of the heart

- AGE Most common in people over the age of 60
- GENDER More common in males
- LIFESTYLE Smoking, a high-fat diet, alcohol abuse, lack of exercise, and excess weight are risk factors
- GENETICS Not a significant factor

Atrial fibrillation is the most common type of rapid, irregular heart rate. It most often occurs in people over 60, and up to 1 in 20 of very elderly people in the UK may be affected by it. In atrial fibrillation, the atria contract weakly at 300–500 beats per minute. Some of the electrical impulses that cause this rapid beating are conducted through the heart to the ventricles (the lower chambers), which also beat more rapidly than normal, at up to 160 beats per minute. Since the atria and ventricles are no longer beating in rhythm, the strength and timing of the heartbeat becomes irregular and less blood is pumped.

The most dangerous complication of atrial fibrillation is stroke (p.532), the risk of which increases with age. Since the atria do not empty properly during contractions, blood stagnates in them and may form a clot. If a part of the clot breaks off and enters the bloodstream, it may block an artery anywhere in the body (*see* THROMBOSIS AND EMBOLISM, p.431). A stroke occurs when part of a clot blocks an artery supplying the brain.

WHAT ARE THE CAUSES?

Atrial fibrillation may occur for no apparent reason, especially in the elderly, but it is usually due to an underlying disorder that causes the atria to enlarge. Such disorders include heart valve disorders (p.421), coronary artery disease (p.405), and high blood pressure (*see* HYPERTENSION, p.403). Smoking, lack of exercise, a high-fat diet, and being overweight are risk factors for many of these disorders. Atrial fibrillation is also common in people with an overactive thyroid gland (*see* HYPERTHYROIDISM, p.679) or low potassium levels in the blood. It may occur in people who drink excessive amounts of alcohol.

WHAT ARE THE SYMPTOMS?

Symptoms do not always develop, but, if they do, their onset is usually sudden. The symptoms may be intermittent or persistent and typically include:

- Palpitations (awareness of an irregular or abnormally rapid heartbeat).
- Light-headedness.
- Shortness of breath.
- Chest pain.

Stroke and acute or chronic heart failure (pp.412–413) may be complications.

WHAT MIGHT BE DONE?

Your doctor may suspect atrial fibrillation if you have a fast, irregular pulse. To confirm the diagnosis, you will have electrocardiography (*see* ECG, p.406) to check your heartbeat. You may have blood tests to look for an underlying cause such as hyperthyroidism or hypertension. If a cause is found, treatment of it often cures the arrhythmia. If atrial fibrillation is diagnosed early, it may be treated successfully using cardioversion (p.420), in which a brief electric shock is applied to the heart.

Atrial fibrillation is usually treated with antiarrhythmic drugs (p.898), such as beta-blocker drugs (p.898) or digitalis drugs (p.901). These drugs slow the conduction of electrical impulses from the atria to the ventricles, giving the ventricles sufficient time to fill with blood between each heartbeat. Other antiarrhythmic drugs are then used to treat the irregular rhythm. You may also be prescribed the anticoagulant drug warfarin, which reduces the risk of blood clot formation (*see* DRUGS THAT PREVENT BLOOD CLOTTING, p.904) and thereby lowers the risk of a stroke.

(WWW) ONLINE SITES: p.1032

Complete heart block

Complete failure of the system that conducts electrical impulses from the the upper to the lower heart chambers

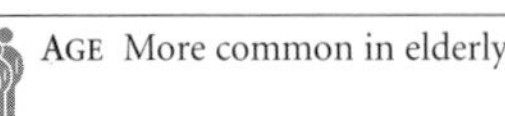
AGE More common in elderly people

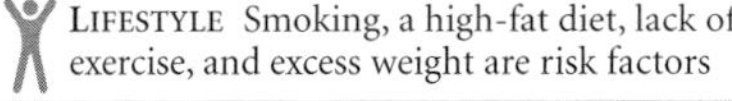
LIFESTYLE Smoking, a high-fat diet, lack of exercise, and excess weight are risk factors

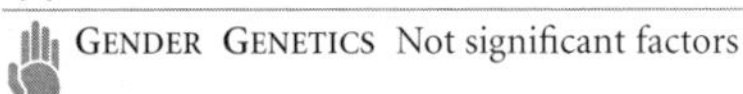
GENDER GENETICS Not significant factors

In complete heart block, damage to the heart's conductive tissue prevents electrical impulses from the atria (the upper chambers) from reaching the ventricles (the lower chambers), so that the ventricles cannot contract normally. Heart muscle contracts automatically in the absence of a regulating signal. In complete heart block, the ventricles contract at about 40 beats per minute instead of the usual rate of 60–80 beats per minute, which greatly reduces the heart's efficiency. In some cases, the heart stops beating altogether for up to 20 seconds.

The tissue damage that causes complete heart block becomes more likely in elderly people and is linked with coronary artery disease (p.405), for which lifestyle factors such as smoking increase the risk. Sudden complete heart block, which may be either temporary or permanent, may follow a heart attack (*see* MYOCARDIAL INFARCTION, p.410).

WHAT ARE THE SYMPTOMS?

The symptoms may come on gradually or suddenly and typically include:

- Palpitations (awareness of an irregular heartbeat).
- Light-headedness, and loss of consciousness if the heart stops beating.
- Shortness of breath.
- Chest pain.

If it is left untreated, complete heart block may lead to acute heart failure (p.412) chronic heart failure (p.413), stroke (p.532), and shock (p.414).

WHAT MIGHT BE DONE?

Complete heart block is usually suspected if you have a very slow heartbeat and is confirmed by electrocardiography (*see* ECG, p.406). Initial treatment may involve the temporary insertion of a pacing wire into the heart, usually through a vein in the chest or groin. The wire transmits electrical impulses that restore a normal heartbeat until an artificial pacemaker can be permanently fitted (*see* CARDIAC PACEMAKER, opposite page) to restore a normal heart rate. However, the general outlook depends on whether there is an underlying disorder, such as coronary artery disease.

(WWW) ONLINE SITES: p.1032

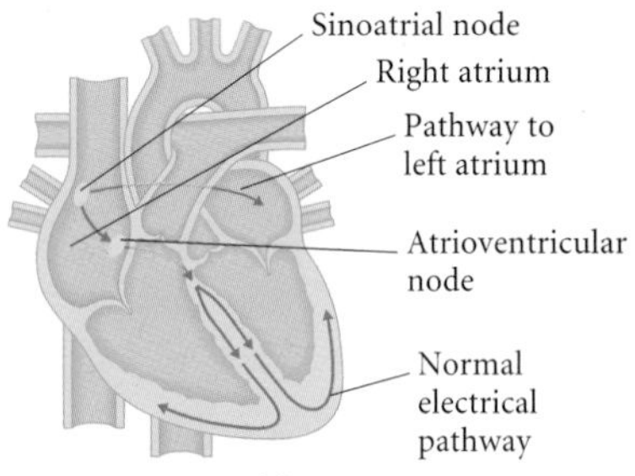

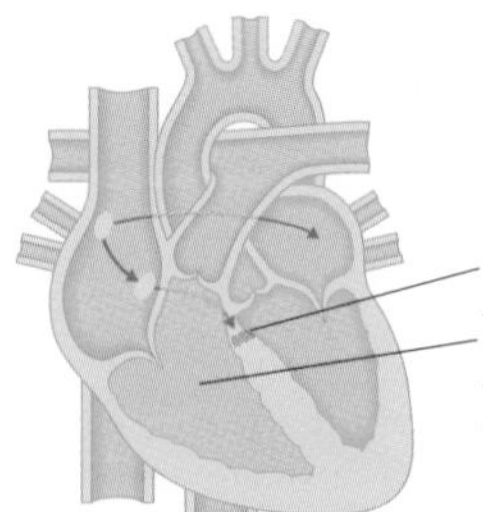

Block in the heart's electrical system
Normally, electrical impulses pass from the sinoatrial node to the atrioventricular node in the right atrium and then to the ventricles. In complete heart block, the impulses cannot reach the ventricles.

(TREATMENT) CARDIAC PACEMAKER

Cardiac pacemakers stimulate the heart with electrical impulses to maintain a regular heartbeat. Pacemakers are used to treat disorders in which the heart's electrical conducting system is faulty, such as complete heart block. Some pacemakers produce impulses continually; others send an impulse only when the heart rate falls too low. Defibrillator pacemakers deliver an electric shock to the heart when ventricular fibrillation (rapid, uncoordinated contraction of the lower chambers of the heart) occurs to restore the normal rate and rhythm.

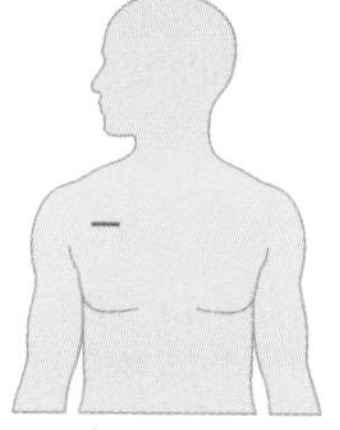

SITE OF INCISION

Insertion of a pacemaker
A pacemaker is inserted just under the skin and stitched into position in the chest wall, usually under local anaesthesia. Two wires from the pacemaker are passed into the large vein above the heart (superior vena cava). One wire is guided into the right atrium and the other into the right ventricle.

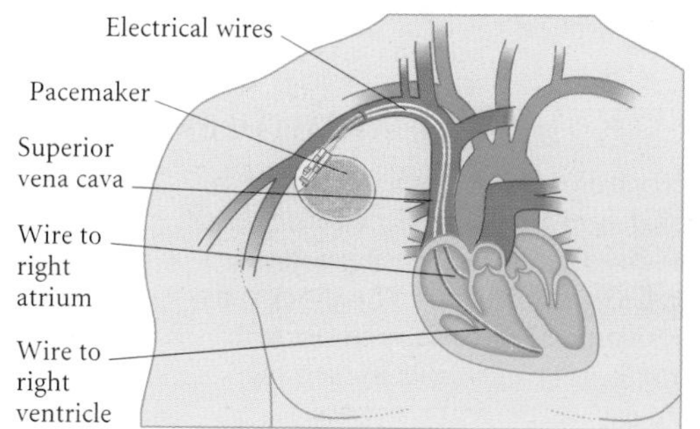
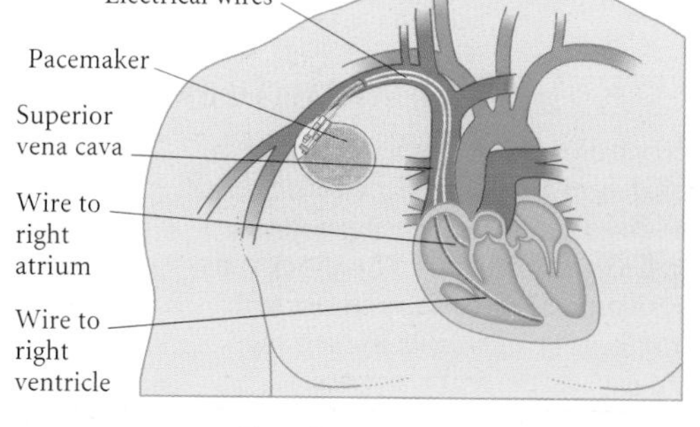

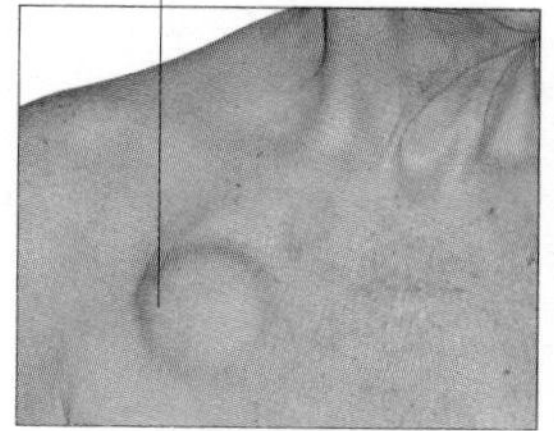

EXTERNAL VIEW

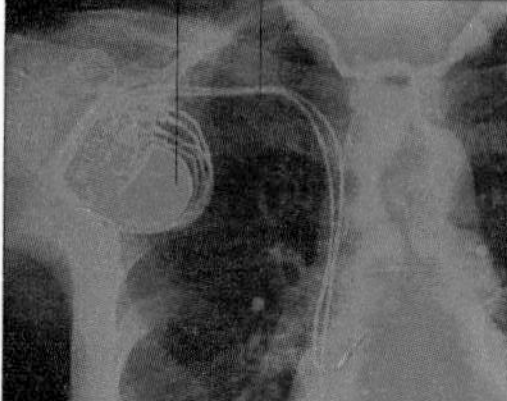

X-RAY IMAGE

Pacemaker in place
The pacemaker is implanted into the chest and appears as a small bulge under the skin. An X-ray image reveals the wires that lead from the pacemaker to the right atrium and ventricle of the heart.

Sick sinus syndrome

Abnormal function of the sinoatrial node, the heart's natural pacemaker

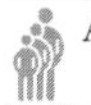
AGE Most common in elderly people

LIFESTYLE Smoking, a high-fat diet, lack of exercise, and excess weight are risk factors

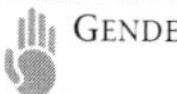
GENDER GENETICS Not significant factors

In sick sinus syndrome, the sinoatrial node, the heart's natural pacemaker, becomes faulty, causing the heart to beat too slowly or to miss a few beats. In some cases, the heart rate alternates between runs of slow and fast beats. Sick sinus syndrome is caused by the degeneration of cells in the sinoatrial node and is most common in elderly people. In most cases, the underlying cause is coronary artery disease (p.405). Sick sinus syndrome may also be due to heart muscle disease (*see* DILATED CARDIOMYOPATHY, p.427). Typically, sick sinus syndrome is a progressive condition with episodes becoming more frequent and prolonged over time.

WHAT ARE THE SYMPTOMS?

Symptoms have a sudden onset and are intermittent. They may include:

- Palpitations (awareness of an irregular heartbeat).
- Brief attacks of light-headedness.
- Loss of consciousness.
- Shortness of breath.

Many of the symptoms are caused by decreased oxygen levels to the brain due to the reduced efficiency of the heart.

WHAT MIGHT BE DONE?

If your doctor suspects sick sinus syndrome, he or she will probably arrange for you to have electrocardiography (*see* ECG, p.406). Since symptoms are intermittent, you may need to have your heartbeat monitored for 24 hours or more while you carry out your everyday activities (*see* AMBULATORY ECG, p.416). Your doctor may also recommend that you have further tests, such as echocardiography (p.425), to look for signs of cardiomyopathy.

Treatment of sick sinus syndrome usually involves inserting a pacemaker to stimulate the heart when it is beating too slowly (*see* CARDIAC PACEMAKER, left). If the heart is alternating between fast and slow rates, antiarrhythmic drugs (p.898) may also be given in order to slow down the fast heart rate. If a pacemaker is required, you will need regular checkups with a doctor or a pacemaker technician.

Sick sinus syndrome can usually be treated successfully with a pacemaker or drugs. However, the general outlook depends on the underlying condition.

(WWW) ONLINE SITES: p.1032

Cardiac arrest

Sudden failure of the heart to pump blood, which is often fatal

AGE More common with increasing age

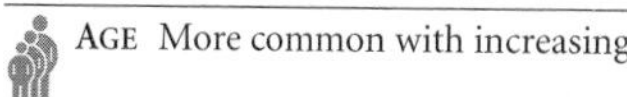
GENDER More common in males

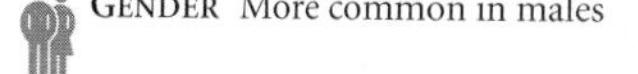
LIFESTYLE Smoking, a high-fat diet, lack of exercise, and excess weight are risk factors

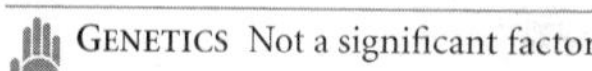
GENETICS Not a significant factor

During cardiac arrest, the heart stops pumping. As a result, the brain and other organs no longer receive oxygenated blood, without which they cannot function. Within 3 minutes of cardiac arrest, the brain will have sustained some damage. Death is likely to occur within 5 minutes if the pumping action of the heart is not restored by emergency treatment or if circulation is not maintained by external cardiac massage.

WHAT ARE THE CAUSES?

Cardiac arrest is commonly caused by one of two types of electrical problem in the heart: ventricular fibrillation, the more common type, and asystole. During ventricular fibrillation, the ventricles (lower chambers of the heart) rapidly contract in an uncoordinated manner, preventing the heart from pumping out blood. Ventricular fibrillation may occur suddenly in people with coronary artery disease (p.405), for which lifestyle factors such as smoking and a high-fat diet increase the risk. It is also a frequent complication of a heart attack (*see* MYOCARDIAL INFARCTION, p.410), usually occurring shortly after the attack. Ventricular fibrillation may also be caused by electrical injuries (p.319), drowning (p.325), and dilated cardiomyopathy (p.427), in which a disease of the heart muscle reduces its pumping efficiency.

Asystole is an electrical problem of the heart in which there is a total failure of the heart muscle to contract, leading to cardiac arrest. Asystole may be due to suffocation or to disorders or injuries that cause massive bleeding.

WHAT ARE THE SYMPTOMS?

Within seconds of a cardiac arrest, these symptoms usually occur:

- Collapse.
- Loss of consciousness.
- Blue lips, fingers, and toes.

An affected person has no pulse and has stopped breathing.

WHAT MIGHT BE DONE?

If you are with a person who has had a cardiac arrest, send for medical help immediately. If you are alone with the affected person, shout for help. At the same time, you should begin resuscitation to maintain blood flow to the brain (*see* FIRST AID: CARDIOPULMONARY RESUSCITATION, p.984).

While continuing cardiopulmonary resuscitation, the paramedic team may conduct electrocardiography (*see* ECG, p.406) to establish whether the cause of cardiac arrest is asystole or ventricular fibrillation. They will then administer the appropriate treatment. Ventricular fibrillation can be treated effectively with a device called an electric defibrillator (*see* CARDIOVERSION, right), which delivers electric shocks to the heart to restore its normal rhythm and rate. Asystole may sometimes be treated successfully by an injection of epinephrine (adrenaline) into a large vein or directly into the heart to start it pumping again.

After resuscitation, monitoring in an intensive care unit will determine if a heart attack has occurred and, if so, whether it was the cause of the cardiac arrest. Monitoring will also detect a recurrence of cardiac arrest. A person with ventricular fibrillation that is not caused by a heart attack may be prescribed antiarrhythmic drugs (p.898) on a long-term basis or have a miniature defibrillator surgically implanted (*see* CARDIAC PACEMAKER, p.419).

WHAT IS THE PROGNOSIS?

If resuscitation has been performed without delay, the chances of survival depend on the underlying cause. In a person who has ventricular fibrillation as a complication of a heart attack, a complete recovery may be possible if the normal heartbeat is restored by cardioversion. The outlook for cardiac arrest caused by asystole depends on whether rapid, effective treatment can be given for the underlying cause and whether the normal heartbeat can be re-established. People are more likely to survive a cardiac arrest that occurs in hospital than one that takes place elsewhere because of prompt recognition of the condition and rapid access to emergency treatment.

(WWW) ONLINE SITES: p.1032

(TREATMENT) CARDIOVERSION

In cardioversion, sometimes known as defibrillation, a brief electric shock is given to the heart using a device called a defibrillator. The shock can return the heartbeat to its normal rhythm. The defibrillator produces an electric current that passes between two metal plates, or paddles, placed on the chest. Cardioversion is performed under general anaesthesia to treat some arrhythmias (abnormal heart rates and rhythms). It is also often performed as an emergency treatment for cardiac arrest.

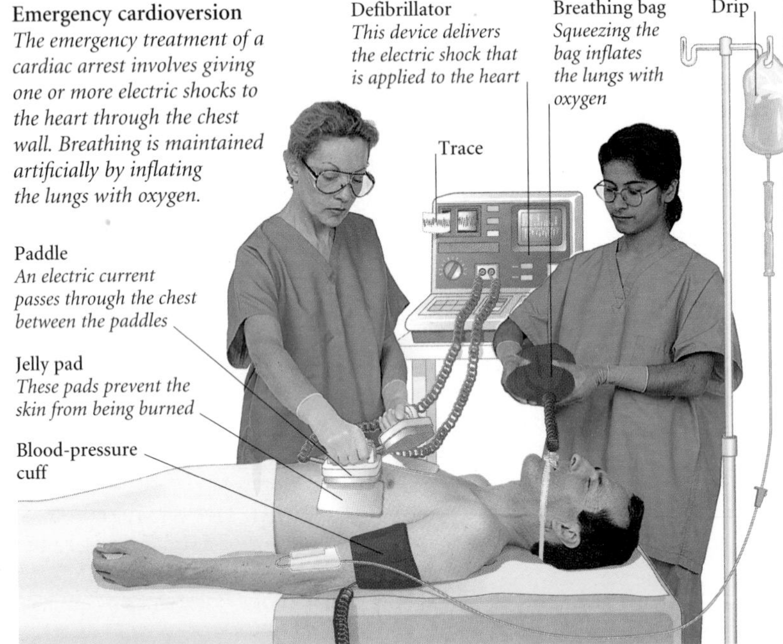

Emergency cardioversion
The emergency treatment of a cardiac arrest involves giving one or more electric shocks to the heart through the chest wall. Breathing is maintained artificially by inflating the lungs with oxygen.

(RESULTS)

Chaotic electrical activity
Electric shock delivered
Normal heartbeat

Effect of defibrillation
This trace shows the heartbeat being returned to its normal rhythm by an electric shock after uncoordinated activity during a cardiac arrest.

HEART VALVE AND MUSCLE DISORDERS

Healthy heart valves and muscle are essential for the heart to pump blood efficiently. Heart valve disorders are less common today in the UK than in the past because a major cause, rheumatic fever, is now rare. Heart muscle disorders often used to be fatal but have a better outlook now because of improved treatments.

The first articles in this section cover heart valve disorders. Blood is pumped around the body at very high pressure by the left side of the heart. The valves on this side, called the aortic and mitral valves, are therefore the ones most often affected by disorders. If a heart valve does not work properly, blood cannot circulate efficiently, and the heart has to pump harder or faster in order to compensate. The next articles discuss disorders of the heart muscle and the lining of the heart (the endocardium).

Any disorder that affects the heart muscle reduces the heart's efficiency and may eventually be fatal. The last article discusses rheumatic fever, a disorder that may damage the heart valves after many years.

Other disorders of the heart muscle, such as heart attack and heart failure, are discussed elsewhere in the book (*see* MAJOR CARDIOVASCULAR DISORDERS, pp.402–414). Congenital heart disease (p.836) is covered in the section on infancy and childhood.

KEY ANATOMY

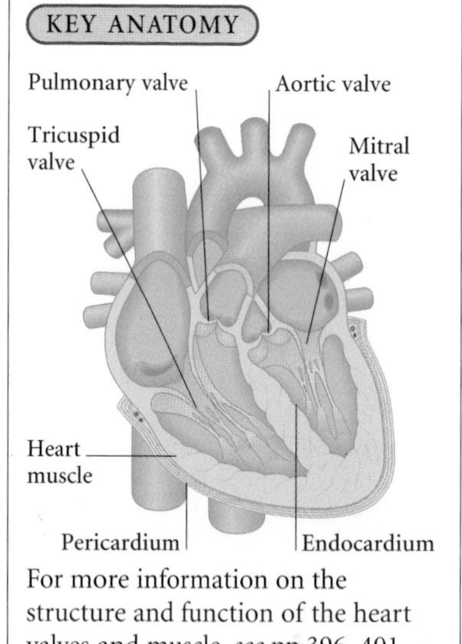

For more information on the structure and function of the heart valves and muscle, *see* pp.396–401.

Heart valve disorders

Abnormalities of the heart valves, which may impair blood flow through the heart

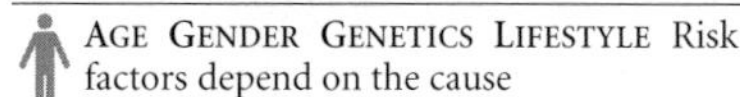

There are four valves in the heart that ensure that blood flows in one direction by opening to let blood through and then closing tightly when the heart muscle contracts. If a heart valve is damaged, blood flow through it may be restricted or blood may leak backwards because a valve fails to close completely. As a result, the heart then has to work harder in order to pump blood around the body. Disorders of the heart valves often do not cause symptoms, but sometimes they result in tiredness and shortness of breath on exertion. Since the efficiency of the heart is impaired, a severe heart valve disorder may result in chronic heart failure (p.413) or an arrhythmia (p.415), in which the heart beats abnormally. Damaged valves are also more susceptible to infection (*see* INFECTIVE ENDOCARDITIS, p.426).

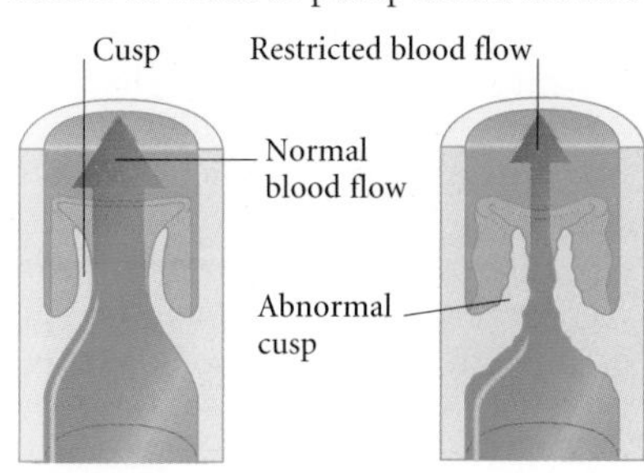

Valve stenosis

If a heart valve is healthy, blood flows through easily when the valve is open. In stenosis, the valve cusps (flaps) do not open fully and blood flow is restricted.

Some heart valve disorders are present at birth. Heart valves may also be damaged later in life by changes due to aging, infection of the heart lining, or a heart attack (*see* MYOCARDIAL INFARCTION, p.410). Rheumatic fever (p.429) was once a major cause of heart valve damage but is now rare in developed countries such as the UK.

WHAT ARE THE TYPES?

The cusps (flaps) inside a heart valve may not open fully, making the opening too narrow (*see* MITRAL STENOSIS, p.424, and AORTIC STENOSIS, p.423). Alternatively, a valve may not form a tight seal when closed, allowing blood to leak back through it (*see* MITRAL INCOMPETENCE, p.423, and AORTIC INCOMPETENCE, p.422). In some cases, both stenosis and incompetence occur in the same valve. Mitral valve prolapse (p.425) is a common, but usually harmless, cause of incompetence; the mitral valve bulges backwards when it is closed and allows slight leakage of blood.

WHAT MIGHT BE DONE?

Valve disorders may be diagnosed in a routine examination or after symptoms have developed. Your doctor listens for sounds, called heart murmurs, that are made by blood flow through abnormal valves. You may have an ECG (p.406) to check the electrical activity of the heart. Chest X-rays (p.490) may also be taken, and the imaging technique echocardiography (p.425) may be used to view the interior of the heart and its blood flow.

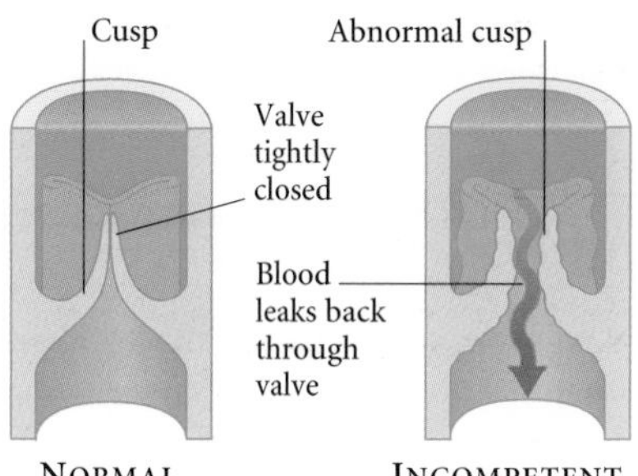

Valve incompetence

Normally, the valve cusps (flaps) meet to stop blood from flowing backwards. An incompetent valve does not close completely and blood leaks backwards.

TREATMENT HEART VALVE REPLACEMENT

Heart valves may need to be replaced if daily activities are affected by symptoms and the valve cannot be repaired by surgery. Replacement heart valves made of tissue may come from a human donor or from a pig's heart. Valves may also be mechanical. Replacing heart valves involves open heart surgery. During the operation, the heart is stopped, and its function is taken over by a heart–lung machine (*see* SURGERY USING A HEART–LUNG MACHINE, p.953). You may need to stay in hospital for 7–14 days after surgery while you recover. If a mechanical valve is used, drugs that prevent blood clotting (p.904) are taken for life to reduce the risk of clots forming on the valve.

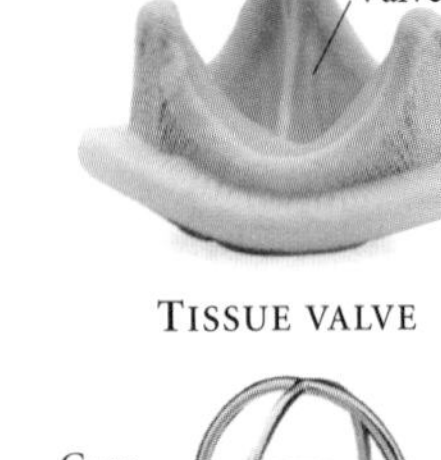

TISSUE VALVE

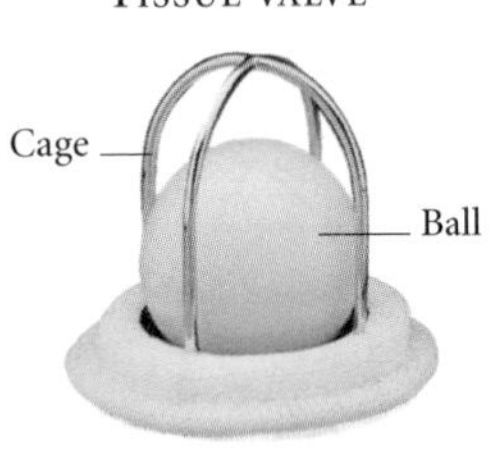

MECHANICAL AORTIC VALVE

Replacement valves
Tissue valves have three cusps that open and close to control blood flow. In one type of mechanical valve, blood flow pushes a ball into a cage to allow blood through the valve.

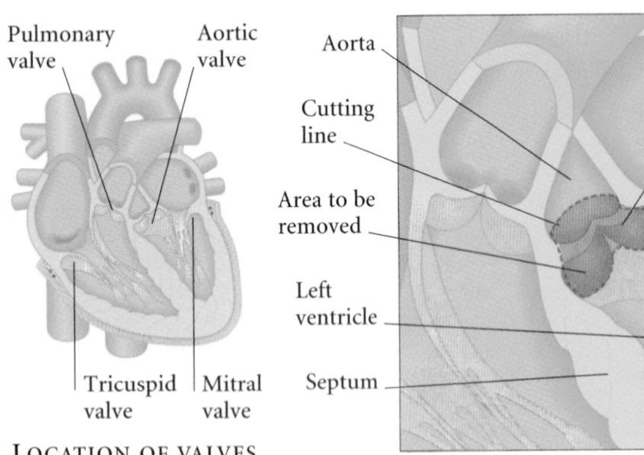

LOCATION OF VALVES

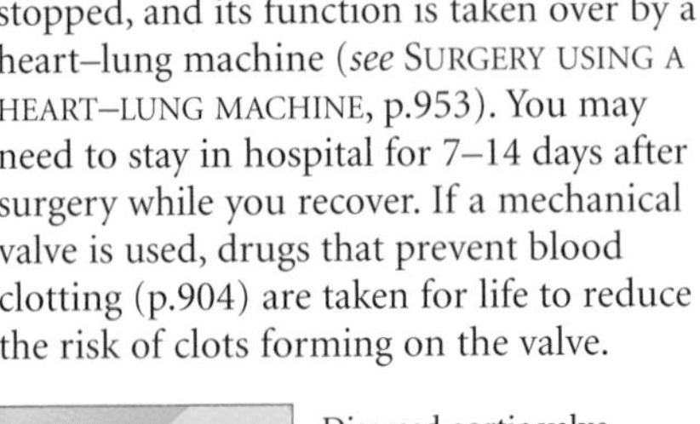

Aortic valve replacement
The aortic valve is the most commonly replaced heart valve. An incision is made in the aorta, the major blood vessel from the heart, to gain access to the valve. The diseased valve is cut out, leaving a ring of tissue to which the replacement aortic valve is then stitched.

If treatment is needed, you may be given drugs to strengthen the heartbeat or relieve the symptoms. In severe valve disorders, surgery may be needed to repair or replace the valve (*see* HEART VALVE REPLACEMENT, above). Your doctor may advise you to take a single dose of an antibiotic (p.885) before you have dental treatment or certain operations, such as those on the digestive tract, that could allow infection into the blood.

(WWW) ONLINE SITES: p.1032

Aortic incompetence

Leakage of blood back through the aortic valve of the heart

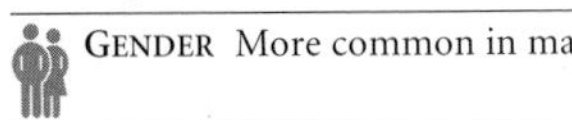
GENDER More common in males

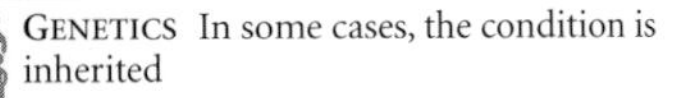
GENETICS In some cases, the condition is inherited

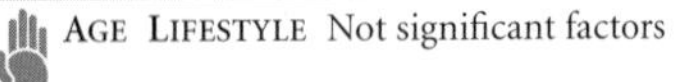
AGE LIFESTYLE Not significant factors

The aortic valve separates the left lower chamber of the heart (the left ventricle) from the aorta, which is the main artery leading from the heart. This valve normally stops blood from flowing back into the heart from the aorta. In aortic incompetence, the valve cusps (flaps) do not close tightly, letting blood leak back from the aorta. As a result, the heart has to pump harder and faster to circulate blood around the body, and this may eventually lead to the development of chronic heart failure (p.413).

WHAT ARE THE CAUSES?

About 1 in 50 boys and 1 in 100 girls are born with an aortic valve with two cusps instead of the normal three. One cause is the rare genetic disorder Marfan's syndrome (p.824). A possible cause of valve damage later in life is infection (*see* INFECTIVE ENDOCARDITIS, p.426). The aortic valve flaps may also become leaky as a result of the rare inflammatory joint disorder ankylosing spondylitis (p.378). Other causes of aortic incompetence include rheumatic fever (p.429) and syphilis, but these diseases are now rare in developed countries due to the widespread use of effective antibiotics.

WHAT ARE THE SYMPTOMS?

If aortic incompetence is mild, it may not cause symptoms for years. If symptoms do develop, they may include:

- Tiredness.
- Shortness of breath during exertion.
- Awareness of the heart beating strongly.

In severe aortic incompetence, heart failure may eventually develop, leading to symptoms such as constant shortness of breath and swollen ankles.

WHAT MIGHT BE DONE?

If there are no symptoms, aortic incompetence is usually discovered during a routine examination. Your doctor may then arrange for electrocardiography (*see* ECG, p.406) to evaluate the electrical activity of the heart. In addition, the heart may be imaged by echocardiography (p.425), which looks at the interior of the heart and can evaluate the movement of the valves. A chest X-ray (p.490) may also be taken to see if the heart has enlarged due to heart failure.

If the aortic incompetence is mild, often no treatment is needed. However, if you have symptoms or if chronic heart failure develops, you may need treatment with drugs such as ACE inhibitors (p.900), which reduce the work that the heart has to do.

If drug treatment fails to relieve your symptoms, surgery may be needed to repair the valve or to replace it with a tissue valve from a human donor or a pig or with a mechanical valve (*see* HEART VALVE REPLACEMENT, above). Surgery is more likely to be successful if it is done before heart failure becomes advanced.

An abnormal or replacement aortic valve is more susceptible to infection than a normal valve. Your doctor may therefore advise you to take a single dose of an antibiotic (p.885) before dental treatment or before operations that carry a risk of introducing bacteria into the bloodstream, such as surgery on the digestive or urinary tracts.

Once the damaged aortic valve has been repaired or replaced, the outlook for the affected person is good and life expectancy should be normal.

(WWW) ONLINE SITES: p.1032

Aortic stenosis

Narrowing of the aortic valve, reducing the flow of blood into the circulation

 AGE May be present at birth but most common in people over the age of 70

 GENDER More common in males

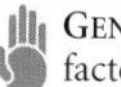 GENETICS LIFESTYLE Not significant factors

The aortic valve separates the left lower chamber (left ventricle) of the heart and the main artery of the body, the aorta. The valve opens to allow blood to flow out of the heart. In aortic stenosis, the opening of the valve is narrowed, reducing the flow of blood through it. The heart then has to pump harder to compensate. Aortic stenosis is the most common valve disorder requiring valve replacement in the UK.

What are the causes?

In young people in developed countries, aortic stenosis is usually the result of a heart abnormality that is present at birth (*see* CONGENITAL HEART DISEASE, p.836). In elderly people, aortic stenosis is often caused by calcium deposits on the valve, which naturally build up over time. Rheumatic fever (p.429) was once a common cause of aortic stenosis. However, rheumatic fever is now rare in developed countries, mainly due to the use of effective antibiotics.

What are the symptoms?

In mild cases of aortic stenosis, there are often no symptoms. In some cases of mild stenosis, tiredness may be the only symptom. Other symptoms may develop in more severe cases, such as:

- Dizziness and fainting.
- Chest pain during exertion.

If the opening through the aortic valve is very narrow, the flow of blood to the coronary arteries that supply blood to the heart muscle is reduced. This will eventually lead to breathlessness due to chronic heart failure (p.413). Abnormal heart rhythms may also develop (*see* ARRHYTHMIAS, p.415), and infection of the valves is more likely.

How is it diagnosed?

Often, mild aortic stenosis is detected during a routine examination. If your doctor suspects that you have aortic stenosis, he or she may arrange for echocardiography (p.425) to image the interior of the heart, including the aortic valve. You may also have a chest X-ray (p.490) because, if there is stenosis, calcium deposits on the valve may be visible on the X-ray. The severity of stenosis can be assessed by a procedure called cardiac catheterization, in which a flexible catheter is inserted into an artery in the arm or groin and passed into the heart. A small device attached to the catheter then measures the pressures on either side of the valve.

What is the treatment?

Mild stenosis is frequently treated with drugs such as diuretics (p.902), which relieve breathlessness by removing excess fluid from the lungs. In severe cases, you may have a balloon valvuloplasty, in which a balloon is inflated in the valve to widen it. However, a heart valve replacement (opposite page) is often needed eventually. You may need to take a single dose of an antibiotic (p.885) before dental treatment or operations that may introduce infection, such as those on the digestive tract. The outlook is good if treatment is given before the heart muscle becomes badly damaged.

(WWW) ONLINE SITES: p.1032

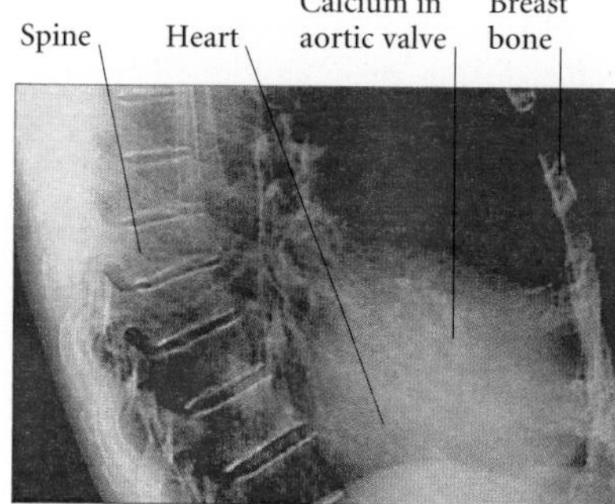

Aortic stenosis

This chest X-ray, taken from the side, shows calcium deposits that have formed in a narrowed aortic valve. The deposits make the valve visible on the X-ray.

Mitral incompetence

Leakage of blood back through the mitral valve of the heart

 GENETICS In some cases, the condition is inherited

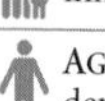 AGE GENDER LIFESTYLE Risk factors depend on the cause

The mitral valve sits between the upper chamber (atrium) and the lower chamber (ventricle) on the left side of the heart. In mitral incompetence, the valve fails to close properly and allows blood to leak back into the atrium. This increases the pressure in the blood vessels leading to that chamber. The left side of the heart has to work harder to pump blood around the body, and eventually chronic heart failure (p.413) develops. Mitral incompetence can occur in conjunction with mitral stenosis (p.424).

What are the causes?

In rare cases, mitral incompetence is present at birth, sometimes as a result of the rare genetic disorder Marfan's syndrome (p.824). Any condition that damages the mitral valve can lead to mitral incompetence. Rheumatic fever (p.429) was once a major cause of the disorder but is now rarely seen in developed countries, mainly because of the widespread use of antibiotics. A more common cause is an infection of the valve (see INFECTIVE ENDOCARDITIS, p.426). Hypertrophic cardiomyopathy (p.428), in which the wall of the left ventricle is thickened, may distort the valve, causing incompetence. The condition can also be a consequence of a heart attack if the heart muscle attached to the valve is affected (*see* MYOCARDIAL INFARCTION, p.410). In some cases, mitral incompetence occurs in conjunction with mitral valve prolapse (p.425).

What are the symptoms?

Symptoms of mitral incompetence usually develop gradually over months or years but may appear suddenly if the cause is a heart attack or valve infection. The symptoms include:

- Unexplained tiredness.
- Shortness of breath during exertion.
- Palpitations (awareness of an irregular or abnormally rapid heartbeat).

Eventually, symptoms of chronic heart failure may occur, such as shortness of breath at rest as well as during exertion, due to fluid in the lungs. The build-up of fluid in the body tissues also causes swelling of the ankles.

ARE THERE COMPLICATIONS?

The backward blood flow into the left atrium may enlarge it, leading to an irregular heartbeat (*see* ATRIAL FIBRILLATION, p.417). If the atrium is so large that it cannot empty fully with each heartbeat, a blood clot may form. If a clot passes into an artery supplying the brain and blocks it, the result may be a stroke (p.532). Another potential complication is infection of the leaky mitral valve after dental treatment or surgery on the digestive or urinary tracts.

WHAT MIGHT BE DONE?

Your doctor may suspect mitral incompetence if he or she hears characteristic sounds known as heart murmurs. Tests to assess the function of the heart and lungs may be carried out, including an ECG (p.406) to monitor the electrical activity of the heart and a chest X-ray (p.490). The interior of the heart may be imaged by echocardiography (opposite page) to confirm the diagnosis. This procedure can show the movements of the mitral valve.

If heart failure develops, drugs such as diuretics (p.902) may be prescribed to relieve the symptoms. If the left atrium becomes enlarged, you may also be given drugs that prevent blood clotting (p.904) to lessen the risk of clots in the atrium. Severe mitral incompetence may need to be treated surgically to repair the valve or implant a heart valve replacement (p.422). If you have a damaged or replacement heart valve, you may be advised to take a single dose of an antibiotic (p.885) before dental treatment and surgical procedures such as those on the digestive or urinary tracts.

The outlook for mitral incompetence is good if treatment is given before the heart has become badly damaged.

(WWW) ONLINE SITES: p.1032

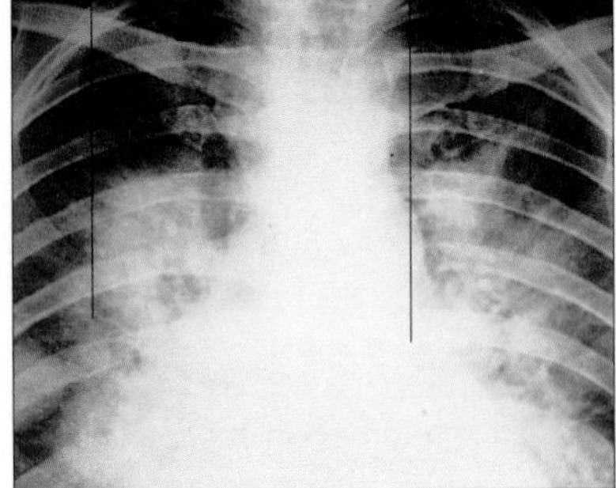

Effects of mitral incompetence
Enlargement of the heart and excess fluid in the lungs, which are indications of heart failure caused by mitral incompetence, can be seen on this chest X-ray.

Mitral stenosis

Narrowing of the mitral valve, resulting in a decrease in blood flow within the heart

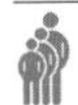 AGE More common after the age of 40

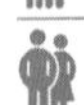 GENDER More common in females

 GENETICS LIFESTYLE Not significant factors

The mitral valve sits between the upper chamber (atrium) and lower chamber (ventricle) on the left side of the heart. In mitral stenosis, the opening of this valve is narrowed, restricting the blood flow through the atrium. The heart works harder to pump blood through the narrow valve, and chronic heart failure (p.413) may eventually develop. Mitral stenosis is more common in females and sometimes occurs with mitral incompetence (p.423).

WHAT ARE THE CAUSES?

Mitral stenosis is almost always due to damage to the valve caused by an earlier attack of rheumatic fever (p.429). This condition is now rare in developed countries, and, in the UK, mitral stenosis is most often found in middle-aged or elderly people who had rheumatic fever during their childhood. In rare cases, mitral stenosis is present at birth.

WHAT ARE THE SYMPTOMS?

Symptoms usually develop gradually in adulthood and may include:

- Unexplained tiredness.
- Shortness of breath, occurring during exertion at first but later also at rest.
- Palpitations (awareness of an irregular or abnormally rapid heartbeat).

As the stenosis becomes worse, the symptoms of heart failure may develop, including swelling of the tissues, which is most noticeable in the ankles.

ARE THERE COMPLICATIONS?

Sometimes, the atria beat irregularly and rapidly (*see* ATRIAL FIBRILLATION, p.417). Blood clots may also form on the wall of the left atrium because it does not empty fully. If fragments of clots break off, they may block a blood vessel elsewhere in the body. If the clot blocks an artery supplying the brain, the result may be a stroke (p.532).

HOW IS IT DIAGNOSED?

Your doctor will examine you and will probably arrange for an ECG (p.406) to assess the electrical activity of the heart. The inside of the heart may be imaged by echocardiography (opposite page), a technique that shows the movement of the heart valves. You may also have a chest X-ray (p.490). The severity of the stenosis may be assessed by a procedure in which a tube called a cardiac catheter is inserted through blood vessels into the heart. The catheter is attached to a device that measures the pressure on either side of the valve.

WHAT IS THE TREATMENT?

In most cases of mitral stenosis, drug treatments are used to help to relieve the symptoms. For example, diuretics (p.902) may be prescribed to remove excess fluid from the body and to relieve shortness of breath. Antiarrhythmic drugs (p.898) may be given to help correct an abnormal heart rhythm. Drugs that prevent blood clotting (p.904) are often prescribed to reduce the risk of blood clots forming in the heart.

If drug treatment is ineffective, a balloon valvuloplasty may be performed, in which a balloon-tipped catheter is passed into the heart and the balloon briefly inflated inside the stenosed valve to widen it. Alternatively, the valve may be repaired or replaced by surgery (*see* HEART VALVE REPLACEMENT, p.422).

An abnormal or replacement valve is susceptible to infection. For this reason, you may be advised to take a single dose of an antibiotic (p.885) before having dental treatment or operations on the digestive or urinary tracts when infection may enter the bloodstream.

Mitral stenosis may recur after a balloon valvuloplasty, often within a year. However, a heart valve replacement is often effective for 10 years or more.

(WWW) ONLINE SITES: p.1032

(TEST) ECHOCARDIOGRAPHY

Echocardiography is a technique that uses ultrasound waves to image the interior of the heart. The test looks at the size and function of the heart and is used to diagnose disorders of the heart and the heart valves. The test is usually performed using an ultrasound transducer (probe) placed on the skin of the chest directly over the heart. In some cases, a small probe is passed down the oesophagus instead so that it is close to the back of the heart. A moving image of the beating heart with its valves and chambers is then produced. The test takes about 20 minutes and is painless.

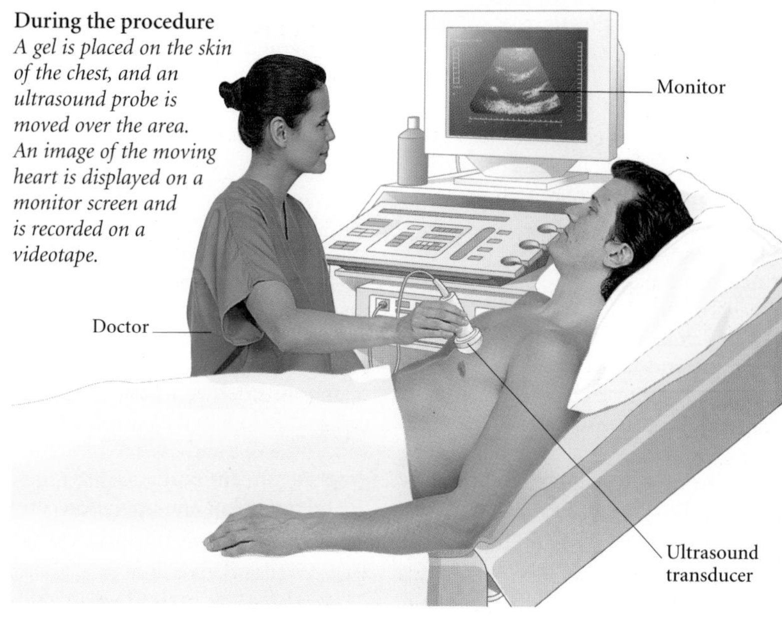

During the procedure
A gel is placed on the skin of the chest, and an ultrasound probe is moved over the area. An image of the moving heart is displayed on a monitor screen and is recorded on a videotape.

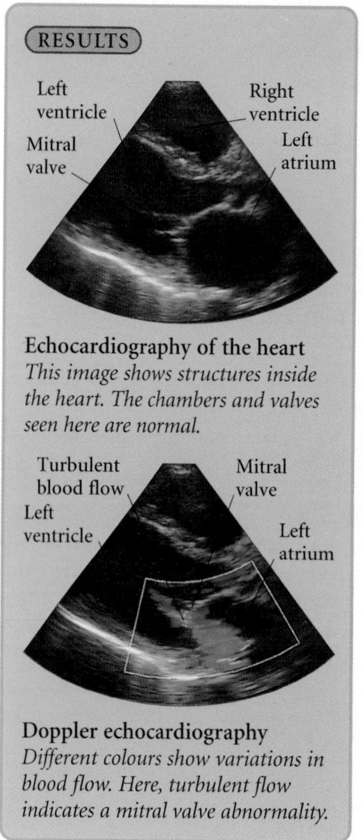

Echocardiography of the heart
This image shows structures inside the heart. The chambers and valves seen here are normal.

Doppler echocardiography
Different colours show variations in blood flow. Here, turbulent flow indicates a mitral valve abnormality.

Mitral valve prolapse

A minor abnormality of the mitral valve, also known as floppy mitral valve

 AGE Most common between the ages of 20 and 40

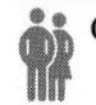 GENDER More common in females

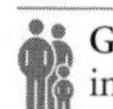 GENETICS In some cases, the condition is inherited

 LIFESTYLE Not a significant factor

The mitral valve sits between the upper chamber (atrium) and the lower chamber (ventricle) on the left side of the heart. This valve normally closes tightly when the heart contracts to pump blood out into the circulation. In the disorder called mitral valve prolapse, the valve is slightly deformed and bulges back into the left atrium. This prolapse may allow a small amount of blood to leak back into the atrium (*see* MITRAL INCOMPETENCE, p.423). Mitral valve prolapse is common, occurring in up to 1 in 20 people. The condition occurs most commonly in young or middle-aged women, but often the cause is not known. In some cases, mitral valve prolapse is associated with the rare genetic disorder Marfan's syndrome (p.824).

WHAT ARE THE SYMPTOMS?

Mitral valve prolapse usually causes no symptoms, and most people are unaware that they have the condition. If symptoms do occur, they are usually intermittent and may include:

- Light-headedness.
- Fainting.
- Sharp, left-sided chest pains.
- Palpitations (awareness of an irregular or abnormally rapid heartbeat).

There is also an increased chance that a floppy valve may become further damaged by an infection (*see* INFECTIVE ENDOCARDITIS, p.426), particularly following dental procedures or surgery on the digestive or urinary tracts.

HOW IS IT DIAGNOSED?

Your doctor may suspect mitral valve prolapse if he or she hears a characteristic clicking sound when listening to your heart with a stethoscope. He or she may arrange for you to have tests, including an ECG (p.406), which monitors the electrical activity of the heart. A diagnosis of mitral valve prolapse is usually confirmed by echocardiography (above), which examines the movements of the valves. If you have palpitations, your heart rhythm may also be monitored over a period of 24 hours while you perform your normal activities (*see* AMBULATORY ECG, p.416).

WHAT IS THE TREATMENT?

Most people with mitral valve prolapse need no treatment. If symptoms such as an irregular heartbeat cause problems, an antiarrhythmic drug (p.898) may be prescribed. You may also be prescribed a single dose of an antibiotic (p.885) before dental treatment or some operations, such as those on the digestive or urinary tracts.

The disorder usually has no effect on life expectancy, but, in very rare cases, mitral incompetence develops, leading to chronic heart failure (p.413). Heart valve replacement (p.422) may then be needed, but the outlook is still good.

(WWW) ONLINE SITES: p.1032

Infective endocarditis

Inflammation of the lining of the heart, particularly affecting the heart valves, caused by an infection

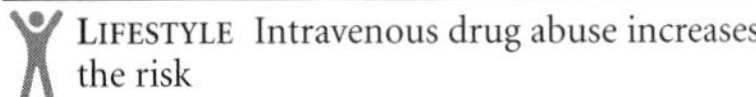

LIFESTYLE Intravenous drug abuse increases the risk

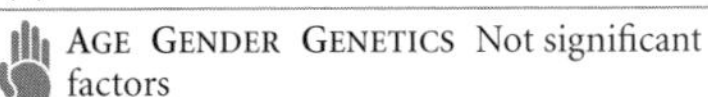

AGE GENDER GENETICS Not significant factors

The internal lining of the heart, the endocardium, may become infected if microorganisms enter the bloodstream and reach the heart. This type of infection causes the lining, especially over the heart valves, to become inflamed, and bacteria and blood clots can accumulate over the inflamed areas. The valves are particularly prone to infection if they are already damaged or if they are replacement valves (*see* HEART VALVE REPLACEMENT, p.422).

In most cases, infective endocarditis is a chronic (long-term) disorder that develops over weeks or months and causes only vague symptoms, such as a fever and aching joints. Rarely, endocarditis is an acute disorder that may rapidly damage one or more of the heart valves. Within days acute endocarditis may cause acute heart failure (p.412), which may be life-threatening.

WHAT ARE THE CAUSES?

The most common causes of infective endocarditis are bacteria and, less often, fungi. Normally harmless microorganisms may enter the blood during dental procedures, especially tooth extraction, and operations on the digestive or urinary tracts. The condition can also occur after a medical procedure, such as the insertion of a catheter into the bladder. Rarely, infective endocarditis develops after cardiac surgery, especially if artificial materials, such as replacement heart valves, are inserted into the heart.

A person with a suppressed immune system is particularly susceptible to infective endocarditis because his or her body is less able to fight the infection. For example, anyone with HIV infection or AIDS (p.297) or who is undergoing treatment with anticancer drugs (p.907) is at increased risk of developing the disorder. People who abuse intravenous drugs are also susceptible to infective endocarditis because microorganisms can be injected into the bloodstream and travel to the heart. There is an even greater risk of infection if needles are shared.

WHAT ARE THE SYMPTOMS?

The symptoms of chronic endocarditis are often generalized and unrelated to heart damage. They may include:

- Abnormal tiredness.
- Fever and night sweats.
- Aching joints.
- Weight loss.

Infected material from the valve may break off and block a vessel elsewhere in the body. For example, small clots may lodge in veins under the fingernails or skin, causing tiny splinter-like haemorrhages. If a clot blocks an artery that supplies blood to the brain, it may result in a stroke (p.532).

The symptoms of acute endocarditis develop suddenly and may include:

- High fever.
- Palpitations (awareness of an irregular or abnormally rapid heartbeat).

These symptoms can rapidly worsen. If acute heart failure develops, there may be other symptoms, such as severe shortness of breath and wheezing.

HOW IS IT DIAGNOSED?

Chronic infective endocarditis is difficult to diagnose because the symptoms are often unrelated to heart damage. Your doctor may suspect the disorder if he or she hears a new heart murmur or a change in an existing heart murmur. The diagnosis may be confirmed by echocardiography (p.425) to image the interior of the heart and detect infected material on the surface of the valves. Blood tests may be done to identify the organism responsible for the infection.

WHAT IS THE TREATMENT?

If you have infective endocarditis, you will usually need treatment with intravenous antibiotics (p.885) for about 6 weeks. You will have regular blood tests to confirm that the infection is clearing up. This treatment is successful in up to 4 in 5 cases. If a valve is badly damaged or if the infection cannot be controlled with drugs, heart valve replacement (p.422) may be necessary.

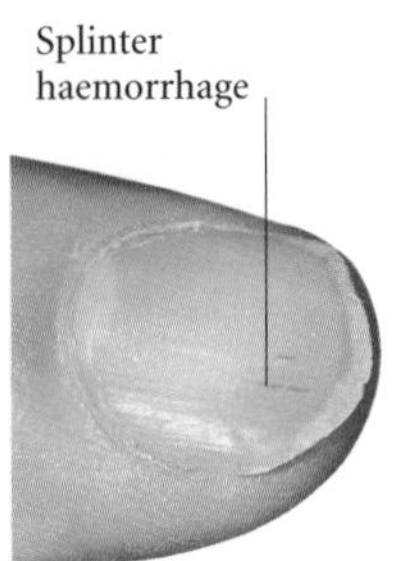

Effect of infective endocarditis
Bleeding under the fingernail, resulting in so-called splinter haemorrhages, can occur in association with the heart disorder infective endocarditis.

If you have a valve disorder or you already have a replacement heart valve, you are at increased risk of developing endocarditis and should be aware of the symptoms. You should contact your doctor immediately if any become apparent. Once you have had one episode of the disorder, you have an increased risk of developing it again. For this reason, you will be advised to take a single dose of an antibiotic (p.885) before dental treatment and operations on the digestive or urinary tracts.

(WWW) ONLINE SITES: p.1032

Myocarditis

Inflammation of the muscle tissue of the heart, usually due to an infection

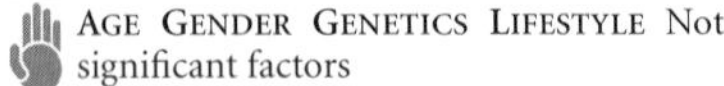

AGE GENDER GENETICS LIFESTYLE Not significant factors

Myocarditis is inflammation of the heart muscle, usually due to an infection. Frequently, the condition goes unrecognized because there are no obvious symptoms. However, severe inflammation of the heart muscle may develop, causing chest pain and leading eventually to heart enlargement and chronic heart failure (p.413).

The most common cause of the disorder is a viral infection, usually with the coxsackie virus. Myocarditis may also be due to rheumatic fever (p.429), although this is now rare in developed countries, mainly due to the widespread use of antibiotics (p.885). Some autoimmune disorders, such as systemic lupus erythematosus (p.461), in which the body attacks its own tissues, may also cause myocarditis.

What are the symptoms?

Myocarditis often causes no symptoms. However, if symptoms do occur, they usually develop over a number of hours or days and may include:

- Fever.
- Tiredness.
- Aching in the chest.
- Palpitations (awareness of an irregular or abnormally rapid heartbeat).

Eventually, breathlessness and swelling of the ankles may develop due to heart failure. Rarely, myocarditis causes sudden death during vigorous exertion.

What might be done?

If your doctor suspects that you have myocarditis, he or she will probably arrange for an ECG (p.406) to monitor the electrical activity of the heart and a chest X-ray (p.490) to see if the heart is enlarged. You may have echocardiography (p.425) to image the interior of the heart. Blood tests may be carried out to check for infection and for the presence of enzymes that can indicate whether or not the heart muscle is damaged.

Myocarditis is usually mild, and the heart should recover within 2 weeks. If severe heart failure does develop, a heart transplant (right) may give the best chance of a return to normal health.

(WWW) ONLINE SITES: p.1032

Dilated cardiomyopathy

Damaged heart muscle, leading to enlargement of the heart

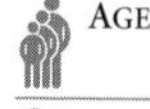 AGE More common over the age of 45

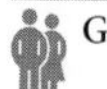 GENDER More common in males

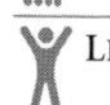 LIFESTYLE Alcohol abuse increases the risk

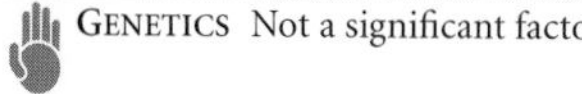 GENETICS Not a significant factor

Healthy heart muscle is vital for the heart to pump blood around the body effectively. In dilated cardiomyopathy, the muscular walls of the heart become damaged. The weakened muscle then stretches, making the heart larger. This weakening and the enlargement of the heart muscle reduce the heart's pumping action, leading to chronic heart failure (p.413). In some cases, dilated cardiomyopathy is caused by alcohol abuse. The disorder may also be due to an autoimmune disorder, in which the body attacks its own tissues, or it may occur after a viral illness. Often, the underlying cause is not found.

The symptoms of dilated cardiomyopathy are similar to those of chronic heart failure. Therefore, before making a diagnosis of dilated cardiomyopathy, your doctor may wish to carry out tests that exclude other disorders that cause heart failure, such as coronary artery disease (p.405) and heart valve disorders. Dilated cardiomyopathy is more common over the age of 45 and in men.

What are the symptoms?

In many cases of mild, dilated cardiomyopathy, there are no symptoms. If symptoms do occur, they usually develop gradually over a number of years and may include:

- Tiredness.
- Shortness of breath during exertion.
- Palpitations (awareness of an irregular or abnormally rapid heartbeat).
- Swelling of the ankles.

As the disorder progresses the heart's pumping efficiency decreases and symptoms, such as shortness of breath, worsen. The heart enlargement may stretch the valves, causing them to become leaky, and may eventually lead to the development of chronic heart failure or an abnormal heart rhythm (*see* ARRHYTHMIAS, p.415). If the chambers in the heart cannot empty fully because they are too large, a blood clot can form, which may break off and block a vessel elsewhere in the body.

How is it diagnosed?

The diagnosis of dilated cardiomyopathy involves a number of tests, many of which are used to exclude other possible causes of your symptoms, such as coronary artery disease. You may have an ECG (p.406) to monitor the heart's electrical activity and echocardiography (p.425) to image the interior of the heart. You may also have a chest X-ray (p.490) to detect enlargement of the heart. Coronary angiography (p.408) is used to exclude coronary artery disease as a cause of symptoms. To exclude valve disease, a cardiac catheter may be passed into the heart from an artery to measure blood pressure inside the heart. If you have palpitations, an ECG

(TREATMENT) Heart transplant

A heart transplant is sometimes the only treatment option if the heart is severely damaged by a disorder such as dilated cardiomyopathy (left). However, there may be a long wait before a suitable donor heart is found. During the operation, the heart's normal function is taken over by a heart–lung machine (*see* SURGERY USING A HEART–LUNG MACHINE, p.953). The operation takes between 3 and 5 hours. You will need lifelong drug treatment to prevent the body from rejecting the donor heart. About 4 in 5 people survive for 5 years or more after having a heart transplant.

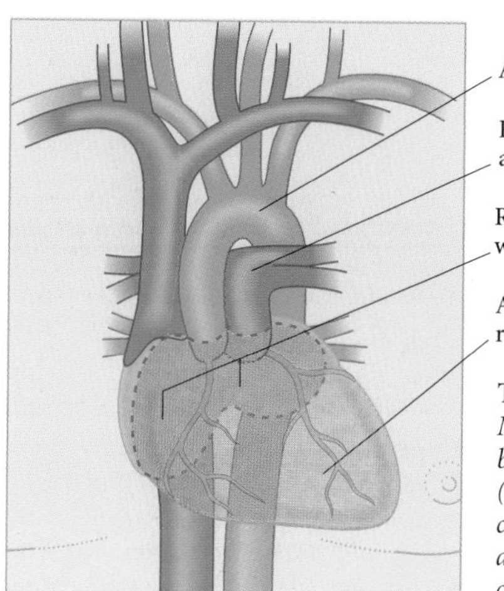

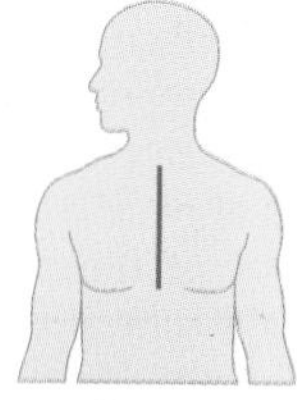

SITE OF INCISION

The procedure

Most of the diseased heart is removed, but the back walls of the upper chambers (atria) are left in place. The lower chambers (ventricles) of the donor heart are then attached to the remaining areas of the recipient's heart.

may be carried out over a period of 24 hours to monitor your heartbeat while you carry out your daily activities (*see* AMBULATORY ECG, p.416).

WHAT IS THE TREATMENT?

If the cause of dilated cardiomyopathy is unknown, no specific treatment can be given. If alcohol abuse is the cause, you must stop drinking. Symptoms of heart failure may be relieved by drugs such as digoxin (*see* DIGITALIS DRUGS, p.901) to improve the function of the heart, diuretic drugs (p.902) to remove excess fluid, and beta-blockers (p.898) and ACE inhibitors (p.900), which may help to prevent deterioration. You may also have drugs that prevent blood clotting (p.904). However, if heart failure worsens in spite of drug treatment, a heart transplant (p.427) may be considered. Without a transplant, only about 3 in 10 people with dilated cardiomyopathy survive for more than 5 years.

(WWW) ONLINE SITES: p.1032

Hypertrophic cardiomyopathy

Abnormal thickening of the muscular walls of the heart, which reduces its pumping efficiency

AGE Usually develops in adolescence but may be delayed until middle age

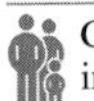
GENETICS In some cases, the condition is inherited

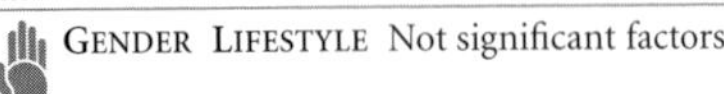
GENDER LIFESTYLE Not significant factors

In hypertrophic cardiomyopathy, the walls of the heart are excessively thick. This thickening prevents the heart from filling properly and may partially block the passage of blood from the heart, both of which reduce the pumping efficiency of the heart. The condition is usually inherited, but the exact cause is unknown. The disorder may cause sudden death in apparently healthy, active young people, but, sometimes symptoms do not develop until middle age.

WHAT ARE THE SYMPTOMS?

Symptoms of the disorder usually develop in adolescence. They first occur during exertion and may include:

- Fainting.
- Shortness of breath.
- Chest pain.
- Palpitations (awareness of an irregular or abnormally rapid heartbeat).

As the disorder progresses, shortness of breath may be present at rest. In some cases, a life-threatening abnormal heart rhythm develops (*see* ARRHYTHMIAS, p.415). Hypertrophic cardiomyopathy may also distort the valve that sits between the left upper and lower chambers of the heart, causing it to leak (*see* MITRAL INCOMPETENCE, p.423).

In severe cases, the thickened heart walls may obstruct the blood flow out of the heart, which results in inadequate blood supply to the rest of the body. This situation is potentially fatal.

HOW IS IT DIAGNOSED?

If your doctor suspects that you may have hypertrophic cardiomyopathy, he or she may arrange for you to have an ECG (p.406) to measure the heart's electrical activity. You may also have echocardiography (p.425) to image the interior of the heart. This shows the size of the heart and the thickness of the heart walls and assesses the degree to which output of blood from the heart is restricted. You may also have your heart rhythm monitored for 24 hours while you carry out your normal activities (*see* AMBULATORY ECG, p.416).

WHAT IS THE TREATMENT?

Treatment is aimed at improving the filling capacity of the heart using drugs such as beta-blockers (p.898) and calcium channel blockers (p.900). If you have an abnormal heart rhythm, it may be treated with antiarrhythmic drugs

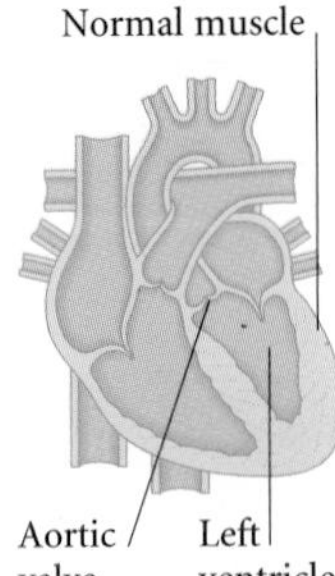

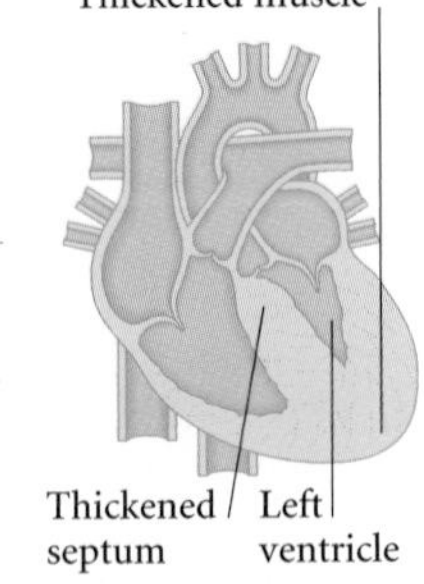

Hypertrophic cardiomyopathy
In this condition, the septum and the muscular wall of the left ventricle become abnormally thick. This thickening prevents the left ventricle from filling properly and obstructs the outflow to the aortic valve.

(p.898). Surgery may be used to remove some of the thickened muscle. In rare cases, a heart transplant (p.427) may be considered. Hypertrophic cardiomyopathy increases your risk of developing an infection of the heart muscle or valve. For this reason, a single dose of an antibiotic (p.885) may be prescribed before dental treatment or some operations, such as those on the digestive tract.

The disorder is sometimes inherited. For this reason, relatives of anyone with hypertrophic cardiomyopathy should be screened with echocardiography to see if they have the condition.

About 1 in 25 affected people die each year. The outlook is better if the symptoms are diagnosed and treated early.

(WWW) ONLINE SITES: p.1032

Pericarditis

Inflammation of the pericardium, the double-layered membrane that envelops the heart

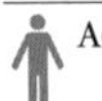
AGE Risk factors depend on the cause

GENDER GENETICS LIFESTYLE Not significant factors

The pericardium is a two-layered membrane that surrounds the heart. In pericarditis, this membrane becomes inflamed, usually due to infection. The inflammation is usually acute with symptoms that are often mistaken for a heart attack (*see* MYOCARDIAL INFARCTION, p.410). The inflammation usually subsides after about a week. However, rarely, the inflammation persists and causes the pericardium to become scarred and thickened and to contract around the heart. As a result, the constricted heart muscle is unable to pump normally. This serious long-term condition is called constrictive pericarditis. In both acute and long-term disorders, fluid may accumulate between the two layers of the pericardium and stop the heart from pumping effectively. This is called a pericardial effusion and may lead to chronic heart failure (p.413).

WHAT ARE THE CAUSES?

In young adults, pericarditis is usually due to a viral infection, although pericarditis may develop as a complication of bacterial pneumonia (p.490). Tuberculosis (p.491) is an important cause of

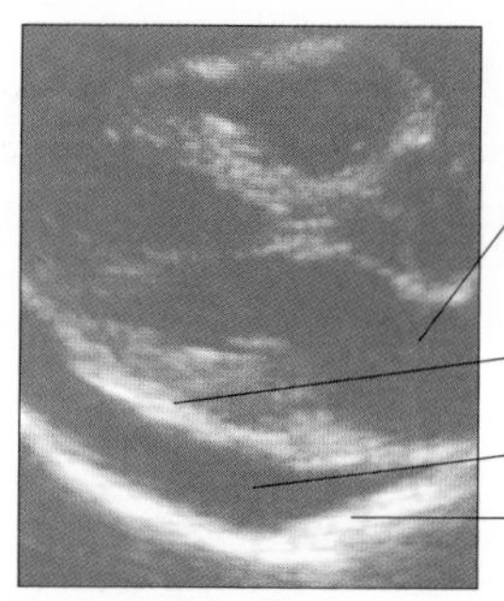

Pericardial effusion

This echocardiogram shows fluid between the two layers of the pericardium, the membrane that surrounds the heart.

pericarditis in some countries. A heart attack can cause pericarditis if the muscle on the surface of the heart is affected. Pericarditis may also develop when a cancerous tumour elsewhere in the body spreads to the pericardium.

Inflammation of the pericardium is also associated with autoimmune disorders, in which the body attacks its own tissues. For example, the conditions rheumatoid arthritis (p.377) and systemic lupus erythematosus (p.461) may sometimes cause pericarditis.

WHAT ARE THE SYMPTOMS?

The symptoms of acute pericarditis develop over a few hours and last for about 7 days. They include:

- Pain in the centre of the chest, which worsens when taking a deep breath and is relieved by sitting forwards.
- Pain in the neck and shoulders.
- Fever.

In chronic constrictive pericarditis or when excess fluid builds up in the pericardium, the heart may be unable to pump blood around the body effectively. Poor circulation may then lead to further symptoms that develop over a few months, such as breathlessness and swelling of the ankles and abdomen. An irregular heartbeat may also develop (*see* ATRIAL FIBRILLATION, p.417).

WHAT MIGHT BE DONE?

Your doctor will probably arrange for you to have a chest X-ray (p.490) and an ECG (p.406) to monitor the heart's electrical activity. Echocardiography (p.425) may be carried out to image the interior of the heart. This technique allows the thickness of the pericardium to be measured and can detect fluid around the heart. Blood tests can check for infection or autoimmune disease.

Pericarditis requires treatment in hospital. You will probably be given nonsteroidal anti-inflammatory drugs (p.894) to relieve chest pain and to help reduce the inflammation.

When pericarditis is caused by a viral infection, the infection should clear up within a week without further treatment. In other cases, the treatment is directed at the underlying cause. For example, antibiotics (p.885) may be prescribed for bacterial infections, corticosteroids (p.930) for autoimmune disorders, and antituberculous drugs (p.886) to treat tuberculosis infection.

Fluid in a pericardial effusion may be withdrawn through a needle passed through the chest wall. If the effusion recurs, a piece of pericardium may be removed, allowing the fluid to drain continuously. In chronic constrictive pericarditis, surgery may be needed to remove most of the pericardium and allow the heart to pump freely.

WHAT IS THE PROGNOSIS?

Most people who have viral pericarditis recover within a week, but about 1 in 10 has a recurrence in the first few months afterwards. Pericarditis may recur if it is due to an autoimmune disorder. Surgery for chronic constrictive pericarditis is successful in only a minority of cases.

(WWW) ONLINE SITES: p.1032

Rheumatic fever

Inflammation of the heart, joints, and skin following bacterial infection

 AGE Most common in people aged 5–15, but effects often not seen until adulthood

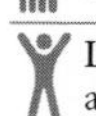 LIFESTYLE Overcrowded living conditions and inadequate nutrition are risk factors

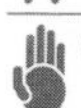 GENDER GENETICS Not significant factors

Fifty years ago, rheumatic fever was a major childhood illness in Europe and North America that left thousands of people with damaged heart valves. The effects of the damage are now being seen in elderly people as heart valve disorders, most commonly as mitral stenosis (p.424). Rheumatic fever is now rare in developed countries, mainly due to the use of antibiotics (p.885) and to improved standards of living, including better nutrition and housing. A few outbreaks have occurred in the US recently but none in the UK. However, the disease still affects many people in developing countries.

Rheumatic fever develops after an infection, usually of the throat, caused by streptococcal bacteria. The condition is caused by the immune system attacking the body's own tissues in response to the infection.

WHAT ARE THE SYMPTOMS?

Rheumatic fever develops 1–4 weeks after the sore throat has cleared up. Symptoms may include:

- High fever.
- Aching and swelling of larger joints, such as the knees, elbows, and ankles.
- Characteristic blotchy pink rash on the trunk and limbs.

If the heart muscle is affected, there may be shortness of breath and chest pain for a few weeks until the inflammation settles. Inflammation of a heart valve causes permanent damage that may lead to thickening and scarring of the valve years later. Valve damage causes symptoms such as excessive tiredness.

WHAT MIGHT BE DONE?

If rheumatic fever is suspected, a swab is taken from the throat and a blood test carried out to look for streptococcal infection. A chest X-ray (p.490) may be taken to look at the size of the heart to see if it is inflamed. An ECG (p.406) may be performed to monitor electrical activity in the heart and echocardiography (p.425) to image the interior of the heart and the valves.

Rheumatic fever is treated with antibiotics to clear up the infection and complete bed rest for about 2 weeks. Nonsteroidal anti-inflammatory drugs (p.894) may be used to reduce fever and joint inflammation, and corticosteroids (p.930) may be prescribed to reduce inflammation of the heart. Low-dose antibiotics often need to be taken for up to 5 years to avoid recurrence.

About 1 in 100 people dies during an initial attack of rheumatic fever. The risk of a recurrence is highest in the first 3 years after the initial infection in young adults and people with damaged heart valves. After 10 years, 2 in 3 people have a detectable heart valve disorder.

(WWW) ONLINE SITES: p.1032, p.1033

PERIPHERAL VASCULAR DISORDERS

The peripheral blood vessels carry blood from the heart to the rest of the body and back to the heart, providing oxygen and nutrients to all parts of the body. If the blood vessels are diseased, oxygen supply to the tissues is reduced, leading to possible tissue damage and even tissue death. Many peripheral vascular disorders are more common in people who smoke and have a high-fat diet.

All of the blood vessels that carry blood around the body, apart from those in the heart and the brain, are known collectively as the peripheral vascular system. The peripheral vascular system consists of arteries, which carry blood away from the heart, and veins, which carry blood towards the heart.

This section begins by discussing aortic aneurysm, which is a potentially life-threatening disorder of the largest artery in the body. The second article examines thrombosis and embolism, in which a peripheral artery or vein becomes blocked. The most common cause of these disorders is a build-up of fatty deposits on the artery walls, which is a factor that also contributes to the development of diabetic vascular disease. All of these disorders reduce blood supply to the tissues, leading to conditions such as lower limb ischaemia and gangrene. Disorders that affect the small blood vessels in the hands and feet are then considered.

The section ends with a discussion of disorders of the peripheral veins. The veins may be blocked by a blood clot, as occurs in deep vein thrombosis and superficial thrombophlebitis, or may develop structural abnormalities, as occurs in varicose veins.

KEY ANATOMY

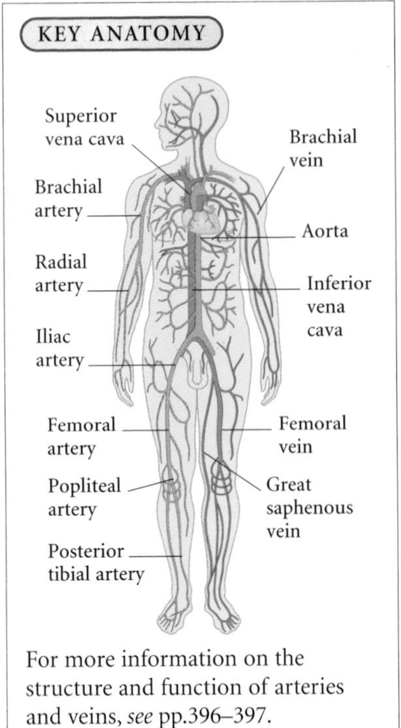

For more information on the structure and function of arteries and veins, *see* pp.396–397.

Aortic aneurysm

Enlargement of a section of the aorta due to weakness in the artery wall

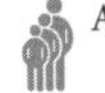
AGE More common over the age of 65

GENDER More common in males

GENETICS Sometimes runs in families

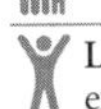
LIFESTYLE Smoking, a high-fat diet, lack of exercise, and excess weight are risk factors

If a section of an artery wall becomes weakened, the pressure of blood in the artery may cause it to bulge out. The bulging section of the artery is called an aneurysm. An aneurysm may occur in any artery in the body, but the aorta, the major artery that transports blood away from the heart, is most commonly involved. Three-quarters of all aortic aneurysms occur in the abdominal section of the aorta below the kidneys, and this type of aneurysm tends to run in families. Aortic aneurysms may also develop in the chest. The risk of having an aneurysm increases with age, and the condition most commonly occurs in men over the age of 65.

Small aortic aneurysms do not usually produce symptoms, although large ones may cause localized pain. In some enlarged aneurysms, known as dissecting aneurysms, the inner layer of the arterial wall tears and peels away from the outer layer, allowing blood to collect in the space between the two. The larger an aneurysm is, the more likely it is to rupture, causing internal bleeding that can rapidly prove fatal.

WHAT ARE THE CAUSES?

The cause of most aneurysms is uncertain, but they are often associated with atherosclerosis (p.402), in which fatty deposits build up in the artery walls. The risk of developing atherosclerosis is increased by some lifestyle factors, such as smoking, eating a diet high in fat, excess weight, and taking little exercise. Aneurysms are also more common in males and people with high blood pressure (*see* HYPERTENSION, p.403).

In rare cases, an injury or an inherited weakness in the artery wall leads to the development of an aneurysm. For example, the genetic disorder Marfan's syndrome (p.824) may lead to the formation of multiple aneurysms.

WHAT ARE THE SYMPTOMS?

Symptoms vary according to the site and usually develop when an aneurysm enlarges. The symptoms of an abdominal aneurysm may include:

- Pain in the abdomen that may spread to the back and can be relieved temporarily by leaning forwards.
- Pulsating sensation in the abdomen.

An aneurysm in the chest may produce symptoms such as:

- Pain in the chest or in the upper back between the shoulder blades.
- Severe cough and wheezing.
- Difficulty swallowing and hoarseness.

If you have symptoms of this kind, you should seek emergency medical help.

ARE THERE COMPLICATIONS?

Sometimes, a blood clot forms at the site of the aneurysm and may obstruct the passage of blood through the aorta. In the case of a dissecting aneurysm, the

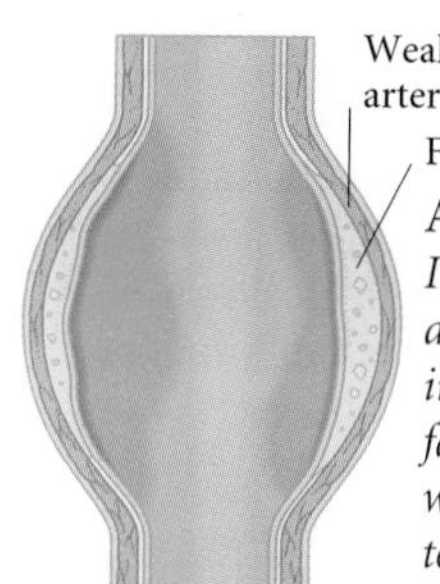

Aneurysm
In an aneurysm, an area of artery wall in which there is a fatty deposit grows weak and bulges due to the pressure of blood in the vessel.

Outer wall
Tear in inner wall
Blood in false channel
Fatty deposit

Dissecting aneurysm
In a dissecting aneurysm, the inner artery wall tears away from the outer wall. Blood then collects in a false channel between the walls.

torn part of the artery wall may block arteries that branch from the aorta close to the aneurysm. In the abdomen, such blockages may result in a reduced blood supply to the intestines or kidneys. If the obstruction occurs in the chest, branches of the aorta leading to the neck or the arms may be affected.

Pressure in the aorta may eventually cause an aneurysm to rupture, allowing blood to leak from the vessel and causing worsening pain. If rupture occurs suddenly, you may have severe pain accompanied by loss of consciousness, a fast pulse, and shock (p.414). Without immediate medical treatment, a ruptured aneurysm is likely to be fatal.

How is it diagnosed?

If there are no symptoms, an aneurysm may be detected during a routine physical examination when a doctor feels a swelling in the abdomen. Sometimes, an aneurysm is seen on an X-ray of the chest or abdomen carried out to check for another disorder. Screening tests for abdominal aortic aneurysm may be advised for some men over the age of 65. If you develop symptoms, ultrasound scanning (p.250) may be carried out at intervals to measure the diameter of the aorta and see if the aneurysm is enlarging. CT scanning (p.247), angiography (*see* CONTRAST X-RAYS, p.245), or MRI (p.248) may be also be performed to image the affected arteries.

What is the treatment?

An aneurysm may be treated by surgery, the aim of which is to repair the artery before the aneurysm dissects or ruptures. Your doctor will consider your age and general state of health, as well as the size and site of the aneurysm, when deciding whether surgery is necessary. Surgery for larger aneurysms involves removing the weakened area of arterial wall and replacing it with a graft of synthetic material. To prevent complications from developing while you are waiting for surgery, you may be given beta-blockers (p.898) to lower blood pressure in the artery. For a dissecting or ruptured aneurysm, you may need to have emergency surgery.

If you are a smoker, you should give up immediately and completely. For anyone who has had an aneurysm, a low-fat diet (*see* A HEALTHY DIET, p.48) and regular exercise will help to slow the progress of atherosclerosis and thus reduce the risk of further aneurysms.

What is the prognosis?

Surgery on an aneurysm offers a good chance of recovery provided the aneurysm has not yet dissected or ruptured. If the aneurysm has dissected or ruptured, between 15 and 50 per cent of people survive, depending on the location of the blood vessel affected.

(WWW) ONLINE SITES: p.1032

Thrombosis and embolism

Obstruction of blood flow in a vessel by a blockage that has formed in that vessel or has travelled from elsewhere in the body

GENETICS Rarely, runs in families

LIFESTYLE Smoking, a high-fat diet, lack of exercise, and excess weight are risk factors

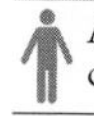
AGE GENDER Risk factors depend on the cause

Both thrombosis and embolism can be serious and potentially fatal conditions. In thrombosis, a blood clot, known as a thrombus, forms in a blood vessel and obstructs the flow of blood. Any blood vessel in the body may become blocked by a thrombus, but thrombosis is more serious in arteries and in deep veins in the legs (*see* DEEP VEIN THROMBOSIS, p.437). In embolism, a plug of material called an embolus travels through the bloodstream until it becomes lodged in an artery. Although some emboli consist of substances such as tissue or fat, most are pieces of blood clot that have become detached from a larger clot elsewhere in the body.

If an artery is blocked by either a thrombus or an embolus, and blood cannot reach the tissues beyond the blockage by an alternative route, those tissues are deprived of oxygen. Unlike thrombosis, which often develops gradually, the effects of embolism usually develop immediately and may be severe if the blood vessel becomes completely obstructed. Blockage of the arteries that supply the brain (*see* STROKE, p.532), the lungs (*see* PULMONARY EMBOLISM, p.495), or the heart (*see* MYOCARDIAL INFARCTION, p.410) often proves fatal.

What are the causes?

Blood flowing through an artery is normally under pressure so that clots are unlikely to form. If the flow of blood in an artery slows down, a clot is more likely to develop. Decreased blood flow through an artery may be caused by narrowing of the vessel due to a gradual build-up of fatty deposits in its walls, known as atherosclerosis (p.402). The long-term risk of developing atherosclerosis, and therefore thrombosis in the arteries, is increased by factors such as smoking and a diet high in fat.

Thrombosis is more likely to develop if there is an increase in the natural tendency of the blood to clot, a condition

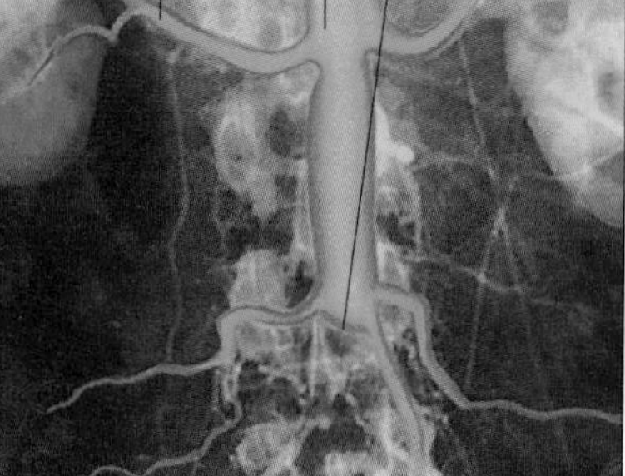

Arterial thrombosis
This contrast X-ray shows blood flow in the aorta and adjacent arteries. A blood clot in the aorta is blocking the flow of blood below the site of the obstruction.

known as hypercoagulability (p.453). In rare cases, the condition is inherited. Hypercoagulability may also occur as a result of taking a combined oral contraceptive (*see* CONTRACEPTION, p.69), being pregnant, or having surgery.

Blood clots sometimes form in the heart when the heartbeat is weak and irregular because the upper chambers (atria) are not totally emptied of blood at each beat (*see* ATRIAL FIBRILLATION, p.417). These blood clots may then be released from the atria into the coronary or peripheral arteries.

WHAT ARE THE SYMPTOMS?

The symptoms caused by thrombosis or embolism vary depending on which blood vessel is blocked. If the blockage affects blood supply to the legs, symptoms may develop within a few hours, and they may be more severe if there is already a reduction in blood supply to this region (*see* LOWER LIMB ISCHAEMIA, p.434). Symptoms include:

- Pain in the legs, even at rest.
- Pale, cold feet.

If the arteries supplying the intestines are affected, symptoms may include:

- Severe abdominal pain.
- Vomiting.
- Fever.

Left untreated, the reduction in blood supply may eventually result in tissue death, which may be life-threatening. The affected tissues will change colour over several days, eventually becoming black (*see* GANGRENE, p.435). If you develop these symptoms, you should seek emergency medical attention.

WHAT MIGHT BE DONE?

If your doctor suspects that you have thrombosis or embolism, he or she will have you admitted to hospital immediately for treatment. The blood flow through your blood vessels may be measured using pulse volume recording and imaging, such as Doppler ultrasound scanning (right). Angiography (*see* CONTRAST X-RAYS, p.245), sometimes combined with MRI (p.248), may be used to obtain detailed images of the blood vessels and look for obstruction.

Depending on the site and size of the clot, you may be given drugs to dissolve it and prevent further clots from forming (*see* DRUGS THAT PREVENT BLOOD CLOTTING, p.904). Emergency surgery may be necessary to remove the clot or to bypass it using a graft made from synthetic material. Alternatively, the affected artery may be widened by angioplasty, a procedure in which a balloon mounted on the tip of a catheter is passed into the artery and then inflated to widen the obstructed area.

After the thrombosis or embolism has been treated, you may need to continue medication for several months to prevent further blood clots from forming. For example, you may be advised to take a low dose of aspirin daily. If you smoke, you should stop immediately. You should also try to eat a low-fat diet (*see* A HEALTHY DIET, p.48) and exercise regularly. If you are taking a combined oral contraceptive, you should consider using another form of contraception.

(WWW) ONLINE SITES: p.1032

(TEST) DOPPLER ULTRASOUND SCANNING

Doppler ultrasound scanning is an imaging technique commonly used to measure the blood flow through a blood vessel in circulatory disorders such as thrombosis and embolism (p.431). It may also be used to measure blood pressure in the limbs. The technique produces an image of the blood flow through the vessel so that narrowing and blockages of the vessel can be detected. A routine Doppler ultrasound scan can take up to 20 minutes to perform and is completely painless and safe.

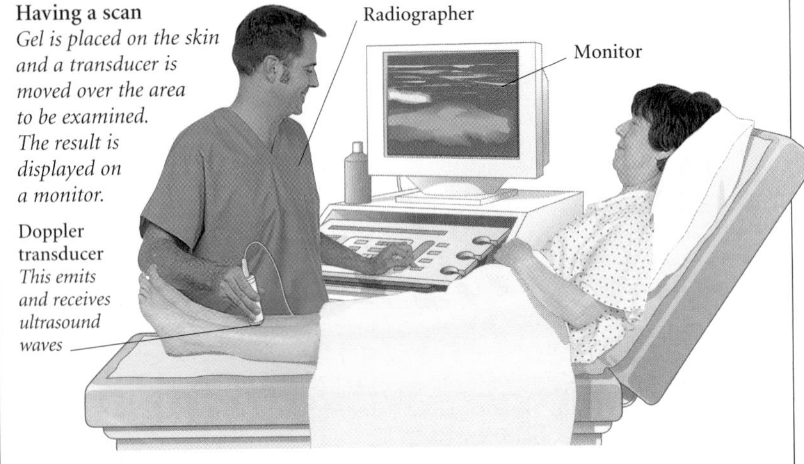

Having a scan
Gel is placed on the skin and a transducer is moved over the area to be examined. The result is displayed on a monitor.

Doppler transducer
This emits and receives ultrasound waves

(RESULTS)

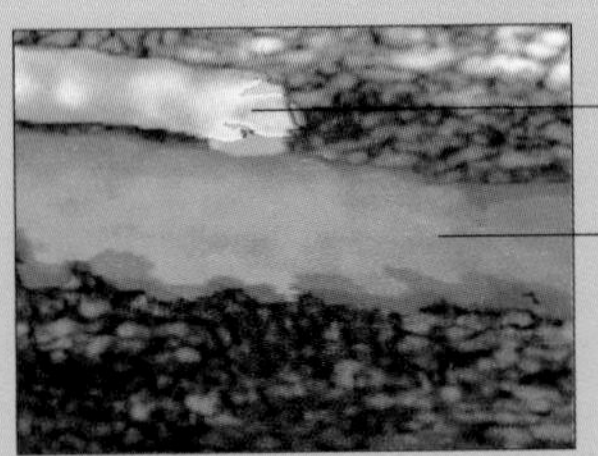

Doppler scan
This ultrasound image shows blood flow through vessels in the leg and confirms a blockage in the artery. Doppler ultrasound scans allow the precise position and severity of a blockage to be determined.

Diabetic vascular disease

Damage to large and small blood vessels throughout the body that can occur in people who have diabetes mellitus

GENETICS The underlying condition sometimes runs in families

LIFESTYLE Smoking, a high-fat diet, lack of exercise, and excess weight are risk factors

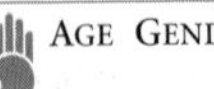
AGE GENDER Not significant factors

Vascular disease is a common long-term complication of diabetes mellitus (p.687), a condition that tends to run in families. There are two types of vascular disease that are more likely to affect people who have diabetes: atherosclerosis (p.402) and small vessel disease.

In atherosclerosis, fatty deposits gradually build up in the walls of larger blood vessels, making these vessels narrower. This condition, which develops to some degree in most people as they become older, is likely to occur earlier and more extensively in people with diabetes.

Diabetic small vessel disease is not fully understood, but it is thought to involve thickening of the walls of the smaller blood vessels as a result of certain chemical changes. This thickening reduces the amount of oxygen passing from blood in the vessels into the surrounding body tissues.

These vascular conditions frequently occur together and each of them may lead to serious complications. The risk of developing either type of diabetic vascular disease is higher the longer a person has had diabetes mellitus. Lifestyle factors such as smoking and a diet that is high in fat increase the risk of developing diabetic vascular disease, as does poor control of blood sugar levels, and it is therefore important that your diabetes is managed effectively (*see* LIVING WITH DIABETES, p.690).

ARE THERE COMPLICATIONS?

Atherosclerosis may eventually lead to blockage of the arteries, causing potentially life-threatening complications, in particular stroke (p.532), heart attack (*see* MYOCARDIAL INFARCTION, p.410), and lower limb ischaemia (p.434).

Damage to small blood vessels may occur in many parts of the body. Small blood vessels in the eyes are commonly damaged (*see* DIABETIC RETINOPATHY, p.579), leading to blurred vision and sometimes even blindness. If the small vessels in the eyes are damaged, similar changes will have occurred in vessels throughout the body. If the blood vessels in the kidneys are affected, kidney function will be impaired (*see* DIABETIC KIDNEY DISEASE, p.705). Kidney damage sometimes leads to high blood pressure (*see* HYPERTENSION, p.403).

Small vessel disease may also lead to nerve damage, most commonly in the feet (*see* DIABETIC NEUROPATHY, p.545). Such damage can reduce sensation in the affected area so that an injury goes unnoticed at first. In addition, the reduced supply of blood slows healing, and persistent skin ulcers (*see* LEG ULCERS, p.350) and even gangrene (p.435) may develop. Some people already have these complications when they are first diagnosed as having diabetes mellitus. In other cases, complications may not develop for many years after diagnosis.

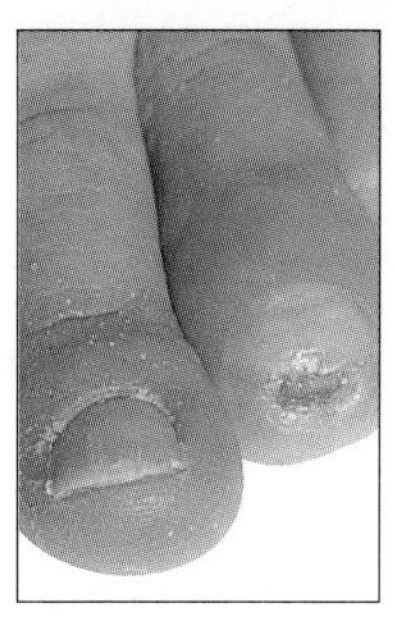

Ulcerated toe
If diabetic vascular disease affects the arteries in the leg, the tissues of the feet may become deprived of oxygen, eventually leading to the formation of a skin ulcer.

WHAT MIGHT BE DONE?

It is essential that diabetes mellitus is diagnosed promptly and managed well. In order to prevent or reduce the effects of diabetic vascular disease on blood vessels, you should try to maintain effective control of your blood sugar

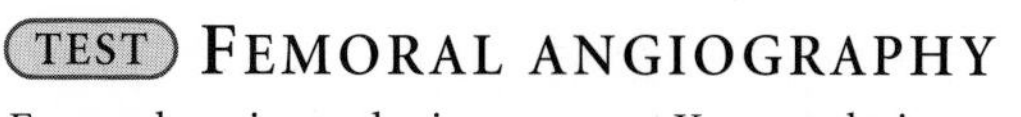

TEST FEMORAL ANGIOGRAPHY

Femoral angiography is a contrast X-ray technique, sometimes combined with MRI (p.248), that is used to diagnose narrowing or blockage of arteries in the legs. During the procedure, which is carried out under local anaesthesia, a contrast medium is injected into the femoral artery. The medium spreads in the circulation to other vessels in the leg. X-rays are then taken of one or more sites. The procedure takes about 30 minutes, and you should be able to return home within 6 hours.

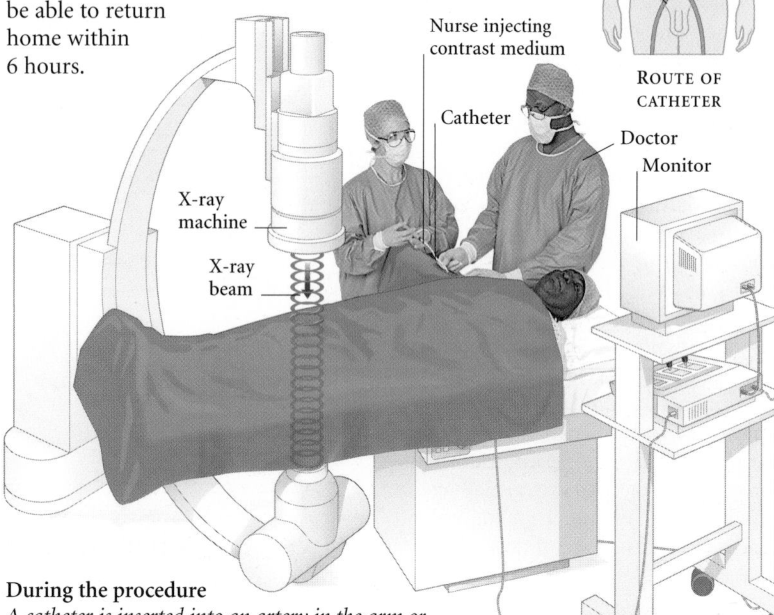

During the procedure
A catheter is inserted into an artery in the arm or leg and guided through the body to the femoral artery. A contrast medium is then injected into the catheter so that the artery can be seen on an X-ray.

RESULTS

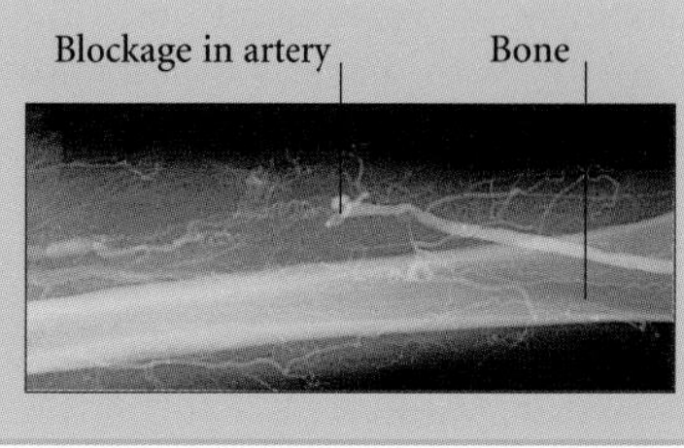

Angiogram of the leg
This contrast X-ray shows a blockage in the main artery in the leg, restricting blood flow to the tissues of the lower leg. If this blockage is not treated, the tissues will be permanently damaged.

levels (*see* MONITORING YOUR BLOOD GLUCOSE, p.689), follow a healthy, low-fat diet (p.48), and avoid smoking. If you have diabetes, your doctor will regularly measure your blood pressure (*see* BLOOD PRESSURE MEASUREMENT, p.404) and the level of cholesterol in your blood (*see* BLOOD CHOLESTEROL TESTS, p.231) to assess your susceptibility to atherosclerosis. Samples of your urine may be tested for protein, the presence of which may be the first sign of kidney disease, and blood tests may be performed to find out if your kidneys are functioning normally. In addition, regular eye checks, using ophthalmoscopy (p.578) and sometimes retinal photography, are carried out to ensure that retinal damage is detected as early as possible since early detection increases the chances of successful treatment.

If you have a high blood cholesterol level, your doctor may prescribe drugs to prevent atherosclerosis from worsening (*see* LIPID-LOWERING DRUGS, p.935). If protein is found in your urine, you may be prescribed ACE inhibitor drugs (p.900), which help to counteract the progression of small vessel damage in the kidneys. Treatment for high blood pressure will be given if necessary (*see* ANTIHYPERTENSIVE DRUGS, p.897).

WHAT IS THE PROGNOSIS?

Diabetic vascular disease is the most common cause of death in people who have diabetes mellitus, and the risk of developing it increases with time.

A person with diabetes is about 10 times more likely to develop lower limb ischaemia than someone without diabetes, four times more likely to have a heart attack, and twice as likely to have a stroke. Damage to small blood vessels in the eyes occurs in about 8 in 10 people with long-term diabetes. However, eye damage is often reversible if it is treated in the early stages. Kidney damage occurs in about 4 in 10 people who have had diabetes mellitus for longer than 15 years. About 3 in 10 people with diabetes develop nerve damage, but only 1 in 10 has severe symptoms.

If your diabetes mellitus is carefully managed and your blood sugar level is well controlled, the progress of diabetic vascular disease will be slowed and the risk of complications will be reduced.

(WWW) ONLINE SITES: p.1030

TREATMENT FEMORAL ARTERY BYPASS GRAFT

This procedure is used to treat blocked or narrowed arteries in the leg, which can cause lower limb ischaemia (below). During the operation, the blocked artery is bypassed using a section of vein from the same leg or, less commonly, an artificial graft. The blocked artery is left in place, but, because blood can flow freely through the bypass, the blood supply to the limb is restored. The cut ends of the vein used for the graft are tied and remain in place, and blood is diverted up other veins in the leg. The operation is performed in hospital under general anaesthesia.

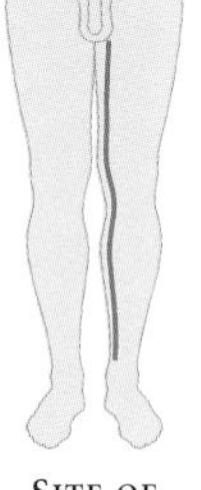
SITE OF INCISION

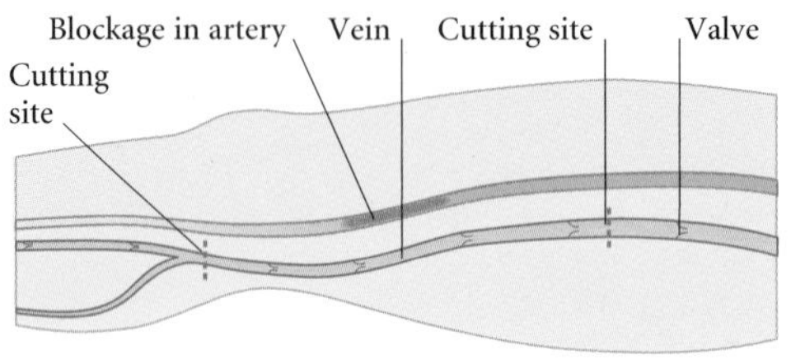

Before surgery
An obstruction in an artery in the leg prevents blood from reaching the lower leg. A small section of a vein from the same leg can be used to create a bypass around this blockage.

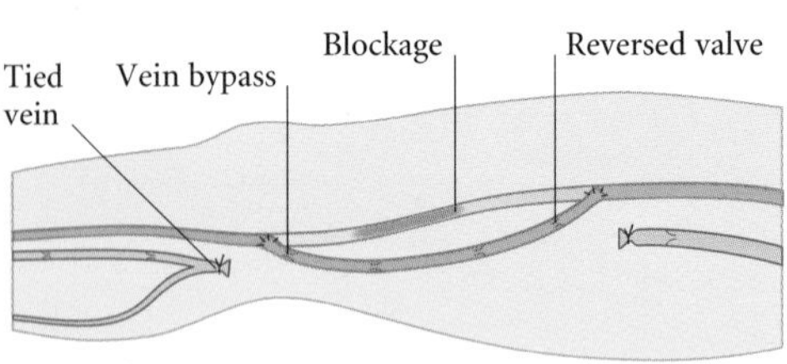

After surgery
A length of vein has been removed and attached above and below the blockage, forming a bypass channel. The vein is reversed so that its valves allow arterial blood flow.

Lower limb ischaemia

A reduced oxygen supply to the tissues of the legs as a result of a poor blood supply

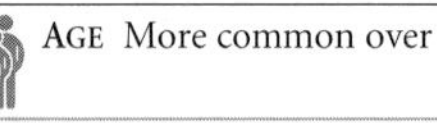
AGE More common over the age of 40

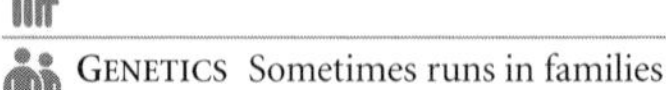
GENDER More common in males

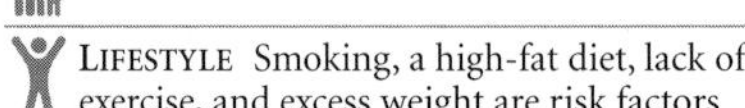
GENETICS Sometimes runs in families

LIFESTYLE Smoking, a high-fat diet, lack of exercise, and excess weight are risk factors

If blood flow to the legs is reduced, the leg tissues may become deprived of oxygen, and this problem may lead to a cramp-like pain on exertion. Reduced blood flow is usually due to atherosclerosis (p.402), a build-up of fatty deposits in artery walls, whose effects are often most noticeable on the lower limbs. People who have an inherited tendency towards high cholesterol levels (*see* INHERITED HYPERLIPIDAEMIAS, p.692) are more likely to develop atherosclerosis, as are those who have had diabetes mellitus (p.687) for a long time. A high-fat diet and smoking also increase the risk. About 9 in 10 people with lower limb ischaemia smoke.

WHAT ARE THE SYMPTOMS?

The symptoms of lower limb ischaemia usually develop gradually over months or years. Symptoms may affect one leg more than the other. In the initial stages of the condition, blood flow to the legs may be adequate to supply the tissues when at rest but not on exertion. The main symptom is a cramp-like pain in the legs with the following features:

- Affects one or both calves when walking and may be severe.
- Consistently appears after walking a particular distance.
- Comes on sooner when walking uphill or in cold temperatures.
- Is relieved by rest and usually disappears after several minutes.

As the disease progresses, the distance a person is able to walk before experiencing pain gradually decreases, so that eventually pain may be present at rest. Additional symptoms of lower limb ischaemia may then include:

- Pale, cold feet.
- Persistent leg or foot ulcers.

If a blockage occurs in blood vessels in the pelvic region, blood flow is reduced to the whole of the lower body, and as a result there may be pain in the buttocks and, in men, impotence. If the blood vessel becomes completely blocked by a clot (*see* THROMBOSIS AND EMBOLISM, p.431), the symptoms may suddenly worsen. Without immediate treatment, death of tissues in the feet and legs may occur (*see* GANGRENE, right).

WHAT MIGHT BE DONE?

Your doctor may suspect that you have lower limb ischaemia from your symptoms and by examining the strength of the pulses in your legs. He or she may arrange for tests such as pulse volume recording and Doppler ultrasound scanning (p.432) to measure the blood flow in your legs and angiography (*see* FEMORAL ANGIOGRAPHY, p.433), which produces detailed images of the vessels, to look for atherosclerosis.

Treatment is aimed at increasing the blood flow to the tissues in the legs. Affected arteries may be widened using a technique known as angioplasty, in which a balloon on the tip of a catheter is passed into the artery and inflated. In some cases, surgery is carried out to bypass affected arteries (*see* FEMORAL ARTERY BYPASS GRAFT, opposite page).

Taking a low dose of aspirin daily may help to prevent blood clots from developing. If a clot has formed, you may be given drugs to dissolve it and to prevent more clots from forming (*see* DRUGS THAT PREVENT BLOOD CLOTTING, p.904). In some cases, the clot needs to be surgically removed. If gangrene has developed, amputation of part or all of the affected limb may be necessary.

If you smoke, it is vital that you stop immediately. The nicotine in cigarettes causes blood vessels to constrict, further reducing blood supply to the legs. Even one cigarette can produce a constricting effect that lasts for several hours, and you need to give up smoking completely to improve the outlook once lower limb ischaemia is diagnosed. If you continue to smoke, the disease is likely to progress, and surgery may be required.

In addition, you should follow a healthy diet (p.48) and try to walk for longer periods each day to build up the amount of exercise you can do without feeling pain (*see* TAKING REGULAR EXERCISE, p.57). Adopting these measures may enable you to prevent the condition from worsening.

WWW ONLINE SITES: p.1032

Gangrene

Tissue death as a result of an inadequate blood supply or infection of a wound

LIFESTYLE Smoking, a high-fat diet, lack of exercise, and excess weight are risk factors

AGE GENDER GENETICS Risk factors depend on the cause

Gangrene involves death of the tissues in a particular area of the body, most commonly the legs and feet, and is a potentially life-threatening condition.

There are two types of gangrene: dry and wet. Dry gangrene occurs when the tissues become deprived of oxygen as a result of a reduced blood supply. Tissue death is localized and does not spread from the affected site. Wet gangrene is less common and occurs when tissue that has been damaged by a wound or by dry gangrene becomes infected with bacteria. Infection is often due to clostridia, which are bacteria that thrive in dead tissues where there is no oxygen and produce a foul-smelling gas. The infection may spread to surrounding healthy tissues and can be fatal.

The reduction in blood supply that leads to gangrene is most often due to a blood clot forming in an artery (*see* THROMBOSIS AND EMBOLISM, p.431), which may already be narrowed by the accumulation of fatty deposits on vessel walls, known as atherosclerosis (p.402). The tissues in the legs and feet are most commonly affected by these underlying conditions (*see* LOWER LIMB ISCHAEMIA, opposite page). The risk of an artery becoming blocked is increased by certain lifestyle factors, such as smoking and a high-fat diet. People with diabetes mellitus (p.687) are more likely to develop gangrene as a result of progressive damage to the small blood vessels (*see* DIABETIC VASCULAR DISEASE, p.432). Frostbite (p.324) may also lead to the development of gangrene.

WHAT ARE THE SYMPTOMS?

The symptoms of dry gangrene may develop gradually or may appear over a few hours, depending on how quickly the blood supply is reduced. If the legs are affected, symptoms include:

- Pain in the leg and foot.
- Pale, cold skin, which becomes red and hot before turning purple and eventually black over several days.

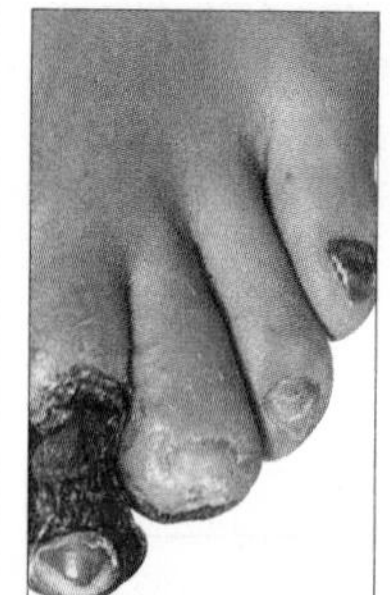

Gangrene
An inadequate supply of blood to the feet may lead to tissue death, also known as gangrene, which causes the toes to turn black. Left untreated, the dead tissue may become infected.

If the gangrene is due to an infection, additional symptoms may be present, including pus around the affected area and fever. Infection may spread to the bloodstream (*see* SEPTICAEMIA, p.299).

WHAT MIGHT BE DONE?

Your doctor will probably be able to diagnose gangrene from its appearance. He or she may arrange for you to have pulse volume recording or Doppler ultrasound scanning (p.432) to measure blood flow in the limb. You may require contrast X-rays (p.245), sometimes combined with MRI (p.248), to look for a blocked artery.

If you have gangrene, you will be admitted to hospital without delay. Intravenous antibiotics (p.885) will be given to prevent or treat infection and, if possible, the blood supply to the gangrenous tissue will be restored. If an artery is obstructed, the vessel may be widened using angioplasty, in which a balloon on the tip of a catheter is passed into the narrowed area and then inflated. Alternatively, surgery may be carried out to remove or bypass the blockage (*see* FEMORAL ARTERY BYPASS GRAFT, opposite page). The gangrenous tissue will be removed, and, if it has become infected, some of the living tissue around the gangrenous area will also be removed to prevent the infection from spreading. In some cases, amputation of a limb is necessary. If you develop wet gangrene, you may be placed in a chamber containing high-pressure oxygen to destroy the bacteria.

The earlier gangrene is diagnosed, the better the outlook, because blood supply to the affected tissues is more likely to be restored. A good blood supply promotes tissue healing after surgery. Gangrene is fatal in about 1 in 5 people, usually because of infection in the bloodstream.

WWW ONLINE SITES: p.1032, p.1033

Buerger's disease

Severe inflammation of the small arteries that is triggered by smoking

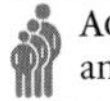
AGE Most common between the ages of 20 and 40

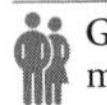
GENDER Three times more common in males

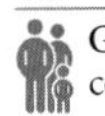
GENETICS Sometimes runs in families; more common in Asians and Eastern Europeans

LIFESTYLE Smoking is a risk factor; exposure to cold aggravates symptoms

Buerger's disease is a rare condition that most frequently affects men who smoke. The condition tends to run in families and is more common in people of Asian or Eastern European descent. The cause is not fully understood, but it is thought that, in people genetically susceptible to the disease, smoking triggers an autoimmune response, in which the immune system produces antibodies that attack the body's own tissues. The arteries in the legs and sometimes those in the arms become inflamed, reducing blood supply to the tissues.

WHAT ARE THE SYMPTOMS?

The initial symptoms of Buerger's disease are often intermittent and include:

- Pale hands or feet, particularly after exposure to the cold.
- Pain in the hands or feet, which may be severe at night and after exercise.
- Numbness, tingling, or a sensation of burning in the fingers or toes.

With time, these symptoms usually become more severe and skin ulcers or gangrene (p.435) may develop on the tips of the toes or fingers.

WHAT MIGHT BE DONE?

If you have the symptoms listed above, your doctor will take your pulse to check if it is weak or absent. If this is so, he or she may suspect Buerger's disease and arrange for angiography (*see* CONTRAST X-RAYS, p.245) and Doppler ultrasound scanning (p.432) to assess blood flow in the small arteries in the hands or feet.

If you are diagnosed with Buerger's disease, the only action you can take to improve the outlook is to stop smoking. In people who continue to smoke, the disease is likely to progress so that amputation of the affected limb may eventually become necessary.

(WWW) ONLINE SITES: p.1032

Raynaud's phenomenon and Raynaud's disease

Sudden, intermittent narrowing of the arteries in the hands or, rarely, the feet

GENDER More common in females

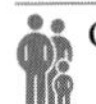
GENETICS Sometimes runs in families

LIFESTYLE Smoking and exposure to cold trigger attacks

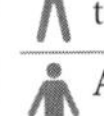
AGE Risk factors depend on the cause

During an attack of Raynaud's phenomenon, the arteries in the hands or feet become narrowed as a result of muscle spasm in the artery walls. This narrowing restricts blood supply to the fingers or toes, causing them to become pale. Numbness or tingling may also develop in the affected fingers or toes.

In about half of all people with Raynaud's phenomenon, the condition is the result of an underlying disorder, particularly the autoimmune disorders scleroderma (p.462), rheumatoid arthritis (p.377), or Buerger's disease (left), all of which run in families. In some people with Raynaud's phenomenon, the condition is linked with hand–arm syndrome (right). Certain drugs, such as beta-blockers (p.898), are known to produce the symptoms of Raynaud's phenomenon as a side effect.

If there is no apparent cause for the condition, it is known as Raynaud's disease. This disorder is most common in women aged between 15 and 45 and is usually mild. Episodes of either condition are triggered by smoking because the nicotine in cigarettes constricts the arteries. Exposure to cold and handling frozen items can also trigger an attack.

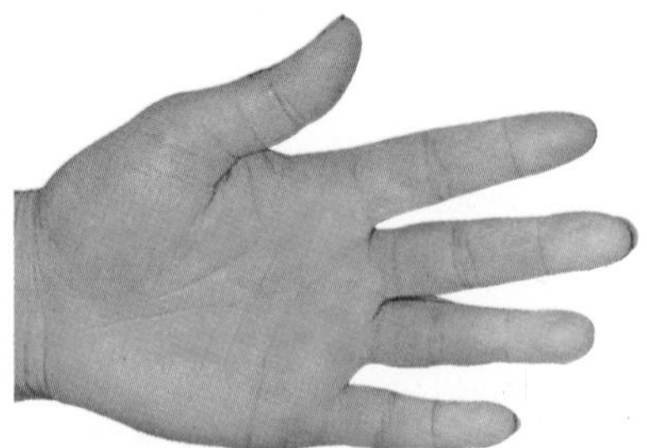

Raynaud's phenomenon
An attack of Raynaud's phenomenon in the hand restricts the blood supply to the tips of the fingers, turning them white.

WHAT ARE THE SYMPTOMS?

The symptoms of Raynaud's phenomenon and Raynaud's disease affect the hands or feet, last from a few minutes to a few hours, and include:

- Numbness and tingling in the fingers or toes that may worsen and progress to a painful burning sensation.
- Progressive change of colour in the fingers or toes, which initially turn pale, then blue, and later red again as blood returns to the tissues.

There may be a marked colour difference between the affected area and the surrounding tissues. In severe cases, skin ulcers or gangrene (p.435) may form on the tips of the fingers or toes.

WHAT MIGHT BE DONE?

Your doctor will carry out tests to look for an underlying cause of your symptoms. For example, blood tests may be performed to look for evidence of an autoimmune disorder.

Immunosuppressant drugs (p.906) may be prescribed to treat an autoimmune disorder. Your doctor may also recommend that you take drugs that dilate the blood vessels during an attack (*see* CALCIUM CHANNEL BLOCKER DRUGS, p.900). If you smoke, you should stop immediately. Wearing thermal gloves and socks in cold weather helps to avoid the onset of symptoms. If symptoms are severe, surgery may be needed to cut the nerves that control arterial constriction.

(WWW) ONLINE SITES: p.1032

Hand–arm syndrome

Painful, pale fingers associated with the use of vibrating tools

GENDER More common in males

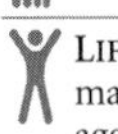
LIFESTYLE Affects people who use vibrating machinery; smoking and exposure to cold aggravate symptoms

AGE GENETICS Not significant factors

Hand–arm syndrome, also known as vibration white finger, causes pain and numbness in parts of the body that are repeatedly exposed to intense vibration from machinery. As the name of the condition implies, the hands, arms, and in particular the fingers are most commonly affected. Prolonged exposure to vibration from the use of mechanical tools causes localized constriction of the small blood vessels and nerve damage. Smoking and exposure to cold, which also constrict the small blood vessels, may trigger or aggravate the symptoms of hand–arm syndrome.

About 3 in 100 people in employment, most of them men, are exposed to machine vibration that may lead to hand–arm syndrome. In the past, the mining and engineering industries were responsible for the majority of cases. The use of chainsaws in the forestry industry is another common cause.

What are the symptoms?

The symptoms of hand–arm syndrome do not appear immediately after exposure to vibration but tend to develop slowly over several years of exposure. Symptoms are often more severe in one hand than the other and may include:

- Pain, numbness, and tingling in the fingers, hands, or arms.
- Pale or blue fingers.
- Difficulty manipulating small objects, such as picking up coins, buttoning clothes, or tying shoelaces.

At first, the symptoms of hand–arm syndrome tend to occur intermittently, but they become more frequent and persistent as the condition progresses.

What might be done?

If you have the symptoms described above and you have been working with vibrating machinery, your doctor may suspect hand–arm syndrome. Once the disorder has been diagnosed, you should avoid exposure to vibration. Your doctor may advise you to change jobs. You should also avoid anything that makes the symptoms worse, such as smoking and exposure to cold. There is no specific treatment, but, if you have severe symptoms, your doctor may prescribe calcium channel blocker drugs (p.900), which dilate the blood vessels.

If you use vibrating machinery, make sure that it is in good working order and that you know how to operate it correctly and safely. In addition, you should always wear approved protective gloves. If you manage to avoid further exposure to vibrating machinery, the symptoms of hand–arm syndrome may improve. However, once numbness has developed, the condition is irreversible.

(WWW) ONLINE SITES: p.1032, p.1036

Deep vein thrombosis

Formation of a blood clot within a deep-lying vein

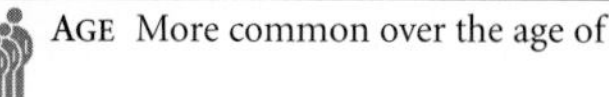
AGE More common over the age of 40

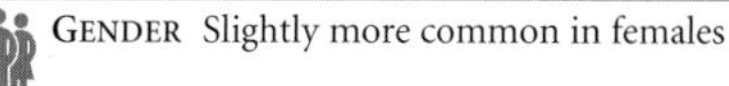
GENDER Slightly more common in females

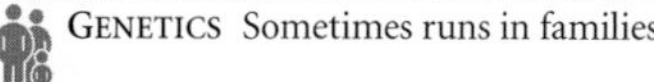
GENETICS Sometimes runs in families

LIFESTYLE Prolonged immobility and excess weight are risk factors

Deep vein thrombosis is a condition in which a blood clot forms in a large vein in a muscle, usually in the leg or pelvic region. It affects half a million people in the UK each year, many of them over 40.

The formation of a clot in a deep vein is usually not dangerous in itself. However, there is a risk that a fragment of the clot may break off and travel through the heart in the circulation. If the fragment lodges in a vessel supplying the lungs, a potentially fatal blockage called a pulmonary embolism (p.495) occurs.

What are the causes?

Deep vein thrombosis is usually caused by a combination of slow blood flow through a vein, an increase in the natural tendency of the blood to clot, and damage to the wall of the vein.

Several factors may slow blood flow and thus increase the risk of deep vein thrombosis. Long periods of immobility, such as those experienced during long flights or car journeys or while bedridden, are a common cause of slow blood flow. Other causes include compression of a vein by the fetus during pregnancy or by a tumour. Leg injury may also slow blood flow and cause a clot to form in the deep veins of the leg.

The blood may clot more easily as a result of an injury, surgery, pregnancy, or taking a combined oral contraceptive (*see* CONTRACEPTION, p.69). Some people have an inherited tendency for the blood to clot too readily (*see* HYPERCOAGULABILITY, p.453).

What are the symptoms?

If a blood clot has formed in a deep-lying vein, it may produce symptoms that include the following:

- Pain or tenderness in the leg.
- Swelling of the lower leg or thigh.
- Enlarged veins beneath the skin.

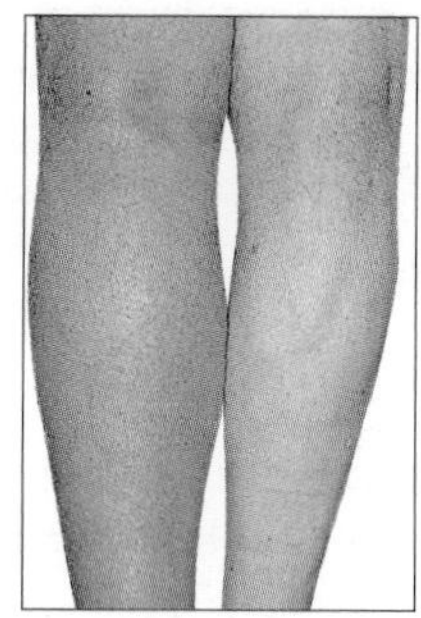

Deep vein thrombosis
The leg on the left is visibly swollen and red compared to the leg on the right, indicating that a blood clot has formed in a deep vein within the leg muscle.

Pulmonary embolism occurs in a small proportion of cases of deep vein thrombosis. The symptoms that occur with pulmonary embolism usually include shortness of breath and chest pain. If the blood supply to the lungs is blocked, the condition is life-threatening.

In some cases, thrombosis causes permanent damage to the vein and varicose veins (p.438) may appear later.

What might be done?

Your doctor may need to carry out various tests to confirm the diagnosis of deep vein thrombosis because the symptoms are often similar to those of other conditions, such as cellulitis (p.352). You may have Doppler ultrasound scanning (p.432) to measure blood flow through the veins and sometimes a venogram, in which dye is injected into a vein and then X-rays are taken to reveal blood clots (*see* CONTRAST X-RAYS, p.245). MRI (p.248) may also be used. A sample of your blood may be taken and analysed to assess how easily it clots.

Thrombolytic drugs (p.904) may be prescribed to dissolve the blood clot in the vein and reduce the risk of a pulmonary embolism. You may also be given injections of anticoagulants to prevent further clots. Although treatment can take place in hospital, you may be able to administer anticoagulant drugs yourself at home. Rarely, surgery is required to remove the clot.

After you have had the initial treatment, your doctor will prescribe drugs to reduce the risk that the condition will recur (*see* DRUGS THAT PREVENT BLOOD CLOTTING, p.904).

Can it be prevented?

Certain surgical procedures carry a risk of deep vein thrombosis, and your susceptibility to developing the condition is assessed beforehand. If there is a high risk, low doses of short-acting anticoagulant drugs will probably be given before and after surgery to prevent the blood from clotting. Your doctor may also advise you to wear special elastic stockings for a few days after the operation to help maintain blood flow in the veins of the leg. Women who use a combined oral contraceptive may need an alternative form of contraception for the 2 or 3 months before surgery.

The risk of deep vein thrombosis can be reduced by avoiding long periods of inactivity. If you are confined to bed, you should regularly stretch your legs and flex your ankles. Your doctor may also recommend that you wear elastic stockings. During a flight, walk around at least once an hour, and, during a long drive, stop regularly to stretch your legs.

WHAT IS THE PROGNOSIS?

Usually, if deep vein thrombosis is diagnosed in its early stages, treatment with thrombolytic drugs and anticoagulants is successful. However, if the affected vein is permanently damaged, persistent swelling of the leg or varicose veins may develop and there is a risk that deep vein thrombosis may recur.

(WWW) ONLINE SITES: p.1032

Varicose veins

Visibly swollen and distorted veins that lie just beneath the skin, mainly in the legs

AGE Rare before the age of 20; more common in elderly people

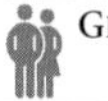
GENDER More common in females

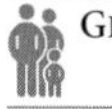
GENETICS Often runs in families

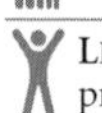
LIFESTYLE Pregnancy, excess weight, and prolonged standing are risk factors

Varicose veins affect about 1 in 5 adults and are more common with increasing age. Although the condition may cause discomfort and appear unsightly, it is not usually harmful to health.

Varicose veins mainly affect the legs. Normally, blood in the legs collects in the superficial veins just below the skin. These veins empty the blood into deep-lying veins through small perforating veins. The deep-lying veins carry blood back towards the heart. Contraction of the leg muscles helps to pump the blood in the veins upwards to the heart, even when you are standing, and the veins have one-way valves to stop blood from flowing backwards into the legs. If the valves in the perforating vein do not close adequately, the blood flows back into the superficial veins. The pressure of returning blood causes these veins to become swollen and distorted, and they are then known as varicose veins. If left untreated, the condition often worsens.

Varicose veins can develop in other parts of the body as a complication of chronic liver disease, which raises blood pressure in the portal veins (*see* PORTAL HYPERTENSION AND VARICES, p.648). The rise in blood pressure may cause veins to become swollen at the lower end of the oesophagus, and, in some cases, around the rectum (*see* HAEMORRHOIDS, p.668).

WHAT ARE THE CAUSES?

Varicose veins may be associated with an inherited weakness of the valves in the veins. The female hormone progesterone, which causes the veins to dilate, may encourage the formation of varicose veins, and the condition is therefore more common in women, especially during pregnancy (*see* COMMON COMPLAINTS OF NORMAL PREGNANCY, p.784). In addition, increased pressure is placed on the veins in the pelvic region during pregnancy as the uterus gradually grows larger. Other factors that increase the risk of developing varicose veins include being overweight and having an occupation that involves standing for long periods with little walking.

Sometimes, varicose veins are caused by a blood clot blocking a deep vein (*see* DEEP VEIN THROMBOSIS, p.437).

WHAT ARE THE SYMPTOMS?

If you develop varicose veins in the legs, you may have the following symptoms:

- Easily visible, blue, swollen, distorted veins that bulge beneath the skin and are more prominent when standing.

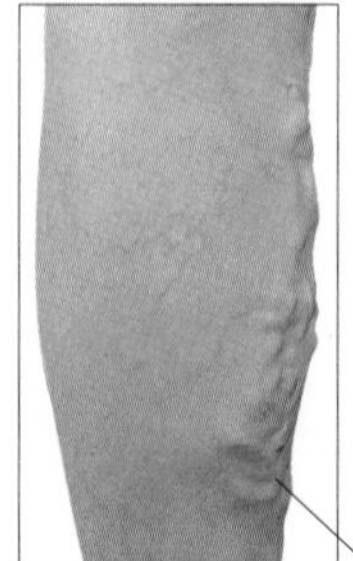

Varicose veins
Abnormal backflow of blood into the superficial veins that lie just beneath the surface of the skin has caused these veins to become swollen and distorted.

- Aching or pain in the affected leg, especially after prolonged standing.

In severe cases, the skin over a varicose vein, usually in the ankle area, becomes thin, dry, and itchy. Eventually, ulceration may occur (*see* LEG ULCER, p.350).

> **SELF-HELP COPING WITH VARICOSE VEINS**
>
> If you have troublesome symptoms caused by varicose veins, the following measures may help:
>
> - Avoid prolonged standing.
> - Take regular walks to exercise the leg muscles and keep blood flowing in the legs.
> - Keep your legs elevated when sitting, if possible.
> - If your doctor has recommended that you wear elastic stockings, put them on before you get out of bed in the morning while your legs are still elevated.
> - Avoid clothing, such as girdles, that may restrict the flow of blood at the top of the legs.
> - If you are overweight, you should try to lose weight.

HOW ARE THEY DIAGNOSED?

Your doctor will examine the affected area while you are standing, when the veins are usually more prominent and easily visible. You may have Doppler ultrasound scanning (p.432) to assess the direction of blood flow in the veins of the leg. If the veins are varicose, the blood will appear to flow backwards.

WHAT IS THE TREATMENT?

In the majority of cases, varicose veins do not require medical treatment, and you may be able to relieve discomfort using self-help measures (*see* COPING WITH VARICOSE VEINS, above).

Treatment is usually carried out only if the veins become painful or especially unsightly or if the skin becomes ulcerated. There are several ways of treating varicose veins (opposite page), and you may need to discuss these options with your doctor. If your varicose veins are small and below the knee, your doctor may recommend that the veins be injected with a solution to make their walls stick together and thus prevent blood from entering them. For varicose veins above the knee, the usual treatment is to tie off the perforating veins so that blood does not enter the varicose vein. If the entire vein is varicose, it may be surgically removed. Even after surgery, varicose veins may recur, and treatment may need to be repeated.

(WWW) ONLINE SITES: p.1032

Superficial thrombophlebitis

Inflammation of a superficial vein (a vein just beneath the surface of the skin) that may cause a blood clot to form

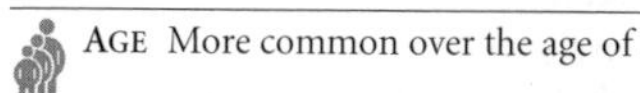
AGE More common over the age of 20

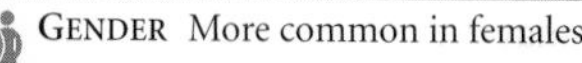
GENDER More common in females

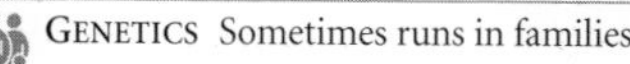
GENETICS Sometimes runs in families

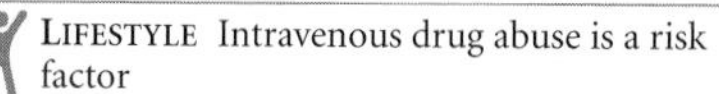
LIFESTYLE Intravenous drug abuse is a risk factor

In superficial thrombophlebitis, a blood clot develops in an inflamed superficial vein. The condition is rarely serious, but it may be painful. Thrombophlebitis can affect any superficial vein but usually occurs in varicose veins (opposite page) in the leg. Superficial thrombophlebitis tends to run in families and is more common in adult women.

Inflammation leading to clot formation may result from damage to a vein, which may be sustained during intravenous drug injection or surgery. The development of blood clots in superficial veins is more common in people who have cancer. In some cases, superficial thrombophlebitis is associated with an increase in the tendency of blood to clot (*see* HYPERCOAGULABILITY, p.453). For example, blood may clot more easily in women who are pregnant or who take a combined oral contraceptive (*see* CONTRACEPTION, p.69). In most cases, however, the cause is unclear.

WHAT ARE THE SYMPTOMS?

The symptoms associated with superficial thrombophlebitis usually develop over 24–48 hours and include:

- Redness of the skin overlying a vein.
- A painful, tender, swollen vein that may feel hard like a cord.
- Mild fever.

Inflammation is usually localized in the area of the blood clot and may spread to the overlying skin. However, in rare cases, thrombophlebitis extends into a deep-lying vein, usually in the leg, leading to deep vein thrombosis (p.437).

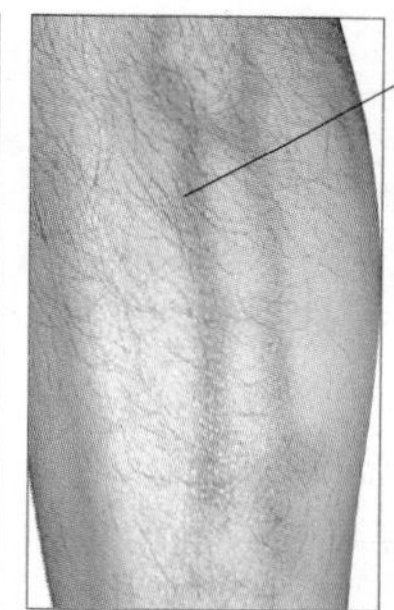

Superficial thrombophlebitis
The skin overlying the affected vein is red and inflamed. The outline of the swollen vein can be seen beneath the surface of the skin.

WHAT MIGHT BE DONE?

Your doctor will probably be able to diagnose superficial thrombophlebitis from your symptoms and the appearance of the vein and the overlying skin.

Most cases improve in a few days without treatment. You may be able to relieve pain by taking a painkiller, such as ibuprofen (*see* NONSTEROIDAL ANTI-INFLAMMATORY DRUGS, p.894), and by keeping the area rested and raised. Warm, moist compresses can also ease discomfort. If the condition is due to hypercoagulability or has resulted in a deep vein thrombosis, your doctor may recommend that you take drugs that prevent blood clotting (p.904). Superficial thrombophlebitis is likely to recur in susceptible people.

(WWW) ONLINE SITES: p.1032

(TREATMENT) TREATING VARICOSE VEINS

There are several methods of treating varicose veins, including injection therapy and surgery. Injection therapy is mainly used to treat small varicose veins below the knee, and surgery is performed to treat larger veins. Surgery may be used to divide faulty perforating veins responsible for the formation of the varicose veins or to remove an entire varicose vein. Treatment may need to be repeated if the varicose veins recur.

DIVISION OF PERFORATING VEINS

Blood normally flows from the superficial veins into the deep veins along perforating veins. If the valves in the perforating veins are not working properly, there is a backflow of blood into the superficial veins, which leads to the formation of varicose veins. During the surgical division of faulty perforating veins, these veins are tied off and cut. Surgery is usually performed in hospital under general anaesthesia.

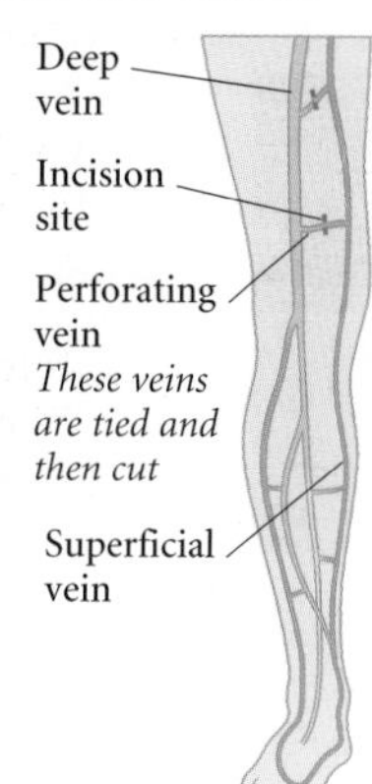

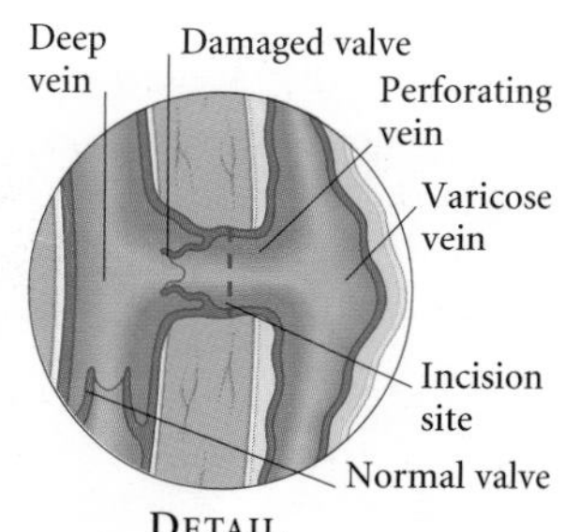

During the procedure
Small incisions are made in the leg, usually in the groin, behind the knee, and sometimes also in the lower leg. The perforating veins are then tied and cut.

INJECTION THERAPY

Injection therapy is used for small varicose veins below the knee. The procedure uses a mild irritant to make the walls of the varicose veins stick together and stop blood from entering them. For a week after the procedure, an elastic bandage is worn around the leg in order to compress the veins and help the vessel walls to stick together.

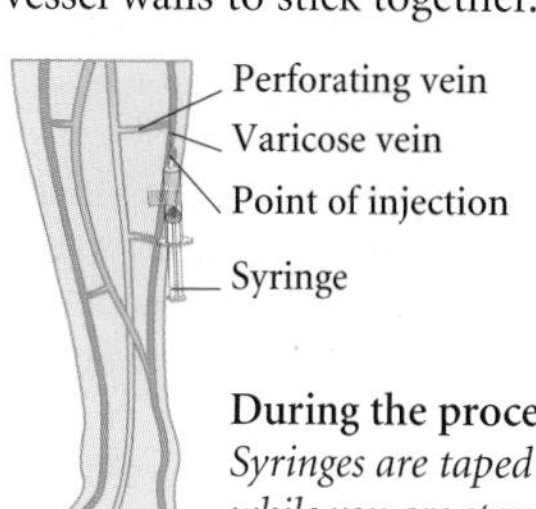

During the procedure
Syringes are taped in place while you are standing. The leg is elevated and the veins are injected at each site. The syringes are then removed.

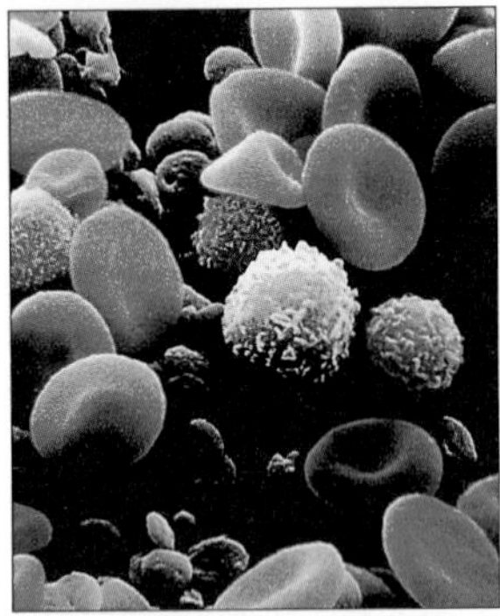

The cells in blood
A magnified view of a drop of blood reveals the various blood cells present: different types of white blood cell, together with red blood cells and platelets.

BLOOD AND THE LYMPHATIC AND IMMUNE SYSTEMS

BLOOD IS THE BODY'S internal transport system, constantly flowing around the body delivering oxygen, nutrients, and other substances to the tissues and removing waste products from them. Running almost parallel with the blood's circulation is the lymphatic system, which collects excess fluid from the tissues and returns it to the blood. Both the blood and the lymphatic system form part of the body's immune system.

Body tissues, such as muscle, brain, heart, and other internal organs, need to have a constant supply of energy to function. The energy is obtained from glucose and oxygen, which are carried to body tissues by the blood in the circulation. Blood circulates around the body in about 1 minute at rest and 20 seconds during vigorous exercise.

CIRCULATORY TRANSPORT

Glucose, a simple sugar that is derived from the breakdown of many foods, is dissolved in the blood and carried in the circulation to every cell within the body. To release its energy, glucose must be "burned" inside the cells, which requires oxygen (a process known as oxidation). The oxygen is transported by red blood cells from the lungs to the body cells, where it is released.

In addition to glucose, the body cells require proteins, fats, vitamins and minerals, and lipids such as cholesterol. These substances are carried in the plasma, the fluid part of the blood, to every cell within the body.

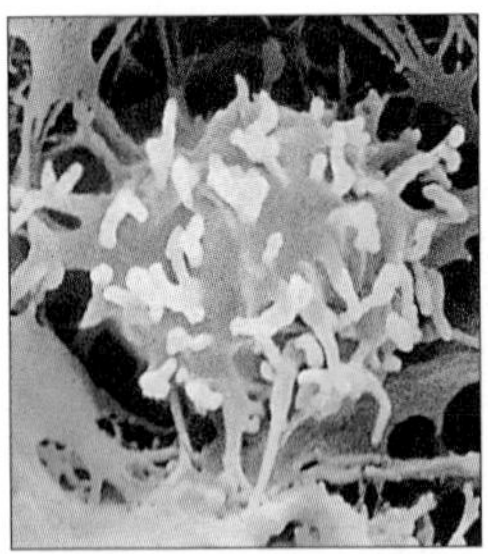

White blood cell
Some white blood cells, such as the one shown, play a particularly important part in the body's defences.

As body cells carry out their various functions, grow, reproduce, and repair damage, they release waste products into the bloodstream. These waste products include carbon dioxide produced from the oxidation of glucose, protein wastes such as urea, and bilirubin from the breakdown of the pigment haemoglobin. The carbon dioxide is eliminated from the blood in the lungs, while the other waste products are mostly processed in the liver before being excreted in the faeces or transported to the kidneys for excretion in the urine.

THE BODY'S DEFENCES

Blood contains colourless cells known as white cells. These are the main components of the immune system, which protects the body against infection, against toxins produced by bacteria, and against some cancers.

Other essential components of the immune system transported in the blood are proteins called antibodies, which help to destroy microorganisms. Blood also contains billions of small cells called platelets, which seal injured blood vessels through blood clotting.

The lymphatic system also forms part of the immune system and helps to protect the body by filtering out and destroying "foreign" particles, such as infectious organisms and cancer cells, that have contaminated body fluids.

(FUNCTION) FORMATION OF BLOOD CELLS

Bone marrow, the soft fatty tissue inside bone cavities, is the source of all the red blood cells and platelets and most of the white blood cells. In adults, blood cells are formed mainly in the bone marrow of flat bones, such as the shoulder blades, ribs, breastbone, and pelvis. All the blood cells are derived from a single type of cell called a stem cell. Production of stem cells is controlled by hormones, including erythropoietin, which is produced by the kidneys; thyroid hormones; corticosteroids secreted by the adrenal glands; and growth hormones from the pituitary gland.

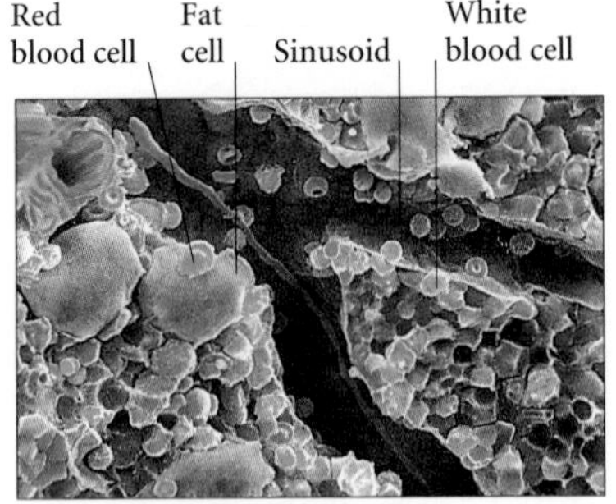

Cells in bone marrow
Blood cells, such as red and white cells, and fat cells are found in bone marrow. Tiny blood vessels called sinusoids supply nourishment and carry away wastes.

STRUCTURE COMPONENTS OF BLOOD

The average person has about 5 litres (9 pints) of blood, which consists of cells and fluid (plasma). Red blood cells, the most numerous blood cells, transport oxygen in the body. White blood cells destroy bacterial organisms, cells infected by viruses, and cancer cells. Platelets are the smallest blood cells; after an injury to a blood vessel, they rapidly clump together to seal the damaged lining. Plasma is mostly water but contains other important substances.

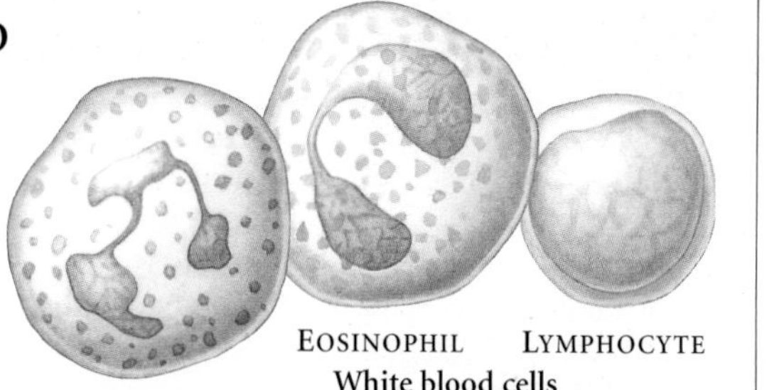

NEUTROPHIL EOSINOPHIL LYMPHOCYTE

White blood cells
There are five main types of white blood cell: neutrophils, eosinophils, lymphocytes, basophils, and monocytes. All have particular roles to play. Some, known as phagocytes, destroy foreign organisms.

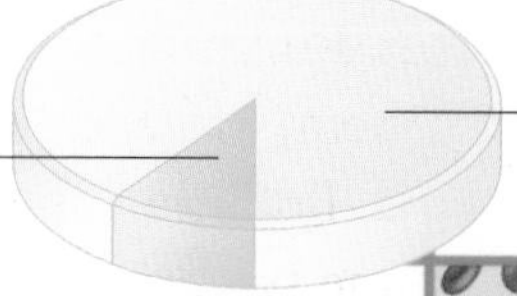

MONOCYTE BASOPHIL

Dissolved substances (10% of plasma)

Water (90% of plasma)

Plasma (55% of blood volume)

White blood cells and platelets (4% of blood volume)

Red blood cells (41% of blood volume)

Plasma
Plasma consists of water, nutrients, salts, hormones, and proteins, including the dissolved protein fibrinogen, which has a key role in blood clotting.

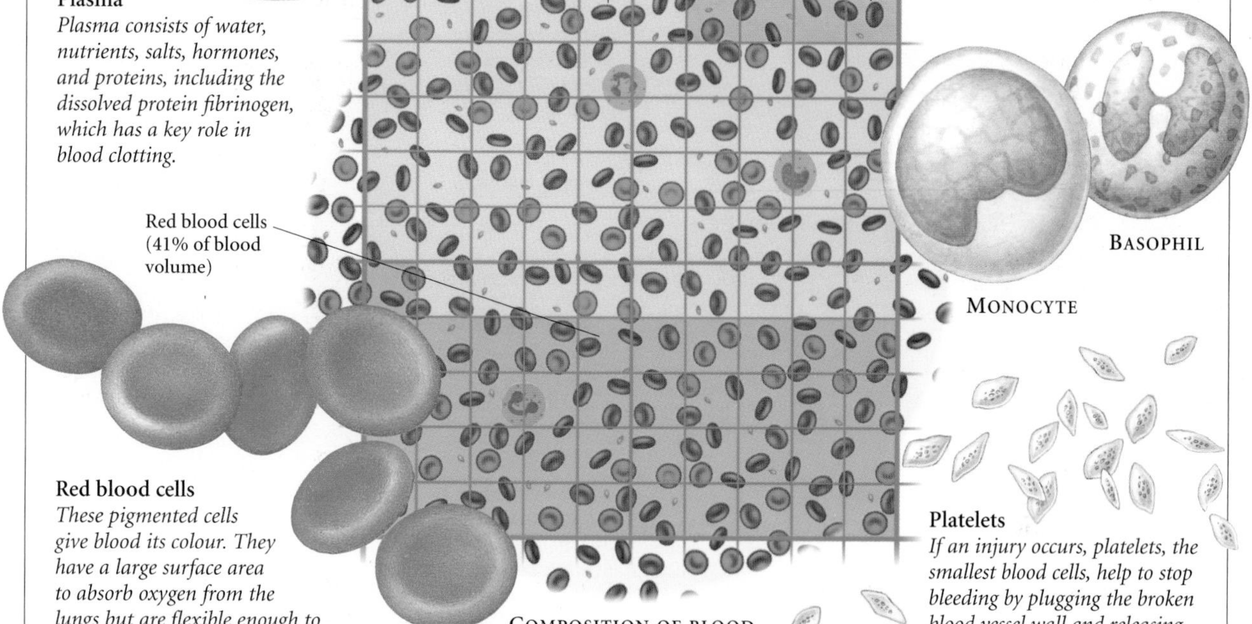

Red blood cells
These pigmented cells give blood its colour. They have a large surface area to absorb oxygen from the lungs but are flexible enough to squeeze through small blood vessels.

COMPOSITION OF BLOOD BY VOLUME

Platelets
If an injury occurs, platelets, the smallest blood cells, help to stop bleeding by plugging the broken blood vessel wall and releasing chemicals that promote clotting.

STRUCTURE BLOOD GROUPS

Each person's red blood cells have proteins called antigens on their surface, which categorize the blood into various groups. Antibodies in the blood are produced against any antigens foreign to the red cells. The ABO system of blood grouping is important when assessing the compatibility of blood to be used in transfusions; if a recipient's blood contains antibodies to antigens in the donor blood, a reaction occurs. The Rhesus (Rh) system is another important method of typing blood.

Blood group A
This group has A antigens on the surface of the red blood cells and anti-B antibodies in the blood.

A antigen

Anti-B antibody

Blood group B
People in this group have red blood cells with B antigens, and anti-A antibodies in their blood.

B antigen

Anti-A antibody

Blood group AB
The rarest blood group, AB, has both antigens on the red cells and neither antibody in the blood.

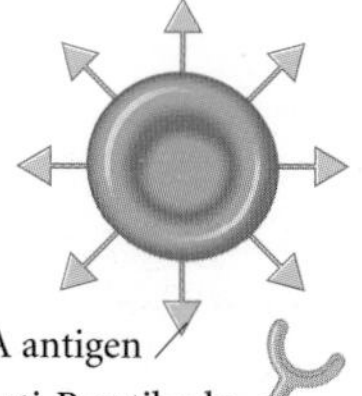

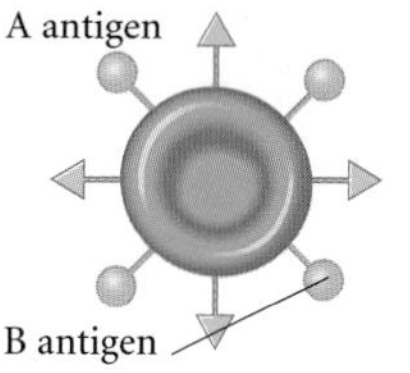

Blood group O
The most common group, O, has no red cell antigens, and anti-A and anti-B antibodies in the blood.

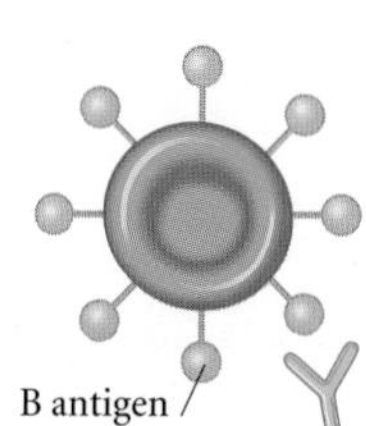
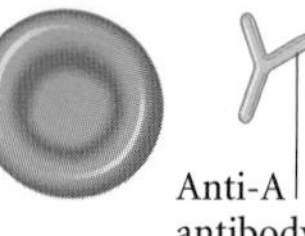

FUNCTION THE ROLES OF BLOOD

One of the main functions of blood is to transport oxygen, cells, proteins, hormones, and other substances around the body to the organs and tissues. Oxygen is carried from the lungs to the body cells, and the waste product carbon dioxide is transported from the cells to the lungs. Blood also has a clotting mechanism that acts to seal damaged blood vessels and prevents internal and external blood loss.

TRANSPORTING OXYGEN

Each red blood cell contains millions of molecules of haemoglobin, each made up of four protein chains (two alpha- and two beta-globin) and four haeme, an iron-bearing red pigment. Haemoglobin combines with oxygen from the lungs to give arterial blood its bright red colour. Once oxygen is released in the tissues, the blood becomes darker, a distinctive feature of venous blood.

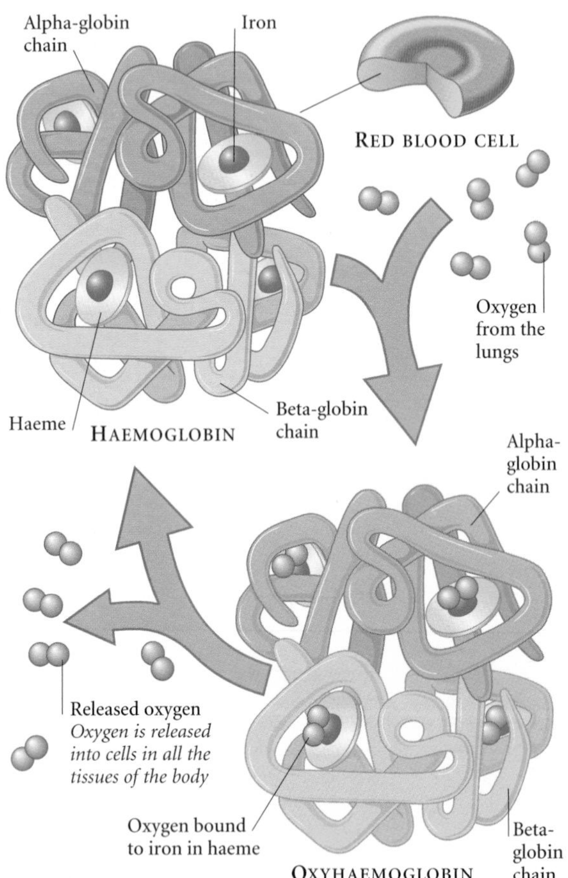

How haemoglobin carries oxygen
The oxygen from the lungs enters the red blood cells in the bloodstream. The oxygen then combines chemically with the haeme within the haemoglobin to form oxyhaemoglobin, which is carried around the body. In areas that need oxygen, the oxyhaemoglobin releases its oxygen and reverts to haemoglobin.

BLOOD CLOTTING

When a blood vessel is cut or torn, the damage triggers a series of chemical reactions that lead to the formation of a blood clot to seal the injury. Clot formation depends on blood cells called platelets, which adhere at the site of injury. The platelets then clump together and release chemicals that activate proteins, called clotting factors.

1 *When a blood vessel is damaged, it constricts at once. Platelets that come into contact with the damaged blood vessel walls are activated. They become sticky and start to adhere to the blood vessel walls near the site of the injury.*

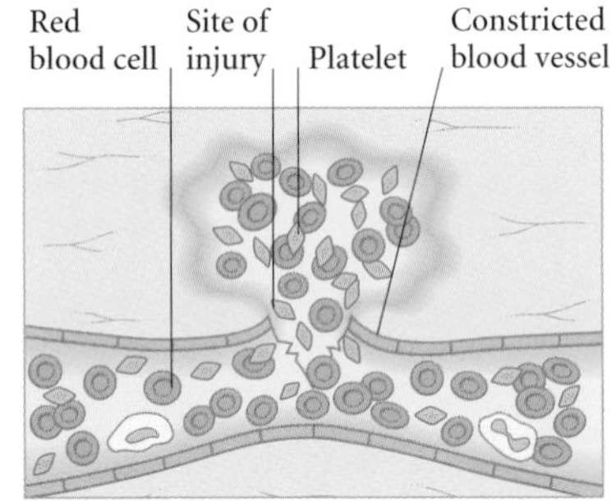

Platelets clumped together

Released chemicals

2 *The platelets clump together. Damaged tissue and activated platelets release chemicals that start a "coagulation cascade", a complex series of reactions involving clotting factors. At each stage, more clotting factors are activated.*

3 *The final stage is conversion of the protein fibrinogen, which is dissolved in the fluid part of the blood, to insoluble fibrin strands. The sticky fibrin threads form a tangled mesh that traps red cells and other blood cells, forming a clot.*

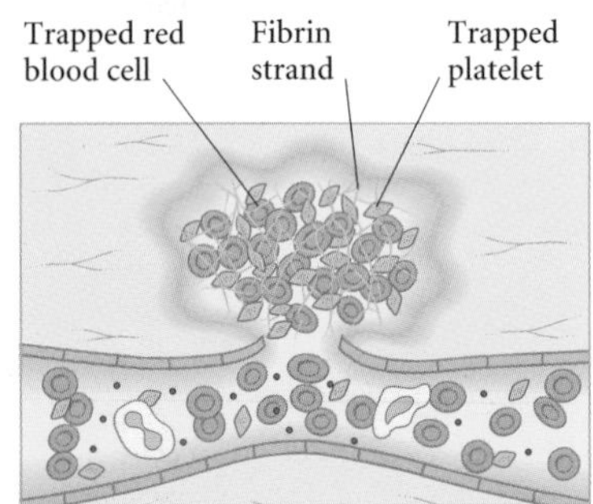

Fibrin strand

Red blood cell

Blood clot
This magnified view shows red blood cells trapped in a mesh of sticky fibrin strands, forming a blood clot. An injured blood vessel is plugged by the clot, which becomes denser as more fibrin strands form. Eventually, the clot will solidify.

STRUCTURE THE LYMPHATIC SYSTEM

A network of lymph vessels, lymphatic tissue, and clumps of bean-shaped lymph nodes (glands) makes up the lymphatic system. The lymph vessels collect fluid (lymph) from the body tissues and return it to the blood, maintaining the fluid balance within the body. Lymph filters through the lymph nodes, which are packed with particular types of white blood cell known as lymphocytes. These cells are produced in the bone marrow, spleen, and thymus, and they help to protect the body against infection.

Incoming lymph vessel
Many of these vessels drain lymph into a single node

Sinus

Valve

Macrophage
This white blood cell engulfs and destroys foreign and dead material

Capsule
The node is covered by fibrous tissue

Germinal centre
This area contains white blood cells called lymphocytes

Artery

Vein

Outgoing lymph vessel
Filtered lymph is carried away by this single vessel

Inside a lymph node
The flow of lymph slows as it moves through the narrow channels in the spaces, called sinuses, in a node. The reduction in flow allows macrophages time to filter disease organisms from the lymph.

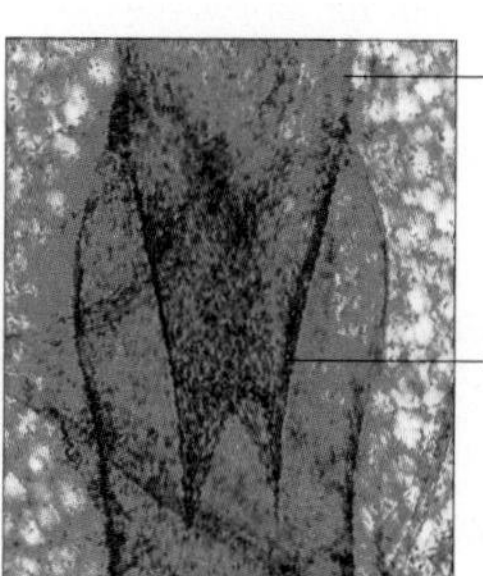

Lymph vessel wall
Thin, specialized walls allow fluid to flow into, but not out of, the vessel

Valve
This structure opens (as here) to let lymph flow through and closes to prevent backflow

Section of a lymph vessel
Lymph vessels have thin walls that allow fluid from the surrounding body tissues (known as lymph) to enter. The lymph is moved through the lymph vessel by the contractions of muscles. Valves in each vessel prevent backflow of fluid.

Fibrous tissue

White blood cell

Lymphatic tissue in a node
This magnified view reveals a fine, fibrous network of lymphatic tissue. White blood cells, a key feature of the body's immune system, are seen entangled within the mesh.

Supratrochlear node

Cervical (neck) nodes
Lymph from the head and neck is filtered here

Axillary (armpit) nodes
These nodes filter lymph from the arms and breasts

Right lymphatic duct
This duct receives lymph that is filtered from the right arm and upper right side of the body

Subclavian vein
This vein, which leads towards the heart, receives filtered lymph from the thoracic and right lymphatic ducts

Thymus gland
The thymus produces vital white blood cells

Thoracic duct
This main duct receives lymph from the majority of lymph vessels

Spleen
This is the largest lymph organ, in which certain types of lymphocytes (white blood cells) are manufactured

Cisterna chyli
This lymph vessel, which narrows into the thoracic duct, receives lymph from the lower body

Peyer's patch
Areas of lymphatic tissue in the intestines are known as Peyer's patches

Deep inguinal (groin) nodes
These nodes filter lymph from the lower part of the body

Popliteal lymph nodes
These nodes, which are situated behind the knees, filter lymph from the legs and feet

Lymph vessel
Many lymph vessels carry lymph from the tissues to the main lymphatic ducts through lymph nodes

FUNCTION THE BODY'S DEFENCES

Several barriers and responses work together to protect the body against infection and the development of cancer. Physical and chemical barriers and the inflammatory response form the first two lines of defence. If invading organisms break through these general lines of defence, the body's immune system fights back with two extremely effective immune responses that are specific to different invaders.

PHYSICAL AND CHEMICAL BARRIERS

The skin and the mucous membranes, which line the body openings and the internal passages, are effective barriers against invading organisms. Saliva, tears, mucus, sebum, sweat, and acid aid these barriers in protecting the different parts of the body.

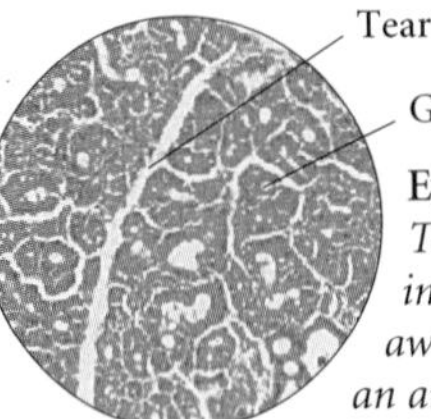

Eyes
Tears from glands in the eyelids wash away dirt and contain an antiseptic substance.

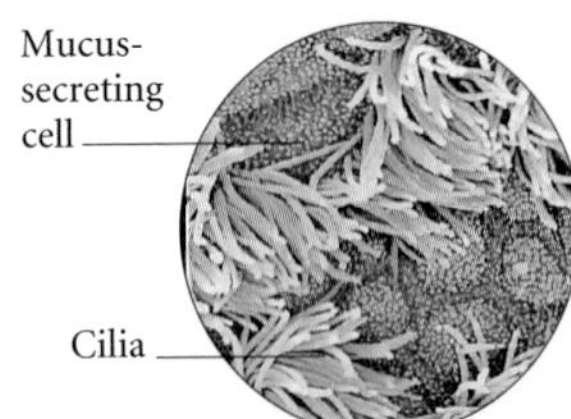

Respiratory tract
The lining of the respiratory tract produces mucus, which traps organisms. Tiny hairs (cilia) move mucus to the throat.

Mouth
Glands in the mouth produce saliva, a mixture of mucus and enzymes that cleans the mouth.

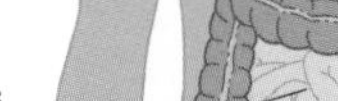

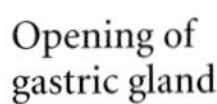

Intestines
Goblet cells in the lining of the intestines produce mucus, which protects the lining from digestive chemicals and harmful organisms.

Stomach
Glands in the stomach lining produce hydrochloric acid, a powerful agent that kills most invading organisms.

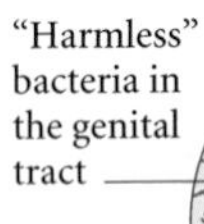

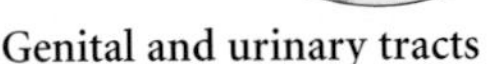

Genital and urinary tracts
"Harmless" bacteria within the genital tract and the flushing action of urine in the urinary tract both help to prevent the growth of harmful organisms.

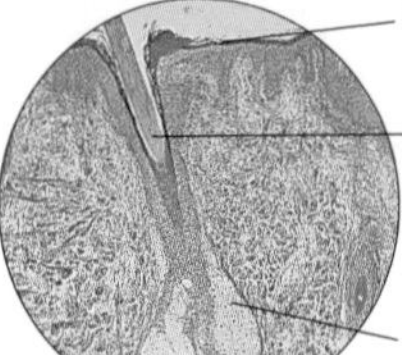

Skin
The skin is protected by an oily substance, sebum, produced by sebaceous glands and by sweat. Both of these are mildly antiseptic.

THE INFLAMMATORY RESPONSE

If foreign organisms such as bacteria overcome the body's physical and chemical barriers, the next line of defence is the inflammatory response, characterized by redness, pain, heat, and swelling at the damaged site.

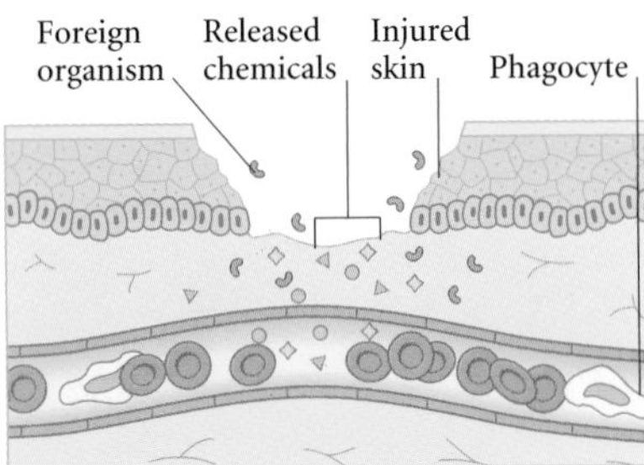

1 *Foreign organisms invade the body through skin that has been broken due to injury. Instantly, the damaged tissue releases specific chemicals that attract specialized white blood cells called phagocytes.*

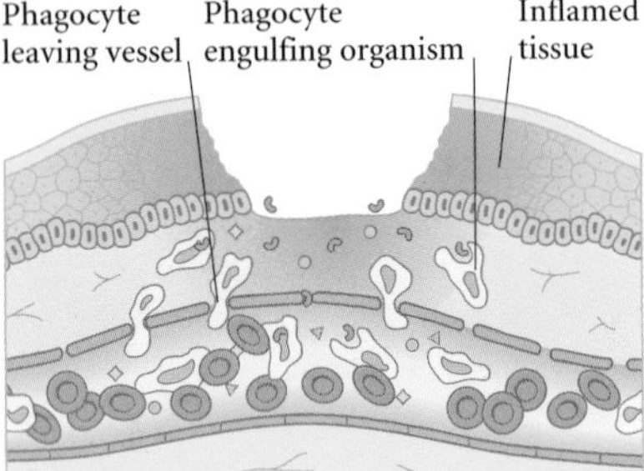
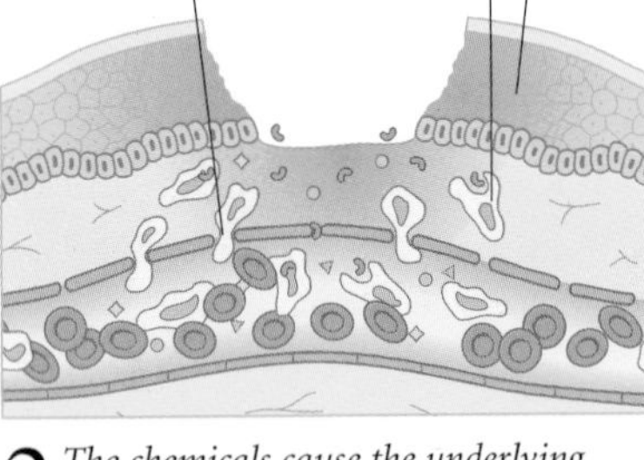

2 *The chemicals cause the underlying blood vessel to widen and the flow of blood to increase, leading to symptoms of inflammation. The vessel walls become slightly porous, allowing phagocytes to reach, engulf, and destroy the foreign organisms.*

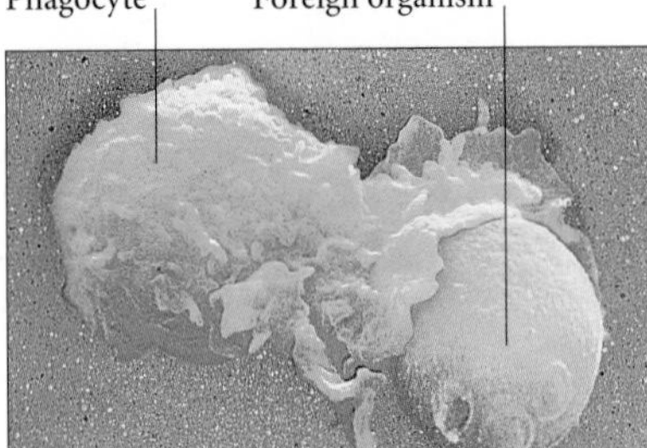

Destroying foreign organisms
Here, a white blood cell called a phagocyte has started to engulf a foreign organism. To destroy the organism, the phagocyte releases enzymes that help to break it down.

The antibody immune response

This specific immune response targets invading bacteria and relies on white blood cells called B-lymphocytes or B-cells. These cells recognize proteins (antigens) of invading bacteria and multiply to produce antibodies. The antibodies seek out the bacteria and lock on to them, causing their destruction.

1 The bacteria enter the body. Some of them are engulfed by cells called phagocytes that bring the bacterial antigens into contact with B-cells, some of which match the antigens.

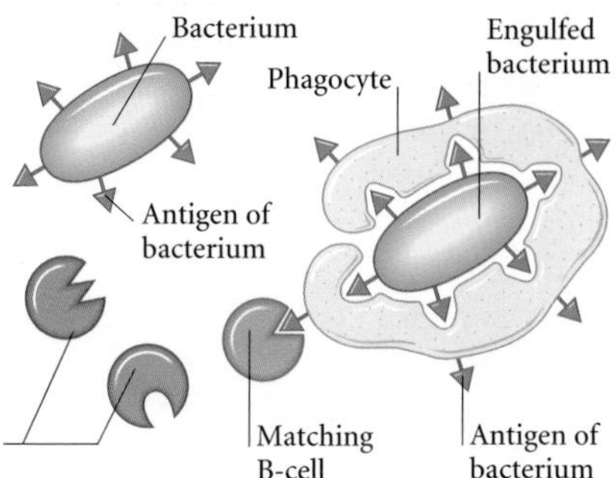

2 The matching B-cell multiplies to produce two types of cell: plasma cells, which produce antibodies to destroy the bacteria, and memory B-cells, which are stored in the body for future use.

Memory B-cell
Second exposure to the same bacteria activates this cell to rapidly produce plasma cells

Plasma cell

Antibody

3 The antibodies that are released by the plasma cells seek out and lock on to bacterial antigens and inactivate the bacteria. The antibodies also attract more phagocytes to the site to destroy the bacteria.

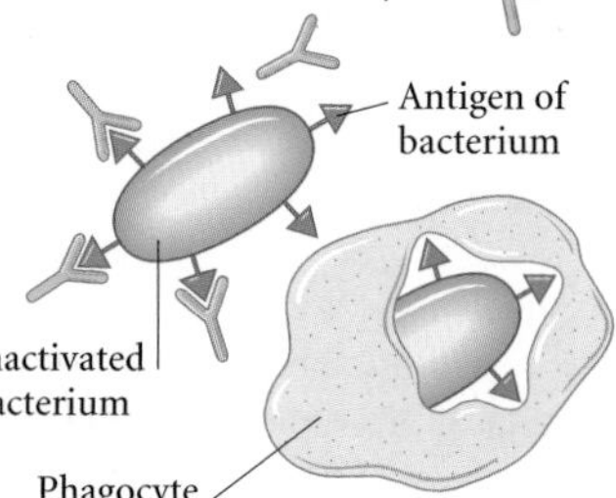

The cellular immune response

This type of specific immune response targets viruses, parasites, and cancer cells. It depends on white blood cells called T-lymphocytes or T-cells. After recognizing a foreign protein (antigen), T-cells multiply and engage in a direct battle against infected cells or cancer cells.

1 Cells that are infected by the invading viruses are engulfed by cells called phagocytes. These bring the viral antigens into contact with T-cells, some of which match up with these antigens.

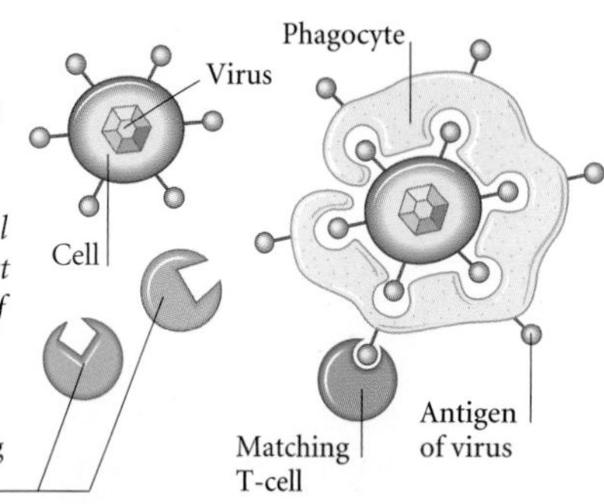

2 The matching T-cell multiplies in order to produce different types of cells, including killer T-cells, which contain toxic proteins, and memory T-cells, stored to protect the body against the virus in the future.

Memory T-cell
Future exposure to the same antigen activates this cell to rapidly produce killer T-cells

Toxic protein

Killer T-cell

3 Killer T-cells lock on to the infected cell bearing the recognized antigen and release their toxic proteins. These proteins then destroy the infected cell. Killer T-cells may then go on to seek out other infected cells.

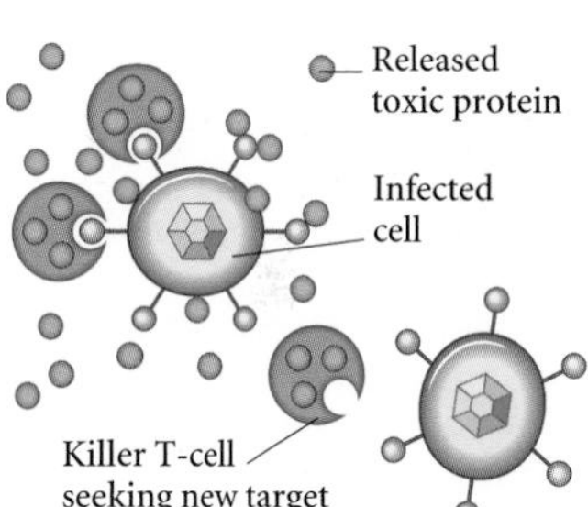

FUNCTION Allergic reactions

An allergy is an inappropriate immune response to a normally harmless substance, called an allergen. On initial exposure to the allergen, the immune system becomes sensitized to it. During subsequent exposures, an allergic reaction occurs. Mast cells, located in the skin, nasal lining, and other tissues, are destroyed, releasing a substance called histamine that causes an inflammatory response, irritating body tissues and producing allergy symptoms.

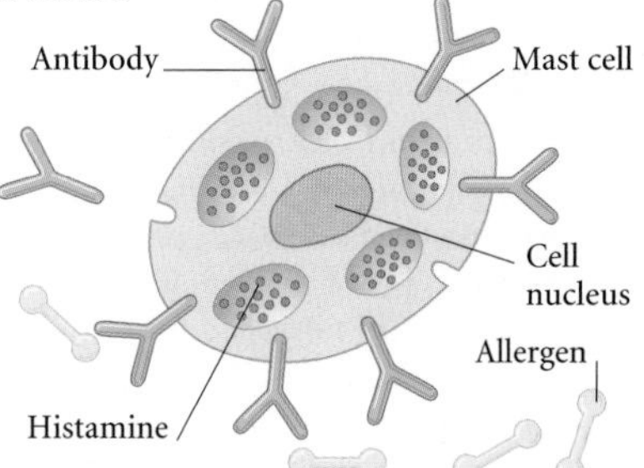

1 On repeat exposure to an allergen, antibodies previously produced in response to it bind to the surface of mast cells, which contain histamine.

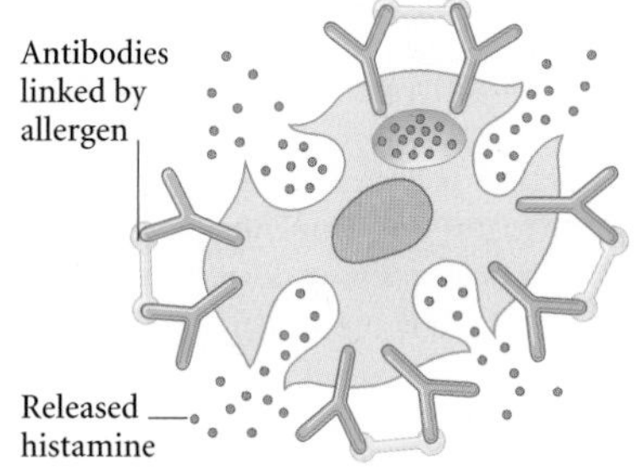

2 The allergens bind to and link two or more antibodies, causing the cell to burst and release the histamine within. Histamine causes the symptoms of allergy.

Blood disorders

Blood transports oxygen and nutrients to all parts of the body and carries away carbon dioxide and other waste materials. Oxygen is carried inside red blood cells, which make up almost half the volume of blood. Other components of blood include white blood cells, which combat infections, and platelets, tiny cells that help to form blood clots to seal damaged blood vessels.

Disorders of the blood may be caused by an abnormality in the number, content, or form of one or more of the different types of blood cell. The first articles in this section deal with the different types of anaemia and with sickle-cell disease. In these disorders, haemoglobin, the oxygen-carrying pigment in red blood cells, is deficient or abnormal, or red cells are destroyed at an accelerated rate. Disorders in which the blood either fails to clot or clots too readily are then discussed. Some of these disorders are inherited, such as haemophilia, Christmas disease, and von Willebrand's disease. In these disorders, the genes that are responsible for producing specific clotting factors are either absent or abnormal. Various cancers of the blood, called leukaemias, are also discussed. These disorders result from an overproduction of white blood cells, which suppresses the production of the normal blood cells in the body. The final article in this section deals with polycythaemia, a condition in which too many red blood cells are produced.

KEY ELEMENTS

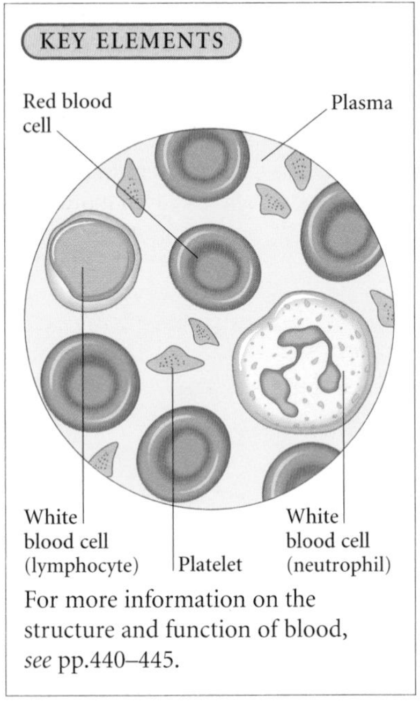

For more information on the structure and function of blood, *see* pp.440–445.

Anaemia

Disorders in which haemoglobin (the oxygen-carrying pigment in red blood cells) is deficient or abnormal

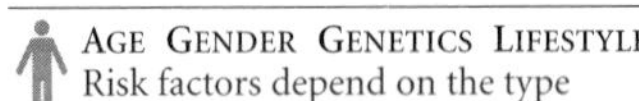

Anaemia is a deficiency or an abnormality of haemoglobin, the component of red blood cells that binds with oxygen from the lungs and carries it through the circulation to the body tissues. The oxygen-carrying capacity of the blood is thus reduced, and the tissues of the body may not receive sufficient oxygen.

Red blood cells are manufactured in the bone marrow and circulate in the bloodstream for about 120 days before they are broken down in the spleen. In a healthy person, the production and destruction of red blood cells are balanced. Anaemia occurs if this balance is upset, reducing the number of healthy cells, or if the haemoglobin is abnormal.

What are the types?

There are four main types of anaemia. The first type is due to a deficiency of one or more of the substances that are essential for the formation of healthy red blood cells. By far the most common form is iron-deficiency anaemia (opposite page), which results from low levels of iron in the body. A much rarer form is megaloblastic anaemia (p.448), which is usually the result of low levels of either vitamin B_{12} or another vitamin, folic acid, in the body.

The second type of anaemia results from inherited abnormalities of haemoglobin production. Examples of this type include sickle-cell disease (p.448) and thalassaemia (p.449). The haemoglobin is abnormal from shortly after birth, but symptoms of anaemia may not develop until later in childhood.

The third type of anaemia is caused by excessively rapid destruction of red blood cells (haemolysis) and is called haemolytic anaemia (p.450).

The fourth type of anaemia, called aplastic anaemia (p.450), is caused by failure of the bone marrow to produce sufficient numbers of red blood cells and often of other types of blood cell as well.

Anaemia may be due to a combination of different causes, and sometimes the exact cause of the condition is not known. In some cases, anaemia develops during a long-term illness, such as cancer or rheumatoid arthritis (p.377).

What are the symptoms?

If your anaemia is mild, your body may be able to make up for a slight reduction in the oxygen-carrying capacity of blood by increasing the blood supply to the tissues. In this case, there may not be any symptoms. Symptoms of more severe anaemia may include:

- Tiredness and a feeling of faintness.
- Pale skin.
- Shortness of breath on mild exertion.

You may also have a rapid heart rate because the heart has to work harder to increase blood supply to the rest of the body. Stress on the heart may result in chronic heart failure (p.413), common symptoms of which are swollen ankles and increasing shortness of breath.

What might be done?

Anaemia is usually confirmed by blood tests to measure the level of haemoglobin and to establish the type and cause of the anaemia. A bone marrow aspiration and biopsy (p.451) may be carried out to obtain tissue samples for examination under a microscope.

Most anaemias respond well to treatment. Severe cases may require blood transfusion (opposite page).

(WWW) ONLINE SITES: p.1027

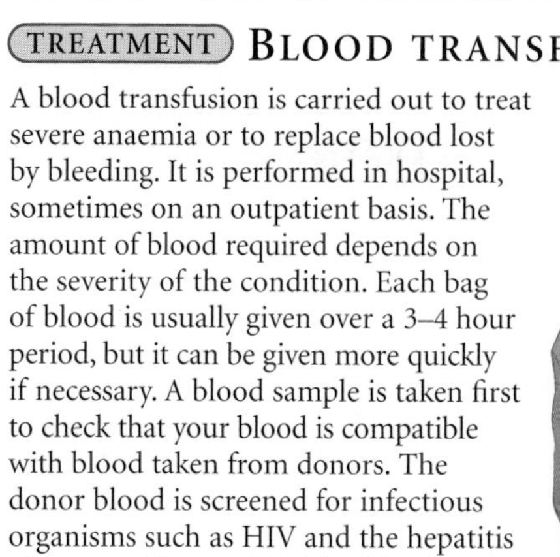

TREATMENT BLOOD TRANSFUSION

A blood transfusion is carried out to treat severe anaemia or to replace blood lost by bleeding. It is performed in hospital, sometimes on an outpatient basis. The amount of blood required depends on the severity of the condition. Each bag of blood is usually given over a 3–4 hour period, but it can be given more quickly if necessary. A blood sample is taken first to check that your blood is compatible with blood taken from donors. The donor blood is screened for infectious organisms such as HIV and the hepatitis viruses and is stored in blood banks.

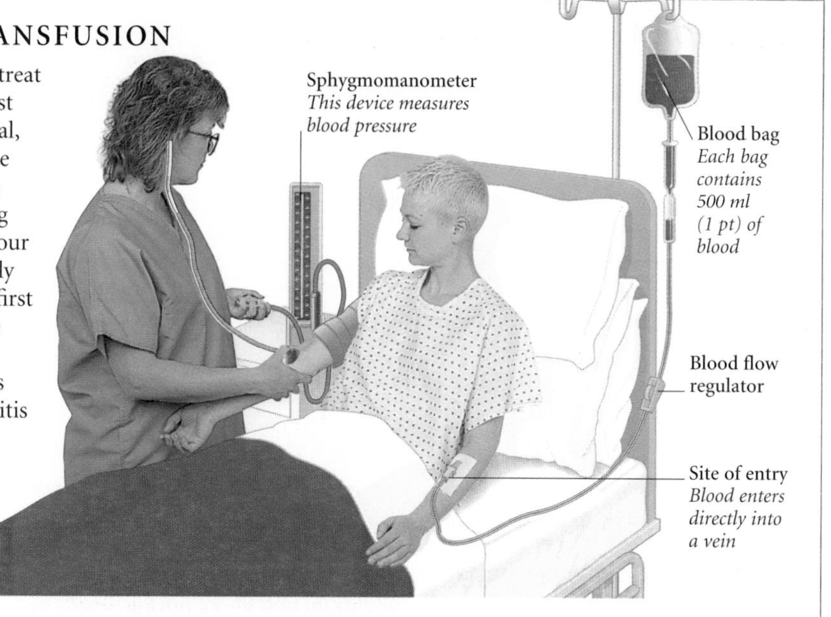

Having a transfusion
A nurse will regularly measure your blood pressure, pulse, and temperature while the blood transfusion is given directly into a vein in your arm.

Iron-deficiency anaemia

A type of anaemia caused by inadequate levels of iron in the body

 GENDER More common in females

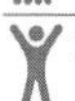 LIFESTYLE A vegan diet is a risk factor

 AGE GENETICS Not significant factors

Iron-deficiency anaemia is the most common form of anaemia (a deficiency of the oxygen-carrying pigment haemoglobin in red blood cells). Iron is an essential component of haemoglobin in the production of blood. If insufficient iron is available, the production of haemoglobin and its incorporation into red blood cells in the bone marrow are reduced. As a result, there is less haemoglobin to bind with oxygen in the lungs and to carry the oxygen to the tissues of the body. Consequently, the tissues may receive insufficient oxygen.

WHAT ARE THE CAUSES?

Iron-deficiency anaemia is most commonly caused by the loss of significant quantities of iron through persistent bleeding. This type of anaemia mainly affects women who experience regular blood loss over a period of time from heavy menstrual bleeding (*see* MENORRHAGIA, p.735). Persistent loss of blood may also be due to stomach ulcers (*see* PEPTIC ULCER, p.640). Prolonged use of aspirin or long-term use of nonsteroidal anti-inflammatory drugs (p.894) is a possible cause of bleeding from the lining of the stomach. In people over the age of 60, a common cause of blood loss is cancer of the bowel (*see* COLORECTAL CANCER, p.665). Bleeding in the stomach or in the upper intestine may go unnoticed, while blood lost from the lower part of the intestine or the rectum may be visible in the faeces.

The second cause of iron-deficiency anaemia is insufficient iron in the diet. People whose diet contains little or no iron, such as vegans, may be at particular risk of developing the condition.

Iron-deficiency anaemia is also more likely to develop when the body needs higher levels of iron than normal and these extra demands are not met by the existing diet. For example, children who are growing rapidly, especially adolescents, and women who are pregnant have an increased risk of developing iron-deficiency anaemia if their diet does not contain plenty of iron.

Some other causes of iron-deficiency anaemia include disorders that prevent absorption of iron from the diet. In the body, iron is absorbed from food as it passes through the small intestine; conditions that cause damage to the small intestine, such as coeliac disease (p.658) or surgery on the small intestine, sometimes result in iron deficiency.

WHAT ARE THE SYMPTOMS?

In addition to any specific symptoms associated with an underlying disorder, you may experience the general symptoms of anaemia, which include:

- Tiredness and a feeling of faintness.
- Pale skin.
- Shortness of breath on mild exertion.

You may also have symptoms that are due to a marked deficiency of iron:

- Brittle, concave-shaped nails.
- Painful cracks in the skin at the sides of the mouth.
- A smooth, reddened tongue.

If your anaemia is severe, you may be at risk of chronic heart failure (p.413) because your heart has to work harder to supply blood to the rest of the body.

WHAT MIGHT BE DONE?

Your doctor will arrange for blood tests to measure the levels of haemoglobin and iron in your blood. If the cause of the iron deficiency is not obvious, other tests may be arranged to look for evidence of internal bleeding. These tests may include upper digestive tract endoscopy (p.641) and colonoscopy (p.661).

If there is an underlying disorder, this will be treated. Your doctor may prescribe iron tablets (syrup for children) or, less commonly, iron injections for several months to replace iron stores (*see* MINERALS, p.929). Severe anaemia may require blood transfusion (above).

(WWW) ONLINE SITES: p.1027, p.1035

Megaloblastic anaemia

A type of anaemia caused by a lack of vitamin B_{12} or folic acid

AGE More common over the age of 40

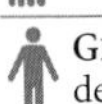

GENDER GENETICS LIFESTYLE Risk factors depend on the cause

Two major vitamins, B_{12} and folic acid, play an essential role in the production of healthy red blood cells. Deficiency of either vitamin may lead to megaloblastic anaemia, in which large, abnormal red blood cells (megaloblasts) are produced by the bone marrow, and the production of normal red blood cells is reduced. The blood may thus be unable to carry sufficient oxygen to the tissues.

WHAT ARE THE CAUSES?

Lack of vitamin B_{12} is rarely due to a dietary deficiency. The problem is usually due to an autoimmune disorder in which antibodies are produced that damage the stomach lining and prevent it from forming intrinsic factor, which is essential for the absorption of vitamin B_{12} from food in the intestines. This type of megaloblastic anaemia, called pernicious anaemia, tends to run in families and is more common in women and in people with other autoimmune disorders, such as Hashimoto's thyroiditis (*see* THYROIDITIS, p.681). Intestinal disorders, such as coeliac disease (p.658), or abdominal surgery can also interfere with vitamin B_{12} absorption.

Folic acid deficiency is often due to a poor diet. People who abuse alcohol are at particular risk because alcohol interferes with the absorption of folic acid in the intestines. Pregnant women may also be at risk of deficiency because folic acid requirements are higher in pregnancy. Disorders causing a rapid turnover of cells, including severe psoriasis (p.332), may also cause folic acid deficiency. In rare cases, the deficiency is a side effect of certain drugs, such as anticonvulsants (p.914) and anticancer drugs (p.907).

WHAT ARE THE SYMPTOMS?

The initial symptoms of megaloblastic anaemia, which are common to all anaemias, develop slowly and may include:

- Tiredness and a feeling of faintness.
- Pale skin.
- Shortness of breath on mild exertion.

These symptoms of megaloblastic anaemia may worsen over time. Although lack of folic acid does not produce additional symptoms, lack of vitamin B_{12} may eventually damage the nervous system, possibly leading to:

- Tingling in the hands and feet.
- Weakness and loss of balance.
- Loss of memory and confusion.

People who have pernicious anaemia may also notice a yellow tinge to their skin due to jaundice (p.643).

WHAT MIGHT BE DONE?

The diagnosis requires blood tests to look for megaloblasts and to measure the levels of vitamin B_{12} and folic acid. You may also have a bone marrow aspiration and biopsy (p.451) to obtain tissue samples for further examination.

Megaloblastic anaemia caused by an inability to absorb vitamin B_{12} may be improved by treating the underlying disorder, but some people, such as those who have pernicious anaemia and malabsorption caused by surgery, require lifelong regular injections of vitamin B_{12} (*see* VITAMINS, p.927). Symptoms should subside within days, but existing damage to the nervous system may be irreversible.

If megaloblastic anaemia is caused by an inadequate diet, the condition usually disappears with an improved diet and a short course of folic acid tablets.

(WWW) ONLINE SITES: p.1027

Sickle-cell disease

An inherited blood disorder in which red blood cells become sickle-shaped

AGE Present from birth; first symptoms appear after about 6 months

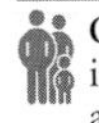

GENETICS Due to an abnormal gene inherited from both parents; mainly affects black people

LIFESTYLE Strenuous exercise and high altitudes may trigger symptoms

GENDER Not a significant factor

Sickle-cell disease is the result of an abnormality of haemoglobin, the pigment within red blood cells that binds to oxygen in the lungs and carries it to the other body tissues. When the amount of oxygen that is bound to the abnormal haemoglobin is reduced, the red blood cells become distorted into an elongated sickle shape. Because these sickle-shaped cells are rigid, they can become lodged in small blood vessels and obstruct the flow of blood, depriving the tissues of oxygen. Sickle-shaped red cells are fragile and may be destroyed prematurely, which can lead to anaemia (p.446).

Sickle-cell disease occurs most commonly in people of African descent, and the condition is less common among people from Mediterranean countries.

WHAT ARE THE CAUSES?

Sickle-cell disease is a genetic disorder in which an abnormal gene is inherited from both parents in an autosomal recessive manner (*see* GENE DISORDERS, p.271). If an abnormal gene is inherited from only one parent, a condition called sickle-cell trait results. Sickle-cell trait does not usually produce symptoms or require treatment. In communities in which sickle-cell disease is particularly common, genetic testing may be recommended for couples planning to have children. If both partners are found to carry the sickle-cell gene, genetic counselling (p.272) will be offered.

WHAT ARE THE SYMPTOMS?

The symptoms of sickle-cell disease are highly variable, even among affected individuals within the same family. In children, the symptoms first appear at about 6 months of age and may include intermittent painful swelling of the fingers and toes and delayed growth.

Distinct episodes of illness, known as sickle-cell crises, occur intermittently throughout childhood and into adult life. These crises may be precipitated by infections, but they can also occur after strenuous exercise, on exposure to cold, or at high altitude. Sickle-cell crises can

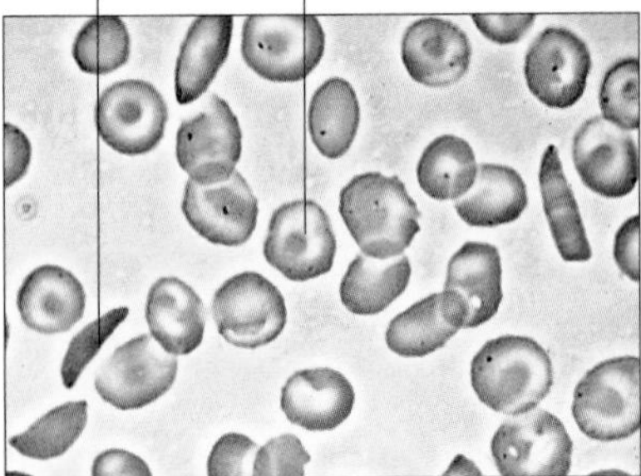

Sickle-shaped red blood cells
In sickle-cell disease, some of the red blood cells become distorted into a distinctive and fragile sickle shape.

produce different groups of symptoms, which may include:

- Pallor, tiredness, breathlessness, and faintness due to severe anaemia.
- Severe pain and swelling around a bone or joint.
- Breathlessness and chest pain.

Sickle-cell crises usually require urgent admission to hospital for treatment, and they can be life-threatening, except for bone pain crises, which although distressing, are never fatal.

Are there complications?

People who have sickle-cell disease are more susceptible to serious infections, such as pneumococcal infection (*see* PNEUMONIA, p.490), and any infection can trigger a sickle-cell crisis. Gallstones (p.651) may develop. The abnormal cells can cause problems by blocking and damaging small blood vessels throughout the body, which may lead to kidney damage (*see* CHRONIC KIDNEY FAILURE, p.706). The risk of transient ischaemic attacks (p.531) and stroke (p.532) is also increased. Women with sickle-cell disease may have decreased fertility, and those who become pregnant face an increased risk of miscarriage (p.791).

What might be done?

To confirm the diagnosis, your doctor may take a sample of blood to look for sickle-shaped cells under a microscope and to test for defective haemoglobin.

If sickle-cell disease is mild, folic acid (*see* VITAMINS, p.927), which is necessary for the production of red blood cells, may be prescribed. If the disease is more severe, you may require long-term drug treatment with hydroxyurea, which reduces the proportion of abnormal red cells in the blood. You may also need to take a preventive antibiotic (p.885) continually and to have vaccination against pneumococcal infection.

Immediate hospital admission is usually necessary for sickle-cell crises. You may be given intravenous fluids to treat dehydration, antibiotics for underlying infections, and painkillers (p.912). People who have recurrent sickle-cell crises may be given exchange transfusions, in which some of their blood is replaced with blood from a healthy donor. In some cases, a bone marrow transplant (p.454) may be considered.

(WWW) ONLINE SITES: p.1027

Thalassaemia

An inherited type of anaemia affecting production of haemoglobin, the oxygen-carrying pigment in red blood cells

AGE Present from birth; age at first appearance of symptoms depends on type

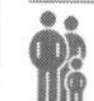
GENETICS Due to an abnormal gene inherited from one or both parents

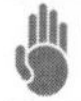
GENDER LIFESTYLE Not significant factors

In thalassaemia, an inherited genetic defect prevents the normal formation of haemoglobin, the oxygen-carrying pigment inside red blood cells. Red cells containing the defective haemoglobin carry less oxygen than normal and are destroyed prematurely, reducing oxygen transport to the body tissues.

The body tries to compensate by producing additional red blood cells throughout the bone marrow and in the liver and spleen, where blood cells are not normally formed. The marrow expands due to overactivity, which may lead to thickening of the bones of the skull and face. The liver and spleen may become enlarged as they produce and, in the case of the spleen, destroy large numbers of the abnormal red blood cells. Thalassaemia mainly affects people from Mediterranean countries, the Middle East, Southeast Asia, and Africa.

What are the causes?

A normal haemoglobin molecule contains four protein (globin) chains: two alpha and two beta chains. Different genes are responsible for the production of each type of chain. Thalassaemia is caused by one or more genetic defects and results in a failure to produce sufficient quantities of either the alpha or the beta globin chains.

Thalassaemia due to abnormal beta chains is more common. If a defective gene for beta-thalassaemia is inherited from only one parent, there may be no symptoms. Inheritance of a defective gene from each parent in an autosomal recessive pattern (*see* GENE DISORDERS, p.271) leads to a more severe condition.

There are two copies of the gene responsible for haemoglobin alpha chains. People who have one abnormal gene for alpha-thalassaemia usually have no symptoms, but a fetus with two defective genes will die before birth.

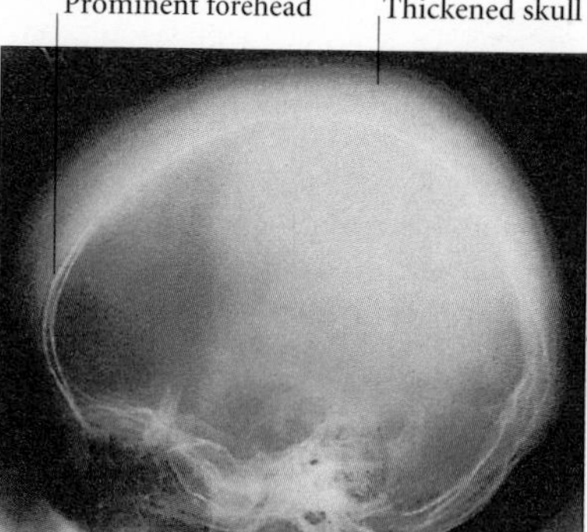

Enlarged skull bones in thalassaemia
In severe thalassaemia, increased bone marrow activity causes the bones of the skull to expand and become thickened, altering the appearance of the face.

Can it be prevented?

In communities in which thalassaemia is particularly common, genetic testing may be offered to couples planning to have children. If a defective gene is identified, they may want to consider genetic counselling (p.272). If a woman or her partner is known to have the disorder, tests can be done to establish whether the fetus has inherited the genetic defect (*see* ANTENATAL GENETIC TESTS, p.787).

What are the symptoms?

People who have alpha-thalassaemia or mild forms of beta-thalassaemia do not usually have symptoms. However, if the defective gene for beta-thalassaemia is inherited from both parents, symptoms of severe anaemia usually appear between 4 and 6 months of age. These symptoms may include:

- Pale skin.
- Shortness of breath on mild exertion.
- Swelling of the abdomen due to an enlarged spleen and liver.

Affected children have slow growth, and sexual development is delayed. The bones of the skull and face may thicken as the bone marrow expands.

What might be done?

If your doctor suspects that you have thalassaemia, he or she may arrange for blood tests to confirm the diagnosis.

If the thalassaemia is mild, you may not require treatment, but you may be advised to take folic acid supplements (*see* VITAMINS, p.927) to help to stimulate the production of red blood cells. If the condition is severe, regular blood transfusions (p.447) may be needed for life. However, frequent blood transfusions can lead to a build-up of iron in the heart, liver, and pancreas, causing progressive damage to these organs. To counteract this build-up, treatment with desferrioxamine (a drug that allows the kidneys to excrete more iron than usual) may be needed. If the spleen is enlarged, it may need to be removed. In severe cases, a bone marrow transplant (p.454) may be considered.

WHAT IS THE PROGNOSIS?

People with mild thalassaemia have a normal life span. Some people who have severe thalassaemia die early in childhood, but life expectancy can be greatly improved with regular transfusions.

(WWW) ONLINE SITES: p.1027

Haemolytic anaemia

A type of anaemia caused by excessive destruction of red blood cells

 GENETICS Risk factors depend on the cause

 AGE GENDER LIFESTYLE Not significant factors

Haemolytic anaemia occurs when the red cells in the blood are broken down more rapidly than they can be replaced. Red blood cells usually have a life span of about 120 days before they are destroyed in the spleen, a process known as haemolysis. The premature destruction of red blood cells may be caused by abnormal immune reactions, inherited disorders, or infections. If the bone marrow cannot replace the red blood cells rapidly, haemolytic anaemia results.

WHAT ARE THE CAUSES?

Haemolytic anaemia is most commonly due to an abnormal immune reaction in which the body produces antibodies that attack red blood cells and encourage their destruction in the spleen. This reaction is often triggered by drugs, including penicillin (*see* ANTIBIOTICS, p.885), methyldopa (*see* ANTIHYPERTENSIVE DRUGS, p.897), or quinine (*see* ANTIMALARIAL DRUGS, p.888). Antibodies that attack red blood cells may also occur in people who have chronic lymphocytic leukaemia (p.455) or an autoimmune disorder such as systemic lupus erythematosus (p.461).

Inherited disorders that affect the red blood cells' chemical make-up or shape may also promote haemolysis. One chemical abnormality, affecting about 100 million people worldwide, is lack of G6PD (glucose-6-phosphate dehydrogenase), an enzyme in the red blood cell membrane. This enzyme helps to process glucose, the red cells' main source of energy. People with the disorder are normally well but have to avoid certain drugs that can trigger haemolysis. In one form of G6PD deficiency, which mostly affects people of Mediterranean origin, severe haemolysis is triggered by a chemical found in broad beans (favism).

There are several inherited disorders that lead to abnormally shaped red blood cells. Such disorders include sickle-cell disease (p.448), in which the red blood cells become sickle-shaped, and spherocytosis, which causes the red blood cells to change to a spherical shape. Both of these disorders may lead to continuous haemolysis from childhood.

Red blood cells may also be destroyed as a result of infections such as malaria (p.305) in which the infective organism multiplies within the red blood cells. Rarely, haemolytic anaemia is due to damage to the red blood cells caused by an artificial heart valve.

WHAT ARE THE SYMPTOMS?

If you have haemolytic anaemia, you may notice the following symptoms, which are common to all anaemias:

- Tiredness and a feeling of faintness.
- Pale skin.
- Shortness of breath on mild exertion.

You may also have symptoms that occur as a result of haemolysis, including:

- Yellowing of the skin and whites of the eyes (*see* JAUNDICE, p.643).
- Swelling of the abdomen caused by enlargement of the spleen as it filters out many damaged red blood cells.

Over a period of several years, you may develop gallstones (p.651), which form from bilirubin, a product of the breakdown of red blood cells.

WHAT MIGHT BE DONE?

Haemolytic anaemia can be diagnosed from blood tests that reveal numerous immature red blood cells and, in some cases, fragmented, abnormally shaped red blood cells. Your doctor may also measure your blood levels of bilirubin, and he or she may arrange for blood tests to look for antibodies to red cells to identify the cause of the anaemia.

Underlying disorders, such as an infection or autoimmune disease, will be treated and any drugs that are causing haemolysis will be stopped. Corticosteroids (p.930) may be given for haemolytic anaemia due to an immune reaction. In some cases of haemolytic anaemia, surgical removal of the spleen is necessary.

(WWW) ONLINE SITES: p.1027

Aplastic anaemia

A type of anaemia caused by failure of the bone marrow to generate new blood cells of all types

 GENETICS Rarely due to an abnormal gene

 LIFESTYLE Exposure to chemicals such as benzene is a risk factor

 AGE GENDER Not significant factors

The blood normally contains red blood cells, white blood cells, and platelets. These components are produced either entirely or mostly in the bone marrow. However, in aplastic anaemia, the bone marrow does not produce stem cells, the initial form of these components, resulting in abnormally low numbers of all these blood cells.

WHAT ARE THE CAUSES?

In many cases of aplastic anaemia, the cause is unknown. However, the condition may result from an autoimmune disorder (p.461) in which antibodies are produced by the immune system that act against and destroy the body's own stem cells. In rare cases, aplastic anaemia is due to an inherited abnormal gene. When the cause of the condition has been established, the term secondary aplastic anaemia is used.

Secondary aplastic anaemia sometimes occurs following a severe viral infection, such as a hepatitis virus infection (*see* ACUTE HEPATITIS, p.644). The disorder may also develop after chemotherapy (p.280) or radiotherapy (p.281), as both treatments may reduce the production of blood cells by the bone marrow. Exposure to certain chemicals, such as benzene, and to some antibiotics (p.885), such as sulphonamides, may also trigger secondary aplastic anaemia.

WHAT ARE THE SYMPTOMS?

Aplastic anaemia may lead to the following symptoms, common to all anaemias and due to the lack of red blood cells:

- Tiredness and a feeling of faintness.
- Pale skin.
- Shortness of breath on mild exertion.

Lack of platelets, the tiny cells involved in blood clotting, may cause symptoms such as easy bruising and excessive bleeding, often from the gums or nose. A deficiency of white blood cells, which form an important part of the immune system, may increase susceptibility to bacterial and fungal infections, which may become life-threatening due to the inadequate immune response.

WHAT MIGHT BE DONE?

To confirm the diagnosis, your doctor may arrange for blood tests to measure blood cell levels and a bone marrow aspiration and biopsy (right) to obtain cell samples for examination.

Treatment of the underlying cause may allow the bone marrow to recover. Immunosuppressant drugs (p.906) or corticosteroids (p.930) may be used to treat autoimmune disorders. During recovery, blood transfusions (p.447) and antibiotics (p.885) may be needed to prevent or treat infection. If these treatments are ineffective, you may be offered a bone marrow transplant (p.454).

WHAT IS THE PROGNOSIS?

If treated early, a person with aplastic anaemia may make a complete recovery. However, in some cases the condition may be fatal. A successful bone marrow transplant can be life-saving.

(WWW) ONLINE SITES: p.1027, p.1036

(TEST) BONE MARROW ASPIRATION AND BIOPSY

Bone marrow aspiration and biopsy is used to diagnose various disorders of the blood, such as leukaemia and severe anaemias. In this procedure, two types of tissue sample are taken for examination: in a bone marrow aspiration, cells are withdrawn with a fine needle and syringe; in a bone marrow biopsy, a core of bone with marrow inside is taken with a large needle. The site may be tender for a few days afterwards. This procedure is usually carried out in hospital, often on an outpatient basis.

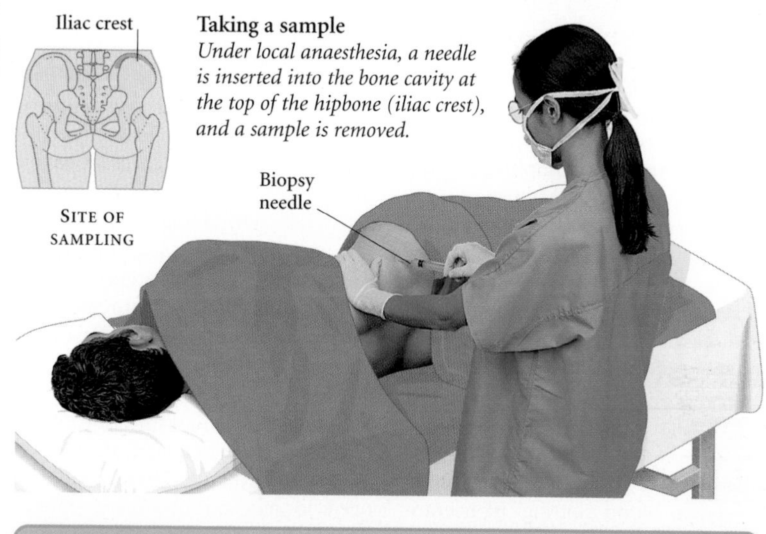

Taking a sample
Under local anaesthesia, a needle is inserted into the bone cavity at the top of the hipbone (iliac crest), and a sample is removed.

(RESULTS)

Bone marrow biopsy sample
This magnified image of a bone marrow sample reveals large numbers of abnormal white blood cells. Chronic myeloid leukaemia is a possible cause of this type of blood cell abnormality.

Bone marrow spaces
Bone marrow containing abnormal cells
Bone

Bleeding disorders

A group of disorders that result in excessive or prolonged bleeding

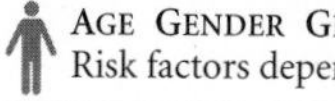

AGE GENDER GENETICS LIFESTYLE
Risk factors depend on the cause

Normally, when there is bleeding a blood clot forms to seal the damaged vessel and prevent further blood loss. A blood clot is formed when chemicals are released from platelets (small blood cells) and react with proteins known as clotting factors. A lack of clotting factors or platelets will disrupt the clotting process, which may lead to easy bruising, prolonged or severe bleeding after even minor injury, or internal bleeding into muscles, organs, and joints.

Many disorders that cause excessive bleeding are inherited, the most important being haemophilia and Christmas disease (p.452) and the related disorder von Willebrand's disease (p.452). These conditions occur when the gene that is responsible for a particular clotting factor is abnormal, resulting in either low levels or a complete absence of the clotting factor in the blood.

In thrombocytopenia (p.453), there are too few platelets in the blood. This condition can occur as a complication of bone marrow disorders, such as leukaemia (p.453) and aplastic anaemia (opposite page), or as a side effect of certain drugs, such as the anticancer drugs used in chemotherapy (p.280). Low platelet levels may result from infections, such as HIV infection (*see* HIV INFECTION AND AIDS, p.297) or sepsis (*see* SEPTICAEMIA, p.299).

Disorders of the liver, where clotting factors are produced, or the intestines, where vitamin K (an essential component of clotting factors) is absorbed, may also result in abnormal bleeding.

WHAT MIGHT BE DONE?

Bleeding disorders due to an absence of one or more clotting factors may be treated by regular injections of the missing factors. If the bleeding disorder is due to a drug, the use of that drug may be stopped. In other cases, treatment is aimed at the underlying disorder.

(WWW) ONLINE SITES: p.1027

Haemophilia and Christmas disease

Inherited deficiencies of blood clotting factors, causing excessive bleeding

GENDER Affect males only

GENETICS Due to abnormal genes, which in some cases are inherited

AGE LIFESTYLE Not significant factors

Normally, a cut or internal injury stops bleeding within 10 minutes, unless it is very serious. In haemophilia, even a small cut may bleed for hours or days, and there are sometimes episodes of spontaneous bleeding. The much rarer Christmas disease has similar features and is named after the person in whom the disease was first diagnosed. Both conditions affect only males.

WHAT ARE THE CAUSES?

Haemophilia and Christmas disease are both due to a deficiency of a protein involved in blood clotting. In haemophilia, the deficient protein is Factor VIII; in Christmas disease, the protein is Factor IX. In both these conditions, the deficiency is the result of a faulty gene. The particular gene involved is different in the two disorders.

In both disorders, the abnormal gene is inherited in a recessive manner and is located on the X chromosome (*see* GENE DISORDERS, p.271). The disorders affect males only; females are unaffected, although women can pass on the faulty gene to their children. Each son of a woman who carries the abnormal gene has a 1 in 2 chance of being affected.

In a third of all cases of haemophilia and Christmas disease, the cause is a spontaneous gene abnormality and there is no family history of the disorders.

WHAT ARE THE SYMPTOMS?

The symptoms are highly variable, and their severity depends on how much Factor VIII or IX is produced. They usually develop in infancy and may include:

- Easy bruising even after minor injury.
- Sudden, painful swelling of muscles and joints due to internal bleeding.
- Prolonged bleeding after an injury or a minor surgical operation.
- Blood in the urine.

Without treatment, prolonged episodes of bleeding into the joints may result in long-term damage and, eventually, may lead to deformity of the joints.

WHAT MIGHT BE DONE?

Your doctor will arrange for tests to see how long your blood takes to clot and to measure the level of Factor VIII or IX (*see* BLOOD CLOTTING TESTS, p.227).

The aim of treatment is to maintain the clotting factors at a high enough level to prevent bleeding. If you have a severe form of either condition, you will probably need regular intravenous injections of Factor VIII or IX to boost the levels of these factors in the blood. If you have a mild form of either condition, you may need injections only after an injury or before surgery. You may also be prescribed desmopressin, which contains a pituitary hormone, to boost the level of Factor VIII in your blood (*see* PITUITARY DRUGS, p.934).

Some people develop antibodies to Factor VIII supplements, which makes treatment difficult. These people may need to take an immunosuppressant drug (p.906) to destroy the antibodies.

WHAT IS THE PROGNOSIS?

If you have haemophilia or Christmas disease, you can lead an active life but need to avoid sustaining any injuries. Activities such as swimming, running, and walking are beneficial, but contact sports, such as wrestling and football, should be avoided. Regular dental care is necessary to avoid the risk of bleeding from inflamed gums.

If you have a family history of either disorder, you should obtain medical advice when planning a pregnancy (*see* GENETIC COUNSELLING, p.24). In the past, some people with haemophilia contracted acute or chronic hepatitis (p.645) or HIV (*see* HIV INFECTION AND AIDS, p.297) after receiving clotting factors contaminated with hepatitis B or C viruses or HIV. Clotting factors are now treated to kill these viruses.

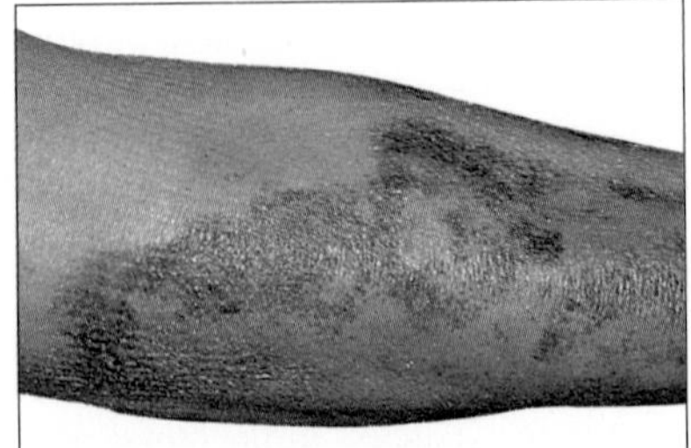

Bruising in haemophilia
In people with haemophilia, severe bruising, as seen on the arm above, can develop after even minor injury because the blood does not clot normally.

(WWW) ONLINE SITES: p.1027

Von Willebrand's disease

An inherited lifelong bleeding disorder similar to haemophilia

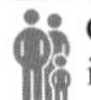
GENETICS Due to an abnormal gene inherited from one parent

AGE GENDER LIFESTYLE Not significant factors

In von Willebrand's disease, a substance called von Willebrand factor is absent from the blood or is present only in very low levels. Von Willebrand factor binds to a blood protein called Factor VIII, which is needed for blood clotting. A deficiency may lead to excessive or prolonged bleeding.

Von Willebrand's disease is a rare disorder caused by a dominant gene (*see* GENE DISORDERS, p.271); a person needs to inherit the gene from only one parent to develop the condition.

The symptoms of von Willebrand's disease include easy bruising, frequent nosebleeds, bleeding gums, heavy menstrual periods in women, and prolonged bleeding from even minor cuts.

WHAT MIGHT BE DONE?

A diagnosis is usually made by determining how long your blood takes to clot and measuring the levels of clotting factors in your blood (*see* BLOOD CLOTTING TESTS, p.227).

In mild cases, treatment is not usually necessary. If you bleed often or are due to have major surgery, you may be prescribed the drug desmopressin (*see* PITUITARY DRUGS, p.934), which raises the levels of von Willebrand factor and Factor VIII in your blood. Women may be advised to take an oral contraceptive to prevent heavy menstrual periods. If bleeding is severe, a blood extract rich in clotting factors may be given intravenously. The condition is usually mild, and, with treatment, the outlook is good.

(WWW) ONLINE SITES: p.1027

Thrombocytopenia

Reduced levels of blood cells called platelets, causing bleeding into the skin and internal organs

AGE GENDER GENETICS LIFESTYLE Not significant factors

In thrombocytopenia, there is a reduction in the number of platelets, the small blood cells that play a vital part in sealing damaged blood vessels, leading to a tendency to bleed abnormally.

Thrombocytopenia may be caused either by a failure of the bone marrow to produce platelets or by excessive destruction of platelets in the spleen. Platelet production in the bone marrow may be affected by disorders such as leukaemia (right) or aplastic anaemia (p.450) or by chemotherapy (p.280). An excessive destruction of platelets is usually due to an abnormal immune reaction in which the body produces antibodies that attack platelets. The cause is often unknown, but it may be triggered by blood transfusions (p.447) or by drugs such as quinine (*see* ANTIMALARIAL DRUGS, p.888) and rifampicin (*see* ANTITUBERCULOUS DRUGS, p.886). In children, the condition is often triggered by a viral infection.

Thrombocytopenia may occur as a result of infection, such as HIV (*see* HIV INFECTION AND AIDS, p.297), or an autoimmune disorder such as systemic lupus erythematosus (p.461). In some cases, it is associated with cancer.

WHAT ARE THE SYMPTOMS?

The symptoms of thrombocytopenia are often mild and may include:

- Easy bruising.
- A rash of many tiny red dots or large purple patches, neither of which fade when pressed (*see* PURPURA, p.339).
- Bleeding gums and heavy nosebleeds.
- In women, heavy menstrual bleeding.

If you have very low levels of platelets, you may be at increased risk of stroke (p.532) due to bleeding in the brain.

WHAT MIGHT BE DONE?

If your doctor suspects from your symptoms that you have thrombocytopenia, he or she may arrange for you to have a blood test to measure your platelet levels. Your doctor may also arrange for you to have a bone marrow aspiration and biopsy (p.451) in order to obtain tissue samples for examination under the microscope.

Mild thrombocytopenia triggered by a viral infection often clears up without treatment. Bleeding due to extremely low platelet levels may be treated with intravenous platelet infusions while the cause is investigated. If you have drug-induced thrombocytopenia, you will be prescribed an alternative drug that does not affect platelets; the level of platelets in the blood should promptly return to normal. When the condition is due to an immune disorder, an oral corticosteroid (p.930) may be prescribed. In severe or recurrent cases due to increased destruction of platelets, removal of the spleen may be necessary for a lasting cure.

(WWW) ONLINE SITES: p.1027

Hypercoagulability

An abnormal tendency for blood to clot inside blood vessels

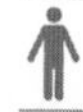
GENDER GENETICS LIFESTYLE Risk factors depend on the cause

AGE Not a significant factor

Blood clotting normally occurs only when a blood vessel is damaged. The clotting process relies on blood cells called platelets and on proteins in the blood known as clotting factors. Other substances in the blood prevent spontaneous blood clotting and help to dissolve clots that have formed. Excessive clotting, termed hypercoagulability, results if the balance of the clotting and anticlotting mechanisms is upset. The risk of abnormal clotting is also increased if blood flow is slowed down.

Increased blood clotting may be life-threatening. A clot that forms in a vein (*see* DEEP VEIN THROMBOSIS, p.437) may break off, travel to the lungs in the bloodstream, and block an artery (*see* PULMONARY EMBOLISM, p.495). Blood clots may also block an artery in the heart, causing a heart attack (*see* MYOCARDIAL INFARCTION, p.410), or in the brain, causing a stroke (p.532).

WHAT ARE THE CAUSES?

Hypercoagulability may be caused by inherited disorders in which a particular anticlotting substance (proteins C or S, or antithrombin III) is deficient. An inherited disorder known as Factor V Leiden, in which an abnormal form of the blood clotting Factor V is produced, may also cause the condition.

Another cause of hypercoagulability is increased "stickiness" of platelets as a result of smoking. The condition may also occur if levels of the female sex hormone oestrogen are raised, as this can affect the clotting factors.

Slowing of the blood flow, leading to hypercoagulability, may be due either to increased levels of red blood cells (*see* POLYCYTHAEMIA, p.457) or to prolonged immobility, such as may occur when confined to bed during an illness.

WHAT MIGHT BE DONE?

If you have a family history of hypercoagulability or if you develop a blood clot, your doctor may arrange for you to have blood clotting tests (p.227) to look for deficient or abnormal anticlotting factors in your blood.

If an inherited disorder such as Factor V Leiden is diagnosed, your doctor may prescribe drugs that prevent blood clotting (p.904). You should avoid smoking or taking drugs that contain oestrogen, such as combined oral contraceptives.

(WWW) ONLINE SITES: p.1027

Leukaemia

A group of bone marrow cancers in which abnormal white blood cells multiply uncontrollably

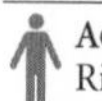
AGE GENDER GENETICS LIFESTYLE Risk factors depend on the type

In every type of leukaemia, cancerous white blood cells multiply rapidly and accumulate within the bone marrow, where all types of blood cell are normally produced. This increase reduces the usual production of normal white blood cells, normal red blood cells, and platelets within the bone marrow.

A reduction in the number of red blood cells reduces the oxygen-carrying capacity of blood (*see* ANAEMIA, p.446). If normal white blood cell levels are lowered, infection becomes a serious risk, while reduced levels of platelets may result in abnormal bleeding (*see* THROMBOCYTOPENIA, left). In most of the leukaemias, the cancerous white blood cells spread, causing the lymph nodes, liver, and spleen to enlarge.

What are the types?

The two main types of leukaemia are acute leukaemia, in which the symptoms develop rapidly, and chronic leukaemia, in which the symptoms can take years to develop. Adults may develop either type of leukaemia, but children usually have the acute form. Acute leukaemia (below) can be divided into acute lymphoblastic and acute myeloid leukaemia, depending on the type of white blood cell involved. Chronic leukaemia also takes two forms: chronic lymphocytic leukaemia (opposite page) and chronic myeloid leukaemia (opposite page).

All leukaemias produce the usual symptoms of anaemia: tiredness, pale skin, and shortness of breath on mild exertion. Other symptoms may include weight loss, fever, night sweats, excessive bleeding, and recurrent infections.

Leukaemia may be diagnosed from a blood test and a bone marrow aspiration and biopsy (p.451). The treatment usually involves chemotherapy (p.280) and, sometimes, radiotherapy (p.281). Blood transfusions (p.447) may also be necessary in some cases.

The outlook varies depending on the type of leukaemia and its severity. Treatment of leukaemia is more likely to be successful in children.

(WWW) ONLINE SITES: p.1027

Acute leukaemia

A cancer in which large numbers of immature, or abnormal, white blood cells are produced by the bone marrow

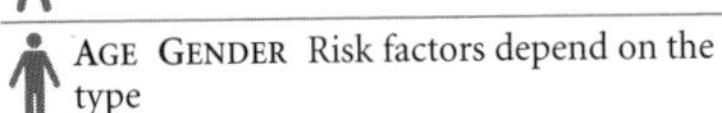
LIFESTYLE Previous exposure to radiation or toxic chemicals is a risk factor

AGE GENDER Risk factors depend on the type

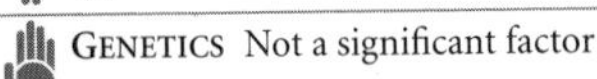
GENETICS Not a significant factor

Acute leukaemia is the most common childhood cancer. Until the 1960s, it was almost always fatal, but now most children survive because of better treatment.

In acute leukaemia, cancerous immature white blood cells multiply rapidly and accumulate in the bone marrow, disrupting the production of normal white blood cells, red blood cells, and platelets. A decrease in the number of normal white blood cells makes the body susceptible to infection. A deficiency of red blood cells reduces the oxygen-carrying capacity of the blood (*see* ANAEMIA, p.446). Fewer platelets, which help to seal damaged blood vessels, may result in abnormal bleeding (*see* THROMBOCYTOPENIA, p.453).

There are two main types of acute leukaemia. In acute lymphoblastic leukaemia (ALL), the abnormal type of white blood cell involved is an immature lymphocyte (lymphoblast). In acute myeloid leukaemia (AML), the type of white blood cell that is abnormal is an immature myeloid cell (myeloblast).

ALL is the most common cancer in children; it occurs more often in boys. AML is more common in people over the age of 60, affecting men and women equally. Left untreated, acute leukaemia can be fatal within a few weeks.

What are the causes?

In most cases of acute leukaemia, no cause can be identified. However, there are some factors that have been found to increase the risk of developing the disorder. For example, previous exposure to high levels of radiation, such as from radiotherapy (p.281), or exposure to some anticancer drugs (*see* CHEMOTHERAPY, p.280) may increase the future risk of acute leukaemia. Exposure to certain toxic chemicals, such as benzene in petrol, may also be a risk factor.

People who have myelodysplasia (a precancerous abnormality of the bone marrow) or certain chromosomal abnormalities, such as Down's syndrome (p.821), also have an increased risk of developing acute leukaemia.

What are the symptoms?

The symptoms of acute leukaemia are caused by abnormal white blood cells overcrowding the bone marrow, which reduces the numbers of normal blood cells of all types. Symptoms are also caused by the invasion of abnormal blood cells into the bloodstream, where they multiply and spread easily to other organs and tissues in the body.

(TREATMENT) Bone marrow transplant

In a bone marrow transplant, cancerous or abnormal bone marrow is replaced with healthy marrow. Before the transplant, the recipient's abnormal bone marrow is eliminated by chemotherapy or radiotherapy. Healthy marrow may have been supplied by a donor or by the patient when the underlying disease was inactive. Up to 1 litre (2 pints) of bone marrow may be extracted from the hipbone with a syringe through a hollow needle.

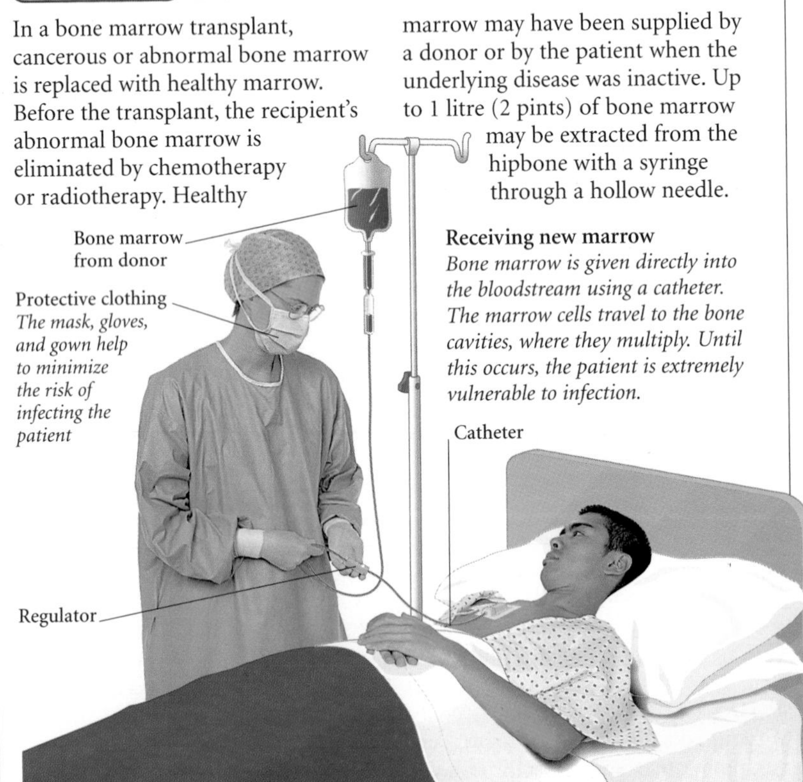

Receiving new marrow
Bone marrow is given directly into the bloodstream using a catheter. The marrow cells travel to the bone cavities, where they multiply. Until this occurs, the patient is extremely vulnerable to infection.

The symptoms of acute leukaemia may develop rapidly and include:

- Tiredness, pale skin, and shortness of breath on exertion due to anaemia.
- Easy bruising and excessive bleeding, often from the gums.
- Bone pain.
- Swelling in the neck, armpits, and groin due to enlarged lymph nodes.
- Swelling of the abdomen due to an enlarged liver and spleen.

Since only immature, nonfunctioning white blood cells are produced, and the cancerous cells are abnormal, susceptibility to infections is increased.

How is it diagnosed?

Your doctor may arrange blood tests to look for abnormal white blood cells, low platelet levels, and reduced numbers of red blood cells. The diagnosis is confirmed by a bone marrow aspiration and biopsy (p.451), a procedure in which tissue samples are obtained for examination under a microscope. You may also need a lumbar puncture (p.527), in which a fluid sample is taken from around the spinal cord, to find out if the disease has spread to the nervous system.

What is the treatment?

If you have acute leukaemia, you will be admitted to hospital, where repeated courses of chemotherapy will be given to kill the abnormal cells in the bone marrow. The aim of this treatment is to induce a remission, a period of time during which the leukaemia is inactive.

You may be given blood transfusions (p.447) to boost the numbers of normal blood cells and antibiotics (p.885) to prevent infection. Some people may need to have radiotherapy to destroy leukaemic cells in the brain.

A bone marrow transplant (opposite page) may be offered if a suitable bone marrow donor can be found. Before the procedure, you will be given either chemotherapy or radiotherapy.

What is the prognosis?

Generally, people with ALL respond better to treatment than those with AML, and the outlook for children is better than for adults. Most children treated for ALL can make a full recovery. About 1 in 3 people under the age of 50 with AML survives longer than 5 years.

(WWW) ONLINE SITES: p.1027

Chronic lymphocytic leukaemia

A bone marrow cancer in which there is uncontrolled production of mature white blood cells called lymphocytes

 AGE Rare under the age of 50; most common between the ages of 60 and 80

 GENDER More common in males

 GENETICS LIFESTYLE Not significant factors

Chronic lymphocytic leukaemia (CLL) is the most common bone marrow cancer in the UK. It mainly affects people over the age of 50 and is more common in men. The cause is unknown.

In CLL, white blood cells called lymphocytes become cancerous as they mature and multiply uncontrollably in the bone marrow, interfering with the production of normal blood cells. A reduced level of normal white blood cells leads to increased susceptibility to infection. Fewer red blood cells results in a reduction in the oxygen-carrying capacity of blood (*see* ANAEMIA, p.446). Reduced levels of platelets, which help to seal damaged blood vessels, may cause prolonged bleeding (*see* THROMBOCYTOPENIA, p.453). The abnormal cells may spread to other tissues such as the lymph nodes, liver, and spleen.

What are the symptoms?

The severity of the disease depends on the red blood cell level and the degree of enlargement of the liver and spleen. Initially, there may be no symptoms; a diagnosis of CLL is often made from a blood test carried out for some other reason. Symptoms are usually mild, develop gradually, and may include:

- Tiredness, pale skin, and shortness of breath on exertion due to anaemia.
- Painless swellings in the armpits, neck, and groin as a result of enlargement of the lymph nodes.
- Swelling of the abdomen due to an enlarged liver and spleen.
- Fever and night sweats.

As the disease progresses, easy bruising and prolonged episodes of bleeding may occur. If you have CLL, you may also have an increased susceptibility to recurrent infections such as shingles (*see* HERPES ZOSTER, p.290).

What might be done?

Following an examination, your doctor may arrange for blood tests to measure your levels of red cells and normal and abnormal white cells. He or she may also arrange for a bone marrow aspiration and biopsy (p.451) to obtain tissue samples for microscopic examination.

Treatment of CLL may not be necessary in the early stages, although any infections should be treated promptly. If the disease is advanced, you may need a course of chemotherapy (p.280).

Most people with mild CLL survive for more than 10 years after diagnosis. People who are severely affected by this form of leukaemia can expect to survive for up to 5 years after diagnosis.

(WWW) ONLINE SITES: p.1027

Chronic myeloid leukaemia

A bone marrow cancer in which white blood cells called granulocytes become abnormal and multiply

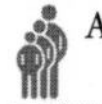 AGE More common over the age of 60

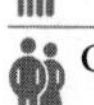 GENDER Slightly more common in males

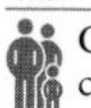 GENETICS May be linked to an abnormal chromosome

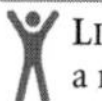 LIFESTYLE Previous exposure to radiation is a risk factor

Chronic myeloid leukaemia (CML) develops when white blood cells known as granulocytes become cancerous and multiply in the bone marrow. This leads to reduced production of red blood cells, normal white blood cells, and platelets in the bone marrow. The consequent shortage of red blood cells leads to a reduction in the oxygen-carrying capacity of blood (*see* ANAEMIA, p.446), and the decreased numbers of platelets, which help to seal damaged blood vessels, may lead to abnormal bleeding (*see* THROMBOCYTOPENIA, p.453).

The cancerous granulocytes are produced mostly in the bone marrow, but also in the liver and the spleen. All of the granulocytes produced function almost normally in fighting infection.

Chronic myeloid leukaemia is more common in people over the age of 60. This type of leukaemia is also slightly more common in men than in women.

TREATMENT SKIN-TUNNELLED CATHETER

A skin-tunnelled catheter is a flexible plastic tube passed through the skin of the chest and inserted into the subclavian vein, which leads to the heart. It is often used in people who have leukaemia or other cancers and need to have regular chemotherapy and blood tests. Using the catheter, drugs can be injected directly into the bloodstream and blood samples can be obtained easily.

The catheter is inserted under local anaesthesia and can remain in position for months. The external end is plugged when not in use. Because the catheter is inserted through the skin some distance away from the site of entry into the vein, the risk of infection is reduced.

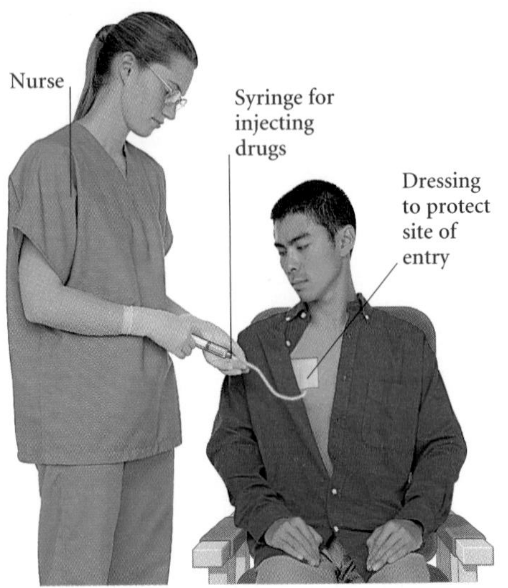

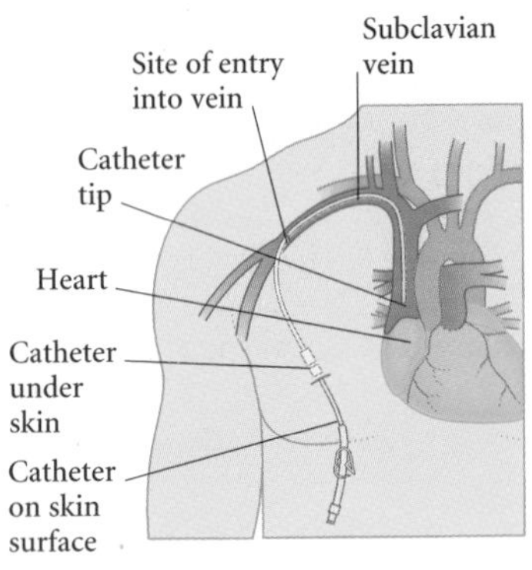

POSITION OF CATHETER

Using the catheter
The catheter is tunnelled under the skin and enters the subclavian vein to lie with its tip in the heart. A syringe can be attached to inject drugs.

WHAT ARE THE CAUSES?

The cause of CML is not known. In almost all people who have the disorder, however, the cancerous cells contain an abnormal chromosome (known as the Philadelphia chromosome), in which part of one chromosome is attached to another. Rarely, CML is linked with past exposure to radiation, such as that used in radiotherapy (p.281).

WHAT ARE THE SYMPTOMS?

There are two phases of CML. In the first, or chronic, phase, lasting for about 3–5 years, the symptoms develop slowly and are often mild. In the second, or acute, phase, symptoms of the disease become more severe. In either phase, you may experience:

- Tiredness, pale skin, and shortness of breath on exertion due to anaemia.
- Swelling of the abdomen due to an enlarged liver and spleen.
- A sensation of fullness due to the enlarged spleen, resulting in loss of appetite and weight loss.
- Night sweats.
- Abnormal bruising and bleeding.

During the acute phase of CML, you may also experience either or both of the following symptoms:

- Fever and abdominal pain.
- Swollen glands in the neck, armpits, and groin.

Rarely, in the acute phase, skin nodules full of abnormal granulocytes appear.

WHAT MIGHT BE DONE?

CML is usually diagnosed by chance during the chronic phase when a blood test is carried out for another reason. In other cases, when the condition is suspected from the symptoms, a blood test will be carried out to measure the levels of blood cells. If you have CML, the test will show high numbers of granulocytes and low numbers of red blood cells and platelets. To confirm the diagnosis, you may need to have a bone marrow aspiration and biopsy (p.451), in which tissue samples are taken for examination under a microscope.

Treatment for CML usually involves oral chemotherapy (p.280). The drug interferon alpha (*see* INTERFERON DRUGS, p.907) may also be used. If your spleen has become enlarged, you may need an operation to remove it.

If CML progresses into the acute phase, you may be admitted to hospital to have intravenous chemotherapy treatment. Anticancer drugs may be injected into the bloodstream through a skin-tunnelled catheter (above).

A bone marrow transplant (p.454) in the chronic phase offers a good chance of a full recovery in some people. Without a transplant, most affected people survive for about 3 years after diagnosis. However, if CML develops into the acute phase, treatment rarely succeeds and the condition is usually fatal within a year.

WWW ONLINE SITES: p.1027

Multiple myeloma

A bone marrow cancer in which abnormal antibody-producing white blood cells multiply uncontrollably

AGE Increasingly common over the age of 40; most common around the age of 70

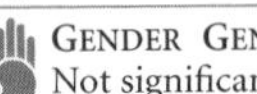
GENDER GENETICS LIFESTYLE Not significant factors

Multiple myeloma is a rare but life-threatening cancer of the bone marrow. The condition affects plasma cells, the white blood cells that normally produce antibodies against infection. In multiple myeloma, a plasma cell undergoes a cancerous change and begins to multiply in an uncontrolled manner, which disrupts the usual production of normal red blood cells, normal white blood cells, and platelets.

The abnormal plasma cells produce abnormal antibodies, and the production of normal antibodies is reduced. As a result, people with myeloma are particularly susceptible to infections. The abnormal plasma cells also destroy bone tissue, releasing excess calcium into the bloodstream.

Low numbers of red blood cells may cause the blood to have a reduced oxygen-carrying capacity (*see* ANAEMIA, p.446). Reduced numbers of platelets, which help to seal damaged blood vessels, may lead to abnormal bleeding (*see* THROMBOCYTOPENIA, p.453).

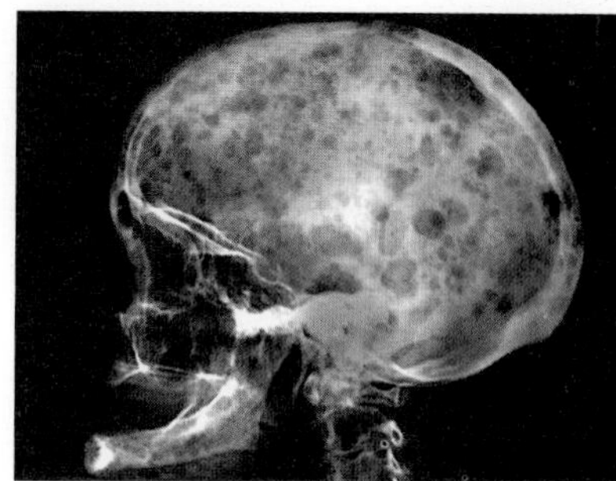

Skull bone loss in multiple myeloma
This X-ray shows the skull of a person with multiple myeloma. The abnormal "pepper-pot" appearance results from areas of localized bone loss.

WHAT ARE THE SYMPTOMS?

The symptoms of multiple myeloma result from the disruption of blood cell production in the bone marrow and the destruction of bone. They include:

- Tiredness, pale skin, and shortness of breath on exertion due to anaemia.
- Bone pain, most often in the spine, as the plasma cells multiply within the bone marrow.
- Repeated infections.
- Bleeding from the nose and gums.
- Easy bruising without injury.
- Thirst, frequent need to pass urine, and constipation due to high calcium levels in the blood.

The loss of calcium from bone tissue may lead to brittle bones that fracture easily. Increased levels of calcium and abnormal antibodies in the blood may lead to kidney failure (p.705).

WHAT MIGHT BE DONE?

Your doctor may arrange for blood tests to measure levels of blood cells and to look for abnormal antibodies. Because these antibodies are excreted in urine, you may also need to have a urine test. Cells may be taken from the bone marrow and examined (*see* BONE MARROW ASPIRATION AND BIOPSY, p.451). You may also have X-rays (p.244) to look for areas of bone loss.

You will probably be treated with oral chemotherapy (p.280) and oral corticosteroids (p.930). The intensity of the treatment depends on the person's age and general health. Radiotherapy (p.281) may be given for severe bone pain, and you may need to have blood transfusions (p.447) for severe anaemia. Infections may be treated with antibiotics (p.885). You may be given bisphosphonates (*see* DRUGS FOR BONE DISORDERS, p.896) to treat high calcium levels. Drinking plenty of fluids will also help to lower the calcium levels.

The outlook varies depending on the severity of the disorder. Most people live for about 2 years after diagnosis, but some have survived for 10 years.

(WWW) ONLINE SITES: p.1028

Polycythaemia

A blood disorder in which there is an increased concentration of red blood cells

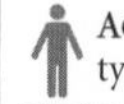
AGE LIFESTYLE Risk factors depend on the type

GENDER GENETICS Not significant factors

In polycythaemia, the concentration of red blood cells is increased. The condition may be due to increased red blood cell production or decreased volume of the fluid part of blood (plasma), leading to a high concentration of red cells.

WHAT ARE THE TYPES?

There are three types of polycythaemia: primary, secondary, and stress.

In primary polycythaemia, which is also known as true polycythaemia or polycythaemia vera, the production of red blood cells in the bone marrow is increased for no known reason. This is a rare disorder, which usually only affects people over the age of 60.

In secondary polycythaemia, there is also increased production of red cells by the bone marrow. In this case, the cause is a low oxygen level in the blood, which can occur for several reasons. For example, it can develop in people living at high altitudes, where oxygen levels are naturally low. It may also occur if the uptake of oxygen by the blood is impaired due to heavy smoking or lung disorders such as chronic obstructive pulmonary disease (p.487).

In stress polycythaemia, production of red cells is normal but the volume of blood plasma is decreased. This change in the composition of blood may result from dehydration. It may also occur in people who are obese or abuse alcohol.

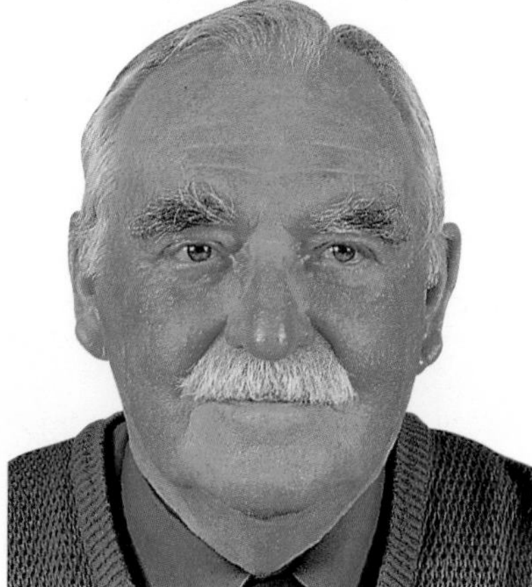

Effect of polycythaemia
This man's ruddy complexion is due to polycythaemia, an abnormally high concentration of red cells in the blood.

WHAT ARE THE SYMPTOMS?

All types of polycythaemia cause similar symptoms, which are due to thickening of the blood. They may include:

- A ruddy complexion, together with bloodshot eyes.
- Headache and ringing in the ears (*see* TINNITUS, p.602).
- Blurred vision and dizziness.

Primary polycythaemia may also produce itching, especially after a hot bath. The spleen may enlarge as it attempts to deal with the increased number of red blood cells, causing abdominal discomfort. There may also be prolonged bleeding or increased blood clotting.

WHAT MIGHT BE DONE?

Your doctor may arrange for a blood test to measure the concentrations of red cells in the blood and a bone marrow aspiration and biopsy (p.451) to look for increased red cell production. You may also have a lung function test (p.488) to look for an underlying cause.

If you have secondary or stress polycythaemia, the treatment is directed at the underlying cause.

Venesection (needle puncture of a vein) may be used to treat primary polycythaemia. At least 300 ml (10 fl oz) of blood are removed from the circulation each week until the levels of red cells are normal. Older people may be given radioactive phosphorus or chemotherapy (p.280) to reduce the production of red cells. With treatment, most people live for 10–15 years following diagnosis. However, primary polycythaemia may develop into another bone marrow disorder, such as acute leukaemia (p.454).

(WWW) ONLINE SITES: p.1027

DISORDERS OF THE LYMPHATIC SYSTEM

The lymphatic system consists of lymph nodes, or glands, connected by a network of lymphatic vessels that extends to all parts of the body. The system drains a fluid called lymph from the body's tissues back into the bloodstream. It also protects the body against infection and the development of cancer by filtering out infectious organisms and cancerous cells from the lymph.

Lymph, a fluid that contains white blood cells called lymphocytes, fats, and protein, flows along the network of lymphatic vessels and ultimately re-enters the bloodstream from which it originally came. Along the way, lymph is filtered through the lymph nodes, which are located in clusters close to the skin's surface in the neck, armpits, and groin. Nodes are also found deep within the abdomen and chest. The lymph nodes contain large numbers of cells and antibodies of the immune system that trap and destroy infectious organisms and cancerous cells that have entered the lymph from the blood and body tissues.

The first article in this section covers lymphadenopathy, in which the lymph nodes become enlarged. A painful swelling of the lymph nodes is not often a cause for concern, but painless swelling may be a sign of a serious underlying disorder, such as cancer. The next articles cover lymphangitis, in which lymphatic vessels are inflamed, and lymphoedema, in which lymph cannot drain from a limb, causing the limb to swell. In developed countries, a common cause of lymphoedema is surgery or radiotherapy for cancer. The final article discusses lymphomas, a group of cancers that may develop in one or more lymph nodes.

KEY ANATOMY

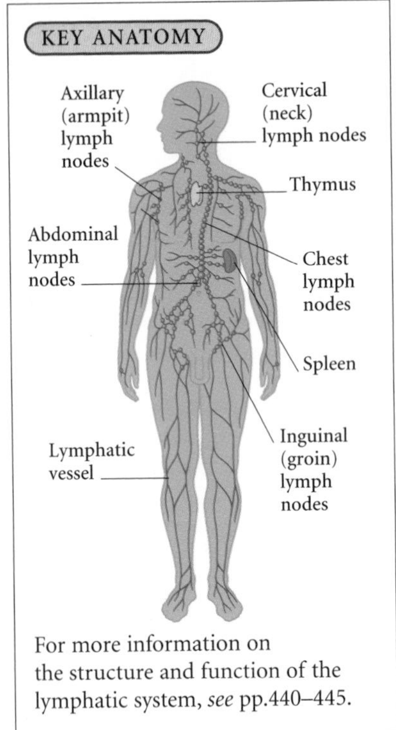

For more information on the structure and function of the lymphatic system, *see* pp.440–445.

Lymphadenopathy

Enlarged lymph nodes, also known as swollen glands, which usually develop as a response to infection

AGE GENDER GENETICS LIFESTYLE
Risk factors depend on the cause

Swelling of the lymph nodes is a common symptom of many conditions. A single node, a group of nodes, or all the lymph nodes may be affected. Lymph nodes most commonly become swollen in response to a bacterial or viral infection. You are more likely to notice a swollen lymph node in the neck, groin, or armpit, because the nodes in these areas lie closest to the skin.

Swelling of a single node or group of lymph nodes is often due to a localized bacterial infection. For example, swollen lymph nodes in the neck are commonly caused by throat infections. In most cases of lymphadenopathy due to an infection, the swelling usually subsides when the infection clears up. Swollen lymph nodes that are the result of an infection are often painful.

Persistent swelling of many, or all, of the lymph nodes may be a result of some types of cancer, such as breast cancer (p.759), lymphoma (opposite page), or leukaemia (p.453). Swollen lymph nodes due to cancer are not normally painful.

In the UK, long-term infections, such as tuberculosis (p.491) and HIV infection (*see* HIV INFECTION AND AIDS, p.297), are an uncommon cause of persistent lymphadenopathy.

You should consult your doctor if a swelling is persistent or if you are worried about accompanying symptoms.

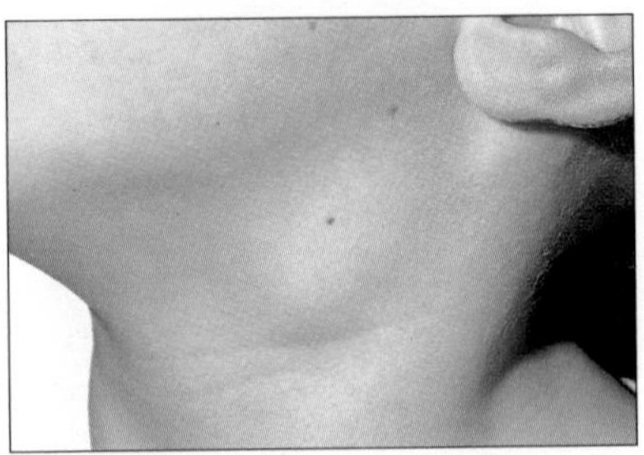

Lymphadenopathy in the neck
A throat infection may cause swelling of the lymph nodes. Here, a swollen lymph node is visible on the side of the neck.

Lymphangitis

Inflammation of the lymphatic vessels as a result of a bacterial infection

AGE GENDER GENETICS LIFESTYLE
Not significant factors

Lymphangitis develops when bacteria spread into lymphatic vessels close to the site of an infection, possibly as a result of an injury. The condition usually affects lymphatic vessels in an arm or a leg and may be accompanied by fever, headache, and a general sense of feeling unwell. The infected lymphatic vessels become inflamed and tender, and hot, red streaks may appear on the skin over the inflamed vessels. Lymph nodes near to the affected area sometimes become swollen (*see* LYMPHADENOPATHY, left). If you develop any of these symptoms following an injury, you should consult your doctor immediately.

In some cases, ulcers form in the skin over an infected lymph vessel. Without treatment, the infection may spread into the blood (*see* SEPTICAEMIA, p.299), which can be life-threatening.

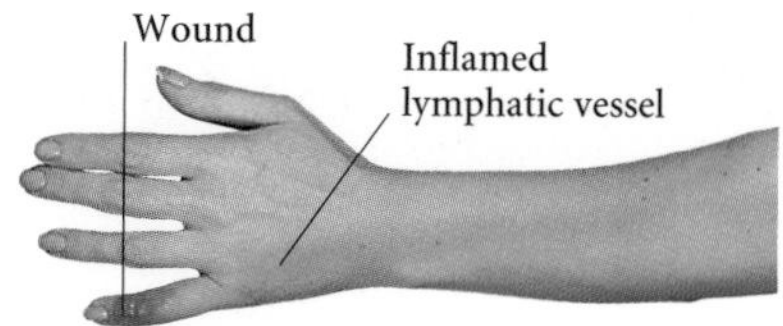

Lymphangitis of the arm
Inflamed lymphatic vessels (lymphangitis) have produced a red streak on the skin. The inflammation is due to bacteria that have spread from a wound on the finger.

If your doctor suspects that you have lymphangitis from your symptoms and after a physical examination, he or she may take a sample of your blood, which will be tested in a laboratory to determine whether the infection has spread into the blood. Antibiotics (p.885) will be prescribed to treat the lymphangitis. The symptoms of the condition usually begin to clear up within 24 hours of starting antibiotic treatment.

Lymphoedema

A localized accumulation of fluid in the lymphatic vessels, causing painless swelling of a limb

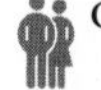 GENDER More common in females

 GENETICS Sometimes runs in families

 AGE LIFESTYLE Not significant factors

Lymphoedema occurs when a defect in the lymphatic vessels prevents drainage of lymph from a limb. Most commonly, lymphoedema is caused by damage to the lymphatic vessels following surgery or radiotherapy (p.281), for example in the treatment of breast cancer (p.759). Rarely, the condition may be due to the blockage of a lymphatic vessel by a cancerous growth in a lymph node.

Lymphoedema can be inherited, in which case it results from incomplete development of the lymphatic vessels. This type is more common in women.

Although the symptoms of lymphoedema may be present from birth, they usually first occur at puberty. The main symptom is painless swelling of a limb. The skin over the affected limb often becomes rough and thickened. Injury to a limb affected by lymphoedema may result in a rapid spread of infection through the tissues. You should contact your doctor immediately if you injure a limb affected by lymphoedema.

In most cases, lymphoedema is a lifelong disorder and treatment is aimed at relieving the symptoms. You can reduce swelling by keeping the affected limb elevated; wearing an elastic stocking or sleeve helps to prevent further swelling.

Lymphoma

Any of several types of cancer arising in the lymphatic system

 GENDER More common in males

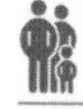 GENETICS Sometimes runs in families

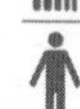 AGE Risk factors depend on the type

 LIFESTYLE Not a significant factor

The lymphomas are a group of diseases in which immune cells become cancerous and multiply uncontrollably in a lymph node. Initially, a single node may be affected, but the cancer may spread to other nodes and also to other tissues, such as the bone marrow.

Lymphomas can be divided into two main categories: Hodgkin's and non-Hodgkin's lymphomas. In Hodgkin's lymphoma, a particular type of cancer cell is present. All the other types of lymphoma are classified as non-Hodgkin's lymphoma. Non-Hodgkin's lymphoma is about three times more common than Hodgkin's lymphoma, and it usually develops in people over the age of 50. Hodgkin's lymphoma most commonly occurs in people who are between the ages of 15 and 30 and the ages of 55 and 70. Different types of lymphoma grow and spread at different rates.

WHAT ARE THE CAUSES?

The cause of lymphoma is not known but the condition sometimes runs in families, suggesting that a genetic factor is involved. Lymphomas are more common if immunity is reduced, such as in people with AIDS (*see* HIV INFECTION AND AIDS, p.297) or those who are taking immunosuppressant drugs (p.906). Some lymphomas may be triggered by a viral infection. For example, Burkitt's lymphoma, which is common in children in equatorial Africa, is associated with the Epstein–Barr virus.

WHAT ARE THE SYMPTOMS?

The symptoms of lymphoma, common to all types, may include:

- One or more persistent and painless swellings in the neck, armpits, or groin caused by enlarged lymph nodes.
- Fever and sweating at night.
- Weight loss.
- Abdominal swelling and discomfort due to enlarged lymph nodes or an enlarged spleen.

Some people with lymphoma develop anaemia (p.446), which causes symptoms such as tiredness, pale skin, and shortness of breath on mild exertion.

WHAT MIGHT BE DONE?

Your doctor may suspect lymphoma from your symptoms and following a physical examination. He or she may arrange for a blood test to check for anaemia. A tissue sample may also be taken from a swollen node to find out whether cancerous cells are present.

If lymphoma is diagnosed, further tests may be needed to find out how far the disease has progressed. These may include imaging techniques, such as CT scanning (p.247), to assess the size of lymph nodes in the chest and abdomen. You may also have bone marrow aspiration and biopsy (p.451) to determine whether your bone marrow is affected.

Treatment depends on the type of lymphoma and how far it has spread. If only one node or one group of nodes is affected, the lymphoma may be treated with local radiotherapy (p.281) alone. When more than one group of lymph nodes is affected, the usual treatment is chemotherapy (p.280), sometimes combined with radiotherapy.

WHAT IS THE PROGNOSIS?

If the cancer is not detectable following treatment, the disease is said to have gone into remission. However, lymphomas sometimes recur, and a second course of treatment may be necessary. If remission continues for 5 years or more, the risk of recurrence is small.

After treatment for Hodgkin's lymphoma, at least 8 in 10 people enter a long-term period of remission and can be assumed to be cured. About half of all people treated for non-Hodgkin's lymphoma enter long-term remission and are considered to be cured.

(WWW) ONLINE SITES: p.1033

IMMUNE DISORDERS

Our immune systems protect us from the threat of infection by microorganisms, such as bacteria and viruses, and parasites, such as worms. The immune system also protects us from certain cancers and helps to repair damaged tissues. We are born with certain built-in defence mechanisms, but much of our immunity is acquired as we are exposed to the organisms that cause disease.

This section begins with an overview of acquired immunodeficiency, one of the major disorders of the immune system. Acquired immunodeficiency is a condition, developing after birth, in which the immune system fails to function properly and is unable to combat microorganisms that invade the body. Such immunodeficiency develops for a variety of reasons. The most widely publicized form of acquired immunodeficiency is AIDS, which develops after infection with the human immunodeficiency virus (*see* HIV INFECTION AND AIDS, p.297). A temporary, mild form of acquired immunodeficiency may appear after infection with other viruses, such as measles (p.293), and may also develop following certain drug treatments.

The second overview article covers autoimmune disorders, which occur when a person's immune system functions abnormally and starts to attack the body's own tissues, causing certain organs to become inflamed and damaged. Individual autoimmune disorders that affect more than one organ are covered next. Such disorders are most common in young adults and can lead to persistent poor health. Their causes are not fully understood, although genetic factors appear to play an important role. Overall, women are affected much more commonly and severely by autoimmune disorders.

Autoimmune disorders that affect specific organs or sites in the body are considered in the relevant sections of this book. For example, rheumatoid arthritis (p.377), which primarily affects the joints, is dealt with in the musculoskeletal disorders section and Hashimoto's thyroiditis (*see* THYROIDITIS, p.681), which causes the underproduction of hormones from the thyroid gland, is covered in the section dealing with metabolic disorders. Immunodeficiency that is present from birth is covered in the section of the book dealing with children's disorders (*see* CONGENITAL IMMUNODEFICIENCY, p.826).

Acquired immunodeficiency

Complete or partial failure of the immune system, developing after birth

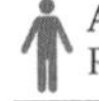
AGE GENDER GENETICS LIFESTYLE
Risk factors depend on the cause

Immunodeficiency is the term used for failure of the immune system to combat infections effectively. As a result of immunodeficiency, infections develop more frequently than normal and are a greater threat to health. Infections that would not normally seriously affect a healthy person may be life-threatening in someone who has immunodeficiency. They include viral infections, such as shingles and chickenpox (p.290), both of which are caused by herpes zoster (p.290) and cause only mild illnesses if the immune system is normal.

Immunodeficiency may be present from birth, in which case it is often inherited (*see* CONGENITAL IMMUNODEFICIENCY, p.826). More commonly, the deficiency in a person's immune system develops later in life, and in such cases the condition is given the name acquired immunodeficiency.

Worldwide, acquired immunodeficiency is most often associated with malnutrition or with infection with the human immunodeficiency virus (*see* HIV INFECTION AND AIDS, p.297).

WHAT ARE THE CAUSES?

In AIDS, the human immunodeficiency virus (HIV) destroys a particular type of white blood cell, and this causes progressive immunodeficiency.

Infections such as influenza (p.289) or measles (p.293) damage the body's ability to fight infection. They do this partly by reducing the number of white blood cells involved in fighting the infection. Usually, this type of immunodeficiency is mild, and the immune system returns to normal once the person has recovered from the infection.

A mild form of immunodeficiency may occur in some long-term disorders, including diabetes mellitus (p.687) and rheumatoid arthritis (p.377). This may occur partly because these diseases put stress on the immune system, reducing its ability to resist other diseases.

Certain types of cancer, particularly tumours of the lymphatic system (*see* LYMPHOMA, p.459), may cause a more severe form of immunodeficiency by damaging the cells of the immune system and by reducing the production of normal white blood cells.

The long-term use of corticosteroids (p.930) suppresses the immune system and has the inevitable effect of causing immunodeficiency. Immunosuppressant drugs (p.906), which may be given to prevent the rejection of an organ following transplant surgery (p.952), also produce immunodeficiency and affect the body's ability to fight infections. Chemotherapy (p.280) can damage the bone marrow, where the majority of blood cells are made, and may also lead to acquired immunodeficiency.

Immunodeficiency may also develop after surgical removal of the spleen, an organ in which some of the white blood cells are produced. Splenectomy may be performed if the spleen has been damaged by an injury, or it may be carried out to treat various disorders including hereditary spherocytosis, which is a type of haemolytic anaemia (p.450).

There are also many rare types of acquired immunodeficiency, the causes of which are not clear. One rare type is immunoglobulin A (IgA) deficiency, in which levels of immunoglobulin A antibodies are lower than normal.

WHAT MIGHT BE DONE?

Your doctor may suspect immunodeficiency if you have recurrent infections. To confirm the diagnosis of acquired immunodeficiency, you may need to have blood tests that measure the levels of white blood cells and antibodies.

If immunodeficiency is due to drug treatment, it may be possible to reduce the dose or stop taking the drug. If the underlying cause cannot be cured or reversed, treatment is aimed at reducing the risk of infection and combating infections as they occur. Your doctor may suggest regular intravenous infusions of immunoglobulin; continual low doses of antibiotics (p.885), antiviral drugs (p.886), and/or antifungal drugs (p.889); and various immunizations, such as the pneumococcus vaccine (*see* VACCINES AND IMMUNOGLOBULINS, p.883) to protect against pneumococcal pneumonia.

The effects of immunodeficiency can usually be controlled by treatment, although immunodeficiency due to HIV infection may worsen over time.

WWW ONLINE SITES: p.1033

Autoimmune disorders

Disorders in which the immune system malfunctions and reacts against the body's own tissues

AGE More common in adults. Less common in childhood and in old age

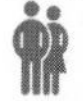
GENDER More common in females

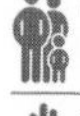
GENETICS Sometimes run in families

LIFESTYLE Not a significant factor

If a person is healthy, the cells of the immune system are able to distinguish between the body tissues and foreign organisms such as bacteria and viruses. If someone has an autoimmune disorder, the immune system mistakenly interprets the body's own tissues as foreign. As a result, antibodies or white blood cells are formed that attack the body tissues and try to destroy them. The underlying cause of this abnormal immune reaction is unclear, but it can run in families. Certain factors, such as some viral infections and reactions to particular drugs, may trigger an autoimmune reaction in susceptible people. Hormonal factors may also play a part, since these disorders occur more often in women than in men. Autoimmune disorders are less common in elderly people and in children.

WHAT ARE THE TYPES?

In some autoimmune disorders, the tissues of a single organ are damaged, preventing normal function. Examples of organs that may be affected by these disorders include the thyroid gland in Hashimoto's thyroiditis (*see* THYROIDITIS, p.681), the pancreas in diabetes mellitus (p.687), the adrenal glands in Addison's disease (p.686), and various joints in rheumatoid arthritis (p.377).

A second group of autoimmune disorders affects connective tissue, the material that holds together the structures of the body (*see* SCLERODERMA, p.462, and SYSTEMIC LUPUS ERYTHEMATOSUS, right). In these disorders, the immune system may react against connective tissue anywhere in the body.

WHAT MIGHT BE DONE?

If your doctor suspects an autoimmune disorder, he or she may arrange for blood tests to assess immune function and look for evidence of inflammation. The treatment of autoimmune disorders depends on which organs are affected. In Hashimoto's thyroiditis or Addison's disease, damage to the affected organs leads to a deficiency in the hormones they normally produce. Replacement of deficient hormones often restores health. In other cases, the aim of treatment is to block the abnormal immune reactions with drugs such as immunosuppressants (p.906) or corticosteroids (p.930) or reduce symptoms with nonsteroidal anti-inflammatory drugs (p.894).

The outlook for people who have autoimmune disorders depends on the amount of damage to the body's tissues and organs. Autoimmune disorders are usually lifelong, but the symptoms can often be controlled with drugs. In some cases, serious complications such as kidney failure (p.705) may develop.

WWW ONLINE SITES: p.1033

Systemic lupus erythematosus

Inflammation of the body's connective tissues, causing damage to the skin, joints, and internal organs

AGE Most common between the ages of 16 and 55

GENDER Much more common in females

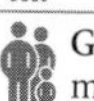
GENETICS Sometimes runs in families; more common in some ethnic groups

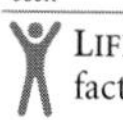
LIFESTYLE Stress and sunlight may be risk factors

In systemic lupus erythematosus (SLE), an autoimmune disorder, the body produces antibodies that react against its own connective tissues. These tissues, which surround body structures and hold them together, become inflamed and swollen. SLE may affect only a few parts of the body or many, and symptoms may range from mild to severe.

The cause of the abnormal immune reaction that occurs in SLE is not known, but it may be triggered by factors such as a viral infection, stress, or sunlight. Hormonal factors may also be involved because many more women than men are affected. SLE sometimes runs in families and appears to be more common in black and Asian women, which suggests that a genetic factor is involved. Symptoms similar to those of SLE may be caused by certain drugs, such as hydralazine (*see* ANTIHYPERTENSIVE DRUGS, p.897) and chlorpromazine (*see* ANTIPSYCHOTIC DRUGS, p.917).

WHAT ARE THE SYMPTOMS?

In typical cases of SLE, the symptoms flare up intermittently for periods of weeks and then become less severe, sometimes for months or even years, but they rarely disappear completely.

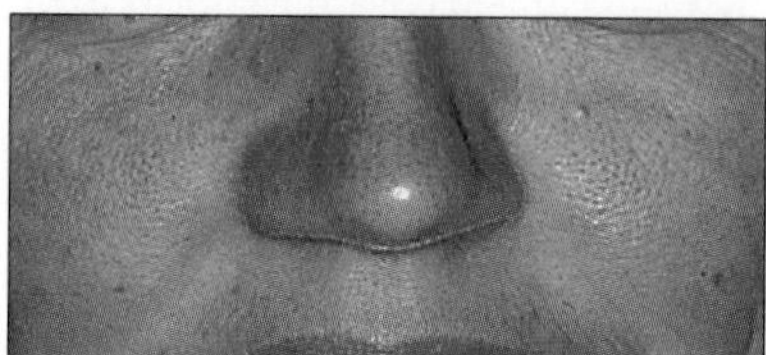

Butterfly-shaped rash in SLE

A common symptom of systemic lupus erythematosus is a red, raised rash that spreads across the nose and the cheeks in a shape that resembles a butterfly.

People who have SLE may have widely varying symptoms. For example, some people suffer from mild symptoms that appear gradually, whereas others report a wide range of more severe symptoms that develop far more rapidly.

The most common symptoms experienced by people with SLE are:

- Aching, swollen joints, which may become increasingly painful.
- Skin rashes – characteristically a raised, red, butterfly-shaped rash on the nose and cheeks.
- Increased sensitivity to sunlight.
- Tiredness and fever.
- Mild depression.

Additionally, there may be less common symptoms of SLE, which include:

- Shortness of breath and chest pain if the membrane covering the lungs is inflamed (*see* PLEURISY, p.493).
- Headaches, seizures, or strokes due to involvement of the nervous system.
- Constant chest pain if the membrane covering the heart is inflamed (*see* PERICARDITIS, p.428).
- Hair loss.
- Pale skin.
- Painless mouth ulcers.

Women who have SLE may find that their symptoms become worse while they are taking oral contraceptive pills or during pregnancy, as a result of hormonal imbalances.

ARE THERE COMPLICATIONS?

SLE may cause damage to the kidneys, which can lead to high blood pressure (*see* HYPERTENSION, p.403) and eventually kidney failure (p.705). In severe cases, problems with painful, swollen joints may cause deformity. SLE may occur in association with polymyositis and dermatomyositis (opposite page).

Although many women with SLE have successful pregnancies, the risk of having an early miscarriage (p.791) is increased. If you have SLE and are planning a pregnancy, you should visit your doctor to ask for advice.

WHAT MIGHT BE DONE?

Since the symptoms of SLE are so varied, they often mimic those of other disorders. However, if your doctor suspects that you may have SLE, he or she may arrange for blood tests to look for antibodies associated with the condition. You may also need to have certain specific tests to determine whether the function of particular organs has been affected by the disorder.

There is no cure for SLE; treatment is aimed at relieving the symptoms and slowing the progression of the condition. However, if you have SLE-like symptoms that are triggered by a particular drug, your doctor will prescribe an alternative treatment if possible, and your symptoms should gradually disappear within a few weeks or months.

If your joints are painful, your doctor may recommend a nonsteroidal anti-inflammatory drug (p.894). You may also be given the drug hydroxychloroquine (*see* ANTIMALARIAL DRUGS, p.888), which is often used to control the symptoms of SLE. A corticosteroid (p.930) may be given to suppress severe inflammation. If the condition fails to respond to corticosteroids, an immunosuppressant drug (p.906) may be prescribed. Physiotherapy (p.961) may be suggested for joint problems. Your doctor may also advise you to avoid direct exposure to the sun and to ensure that infections are treated without delay.

Most people with SLE can lead an active life. Only in the most severe cases may life expectancy be shortened.

(WWW) ONLINE SITES: p.1033

Scleroderma

Thickening and hardening of the connective tissues in the skin, joints, and internal organs

 AGE Most common between the ages of 20 and 50

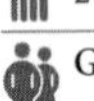 GENDER More common in females

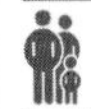 GENETICS Sometimes runs in families; more common in black people

 LIFESTYLE Not a significant factor

Scleroderma, also known as systemic sclerosis, is a rare disorder in which the connective tissues that hold together the structures of the body become inflamed, damaged, and thickened. The tissues, particularly those in the skin, then contract and harden.

This condition is an autoimmune disorder in which the body produces antibodies that attack and damage its own connective tissues. The reason for this reaction is unknown, but genetic factors may play a part since the condition sometimes runs in families and is more common in black people. Scleroderma is approximately four times more common in women than it is in men and occurs most commonly in adults under the age of 50.

WHAT ARE THE SYMPTOMS?

Scleroderma commonly affects the skin and the joints, but other organs may be involved. Symptoms vary from mild to severe and may include:

- Fingers or toes that are sensitive to the cold, becoming white and painful (*see* RAYNAUD'S PHENOMENON AND RAYNAUD'S DISEASE, p.436).
- Ulcers and small, hardened areas that appear on the fingers.
- Swollen fingers or hands.
- Pain in the joints, especially the joints in the hands.
- Thickening and tightening of the skin, which is most severe on the limbs but may affect the trunk and face.
- Muscle weakness.
- Difficulty swallowing due to stiffening of the tissues of the oesophagus (the tube that runs from the mouth to the stomach).

If the lungs are affected, shortness of breath may develop. In some people, scleroderma causes high blood pressure (*see* HYPERTENSION, p.403) and eventually kidney failure (p.705).

WHAT MIGHT BE DONE?

Your doctor may be able to make a diagnosis from your symptoms and from a physical examination. He or she may also arrange for blood tests to look for certain antibodies. A small skin sample may also be taken for examination.

There is no cure for scleroderma, but treatment can slow the progression of the condition, reducing the damage to

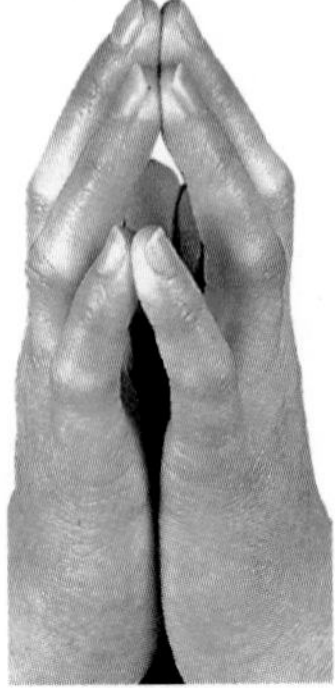

Effects of scleroderma
In a person with scleroderma, the skin on the fingers and hands may become thickened and swollen, making it difficult to straighten the fingers.

body organs and relieving symptoms. Thickening of the skin may be slowed down by drugs such as D-penicillamine (*see* ANTIRHEUMATIC DRUGS, p.895). If the lungs are affected, an immunosuppressant (p.906) may be prescribed. A corticosteroid (p.930) may be given to relieve joint pain. Your doctor may advise you to wear gloves and socks to protect your fingers and toes against the cold.

The course of scleroderma is variable. The condition may remain mild or, if severe, may improve spontaneously. In some rare cases, scleroderma progresses rapidly and is fatal.

(WWW) ONLINE SITES: p.1033

Sjögren's syndrome

Damage to glands, including the tear and salivary glands, causing dryness of the eyes and mouth

 AGE Most common between the ages of 40 and 60, but may occur at any age

 GENDER More common in females

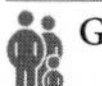 GENETICS Sometimes runs in families

 LIFESTYLE Not a significant factor

Sjögren's syndrome is a lifelong disorder in which damage to the tear and salivary glands causes the eyes and mouth to become very dry. Glands that lubricate the skin, nasal cavity, throat, and vagina may also be affected.

The syndrome is an autoimmune disorder in which gland tissues are attacked by the body's own antibodies and become inflamed and damaged. The cause is not known, but genetic factors may play a role. The condition is nine times more common in women and usually occurs between the ages of 40 and 60.

The main symptoms usually develop over several years and include gritty, red, dry eyes and dry mouth. Lack of saliva often leads to difficulty swallowing dry foods and to dental problems (*see* DENTAL CARIES, p.609). Some people develop joint problems similar to mild rheumatoid arthritis (p.377).

What might be done?

Your doctor may be able to make a diagnosis from your symptoms and an examination. He or she may arrange for blood tests to look for antibodies. You

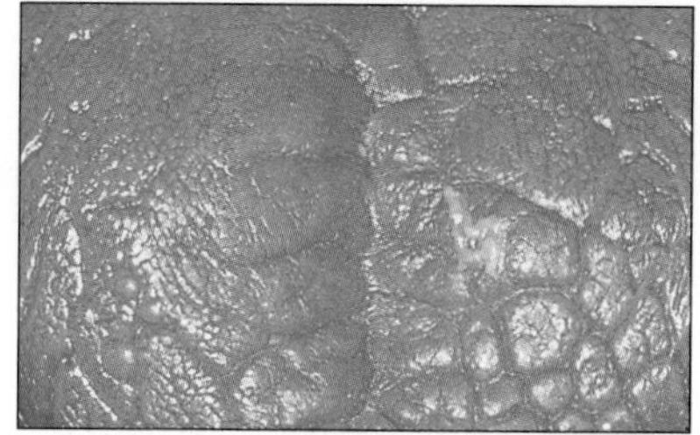

Dry tongue in Sjögren's syndrome
The salivary glands become inflamed in Sjögren's syndrome, preventing normal saliva production. As a result, the mouth and the tongue become very dry.

may also need to have tests to measure the quantity of tears your eyes produce, and a small sample of tissue may be removed from your salivary glands to look for damaged cells.

There is no cure for this disorder, but symptoms can be controlled, usually with lifelong treatment. Artificial tears may be prescribed or, occasionally, tear ducts will be plugged by an ophthalmologist to decrease tear drainage. You will be advised to drink plenty of liquids and to visit your dentist regularly. If symptoms are severe, a corticosteroid (p.930), an immunosuppressant (p.906), or the drug hydroxychloroquine (*see* ANTIMALARIAL DRUGS, p.888) may be given to reduce the inflammation.

(WWW) ONLINE SITES: p.1033

Polymyositis and dermatomyositis

Muscle inflammation (polymyositis), sometimes with a rash (dermatomyositis)

 AGE Most common in children aged 5–15 and adults aged 40–60

 GENDER More common in females

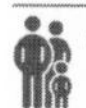 GENETICS Sometimes runs in families

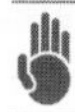 LIFESTYLE Not a significant factor

In polymyositis, inflammation of the muscles causes muscle weakness and wasting, particularly around the shoulders and pelvis. If a rash also occurs, the disorder is known as dermatomyositis. Both conditions are rare autoimmune disorders in which tissues are attacked by the body's own antibodies. The cause of this abnormal immune reaction is not known, although its onset may be triggered by a viral infection. In adults, these diseases may be associated with cancer. They can also occur in association with other autoimmune disorders, such as systemic lupus erythematosus (p.461). Polymyositis and dermatomyositis sometimes run in families, which suggests that genetic factors may be involved. Both disorders are more common in women and tend to occur in childhood and middle age.

What are the symptoms?

The symptoms of polymyositis and dermatomyositis may develop rapidly, particularly in children; in adults, the symptoms usually develop over several weeks. Symptoms may include:

- Weakness of affected muscles, leading, for example, to difficulty raising the arms or getting up from a sitting or squatting position.
- Painful, swollen joints.
- Tiredness.
- Difficulty swallowing if the muscles of the throat are affected.
- Shortness of breath if the heart or chest muscles are involved.

In dermatomyositis, the above symptoms may be preceded, accompanied, or followed by:

- A red rash, often on the face, chest, or backs of the hands over the knuckles.
- Swollen, reddish-purple eyelids.

About half of all children who have dermatomyositis develop skin ulcers.

What might be done?

If polymyositis or dermatomyositis is suspected, your doctor may arrange for blood tests to investigate inflammation and to look for antibodies that are specific to these conditions. You may also have electromyography (*see* NERVE AND MUSCLE ELECTRICAL TESTS, p.544) to measure electrical activity in the muscle, and a muscle biopsy, in which a sample of muscle tissue is removed for examination. An ECG (p.406) may be carried out to check for involvement of the heart muscle. You may also have a chest X-ray (p.490) and other tests to exclude the possibility of an underlying cancer.

There is no cure for polymyositis or dermatomyositis. However, the symptoms can usually be controlled. You will probably be prescribed high doses of corticosteroids (p.930) to help to reduce the inflammation. If there is no marked improvement, an immunosuppressant drug (p.906) or a drug that is normally used to treat cancer (*see* ANTICANCER DRUGS, p.907), may be given to slow the progression of the disorder. If dermatomyositis does not respond to these drugs, injections of immunoglobulins (antibodies) may be given. Physiotherapy (p.961) may help to prevent muscle stiffness and restore strength.

WHAT IS THE PROGNOSIS?

The outlook for both polymyositis and dermatomyositis is better in children than in adults. About 7 in 10 affected children recover completely in 2 years. Adults with polymyositis or dermatomyositis may need corticosteroid drugs for several years. In people who have cancer, the autoimmune disorder may improve if the cancer can be treated.

(WWW) ONLINE SITES: p.1033

Polymyalgia rheumatica

Pain and stiffness in the muscles around the shoulders and hips

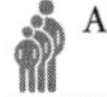 AGE Rare under the age of 60

 GENDER Twice as common in females

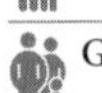 GENETICS Sometimes runs in families

 LIFESTYLE Not a significant factor

In polymyalgia rheumatica, inflammation of tissues causes pain and stiffness in the shoulder and pelvic muscles and may be associated with a general sense of feeling unwell and loss of energy.

Polymyalgia rheumatica is an autoimmune disorder in which the immune system attacks the body's own tissues. The condition is rare, can run in families, and is more common in older women. It may occur in association with the disorder temporal arteritis (right).

WHAT ARE THE SYMPTOMS?

The symptoms usually appear over a few weeks but sometimes develop suddenly. They may include:

- Painful, stiff muscles, often causing difficulty getting out of bed.
- Tiredness.
- Persistent or intermittent fever and night sweats.
- Weight loss.
- Depression (p.554).

The symptoms may be accompanied by those of temporal arteritis, such as severe headaches on one or both sides of the head and tenderness of the scalp.

WHAT MIGHT BE DONE?

Your doctor will probably be able to make a diagnosis based on a physical examination and the results of blood tests to look for inflammation. In some cases, additional blood tests will be performed to exclude other disorders, such as rheumatoid arthritis (p.377).

Your doctor will probably prescribe an oral corticosteroid (p.930) to reduce the inflammation. If you also have temporal arteritis, the initial doses of this drug may be higher. In either case, the dose will be reduced to a maintenance level once the symptoms subside.

Symptoms are usually relieved soon after starting corticosteroid treatment. However, polymyalgia rheumatica may persist for a longer period, in which case you need to continue taking low doses of a corticosteroid to control symptoms.

(WWW) ONLINE SITES: p.1033

Temporal arteritis

Inflammation of the blood vessels around the head and scalp

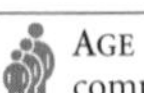 AGE Rare under the age of 55; increasingly common with age

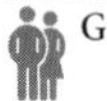 GENDER More common in females

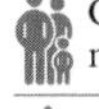 GENETICS Sometimes runs in families; more common in white people

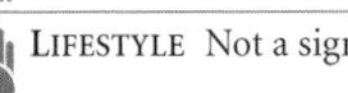 LIFESTYLE Not a significant factor

In temporal arteritis, also called giant-cell arteritis, particular arteries become inflamed and narrowed, reducing the blood flow through them. The disorder mainly affects blood vessels in the head and scalp, such as the temporal arteries (the arteries on the sides of the forehead). In some cases, the arteries that supply blood to the eyes are affected.

The cause of temporal arteritis is not known, but it may be due to an autoimmune reaction in which the immune system attacks the arteries. Temporal arteritis may be accompanied by polymyalgia rheumatica (left), and it sometimes runs in families, suggesting that genetic factors may be involved. Temporal arteritis occurs more commonly in women and older people.

WHAT ARE THE SYMPTOMS?

If you have temporal arteritis, you may notice the following symptoms:

- Severe headaches affecting either one or both sides of the head.
- Tenderness of the scalp.
- Pain in the sides of the face, which becomes worse on chewing.
- Prominent, tender temporal arteries.
- Tiredness.
- Loss of appetite and weight loss.

These symptoms may be accompanied by those of polymyalgia rheumatica, such as pain and stiffness in the muscles of the shoulders and pelvis. In rare cases, a stroke (p.532) may occur. If you also develop visual disturbances, you should consult your doctor at once because untreated temporal arteritis can lead to loss of an area of vision or even blindness.

WHAT MIGHT BE DONE?

Your doctor may be able to diagnose temporal arteritis from your description of the headache and by a physical examination. He or she may arrange for an urgent blood test to look for inflammation. You may also have a biopsy of the temporal artery, in which a tissue sample is taken for examination.

To reduce inflammation, a high dose of an oral corticosteroid (p.930) will be prescribed immediately. The symptoms of temporal arteritis usually improve within 24 hours of starting treatment. Once the condition begins to improve, the initial high dose of corticosteroid

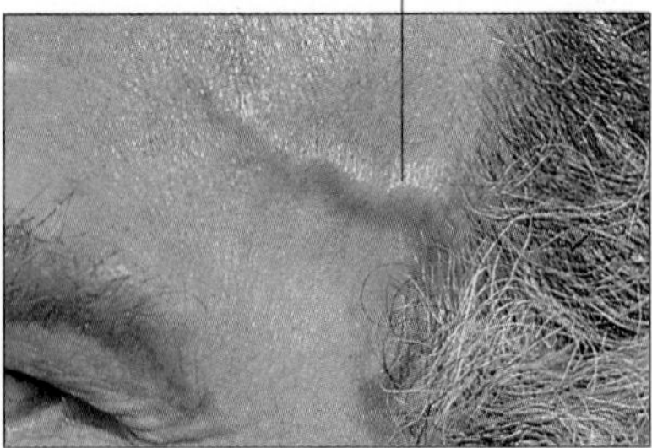

Temporal arteritis
The temporal artery shown above is prominent and inflamed due to temporal arteritis. Headaches and tenderness of the scalp are common with this disorder.

will be reduced, although it may be necessary for you to continue taking smaller doses for 2–3 years.

Your doctor will probably recommend that you have regular blood tests to monitor the course of the disorder. He or she may prescribe an immunosuppressant (p.906) as an alternative drug if there is little or no improvement in your condition or if you develop side effects with the corticosteroid.

WHAT IS THE PROGNOSIS?

In some cases, temporal arteritis may clear up completely with treatment, but in other cases the symptoms may recur. If you already have vision impairment due to temporal arteritis, your sight may not improve with treatment. However, it may be possible to prevent further deterioration of your vision.

(WWW) ONLINE SITES: p.1033

Polyarteritis nodosa

Widespread tissue damage as a result of patchy inflammation of the arteries

 AGE Can occur at any age, but most common between the ages of 40 and 60

 GENDER Twice as common in males

 GENETICS LIFESTYLE Not significant factors

In polyarteritis nodosa, segments of small- to medium-sized arteries are inflamed, reducing the blood supply to muscles, joints, and many of the internal organs. If the arteries that supply the heart or kidneys are affected, the condition may be life-threatening.

Polyarteritis nodosa is an autoimmune disorder in which the immune system attacks the body's own arteries. The cause of the abnormal immune reaction is not known, but the hepatitis B and C viruses (*see* ACUTE HEPATITIS, p.644) have been found in some people who have polyarteritis nodosa, suggesting that these viruses may trigger the disorder. Polyarteritis nodosa is more common in middle-aged men.

WHAT ARE THE SYMPTOMS?

The number and severity of symptoms vary depending on which organs are affected. The symptoms may include:

- Tiredness.
- Weight loss.

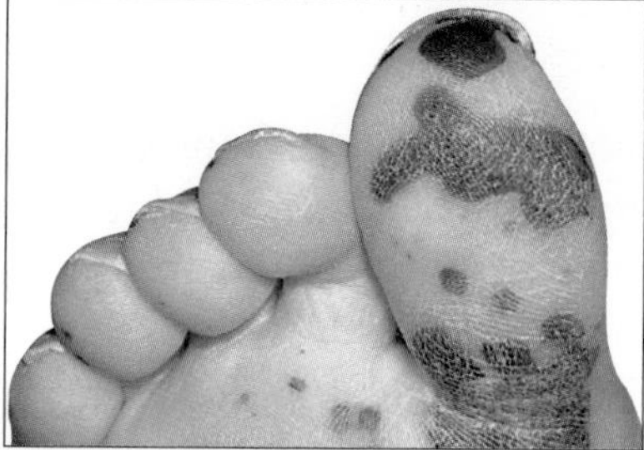

Rash of polyarteritis nodosa
This rash is due to polyarteritis nodosa, in which the blood vessels are inflamed and blood flow to the tissues is restricted.

- Fever.
- Abdominal pain or discomfort.
- Joint pain and muscle weakness.
- Tingling and numbness in the fingers and toes.
- A red-purple patchy rash on the skin that does not fade with pressure.
- Skin ulcers.

Polyarteritis nodosa commonly leads to increased blood pressure (*see* HYPERTENSION, p.403). In some people, there is severe damage to the kidneys, leading to kidney failure (p.705). Less commonly, polyarteritis may cause lung damage, a heart attack (*see* MYOCARDIAL INFARCTION, p.410), or a stroke (p.532).

HOW IS IT DIAGNOSED?

Your doctor may arrange for you to have blood tests to check for inflammation and to look for the hepatitis B or C viruses. To confirm the diagnosis, you may have a biopsy, in which a sample of an affected artery or organ is removed and examined under a microscope. You may also have angiography, in which an X-ray of the arteries is taken to look for abnormal areas in the blood vessels (*see* FEMORAL ANGIOGRAPHY, p.433).

WHAT IS THE TREATMENT?

Polyarteritis nodosa cannot be cured; the aim of treatment is to relieve symptoms and to prevent tissue injury. Your doctor may initially prescribe a high dose of a corticosteroid (p.930), which will be reduced once the symptoms subside. If there is no improvement, an immunosuppressant drug (p.906) may be prescribed. Without treatment, the condition may be life-threatening; with treatment, life expectancy is normal in about half of all cases.

(WWW) ONLINE SITES: p.1033

Behçet's syndrome

An inflammatory disorder producing recurrent mouth and genital ulcers

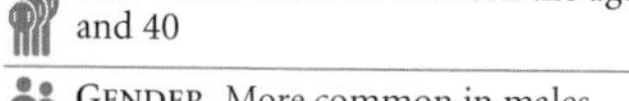 AGE Most common between the ages of 20 and 40

GENDER More common in males

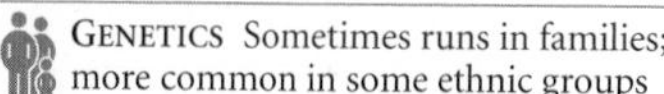 GENETICS Sometimes runs in families; more common in some ethnic groups

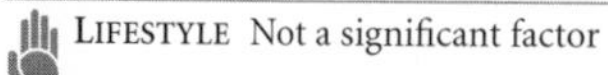 LIFESTYLE Not a significant factor

Behçet's syndrome is a rare disorder that varies in severity. The effects range from difficulty in eating to significant disability. Painful ulcers usually recur in the mouth and on the genitals. Other symptoms include eye inflammation (*see* UVEITIS, p.574), an acne-like rash, and small, tender lumps on the shins. The brain, spinal cord, and joints (*see* ARTHRITIS, p.374) may be affected, and the blood has an increased tendency to clot.

Behçet's syndrome is an autoimmune disorder in which the body produces antibodies that attack its own tissues. The cause of this abnormal immune reaction is unknown, but it may be triggered by viral infection. The syndrome sometimes runs in families and occurs more often in people of Mediterranean or Japanese origin, which suggests that genetic factors may be involved. Behçet's syndrome is twice as common in men as in women and most often occurs in people under the age of 40.

WHAT MIGHT BE DONE?

Your doctor may suspect Behçet's syndrome from your symptoms and a physical examination. It may take some time to confirm the diagnosis because there are no specific tests for the condition and many other disorders with similar symptoms need to be excluded. Some of the symptoms may disappear of their own accord, but your doctor may prescribe a topical corticosteroid (p.892) for the ulcers and eyedrops for eye inflammation (*see* DRUGS ACTING ON THE EYE, p.919). In severe cases, oral corticosteroids (p.930) and/or immunosuppressants (p.906) may be needed.

Behçet's syndrome is a lifelong condition with symptom-free periods that may last weeks, months, or even years. It rarely affects life expectancy.

(WWW) ONLINE SITES: p.1033

ALLERGIES

An allergy is an abnormal reaction of the body's immune system to a foreign substance. In most people, the substance produces no symptoms, but in a susceptible person it triggers an allergic reaction. Most allergies are mild and merely unpleasant, and they are easily treated with drugs and self-help remedies. However, sometimes allergies can be life-threatening.

In this section, allergic reactions due to foreign substances such as pollen, food, and certain drugs are discussed first. The trigger substance, called an allergen, causes no symptoms on initial contact. However, the body's immune system begins to form antibodies against the allergen, and certain types of white blood cells become sensitive to it. Later contact with the allergen may then stimulate specialized cells called mast cells to release histamine, the chemical that triggers the allergic response. In some cases, allergic reactions may lead to urticaria or angioedema, which are discussed next. The last article covers anaphylaxis, a severe and potentially life-threatening reaction to an allergen.

Allergies often develop in childhood and may either persist or disappear in adulthood. Conditions such as asthma (p.483) and eczema (p.333), which may have an allergic basis, are dealt with in the sections of the book that cover the relevant body systems.

KEY STRUCTURES

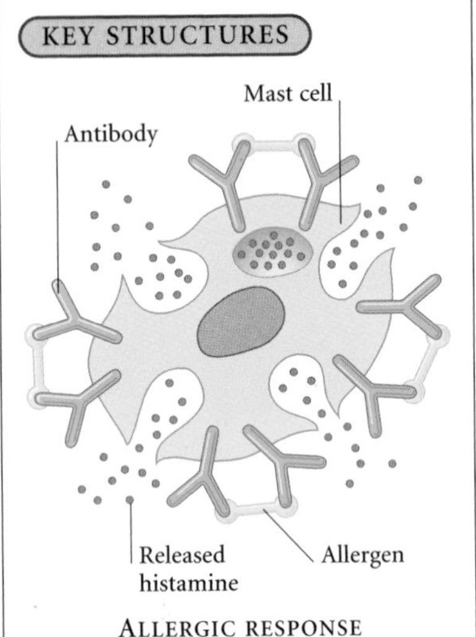

ALLERGIC RESPONSE

For more information on the allergic response, *see* p.445.

Allergic rhinitis

Inflammation of the membrane lining the nose and throat due to an allergic reaction

GENETICS Sometimes runs in families

AGE GENDER LIFESTYLE Not significant factors

Allergic rhinitis is a condition in which the membrane lining the nose and the throat becomes inflamed. It affects people who experience an allergic reaction after they inhale specific airborne substances (allergens). Allergic rhinitis may occur only in the spring and summer, in which case it is known as seasonal allergic rhinitis or hay fever, or it may be perennial and occur all year round. Allergic rhinitis is more common in people who also have other allergic disorders, such as asthma (p.483).

WHAT ARE THE CAUSES?

Seasonal allergic rhinitis is usually due to grass, tree, flower, or weed pollens; it occurs mostly during the spring and summer when pollen counts are high. The most common allergens that provoke perennial allergic rhinitis include house dust and dust mites, animal fur and dander, feathers, and mould spores.

WHAT ARE THE SYMPTOMS?

The symptoms of both forms of allergic rhinitis usually appear soon after contact with the allergen but tend to be more severe in hay fever. They include:

- Itchy sensation in the nose.
- Frequent sneezing.
- Blocked, runny nose.
- Itchy, red, watery eyes.

Some people may develop a headache. If the lining of the nose is severely inflamed, nosebleeds may occur.

WHAT MIGHT BE DONE?

Your doctor will probably recognize allergic rhinitis from your symptoms, particularly if you are able to identify the substance that triggers a reaction.

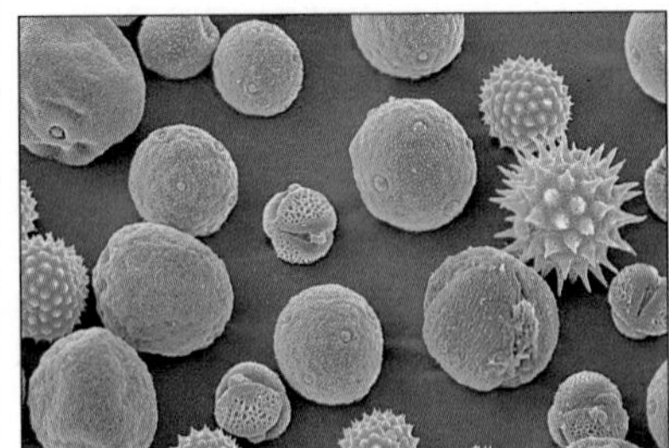

Possible allergens in allergic rhinitis
This magnified view reveals a variety of grain pollens that can cause seasonal allergic rhinitis in susceptible people.

A skin prick test (p.468) may be carried out to identify the allergen that causes the allergic rhinitis. In some cases, the allergen cannot be found.

If you are able to avoid the allergens that affect you, your symptoms will subside (*see* PREVENTING ALLERGIC RHINITIS, opposite page). Many antiallergy drugs (p.905) are available over the counter or on prescription. For example, allergies can be blocked by nasal sprays that contain sodium cromoglicate. Alternatively, corticosteroid drugs (*see* CORTICOSTEROIDS FOR RESPIRATORY DISEASE, p.911) are effective for hay fever but may take a few days to work. Nasal sprays containing decongestants (p.909) can relieve the symptoms but should not be used regularly. Oral antihistamines (p.906) may be combined with decongestants to relieve inflammation and itching. Eyedrops may help to relieve eye symptoms. Rarely, if symptoms are severe, your doctor may prescribe an oral corticosteroid (p.930).

The most specific treatment for allergic rhinitis is immunotherapy, in which you are injected with gradually increasing doses of allergen with the aim of desensitizing the immune system. This treatment, which typically takes as long as 3–4 years, is not always successful.

(WWW) ONLINE SITES: p.1027

SELF-HELP PREVENTING ALLERGIC RHINITIS

The following measures are all aimed at maintaining an allergen-free environment in your home. Tips on preventing perennial allergic rhinitis include:

- Avoid keeping furry animals as pets if you are allergic to them.
- Replace pillows and quilts containing animal materials such as duck feathers with those containing synthetic stuffing.
- Cover mattresses with plastic.
- Remove dust-collecting items such as upholstered furniture and curtains if possible.

To help prevent the symptoms of seasonal allergic rhinitis, also known as hay fever, the following measures may be effective:

- Avoid areas with long grass or where grass is being cut.
- In summer, keep doors and windows closed and spend as much time as possible in air-conditioned buildings.
- Try to stay inside during late morning and early evening when the pollen count is highest.
- Make sure your car is fitted with an effective pollen filter.
- When outside, wear sunglasses to help to prevent eye irritation.

Food allergy

An abnormal reaction of the immune system to certain foods

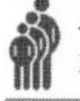
AGE Affects all ages, but most common in infants and children

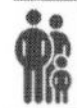
GENETICS Sometimes runs in families

GENDER LIFESTYLE Not significant factors

Food allergy is an uncommon condition in which the immune system reacts in an inappropriate or an exaggerated way to a specific food or foods, causing the development of various symptoms such as an itchy rash. This condition should not be confused with food intolerance (p.657), which often causes abdominal discomfort and indigestion but does not involve the immune system.

WHAT ARE THE CAUSES?

Although allergic reactions can occur in response to any food, nuts (especially peanuts) are probably the most common cause. Other relatively common causes of food allergy include seafood, strawberries, and eggs. Food colourings and preservatives rarely cause reactions, but intolerance to the food additive monosodium glutamate (MSG) is common.

Wheat may cause a condition known as coeliac disease (p.658) and an allergic reaction to the protein in cows' milk is especially common in infants and young children (*see* COWS' MILK PROTEIN ALLERGY, p.864). These conditions differ from immediate sensitivity to nuts or other foods in that they produce less severe but more persistent symptoms.

Food allergy is more common in people with other allergy-related conditions such as asthma (p.483), eczema (p.333), or allergic rhinitis (opposite page). If a close relative is allergic to a particular food, there is a greater risk that you will also develop an allergy to that food.

WHAT ARE THE SYMPTOMS?

Symptoms may appear almost immediately after eating the food or develop over a few hours. They may include:

- Itching and swelling affecting the lips, mouth, and throat.
- An itchy, red rash anywhere on the body (*see* URTICARIA, p.468).
- Nausea, vomiting, and diarrhoea.

If you have a severe reaction, the following symptoms may also be present:

- Nonitchy swelling anywhere on the body, especially the face, mouth, and throat (*see* ANGIOEDEMA, p.469).
- Shortness of breath or wheezing.

Sometimes, a food allergy may lead to anaphylaxis (p.469), a life-threatening allergic response that causes sudden difficulty in breathing and collapse. If you develop the symptoms of a severe reaction, seek immediate medical help.

WHAT MIGHT BE DONE?

You may be able to diagnose food allergy yourself if the symptoms occur soon after eating a particular food. However, you should consult your doctor if you suspect you have an allergy. If he or she is unsure what has caused the reaction, you may have a skin prick test (p.468).

Your doctor may advise you to follow an exclusion diet for 1 or 2 weeks. If your symptoms improve substantially while you are on the diet, this may indicate that you have one or more allergies to the foods that have been excluded. You can then gradually add foods to the exclusion diet, but if symptoms recur when a particular food is introduced, you should avoid it in the future. You should not embark on an exclusion diet without first consulting your doctor and you should not follow a nutritionally restricted diet for more than 2 weeks. Interpreting the results of an exclusion diet is often difficult.

Avoiding the problem food is the only effective treatment. Always ask about ingredients when eating out, and check labels on packaged foods. Consult a diet or nutrition counsellor if you need to exclude a food that is a major part of a normal diet, such as wheat. If a major permanent dietary change is needed, be sure to maintain a balanced diet.

WHAT IS THE PROGNOSIS?

Many food allergies, particularly nut allergies, are permanent, and people must avoid the relevant foods throughout their lives. Some food allergies may disappear. Children under the age of 4 who completely avoid problem foods, such as wheat, for 2 years have an excellent chance of outgrowing their allergy.

(WWW) ONLINE SITES: p.1027, p.1035

Drug allergy

An abnormal reaction to a drug, most commonly an antibiotic

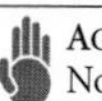
AGE GENDER GENETICS LIFESTYLE Not significant factors

Both over-the-counter and prescription drugs can cause various problems. Most symptoms, such as nausea or diarrhoea, are not allergies but side effects that can affect anyone taking the drug. A drug allergy occurs when the immune system produces an abnormal reaction to a specific drug. Often, the reactions are mild, but some can be life-threatening.

WHAT ARE THE CAUSES?

A drug may provoke an allergic reaction the first time you use it. It is also possible to develop an allergic reaction to a drug that you have been taking for some time. In the latter case, your body will gradually become more and more sensitive to the drug. Allergic reactions may occur with any drug but are most common with antibiotics (p.885). Your doctor will ask you about any known allergies before prescribing drugs.

WHAT ARE THE SYMPTOMS?

An allergic reaction to a drug may give rise to the following symptoms:

- Wheezing.
- Swelling anywhere on the body, but typically affecting the face and throat (*see* ANGIOEDEMA, opposite page).
- Nausea and diarrhoea.
- An itchy rash consisting of red, raised areas and, occasionally, white lumps (*see* URTICARIA, right).

If you develop these symptoms and suspect that they are due to a prescription or over-the-counter drug, contact your doctor at once before taking the next dose. Rarely, a drug allergy may lead to a severe and potentially fatal reaction called anaphylaxis (opposite page).

WHAT MIGHT BE DONE?

If your doctor suspects that you are allergic to a particular drug, he or she will advise you to stop taking it and may prescribe an alternative. Usually, mild symptoms disappear without treatment within a few days of stopping the drug. Itchy rashes can be treated with over-the-counter products such as calamine lotion or oral antihistamines (p.906). A drug allergy is usually lifelong. It is therefore important to inform any doctor who treats you that you have an allergy to a certain drug. If the reaction was severe, you will be advised to carry a card or bracelet with you at all times to alert other people to your drug allergy in case you need emergency treatment.

(WWW) ONLINE SITES: p.1027, p.1030

Urticaria

Areas of swelling on the skin, often known as hives, that occur as the result of an allergic reaction

AGE Affects all ages, but less common in elderly people

GENETICS Sometimes runs in families

GENDER LIFESTYLE Not significant factors

Urticaria
This rash, known as urticaria, consists of white lumps and red, inflamed areas. It is usually caused by an allergic reaction.

Urticaria, also known as hives, is an intensely itchy rash that may affect the whole body or just a small area of skin. The rash consists of raised, red areas and, sometimes, white lumps. The inflamed areas usually vary in size and may merge to involve very large areas of skin. Urticaria typically lasts for only a few hours (acute urticaria), but in some cases it may persist for up to several months (chronic urticaria). Both the acute and chronic forms of urticaria may recur. Sometimes, urticaria occurs at the same time as the more serious condition called angioedema (opposite page). Urticaria is also sometimes an early symptom of anaphylaxis (opposite page), a severe and potentially fatal allergic reaction to a substance.

WHAT ARE THE CAUSES?

Urticaria can occur as a result of an allergic reaction to a particular food, such as nuts (*see* FOOD ALLERGY, p.467). The condition may also be due to a drug allergy (p.467) or an allergy to plants, or it may develop after an insect bite or sting. However, when urticaria occurs for the first time in an adult, it is often difficult to identify the cause. The tendency to develop urticaria may sometimes run in families.

WHAT MIGHT BE DONE?

Acute urticaria usually disappears without any treatment within a few hours. The chronic form of the condition may take several weeks or months to clear up. Over-the-counter products such as calamine lotion and oral antihistamines (p.906) may help to relieve itching.

If your symptoms persist or recur and the cause of the problem is not obvious, you should consult your doctor. He or she may arrange for a skin prick test (left) to try to identify the substances to which you are allergic (allergens). When the substance causing your urticaria has been identified, you should take all possible steps to avoid coming into contact with it in the future in order to prevent a recurrence of the condition.

(WWW) ONLINE SITES: p.1027, p.1036

(TEST) SKIN PRICK TEST

A skin prick test is a simple and painless procedure undertaken to find out which substances (allergens) cause allergic reactions in an affected person. Dilute solutions are made from extracts of allergens, such as pollen, dust, dander, and food, that commonly cause allergic reactions.

A drop of each solution is placed on the skin, which is then pricked with a needle. The skin is observed for a reaction, which usually occurs within 30 minutes of applying the solution. Antihistamines should not be taken on the day of the test because they may prevent any reaction.

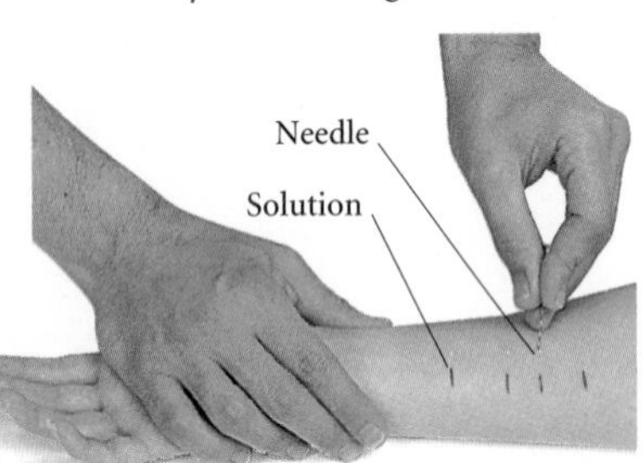

1 *Drops from 8–10 solutions containing different allergens are placed on the skin. The skin underneath is then pricked with a needle and observed for a reaction.*

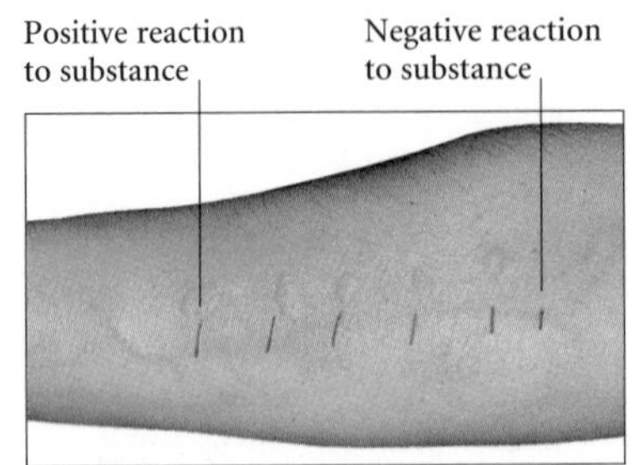

2 *If a person is allergic to one of the substances applied to the skin, a red lump, indicating a positive reaction, appears at the site of the needle prick.*

Angioedema

Swelling of body tissues, particularly around the face, usually due to an allergic reaction

 GENETICS Sometimes runs in families

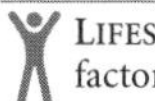 LIFESTYLE In some cases, stress is a trigger factor

 AGE GENDER Not significant factors

Angioedema is a condition in which the mucous membranes and tissues under the skin suddenly become swollen. The face and neck are usually affected.

The most common cause of angioedema is an allergic reaction to a type of food, such as seafood, nuts, or strawberries (*see* FOOD ALLERGY, p.467). Less commonly, the condition may result from an allergic reaction to a drug (*see* DRUG ALLERGY, p.467), most often to an antibiotic (p.885). Angioedema may also develop after an insect bite.

Rarely, a person may inherit a tendency to develop angioedema that is unrelated to an allergy. In such cases, episodes of unexplained angioedema may begin in childhood and may be triggered by stressful events, such as an injury or a dental extraction.

It is not unusual for people to have only a single episode of angioedema, for which no cause can be determined.

WHAT ARE THE SYMPTOMS?

Swelling usually develops within a few minutes and is often asymmetrical; for example, only one side of a lip may be affected. The main symptoms are:

- Swelling of any part of the body, most commonly the face, lips, and genitals.
- Sudden difficulty in breathing, speaking, or swallowing due to swelling of the tongue, mouth, and airways.
- In about half of all cases, an itchy rash affecting areas that are not swollen (*see* URTICARIA, opposite page).

The swelling may affect the larynx (voice box) and can be life-threatening if the airway becomes blocked. Angioedema may occur at the same time as anaphylaxis (right), a potentially fatal allergic reaction that requires urgent medical attention. If you develop the symptoms of angioedema above or you experience difficulty in breathing, you should seek medical help immediately.

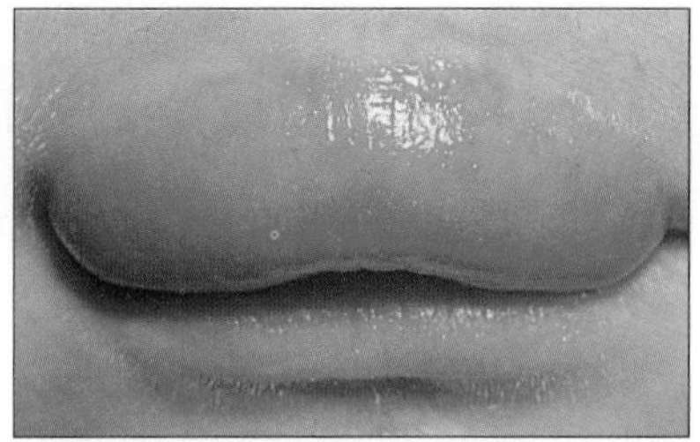

Angioedema of the upper lip
Sudden, severe swelling of the face, lips, or neck is known as angioedema, which is usually caused by an allergic reaction.

WHAT MIGHT BE DONE?

Severe angioedema requires an urgent injection with the drug epinephrine (adrenaline), followed by observation in hospital. In milder cases, a corticosteroid (p.930) or an antihistamine (p.906) may be given to reduce the swelling; this may take hours or days to subside.

Your doctor may carry out tests to determine the cause of the angioedema. If a food allergy is suspected, a skin prick test (opposite page) and/or an exclusion diet may be used to identify the substances to which you are allergic. If you suffer from severe angioedema, your doctor may teach you how to self-inject epinephrine (*see* EMERGENCY AID FOR ANAPHYLAXIS, right).

(WWW) ONLINE SITES: p.1027, p.1036

Anaphylaxis

A severe, potentially fatal allergic reaction to certain substances

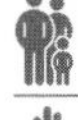 GENETICS Sometimes runs in families

 AGE GENDER LIFESTYLE Not significant factors

Anaphylaxis, also known as anaphylactic shock, is a rare and severe type of allergic reaction that occurs in people who have developed an extreme sensitivity to a specific substance (allergen). The reaction spreads throughout the body, causing a sudden drop in blood pressure and narrowing of the airways, and it can be fatal unless immediate treatment is available. Anaphylaxis is most commonly triggered by insect stings or by certain drugs such as the antibiotic penicillin (*see* DRUG ALLERGY, p.467). Foods such as nuts or strawberries may also trigger this serious form of allergic reaction (*see* FOOD ALLERGY, p.467).

WHAT ARE THE SYMPTOMS?

If you have an extreme sensitivity to a substance, you may experience some or all of the following symptoms as soon as you are exposed to it:

- Sudden feeling of extreme anxiety.
- Swollen face, lips, and tongue.
- Wheezing and difficulty breathing.
- In some cases, an itchy, red rash (*see* URTICARIA, opposite page) and flushing of the skin.
- Light-headedness or, in some cases, loss of consciousness.

If either you or anyone you are with develops these symptoms, you should call an ambulance immediately.

WHAT IS THE TREATMENT?

Emergency treatment for anaphylaxis is an immediate injection of epinephrine (adrenaline). Antihistamines (p.906) or corticosteroids (p.930), together with fluids, are also given intravenously.

You should avoid any substance to which you are sensitive, especially if you have had a previous anaphylactic reaction. You may be given epinephrine to self-inject (*see* EMERGENCY AID FOR ANAPHYLAXIS, below). You will also be advised to carry an emergency card or bracelet to alert others to your allergy.

(WWW) ONLINE SITES: p.1027, p.1032

(TREATMENT) EMERGENCY AID FOR ANAPHYLAXIS

If you have previously experienced anaphylaxis or severe angioedema, your doctor may provide you with syringes of injectable epinephrine (adrenaline). Keep one at home and one at work, and carry one with you at all times. In the event of anaphylaxis, inject epinephrine immediately, then call for an ambulance.

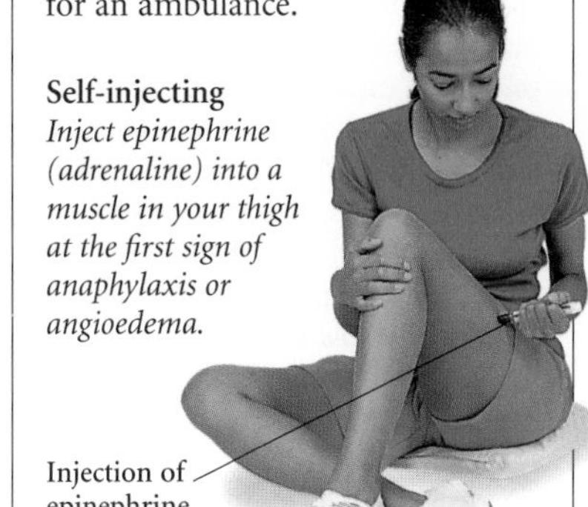

Self-injecting
Inject epinephrine (adrenaline) into a muscle in your thigh at the first sign of anaphylaxis or angioedema.

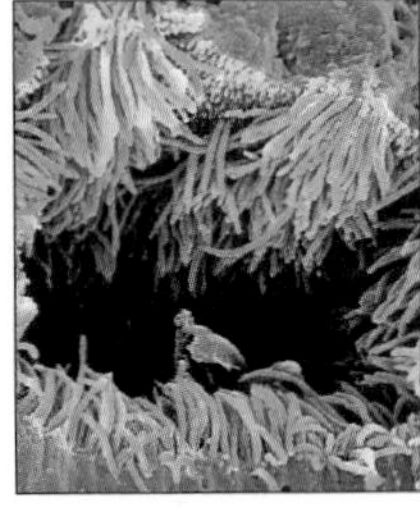

A filtering system
Fine hair-like strands, known as cilia, line the airways and trap foreign particles as the air passes through.

Respiratory System

EVERY LIVING CELL IN THE BODY needs a constant supply of oxygen to survive. Cells must also dispose of their primary waste product, carbon dioxide. The role of the respiratory system, together with the circulatory system, is to deliver oxygen from the lungs to the cells and to remove carbon dioxide and return it to the lungs to be exhaled. This exchange of oxygen and carbon dioxide is very effective because of the combination of the vast surface area of the lungs, which is about 40 times greater than that of the body, and the fact that all of the blood passes through the lungs every minute.

The exchange of oxygen and carbon dioxide between the air, blood, and body tissues is known as respiration. Air enters and leaves the body by the respiratory system, which is made up of the mouth, nose, throat, branching airways, and lungs. The circulatory system, which consists of the heart and blood vessels, ensures that oxygen is delivered to the cells and carbon dioxide is carried away.

Respiratory processes

Healthy lungs take in about 500 ml (1 pint) of air 12–15 times each minute. Breathing is an automatic process that is controlled by the respiratory centre in the brain; we only become aware of breathing when it is difficult, such as during exercise. When we inhale, air enters the body through the mouth or nose and is warmed and moistened. Air passes down the pharynx (throat) and larynx (voice box) and into the trachea (windpipe). A small flap of cartilage called the epiglottis covers the trachea during swallowing to prevent food from entering the airways.

In the lungs, oxygen from the air passes into the surrounding blood vessels. There, it binds to the molecule haemoglobin in the red blood cells. The oxygen-rich blood then travels from the lungs to the heart and the body tissues, where oxygen is released. At the same time, carbon dioxide waste from the tissues passes into the blood and dissolves in the plasma, the fluid part of blood. This carbon dioxide is returned to the lungs and exhaled.

Sometimes, infectious organisms or foreign particles enter the body when we inhale. The respiratory system has several ways of protecting the lungs from damage. Situated in the walls of the pharynx are collections of tissue called the tonsils and the adenoids. These help to destroy some infectious organisms as they travel towards the lungs. Airborne particles may also be trapped by mucus in the airways and then directed away from the lungs by tiny hairs called cilia. Finally, foreign particles or excess mucus that irritate the airways or lungs can be expelled by a sneeze or a cough.

Speech production

The respiratory system also contains the vocal cords, the organs that are responsible for speech production. Sounds are formed when the vocal cords are partially closed and air from the lungs causes them to vibrate. Using these vibrations, we can produce a remarkable range of sounds.

(STRUCTURE) Sinuses

Several air-filled cavities, known as sinuses, are situated in the skull bones around the nose and the eyes. The size and shape of these sinuses vary between individuals. Sinuses are not present at birth but gradually develop throughout childhood. They help to lighten the skull bones and give the voice resonance. Within the lining of the sinuses are many mucus-secreting glands. Mucus passes continuously through narrow channels that lead from the sinuses to the back of the nose. The mucus traps small airborne particles and moistens inhaled air as it passes though the airways.

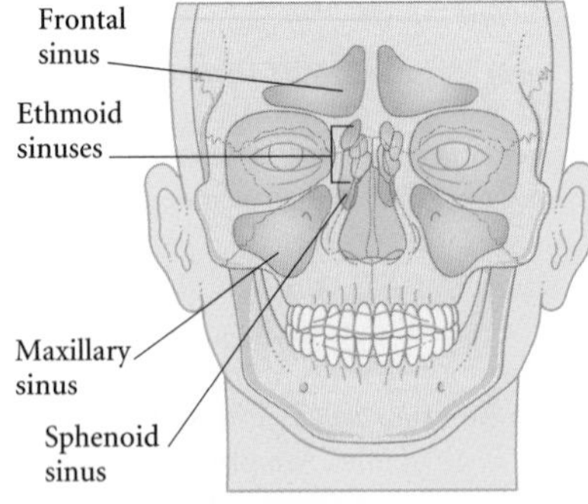

Front view of the sinuses
Sinuses are named after the bones in which they are found. The sinuses in the front of the skull are the frontal and maxillary sinuses.

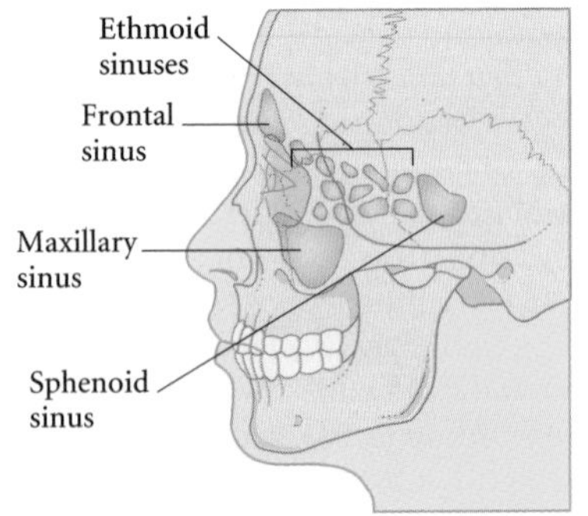

Side view of the sinuses
The two sphenoid sinuses are situated deep in the skull. In front of them lie the numerous ethmoid sinuses.

STRUCTURE RESPIRATORY SYSTEM

The upper part of the respiratory system includes the nasal passages, the pharynx (throat), the larynx (voice box), and the main airway, which is called the trachea or windpipe. The two lungs and the lower airways (the bronchi and the smaller bronchioles) are encased in a bony cage formed by the ribs. The airways terminate in millions of balloon-like sacs called alveoli. The alveoli provide a vast surface area for gas exchange with the large numbers of tiny blood vessels that surround them.

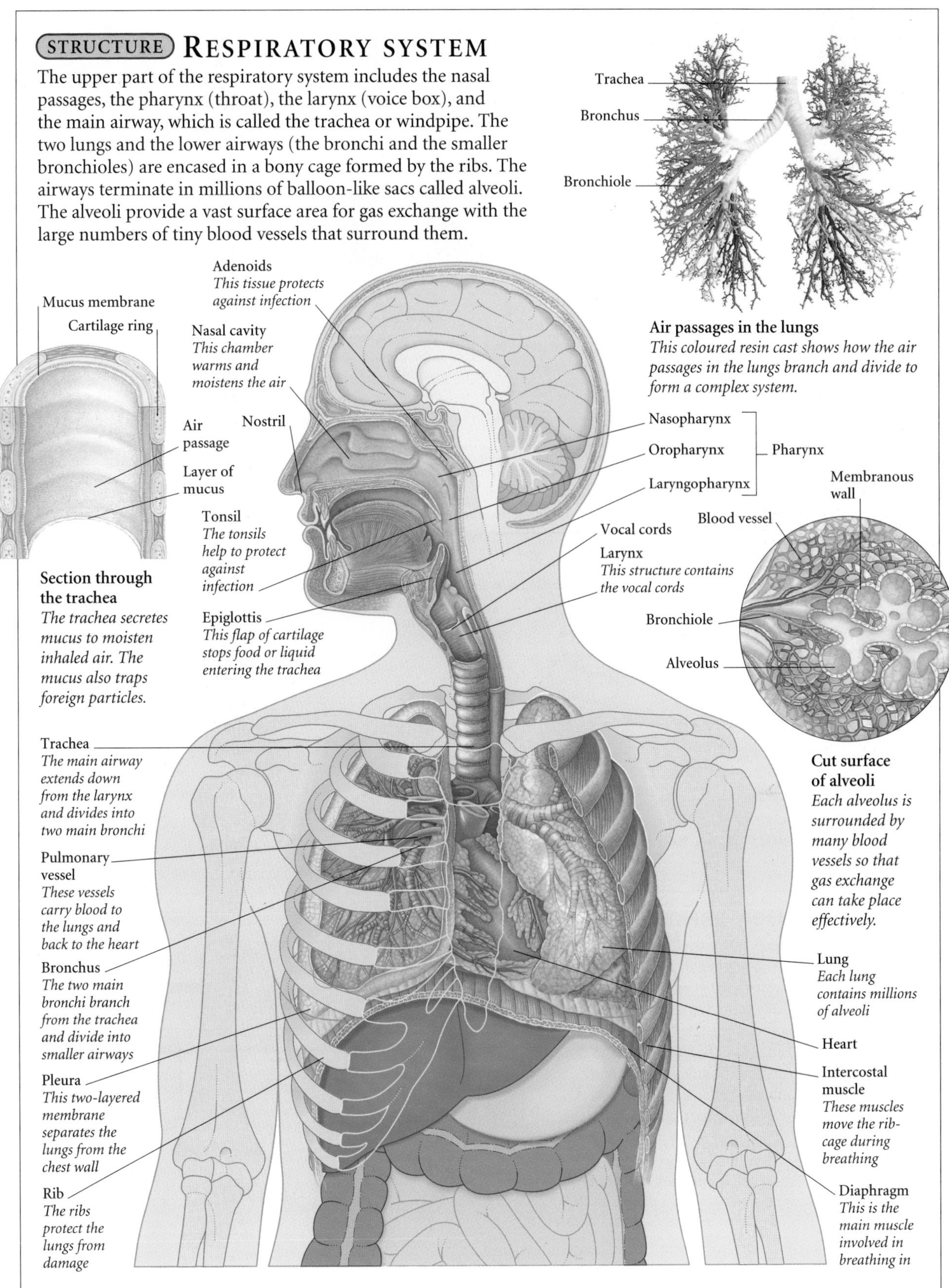

FUNCTION BREATHING AND RESPIRATION

Air constantly enters and leaves the lungs, enabling the tissues of the body to receive an adequate supply of oxygen and to dispose of their waste product, carbon dioxide. Breathing is controlled by the respiratory centre in a part of the brain known as the medulla. The respiratory centre stimulates the intercostal muscles around the chest cavity to contract and relax so that we breathe in and out.

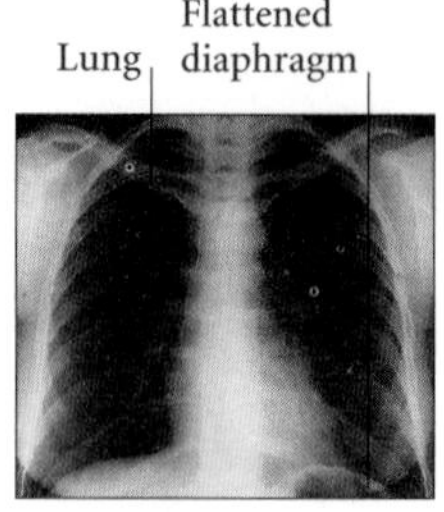

INHALATION

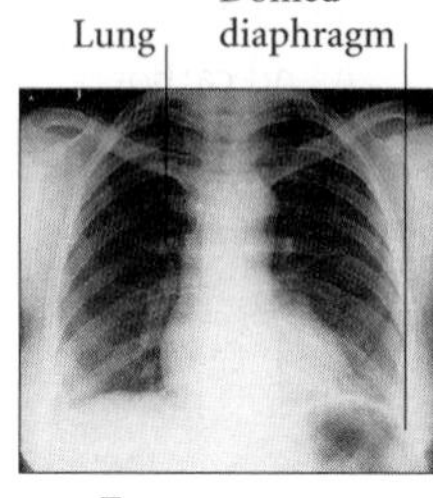

EXHALATION

Chest X-rays
These normal chest X-rays show the volume of air in the lungs during inhalation and exhalation, which is achieved by changes in the position of the ribs and diaphragm.

HOW BREATHING WORKS

During breathing, air moves from areas of high pressure to areas of low pressure. When the pressure in the lungs is lower than the pressure in the atmosphere, air enters the airways. If the pressure in the lungs increases, air moves out of the lungs and is then exhaled.

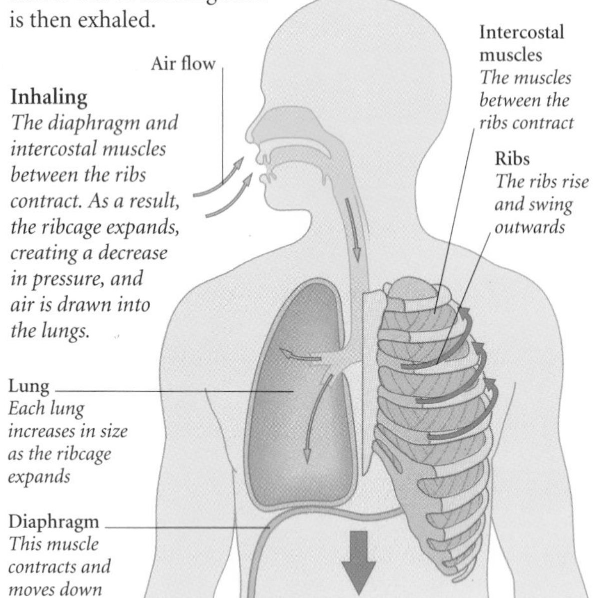

Inhaling
The diaphragm and intercostal muscles between the ribs contract. As a result, the ribcage expands, creating a decrease in pressure, and air is drawn into the lungs.

Exhaling
After breathing in, the diaphragm and intercostal muscles relax and the rib-cage contracts. Pressure inside the lungs increases and air moves out of the lungs in order to be exhaled.

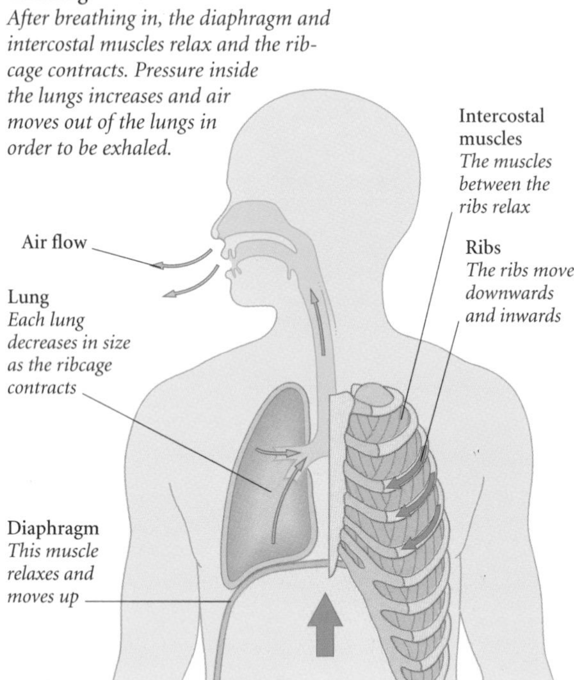

FUNCTION HOW BREATHING IS REGULATED

Even while we sleep, our basic breathing rhythm is controlled by a collection of nerve cells in the brain called the respiratory centre. From there, messages travel down nerves to the diaphragm and rib muscles and stimulate them so that we continue breathing. As activity changes, so does the amount of carbon dioxide in the blood. Receptors in some of the large arteries detect the changes and send instructions to the brain.

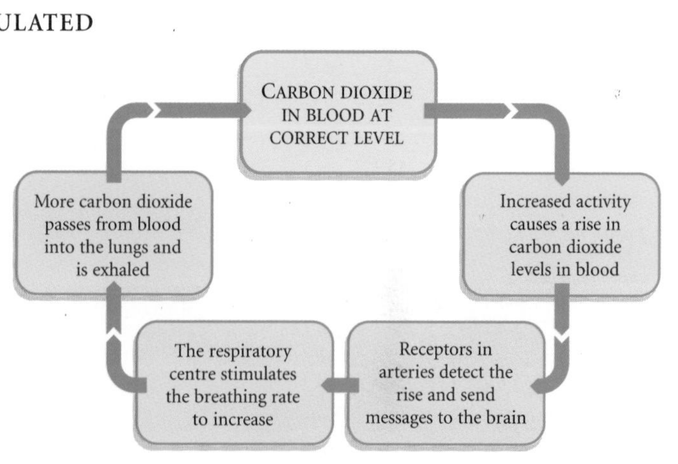

How carbon dioxide influences breathing
Nerve cells in arteries and in the brain's respiratory centre are sensitive to levels of carbon dioxide in the blood. A slight rise in the carbon dioxide level increases the breathing rate to return the level to normal.

GAS EXCHANGE IN THE BODY

The exchange of oxygen and carbon dioxide gases occurs constantly throughout the body. In the lungs, oxygen crosses the delicate walls of the alveoli (air sacs) and enters tiny blood vessels (capillaries), where it binds to the molecule haemoglobin in the red blood cells. At the same time, carbon dioxide is released from the blood into the alveoli and exhaled through the mouth or nose. In tissue cells, blood from the lungs exchanges its supply of oxygen for carbon dioxide.

Exchange of gases
Body cells require a constant supply of oxygen in order to obtain energy to survive. In addition, waste products from the body cells, mainly carbon dioxide, must be transported away from the cells.

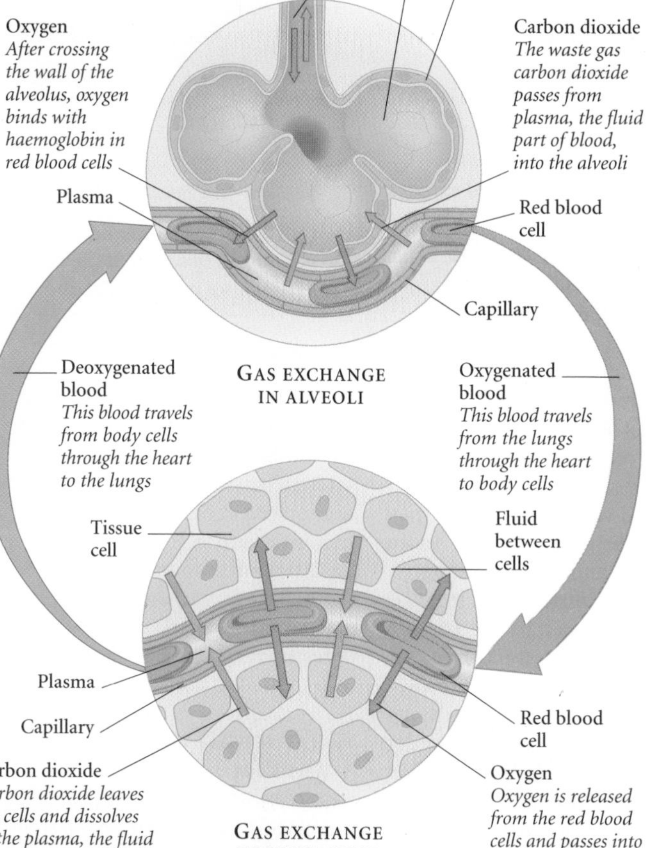

Bronchiole (small air passage)

Air space of alveolus

Wall of alveolus

Oxygen
After crossing the wall of the alveolus, oxygen binds with haemoglobin in red blood cells

Carbon dioxide
The waste gas carbon dioxide passes from plasma, the fluid part of blood, into the alveoli

Plasma

Red blood cell

Capillary

Deoxygenated blood
This blood travels from body cells through the heart to the lungs

GAS EXCHANGE IN ALVEOLI

Oxygenated blood
This blood travels from the lungs through the heart to body cells

Tissue cell

Fluid between cells

Plasma

Capillary

Red blood cell

Carbon dioxide
Carbon dioxide leaves the cells and dissolves in the plasma, the fluid part of blood

GAS EXCHANGE IN BODY CELLS

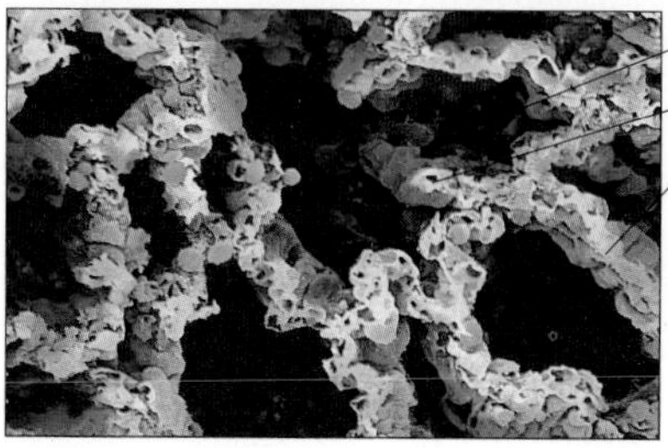

Oxygen
Oxygen is released from the red blood cells and passes into the tissue cells

Air space

Blood vessel

Membranous wall

Cross section of alveoli
This magnified view of lung tissue shows the alveolar air spaces and their thin walls. The tiny holes seen in the walls are blood vessels.

FUNCTION SPEECH

The larynx (voice box) is responsible for voice production. Sounds are made when air from the lungs passes across two fibrous bands within the larynx, known as vocal cords. The sounds produced by the vibrating cords are formed into speech by the mouth and tongue.

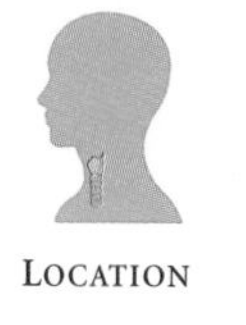
LOCATION

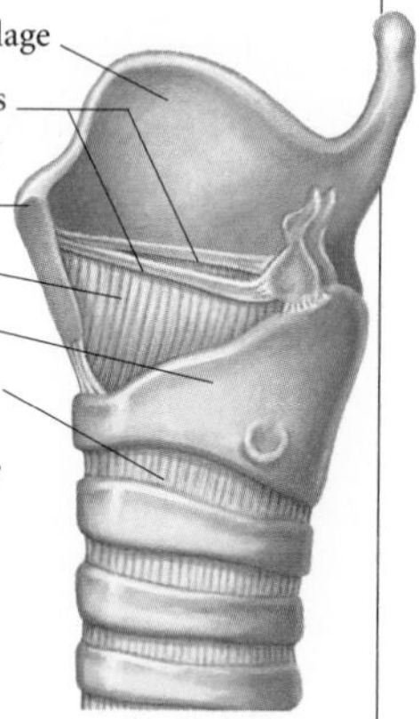

Thyroid cartilage

Vocal cords

Cut edge of cartilage

Ligament

Cricoid cartilage

Trachea

Side view of the larynx
The larynx is composed of the vocal cords and the thyroid and cricoid cartilages, which are connected by ligaments. The organ is located in the neck, above the trachea.

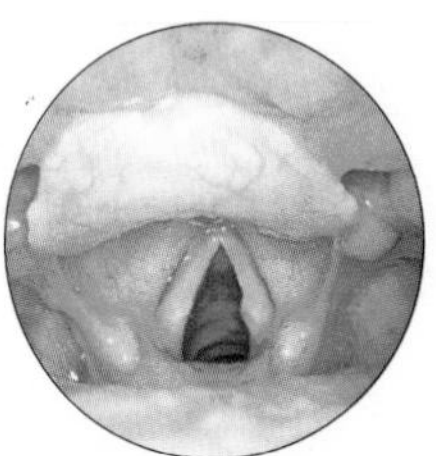
OPEN VOCAL CORDS

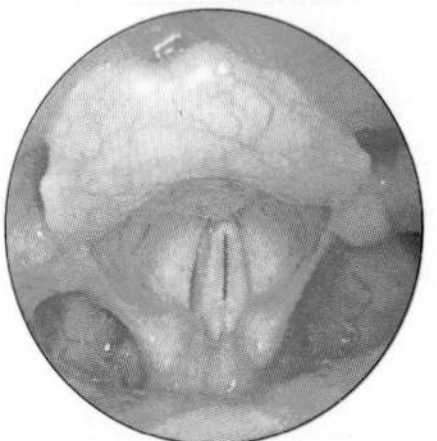
CLOSED VOCAL CORDS

Movements of the vocal cords
The vocal cords are held open during breathing, but during speech they pull together and vibrate as air from the lungs passes between them. Sounds vary according to the exact position of the cords.

FUNCTION THE COUGH REFLEX

If substances such as dust or excess mucus irritate the lungs or airways, they may be removed by the familiar reaction known as a cough. The irritation stimulates nerve cell receptors in the airways, sending signals to the brain, which then triggers the cough reflex.

The cough
During a cough, air, moisture, and foreign particles are noisily and forcefully expelled. This reflex action helps to clear irritant material from the airways, preventing it from causing damage.

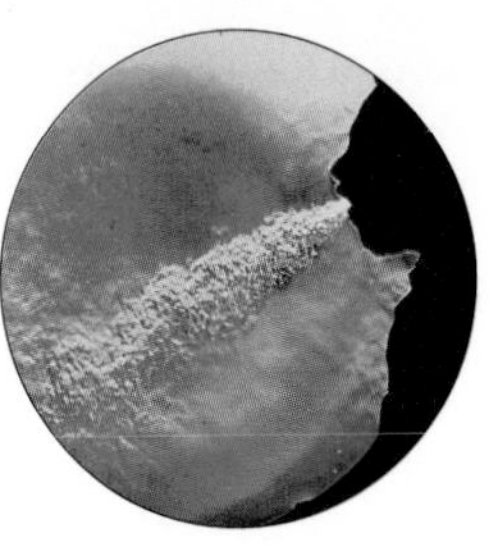

NOSE AND THROAT DISORDERS

The upper part of the respiratory system is made up of the nose and throat and structures associated with them. These include the sinuses (the air-filled cavities in the front of the skull) and the larynx, also known as the voice box. The upper respiratory system can be affected by a variety of disorders ranging from common complaints, such as nosebleeds, snoring, and laryngitis, to rare conditions such as cancers of the throat and larynx.

Disorders that affect the nose and the sinuses are covered first in this section. These conditions include nosebleeds, which are often a symptom of a minor injury but are sometimes due to a serious underlying disorder, and sinusitis, inflammation of the sinuses, which is usually caused by a viral infection such as the common cold.

Obstruction in the nasal passages may cause problems with sleep, and two such disorders, snoring and sleep apnoea, are covered here. Articles follow on common conditions that involve inflammation of the throat or larynx, such as pharyngitis, tonsillitis, and laryngitis. Finally, noncancerous growths in the larynx, known as vocal cord nodules, and cancers of the throat and larynx are discussed.

Infections that affect the nose and the throat are described elsewhere (*see* INFECTIONS AND INFESTATIONS, pp.284–313), as is allergic rhinitis (p.466), a common disorder of the nose. Disorders of the nose and throat that are common in children, such as enlarged adenoids, are covered in another section (*see* INFANCY AND CHILDHOOD, pp.836–843).

KEY ANATOMY

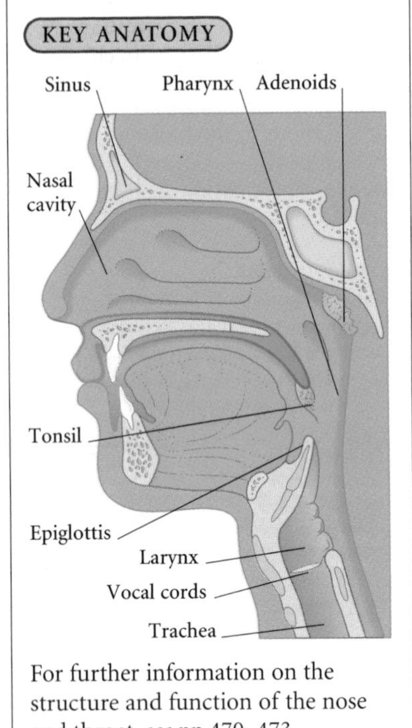

For further information on the structure and function of the nose and throat, *see* pp.470–473.

Nosebleed

Bleeding from the nose, usually from one nostril only

AGE Most common in children and in adults over the age of 50

GENDER GENETICS LIFESTYLE Not significant factors

Nosebleeds are common in children, but the bleeding usually stops by itself and is minor. Nosebleeds are also common, but sometimes serious, in people over the age of 50. In this age group, bleeding may come from the back of the nose and be hard to stop. If the blood is swallowed, bleeding may not be seen.

WHAT ARE THE CAUSES?

Nosebleeds commonly occur spontaneously. In dry environments or during winter months, the membranes lining the nose may become dry and cracked, causing bleeding to occur. Nosebleeds may also occur if the lining of the nose is injured by a blow to the nose or by nose-picking or forceful nose-blowing. In children, nosebleeds often occur as a result of rough play. A foreign body in the nose or an infection in the upper respiratory tract may also result in a nosebleed. In people over the age of 50, the small blood vessels in the nose may be more fragile and therefore more likely to rupture and cause bleeding.

In rare cases, nosebleeds may be associated with cancer in the passage connecting the nose to the throat (*see* CANCER OF THE NASOPHARYNX, p.480) or may indicate another underlying disease, such as the bleeding disorder thrombocytopenia (p.453) or a liver disease that affects blood clotting. Nosebleeds may also be caused by drugs that prevent blood clotting (p.904). A nosebleed is more likely to be prolonged if you have high blood pressure (*see* HYPERTENSION, p.403).

WHAT CAN I DO?

If you have a nosebleed, you should put direct pressure on the soft part of your nose by pressing both sides together for at least 15 minutes while breathing through your mouth. You should try to avoid sniffing and/or blowing your nose afterwards because you may dislodge the blood clot that has formed and cause another nosebleed. Self-help measures are usually successful in stopping a nosebleed. If bleeding persists for half an hour or more, you should seek medical attention. If membranes in the nose are dry and cracked, rubbing water-based ointment in your nose a few times a day or using a saline spray may help to prevent recurrent nosebleeds.

WHAT MIGHT THE DOCTOR DO?

A persistent nosebleed will probably require hospital treatment. Your doctor may pack your nose with nasal sponges, which are left in place for about 2 days. Alternatively, a flexible tube with a small balloon at the tip may be inserted into the back of your nose and inflated to stop the bleeding by applying pressure to leaking vessels. Bleeding vessels may also be cauterized (sealed using heat) under local anaesthesia.

If the cause is not obvious, your doctor may arrange for you to have endoscopy of the nose (*see* ENDOSCOPY OF THE NOSE AND THROAT, p.476), in which an optical instrument is passed into each nostril in turn to look for ruptured vessels or a tumour. Rarely, CT scanning (p.247) or MRI (p.248) may be carried out to rule out a tumour. Blood tests may also be arranged to check how efficiently the blood clots.

Recurrent bleeding that is not caused by a tumour may be investigated by injecting a contrast medium into the blood vessels and taking contrast X-rays (p.245). A special substance is then injected into the leaking blood vessel to block it and prevent further blood loss. In other cases, surgery may be required to tie off the leaking blood vessels.

(WWW) ONLINE SITES: p.1031

Sinusitis

Inflammation of any of the sinuses (the air-filled cavities in the bones around the nose)

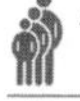

AGE More common in adults

GENETICS Risk factors depend on the cause

GENDER LIFESTYLE Not significant factors

The sinuses are air-filled cavities in the skull situated behind the nose and eyes and in the cheeks and forehead. They are lined with a mucus-secreting membrane and are connected to the nasal cavity by a number of narrow channels. Inflammation of the sinuses, known as sinusitis, may be acute (developing and clearing up rapidly) or chronic (long-term). Sinusitis rarely occurs in children under the age of 5, partly because their sinuses are not fully developed.

What are the causes?

The most common cause of sinusitis is a viral infection, such as the common cold (p.288). If the channels connecting the nose to the sinuses become blocked due to the viral infection, mucus collects in the sinuses. In some cases, the mucus becomes infected with bacteria.

Blockage of the channels is more likely in people with an abnormality in the nose, such as a deviated nasal septum (p.476) or nasal polyps (p.476). In addition, people with allergic rhinitis (p.466) or a disorder such as the inherited condition cystic fibrosis (p.824) are more likely to develop sinusitis. Rarely, the channels are blocked by a tumour (*see* CANCER OF THE NASOPHARYNX, p.480). People with reduced immunity, such as those with HIV infection (*see* HIV INFECTION AND AIDS, p.297) and those taking immunosuppressant drugs (p.906), are more susceptible to infections that lead to sinusitis.

What are the symptoms?

Symptoms depend on which sinuses are affected and may include:

- Headache.
- Pain and tenderness in the face that tends to worsen when bending down.

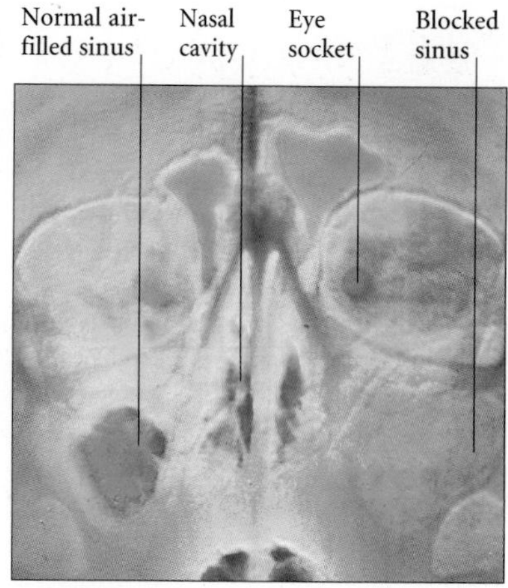

Sinusitis
This colour-enhanced facial X-ray shows a normal air-filled sinus and a sinus filled with mucus, indicating sinusitis.

- Toothache, if the sinuses behind the cheeks are affected.
- Discoloured nasal discharge.
- Nasal congestion or obstruction.

In a few cases, the infection spreads and may cause redness and swelling of the tissue around an eye.

What can I do?

In many cases, sinusitis clears up without treatment. Painkillers (p.912) and decongestants (p.909), both available over the counter, may alleviate symptoms. Steam inhalation (left), which usually helps to clear the nose, may also relieve symptoms. If symptoms become worse or do not improve within 3 days, you should consult a doctor.

What might the doctor do?

Your doctor may prescribe antibiotics (p.885) to clear up secondary bacterial infection. If sinusitis recurs or does not clear up completely, you may have X-rays (p.244) to look for thickening of the lining of the sinuses and excess mucus. Your doctor may also perform endoscopy of the nose (*see* ENDOSCOPY OF THE NOSE AND THROAT, p.476) and arrange for CT scanning (p.247) to look for a specific cause, such as nasal polyps or a tumour. Surgery may be necessary to enlarge drainage channels from the sinuses to the nose or create new ones. Acute sinusitis usually clears up in a few weeks, but the symptoms of chronic sinusitis may last for a couple of months.

(WWW) ONLINE SITES: p.1031

(SELF-HELP) Steam inhalation

Inhaling steam from a bowl of hot water can be used to relieve some of the symptoms of colds, sore throats, sinusitis, and laryngitis. The moisture in the steam helps to loosen secretions in congested lungs and in the nose and throat, making them easier to clear. Alternatively, you can run hot water while you are in the bathroom and inhale the steam. Children should not carry out steam inhalation unless they are supervised by an adult.

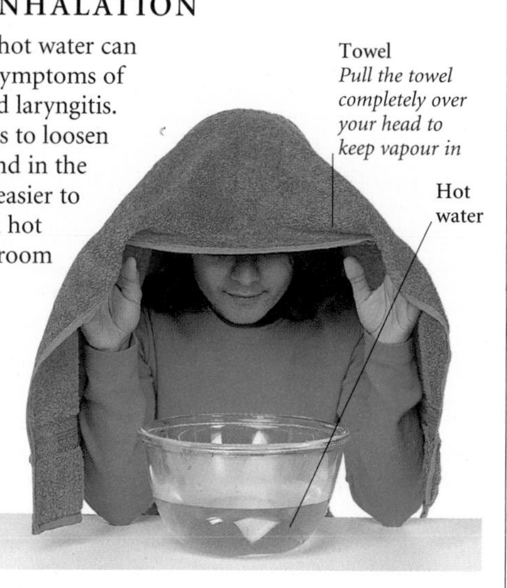

Inhaling steam
Fill a bowl one-third full with hot water. Lean forwards, pull a towel completely over your head and the bowl, and inhale steam for several minutes.

TEST ENDOSCOPY OF THE NOSE AND THROAT

Endoscopy can be used to look at the internal structures of the nose and throat as well as to diagnose disorders such as nasal polyps or cancer of the larynx. During the procedure, an endoscope is inserted up each nostril in turn and into the nasal cavity. The instrument may be flexible or rigid; flexible endoscopy is mainly used to examine the back of the throat and the larynx. Endoscopy is carried out under local anaesthesia. The procedure can be repeated easily to monitor the progress of a disorder or treatment.

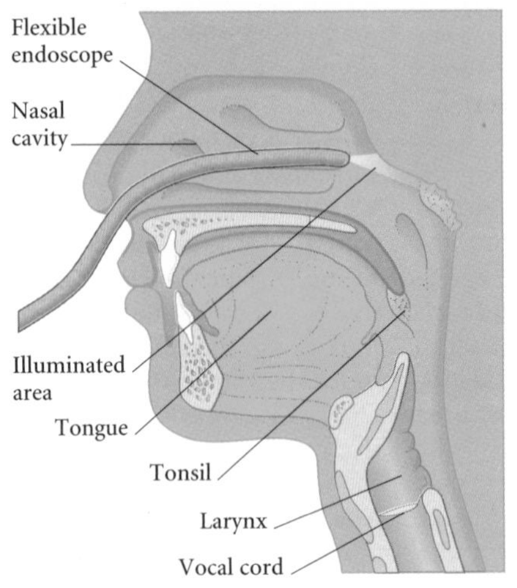

During the procedure
The endoscope is used to examine the nasal cavity and sometimes also the larynx. Instruments inserted through the endoscope can collect tissue samples or remove minor abnormalities, such as polyps.

VIEW

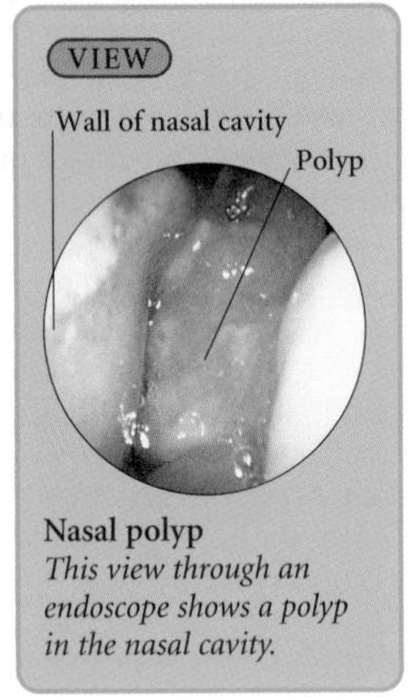

Nasal polyp
This view through an endoscope shows a polyp in the nasal cavity.

Deviated nasal septum

An abnormality of the partition that separates the nostrils

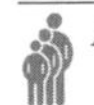 AGE Often present at birth

 GENDER More common in males

 LIFESTYLE Playing contact sports, such as football, is a risk factor

 GENETICS Not a significant factor

Sometimes, the wall of cartilage and bone that divides the nostrils, called the nasal septum, is slightly misshapen or deviated but causes no problems. However, in some people, the nasal septum is very misshapen and blocks one side of the nose, impairing breathing. The defect is sometimes associated with snoring (opposite page).

A mildly deviated nasal septum is often present from birth. In other cases, the condition results from a blow to the nose, usually due to a fall or an athletic injury. A deviated septum occurs more commonly in men because men are more likely to participate in contact sports that may lead to this type of injury. A severely deviated nasal septum may increase the risk of infections in the sinuses (*see* SINUSITIS, p.475).

If you have a deviated septum that causes recurrent sinusitis or breathing difficulties, your doctor may recommend surgery. The deviated septum is straightened by realigning the cartilage and bone or by removing them. Surgery is carried out under local or general anaesthesia and is usually successful.

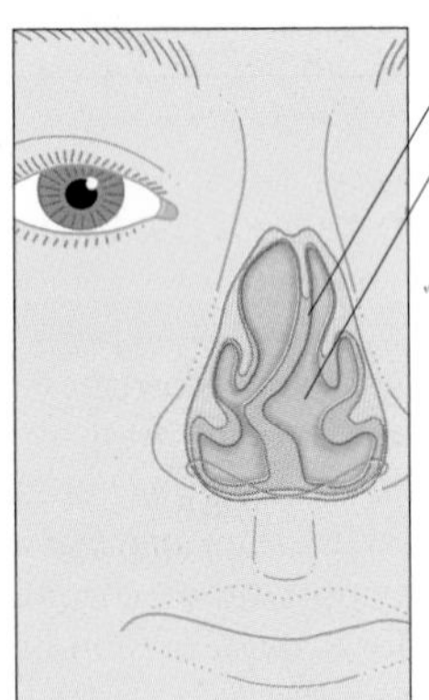

Deviated nasal septum
A misshapen nasal septum is not usually a problem, but a severe deviation may obstruct breathing.

WWW ONLINE SITES: p.1031

Nasal polyps

Fleshy growths of the mucus-secreting lining of the nose

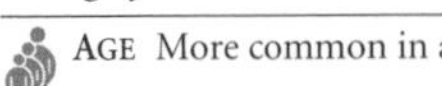 AGE More common in adults

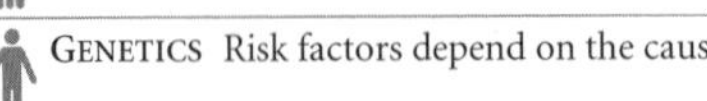 GENETICS Risk factors depend on the cause

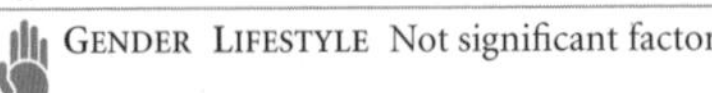 GENDER LIFESTYLE Not significant factors

Growths that develop in the mucus-secreting lining of the nose are known as nasal polyps. The exact cause of nasal polyps is not known. However, they are more common in people who have asthma (p.483) or rhinitis, a condition in which the membrane that lines the nose and throat becomes inflamed. Although polyps rarely occur in children, they do sometimes develop in children who have the inherited condition cystic fibrosis (p.824).

WHAT ARE THE SYMPTOMS?

The symptoms of nasal polyps often develop gradually over months. The severity of the symptoms depends on the number and the size of the polyps. Symptoms may include:

- Blocked nose due to obstruction by the polyps.
- Decreased sense of smell.
- In some cases, a runny nose due to excess secretion of mucus.

Nasal polyps may lead to recurrent sinusitis (p.475) if the narrow channels that drain mucus from the sinuses become blocked by the polyps and the sinuses become inflamed.

WHAT MIGHT BE DONE?

If your doctor suspects that you have nasal polyps but cannot see them easily, he or she may arrange for you to have endoscopy of the nose (*see* ENDOSCOPY OF THE NOSE AND THROAT, above). You may also have CT scanning (p.247) if the number and size of the polyps cannot be assessed with an endoscope. If there is a single polyp, a small sample of the polyp may be removed and examined under a microscope to exclude cancer.

Small nasal polyps may be treated by using a corticosteroid nasal spray, which shrinks the polyps over a few weeks.

Larger polyps may be removed during an endoscopic procedure. A corticosteroid spray may also be necessary for several months after surgery to prevent the polyps from recurring. In more severe cases, a course of oral corticosteroids (p.930) may also be prescribed.

(WWW) ONLINE SITES: p.1031

Snoring

Noisy breathing during sleep, which may be a symptom of the more serious disorder sleep apnoea

 AGE Most common in children and in adults between the ages of 40 and 60

 GENDER More common in males

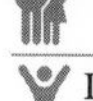 LIFESTYLE Being overweight, drinking alcohol, and smoking are risk factors

 GENETICS Not a significant factor

Snoring is the sound made by the vibration of the soft tissues at the back of the mouth. Although it is often considered to be an insignificant problem, the disturbance and loss of sleep caused by snoring can be distressing both to the people who are affected and their partners. Loud snoring may also be an early symptom of sleep apnoea (right). The condition is most common in children and adults between the ages of 40 and 60 and particularly affects men.

WHAT ARE THE CAUSES?

Vibration of the soft palate may be caused by an obstruction or narrowing of the nasopharynx (the passage leading from the back of the nasal cavity to the throat). The nasopharynx may become obstructed if you are overweight. Sleeping on your back can make snoring worse because the nasopharynx is more likely to become partly blocked if you lie in this position.

Other causes of snoring include narrowing of the nasopharynx caused by relaxation or swelling of the tissues of the soft palate. Relaxation may be the result of drinking alcohol or taking sedatives. Swelling may be caused by a throat infection or irritation of the soft palate by tobacco smoke.

Snoring also occurs because of congestion due to a common cold (p.288). In some cases, an anatomical abnormality such as a deviated nasal septum (opposite page) may be associated with snoring. In children, the condition usually occurs as a result of enlarged tonsils and adenoids (p.842).

WHAT CAN I DO?

If you have other symptoms, such as daytime sleepiness or lack of concentration, you should consult your doctor in case you have sleep apnoea. Otherwise, the following self-help measures may bring relief. You may be able to prevent snoring by making it uncomfortable to sleep on your back, perhaps by sewing a small object, such as a tennis ball, into the back of your night clothes. If you are overweight, it will help to lose weight. You should also give up smoking, reduce alcohol consumption, and avoid taking sedatives or drinking alcohol before going to bed.

(WWW) ONLINE SITES: p.1031

Sleep apnoea

Repeated temporary interruption of breathing during sleep

 AGE Most common in children and in adults between the ages of 40 and 60

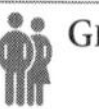 GENDER More common in males

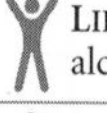 LIFESTYLE Being overweight, drinking alcohol, and smoking are risk factors

GENETICS Not a significant factor

In sleep apnoea, breathing stops during sleep for at least 10 seconds at least five times an hour. Mild sleep apnoea causes few symptoms, but severe sleep apnoea may lead to low oxygen levels, which can cause serious symptoms. Sleep apnoea is more common in people who smoke, drink alcohol, or are overweight. It may occur at high altitudes.

(TEST) SLEEP STUDIES

Sleep studies monitor the changes in body processes during a period of normal sleep. Variables that are usually monitored during sleep include oxygen levels in the blood, brain activity, heart rate, blood pressure, airflow in the respiratory passages, and movement of the chest wall and the abdomen. If you undergo testing in a sleep laboratory, you may need to stay overnight.

Monitor

Control panel

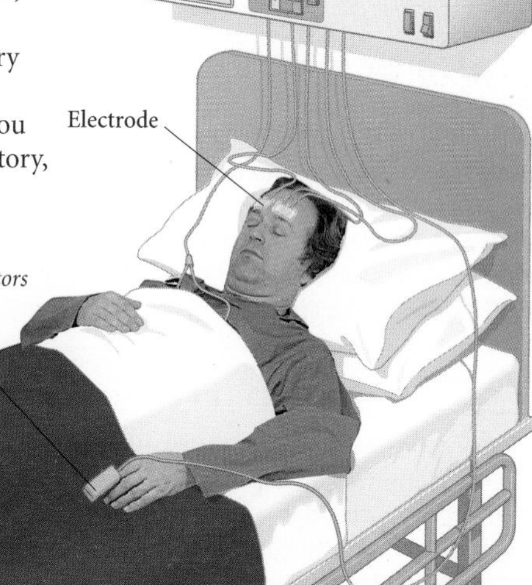

In the sleep laboratory *You will be attached to instruments that will continuously monitor various body functions while you are sleeping.*

Oximeter *This monitors oxygen levels*

(RESULTS)

Trace indicating sleep apnoea *A trace of a 2.5 minute period of sleep shows oxygen levels falling each time breathing temporarily stops, indicating sleep apnoea. The heart rate rises in response to the lower oxygen levels.*

Oxygen level (%): 100, 90, 80, 70, 60, 50, 40
Heart rate (beats/min): 150, 100, 50
Time (minutes): 0, 0.5, 1, 1.5, 2, 2.5
Normal oxygen level
Low oxygen level
Raised heart rate

What are the types?

Sleep apnoea can be divided into two types: obstructive sleep apnoea (OSA), which is common and due to blockage of the airway, and central sleep apnoea, which is rare and caused by a problem with the nerves that control breathing. In some cases, a mixture of both types of sleep apnoea occurs.

OBSTRUCTIVE SLEEP APNOEA This condition mainly affects men aged between 40 and 60. OSA occurs when the air passages in the upper respiratory tract become obstructed during sleep. Most commonly, obstruction is caused by the soft tissue of the pharynx relaxing and blocking the flow of air. The obstruction prevents breathing until the low levels of oxygen in the blood cause a person to respond by waking up and taking a deep, snorting breath. Being overweight (particularly around the neck area) or having a large tongue or a small mouth can also cause or contribute to the obstruction. In children, enlarged tonsils (*see* TONSILLITIS, p.843) or enlarged adenoids (p.842) are the most common causes of obstruction that can lead to OSA.

CENTRAL SLEEP APNOEA In this rare type of sleep apnoea, the region of the brain and the nerves that regulate breathing do not function normally, and this causes breathing to be impaired. Causes of central sleep apnoea include brain damage following a head injury (p.521) or a stroke (p.532).

What are the symptoms?

The symptoms of OSA develop gradually, and it may be a partner or another member of your family who first notices your disturbed sleep. Central sleep apnoea may develop suddenly, depending on the cause. Symptoms of both types may include:

- Restless, unrefreshing sleep.
- Daytime sleepiness.
- Poor memory and concentration.
- Headache in the morning.
- Loud snoring (p.477).
- Change in personality.
- In men, impotence (p.770).
- Frequent passing of urine at night.

In severe cases, daytime sleepiness may result in accidents, such as when driving. Taking sleeping drugs (p.915) and drinking alcohol may aggravate the symptoms. Left untreated, complications may develop, such as an irregular heartbeat (*see* ARRHYTHMIAS, p.415) and pulmonary hypertension (p.505). There is also an increased risk of high blood pressure developing (*see* HYPERTENSION, p.403). Severe sleep apnoea may eventually be life-threatening.

How is it diagnosed?

If your doctor suspects that you have sleep apnoea, he or she will examine your nose and throat to look for an obvious cause of obstruction to your breathing. You may also have an endoscopy of the nose and throat (p.476) and X-rays (p.244) or CT scanning (p.247) of the head and neck. To confirm the diagnosis, you may be asked to undergo sleep studies (p.477), in which variables such as your breathing, oxygen levels in your blood, and your heart rate are measured while you are asleep. Sleep studies may also help in assessing the severity of sleep apnoea.

What is the treatment?

If you have mild OSA, you should avoid sleeping drugs and alcohol. If you are overweight, losing weight often helps. You should also try to sleep on your side, which may relieve the symptoms. If it is caused by high altitudes, sleep apnoea should disappear when you acclimatize or return to lower altitudes.

The first choice of treatment for OSA is usually positive pressure ventilation (below). In this procedure, air is steadily pumped through a tightly-fitting nasal mask. The increased air pressure keeps the airways open so that breathing is easier. The treatment is easy to use, but some people find the mask difficult to tolerate. If positive pressure ventilation is not effective, surgery to reconstruct the soft palate may be considered. If OSA is caused by enlarged tonsils or adenoids, surgery may be necessary to remove them (*see* TONSILLECTOMY AND ADENOIDECTOMY, p.843).

Treatment for OSA is usually successful. Central sleep apnoea is more difficult to treat because, in most cases, the underlying causes are less likely to be reversed. However, for some people, drugs that act on the brain to stimulate breathing may be helpful.

(WWW) ONLINE SITES: p.1031, p.1036

TREATMENT Positive pressure ventilation

During positive pressure ventilation, a steady supply of air is pumped to the nose during sleep through a tube and mask. The high pressure of the pumped air keeps the upper airways open. Positive pressure ventilation may be used to treat people with sleep apnoea, in which breathing repeatedly ceases for short periods of time during sleep. The treatment needs to be carried out every night during sleep, and it can be given easily at home.

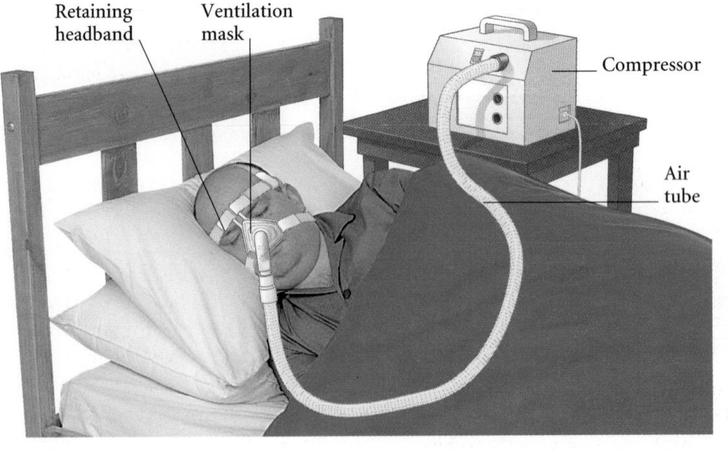

Wearing the mask

A compressor supplies a flow of air at high pressure to the nose through a tube and mask. The mask is held in place by straps around the back of the head above and below the ears.

Pharyngitis and tonsillitis

Inflammation of the pharynx (throat) and/or the tonsils

AGE Pharyngitis more common in adults; tonsillitis more common in children

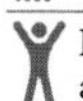
LIFESTYLE Smoking and drinking alcohol are risk factors

GENDER GENETICS LIFESTYLE Not significant factors

Pharyngitis and tonsillitis are common disorders, which are often described as a sore throat. The pharynx connects the back of the mouth and nose to the larynx (voice box) and the oesophagus. The tonsils lie at the top of the pharynx and help to defend against infection. Tonsillitis (p.843) is much more common in children because they have large tonsils, which shrink substantially as children get older. Adults tend to get pharyngitis. However, pharyngitis and tonsillitis can occur together in adults and children.

WHAT ARE THE CAUSES?

Pharyngitis and tonsillitis are usually the result of a viral infection, such as a common cold (p.288). Other causes include bacterial infections, such as with streptococcal bacteria, and fungal infections, such as candidiasis (p.309). Smoking and drinking alcohol may lead to pharyngitis in adults.

WHAT ARE THE SYMPTOMS?

Pharyngitis and tonsillitis have similar symptoms that tend to become worse over about 12 hours. They may include:

- Sore throat.
- Difficulty in swallowing.

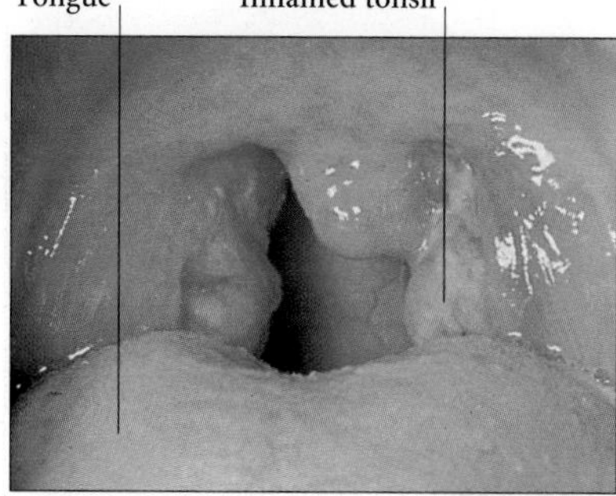

Tonsillitis
The tonsils shown here have become inflamed and covered with a white coating, a condition known as tonsillitis.

> **SELF-HELP SOOTHING A SORE THROAT**
>
> A sore throat may be caused by pharyngitis, tonsillitis, or both. The following measures may help to relieve the discomfort:
>
> - Drink plenty of fluids, especially hot or very cold drinks.
> - Eat ice cream and ice lollies.
> - Gargle warm salt water.
> - Take painkillers (p.912), such as paracetamol, in the recommended dose.
> - Suck throat lozenges containing a local anaesthetic (these are only suitable for adults).
> - Install a humidifier or place bowls of water near radiators to keep the air moist.

- Pain in the ear, which may be worse on swallowing.
- Enlarged and tender lymph nodes in the neck.

Pharyngitis and tonsillitis may also be associated with a fever and feeling unwell, especially if the conditions are caused by a bacterial infection.

ARE THERE COMPLICATIONS?

In severe cases, the pharynx and/or the tonsils may become so swollen that difficulties with breathing gradually develop. Occasionally, an abscess forms next to a tonsil, a condition known as a peritonsillar abscess. Rarely, if pharyngitis and/or tonsillitis is caused by a streptococcal infection, the kidney disorder glomerulonephritis (p.699) may develop some weeks later.

WHAT MIGHT BE DONE?

There are several self-help measures that you can take to ease a sore throat, such as drinking plenty of hot or very cold fluids and eating ice cream (*see* SOOTHING A SORE THROAT, above). Both pharyngitis and tonsillitis normally clear up with these measures after a few days. However, if the pain is severe or has not improved after about 48 hours, or if you have difficulty breathing or swallowing, you should seek medical advice.

Your doctor may take a blood sample to test for infectious mononucleosis. If the doctor suspects that you have a bacterial infection, you may be given antibiotics (p.885). A peritonsillar abscess may be treated with intravenous antibiotics. Alternatively, it may need to be drained under general anaesthesia. In some circumstances, it may be necessary to remove the tonsils.

Tonsillitis rarely recurs in adults, but children may have repeated attacks. Pharyngitis may recur throughout life.

WWW ONLINE SITES: p.1031

Laryngitis

Inflammation of the larynx (voice box), usually caused by infection and producing hoarseness

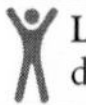
LIFESTYLE Smoking is a risk factor; drinking alcohol aggravates the condition

AGE GENDER GENETICS Not significant factors

Laryngitis is inflammation of the larynx, which lies between the throat and the trachea (windpipe) and contains the vocal cords. The condition may be acute, lasting for only a few days, or be chronic and persist for months. It is rarely serious but can cause breathing difficulties in children (*see* CROUP, p.841).

Acute laryngitis is usually caused by a viral infection, such as a common cold (p.288), but it may occur after straining the voice. Chronic laryngitis may be caused by smoking and long-term overuse of the voice, which may damage the larynx. Drinking alcohol, particularly spirits, may aggravate laryngitis.

WHAT ARE THE SYMPTOMS?

The symptoms of laryngitis usually develop over a period of 12–24 hours and vary depending on the underlying cause. Symptoms may include:

- Hoarseness.
- Gradual loss of the voice.
- Pain in the throat, especially when using the voice.

Sometimes, laryngitis is associated with vocal cord nodules (p.480).

WHAT CAN I DO?

Acute laryngitis that is caused by a viral infection usually clears up without treatment. There is no specific treatment for chronic laryngitis. For both forms of the condition, resting your voice can help to relieve pain and to avoid further damage to the vocal cords.

Inhaling steam while under a towel may also help to relieve symptoms (*see* STEAM INHALATION, p.475). To prevent a recurrence of chronic laryngitis, you should try not to overuse your voice. If you smoke, you should try to stop completely, and, if you drink heavily, you should reduce your intake of alcohol.

Since hoarseness can be a symptom of cancer of the larynx (opposite page), you should consult your doctor if a voice change persists for more than 2 weeks. He or she will probably arrange for you to go to hospital for mirror laryngoscopy (opposite page).

(WWW) ONLINE SITES: p.1031

Vocal cord nodules

Small, noncancerous lumps on the vocal cords, causing hoarseness

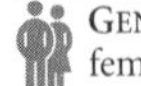 GENDER More common in boys and adult females

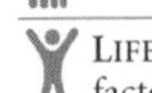 LIFESTYLE Excessive use of the voice is a risk factor

 AGE GENETICS Not significant factors

Constant strain on the voice sometimes leads to the formation of small, greyish-white nodules on the vocal cords of the larynx (voice box). Vocal cord nodules are noncancerous. The size of the nodules ranges from that of a pinhead to a grape seed. They sometimes cause scarring of the vocal cords.

The condition is common in people who tend to overuse their voices over a long period of time. For example, singers and teachers may be affected by vocal cord nodules. Drinking alcohol and smoking aggravate the symptoms. Nodules sometimes occur in persistently noisy children, especially boys.

The symptoms include increasing hoarseness, which develops suddenly or gradually, and rapid voice loss. You should consult a doctor if symptoms last more than 2 weeks because some types of cancer of the larynx (opposite page) have similar symptoms.

WHAT MIGHT BE DONE?

Your doctor will probably arrange for you to go to hospital for mirror laryngoscopy (opposite page) and possibly for a biopsy, in which a sample of tissue is removed using an endoscope (*see* ENDOSCOPY OF THE NOSE AND THROAT, p.476). If the nodules are small, you may be taught how to avoid straining your voice by a speech therapist (*see* SPEECH THERAPY, p.963). The nodules may then shrink or gradually disappear. Your doctor may suggest that you have larger nodules removed using laser treatment (p.951) or microsurgery (p.950). Sometimes the condition recurs.

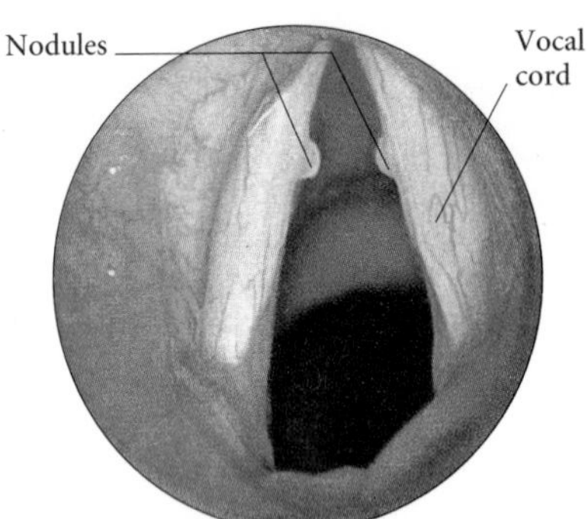

Vocal cord nodules
This view of the larynx (voice box) through an endoscope shows the vocal cords. A nodule can be seen on each vocal cord.

(WWW) ONLINE SITES: p.1031

Cancer of the nasopharynx

A cancerous growth in the nasopharynx, the passage connecting the back of the nose to the throat

 AGE Most common between the ages of 50 and 60

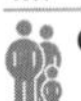 GENETICS More common in Chinese people

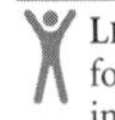 LIFESTYLE Smoking, alcohol abuse, eating foods containing certain chemicals, and inhaling some dusts are risk factors

 GENDER Not a significant factor

Cancer of the nasopharynx is a rare condition in which a tumour originates in the nasopharynx, the passage connecting the nasal cavity to the throat. This type of cancer occurs most frequently in Chinese people. The precise reason for this is unknown, but it may involve genetic factors or certain chemicals present in foods such as salted fish and fermented dishes.

Other factors that may increase the risk of cancer of the nasopharynx include smoking or using snuff, alcohol abuse, and a viral infection, especially with the Epstein–Barr virus (*see* INFECTIOUS MONONUCLEOSIS, p.291). People who inhale hardwood dust or nickel dust over a long period may also be at risk. If cancer of the nasopharynx is diagnosed early, it is usually easily treated. However, if the cancer is not diagnosed at an early stage, it may spread to the lymph nodes of the neck and to other parts of the body and in some cases can be fatal.

WHAT ARE THE SYMPTOMS?

Initially, cancer of the nasopharynx may not cause symptoms and may not be noticed until the tumour spreads to a lymph node, causing a painless swelling in the neck. If symptoms do develop, they may include:

- Facial pain and swelling.
- Earache and loss of hearing.
- Loss of sense of smell.
- Repeated nosebleeds.
- Blocked or runny nose, usually affecting one nostril only.
- Discomfort on swallowing.
- Repeated infection and inflammation of the sinuses (*see* SINUSITIS, p.475).

Left untreated, the cancer may spread to other areas such as nearby nerves, causing your voice to change or one side of your face to become paralysed.

WHAT MIGHT BE DONE?

You may have endoscopy of the nose and throat (p.476). If a tumour is found, you may have a biopsy, in which a sample of tissue is removed from the growth and examined for signs of cancer. You may have CT scanning (p.247) or MRI (p.248) to assess the size of the tumour and to see if the cancer has spread.

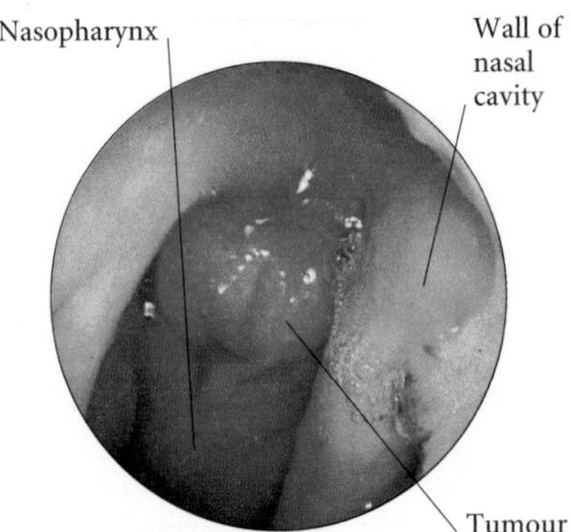

Cancer of the nasopharynx
This view through an endoscope shows a tumour in the nasopharynx, the passage connecting the nasal cavity and throat.

If cancer is diagnosed early, a cure is possible. The usual treatment is radiotherapy (p.281), although if the lymph nodes in the neck are affected, surgery may be required. Both procedures may also be used to relieve symptoms. The outlook depends on how far the cancer has advanced. If treated early, a third of people survive for more than 5 years.

(WWW) ONLINE SITES: p.1028, p.1031

Cancer of the larynx

Cancer of the larynx (voice box), often causing persistent hoarseness

 AGE Most common between the ages of 55 and 65

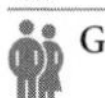 GENDER Five times more common in males

 LIFESTYLE Smoking and alcohol abuse are risk factors

 GENETICS Not a significant factor

Cancer of the larynx accounts for about 1 in 100 cases of cancer in men, usually in those aged 55–65. In about 6 in 10 cases, cancer develops on the vocal cords; in the remainder, it begins above or below the cords. If the cancer is on the cords, symptoms develop early, allowing prompt diagnosis and treatment. If cancer develops elsewhere in the larynx, it is more likely to be fatal.

The cause of laryngeal cancer is not known, but it may be associated with smoking, particularly when combined with alcohol abuse. Without treatment, cancer of the larynx may spread to the lymph nodes in the neck and eventually to other parts of the body.

What are the symptoms?

If a tumour develops on the vocal cords, the first noticeable symptom is hoarseness. If the tumour is not detected, it may spread above and below the vocal cords, causing symptoms such as:

- Loud breathing.
- Difficulty in breathing.
- Difficult and painful swallowing.

These symptoms may also occur if cancer develops above or below the vocal cords, although often these tumours do not produce symptoms at first. Tumours developing anywhere in the larynx may spread to the lymph nodes in the neck, causing them to become enlarged.

How is it diagnosed?

Your doctor will examine your throat (*see* MIRROR LARYNGOSCOPY, below). If cancer is suspected, you will have a further examination known as direct laryngoscopy. In this procedure, which is usually carried out under general anaesthesia, a tissue sample is removed. If the lymph nodes in the neck are enlarged, fine needle aspiration may be performed, in which a tissue sample is taken from a lymph node using a needle attached to a syringe. You may also have CT scanning (p.247) or MRI (p.248) to see how far the cancer has spread.

What is the treatment?

Treatment will depend on how far the cancer has spread. You may be offered radiotherapy (p.281), and you will possibly be given surgery at a later stage. If surgery to remove the entire larynx is necessary, you will need a permanent laryngectomy, in which a hole (stoma) is made in the windpipe (trachea) to maintain an airway for breathing. You may need a similar procedure called a tracheostomy temporarily while you are having radiotherapy, but it can be reversed when treatment is completed.

If the larynx has to be removed, normal speech will no longer be possible. However, several techniques have been developed that allow speech without a larynx. A speech therapist (*see* SPEECH THERAPY, p.963) may teach you to speak using your oesophagus, or a small device known as a tracheo-oesophageal valve may be fitted to help you to speak. Alternatively, you may be taught to speak using a hand-held electromechanical device that generates sounds.

In more than 9 in 10 cases in which the tumour develops on the vocal cords and is detected and treated early, treatment is successful. The chances of a cure are reduced if the cancer originates elsewhere in the larynx because symptoms appear later and the cancer may have already spread. In these cases, treatment may be given only to relieve symptoms, and survival rates are much lower.

(WWW) ONLINE SITES: p.1028, p.1031

(TEST) Mirror laryngoscopy

Mirror laryngoscopy is simple, quick, and painless and is used to detect disorders of the larynx (voice box), such as vocal cord nodules and cancer of the larynx. The procedure, for which a local anaesthetic is sometimes given, involves viewing the larynx by shining a light on to an angled mirror held at the back of the palate. You should not eat or drink until the anaesthetic has worn off to avoid inhaling food or fluids. If tissue samples need to be taken, you may need direct laryngoscopy.

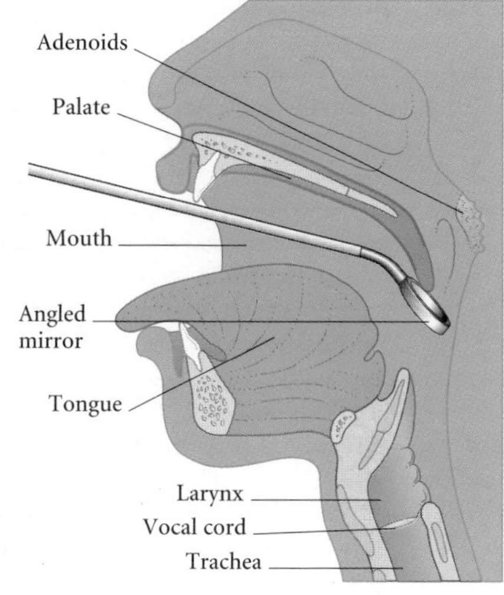

Viewing the larynx
After spraying your throat with a local anaesthetic, the doctor places an angled mirror at the back of the palate. This enables the doctor to examine the larynx and vocal cords for abnormalities.

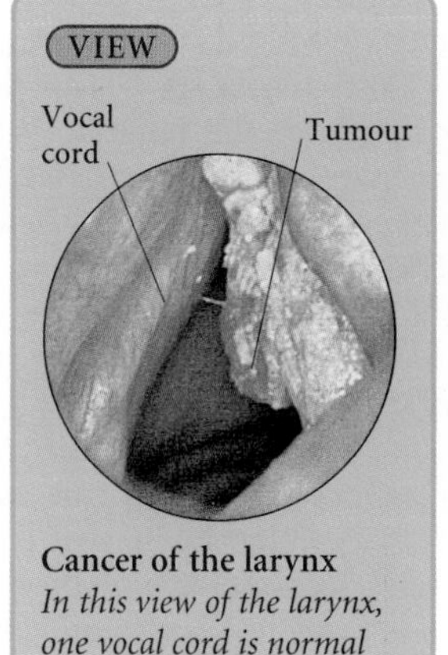

Cancer of the larynx
In this view of the larynx, one vocal cord is normal and the other vocal cord has a cancerous tumour.

LUNG DISORDERS

The lower part of the respiratory system consists of the trachea, which divides into the two bronchi and then into smaller air passages, and the lungs. The lungs can be damaged by many factors, such as inhaled smoke and dust, infections, and allergies. The resulting disorders vary in severity from mild conditions, such as a cough, to life-threatening illnesses, such as lung cancer.

This section starts with two common symptoms, cough and hiccups, both of which often clear up before a cause is found. More serious disorders of the airways are discussed next, including asthma, an increasingly common long-term disorder in developed countries.

Many common lung diseases, such as pneumonia and tuberculosis, are caused by infections. After discussion of these disorders, articles follow on disorders of the pleura, the double-layered membrane that surrounds the lungs. Occupational lung diseases caused by exposure to substances in the workplace, such as asbestos, silica, and coal dust, are then covered.

The next article discusses primary lung cancer, one of the most common types of cancer in the world and the most likely to prove fatal. Lung cancer is almost always caused by smoking. The final articles cover acute, potentially life-threatening lung disorders, such as acute respiratory distress syndrome.

Lung diseases specific to children are dealt with elsewhere (*see* INFANCY AND CHILDHOOD, pp.836–843).

KEY ANATOMY

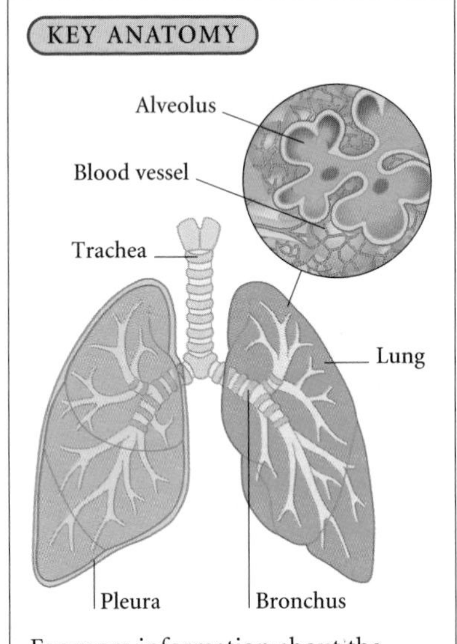

For more information about the structure and function of the lungs, *see* pp.470–473.

Cough

A reflex response to irritation or infection of the respiratory tract

 LIFESTYLE More common in smokers

 AGE GENDER GENETICS Not significant factors

A cough is a protective reflex action that helps to clear irritants or blockages from the airways. If sputum is produced, the cough is termed productive; if no sputum is produced, the cough is called dry.

Most coughs are due to short-term irritation of the respiratory tract and generally disappear spontaneously. In other cases, coughing may be a sign of a serious disorder of the lungs that requires medical treatment.

WHAT ARE THE CAUSES?

Many coughs are caused by irritation of the upper airways (the throat and trachea), either by inhaled particles or by mucus dripping from the back of the nose. Coughing is also often caused by inflammation of the upper airways, usually as a result of a viral infection such as influenza (p.289) or the common cold (p.288). Less commonly, a small foreign object, for example a peanut, is inhaled and causes violent coughing. Gastro-oesophageal reflux (p.636), a disorder in which acidic fluid from the stomach is regurgitated into the oesophagus, may result in a persistent cough.

More severe coughing may indicate damage to the lungs caused by inflammation associated with infections such as pneumonia (p.490), which is usually caused by bacterial infection, and acute bronchitis (p.486). In asthma (opposite page), the airways in the lungs become narrowed and inflamed, producing a cough that is often worse at night or following exercise. The lungs may also be damaged by smoking, which provokes a characteristic "smoker's cough". Such a cough may indicate the development of chronic obstructive pulmonary disease (p.487). A smoker's cough is frequently much worse in the morning before the chest has been cleared of mucus that has accumulated overnight. Smoking-induced damage to the cilia (tiny hairs) that line the airways interferes with the normal process by which the lungs are cleared of excess mucus.

If a long-term smoker's cough suddenly becomes more intense or occurs more frequently than usual, this change may indicate the development of primary lung cancer (p.503) and requires immediate medical investigation.

A cough may also develop as a side effect of ACE inhibitor drugs (p.900), which are used in the treatment of high blood pressure and heart disease.

WHAT CAN I DO?

The majority of coughs clear up after a few days without requiring treatment. However, you should consult your doctor as soon as possible if you develop a cough that persists for more than about 2 weeks. You should also seek medical advice if the cough is severe or painful, produces bloody or discoloured sputum, or is accompanied by symptoms such as chest pain or shortness of breath.

You may be able to relieve a mild cough with an over-the-counter remedy (*see* COUGH REMEDIES, p.909). For example, some coughs may be relieved by taking a cough suppressant, which works by inhibiting the cough reflex. However, cough suppressants should not be used to treat a productive cough because coughing is the body's natural mechanism for clearing excess mucus from the lungs. Steam inhalation (p.475) may help to loosen the mucus.

WHAT MIGHT THE DOCTOR DO?
Your doctor may be able to diagnose the cause by listening to your cough and examining your chest. Sometimes, chest X-rays (p.490) or lung function tests (p.488) are necessary to confirm the diagnosis. Drugs can relieve a cough, but the cause may require specific treatment. For example, antibiotics (p.885) may be used to treat bacterial infection.

(WWW) ONLINE SITES: p.1034

Hiccups
A sudden and involuntary intake of air, producing an unmistakable sound

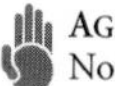
AGE GENDER GENETICS LIFESTYLE Not significant factors

Almost everyone has occasional attacks of hiccups. Usually, they last for only a few minutes and are no cause for concern. When you have hiccups, the muscles you use in order to breathe in, primarily the diaphragm, contract suddenly, causing a sharp intake of breath. This is interrupted almost immediately by an involuntary closure of the throat, which causes the characteristic sound of a hiccup. Hiccups occur even before birth; babies hiccup inside the uterus, possibly in preparation for breathing.

WHAT ARE THE CAUSES?
In most cases, there is no obvious cause for hiccups. If they are persistent, hiccups may be due to physical irritation of the diaphragm or the nerves that supply it. Such irritation may be caused by a gastrointestinal problem, such as abnormal stretching of the stomach as a result of an obstruction. In rare cases, hiccups are a symptom of a severe imbalance in body chemistry caused by disorders such as kidney failure (p.705) or liver failure (p.650).

WHAT MIGHT BE DONE?
There are a vast number of popular home remedies for hiccups, such as holding your breath or drinking a glass of water rapidly. If your hiccups are persistent, your doctor may prescribe a drug that relaxes your diaphragm, such as chlorpromazine (*see* ANTIPSYCHOTIC DRUGS, p.917). In rare cases, it may be necessary to paralyse the diaphragm by injecting a drug around the nerves that supply it or by cutting them.

Asthma
Intermittent narrowing of the airways, causing shortness of breath and wheezing

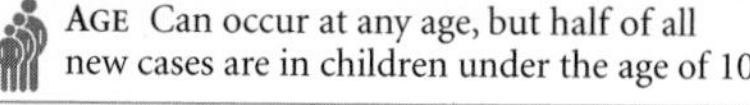
AGE Can occur at any age, but half of all new cases are in children under the age of 10

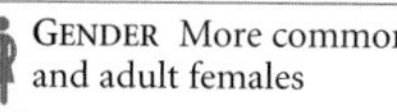
GENDER More common in male children and adult females

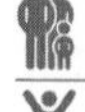
GENETICS Sometimes runs in families

LIFESTYLE Exposure to tobacco smoke and house dust mites are risk factors

People with asthma have attacks of wheezing and shortness of breath that vary in severity from day to day and from month to month. Some people have only occasional mild attacks, while others may experience severe disabling symptoms on most days. Most people have symptoms that fall somewhere between these two extremes, but, when their asthma attacks occur, they tend to be unpredictable in length and severity. Severe attacks of asthma are potentially life-threatening if they are not given immediate medical treatment.

Although asthma can begin at any age, most adults with the condition developed it as children. More boys than girls are affected but, in adults, asthma is more common in women. The problems associated with asthma and its management are different in children. For this reason, there is a separate article on asthma in children (p.839) in the section on childhood disorders.

HOW COMMON IS IT?
In the past 20 years, asthma has become more common in all developed countries. In the UK, asthma cases and deaths as a result of asthma have doubled since the mid-1980s for reasons that are unclear. Asthma now affects about 1 in 25 adults and 1 in 7 children. Each year in the UK, there are more than 85,000 admissions to hospital for the treatment of asthma, and about 100,000 people attend hospital for outpatient consultations for the disorder.

WHAT ARE THE CAUSES?
During an asthma attack, the muscle in the walls of the bronchi (airways) contracts, causing narrowing. The linings of the airways also become swollen and inflamed, producing excess mucus that can block the smaller airways.

In some people, an allergic response triggers the airway changes. This allergic type of asthma tends to occur in childhood, and may develop in association with eczema or certain other allergic conditions, such as hay fever (*see* ALLERGIC RHINITIS, p.466). Susceptibility to these conditions frequently runs in families and may be inherited.

Some substances, called allergens, are known to trigger attacks of allergic asthma. They include pollen, house dust mites, mould, and dander and saliva from furry animals, such as cats and dogs. Rarely, certain foods, such as milk, eggs, nuts, and wheat, provoke an allergic asthmatic reaction. Some people who have asthma are sensitive to aspirin and taking it may trigger an attack.

When asthma starts in adulthood, there are usually no identifiable allergic triggers. The first attack is sometimes brought on by a respiratory infection.

Factors that can provoke attacks in a person with asthma include cold air, exercise, smoke, and occasionally emotional factors such as stress and anxiety. Although industrial pollution and exhaust emissions from motor vehicles do not normally cause asthma, they do

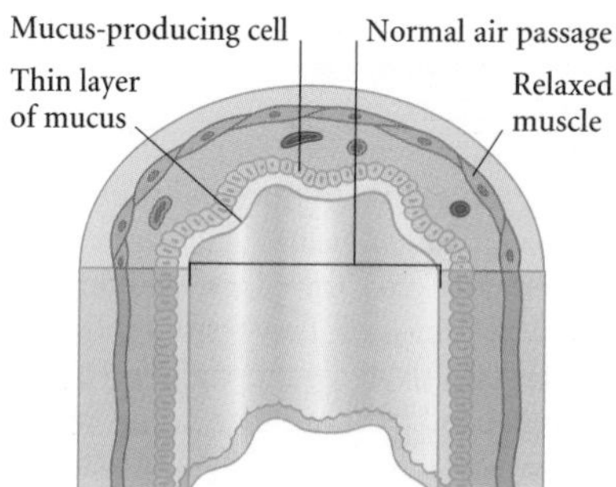

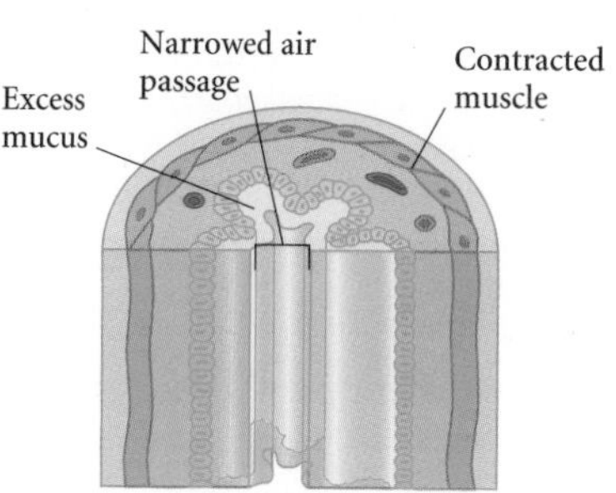

The effect of asthma on the airways
Normally, air flows freely through the airways. In an asthma attack, the muscles of the bronchi walls contract, and excess mucus collects, restricting the flow of air.

appear to worsen symptoms in people who already have the disorder. Pollution in the atmosphere may also trigger asthma in susceptible people.

In some cases, a substance that is inhaled regularly in the work environment can cause a previously healthy person to develop asthma. This is called occupational asthma and is one of the few occupational lung diseases (p.499) that is still increasing in incidence. If you develop wheezing and shortness of breath that improve when you are not in your work environment, you may have occupational asthma.

There are currently about 200 substances used in the workplace that are known to trigger symptoms of asthma, including glues, resins, latex, and some chemicals, especially isocyanate chemicals that are used in spray-painting. However, occupational asthma can be difficult to diagnose because a person may be regularly exposed to a particular trigger substance for weeks, months, or even years before the symptoms of asthma begin to appear.

WHAT ARE THE SYMPTOMS?

The symptoms of asthma may develop gradually and may not be noticed until a trigger provokes the first severe attack. For example, exposure to an allergen or a respiratory tract infection may cause the following symptoms:

- Wheezing.
- Painless tightening in the chest.
- Shortness of breath.
- Difficulty exhaling.
- Dry, persistent cough.
- Feelings of panic.
- Sweating.

These symptoms often become considerably worse at night and in the early hours of the morning.

Some people find that they develop mild wheezing during a common cold or a chest infection, but usually this does not indicate asthma. The main feature that distinguishes asthma from other respiratory conditions is its variability.

If asthma becomes severe, the following symptoms may develop:

- Wheezing that is inaudible because so little air flows through the airways.
- Inability to complete a sentence due to shortness of breath.
- Blue lips, tongue, fingers, and toes due to lack of oxygen.
- Exhaustion, confusion, and coma.

If you are with someone who is having a severe attack of asthma or your own symptoms continue to worsen, you need to call an ambulance.

HOW IS IT DIAGNOSED?

If you have had breathing problems recently but are free of symptoms when you consult the doctor, he or she will ask you to describe your symptoms and will examine you. Your doctor may also arrange for you to have various tests, such as spirometry, to measure how efficiently your lungs work (*see* LUNG FUNCTION TESTS, p.488). As part of these tests, your doctor may ask you to exercise for a few minutes in an attempt to induce a mild attack of asthma. Less commonly, the doctor will measure how irritable your airwaves are by getting you to breathe in a small dose of a test chemical. If you do have an asthma attack as a result of these tests, you will be given medication to relieve it.

If you are having a mild attack when you consult your doctor, he or she may measure the speed at which you exhale using a device called a peak flow meter (*see* MONITORING YOUR ASTHMA, left) and then ask you to inhale a bronchodilator (p.910), which relaxes the airways. Your doctor may be able to diagnose asthma if your peak flow rate increases substantially after you have inhaled the bronchodilator drug.

If you have a severe attack of shortness of breath, you may be treated and sent to hospital for assessment. Once you are admitted to hospital, the oxygen level in your blood will be assessed (*see* MEASURING BLOOD GASES, p.501), and you may have a chest X-ray (p.490) to rule out other serious lung disorders, such as a pneumothorax (p.496).

If you are diagnosed with asthma, your doctor may suggest that you have further tests at a later date to check for allergies to substances that are known to trigger attacks. If the timing and occurrence of your symptoms suggests that you have occupational asthma, your doctor will ask about substances used in your workplace to try to identify a specific trigger for your asthma.

(TEST) MONITORING YOUR ASTHMA

The best way to monitor your asthma is with a peak flow meter, which is used every morning and evening to measure the maximum rate at which you can exhale in litres per minute. The reading indicates whether your airways are narrowed. Plotted on a chart, your peak flow results show how effectively your asthma is being controlled. You can then adjust your treatment, following advice given to you previously by your doctor.

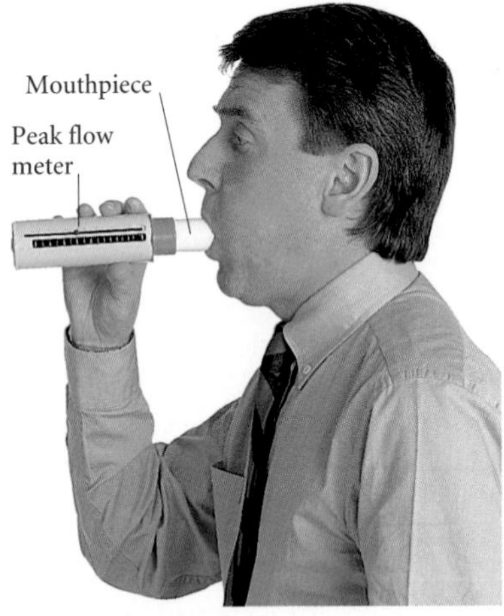

Using a peak flow meter
You should take a full breath in, seal your lips around the mouthpiece, and exhale as hard as you can. The pointer on the side of the meter shows your peak flow result.

(RESULTS)

Charting your peak flow
This chart shows twice-daily peak flow readings with marked variations between the morning and evening readings. These variations indicate that the asthma is poorly controlled.

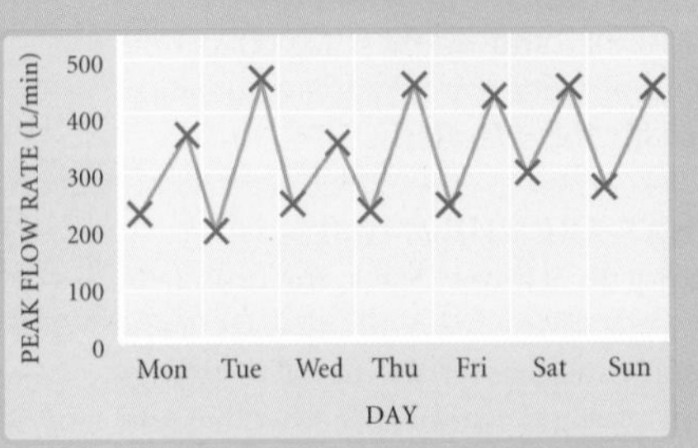

SELF-HELP TAKING INHALED ASTHMA DRUGS

Drugs to prevent or treat asthma are often inhaled. Inhaled drugs reach the lungs quickly and have few side effects because only a small amount of drug enters the circulation. A metered-dose inhaler delivers a precise dose when the inhaler is pressed. A spacer can be used to hold the dose before it is inhaled. For treatment of a severe asthma attack, a nebulizer, which enables the delivery of large drug doses, may be used. Different devices are available for children (*see* GIVING INHALED DRUGS TO CHILDREN, p.839).

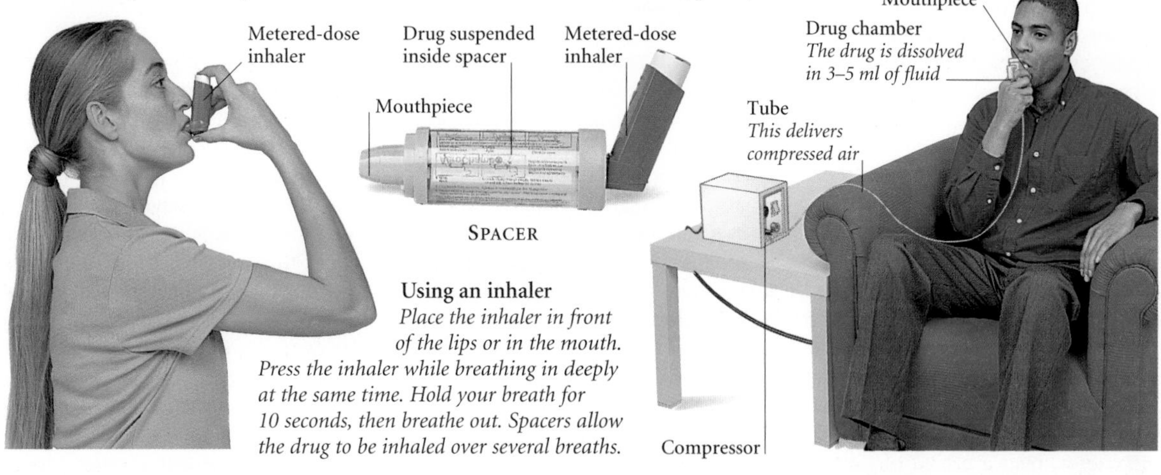

Using an inhaler
Place the inhaler in front of the lips or in the mouth. Press the inhaler while breathing in deeply at the same time. Hold your breath for 10 seconds, then breathe out. Spacers allow the drug to be inhaled over several breaths.

Using a nebulizer
A nebulizer creates a fine mist of drugs by forcing compressed air or oxygen through a liquid dose of the drug. The drug in mist form is then inhaled, through either a mouthpiece or a face mask.

WHAT IS THE TREATMENT?

Some people with asthma do not need treatment if they manage to avoid the factors that trigger their symptoms (*see* LIVING WITH ASTHMA, p.486). However, there are so many triggers that it is very difficult to avoid them all, and for this reason treatment is often necessary.

Today, asthma attacks can usually be treated with short-acting drugs. In addition, long-term maintenance treatment can prevent asthma attacks developing. The current approach to asthma treatment is to give you the knowledge and confidence to be able to manage the condition yourself on a day-to-day basis, in partnership with your doctor. The most important aspects of controlling your asthma effectively are the careful planning of drug treatment and regular monitoring of your condition.

The aim of all drug treatment is to eliminate symptoms and reduce the frequency and severity of asthma attacks so that visits to an accident and emergency department are no longer needed. Severe, potentially fatal attacks rarely develop without warning. Recognizing a serious change in your condition and taking prompt action by adjusting your treatment or contacting your doctor are essential to prevent an attack occurring.

TYPES OF DRUGS The drugs that are used to treat asthma fall into two distinct categories: quick-relief drugs (relievers), which are used to relieve an attack of wheezing; and preventer drugs, which help to prevent attacks occurring. Most relievers are bronchodilators. There are several different types of bronchodilator, all of which relax the muscles that narrow the airways and treat breathing problems as they occur. Relievers are usually effective within a few minutes if they are inhaled, but their effect lasts for only a few hours. They should be used as soon as symptoms develop or, if recommended by your doctor, before you start to exercise.

Most preventers of asthma are corticosteroid drugs (*see* CORTICOSTEROIDS FOR RESPIRATORY DISEASE, p.911), which slow the production of mucus, reduce inflammation in the airways, and make the airways less likely to narrow when they are exposed to a trigger substance. Nonsteroidal preventers, such as sodium cromoglicate and leukotriene antagonist drugs (*see* ANTIALLERGY DRUGS, p.905), are sometimes used to reduce the allergic response and to prevent narrowing of the airways. This type of treatment must be used on a daily basis and can take several days to become effective.

Both relievers and preventers are usually inhaled from a special device called a metered-dose inhaler, which delivers a fixed dose of the drug. Your doctor will show you how to use an inhaler. For acute asthma attacks, some people find drugs are most effective when inhaled using a spacer attached to the inhaler or through a device called a nebulizer. This device produces a fine mist of drugs to be inhaled through a mouthpiece or face mask (*see* TAKING INHALED ASTHMA DRUGS, above). Spacers are also useful if you find it difficult to coordinate releasing the drug and inhaling. Children may need to use spacers.

People with long-term severe asthma may be given preventers in the form of low-dose oral corticosteroids rather than inhaled drugs. Oral corticosteroids may also be given to relieve severe attacks.

DAY-TO-DAY MANAGEMENT Nowadays, adults with asthma are encouraged to take as much responsibility as possible for managing their condition. Asthma may vary in severity from day to day or over longer periods. For this reason, you and your doctor will probably develop an asthma management plan which helps you to assess your symptoms and make adjustments to your treatment accordingly. The key to controlling asthma is regular monitoring of symptoms and self-assessment using a symptom diary and a peak flow meter, which determines the rate at which you are able to exhale.

As you follow your management plan, your asthma treatment will move up a level, down a level, or stay the same, depending on your most recent symptoms and peak flow readings. A different level of treatment may involve altering a drug dosage; taking the medicine in another way, such as orally instead of by inhaling; taking a different drug; and/or using the treatment more or less frequently. If one level of treatment is not controlling your asthma, you move up to the next level.

If you are an adult newly diagnosed with asthma, treatment may start with a reliever drug only. Preventers may be added gradually if you find that you are using relievers more than a few times a week. Your doctor will closely monitor your progress over a period of time to determine whether your treatment plan needs to be changed. If you use your peak flow meter to monitor your asthma every day, you will get an early warning sign of worsening of your condition and can adapt your treatment in accordance with the prescribed plan. Discuss your treatment plan with your doctor and ensure that you understand it. Your plan should include specific advice on what to do if you experience a severe attack of asthma.

SELF-HELP LIVING WITH ASTHMA

Without doubt, the single most important aspect of controlling your asthma is the careful and planned use of drug treatments. However, there are several things that you can do to reduce your risk of an attack and to decrease the severity of your symptoms:

- Do not smoke and try to avoid polluted or smoky atmospheres.
- Take regular exercise to improve your stamina. Swimming is a particularly beneficial form of exercise. Avoid exercising outside when it is cold because this may provoke an attack.
- Avoid substances that are likely to provoke an allergic response; do not keep furry animals as pets if you are allergic to them.
- Always carry an inhaler, and be sure that you take medication with you on holiday.
- If your attacks are triggered by stress, try to practise relaxation exercises (p.75).

EMERGENCY TREATMENT If you have a sudden, severe attack of asthma, you should use your reliever inhaler as instructed by your doctor. If this treatment does not appear to be working, call for an ambulance immediately. If you have been given a reserve supply of corticosteroids as part of your treatment plan, taken them as advised by your doctor. You should try to stay calm and sit in a comfortable position. Place your hands on your knees to help to support your back; do not lie down. Try to slow down the rate of your breathing to prevent yourself from becoming exhausted.

Once you are in hospital, you will probably be given oxygen and corticosteroids and also bronchodilators at a high dose, either through a nebulizer or using a spacer. On the rare occasions when emergency drug treatment is not immediately effective, mechanical ventilation to force oxygen-enriched air into the lungs may be needed. Mechanical ventilation may have to be continued until the drugs begin to take effect and the airways relax.

WHAT IS THE PROGNOSIS?

The majority of children and adults with asthma are able to lead normal lives if they receive medical advice for their condition and then follow their treatment plans. Asthma that begins in childhood disappears by the age of 20 in at least half of all cases.

Generally, the outlook is excellent for adults who have asthma but are otherwise healthy as long as there is careful monitoring of their condition.

In spite of this encouraging outlook, more than 1,600 people in the UK die from severe asthma attacks every year. In most cases, the cause of death is a delay in recognizing the severity of an asthma attack and consequently a delay in getting to hospital.

(WWW) ONLINE SITES: p.1027

Acute bronchitis

Short-term inflammation of the airways, most often due to a viral infection

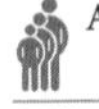
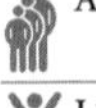
AGE More common in adults

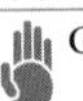
LIFESTYLE Smoking and air pollution are risk factors

GENDER GENETICS Not significant factors

In otherwise healthy adults, acute bronchitis may develop as a complication of respiratory infection. It is a recurrent problem for people with chronic obstructive pulmonary disease (opposite page), who often have several episodes each winter. In acute bronchitis, the lining of the bronchi (the main airways of the lungs), becomes inflamed, often due to infection. The inflammation produces a large amount of mucus, which is usually coughed up as sputum. In adults who are otherwise well, acute bronchitis does not usually cause permanent damage, but in older people or those who have a heart or lung disorder, infection may spread further into the lungs, causing pneumonia (p.490).

Acute bronchitis is often caused by a viral infection, such as a common cold (p.288) that has spread from the nose, throat, or sinuses. Smokers, people who have an existing lung disorder, or those who are exposed to high levels of air pollution are more prone to attacks.

WHAT ARE THE SYMPTOMS?

The symptoms of acute bronchitis usually develop quickly over 24–48 hours and may include the following:

- Irritating, persistent cough that produces clear sputum.
- Central chest pain on coughing.
- Tightness of the chest and wheezing.
- Mild fever.

If you have a long-term heart or lung disease and develop the above symptoms, or if you cough up discoloured sputum, indicating a secondary infection, contact your doctor promptly. If you have a reserve supply of antibiotics, take them as instructed by your doctor.

WHAT MIGHT BE DONE?

In a person who is otherwise in good health, acute bronchitis caused by a viral infection usually clears up within a few days. Taking an over-the-counter painkiller (p.912), such as paracetamol, may help to bring down your temperature. If you smoke, give up immediately.

If your doctor suspects that you have developed a secondary bacterial infection, he or she will probably prescribe antibiotics (p.885). You should make a full recovery within 2 weeks of starting treatment. If acute bronchitis persists, your doctor may arrange for you to have additional investigations, such as a chest X-ray (p.490), to look for an underlying lung disorder.

(WWW) ONLINE SITES: p.1033, p.1034

Chronic obstructive pulmonary disease

Progressive damage to the lungs, usually caused by smoking, resulting in wheezing and shortness of breath

 AGE More common over the age of 40

 GENDER Twice as common in males

 GENETICS Rarely, due to an abnormal gene inherited from both parents

 LIFESTYLE Smoking especially, and air pollution are risk factors

In chronic obstructive pulmonary disease (COPD), the airways and tissues of the lungs gradually become damaged over time, causing increasing shortness of breath. Eventually, some people with COPD become so short of breath that they are seriously disabled and unable to carry out even simple daily activities. COPD is twice as common in men and is almost always caused by smoking.

People with COPD usually have two separate lung conditions, chronic bronchitis and emphysema. Either one may be dominant. In chronic bronchitis, the bronchi (airways) become inflamed, congested, and narrowed, and this obstructs the flow of air through them. In emphysema, the alveoli (air sacs) in the lungs become enlarged and damaged, making them less efficient in transferring oxygen from the lungs to the bloodstream. Damage to the lungs caused by bronchitis and emphysema is usually irreversible, although coughing and sputum production may lessen after a person gives up smoking. COPD affects about 1 in 6 people over 40 in the UK, and is a leading cause of death.

What are the causes?

The main cause of both chronic bronchitis and emphysema, and hence of COPD, is smoking. Atmospheric pollution also contributes to the condition. For this reason, COPD is more common in industrialized areas where there is a high percentage of smokers in the population. Occupational exposure to dust, noxious gases, or other lung irritants can worsen existing COPD.

In chronic bronchitis, the linings of the airways of the lungs respond to smoke irritation by becoming thickened, narrowing the passages that carry air into and out of the lungs. Mucus glands in the bronchial linings multiply so that more mucus is produced, and the normal mechanism for clearing the airways and coughing up excess mucus as sputum is impaired. As the disease progresses, retained mucus in the airways easily becomes infected, which may lead to further damage. Repeated infections eventually cause the linings of the airways to become permanently thickened and scarred.

In emphysema, tobacco smoke and other airborne pollutants damage the tissues of the air sacs. The sacs eventually lose their elasticity, and the lungs become distended. Eventually, the air sacs tear and merge together, reducing their total surface area, and air becomes trapped in the dilated sacs. As a result, the amount of oxygen that enters the blood with each breath is reduced. In rare cases, the main cause of emphysema is an inherited condition called alpha$_1$-antitrypsin deficiency (p.489). In such cases, damage occurs whether or not the person smokes, but smoking accelerates the disease.

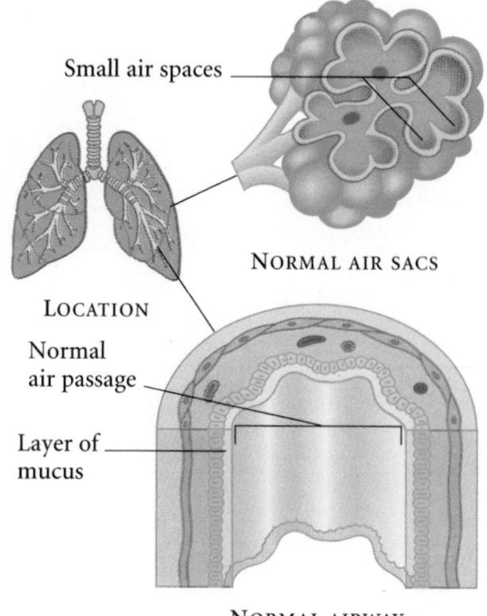

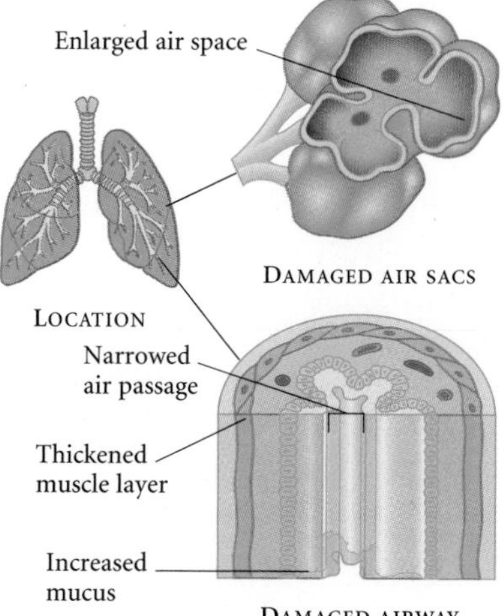

Damage to the lungs from COPD
In chronic obstructive pulmonary disease, the lungs are damaged in two ways. The air sacs of the lungs become stretched, reducing the area over which oxygen is absorbed, and the air passages narrow due to thickened walls and increased mucus.

What are the symptoms?

The symptoms of COPD may take many years to develop. When they do appear, symptoms often occur in this order:

- Coughing in the morning that produces sputum.
- Coughing throughout the day.
- Increasing production of sputum.
- Frequent chest infections, especially in the winter months, producing yellow or green sputum.
- Wheezing, especially after coughing.
- Shortness of breath on mild exertion, becoming progressively worse so that eventually breathlessness occurs even when at rest.

Cold weather and infections such as influenza (p.289) cause symptoms to worsen. Some people with emphysema develop a barrel-shaped chest as their lungs become distended. Respiratory failure (p.507) may develop, in which lack of oxygen causes the lips, tongue, fingers, and toes to turn blue. In addition, there may be swelling of the ankles caused by reduced kidney function and chronic heart failure (p.413). Some people with severe narrowing of

TEST LUNG FUNCTION TESTS

Two tests are used to detect airflow problems in the lungs: spirometry, which measures how quickly the lungs fill and empty, and the lung volume test, which shows how much air the lungs can hold. These tests distinguish between disorders that narrow the airways and those that cause lung shrinkage. Gas transfer tests (not shown) use a small amount of inhaled carbon monoxide to determine how fast a gas is absorbed from the lungs into the blood.

SPIROMETRY

A spirometer is used to measure the volume of air (in litres) that you can inhale and exhale over a period of time. The results show whether the airways are narrowed as a result of lung disorders such as asthma. Spirometry can also be used to monitor the effectiveness of certain treatments for lung disorders, such as bronchodilator drugs, which widen the airways.

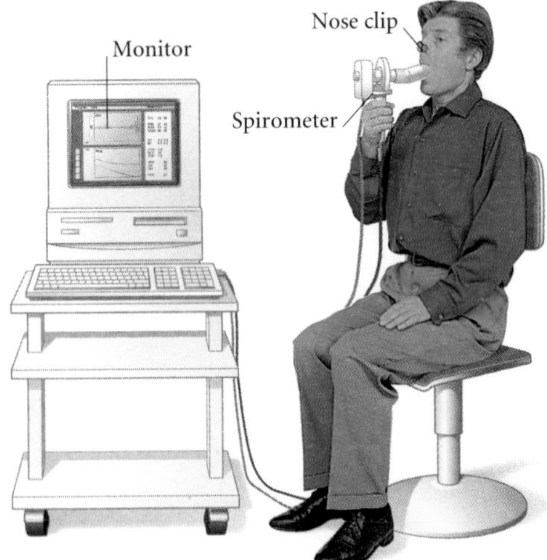

Using the spirometer
You will be asked to inhale and exhale fully through a mouthpiece several times. The volume of air inhaled and exhaled is displayed on the monitor.

RESULTS

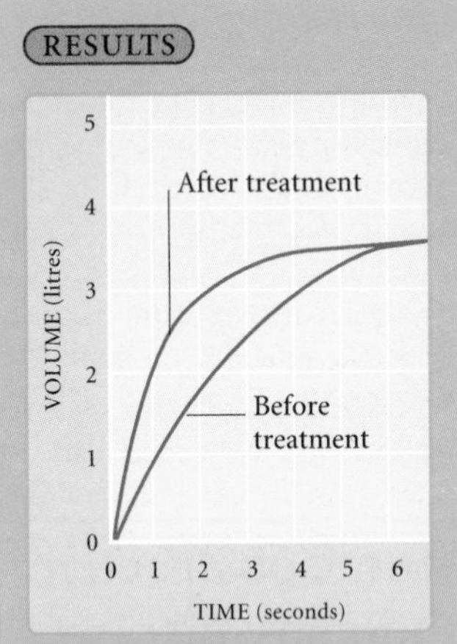

Spirometry graph
This graph shows the effect of drug treatment to widen the air passages in a person with asthma. The volume of air that is exhaled in 1 second rises from about 1 litre to 2 litres soon after the drugs have been taken.

LUNG VOLUME TEST

This test measures the volume of air (in litres) that can be taken in with a full breath and the volume of air that remains in the lungs when the breath is fully exhaled. The lung volume test is used to help diagnose disorders such as chronic obstructive pulmonary disease that affect the volume of air retained by the lungs after breathing out.

During the test
You will be asked to sit in an airtight booth and breathe in and out through a tube as fully as you can. The volume of air you can inhale and exhale is displayed as a graph on a monitor.

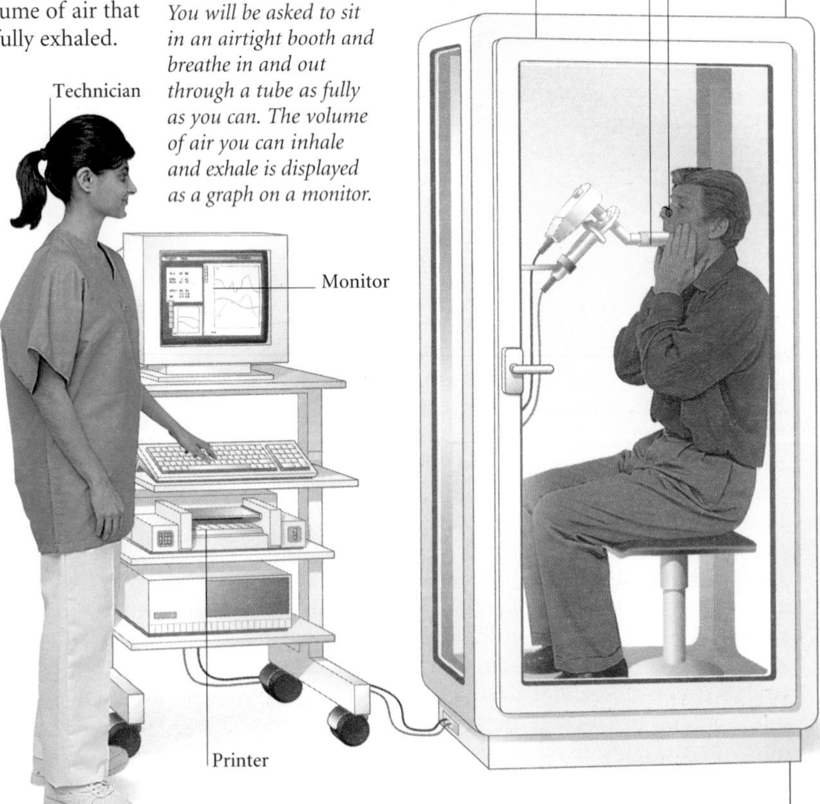

RESULTS

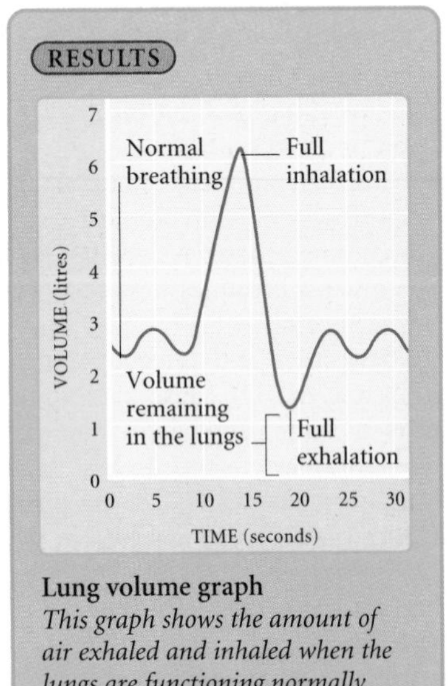

Lung volume graph
This graph shows the amount of air exhaled and inhaled when the lungs are functioning normally.

the airways compensate by working hard at breathing and manage to keep their oxygen levels within a normal range when they are at rest. They tend to have a rosy flush to the skin and may be thin because of the amount of energy they need to expend on breathing and because they find it difficult to eat and breathe at the same time. Other people with severe COPD can only manage shallow, ineffective breathing and consequently carbon dioxide builds up in the blood and oxygen levels fall. These people tend to have a blue complexion and tissue swelling in the feet and legs because there is insufficient oxygen reaching the kidneys. Their condition is often compounded by heart failure.

How is it diagnosed?

If you have a history of smoking, the doctor may suspect COPD from your symptoms and a physical examination. He or she may arrange for you to have lung function tests (opposite page) to assess the extent of damage to the lungs. You may have a chest X-ray (p.490) or CT scanning (p.247) to exclude other disorders and look for evidence of lung tissue damage. Part of the assessment of lung function may involve taking samples of your blood to check the levels of both oxygen and carbon dioxide (*see* MEASURING BLOOD GASES, p.501).

If members of your family have developed COPD before the age of 60, you may need a blood test to check the levels of the enzyme alpha$_1$-antitrypsin to look for a deficiency. Your doctor may take a sample of sputum to check for infection, and you may also have electrocardiography (*see* ECG, p.406) or echocardiography (p.425) to see if your heart is working unusually hard to pump blood through the lungs.

Chronic asthma (p.483) can produce similar symptoms to those of COPD. If your doctor suspects that you have asthma, you may be prescribed corticosteroid drugs (*see* CORTICOSTEROIDS FOR RESPIRATORY DISEASE, p.911). If your symptoms improve, this suggests that you have asthma rather than COPD.

What can I do?

If you develop COPD and you smoke, giving up permanently is the only action that can delay the progress of COPD. Simply cutting down on your smoking will have little or no effect on the progress of the disorder. Your environment should be kept as free as possible from smoke, pollution, dust, dampness, and cold. Gentle exercise may help to build up your tolerance to exercise, but it will not improve the function of your lungs. You should ask your doctor whether there is a pulmonary rehabilitation programme at a hospital near you.

How might the doctor treat it?

The damage caused by COPD is largely irreversible, but there are treatments that may ease the symptoms. Your doctor may prescribe an inhaler containing a bronchodilator drug (p.910) to open up the airways of the lungs by relaxing muscle in the bronchial walls. Some people may be offered continuous home oxygen therapy (p.507) to relieve shortness of breath. Low-dose oxygen must be used continuously for at least 15 hours each day to help to prevent heart failure and improve life expectancy.

If you have swollen ankles, your doctor may prescribe diuretics (p.902) to reduce the build-up of fluid. Antibiotics (p.885) may be prescribed if a chest infection develops. You should be immunized against influenza each winter, and you may also be given a further vaccine to protect against infection with the bacterium *Streptococcus pneumoniae.* Both of these infections are likely to be serious in people with COPD.

If the lungs are very distended, part of the lung tissue may be removed to allow the lungs to inflate and deflate more easily and increase oxygen in the blood. This procedure, called lung volume reduction surgery, is still being evaluated for its effectiveness.

What is the prognosis?

If your COPD is mild and has been diagnosed at an early stage, you may be able to avoid severe, progressive lung damage by giving up smoking at once. However, most people with COPD do not realize they have the condition until it is well advanced. For these people, the outlook is poor. They often need to retire from work early and may become inactive and housebound by shortness of breath. Fewer than 1 in 20 people with COPD survives for longer than 10 years.

(WWW) ONLINE SITES: p.1034

Alpha$_1$-antitrypsin deficiency

A rare inherited disorder that results in damage to the lungs and liver

AGE Present from birth, but effects usually appear after the age of 50

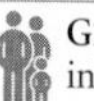
GENETICS Due to an abnormal gene inherited from both parents

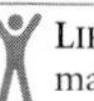
LIFESTYLE Smoking and drinking alcohol may hasten onset of symptoms

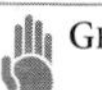
GENDER Not a significant factor

The enzyme alpha$_1$-antitrypsin prevents other enzymes in the body from destroying tissues, mainly those in the lungs and liver. People with alpha$_1$-antitrypsin deficiency lack this protective enzyme. The condition is rare and is inherited in an autosomal recessive pattern, which means that a person must inherit one abnormal gene from each parent to develop it (*see* GENE DISORDERS, p.271).

In severe cases, alpha$_1$-antitrypsin deficiency causes jaundice in newborn babies (*see* NEONATAL JAUNDICE, p.817). However, the effects of the disorder most often appear after the age of 50 and include damage to the air sacs (alveoli) in the lungs (*see* CHRONIC OBSTRUCTIVE PULMONARY DISEASE, p.487) and, less commonly, inflammation of the airways (*see* BRONCHIECTASIS, p.496). Liver cirrhosis (p.647) may also develop.

What might be done?

The diagnosis is made by measuring levels of the enzyme in the blood, and a blood test should establish if you have the abnormal gene. Other family members may also need to be tested. If you are planning to start a family, you may wish to consult your doctor about having genetic counselling (p.272).

At present, no specific treatment for alpha$_1$-antitrypsin deficiency is available, but trials of enzyme replacement therapy are in progress. Your doctor may prescribe inhaled bronchodilator drugs (p.910) to assist your breathing. People with severe lung or liver disease may be helped by an organ transplant. You should not smoke or drink alcohol if you have alpha$_1$-antitrypsin deficiency because these activities may cause lung and liver disease to worsen.

(WWW) ONLINE SITES: p.1034

Pneumonia

Inflammation of the alveoli (air sacs) of the lungs, usually resulting from infection

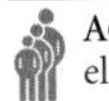
AGE Most common in infants, children, and elderly people

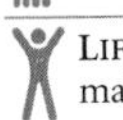
LIFESTYLE Smoking, alcohol abuse, and malnutrition are risk factors

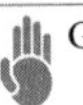
GENDER GENETICS Not significant factors

In pneumonia, some of the alveoli (air sacs) in the lungs become inflamed and fill with white blood cells and secretions. As a result, it is more difficult for oxygen to pass across the walls of the alveoli into the bloodstream. Usually, only part of one lung is affected, but, in some severe cases, pneumonia affects both lungs and can be life-threatening.

The cause of the inflammation is usually a bacterial infection, but other organisms, including viruses, protozoa, and fungi, may also cause pneumonia. Less commonly, inhaling certain substances, such as chemicals or vomit, causes inflammation, which may lead to a serious condition called acute respiratory distress syndrome (p.506).

Pneumonia used to be a major cause of death in young adults, but the great majority of people with the disorder now recover completely due to more effective antibiotics. However, pneumonia can still be fatal in elderly people or people with another illness, and it results in about 27,000 deaths each year in the UK. Some forms of pneumonia are becoming more difficult to treat due to the increasing resistance to antibiotics of some of the organisms responsible for the disease. For this reason, pneumonia is now the most common fatal infection acquired in hospital.

Infants, elderly people, and people who are already seriously ill or have a long-term disease, such as diabetes mellitus (p.687), are at the greatest risk of developing pneumonia. Other people more likely to develop pneumonia are those who have lowered immunity as a result of a serious disease such as AIDS (*see* HIV INFECTION AND AIDS, p.297). Impaired immunity can also occur during treatment with immunosuppressant drugs (p.906) or chemotherapy (p.280). People who smoke, abuse alcohol, or who are malnourished are also at increased risk of pneumonia.

WHAT ARE THE CAUSES?

Most cases of pneumonia in adults are caused by infection with a bacterium, most commonly *Streptococcus pneumoniae*. This type of pneumonia may develop as a complication of a viral infection in the upper respiratory tract, such as a common cold (p.288). Other common causes of bacterial pneumonia in healthy adults include infection with the bacteria *Haemophilus influenzae* and *Mycoplasma pneumoniae*.

The bacterium known as *Legionella pneumophila* causes a form of pneumonia called Legionnaires' disease, which can be spread through air-conditioning systems. Legionnaires' disease may also lead to liver and kidney disorders.

Pneumonia caused by the bacterium *Staphylococcus aureus* usually affects people who are already in hospital with another illness, particularly very young children and the elderly. This type of pneumonia can also develop as a serious complication of influenza (p.289). Other causes of pneumonia that are acquired in hospital include infection with klebsiella and pseudomonas bacteria. Viral causes of pneumonia include the organisms that are responsible for influenza and chickenpox (p.290).

In some cases, pneumonia is due to other organisms, such as fungi and protozoa. These infections tend to be rare and mild when they occur in otherwise healthy adults but are more common and potentially more serious in those with reduced immunity. For example, *Pneumocystis carinii* may live harmlessly in healthy lungs but can cause severe pneumonia in people who have AIDS (*see* PNEUMOCYSTIS INFECTION, p.308).

TEST CHEST X-RAY

A chest X-ray is often one of the first tests used to investigate lung and heart conditions because it is painless, quick, and safe. To create the image, X-rays are passed through your chest on to photographic film. Dense tissues, such as the bones, absorb X-rays and appear white; soft tissues appear grey; and air appears black. Damaged or abnormal lung tissue or excess fluid in the chest shows up as a white area because it does not contain air as it should. Chest X-rays are usually taken from behind, although side views may also be required.

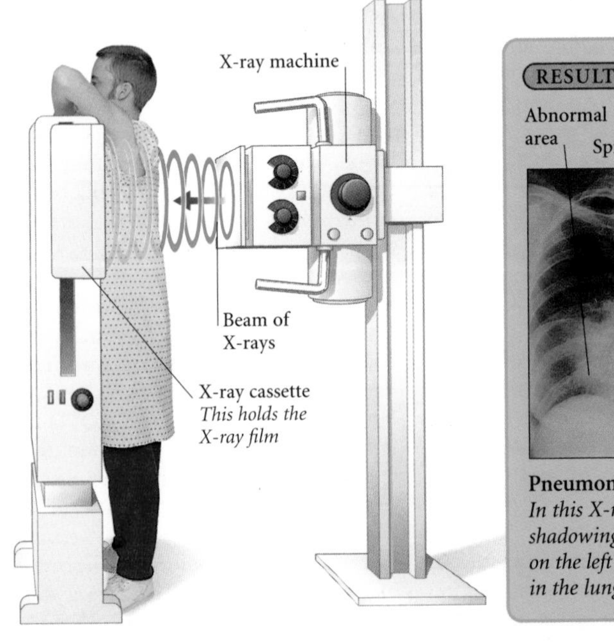

Having a chest X-ray
You will be asked to raise your arms to move your shoulder blades away from your lungs and to take a deep breath. While the X-ray is being taken, you must remain still to prevent the image from blurring.

RESULTS

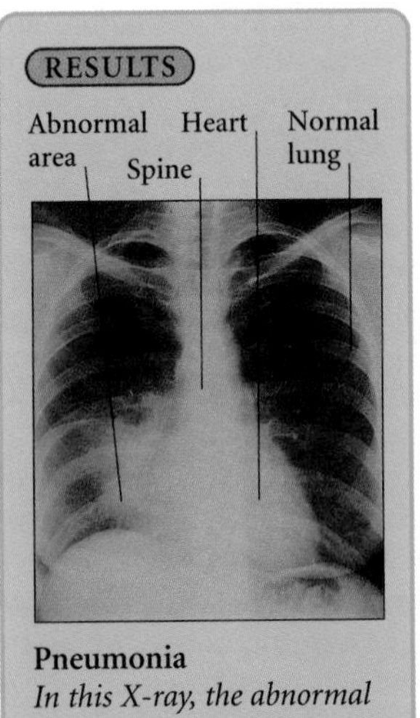

Pneumonia
In this X-ray, the abnormal shadowing in the lung seen on the left is due to infection in the lung tissue.

A rare type of pneumonia, known as aspiration pneumonia, may be caused by the accidental inhalation of vomit. Aspiration pneumonia is most likely to occur in people who have no cough reflex, often because they are unconscious after consuming an excessive amount of alcohol, taking a drug overdose, or sustaining a head injury (p.521).

WHAT ARE THE SYMPTOMS?

Bacterial pneumonia usually has a rapid onset, and severe symptoms generally develop within a few hours. You may experience the following symptoms:

- Cough that may produce bloody or rust-coloured sputum.
- Chest pain that becomes worse when you inhale.
- Shortness of breath at rest.
- High fever, delirium, or confusion.

When pneumonia is caused by organisms other than bacteria, it produces less specific symptoms that may develop gradually. You may feel generally unwell for several days and develop a fever, and you may lose your appetite. Coughing and shortness of breath may be the only respiratory symptoms.

The symptoms associated with all types of pneumonia are often less obvious in infants, children, and elderly people. Infants may initially vomit and can develop a high fever that may cause a convulsion. Elderly people may have no respiratory symptoms but often become progressively confused.

ARE THERE COMPLICATIONS?

Inflammation as a result of pneumonia may spread from the alveoli in the lungs to the pleura (the two-layered membrane that separates the lungs from the chest wall), causing pleurisy (p.493). Fluid may accumulate between the two pleura (*see* PLEURAL EFFUSION, p.494), compressing the underlying lung and making breathing difficult.

In severe cases, the microorganism that initially caused the infection may enter the bloodstream, leading to blood poisoning (*see* SEPTICAEMIA, p.299). In some vulnerable people, such as young children, elderly people, or those with a weakened immune system, the inflammation caused by pneumonia may spread widely into the lung tissue and result in respiratory failure (p.507), which is a life-threatening condition.

HOW IS IT DIAGNOSED?

If your doctor suspects pneumonia, the diagnosis may be confirmed by a chest X-ray (opposite page), which will show the extent of infection in the lung. A sample of sputum may be collected and tested to identify the organism that has caused the infection. The doctor may also arrange for you to have blood tests to help to reach a precise diagnosis.

WHAT IS THE TREATMENT?

If you are otherwise healthy and have a mild form of pneumonia, you can probably be treated at home. Painkillers (p.912) should help to reduce fever and chest pain. If a bacterial infection is the cause of the pneumonia, your doctor will treat it with antibiotics (p.885). If pneumonia is caused by a fungal infection, antifungal drugs (p.889) may be prescribed. No drug treatment is usually needed for mild viral pneumonia.

Hospital treatment will probably be needed in severe cases of pneumonia and also for infants, children, elderly people, and people whose immune systems are suppressed. In all these cases, drug treatment is essentially the same as for people treated at home. Severe pneumonia caused by a viral infection, such as infection by the varicella zoster virus that causes chickenpox, may be treated with oral or intravenous aciclovir (*see* ANTIVIRAL DRUGS, p.886).

If the oxygen levels in your blood are low or if you are short of breath, you will be given oxygen through a face mask. Less commonly, mechanical ventilation in an intensive care unit (p.958) may be required. You may have chest physiotherapy (p.962) regularly while you are in hospital to help to loosen excess mucus in the airways so that it can be coughed up as sputum.

WHAT IS THE PROGNOSIS?

Young people who are in good health are generally able to recover from most types of pneumonia within 2–3 weeks, and there is no permanent damage to the lung tissue. Recovery from bacterial pneumonia usually begins within a few hours of starting treatment with antibiotics. However, some severe types of pneumonia, such as Legionnaires' disease, may be fatal, especially in people whose immune systems are weakened.

(WWW) ONLINE SITES: p.1033, p.1034

Tuberculosis

A bacterial infection that most often affects the lungs but may also affect many other parts of the body

 AGE Most common in children and in adults over the age of 60

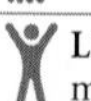 LIFESTYLE Overcrowded conditions and malnutrition are risk factors

 GENDER GENETICS Not significant factors

Tuberculosis (TB) is a slow-developing bacterial infection that usually begins in the lungs but can spread to many other parts of the body. TB can now be treated very effectively using oral antibiotics (*see* ANTITUBERCULOUS DRUGS, p.886), but, left untreated, it may cause long-term ill health and can be fatal.

Worldwide, TB causes more deaths among adults than any other bacterial infection. The disease is still common in developing countries. In developed countries, the number of cases steadily decreased during most of the 20th century due to improved health care, diet, and housing. However, since 1985 there has been a worldwide increase in the number of cases of TB. In the late 1990s, about 6,000 cases were being reported in the UK each year. This rise in TB is associated with an increase in travel and with the spread of strains of TB bacteria that are resistant to antibiotic treatment. Another factor is the emergence of HIV infection and AIDS (p.297), which lowers immunity, making people more susceptible to infection.

WHAT IS THE CAUSE?

The bacterium *Mycobacterium tuberculosis* causes most cases of TB and is usually transmitted in airborne droplets that are produced when an infected person coughs. Although many people are infected with the bacterium at some point in their lives, only a small proportion of these people develop TB.

When the bacteria are inhaled, an initial minor infection develops in the lungs. The outcome of this initial lung infection will depend on the strength of a person's immune system. In many healthy people, the infection does not progress. However, some TB bacteria lie dormant in the lungs, and the disease may be reactivated years later if a person's immunity is reduced.

In some cases, the bacteria enter the bloodstream and spread to other sites in the body. Rarely, the infection does not begin in the lungs but in another part of the body. For example, TB may affect the gastrointestinal tract if a person drinks unpasteurized milk from a cow infected with TB.

WHO IS AT RISK?

People with reduced immunity are more likely to develop TB. This includes people who are infected with HIV, those who have diabetes mellitus (p.687), and those who are taking immunosuppressant drugs (p.906). Others at risk of TB include people with long-term lung disease and those living in overcrowded conditions with poor sanitation or who have a poor diet. Generally, elderly people and children are more susceptible.

WHAT ARE THE SYMPTOMS?

During the initial stages of the infection, many people have no symptoms. However, some people may experience:

- Cough, which may be dry.
- Generally feeling unwell.

If the disease progresses, further symptoms usually appear over 2–6 weeks, but progression may be more rapid. Later symptoms may include:

- Persistent cough, which may produce greenish or yellowish sputum that is sometimes blood-streaked.
- Chest pain when inhaling deeply.
- Shortness of breath.
- Fever.
- Poor appetite and weight loss.
- Excessive sweating at night.
- Tiredness.

Untreated TB that begins in the lungs can spread directly to the tissue covering the heart (*see* PERICARDITIS, p.428). The infection may also be carried in the blood to the brain (*see* MENINGITIS, p.527), the bones, the lymph nodes, and many other parts of the body.

The onset of TB in areas of the body other than the lungs is very slow, and symptoms are not specific, making the condition difficult to diagnose. For example, the symptoms of gastrointestinal tuberculosis may be similar to those of Crohn's disease (p.658).

Abnormal area in lung | Heart | Normal lung

Chest X-ray in tuberculosis
This X-ray image shows an abnormal area at the top of the lung seen on the left due to an infection with tuberculosis.

HOW IS IT DIAGNOSED?

Your doctor may suspect TB from your symptoms and a physical examination. He or she may also arrange for you to have a chest X-ray (p.490) and possibly CT scanning (p.247) to look for evidence of lung damage.

If you are coughing up sputum, a sample will be sent to the laboratory so that it can be examined for bacteria and tested for sensitivity to particular drugs (*see* CULTURE AND TESTS FOR DRUG SENSITIVITY, p.234). In the meantime, you will be treated with a combination of antituberculous drugs.

Sometimes, a bronchoscopy (p.504) may be necessary to obtain lung tissue samples for examination. In addition, if your doctor suspects that you may have infection in a part of the body other than the lungs, such as in the lymph nodes, a sample of tissue may be taken from the area to look for TB.

If you have recently been in close contact with someone with TB bacteria in his or her sputum, you need to be screened. A chest X-ray may be carried out to look for signs of infection, along with a TB skin test, in which a substance extracted from TB bacteria is injected under the skin. The injection site is checked for a reaction 2 or 3 days later. A reaction indicates that you have been exposed to TB or immunized against it.

WHAT IS THE TREATMENT?

If you have TB, you will probably be treated at home unless you are very ill. You will be prescribed a combination of antituberculous drugs, which should be taken for at least 6 months. Using a combination of drugs helps to prevent the development of bacterial resistance to antibiotics. The drugs that are used depend on the antibiotic sensitivity of the bacteria and whether the infection has spread to other areas of the body. TB affecting areas that drugs do not penetrate easily, such as the bones, generally needs treatment for a longer period.

It is important to complete the full course of antituberculous drugs. Since it is very easy to forget to take the drugs, some people need help with their treatment using directly observed therapy, in which they attend a health centre regularly to be given the drugs under medical supervision. While you are undergoing treatment for TB, you will probably need to have chest X-rays and blood tests repeated on a regular basis to make sure that the infection is responding to treatment and to detect side effects of the drugs.

A BCG vaccine against TB is available, and immunization is routinely carried out in most parts of the UK at around the age of 13 (*see* ROUTINE IMMUNIZATIONS, p.45). Newborn babies in areas where there is a high risk of contracting the disease may also be immunized.

WHAT IS THE PROGNOSIS?

Most people make a full recovery from TB if antituberculous medication is taken regularly as directed. However, in people who have a type of TB that is resistant to two or more drugs, in those whose immunity is severely weakened, or in people with widespread TB, the disease may be fatal.

(WWW) ONLINE SITES: p.1033, p.1034

Pertussis

A bacterial infection, also called whooping cough, that causes bouts of coughing

AGE Can occur at any age but more common under the age of 5

GENDER GENETICS LIFESTYLE Not significant factors

Pertussis is a distressing and extremely infectious disease that is caused by the *Bordetella pertussis* bacterium, which infects and inflames the trachea (windpipe) and the bronchi (airways) in the lungs. The bacteria are transmitted in the airborne droplets that are produced when infected people cough and sneeze. Pertussis brings about violent fits of coughing that often end in a characteristic high-pitched "whoop" when the affected person inhales.

Pertussis is most serious in children under the age of 12 months, when the disease can be life-threatening. Before the introduction of a reliable vaccine, pertussis was responsible for a considerable proportion of childhood deaths in the UK. The incidence of pertussis has been greatly reduced by routine childhood immunization, and the number of cases of the disease reported each year in the UK is now fewer than 2,000.

What are the symptoms?

The first symptoms usually appear 2–3 weeks after infection. These symptoms are mild and resemble those of a common cold, typically a dry cough, runny nose, and sneezing. During this initial stage, which lasts about 7–14 days, the disease is highly infectious. Following this period, symptoms worsen and may include the following:

- Attacks of coughing followed by a sharp intake of breath that may produce a whooping sound. Bouts of coughing are often much worse during the night.
- Production of large amounts of sputum during coughing fits.
- Vomiting, which is caused by severe, repeated fits of coughing.

Episodes of prolonged coughing may cause small blood vessels to burst, resulting in a rash, especially around the face, hairline, and eyes. Nosebleeds may also occur if vessels in the nose burst.

Complications include pneumonia (p.490) and bronchiectasis (p.496), in which the airways become abnormally widened. Infants may stop breathing temporarily after a severe coughing spasm, and the resulting lack of oxygen may cause seizures and brain damage.

What might be done?

The doctor will probably be able to diagnose the condition in a child from the characteristic sound of the cough. However, in adults, the symptoms may not be so obvious. The diagnosis can be confirmed by taking nose or throat swabs to look for the pertussis bacteria under the microscope. Pertussis is normally treated with antibiotics (p.885). Antibiotics are effective in fighting the infection only when they are given early in its course. However, when given in the later stages, antibiotics are still useful because they ensure that infection cannot be passed to others. Seriously ill children need to be admitted to hospital for monitoring, and they may be given oxygen therapy and intravenous fluids along with antibiotics. To prevent the infection from spreading further, antibiotics may also be prescribed for people who have been in close contact with an infected person.

The symptoms of pertussis usually improve within 4–10 weeks if there are no complications, but a dry cough may persist for several months.

Can it be prevented?

The pertussis vaccine is usually given routinely in early childhood as part of the DTP (diphtheria, tetanus, and pertussis) triple vaccine (*see* VACCINES AND IMMUNOGLOBULINS, p.883).

Pertussis immunization may carry a small risk of inflammation of the brain, and your doctor will advise you if he or she believes your child is at risk of developing this condition. It should be kept in mind that the disease itself presents a far greater risk than the risks of immunization. Your child should receive the complete course of immunization, including the preschool dose.

(WWW) ONLINE SITES: p.1033, p.1034, p.1028

Pleurisy

Inflammation of the pleura, the two-layered membrane separating the lungs from the chest wall

AGE GENDER GENETICS LIFESTYLE
Risk factors depend on the cause

Normally, when people breathe, the two layers of the pleura (the membrane that separates the lungs from the chest wall) slide over each other, allowing the lungs to inflate and deflate smoothly. In pleurisy, inflammation of the pleura prevents the layers from moving over each other easily, and they grate as they rub against each other, causing sharp, severe chest pain when inhaling.

What are the causes?

Pleurisy may be caused by a viral illness, such as influenza (p.289), which affects the pleura itself. However, the disorder is often a reaction to damage to the lung just beneath the pleura. This lung damage may be due to pneumonia (p.490) or pulmonary embolism (p.495), in which the blood supply to part of the lung is blocked by a blood clot. The pleura can also be affected by primary lung cancer (p.503). Occasionally, an autoimmune disorder, such as rheumatoid arthritis (p.377) or systemic lupus erythematosus (p.461), in which the immune system attacks healthy tissues, affects the pleura and leads to pleurisy.

What are the symptoms?

If an infection or a pulmonary embolism is the cause of the inflammation, the symptoms usually develop rapidly over 24 hours. In other cases, the symptoms occur gradually. They may include:

- Sharp chest pain that causes you to catch your breath on inhaling.
- Difficulty in breathing.

The pain is often restricted to the side of the chest affected by the underlying inflamed pleura. In some cases, fluid accumulates between the layers of the pleura (*see* PLEURAL EFFUSION, p.494). This condition may actually lessen the pain because it eases the movements of the pleural layers over each other.

What might be done?

If you suspect that you have pleurisy, you should consult your doctor within 24 hours. He or she may be able to hear the layers of the pleura rubbing against each other when listening to your chest with a stethoscope. You may need a chest X-ray (p.490) to check for a problem in the underlying lung or for the presence of a pleural effusion.

You may be prescribed nonsteroidal anti-inflammatory drugs (p.894) to relieve the pain and inflammation. You may also find that holding the affected side while coughing helps to relieve the discomfort. In addition, you will probably need treatment for the underlying condition that is causing the pleurisy. For example, if a lung infection is the cause, you may be prescribed a course of antibiotics (p.885). If you have a pulmonary embolism, you will probably be given anticoagulant drugs (*see* DRUGS THAT PREVENT BLOOD CLOTTING, p.904). In the majority of affected people, the condition clears up within 7–10 days of the start of treatment.

(WWW) ONLINE SITES: p.1034

Pleural effusion

An accumulation of fluid between the layers of the pleura, the membrane that separates the lungs from the chest wall

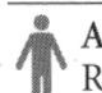
AGE GENDER GENETICS LIFESTYLE
Risk factors depend on the cause

A pleural effusion occurs when fluid accumulates between the layers of the pleura, the two-layered membrane separating the lungs from the chest wall. As fluid accumulates, the lung underneath becomes compressed, gradually causing shortness of breath. In some cases, the amount of fluid accumulated may be as much as 2–3 litres (4–6 pints).

WHAT ARE THE CAUSES?

In most cases of pleural effusion, the pleura itself is inflamed and produces fluid (*see* PLEURISY, p.493). The inflammation may be due to a lung infection, such as pneumonia (p.490) or tuberculosis (p.491), or to other disorders that affect the lung, such as lung cancer (*see* PRIMARY LUNG CANCER, p.503) or cancer that has spread to the pleura from elsewhere in the body, for example from the breast, ovary, or bowel. Less often, the cause may be an autoimmune disorder, such as systemic lupus erythematosus (p.461), in which the immune system attacks the body's own tissues.

In some cases, the pleura itself is not the cause of the effusion. Instead, fluid leaks into the space between the pleural layers as a result of a serious underlying disorder such as heart failure (*see* ACUTE HEART FAILURE and CHRONIC HEART FAILURE, pp. 412–413), cirrhosis (p.647), or kidney disease. In these cases, a pleural effusion is often associated with a build-up of fluid elsewhere in the body, such as in the ankles or abdomen.

A pleural effusion that produces little fluid may not cause symptoms. In severe cases, a large amount of fluid between the pleural layers compresses the lungs and may result in shortness of breath.

WHAT MIGHT BE DONE?

Your doctor may be able to detect a pleural effusion while examining your chest. You may also have a chest X-ray (p.490) to confirm the diagnosis and to assess the severity of the effusion. In order to identify the underlying cause, your doctor may take a sample of fluid by inserting a needle through the chest wall under local anaesthesia. A sample of the pleura may also be removed. The sample is examined under a microscope to look for evidence of infection or cancer. A sample of blood may be taken for testing to exclude other problems, such as kidney disorders.

Shortness of breath due to a severe pleural effusion may be relieved by removing some of the fluid through a tube inserted into the chest under local anaesthesia. Your doctor may prescribe antibiotics (p.885) if a bacterial infection is the cause of the effusion. Diuretic drugs (p.902) may be given to reduce the volume of fluid in the body. An effusion

TEST RADIONUCLIDE LUNG SCANNING

Radionuclide lung scanning is used to diagnose pulmonary embolism. It involves two scans that are performed simultaneously: one to assess blood flow through the lungs and the other, which is called a ventilation scan, to assess airflow. A diagnosis can be made by comparing the ventilation scan and the blood flow scan because many lung disorders disrupt the flow of both blood and air in a specific area, whereas a pulmonary embolism disrupts only blood flow. The procedure usually takes about 20 minutes to perform.

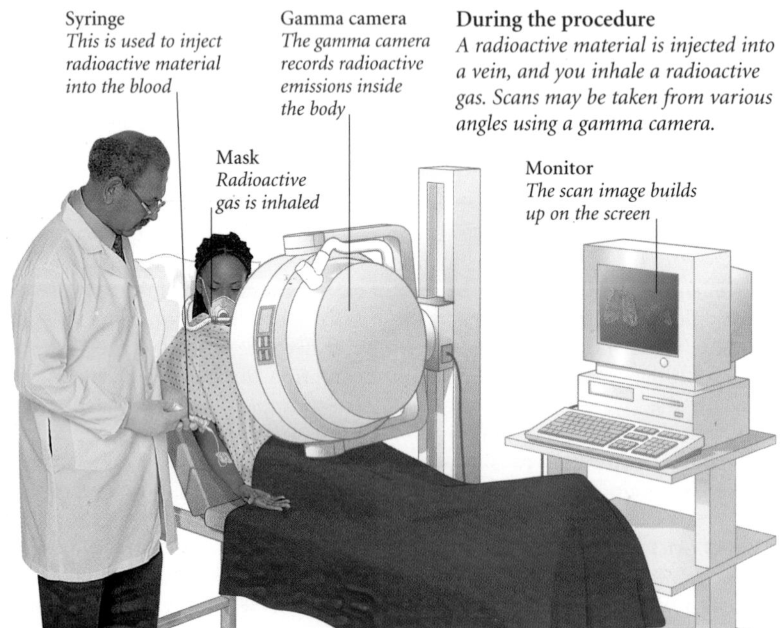

During the procedure
A radioactive material is injected into a vein, and you inhale a radioactive gas. Scans may be taken from various angles using a gamma camera.

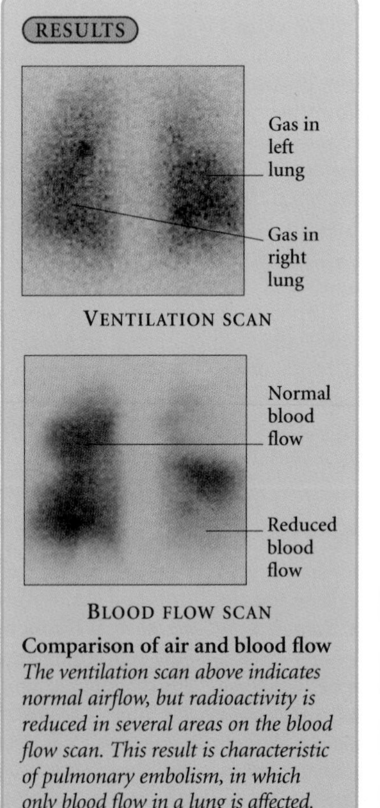

Comparison of air and blood flow
The ventilation scan above indicates normal airflow, but radioactivity is reduced in several areas on the blood flow scan. This result is characteristic of pulmonary embolism, in which only blood flow in a lung is affected.

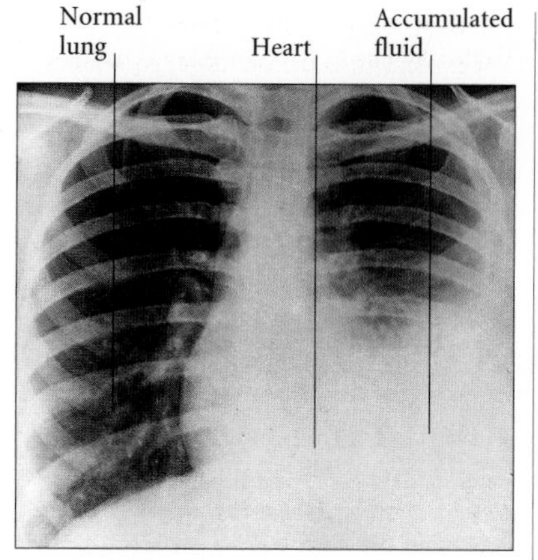

Pleural effusion
In this X-ray, the left lung (on the right of the image) is partly obscured by the accumulated fluid of a pleural effusion.

that is associated with lung cancer may be treated by chemotherapy (p.280), in which anticancer drugs are injected between the pleural layers, or occasionally by radiotherapy (p.281). Usually, the excess fluid slowly disappears once the underlying cause has been treated.

In some people, particularly those who have lung cancer, pleural effusion may recur. If the effusion does recur, a chemical can be injected into the chest cavity to make the two layers of the pleura stick together.

(WWW) ONLINE SITES: p.1034

Pulmonary embolism

Obstruction of the blood flow to the lungs by one or more blood clots

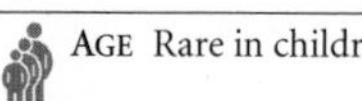
AGE Rare in children

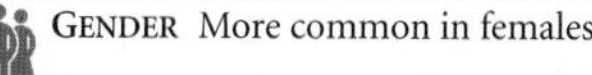
GENDER More common in females

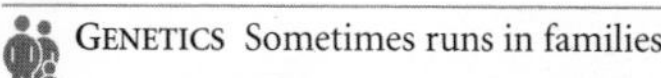
GENETICS Sometimes runs in families

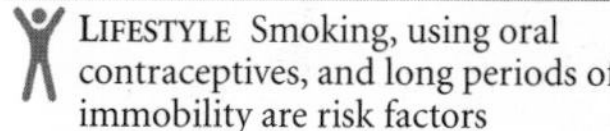
LIFESTYLE Smoking, using oral contraceptives, and long periods of immobility are risk factors

In pulmonary embolism, a piece of a blood clot (embolus) becomes lodged in an artery in the lungs and partially or completely blocks blood flow in the affected area. Usually, the clot has broken off from a larger clot in the veins of the legs or the pelvic region (*see* DEEP VEIN THROMBOSIS, p.437) and travelled to the lungs in the bloodstream. Pulmonary embolism may be mild if the blocked artery is small, but blockage of a major artery may suddenly cause severe symptoms and can be fatal. Rarely, small clots can block numerous small arteries in the lungs over months or years, and symptoms may not appear for some time. This condition is called recurrent pulmonary embolism.

Pulmonary embolism is most likely to occur in people who have developed deep vein thrombosis as a result of a period of immobility, such as that following childbirth or surgery (especially repair of fractures or pelvic surgery) or, rarely, during a long journey. A tendency to develop blood clots (*see* HYPERCOAGULABILITY, p.453) increases the risk of deep vein thrombosis, as does smoking and using combined oral contraceptives.

What are the symptoms?

The symptoms depend on the extent of blockage to the flow of blood. Massive pulmonary embolism, in which a large blood clot blocks a major pulmonary artery, may cause sudden death without warning. Single small clots may not produce symptoms. However, in most cases the symptoms develop over only a few minutes and may include:

- Shortness of breath.
- Sharp chest pain that is often much worse when inhaling.
- Coughing up blood.
- Feeling faint.
- Palpitations.

In some cases of recurrent pulmonary embolism, shortness of breath that worsens over months is the only symptom. Eventually, so many vessels may become blocked that pressure in the pulmonary arteries is increased (*see* PULMONARY HYPERTENSION, p.505) and chronic heart failure (p.413) may then develop.

How is it diagnosed?

If your doctor suspects that you have pulmonary embolism, you will be admitted to hospital as an emergency. You may be given tests to measure the levels of oxygen and carbon dioxide in your blood (*see* MEASURING BLOOD GASES, p.501). You may also have a chest X-ray (p.490) to exclude other lung conditions and radionuclide lung scanning (opposite page) to look at the flow of blood in the lungs. The blood flow in the veins of your legs may be measured by using Doppler ultrasound scanning (p.432). If the diagnosis is not clear, you may need to have CT scanning (p.247) or contrast X-rays (p.245) to image the blood vessels in the lungs and to pinpoint the exact location of blockages. Blood tests may also be carried out to check if you have a clotting disorder.

What is the treatment?

Treatment depends on the severity of the blockage. You may have a continuous intravenous infusion or injections of heparin, an anticoagulant drug that acts immediately to prevent the existing clots from enlarging and new clots from developing (*see* DRUGS THAT PREVENT BLOOD CLOTTING, p.904). At the same time, you may be started on an oral anticoagulant drug, such as warfarin, which also prevents further clotting by thinning the blood but takes a few days to become effective. Anticoagulant drug treatment may last for 3 months if pulmonary embolism followed a single period of immobility. If the embolism is due to a long-term condition, such as hypercoagulability, you may need drug treatment indefinitely. Treatment is usually monitored with regular blood tests to check your blood clotting, and the drug dosage is altered as necessary.

In severe cases, thrombolytic drugs (p.904) may be used to dissolve the clot. If the main artery supplying the lungs is affected, life-saving emergency surgery may be necessary to remove the clot. If clots recur despite anticoagulant drug therapy, you may need to have surgery in which a filter to trap blood clots is placed in the main vein that leads from the lower half of the body to the heart.

What is the prognosis?

Massive pulmonary embolism is fatal in about 1 in 3 cases. However, if you survive the first few days, you are likely to make a full recovery. People who have recurrent pulmonary embolism may remain short of breath.

If you have already had pulmonary embolism, you have a higher than average risk of further episodes and should avoid periods of prolonged immobility, such as sitting down continually during a long journey. You may need to have preventive treatment, such as heparin injections, after any surgery that involves prolonged immobility.

(WWW) ONLINE SITES: p.1034

Bronchiectasis

Abnormal widening of the larger airways in the lungs (bronchi), causing a persistent cough with large amounts of sputum

 AGE May begin in childhood but may not become apparent until after the age of 40

 GENETICS In some cases, the underlying cause is inherited

 GENDER LIFESTYLE Not significant factors

In bronchiectasis, the larger branches of the airways in the lungs (the bronchi) become abnormally wide, and their lining is damaged. Bronchiectasis usually starts in childhood as a result of a lung infection, but the symptoms of the disorder may not appear until after the age of 40. The main symptoms are a persistent cough that produces large amounts of sputum and shortness of breath that becomes progressively more severe. The disorder was once fairly common, but it is now rare in the developed world due to the greatly reduced incidence of childhood lung infections.

What are the causes?

Childhood infections such as whooping cough (*see* PERTUSSIS, p.492) and measles (p.293) were once very common causes of bronchiectasis. Today, the main cause is repeated bacterial infections of the lungs in people with the inherited condition cystic fibrosis (p.824), in which the mucus produced by the lining of the airways is thicker than normal and tends to collect in the lungs. The repeated infections damage the bronchi, which become distorted so that small pockets form in the tissue. Stagnant mucus then builds up in the pockets, where it may become infected. Bronchiectasis may also occur in alpha$_1$-antitrypsin deficiency (p.489). When the condition is confined to just one area of the lung it may be caused by a blockage in one of the bronchi, which may be due to an inhaled object, such as a peanut.

What are the symptoms?

The symptoms of bronchiectasis gradually worsen over a period of several months or years and may include:

- A persistent cough that produces very large quantities of dark green or yellow sputum. The cough is often worse when lying down.

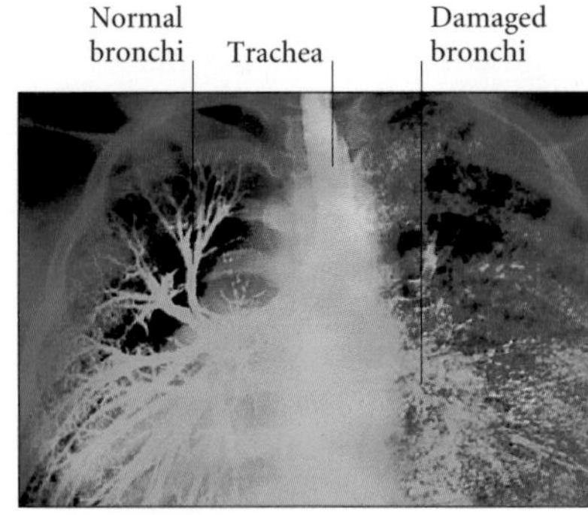

Bronchiectasis
In this specialized X-ray, obtained using radiopaque dye to visualize the airways, the bronchi (large airways) seen on the right have become damaged and distorted.

- Coughing up blood.
- Bad breath.
- Wheezing and shortness of breath.
- Enlarged fingertips with abnormal fingernails, known as clubbing (*see* NAIL ABNORMALITIES, p.360).

Eventually, an affected person will also experience the effects of long-term infection, such as weight loss and anaemia (p.446). Bronchiectasis may affect an increasing number of bronchi, causing extensive damage to a large area of the lung tissue, and may finally lead to respiratory failure (p.507).

How is it diagnosed?

Your doctor may suspect that you have bronchiectasis from the large amount of sputum that you cough up. Your sputum may be tested in order to identify an infection, and you may also have a chest X-ray (p.490) and lung function tests (p.488). CT scanning (p.247) may be used to assess airway damage.

What might be done?

If you have bronchiectasis, you should not smoke, and you should avoid smoky atmospheres and dust.

A family member or friend may be taught how to give you chest physiotherapy (p.962), which ideally should be carried out every day. This technique helps mucus to drain from the lungs. You lie on a bed or other flat surface with your head and chest hanging over the edge so that the mucus can drain into your windpipe. A relative or friend then taps your back with cupped hands to help to free the mucus in your lungs. Keeping the lungs as clear of mucus as possible reduces the risk of infections that may cause further lung damage.

You may be prescribed inhaled bronchodilator drugs (p.910) to help you to breathe more easily. If an infection develops, it will be treated with antibiotics (p.885). In severe cases, a heart and lung transplant may be considered.

(WWW) ONLINE SITES: p.1034, p.1029

Pneumothorax

Presence of air between the layers of the pleura, the two-layered membrane that separates the lungs from the chest wall

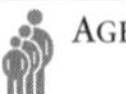 AGE Most common in young people

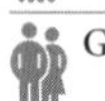 GENDER Much more common in males

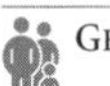 GENETICS Sometimes runs in families

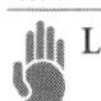 LIFESTYLE Not a significant factor

In a pneumothorax, air enters between the two layers of the pleura, the membrane that separates the lungs from the chest wall. A pneumothorax may cause the lung beneath it to collapse, which can then lead to chest pain and shortness of breath. The air that produces a pneumothorax can come from within the lungs or outside the body, depending on the cause. The condition often affects only one side of the chest.

The amount of air between the layers of the pleura may be small, and in such cases breathing is not severely affected.

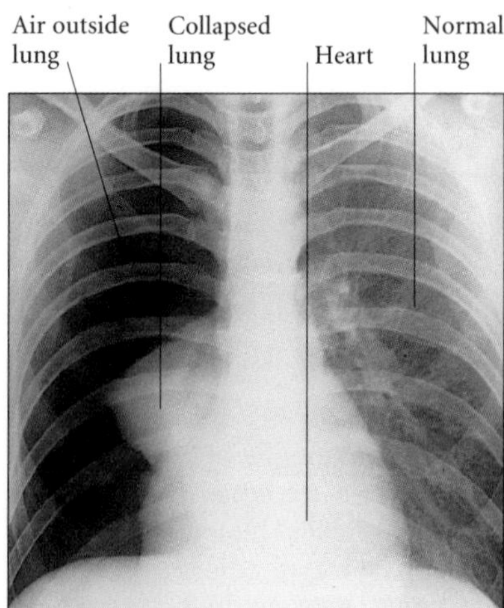

Pneumothorax
A large volume of trapped air can be seen on the left side of this X-ray image. It has caused the lung beneath it to collapse.

(TREATMENT) CHEST DRAIN

A chest drain is used to treat a pneumothorax, in which air enters between the layers of the pleura (the membrane that separates the lungs from the chest wall). It may also be needed following chest surgery. A tube is inserted between the layers of the pleura, allowing air to escape. The tube may be connected to a pump that extracts the air. A chest drain must remain in place until the lung heals, which takes from 1–21 days.

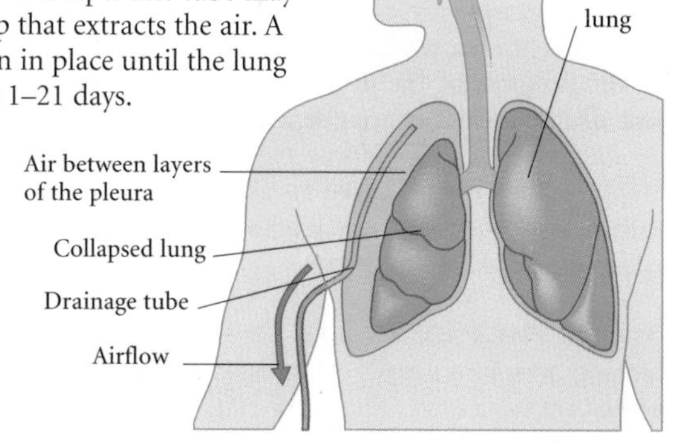

Insertion of a chest drain
A local anaesthetic is applied to the skin and an incision made in the chest wall. A drainage tube, often with a one-way valve to control airflow, is then inserted.

However, a large pneumothorax may cause severe shortness of breath. In a tension pneumothorax, air that enters between the layers of the pleura cannot get back out and causes the pressure inside the pleural layers to rise. This condition also causes severe shortness of breath and can be fatal. It requires immediate medical treatment.

WHAT ARE THE CAUSES?

In most cases, the cause of a pneumothorax is the spontaneous rupture of an abnormally dilated alveolus (air sac), known as a bulla, on the surface of the lung. Most bullae are present from birth. Rupture of a bulla is often caused by vigorous exercise but can sometimes occur at rest. A pneumothorax due to the rupture of a bulla occurs most frequently in tall, thin young men.

A pneumothorax may develop as a complication of lung disorders such as asthma (p.483) and chronic obstructive pulmonary disease (p.487). Repeated pneumothoraces may be associated with Marfan's syndrome (p.824), a rare inherited disorder that affects connective tissue and results in abnormalities of the bones, heart, and eyes.

Other possible causes of a pneumothorax include a penetrating chest wound that allows air to enter between the layers of the pleura from outside the body, fractured ribs that tear the lung beneath them, or surgical procedures performed on the chest.

WHAT ARE THE SYMPTOMS?

Symptoms of a pneumothorax usually develop rapidly and may include:

- Chest pain, which may be felt as sudden and sharp or may cause only slight discomfort.
- Shortness of breath or a sudden worsening of pre-existing shortness of breath in someone with a long-term respiratory disorder.
- Tightness across the chest.

In a tension pneumothorax, there is severe pain and shortness of breath. The high pressure caused by a tension pneumothorax prevents blood from returning to the heart from the lungs, which in turn causes low blood pressure, fainting, and shock (p.414).

WHAT MIGHT BE DONE?

If your doctor suspects that you have a pneumothorax, a chest X-ray (p.490) will be carried out to confirm the diagnosis. A small pneumothorax usually disappears by itself over the course of a few days as the leak that created it heals and the air is gradually absorbed by the body. If the pneumothorax is larger or you have an underlying lung disorder such as asthma, you may need hospital treatment. The doctor will either withdraw some air with a needle or insert a drainage tube through the chest wall under local anaesthesia to enable air to escape (*see* CHEST DRAIN, above).

A tension pneumothorax is a medical emergency. It is treated by inserting a large, hollow needle directly into the affected side of the chest to allow air to escape. This procedure provides immediate relief of symptoms.

If an air leak persists or returns, a technique known as pleurodesis may be used to prevent further lung collapse. This procedure introduces a chemical irritant between the two layers of the pleura to make them stick together. However, pleurodesis is not always successful and, rarely, surgery may be required to repair the damaged area.

With appropriate treatment, most people with a pneumothorax recover completely. However, in 1 in 5 cases the condition recurs, usually within a year.

(WWW) ONLINE SITES: p.1034

Fibrosing alveolitis

Progressive thickening of the walls of the air sacs of the lungs, resulting in shortness of breath

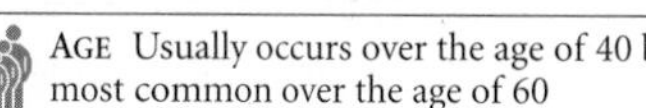
AGE Usually occurs over the age of 40 but is most common over the age of 60

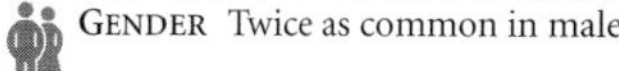
GENDER Twice as common in males

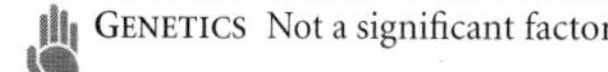
GENETICS Not a significant factor

Inflammation and thickening of the walls of the alveoli (air sacs) in the lungs is called fibrosing alveolitis. As a result of this condition, it is difficult for oxygen to pass into the bloodstream, and the level of oxygen in the blood falls. In addition, the alveoli begin to lose their elasticity, causing shortness of breath.

Usually, fibrosing alveolitis is a long-term disorder, developing over months or years. Rarely, an acute form develops rapidly over a few days or weeks. Both forms tend to become progressively worse and are difficult to treat successfully. The condition most commonly occurs in people over the age of 60 and is more common in men.

WHAT ARE THE CAUSES?

In some cases, fibrosing alveolitis is the result of an autoimmune disorder, in which the immune system attacks the body's own healthy tissues. For example, the condition may be associated with rheumatoid arthritis (p.377) or systemic lupus erythematosus (p.461). Other possible causes include radiotherapy (p.281) of the organs in the chest and certain drugs that are used in the treatment of cancer (*see* ANTICANCER DRUGS, p.280). In about half of all cases, no cause can be found, and the condition is then known as idiopathic pulmonary fibrosis.

WHAT ARE THE SYMPTOMS?

In long-term fibrosing alveolitis, symptoms worsen gradually over months or years. When the disorder has a sudden onset, they worsen over a few days. Symptoms may include the following:

- Shortness of breath.
- Persistent, dry cough.
- Joint pains.

As the condition progresses, breathing becomes increasingly difficult, especially during vigorous exercise. In severe cases, there is an increased risk of respiratory failure (p.507) and chronic heart failure (p.413). Some people with the disorder are more susceptible to lung cancer (*see* PRIMARY LUNG CANCER, p.503).

HOW IS IT DIAGNOSED?

Your doctor may suspect that you have fibrosing alveolitis from your symptoms and medical history and from listening to your chest with a stethoscope. You may have a chest X-ray (p.490) or CT scanning (p.247) to look for thickened lung tissue. Your doctor may also arrange for you to have a blood test to check the levels of oxygen and carbon dioxide in your blood (*see* MEASURING BLOOD GASES, p.501) and lung function tests (p.488). A small sample of lung may be taken using a bronchoscope (*see* BRONCHOSCOPY, p.504) to exclude other disorders. A positive diagnosis of fibrosing alveolitis may be made by taking a lung sample surgically.

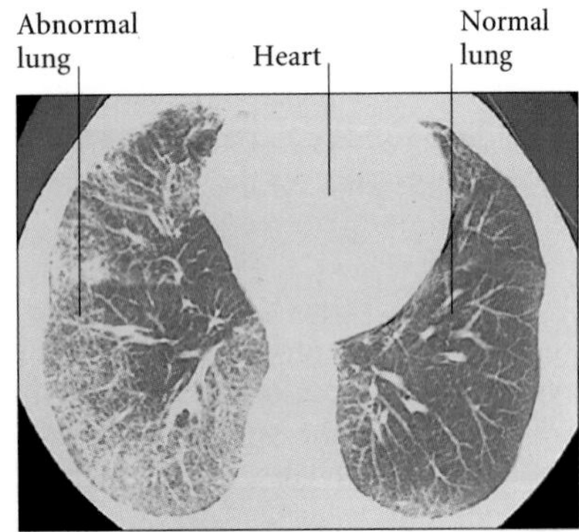

Fibrosing alveolitis
This horizontal CT scan through the chest shows multiple areas of thickening within the tissue of the lung on the left.

WHAT IS THE TREATMENT?

Sometimes, fibrosing alveolitis remains stable for months or years and does not need treatment. In this case, it will be monitored regularly. If it is progressing, high-dose corticosteroids (*see* CORTICOSTEROIDS FOR RESPIRATORY DISEASE, p.911) combined with other immunosuppressant drugs (p.906) may be used to suppress the immune system and slow the progress of the lung damage. These drug treatments are effective in only about 1 in 4 cases. Home oxygen therapy (p.507) may be used to assist breathing, but the treatment has to be used for at least 15 hours a day.

WHAT IS THE PROGNOSIS?

Fibrosing alveolitis usually progresses, making breathing increasingly difficult. Only about half of those with the condition survive for longer than 5 years. For some people, a lung transplant may be life-saving. About 1 in 10 people with the condition develops lung cancer.

(WWW) ONLINE SITES: p.1034

Sarcoidosis

Inflammation of tissue in one or many parts of the body, most often affecting the lungs, lymph nodes, skin, and eyes

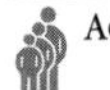 AGE Most common in young adults

 GENDER More common in females

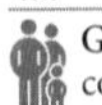 GENETICS Sometimes runs in families; more common in black people

 LIFESTYLE Not a significant factor

In sarcoidosis, areas of inflammation develop on one or more parts of the body, frequently in the lungs. In some cases, only a single type of tissue is affected; in others, the condition affects several different organs. Sarcoidosis is thought to be caused by an abnormal, exaggerated response of the immune system. The trigger for this response is not fully understood, but it is thought that an infection may be involved.

Sarcoidosis may not produce symptoms. If symptoms do develop, they either appear suddenly over a few days (acute sarcoidosis) or progress slowly over several years (chronic sarcoidosis). There is no cure, but symptoms disappear spontaneously in some cases. The condition, particularly in its acute form, is five times more common in women than in men. Sarcoidosis sometimes runs in families and is much more common among black people.

WHAT ARE THE SYMPTOMS?

Some people who have sarcoidosis never develop symptoms. However, those who have acute sarcoidosis may experience the following symptoms:

- Cough.
- Fever and excessive sweating at night.
- Weight loss.
- Tiredness.
- Pain in the joints.
- Painful red lesions on the shins (*see* ERYTHEMA NODOSUM, p.348).

People with chronic sarcoidosis may not experience symptoms initially, but they may gradually develop:

- Increasing shortness of breath.
- Cough.

Both acute and chronic sarcoidosis may cause redness of the eyes, blurred vision (*see* UVEITIS, p.574), skin lesions on the nose and face, and swelling of the lymph nodes. There may also be high levels of calcium in the blood and/or urine, which may cause nausea and constipation and eventually lead to kidney damage.

HOW IS IT DIAGNOSED?

If there are no symptoms, chronic sarcoidosis is usually discovered only after a chest X-ray (p.490) has been taken for another reason. Sarcoidosis may also be diagnosed by an X-ray taken to investigate symptoms such as coughing and shortness of breath. The X-ray usually shows swollen lymph nodes in the chest or shadows on the lungs. Sarcoidosis may also be diagnosed by the presence of skin lesions and confirmed by an examination of affected tissue from a skin sample or a biopsy taken from the lung or airways during bronchoscopy (p.504). You may also have lung function tests (p.488) and blood tests to measure your calcium levels.

WHAT IS THE TREATMENT?

There is no cure for sarcoidosis, but your symptoms may be relieved by using corticosteroids (*see* CORTICOSTEROIDS FOR RESPIRATORY DISEASE, p.911). These drugs are usually effective, although you may need low-dose treatment for several years if you have chronic sarcoidosis.

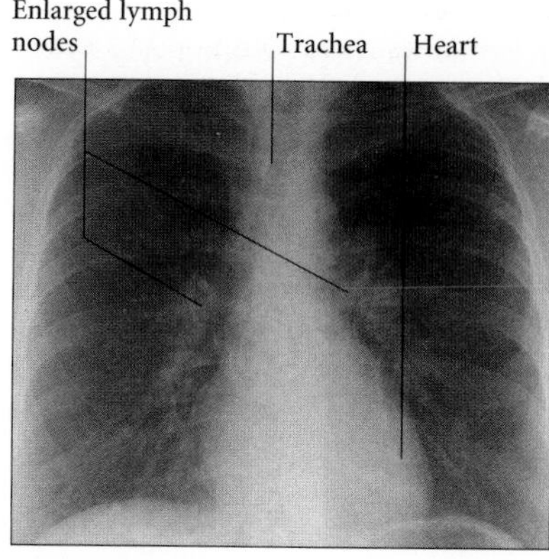

Sarcoidosis
This chest X-ray shows enlarged lymph nodes due to sarcoidosis, a disorder causing inflammation of various body tissues.

Corticosteroids (p.930) may be used for serious complications such as uveitis. You may need regular blood tests, chest X-rays, and lung function tests to monitor your response to treatment.

What is the prognosis?

In about 8 in 10 affected people, most commonly those with acute sarcoidosis, the disorder clears up spontaneously within 3 years. Sarcoidosis is progressive in only about 1 in 10 people with the disorder, and it proves fatal in only about 2 in 100 people.

(WWW) ONLINE SITES: p.1033

Occupational lung diseases

A variety of disorders caused by inhaling damaging dusts or gases at work

 AGE More common over the age of 40

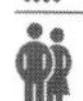 GENDER More common in males due to increased risk of occupational exposure

 LIFESTYLE Smoking causes some disorders to progress more quickly

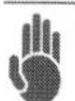 GENETICS Not a significant factor

In developed countries, the number of cases of most occupational lung diseases is decreasing. This is partly due to the improved measures now used to protect workers, such as masks and protective clothing. In addition, regulations are in place that limit the maximum exposure levels for inhaled substances. A decline in the number of workers in industries such as mining in developed countries has also led to a reduction in occupational lung diseases. However, the diseases are still common in developing countries where workers are less likely to have adequate protection.

Occupational lung diseases are initiated by the body's reaction to small solid particles or gases that are breathed into the lungs while a person is in the workplace. The nature of the lung disorder depends on the type and amount of particles that are inhaled.

What are the types?

Occupational lung diseases associated with mineral dusts include coalworkers' pneumoconiosis (right), silicosis (p.500), and asbestosis (*see* ASBESTOS-RELATED DISEASES, p.501). In the most severe cases, these disorders can result in irreversible scarring of lung tissue. Asbestos can also cause thickening of the pleura (the two-layered membrane that separates the lungs from the chest wall) and mesothelioma, a form of cancer that affects the pleura. Silicosis and coalworkers' pneumoconiosis are rare in developed countries. However, the incidence of mesothelioma is still increasing because it takes many years for symptoms to develop. Workers who have been exposed to asbestos before the introduction of safer working practices are still at risk of developing the disease at a later date.

Exposure to certain biological dusts, spores, and chemicals may induce allergic reactions, causing inflammation of the alveoli (air sacs) inside the lungs (*see* EXTRINSIC ALLERGIC ALVEOLITIS, p.502) or asthma (p.483). Although occupational asthma has probably been occurring for centuries, doctors have only recently begun to recognize the extent of the disorder. There is a growing list of substances known to trigger asthma and an increasing number of reported cases each year.

What might be done?

If you have respiratory symptoms, such as shortness of breath or a persistent cough, you should consult your doctor. Tell the doctor if your past or current occupation has involved working with dust or other irritants that could be causing your symptoms. He or she may arrange for you to have a chest X-ray (p.490) and lung function tests (p.488) to look for evidence of lung damage.

If your doctor suspects that you have occupational asthma, he or she will need to identify a trigger substance and confirm its presence in your workplace.

It is vital that you have no further contact with the substance that is causing your symptoms. If you are not able to do this, you will have to consider changing your occupation to prevent a deterioration in your condition. Avoiding these triggers should help to relieve symptoms. Otherwise, treatment is the same as for other forms of asthma.

(WWW) ONLINE SITES: p.1034, p.1036

Coalworkers' pneumoconiosis

Scarring of the lung tissue caused by long-term exposure to coal dust, also known as black lung

 AGE More common over the age of 40

 GENDER More common in males due to increased risk of occupational exposure

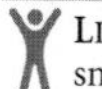 LIFESTYLE Caused by exposure to coal dust; smoking aggravates the disease

 GENETICS Not a significant factor

Coalworkers' pneumoconiosis is a serious lung disorder caused by inhaling coal dust. The dust causes a gradual build-up of scar tissue in the lungs over many years, which leads to progressive and disabling shortness of breath. The severity of the condition depends on the degree to which a person has been exposed to coal dust. Pneumoconiosis was once a common disease in coal-mining areas. However, the decline of the coal industry and improved safety practices have made it increasingly rare in developed countries.

What are the causes?

In pneumoconiosis, minute particles of coal dust are inhaled into the lungs, where they reach the alveoli (air sacs). Over many years of exposure, the dust causes irritation of the lung tissue. This form of the disorder is known as simple pneumoconiosis. Continuing exposure to the dust results in a serious complication known as progressive massive fibrosis (PMF). In this condition, lung

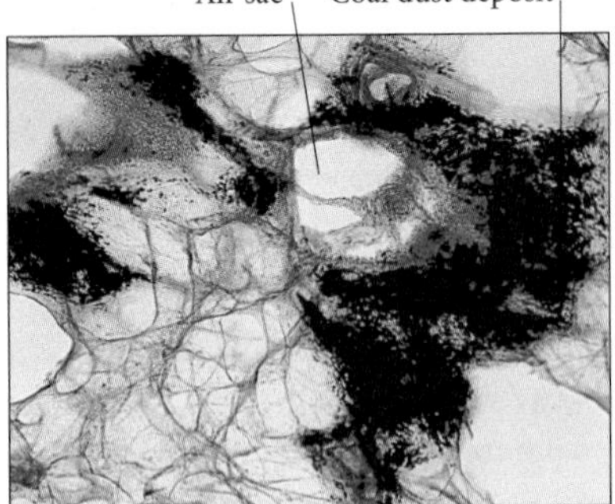

Coalworkers' pneumoconiosis
This magnified view of lung tissue shows black deposits of coal dust in and around the alveoli (air sacs). Eventually, the coal dust deposits cause scarring of lung tissue.

tissue becomes heavily scarred. The disorder is likely to be worse if the coal dust contains a high level of silica (*see* SILICOSIS, right). Smoking causes the condition to progress more rapidly.

WHAT ARE THE SYMPTOMS?

Although the condition does not initially produce symptoms, the following symptoms of simple pneumoconiosis and PMF may develop over time:

- Coughing up black sputum.
- Shortness of breath on exertion that becomes progressively worse.

People with simple pneumoconiosis or PMF are also more susceptible to many other lung disorders, including chronic bronchitis (*see* CHRONIC OBSTRUCTIVE PULMONARY DISEASE, p.487) and tuberculosis (p.491). Coalworkers who also have rheumatoid arthritis (p.377) may develop Caplan's syndrome, in which inflamed nodules form in the lungs.

As simple pneumoconiosis or PMF progresses, breathing difficulties may become so severe that respiratory failure (p.507) develops.

HOW IS IT DIAGNOSED?

Your doctor will probably base the diagnosis on your occupational history and symptoms. He or she may arrange for a chest X-ray (p.490) and lung function tests (p.488) to confirm the diagnosis and assess existing damage to the lungs. You will probably also have tests that measure the levels of oxygen and carbon dioxide in your blood (*see* MEASURING BLOOD GASES, opposite page). These tests show how effectively oxygen from your lungs is reaching the bloodstream.

WHAT IS THE TREATMENT?

You should not smoke and should avoid further exposure to coal dust as far as possible. If you have simple pneumoconiosis and are no longer exposed to the dust, no treatment is necessary because the disease will not progress. If you have PMF, the symptoms may get worse even after exposure to the dust has stopped. Although there is no complete cure for PMF, your doctor may prescribe bronchodilator drugs (p.910) and oxygen therapy (*see* HOME OXYGEN THERAPY, p.507) to help to relieve your symptoms. You may also need to have chest physiotherapy (p.962) regularly to help to remove mucus from the airways, and a friend or member of the family may be taught how to do this.

CAN IT BE PREVENTED?

In most developed countries, there are regulations governing the coal-mining industry that require adequate ventilation in the workplace and other safety measures. Appropriate face masks and equipment to control dust may also be needed for people who work underground. Workers exposed to coal dust should have a chest X-ray every few years to detect the presence of simple pneumoconiosis before PMF develops.

(WWW) ONLINE SITES: p.1034, p.1036

Silicosis

Scarring of the lung tissue caused by inhaling dust containing silica

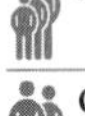 AGE More common over the age of 40

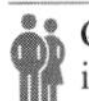 GENDER More common in males due to increased risk of occupational exposure

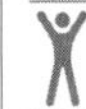 LIFESTYLE Caused by exposure to silica dust; smoking aggravates the disease

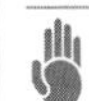 GENETICS Not a significant factor

Once common in developed countries, silicosis is a disorder that leads to irreversible lung damage. It tends to affect people who work with sandstone, granite, slate, and coal, as well as foundry workers, potters, and sandblasters. The number of new cases of silicosis diagnosed each year in the UK is now less than 100, due to safer working practices.

Most people with silicosis have the long-term form of the disease, which usually develops following 20–30 years of exposure to silica dust. The acute form of silicosis, which tends to develop suddenly after only a few months' exposure to a high level of silica dust, can lead to death in less than a year.

Unlike most other dust particles that are breathed into the lungs, silica dust causes a strong inflammatory response in lung tissue. Over time, the inflammation causes thickening and scarring, and the lungs become less efficient in supplying oxygen to the blood. Symptoms of silicosis may be more severe and the condition may progress more rapidly in people who smoke.

WHAT ARE THE SYMPTOMS?

The symptoms of chronic and acute silicosis are the same but develop over different time periods. They include:

- Coughing up sputum.
- Shortness of breath on exertion.
- Tightness of the chest.

A complication of both forms of silicosis is an increased susceptibility to tuberculosis (p.491). Even without further exposure to silica dust, silicosis may progress and may eventually lead to respiratory failure (p.507).

WHAT MIGHT BE DONE?

You should tell your doctor if your past or current work has involved handling materials that produce silica dust. He or she will probably arrange for a chest X-ray (p.490) and for lung function tests (p.488) to assess the level of damage to the lungs. There is no treatment for silicosis, but avoiding further exposure to the dust may slow the progress of the disease. If you have silicosis, you should not smoke, and, if you cannot avoid exposure to silica dust at work, your doctor may advise you to change your job. If you have severe silicosis, you may be given home oxygen therapy (p.507) to ease your breathing.

CAN IT BE PREVENTED?

If you think that you are at risk of silicosis, you should discuss the matter with your doctor and your employer. It is very important that you and your employer take immediate measures to reduce the amount of silica dust that you inhale. Appropriate ventilation, dust-control facilities, face masks, and showers should all be used.

(WWW) ONLINE SITES: p.1034, p.1036

Asbestos-related diseases

Serious lung disorders that develop as a result of inhaling asbestos fibres many years earlier

AGE Rare under the age of 40; more common with increasing age

GENDER More common in males due to increased risk of occupational exposure

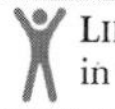
LIFESTYLE Caused by exposure to asbestos in the workplace or at home

GENETICS Not a significant factor

Asbestos is a fibrous mineral that can cause serious lung damage if inhaled. Inhaling even very small numbers of asbestos fibres can lead to problems decades later, but those with the heaviest exposure are at greatest risk. The damage caused by inhaling asbestos fibres is irreversible, and preventing exposure to the dust is very important. The families of people who are exposed to asbestos at work may also be at risk of developing asbestos-related diseases because fibres from the workplace may be brought into the home on clothing.

Over the past 25 years, there has been a general decline in the use of asbestos and safer working practices have been introduced. However, the number of people with asbestos-related diseases is continuing to rise because there is a time lag of up to 50 years between first exposure to asbestos and the development of lung disease.

What is the cause?

Asbestos fibres are needle-shaped. They are therefore drawn deep into the lungs when inhaled, where they can penetrate the lung tissue. The asbestos fibres then trigger a reaction from the defensive white blood cells in the lungs, which try to engulf the fibres. However, the fibres usually destroy the white blood cells, and inflammation and eventual scarring of the lung tissue may follow.

Asbestos fibres are divided into three main types: white, blue, and brown, all of which are dangerous. White asbestos is the type most commonly used for commercial purposes. Blue and brown asbestos fibres are less common, but they are particularly dangerous and are the most likely to trigger the development of asbestos-related diseases.

What are the types?

The inhalation of asbestos fibres can result in three different types of disease: asbestosis; diffuse pleural thickening, in which the pleura (the membrane that separates the lungs from the chest wall) becomes abnormally thickened; and mesothelioma, a cancerous tumour of the pleura. Often, more than one type of asbestos-related disease occurs simultaneously in one person.

ASBESTOSIS In this condition, widespread fine scarring occurs in the lung tissue. The disease may progress even when exposure to asbestos is discontinued. Asbestosis tends to develop among people who have been heavily exposed to asbestos, such as asbestos miners, people who work in asbestos factories, and workers who regularly handle insulation materials that contain asbestos.

The period of time between first exposure to asbestos and development of symptoms is usually at least 20 years and is often longer. The main symptom is shortness of breath on exertion, which may eventually become disabling. Other symptoms include a dry cough, an abnormal shape to the fingernails known as clubbing (*see* NAIL ABNORMALITIES, p.360), and a bluish tinge to the complexion. Some people with asbestosis develop primary lung cancer (p.503).

DIFFUSE PLEURAL THICKENING Pleural thickening may develop after only a brief exposure to asbestos. Usually, the condition produces no obvious symptoms and is detected only if a chest X-ray (p.490) is performed for another reason. However, in some cases, pleural thickening is severe and widespread, and the ability of the lungs to expand is restricted, causing shortness of breath.

MESOTHELIOMA This disorder is a cancerous tumour of the pleura or less often of the peritoneum (the thin membrane that lines the abdominal cavity). Mesotheliomas most commonly result from working with blue or brown asbestos. It may take 30–50 years from the initial exposure for symptoms to first appear.

(TEST) Measuring blood gases

Measuring the levels of oxygen and carbon dioxide in the blood helps in the diagnosis and monitoring of many lung disorders. To measure these gases, a blood sample is taken from an artery, usually in the wrist. This test also measures blood acidity (pH), which may be abnormal in conditions such as diabetes mellitus and in some forms of poisoning. Oxygen levels in the blood can also be measured continuously using a pulse oximeter, which detects changes in the amount of light that blood absorbs.

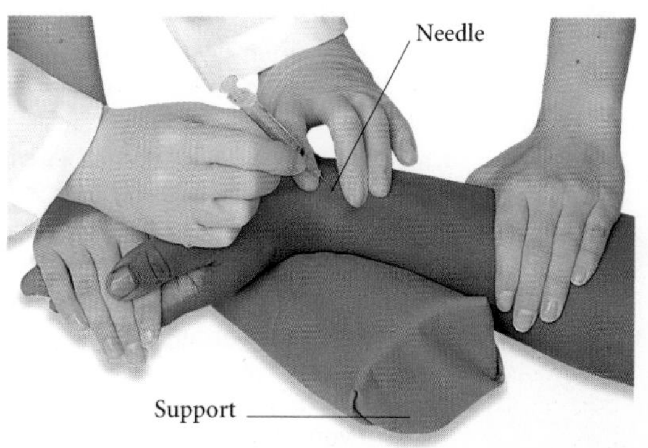

Taking blood
To obtain a blood sample, the skin is cleaned and a local anaesthetic may be given before the blood is withdrawn from an artery with a needle and syringe. The procedure may be uncomfortable, but it is quick. Pressure must be applied for a few minutes afterwards to prevent bleeding.

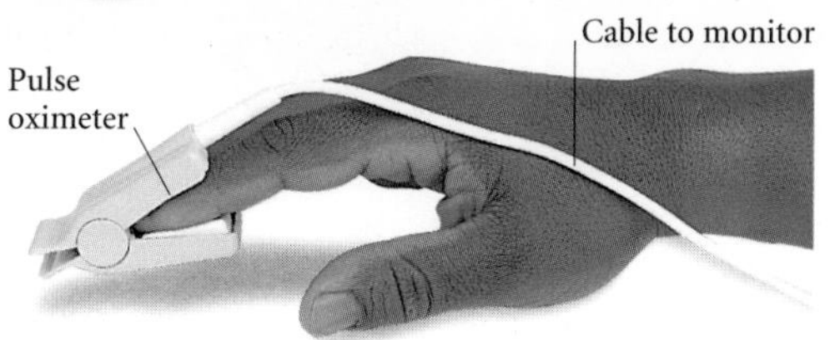

Pulse oximeter
A machine called a pulse oximeter shines a light through the soft tissues of the finger or earlobe to measure oxygen levels in the blood painlessly.

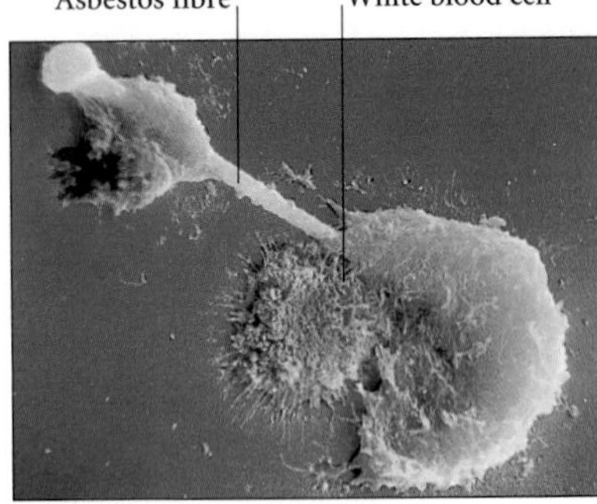

Asbestos fibre in the lungs
Fibres of asbestos inhaled into the lungs are engulfed by white blood cells, as shown above, but destroy the cells. The result is scarring of the lungs called asbestosis.

Mesotheliomas that affect the pleura usually cause chest pain and shortness of breath. In the peritoneum, they may cause an intestinal obstruction (p.663), resulting in symptoms such as abdominal pain, vomiting, and weight loss.

ARE THERE COMPLICATIONS?

People with asbestos-related diseases are particularly susceptible to developing primary lung cancer (opposite page). People who smoke and who also have an asbestos-related disease are considered 75–100 times more likely to develop lung cancer than people with neither factor. Asbestos-related diseases may also increase a person's susceptibility to other serious lung conditions, including tuberculosis (p.491) and chronic obstructive pulmonary disease (p.487).

HOW IS IT DIAGNOSED?

If your doctor suspects that you have an asbestos-related disease, he or she will ask you about your current occupation and work history. Asbestos-related disease is usually diagnosed using a chest X-ray (p.490) to look for signs of thickening of the pleura. Your doctor may also listen to your chest for abnormal sounds and may arrange for lung function tests (p.488) to assess the extent of your breathing problems. A sample of sputum from the lungs may be examined for evidence of asbestos fibres. If a mesothelioma is suspected, CT scanning (p.247) or MRI (p.248) may be performed. To confirm the diagnosis of mesothelioma, a sample of tissue may be taken from the pleura under local anaesthesia to check for cancerous cells.

WHAT IS THE TREATMENT?

No treatment can reverse the progress of an asbestos-related disease. However, further exposure to asbestos may cause the condition to worsen more rapidly and should therefore be avoided. If you have asbestosis, you may be given oxygen (*see* HOME OXYGEN THERAPY, p.507) to relieve shortness of breath. Diffuse pleural thickening requires no specific treatment because the condition rarely causes severe symptoms. Mesothelioma cannot be treated effectively, but radiotherapy (p.281) may relieve pain.

CAN IT BE PREVENTED?

The only way to prevent asbestos-related diseases is to minimize your exposure to asbestos fibres in the workplace and at home. Since the 1970s, the use of asbestos has been severely restricted, and industries that use asbestos have improved fibre-control measures. Most cases of asbestos-related diseases now being diagnosed are the result of working practices that were in effect before the 1970s. If you are carrying out repair work on a house that was constructed before 1970, you should check for the presence of asbestos. If you find asbestos, you should seek professional advice before you continue the work.

WHAT IS THE PROGNOSIS?

About 4 in 10 people with asbestosis or diffuse pleural thickening will eventually die of lung cancer, and smoking should be avoided to lower this risk. Only a few people with asbestos-related mesothelioma survive for longer than 2 years after the diagnosis.

(WWW) ONLINE SITES: p.1034, p.1036

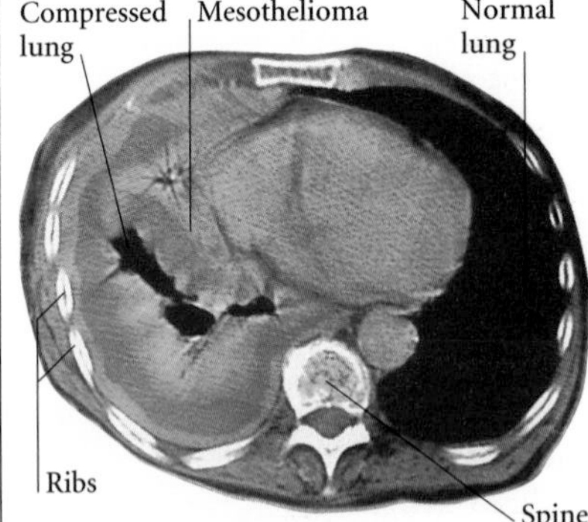

CT scan of mesothelioma
The lung seen on the left is encased in a mesothelioma, a cancerous tumour, which consists of a mass of thickened pleura.

Extrinsic allergic alveolitis

An allergic reaction to inhaled dusts or chemicals, causing cough and fever

 AGE More common in adults

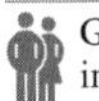 GENDER More common in males due to increased risk of occupational exposure

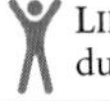 LIFESTYLE Exposure to certain organic dusts and chemicals is a risk factor

 GENETICS Not a significant factor

In some people, inhaling certain dusts or chemicals containing organic substances, such as proteins and fungal spores, triggers an allergic reaction that causes inflammation of lung tissue and shortness of breath. This condition is known as extrinisic allergic alveolitis. The dusts, fungal spores, and chemicals that cause it may be found in the workplace and can affect people in a variety of different occupations.

WHAT ARE THE CAUSES?

Many substances in the workplace can trigger the allergic response that results in extrinsic allergic alveolitis. There are several forms of the disorder, which tend to be named according to the occupation that typically causes them. For example, in farmer's lung, the allergic reaction is triggered by fungal spores from mouldy hay. If particles from bird droppings are the cause, the disorder is known as bird fanciers' lung. Other substances that can trigger extrinsic allergic alveolitis include cheese mould, coffee dust, mushroom soil, and certain chemicals that are used in manufacturing products such as insulation and packing materials. Certain microorganisms that may be in air-conditioning systems and humidifiers can trigger the disorder in office environments.

The allergic reaction causes inflammation of the alveoli (air sacs) and small airways in the lungs. The walls of the alveoli thicken, reducing their efficiency in transferring oxygen to the blood, and the airways narrow. Not everyone who is exposed to these dusts and chemicals will develop an allergic reaction if they inhale them. However, some people are particularly susceptible to allergies, and, in such people, exposure to these substances provokes a sudden acute attack. If exposure to the trigger substance continues after the allergy has become established, some people may go on to develop a long-term form of the disorder, which may cause permanent damage to the lungs.

WHAT ARE THE SYMPTOMS?

The symptoms of an acute attack of extrinsic allergic alveolitis have a rapid onset and are similar to those of influenza. They usually develop 4–8 hours after initial exposure and may include:

- Fever and chills.
- Coughing and wheezing.
- Tightness in the chest and, in some people, shortness of breath.

If exposure to the substance stops, these symptoms usually begin to clear up spontaneously within 12–24 hours and often disappear completely within 48 hours. If there is further exposure to the substance, sudden attacks are eventually followed by continuous symptoms.

In long-standing (chronic) extrinsic allergic alveolitis, symptoms develop over time and include:

- Coughing that may become progressively worse over time.
- Progressive shortness of breath.
- Loss of appetite and weight loss.

In chronic extrinsic allergic alveolitis, symptoms may continue even after exposure to the substance has stopped. If exposure to the substance continues, progressive lung damage may eventually lead to respiratory failure (p.507).

WHAT MIGHT BE DONE?

Your work or hobbies may alert your doctor to the diagnosis, which can be confirmed by blood tests to look for antibodies against the substance causing the allergic reaction. Your doctor may also arrange for a chest X-ray (p.490) and lung function tests (p.488) to look for evidence of lung damage.

If you have a severe, sudden attack of extrinsic allergic alveolitis, you may be given corticosteroids (*see* CORTICOSTEROIDS FOR RESPIRATORY DISEASE, p.911) to help to reduce inflammation in the lungs and bronchodilator drugs (p.910) to help to widen the airways. If the lung damage is severe, you may also be given oxygen (*see* HOME OXYGEN THERAPY, p.507). In most acute attacks, the symptoms clear up once exposure to the dust has stopped. In long-term cases, continued treatment that includes corticosteroids may be necessary even after exposure to the trigger has ended.

CAN IT BE PREVENTED?

If you become sensitive to substances in your workplace, you should wear a protective mask. Employers should store materials safely and ensure that air conditioners are serviced regularly. You may consider changing your lifestyle or finding alternative employment to prevent the allergy from becoming persistent.

(WWW) ONLINE SITES: p.1034, p.1033

Primary lung cancer

A cancerous tumour that develops in the tissue of the lungs

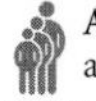 AGE Most common between the ages of 50 and 70

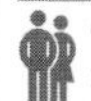 GENDER More common in males but increasingly common in women

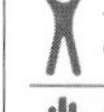 LIFESTYLE Smoking and certain occupations are risk factors

 GENETICS Not a significant factor

Since 1900, the number of cases of primary lung cancer has risen faster than that of any other form of cancer. Primary lung cancer, in which a tumour develops in lung tissue, is now the most common type of cancer after skin cancer and the leading cause of death due to cancer. Although more common in men, incidence is increasing in women, and, in many areas, lung cancer is now more common in women than breast cancer. Lung cancer usually develops between the ages of 50 and 70. In the UK, there are about 80,000 new cases a year.

Smoking is the main cause of lung cancer. The rise in the incidence of the disease over the last hundred years is largely due to a dramatic increase in the number of smokers. Although smoking is becoming less common in developed countries, the incidence of lung cancer in these countries is not expected to decrease for some decades because lung cancer can take many years to develop. The more cigarettes you smoke, the sooner you may develop cancer. For example, if you smoke 20 cigarettes a day, you may develop lung cancer after 20 years; if you smoke 40 a day, you may develop the disease after only 10 years.

WHAT ARE THE TYPES?

The type of cancer that develops depends on the type of cell in the lungs that becomes cancerous. Most lung cancers fall into one of four categories. The most common types are squamous cell carcinoma and small cell carcinoma, with adenocarcinoma and large cell carcinoma accounting for the remainder. Most of these cancers begin in the cells that line the bronchi, the airways that lead to the lungs.

Each type of cancer has a different growth pattern and response to treatment. In general terms, squamous cell carcinoma grows more slowly than the other types of lung cancer and spreads to other parts of the body late in the course of the disease. Small cell carcinoma is the most highly malignant (cancerous) type; this type of cancer grows rapidly and spreads very quickly

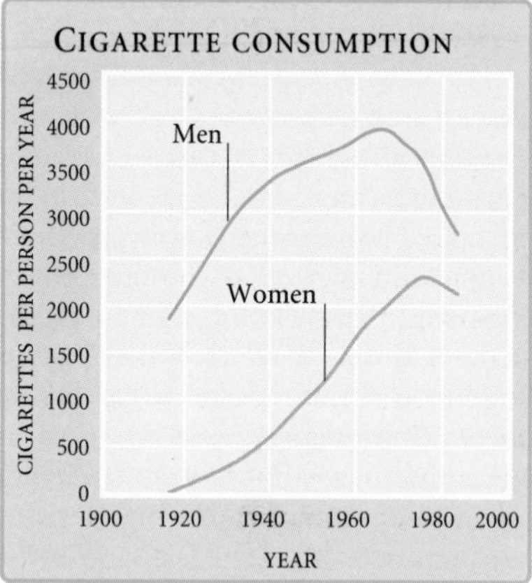

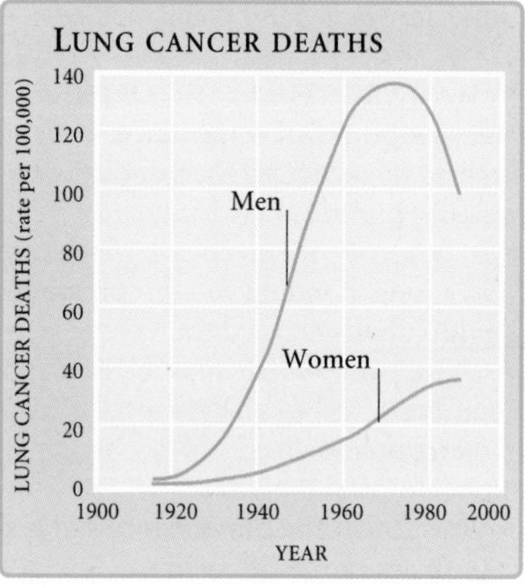

Lung cancer and smoking

The rise in cigarette smoking in men in the UK early in the century was followed by a dramatic rise in lung cancer deaths in the 1940s and 50s. Smoking and lung cancer deaths in women have risen more recently.

throughout the body. Adenocarcinoma and large cell carcinoma both develop at a rate somewhere between that of squamous and small cell carcinomas.

Lung metastases (opposite page) are cancers that have spread to the lung from a tumour in another part of the body. Lung tissue is a common site for metastases because all circulating blood passes through the lungs, allowing cancerous cells to pass into lung tissue.

WHAT ARE THE CAUSES?

Smoking is the cause of lung cancer in approximately 80–90 per cent of cases, and about 1 in 7 smokers is likely to develop the disease by the age of 70. The risk is greatest for people who have smoked more than 20 cigarettes a day since early adulthood. For people who have never smoked, the risk of lung cancer is small, but it increases slightly for anyone who is exposed to other people's cigarette smoke on a regular basis.

Working with particular substances, such as radioactive materials, asbestos (*see* ASBESTOS-RELATED DISEASES, p.501), chromium, and nickel, may lead to an increased risk of lung cancer, especially when the exposure is combined with smoking. Exposure to radon, a radioactive gas that is released slowly from granite rock, also leads to a slightly increased risk for people who live in areas that have a lot of granite. Living in an environment with a high level of air pollution may be a factor in some cases of lung cancer, but it is far less important as a cause than smoking.

WHAT ARE THE SYMPTOMS?

The symptoms of lung cancer depend on how far advanced the tumour is, but initial symptoms may include:

- A new, persistent cough or change in a long-standing cough, sometimes with blood-streaked sputum.
- Chest pain, which may be felt as a dull ache or as a sharp pain that is worse on inhaling.
- Shortness of breath.
- Wheezing if the tumour is positioned so that it blocks an airway.
- Abnormal curvature of the fingernails, known as clubbing (*see* NAIL ABNORMALITIES, p.360).

Some lung cancers do not produce any symptoms until they are advanced, when they may cause shortness of breath.

You should consult your doctor as soon as possible if you develop a new cough that is persistent, experience a change in a long-term cough, or develop any of the other symptoms associated with lung cancer listed above.

ARE THERE COMPLICATIONS?

In some cases, pneumonia (p.490) may develop in an area of the lung if an airway is blocked by a tumour. This may be the first indication of lung cancer. A tumour may also cause fluid to accumulate between the layers of the pleura, the thin membrane that separates the lungs from the wall of the chest (*see* PLEURAL EFFUSION, p.494), which may lead to increased shortness of breath. Later, as the disease progresses, loss of appetite followed by weight loss and weakness may develop. A tumour at the top of the lung may affect the nerves that supply the arm, making the arm painful and weak. Small cell carcinomas may produce chemicals that mimic different hormones in the body and upset body chemistry as a result.

In addition, there may be symptoms from tumours that have spread from the lungs to other parts of the body. For example, headaches may result from cancer that has spread to the brain.

TEST AND TREATMENT BRONCHOSCOPY

Bronchoscopy is used to diagnose or treat lung disorders, such as lung cancer and tuberculosis. A rigid or flexible tube called a bronchoscope is used to view the bronchi (airways). The rigid type is passed through the mouth into the lungs under general anaesthesia. The flexible type is passed into the lungs through the nose or mouth, which are first numbed by a local anaesthetic. Instruments to take tissue samples and perform laser surgery can be introduced through the tube.

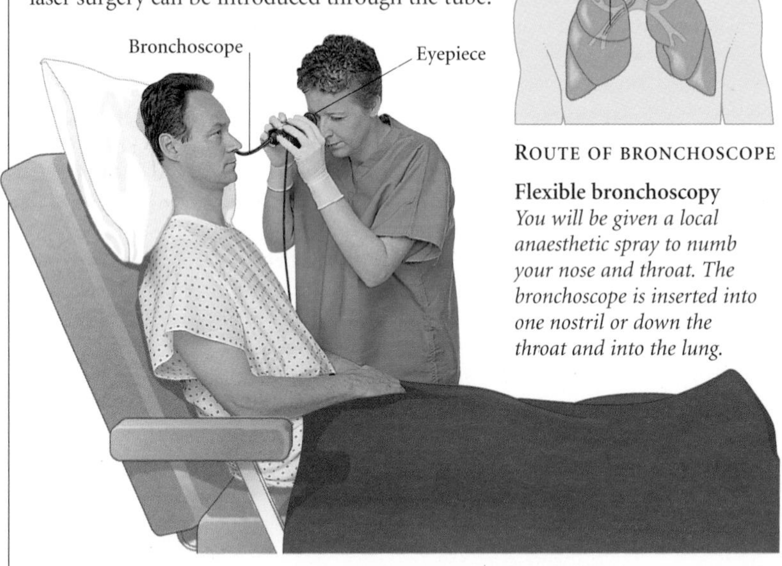

ROUTE OF BRONCHOSCOPE

Flexible bronchoscopy
You will be given a local anaesthetic spray to numb your nose and throat. The bronchoscope is inserted into one nostril or down the throat and into the lung.

RESULTS

Tumour in the bronchus
This view down a bronchoscope clearly shows a tumour almost completely blocking a bronchus. During bronchoscopy, cell and tissue samples can be taken through the bronchoscope for laboratory analysis.

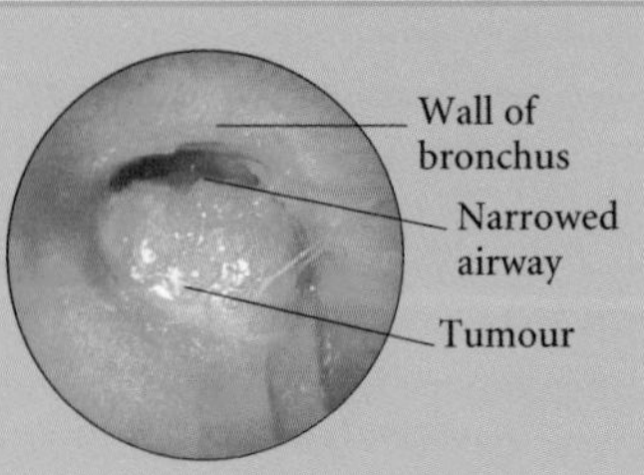

How is it diagnosed?

A chest X-ray (p.490) is often one of the first investigations used when a person has a lung problem. A tumour is usually visible as a shadow on the X-ray.

Samples of sputum may be taken to look for cancerous cells, and your doctor may also perform a bronchoscopy (opposite page) to examine your airways. If a tumour is found during the procedure, a sample will be removed and examined under the microscope. If the tumour is cancerous, tests may be carried out to determine whether cancerous cells have spread to other parts of the body. In addition to blood tests, CT scanning (p.247) and MRI (p.248) of the brain, chest, and abdomen may be used to assess the extent of cancer spread. Radionuclide scanning (p.251) may be performed to determine whether the cancer has spread to the bones.

What is the treatment?

Treatment of lung cancer depends on the type of cancer and whether it has spread to other parts of the body.

Surgery to remove a tumour in the lung is considered as an option only if the cancer has not spread. Surgery normally involves removal of the whole lung or a major part of it.

In 4 out of 5 cases, the cancer has already spread to other organs, and surgery is not an option. The size or location of the tumour or the presence of another serious disorder, such as chronic obstructive pulmonary disease (p.487) may also make surgery inadvisable.

Small cell carcinoma is rarely treated with surgery because it is highly malignant and has usually spread beyond the lungs by the time it is diagnosed. This type of cancer is usually treated with chemotherapy (p.280). Radiotherapy (p.281) may be used to treat metastases.

If a tumour cannot be removed surgically and is not a small cell carcinoma, radiotherapy is usually given initially. Although this does not destroy all cancerous cells, it does slow tumour growth.

What is the prognosis?

The outlook is best for people whose cancer is detected early. Only about 1 in 20 people with lung cancer survives for 5 years or more after it is diagnosed. About 3 in 4 people who have surgery to remove a tumour survive for 2 years.

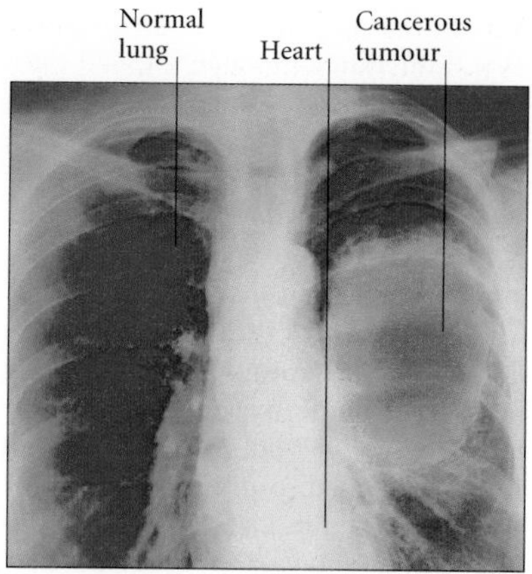

Lung cancer
In this colour-enhanced chest X-ray, a large cancerous tumour can be seen in one lung. The other lung is normal.

People with small cell carcinoma usually survive for only 2–10 months after diagnosis. Surgery, radiotherapy, and chemotherapy may not prolong life in all cases, but they can alleviate symptoms and improve quality of life.

Can it be prevented?

Lung cancer is closely linked to smoking. People who stop smoking greatly improve their chances of avoiding lung cancer, and long-term ex-smokers have only a slightly greater risk of developing lung cancer than nonsmokers.

(WWW) ONLINE SITES: p.1028, p.1034

Lung metastases

Cancerous tumours in lung tissue that have spread from another part of the body

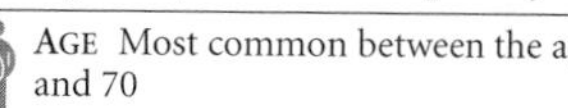
AGE Most common between the ages of 50 and 70

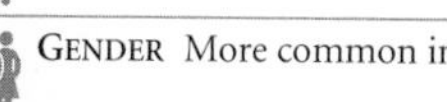
GENDER More common in females

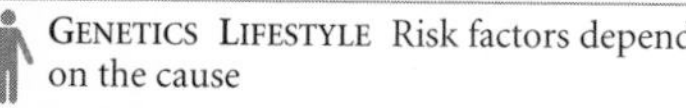
GENETICS LIFESTYLE Risk factors depend on the cause

Lung metastases, also known as secondary lung cancer, are tumours that have spread to the lungs from other parts of the body. Lung tissue is a very common site for metastases because all circulating blood passes through the lungs, allowing cancerous cells to be carried into lung tissue from other parts of the body. The primary (original) cancers that spread most often to the lungs include cancers of the breast, colon, prostate gland, and kidney.

Secondary lung cancers may not cause symptoms. However, if many secondary tumours have formed in the lung, you may feel short of breath. You may also develop a cough, which can produce blood if a tumour is blocking an airway.

What might be done?

If cancer has already been diagnosed elsewhere in your body, your doctor may arrange for you to have a chest X-ray (p.490) to check whether the cancer has spread to your lungs. If the site of the original cancer has not been confirmed, further tests may be carried out to locate it. For example, women will probably have a breast X-ray (*see* MAMMOGRAPHY, p.759) to look for evidence of a breast tumour.

Treatment is aimed at destroying the primary cancer. Chemotherapy (p.280), radiotherapy (p.281), or hormonal treatment (*see* ANTICANCER DRUGS, p.907) may be used, depending on the type and extent of the primary tumour. To some extent, the overall outlook depends on the type of primary cancer. However, by the time lung metastases have been detected, there are usually several tumours, and treatment is difficult.

(WWW) ONLINE SITES: p.1028, p.1034

Pulmonary hypertension

Abnormally high pressure in the blood vessels supplying the lungs

AGE More common over the age of 40

LIFESTYLE Risk factors depend on the cause

GENDER GENETICS Not significant factors

Blood is normally pumped through the lungs by the heart at a lower pressure than blood is pumped around the rest of the body. In pulmonary hypertension, the pressure of the blood in the arteries supplying the lungs is abnormally high. Consequently, the right side of the heart, which pumps the blood through the lungs, must contract much more vigorously than normal to maintain an adequate flow of blood through the arteries of the lungs. This causes enlargement of the muscle wall on the right side of the heart.

WHAT ARE THE CAUSES?

There are various lung and heart conditions that may result in pulmonary hypertension. For example, in chronic obstructive pulmonary disease (p.487), resistance to blood flow in the lungs is caused by destruction of lung tissue. In diseases that cause extensive scarring of the tissue in the lungs, such as fibrosing alveolitis (p.497), blood vessels in the lungs are destroyed, making blood flow more difficult. Blood clots in the lungs (*see* PULMONARY EMBOLISM, p.495) may obstruct the flow of blood and lead to pulmonary hypertension. Narrowing of the mitral valve in the heart prevents blood from leaving the lungs, causing back pressure (*see* MITRAL STENOSIS, p.424) and pulmonary hypertension.

In some forms of congenital heart disease (p.836), the heart pumps more blood than is normal into the lungs, and as a result the pressure rises.

Rarely, sleep apnoea (p.477) leads to pulmonary hypertension. Occasionally, there is no obvious cause for the condition, and it is then known as primary pulmonary hypertension.

WHAT ARE THE SYMPTOMS?

Many people who develop pulmonary hypertension already have symptoms of a long-term heart or lung disorder. The additional symptoms associated with pulmonary hypertension may include:

- Shortness of breath that tends to become worse on exertion.
- Tiredness.

As the disease progresses, shortness of breath becomes increasingly severe until it may occur at rest. Eventually, the right side of the heart, which pumps blood through the lungs, may fail, leading to tissue oedema (swelling caused by fluid build-up), especially around the ankles.

WHAT MIGHT BE DONE?

If you have an existing long-term heart or lung disorder and your symptoms suddenly become worse, your doctor may suspect that you are developing pulmonary hypertension. He or she may arrange for a chest X-ray (p.490) to look for enlarged arteries. An echocardiogram (*see* ECHOCARDIOGRAPHY, p.425) and an electrocardiogram (*see* ECG, p.406) may be carried out to look for signs of heart disease, and lung function tests (p.488) are useful to assess the extent of lung damage. If the diagnosis is still unclear, a procedure called right heart catheterization may be used. This involves passing a tube through a vein in the arm or leg into the right side of the heart to measure blood pressure there.

If you have already developed pulmonary hypertension, treatment will first be directed at the underlying cause if one is found. Your doctor may advise long-term home oxygen therapy (opposite page) if you have low oxygen levels due to a disorder such as chronic obstructive pulmonary disease. Drugs that prevent blood clotting (p.904) may be prescribed if the blood vessels in the lungs have become blocked by clots. You may also be prescribed drugs to dilate blood vessels in the lungs and lower the pressure in them. If heart failure has developed, you may be given diuretic drugs (p.902) to reduce excess fluid.

WHAT IS THE PROGNOSIS?

If the underlying cause of pulmonary hypertension is identified and can be treated successfully, it is possible that the condition may improve. However, in most cases, pulmonary hypertension becomes progressively worse.

In primary pulmonary hypertension and cases in which the underlying cause is untreatable, the disorder may progress to chronic heart failure (p.413), which may be life threatening. For this reason, if you have pulmonary hypertension, are under the age of 55, and are otherwise in good health, you may be considered for a heart and lung transplant.

(WWW) ONLINE SITES: p.1034

Acute respiratory distress syndrome

Inflammatory response of the lungs to severe disease or injury

AGE GENDER GENETICS LIFESTYLE
Not significant factors

Acute respiratory distress syndrome (ARDS) is a serious lung disorder that develops suddenly as a result of severe damage either to the lungs or elsewhere in the body. In ARDS, the tiny blood vessels (capillaries) in the lungs leak fluid into the alveoli (air sacs), reducing the amount of oxygen that reaches the blood and preventing the lungs from expanding fully. This in turn can lead to the failure of other vital organs, including the kidneys and liver. ARDS is a life-threatening disorder that requires emergency medical treatment.

WHAT ARE THE CAUSES?

ARDS can develop after any serious illness or injury. A third of cases result from widespread bacterial infection of the blood (*see* SEPTICAEMIA, p.299). In other cases, major trauma such as multiple fractures, crushed internal organs, or severe burns are the cause. Less commonly, ARDS results from pneumonia (p.490), obstetric emergencies, inhaling vomit, or an overdose of an opioid drug such as heroin. How these conditions and emergencies cause leakage in the lungs remains unclear.

WHAT ARE THE SYMPTOMS?

The symptoms of ARDS usually begin 24–48 hours after the injury or onset of the disease that brings about the condition and may include the following:

- Severe shortness of breath.
- Wheezing.
- Mottled blue skin.
- Confusion or unconsciousness.

These symptoms develop in addition to those related to the underlying disorder that has caused the lung damage. As well as being a possible cause of ARDS, pneumonia may develop as a complication. Other complications, such as acute kidney failure (p.706), may also occur.

WHAT MIGHT BE DONE?

A doctor will probably suspect ARDS if a person who is already seriously ill develops sudden, unexpected breathing difficulties. The diagnosis can often be confirmed by a chest X-ray (p.490), which is used to look for evidence of fluid in the alveoli, and analysis of the oxygen levels in the blood (*see* MEASURING BLOOD GASES, p.501).

People with ARDS are usually treated in an intensive care unit (p.958). High concentrations of oxygen are given using artificial ventilation in order to increase the amount of oxygen that passes from the lungs into the blood. Diuretic drugs (p.902) may be given to reduce the amount of fluid in the lungs. The underlying cause and any complications are treated, and the condition of major organs is monitored.

What is the prognosis?

Only 1 in 2 people who develop ARDS survive. In those who recover, symptoms usually improve over 7–10 days. There is often little or no permanent damage to the lungs, and the majority of people who do make a recovery experience no further problems.

(WWW) ONLINE SITES: p.1034

Respiratory failure

Abnormally low levels of oxygen in the blood, resulting from lung damage

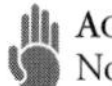

AGE GENDER GENETICS LIFESTYLE
Not significant factors

Respiratory failure occurs if the amount of oxygen that enters the bloodstream from the lungs is greatly reduced, leading to severe shortness of breath and eventually to profound confusion or unconsciousness. Simultaneously, there may be an excess of carbon dioxide in the blood. Respiratory failure is a life-threatening condition that should be treated promptly to prevent damage to other organs, such as the heart, which need an adequate supply of oxygen to maintain their function.

What are the causes?

There are two broad groups of conditions that lead to respiratory failure. In the first group of disorders, there is no difficulty in moving air into and out of the lungs, but less oxygen than normal is transferred to the blood as a result of damage to the alveoli (air sacs) in the lungs. The most common causes of this type of respiratory failure are long-term lung disorders such as fibrosing alveolitis (p.497). Less commonly, the alveoli may become filled with fluid, as occurs in acute respiratory distress syndrome (opposite page). In this case, the levels of oxygen in the blood are low, but carbon dioxide levels are usually normal.

The second group of conditions consists of ventilation disorders, in which a person cannot move sufficient air into and out of the lungs. A ventilation disorder may develop suddenly after a stroke (p.532) or an injury to the area of the brain that controls breathing. A drug overdose (*see* DRUG OVERDOSE AND ACCIDENTAL INGESTION, p.321) or injury to the chest wall may also reduce breathing. In addition, breathing difficulties may result from particular disorders, such as myasthenia gravis (p.549), in which the muscles involved in breathing become progressively weakened. Ventilation problems usually lead to low levels of oxygen and high levels of carbon dioxide in the blood.

What are the symptoms?

Disorders that involve damage to the alveoli are usually long-term conditions, and symptoms develop gradually. In ventilation disorders, symptoms of respiratory failure may develop either suddenly or gradually over a period of time, depending on the cause.

Whatever the underlying cause, the symptoms of respiratory failure are mainly due to low levels of oxygen in the blood and may include:

- Shortness of breath.
- A bluish tinge to the lips and tongue, a condition known as cyanosis.
- Anxiety.
- Agitation.
- Confusion.
- Sweating.

In addition to the symptoms listed above, ventilation disorders cause symptoms, such as headache and drowsiness, due to the high concentration of carbon dioxide in the blood.

What might be done?

Respiratory failure can usually be diagnosed from the symptoms, and its severity can be assessed by measuring the levels of oxygen and carbon dioxide in blood (*see* MEASURING BLOOD GASES, p.501). If the cause is not obvious, you may need further tests.

Respiratory failure due to permanent damage to the alveoli cannot be treated except with a lung transplant. However, symptoms may be relieved by long-term home oxygen therapy (below), which needs to be used continuously for at least 15 hours a day to prevent chronic heart failure (p.413).

If you develop respiratory failure caused by a ventilation disorder, you may need help from a ventilator to breathe. This is usually performed in hospital at first, but, if long-term ventilation is required, it may be possible to continue the treatment at home.

If respiratory failure occurs suddenly due to a ventilation disorder, recovery is possible if the underlying cause can be treated successfully. Cases of gradual respiratory failure are less likely to show significant improvement, but the symptoms can be controlled effectively with long-term oxygen therapy.

(WWW) ONLINE SITES: p.1034

(TREATMENT) Home oxygen therapy

Oxygen therapy can be used at home to relieve symptoms of many lung disorders that lead to low blood oxygen levels. You can use either oxygen cylinders or an oxygen concentrator. In people with chronic respiratory failure, the treatment improves symptoms and can delay the development of complications and prolong life if used for at least 15 hours a day. Smaller, portable oxygen cylinders can be used when outside, enabling you to move around freely while receiving extra oxygen.

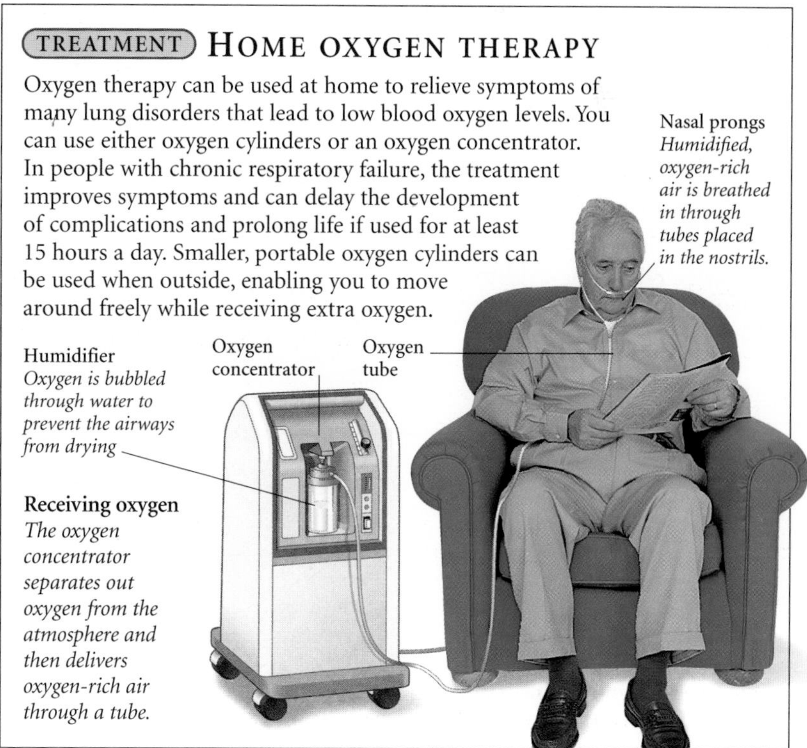

Receiving oxygen *The oxygen concentrator separates out oxygen from the atmosphere and then delivers oxygen-rich air through a tube.*

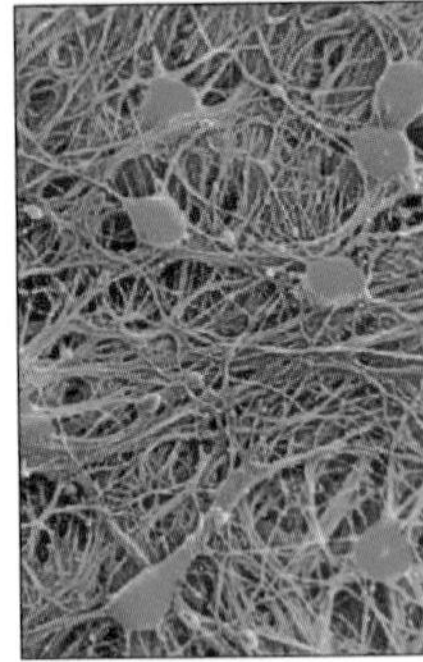

Nerve fibres
Brain tissue consists of networks of nerve fibres along which electrical signals travel.

NERVOUS SYSTEM AND MENTAL FUNCTION

THE NERVOUS SYSTEM IS THE MOST complex system in the body and regulates hundreds of activities simultaneously. It is the source of our consciousness, intelligence, and creativity and allows us to communicate and experience emotions. It also monitors and controls almost all bodily processes, ranging from automatic functions of which we are largely unconscious, such as breathing and blinking, to complex activities that involve thought and learning, such as playing a musical instrument and riding a bicycle.

The nervous system has two parts: the central nervous system (CNS), which consists of the brain and spinal cord; and the peripheral nervous system (PNS), which is made up of of all the nerves that emerge from the CNS and branch throughout the body. Nerve signals are processed and coordinated by the CNS, while the PNS transmits nerve signals to and from the CNS and other parts of the body.

The nervous system has immediate control over our voluntary actions, such as walking, and our automatic body functions, such as salivation.The longer-term control of automatic body activities, such as maintaining normal blood pressure and temperature, is aided by some of the hormones produced by the endocrine system.

HOW THE NERVOUS SYSTEM WORKS

Most of the activity of the nervous system is carried out by cells called neurons. Each neuron typically has a long projection known as a nerve fibre (axon), which relays information in the form of electrical signals. When a signal reaches the end of a nerve fibre, it is carried in chemical form to the next neuron or to another kind of cell. In the PNS, nerve fibres form bundles called nerves, and these carry messages concerning the outside world and the inside of the body. For example, information about sound is detected by sensory receptors in the ear and converted into nerve impulses. These signals travel along nerve fibres towards the brain. In response to these nerve impulses, the CNS then transmits signals to the motor nerves in the PNS, which communicate with glands, organs, or muscles to produce an appropriate response to the original stimuli. The CNS also receives a constant stream of data concerning the inner organs and bodily functions, such as blood pressure and body temperature, from other sensory organs throughout the body. This information is monitored continuously and elicits appropriate responses, often without any input from the conscious mind.

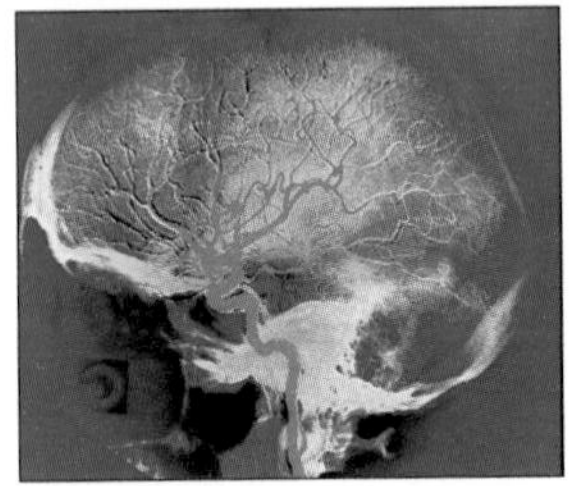

Arteries supplying the brain
Four arteries branch at the base of the brain to supply it with about one-fifth of the body's total supply of blood.

COMPLEX ACTIVITIES

Many complex activities and functions, including creativity and logic, involve conscious thought. However, some activities that require the coordination of several physical tasks are regulated unconsciously. For example, your first attempts to ride a bicycle require a conscious effort but when you have learned and memorised the necessary skills you can cycle without conscious thought. However, you still remain conscious of sensory stimuli, such as sight and sound, that aid navigation.

(FUNCTION) NERVOUS SYSTEM ORGANISATION

The nervous system is divided into two parts: the central nervous system (CNS), which regulates bodily activity; and the peripheral nervous system (PNS), which transmits signals between the body and the CNS. The PNS is divided into nerves that control voluntary actions or transmit sensations, and nerves that regulate internal functions.

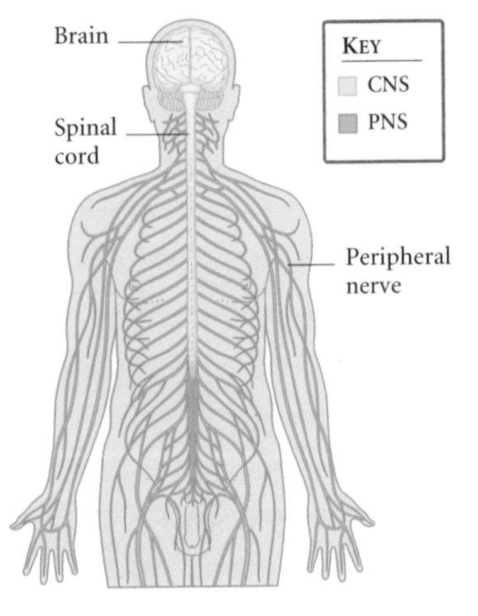

Nerve links between brain and body
Nerve fibres leave the brain and enter the spinal cord to form a thick bundle of nerves. Individual nerves then emerge from the spinal cord and branch out through the body, supplying every tissue.

STRUCTURE NERVOUS SYSTEM

The brain and spinal cord form the central nervous system and are protected by the bones of the skull and the vertebral column. Inside these hard outer coverings, further protection is provided by three membranes called the meninges and a clear liquid known as cerebrospinal fluid. The cranial nerves emerge directly from the brain, and the spinal nerves from the spinal cord. Together, these form the peripheral nerves that branch to every part of the body.

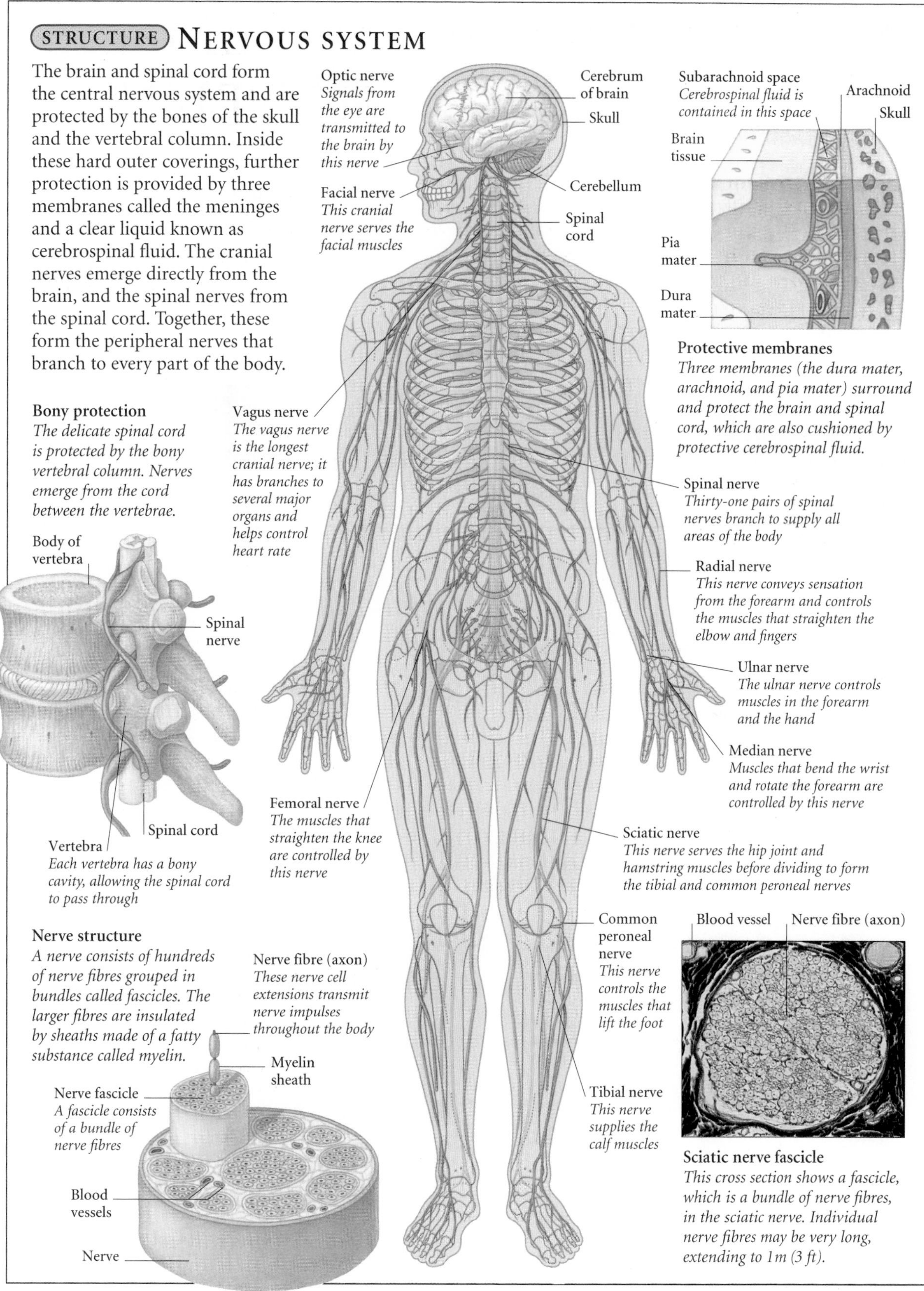

Protective membranes
Three membranes (the dura mater, arachnoid, and pia mater) surround and protect the brain and spinal cord, which are also cushioned by protective cerebrospinal fluid.

Bony protection
The delicate spinal cord is protected by the bony vertebral column. Nerves emerge from the cord between the vertebrae.

Nerve structure
A nerve consists of hundreds of nerve fibres grouped in bundles called fascicles. The larger fibres are insulated by sheaths made of a fatty substance called myelin.

Sciatic nerve fascicle
This cross section shows a fascicle, which is a bundle of nerve fibres, in the sciatic nerve. Individual nerve fibres may be very long, extending to 1m (3 ft).

STRUCTURE AND FUNCTION

BRAIN, SPINAL CORD, AND NERVES

The brain contains more than 100 billion neurons and weighs about 1.4 kg (3 lb). The brain and spinal cord contain two main types of tissue: grey matter, which originates and processes nerve impulses; and white matter, which transmits them. The largest structure in the brain is the cerebrum, which is divided into two halves or hemispheres. Other structures include the cerebellum, the brain stem, and a central region that includes the thalamus and hypothalamus. The spinal cord is an extension of the brain stem and continues downwards from the base of the skull.

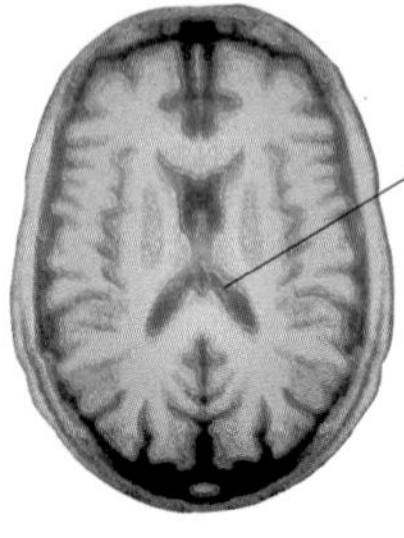

Lateral ventricles
The left and right lateral ventricles appear X-shaped when viewed in cross section

MRI scan of the brain
Protective cerebrospinal fluid is made in four ventricles, or cavities, in the brain. This section of the brain shows the lateral ventricles.

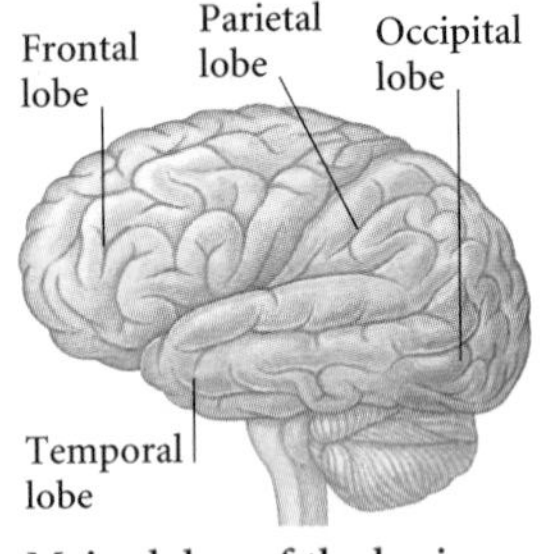

Major lobes of the brain
The brain is divided into several lobes that take their names from the skull bones that cover them.

Cerebrum
The cerebrum consists of grey and white matter. It is the largest part of the brain and links to every part of the body

Meninges
Surrounding the brain and the spinal cord are three protective membranes called the meninges

Cerebral cortex
This outer layer of the cerebrum governs higher brain functions, including thought. It receives and processes sensations and initiates movement

Subarachnoid space
This region contains cerebrospinal fluid, which protects the brain and spinal cord as it circulates around them before draining back into the venous sinuses

Arachnoid granulation
Cerebrospinal fluid is absorbed from here into the blood

Skull

Venous sinus
This is one of several major blood vessels that drain blood away from the brain

Corpus callosum
This large bundle of about 300 million nerve fibres connects the two cerebral hemispheres

Choroid plexus
This area is involved in producing cerebrospinal fluid

Hypothalamus
The hypothalamus controls the endocrine system. It regulates sleep, sexual function, body temperature, and water content

Thalamus
Sensory nerve impulses pass through the thalamus on their way to the cerebral cortex

Pituitary
This gland regulates other glands throughout the body

Cerebellum
This area is involved in balance and the control of muscle movement

Grey matter
Grey matter consists mainly of neuron cell bodies, from which nerve impulses originate

Basal ganglia
These islands of grey matter help to coordinate movement

White matter
White matter consists largely of nerve fibres; its main role is to transmit nerve impulses

Midbrain
Pons
Medulla

Brain stem
The brain stem relays nerve impulses between the spinal cord and the brain; it controls vital functions such as heart rate and breathing

Brain stem
The main motor pathways cross over in the brain stem to the opposite sides of the spinal cord

Spinal cord
Nerve impulses sent between the brain and the peripheral nerves travel along nerve fibres that run through tracts (pathways) in the spinal cord

Cerebellum

Brain tissue
The outer layer of the brain, the cerebral cortex, is made of grey matter. Beneath are white matter and islands of grey matter.

Cranial nerves

Twelve pairs of cranial nerves emerge directly from the underside of the brain. Most of these nerves supply the head, face, neck, and shoulders. Certain organs in the chest and abdomen, including the heart, lungs, and much of the digestive system, are supplied by the vagus nerve.

Olfactory nerve
This nerve relays information about smell from the nose

Optic nerve
This nerve transmits information about visual images

Oculomotor, trochlear, and abducent nerves
These nerves supply muscles that move the eyes

Trigeminal nerve
Sensations from the face are relayed by this nerve, which also controls muscles used in chewing

Vestibulocochlear nerve
Fibres in this nerve carry information about sound and balance from the ear

Facial nerve
This nerve transmits information from the taste buds and controls facial expression

Glossopharyngeal and hypoglossal nerves
These nerves carry information about taste in addition to controlling movements of the tongue

Spinal accessory nerve
This nerve controls some movements of the head and shoulder muscles

Vagus nerve
This nerve performs many roles, such as regulation of heart rate and speech

Cranial nerve functions
The cranial nerves contain sensory and/or motor fibres, which control various conscious and unconscious functions.

Left optic nerve

Crossover point

Right optic nerve

MRI scan of optic nerves
The optic nerves from the left and the right eyes merge and then diverge in the centre of the brain so that each cerebral hemisphere receives data from both eyes.

Spinal nerves

Thirty-one pairs of spinal nerves emerge from the spinal cord and extend through the protective, bony spinal column. These nerves divide to supply all parts of the trunk and the limbs. Before reaching the limbs, bundles of nerves converge to form braid-like plexuses, called the brachial and lumbar plexuses, which then branch further along.

Brain stem
The brain stem connects the spinal cord to other parts of the brain

Cervical nerves
Eight pairs of cervical nerves supply the head, neck, shoulders, arms, and hands

Thoracic nerves
The twelve pairs of thoracic nerves connect to parts of the upper abdomen and to muscles in the back and chest

Spinal cord
Nerve impulses are carried between the spinal nerves and the brain along this column of nervous tissue

Lumbar nerves
Five pairs of lumbar nerves supply the area of the lower back and the legs

Sacral region
Five pairs of sacral nerves and a pair of coccygeal nerves supply the buttocks, legs, feet, anal, and genital areas

Role of the spinal nerves
The spinal nerves (shown here from the front) carry sensory nerve impulses towards the spinal cord and brain. They also carry motor nerve impulses from the brain to the rest of the body.

Structure of the spinal cord

The spinal cord has a core of grey matter containing nerve cell bodies, dendrites, and supporting cells. Surrounding the grey matter is white matter containing columns of nerve fibres that carry signals to and from the brain along the length of the spinal cord.

Sensory nerve root
These sensory fibres carry data about sensations and enter the rear of the cord

Motor nerve root
These motor nerve fibres control movement and leave the front of the spinal cord

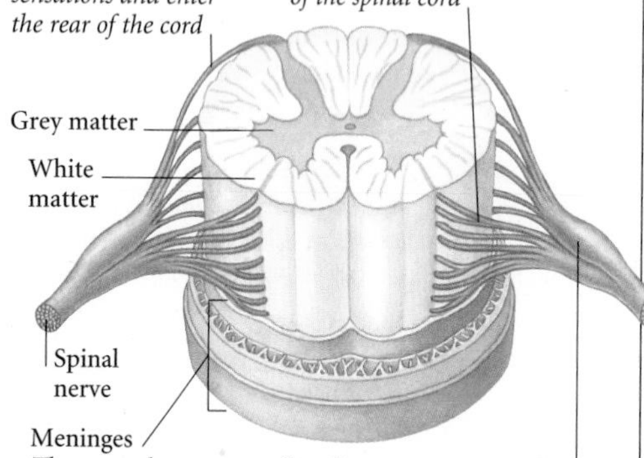

Meninges
These membranes protect the spinal cord

Ganglion
This nodule contains the cell bodies of sensory nerve fibres

Nerve root pathways
Each spinal nerve has motor and sensory nerve roots. The sensory nerve roots enter the back of the spinal cord to join fibres that lead to the brain. Nerve fibres carrying signals from the brain join motor nerve roots leaving the front of the cord.

STRUCTURE AND FUNCTION — NERVE CELLS

Neurons are nerve cells that originate, process, transmit, and receive nerve impulses. They are connected to other neurons or to cells in muscles, organs, or glands. Nerve impulses travel electrically along the neuron and are transmitted by chemical messengers (neurotransmitters) to the next neuron across a tiny gap, called a synapse, between the neuron and the adjacent cell, which is known as the target cell. In addition to neurons, the nervous system contains large numbers of other types of cell, called neuroglia, which protect, nourish, and support neurons.

Cell body of neuron

Nerve fibre (axon)

Neural connection
This magnified image shows two neurons. The nerve fibre of one neuron links to the cell body of the other.

NEURONS

In addition to features common to all cells, such as a nucleus, neurons have specialised projections, known as nerve fibres (axons), that carry nerve signals. Neurons in the brain form densely packed clusters. Neurons in the spinal cord and around the body form long communication tracts.

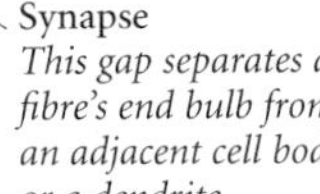

Node of Ranvier
These gaps in the myelin sheath help the conduction of nerve impulses

Myelin sheath
Some fibres have this fatty coating, which speeds up nerve impulse transmission

Nerve fibre (axon)
Nerve fibres may link to the cell bodies or the dendrites of other neurons or to other cells

Dendrite
A neuron may have up to 200 of these short, branching projections

Synapse
This gap separates a fibre's end bulb from an adjacent cell body or a dendrite

Synaptic end bulb
This swelling at the end of the nerve fibre holds chemicals that are able to travel across the synapse

Nucleus

Neuron cell body

Neuron structure
A typical neuron has one or two long nerve fibres and many dendrites. Nerve fibres carry signals away from a neuron's cell body, and dendrites carry signals toward it.

CONDUCTION OF NERVE SIGNALS

Nerve impulses travel along neurons in the form of electrical signals. These signals cross the synapses (tiny gaps) between one neuron and the next in chemical form before being transmitted again in electrical form. Signals are also chemically transmitted to other target cells, such as those in muscles, which make appropriate responses.

Electrical and chemical conduction
When an electrical signal arrives at the end of a nerve fibre, it triggers the release of neurotransmitter molecules, which transmit the signal in chemical form to the next cell.

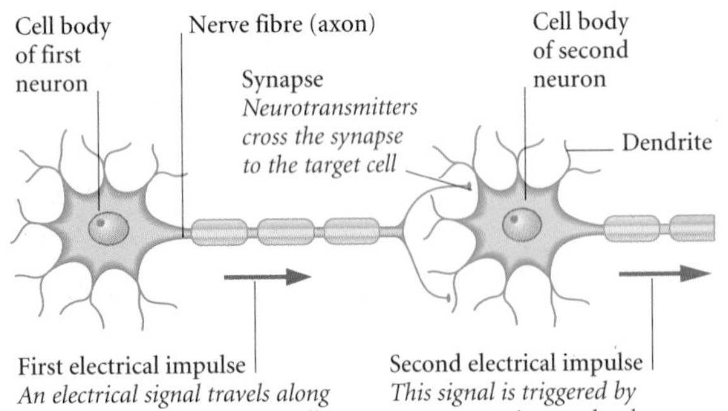

HOW NEUROTRANSMITTERS WORK

More than 50 neurotransmitters have been identified. Their task is to carry nerve impulses across the synapse (a tiny gap) between neurons and target cells. Neurotransmitters either stimulate or inhibit electrical impulses in target cells.

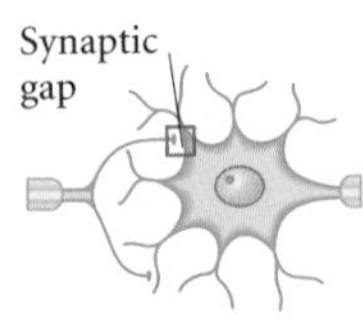

LOCATION

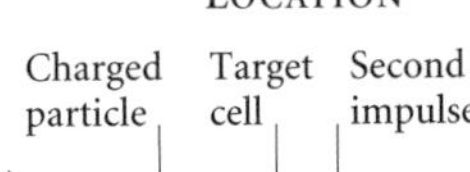

Open channel
Neurotransmitters open channels in the target cell to let charged particles through

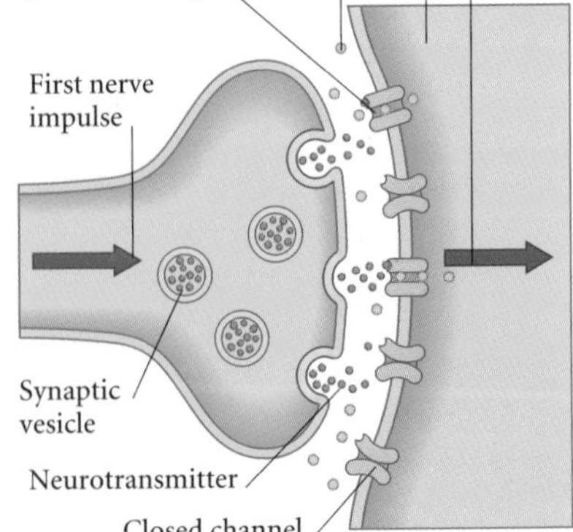

Crossing the synapse
Arrival of a nerve impulse stimulates the release of neurotransmitters from vesicles. They pass across the synapse and open channels in the target cell. Charged particles can then enter and trigger a second impulse.

STRUCTURE AND FUNCTION

SENSORY RECEPTORS

Sensory receptors respond to stimuli and transmit data about them to the brain. In the skin, receptors detect touch, pressure, vibration, temperature, and pain. Elsewhere in the body, more specialised receptors detect light (*see* HOW THE EYE WORKS, p.568), sound (*see* THE MECHANISM OF HEARING, p.594), smell, and taste. Internal receptors called proprioceptors sense body position and the location of body parts in relation to each other.

TOUCH

Touch receptors are found all over the body. The most common are free nerve endings, which sense pain, pressure, and temperature in addition to touch. Other touch receptors include Merkel's discs and Meissner's corpuscles, which detect light touch, and Pacinian corpuscles, which sense deep pressure and vibration.

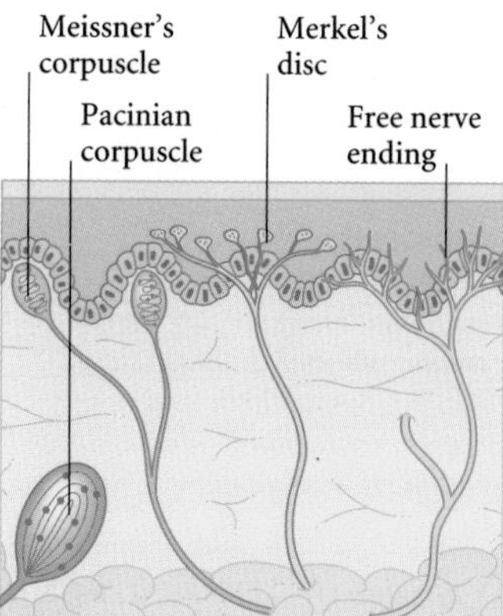

Receptors in the skin
Merkel's discs and Meissner's and Pacinian corpuscles end in a capsule. Free nerve endings are uncovered.

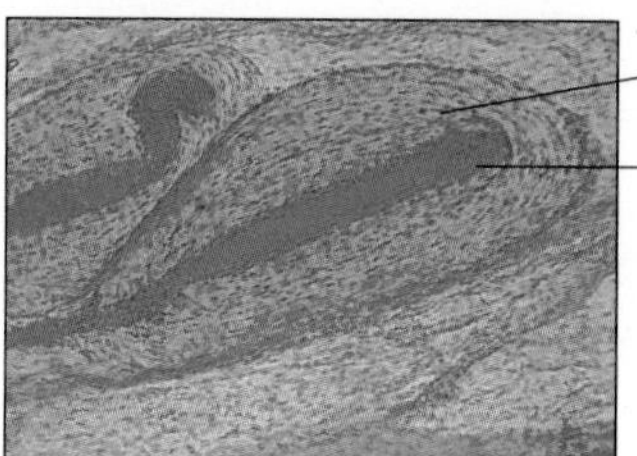

Pacinian corpuscle
This receptor consists of a nerve ending surrounded by layered membranes. Pacinian corpuscles are found in the palms, soles, genitals, and nipples.

SMELL

Olfactory receptors in the roof of the nasal cavity are stimulated by odours. Nerve impulses from these receptors travel to the olfactory bulb (the end of the olfactory nerve) and then to the olfactory centres in the brain. Our sense of smell is thousands of times more sensitive than our sense of taste, and we can detect more than 10,000 odours.

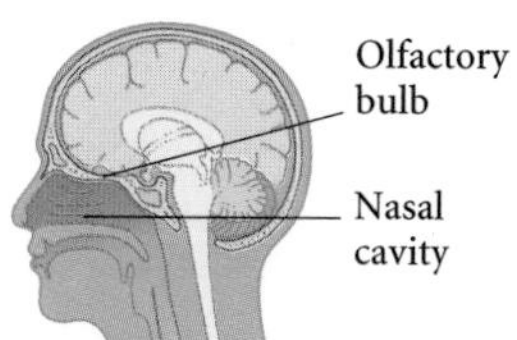

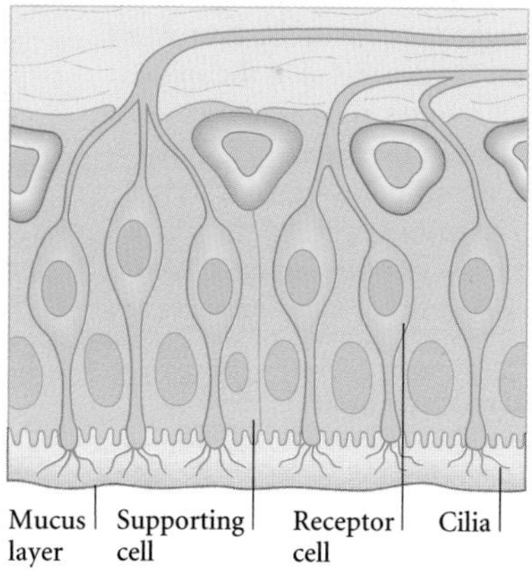

Olfactory receptors
When odour molecules enter the nose, they stimulate the cilia (tiny hairs) attached to receptor cells, causing nerve impulses to pass to the olfactory bulb and then to the brain.

TASTE

There are about 10,000 taste buds on the upper surface of the tongue. Each bud contains about 25 sensory receptor cells, on which tiny taste hairs are exposed to drink and food dissolved in saliva. Buds in different parts of the tongue sense the four basic tastes: bitter, sour, salty, and sweet. A combination of odours and these basic tastes produce more subtle tastes.

Taste bud structure
Substances in the mouth come into contact with taste hairs on the tongue. These tiny hairs generate nerve impulses that travel along nerve fibres to a specialised area of the brain.

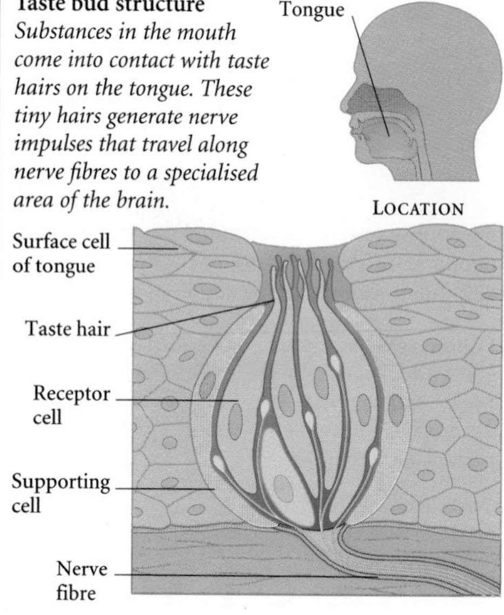

PROPRIOCEPTORS

Proprioceptors are types of internal sensory receptors that monitor the degree of stretch of muscles and tendons around the body. This information gives us our sense of balance and our awareness of the position of various parts of the body in relation to each other.

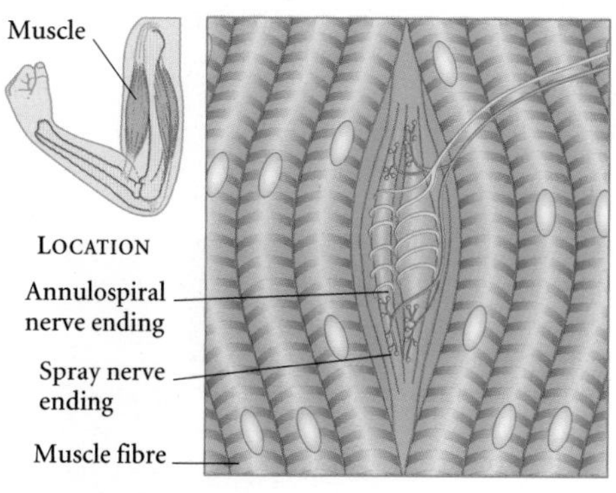

Muscle proprioceptors
Two types of muscle proprioceptor are annulospiral sensory endings, which wind around the muscle fibres, and spray endings, which lie on top of the fibres.

FUNCTION VOLUNTARY AND INVOLUNTARY RESPONSES

The responses of the nervous system to stimuli may be voluntary or involuntary. Voluntary responses are mainly under conscious control, but some voluntary movements, such as walking, require less conscious attention. There are two types of involuntary response, autonomic and reflex. Autonomic responses regulate the body's internal environment. Reflexes mainly affect those muscles that are normally under voluntary control.

VOLUNTARY RESPONSES

All voluntary activities involve the brain, which sends out the motor impulses that control movement. These motor signals are initiated by thought and most also involve a response to sensory stimuli. For example, people use sight and sense of position to help them coordinate the action of walking.

Voluntary pathways
The sensory impulses that trigger voluntary responses are dealt with in many parts of the brain.

Cerebral cortex
The cortex processes sensory data and sends impulses to the muscles

Cerebellum
The cerebellum monitors sensory data on body position, fine-tuning motor nerve impulses from the cerebral cortex to coordinate movement

Basal ganglia
These masses of grey matter help to control coordinated movements, such as walking

Sensory nerve impulse

Motor nerve impulse

Spinal cord

Nerve–muscle junction
At this junction, a nerve fibre transmits signals to produce a response from muscle fibres.

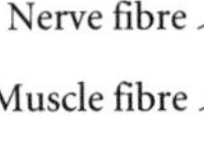

Nerve fibre

Muscle fibre

AUTONOMIC RESPONSES

The autonomic nervous system controls the body's internal environment without conscious intervention and helps to regulate vital functions, such as blood pressure. The two types of autonomic nerves, sympathetic and parasympathetic, have opposing effects but balance each other most of the time. At certain times, such as during stress or exercise, one system dominates.

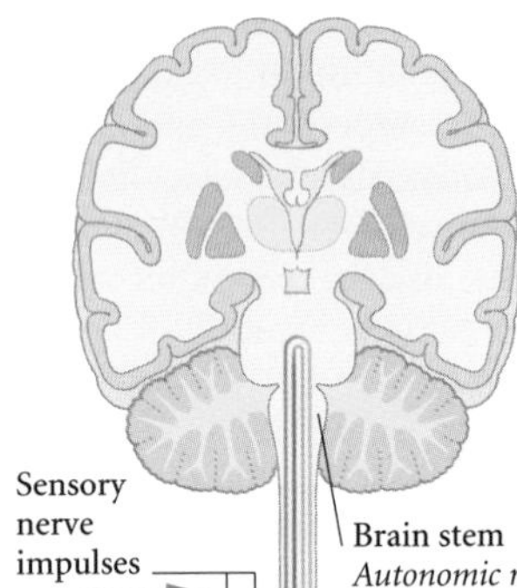

Autonomic pathways
Information collected by internal receptors travels along sensory nerves to the spinal cord and the brain stem for processing. Sympathetic and parasympathetic response signals have separate pathways.

DIVISIONS OF THE AUTONOMIC SYSTEM

AFFECTED ORGAN	SYMPATHETIC RESPONSE	PARASYMPATHETIC RESPONSE
Eyes	Pupils dilate	Pupils constrict
Lungs	Bronchial tubes dilate	Bronchial tubes constrict
Heart	Rate and strength of heartbeat increase	Rate and strength of heartbeat decrease
Stomach	Enzymes decrease	Enzymes increase
Liver	Releases glucose	Stores glucose

Two types of responses
Sympathetic and parasympathetic nerves each produce different responses in a particular organ. The sympathetic responses prepare the body to cope at times of stress. Parasympathetic responses help conserve or restore energy.

REFLEXES

A reflex is an involuntary response to a stimulus, such as withdrawing your hand from a hot surface before you become aware of the heat. Most reflexes are processed in the spine, although some, such as blinking, are processed in the brain. In a spinal reflex, the stimulus signal travels along a sensory nerve to the spinal cord, and a response signal travels back by means of a motor nerve.

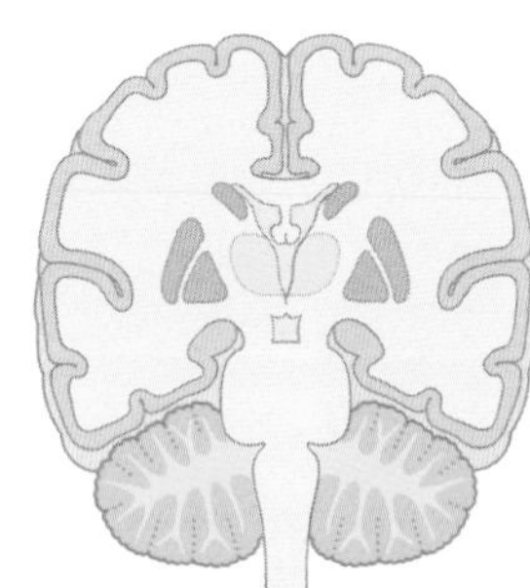

Spinal reflex pathway
Spinal reflexes involve the simplest nerve pathways: the sensory and motor neurons are directly linked together in the spinal cord.

FUNCTION INFORMATION PROCESSING

Different types of sensory information are processed in different parts of the nervous system, which sends out appropriate response signals. Complex information, such as data about music and emotion, is processed in the cerebral cortex, which is known as the "higher" part of the brain. Some specialized functions, such as the interpretation of language, are processed mainly in one side of the brain, the "dominant hemisphere". The left hemisphere is dominant in more than 9 out of 10 people.

Broca's area in right hemisphere

Broca's area in left hemisphere

Wernicke's area in left hemisphere

Language interpretation in the brain
The coloured areas in this PET scan show the regions of the brain that are most active while interpreting language. There is more activity in the left dominant hemisphere than in the right hemisphere.

PROCESSING HIGHER FUNCTIONS

Neuroscientists can now pinpoint those parts of the brain's cortex that process nerve impulses concerned with higher human functions, such as intellect and memory. Areas of the cortex that are mainly concerned with detecting nerve impulses are known as primary areas; the parts that are concerned with analysing impulses are known as association areas.

Motor cortex
The motor cortex sends signals to muscles to cause voluntary movements

Premotor cortex
This part of the cortex coordinates complex movement sequences, such as piano playing

Prefrontal cortex
The prefrontal cortex deals with various aspects of behaviour and personality

Broca's area
This area is vital for the formation of speech

Primary auditory cortex
This area detects discrete qualities of sound, such as pitch and volume

Auditory association cortex
This area analyses data about sound. Data about individual sounds are combined, so that words or melodies can be recognized

Primary sensory cortex
This area receives data about sensations in skin, muscles, joints, and organs

Sensory association cortex
Data about sensations are analysed here

Visual association cortex
Images are formed once visual data have been analysed here

Primary visual cortex
This part of the cortex receives nerve impulses from the eye

Wernicke's area
This area interprets spoken and written language

The brain map
Different areas of the cortex have specific functions. Many areas of the cortex are involved in complex functions such as learning.

MOVEMENT AND TOUCH

Each side of the brain has its own motor and sensory cortices, which control movement and sense touch in the opposite side of the body. Movement signals are processed by a particular region at the top of the cerebrum in the motor cortex. An adjacent area, known as the sensory cortex, processes touch signals. Movements that involve great complexity or body parts that are extremely sensitive to touch are allocated a larger proportion of motor or sensory cortex. In general, those parts of the body capable of complex movement are also highly sensitive to touch.

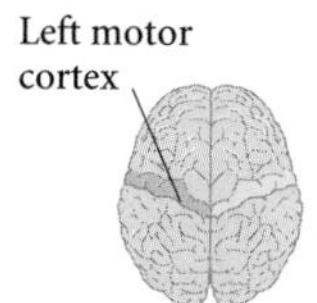

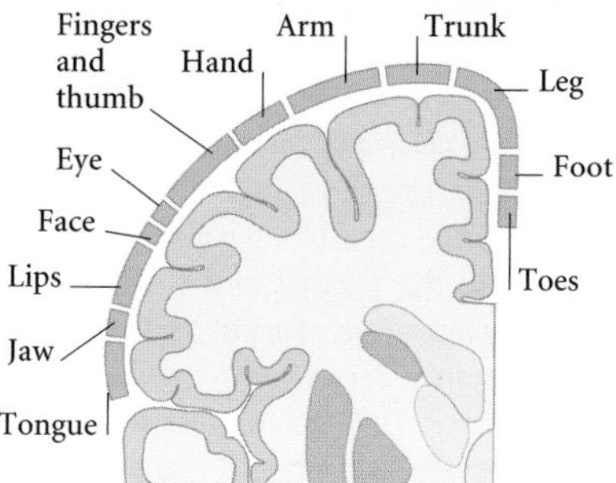

Motor map of the brain
Areas of the body that require great skill and precision of movement, such as the hands, are allocated relatively large areas of the motor cortex.

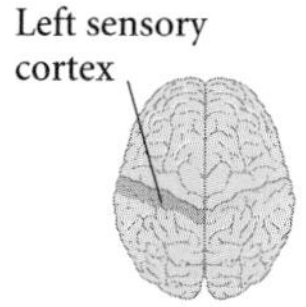

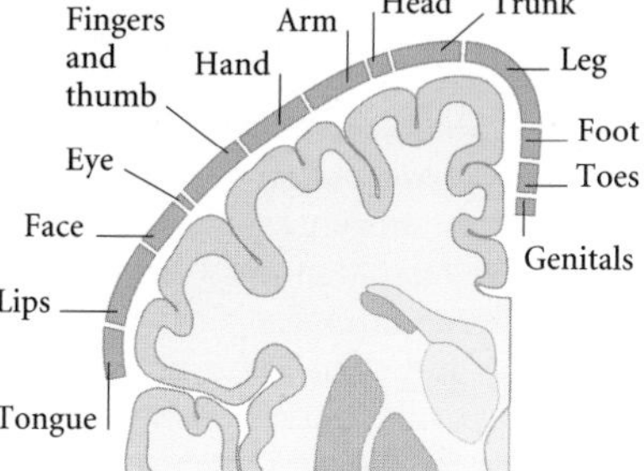

Touch map of the brain
Very sensitive areas of the body, such as the fingers, lips, and genitals have disproportionately large areas of the sensory cortex allocated to them.

General Nervous System Disorders

The nervous system is composed of the brain and spinal cord, together known as the central nervous system, and a vast array of peripheral nerves that transmit information to and from these central structures. The nervous system may be damaged by infection, injury, or vascular problems. However, the causes of many general nervous system disorders are not fully understood.

The first article in this section deals with pain. Most people feel pain when injured, and it is a common symptom of many disorders. A description of the pain, including information about where it occurs and its nature, often helps in the diagnosis of a disorder. Fortunately, the advent of effective painkillers and new treatments, such as transcutaneous electrical nerve stimulation (TENS), means that prolonged, unbearable pain can be effectively treated and/or controlled.

The different types of headache are discussed next. Tension headaches cause discomfort and pain to millions of people every year, often due to stress or tension. Migraine is also relatively common, while cluster headaches are a severe but less common type of headache that occur in a characteristic pattern. A headache can be a sign of an underlying disorder, and persistent or severe headaches associated with other symptoms, such as vomiting, should be assessed by a doctor without delay.

The final article in this section discusses chronic fatigue syndrome, a complex and debilitating condition.

Headaches and migraine in children are covered elsewhere (*see* INFANCY AND CHILDHOOD, pp.844–850).

KEY ANATOMY

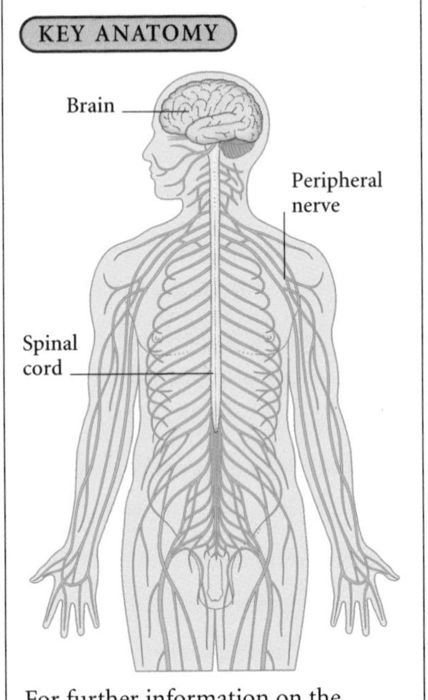

For further information on the structure and function of the nervous system, *see* pp.508–515.

Pain

An unpleasant sensation often felt as a result of tissue disease or damage

AGE GENDER GENETICS LIFESTYLE Not significant factors

Pain is the body's response to an injury or a disease that results in tissue damage. Pain usually functions as a protective warning mechanism that helps to prevent further damage, although chronic (long-term) pain often seems to serve no useful function. Everyone has experienced pain, but its type and severity depend to some extent on the cause. For example, pain that results from a sports injury may be less severe than that of a similar injury caused by a violent assault. Mood and personality also affect the way we perceive pain. For example, fear or anxiety can make pain worse, while relaxation may help to relieve it to a certain extent.

The brain and spinal cord produce their own painkillers, known as endorphins, in response to pain. Endorphins are natural chemicals that are closely related to morphine and act as highly effective pain relievers for short periods but are less effective for chronic pain.

Most forms of pain can now be controlled as a result of improvements in treatment, and it is rare for someone to have to live with persistent pain.

What are the causes?

When tissue is damaged by trauma, infection, or a problem with its blood supply, specialized nerve endings called pain receptors are stimulated. Electrical signals travel along the nerves and through the spinal cord to the brain, which interprets them as pain. While this is happening, the damaged tissues release chemicals known as prostaglandins, which cause inflammation and swelling. The prostaglandins further stimulate the pain receptors. The skin and other sensitive parts of the body, such as the tongue and the eyes, have a large number of pain receptors and are therefore very sensitive to painful stimuli. The internal organs of the body have fewer pain receptors and are insensitive to most types of injury.

What are the types?

Although each individual may describe the character or the site of pain in a different way, there are some types of pain that usually result from specific problems. For example, throbbing pain is often due to increased blood flow, either as a result of widening of the blood vessels, as may occur in migraine (p.518), or because of an increase in blood flow through injured tissues. Severe, shooting pains, such as sciatica (p.546), can be caused by pressure or irritation of the nerve at the point where it emerges from the spinal cord. Colicky pain is caused by intermittent stretching and contraction of muscles in the walls of the intestines, or in other parts of the body such as the bile ducts, which lead from the liver to the intestine.

The location of the pain usually acts as a good guide to its source. However, in some cases, overlapping nerve pathways can result in a confused message, causing pain to be felt in a different area of the body from the site where it originates. This type of pain, known as referred pain, occurs when the nerves carrying the sensation of pain merge with other nerves before they reach the brain. For example, hip problems may be felt as knee pain, while problems with a tooth may be felt as earache. Heart problems can cause pain across the chest, into the neck, and in one or both arms. Pain due to problems in the intestines tends to be felt in the centre of the abdomen and is felt locally only when the abdominal wall is affected, as in the late stages of appendicitis (p.664).

Sudden (acute), severe pain may be associated with other symptoms, such as pale skin, sweating, nausea or vomiting, rapid pulse, and dilated pupils, and may even result in fainting. Prolonged periods of severe pain that continue for weeks or months may lead to depression (p.554), loss of weight as a result of decreased appetite, and disturbed sleep (*see* INSOMNIA, p.554).

TREATMENT PAIN RELIEF USING TENS

Transcutaneous electrical nerve stimulation (TENS) is sometimes useful for relieving severe, persistent pain, such as back pain. In TENS, electrical impulses are relayed from an impulse generator to electrodes placed on the skin in the area of the pain. After about 30 minutes, pain may be significantly reduced. Relief may last for several hours. TENS can be used while pursuing normal activities.

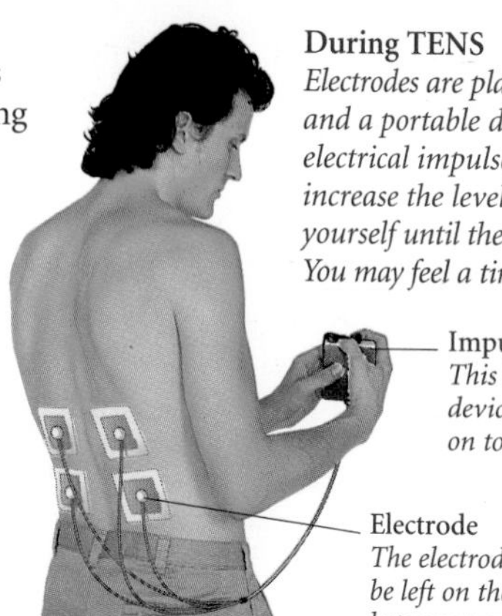

During TENS
Electrodes are placed on the skin, and a portable device generates electrical impulses. You can increase the level of stimulation yourself until the pain is relieved. You may feel a tingling sensation.

Impulse generator
This battery-operated device can be clipped on to a belt

Electrode
The electrodes can be left on the skin between treatments

WHAT MIGHT BE DONE?

If you experience severe or recurrent unexplained pain, you should see your doctor who may be able to establish the cause of pain after a physical examination. Further investigations, including blood tests and imaging tests such as ultrasound scanning (p.250), may be necessary if there is no obvious cause.

Since it is difficult to measure the severity of pain, your doctor may ask how the pain affects your sleep and your ability to cope with daily activities. You may also be asked to describe the severity of the pain on a scale of 1 to 10, using 1 for slight discomfort and 10 for almost unbearable pain.

The most effective remedy for pain is treatment of the underlying cause, if possible. However, pain relief is also important until treatment of the cause takes effect. There are many different ways to relieve pain, including drugs and physical methods. The form of pain relief chosen depends on the cause and type of pain you experience.

Since pain, especially persistent pain, is influenced by other factors such as personality and levels of stress, treatment has to be tailored to the individual.

DRUG TREATMENT Virtually all short-lived pain and much long-term pain can be relieved by painkillers (p.912). When pain is caused partly by local prostaglandin release, treatment with a nonsteroidal anti-inflammatory drug (p.894) such as ibuprofen often works well because these drugs limit the release of prostaglandins.

Opioid drugs, such as morphine and codeine, act directly on the part of the brain that perceives pain and are usually highly effective. Opioid drugs may be needed to relieve intense pain, such as that following surgery, and the severe pain associated with some cancers (*see* PAIN RELIEF FOR CANCER, p.283). The risk of addiction to these drugs is small when they are used for short periods, and dependence is not a cause for concern when they are used in caring for a terminally ill person (p.965).

In addition to painkillers, a number of other drugs are prescribed for certain types of pain. These include local anaesthetics (p.914) and drugs that affect the transmission of nerve impulses, such as antidepressant drugs (p.916) and anticonvulsant drugs (p.914). Pain that is caused by muscle tension may be relieved by small doses of antidepressants. Anticonvulsant drugs are often used to treat pain associated with neuropathies, such as trigeminal neuralgia (p.546).

Nerve endings

Nerve fibre

Nerve endings
Branching nerve endings, as shown here, may respond to tissue damage by sending electrical signals to the brain. These signals are then interpreted as pain.

PHYSICAL TREATMENT A wide range of nondrug therapies is available to help to relieve pain, including gentle massage and the use of hot or cold compresses. These treatments both alter blood flow through damaged tissues and stimulate other nerve endings, blocking pain.

Acupuncture (p.973) is helpful for some types of pain and may be used to relieve pain after operations or for persistent pain that does not respond to other types of treatment. Acupuncture is believed to work by causing the brain to release endorphins or by stimulating nerve endings near the site of the pain so that they stop sending pain messages.

If your pain is due to damaged ligaments or muscles, your doctor may offer ultrasound treatment, in which sound waves produce vibrations in the tissues and generate heat. Transcutaneous electrical nerve stimulation (*see* PAIN RELIEF USING TENS, above) uses electric impulses to reduce pain by stimulating the nerves and is sometimes used for lower back pain (p.381) or during labour.

WHAT IS THE PROGNOSIS?

Almost all pain can be relieved to some degree, even if the underlying cause of the pain cannot be definitively treated. However, persistent pain is often more difficult to control than acute pain.

WWW ONLINE SITES: p.1035

Headache

Pain in the head of variable severity due to a variety of causes

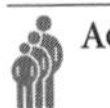 AGE More common over the age of 20

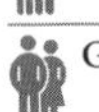 GENDER More common in females

 LIFESTYLE Stress is a risk factor

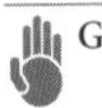 GENETICS Not a significant factor

In the UK, 8 in 10 people have at least one headache each year. The majority of headaches last for only a few hours, but some persist for weeks.

Pain may occur in only one part of the head, such as above the eyes, or it may be spread across the entire head. The type of pain varies; it may be sharp and sudden or dull and constant. Sometimes, other symptoms, such as nausea, occur at the same time.

WHAT ARE THE CAUSES?

There are many possible causes of headache that determine the site and nature of the pain. About 3 in 4 of all headaches are caused by tension in the scalp or neck muscles. Tension headaches (right) tend to recur frequently and cause moderate pain that affects both sides of the head. Other types of headache, including migraine (right) and cluster headaches (opposite page), have a variety of possible causes.

Very few headaches have a serious underlying cause (*see* SYMPTOM CHART: HEADACHE, p.110), but those that do require urgent medical attention. For example, a severe headache may be a sign of meningitis (p.527), a condition in which the membranes covering the brain and spinal cord become inflamed, or subarachnoid haemorrhage (p.534), in which there is bleeding between the membranes covering the brain. In an elderly person, a headache with tenderness of the scalp or temple may be due to temporal arteritis (p.464), an inflammation of the blood vessels in the head. Occasionally, headache results from prolonged use of strong painkillers (p.912).

If your headache is severe, lasts more than 24 hours, or is accompanied by other symptoms, such as problems with your vision or vomiting, you should seek medical advice without delay.

WHAT MIGHT BE DONE?

You will be physically examined by your doctor. If it appears that an underlying disorder is causing your headache, you may have tests, such as CT scanning (p.247) or MRI (p.248) of your brain.

Treatment depends on the cause of the headache. A tension headache will usually clear up with rest and painkillers. Cluster headaches and migraine headaches can be treated with a specific drug, such as a triptan drug or ergotamine (*see* ANTIMIGRAINE DRUGS, p.913).

(WWW) ONLINE SITES: p.1032

Tension headaches

Moderate or severe pain, affecting one or more areas around the head, often as a result of stress

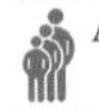 AGE More common over the age of 20

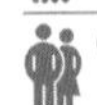 GENDER More common in females

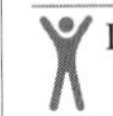 LIFESTYLE Stress is a risk factor

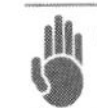 GENETICS Not a significant factor

Tension headaches are often the result of stress (p.74) or bad posture, which causes a tightening of the muscles in the neck and scalp. Tension headaches usually last only a few hours, but some people may have persistent headaches that last for several days or weeks. Recurrent tension headaches often affect people with depression (p.554) or those who are under continuous stress due to difficulties at work or at home. Tension headaches are often made worse by noise and hot, stuffy environments. This type of headache occurs most commonly in women over the age of 20.

WHAT ARE THE SYMPTOMS?

Symptoms often begin late in the morning or in the early afternoon and may persist for several hours. They include:

- Pain that is usually constant and may be throbbing. Pain is felt above the eyes or more generally over the head.
- Feeling of pressure behind the eyes.
- Tightening of neck muscles.
- Feeling of tightness around the head.

People who have persistent headaches often find it difficult to sleep (*see* INSOMNIA, p.554). They may also become depressed and feel depleted of energy.

WHAT CAN I DO?

Taking an over-the-counter painkiller (p.912) such as paracetamol may help to relieve a tension headache. However, the prolonged use of painkilling drugs may cause headaches eventually. If you have a severe headache that lasts for more than 24 hours, does not respond to self-help measures, or is associated with symptoms such as vomiting or blurred vision, consult your doctor immediately.

WHAT MIGHT THE DOCTOR DO?

Your doctor will ask about the severity and frequency of your headaches and may look for signs of stress or depression. A diagnosis of tension headache is often clear from the symptoms, but you may need further tests, such as MRI (p.248) or CT scanning (p.247) of the brain, to check for an underlying cause.

Your doctor may recommend ways for you to deal with stress, such as yoga or relaxation exercises (p.75). If you are suffering from depression, he or she may prescribe antidepressant drugs (p.916). Once your stress or depression has been relieved, tension headaches usually clear up, but they may recur in the future.

(WWW) ONLINE SITES: p.1032

Migraine

A severe headache often associated with visual disturbances and nausea or vomiting

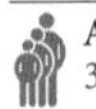 AGE First attack usually occurs by the age of 30; incidence decreases with age

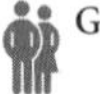 GENDER More common in females

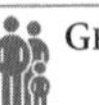 GENETICS Sometimes runs in families

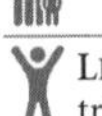 LIFESTYLE Stress and certain foods can trigger an attack

Each year about 1 in 10 people in the UK has a migraine. Migraine is more common in women, and people usually have their first attack before the age of 30. First attacks can occur in children as young as 2 years old (*see* MIGRAINE IN CHILDREN, p.847) but their onset is rare in people over the age of 50. Migraine headaches recur at varying intervals. Some people have attacks several times a month; others have fewer than one a year. Most people find that migraine attacks occur less frequently and become less severe as they get older.

There are two major types of migraine: migraine with aura and migraine without aura. Aura is the term used for a group of symptoms, including visual disturbances, that develop before the onset of the main headache. Migraine with aura accounts for about 1 in 5 of all migraine cases. Some people have attacks of both types of migraine.

What are the causes?

The underlying cause of migraine is unknown, but increased blood flow as a result of widening of the blood vessels in the brain is known to occur during a migraine. About 8 in 10 people who have migraine have a close relative with the disorder. Stress (p.74) and depression (p.554) may be trigger factors, as may the relief of stress, such as relaxing after a difficult day. Other potential triggers include missed meals, lack of sleep, and certain foods, such as cheese or chocolate. Many women find that their migraines tend to occur around the time of menstruation.

What are the symptoms?

Migraine headaches, either with or without aura, are sometimes preceded by a group of symptoms that are collectively known as a prodrome. These prodrome symptoms tend to appear about an hour before the main symptoms begin. The prodrome often includes:

- Anxiety or mood changes.
- Altered sense of taste and smell.
- Either an excess or a lack of energy.

People who have a migraine with aura experience a number of further symptoms before the migraine, including:

- Visual disturbances, such as blurred vision and bright flashes.
- Pins and needles, numbness, or a sensation of weakness on the face or on one side of the body.

The main symptoms, common to both types of migraine, then develop. These symptoms include:

- Headache that is severe, throbbing, made worse by movement, and usually felt on one side of the head, over one eye, or around one temple.
- Nausea or vomiting.
- Dislike of bright light or loud noises.

A migraine may last for anything from a few hours to a few days but eventually clears up. After a migraine, you may feel tired and unable to concentrate.

What might be done?

Your doctor will usually be able to diagnose a migraine from your symptoms. Rarely, tests such as MRI (p.248) or CT scanning (p.247) of the brain may be carried out to rule out more serious causes such as a brain tumour (p.530).

Once migraine has been diagnosed, your doctor may prescribe drugs that reduce the duration of the attacks, help to treat the symptoms, or prevent further migraines occurring. For example, he or she may prescribe an antimigraine drug (p.913), such as a triptan drug that, if taken in the early stages of an attack, will usually prevent the migraine from developing further. Ergotamine, another antimigraine drug, may also be given to help to relieve an attack but should not be taken for long periods of time.

If a full-blown migraine develops, painkillers (p.912) or nonsteroidal anti-inflammatory drugs (p.894) may help to relieve the pain. If you also experience nausea and vomiting, antiemetic drugs (p.922) may provide relief.

Self-help measures may be useful in preventing further migraines (*see* Preventing a migraine, below). If you experience severe migraines or you have more than four attacks a month, your doctor may prescribe a drug such as propranolol (*see* Beta-blockers, p.898) to take every day to prevent attacks.

(WWW) ONLINE SITES: p.1032

SELF-HELP Preventing a migraine

Many factors are known to trigger a migraine. You need to identify the ones that affect you. Avoiding these factors may reduce the frequency and severity of attacks.

- Keep a diary for a few weeks to help to pinpoint trigger factors.
- Avoid any food that brings on an attack. Common dietary triggers of migraine include red wine, chocolate, and cheese (especially matured cheese).
- Eat regularly, because missing a meal may trigger an attack.
- Follow a regular sleep pattern if possible, because changing it may trigger an attack.
- If stress is a trigger, try relaxation exercises (p.75).

Cluster headaches

Severe short-lived headaches that recur over a few days

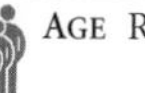
Age Rare under the age of 30

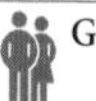
Gender More common in males

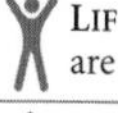
Lifestyle Smoking and drinking alcohol are risk factors

Genetics Not a significant factor

Cluster headaches are brief episodes of often excruciating pain experienced in one part of the head. They occur in a characteristic pattern, usually between one and four times a day, and there may be gaps of months or years between each group of headaches. However, a few people have persistent cluster headaches that occur at regular intervals with very few remission periods between attacks. Like migraines (opposite page), cluster headaches are likely to be related to an increase in blood flow as a result of widening of the blood vessels in the brain. These headaches affect about 1 in 100 people in the UK and tend to be more common in men. Smoking and drinking alcohol increase the risk.

What are the symptoms?

Cluster headaches often develop early in the morning. The major symptoms, which appear suddenly and affect one side of the head or face, include:

- Severe pain around one eye or temple.
- Watering and redness of the eye.
- Drooping of the eyelid.
- Stuffiness in the nostril and, sometimes, a runny nose on one side.
- Flushing of one side of the face.

Individual episodes of pain may last from a few minutes to about 3 hours. The average attack lasts 15–30 minutes. If you have a sudden, severe headache for the first time or if you have symptoms that are different from those of previous headaches, you should consult your doctor at once so that a more serious underlying cause can be excluded.

What might be done?

Your doctor may prescribe an antimigraine drug (p.913) to help to reduce the length and severity of a cluster attack. In a sudden, severe attack, oxygen inhaled through a mask may bring relief. If the attacks continue, lithium (*see* MOOD-STABILISING DRUGS, p.918) and calcium channel blockers (p.900) are sometimes effective.

If the cluster is prolonged, a short course of corticosteroids (p.930) may help to prevent the headaches recurring. These drugs should be gradually reduced in dose, as advised by your doctor, as the headaches disappear.

If you are prone to cluster headaches, you should not smoke or drink even small amounts of alcohol because both increase the risk of an attack.

Cluster headaches may continue for the rest of your life, but you may have prolonged periods of remission.

(WWW) ONLINE SITES: p.1032

Chronic fatigue syndrome

Prolonged fatigue and a wide range of other symptoms, lasting at least 6 months

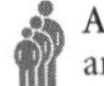
AGE Most common between the ages of 25 and 45

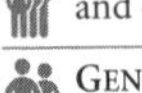
GENDER More common in females

GENETICS LIFESTYLE Not significant factors

Chronic fatigue syndrome is a complex illness that produces extreme fatigue over a prolonged period. The condition has also been called post-viral fatigue syndrome, myalgic encephalomyelitis (ME), or chronic fatigue and immune dysfunction syndrome. The condition can be extremely debilitating and may continue for months or years.

Since the symptoms are so variable, chronic fatigue syndrome is often unrecognised or misdiagnosed. This makes it difficult to estimate the number of people affected, but it is thought to be about 150,000 in the UK. The condition is most often seen in women aged between 25 and 45, but it can affect children or adults of any age and people from all ethnic groups.

WHAT ARE THE CAUSES?

The cause of chronic fatigue syndrome is unknown, although it is believed that several different factors are likely to be involved. In some cases, chronic fatigue syndrome develops after recovery from a viral infection or after an emotional trauma, such as bereavement. In other cases, there is no specific preceding illness or life event. Sometimes, chronic fatigue syndrome is associated with depression (p.554), although it is unclear whether depression is a result of the condition or a cause of it.

WHAT ARE THE SYMPTOMS?

Although the number and severity of symptoms may vary, the major symptoms of chronic fatigue syndrome are:

- Extreme tiredness lasting at least 6 months.
- Impairment of short-term memory or concentration.
- Sore throat.
- Tender lymph nodes.
- Muscle and joint pain without swelling or redness.
- Unrefreshing sleep.
- Headaches.
- Prolonged muscle fatigue and feeling ill after even mild exertion.

Many people who have chronic fatigue syndrome also develop symptoms of depression, such as loss of interest in their work and leisure activities, or of anxiety (*see* ANXIETY DISORDERS, p.551). Conditions involving an allergic reaction, such as eczema (p.333) and asthma (p.483), may become worse in people who have chronic fatigue syndrome.

HOW IS IT DIAGNOSED?

Your doctor may suspect chronic fatigue syndrome if you have had prolonged fatigue for more than 6 months with no obvious cause and you also have at least four of the other symptoms listed above. However, since persistent tiredness is a symptom of many other disorders, including an underactive thyroid gland or adrenal glands (*see* HYPOTHYROIDISM, p.680, and ADDISON'S DISEASE, p.686) and anaemia (p.446), your doctor will try to exclude other causes first.

Your doctor will probably perform a general physical examination, and he or she may ask you questions to find out if you have psychological problems, such as depression. Blood tests may also be arranged. If no underlying cause is identified, a diagnosis of chronic fatigue syndrome will be made if your symptoms meet the criteria. Since there is no specific diagnostic test for chronic fatigue syndrome, confirmation of the disorder can take some time.

(SELF-HELP) COPING WITH CHRONIC FATIGUE SYNDROME

If you develop chronic fatigue syndrome, you are likely to have fluctuating energy levels. You will need to be flexible and adjust your lifestyle to help you to live with the condition. The following self-help measures may be useful:

- Try to divide the day into sessions of rest and work.
- Graded exercise may be useful. Try to set yourself a progressive increase in activity week by week.
- Set realistic goals for yourself.
- Make dietary changes: in particular, reduce your intake of alcohol and cut out drinks containing caffeine.
- Try to reduce stress (*see* RELAXATION EXERCISES, p.75).
- Join a support group so that you do not feel isolated.

WHAT IS THE TREATMENT?

Although there is no specific treatment for chronic fatigue syndrome, there are a number of self-help measures that may help you to cope with the condition (*see* COPING WITH CHRONIC FATIGUE SYNDROME, above). Your doctor may give you drugs to help to relieve some of your symptoms. For example, headaches and muscle and joint pain may be relieved by painkillers (p.912) or nonsteroidal anti-inflammatory drugs (p.894). Antidepressant drugs (p.916) may produce an improvement in your condition even if you have not developed symptoms of depression. You may find cognitive therapy (p.970) and behaviour therapy (p.969) beneficial. A course of physiotherapy (see p.961) will help to build up your stamina. Your doctor may suggest counselling (p.971) to help you to cope with your illness, and joining a support group may also be helpful.

WHAT IS THE PROGNOSIS?

Chronic fatigue syndrome is a long-term disorder, but there may be periods of relief from some symptoms. Many people find symptoms are worst in the first 1–2 years. In more than half of all cases, the condition clears up after several years.

(WWW) ONLINE SITES: p.1035

DISORDERS OF THE BRAIN AND SPINAL CORD

The brain and spinal cord process all incoming information from different sense organs throughout the body and coordinate appropriate responses. Both the brain and the spinal cord are connected to other parts of the body by the peripheral nerves. The brain and spinal cord are protected by overlying membranes as well as by the skull and the flexible, bony vertebral column.

The first articles in this section cover head injuries and different states of unconsciousness, such as coma. Spinal injuries, often caused by whiplash in road accidents, are described next.

Disorders associated with abnormal brain function, such as epilepsy and narcolepsy, which causes an irresistible tendency to sleep. are then discussed. The next articles focus on infectious disorders affecting the brain, such as meningitis, in which the membranes surrounding the brain and spinal cord are inflamed, and viral encephalitis, in which the brain becomes inflamed. Cancerous and noncancerous brain tumours are then detailed.

Different types of stroke and brain haemorrhages, all of which may affect speech, mobility, or mental ability, are discussed next. The final articles in this section deal with degenerative disorders, such as types of dementia and motor neuron disease.

General disorders that affect the brain, such as headache, are discussed elsewhere (*see* GENERAL NERVOUS SYSTEM DISORDERS, pp.516–520).

KEY ANATOMY

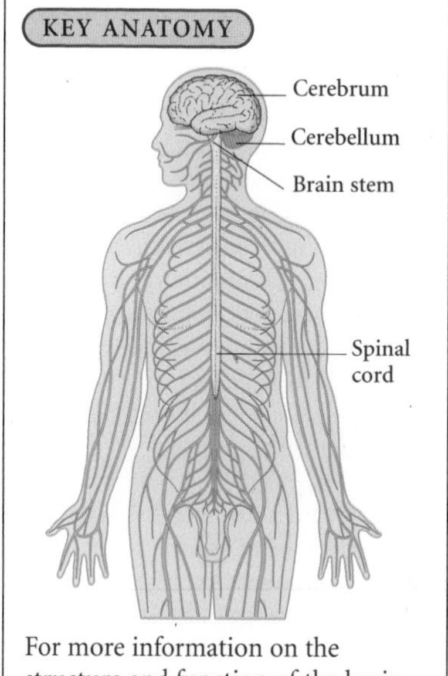

For more information on the structure and function of the brain and spinal cord, *see* pp.508–515.

Head injuries

Damage to the scalp, skull, or brain that can vary in severity from minor to life-threatening

 AGE More common under the age of 35

 GENDER More common in males

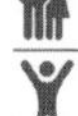 LIFESTYLE Drinking and driving and certain sports are risk factors

 GENETICS Not a significant factor

Many people sustain a head injury at some time in their lives, but most are minor with no long-term consequences. For example, from time to time most children fall over and bump their heads. However, head injuries can be serious and are a major cause of death in young men. About 1 million people in the UK attend hospital each year as a result of a head injury, and more than a quarter require admission. Road accidents are the single largest cause of head injuries, while sports injuries, falls, and assaults, account for most of the remainder.

The severity of a head injury should not be judged simply by appearance because serious brain damage can occur with no sign of damage to the scalp or skull.

WHAT ARE THE TYPES?

Head injuries vary in severity and can damage the scalp, skull, or brain, or a combination of all three. In some head injuries, the eyes may also be damaged (*see* EYE INJURIES, p.582).

Scalp injuries alone are usually minor and have no long-term harmful consequences. However, a small cut to the scalp may result in profuse bleeding because many of the blood vessels are close to the skin surface. As a result, the injury often appears worse than it is.

Fractures of the skull may result from a blow to the head. There may be no bleeding from the scalp, but fractures are sometimes associated with bleeding inside the skull or damage to the brain.

The brain can be damaged directly or indirectly. Direct damage usually occurs in conjunction with a skull fracture or after a penetrating injury, such as a stab wound. Indirect damage tends to occur as a result of a hard blow to the head that does not damage the skull. For example, if the head is struck on one side, the brain can be bruised as it is shaken violently within the skull. The brain may also be damaged by pressure inside the skull caused by a build-up of fluid in the brain after an injury. Bleeding between the membranes that cover the brain (*see* SUBDURAL HAEMORRHAGE, p.535) may also cause dangerous compression of brain tissue.

WHAT ARE THE SYMPTOMS?

Initial symptoms often develop soon after a head injury and, in minor cases, usually include a mild headache and a lump, bruise, or cut on the scalp. However, an injured person may appear well at first, and then symptoms that can be indications of a more serious head injury develop hours or even days later. These symptoms include:

- Blurred or double vision.
- Loss of consciousness.
- Headache accompanied by nausea and vomiting.
- Confusion or drowsiness.

- Slurred speech.
- Vomiting.
- Blood or clear fluid leaking from the nose or ears.

In severe cases, the person may be persistently unconscious (*see* COMA, right). Sometimes, a very serious head injury is immediately fatal.

If you have a severe headache or a cut that requires stitches or if additional symptoms develop, you must go to hospital or get medical help at once. A very young child who is unable to describe his or her symptoms should be watched closely after a head injury. If the child vomits or becomes distressed or drowsy, you should seek medical attention immediately. A head injury that causes loss of consciousness should be assessed in hospital without delay.

ARE THERE COMPLICATIONS?

Following a head injury, a few people develop long-term problems that continue for several months or more. These problems include frequent headaches, dizziness, poor concentration, and loss of balance. Persistent ringing in the ears (*see* TINNITUS, p.602) may also develop. People such as boxers who sustain repeated head injuries may eventually develop parkinsonism (*see* PARKINSON'S DISEASE AND PARKINSONISM, p.539).

If a head injury results in an open wound, bacteria can enter the skull and cause an infection (*see* BRAIN ABSCESS, p.529). Rarely, brain damage may affect speech, movement, or mental ability. Some injuries may result in recurrent seizures (*see* EPILEPSY, p.524).

WHAT CAN I DO?

If you have sustained a blow to the head but have not lost consciousness and have only a mild headache, it is safe to take paracetamol (*see* PAINKILLERS, p.912) to relieve the pain. However, painkillers such as aspirin and other nonsteroidal anti-inflammatory drugs (p.894) should not be taken because they may make bleeding worse.

If you are with someone who has a head injury, you should carry out relevant first-aid treatment (*see* FIRST AID: HEAD INJURY, p.991). If the person has lost consciousness, however briefly, or if you are concerned about the severity of the injury, you should seek medical advice immediately.

WHAT MIGHT THE DOCTOR DO?

Your doctor will examine you and, if necessary, will arrange for you to have tests at a hospital. These may include X-rays (p.244) to look for a fracture and MRI (p.248) or CT scanning (p.247) to look for swelling or bleeding. You may also need to be admitted to hospital overnight for observation.

If you have a minor injury, your doctor may advise you to rest at home. However, you must seek medical attention if further symptoms develop. A person with a severe head injury is usually admitted to an intensive care unit (p.958), where continuous monitoring can be carried out. If there is swelling of the brain, corticosteroids (p.930) may be given. Antibiotics (p.885) are given if there is a risk of infection. Surgery may be needed to relieve pressure on the brain caused by a build-up of fluid or from the skull pressing on it. You may also need surgery to remove a blood clot.

If brain damage has affected speech or movement, speech therapy (p.963), physiotherapy (p.961), and occupational therapy (p.962) may be required.

WHAT IS THE PROGNOSIS?

Most people with a minor head injury recover completely within a few days. The outcome of a serious head injury is often difficult to predict. About 1 in 2 people survives such an injury, although recovery may take up to 2 years, and some impairment, such as speech problems, may remain. In the most severe cases of head injury, there may be paralysis, coma, persistent loss of consciousness (*see* PERSISTENT VEGETATIVE STATE, opposite page), or death.

(WWW) ONLINE SITES: p.1032, p.1035

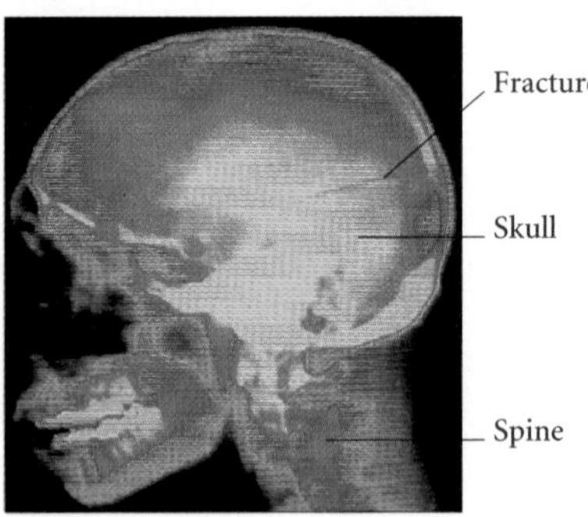

Skull fracture
This colour-enhanced X-ray shows a long horizontal line in the skull, which is a fracture caused by a head injury.

Coma

A state of unconsciousness in which a person's responses to stimuli are absent or reduced

AGE GENDER GENETICS LIFESTYLE
Not significant factors

Coma is an unconscious state in which a person does not respond to outside stimuli such as sound, light, or touch. There are varying depths of coma. In less severe forms, a person may still respond to certain stimuli, move his or her eyes, cough, and murmur occasionally. A person who is deeply comatose does not make any movements or respond to any form of stimulation.

In the past, being in a state of coma was usually fatal within a short time. Nowadays, recovery is possible because vital functions, such as breathing, can be sustained with life-support machines (*see* INTENSIVE CARE UNIT, p.958).

In severe cases of coma, some people lose all automatic functions irreversibly (*see* BRAIN DEATH, opposite page). Other people still retain these basic functions but are otherwise unresponsive. This condition is called a persistent vegetative state (opposite page).

WHAT ARE THE CAUSES?

A state of coma is caused by damage to the brain. Although such damage is often treatable, very severe damage may be irreversible and is sometimes fatal.

A serious head injury (p.521) or a disorder that prevents blood flow to the brain, such as a stroke (p.532) or cardiac arrest (p.419), may damage enough brain tissue to result in a state of coma. Other causes of coma include infections that affect the brain, such as meningitis (p.527) and viral encephalitis (p.528).

Excessively high or low levels of certain substances in the blood may result in a state of coma. For example, a person with diabetes mellitus (p.687) may become comatose if his or her blood glucose (sugar) level rises or falls excessively. In such circumstances, it is usually possible to reverse the condition with appropriate treatment. A state of coma may also be caused by a drug overdose (*see* DRUG OVERDOSE AND ACCIDENTAL INGESTION, p.321) or by drinking an excessive amount of alcohol or be associated with kidney or liver failure.

How is it diagnosed?

A person who is unconscious on admission to hospital will be examined for evidence of injury and to assess nervous system function. Family members and friends will be asked about possible causes. Coma is diagnosed when a person is persistently unconscious, and the depth of coma is assessed by measuring the person's response to stimuli such as pain. For example, the doctor may rub the sternum (breastbone) or press hard at the base of a nail bed. Blood tests are used to look for an underlying cause, such as a drug overdose, high levels of alcohol, or abnormal levels of glucose. Imaging tests, such as MRI (p.248) or CT scanning (p.247), may be carried out to look for brain damage.

If meningitis is suspected, a lumbar puncture (p.527) may be performed. In this test, a sample of fluid from around the spinal cord is taken and tested for evidence of an infection.

What is the treatment?

A person who is comatose is likely to need care in an intensive care unit, and mechanical ventilation may be necessary if breathing is impaired. If possible, underlying causes are treated immediately. For example, antibiotics (p.885) are given for an infection. The level of consciousness is assessed at regular intervals. Monitoring the pressure inside the skull may also be necessary because a state of coma may be associated with raised pressure. If the pressure rises, drugs can be given to reduce it.

What is the prognosis?

If brain damage is minor or reversible, a person may come out of a state of coma and make a full recovery. However, sometimes it is difficult for doctors to predict the likelihood of a complete recovery. Deep coma caused by severe head trauma often leads to long-term neurological problems. Problems may include muscle weakness or changes in behaviour for which long-term treatments such as physiotherapy (p.961) or occupational therapy (p.962) may be needed. If the damage to the brain is severe and irreversible, particularly if the brainstem has been affected, the person is unlikely to recover, and death may be the eventual outcome.

(WWW) ONLINE SITES: p.1035

Persistent vegetative state

A long-term state of unconsciousness caused by damage to the brain

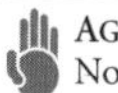
AGE GENDER GENETICS LIFESTYLE
Not significant factors

If large areas of both sides of the brain or the brainstem are damaged, coma (opposite page) may result. In persistent vegetative state, the parts of the brain that control higher mental functions, such as thought, are damaged. However, the areas that control vital automatic functions, such as heart rate and breathing, are intact. Although the affected person is physically and mentally unresponsive to noise, light, and other stimuli, he or she can breathe without any assistance. Random movements of the head or limbs may occur.

People in a persistent vegetative state appear to have normal sleep patterns, with their eyes closing and opening as if sleeping and waking. However, they do not appear to feel physical sensations, such as pain, or experience emotional distress. Since areas of the brain that control breathing and other vital functions are intact, a person in a persistent vegetative state can remain alive for months or even years, provided appropriate medical treatment is given.

The most common cause of the condition is a severe head injury (p.521). It can also be caused by an infection of the brain, such as viral encephalitis (p.528), or by oxygen deprivation of the brain as a result of near-drowning or cardiac arrest (p.419).

What might be done?

The diagnosis of persistent vegetative state is made if a person who is unconscious fails to respond to stimulation or to communicate, but vital functions, such as breathing, are maintained. There is no evidence that the mind of the person is functioning consciously.

There is no treatment for persistent vegetative state. However, general supportive measures and nursing care will ensure that an affected person is kept as comfortable as possible. A person in a persistent vegetative state can live for several years, but recovery is unlikely.

(WWW) ONLINE SITES: p.1035

Brain death

Irreversible cessation of the functions of the brain and brainstem

AGE GENDER GENETICS LIFESTYLE
Not significant factors

When a person does not respond to external stimuli because of brain damage, he or she is in a state of coma (opposite page). In some cases, damage may affect the whole brain, including the brainstem. This part of the brain controls many of the body's vital automatic functions, such as heart rate and breathing. If the brainstem is severely damaged, such as after a head injury (p.521), these vital functions may be affected; if this damage is irreversible, the person may be certified as brain dead.

A person who is brain dead is unable to respond to any stimuli and cannot breathe independently. Without a life-support machine (*see* INTENSIVE CARE UNIT, p.958), death occurs within a few minutes and, even with life support, death occurs within a few days.

What might be done?

If doctors believe that brain death has occurred, a series of tests is carried out by two experienced medical consultants to confirm the diagnosis. These tests check the person's response to stimuli and the functions that are controlled by the brainstem. They include testing the ability to breathe independently without a life-support machine.

A diagnosis of brain death is made only if doctors confirm that brain and brainstem functions have been lost, and that the cause has been identified but cannot be reversed, in spite of everything possible having been done.

Someone with brain death will not survive for more than a few days, even with care in an intensive care unit. Full medical support, including mechanical ventilation, will continue while relatives are given counselling. Doctors will discuss the situation fully with the family, and involve family members as much as possible in the decision of when to switch off the life-support machine.

Depending on the age and previous health of the person and the cause of death, relatives may be asked about their wishes regarding organ donation.

(WWW) ONLINE SITES: p.1035

Spinal injuries

Damage to the back or neck that may involve the spinal cord

 AGE More common under the age of 30

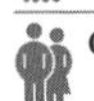 GENDER More common in males

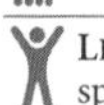 LIFESTYLE Drinking and driving and certain sports are risk factors

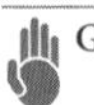 GENETICS Not a significant factor

Injuries to the neck and back are most commonly caused by traffic accidents. The areas most often damaged are the muscles of the back and neck, the bones of the spine (vertebrae), and the ligaments that hold the bones together.

Injuries to the spine may also damage the spinal cord, which lies in a narrow canal in the vertebrae and carries all the major nerve pathways connecting the limbs and trunk to and from the brain. Damage to the spinal cord may cause numbness and weakness in part of the body. If damage is severe, it can result in paralysis, which may be permanent and even life-threatening. Spinal injuries occur more commonly in young men, often as a result of risk-taking behaviour or playing contact sports.

What are the types?

The most common type of spinal injury is whiplash, in which the ligaments and muscles of the neck are damaged. The spinal cord is not usually affected by this type of injury. Whiplash is caused by sudden, extreme bending of the spine when the neck is "whipped" back, usually as the result of a road accident.

A spinal injury may dislocate or fracture one or more of the vertebrae. The vertebrae may be damaged by an impact, such as being hit by a car, or by compression, usually due to a fall from a considerable height. The spinal cord may be damaged by dislocated or broken vertebrae or by a penetrating injury.

What are the symptoms?

Symptoms of a spinal injury depend on the type and severity of the damage and on which part is injured. A whiplash injury may lead to one or more of the following symptoms:

- Headache.
- Neck pain and stiffness.
- Swelling of the affected area.
- Shoulder pain.

Displacement or damage to vertebrae, including compression of a disc, may cause pain and inflammation. If there is damage to the spinal cord, symptoms occur in other parts of the body. These symptoms may include:

- Loss of sensation.
- Weakness.
- Inability to move the affected part.
- Problems with control of the bladder and bowels.
- Difficulty in breathing.

The areas of the body that are affected by symptoms depend on which part of the spinal cord has been damaged. The higher up the spinal cord the damage has occurred, the more parts of the body will be affected. For example, damage to the mid-chest area of the spine may cause weakness and numbness in the legs but will not affect the arms. If the spinal cord is severely damaged in the neck area, there may be total paralysis of all four limbs (quadriplegia), the trunk, and the muscles that control breathing, and death may result.

Anyone who has a suspected neck or spinal injury must not be moved without medical supervision. Emergency first-aid measures should be carried out (*see* FIRST AID: SPINAL INJURY, p.990) and medical help sought at once.

How are they diagnosed?

Once the injured person is in hospital, a full neurological assessment will be performed. This will include measuring the person's responses to different kinds of stimuli, which helps to assess whether the spinal cord has been damaged. If there is damage, CT scanning (p.247) or MRI (p.248) may be used to determine its nature and extent. If a fracture of the vertebrae is suspected, X-rays (p.244) of the spine may be taken.

What is the treatment?

If there is ligament and muscle damage, but the vertebrae are undamaged and unlikely to become displaced, bed rest and regular monitoring will probably be the only treatments that are needed. Nonsteroidal anti-inflammatory drugs (p.894) may be used to relieve pain and swelling of tissues, and physiotherapy (p.961) may be required to strengthen the damaged muscles. If the injury has caused vertebrae to become displaced or damaged, the affected bones will need to be stabilized. Surgery may be carried out to realign damaged vertebrae and prevent possible damage to the spinal cord. People who have irreversible damage to the spinal cord may be paralysed. Sometimes, early treatment with drugs reduces inflammation and limits the extent of the damage. Long-term physiotherapy is necessary to maintain muscle strength.

What is the prognosis?

Recovery from a spinal injury involving only muscles and ligaments is likely to take 4–6 weeks. Fractures usually heal in 6–8 weeks. If the spine is stable and there is no damage to the spinal cord, the person usually makes a complete recovery. When paralysis occurs, a long period of rehabilitation is needed. If there is no improvement after 6 months, the paralysis is likely to be permanent.

(WWW) ONLINE SITES: p.1032, p.1035

Epilepsy

A disorder of brain function causing recurrent seizures

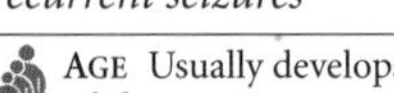 AGE Usually develops in children and young adults

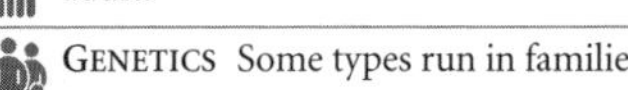 GENETICS Some types run in families

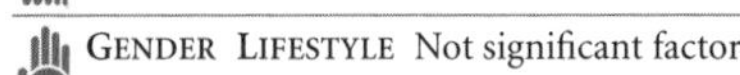 GENDER LIFESTYLE Not significant factors

In a person who has epilepsy, recurrent seizures or brief episodes of altered consciousness are caused by abnormal electrical activity in the brain. Epilepsy is a common disorder, affecting about 1 in 130 people in the UK.

The condition usually develops in childhood but may gradually disappear. However, elderly people are also at risk of developing epilepsy because they are more likely to have conditions that can cause it, such as stroke (p.532).

Many people with epilepsy lead normal lives. However, people who have recurrent seizures may have to limit particular aspects of their lifestyle.

What are the causes?

In 6 out of 10 people with epilepsy, the underlying cause is not clear, although a genetic factor may be involved. In other cases, recurrent seizures may be the result of disease or damage to the brain caused by an infection such as meningitis (p.527), a stroke, a brain tumour (p.530), or scarring following a severe head injury (p.521).

In people with epilepsy, seizures may be triggered by lack of sleep or by missing a meal. Other trigger factors include drinking excessive alcohol and visual effects such as flashing lights and flickering television and computer screens.

A single seizure is not labelled as epilepsy. For example, high fever in a child can result in a single febrile convulsion (p.849). People who abuse alcohol over a long period may have a seizure, either while drinking heavily or during withdrawal from alcohol (*see* ALCOHOL DEPENDENCE, p.564). Very low blood glucose levels, which can occur as a result of treatment for diabetes mellitus (p.687), can also trigger a seizure.

TEST EEG

Electroencephalography (EEG) is used to diagnose conditions, such as epilepsy, that are associated with abnormal electrical activity in the brain. Electrodes are attached to a person's scalp, and recordings are made of brain activity with the eyes open and closed. A strobe light may be switched on for short periods to see if brain activity changes. The procedure takes approximately 20–30 minutes and is painless.

During the procedure
With the electrodes attached to your scalp, you relax on a bed while a continuous recording of your brain activity is made.

RESULTS

Electroencephalogram
These three EEG traces taken from a multitrace recording show an episode of abnormal electrical activity in the brain of a person who has had recurrent seizures.

WHAT ARE THE TYPES?

Epileptic seizures may be generalized or partial, depending on how much of the brain is affected by abnormal electrical activity. During a generalized seizure, all areas of the brain are affected at the same time, whereas during a partial seizure only one part of the brain is affected. Generalized seizures fall into two categories: tonic–clonic seizures and petit mal seizures. There are also two types of partial seizure: simple partial seizures and complex partial seizures. Both simple partial and complex partial seizures can become generalized.

TONIC–CLONIC SEIZURES This type of seizure may be preceded by a warning of an attack, known as an aura. This aura lasts for a few seconds and gives people an opportunity to sit or lie down before they lose consciousness and fall. Auras may consist of a sensation of fear or unease. During the first 30 seconds of a seizure, the body stiffens and breathing may become irregular or stop briefly. This stage is followed by several minutes of uncontrolled movement of the limbs and trunk. After the seizure, consciousness is regained, breathing returns to normal, and the muscles relax. Relaxation of the muscles in the bladder can cause incontinence. The person may be confused and disoriented for a few hours afterwards and may develop a headache. After a tonic–clonic seizure, the person affected usually has no memory of what has happened.

Status epilepticus is a serious condition in which a person has repeated tonic–clonic seizures without regaining consciousness in between. The condition can be life-threatening, and medical attention should be sought urgently.

PETIT MAL SEIZURES These seizures are sometimes known as absence seizures. They start in childhood and may continue into adolescence. Petit mal seizures are rare in adults. During an attack, the child loses touch with his or her surroundings and seems to be daydreaming because his or her eyes remain open and staring. Each attack lasts for between 5 and 30 seconds, and the child is usually unaware afterwards that anything was wrong. Since the seizures are almost never associated with abnormal movements or the child falling down, they may not be noticed. However, frequent attacks can affect schoolwork.

SIMPLE PARTIAL SEIZURES During a simple partial seizure, the affected person remains conscious. The head and the eyes may turn to one side, the hand, arm, and one side of the face may twitch, or the person may feel a tingling sensation in some of these areas. Temporary weakness or paralysis of one side of the body may follow an attack. The person may also have strange sensations, such as odd smells, sounds, and tastes.

COMPLEX PARTIAL SEIZURES Before this type of seizure, an affected person may experience odd tastes or smells or have a feeling of having already experienced what is happening (déjà vu). A brief dream-like state follows during which the person may be uncommunicative. During the attack, there may be smacking of the lips, grimacing and fidgeting. Afterwards, the person may not remember what has happened. Sometimes, a generalized seizure occurs as a progression of the complex partial seizure.

HOW IS IT DIAGNOSED?

You should consult a doctor if you lose consciousness for an unknown reason or if someone witnesses you having a seizure. If your child has a seizure, you should also seek medical advice immediately. It is helpful if you can obtain full details of your seizure from a witness so that you are able to give the doctor a reliable account of what happened. The doctor may arrange tests to look for an underlying cause of the seizure, such as a brain tumour or an infection such as meningitis. If no cause is found or if you have recurrent seizures, you may have an EEG (p.525) to look for abnormal electrical activity in the brain. An EEG also helps to diagnose the particular type of epilepsy because some forms produce a distinctive pattern of electrical activity. Your doctor may also arrange for CT scanning (p.247) or MRI (p.248) of the brain to look for structural abnormalities that may be causing epilepsy.

(SELF-HELP) LIVING WITH EPILEPSY

If you have recently been diagnosed as having epilepsy, the following points may be helpful:

- Avoid anything that has previously triggered or may trigger a seizure, such as flashing lights.
- Learn relaxation exercises (p.75) to help you cope with stress, which may trigger seizures.
- Eat and sleep at regular times.
- Avoid drinking too much alcohol.
- Check with your doctor before taking medications that may interact with anticonvulsant drugs.
- Make sure that you have someone with you if you are swimming or playing water sports.
- Wear protective headgear when participating in contact sports.
- Before applying for a driving licence, talk to your doctor and contact the Driver and Vehicle Licensing Agency for regulations.
- Consult an adviser before choosing a career because some types of employment may not be suitable.
- Seek advice from your doctor if you plan to become pregnant.

HOW MIGHT THE DOCTOR TREAT IT?

If only one seizure has occurred, treatment may not be needed. However, an underlying problem, such as poor control of diabetes, may need to be treated. If you have had recurrent seizures, you will probably be treated with anticonvulsant drugs (p.914). Usually, the dose of the drugs is gradually increased until the seizures are controlled. Occasionally, a second anticonvulsant is needed.

You will probably have regular blood tests to monitor drug levels. If you have no seizures for 2–3 years, it may be possible to reduce the drug treatment or even stop it, depending on a number of factors including the results of the EEG tests and the brain scan. However, any changes in dosage must be carried out under medical supervision. Up to 1 in 2 people who stop taking anticonvulsant drugs have seizures again within 2 years. If drugs do not control the seizures and a small area of brain tissue is found to be their cause, it may be removed surgically.

People with status epilepticus need to be admitted to hospital immediately, where they will be given intravenous drugs to control the seizures.

WHAT CAN I DO?

If you have epilepsy, you should avoid anything that triggers an attack, such as stress or lack of sleep (*see* LIVING WITH EPILEPSY, left). You should carry identification that will alert others to your condition in case you have a seizure.

If you witness someone having an epileptic seizure, you can help by turning the person onto his or her side and protecting him or her from self-injury (*see* FIRST AID: MAJOR SEIZURES, p.989). If the seizure lasts for more than 5 minutes, you should call an ambulance.

WHAT IS THE PROGNOSIS?

About 1 in 3 people who have a single seizure will have another one within 2 years. The risk of recurrent seizures is highest in the first few weeks after an attack. However, the outlook for most people with epilepsy is good, and more than 7 in 10 people go into long-term remission within 10 years.

(WWW) ONLINE SITES: p.1031

Narcolepsy

An extreme tendency to fall asleep during normal waking hours

 AGE Usually develops before the age of 20

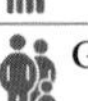 GENETICS Sometimes runs in families

 GENDER LIFESTYLE Not significant factors

People with narcolepsy fall asleep at any time of the day, often when carrying out a monotonous task. Sleep may also occur at inappropriate times, such as while eating. Affected people can be awakened easily but may fall asleep again soon afterwards. Narcolepsy can seriously interfere with daily life.

Some people with narcolepsy have vivid hallucinations just before falling asleep. Others find that they are unable to move while they are falling asleep or waking up (sleep paralysis). About 3 in 4 people with narcolepsy also have cataplexy, in which there is a temporary loss of strength in the limbs that causes the person to fall to the ground. Cataplexy is sometimes triggered by an emotional response, such as fear or laughter.

The cause of narcolepsy is unknown, but it can run in families. It affects about 1 in 1,000 people in the UK, usually developing before the age of 20.

WHAT MIGHT BE DONE?

Your doctor will probably diagnose narcolepsy from your symptoms. EEG (p.525) may also be used to record the electrical activity of your brain. These tests may be carried out while you are asleep in a hospital clinic.

You should take regular, short naps during the day and keep busy while you are awake. Your doctor may prescribe amphetamines (*see* CENTRAL NERVOUS SYSTEM STIMULANT DRUGS, p.918), to help you to keep awake. Certain tricyclic antidepressant drugs (p.916) are useful in treating people with cataplexy.

Although narcolepsy is usually a lifelong condition, in some cases, there is a spontaneous improvement over time.

(WWW) ONLINE SITES: p.1035, p.1036

Meningitis

Inflammation of the meninges, the membranes that cover the brain and spinal cord, due to an infection

AGE LIFESTYLE Risk factors depend on the cause

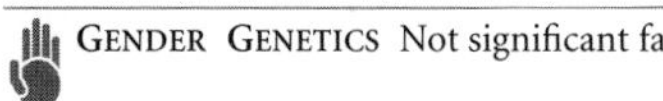

GENDER GENETICS Not significant factors

In meningitis, the meninges, the membranes that cover the brain and spinal cord, are inflamed. The disease is most often caused by a viral or bacterial infection. The viral form of meningitis is the more common and is usually not as severe as bacterial meningitis. The bacterial form is rarer but can be life-threatening. Although both forms of meningitis can occur at any age, bacterial meningitis occurs predominantly in children (*see* MENINGITIS IN CHILDREN, p.848), and viral meningitis is most common in young adults. In rare cases, meningitis may be caused by a fungal infection. This type predominates in people with AIDS (*see* HIV INFECTION AND AIDS, p.297) and in those with other disorders that impair the immune system, such as leukaemia.

(TEST) LUMBAR PUNCTURE

A lumbar puncture is usually performed to look for evidence of meningitis or other nervous system disorders, such as multiple sclerosis. The procedure is carried out under local anaesthesia and takes about 15 minutes. During the procedure, the pressure of the cerebrospinal fluid is checked, and a sample is taken for analysis. You should remain lying down and rest for an hour afterwards to prevent a severe headache.

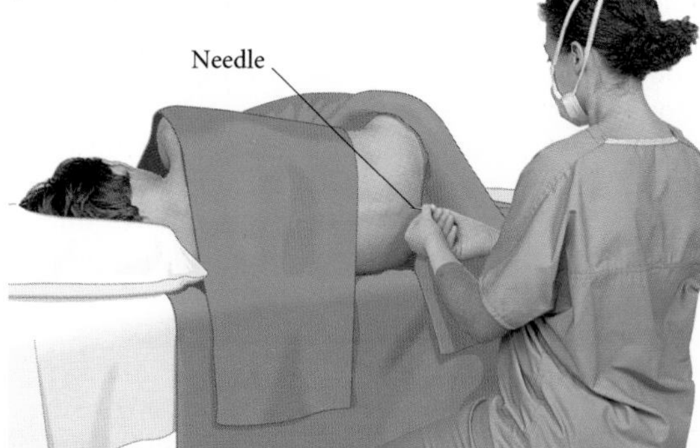

During the procedure
A hollow needle is inserted between two vertebrae near the base of the spine and into the cerebrospinal fluid. A small sample of the fluid is removed for analysis.

(RESULTS)

Evidence of meningitis
This magnified view of a sample of cerebrospinal fluid shows several meningococcal bacteria, which confirm meningitis. The large numbers of white blood cells are a response to the infection.

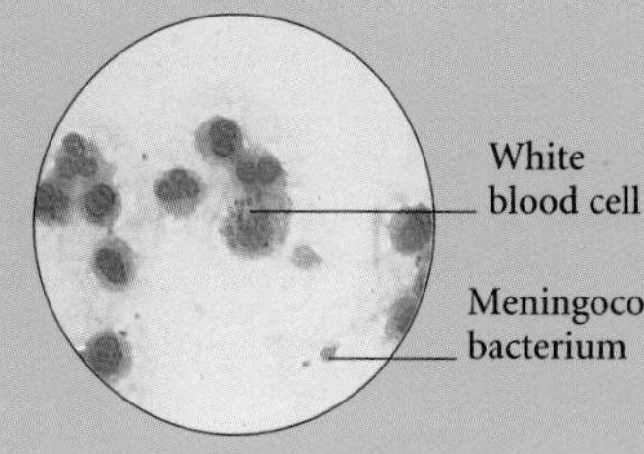

WHAT ARE THE CAUSES?

Many different viruses can result in meningitis. Among the most common are enteroviruses, such as the coxsackie virus, which can cause sore throats or diarrhoea, and, more rarely, the virus that causes mumps (p.293). Viral meningitis tends to occur in small outbreaks, most commonly in summer.

Bacterial meningitis most commonly occurs as a result of infection of the meninges with the bacterium *Neisseria meningitidis* in an otherwise healthy child or teenager. This bacterium is the cause of meningococcal meningitis and has three main types: A, B, and C. Type B is the most common in the UK. Although many people carry *Neisseria meningitidis* bacteria in the back of their throats, only a fraction develop meningitis. Other bacteria that can cause the disease include *Haemophilus influenzae* (Hib) and *Streptococcus pneumoniae,* both of which can also cause infections in the lungs and the throat.

Less often, bacterial meningitis is a complication of an infection that has already developed elsewhere in the body. For example, the bacterium that causes tuberculosis (p.491) can spread from the lungs to the meninges.

Bacterial meningitis usually occurs as single cases only. However, there may be small outbreaks, especially in institutions such as schools and colleges. This form of meningitis is most common during the winter.

People who have a weakened immune system as a result of an existing illness or a particular treatment, such as people with HIV infection or those having chemotherapy (p.280), are at increased risk of all types of meningitis.

WHAT ARE THE SYMPTOMS?

Initially, meningitis may produce vague flu-like symptoms, such as mild fever and aches and pains. More pronounced symptoms may then develop. Symptoms are the most severe in bacterial meningitis and may develop rapidly, often within a few hours.

The symptoms of viral meningitis may take a few days to develop, while in fungal and tuberculosis meningitis, symptoms develop slowly and may take several weeks to become pronounced.

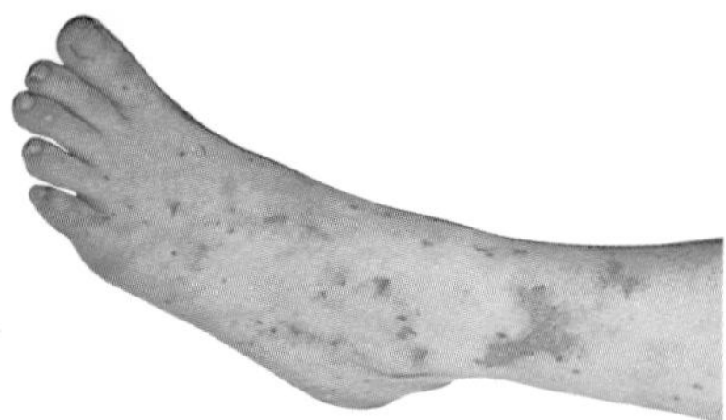

Meningococcal rash
In meningococcal meningitis, dark red or purple spots may appear that develop into blotches. The rash does not fade when pressed and viewed under a glass.

In adults, the main symptoms of meningitis may include the following:

- Severe headache.
- Fever.
- Stiff neck.
- Dislike of bright light.
- Nausea and vomiting.
- In meningococcal meningitis, a rash of flat, reddish-purple lesions, varying in size from pinheads to large patches, that do not fade when pressed (*see* CHECKING A RED RASH, p.129).

Unless prompt treatment is given, bacterial meningitis may lead to seizures, drowsiness, and coma (p.522). In some cases, pus collects (*see* BRAIN ABSCESS, opposite page), which results in compression of nearby tissue.

WHAT MIGHT BE DONE?

If meningitis is suspected, immediate medical attention and admission to hospital is necessary. Intravenous antibiotics (p.885) are started immediately. A sample of fluid from around the spinal cord is then taken and tested for evidence of infection (*see* LUMBAR PUNCTURE, p.527). CT scanning (p.247) or MRI (p.248) may also be carried out to look for a brain abscess.

If bacterial meningitis is confirmed by the lumbar puncture test, antibiotics are continued for at least a week. If meningitis is found to be caused by tuberculosis bacteria, antituberculous drugs (p.886) will be given. In cases of bacterial meningitis, continuous monitoring in an intensive care unit (p.958) is often needed. Intravenous fluids, anticonvulsant drugs (p.914), and drugs to reduce inflammation in the brain, such as corticosteroids (p.930), may be given.

There is no specific treatment for viral meningitis. As long as bacterial meningitis has been excluded by tests, people with viral meningitis are usually allowed to go home if they are well enough. They may be given drugs to relieve symptoms, such as painkillers (p.912) for headaches. Fungal meningitis is treated with intravenous antifungal drugs (p.889) in hospital.

WHAT IS THE PROGNOSIS?

Recovery from viral meningitis is usually complete within 1–2 weeks. It may take weeks or months to make a complete recovery from bacterial meningitis. Occasionally, there may be long-term problems, such as impaired hearing or memory impairment due to damage to a part of the brain. About 1 in 10 people with bacterial meningitis dies despite treatment. Deaths most commonly occur in infants and elderly people.

CAN IT BE PREVENTED?

People in close contact with someone with meningococcal meningitis are usually given antibiotics for 2 days. This treatment kills any meningococcal bacteria that may be present in the back of the throat and prevents their spread to other people. Children are immunized against *Haemophilus influenza* type b (Hib) and *Neisseria meningitidis* type C (*see* ROUTINE IMMUNIZATIONS, p.45). Teenagers are also immunized against *Neisseria meningitidis* type C unless they have been immunized previously. No vaccine is yet available against type B meningoccal meningitis. People travelling to high-risk areas, such as Africa, may be immunized against types A and C (*see* TRAVEL IMMUNIZATIONS, p.86).

(WWW) ONLINE SITES: p.1033, p.1035

Viral encephalitis

Inflammation of the brain as a result of a viral infection

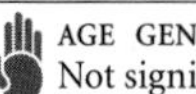

AGE GENDER GENETICS LIFESTYLE
Not significant factors

Viral encephalitis is a rare condition in which the brain becomes inflamed as a result of a viral infection. Often, the meninges, the membranes surrounding the brain and spinal cord, are also affected. Viral encephalitis varies in severity. An attack can be so mild that it causes almost no symptoms and is barely noticeable. However, occasionally it is serious and potentially life-threatening.

WHAT ARE THE CAUSES?

Many different viruses can cause viral encephalitis. Mild cases are sometimes the result of infectious mononucleosis (p.291). In addition, viral encephalitis still occurs as a complication of some childhood infections, such as measles (p.293) and mumps (p.293), although routine immunization (p.45) has made these disorders much less common.

The most common cause of life-threatening viral encephalitis is the herpes simplex virus (*see* HERPES SIMPLEX INFECTIONS, p.291), particularly in people with HIV infection (*see* HIV INFECTION AND AIDS, p.297). In tropical countries, viral encephalitis can be caused by mosquito- and tick-borne infections, such as yellow fever (p.296).

In the past, the disorder was frequently caused by infection with the polio virus. However, this disease is now rare in developed countries as a result of routine immunization.

WHAT ARE THE SYMPTOMS?

Mild cases of viral encephalitis usually develop gradually over several days and may cause only a slight fever and mild headache. However, in severe cases, the symptoms usually develop quickly over 24–72 hours and may include:

- High fever.
- Intense headache.
- Nausea and vomiting.
- Problems with speech, such as slurring of words.
- Weakness or paralysis in one or more parts of the body.
- Memory impairment.
- Hearing loss.

If the membranes that surround the brain become inflamed (*see* MENINGITIS, p.527), other symptoms such as a stiff neck and intolerance of bright light

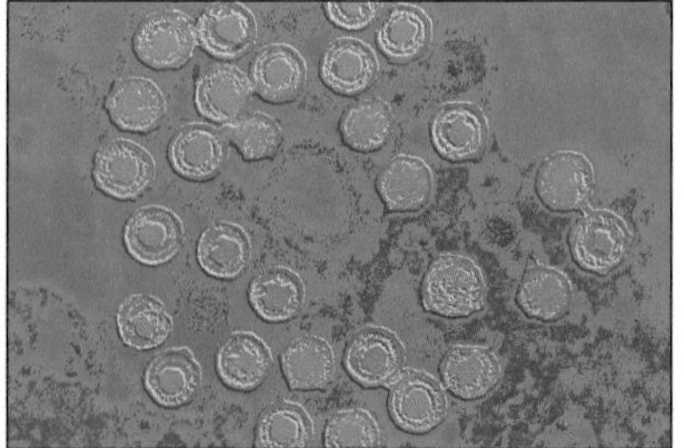

Herpes simplex virus
This highly magnified view shows the herpes simplex virus, the most common cause of life-threatening viral encephalitis.

may develop. The person affected may have seizures. In some cases, there is confusion, which may then progress to drowsiness, a gradual loss of consciousness, and coma (p.522).

How is it diagnosed?

If viral encephalitis is suspected, you will be admitted to hospital. Your doctor may arrange for a blood test to look for signs of viral infection. You may also have CT scanning (p.247) or MRI (p.248) to look for areas of brain swelling caused by inflammation and to exclude other possible reasons for the symptoms, such as a brain abscess (right). A sample of the fluid surrounding the brain and spinal cord may be taken (*see* LUMBAR PUNCTURE, p.527) to look for evidence of infection. You may have an EEG (p.525) to look for abnormal electrical activity in the brain, which is frequently a sign of viral encephalitis. Rarely, a brain biopsy is performed, in which a sample of tissue is taken from the brain under general anaesthesia and then examined to confirm the diagnosis.

What is the treatment?

Viral encephalitis that is caused by the herpes simplex virus can be treated with intravenous doses of aciclovir (*see* ANTIVIRAL DRUGS, p.886) and possibly also with corticosteroids (p.930) to reduce inflammation of the brain. In severe cases, intravenous aciclovir may be given, even if the cause has not been identified. Anticonvulsant drugs (p.914) may be prescribed if seizures develop. Severely affected people may need to be treated in an intensive care unit (p.958).

What is the prognosis?

It is often difficult to predict the outcome of viral encephalitis. People who have mild encephalitis usually make a full recovery over several weeks, but occasional headaches may occur for a few months. However, in severe cases, the condition may be fatal. Encephalitis caused by the herpes simplex virus often produces long-term effects, such as memory problems or muscle weakness. In children, herpes simplex viral encephalitis may cause learning difficulties. The effects of this type of viral encephalitis can usually be minimized if treatment is begun early.

(WWW) ONLINE SITES: p.1033, p.1035

Brain abscess

A pus-filled swelling in the brain caused by bacterial or fungal infection

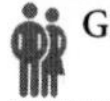

GENDER More common in males

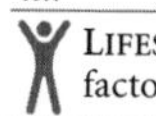

LIFESTYLE Intravenous drug abuse is a risk factor

AGE GENETICS Not significant factors

Brain abscesses are collections of pus. They are rare and, if left untreated, can be life-threatening. Pus may collect to form a single abscess or may form several abscesses in different parts of the brain. Brain tissue around the abscess or abscesses becomes compressed, and the brain itself may swell, increasing pressure inside the skull.

People who have impaired immunity, including those with HIV infection (*see* HIV INFECTION AND AIDS, p.297) and those having chemotherapy (p.280), are more likely to develop a brain abscess. The risk of a brain abscess is also higher in intravenous drug users than in other people because reused needles may be contaminated with infectious microorganisms. Men are twice as likely as women to develop a brain abscess.

What are the causes?

Most brain abscesses are caused by a bacterial infection that has spread to the brain from an infection in nearby tissues in the skull. For example, the infection may spread from a dental abscess (p.611) or from an infection in the sinuses (*see* SINUSITIS, p.475). If the skull is penetrated (*see* HEAD INJURIES, p.521), bacteria may enter the brain and cause infection. Bacterial infection can also be carried in the bloodstream to the brain from an infection in another part of the body, such as the lungs (*see* PNEUMONIA, p.490) or the heart (*see* INFECTIVE ENDOCARDITIS p.426). In 1 in 10 cases, the source of the infection cannot be found. Occasionally, a brain abscess may be the result of a fungal infection.

What are the symptoms?

The symptoms of a brain abscess may develop in a few days or gradually over a few weeks. They may include:

- Headache.
- Fever.
- Nausea and vomiting.

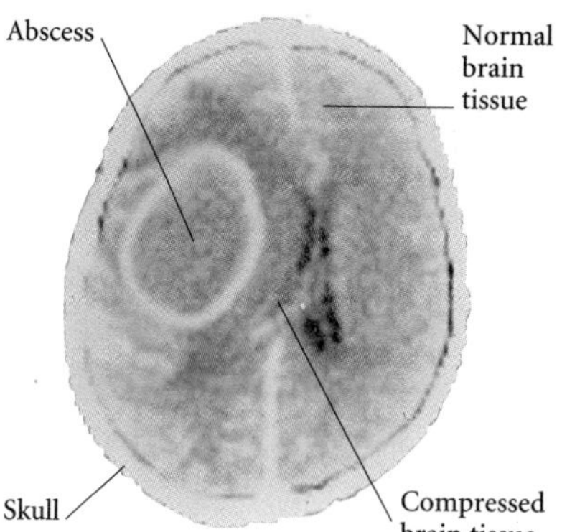

Brain abscess
This CT scan shows a large brain abscess caused by bacterial infection compressing and displacing brain tissue.

- Stiff neck.
- Seizures.

Other symptoms, including speech and vision problems or weakness of one or more limbs, may develop depending on which part of the brain is affected. Without treatment, consciousness may be impaired and may lead to coma (p.522).

What might be done?

If your doctor suspects a brain abscess, you will be admitted to hospital immediately. The diagnosis can be confirmed by MRI (p.248) or CT scanning (p.247) of the head. You may have blood tests to identify the infecting organism and X-rays (p.244) to look for its source.

Brain abscesses caused by bacterial infections are treated with high doses of antibiotics (p.885), given intravenously at first and then orally for about 6 weeks. If the abscess is large or causing considerable brain swelling, a small hole may be drilled through the skull under general anaesthesia to allow pus to drain. The pus is then analysed to identify the infecting organism. You may have corticosteroids (p.930) to control swelling of the brain. Anticonvulsant drugs (p.914) may be prescribed to reduce the risk of seizures. In severe cases, mechanical ventilation in an intensive care unit (p.958) may be needed.

What is the prognosis?

Up to 8 in 10 people recover from a brain abscess if treatment is begun early. However, some have persistent problems, such as seizures, slurred speech, or weakness of a limb.

(WWW) ONLINE SITES: p.1033, p.1035

Brain tumours

Abnormal growths developing in brain tissue or the coverings of the brain

 AGE Most common between the ages of 60 and 70. Some types occur only in children

 GENDER More common in males

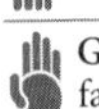 GENETICS LIFESTYLE Not significant factors

Brain tumours may be cancerous or noncancerous. Unlike most tumours in other parts of the body, cancerous and noncancerous brain tumours can be equally serious. The seriousness of a tumour depends on its location, size, and rate of growth. Both types of tumour can compress nearby tissue, causing pressure to build up inside the skull.

Tumours that first develop in brain tissues are called primary tumours. They may arise from support cells in the brain (gliomas) or from meningiomas, cells in the meninges (the membranes covering the brain). Gliomas are often cancerous, but most meningiomas are noncancerous. Primary brain tumours are slightly more common in men and usually develop between the ages of 60 and 70. Some types only affect children (*see* BRAIN AND SPINAL CORD TUMOURS IN CHILDREN, p.850). Tumours that arise in the pituitary gland, at the base of the brain, are discussed in the article on pituitary tumours (p.676).

Secondary brain tumours (metastases) are more common than primary tumours. They are always cancerous, having developed from cells that have been carried in the blood from cancerous tumours in areas such as the breast or the lungs. Several metastases may develop in the brain simultaneously.

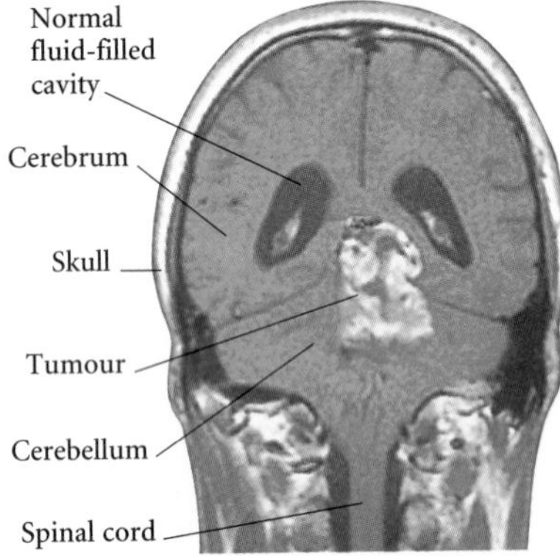

Brain tumour

This MRI scan shows a brain tumour in the cerebellum, the part of the brain that helps to maintain posture and control movement. Balance and coordination are affected when the cerebellum is damaged.

WHAT ARE THE SYMPTOMS?

Symptoms usually occur when a primary tumour or metastasis compresses part of the brain or raises the pressure inside the skull. They may include:

- Headache that is usually more severe in the morning and is worsened by coughing or bending over.
- Nausea and vomiting.
- Blurred vision.

Other symptoms tend to be related to whichever area of the brain is affected by the tumour and may include:

- Slurred speech.
- Unsteadiness.
- Double vision.
- Difficulty in reading and writing.
- Change of personality.
- Numbness and weakness of the limbs on one side of the body.

A tumour may also cause seizures (*see* EPILEPSY, p.524). Sometimes, a tumour blocks the flow of the cerebrospinal fluid, which circulates in and around the brain and spinal cord. As a result, the pressure inside the ventricles (the fluid-filled spaces inside the brain) increases and causes further compression of brain tissue. Left untreated, drowsiness can develop, which may eventually progress to a state of coma (p.522) and death.

HOW ARE THEY DIAGNOSED?

If your doctor suspects a brain tumour, he or she will refer you to hospital for immediate assessment by a neurologist. You will have CT scanning (p.247) or MRI (p.248) of the brain to look for a tumour and check its location and size. If these tests suggest that a tumour has spread from a cancer elsewhere in the body, you may need to have other tests, such as chest X-rays (p.490) or mammography (p.759), to check for tumours in the lungs or breasts. Cerebral angiography (p.533) may be performed to look at blood flow around the tumour. You may also need to have a brain biopsy, in which a sample of the tumour is removed surgically under general anaesthesia. The sample is then examined in a laboratory to find the type of cell from which the tumour has arisen.

WHAT IS THE TREATMENT?

Treatment for brain tumours depends on whether there is one tumour or several, the precise location of the tumour, and the type of cell affected. Primary brain tumours may be treated surgically. The aim of surgery is to remove the entire tumour, or as much of it as possible, with minimal damage to the surrounding brain tissue. Surgery will probably not be an option for tumours located deep within the brain tissue. Radiotherapy (p.281) may be used in addition to surgical treatment, or as an alternative to it, for both cancerous and noncancerous primary tumours.

As brain metastases are often multiple, surgery is not usually an option. However, in cases where there is a single metastasis, surgical removal may be successful. Multiple tumours are usually treated with radiotherapy or, less commonly, with chemotherapy (p.280).

Other treatments may be necessary to treat the effects of brain tumours. For example, the drug dexamethasone (*see* CORTICOSTEROIDS, p.930) may be given to reduce the pressure inside the skull, and anticonvulsant drugs (p.914) may also be prescribed to prevent or treat seizures. If a tumour blocks the flow of cerebrospinal fluid in the brain and fluid builds up in the ventricles, a small tube may be inserted through the skull to bypass the blockage.

You may also benefit from treatments for the physical effects of the tumour, such as physiotherapy (p.961) to help with mobility problems or speech therapy (p.963) for speech problems.

WHAT IS THE PROGNOSIS?

The general outlook for brain tumours depends on their location, size, and rate of growth. The outcome is usually better for a noncancerous tumour that grows slowly; many people with this type are completely cured by surgery.

The outlook for other tumours depends on the type of cell they affect and whether they can be surgically removed. About 1 in 4 people is alive 2 years after diagnosis of a primary cancerous brain tumour, but few people live longer than 5 years. Most people with brain metastases do not live longer than 6 months, although in rare cases, a person with a single metastatic tumour may be cured.

(WWW) ONLINE SITES: p.1028

Transient ischaemic attacks

Episodes of temporary loss of function in one area of the brain resulting from a reduced blood supply to the brain

AGE More common over the age of 45

GENDER More common in males

GENETICS Sometimes runs in families

LIFESTYLE Smoking and a high-fat diet are risk factors

In a transient ischaemic attack, part of the brain suddenly and briefly fails to function properly because it is temporarily deprived of oxygen by blockage of its blood supply. Transient ischaemic attacks can last for anything from a few seconds to 1 hour and have no after-effects. However, if the symptoms persist for longer than 24 hours, the attack is classified as a stroke (p.532).

In the UK, about 1 in 2,000 people has a transient ischaemic attack, more commonly after the age of 45. Attacks are three times more common in men. It is important that a transient ischaemic attack is not ignored because there is a strong possibility that it may be followed by a stroke. Without treatment, about 1 in 3 people who has an attack goes on to have a stroke later on.

WHAT ARE THE CAUSES?

Two conditions can lead to blockage of an artery supplying the brain. A blood clot, called a thrombus, may develop in an artery, or a fragment from a blood clot, called an embolus, may detach itself from elsewhere in the body and travel in the blood to block an artery (*see* THROMBOSIS AND EMBOLISM, p.431).

A thrombus usually forms in blood vessels that are affected by atherosclerosis (p.402), a condition in which fatty deposits build up in the vessel wall. People at increased risk of atherosclerosis include smokers and those who have a high-fat diet. People who have an inherited tendency towards high levels of fat (*see* INHERITED HYPERLIPIDAEMIAS, p.692) or people with diabetes mellitus (p.687) are at risk. High blood pressure (*see* HYPERTENSION, p.403) increases the risk of atherosclerosis.

The emboli that cause transient ischaemic attacks usually originate in the heart, the aorta (the main artery of the body), or the carotid arteries in the neck. Blood clots are more likely to form in the heart if it has been damaged by a heart attack (*see* MYOCARDIAL INFARCTION, p.410), if the heartbeat is irregular (*see* ATRIAL FIBRILLATION, p.417), or if the heart valves are damaged or have been replaced (*see* HEART VALVE DISORDERS, p.421). Sickle-cell disease (p.448) can also increase the risk of transient ischaemic attacks because abnormally shaped red blood cells tend to clump together and block blood vessels.

WHAT ARE THE SYMPTOMS?

The symptoms of a transient ischaemic attack usually develop suddenly and are often short-lived, lasting for only a few minutes. Symptoms vary depending on which part of the brain is affected and may include the following:

- Loss of vision in one eye or blurred vision in both.
- Slurred speech.
- Difficulty in finding the right words.
- Problems understanding what other people are saying.
- Numbness on one side of the body.
- Weakness or paralysis on one side of the body, affecting one or both limbs.

TEST CAROTID DOPPLER SCANNING

Carotid Doppler scanning uses ultrasound to look at the flow of blood through blood vessels in the neck. The procedure is generally used to investigate disorders such as transient ischaemic attacks or stroke. Ultrasound waves from a transducer produce a picture of the blood flow, which can reveal narrowing of the carotid blood vessels in the neck. The procedure takes about 20 minutes and is painless and safe.

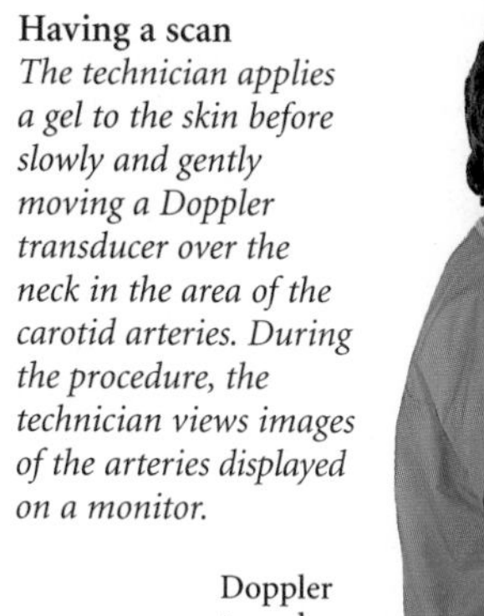
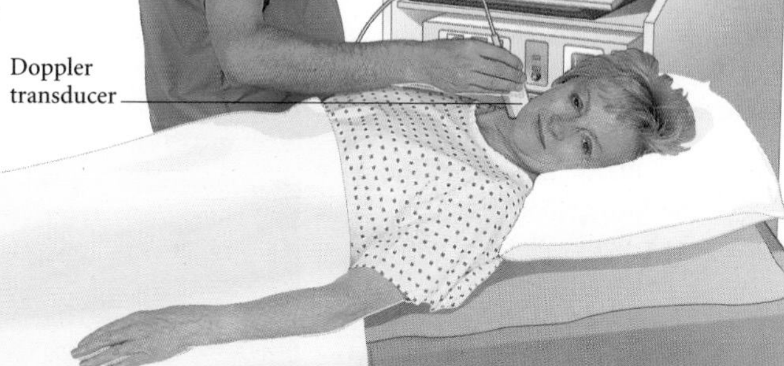

Having a scan
The technician applies a gel to the skin before slowly and gently moving a Doppler transducer over the neck in the area of the carotid arteries. During the procedure, the technician views images of the arteries displayed on a monitor.

RESULTS

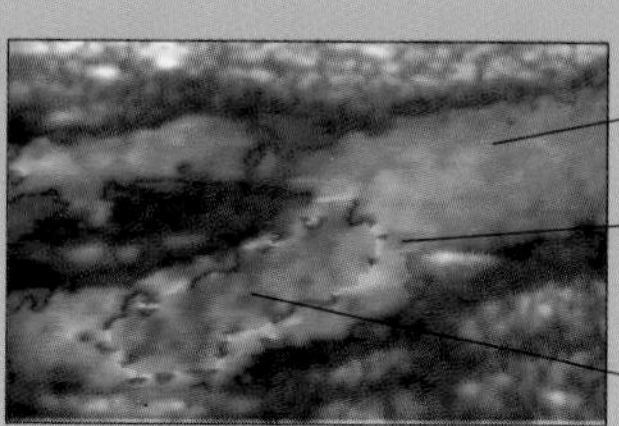

Carotid Doppler scan
This ultrasound image shows the blood flow through a branched carotid artery. After the blood passes through a narrowed section of the artery, the flow becomes disrupted.

- Feeling of unsteadiness and general loss of balance.
- Brief loss of consciousness.

Although the symptoms of transient ischaemic attacks disappear within an hour, attacks tend to recur. People may have a number of attacks in one day or over several days. Sometimes, several years may elapse between attacks.

How are they diagnosed?

Your doctor will carry out a physical examination, which will include checking your blood pressure, heart rhythm, and neurological function. He or she may arrange for CT scanning (p.247) or MRI (p.248) of your brain to look for other causes of your symptoms. You might also have ultrasound scanning of the arteries in your neck (*see* CAROTID DOPPLER SCANNING, p.531) to look for narrowing. If these arteries are significantly narrowed, further imaging tests will be carried out to assess the severity of the narrowing. For example, you may have cerebral angiography (opposite page), in which X-rays are taken of the arteries that supply the brain.

Tests to look for the source of the blood clots include echocardiography (p.425), which is used to look at the structure of your heart and the movement of its valves. Your heart rate may also be monitored for 24 hours to look for irregularities in your heart rhythm (*see* AMBULATORY ECG, p.416).

You may have blood tests to look for other factors that increase the risk of having a transient ischaemic attack, such as diabetes mellitus and hyperlipidaemias. Blood tests may also be used to check for blood disorders that increase the risk of a clot forming.

What is the treatment?

Once a transient ischaemic attack has been diagnosed, the aim of treatment is to reduce your risk of having a stroke in the future. You will be advised to reduce the amount of fat in your diet and, if you smoke, you should stop. If you have diabetes mellitus, you should make sure your blood glucose levels are well controlled. Your doctor will prescribe appropriate drugs to treat high blood pressure (*see* ANTIHYPERTENSIVE DRUGS, p.897) or an irregular heartbeat (*see* ANTIARRHYTHMIC DRUGS, p.898) if you have either of these conditions. Treatment after a transient ischaemic attack can be as simple as taking half an aspirin daily to help to prevent blood clots from forming inside blood vessels. Other drugs that help to prevent blood clotting (p.904), such as warfarin, may be prescribed if emboli originate from clots that have formed in the heart.

If your doctor finds that the arteries in your neck are severely narrowed, he or she may suggest that you have a surgical procedure called a carotid endarterectomy to clear fatty deposits from the narrowed arteries. Alternatively, you may be referred for a surgical procedure called balloon angioplasty, in which a small balloon is inserted into the affected artery or arteries. Once in place, the balloon is inflated to open up the narrowed section of artery. Both of these procedures increase the diameter of the blood vessel and improve the blood supply to the brain.

What is the prognosis?

Transient ischaemic attacks may occur intermittently over a long period or they may stop spontaneously. Of those people who have a transient ischaemic attack, about 1 in 5 will have a stroke within a year. The more frequently you have transient ischaemic attacks, the higher your risk of having a stroke in the future. However, if you take appropriate steps to change aspects of your lifestyle, such as giving up smoking and adopting a low-fat diet, you will reduce the risk of having further transient ischaemic attacks or a stroke.

(WWW) ONLINE SITES: p.1037

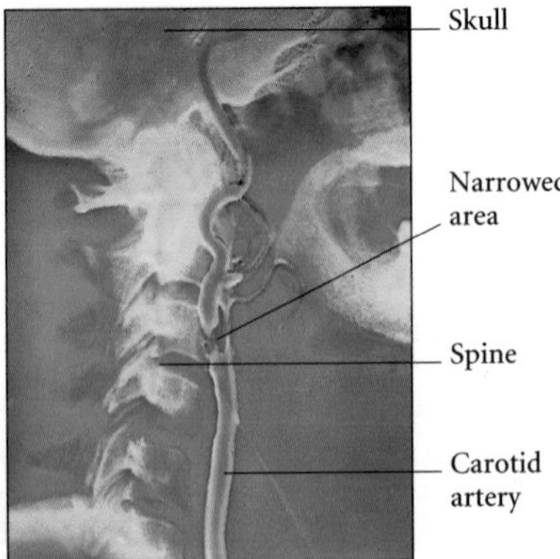

Narrowed carotid artery
This coloured X-ray shows a narrowed area in the carotid artery, which supplies blood to the brain. This narrowing may result in transient ischaemic attacks.

Stroke

Damage to part of the brain caused by an interruption in its blood supply, sometimes called a brain attack

AGE More common over the age of 70

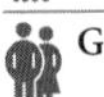
GENDER More common in males

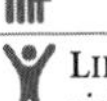
LIFESTYLE Smoking and a high-fat diet are risk factors

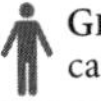
GENETICS Risk factors depend on the cause

If the blood supply to part of the brain is interrupted, the affected region no longer functions normally. This condition is called a stroke, although today it is often described as a "brain attack" to highlight the need for urgent medical attention. A stroke may be due to either a blockage or bleeding from one of the arteries supplying the brain.

There is usually little or no warning of a stroke. Immediate admission to hospital for assessment and treatment is essential if there is to be a chance of preventing permanent brain damage. The after-effects of a stroke vary depending on the location and extent of the brain tissue affected. They range from mild, temporary symptoms, such as blurred vision, to lifelong disability or death.

If the symptoms disappear within 24 hours, the condition is known as a transient ischaemic attack (p.531), which is a warning sign of a possible future stroke.

How common is it?

Each year, about 120,000 people in the UK have a stroke. The condition is more common in men and in older people. A 70-year-old living in the UK is about 100 times more likely to have a stroke than a 40-year-old. Although the number of deaths from stroke has fallen over the last 50 years, stroke is still the third most common cause of death in the UK after heart attacks and cancer.

What are the causes?

About half of all strokes occur when a blood clot forms in an artery in the brain, a process called cerebral thrombosis. Other major causes are cerebral embolism and cerebral haemorrhage (bleeding). Cerebral embolism occurs when a fragment of a blood clot that has formed in another part of the body,

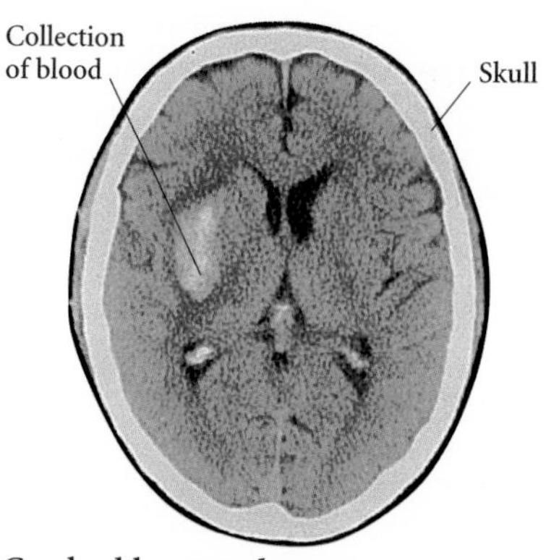

Cerebral haemorrhage
Bleeding into the brain tissue, as shown in this CT brain scan, is known as a cerebral haemorrhage and is one cause of stroke.

such as in the heart or the main arteries of the neck, travels in the blood and lodges in an artery supplying the brain. Just under one-third of all strokes are caused by cerebral embolism. Cerebral haemorrhage, which causes about one-fifth of all strokes, occurs when an artery supplying the brain ruptures and blood seeps out into the surrounding tissue.

The blood clots that lead to cerebral thrombosis and cerebral embolism are more likely to form in an artery that has been damaged by atherosclerosis (p.402), a condition in which fatty deposits build up in artery walls. Factors that increase the risk of atherosclerosis developing are a high-fat diet, smoking, diabetes mellitus (p.687), and high levels of lipids in the blood (*see* INHERITED HYPERLIPIDAEMIAS, p.692).

Cerebral embolism may be a complication of heart rhythm disorders (*see* ARRHYTHMIAS, p.415), heart valve disorders (p.421), and recent myocardial infarction (p.410), all of which can cause blood clots to form in the heart. The risk of cerebral embolism, thrombosis, or haemorrhage is increased by high blood pressure (*see* HYPERTENSION, p.403). Sickle-cell disease (p.448), an abnormality of the red blood cells, also increases the risk of cerebral thrombosis because abnormal blood cells tend to clump together and block blood vessels. Less commonly, thrombosis is caused by narrowing of the arteries supplying the brain due to inflammation. The inflammation may be due to an autoimmune disorder, such as polyarteritis nodosa (p.465), in which the immune system attacks the body's own healthy tissues.

What are the symptoms?

In most people, the symptoms develop rapidly over a matter of seconds or minutes. The exact symptoms depend on the area of the brain affected. The symptoms may include:

- Weakness or inability to move on one side of the body.
- Numbness on one side of the body.
- Clumsiness, or loss of control of fine movements.
- Visual disturbances, such as blurred vision or loss of vision in one eye.
- Slurred speech.
- Difficulty in finding words and understanding what others are saying.
- Vomiting, and difficulty in maintaining balance.

If the stroke is severe, areas of the brain that control breathing and blood pressure may be affected or the person may lapse into coma (p.522). In these circumstances, the outcome can be fatal.

How is it diagnosed?

If you suspect that a person has had a stroke, he or she should be taken to hospital immediately so that a cause can be identified and treatment can begin.

Imaging of the brain, such as CT scanning (p.247) or MRI (p.248), may be used to find out whether the stroke was caused by bleeding or a blockage in a vessel. Cerebral angiography (below) or carotid Doppler scanning (p.531) may be performed to help to identify

(TEST) Cerebral angiography

Cerebral angiography uses X-rays to look for abnormalities of the vertebral or carotid arteries, which supply blood to the brain. It is often used to investigate transient ischaemic attacks and stroke. Under local anaesthesia, a thin, flexible tube called a catheter is inserted into an artery, usually at the groin or elbow, and guided to an artery in the neck. A dye that shows up on X-rays is then injected through it. The outline of blood flow through the arteries is then seen on the X-ray (angiogram).

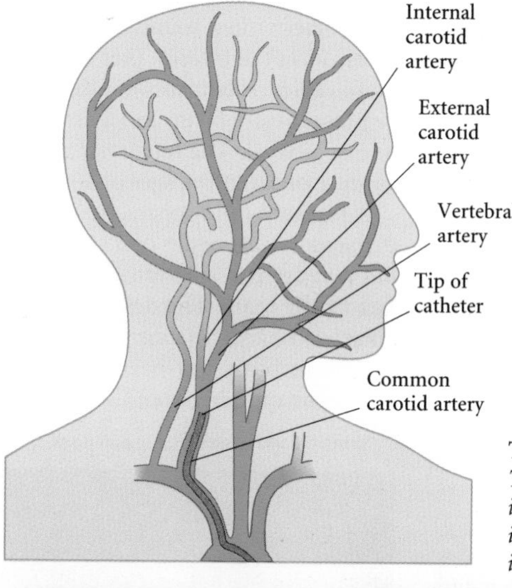

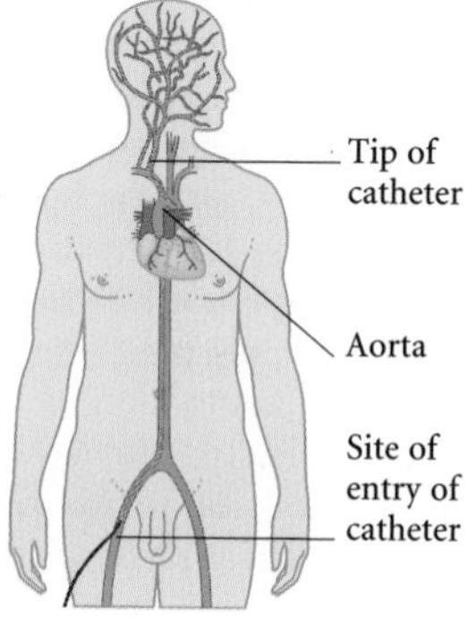

The procedure
The tip of the catheter is guided into the artery being investigated, in this case, the carotid artery. Dye is injected, and X-rays are taken.

(RESULTS)

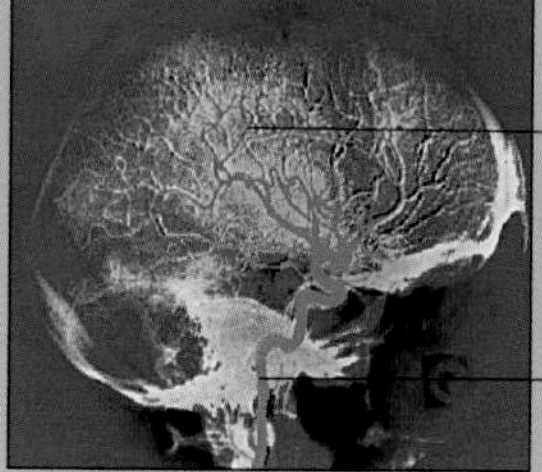

Angiogram
This colour-enhanced contrast X-ray, called an angiogram, shows the internal carotid artery, a main artery supplying the brain, branching into many smaller blood vessels. In this angiogram, the artery is normal.

narrowed areas of arteries that can be corrected by surgery. Further tests may be carried out to look for the source of an embolus. These tests may include echocardiography (p.425) to assess the heart valves and heart monitoring (*see* ECG, p.406) to check the heart rhythm.

What is the treatment?

The initial treatment following a stroke is close monitoring and nursing care to protect the person's airways during recovery. If CT scanning reveals a clot in a blood vessel, immediate treatment with thrombolytic drugs (p.904) to dissolve the clot may be considered. This treatment may improve the outcome, but it is not given routinely because it increases the risk of bleeding within the brain.

Long-term treatment to reduce the risk of further strokes will depend on the cause of the stroke. If the cause was a cerebral embolism, you may be given drugs such as aspirin or warfarin, which act on clotting factors in the blood to reduce the risk of further clots (*see* Drugs that prevent blood clotting, p.904). If a narrowed artery has been identified, it may be widened surgically. After a cerebral haemorrhage, treatment tends to be focused on the underlying cause, although in a few cases, surgery to remove a clot from the brain is carried out first. Long-term treatment may include antihypertensive drugs (p.897) to lower blood pressure. If the stroke is the result of inflammation of the arteries, corticosteroids (p.930) may be given.

In all cases of stroke, rehabilitative therapies, such as physiotherapy (p.961) and speech therapy (p.963), provided in hospital or at home, are essential. Lifestyle changes, such as reducing fat in your diet and giving up smoking, can reduce the risk of another stroke.

What is the prognosis?

The outlook after a stroke is often difficult to predict at first and depends to some extent on the cause. Following a stroke, about one-third of people make a full or almost full recovery. Another third have some disability, and some of these may need long-term care in a nursing home. Symptoms that persist for more than 6 months are likely to be permanent. About 1 in 5 people dies within a month of the stroke.

(WWW) ONLINE SITES: p.1037

Subarachnoid haemorrhage

Bleeding into the space between the two inner membranes covering the brain

Age Most common between the ages of 40 and 60

Gender Genetics Lifestyle Not significant factors

A subarachnoid haemorrhage occurs when an artery near the brain ruptures spontaneously and leaks blood into the subarachnoid space, the area between the middle and innermost of the three membranes that cover the brain. When this happens, the immediate symptom is an intensely painful headache.

Subarachnoid haemorrhage is rare, affecting only about 1 in 10,000 people in the UK each year. When the condition does occur, it is life-threatening and needs emergency medical attention.

What are the causes?

About 7 in 10 subarachnoid haemorrhages are caused by the rupture of a berry aneurysm, an abnormal swelling in an artery often found at a Y-shaped junction in the arteries that supply the brain. Berry aneurysms are thought to be present from birth, and there may be one or several. The aneurysms usually rupture between the ages of 40 and 60.

A further 1 in 10 subarachnoid haemorrhages are the result of a rupture of a knot of arteries and veins on the surface of the brain. The defect, known as an arteriovenous malformation, is present from birth, but haemorrhages do not occur until between the ages of 20 and 40. The cause of 2 in 10 subarachnoid haemorrhages is unknown.

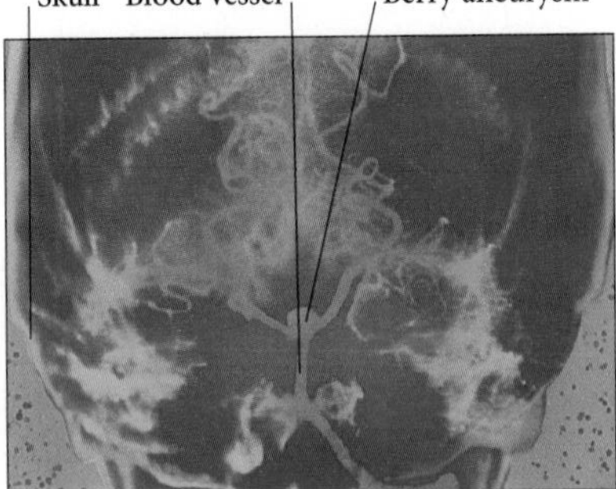

Berry aneurysm
This contrast X-ray shows a small swelling called a berry aneurysm at the base of the brain. Rupture of an aneurysm can result in a subarachnoid haemorrhage.

In people who are at risk, subarachnoid haemorrhage may be triggered by intense exertion. The disorder is more common in people who have high blood pressure (*see* Hypertension, p.403).

What are the symptoms?

The onset of symptoms is usually sudden and without warning. However, in a minority of cases, a headache comes on gradually a few hours before the haemorrhage occurs. Typical symptoms may include the following:

- Sudden, severe headache.
- Nausea and vomiting.
- Stiff neck.
- Dislike of bright light.
- Irritability.

In a few minutes, these may lead to:

- Confusion and drowsiness.
- Seizures.
- Loss of consciousness.

The body may react to the haemorrhage by constricting the arteries in the brain. As a result, the supply of oxygen to the brain is further reduced, and this may cause a stroke (p.532), possibly resulting in muscle weakness or paralysis.

What might be done?

If a subarachnoid haemorrhage is suspected, the affected person should be admitted to hospital immediately. CT scanning (p.247) is usually carried out to identify the location and extent of bleeding. A lumbar puncture (p.527) may need to be performed to look for signs of bleeding into the fluid surrounding the brain and spinal cord. MRI (p.248) or cerebral angiography (p.533) may also be performed to look at the blood vessels of the brain.

If a subarachnoid haemorrhage is confirmed, drugs called calcium channel blockers (p.900) are usually given to reduce the risk of a stroke.

If cerebral angiography shows that one or more berry aneurysms are present, surgery will probably be required. During the operation, clips are applied to the affected arteries to prevent them from bleeding again at a later time. If surgery is carried out early, there is a good chance of recovery. Sometimes, knotted or distended vessels are blocked and made safe without the need for surgery by inserting coils or glue during angiography. If damage to the brain has caused persistent symptoms, such as muscle weakness as a result of a stroke, physiotherapy (p.961) may be arranged.

WHAT IS THE PROGNOSIS?

Nearly half of all people with a subarachnoid haemorrhage die before they reach hospital. Of those people admitted to hospital, about half are treated successfully, but the remainder have another subarachnoid haemorrhage. If there is no further haemorrhage within the next 6 months or if surgery is successful, further bleeding is unlikely.

(WWW) ONLINE SITES: p.1035

Subdural haemorrhage

Bleeding inside the skull between the two outer membranes that surround the brain

AGE One type is more common in elderly people

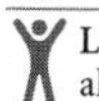
LIFESTYLE Contact sports and excessive alcohol consumption are risk factors

GENDER GENETICS Not significant factors

In a subdural haemorrhage, a vein in the subdural space is torn due to a head injury. The subdural space lies between the two outer membranes of the three membranes that surround the brain. Subsequent bleeding into the subdural space causes a blood clot, known as a haematoma, to form. As the blood clot enlarges, it compresses the surrounding brain tissue, causing symptoms such as headache and confusion.

A subdural haemorrhage is a potentially life-threatening condition that requires prompt medical treatment. It is the most common cause of death from contact sports such as boxing.

WHAT ARE THE TYPES?

After a head injury, bleeding may occur within minutes (acute subdural haemorrhage) or blood may build up slowly over a period of days or even weeks (chronic subdural haemorrhage).

An acute subdural haemorrhage may follow a severe blow to the head, the type of injury sustained in a road accident or while playing contact sports. Bleeding occurs immediately, and the blood clot enlarges quickly.

A chronic subdural haemorrhage can result from an apparently trivial head injury, especially in the elderly. Bleeding is slow, and it may be several months before the blood clot begins to cause symptoms. Chronic subdural haemorrhage often affects people who have frequent falls and therefore occurs more commonly in elderly people or in people who drink excessive amounts of alcohol. Disorders or treatments that impair blood clotting, such as treatment with drugs that prevent blood clotting (p.904), also increase the risk of chronic subdural haemorrhage.

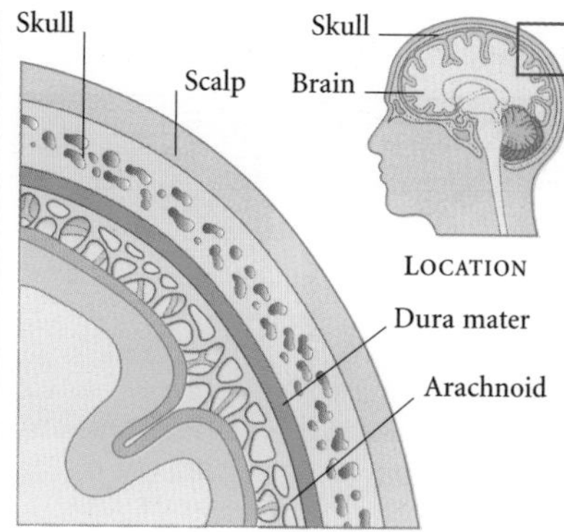

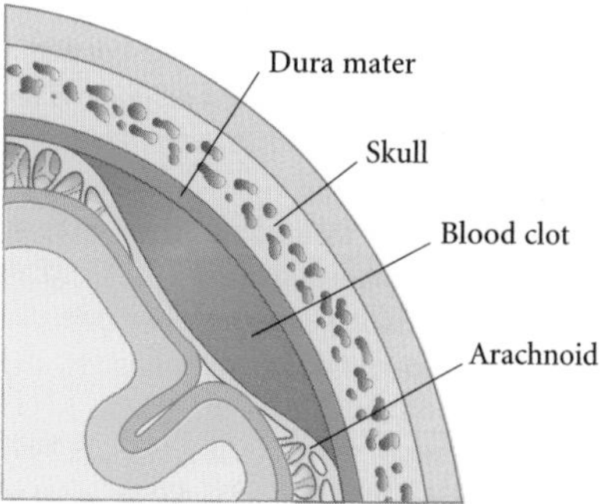

Subdural haemorrhage

Bleeding (haemorrhage) between two of the membranes that cover the brain, the dura mater and the arachnoid, leads to the formation of a blood clot.

WHAT ARE THE SYMPTOMS?

Symptoms may develop at any time between a few hours and a few months after the head injury, depending on whether the subdural haemorrhage is acute or chronic. In both types, symptoms are variable and often fluctuate in severity. The symptoms of acute subdural haemorrhage may include:

- Drowsiness.
- Confusion.
- Coma.

The symptoms of a chronic subdural haemorrhage may include:

- Headaches.
- Gradually developing confusion and drowsiness.
- Visual disturbances.

In acute and chronic subdural haemorrhage, the symptoms may also include seizures, vomiting, and progressive muscle weakness or paralysis on one side of the body. If these symptoms develop, seek medical attention immediately.

WHAT MIGHT BE DONE?

If your doctor suspects that you have a subdural haemorrhage, he or she will arrange for CT scanning (p.247) or MRI (p.248) of your brain to look for a clot. If the condition is confirmed, a surgical procedure in which blood is drained through small holes made in the skull will probably be necessary.

If a chronic subdural haemorrhage is small and produces few symptoms, the affected person may be monitored with regular scans, and the clot may clear without the need for surgery.

In all cases, the prognosis is determined by the size and location of the clot. Many people recover rapidly, but some residual symptoms, such as weakness, may persist. If the haemorrhage has affected a large area of brain, the condition may be fatal.

(WWW) ONLINE SITES: p.1032, p.1035

Dementia

A deterioration in mental ability due to disorders affecting the brain

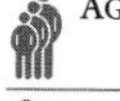
AGE More common over the age of 65

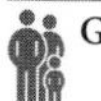
GENETICS Sometimes runs in families

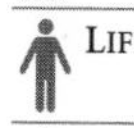
LIFESTYLE Risk factors depend on the cause

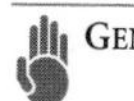
GENDER Not a significant factor

Dementia is a combination of memory loss, confusion, and general intellectual decline. The affected person may not realize that there is anything wrong, but his or her condition is usually distressing for close friends and family. Poor memory alone is not a sign of dementia because some memory impairment is a natural part of aging. Dementia is relatively common in elderly people, with about 1 in 10 people in the UK over the age of 65 affected to some degree. Although dementia is usually progressive and cannot be treated, in about 1 in 10 cases the underlying cause is treatable. An elderly person with severe depression (p.554) may seem to have dementia because the conditions have similar features, such as forgetfulness.

WHAT ARE THE CAUSES?

The underlying abnormality in dementia is a decline in the number of brain cells, resulting in shrinkage of brain tissue. Alzheimer's disease (right), which occurs mainly in people over 65 and may run in families, is the most common cause of dementia. In multi-infarct dementia (opposite page), blood flow in the small vessels of the brain is blocked by blood clots. Less common causes of dementia include other brain disorders, such as Huntington's disease (p.538), Parkinson's disease (p.539), and Creutzfeldt–Jacob disease (p.540).

Dementia may also occur in young people. For example, people with AIDS (*see* HIV INFECTION AND AIDS, p.297) may eventually develop AIDS-related dementia. Long-term abusers of alcohol are at risk of dementia because of direct damage to the brain tissue and because their poor diet often leads to vitamin B_1 deficiency. Severe vitamin B_1 deficiency can cause the brain disorder Wernicke–Korsakoff syndrome (p.538). In pernicious anaemia (*see* MEGALOBLASTIC ANAEMIA, p.448), there is a deficiency of vitamin B_{12} due to impaired absorption in the digestive tract. A severe deficiency can result in dementia. The disorder may also follow a serious head injury (p.521).

Certain drugs, such as anticonvulsant drugs (p.914) and mood-stabilizing drugs (p.918), may cause memory impairment similar to that of dementia.

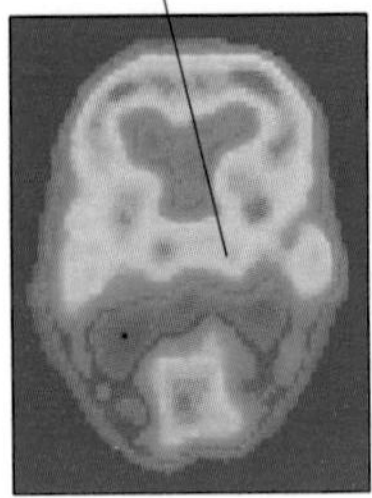

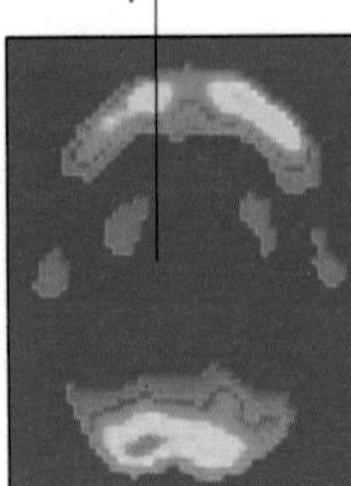

Brain activity in dementia
These PET scans show a large area of normal activity in the brain of a normal person compared to reduced activity in the brain of a person who has dementia.

(SELF-HELP) CARING FOR SOMEONE WITH DEMENTIA

If you are taking care of someone with dementia, you need to balance his or her needs with your own. In the early stages, it is important to allow the person to remain as independent and active as possible. As the disorder progresses, there are several measures you can take which help to compensate for the person's failing memory, loss of judgment, and unpredictable behaviour:

- Put up a bulletin board with a list of things that need to be done during each day.
- If wandering is a problem, persuade the person to wear a badge with your contact details and phone number on it.
- Place notes around the house that help the person to remember to turn off appliances.
- Consider installing bath aids to make washing easier.
- Try to be patient. It is common for people with dementia to have frequent mood changes.
- Give yourself a break whenever you can by finding someone who can help for a few hours.
- Join a carers' support group and investigate day centres and respite care options.

WHAT ARE THE SYMPTOMS?

The symptoms may develop gradually over a few months or years, depending on the cause. They may include:

- Impairment of short-term memory.
- Gradual loss of intellect, affecting reasoning and understanding.
- Difficulty engaging in conversations.
- Reduced vocabulary.
- Emotional outbursts.
- Wandering and restlessness.
- Neglect of personal hygiene.
- Urinary incontinence.

In the early stages of the disorder, a person is prone to becoming anxious (*see* ANXIETY DISORDERS, p.551) or depressed due to awareness of the memory loss. As the dementia gets worse, the person may become more dependent on others.

WHAT MIGHT BE DONE?

The doctor may arrange for the person to have tests to look for the underlying cause and to exclude other disorders. If memory loss is due to a deficiency of one or more of the B vitamins, injections of vitamin supplements (*see* VITAMINS, p.927) may be given. Symptoms that are caused by certain drugs may be relieved by a change of medication. Most other causes of dementia cannot be treated, but drugs may relieve some symptoms. For example, depression may be treated with antidepressants (p.916).

A person who has dementia usually needs support at home and may eventually need full-time care in a nursing home. Carers may also need support (*see* CARING FOR SOMEONE WITH DEMENTIA, left, and HOME CARE, p.960).

(WWW) ONLINE SITES: p.1026, p.1027, p.1035

Alzheimer's disease

A progressive deterioration in mental ability due to degeneration of brain tissue

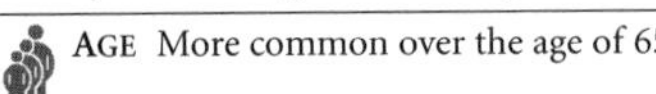
AGE More common over the age of 65

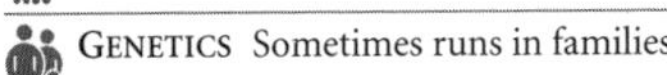
GENETICS Sometimes runs in families

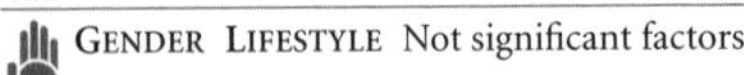
GENDER LIFESTYLE Not significant factors

It is normal to become mildly forgetful with increasing age, but severe impairment of short-term memory may be a sign of Alzheimer's disease. In this disorder, brain cells gradually degenerate and deposits of an abnormal protein build up in the brain. As a result, the brain tissue shrinks, and there is a progressive loss of mental abilities, known as dementia (p.535).

Alzheimer's disease is the most common cause of dementia. In developed countries, the condition affects about 7 in 100 people by the age of 65 and 3 in 10 people by the age of 85. Sometimes, younger people are affected. The underlying cause of the tissue destruction is unknown, although genetic factors may be involved. Studies have found that 15 in 100 people with Alzheimer's disease have a parent affected by the disorder.

WHAT ARE THE SYMPTOMS?

The first symptom of Alzheimer's disease is usually forgetfulness. The normal deterioration of memory that occurs in old age becomes much more severe and begins to affect intellectual ability. Memory loss is eventually accompanied by other symptoms, which may include:

- Poor concentration.
- Difficulty in understanding written and spoken language.
- Wandering and getting lost, even in familiar surroundings.

In the early stages of the disease, people are usually aware that they have become more forgetful. This may lead to depression (p.554) and anxiety (*see* ANXIETY DISORDERS, p.551). Over a longer period, the existing symptoms may get worse and additional symptoms may develop. These may include:

- Slow movements and unsteadiness when walking.
- Rapid mood swings from happiness to tearfulness.
- Personality changes, aggression, and feelings of persecution.

Sometimes people find it difficult to sleep (*see* INSOMNIA, p.554) and become restless at night. After several years, most people with the disease cannot look after themselves and need full-time care.

HOW IS IT DIAGNOSED?

There is no single test that can be used to diagnose Alzheimer's disease. The doctor will discuss the symptoms with the affected person and his or her family. Tests may be arranged to exclude other possible causes of dementia. For example, blood tests may be carried out to check for vitamin B deficiencies. CT scanning (p.247), PET scanning (p.253), or MRI (p.248) may be carried out to exclude other brain disorders, such as multi-infarct dementia (below), subdural haemorrhage (p.535), or a brain tumour (p.530). An assessment of mental ability, which may include memory and writing tests, may be used to determine the severity of the dementia.

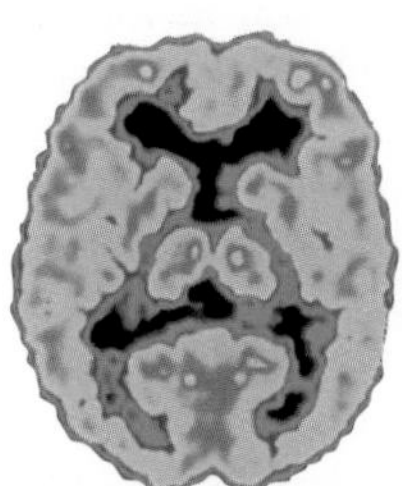

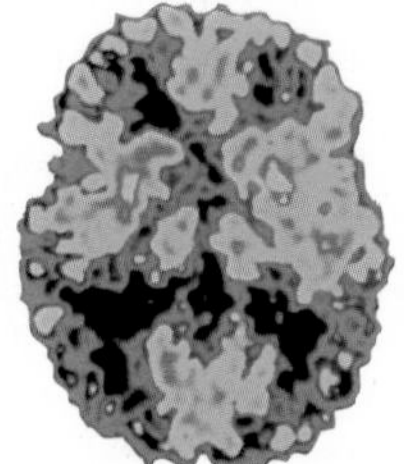

NORMAL BRAIN — BRAIN IN ALZHEIMER'S DISEASE

Effect of Alzheimer's disease

PET scans show a pattern of large, bright areas of high activity and small, dark areas of low activity in a normal brain compared to patchy activity in the brain of a person with Alzheimer's disease.

WHAT IS THE TREATMENT?

There is no cure for Alzheimer's disease, but drugs such as donepezil may slow the loss of mental function in mild to moderate cases. Some of the symptoms that are sometimes associated with Alzheimer's disease, such as depression and sleeping problems, can be relieved by antidepressant drugs (p.916). A person who is agitated may be given a sedative drug to calm him or her down.

Eventually, full-time care may be necessary, either at home (*see* HOME CARE, p.960, and CARING FOR SOMEONE WITH DEMENTIA, opposite page) or in a nursing home. Caring for a person who has Alzheimer's disease is often stressful, and carers need practical and emotional support, especially if the affected person starts to become hostile and aggressive. Support groups can help a person to cope with caring for an elderly relative with the disease. Most people with Alzheimer's disease survive for up to 10 years from the time of diagnosis.

(WWW) ONLINE SITES: p.1027

Multi-infarct dementia

A deterioration in mental ability due to blood clots in small blood vessels in the brain that cause tissue damage

AGE More common over the age of 60

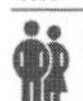
GENDER More common in males

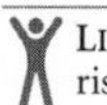
LIFESTYLE Smoking and a high-fat diet are risk factors

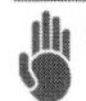
GENETICS Not a significant factor

Multi-infarct dementia, also known as vascular dementia, occurs when blood flow in the small blood vessels supplying the brain is obstructed by blood clots. Each of these clots prevents oxygen from reaching a small part of the brain, and this causes tissue death (infarcts) in the affected parts. Infarcts occur in a number of distinct episodes. People who have multiple small infarcts are at increased risk of a major stroke (p.532), which can be life-threatening.

The risk of multi-infarct dementia is increased by atherosclerosis (p.402), in which fatty deposits build up in the artery walls, causing them to become narrowed and increasing the risk of clots forming. The risk of atherosclerosis is increased if a person has high blood pressure (*see* HYPERTENSION, p.403). Lifestyle factors, such as eating a high-fat diet and smoking, can also contribute to the development of atherosclerosis. Multi-infarct dementia is more common in men and is more likely to occur in people over the age of 60.

WHAT ARE THE SYMPTOMS?

Symptoms of multi-infarct dementia vary from one individual to another because they depend on the part of the brain affected. Unlike other types of dementia, multi-infarct dementia gets incrementally worse following each separate episode. Symptoms are similar to those that occur with other forms of dementia and include:

- Poor memory, particularly when trying to recall recent events.
- Difficulty in making decisions.
- Problems with simple, routine tasks, such as getting dressed.
- Tendency to wander and get lost in familiar surroundings.

It is common for a person with multi-infarct dementia to develop depression (p.554) and have episodes of agitation. There may be other symptoms, depending on which part of the brain is affected. These may include partial loss of sight and slow, sometimes slurred, speech. Some people begin to walk with very small steps, or develop a weakness or partial paralysis in one leg that can make walking difficult.

WHAT MIGHT BE DONE?

Diagnosis of multi-infarct dementia is usually possible from the symptoms, although various tests, such as blood tests, may also be carried out to rule out other types of dementia. The doctor may arrange for CT scanning (p.247) or MRI (p.248) of the brain to look for evidence of multiple small infarcts.

Although the dementia itself cannot be cured, treatment can help to prevent further infarcts that would make the condition worse. A person with multi-infarct dementia should eat a low-fat diet and take regular exercise. Smokers should stop smoking immediately. Antihypertensive drugs (p.897), which help to control raised blood pressure, and a daily dose of aspirin, which reduces the risk of blood clots, may be prescribed.

Weakness and loss of movement can be treated with physiotherapy (p.961), and speech therapy (p.963) can help to alleviate speech problems. Antidepressants (p.916) and counselling (p.971) may be used to treat depression.

WHAT IS THE PROGNOSIS?

Many people with multi-infarct dementia find that their symptoms improve for short periods of time but later become worse again. Early recognition of the condition and treatment of risk factors, such as high blood pressure, may prevent further progression of the disorder and increasing disability and reduce the risk of a future, potentially fatal stroke.

(WWW) ONLINE SITES: p.1026, p.1035

Wernicke–Korsakoff syndrome

A brain disorder caused by severe vitamin B_1 deficiency, usually the result of long-term alcohol abuse

 AGE More common over the age of 45

 GENDER More common in males

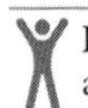 LIFESTYLE Long-term alcohol abuse is a risk factor

 GENETICS Not a significant factor

Wernicke–Korsakoff syndrome is a rare disorder of the brain, causing dementia, abnormal eye movements, and an abnormal gait. The condition develops rapidly and is due to a severe deficiency of vitamin B_1. It is a medical emergency. If untreated, coma (p.522) and death may occur. About 2 in 10 individuals with the disorder die within 5 days. Vitamin B_1 deficiency is usually caused by many years of severe alcohol abuse, but it may be due to extreme malnutrition or starvation. The disorder is most common in people over the age of 45 and affects more men than women.

WHAT ARE THE SYMPTOMS?

Symptoms may start gradually or suddenly, sometimes after heavy drinking, and are easily mistaken for drunkenness. They include the following:

- Abnormal movements of the eyes, which often result in double vision.
- Unsteadiness when walking.
- Confusion and restlessness.

Unless the individual is given urgent treatment, he or she will develop severe memory loss, become drowsy, go into a coma, and eventually die.

WHAT MIGHT BE DONE?

A person with Wernicke–Korsakoff syndrome needs immediate admission to hospital for intravenous treatment with high-dose vitamin B_1. After treatment, many of the symptoms may be reversed within days, but memory loss may persist. If untreated, the disorder is fatal.

(WWW) ONLINE SITES: p.1026, p.1035

Huntington's disease

An inherited brain disorder that causes personality changes, involuntary movements, and dementia

 AGE More common over the age of 30

 GENETICS Due to an abnormal gene inherited from one parent

 GENDER LIFESTYLE Not significant factors

Huntington's disease is an inherited disorder that causes degeneration of a particular part of the brain. Also known as Huntington's chorea, the condition causes jerky, involuntary movements, clumsiness, and progressive dementia. Huntington's disease is rare, affecting only about 6,000 people in the UK. The symptoms commonly develop between the ages of 30 and 50.

Huntington's disease is caused by an abnormal dominant gene. To develop the disease, an affected person has to inherit the abnormal gene from only one parent (*see* GENE DISORDERS, p.271). People who have the gene have a 1 in 2 chance of passing it on to each of their children. Since the symptoms do not develop until later in life, an abnormal gene may be passed on to children before the affected parent becomes aware that he or she has Huntington's disease. However, a genetic test can be carried out at any age to find out if an individual has inherited the abnormal gene from a parent (*see* TESTS FOR ABNORMAL GENES, p.239).

WHAT ARE THE SYMPTOMS?

Symptoms develop gradually over a period of months or years. Initially, they may include the following:

- Jerks and spasms of the face, arms, and trunk.
- Clumsiness.
- Mood swings, including outbursts of aggressive, antisocial behaviour.
- Poor memory, especially for events that have occurred recently.

As the disease progresses, further symptoms of dementia, such as losing the ability to think rationally, may develop. There may be difficulty in speaking and swallowing, and problems with urinary incontinence (p.710). Anxiety and depression (p.554) may also occur.

WHAT MIGHT BE DONE?

Unless the condition has already been diagnosed within the family, it may not be recognized during its early stages. Usually, a member of the affected person's family first realizes that there is a problem. The affected person may be suspicious of others and refuse help. Diagnosis is usually made from the symptoms and by CT scanning (p.247) or MRI (p.248) of the brain, which may show distinct patterns of abnormality.

There is no cure for Huntington's disease, but drugs may relieve certain symptoms. For example, antipsychotic drugs (p.917) help to control jerks and spasms. Speech therapy (p.963) and occupational therapy (p.962) are used to help an affected person to lead as normal a life as possible. However, care in a nursing home may be necessary if the person is unable to live at home or when carers need a period of respite.

Members of the family may decide to have a blood test to determine whether they have the abnormal gene themselves (*see* TESTS FOR ABNORMAL GENES, p. 239). These tests are performed after genetic counselling because the results are likely to have a bearing on whether or not they decide to have children.

Huntington's disease has a slow progression; a person may live for 15–20 years after the onset of symptoms.

(WWW) ONLINE SITES: p.1032, p.1035

Parkinson's disease and parkinsonism

A progressive brain disorder causing shaking and problems with movement

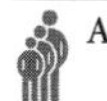 **AGE** More common over the age of 60

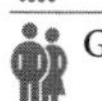 **GENDER** More common in males

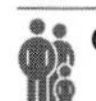 **GENETICS** Sometimes runs in families

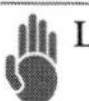 **LIFESTYLE** Not a significant factor

Parkinson's disease results from degeneration of cells in a part of the brain called the basal ganglia, which controls the smoothness of muscle movements. Normally, these cells produce a neurotransmitter (a chemical that transmits nerve impulses) called dopamine, which acts with acetylcholine, another neurotransmitter, to fine-tune muscle control. In Parkinson's disease, the level of dopamine relative to acetylcholine is reduced, adversely affecting muscle control.

About 1 in 200 people in the UK has Parkinson's disease. The disorder tends to occur after the age of 60 and is more common in men. Although the cause is not known, genetic factors may be involved. About 3 in 10 affected people have a family member with the disorder.

Parkinsonism is the term used for symptoms of Parkinson's disease when they are due to an underlying disorder or certain drugs. Repeated head injuries (p.521) may cause parkinsonism, as may some antipsychotic drugs (p.917) used to treat severe psychiatric illness.

What are the symptoms?

The main symptoms of Parkinson's disease develop gradually over months or even years. Parkinsonism may have a gradual or sudden onset depending on the cause. Symptoms include:

- Tremor of one hand, arm, or leg, usually when resting, that later occurs on both sides.
- Muscle stiffness, making it difficult to start moving.
- Slowness of movement.
- Shuffling walk with loss of arm swing.
- Expressionless or mask-like face.
- Stooped posture.

As the disease progresses, stiffness, immobility, and constant trembling of the hands may make some daily tasks difficult to perform. Speech may become slow and hesitant, and swallowing may be difficult. Many people with the disorder develop depression (p.554). About 3 in 10 people with the disease eventually develop dementia (p.535).

How is it diagnosed?

Since Parkinson's disease begins gradually, it is often not possible to diagnose the condition immediately. Your doctor will examine you and may arrange tests such as CT scanning (p.247) or MRI (p.248) to exclude other possible causes. If a specific underlying disorder is found to be causing your symptoms, you will be diagnosed as having parkinsonism rather than Parkinson's disease.

How might the doctor treat it?

There is no specific cure for Parkinson's disease, but drugs, physical treatments, and, more rarely, surgery can relieve symptoms. If you have parkinsonism due to medications, your doctor may change your drugs. Symptoms then usually disappear within 8 weeks. If the symptoms persist, you may need to be treated with antiparkinsonism drugs.

DRUG TREATMENT In the early stages of Parkinson's disease when symptoms are mild, treatment may not be necessary because drugs cannot change the progression of the disease. Later on, drugs are used to relieve symptoms and reduce disability by correcting chemical imbalances in the brain, either by boosting dopamine levels or by blocking some of the effects of acetylcholine or a combination of both. The choice and dosage of drugs is tailored to the individual's particular problems and adjusted to reduce side effects.

Often, an anticholinergic drug such as trihexyphenidyl (benzhexol) is given initially to reduce shaking and stiffness. Anticholinergic drugs can be effective for several years, but they may cause dry mouth, blurred vision and difficulty in passing urine.

The main treatment for Parkinson's disease is with levodopa, which boosts the level of dopamine within the brain. Levodopa controls major symptoms such as mobility problems but may initially cause side effects, such as nausea and vomiting. For this reason, the drug is increased gradually and is usually prescribed with other drugs, such as carbidopa or benserazide, which reduce the amount of levodopa that is needed. However, some people develop involuntary jerky or writhing movements as a side effect of this treatment. Levodopa is usually effective for 2–5 years, but long-term use may be associated with abrupt changes in symptoms known as the "on–off" effect of levodopa. The affected person has periods of normal mobility punctuated by unpredictable episodes of weakness and difficulty in moving.

When levodopa is no longer effective, seligiline, a drug that slightly increases dopamine activity in the brain, may be tried, and, later, other drugs, including dopamine agonists such as bromocriptine, may be used. Such drugs may cause confusion, hallucinations, and, occasionally, aggressive behaviour. Although there is no wholly successful therapy for symptoms of this disease, new drugs are always being developed.

PHYSICAL TREATMENT The doctor may arrange for physiotherapy (p.961) to help with mobility problems or speech therapy (p.963) for speech and swallowing problems. If you are finding it difficult to cope at home, an occupational therapist (p.962) may suggest changes, such as installing hand-rails to make it easier for you to move around.

SURGICAL TREATMENT Younger people who are otherwise in good health may have surgery if the tremor cannot be controlled by drugs. Surgery involves destroying a part of the brain tissue responsible for the tremor. Therapies still being assessed include replacement of damaged brain cells with transplanted tissue and deep brain stimulation with electrical impulses to reduce tremor. Deep brain stimulation, in particular, holds promise as a future treatment.

What can I do?

It is important to pay attention to your general health. Taking a walk each day and doing simple stretching exercises will help you to maintain strength and mobility. You should also rest during the day to avoid getting tired. Emotional and practical help from family, friends, and support groups is important.

What is the prognosis?

The course of the Parkinson's disease is variable, but drugs can be effective in treating the symptoms and improving the quality of life. People can lead active lives for many years after being diagnosed. However, most people with the disorder need daily help eventually, and their symptoms may be increasingly hard to control with drugs.

(WWW) ONLINE SITES: p.1035

Creutzfeldt–Jakob disease

A progressive, degenerative disease of brain tissue due to an infection

Age More common over the age of 50

Genetics Sometimes runs in families

Lifestyle Risk factors depend on the cause

Gender Not a significant factor

Creutzfeldt–Jacob disease (CJD) is an extremely rare condition in which brain tissue is progressively destroyed by an unusual infectious agent. The disorder leads to a general decline in all areas of mental and physical ability and ultimately to death. CJD affects about one person in a million each year worldwide.

What is the cause?

CJD is caused by an infectious agent known as a prion, which replicates in the brain and causes brain damage. One type of CJD, accounting for 15 in 100 cases, has been found to run in families.

Most people who develop CJD are over the age of 50. Usually, the source of the infection is unknown, but in about 1 in 20 people it can be traced to earlier treatment with products derived from human tissue. Before the use of artificial growth hormones to treat growth disorders, human growth hormone injections were one source of infection.

In the mid 1990s, a new, rare variant of CJD that affects people in their teens or 20s was discovered in the UK. By the year 2000, about 50 cases had been reported. This variant is believed to be linked with eating contaminated meat from cattle with a disease called bovine spongiform encephalopathy (BSE).

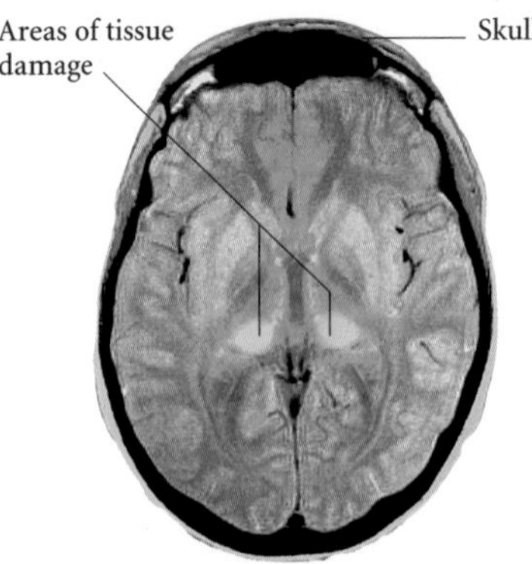

Brain in Creutzfeldt–Jakob disease
This colour-enhanced MRI scan of a brain affected by Creutzfeldt–Jakob disease shows generalized shrinkage of brain tissue and areas of particular damage.

What are the symptoms?

It is thought that CJD is present for 2–15 years before symptoms begin to develop gradually. They may include:

- Depression.
- Poor memory.
- Unsteadiness and poor coordination.

Other symptoms develop as the condition progresses and include:

- Sudden muscle contractions.
- Seizures.
- Weakness or paralysis on one side of the body.
- Progressive dementia.
- Impaired vision.

In the later stages of CJD, a person may be unable to move and talk. Those who are confined to bed are prone to serious lung infections (*see* Pneumonia, p.490).

What might be done?

CJD is usually diagnosed from a person's symptoms because no specific test is yet available. Anyone suspected of having CJD will have extensive tests, such as MRI (p.248), to exclude other treatable causes, and EEG (p.525) to look for characteristic changes in electrical activity in the brain. A brain biopsy, in which a small piece of tissue is surgically removed for examination, may be performed. There is no cure for CJD, but drugs can relieve some symptoms. For example, symptoms of depression may be treated with antidepressant drugs (p.916), and muscle contractions may be controlled by muscle relaxant drugs (p.896). However, the disorder is usually fatal within 3 years.

(WWW) ONLINE SITES: p.1033, p.1035

Motor neuron disease

Progressive degeneration of the nerves in the brain and spinal cord that control muscular activity

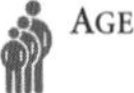
Age More common over the age of 40

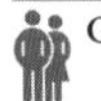
Gender More common in males

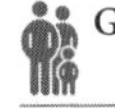
Genetics Sometimes runs in families

Lifestyle Not a significant factor

Motor neuron disease is rare, affecting 1–2 people in every 100,000 worldwide each year. In this disease, also known as amyotrophic lateral sclerosis, degeneration of the nerves involved in muscular activity results in progressive wasting of the muscles and weakness. There are several types of motor neuron disease. Some affect mainly the spinal nerves, while other types also affect the brain. The condition is not painful, does not affect bowel or bladder function, and does not usually affect the intellect or the senses, such as sight.

The cause of motor neuron disease is unknown. Genetic factors are involved because, in about 1 in 10 cases, the disease runs in the family. The disease is slightly more common in men and usually develops after the age of 40.

What are the symptoms?

Initially, weakness and wasting develop over a few months and usually affect the muscles of the hands, arms, or legs. Other early symptoms may include:

- Twitching movements in the muscles.
- Stiffness and muscle cramps.
- Difficulty in carrying out twisting movements, such as unscrewing bottle tops and turning keys.

As the disease progresses, other symptoms may include:

- Dragging one foot or a tendency to stumble when walking.
- Difficulty in climbing stairs or getting up from low chairs.

Less commonly, the muscles of the mouth and throat are involved, and may cause slurred speech, hoarseness, and difficulty in swallowing.

An affected person may have mood swings and may become anxious and depressed. If the muscles involved in breathing and swallowing are affected, small particles of food may enter the lungs and cause recurrent chest infections and possibly pneumonia (p.490). The head may fall forwards because the muscles in the neck are too weak to support it. Eventually, weakness of the muscles that control respiration may cause difficulty in breathing.

How is it diagnosed?

There is no specific test to diagnose motor neuron disease. However, electromyography (*see* Nerve and muscle electrical tests, p.544) may be carried out to detect a decrease in electrical activity in the muscles. Additional tests may be used to exclude other possible causes of the symptoms. For example, MRI (p.248) or CT scanning (p.247) of the brain and neck may be used to exclude a local problem such as a tumour or cervical spondylosis (p.376).

What is the treatment?

At present, no treatment can significantly slow down the progression of motor neuron disease, although a new drug called riluzole may have a small effect. Treatment for symptoms may include antidepressants (p.916) to relieve depression and antibiotics (p.885) to treat chest infections. If the person is having difficulty in swallowing, a gastrostomy may be created surgically. This is an opening through which a permanent feeding tube is inserted directly into the stomach or the small intestine.

Usually, a team of specialists provide support and care for an affected person and members of the family. Counselling (p.971) may be offered to both. The person affected by the disease may have physiotherapy (p.961) to keep joints and muscles supple and may be given aids to help with activities such as eating and walking (*see* Occupational therapy, p.962). A speech therapist (*see* Speech therapy, p.963) can supply communication aids to help with speech difficulties and advise on swallowing problems. Joining a self-help group is often helpful to the person with motor neuron disease and his or her family.

The outlook for motor neuron disease is variable, with approximately 2 in 10 affected people alive 5 years after diagnosis. About 1 in 10 affected people survives more than 10 years.

Multiple sclerosis

A progressive disease of nerves in the brain and spinal cord causing weakness and problems with sensation and vision

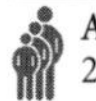
Age Usually develops between the ages of 20 and 40

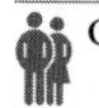
Gender More common in females

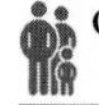
Genetics Sometimes runs in families

Lifestyle Stress and heat may aggravate symptoms

Multiple sclerosis (MS) is the most common nervous system disorder affecting young adults. In this condition, nerves in the brain and spinal cord are progressively damaged, causing a wide range of symptoms that affect sensation, movement, body functions, and balance. Specific symptoms may relate to the particular areas that are damaged and vary in severity between individuals. For example, damage to the optic nerve may cause blurred vision. If nerve fibres in the spinal cord are affected, it may cause weakness and heaviness in the legs or arms. Damage to nerves in the brain stem, the area of the brain that connects to the spinal cord, may affect balance.

In many people with MS, symptoms occur intermittently and there may be long periods of remission. However, some people have chronic (long-term) symptoms that gradually get worse.

In the UK, about 85,000 people are affected by MS. People who have a close relative with MS are more likely to develop the disorder. The condition is much more common in the northern hemisphere, which suggests that environmental factors also play a part. MS is more common in females and the disorder is more likely to develop between early adulthood and middle age.

What are the causes?

MS is an autoimmune disorder, in which the body's immune system attacks its own tissues, in this case those of the nervous system. Many nerves in the brain and spinal cord are covered by a protective insulating sheath of material called myelin. In MS, small areas of myelin are damaged, leaving holes in the sheath, a process known as demyelination. Once the myelin sheath has been damaged, impulses cannot be conducted normally along nerves to and from the brain and spinal cord. At first, the damage may be limited to only one nerve, but myelin covering other nerves may become damaged over time. Eventually, damaged patches of myelin insulation are replaced by scar tissue.

It is thought that MS may be triggered by external factors such as a viral infection during childhood in genetically susceptible individuals.

What are the types?

There are two types of MS. In the most common, known as relapsing–remitting MS, symptoms last for days or weeks and then clear up for months or even years. However, some symptoms may eventually persist between the attacks. About 3 in 10 people with MS have a type known as chronic–progressive MS, in which there is a gradual worsening of symptoms with no remission. A person with relapsing–remitting MS may go on to develop chronic–progressive MS.

What are the symptoms?

Symptoms may occur singly in the initial stages and in combination as the disorder progresses. They may include:

- Blurred vision.
- Numbness or tingling in any part of the body.
- Tiredness, which may be persistent.
- Weakness and a feeling of heaviness in the legs or arms.
- Problems with coordination and balance, such as an unsteady gait.
- Slurred speech.

Stress and heat sometimes make symptoms worse. About half of the people

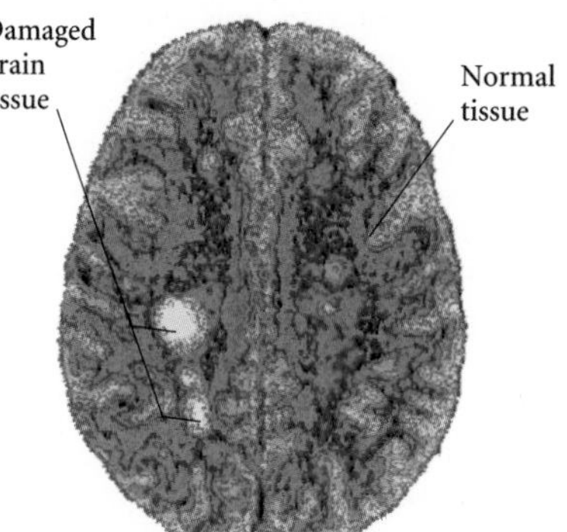

Damage due to multiple sclerosis
This MRI scan of the brain of a person with multiple sclerosis shows damaged brain tissue caused by the destruction of the sheaths that surround nerve fibres.

who have MS find it hard to concentrate and experience memory lapses. Depression (p.554) is common. Later in the course of the disease, some people with muscle weakness develop painful muscle spasms. Spinal cord damage can lead to urinary incontinence (p.710), and men may have increasing difficulty in achieving an erection (*see* IMPOTENCE, p.770). Eventually, damage to myelin covering nerves in the spinal cord may cause partial paralysis, and an affected person may need a wheelchair.

HOW IS IT DIAGNOSED?

There is no single test to diagnose MS, and, because symptoms are so wide-ranging, a diagnosis is only made once other possible causes of the symptoms have been excluded. Your doctor will take your medical history and carry out a physical examination. If you are having visual problems, such as blurred vision, you may be referred to an ophthalmologist, who will assess the optic nerve, which is commonly affected in the early stages of the disorder (*see* OPTIC NEURITIS, p.581). Your doctor may arrange for tests to find out how quickly your brain receives messages when particular nerves are stimulated. The most common test measures damage to the visual pathways (*see* VISUAL EVOKED RESPONSES, right). You will probably also have an imaging test of the brain, such as MRI (p.248), to see if there are areas of demyelination.

Your doctor may arrange for a lumbar puncture (p.527), a procedure in which a small amount of the fluid that surrounds the spinal cord is removed for microscopic analysis. Abnormalities in this fluid may confirm the diagnosis.

WHAT IS THE TREATMENT?

There is no cure for MS, but if you have relapsing–remitting MS, interferon beta (*see* INTERFERON DRUGS, p.907) may help to lengthen remission periods and shorten the length of attacks. Your doctor may also prescribe corticosteroids (p.930) to shorten the duration of a relapse. However, at present, there is no specific treatment to halt the progression of chronic–progressive MS.

Many of the more common symptoms that occur in all types of MS can be relieved by drugs. For example, your doctor may treat muscle spasms with a drug that relaxes muscles (*see* MUSCLE RELAXANTS, p.896). Similarly, incontinence can often be improved by drugs (*see* DRUGS THAT AFFECT BLADDER CONTROL, p.939). Problems in getting an erection may be helped by a drug treatment such as sildenafil. If you have mobility problems, your doctor may arrange for you to have physiotherapy (p.961). Occupational therapy (p.962) may make day-to-day activities easier.

WHAT CAN I DO?

If you are diagnosed with MS, you and your family will need time and possibly counselling (p.971) to come to terms with the disorder. You should minimize stress in your life and avoid exposure to high temperatures if heat tends to make your symptoms worse. Regular, gentle exercise, such as swimming, will help to keep your muscles strong without the risk of overstraining them.

WHAT IS THE PROGNOSIS?

The progression of MS is extremely variable, but people who are older when the disease first develops tend to fare less well. About 7 in 10 people with MS have active lives with long periods of remission between relapses. However, some people, particularly those with chronic–progressive MS, become increasingly disabled. Half of all people with MS are still leading active lives 10 years after diagnosis, and the average lifespan from diagnosis is 25–30 years.

(WWW) ONLINE SITES: p.1035

(TEST) VISUAL EVOKED RESPONSES

A visual evoked response test measures the function of the optic nerve, the nerve that transmits messages from the eye to the brain. The test is most often used in the diagnosis of multiple sclerosis and can detect abnormalities even if visual symptoms are not apparent. The test records brain activity in response to a visual stimulus to find out the speed at which messages from the eye reach the brain. The test takes 20–30 minutes.

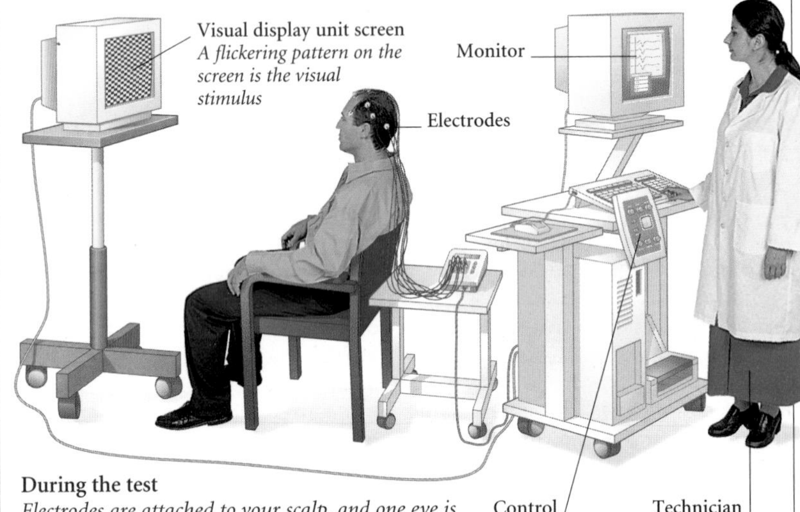

During the test
Electrodes are attached to your scalp, and one eye is covered. You are asked to focus on a fixed dot of light while the checkered pattern flickers on the screen.

(RESULTS)

Visual evoked responses
This normal tracing shows electrical activity in an area of the brain as it receives messages from the eye. The first spike on the trace shows the moment of visual stimulus. The time taken for the signal to reach the brain is measured.

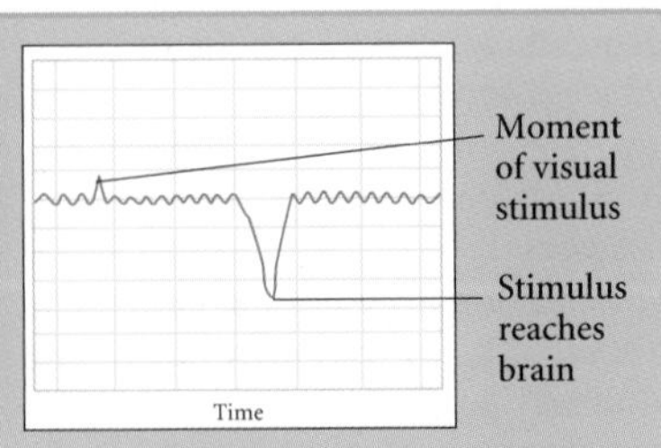

PERIPHERAL NERVOUS SYSTEM DISORDERS

The peripheral nervous system is composed of nerves that branch from the brain and spinal cord and then divide repeatedly to supply every part of the body. The nerves transmit information necessary for sensation, muscle stimulation, and the regulation of unconscious functions. Disorders of these nerves may be painful, cause loss of sensation, or lead to paralysis.

This section starts with an overview of peripheral neuropathies, in which one or more peripheral nerves are damaged. Peripheral neuropathies are relatively common and have many causes, including injuries, infection, nutritional deficiencies, and disorders such as diabetes mellitus. Diabetic neuropathy, the most common cause of peripheral nerve damage, is covered next. This is followed by an article on nutritional neuropathies, in which deficiency of essential nutrients in the diet, especially the vitamin B complex, causes the nerve damage.

The next articles cover disorders such as sciatica, carpal tunnel syndrome, and facial palsy, all of which may be caused by compression of a nerve. Rarer disorders that affect peripheral nerves are covered next. Such disorders include myasthenia gravis, in which the immune system affects the body's ability to transmit impulses from the nerves to muscles, and Guillain–Barré syndrome, which is the result of an abnormal response of the immune system after an infection. The final article covers nervous tics, which are often caused by stress.

KEY ANATOMY

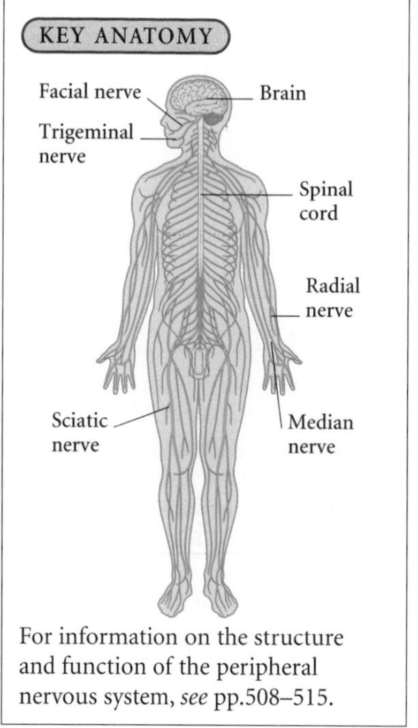

For information on the structure and function of the peripheral nervous system, *see* pp.508–515.

Peripheral neuropathies

Disorders of one or more of the nerves outside the brain and spinal cord, known as the peripheral nerves

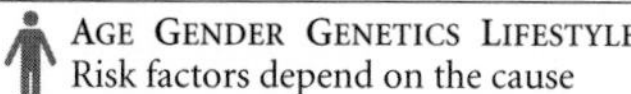
AGE GENDER GENETICS LIFESTYLE
Risk factors depend on the cause

Disorders of the peripheral nerves, the nerves that branch from the brain and spinal cord to the rest of the body, are called neuropathies. Depending on the nerves affected, peripheral neuropathies may affect sensation, movement, or automatic functions, such as bladder control. Rarely, a peripheral neuropathy may be life-threatening.

WHAT ARE THE CAUSES?

In developed countries, the most common cause of damage to the peripheral nerves is diabetes mellitus (*see* DIABETIC NEUROPATHY, p.545). Vitamin B complex deficiencies and some nutritional disorders may also result in nerve damage (*see* NUTRITIONAL NEUROPATHIES, p.545). In the developed world, nutritional neuropathy is often the result of a poor diet in people who abuse alcohol. Drinking too much alcohol may also damage peripheral nerves directly.

Damage to a single nerve may occur as a result of an injury (*see* PERIPHERAL NERVE INJURIES, p.548) or because of compression. For example, in carpal tunnel syndrome (p.547), the median nerve, which supplies part of the hand, is compressed at the wrist.

Neuropathy may also be associated with an infection, such as Hansen's disease (p.302) or HIV infection (*see* HIV INFECTION AND AIDS, p.297). Guillain–Barré syndrome (p.550), a neuropathy that is rapidly progressive, is caused by an abnormal immune response that sometimes occurs after an infection.

Autoimmune disorders such as systemic lupus erythematosus (p.461), in which the immune system attacks the body's tissues, may cause nerve damage. Occasionally, a disorder such as polyarteritis nodosa (p.465) may damage nerves by causing inflammation of the blood vessels that supply them. Neuropathy may also result from certain cancers, particularly primary lung cancer (p.503) and lymphoma (p.459). Occasionally, neuropathy is caused by amyloidosis (p.693), in which an abnormal protein is deposited in the body.

Some drugs, such as isoniazid (*see* ANTITUBERCULOUS DRUGS, p.886), may cause nerve damage, as may exposure to certain toxic substances, such as lead. In some cases, the cause is unknown.

WHAT ARE THE TYPES?

Peripheral neuropathies may affect the nerves that transmit sensory information (sensory nerves), the nerves that stimulate the muscles (motor nerves), and/or the nerves that control automatic functions (autonomic nerves).

SENSORY NERVE NEUROPATHIES These neuropathies first affect the hands and feet and then spread towards the centre of the body. The symptoms may include tingling, pain, and numbness in the affected area. If the fingertips are numb, everyday tasks may become difficult. This type of neuropathy is most often caused by nutritional disorders or drugs.

MOTOR NERVE NEUROPATHIES If the motor nerves are damaged, the muscles they supply become weak, and wasting occurs eventually. In severe cases, mobility may become restricted, and, very rarely, breathing may have to be assisted by mechanical ventilation (*see* INTENSIVE CARE UNIT, p.958). Lead poisoning may result in a neuropathy that affects the motor nerves only.

AUTONOMIC NERVE NEUROPATHIES A neuropathy that is affecting one or more autonomic nerves may result in constipation (p.628), fainting due to low blood pressure (*see* HYPOTENSION, p.414), diarrhoea (p.627), urinary incontinence (p.710), or impotence (p.770). This type of neuropathy is often caused by long-standing diabetes mellitus.

WHAT MIGHT BE DONE?

Your doctor may be able to tell which nerves are affected from your symptoms and an examination. If the cause of your neuropathy is not clear, he or she will probably arrange for blood tests to look for evidence of an underlying disorder, such as nutritional deficiencies or an autoimmune disorder. If there is evidence of compression of a nerve, you may also have CT scanning (p.247) or MRI (p.248) to assess the severity and extent of nerve damage. Special tests to assess the function of the nerves (*see* NERVE AND MUSCLE ELECTRICAL TESTS, below) may also be carried out.

The treatment of a peripheral neuropathy depends on the cause and the type of nerve affected. For example, careful control of diabetes mellitus may

(TEST) NERVE AND MUSCLE ELECTRICAL TESTS

Nerve and muscle electrical tests consist of nerve conduction studies and electromyography (EMG). Nerve conduction studies are used to assess how well a nerve is conducting electrical impulses. They are often followed by EMG to see whether symptoms, such as weakness, are due to a disorder of the muscle or the nerve supplying it. Both tests are usually done on an outpatient basis. Each takes about 15 minutes and may cause discomfort.

NERVE CONDUCTION STUDIES

Nerve conduction studies are carried out to assess nerve damage in disorders such as peripheral neuropathies. A nerve is stimulated by an electrical impulse, and the response to the stimulus and the speed at which this response travels along the nerve indicates whether the nerve is damaged and the nature and extent of the damage.

Control panel

Monitor *The results are displayed here as a trace*

Technician

Stimulator

Recording electrode

During the procedure
A probe is held against the skin to stimulate the nerve to be tested. The signal that is produced by the nerve is picked up by a recording electrode placed further along the nerve on the skin.

(RESULTS)

Moment of stimulation

Response to stimulus

Nerve conduction trace
This trace shows a normal electrical impulse through a nerve. The nerve is stimulated, and the speed at which the impulse travels through the nerve is measured.

ELECTROMYOGRAPHY

EMG is used to differentiate between nerve and muscle disorders and to diagnose disorders such as muscular dystrophy. A fine needle is used to record the electrical activity of a muscle at rest and when contracting. The results are recorded on a trace.

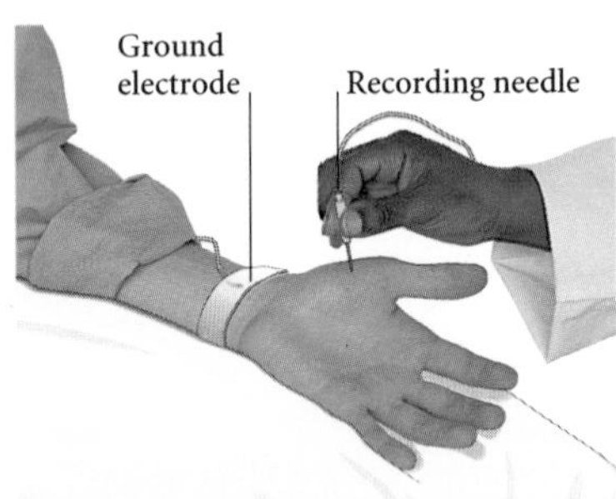

During the procedure
A needle placed in or on the muscle records electrical activity at rest and when you contract the muscle. A ground electrode eliminates background electrical activity.

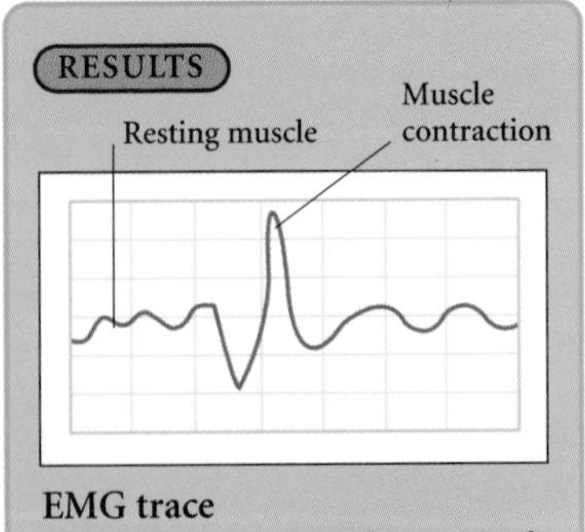

EMG trace
This trace shows normal patterns of electrical activity in a muscle at rest and when contracting.

keep diabetic neuropathy from worsening, and vitamin B complex injections (*see* VITAMINS, p.927) may help a nutritional neuropathy. If motor nerves are affected, you may have physiotherapy (p.961) to help to maintain muscle tone. Wearing a foot splint may assist walking. Sometimes, the underlying cause can be treated, but long-standing nerve damage may be irreversible.

(WWW) ONLINE SITES: p.1026, p.1035

Diabetic neuropathy

Damage to one or more of the peripheral nerves caused by diabetes mellitus

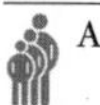 AGE More common over the age of 40

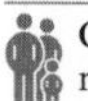 GENETICS Diabetes mellitus sometimes runs in families

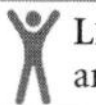 LIFESTYLE Poor control of diabetes mellitus and smoking are risk factors

 GENDER Not a significant factor

In diabetic neuropathy, one or more of the peripheral nerves that branch from the brain and spinal cord to the rest of the body are damaged as a result of diabetes mellitus (p.687). Diabetic neuropathy is the most common cause of peripheral neuropathy in developed countries. If diabetes is poorly controlled, it results in high levels of glucose in the blood that damage the peripheral nerves directly and the blood vessels that supply them (*see* DIABETIC VASCULAR DISEASE, p.432). Good control of diabetes reduces this risk by up to half.

About 3 in 10 people with diabetes mellitus have damage to one or more peripheral nerves, but only 1 of these 3 people develops significant symptoms.

People with diabetes mellitus who smoke increase the risk of damaging the blood vessels that supply the nerves.

WHAT ARE THE SYMPTOMS?

The symptoms of diabetic neuropathy usually develop slowly over a number of years. Rarely, they develop rapidly over days or weeks. Symptoms vary depending on which nerves are involved, but the feet are frequently affected. Less commonly, diabetic neuropathy may affect the larger nerves, mainly in the thighs. Symptoms may include:

- Pins and needles.
- Numbness.
- Pain, which is often worse at night.
- Muscle weakness and wasting.

If sensation is lost, a minor injury to the foot, such as rubbing by badly fitting shoes, may not be noticed. Slow healing due to poor blood supply may lead to infection. If left untreated, ulcers may develop (*see* LEG ULCER, p.350) and, in severe cases, gangrene (p.435) occurs.

Eventually, diabetic neuropathy may also affect the autonomic nerves that regulate automatic body functions such as blood pressure control and digestion. Damage to these nerves causes symptoms such as dizziness when standing (*see* HYPOTENSION, p.414), diarrhoea (p.627), and impotence (p.770).

WHAT MIGHT BE DONE?

Careful control of diabetes reduces the risk of developing diabetic neuropathy. However, if you develop symptoms of nerve damage, you should consult your doctor. He or she will probably be able to diagnose the condition from your symptoms. However, nerve conduction tests may need to be carried out in hospital to confirm which nerves are affected and to assess the severity of the damage (*see* NERVE AND MUSCLE ELECTRICAL TESTS, opposite page).

The goal of treatment of diabetic neuropathy is to prevent further nerve damage and the development of complications. Your doctor will help you to monitor your blood sugar level carefully and advise you about good foot care (*see* LIVING WITH DIABETES, p.690). For example, you should check your feet regularly for cuts or abrasions, particularly if you have been wearing new shoes. You should avoid wearing open-toed sandals or walking barefoot. If you smoke, you should try to give up.

To relieve pain, particularly at night, certain anticonvulsant drugs (p.914), such as carbamazepine and phenytoin, or an antidepressant drug (p.916), such as amitriptyline, may be prescribed.

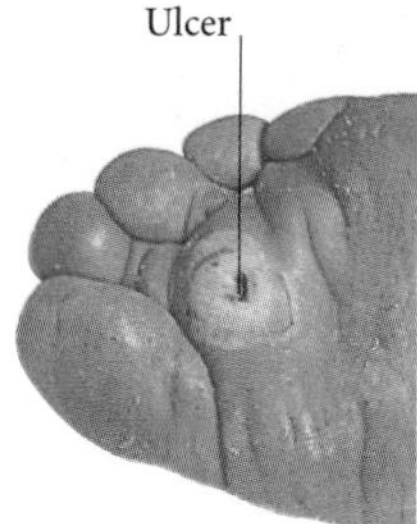

Foot ulcer
If nerves are damaged as a result of diabetic neuropathy, a painless ulcer, such as shown here on the sole, may develop.

WHAT IS THE PROGNOSIS?

Good control of blood glucose levels in diabetes mellitus not only reduces the risk of developing diabetic neuropathy but may also halt further progression of the disease. However, in most cases, nerve damage is irreversible.

(WWW) ONLINE SITES: p.1030

Nutritional neuropathies

Damage to peripheral nerves caused by nutritional deficiency

 LIFESTYLE Poor diet and excessive alcohol consumption are risk factors

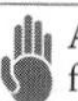 AGE GENDER GENETICS Not significant factors

In nutritional neuropathies, the peripheral nerves, which branch from the brain and spinal cord, are damaged by deficiencies of essential nutrients, particularly those of the vitamin B complex (*see* NUTRITIONAL DEFICIENCIES, p.630).

Worldwide, nutritional neuropathies are generally caused by malnutrition. In developed countries, such neuropathies are more commonly associated with excessive alcohol consumption. People who drink heavily often also have a poor diet, which can cause a vitamin B_1 deficiency. In addition, alcohol may directly damage the peripheral nerves. A person who has been drinking heavily for 10 years or more has a greatly increased risk of developing a nutritional neuropathy.

Nutritional deficiencies may occur in people with eating disorders, such as anorexia nervosa (p.562). People with long-term conditions that affect absorption of nutrients from the intestines (*see* MALABSORPTION, p.655) may also develop nutritional deficiencies.

WHAT ARE THE SYMPTOMS?

Nutritional neuropathies usually first affect the tips of the fingers and the toes. The symptoms appear gradually over several months or years and slowly progress up the limbs to the trunk. Symptoms may include:

- Loss of sensation.
- Pins and needles.
- Pain in the feet and/or the hands.

Walking may be clumsy as a result of the loss of sensation in the feet and legs.

If the motor nerves (nerves that stimulate the muscles) are affected, muscle weakness and wasting may develop and further affect the ability to walk.

What might be done?

Your doctor will examine you by checking your reflexes and your ability to feel sensation such as a pin prick. He or she may arrange for blood tests to look for a vitamin deficiency or for evidence of liver damage caused by excessive alcohol consumption. Your doctor may also arrange for tests that measure the extent of the nerve damage (*see* Nerve and muscle electrical tests, p.544).

Nutritional neuropathies are treated by replacing the missing nutrients. This is done either by giving a course of oral supplements or, in some cases, by injections (*see* Vitamins, p.927). Your doctor may also prescribe anticonvulsant drugs (p.914) or antidepressants (p.916) to help to control the symptoms. You may also be prescribed painkillers (p.912) to relieve any discomfort.

Nerve damage is usually irreversible, but with treatment the progression of the disease can usually be halted.

(WWW) ONLINE SITES: p.1026, p.1035

Trigeminal neuralgia

Severe pain on one side of the face due to compression, inflammation, or damage to the trigeminal nerve

 Age More common over the age of 50

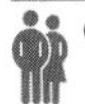 Gender More common in males

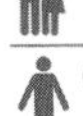 Genetics Risk factors depend on the cause

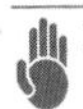 Lifestyle Not a significant factor

The trigeminal nerve transmits sensation from parts of the face to the brain and controls some of the muscles that are involved in chewing. Damage to this nerve causes repeated bursts of sharp, stabbing pain, known as trigeminal neuralgia, in the lip, gum, or cheek on one side of the face. Attacks may last for a few seconds or several minutes and may become more frequent over time. In severe cases, the pain may be so intense that the affected person is unable to do anything during the attack. Afterwards, the pain usually disappears completely. An attack may occur spontaneously or be triggered by certain facial movements, such as chewing, or by touching a trigger spot on the face. Attacks rarely occur at night.

Trigeminal neuralgia affects about 1 in 25,000 people in the UK. The disorder is most common in men over the age of 50. The cause of trigeminal neuralgia is usually unknown. However, in people under 50, symptoms may be an early sign of multiple sclerosis (p.541). Rarely, the nerve is compressed by a tumour or by a dilated blood vessel.

What might be done?

There are no specific tests to diagnose trigeminal neuralgia. Your doctor will examine you to rule out any other causes of facial pain, such as toothache or sinusitis (p.475). He or she may also arrange for you to have MRI (p.248) to look for the presence of a tumour.

Your doctor may prescribe painkillers (p.912), such as paracetamol or ibuprofen. However, if the pain persists, your doctor may prescribe anticonvulsant drugs (p.914), such as carbamazapine, or certain antidepressants (p.916), all of which have been shown to be effective in treating trigeminal neuralgia. Unlike painkillers, which are taken only when the pain is present, both anticonvulsants and antidepressants need to be taken every day to prevent attacks.

If a tumour is found, surgery may be necessary to remove it. Surgery may also be used to separate the trigeminal nerve from a blood vessel if the vessel is compressing the nerve. Rarely, people who have persistent, severe pain that does not respond to drugs are offered treatment to numb the affected side of the face. For example, pain can be alleviated by using a heated probe to destroy the nerve. Alternatively, the trigeminal nerve may be cut, or alcohol may be injected into the nerve to deaden it. Trigeminal neuralgia will not recur after treatment to numb the face, but you will need to take care when consuming hot food or drinks because of the lack of sensation in your face.

Attacks of neuralgia may stop spontaneously, become more frequent, or persist unchanged for months or years. However, symptoms usually improve significantly with treatment.

(WWW) ONLINE SITES: p.1035

Sciatica

Pain in the buttock and down the back of the leg, occurring when the sciatic nerve or its roots are compressed or damaged

 Age Gender Lifestyle Risk factors depend on the cause

 Genetics Not a significant factor

Sciatica is a form of nerve pain that may be felt anywhere along the course of one of the sciatic nerves, the two largest nerves in the body and the main nerve in each leg. The sciatic nerves are formed from nerve roots in the lower part of the spinal cord. They run from the base of the spine down the backs of the thighs to above the knees, where they divide into branches that supply the front and back of the leg and foot. The pain of sciatica is caused by compression of or damage to the sciatic nerve, usually where it leaves the spinal cord. Many people have at least one episode of sciatica during their lives. Often, only one leg is affected. In most cases, the pain disappears gradually over about 1–2 weeks, but it may recur.

What are the causes?

Sometimes, the cause of sciatica is unknown. However, in people aged 20 to 40, the most common cause is a prolapsed or herniated disc (p.384) in the spinal column that presses on a spinal

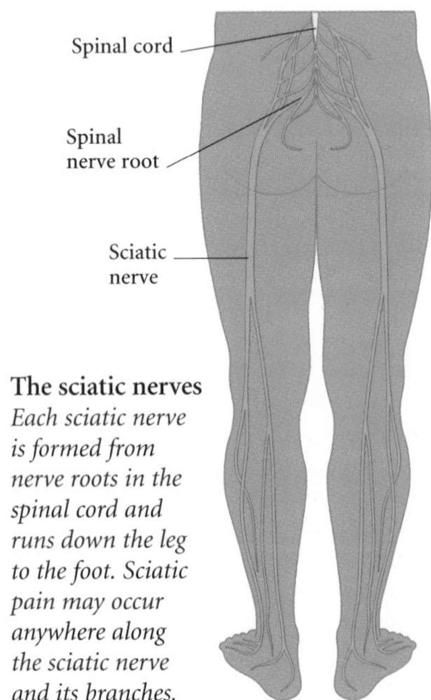

The sciatic nerves
Each sciatic nerve is formed from nerve roots in the spinal cord and runs down the leg to the foot. Sciatic pain may occur anywhere along the sciatic nerve and its branches.

nerve root. Sciatica may also develop from spondylolisthesis (p.385), in which a vertebra (bone in the spine) slips out of position. In older people, sciatica may be caused by changes in the spine as a result of various conditions, such as osteoarthritis (p.374). Women may develop sciatica during the last months of pregnancy because of posture changes that cause increased pressure on the sciatic nerve (*see* COMMON COMPLAINTS OF NORMAL PREGNANCY, p.784).

Muscle spasm and sitting in an awkward position for long periods of time are relatively common causes of brief episodes of sciatica in all age groups.

Less commonly, sciatica may be the result of an injection into the buttock muscles that was mistakenly given too close to one of the sciatic nerves. Rarely, a tumour on the spinal cord may press on the sciatic nerve roots.

WHAT ARE THE SYMPTOMS?

The symptoms can be mild or severe, with spasmodic or persistent pain in the affected leg. Symptoms may include:

- Pain that is made worse by movement or by coughing.
- Tingling or numbness.
- Muscle weakness.

If sciatica is severe, you may have difficulty in lifting the foot on the affected side because of muscle weakness, and you may be unable to stand upright. Some people have difficulty in walking.

WHAT MIGHT BE DONE?

The doctor will examine you and test your leg reflexes, muscle strength, and sensation. You may be advised to rest in bed on a firm mattress for a couple of days and be given painkillers (p.912) to relieve discomfort. If symptoms persist, you may have tests, such as MRI (p.248) of the spine, to look for changes in the bones or a prolapsed disc.

Sciatica as a result of pregnancy will usually disappear after childbirth. Pain caused by muscle spasm or sitting awkwardly also tends to clear up without treatment. Occasionally, the condition can be helped by regular physiotherapy (p.961), exercise (*see* PREVENTING BACK PAIN, p.382), or chiropractic treatments (p.973). However, sciatica can recur. In some cases, surgery may be necessary to relieve pressure on the nerve.

(WWW) ONLINE SITES: p.1027, p.1035

Carpal tunnel syndrome

Tingling and pain in the hand and forearm due to a compressed nerve at the wrist

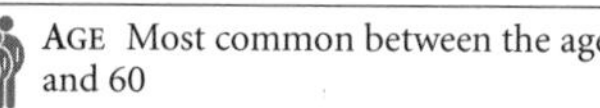

AGE Most common between the ages of 40 and 60

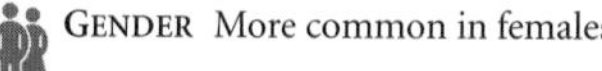

GENDER More common in females

LIFESTYLE Work that involves repetitive hand movements is a risk factor

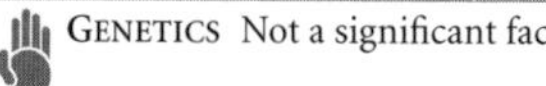

GENETICS Not a significant factor

The carpal tunnel is the narrow space formed by the bones of the wrist (carpal bones) and the strong ligament that lies over them. In carpal tunnel syndrome, the median nerve, which controls some hand muscles and conveys sensation from nerve endings in part of the hand, is compressed where it passes through the tunnel. This compression causes painful tingling in the hand, wrist, and forearm. Carpal tunnel syndrome is a common disorder, especially in women aged 40–60, and often affects both hands.

WHAT ARE THE CAUSES?

In some cases, the underlying cause of nerve compression is not known. In others, it occurs because the soft tissues within the carpal tunnel swell, compressing the median nerve at the wrist. Such swelling may be due to diabetes mellitus (p.687), or it may occur during pregnancy. The carpal tunnel may also be narrowed by a joint disorder, such as rheumatoid arthritis (p.377), or by a wrist fracture. The syndrome is associated with work that involves repetitive hand movements, such as typing, which can result in inflammation of the tendons in the wrist (*see* TENDINITIS AND TENOSYNOVITIS, p.390).

WHAT ARE THE SYMPTOMS?

Symptoms mainly affect specific areas of the hand, such as the thumb, the first and middle fingers, the inner side of the ring finger, and the palm of the hand. Initially, symptoms may include:

- Burning and tingling in the hand.
- Pain in the wrist and up the forearm.

As the condition worsens, other symptoms may gradually appear including:

- Numbness of the hand.
- Weakened grip.

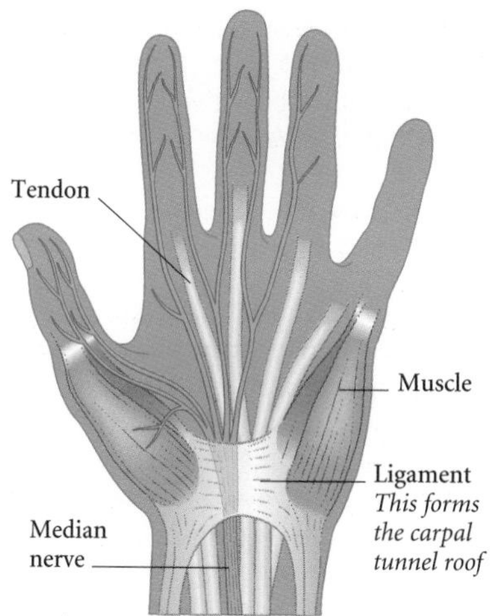

Carpal tunnel
The carpal tunnel is formed by the bones of the wrist and the ligament over them. Compression of the median nerve in the tunnel causes carpal tunnel syndrome.

- Wasting of some hand muscles, particularly at the base of the thumb.

Symptoms may be more severe at night, and pain may interrupt sleep. Shaking the affected arm may temporarily relieve symptoms, but the numbness may become persistent if left untreated.

WHAT MIGHT BE DONE?

Your doctor may suspect carpal tunnel syndrome from your symptoms. He or she will examine your wrists and hands and may tap the inside of your wrists to check if a tingling sensation occurs. Nerve conduction studies (*see* NERVE AND MUSCLE ELECTRICAL TESTS, p.544) may be carried out to confirm the diagnosis. If pregnancy is the cause of carpal tunnel syndrome, the symptoms usually disappear after childbirth. In other cases, treating the cause, if it can be identified, usually relieves symptoms.

The symptoms of carpal tunnel syndrome may be relieved temporarily by nonsteroidal anti-inflammatory drugs (p.894) or by wearing a wrist splint, particularly at night. In some cases, a corticosteroid injection (*see* LOCALLY ACTING CORTICOSTEROIDS, p.895) under or around the ligament may reduce swelling. If symptoms persist or recur, you may have surgery under local anaesthesia to cut the ligament and release pressure on the nerve. After surgery, there are usually no further symptoms.

(WWW) ONLINE SITES: p.1035

Facial palsy

Weakness or paralysis of the facial muscles on one side of the face due to damage to one of the facial nerves

AGE GENDER GENETICS LIFESTYLE
Not significant factors

The facial nerve controls the muscles of expression and emotion in the face and carries taste sensations from the front of the tongue to the brain. In facial palsy, one of the two facial nerves is damaged, compressed, or inflamed, and this results in weakness of the facial muscles, causing the eyelid and corner of the mouth to droop on one side of the face. People with facial palsy are often concerned that they have had a stroke (p.532), but this is unlikely if only the face is affected because a stroke is usually also associated with muscle weakness in other parts of the body.

Facial palsy is usually temporary, but a full recovery may take several months. The disorder affects about 1 in 4,000 people in the UK each year.

WHAT ARE THE CAUSES?

The most common form of facial palsy is Bell's Palsy. This type of palsy occurs for no known reason, although a viral infection is believed to play a part.

In other types of facial palsy, there are known causes of damage to the facial nerve. These include the viral infection shingles (*see* HERPES ZOSTER, p.290) and the bacterial infection Lyme disease (p.303). In addition, the facial nerve sometimes becomes inflamed as a result of a middle-ear infection (*see* OTITIS MEDIA, p.597). In rare cases, the facial nerve may be compressed by a tumour called an acoustic neuroma (p.605). Facial palsy can also result from damage to the nerve from a tumour of the parotid salivary gland (p.635).

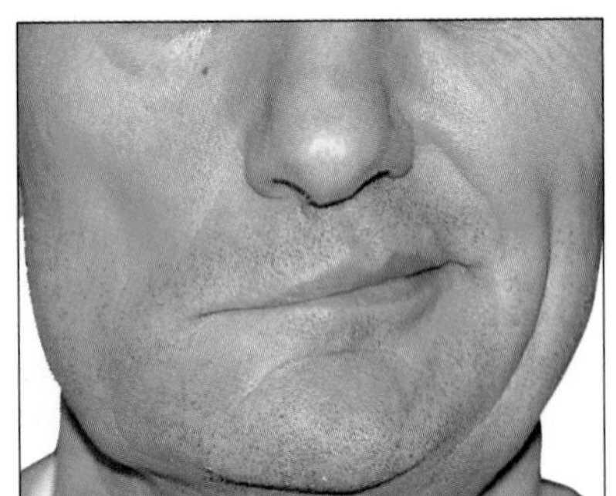

Facial palsy
Facial palsy caused by nerve damage has affected the muscles on the right side of this man's face, causing a lopsided smile.

WHAT ARE THE SYMPTOMS?

In some cases, such as in Bell's palsy, the symptoms of facial palsy appear suddenly over about 24 hours. In other cases, including facial palsy caused by an acoustic neuroma, symptoms may develop slowly. The symptoms include:

- Partial or complete paralysis of the muscles on one side of the face.
- Pain behind the ear on the affected side of the face.
- Drooping of the corner of the mouth, sometimes associated with drooling.
- Inability to close the eyelid on the affected side and watering of the eye.
- Impairment of taste.

If facial palsy is very severe, you may have difficulty in speaking and eating, and, occasionally, sounds may seem unnaturally loud in the ear on the affected side. If the eyelid cannot be closed, the eye may become infected, leading to ulceration of the cornea, the transparent front part of the eye. In facial palsy due to shingles, you will also have a rash of crusting blisters on your ear.

HOW IS IT DIAGNOSED?

Your doctor will probably be able to diagnose facial palsy from your symptoms alone. A rapid onset over about 24 hours suggests Bell's palsy. Symptoms that develop more slowly usually indicate another cause.

If your doctor suspects a tumour may be compressing the facial nerve, he or she may arrange for you to have CT scanning (p.247) or MRI (p.248). Nerve and muscle electrical tests (p.544) may also be arranged to assess nerve damage. If you live in a part of the UK where Lyme disease is common, you may have a blood test to look for evidence of this disorder.

WHAT MIGHT BE DONE?

If your symptoms have appeared in the last 48 hours, your doctor may prescribe corticosteroids (p.930) for up to 2 weeks to reduce inflammation of the nerve. He or she may also recommend that you take painkillers (p.912). To prevent damage to the cornea, you may be given artificial tears (*see* DRUGS ACTING ON THE EYE, p.919), and you will probably be advised to tape the affected eye shut when you go to sleep.

Bell's palsy usually clears up without further treatment. If facial palsy has an underlying cause, it will be treated if possible. For example, if facial palsy is due to shingles, antiviral drugs (p.886), such as aciclovir, will be prescribed. To be effective, treatment with aciclovir should begin as soon as the rash appears. If you have an acoustic neuroma, it will be removed surgically to relieve compression of the facial nerve.

If muscle paralysis persists, plastic surgery (p.952) may be used to reroute another nerve to the face. Facial exercises and massage may help to maintain tone (*see* PHYSIOTHERAPY, p.961).

WHAT IS THE PROGNOSIS?

With appropriate treatment, facial palsy usually improves within about 2 weeks. However, a full recovery may take up to 3 months. Some people are left with weakness, and facial palsy may recur.

(WWW) ONLINE SITES: p.1035

Peripheral nerve injuries

Damage to a nerve outside the brain or spinal cord as a result of physical injury

AGE GENDER GENETICS LIFESTYLE
Not significant factors

Any of the peripheral nerves, which connect the brain and the spinal cord to the rest of the body, may be damaged by physical injury. This damage may cause weakness and loss of sensation in the part of the body that the nerve supplies. A peripheral nerve may be partially or completely severed, or it may be compressed. Damage may not be permanent because peripheral nerves can regenerate if they are not completely cut.

WHAT ARE THE SYMPTOMS?

The part of the body affected depends on which peripheral nerve is damaged. Symptoms usually include:

- Tingling and numbness.
- Muscle weakness or paralysis.
- Eventually, muscle wasting.

The severity of the symptoms depends on whether the nerve is damaged or completely severed.

WHAT MIGHT BE DONE?

Your doctor will check for loss of sensation, test your reflexes, and assess the strength of your muscles. You may also have nerve and muscle electrical tests (p.544), in which the function of the affected nerve is tested to assess how severely it has been damaged.

Treatment is often unnecessary if a peripheral nerve is only compressed or partially severed. After a few weeks, nerve and muscle tests may be repeated to see if there has been an improvement in your condition. If the nerve is totally severed, it cannot regenerate by itself, and you may be offered microsurgery (p.950) to try to repair it. After the operation, you may have physiotherapy (p.961) to help to regain lost muscle strength and coordination. However, even with the most skilled surgery, full recovery may not be possible, and you may continue to have symptoms.

(WWW) ONLINE SITES: p.1035, p.1036

Myasthenia gravis

Long-term muscle weakness, especially of the muscles of the face, throat and around the eyes, due to an immune disorder

AGE Most common between the ages of 20 and 40 in females and 50 and 70 in males

GENDER More common in females

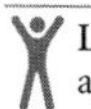
LIFESTYLE Stress and tiredness may aggravate the symptoms

GENETICS Not a significant factor

Myasthenia gravis is a rare autoimmune disorder in which the immune system produces antibodies that attack and slowly destroy the receptors in muscles that receive nerve impulses. As a result, the affected muscles fail to respond or respond only weakly to nerve impulses. The muscles of the face, the throat, and around the eyes are most often affected, causing speech and vision problems. However, other muscles may be affected, including those in the arms and legs and, rarely, the respiratory muscles.

Myasthenia gravis is a long-term condition that varies in severity. It is more common in women, especially in those aged 20 to 40 years. In men, the disorder tends to occur between the ages of 50 and 70. In the UK, about 1 in 20,000 people are diagnosed annually.

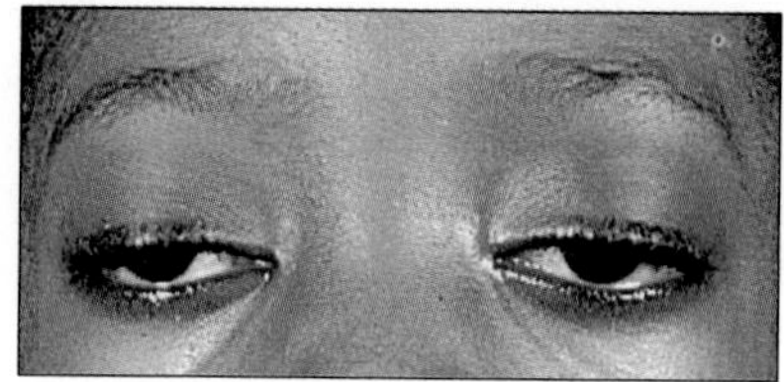

Myasthenia gravis
The rare immune disorder myasthenia gravis has affected the muscles controlling the eyelids, causing them to droop.

WHAT ARE THE CAUSES?

In most cases, the cause of the disorder is not known. However, about 3 in 4 affected people have an abnormality of the thymus gland, which is part of the body's immune system and is located at the base of the neck just underneath the breastbone. In a number of these people, myasthenia gravis is associated with a thymoma, a noncancerous tumour of the thymus gland. Other causes of the condition include certain drugs, such as penicillamine (*see* ANTIRHEUMATIC DRUGS, p.895). Myasthenia gravis may also be associated with other autoimmune disorders, such as the joint disorder rheumatoid arthritis (p.377).

WHAT ARE THE SYMPTOMS?

The symptoms of myasthenia gravis usually develop gradually over several weeks or months and tend to fluctuate. In some cases, symptoms appear suddenly. Symptoms may include:

- Drooping eyelids.
- Double vision.
- Slurred speech.
- Difficulty chewing and swallowing.
- Weakness in the arm and leg muscles.

Symptoms usually improve with rest but worsen when the affected muscles are used. Symptoms may also be made worse by stress and, in women, by menstruation. Rarely, if respiratory muscles are weakened, life-threatening breathing difficulties may develop.

About 1 in 7 babies born to mothers with myasthenia gravis develops symptoms immediately after birth, but these usually disappear over a few weeks.

HOW IS IT DIAGNOSED?

Your doctor may suspect myasthenia gravis from your symptoms. To confirm the diagnosis, you will probably be given an injection that increases the levels of neurotransmitters, the chemicals responsible for conveying nerve impulses from nerves to muscle receptors. If the injection produces a rapid but only temporary improvement in muscle strength, you probably have myasthenia gravis. You may also have blood tests to search for the particular antibodies that attack the receptors in muscles and electromyography (*see* NERVE AND MUSCLE ELECTRICAL TESTS, p.544) to look for muscle weakness by measuring electrical activity. In some people, CT scanning (p.247) of the chest may be carried out to look for a thymoma.

WHAT IS THE TREATMENT?

Your doctor may prescribe drugs that raise the levels of neurotransmitters. If your symptoms are mild, this treatment may control them sufficiently for you to resume normal activities. If your symptoms are more persistent, you may be prescribed oral corticosteroids (p.930) or other immunosuppressant drugs (p.906), such as azathioprine, to reduce antibody production. Treatment with oral corticosteroids may be started in hospital because the drugs may have an adverse effect initially, and symptoms may become worse.

In severe cases, regular plasmapheresis may be necessary. In this procedure, plasma (the fluid part of the blood) is taken from the body and replaced with fresh, donated plasma. If breathing becomes difficult, mechanical ventilation may be necessary (*see* INTENSIVE CARE UNIT, p.958) until the person is able to breathe independently.

If a tumour of the thymus is found, surgery will be performed to remove the thymus gland. Some people under the age of 45 with severe symptoms but no thymoma may also benefit from surgical removal of the thymus gland.

People with myasthenia gravis should avoid extremes of temperature, infections, stress, and becoming overtired, all of which intensify muscle weakness.

WHAT IS THE PROGNOSIS?

About 8 in 10 people with myasthenia gravis can be cured or their symptoms substantially improved with treatment. In a few people, the symptoms disappear spontaneously after about a year. Rarely, if the respiratory muscles are involved, the disorder may be fatal.

(WWW) ONLINE SITES: p.1035

Guillain–Barré syndrome

A disorder in which damage to the peripheral nerves results in weakness that spreads upwards from the legs

AGE GENDER GENETICS LIFESTYLE Not significant factors

Guillain–Barré syndrome is a rare and potentially life-threatening disorder that causes progressive loss of feeling and weakness that can rapidly lead to paralysis. The condition is the result of an abnormal immune response that develops 2–3 weeks after certain infections, such as infection with *Campylobacter jejuni* bacteria (*see* FOOD POISONING, p.629). Rarely, Guillain–Barré syndrome may develop as a complication following an immunization.

In Guillain–Barré syndrome, antibodies that are produced in response to an infection or vaccine attack the peripheral nerves, causing the nerves to become inflamed. Initially, the legs are affected, followed by the trunk, arms, and head. The condition is often mild, but, if severe, Guillain–Barré syndrome may cause difficulty in swallowing and breathing. In such circumstances, the affected person may need to have artificial feeding and mechanical ventilation. Each year in the UK about 900 people are affected by the syndrome.

What are the symptoms?

The symptoms may develop in a few days or weeks and include:

- Weakness in the legs, which may spread up the trunk and to the arms.
- Numbness and tingling of the limbs.

Usually, no further symptoms develop, but, in severe cases, symptoms become progressively worse and include:

- Paralysis of the limbs.
- Difficulty in speaking and swallowing.

If the muscles of the ribcage and diaphragm are affected, serious breathing difficulties may develop.

How is it diagnosed?

Your doctor will probably diagnose Guillain–Barré syndrome from your symptoms. However, you may have tests to confirm the diagnosis, including nerve conduction studies (*see* NERVE AND MUSCLE ELECTRICAL TESTS, p.544). You may also have a lumbar puncture (p.527), in which a sample of fluid from around the spinal cord is removed under local anaesthesia for analysis.

What is the treatment?

During the early stages of Guillain–Barré syndrome, you will be admitted to hospital for continuous monitoring. If you develop breathing difficulties, mechanical ventilation may be necessary (*see* INTENSIVE CARE UNIT, p.958). If you have difficulty in swallowing, you may be given fluids intravenously or through a tube. Severe episodes have been found to respond to intravenous immunoglobulin. An alternative treatment is plasmapheresis, in which plasma (the fluid part of the blood) is withdrawn and replaced with fresh, donated plasma. While you are recovering, you may have physiotherapy (p.961) to help to maintain muscle tone.

What is the prognosis?

Most people with Guillain–Barré syndrome recover without needing specific treatment. Mild symptoms usually disappear in a few weeks, but people who have severe symptoms may take several months to recover and may be left with some weakness in affected areas. The syndrome is fatal in 3 in 100 cases.

(WWW) ONLINE SITES: p.1035

Nervous tics

Involuntary repeated contraction of one or more muscles

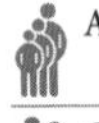
AGE More common in children

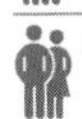
GENDER More common in males

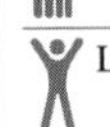
LIFESTYLE Stress is a risk factor

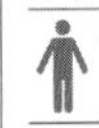
GENETICS Risk factors depend on the cause

Nervous tics occur when a muscle or a group of muscles controlled by peripheral nerves contracts repeatedly and involuntarily. The condition most often affects the facial muscles, but sudden, uncontrolled movements of the limbs and sounds such as grunts and throat clearing can also occur. Typical nervous tics include repetitive blinking, mouth twitching, and shrugging. Tics are common, recurrent, and painless. However, they may result in self-consciousness and teasing by others. Nervous tics usually develop during childhood and occur more commonly in boys than girls.

Often, the cause is unknown, but tics may be associated with stress because they tend to occur when children are tired or upset. In Tourette's syndrome, a rare genetic disorder that occurs more frequently in boys, there may be uncontrolled movements of the head, arms, and legs and repetitive shouts, noises, grimaces, and spoken obscenities.

What are the symptoms?

A tic usually lasts only a fraction of a second. The muscle contraction may occur repeatedly and may cause:

- Rapid, uncontrolled blinking.
- Twitching of the muscles around the mouth.
- Shrugging of the shoulders or jerking movements of the neck.
- Involuntary contractions of the diaphragm, causing grunting or hiccups.

Nervous tics may be suppressed for a short period, but, in doing this, people often become more tense. When children are absorbed in an activity or asleep, tics usually disappear. Tourette's syndrome may be associated with phobias (p.552) and learning disabilities.

What might be done?

You should consult your doctor if you or your child has persistent nervous tics. Often, no treatment is necessary. In other cases, your doctor may suggest one or more psychological therapies (pp.968–971) to help to relieve stress. If symptoms are severe, your doctor may prescribe an antianxiety drug (p.916) for short periods of time. In some cases, nervous tics produced by Tourette's syndrome can be suppressed by antipsychotic drugs (p.917), such as haloperidol. Some of the other problems that are associated with Tourette's syndrome, such as phobias and learning disabilities, may need specialist psychological treatment.

Nervous tics, particularly those that occur in children, will usually disappear within about a year of the disorder first developing. However, in a few children, nervous tics tend to persist and continue in adulthood. Tourette's syndrome is always a lifelong condition.

(WWW) ONLINE SITES: p.1028, p.1035

MENTAL HEALTH DISORDERS

Few people hesitate to seek treatment for a physical illness, but many find it hard to accept that they may have a mental health problem. However, disorders such as depression and anxiety and irrational fears are common, well understood, and, in many cases, treatable. No one needs to feel embarrassed about a mental illness or believe that he or she must deal with it alone.

This section begins with anxiety disorders, which are among the most common mental health problems in the UK. Feeling worried is a natural reaction to problems and stress. However, persistent anxiety, often with no obvious cause, needs treatment to prevent it from becoming a long-term problem. Phobias, irrational fears of anything from spiders to confined spaces, can dominate many areas of a person's life. Other anxiety-related illnesses include post-traumatic stress disorder, a response to events such as serious accidents and natural disasters.

Insomnia, a symptom of many mental illnesses, particularly anxiety and depression, is covered next. Depression, a very common disorder that affects 1 in 10 people at some time in their lives, is described in the article that follows. The condition requires prompt treatment to relieve symptoms and prevent persistent feelings of despair and possibly even suicide. The two eating disorders described next, anorexia nervosa and bulimia, are most common in teenage girls and young women, but they can also affect younger children and boys.

The common factor in the next group of disorders, which includes somatization and hypochondriasis, is the relationship between the mind and physical symptoms. Discussion of schizophrenia, a severe mental illness that may cause disturbed emotions and a break with reality, follows.

The final articles focus on drug and alcohol dependence and compulsive gambling. Treatment for these disorders begins when a person is able to acknowledge that there is a problem and is motivated to overcome it.

Anxiety disorders

Intense apprehension that may or may not have an obvious cause

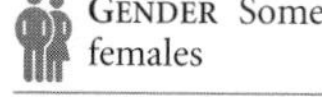
GENDER Some types more common in females

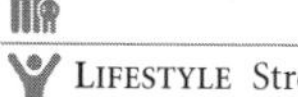
GENETICS Some types run in families

LIFESTYLE Stress is a risk factor

AGE Risk factors depend on the type

Temporary feelings of nervousness or worry in stressful situations are natural and appropriate. However, when anxiety becomes a general response to many ordinary situations and causes problems in coping with normal everyday life, it is considered a disorder.

Anxiety disorders occur in a number of different forms. The most common is persistent anxiety state or generalized anxiety disorder, characterized by excessive and persistent anxiety that is difficult to control. Another type of anxiety disorder is panic disorder, in which there are recurrent panic attacks of intense anxiety and alarming physical symptoms. These attacks occur unpredictably and usually have no obvious cause. Panic attacks may also feature in persistent anxiety state. In another type of anxiety disorder known as phobia, severe anxiety is provoked by an irrational fear of a situation, activity, creature, or object (*see* PHOBIAS, p.552).

Persistent anxiety state affects about 2–4 per cent of people every year in the UK. The condition usually begins in middle age and affects more women than men. Sometimes, anxiety disorders exist alongside other mental health disorders, such as depression (p.554) or schizophrenia (p.560).

WHAT ARE THE CAUSES?

An increased susceptibility to anxiety disorders may be inherited or may be due to experiences in childhood. For example, poor bonding between a parent and child and abrupt separation of a child from a parent have been shown to play a part in some anxiety disorders. Persistent anxiety state may develop after a stressful life event, such as the death of a close relative. However, frequently the anxiety has no particular cause. Similarly, panic disorder often develops for no obvious reason.

WHAT ARE THE SYMPTOMS?

People with persistent anxiety state and panic disorder experience both physical and psychological symptoms. However, in persistent anxiety state, the psychological symptoms tend to be persistent while physical symptoms are intermittent. During panic attacks, psychological and physical symptoms develop together suddenly and unpredictably. The psychological symptoms of persistent anxiety state include:

- A sense of foreboding with no obvious reason or cause.
- Being on edge and unable to relax.
- Impaired concentration.
- Repetitive worrying thoughts.
- Disturbed sleep (*see* INSOMNIA, p.554) and, sometimes, nightmares.

In addition, you may have symptoms of depression, such as early waking or a general sense of hopelessness. Physical symptoms of the disorder, which occur intermittently, include:

- Headache.
- Abdominal cramps, sometimes with diarrhoea, and vomiting.
- Frequent passing of urine.
- Sweating, flushing, and tremor.
- A feeling of something being stuck in the throat.

Psychological and physical symptoms of panic attacks include the following:

- Shortness of breath.
- Sweating, trembling, and nausea.
- Palpitations (awareness of an abnormally rapid heartbeat).
- Dizziness and fainting.

- Fear of choking or that death may be imminent.
- A sense of unreality and fears about loss of sanity.

Many of these symptoms can be misinterpreted as signs of a serious physical illness, and this may increase your level of anxiety. Over time, fear of having a panic attack in public may lead you to avoid situations such as eating out in restaurants or being in crowds.

WHAT MIGHT BE DONE?

You may be able to reduce your anxiety levels yourself using methods such as relaxation exercises (p.75). If you are unable to deal with or identify a specific cause for your anxiety, you should consult your doctor. It is important to see a doctor as soon as possible after a first panic attack to prevent repeated attacks developing. There are several measures you can try to help to control a panic attack, such as breathing into a bag (*see* COPING WITH A PANIC ATTACK, below). For any anxiety disorder, your doctor may suggest counselling (p.971) to help you to manage stress or offer cognitive therapy (p.970) or behaviour therapy (p.969) to help you to control anxiety. A self-help group may also be useful.

If you are undergoing a particularly stressful period in your life, your doctor may prescribe a benzodiazepine (*see* ANTIANXIETY DRUGS, p.916), but these drugs are usually prescribed for only a short period of time because there is a danger of dependence. You may be prescribed beta-blocker drugs (p.898) to treat the physical symptoms of anxiety. If you have symptoms of depression, you may be given antidepressant drugs (p.916), some of which are also useful in the treatment of panic attacks.

In most cases, the earlier anxiety disorders are treated, the quicker their effects can be reduced. Without treatment, an anxiety disorder may develop into a lifelong condition.

(WWW) ONLINE SITES: p.1029, p.1034

(SELF-HELP) COPING WITH A PANIC ATTACK

Rapid breathing in a panic attack reduces carbon dioxide levels in the blood and may cause tingling in the fingers. You can control these symptoms by breathing through the mouth into a paper bag. By doing this, you rebreathe air with more carbon dioxide and restore the body's levels to normal.

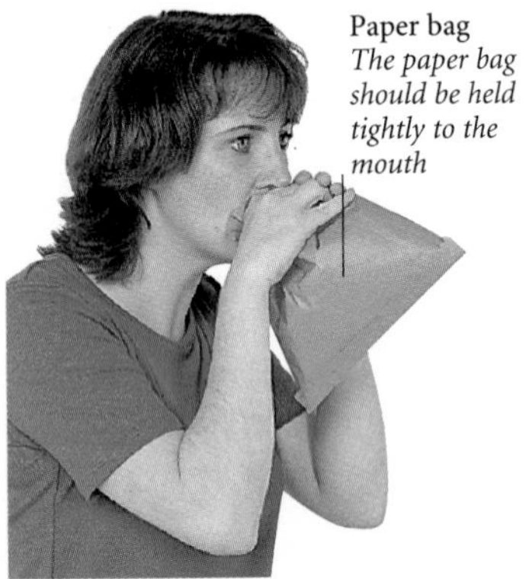

Paper bag
The paper bag should be held tightly to the mouth

Rebreathing from a bag
Breathe in and out slowly into a paper bag about 10 times and then breathe normally for 15 seconds. Continue until you no longer need to breathe rapidly.

Phobias

Persistent and irrational fears of, and a compelling desire to avoid, particular objects, activities, or situations

 AGE Most commonly develop from late childhood to early adulthood

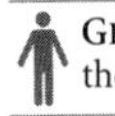 GENDER GENETICS Risk factors depend on the type

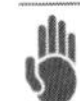 LIFESTYLE Not a significant factor

Many people have particular fears, such as a fear of dogs or heights, that are upsetting occasionally but do not disrupt their everyday activities. A phobia is a fear or anxiety that has been carried to extremes. A person with a phobia has such a compelling desire to avoid contact with a feared object or situation that it interferes with normal life.

Being exposed to the subject of the phobia causes a panic reaction of severe anxiety, sweating, and a rapid heartbeat. A person with a phobia is aware that this intense fear is irrational but still feels anxiety that can be alleviated only by avoiding the feared object or situation. The need to do this may disrupt routines and limit the person's capacity to take part in new experiences. About 1 in 10 people in the UK has a phobia. Phobias usually develop in late childhood, adolescence, or early adult life.

WHAT ARE THE TYPES?

Phobias take many different forms, but they can be broadly divided into two types: simple and complex phobias.

SIMPLE PHOBIAS Phobias specific to a single object, situation, or activity, such as a fear of spiders, heights, or air travel, are called simple phobias. For example, claustrophobia, a fear of enclosed spaces, is a simple phobia. A fear of blood is a common simple phobia that affects more men than women.

COMPLEX PHOBIAS More complicated phobias that have a number of component fears are described as complex phobias. Agoraphobia is an example of a complex phobia that involves multiple anxieties. These fears may include being alone in an open space or being trapped in a public area with no exit to safety. The kind of situations that provoke agoraphobic anxiety include using public transport and lifts, and visiting crowded shops. Tactics to avoid these situations may disrupt work and social life, so that a person with severe agoraphobia may eventually become unable to leave the house. Agoraphobia occasionally develops in middle age and is more common in women.

Social phobias are also classified as complex phobias. People with a social phobia have an overwhelming fear of embarrassing themselves or of being humiliated in front of other people in social situations, such as when they are eating or speaking in public.

WHAT ARE THE CAUSES?

Often, there is no reasonable explanation for the phobia, but occasionally a simple phobia can be traced to an earlier experience. For example, being trapped temporarily in a confined enclosed space during childhood may lead to claustrophobia in later life. Simple phobias appear to run in families, but this is thought to be because children "learn" rather than inherit their fear from a family member with a similar phobia.

The causes of complex phobias, such as agoraphobia and social phobia, are unclear, but they may develop from a general tendency to be anxious. Agoraphobia sometimes develops after an unexplained panic attack. Some people recall a stressful situation as the trigger for their symptoms and then become conditioned to be anxious in similar circumstances. Most social phobias also begin with a sudden episode of intense anxiety in a social situation, which then becomes the main focus of the phobia. A person who is lacking in self-esteem generally is more likely to develop agoraphobia or a social phobia.

WHAT ARE THE SYMPTOMS?

Exposure to or simply thinking about the object, creature, or situation that generates the phobia leads to intense anxiety accompanied by:

- Dizziness and feeling faint.
- Palpitations (awareness of an abnormally rapid heartbeat).
- Sweating and trembling.
- Nausea.
- Shortness of breath.

A factor that is common to every phobia is avoidance. Activities may become limited because of fear of unexpectedly encountering the subject of the phobia, and this may lead to depression (p.554). Anxiety and panic attacks (*see* ANXIETY DISORDERS, p.551) may develop. Sometimes, a person with a phobia attempts to relieve fear by drinking too much alcohol or abusing drugs.

WHAT MIGHT BE DONE?

If you have a phobia that interferes with your life, you should seek treatment. Many simple phobias can be treated effectively using a form of behaviour therapy (p.969), such as desensitization (*see* DESENSITIZATION THERAPY, p.969). During treatment, a therapist gives support while you are safely and gradually exposed to the object or situation that you fear. Inevitably, you will experience some anxiety, but exposure is always kept within bearable limits.

Members of your family may be given guidance on how to help you cope with your phobia. You may also benefit from contacting a self-help group.

WHAT IS THE PROGNOSIS?

A simple phobia often resolves itself as a person gets older. However, complex phobias, such as social phobias and agoraphobia, tend to persist unless they are treated. More than 9 in 10 people with agoraphobia are treated successfully with desensitization therapy.

(WWW) ONLINE SITES: p.1029, p.1034

Post-traumatic stress disorder

A prolonged emotional response to an extreme personal experience

 AGE Most common in children and elderly people

 GENDER GENETICS LIFESTYLE Not significant factors

Post-traumatic stress disorder (PTSD) occurs when a person is involved in a stressful event that triggers persistent intense emotions for some time afterwards. Experiencing an event in which life and personal safety are perceived to be at risk or simply witnessing a traumatic event is often enough to trigger the disorder. The kind of events that result in PTSD include natural disasters, accidents, and being assaulted.

About 1 in 10 people experiences PTSD. Children and elderly people are more susceptible, as are people who lack emotional support or who have a history of anxiety disorders (p.551).

WHAT ARE THE SYMPTOMS?

The symptoms of PTSD occur soon after the event or develop weeks, months, or, rarely, years later. They may include:

- Involuntary thoughts about and repeated reliving of the experience.
- Daytime flashbacks of the event.
- Panic attacks with symptoms such as shortness of breath and fainting.
- Avoidance of reminders of the event and refusal to discuss it.
- Sleep disturbance and nightmares.
- Poor concentration.
- Irritability.

People with PTSD often feel emotionally "numb", detached from events, and estranged from family and friends. After a while, they may lose interest in their normal everyday activities. Other psychological disorders, such as depression (p.554) and anxiety, may coexist with PTSD. Occasionally, the disorder leads to alcohol or drug abuse.

WHAT MIGHT BE DONE?

The doctor will assess the severity of symptoms and ask whether there have been mental health problems in the past. Counselling (p.971) may help the person to talk about his or her experiences, and support for the individual and family members is frequently an important part of treatment. Drugs such as antidepressants (p.916) may be used together with counselling. Although this approach often produces an improvement within 8 weeks, drugs may need to be taken for at least a year. Often, most of the symptoms of PTSD disappear after a few months of treatment, but some symptoms may persist for years. Once a person has experienced PTSD, there is an increased likelihood of it recurring following another traumatic event.

(WWW) ONLINE SITES: p.1029, p.1034

Obsessive–compulsive disorder

Uncontrollable thoughts that are often accompanied by irresistible urges to carry out acts or rituals to relieve anxiety

 AGE Usually develops in adolescence

 GENETICS Sometimes runs in families

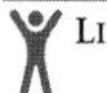 LIFESTYLE Stress is a risk factor

 GENDER Not a significant factor

A person with obsessive–compulsive disorder feels dominated by unwanted thoughts that enter the mind repeatedly. Obsessive thoughts are frequently accompanied by a form of compulsive ritual, in which a behaviour or action, such as checking that keys are still in a pocket, is repeated again and again. The affected person does not want to perform these actions but feels driven to do so. Thoughts may be concerns about hygiene, personal safety, or security of

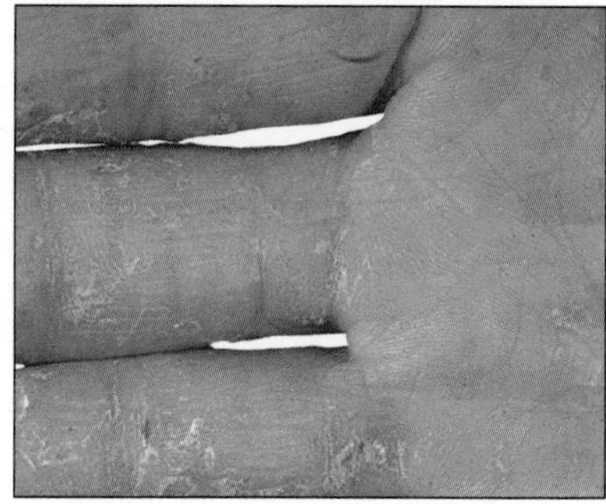

Effects of compulsive handwashing
Repeated handwashing in a person with obsessive–compulsive disorder has made the skin of the hands raw and chapped.

possessions. Alternatively, there may be violent and obscene thoughts that are completely out of character. Examples of common compulsions include hand-washing, checking that windows and doors are locked, and arranging objects on a desk in precise patterns. Carrying out the ritual brings short-lived relief, but, in severe cases, the ritual is performed hundreds of times a day and interferes with work and social life.

About 1 in 100 people in the UK have obsessive–compulsive disorder, which sometimes runs in families. Having an obsessive–compulsive personality (*see* PERSONALITY DISORDERS, p.561) tends to increase the risk of the disorder. Stressful life events may trigger the condition.

WHAT ARE THE SYMPTOMS?

An obsession or compulsion can focus on any object, event, or idea. The most common symptoms include:

- Intrusive, irrational mental images.
- Repeated attempts to resist thoughts.
- Repetitive behaviour.

The person may be aware that the behaviour is irrational and be distressed by it but cannot control the compulsions.

TEST PSYCHOLOGICAL ASSESSMENT

To help diagnose a mental health disorder, your doctor may arrange for you to have a psychological assessment. You will be asked a series of questions to establish the nature of your problem and its effect on your life. Areas of discussion include your family, your history, how life was before you became ill, and factors that might have triggered the disorder, such as a bereavement.

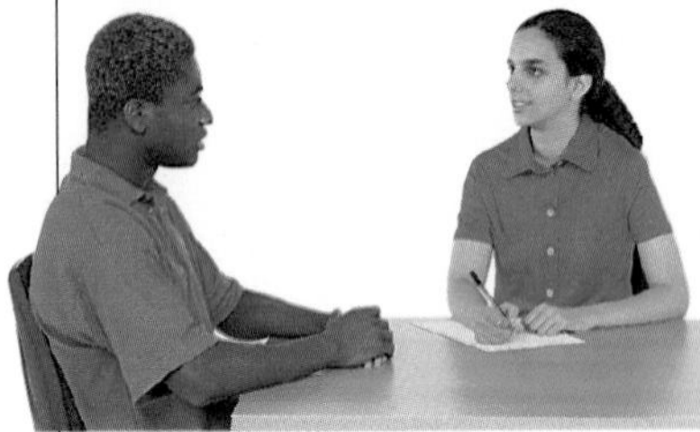

Having an assessment
Although questions are intimate and personal, they are part of a standard assessment procedure. The doctor usually records answers on a checklist.

WHAT MIGHT BE DONE?

Your doctor will probably be able to diagnose obsessive–compulsive disorder from your symptoms. To help you confront your compulsion to carry out rituals, your doctor may suggest treatment with a form of psychotherapy, such as behaviour therapy (p.969). He or she may prescribe an antidepressant drug (p.916) because drugs combined with psychotherapy usually offer the best chance of success. Initially, behaviour therapy may make your anxiety and your compulsion to perform rituals worse, but, given time, therapy may help you to resist compulsive urges.

As part of your treatment, you may want to involve a family member or friend to encourage you. You should also try to identify stress factors that may contribute to your condition and seek ways to reduce them. Many people find joining a self-help group is beneficial.

More than 9 in 10 people begin to improve within a year of starting treatment. Other people, particularly those who have an obsessive–compulsive personality, have a long-term illness that fluctuates in severity.

(WWW) ONLINE SITES: p.1029, p.1034

Insomnia

A regular inability to fall asleep or stay asleep, leading to excessive tiredness

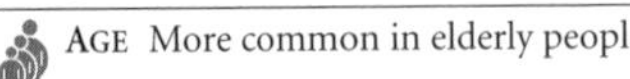

AGE More common in elderly people

GENDER More common in females

LIFESTYLE Stress and a high intake of caffeine or alcohol are risk factors

GENETICS Not a significant factor

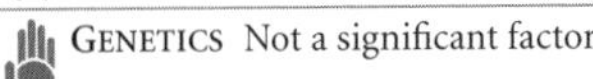

At some point in their lives, about 1 in 3 people has regular difficulty in sleeping, known as insomnia. Problems include difficulty in falling asleep and waking during the night and being unable to get back to sleep. Insomnia is distressing and may lead to excessive tiredness and a general inability to cope. Sleep problems are more common in women and in elderly people of both sexes.

Sleeping difficulties most commonly start when a person is worried or anxious. A high intake of caffeine or alcohol during the day may also lead to sleeplessness. Often, not sleeping properly then becomes persistent because good sleep habits are lost. Insomnia may be caused by an illness with symptoms that cause problems at night, such as asthma (p.483) or the metabolic disorder hyperthyroidism (p.679). Insomnia is often associated with mental health problems such as depression (below) and anxiety disorders (p.551).

WHAT MIGHT BE DONE?

Your doctor will first treat any physical and mental problems that may be causing your insomnia. For example, if you are depressed, the doctor may prescribe antidepressant drugs (p.916). However, if there is no obvious cause for your insomnia, your doctor may arrange for you to be assessed during sleep at a sleep clinic. Tests often show that many people sleep more hours than they think they do but wake frequently. Reassurance that you are getting sufficient sleep may be all that is needed.

Your doctor may suggest changes to your lifestyle, such as taking more exercise or cutting out caffeinated drinks (*see* SLEEP, p.73). Elderly people in particular may be advised to avoid taking daytime naps because they reduce the need for sleep at night. Rarely, the doctor may prescribe sleeping drugs (p.915) for a few days to help to restore a normal sleep pattern. Sleeping drugs should not be taken for a longer period because of the risk of dependence.

(WWW) ONLINE SITES: p.1034, p.1036

Depression

Feelings of sadness, often accompanied by loss of interest in life as a whole and reduced energy

AGE More common from the late 20s onwards

GENDER More common in females

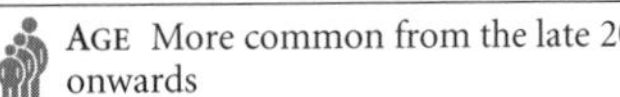

GENETICS Sometimes runs in families

LIFESTYLE Social isolation is a risk factor

Sadness is an expected reaction to adversity or personal misfortune and may last for a considerable time. Depression exists when feelings of unhappiness intensify and daily life becomes difficult. Depression is one of the most common mental health disorders in the UK. It affects about 1 in 10 people, most often from the late 20s onwards. Women are twice as likely to report symptoms of depression as men. In some cases, the disorder lifts spontaneously after days or weeks. However other people may need professional help and support. In severe cases of depression, hospital admission may be necessary to protect a person from neglect or self-harm.

Depression is often accompanied by symptoms of anxiety (*see* ANXIETY DISORDERS, p.551). For example, there may be a persistent sense of foreboding and repetitive, worrying thoughts.

WHAT ARE THE CAUSES?

Depression may develop when a person has to face one or more stressful life events. The trigger is often some form of loss, such as the breakdown of a close relationship or a bereavement.

A traumatic experience in childhood, such as the death of a parent, may increase susceptibility to depression later on. A tendency towards the disorder may also run in families.

Several physical illnesses may cause depression. These include some infections, such as infectious mononucleosis (p.291); neurological disorders, such as Parkinson's disease (p.539); and hormonal disorders, such as Cushing's syndrome (p.684). Hormonal changes at the menopause or after childbirth may also trigger the disorder (*see* DEPRESSION AFTER CHILDBIRTH, p.807).

A number of mental health disorders may lead to depression. They include phobias (p.552), the eating disorder anorexia nervosa (p.562), alcohol dependence (p.564), and drug dependence (p.564). Some people feel generally low and become depressed only during the winter months, a condition known as seasonal affective disorder. Depression can also be a side effect of certain drugs, such as oral contraceptives and beta-blockers (p.898). However, often depression has no identifiable cause.

WHAT ARE THE SYMPTOMS?

A typical sign of depression is a feeling of sadness, even misery, that is worse in the morning and lasts for most of the day. Other common symptoms include:

- Loss of interest in and enjoyment of work and leisure activities.
- Diminished energy levels.
- Poor concentration.
- Reduced self-esteem.
- Feelings of guilt.
- Tearfulness.
- Inability to make decisions.
- Early waking and inability to resume sleep (*see* INSOMNIA, opposite page) or an excessive need to sleep.
- Loss of hope for the future.
- Recurrent thoughts of death.
- Weight loss or increase in weight.
- Decreased sex drive (p.769).

In an elderly person, other symptoms may occur, including confusion, forgetfulness, and personality changes, that may be mistakenly attributed to dementia (p.535). Neglect of personal hygiene and diet in an elderly person may also be an indication of underlying depression. Sometimes, depressive illness manifests itself as a physical symptom, such as tiredness (*see* SOMATIZATION, p.559), or may cause associated physical problems, such as constipation or headache.

Severely depressed people may see or hear things that are not there. Irrational delusions may also occur. For instance, a depressed person may become convinced that his or her partner is having a sexual relationship with someone else.

Depression may also alternate with periods of euphoria in a person who has manic depression (*see* BIPOLAR AFFECTIVE DISORDER, p.557).

ARE THERE COMPLICATIONS?

Rarely, if the condition is not treated, a depressive stupor may develop, in which speech and movement are greatly reduced. Left untreated, depression can delay recovery from a physical illness and intensify pain whatever the cause, which then increases the depression. A person who is severely depressed may contemplate or attempt suicide (*see* ATTEMPTED SUICIDE AND SUICIDE, p.556).

WHAT MIGHT BE DONE?

If your depression is mild, your symptoms may disappear spontaneously if you are given sympathy and support from those close to you.

However, if you do need help for depression, it can almost always be treated effectively, and you should not put off seeing your doctor if you continue to feel low. He or she may examine you and arrange for blood tests to make sure that your low energy levels and mood are not caused by a physical illness. You may be asked to have a psychological assessment (opposite page) in case there are other mental health problems that may be causing or contributing to your depression.

If depression is diagnosed, you may be treated with drugs, a psychological therapy (pp.968–971), or therapy and drugs. Rarely, severe cases are treated with electroconvulsive therapy.

DRUG TREATMENTS The doctor usually prescribes a course of antidepressant drugs (p.916). There are several different types, and your doctor will choose the one most suitable for your needs. Although some have undesirable side effects, other side effects may be useful. For example, an antidepressant drug that is mildly sedating may relieve a sleeping problem. Your mood usually improves after you have been taking an antidepressant for 2–4 weeks, although some of your symptoms may improve more quickly. If your depression shows little improvement after a month or if you have troublesome side effects from your treatment, your doctor may adjust the dosage or prescribe an alternative

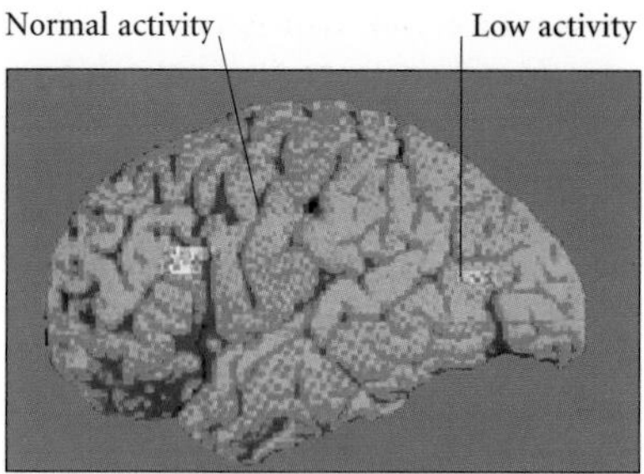

BRAIN OF NORMAL PERSON

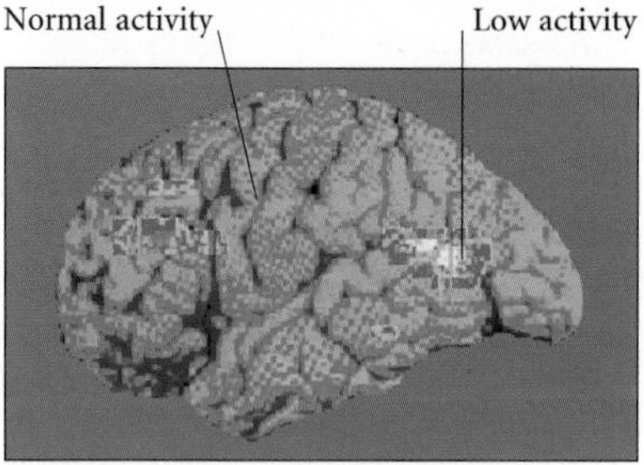

BRAIN OF DEPRESSED PERSON

Reduced brain activity in depression
These images show large areas of low activity in the brain of a depressed person compared with small areas of low activity in the brain of a normal person.

drug. Once your depression has lifted, you should continue taking antidepressants for as long as your doctor suggests. Treatment usually lasts for a minimum of 6 months, but the length of time depends on how quickly the depression responds to treatment and whether you have had previous episodes of depression. There is no risk of addiction with antidepressants, but depression may recur if they are stopped suddenly.

PSYCHOLOGICAL TREATMENTS Support from your doctor or other health professionals is essential while you are depressed. Your doctor may refer you to a therapist for treatments such as cognitive therapy (p.970) to help you to change negative patterns of thinking or psychoanalytic-based psychotherapy (p.968) to look into the reasons for your depression. Counselling (p.971), either on an individual basis or as part of a group, may help you to identify your feelings and make sense of them.

SELF-HELP RECOVERING FROM DEPRESSION

There are a number of strategies that help you to rebuild your self-confidence and regain control of your life while you are recovering from depression. Try to plan your day so that any potentially difficult tasks become easier to deal with, and practice relaxation techniques on a regular basis. You might like to try some of the following ideas:

- Make a list of things that you have to do each day, beginning with the most important.
- Tackle one task at a time, and reflect on what you have achieved when each is done.
- Set aside a few minutes each day to relax by breathing deeply or stretching (*see* RELAXATION EXERCISES, p.75).
- Exercise regularly to help to reduce feelings of stress (*see* THE BENEFITS OF EXERCISE, p.55).
- Eat a healthy diet (p.48).
- Take up a pastime or hobby that distracts you from worries.
- Join a support group where you can meet other people who have had similar experiences.

ELECTROCONVULSIVE THERAPY In rare cases, treatment with electroconvulsive therapy (ECT) is given for severe depression. In this procedure, which is carried out under general anaesthesia, an electrical stimulus that causes a brief seizure in the brain is given by placing two electrodes on the head. Between 6 and 12 treatments may be given over a period of about 1 month. ECT is particularly useful for treating depression that is accompanied by delusions. After treatment, antidepressants are given for at least a few months to prevent relapse.

WHAT IS THE PROGNOSIS?

Antidepressants are effective in treating about 3 in 4 people with depression. When drug treatments and psychological therapy are used in combination, the symptoms of depression can often be relieved completely in 2–3 months. Of the small number of people who are treated with ECT, about 9 in 10 make a successful recovery. However, for some people, depression can last for years or recur with no obvious trigger.

WWW ONLINE SITES: p.1029, p.1030

Attempted suicide and suicide

An attempt to end one's life that may have a nonfatal or fatal outcome

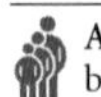
AGE More young people attempt suicide, but more elderly people die from an attempt

GENDER More females attempt suicide, but more males die from an attempt

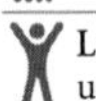
LIFESTYLE Social isolation and living in urban areas are risk factors

GENETICS Not a significant factor

Most people who attempt suicide are in their teens or are elderly. Among those who attempt suicide, some are certain that they wish to die while others use the attempt to signal their desperation rather than end their lives. More than half of all suicides and suicide attempts involve a drug overdose (*see* DRUG OVERDOSE AND ACCIDENTAL INGESTION, p.321), most commonly of a painkiller (p.912) such as paracetamol.

The suicide rate in the UK is about 7 in 100,000. About 4,000 deaths each year are attributed to suicide, but the exact number of suicides is unknown because some are recorded as deaths from other causes. Nevertheless, suicide is estimated as the eighth leading cause of death in the UK and is the second most common cause of death after accidents in young men. Women are three times more likely than men to attempt suicide. However, men are four times more likely to die as a result of a suicide attempt because they use methods, such as hanging, that have a greater potential to kill.

WHAT ARE THE CAUSES?

The majority of suicides in people of all ages are associated with an underlying mental health disorder. About half of all suicide attempts are a consequence of depression (p.554) or bipolar affective disorder (opposite page).

Teenage suicide attempts are often impulsive and may follow family quarrels or the breakup of a relationship. These attempts rarely indicate a wish to die, but a fatal dose of tablets may be taken by mistake. Suicide in elderly people is often the result of depression caused by bereavement and loneliness. Incurable physical illnesses lead to 1 in 5 suicides of people over the age of 65.

Other mental health disorders associated with suicide are schizophrenia (p.560), drug dependence (p.564), and alcohol dependence (p.564).

WHAT MIGHT BE DONE?

If suicide has been attempted, admission to hospital is usually necessary for assessment and treatment. In the case of an overdose, as much of the ingested substance as possible is removed from the body to prevent it from being absorbed. If the substance is identifiable, an antidote will be given if there is one available. Any physical effects of an attempted suicide, such as cuts to the wrists, are treated appropriately.

Treatment for underlying psychiatric problems is particularly important to prevent future suicide attempts. Drugs such as antidepressants (p.916) may be prescribed, and a form of psychotherapy or counselling (*see* PSYCHOLOGICAL THERAPIES, pp.968–971) may be recommended. Any problems that may have precipitated the suicide attempt will be identified and, if possible, help offered to resolve them. After a first attempt, there is an increased risk of future ones.

Can it be prevented?

Some people talk about their wish to kill themselves before they attempt suicide, and these threats should be taken seriously. Family and friends should try to remove any available means and seek professional help urgently. If there is a high risk of suicide, it may be necessary to admit the person to hospital, with, or possibly without his or her consent.

After a suicide attempt, treatment for any underlying mental health problems and family support and vigilance may prevent further attempts. However, a person who has a strong desire to die may try to prevent discovery during an attempt and is more likely to choose a method that will prove fatal.

(WWW) ONLINE SITES: p.1029, p.1034

Bipolar affective disorder

A disorder in which mood fluctuates between extremes of highs and lows

 AGE Usually develops in the early 20s

 GENETICS Sometimes runs in families

 GENDER LIFESTYLE Not significant factors

About 8 in 1,000 people in the UK have bipolar affective disorder, also known as manic depression. In this disorder, episodes of elation and abnormally high activity levels (mania) tend to alternate with episodes of low mood and abnormally low energy levels (depression). More than half of all people with bipolar affective disorder have repeated episodes. The factors that trigger manic and depressive episodes are not generally known, although episodes are sometimes brought on in response to a major life event, such as a marital breakup or bereavement. Bipolar affective disorder usually develops in the early 20s and can run in families, but exactly how it is inherited is not known.

What are the symptoms?

Symptoms of mania and depression tend to alternate, each episode lasting an unpredictable length of time. Between periods of mania and depression, mood and behaviour are generally normal. However, occasionally, a manic phase may be followed immediately by depression. Sometimes, either depression or mania predominates to the extent that there is little evidence of a pattern of changing moods. Occasionally, symptoms of depression and mania are present during the same period. During a manic episode of the disorder, the symptoms may include:

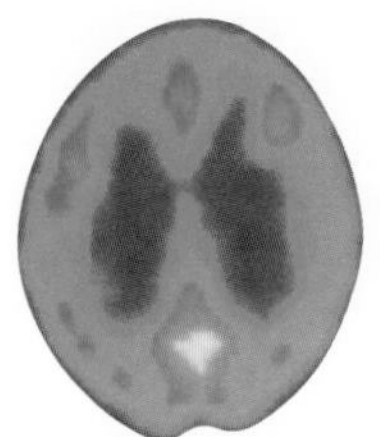

BRAIN IN NORMAL PERIODS

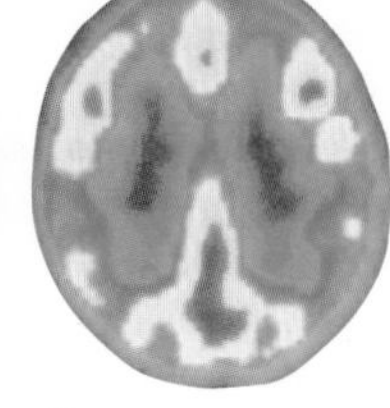

BRAIN IN MANIC PHASE

Increased brain activity in bipolar affective disorder

These PET scans of the brain of a person with bipolar affective disorder show high levels of activity during a manic episode.

- Elated, expansive, or sometimes irritable mood.
- Inflated self-esteem, which may lead to delusions of great wealth, accomplishment, creativity, and power.
- Increased energy levels and decreased need for sleep.
- Distraction and poor concentration.
- Loss of social inhibitions.
- Unrestrained sexual behaviour.
- Spending excessive sums of money on luxuries and holidays.

Speech may be difficult to follow because the person tends to speak rapidly and change topic frequently. At times, he or she may be aggressive or violent and may neglect diet and personal hygiene.

During an episode of depression, the main symptoms include:

- Feeling generally low.
- Loss of interest and enjoyment.
- Diminished energy level.
- Reduced self-esteem.
- Loss of hope for the future.

While severely depressed, a person affected by the disorder may not care whether he or she lives or dies. About 1 in 10 people with bipolar disorder eventually attempts suicide (*see* ATTEMPTED SUICIDE AND SUICIDE, opposite page).

In severe cases of bipolar affective disorder, delusions of power during manic episodes may be made worse by hallucinations. When manic, the person may hear imaginary voices praising his or her qualities. In his or her depressive phase, these hallucinatory voices may describe the person's inadequacies and failures. In such cases, the disorder may resemble schizophrenia (p.560).

What might be done?

During a manic phase, people usually lack insight into their condition and may not be aware of the fact that they are ill. Often, a person's erratic behaviour is first noticed by a relative or friend, who seeks professional advice. A diagnosis of bipolar affective disorder is based on the full range of the person's symptoms, and treatment will depend on whether the person is in a manic or a depressive phase. For the depressive phase, antidepressants (p.916) are prescribed, but their effects have to be monitored to ensure that they do not precipitate a manic phase. During the first days or weeks of a manic phase, symptoms may be controlled initially by antipsychotic drugs (p.917).

Some people may need to be admitted to the secure environment of a hospital for assessment and treatment during a manic phase or a severe depressive phase. They may feel creative and energetic when manic and may be reluctant to accept long-term medication because it makes them feel "flat".

Most people make a good recovery from manic–depressive episodes, but recurrences are common. For this reason, initial treatments for depression and mania may be gradually replaced with lithium (*see* MOOD-STABILIZING DRUGS, p.918), a drug that has to be taken continuously to prevent relapse. If lithium is not fully effective, other types of drug, including certain anticonvulsant drugs (p.914), may be given. In severe cases in which drugs have no effect, electroconvulsive therapy (ECT) may be used to relieve symptoms by inducing a brief seizure in the brain under a general anaesthetic.

Once symptoms are under control, the person will need regular checkups to look for signs of mood changes. A form of psychotherapy (*see* PSYCHOLOGICAL THERAPIES, pp.968–971) may help the person come to terms with the disorder and reduce stress factors in his or her life that may contribute to it.

(WWW) ONLINE SITES: p.1029, p.1034

Mental problems due to physical illness

One or more psychological conditions resulting from a physical illness

 LIFESTYLE Unsettled domestic or financial circumstances are risk factors

 AGE GENDER GENETICS Not significant factors

Changes in mental state are a common response to a physical illness. A serious physical illness may cause anxiety (*see* ANXIETY DISORDERS, p.551), depression (p.554), anger, or denial of the problem. Usually, reactions are transient and disappear when the person adjusts to the change in his or her physical condition. However, illnesses that may be fatal or long-term disorders that involve lengthy or unpleasant treatment may cause persistent mood problems. People who have had previous psychiatric disorders are more at risk, as are people who are subject to additional stresses, such as an unstable home life or financial problems, or those who generally find it hard to deal with adversity.

Mood problems are sometimes a recognized symptom of a physical illness. For example, anxiety is a symptom of the hormonal disorder hyperthyroidism (p.679), and depression is associated with multiple sclerosis (p.541) and also Parkinson's disease (*see* PARKINSON'S DISEASE AND PARKINSONISM, p.539).

WHAT ARE THE SYMPTOMS?

The psychological symptoms that may result from a physical illness include:

- Feelings of anxiety, ranging from mild apprehension to fear and panic.
- Depressive symptoms, such as a sense of hopelessness and worthlessness.
- Irritability and anger.

In extreme cases, there may be social withdrawal and drug or alcohol abuse.

WHAT MIGHT BE DONE?

If your doctor thinks you are at risk of developing a psychological problem as a result of illness, you will be offered support and counselling (p.971) to help you adjust. If there are signs that you are avoiding coming to terms with an illness, your doctor will encourage you to ask questions and talk about possible anxieties. Home and work problems may be discussed, and your doctor will want to know if you have a history of depression or anxiety disorders.

A person who has developed psychological problems as a result of illness may not be aware of the fact, and a family member or friend may first contact the doctor on his or her behalf. The doctor may prescribe antidepressant drugs (p.916). Less commonly, an anti-anxiety drug (p.916) may be given for a short time. The person may be referred to a psychologist, who will encourage a problem-solving approach to illness that concentrates on seeking solutions rather than focusing on difficulties.

The outlook for a mental problem resulting from physical illness depends on how well the person develops an ability to cope with the demands of his or her illness. Given continued support, most people are able to recognize and deal with mood problems, which gradually diminish as a result.

(WWW) ONLINE SITES: p.1029, p.1034

Munchausen's syndrome

A condition in which medical care is sought repeatedly for nonexistent or self-induced symptoms

 AGE Usually begins in early adulthood

 GENDER More common in males

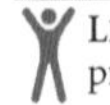 LIFESTYLE Working in a health-related profession is a risk factor

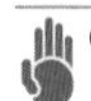 GENETICS Not a significant factor

Munchausen's syndrome is a rare condition in which a person claims to have symptoms of illness, usually abdominal pain, blackouts, and fever, and may repeatedly seek treatment from a number of hospitals. This unexplained desire to assume the role of a patient is seen as an attempt to escape from everyday life and be cared for and protected.

The syndrome usually develops in early adulthood and is more common in men. Those affected tend to have some knowledge of symptoms and hospital procedures, which may have been acquired through working in a health-related profession. For this reason, their bogus claims to illness may be taken seriously until test results prove negative or exploratory surgery is carried out. People with the disorder tend to conceal personal details or give extraordinary accounts of their circumstances. If challenged, they may accuse doctors of incompetence and leave the hospital.

In factitious disorder, a variant of Munchausen's syndrome, a person aggravates an existing condition or causes deliberate self-injury. The disorder occurs most often in health professionals. In another related condition, Munchausen's syndrome by proxy, a parent, often the mother, repeatedly claims her child is ill and in need of treatment.

WHAT ARE THE SYMPTOMS?

Munchausen's syndrome and factitious disorder have similar typical patterns of behaviour, which may include:

- Dramatic presentation of symptoms and their history.
- Histrionic and argumentative behaviour towards medical staff.
- Wide knowledge of medical terms and medical procedures.

There may be evidence of multiple surgical operations, such as a number of scars on the abdomen. An affected person may demand strong painkillers, possibly because he or she has an addiction. In Munchausen's syndrome by proxy, the parent may fake physical signs of illness in a child and give a false description of symptoms. The child may be repeatedly admitted to hospital for unnecessary tests or treatment.

WHAT MIGHT BE DONE?

Treatment is difficult because as soon as staff begin to suspect that a person is feigning symptoms, he or she may leave the hospital to avoid being discovered.

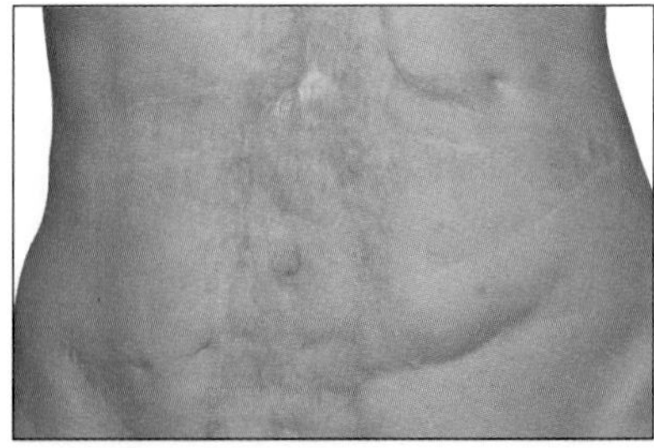

Scars due to Munchausen's syndrome
The numerous scars on the abdomen of this person with Munchausen's syndrome are the result of multiple operations to investigate fictitious symptoms.

Munchausen's syndrome may be identified only with hindsight.

It is often difficult to treat Munchausen's syndrome and related conditions because deception is a characteristic of the disorders. The doctor will try to prevent further unnecessary treatments and tests by building a calm and supportive relationship with the person. In cases of Munchausen's syndrome by proxy, a social worker should be alerted in case a child needs to be placed in foster care.

(WWW) ONLINE SITES: p.1034

Somatization

The expression of psychological problems as physical symptoms

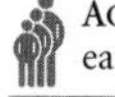 AGE Usually develops in adolescence or early adulthood

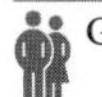 GENDER More common in females

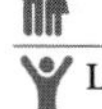 LIFESTYLE Stress is a risk factor

 GENETICS Not a significant factor

Somatization describes a process in which a psychological problem manifests itself as a physical symptom or a range of physical symptoms. Although occasionally bizarre, these symptoms are not fabricated and may be frightening if they are interpreted as signs of a progressive or potentially fatal disease. The condition is related to hyponchondriasis (right), a condition in which there are constant, unfounded worries that minor symptoms are caused by a serious underlying disorder. However, in somatization, psychological problems generate actual physical changes, which cause debilitating symptoms.

People with somatization may make repeated visits to their doctor to ask for investigations into their symptoms and treatment. When test results are normal, and reassurance is given that there is no underlying physical illness, an affected person feels no relief and may consult other doctors to find a physical cause for the symptoms. In extreme cases of somatization, life is continually disrupted by numerous follow-up medical appointments, and health is placed at risk by invasive tests and investigations.

Several psychiatric illnesses may be associated with somatization, including anxiety disorders (p.551) and depression (p.554). A person with the condition may have an underlying personality disorder (p.561) marked by self-absorption and reliance on others. Somatization usually develops in adolescence or early in adult life and may become a lifelong problem. It is more common in women and is often associated with stress

What are the symptoms?

A person who has a somatization disorder may have a long history of varying physical symptoms that fluctuate in severity and have no identifiable medical cause. Symptoms that sometimes have psychological causes include:

- Headaches.
- Chest pain, often accompanied by shortness of breath and palpitations.
- Abdominal pain and nausea.
- Tiredness.
- Itching of the skin.
- Partial weakness of a limb.
- Difficulty in swallowing.

In addition, there may be psychological symptoms of anxiety, depression, and substance abuse. Severely affected people may attempt suicide (*see* ATTEMPTED SUICIDE AND SUICIDE, p.556).

What might be done?

The doctor will first carry out a physical examination and may arrange for blood and urine tests to exclude a physical illness. Medical records will give a picture of past symptoms and investigations.

Treating somatization is often difficult because the affected person may be convinced there is a physical illness in spite of normal test results. The doctor may prescribe treatment for symptoms, such as painkillers (p.912) for headaches, but will try to avoid further tests and investigations by offering reassurance that physical symptoms are taken seriously and explaining how they may be caused by psychological problems.

The doctor may recommend a psychological assessment (p.554) to look for an underlying mental health disorder, but this may be resisted by the person. Cognitive therapy (p.970) and behaviour therapy (p.969) can be particularly helpful for some people.

If depression is causing somatization, it may be treated with antidepressant drugs (p.916) and a form of psychological therapy (pp.968–971).

(WWW) ONLINE SITES: p.1029, p.1034

Hypochondriasis

A deep, worrying, and unfounded suspicion of being seriously ill

 AGE Most common between the ages of 20 and 30

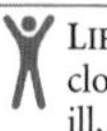 LIFESTYLE Long-term illness in childhood, close contact with people who are seriously ill, and stress are risk factors

 GENDER GENETICS Not significant factors

People who suffer from hypochondriasis are constantly anxious about their health and interpret all symptoms, no matter how minor, as indications of serious illness. They may be concerned about a combination of symptoms or a single symptom, such as a headache.

Inevitably, the disorder leads to frequent visits to the doctor to have tests. Even when the results are negative, people affected by hypochondriasis remain convinced that they are seriously ill. They may reject the doctor's findings and react with strong feelings of frustration and hostility. Frequently, their anxiety about illness causes problems with relationships, work, and social life.

Somatization (left) is a related condition in which psychological problems are expressed as physical symptoms.

Hypochondriasis is most common between the ages of 20 and 30 and may be a complication of other psychological disorders, such as depression (p.554) or anxiety (*see* ANXIETY DISORDERS, p.551). Often, the cause is unknown, but people who were very ill in childhood or who have prolonged contact with someone with a long-term illness are more susceptible. Stress increases the risk of the disorder developing.

What might be done?

The doctor will first look for and treat any underlying psychological disorders. For example, he or she may prescribe antidepressant drugs (p.916) for depression. The doctor will avoid unnecessary tests by reassuring the person that he or she does not have a serious illness and will explain normal body reactions if the person is mistaking responses, such as rapid heartbeats during exercise, for signs of serious illness. In some people, cognitive therapy (p.970) and behaviour therapy (p.969) can be helpful.

(WWW) ONLINE SITES: p.1034

Schizophrenia

A serious mental disorder in which there is loss of a sense of reality and an inability to function socially

AGE Usually develops in males aged 18–25 and females aged 26–45

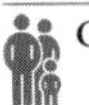
GENETICS Sometimes runs in families

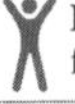
LIFESTYLE Stressful life events are risk factors

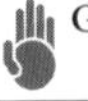
GENDER Not a significant factor

Schizophrenia is a severe and disruptive mental illness that occurs in all cultures and affects about 1 in 100 people worldwide. Although the term is sometimes used mistakenly to refer to a split personality, schizophrenia is actually an impairment of a person's sense of reality that leads to irrational behaviour and disturbed emotional reactions. People with schizophrenia may hear voices, and this may contribute to their bizarre behaviour. In addition, they are usually unable to function at work or maintain relationships with other people.

Without proper support and treatment, people with schizophrenia are likely to neglect or harm themselves. About 1 in 10 people with the condition commits suicide (*see* ATTEMPTED SUICIDE AND SUICIDE, p.556).

WHAT ARE THE CAUSES?

No single cause of schizophrenia has been identified, but genetic factors are known to play a part. A person who is closely related to someone with schizophrenia has a significantly increased risk of developing the disorder. In addition, a stressful life event, such as a serious illness or a bereavement, may trigger the disorder in a person who is susceptible. Evidence also points to abnormalities in brain structure, such as enlarged fluid-filled cavities that suggest loss of brain tissue.

WHAT ARE THE SYMPTOMS?

Schizophrenia tends to develop in men during their teens or early 20s, but the onset in women may be 10–20 years later. The condition usually develops gradually, with the person losing energy and personal motivation and becoming increasingly withdrawn over a period of months or years. In other cases, the

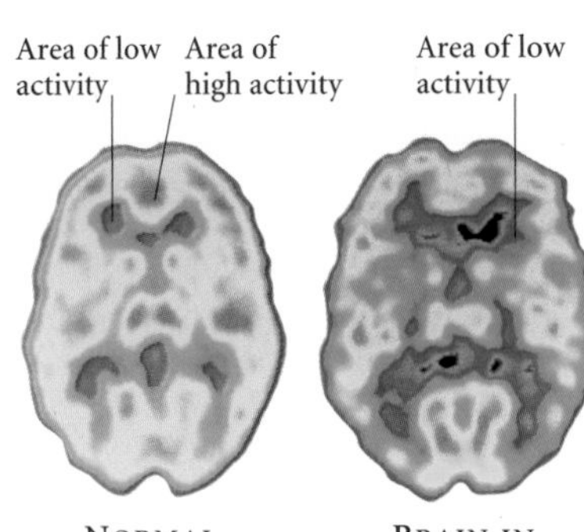

Brain activity in schizophrenia
PET scans show a distinctive pattern of large areas of low activity in the brain of a person with schizophrenia when compared with the brain of an unaffected person.

illness is more sudden and may be a response to an episode of stress. Some people have clear-cut episodes of illness and recover completely in between. In other cases, the disorder is more or less continuous. Symptoms may include:

- Hearing hallucinatory voices.
- Having irrational beliefs, in particular that thoughts and actions are being controlled by an outside force.
- Delusions of persecution or a conviction that trivial objects and events have deep significance.
- Expression of inappropriate emotions, such as laughing at bad news.
- Rambling speech with rapid switching from one topic to another.
- Impaired concentration.
- Slow movement and thought.
- Agitation and restlessness.

A person with schizophrenia may be depressed, lethargic, and socially withdrawn. He or she may begin to neglect personal care and become increasingly isolated. In rare cases, violence towards other people may occur.

HOW IS IT DIAGNOSED?

If you are worried that a close friend or family member is suffering from schizophrenia, you should contact a doctor. Normally, the doctor will look for evidence of a profound break with reality, disturbed emotions, and strange beliefs lasting for several months before considering a diagnosis of schizophrenia. He or she will carry out a full physical examination, and blood or urine tests may be arranged to exclude other possible causes of abnormal behaviour, such as alcohol or drug abuse. The doctor may arrange for imaging of the brain by CT scanning (p.247) or MRI (p.248) to exclude an underlying physical disorder, such as a brain tumour (p.530).

WHAT IS THE TREATMENT?

If schizophrenia is suspected, it will be necessary to admit the person to hospital for further assessment and to begin treatment. Antipsychotic drugs (p.917) are prescribed to help to calm the affected person. About 3 weeks of treatment may be needed to reduce the more obvious symptoms of schizophrenia. Some drugs may cause serious side effects, such as tremors, although these are less likely to occur with newer drugs. However, doses may have to be reduced or other drugs prescribed to minimize these effects. Treatment with adjusted doses of drugs usually continues after symptoms have subsided.

After assessment and treatment, people with schizophrenia are usually sent home, but it is essential that they have support and a calm and unthreatening home environment. People who have schizophrenia need to be protected from stressful situations because anxiety may trigger symptoms. They also need frequent, regular contact with community mental health service workers, who will supervise their progress and well-being after they leave hospital.

Counselling (p.971) may be offered both to the person with schizophrenia and to family members. People close to the affected person should watch for signs of relapse and indications that the person is sinking into a general state of apathy and self-neglect.

WHAT IS THE PROGNOSIS?

For most affected people, schizophrenia is a long-term illness. However, about 1 in 5 of those affected have one sudden episode from which they recover and lead a normal life. The majority have a number of episodes of severe symptoms that may require hospital stays, interspersed with periods of recovery. Drugs have improved the outlook for people with schizophrenia, but adequate community care and support is essential to prevent relapse. The outlook is worse for people who develop schizophrenia gradually while they are young.

(WWW) ONLINE SITES: p.1034

Delusional disorders

The development of one or more persistent delusions of persecution or jealousy

AGE More common over the age of 40

GENDER More common in females

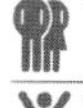
LIFESTYLE Stress may be a risk factor

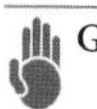
GENETICS Not a significant factor

Delusional disorders are rare, affecting only about 3 in 10,000 people worldwide. The main characteristic of these disorders is an irrational belief or set of beliefs that is not associated with other symptoms or caused by another mental illness, such as schizophrenia (opposite page). These beliefs or delusions persist in spite of all rational arguments and evidence to the contrary. However, apart from behaviour related to the delusion, the person appears well, and work and relationships may not be affected.

There are several different types of delusion, the most common of which is persecutory. People with this type of delusion believe they are being hounded, chased, or spied upon. Extreme jealousy, in which a person has the unreasonable belief that his or her partner is unfaithful, is another common form.

Major life events, such as moving to another country, and long-term stress factors, such as poverty, may contribute to the development of delusions. A person who has a paranoid personality (*see* PERSONALITY DISORDERS, right) is at an increased risk of delusions, as is a person who is alcohol dependent (p.564).

Delusional disorders usually develop suddenly, most often in middle age or late in life, and tend to occur more commonly in women than in men.

WHAT MIGHT BE DONE?

People with a delusional disorder are often suspicious or dismissive of others who are trying to help them. They may be reluctant to discuss their beliefs and unable to recognize that their delusions are irrational. Family members often seek medical advice on their behalf.

The doctor will look for additional symptoms in case delusions are being caused by another psychological illness, such as schizophrenia. The doctor will try to find out how firmly held or "fixed" the delusions are and whether the person is likely to act on them. If there is a risk of violence or self-harm, the person may need to be admitted to hospital, possibly without his or her consent.

Occasionally, an antipsychotic drug (p.917) is used to reduce the intensity of severe delusions. Counselling (p.971) may bring about a shift in perspective. Generally, delusional disorders tend to persist but without causing major disruption, although delusions of jealousy may pose a risk of violence to a partner.

(WWW) ONLINE SITES: p.1029, p.1034

Personality disorders

A group of disorders in which habitual patterns of thought and behaviour cause persistent life problems

AGE Develop in adolescence or early adulthood

GENDER GENETICS LIFESTYLE Risk factors depend on the type

People with personality disorders have ingrained patterns of thought and behaviour that prevent them from fitting in with society. An affected person often fails to see that his or her personality is unusual but is aware that it is causing problems in daily life. Although many people have strong personalities, this is not the same as a personality disorder. People with personality disorders are inflexible and unable to adapt.

Personality disorders tend to develop in adolescence and early adulthood but may not be properly diagnosed until later in life. The cause of most of these disorders is unknown.

WHAT ARE THE TYPES?

Personality disorders are divided into three broad groups: emotional or erratic, eccentric or odd, and anxious or fearful. Each group has its own pattern of thought processes and behaviour, although they may overlap.

EMOTIONAL OR ERRATIC This personality disorder further divides into four different types: antisocial, borderline, histrionic, and narcissistic.

An antisocial personality is typified by impulsive, destructive behaviour that often disregards the feelings and rights of others. A person with an antisocial personality lack a sense of guilt and cannot tolerate frustration. He or she may have problems with relationships and may often be in trouble with the law.

A person with a borderline personality has multiple abnormalities that may include an uncertainty about personal identity and an inability to form stable relationships. People who have this disorder are habitually bored and may indulge in promiscuity, reckless spending, or substance abuse. They may harm themselves or threaten suicide.

People with a histrionic personality have emotions that are exaggerated and shallow. They are self-centred, inconsiderate, and easily bored and constantly demand reassurance and approval.

People with a narcissistic personality believe themselves to be unique, special, and superior to others. They constantly seek attention and admiration and lack concern for the problems of others.

ECCENTRIC OR ODD This group of disorders can be further divided into three separate types of personality: paranoid, schizoid, and schizotypal.

A person with a paranoid personality tends to be mistrustful, jealous, and self-important. He or she readily interprets other people's actions as hostile and may feel continually rebuffed.

People who have a schizoid personality are emotionally cold and indifferent to others. They tend to be prone to fantasy and ill at ease in company. This disorder is not related to the mental illness schizophrenia (opposite page).

People with a schizotypal personality display eccentric and suspicious behaviour, often accompanied by odd ideas, such as a belief in magic or telepathy. They may have an unkempt appearance and vague, abstract speech patterns and may talk to themselves.

ANXIOUS OR FEARFUL The four different types of personality that make up the anxious or fearful group of disorders are: avoidant, passive–aggressive, obsessive–compulsive, and dependent.

A person with an avoidant personality is timid, oversensitive to rejection, and cautious of new experiences and responsibilities. He or she is generally ill at ease in social situations.

People with a passive–aggressive personality react to any demands made on them by being stubborn and argumentative. They put off tasks at work and at home and are deliberately inefficient and critical of people in authority.

An obsessive–compulsive personality is marked by a continual striving for perfection that disregards the feelings of other people. Generally, people with this disorder are inflexible, judgmental, and narrow-minded.

People with a dependent personality are weak-willed and submissive. They appear helpless, lack self-reliance, and leave decisions to other people.

What might be done?

A person with a personality disorder is often aware that he or she does not fit in, but it may be a family member who contacts the doctor. The doctor will first assess the person's behaviour and how it affects others and then look for provoking factors. If drug or alcohol abuse is contributing to difficulties, part of the treatment plan will include advice on overcoming the problem.

People in whom relationship difficulties or low self-esteem are the main problems may benefit from a form of psychological therapy (pp.968–971). A few people with severe problems may have prolonged treatment in a special community where they can learn to deal with day-to-day experiences.

Generally, an abnormal personality tends to improve as people get older.

(WWW) ONLINE SITES: p.1029, p.1034

Anorexia nervosa

Extreme concern about body size that results in a long-term refusal to eat and severe loss of weight

 **AGE** Usually develops in early adolescence

 **GENDER** More common in females

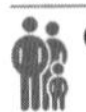 **GENETICS** Sometimes runs in families

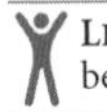 **LIFESTYLE** Social and job-related pressure to be slim is a risk factor

People with anorexia nervosa tend to be obsessively preoccupied with their body shape and weight. Often they are convinced, against all evidence to the contrary, that they are fat, even when they are terribly thin. They deliberately lose weight by a number of means, including dieting, exercising excessively, vomiting, and using laxatives. Those affected often go to great lengths to conceal these strategies and hide their weight loss from family and friends.

The condition can cause changes in hormone levels that may affect growth during adolescence and menstruation in girls and women. In severe cases, the loss of weight may be life-threatening.

Anorexia nervosa occurs mainly in the developed world, especially in the middle and upper social classes. The vast majority of people with the condition are teenage girls between the ages of 12 and 18. Up to 1 in 100 girls in this age group develops the disorder. Nevertheless, an increasing number of boys and younger children are being affected. Anorexia nervosa may run in families and may be associated with the binge-eating disorder bulimia (opposite page).

What are the causes?

Anorexia nervosa often develops following a normal weight-loss diet. In Western culture, the importance placed on having a slim body leads many people of normal size to diet unnecessarily, particularly if they lack self-confidence. Sometimes, the condition is triggered by stress (p.74) or depression (p.554).

Anorexia nervosa often affects young people who are under pressure to succeed in a family that over-emphasizes achievement. In these circumstances, a teenager may feel driven to take control over an aspect of his or her life by refusing to eat. The condition has become an occupational hazard for people such as models, gymnasts, and ballet dancers, who are required to be extremely slim to succeed in their profession.

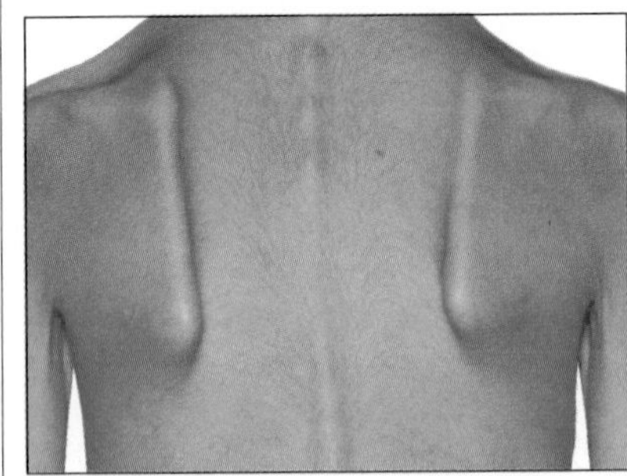

Wasting due to anorexia nervosa
The prominent shoulder blades and spine of this person with anorexia nervosa are signs of the extreme weight loss that is associated with the disorder.

What are the symptoms?

Almost everyone attempts to lose some weight from time to time, and teenagers are usually especially anxious to be slim. However, normal dieting needs to be distinguished from anorexia nervosa, in which a person who is already of average or low weight follows a weight-loss diet for a prolonged period. Symptoms and behaviour patterns that may be apparent early in the disorder include:

- Refusal to eat, particularly foods that are high in calories.
- An obsessional interest in the subject of food.
- Preoccupation with body weight and body size.
- Weight loss that may be concealed by wearing baggy clothes.
- A conviction that one is overweight.
- Use of appetite suppressants and laxative drugs.
- Exercising excessively.

Depression may develop as a complication and lead to self-harm and suicide attempts (*see* ATTEMPTED SUICIDE AND SUICIDE, p.556). Physical symptoms may appear gradually over weeks or months and become more obvious and extreme as the condition develops. They include:

- Extreme weight loss.
- Muscle wasting.
- Swollen ankles.
- Fine body hair on trunk and limbs.
- In women, an absence of menstrual periods (*see* AMENORRHOEA, p.735).

If anorexia nervosa develops before or around the onset of puberty, the development of adult sexual characteristics may be delayed or stop (*see* ABNORMAL PUBERTY IN FEMALES, p.739).

If there is a continued refusal to eat, extreme weight loss leads to complications such as chemical imbalances in the blood, nutritional deficiencies (p.630), loss of bone density (*see* OSTEOPOROSIS, p.368), infertility, chronic heart failure (p.413), and eventually death.

How is it diagnosed?

A person with anorexia nervosa is usually reluctant to admit that there is a problem. Often a concerned parent or friend consults the doctor first. The doctor will examine the affected person to assess the degree of weight loss and exclude other causes of weight loss, such as a digestive disorder or cancer. He or she will arrange for blood tests to see if an imbalance of chemicals in the blood has developed. The doctor will also look for an underlying or associated psychological disorder, such as depression.

What is the treatment?

Treatment is often difficult because of the person's refusal to acknowledge the illness. If weight loss is very severe or there is a risk of self-harm, the person will be admitted to hospital. Otherwise, treatment can be carried out at home under the doctor's supervision. Initially, the doctor sets a healthy weight target and monitors weight gain on a weekly basis. A dietitian will talk to the person about the importance of nutrition in general health and plan a healthy, balanced diet. In hospital, a person with anorexia nervosa is sometimes asked to stay in bed while eating habits are monitored and modified until a mutually agreed upon weight has been achieved. At home, family members or a friend will be asked to monitor the person's diet in a calm, supportive atmosphere.

People with anorexia nervosa are usually referred for psychological therapy. The doctor may suggest cognitive therapy (p.970) to help an affected person develop a more realistic self-image or behaviour therapy (p.969) to bring about changes in abnormal behaviour. Family therapy may be arranged if it appears that family problems are contributing to the disorder. Antidepressant drugs (p.916) may be given if there are symptoms of depression.

What is the prognosis?

About 1 in 5 people makes a complete recovery following treatment, but the same number remain severely ill. Even when a person has achieved his or her weight target, he or she needs continued professional support to maintain it.

For the remaining 3 in 5 people, the disorder persists but fluctuates in severity. Some people gain enough weight to recover but retain abnormal eating habits. Symptoms may also recur in response to stress. In some cases, bulimia develops up to 5 years after anorexia nervosa is first diagnosed.

About 1 in 20 people with anorexia nervosa dies from complications caused by malnutrition or commits suicide as a result of severe depression.

(WWW) ONLINE SITES: p.1029, p.1030, p.1034

Bulimia

Episodes of binge-eating followed by strategies to avoid weight gain

AGE Usually develops in early adulthood

GENDER More common in females

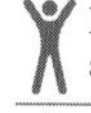
LIFESTYLE Episodes can be brought on by stress

GENETICS Not a significant factor

People with bulimia worry excessively about their weight, body shape, and self-image. Rather than dieting moderately, they starve themselves for a day or two and then eat uncontrollably (binge) on high-calorie foods, such as ice cream or chocolate. After binge-eating, they use methods to avoid weight gain, such as self-induced vomiting, using laxatives (p.924), and excessive exercising.

A person affected by bulimia is usually of average weight, and binge-eating and purging by vomiting and using laxatives are carried out secretly. He or she may have had anorexia nervosa (opposite page) in the past or may alternate between the two conditions. The disorder is more common in women and usually develops between the ages of 18 and 30. The person may have poor self-control and low self-esteem and may also indulge in substance abuse. Bouts of bulimia may be triggered by stress.

What are the symptoms?

Binge-eating followed by vomiting may occur once or several times a day. Over time, bulimia causes psychological and physical symptoms. The psychological symptoms include:

- A constant craving for food.
- Feelings of isolation as a result of eating alone and in secret.
- Guilt and disgust after binge-eating.

There may also be symptoms of depression (p.554) and anxiety (*see* ANXIETY DISORDERS, p.551). The physical symptoms caused by repeated episodes of binge-eating and vomiting include:

- Severe abdominal pain and swelling immediately following a binge.
- Physical weakness.
- Erosion of tooth enamel by stomach acids contained in vomit.
- Lesions on the knuckles from using fingers to induce vomiting.

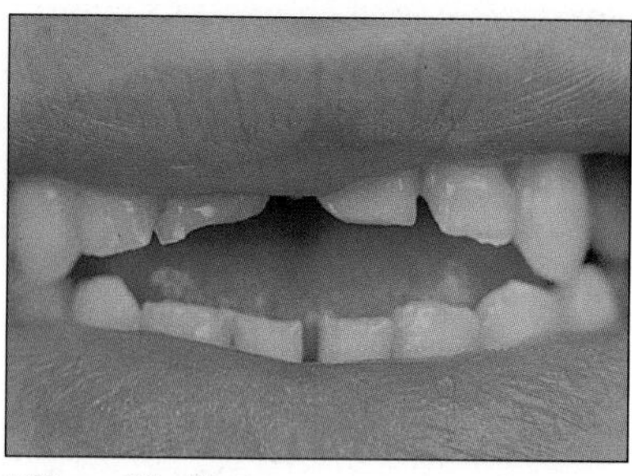
Effect of bulimia
Frequent self-induced vomiting leads to erosion of tooth enamel by stomach acid and eventually to the loss of front teeth.

- Bleeding from injuries to the lining of the oesophagus caused by vomiting.

Bulimia is unlike anorexia nervosa in that it rarely leads to severe weight loss. However, repeated excessive vomiting may cause dehydration and chemical imbalances in the blood. These imbalances sometimes lead to irregular heart rhythms (*see* ARRHYTHMIAS, p.415) that, very rarely, cause sudden death.

What might be done?

People with bulimia may be distressed by their behaviour and seek medical help themselves, or a family member or friend may encourage a person to see a doctor. The doctor will establish the severity of the illness by asking the person about his or her attitude to food. The doctor will look for signs of psychological problems, such as depression, anxiety, and substance abuse, and may arrange for blood tests to look for chemical imbalances in the blood.

The doctor may recommend a psychological therapy, such as cognitive therapy (p.970), with a therapist who specializes in eating disorders. The goal of treatment is to boost self-esteem and help develop a rational approach to eating, while establishing a regular eating pattern. The doctor may prescribe antidepressant drugs (p.916) because they can be helpful even if a person with bulimia does not feel depressed.

What is the prognosis?

It is rare for bulimia to disappear spontaneously. In many cases, there is a risk of relapse weeks or even months after treatment is completed. However, in about 4 out of 5 cases, the frequency of binge-eating is reduced by therapy.

(WWW) ONLINE SITES: p.1029, p.1030, p.1034

Drug dependence

Compulsive use of drugs, producing withdrawal symptoms when stopped

 AGE Usually develops in adolescence

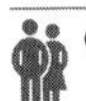 GENDER More common in males

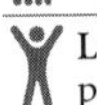 LIFESTYLE Stress, social factors, and peer pressure, are risk factors

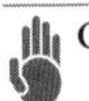 GENETICS Not a significant factor

Drug dependence, or addiction, is the excessive and compulsive use of drugs for their effects on mental state. Often, increasing quantities of the drug are needed to produce the desired effect, and physical symptoms may develop if use stops or is delayed. Some drugs, such as LSD, do not cause this physical addiction but may cause psychological craving (*see* DRUGS AND HEALTH, p.65).

Drugs that may produce dependence include those obtained illegally, such as heroin and cocaine, and drugs that are prescribed by a doctor, such as benzodiazepines (*see* SLEEPING DRUGS, p.915) and painkillers (p.912). Two common types of dependence are nicotine dependence (*see* TOBACCO AND HEALTH, p.63) and alcohol dependence (right). Nicotine dependence rarely affects work and social life, but alcohol dependence is often damaging. Drug addictions may lead to debt, loss of work, and breakdown in close relationships.

WHAT ARE THE CAUSES?

Initially, drugs may be taken for the psychological "high" they produce and because they relieve symptoms such as anxiety (*see* ANXIETY DISORDERS, p.551) and insomnia (p.554). People who find it difficult to cope with stress may be more susceptible, as may people who have a parent who has abused drugs or alcohol. Dependence is more common in men than in women. Peer pressure in adolescence and readily available illegal drugs make young people particularly susceptible. The risk of dependence developing depends on which drug is taken. For example, heroin may cause dependence after only a few doses.

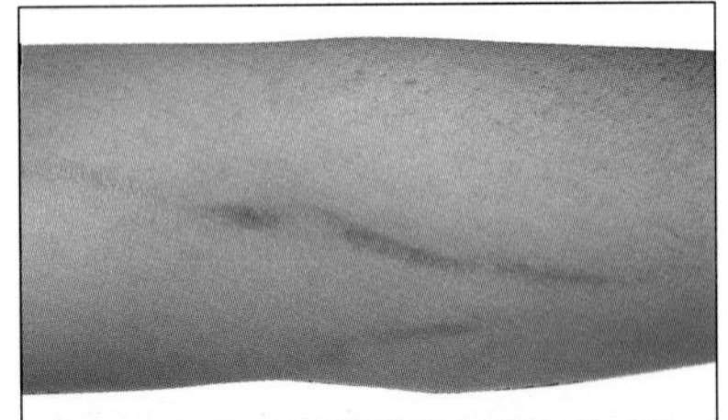

Needle tracks from drug injections

When a drug-dependent person repeatedly injects drugs, the veins can be damaged. In this picture, the damage is visible as needle tracks on the inside of the arm.

WHAT ARE THE SYMPTOMS?

There are different symptoms for each drug. However, certain areas of behaviour tend to be altered by most drugs that cause dependence. Symptoms of drug dependence often include:

- Mood changes.
- Changes in concentration levels.
- Altered energy levels.
- Faster or slower speech rate.
- Increased or decreased appetite.

Typically, withdrawal symptoms develop within 12 hours of last using or taking a drug. Effects range from mild to extremely severe and may include:

- Anxiety and restlessness.
- Overheating and sweating, alternating with chills and shivering.
- Confusion and hallucinations.
- Muscle aches and abdominal cramps.
- Diarrhoea and vomiting.
- Seizures.

Rarely, withdrawal from opioid drugs, such as heroin, may lead to coma (p.522). If drugs are injected, sharing needles may transmit diseases such as HIV infection (*see* HIV INFECTION AND AIDS, p.297) and hepatitis B and C (ACUTE HEPATITIS, p.644). Drug dependence often leads to depression (p.554).

WHAT MIGHT BE DONE?

People who are dependent on drugs may not accept that they need help, and a member of their family or a friend may consult a doctor on their behalf. The doctor will ask which drugs are used and about the length and pattern of use.

Once a person has accepted that he or she needs treatment, withdrawal from the drug can begin. If the symptoms of withdrawal are likely to be severe or if there have been failed attempts in the past, admission to hospital or a drug rehabilitation centre will be arranged. Otherwise, withdrawal may be closely supervised at home. Withdrawal symptoms are usually treated with substitute drugs that are less likely to cause dependence. For example, benzodiazepines (*see* ANTIANXIETY DRUGS, p.916) may be used to treat symptoms of withdrawal from barbiturates. The doctor will offer support and specialized drug services for long-term counselling (p.971).

WHAT IS THE PROGNOSIS?

Treatment of drug dependence is difficult and often unsuccessful. Sometimes there are several withdrawal attempts before dependence is overcome. Success is most likely if the person is strongly motivated and has good support from family, friends, and counselling services. Joining a support group also increases the chance of overcoming dependence.

(WWW) ONLINE SITES: p.1029, p.1030

Alcohol dependence

Compulsive regular consumption of alcohol, producing withdrawal symptoms when intake is stopped

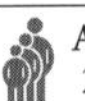 AGE Most common between the ages of 20 and 40

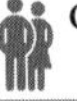 GENDER More common in males

 GENETICS Sometimes runs in families

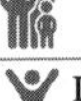 LIFESTYLE Stress and occupations that are associated with social drinking are risk factors

A person who is dependent on alcohol has an irresistible compulsion to drink, which takes priority over almost everything else in life. This craving for drink, coupled with withdrawal symptoms when drinking stops, is what separates alcohol dependence from alcohol abuse, a term used to describe regular drinking to excess (*see* ALCOHOL AND HEALTH, p.62). About 1 million people in the UK abuse or are dependent on alcohol. Drinking problems are more common in men, particularly between the ages of 20 and 40. In addition to causing damage to the liver and brain, the need to drink to excess regularly is damaging to mental health and may destroy a person's family and social life and career.

WHAT ARE THE CAUSES?

Alcohol dependence is often the result of a combination of factors. Sometimes, alcohol dependence runs in families, partly as a result of children growing up in an environment of heavy drinking and partly because of an inherited predisposition. People who are shy, anxious, or have a social phobia (*see* ANXIETY DISORDERS, p.551) or depression (p.554) may rely heavily on alcohol. Working in an occupation that is associated with social drinking increases the risk of dependence. Stressful events may turn a moderate drinker into a heavy one.

WHAT ARE THE SYMPTOMS?

Alcohol dependence may develop after a number of years of moderate to heavy drinking. Symptoms may include:

- A compulsion to drink and loss of control over the amount consumed.
- Increased tolerance to the effects of alcohol, leading to greater consumption to achieve the desired effects.
- Withdrawal symptoms, such as nausea, sweating, and tremor, that start a few hours after the last drink.

In severe cases, withdrawal seizures develop after alcohol is stopped. After a few days without alcohol, delirium tremens may develop with symptoms of fever, shakes, seizures, disorientation, and hallucinations. Symptoms last for 3 to 4 days and are usually followed by a deep, prolonged sleep. In extreme cases, shock (p.414) occurs and may be fatal.

ARE THERE COMPLICATIONS?

Alcohol has direct effects on the body and may cause many diseases. Long-term alcohol dependence is the most common cause of severe liver disease (*see* ALCOHOL-RELATED LIVER DISEASE, p.646) and may damage the digestive system, causing peptic ulcers (p.640).

Heavy drinkers often have a poor diet, which may lead to a deficiency in vitamin B_1 (thiamine) that may eventually cause dementia (p.535). Rarely, severe thiamine deficiency leads to Wernicke–Korsakoff syndrome (p.538), a severe brain disorder that causes confusion and amnesia and may lead to coma. If excessive drinking continues for a prolonged period of time, damage to vital organs may be life-threatening.

Psychiatric problems associated with alcohol dependence include anxiety, depression, delusional disorders (p.561), and suicidal behaviour (*see* ATTEMPTED SUICIDE AND SUICIDE, p.556). Generally, heavy drinkers tend to be self-centred and lack concern for family and friends.

HOW IS IT DIAGNOSED?

Before the doctor can make a diagnosis, a person may need to be persuaded to seek help. The doctor will ask about the extent of the person's drinking and look for evidence of dependence. Blood tests to assess possible damage to the liver and other organs may be arranged.

WHAT IS THE TREATMENT?

Gradual reduction of alcohol intake or limiting alcohol consumption to social drinking is rarely possible. Instead, the person will be asked to stop drinking completely. In mild to moderate cases, withdrawal can take place at home, provided that adequate support is available. Antianxiety drugs (p.916), such as a benzodiazepine, may be prescribed for a short time to reduce agitation and other physical effects of withdrawal.

When heavy drinking is stopped suddenly, withdrawal seizures or delirium tremens may develop. The symptoms of delirium tremens are potentially life-threatening and require admission to hospital or a detoxification unit. Withdrawal symptoms are usually treated with antianxiety drugs.

Treatment for physical problems as a result of long-term alcohol dependence includes ulcer-healing drugs (p.923) for peptic ulcers and vitamin B_1 injections for a thiamine deficiency.

When the symptoms of withdrawal have been treated, the doctor may prescribe drugs that reduce cravings for alcohol or cause unpleasant reactions when it is consumed. Support is given to help prevent a relapse. Individual counselling (p.971) or group therapy (p.970) help people to address the problems that contribute to alcohol dependence.

WHAT IS THE PROGNOSIS?

Accepting that there is a problem and receiving emotional support during the effort to give up drinking greatly improve a person's chance of recovery. Attending a self-help group, such as Alcoholics Anonymous, reduces the risk of relapse. However, after a long period of dependence, several attempts at detoxification may be needed before a person abstains from alcohol altogether.

In about 1 in 5 cases in which delirium tremens develops and is untreated, the condition proves fatal.

(WWW) ONLINE SITES: p.1027, p.1029

Compulsive gambling

Frequent gambling that dominates a person's life

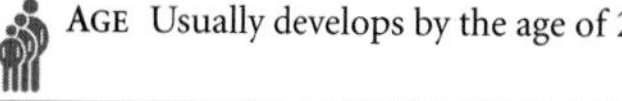
AGE Usually develops by the age of 25

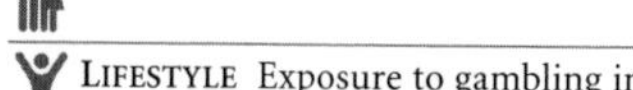
GENDER More common in males

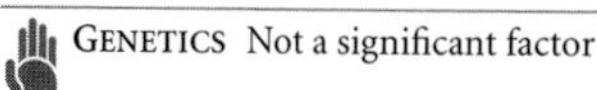
LIFESTYLE Exposure to gambling in adolescence is a risk factor

GENETICS Not a significant factor

In compulsive gambling or pathological gambling, a person has an intense urge to gamble that dominates his or her life. Compulsive gamblers continually increase their spending to achieve their desired intensity of excitement. They build up large debts and may lie, steal, and defraud to continue gambling. This behaviour continues regardless of its effects on family and social life and jeopardizes work and relationships.

Compulsive gambling is more common in men and usually develops before the age of 25. Growing up with a parent who gambles compulsively or who is dependent on alcohol has been shown to increase the risk. Adolescents who gamble are at an increased risk of developing a gambling problem. A person who gambles compulsively often appears optimistic and full of confidence. However, the disorder may be associated with mood disorders, such as anxiety (*see* ANXIETY DISORDERS, p.551) and depression (p.544), and with an antisocial personality disorder (p.561).

WHAT MIGHT BE DONE?

If a person is gambling excessively, a family member or friend may consult the doctor. The person will be assessed and treated for any underlying psychological disorders, such as anxiety or depression. Most self-help groups offer valuable support and encouragement, and a number of groups also give support to family and friends in their efforts to help a compulsive gambler.

Psychological therapies (pp.968–971) may be beneficial once the person has managed to refrain from gambling for a period of at least 3 months. Generally, therapy works best when a person has managed to gain some control over the compulsion to gamble.

(WWW) ONLINE SITES: p.1029, p.1034

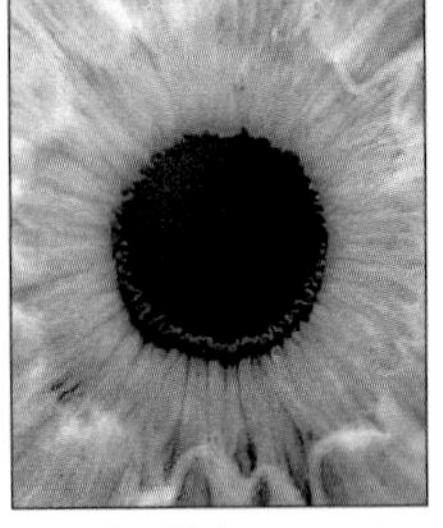

Detail of iris
The colour of the iris depends on the amount of pigment it contains.

EYES AND VISION

THE HUMAN EYE is a remarkable organ, and our visual capabilities are among the most sophisticated of any living creature. We can judge speed and distance well enough to catch a fast-moving ball. Close up, we can see an incredible level of detail, allowing us to thread a needle or read small print. We can detect a vast range of colours, and, when we look rapidly from a close to a distant object or move from bright to dim light, our eyes automatically adjust. The eyes are protected by the eyelids and by tears, which flush out dirt and foreign matter.

For most humans, vision dominates their conscious perception from the moment of birth. Working with but often overshadowing our other senses, vision supplies vast quantities of information about our surroundings and enables us to interact with our environment and the people within it.

The eye acts as a highly sophisticated biological video camera, focusing light from everything around us to form sharp images on a light-sensitive layer, the retina, at the back of the eye. Cells within the retina convert the images into electrical signals that travel along the optic nerve to the brain.

Visual perception depends not only on the eye but also on highly complex processing within the brain. In certain areas of the cortex (the outer layer of the brain), signals from both eyes are merged to provide three-dimensional vision. Also in the brain, signals from the eyes are combined with other information, such as memories and nerve impulses from other senses, to give meaning and structure to the visual world.

FORMING AN IMAGE

For us to see clearly, light rays entering the eye must be focused precisely on the retina. The first part of the eye to focus is the cornea, the transparent part of the front of the eye. The lens of the eye then fine-focuses the light rays by adjusting its focusing power automatically to create clear and sharp images of near and distant objects. The image formed on the retina is upside down, but the brain interprets the image so that we see the world the right way up.

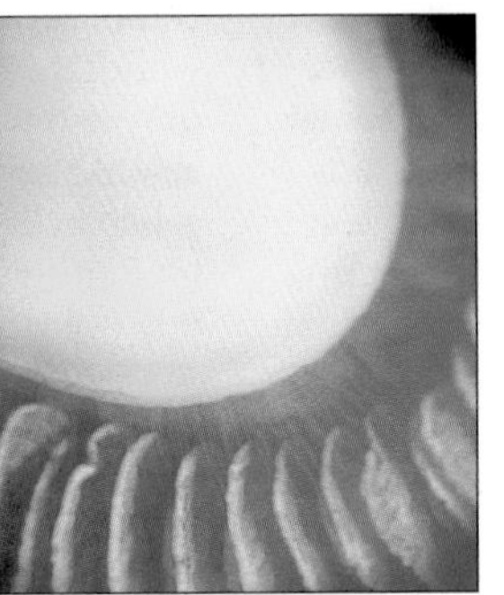

Inside the eye, looking out
This magnified view of the eye shows the delicate fibres that support the eye's elastic lens.

When light falls on the retina, light-sensitive cells called rods and cones produce tiny electrical impulses in a pattern corresponding to the visual image. Each cone responds to one of the primary colours of light (red, green, or blue), and together these cells allow us to see a wide range of colours.

Our visual acuity (the level of detail we can see) is determined by the density of the light-sensitive cells in the retina. Compared with animals, our visual acuity is very good. However, birds of prey have a much higher density of both rods and cones, which gives them much greater visual acuity. For example, an eagle could spot an object at 5 km (3 miles) that we would struggle to see from a distance of 1 km (½ mile).

The electrical impulses from all of the cells in the retina form the visual signal, which travels from the eye to the brain along the optic nerve. Impulses from both eyes are sent to a part at the back of the brain called the occipital, or visual, cortex. Here, the visual signals are integrated, giving a complete view of the visual field.

PROTECTING THE EYES

The eyes are protected by the eyelids and by tears. The eyelids have the ability to close together to prevent harmful material from entering the eyes, while tears help to stop infection by washing away potentially dangerous materials that might damage the eye. Tears also contain a natural antiseptic.

(FUNCTION) THE TEAR APPARATUS

Tears are produced by the lacrimal (tear) glands, which are situated above each eyeball. The glands continually secrete a small amount of salty fluid that is distributed over the surface of the eyes through the action of blinking and drain into the nose. Tears form a protective film that lubricates the eye and flushes out any dust and dirt. They also contain an antibacterial ingredient. Tear production increases when you cry or if the eye is irritated by a chemical or foreign particle.

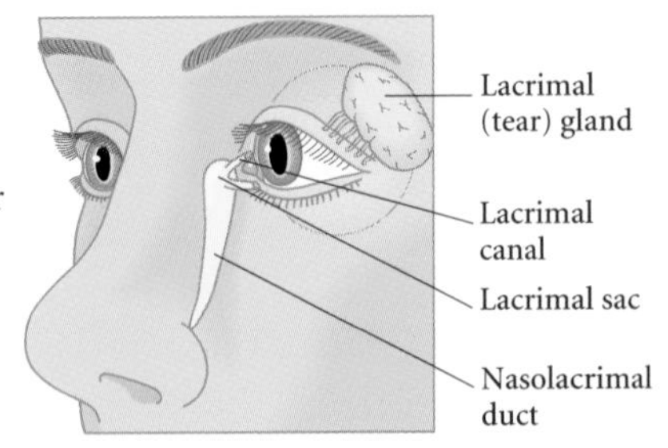

Drainage of tears
Tears drain away through the lacrimal canals into the lacrimal sac and then into the nose via the nasolacrimal duct.

STRUCTURE STRUCTURE OF THE EYE

Each eyeball is roughly spherical, about 2.5 cm (1 in) in diameter, and lies in a protective bony socket in the skull. The eyeball has a tough outer coat called the sclera that maintains its shape. The choroid, which supplies the eye with nutrients, lies inside the sclera. The innermost layer, the retina, contains two types of light-sensitive cells: rods, which respond to dim light; and cones, which detect colour.

View of the retina
Blood vessels and nerve fibres leave the retina via an area called the optic disc. The area of the retina responsible for the most detailed vision is the macula.

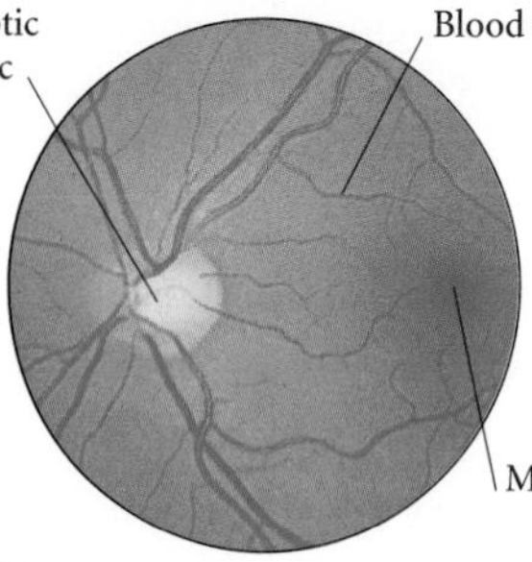

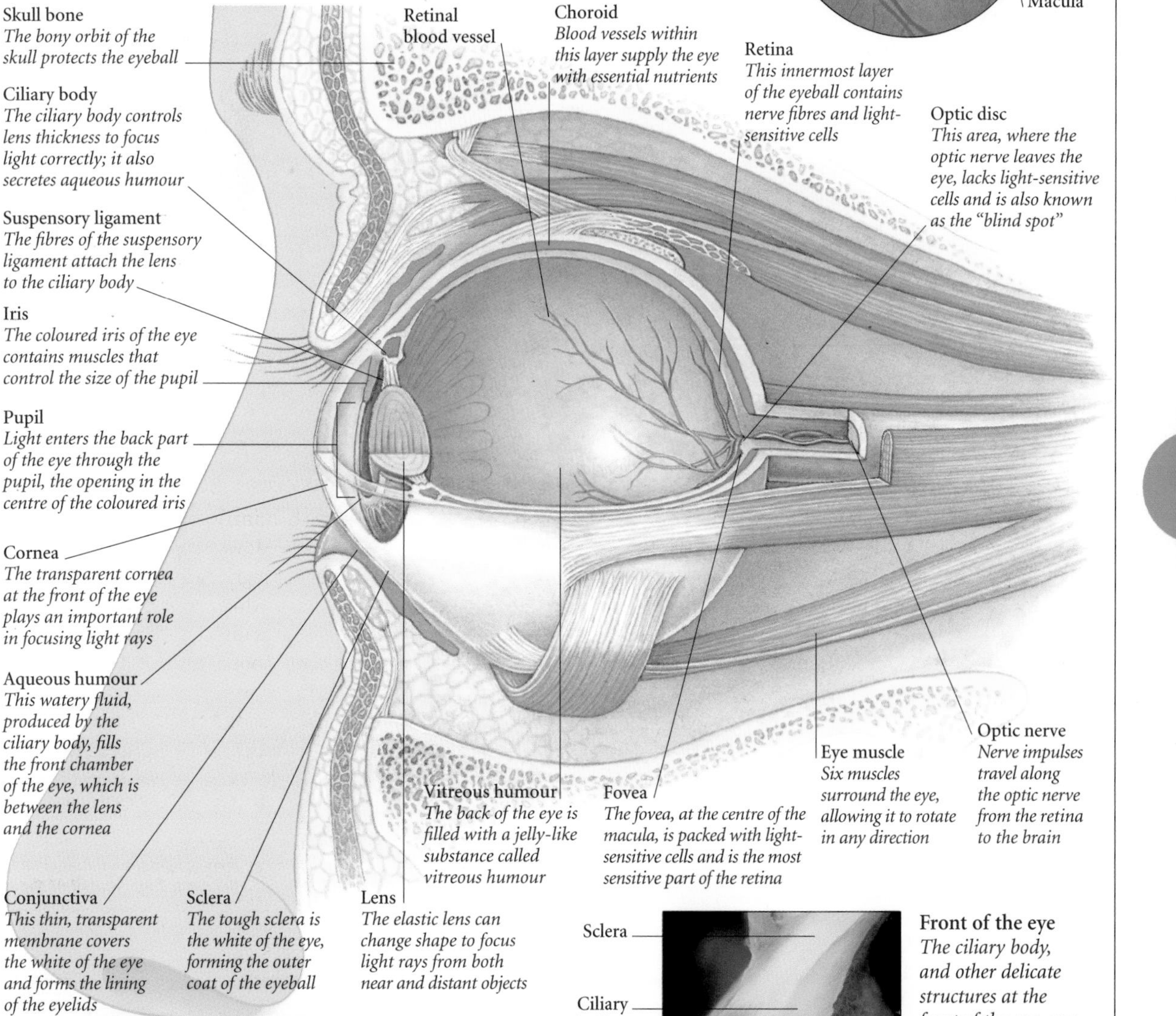

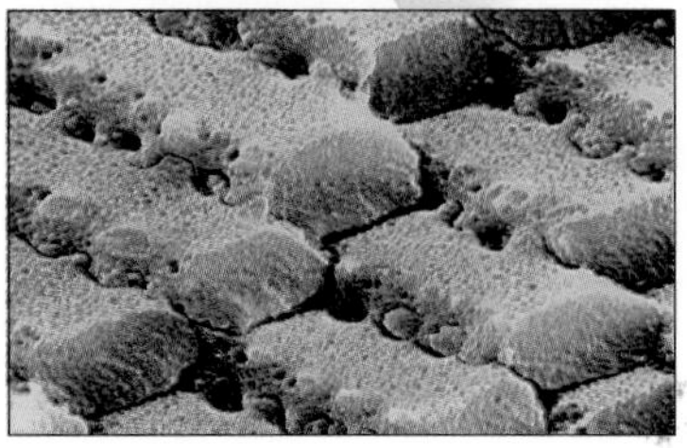

Lens structure
This highly magnified view shows the precise arrangement of the fibre-like cells that make up the lens. The cells have no nuclei; this feature helps to make the lens transparent.

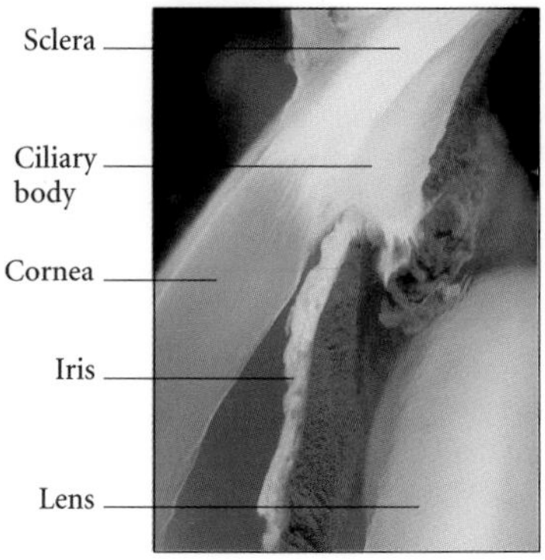

Front of the eye
The ciliary body, and other delicate structures at the front of the eye, can be seen in detail in this magnified image. The ciliary body alters the shape of the eye's lens so that light from either near or distant objects can be focused correctly.

STRUCTURE AND FUNCTION

HOW THE EYE WORKS

When you look at an object, light rays reflected from the object hit the transparent cornea at the front of your eye. The rays are partly focused and pass through the pupil, which enlarges or constricts depending on light conditions. The lens varies its focusing power for near and distant objects and fine-focuses the rays to create a sharp image on the fovea, the most responsive area of the light-sensitive retina at the back of the eye.

THE MECHANISM OF VISION

Light rays focused by the cornea and lens produce an image on the retina that is upside down. Electrical signals from stimulated cells in the retina travel along the optic nerve to the brain, where the image is interpreted as being upright.

Blood vessel
Retinal arteries and veins supply nutrients and remove waste from the retina

Ciliary body
The muscles of the ciliary body control the shape and focusing power of the lens

Lens
The lens provides fine focusing of light rays

Cornea
Incoming light rays are initially refracted (bent) by the cornea

Object
Light reflected from an object travels in all directions. Some rays enter the eye

Pupil
Light rays enter the pupil to reach the retina

Iris
The ring of muscles in the iris controls the pupil's size to allow in more or less light

Retina
Light-sensitive cells (rods and cones) in the retina transform light into nerve signals

Macula
The macula, the area of the retina surrounding the fovea, is responsible for detailed vision

Fovea
The fovea contains the highest density of cells

Optic nerve
Fibres of the optic nerve carry impulses from the retina to the brain

Inverted image
The image on the retina is upside down

Light rays
Rays of light from the object cross in the eye and are focused on the retina

ACTION OF THE PUPIL

In dim conditions, the pupil widens (dilates) to allow the maximum amount of light to reach the light-sensitive retina. In bright light, the pupil constricts. Two sets of muscles in the coloured iris control these processes.

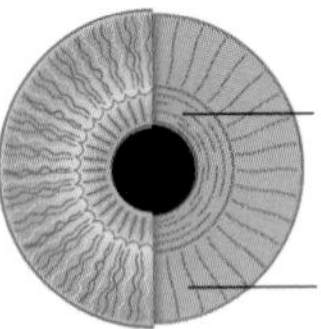

CONSTRICTED

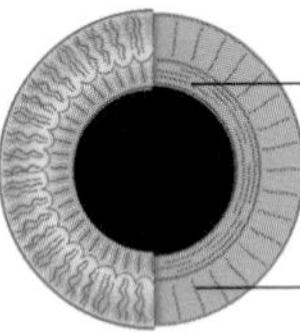

DILATED

Changes in pupil size
To make the pupil constrict, the circular muscles contract; and to widen (dilate) it, the radial muscles contract.

ACCOMMODATION

The eye adjusts for near and distant vision by changing the shape of its lens. This varies the extent to which incoming light is refracted (bent). To create a sharp image on the retina, light rays from near objects must be bent more than those from distant objects. This process is called accommodation.

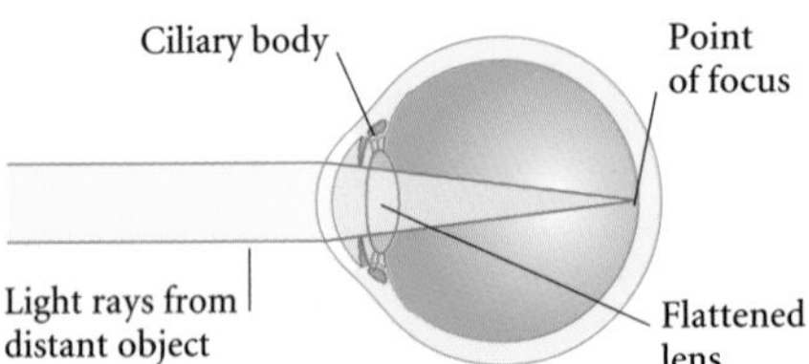

Focusing for distant objects
When you look at an object in the distance, muscles in the ciliary body relax and the lens assumes a flatter shape.

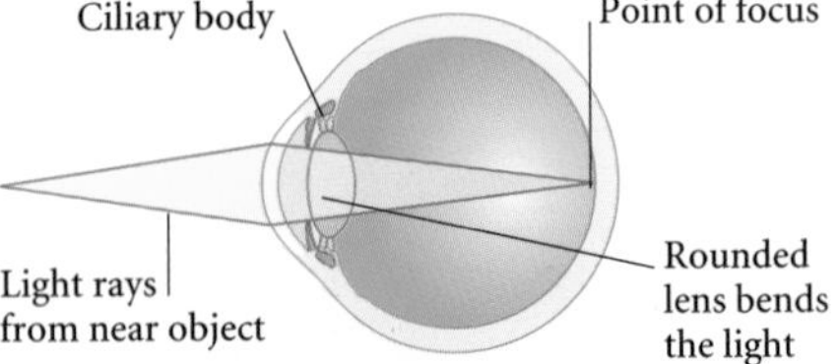

Focusing for near objects
When you look at a close object, muscles in the ciliary body contract, allowing the elastic lens to spring into a more spherical shape.

Visual pathways

Electrical signals from each retina pass along the optic nerves, which meet at a junction called the optic chiasm. Here, half of the nerve fibres from the left eye cross to the right side and vice versa, and the fibres continue along the optic tracts to the brain. Information from the right half of each retina passes to the right visual cortex; information from the left half of each retina goes to the left visual cortex. The brain then integrates these messages into a complete visual picture.

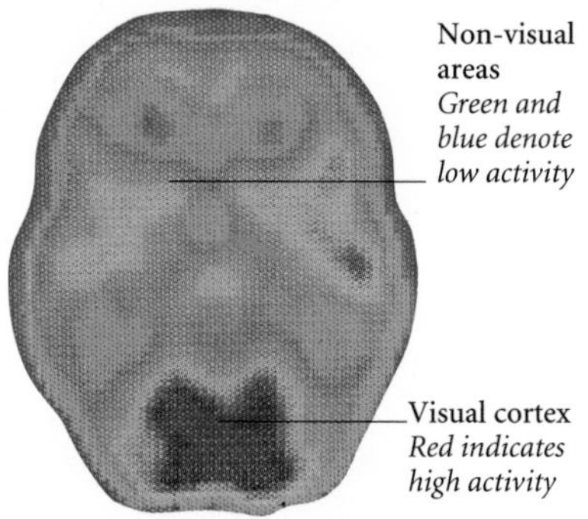

Brain during visual stimulation
The visual cortex, which is located at the back of the brain, exhibits high activity compared with the rest of the brain when a detailed coloured picture is observed.

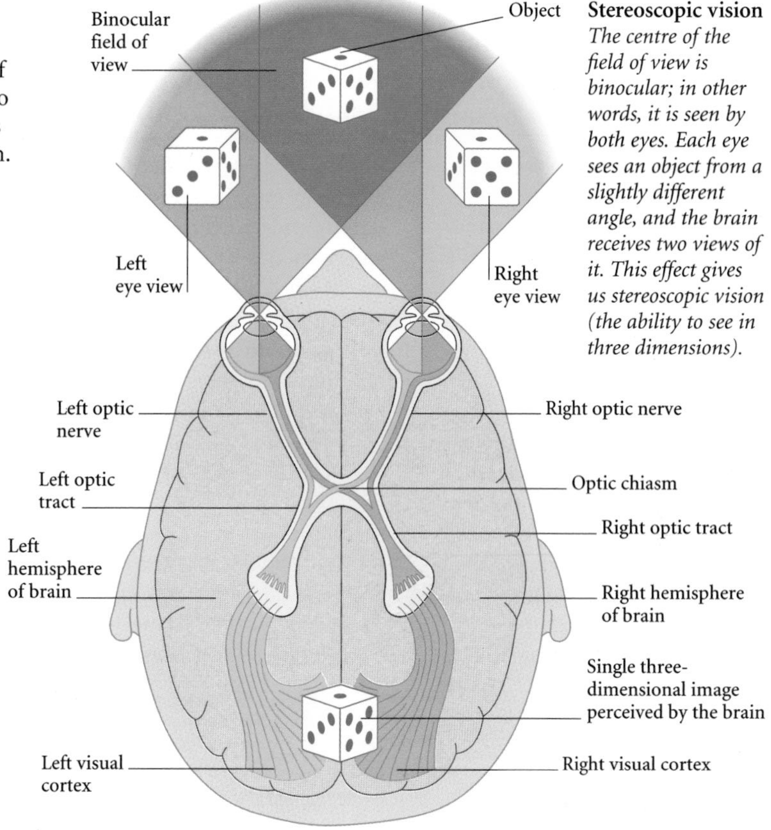

Stereoscopic vision
The centre of the field of view is binocular; in other words, it is seen by both eyes. Each eye sees an object from a slightly different angle, and the brain receives two views of it. This effect gives us stereoscopic vision (the ability to see in three dimensions).

Rods and cones

There are two types of light-sensitive cells in the retina: rods and cones. Up to 120 million rods are distributed throughout the retina. Although rods are sensitive to all visible light, they contain only one type of pigment and cannot distinguish colours. They are therefore responsible mainly for night vision. In contrast, the 6.5 million cones provide detailed and colour vision. Every cone responds to red, green, or blue light, working only in bright light. They are most concentrated in the central part of the retina, the fovea.

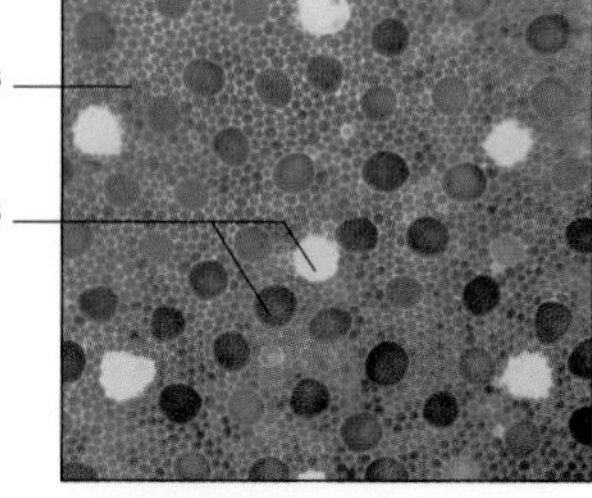

Rods and cones
This magnified view of the retina shows that rods greatly outnumber cones. Here, the cones are shown in two colours.

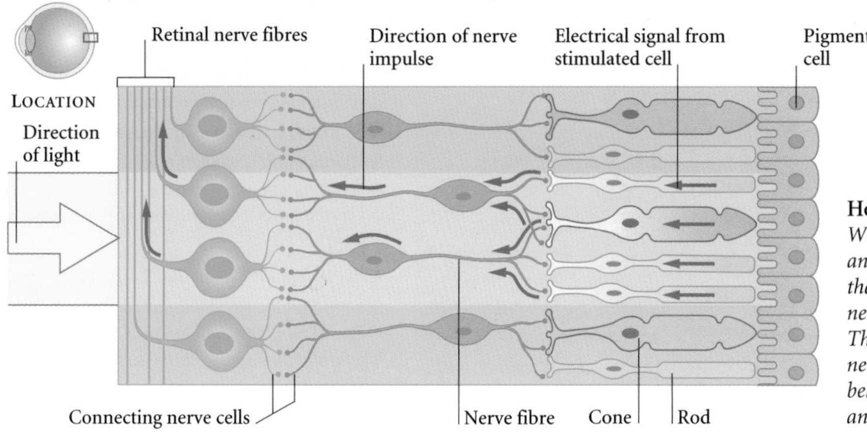

How the retina responds to light
When light strikes the retina, the rods and cones produce electrical signals that trigger further impulses in the nerve cells to which they are connected. These signals travel along the optic nerve to the brain. Pigment cells behind the rods and cones absorb light and prevent reflection inside the eye.

EYE DISORDERS

The eye is a complex organ made up of several highly specialized components. Many eye disorders do not threaten sight, but a few serious conditions may damage the eye's components and lead to loss of vision. Eye disorders are very common, but early diagnosis usually leads to successful treatment.

This section covers disorders caused by disease, structural abnormality, or injury to the eye. Conditions that involve the front covering of the eye (the conjunctiva and cornea) are described first, followed by disorders that affect the front chamber of the eye and the structures within it, including the iris and lens.

The next group of articles discusses disorders of the light-sensitive retina at the back of the eye and conditions affecting the optic nerve, which carries nerve signals from the retina to the brain. The final articles in this section cover conditions in which the eye is displaced or injured in some way.

Impaired vision, whether occurring in healthy eyes or as a consequence of serious underlying causes, is described separately (*see* VISION DISORDERS, pp.586–591), as are disorders of the eyelid and tear system (pp.583–585) and eye disorders that usually or only affect children. These include congenital blindness (p.856), cancer of the retina (*see* RETINOBLASTOMA, p.858), and misalignment of the gaze of the eyes (*see* STRABISMUS, p.857).

Many major eye disorders that in the past would have ultimately progressed to blindness can now be treated successfully if detected early. For example, diabetic retinopathy is often now treated by laser surgery to prevent further sight loss. Regular eye examinations are therefore important, especially for people over the age of 40.

KEY ANATOMY

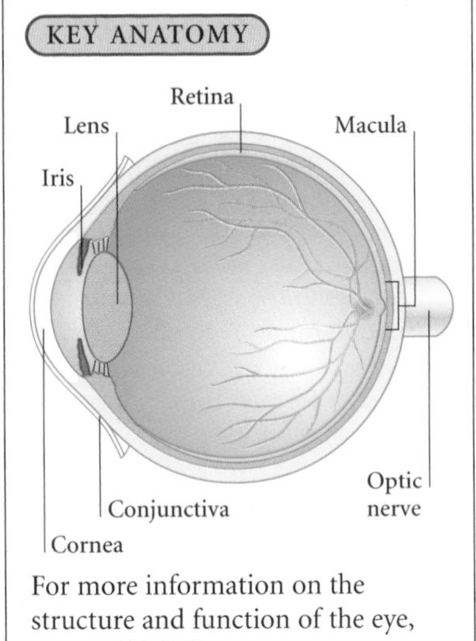

For more information on the structure and function of the eye, *see* pp.566–569.

Conjunctivitis

Inflammation of the conjunctiva, the membrane covering the white of the eye and the inside of the eyelids

LIFESTYLE Wearing contact lenses and using cosmetics or eyedrops are risk factors

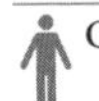
GENETICS Risk factors depend on the type

AGE GENDER Not significant factors

Conjunctivitis, also called pink eye, is a common condition in which the conjunctiva, the clear membrane covering the white of the eye and lining the eyelids, becomes inflamed. The affected eye becomes red and sore and may look alarming, but the condition is rarely serious. One or both of the eyes may be affected, and in some cases it begins in one eye then spreads to the other.

WHAT ARE THE CAUSES?

Conjunctivitis may be caused by a bacterial or viral infection, or result from an allergic reaction or irritation of the conjunctiva for example, by smoke, pollution, or ultraviolet light.

Bacterial conjunctivitis is common, and may be due to several types of bacteria. Viral conjunctivitis can occur in epidemics caused by one of the viruses that causes the common cold (p.288). One viral form of conjunctivitis, called herpes keratoconjunctivitis, results from a herpes simplex infection (p.291). Conjunctivitis due to viruses or bacteria can be spread by hand-to-eye contact and is highly contagious.

Newborn babies sometimes develop conjunctivitis. This can happen if an infection is transmitted to the baby's eyes from the mother's vagina during the birth. This form of conjunctivitis is usually caused by the microorganisms responsible for certain sexually transmitted infections, including chlamydial infection (p.765), gonorrhoea (p.764), and genital herpes (p.767).

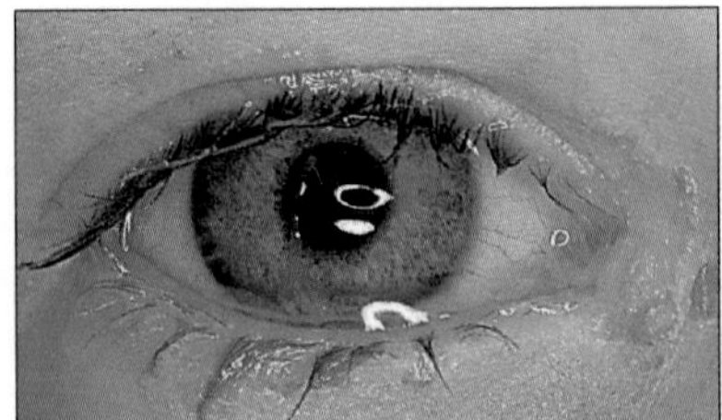

Conjunctivitis
This eye shows signs of conjunctivitis, including swollen eyelids, a discharge, and redness over the white of the eye.

Allergic conjunctivitis is a common feature of hay fever and of allergy to dust, pollen, and other airborne substances (*see* ALLERGIC RHINITIS, p.466). The condition may also be triggered by chemicals found in eyedrops, cosmetics, or contact lens solutions. Allergic conjunctivitis often runs in families.

WHAT ARE THE SYMPTOMS?

The symptoms of conjunctivitis usually develop over a few hours and are often first experienced on waking. The symptoms generally include:

- Redness of the white of the eye.
- Gritty and uncomfortable sensation in the eye.
- Swelling and itching of the eyelids.
- Discharge that may be yellowish and thick or clear and watery.

The discharge may dry out during sleep and form crusts on the eyelashes and eyelid margins. As a result, the eyelids sometimes stick together on waking.

WHAT CAN I DO?

The symptoms can be relieved by bathing the eye with artificial tears, which are available over the counter. To avoid spreading infection, wash your hands after touching the eye and do not share towels or facecloths. Once conjunctivitis has cleared up, sight is rarely affected.

If you are susceptible to allergic conjunctivitis, avoid exposure to triggering substances. Antiallergy eyedrops can be used to ease the symptoms (*see* DRUGS ACTING ON THE EYE, p.919). If an eye becomes painful and red, you should consult your doctor to rule out the possibility of a more serious condition.

WHAT MIGHT THE DOCTOR DO?

Your doctor will probably make a diagnosis from your symptoms. If infection is suspected, he or she may take a sample of the discharge to identify the cause.

Bacterial conjunctivitis is treated by applying antibiotic drops or ointment. In such cases, the symptoms usually clear up within 48 hours. However, the treatment should be continued for 2–10 days, even if the symptoms improve, to ensure the infection is eradicated. Viral conjunctivitis that occurs because of a herpes infection may be treated with eyedrops containing an antiviral drug (p.886). Although other types of viral conjunctivitis cannot be treated, their symptoms usually clear up within 2–3 weeks. Your doctor may prescribe eyedrops or oral antiallergy drugs if you have allergic conjunctivitis.

(WWW) ONLINE SITES: p.1027

Subconjunctival haemorrhage

Bleeding between the white of the eye and the conjunctiva, the membrane covering the white of the eye and lining the eyelids

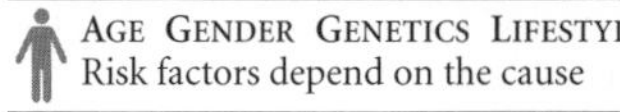

Ruptured blood vessels in the conjunctiva, the clear membrane covering the white of the eye and lining the eyelids, cause bleeding under the membrane. The condition, called subconjunctival haemorrhage, is common because the blood vessels in the conjunctiva are easily damaged. The bleeding causes a red area over the white of the eye.

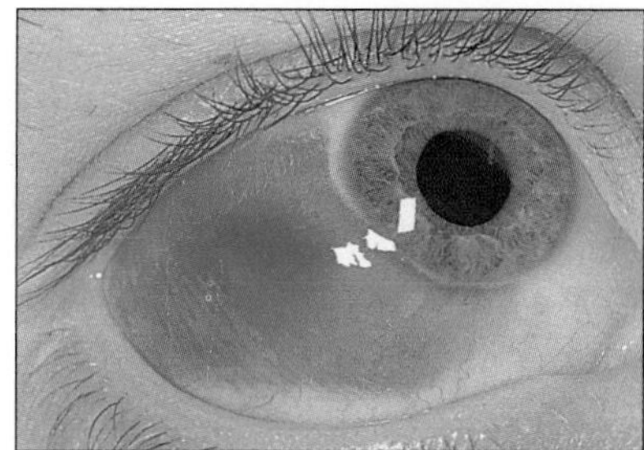

Subconjunctival haemorrhage
The red area on this eye is caused by bleeding under the conjunctiva, the outer membrane covering the white of the eye.

The condition may result from a minor eye injury (p.582), sneezing, coughing, or, rarely, a bleeding disorder (p.451). Most often, it is spontaneous, especially in elderly people. Although the haemorrhage looks dramatic, it is generally painless and usually clears up without treatment within 2–3 weeks. If the eye is painful or the redness persists, you should consult your doctor.

Corneal abrasion

A scratch on the surface of the cornea, the transparent front part of the eye

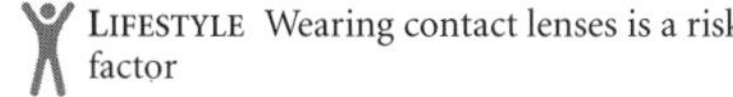

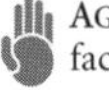

The cornea, situated at the front of the eye, is susceptible to minor damage. For example, if it is scraped by the edge of a newspaper or by a foreign particle such as a speck of dirt, an injury known as a corneal abrasion may occur. People who wear soft contact lenses and rub their eyes excessively are particularly at risk of damage because tiny particles can become stuck behind a lens and scratch the surface of the cornea.

WHAT ARE THE SYMPTOMS?

The symptoms of a corneal abrasion usually occur suddenly. They include:

- Pain in the eye.
- Redness and watering of the eye.
- Blurred vision.
- Sensitivity to bright light.
- Frequent blinking.

A corneal abrasion is not usually serious. However, there is a risk that the abrasion may become infected and a corneal ulcer (right) may develop.

WHAT MIGHT BE DONE?

Painkillers (p.912) will relieve the discomfort of an abrasion, but you should consult your doctor or go to an accident and emergency department for treatment. The doctor will place drops containing fluorescein dye in your eyes and examine them with an instrument known as a slit lamp (*see* SLIT-LAMP EXAMINATION, p.574). If an abrasion is highlighted by the dye, your doctor may recommend an eye patch and also prescribe antibiotic eyedrops to prevent infection and ulceration (*see* DRUGS ACTING ON THE EYE, p.919). A corneal abrasion usually heals within a few days.

(WWW) ONLINE SITES: p.1031, p.1036

Corneal ulcer

A deep erosion in the cornea, the transparent front part of the eye

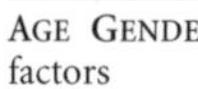

LIFESTYLE Wearing contact lenses is a risk factor

AGE GENDER GENETICS Not significant factors

An eroded area in the cornea, the transparent outer part of the front of the eye, is known as a corneal ulcer. These ulcers can be very painful and, if left untreated, may cause scarring and lead to permanently impaired vision, blindness (p.591), or even loss of the eye. People who wear contact lenses are at increased risk of corneal ulcers.

WHAT ARE THE CAUSES?

Corneal ulcers may be caused by an eye injury, an infection, or a combination of both. A relatively small injury, such as a corneal abrasion (left), can develop into a corneal ulcer if the damaged area becomes infected. A more severe injury,

Normal area of the cornea | Ulcerated area

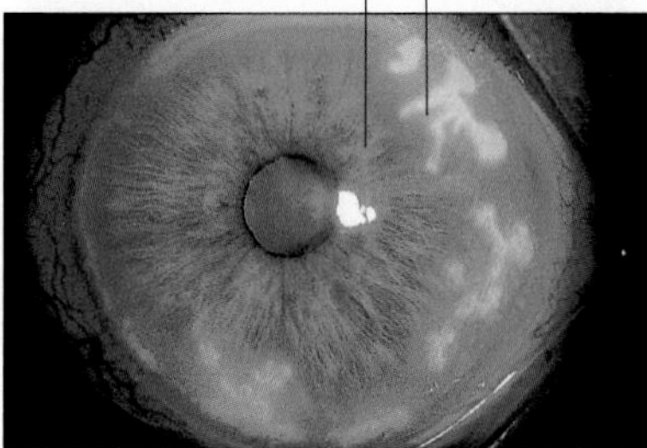

Corneal ulcer
Fluorescein eyedrops placed in this eye revealed an ulcerated cornea. These ulcers are due to a herpes simplex infection.

such as that caused by a caustic chemical, can produce an ulcer in the absence of infection. However, an ulcer that becomes infected may enlarge and penetrate more deeply into the cornea. Only rarely do infections cause corneal ulcers without prior injury. The most common of these infections are herpes zoster (p.290), known as shingles, and herpes simplex infections (p.291).

What are the symptoms?

If you have a corneal ulcer, you may experience the following symptoms:

- Intense pain in the eye.
- Redness and discharge from the eye.
- Blurred vision.
- Increased sensitivity to light.

With an untreated infected ulcer, the infection may spread and permanently impair vision and cause damage to the eye itself. You should consult a doctor immediately if you develop a painful, red eye together with blurred vision.

What might be done?

The doctor may place fluorescein eyedrops in the affected eye and examine it under blue light with a slit lamp (*see* SLIT-LAMP EXAMINATION, p.574). He or she may also take a swab to identify the cause. If the dye reveals an ulcer, you may be given antibiotic or antiviral eyedrops to treat the infection (*see* DRUGS ACTING ON THE EYE, p.919). Even severe ulcers usually clear up within 1–2 weeks of treatment, but they can leave scars that permanently affect vision.

(WWW) ONLINE SITES: p.1031

Hyphaema

A pool of blood in the front chamber of the eye, behind the transparent cornea

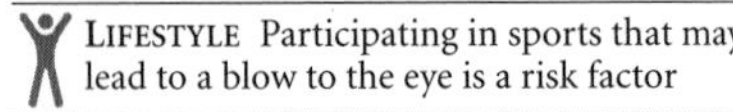
LIFESTYLE Participating in sports that may lead to a blow to the eye is a risk factor

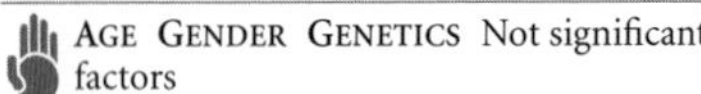
AGE GENDER GENETICS Not significant factors

A blow to the eye may rupture a blood vessel in the iris (the coloured part of the eye) or in the ciliary body, the ring of muscle behind the iris. The damaged blood vessel may bleed into the chamber between the lens and the cornea, the transparent front part of the eye, forming a pool of blood known as a hyphaema. Initially, the blood mixes with the clear fluid behind the cornea, resulting in severely blurred vision, but within a few hours the blood cells sink to the bottom of the chamber, which enables the vision to return to normal.

If you have an eye injury, first take immediate emergency action (*see* FIRST AID: EYE WOUND, p.993). If you experience blurred vision, you should consult your doctor immediately or go to hospital. Hyphaema blood usually disappears in less than a week, and restricting your activities may stop further bleeding. If bleeding recurs, the pressure in the eye can rise and cause acute glaucoma (p.575), which needs urgent treatment.

(WWW) ONLINE SITES: p.1031

Trachoma

A persistent eye infection that often causes damage to the cornea, the transparent front part of the eye

AGE Particularly common in children

LIFESTYLE Living in an area with limited water and poor hygiene is a risk factor

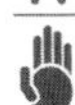
GENDER GENETICS Not significant factors

Trachoma is a serious, persistent eye infection that often causes permanent scarring of the cornea, the transparent front part of the eye. Although rare in developed countries, trachoma is one of the world's main causes of blindness. It affects about 400 million people, of whom about 6 million are blind.

Trachoma is due to the bacterium *Chlamydia trachomatis*, which is spread to the eyes by direct contact with contaminated hands or by flies. Trachoma is common in poor parts of the world, particularly in hot, dry countries that have poor sanitation and limited water supplies. Overcrowding encourages the spread of the trachoma infection.

To avoid becoming infected in a high-risk area, you should wash your hands and face regularly and avoid touching your eyes with dirty fingers.

What are the symptoms?

Initially, trachoma causes inflammation of the conjunctiva, the membrane that covers the white of the eye and lines the eyelids (*see* CONJUNCTIVITIS, p.570). Later symptoms include:

- Thick discharge from the affected eye that contains pus.
- Redness of the white of the eye.
- Gritty sensation in the eye.

Over time, repeated episodes of trachoma can cause scarring on the inside of the eyelids. The scars may pull the eyelids inwards and cause the eyelashes to rub against the delicate cornea (*see* ENTROPION, p.584). Left untreated, the condition can lead to blindness.

What is the treatment?

In the early stages, trachoma is treated with antibiotic eyedrops or ointment (*see* DRUGS ACTING ON THE EYE, p.919). If the cornea has become scarred, sight may be restored by an operation called a corneal graft, in which a cornea from a donor is used to replace the scarred one.

(WWW) ONLINE SITES: p.1033

Keratoconus

Progressive change in the shape of the cornea, the transparent front part of the eye, causing blurred vision

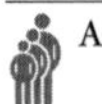
AGE Usually develops around puberty

GENDER More common in females

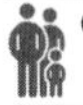
GENETICS Sometimes runs in families

LIFESTYLE Not a significant factor

In keratoconus, the central area of the transparent cornea that forms the front of the eye grows abnormally, becoming cone-shaped and thin. This rare, sometimes inherited condition, also known as conical cornea, is more common in females and usually begins at puberty.

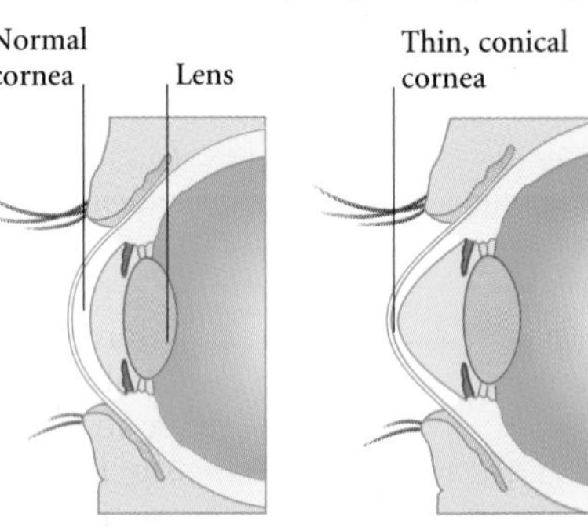

Effects of keratoconus

The normal cornea has an even, spherical curvature. Keratoconus causes the cornea to grow abnormally, becoming thinner and bulging forwards in a conical shape.

The condition may affect one or both eyes. As the shape of the cornea changes, vision becomes blurred, and shortsightedness develops (*see* MYOPIA, p.586). These symptoms worsen, in some cases quite rapidly, as the distortion of the cornea progresses.

WHAT MIGHT BE DONE?

A slit lamp may be used to examine your eyes (*see* SLIT-LAMP EXAMINATION, p.574). If keratoconus is detected in its early stages, your vision can be corrected by glasses or hard contact lenses (*see* GLASSES AND CONTACT LENSES, p.588). However, if your vision has seriously deteriorated, your doctor may suggest a corneal graft, an operation in which the abnormal cornea is replaced with a healthy one from a donor. This operation will usually restore normal vision permanently.

(WWW) ONLINE SITES: p.1031

Cataract

Clouding of the lens of the eye, causing loss of vision

 AGE More common after the age of 75 but may be present from birth

 GENETICS Sometimes due to an abnormal chromosome

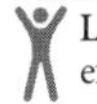 LIFESTYLE Contact sports and frequent exposure to the sun are risk factors

 GENDER Not a significant factor

If you have a cataract, the normally transparent lens of the eye is cloudy as a result of changes in protein fibres in the lens. The clouding affects the transmission and focusing of light entering the eye, reducing clarity of vision.

If cataracts are present from birth, total loss of vision (*see* CONGENITAL BLINDNESS, p.856) may result. However, cataracts do not usually affect children or young adults. Most people over the age of 75 have some cataract formation, but visual loss is often minimal as only the outer edges of the lens are affected.

Cataracts usually develop in both eyes, but generally one eye is more severely affected. A cataract in the central part of the lens or one that affects the whole lens can cause total loss of clarity and detail in vision. However, the affected eye will still be able to detect light and shade.

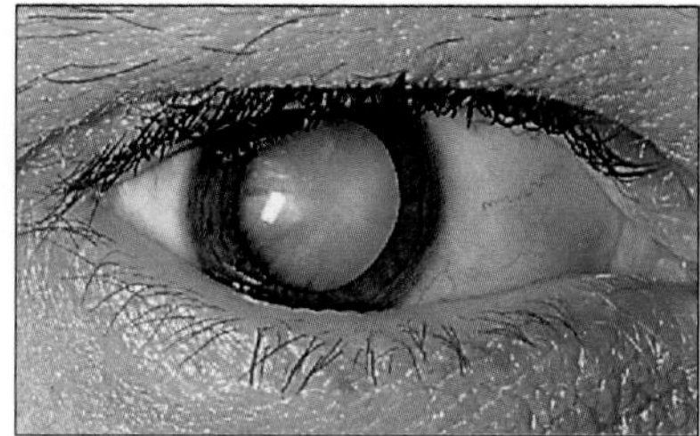

Severe cataract
This cataract, seen as a cloudy area behind the pupil, affects a large part of the lens. Cataracts cause visual impairment.

WHAT ARE THE CAUSES?

All cataracts occur as a result of structural changes to protein fibres within the lens. These changes cause part or all of the lens to become cloudy.

Changes in the protein fibres are a normal part of aging, but cataracts that develop in young adults may be the result of an eye injury (p.582) or prolonged exposure to sunlight. They may also develop due to diabetes mellitus (p.687), uveitis (p.574), or long-term treatment with corticosteroids (p.930). Cataracts are a common disorder in people with the chromosome disorder Down's syndrome (p.821).

WHAT ARE THE SYMPTOMS?

Cataracts usually develop over a period of months or years. In most cases, they are painless and usually cause only visual symptoms, such as:

- Blurred or distorted vision.
- Star-shaped scattering of light from bright lights, particularly at night.
- Altered colour vision: objects appear reddish or yellow.
- In longsighted people, temporary improvement in near vision.

A severe cataract may make the pupil of the eye appear cloudy.

WHAT MIGHT BE DONE?

The doctor may examine your eyes with a slit lamp (*see* SLIT-LAMP EXAMINATION, p.574) and an ophthalmoscope (*see* OPHTHALMOSCOPY, p.578). If your vision is affected significantly, he or she may recommend that the cataract is removed surgically and an artificial lens put in the eye (*see* CATARACT SURGERY, below). If there is no other reason for your visual deterioration, your sight should improve greatly after the operation. However, you may still need to wear glasses afterwards.

(WWW) ONLINE SITES: p.1027, p.1031

(TREATMENT) CATARACT SURGERY

A cataract is an opaque region in the lens of the eye causing loss of vision. During cataract surgery, the affected lens is removed and replaced with an artificial lens. The operation is usually performed under a local anaesthetic, and you will probably be able to go home the same day. In the technique shown here, the lens is first softened by an ultrasound probe. The softened tissue is extracted, and a new lens is inserted.

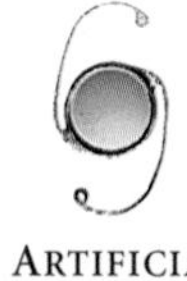

ARTIFICIAL LENS (actual size)

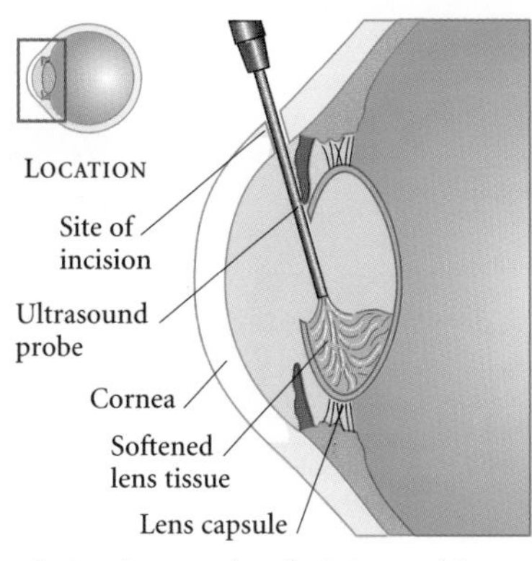

1 *An ultrasound probe is inserted into the lens through a small incision in the cornea. The probe softens the lens by emitting sound waves, and the softened tissue is then sucked out.*

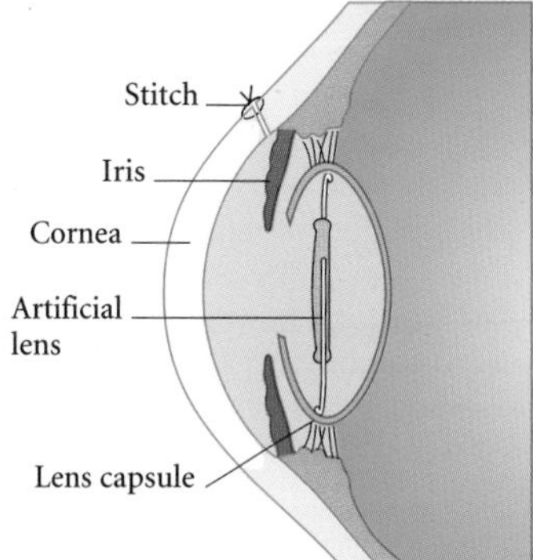

2 *The back of the natural lens capsule is left in place, and an artificial lens is placed inside it. The incision in the cornea is either closed with surgical stitches or left to seal itself without stitching.*

Scleritis

Inflammation of the sclera, the tough, white, outer covering of the eye

GENDER More common in females

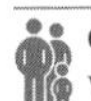
GENETICS May run in families if associated with rheumatoid arthritis

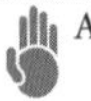
AGE LIFESTYLE Not significant factors

Scleritis is a rare, serious condition in which the sclera (the white outer coat of the eye) becomes inflamed. The condition is more common in women and is frequently associated with inflammatory disorders, such as rheumatoid arthritis (p.377). The main symptoms are severe pain in the eye, redness of the white of the eye, and excessive watering. If scleritis is linked with rheumatoid arthritis, you may experience repeated attacks. Rarely, severe cases of scleritis may cause perforation of the sclera and blindness (p.591) in the affected eye.

If you have any of these symptoms, contact your doctor immediately. Mild cases may need only anti-inflammatory eyedrops (*see* DRUGS ACTING ON THE EYE, p.919), but if rheumatoid arthritis is the cause, immunosuppressant drugs (p.906) can help both conditions.

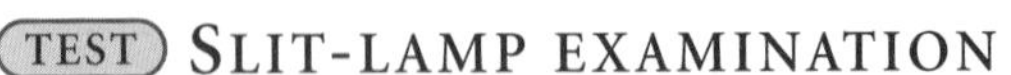
(WWW) ONLINE SITES: p.1031

Uveitis

Inflammation of any part of the uveal tract, which is a group of connected structures inside the eye

AGE GENDER GENETICS LIFESTYLE Risk factors depend on the cause

The uveal tract consists of several connected structures: the iris (the coloured part of the eye); the ciliary body (a ring of muscle behind the iris); and the choroid (a layer of tissue that supports the light-sensitive retina). Inflammation of any part of the uveal tract is called uveitis. The condition may involve the iris and/or the ciliary body (anterior uveitis or iritis) or the choroid (posterior uveitis). If uveitis is not treated, vision can be seriously impaired.

WHAT ARE THE CAUSES?

Uveitis is most commonly caused by an autoimmune disorder, in which the body attacks its own tissues, such as juvenile chronic arthritis (p.835). There may be links with some inflammatory disorders, such as sarcoidosis (p.498), ankylosing spondylitis (p.378), Crohn's disease (p.658), and ulcerative colitis (p.659). The condition may also occur with certain infectious diseases, including tuberculosis (p.491).

WHAT ARE THE SYMPTOMS?

Both anterior and posterior uveitis may affect only one eye. In anterior uveitis, the following symptoms may develop gradually over hours or days:

- Redness and watering of the eye.
- Sensitivity to bright light.
- Blurred vision.
- Aching in the eye.
- Small, irregularly shaped pupil.

Symptoms of posterior uveitis develop rapidly and include:

- Blurred vision.
- Spots or haziness in the visual field.

Consult your doctor at once if your eye becomes red and painful or if you develop blurred vision.

The main danger in anterior uveitis is that the inflamed iris may stick to the lens. This prevents normal drainage of fluid through the pupil and increases the pressure inside the eye (*see* ACUTE GLAUCOMA, opposite page). If this rise in pressure is not treated promptly, it can lead to blindness (p.591). The condition may also increase the risk of developing a cataract (p.573). Repeated attacks can lead to permanent damage to the iris and deterioration in vision.

Occasionally, parts of the retina may be damaged irreversibly by posterior uveitis, resulting in partial or total loss of vision in the affected eye.

(TEST) SLIT-LAMP EXAMINATION

The slit lamp is used to examine structures at the front of the eye: the transparent cornea, which covers the front part of the eye; the coloured iris; the lens; and the front chamber, which lies between the cornea and the lens. The slit lamp produces a long, narrow beam of brilliant light that is focused onto the eye. Although the examination is painless, eye drops used to dilate the pupil may make your vision blurred for a few hours afterwards.

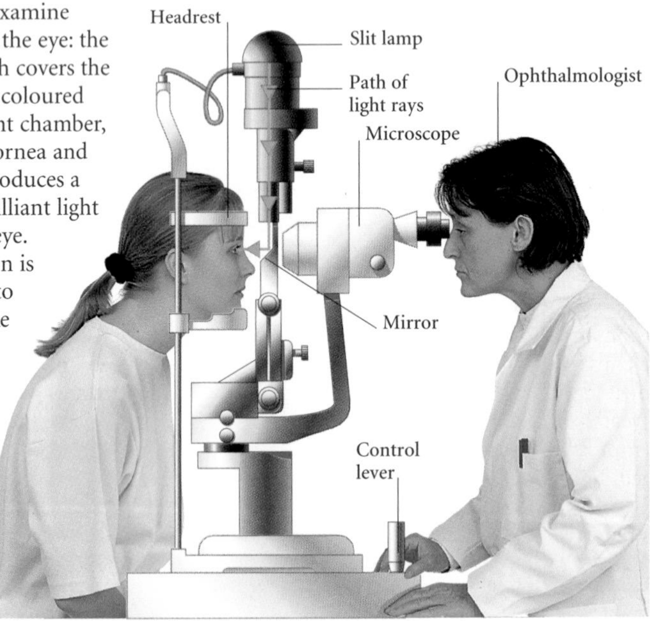

During the examination
As the ophthalmologist moves the light beam across your eye using a control lever, a headrest and chin support keep your head still.

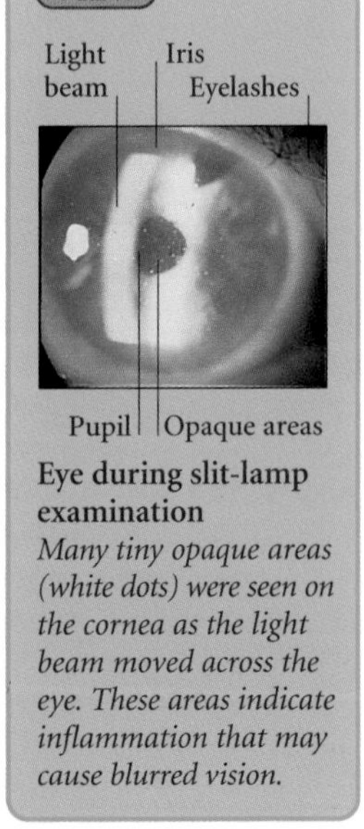

Eye during slit-lamp examination
Many tiny opaque areas (white dots) were seen on the cornea as the light beam moved across the eye. These areas indicate inflammation that may cause blurred vision.

What might be done?

If uveitis is suspected, you may have a slit-lamp examination (opposite page) and ophthalmoscopy (p.578), which examines the inside of your eye. If this is your first attack of uveitis, you will probably have other diagnostic tests to establish the underlying cause.

Your doctor may prescribe eyedrops to dilate the pupil and stop the iris from sticking to the lens, or corticosteroid eyedrops to reduce the inflammation (*see* DRUGS ACTING ON THE EYE, p.919). Treatment of uveitis is usually effective, but the condition tends to recur.

(WWW) ONLINE SITES: p.1031, p.1033

Glaucoma

Abnormally high pressure of the fluid inside the eye

 AGE Rare under the age of 40; more common over the age of 60

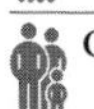 GENETICS Some types run in families

 GENDER LIFESTYLE Not significant factors

Fluid continually moves into and out of the eye to nourish its tissues and maintain its shape. In glaucoma, the flow of fluid out of the eye becomes blocked and pressure rises inside the eye. This high pressure may permanently damage nerve fibres in the light-sensitive retina and in the optic nerve, which carries nerve signals from the retina to the brain. Glaucoma becomes more common with age, and mainly affects people over the age of 60. If untreated, the condition may cause blindness (p.591).

What are the types?

There are two common types of glaucoma (acute and chronic) and two rare types (congenital and secondary). Acute glaucoma (right) develops suddenly, causing rapid loss of vision and severe eye pain. In contrast, chronic glaucoma (p.576) develops slowly and painlessly, often over many years. It may not cause noticeable symptoms until the eyes are badly damaged. Both types can run in families.

Secondary glaucoma occurs because of an underlying disorder, such as uveitis (opposite page), or from using certain drugs such as corticosteroid eyedrops (*see* DRUGS ACTING ON THE EYE, p.919). The other rare form, congenital glaucoma, is due to a defect in the drainage apparatus of the eye. Congenital glaucoma is present from birth and can lead to blindness (*see* CONGENITAL BLINDNESS, p.856). Secondary glaucoma can also result in blindness.

Glaucoma is diagnosed by measuring pressure in the eye using an instrument called a tonometer (*see* TONOMETRY, p.576). Treatment should always be given immediately. Eyedrops are used first to reduce pressure in the eye (*see* DRUGS FOR GLAUCOMA, p.920). In some cases, surgery is necessary to increase drainage of fluid and prevent build-up of pressure in the eye (*see* LASER IRIDOTOMY, p.576, and TRABECULECTOMY, p.577). Correct treatment normally prevents further vision loss.

(WWW) ONLINE SITES: p.1031

Acute glaucoma

An abrupt blockage of the drainage system in the eye, causing a painful, rapid rise in fluid pressure

 AGE Rare under the age of 40; more common over the age of 60

 GENDER More common in females

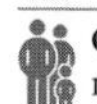 GENETICS Sometimes runs in families; more common in people of Asian descent

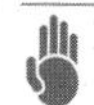 LIFESTYLE Not a significant factor

Normally, the fluid that is secreted into the front of the eye to maintain the eye's shape and nourish the tissues drains away continuously. However, in acute (narrow-angle) glaucoma, the drainage system suddenly develops a blockage, and the fluid pressure inside the eye rises rapidly. Acute glaucoma is a medical emergency requiring prompt treatment. Left untreated, the eye can swiftly become damaged and a permanent reduction in vision can result.

What are the causes?

The fluid in the front part of the eye is produced continuously by a ring of tissue called the ciliary body, behind the eye's coloured iris. Normally the fluid flows out through the pupil and drains away through the trabecular meshwork, which surrounds the iris. This sieve-like meshwork is situated behind the drainage angle, which is found between the outer rim of the iris and the edge of the cornea. In acute glaucoma, the iris bulges forwards and closes the drainage angle, trapping fluid within the eye. The pressure inside the eye rises as more fluid is secreted. As the pressure rises, it may damage the nerves in the light-sensitive retina and in the optic nerve, which carries nerve signals to the brain, causing reduced vision.

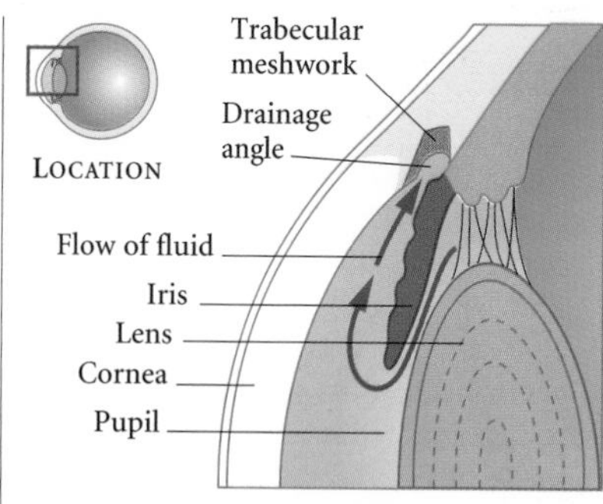

NORMAL EYE

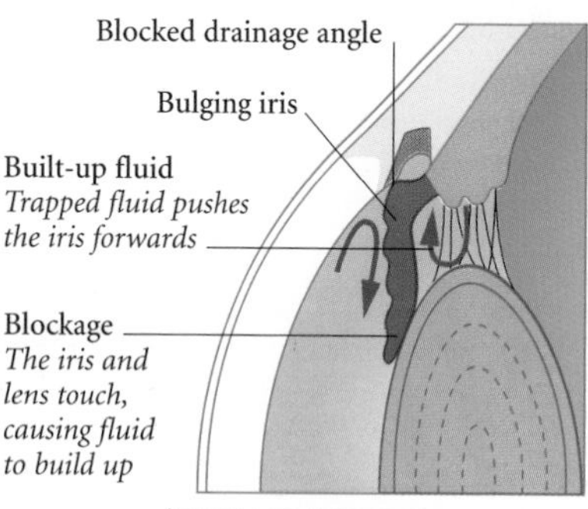

ACUTE GLAUCOMA

Mechanism of acute glaucoma

Fluid normally flows out through the pupil and drains out of the meshwork at the back of the drainage angle. If the iris and lens touch, fluid becomes trapped and the iris bulges forwards. This blocks the drainage angle, causing acute glaucoma.

Having a smaller eyeball than usual is a common cause of longsightedness (*see* HYPERMETROPIA, p.586) and increases the risk of developing acute glaucoma. The disorder is more common in older people because the lens of the eye grows throughout life and may eventually press against the iris. Fluid builds up behind the iris, which bulges forwards and blocks the drainage angle. Acute glaucoma can be triggered when dim light causes the pupil to widen. The iris thickens and the drainage angle can close. Acute glaucoma sometimes runs in families and is more common in women and in people of Asian descent.

TEST TONOMETRY

The eye condition glaucoma, in which the pressure inside the eye is elevated, can be detected using an instrument called a tonometer. Anaesthetic drops are put into your eye, then the tonometer is pressed gently against the cornea, the transparent front part of the eye, and the force needed to flatten the cornea is measured. The test takes only a few seconds and is painless.

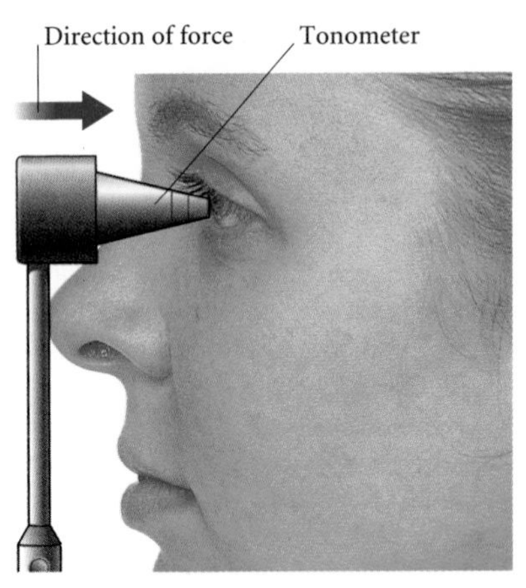

During the test
The tonometer is held against the cornea. As the internal pressure is measured, the pressure on your eye will increase slightly.

WHAT ARE THE SYMPTOMS?

A full-blown attack of acute glaucoma may be preceded by mild attacks in the weeks before. Mild attacks usually take place in the evening. Symptoms include pain in the eyes and haloes appearing around lights and are relieved by sleeping. If you have these symptoms, you should consult your doctor at once. Full-blown attacks develop suddenly. Symptoms include:

- Rapid deterioration of vision.
- Intense pain in the eye.
- Redness and watering of the eye.
- Sensitivity to bright light.
- Haloes appearing around lights.
- Nausea and vomiting.

If you develop a painful eye or your vision deteriorates suddenly, go to an accident and emergency department or consult your doctor immediately.

WHAT MIGHT BE DONE?

The pressure inside the eye is measured using a technique such as tonometry (above). If acute glaucoma is detected, you will be given immediate drug treatment by intravenous injection, as eyedrops, and possibly also by mouth to reduce the pressure in the eye (*see* DRUGS FOR GLAUCOMA, p.920). Laser iridotomy (below) will probably be performed as soon as the pressure falls. In this technique, a laser is used to make a small hole in the iris so that fluid can be released. The unaffected eye may also be treated as a precaution.

After surgery, most people are symptom-free, but some loss of the outer edges of vision may remain. Long-term drug treatment or a second operation may be needed to prevent loss of sight.

(WWW) ONLINE SITES: p.1031

Chronic glaucoma

A gradual, painless increase in the fluid pressure inside the eye

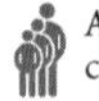 AGE Rare under the age of 40; more common over the age of 60

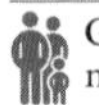 GENETICS Sometimes runs in families; more common in people of African descent

 GENDER LIFESTYLE Not significant factors

Chronic glaucoma is also known as open-angle glaucoma. The condition causes a gradual deterioration of sight due to a progressive build-up of fluid pressure inside the eye over a period of several years. There are often no symptoms until late in the disease, and loss of vision is permanent. Although the condition can lead to total blindness (p.591), early treatment can prevent severe damage. In most cases, both eyes are affected, although symptoms may occur only in one eye initially.

WHAT ARE THE CAUSES?

Fluid is continually secreted into the front of the eye to nourish the tissues and maintain the shape of the eye. Normally, this fluid drains away through the trabecular meshwork, a sieve-like structure at the back of the angle that is formed between the iris and the edge of the cornea (called the drainage angle).

However, in chronic glaucoma, a gradual blockage develops in the meshwork. Although the drainage angle remains open, fluid is prevented from draining normally, and the pressure in the eye gradually rises. The increasing

TREATMENT LASER IRIDOTOMY

This technique is used to treat acute glaucoma, in which pressure in the eye rises suddenly due to blockage in the outflow of fluid. The pressure is reduced using eyedrops, intravenous drugs, and, sometimes, oral drugs. Anaesthetic eyedrops are then put into the eye, and a thick contact lens is placed in front of it to focus a laser beam onto the bulging iris. The laser cuts a small hole in the iris, releasing the fluid behind it. The iris flattens, opening the drainage angle and letting trapped fluid out. The hole remains in the eye with no ill effects.

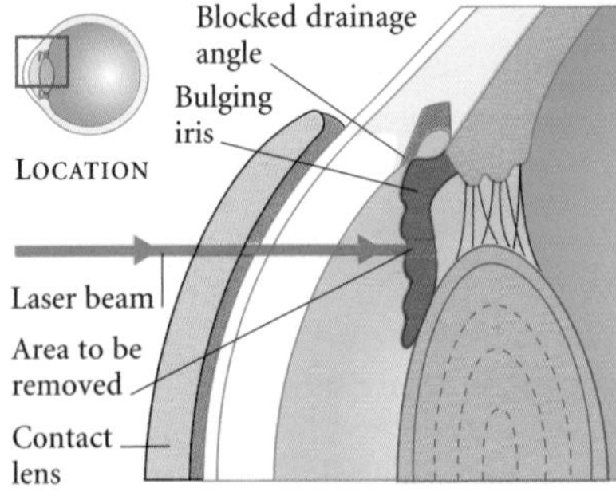

1 *A thick contact lens is held in front of the eye, and a laser beam is focused through it onto the bulging iris. The laser then cuts a small hole right through the iris.*

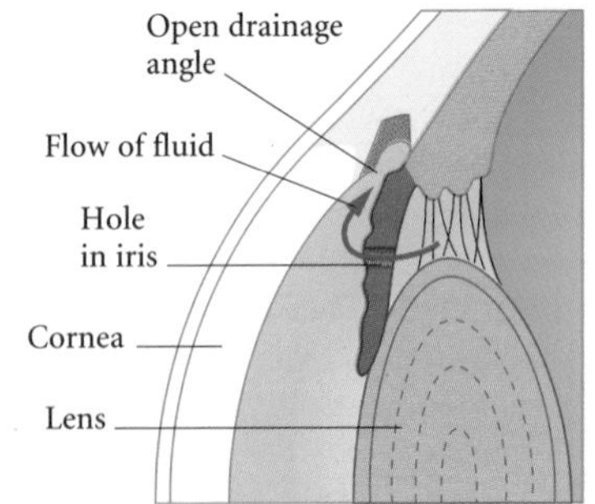

2 *Fluid trapped behind the iris flows through the hole. The iris returns to its normal shape, and the drainage angle opens, allowing the eye to drain normally.*

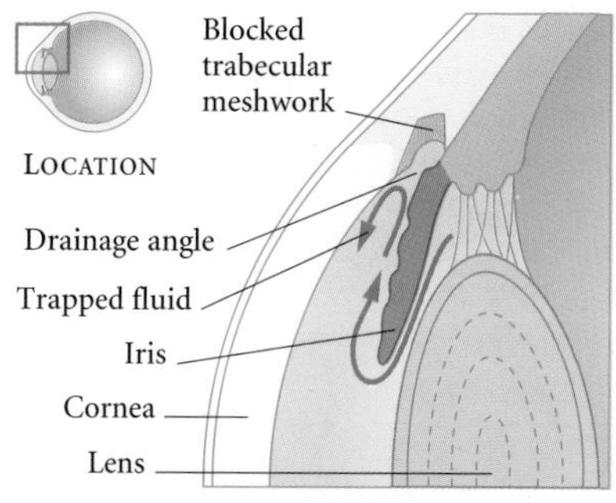

Fluid flow in chronic glaucoma
Normally, fluid flows out of the eye through the meshwork around the iris. In chronic glaucoma, the meshwork is blocked, and pressure builds up.

fluid pressure progressively damages the nerve fibres situated in the light-sensitive retina at the back of the eye and in the optic nerve, which carries nerve signals from the retina to the brain, causing loss of vision.

The underlying reason for the problem in the drainage system is not yet fully understood. Genetic factors may be involved and the condition sometimes runs in families. It is also more common in people of African descent. There is also an increased risk of developing chronic glaucoma if you are very shortsighted (*see* MYOPIA, p.586).

WHAT ARE THE SYMPTOMS?

Chronic glaucoma often has no symptoms until late in the disease, by which time it is probable that your vision has been permanently affected. During the later stages, the symptoms may include:

- Bumping into objects because of loss of the outer edges of vision (peripheral vision).
- Eventual blurring of objects that are straight ahead.

Always consult your doctor promptly if you notice a change in your vision. Because the risk of chronic glaucoma increases beyond middle age, everyone over the age of 40 should be tested for the condition every 2 years. If you are in a high-risk group, you should be tested regularly whatever your age.

HOW IS IT DIAGNOSED?

Chronic glaucoma can be detected at an early stage during a routine eye examination. Ophthalmologists often use a technique known as tonometry (opposite page) to measure the pressure inside the eye. The retina may also be examined using ophthalmoscopy (p.578). This is a technique that will reveal damage to the optic nerve resulting from the high pressure. Your ophthalmologist may also perform a visual field test (p.590) to check for loss of peripheral vision.

WHAT IS THE TREATMENT?

If chronic glaucoma is diagnosed early, eyedrops to reduce the pressure in the eye will probably be prescribed (*see* DRUGS FOR GLAUCOMA, p.920). You will probably have to continue using these eyedrops for the rest of your life.

If the condition is advanced, or if eyedrops do not lower the pressure sufficiently, surgery may be needed to make a drainage channel in the white of the eye (*see* TRABECULECTOMY, below). In another surgical technique, called laser trabeculoplasty, a laser beam is used to increase flow through the trabecular meshwork, allowing fluid to drain away. Both procedures usually eliminate the symptoms and prevent sight loss. If the condition affects only one eye, the other will probably also need treatment eventually.

WWW ONLINE SITES: p.1031

Floaters

Dark specks that appear to float and move in front of the eye

AGE GENDER GENETICS LIFESTYLE Not significant factors

It is quite common to see small specks, known as floaters, that appear to float in the field of vision. Although floaters seem to lie in front of the eyes, they are in fact fragments of tissue in the jelly-like vitreous humour that fills the back of the eye. These fragments cast shadows on the light-sensitive retina at the back of the eye. They move rapidly with any eye movement, but, when the eyes are still, they drift slowly.

The reason for most floaters is not known. They rarely affect vision, but you should consult your doctor immediately if floaters suddenly appear in large numbers or interfere with vision. A sudden increase in the number of floaters may indicate a serious eye disorder that requires urgent treatment, such as separation of the retina from its underlying tissue (*see* RETINAL DETACHMENT, p.578), or a leakage of blood into the vitreous humour (*see* VITREOUS HAEMORRHAGE, p.578).

TREATMENT TRABECULECTOMY

This surgical technique is used to treat chronic glaucoma, in which the pressure in the eye gradually rises due to a blockage of the trabecular meshwork, a sieve-like structure through which the fluid in the eye normally drains. Trabeculectomy may be carried out under a general or local anaesthetic and involves cutting out a section of the blocked meshwork so that fluid can flow out freely. Your doctor may advise you to wear an eye shield for a few days while the eye heals. You should also avoid strenuous activity for several weeks after the procedure.

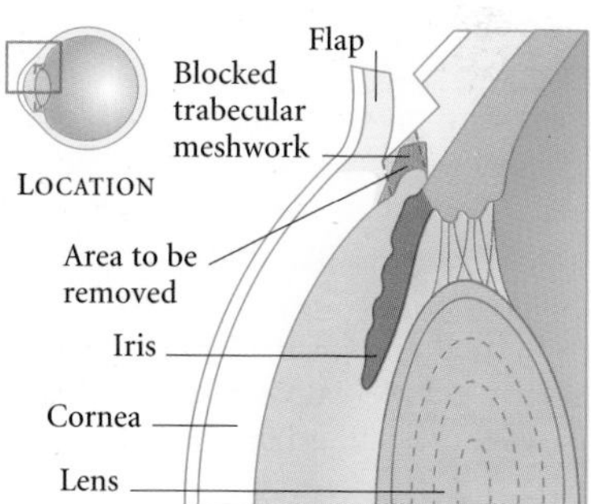

1 *An incision is made in the white of the eye over the area where fluid normally drains away. The flap is pulled back to expose the trabecular meshwork, and a section of the blocked meshwork is cut out.*

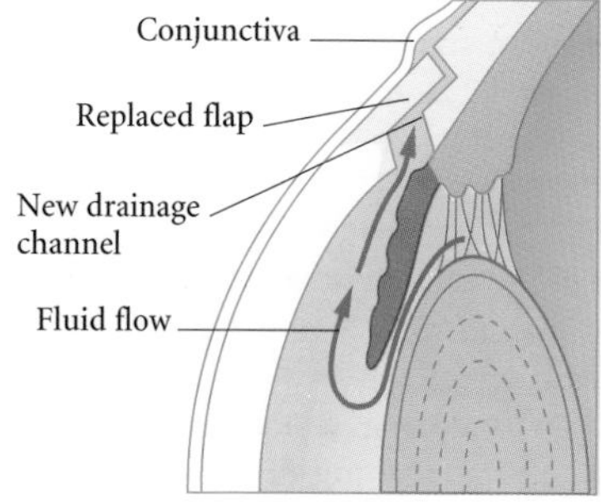

2 *The flap in the white of the eye is replaced. Fluid can now drain around the edges of the flap and under the clear conjunctiva that covers the white of the eye. Pressure in the eye is then relieved.*

TEST OPHTHALMOSCOPY

In this technique, an instrument called an ophthalmoscope is used to examine the inside of the eye. You will be asked to focus on a distant object while the instrument directs a beam of light into your eye. Through the lenses in the ophthalmoscope, the ophthalmologist can examine the light-sensitive retina; the retinal blood vessels; the head of the optic nerve, which carries nerve signals from the eye to the brain; and the jelly-like vitreous humour, which fills the back of the eye. Ophthalmoscopy is painless, but if eyedrops are used to dilate the pupils, your vision may become temporarily blurred.

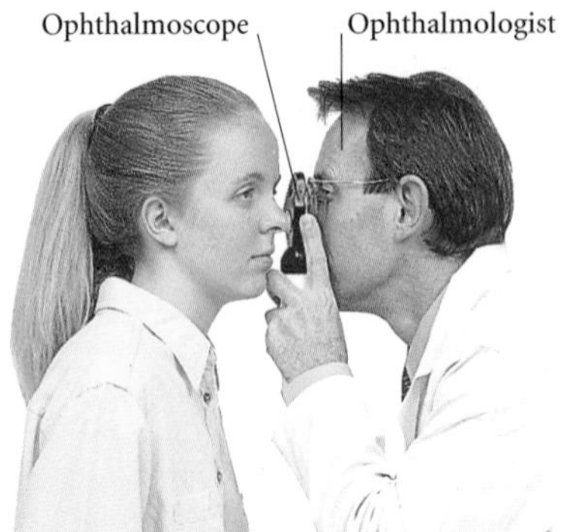

During the examination
The ophthalmologist looks through the lens of the ophthalmoscope to examine the structures inside the eye.

Vitreous haemorrhage

Bleeding into the vitreous humour, the jelly-like substance that fills the back part of the eye, due to ruptured blood vessels

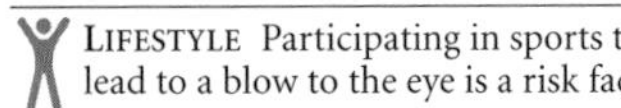
LIFESTYLE Participating in sports that may lead to a blow to the eye is a risk factor

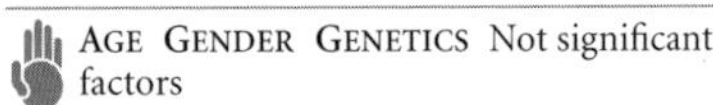
AGE GENDER GENETICS Not significant factors

If blood vessels in the light-sensitive retina at the back of the eye rupture, blood leaks into the jelly-like vitreous humour. This bleeding is known as a vitreous haemorrhage. The rupture may be due to a blow to the eye; a blocked vein in the retina (*see* RETINAL VEIN OCCLUSION, right); or the growth of abnormally fragile blood vessels in the retina because of other disorders, such as diabetic retinopathy (opposite page).

If the bleeding is minor, the only symptom may be the sudden appearance of large numbers of specks that seem to float in front of the eye (*see* FLOATERS, p.577). More severe bleeding can cause sudden loss of vision. Rarely, the blood in the vitreous humour clots, forming fibrous strands. Over a long period of time, new blood vessels may grow along these strands and pull on the retina, resulting in retinal detachment (right) and blindness (p.591).

You should call your doctor immediately if you have sudden loss of vision or if floaters appear in your eye in large numbers. He or she will examine the eye using ophthalmoscopy (above). In mild cases, floaters disappear within a few days but a large haemorrhage may take several weeks to clear, and, in severe cases, an operation may be needed to remove the affected vitreous humour and seal leaking blood vessels.

(WWW) ONLINE SITES: p.1031

Retinal vein occlusion

Blockage of a vein in the light-sensitive retina at the back of the eye

AGE Increasingly common over the age of 50

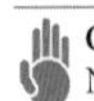
GENDER GENETICS LIFESTYLE Not significant factors

Retinal vein occlusion (an obstructed vein in the eye's light-sensitive retina) is usually caused by a blood clot in the vein, preventing blood from draining away from the retina. The condition may cause the blocked vein to burst, or the rising pressure may cause bleeding throughout the retina. Blockage of a small vein may not cause symptoms, but, if a large vein is affected, vision may deteriorate over a few hours.

Retinal vein occlusion affects mostly elderly people whose blood vessels are narrowed by atherosclerosis (p.402). It is also more common in people with glaucoma (p.575), high blood pressure (*see* HYPERTENSION, p.403), or a disorder that makes blood clot easily (*see* HYPERCOAGULABILITY, p.453).

The blockage of a small vein is often detected during a routine examination of the eye by ophthalmoscopy (left), but, if your vision deteriorates suddenly, see a doctor at once. There is no treatment for the condition, but treating the underlying cause will stop the problem recurring. Your vision may improve but rarely returns to normal.

(WWW) ONLINE SITES: p.1031

Retinal detachment

Separation of the light-sensitive retina at the back of the eye from the supporting tissues underneath

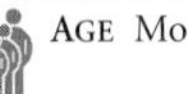
AGE More common over the age of 50

GENETICS Sometimes runs in families

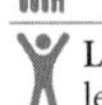
LIFESTYLE Participating in sports that may lead to a blow to the eye is a risk factor

GENDER Not a significant factor

The light-sensitive retina of the eye is normally attached to the underlying tissue, but in retinal detachment part of the retina peels away from this tissue. The condition usually affects one eye only but, without rapid treatment, can cause partial or total blindness (p.591).

Retinal detachment usually begins with a small tear in the retina. Fluid is then able to pass through the hole and separates the retina from the supporting tissues underneath. Tears may be caused by disorders such as severe shortsightedness (*see* MYOPIA, p.586) or eye injuries. In some people, tears appear as a result of scarring after a vitreous haemorrhage (left). Retinal detachment sometimes runs in families.

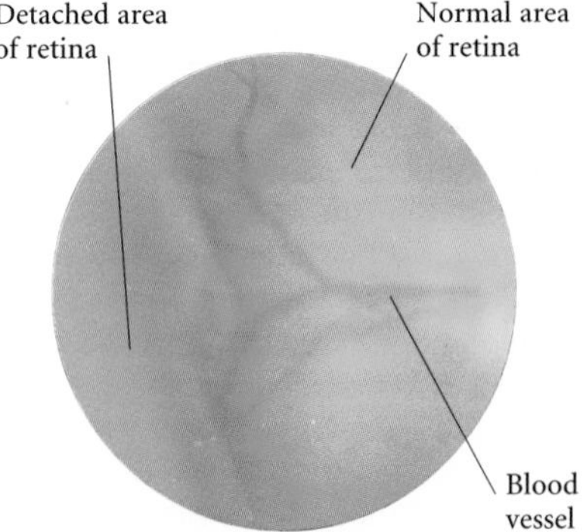

Detached retina
In this view through an ophthalmoscope, the area of detached retina can be clearly distinguished from the normal area of retinal tissue seen on the right.

WHAT ARE THE SYMPTOMS?

Retinal detachment is painless, but its visual symptoms may include:

- Flashing lights in the corner of the eye.
- Large numbers of dark spots in the field of vision (*see* FLOATERS, p.577).

If a large area of the retina has become detached, you may experience a cloudy ring or a black area across your field of vision. If you experience any of these symptoms, you should go to an accident and emergency department or call your doctor immediately.

WHAT MIGHT BE DONE?

Retinal detachment is diagnosed by using a special head-mounted ophthalmoscope to examine the eye's internal structures. If only a small area of retina has detached, the tear may be sealed by laser treatment (p.951) under a local anaesthetic. However, if a large area has detached, an operation under a general anaesthetic is necessary. If treated early, normal vision may be restored, but delayed treatment is less effective.

(WWW) ONLINE SITES: p.1031

(TREATMENT) LASER SURGERY FOR RETINOPATHY

Laser surgery is used in diabetic retinopathy to destroy abnormal blood vessels growing out from the retina and to prevent abnormal vessels from forming. Treatment is performed under a local anaesthetic, usually over several sessions. The laser makes thousands of tiny burns that destroy parts of the peripheral retina and associated blood vessels but leave the macular area of the retina intact. Some outer vision may be lost, but blindness is prevented.

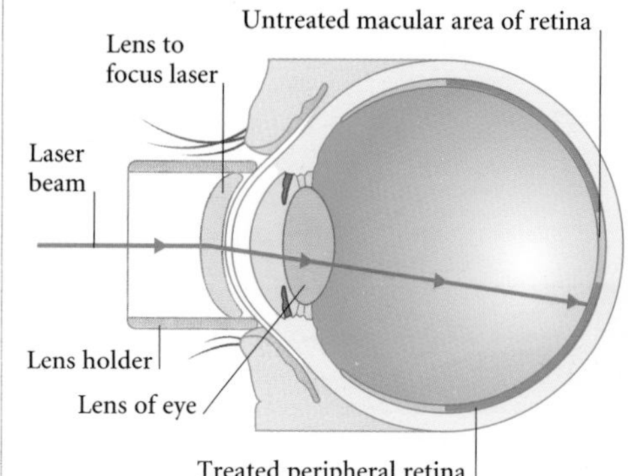

During surgery
A special lens held in front of your eye focuses the laser beam. Treatment is virtually painless, but you will see flashes of light as the laser strikes the retina.

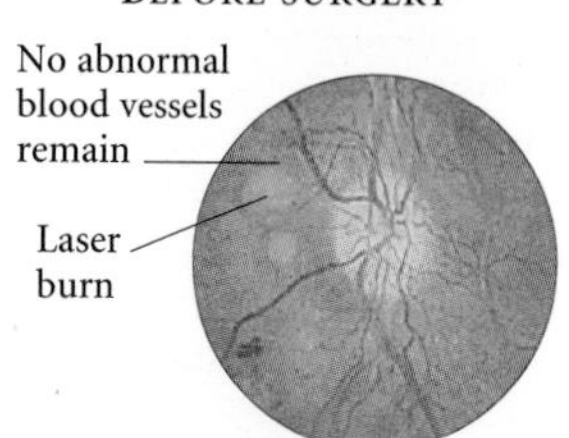

Results of laser treatment
Before laser surgery, new, abnormal blood vessels, which were formed on the surface of the light-sensitive retina, are visible. The laser surgery destroys these abnormal blood vessels. Following surgery, the outer area of the retina appears much paler.

Retinopathy

Damage to the small blood vessels in the retina, the light-sensitive membrane at the back of the eye

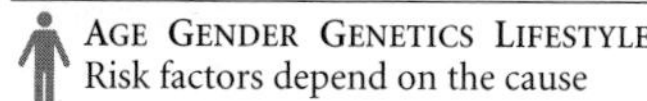
AGE GENDER GENETICS LIFESTYLE
Risk factors depend on the cause

Some long-standing diseases can damage small blood vessels throughout the body. If the blood vessels in the retina (the light-sensitive membrane at the back of the eye) are affected, the damage is known as retinopathy. Retinal damage varies according to the underlying disorder but can include leakage of blood from damaged vessels, loss of blood flow to some areas, and abnormal development of new blood vessels. Retinopathy may cause loss of vision.

One of the most common causes of retinopathy is diabetes mellitus (*see* DIABETIC RETINOPATHY, right). The condition can also occur as a result of high blood pressure (*see* HYPERTENSION, p.403), although vision is not usually affected in this case. Less frequently, retinopathy may be caused by AIDS (*see* HIV INFECTION AND AIDS, p.297), oxygen therapy in premature babies (*see* PROBLEMS OF THE PREMATURE BABY, p.816), or by sickle-cell disease (p.448). Usually, only the underlying disease is treated. However, in diabetic retinopathy, laser treatment of the retina itself (*see* LASER SURGERY FOR RETINOPATHY, above) can save vision.

(WWW) ONLINE SITES: p.1031

Diabetic retinopathy

Damage to blood vessels in the retina, caused by diabetes mellitus

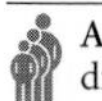
AGE Usually occurs in adults who have had diabetes mellitus for many years

GENETICS Sometimes runs in families

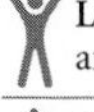
LIFESTYLE Poor control of diabetes mellitus and smoking are risk factors

GENDER Not a significant factor

If you have diabetes mellitus (p.687), you have an increased risk of developing retinopathy. Diabetes mellitus can lead to abnormalities in small blood vessels anywhere in the body. If the damage affects vessels in the retina, the light-sensitive membrane at the back of the eye, diabetic retinopathy develops. The condition usually affects both eyes. At first, small blood vessels in the retina leak. Later, fragile new blood vessels may grow out into the jelly-like vitreous humour. Loss of vision may result if the condition is left untreated, and blindness (p.591) may eventually follow.

The longer people have had diabetes and the less tightly the disorder is controlled, the greater the risk. Only a few people with type 1 diabetes mellitus develop retinopathy within the first 10 years after diabetes is diagnosed but, once retinopathy is established, it can progress rapidly. The condition may be present to some extent in type 2 diabetes mellitus by the time the diabetes has been recognized.

WHAT ARE THE SYMPTOMS?

Symptoms of diabetic retinopathy may not be noticeable until damage to the retina is severe, although there may be areas of blurred vision. As the disease progresses, vision may suddenly be lost in one eye due to rupture of one of the fragile new blood vessels in the retina

TEST FLUORESCEIN ANGIOGRAPHY

This technique is used to study the blood vessels in the light-sensitive retina of the eye. A fluorescent dye (fluorescein) is injected into the circulatory system through one of the veins in the arm. As the dye passes through the retinal vessels, a series of photographs (fluorescein angiograms) is taken to define any underlying abnormalities. The ophthalmologist can then assess the extent of the damage. The test is painless, but your skin and urine may turn dark yellow until all the dye has been excreted.

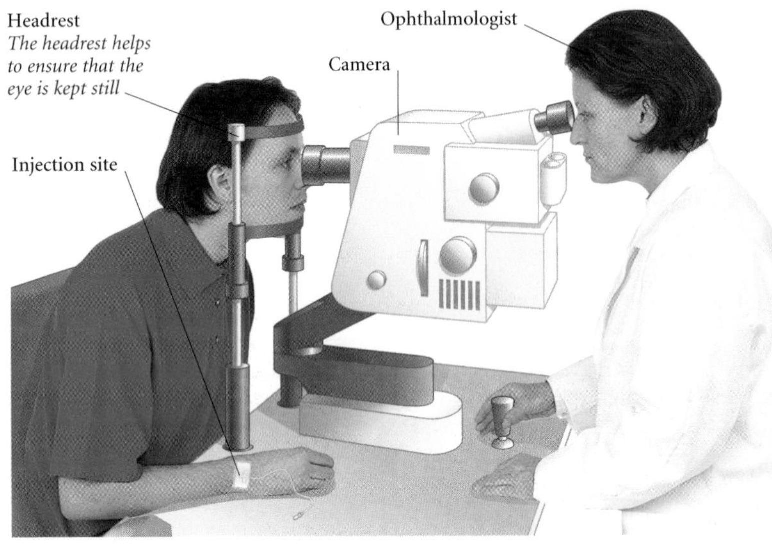

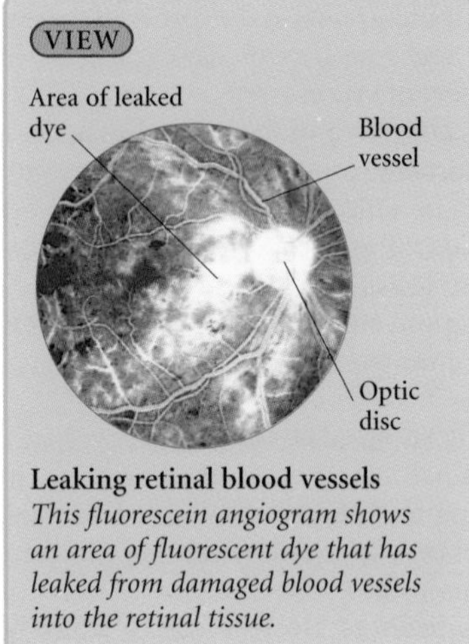

Leaking retinal blood vessels
This fluorescein angiogram shows an area of fluorescent dye that has leaked from damaged blood vessels into the retinal tissue.

During the test
The pupils are dilated with eyedrops, and fluorescein dye is injected into a vein in your arm. When the dye reaches your eye, the ophthalmologist observes it moving through the retinal blood vessels, and a series of photographs is taken over a period of time.

(*see* VITREOUS HAEMORRHAGE, p.578) or the separation of the retina from the underlying tissue (*see* RETINAL DETACHMENT, p.578). If you have diabetes mellitus, your eyes should be examined by an ophthalmologist at least once a year. Consult your doctor immediately if you experience sudden loss of vision.

WHAT MIGHT BE DONE?

Established diabetic retinopathy can be identified by studying the retina with an instrument called an ophthalmoscope (*see* OPHTHALMOSCOPY, p.578). If your doctor suspects early retinopathy, he or she may arrange for fluorescein angiography (above), in which dye is injected into the circulatory system to show the retinal blood vessels in detail.

Laser surgery can be used to treat the condition by destroying abnormal parts of the retina and preventing new blood vessels from forming (*see* LASER SURGERY FOR RETINOPATHY, p.579). Visual loss due to diabetic retinopathy is usually permanent. Laser surgery should prevent further loss of sight, but it may be necessary to have repeat treatments.

WWW ONLINE SITES: p.1030, p.1031

Macular degeneration

Progressive damage to the macula, the area near the centre of the light-sensitive retina that is responsible for detailed vision

- AGE Increasingly common with age, especially over the age of 70
- GENDER More common in females
- GENETICS Sometimes runs in families
- LIFESTYLE Smoking and excessive exposure to sunlight are risk factors

Gradual deterioration of the macula, the most sensitive region of the light-sensitive retina at the back of the eye, is known as macular degeneration. The condition leads to progressive loss of central and detailed vision. Affected people become unable to read or to recognize faces. However, the edges of their vision (peripheral vision) remain clear, so that they can still move around safely. Usually both eyes are affected.

Macular degeneration is more common in females and sometimes runs in families. The condition usually develops after the age of 70, although there are some rare forms that affect younger people. The risk of developing macular degeneration is increased by excessive exposure to sunlight and smoking.

WHAT ARE THE TYPES?

There are two main types of macular degeneration, but their causes are not known. In dry macular degeneration, light-sensitive cells in the macula and cells in the supporting layer underneath die. In wet macular degeneration, fragile new blood vessels grow underneath the macula. If the blood vessels leak fluid or bleed, the light-sensitive cells in the macula are damaged.

WHAT ARE THE SYMPTOMS?

Macular degeneration causes progressive visual loss over several months. Symptoms may include:

- Difficulty in reading, watching television, and recognizing faces.
- Distortion of vision so that objects appear larger or smaller than normal, or straight lines appear wavy.

Wet macular degeneration occasionally causes sudden loss of central vision due to rupture of an abnormal blood vessel.

Although the fluid or blood from the ruptured vessel gradually disappears, the damaged macula becomes scarred, causing permanent visual impairment.

WHAT MIGHT BE DONE?

Diagnosis of the condition is made by vision tests (p.587) and by examination of the retina with an ophthalmoscope (*see* OPHTHALMOSCOPY, p.578). If there is a possibility of wet macular degeneration, then fluorescein angiography (opposite page) may be carried out to check for abnormal blood vessels.

Dry macular degeneration cannot be treated. The early stages of wet macular degeneration can sometimes be treated by laser surgery, which seals off any abnormal blood vessels and can prevent further loss of vision. If abnormal blood vessels continue to develop, the process may need to be repeated.

If sight becomes severely affected, aids such as magnifying glasses may help with tasks such as reading.

(WWW) ONLINE SITES: p.1031

Retinitis pigmentosa

An inherited progressive degeneration in the retina, the light-sensitive membrane at the back of the eye

 AGE Most commonly begins in young adults

 GENDER More common in males

 GENETICS Due to an abnormal gene inherited from one or both parents

 LIFESTYLE Not a significant factor

Retinitis pigmentosa is a rare disorder in which the cells in the light-sensitive retina in the eye are progressively lost. Dark patches of pigment form on the retina, and vision deteriorates. The disorder is more common in males and is inherited, usually in an autosomal recessive manner (*see* GENE DISORDERS, p.271). It may not cause symptoms until early in adult life. Both eyes are affected equally.

If you have retinitis pigmentosa, the first symptom you may notice is poor vision in dim light. Later, the outer edges of vision, known as peripheral vision, are lost, and sight deteriorates progressively inwards until only a small area of central vision remains (this is known as tunnel vision). Rarely, tunnel vision

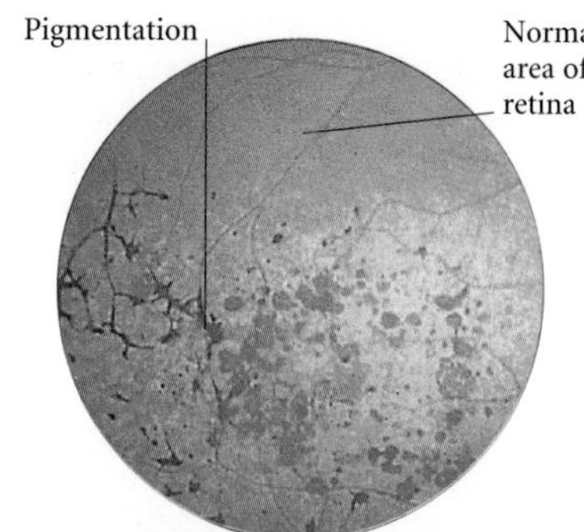

Retinitis pigmentosa
In this view through an ophthalmoscope, areas of pigmentation caused by retinitis pigmentosa are visible on part of the retina. The disorder leads to loss of vision.

can cause blindness (p.591). Retinitis pigmentosa is diagnosed by examining the retina with an ophthalmoscope (*see* OPHTHALMOSCOPY, p.578), an instrument which directs a beam of light into the eye. Although the condition is untreatable, special glasses may help to widen the field of vision if your visual loss becomes severe. If you plan to have children, you may wish to have genetic counselling (p.272) to assess the risk of the abnormal gene being inherited.

(WWW) ONLINE SITES: p.1031, p.1032

Optic neuritis

Inflammation of the optic nerve, which carries signals from the light-sensitive retina to the brain

 AGE Mainly affects young adults

 GENDER Three times more common in females

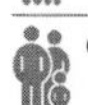 GENETICS Sometimes runs in families

 LIFESTYLE Not a significant factor

The optic nerve carries signals from the light-sensitive retina, found at the back of the eye, to the brain. Optic neuritis causes the nerve to become inflamed, resulting in pain and blurred vision. Usually, only one eye is affected.

Optic neuritis is most often caused by degeneration of the protective fatty sheath that surrounds the optic nerve fibres. This process, called demyelination, can be caused by a variety of conditions, including multiple sclerosis (p.541). Optic neuritis can also occur as a result of poisoning with chemicals, such as lead and methanol, or some viral infections, such as chickenpox (p.290). The condition can also occur for no obvious reason, most commonly in women in their late teens or twenties.

WHAT ARE THE SYMPTOMS?

Optic neuritis usually causes vision to deteriorate over hours or days. You may notice various symptoms, including:

- Loss of visual detail, making it difficult to read or to recognize faces.
- Loss of the central area of vision.
- Pain in the back of the eye that gets worse with eye movement.

If you experience a rapid deterioration in your vision, you should consult your doctor immediately.

WHAT MIGHT BE DONE?

Your doctor will use an ophthalmoscope (*see* OPHTHALMOSCOPY, p.578) to examine your eye and may also carry out vision tests (p.587). The optic nerve and other parts of the nervous system may be tested for signs of multiple sclerosis (*see* VISUAL EVOKED RESPONSES p.542) because optic neuritis may be the first sign of this disorder.

If you have optic neuritis, you may be given oral corticosteroids (p.930) to relieve inflammation. Although vision often improves in 3–6 weeks, optic neuritis often recurs, and visual damage may be permanent. About half of all people who have optic neuritis develop multiple sclerosis within 5 years.

(WWW) ONLINE SITES: p.1031

Papilloedema

Swelling of the optic disc, the area on the light-sensitive retina where the optic nerve enters the eye

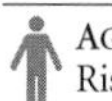 AGE GENDER GENETICS LIFESTYLE Risk factors depend on the cause

When the eye sends a signal to the brain, the signal travels along the optic nerve. The point on the light-sensitive retina where the optic nerve enters the eye is known as the optic disc, which can swell if pressure inside the skull increases. This condition is called papilloedema or optic disc oedema. There are several causes, including raised blood pressure (*see* HYPERTENSION, p.403), head injuries (p.521), a brain tumour

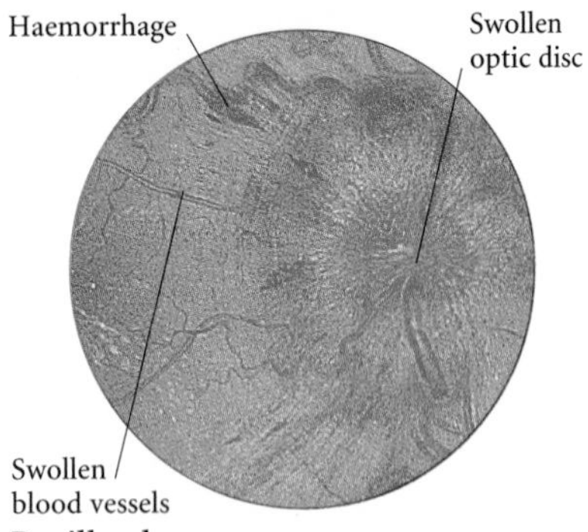

Papilloedema

This view through an ophthalmoscope shows a swollen optic disc (papilloedema) and distended retinal blood vessels caused by raised pressure inside the skull.

(p.530), or inflammation of the membranes that surround the brain (*see* MENINGITIS, p.527). The disorder itself does not cause pain, but the raised pressure of blood inside the head often causes headaches and vomiting.

Papilloedema is diagnosed with an instrument called an ophthalmoscope (*see* OPHTHALMOSCOPY, p.578). MRI (p.248) or CT scanning (p.247) may be used to look for an underlying cause of the disorder. In the meantime, corticosteroids (p.930) may be given to reduce pressure in the skull and prevent lasting damage to the optic nerve.

(WWW) ONLINE SITES: p.1031, p.1035

Exophthalmos

Bulging of one or both eyes, making them look abnormally prominent

GENDER More common in females

AGE GENETICS LIFESTYLE Not significant factors

If the tissue in the eye socket swells, the eyeball can protrude, causing a staring appearance known as exophthalmos. The condition usually affects both eyes and is more common in women. It is often linked with an overactive thyroid gland (*see* HYPERTHYROIDISM, p.679). Less commonly, the cause may be bleeding or infection behind the eye, a tumour, or a cyst. In these cases, usually only one eye is affected.

Severe exophthalmos can result in blurred vision because of pressure on the eye. Abnormal eye movement may lead to a change in the position of the eye, which can result in double vision (p.589). Exophthalmos may keep the eyelids from closing properly, causing the front of the eye to dry out, increasing the risk of damage to the cornea.

WHAT IS THE TREATMENT?

Exophthalmos may be corrected by dealing with the underlying cause, such as by treating a bacterial infection with antibiotics (p.885). However, if the exophthalmos is due to hyperthyroidism, it often remains after the underlying condition has been treated.

If exophthalmos persists, you may need surgery to make more room for the eye by removing part of the socket.

(WWW) ONLINE SITES: p.1031 p.1033

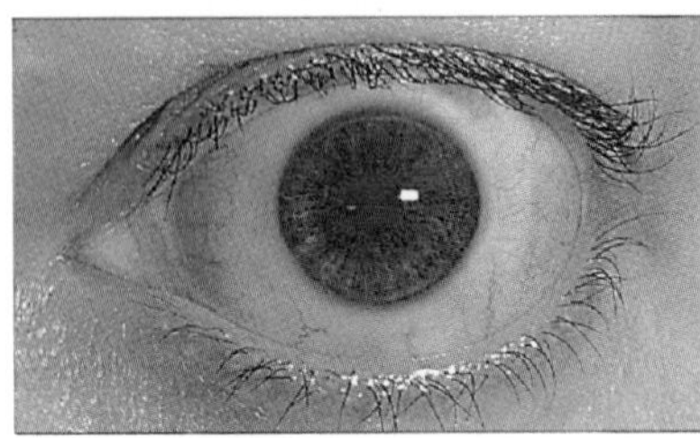

Exophthalmos

The staring appearance of this eye is due to swelling of tissues in the eye socket, making the eye bulge forwards (exophthalmos).

Eye injuries

Physical damage to the structures of the eye

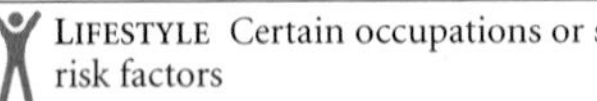
LIFESTYLE Certain occupations or sports are risk factors

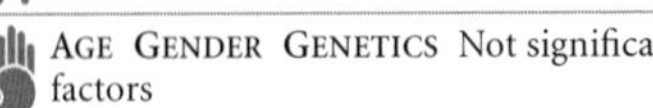
AGE GENDER GENETICS Not significant factors

The eyelid-closing reflex and the bony socket around the eye help to protect the eye from injuries. However, eye injuries are still common, and in some cases blindness may result if treatment is not given promptly.

The most common injury to the eye is a scratch on the transparent cornea caused by a foreign body in the eye (*see* CORNEAL ABRASION, p.571). Minor injuries of this type rarely damage vision permanently unless an infection develops and remains untreated. However, penetrating injuries in which the eye is pierced by a tiny, fast-moving object, such as a metal chip from machinery, can lead to total loss of sight. Blunt injuries, such as those caused by a blow from a fist or ball, may also endanger vision. Injuries can also occur when using caustic chemicals or while looking directly at the sun.

Most eye injuries can be prevented by the use of protective eyewear when working with dangerous machines or chemicals or when participating in athletic activities. Never look directly at the sun, even while wearing sunglasses.

WHAT ARE THE SYMPTOMS?

The symptoms of eye injuries differ according to the type and severity of damage, but symptoms may include:

- Pain and watering of the eye.
- Inability to open the eye.
- Bleeding under the front surface of the eye (*see* SUBCONJUNCTIVAL HAEMORRHAGE, p.571).
- Bruising and swelling of the skin around the eye.
- Reduced vision in the affected eye.

In the majority of minor eye injuries, first aid will often be helpful (*see* FIRST AID: EYE WOUND, p.993), but you should always seek medical attention for any eye injury. If the injury was caused by a blow to the eye, involves a penetrating foreign body, or results in reduced vision, hold a clean, dry cloth over the injured eye and go to the nearest accident and emergency department.

WHAT MIGHT BE DONE?

Your doctor will probably assess the eye by ophthalmoscopy (p.578) and a slit-lamp examination (p.574). Ultrasound scanning (p.250) may also be used to look for a foreign body in the eye.

Most eye injuries can be treated under a local anaesthetic, although some will require surgery under a general anaesthetic. Chemical injuries may be treated with corticosteroids (*see* DRUGS ACTING ON THE EYE, p.919).

Most eye injuries heal completely with prompt treatment. Sometimes corneal injuries leave a scar, and, if the lens is damaged, part of it may become cloudy (*see* CATARACT, p.573). Sunlight may cause permanent damage to the retina, and separation of the retina from its underlying layer (*see* RETINAL DETACHMENT, p.578) due to a heavy blow requires urgent treatment to prevent loss of sight. A serious eye injury can cause permanent blindness.

(WWW) ONLINE SITES: p.1031, p.1036

EYELID AND TEAR SYSTEM DISORDERS

Eyelids and tears work together to protect the eye against damage. The eyelids act as shutters, closing to stop material from entering the eyes. Tears keep the surface of the eyes moist and help to prevent infection. Disorders of the eyelids or tear system can damage the eyes, but most are easily treated if detected early.

KEY ANATOMY

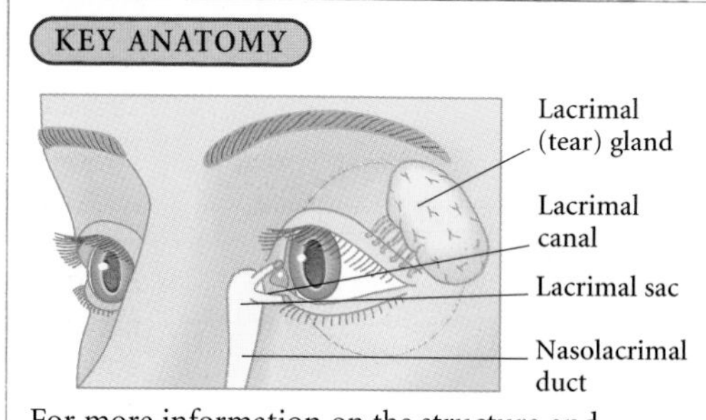

For more information on the structure and function of the eye, *see* pp.566–569.

The upper and lower eyelids provide essential protection for the eyes. If anything approaches the eye or face rapidly, the eyelids close together almost instantaneously as a reflex action. Furthermore, each eyelid has two or three rows of eyelashes, which help to prevent small particles from entering the eye.

Tears are another important part of the eyes' defences. They are made up of a salty fluid produced by the lacrimal (tear) glands, which are located above the upper eyelids. Tears lubricate the exposed surface of the eye and wash away potentially harmful materials, such as dust and chemicals. Tears also contain a natural antiseptic that helps to protect the eye against infection.

The initial articles in this section focus on conditions that affect the eyelids. These conditions include infections of the eyelid and disorders that alter the physical shape of the eyelids. The section then discusses disorders that affect the tear system, which include blockage of the tear drainage channels and problems with tear production. Disorders that affect the physical structures of the eye itself are covered elsewhere in the book (*see* EYE DISORDERS, pp. 570–582).

Stye

A painful, pus-filled swelling at the root of an eyelash due to a bacterial infection

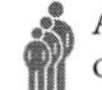
AGE More common in children but can occur at any age

LIFESTYLE Wearing contact lenses and using eye make-up may be risk factors

GENDER GENETICS Not significant factors

An infection at the root of an eyelash may result in the formation of a pus-filled swelling called a stye. Most styes are caused by *Staphylococcus aureus*, a bacterium found on the skin of many healthy people. Adults are less likely than children to develop styes, but, if you use eye make-up or wear contact lenses, you may be at increased risk.

A stye begins as a red lump on the edge of the eyelid. Over the next few days, the eyelid becomes swollen and tender, and a yellow spot may form at the centre of the swelling.

WHAT IS THE TREATMENT?

Styes usually rupture, drain, and heal in a few days without treatment. You may be able to speed the process by placing a clean, warm, damp cloth on the stye for about 20 minutes four times a day.

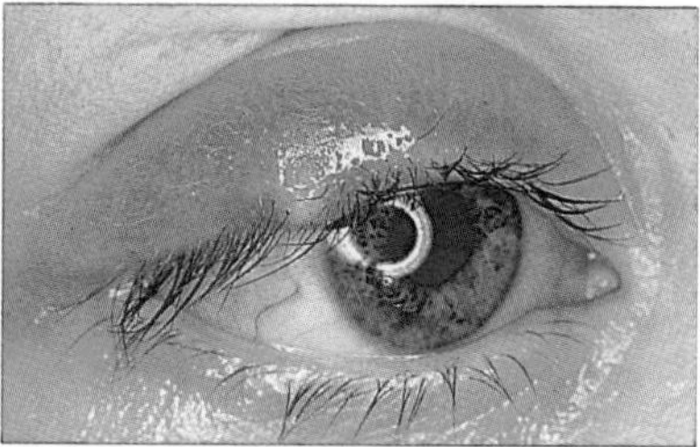

Stye on the upper eyelid
The swelling and redness of this eyelid are due to a stye, caused by a pus-producing infection at the root of an eyelash.

To avoid infecting other people or reinfecting yourself, always wash your hands after touching the infected eyelid and avoid sharing or reusing personal items such as towels or facecloths.

If a stye does not heal in a few days or if the swelling becomes worse, see your doctor. He or she may prescribe a topical antibiotic, which should be put directly on the stye and the skin surrounding it (*see* DRUGS ACTING ON THE EYE, p.919). However, if the stye persists, you may also need to take an oral antibiotic (p.885). The stye should clear up within 2–3 days of taking the antibiotic. Styes are unlikely to cause long-term damage, but they tend to recur in some people who are prone to them.

Blepharitis

Inflammation of the margin of the upper or lower eyelid or both

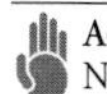
AGE GENDER GENETICS LIFESTYLE Not significant factors

Blepharitis, in which the margin of one or both eyelids becomes inflamed, is often associated with the skin disorder seborrhoeic dermatitis (p.335). Blepharitis may also be due to a bacterial infection or an allergy to cosmetics.

If you have blepharitis, your eyelids will be swollen, red, and itchy. The margins of the eyelids may be covered with soft, greasy scales that dry into crusts, sticking the eyelashes together. In some cases, the roots of the eyelashes become infected, causing small ulcers or styes (left) to form.

WHAT IS THE TREATMENT?

You can relieve the symptoms by holding a clean, warm, damp cloth against the eyelid. The healing process may be helped by gently cleaning the eyelids twice a day with baby shampoo diluted half-and-half with water. If you have seborrhoeic dermatitis, treating it with a dandruff shampoo that contains an antifungal agent should also help the blepharitis. If the blepharitis recurs repeatedly, see your doctor, who may prescribe topical antibiotics (*see* DRUGS ACTING ON THE EYE, p.919) or a corticosteroid (p.930). The condition often clears up after 2 weeks of treatment, but it may recur. Allergic blepharitis usually improves on its own if you avoid contact with the trigger substance.

(WWW) ONLINE SITES: p.1036

Chalazion

A swelling in the eyelid that may be painless

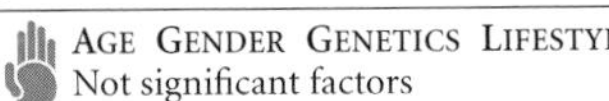

AGE GENDER GENETICS LIFESTYLE
Not significant factors

If an oil-secreting gland in the eyelid becomes blocked, the gland enlarges, creating a swelling called a chalazion. A chalazion may at first look like a stye (p.583), but, unlike a stye, it is not on the eyelid margin. Usually, the pain and redness associated with a chalazion disappear after a few days. However, if the swelling is large, it may cause long-term discomfort, and pressure on the front of the eye can interfere with vision.

WHAT MIGHT BE DONE?

If your doctor diagnoses a chalazion, he or she will probably wait for several weeks before arranging any treatment because it will probably disappear on its own. Meanwhile, if the chalazion is painful or irritating, holding a clean, warm, damp cloth against it may help.

A persistent chalazion can be treated by a simple operation in which a small cut is made in the inner surface of the eyelid and the contents of the swelling removed. The procedure is performed with local anaesthesia and is painless.

(WWW) ONLINE SITES: p.1031

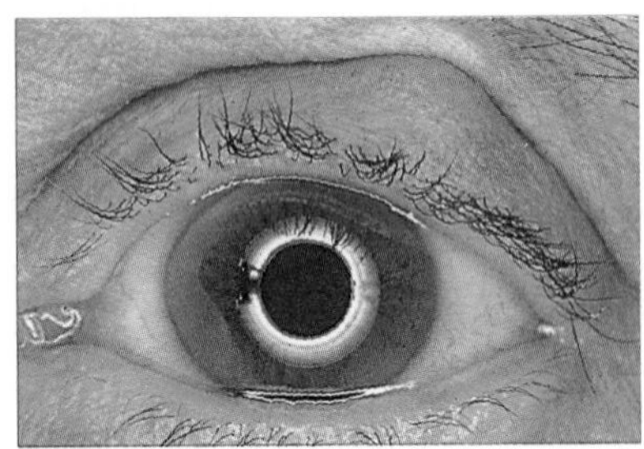

Chalazion
The swelling in the upper eyelid of this eye is a chalazion, caused by blockage of an oil-secreting gland.

Ptosis

Abnormal drooping of one or both upper eyelids

AGE GENDER HEREDITY LIFESTYLE
Risk factors depend on the cause

Drooping of the upper eyelid due to weakness of the muscle that raises it is called ptosis. The condition may be the result of a problem with the muscle or nerve that controls the eyelid. The sagging lid may partly or totally close the eye. One or both eyes may be affected.

Ptosis is occasionally present from birth. If a baby's eyelid droops and it covers the pupil, his or her vision may not develop normally (*see* AMBLYOPIA, p.858) and early treatment is vital.

Ptosis in adults can occur as a part of the aging process, or it may be a symptom of myasthenia gravis (p.549), which causes progressive muscle weakness. If ptosis starts suddenly, it may be due to a brain tumour (p.530) or a defective blood vessel in the brain. If you develop ptosis, see your doctor to rule out a serious underlying disorder.

WHAT IS THE TREATMENT?

Ptosis in babies can be corrected by surgically tightening the eyelid muscle. If treatment is carried out early, the child's vision should develop normally.

In adults, surgery for ptosis should be carried out only after any possible significant underlying disorders have been ruled out. Surgery is very effective for ptosis caused by the aging process.

(WWW) ONLINE SITES: p.1031, p.1035

Entropion

Inward turning of the margin of the upper or lower eyelid or both

AGE More common in elderly people

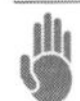

GENDER GENETICS LIFESTYLE
Not significant factors

In entropion, the eyelid turns inwards. The eyelashes rub against the cornea (the transparent front part of the eye) and the conjunctiva (which covers the white of the eye). Although the conjunctiva also lines the eyelids, this area is unaffected. Typical symptoms of the condition are pain in the eye area, watery eye (opposite page) and irritation. Left untreated, the cornea may become damaged (*see* CORNEAL ULCER, p.571), leading to loss of vision.

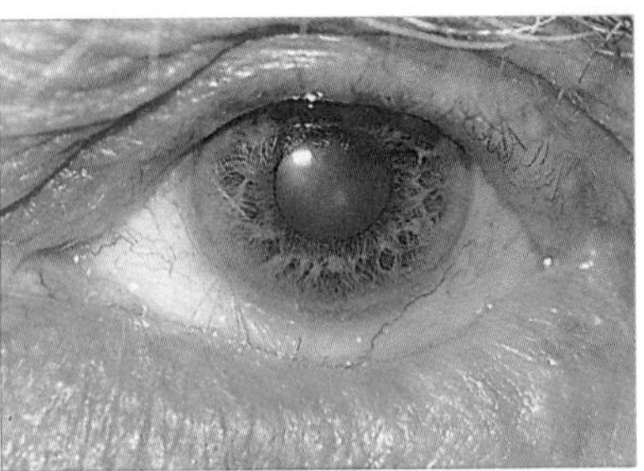

Entropion
This eye's lower lid has turned inwards, causing the eyelashes to rub against the eye. This condition is called entropion.

In developed countries, entropion mainly affects elderly people because of the natural weakening of the muscles around the eyelids that takes place with increasing age. In developing countries, entropion most often follows bouts of the eye infection trachoma (p.572), which causes scar tissue to form on the inner surface of the eyelids. Eventually, this tissue may shrink, making the eyelids turn inwards.

A minor operation can be carried out to realign the eyelid. This procedure usually corrects the condition and prevents any further damage to the eye.

(WWW) ONLINE SITES: p.1031

Ectropion

Outward turning of the margin of the lower eyelid

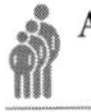

AGE More common in elderly people

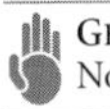

GENDER GENETICS LIFESTYLE
Not significant factors

If the edge of the lower eyelid turns outwards and the eyelid hangs away from the eye, the exposed inner surface of the lid becomes dry and sore. This condition is known as ectropion and may stop tears from entering the nasolacrimal duct, which runs from the eye to the nose, causing the eye to water continuously. Since the eyelids cannot close fully, the transparent cornea at the front part of the eye is constantly exposed and may become damaged (*see* CORNEAL ABRASION, p.571) or repeatedly infected. The condition most often occurs in elderly people as a result of weakness of the lower eyelid that may occur with increasing age. Both eyes are usually affected. Ectropion may also be caused by contraction of a scar on the eyelid or cheek or by facial palsy (p.548), in which the muscles around the eye (and other facial muscles on the affected side) are paralysed. In these cases, only one eye is usually involved.

What is the treatment?

If you think that you have ectropion, you should consult your doctor as soon as you can because treatment of the disorder is most successful when it is carried out early. Your doctor will probably recommend a straightforward surgical operation, performed under local anaesthesia, in which the skin and muscles around the eyelid are tightened. In severe cases, more complex plastic surgery (p.952) may be necessary.

(WWW) ONLINE SITES: p.1031

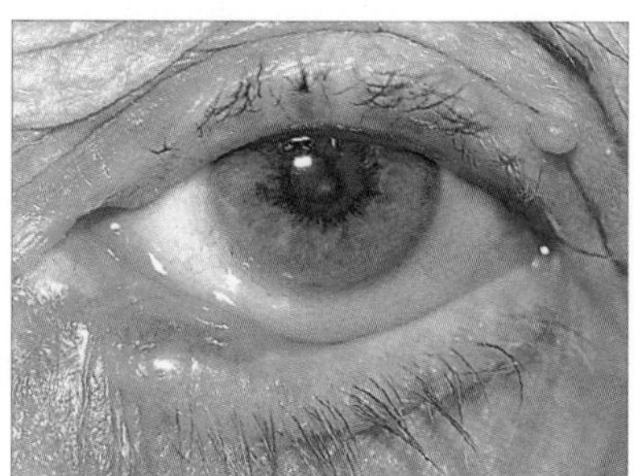

Ectropion
The lower eyelid of this eye has turned outwards (ectropion), exposing the inner surface and preventing drainage of tears.

Watery eye

Overflow of tears from the eye due to overproduction or poor drainage

 AGE Most common in babies and elderly people

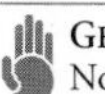 GENDER GENETICS LIFESTYLE Not significant factors

Watery eye usually results from irritation of the eye by a foreign body such as a particle of dirt. Older people often have watery eye as a result of entropion (opposite page), in which the eyelashes rub against the eye, or ectropion (opposite page), in which tears do not drain away normally. The watering usually stops when the irritant is removed or the underlying condition is corrected. Watery eye may also occur as a result of a blocked nasolacrimal system (which drains tears), possibly caused by an infection of the eye or sinus infection.

Babies may have watery eyes because the nasolacrimal system is underdeveloped. Gently massaging between the corner of the eyelid and the nose may help. The condition usually corrects itself by the age of 6 months. Persistent blockages, at any age, must be treated by a doctor, who may clear the tear duct by inserting a fine probe.

Dacryocystitis

Painful swelling of the lacrimal (tear) sac, into which fluid drains from the surface of the eye

 AGE Most common in babies and elderly people

 GENDER GENETICS LIFESTYLE Not significant factors

Normally, tears from the eyes drain into the lacrimal sacs on either side of the nose. An infection of the lacrimal sacs is known as dacryocystitis. The condition is usually caused by a bacterial infection and most commonly results from a blockage in the nasolacrimal duct, which normally carries tears from the lacrimal sac to the nose. Nasolacrimal blockage is common in babies because the ducts are not fully developed until a year after birth. Elderly people may develop a blockage with no apparent cause, although it may be due to previous injury or inflammation.

Dacryocystitis usually starts with a red, watery eye. The area beside the nose just below the eye then becomes tender, red, and swollen. Pus may be discharged into the eye. Dacryocystitis usually affects only one eye at a time, but it can recur in either eye.

What might be done?

In adults, warm compresses and oral antibiotics (p.885) may help to clear the infection. If the problem continues, a probe may be inserted to clear the nasolacrimal duct or surgery may be required to correct the damage. In babies, gentle massage of the lacrimal sac may help to relieve the condition. Antibiotics may also be given. As with adults, the blockage may be cleared by the insertion of a tiny probe.

(WWW) ONLINE SITES: p.1031

Keratoconjunctivitis sicca

Persistent dryness of the eye due to insufficient production of tears, also known as dry eye

 AGE Increasingly common over the age of 35

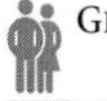 GENDER More common in females

 GENETICS LIFESTYLE Not significant factors

Insufficient tear production, known as keratoconjunctivitis sicca or dry eye, results from damage to the lacrimal (tear) glands. The condition causes eye irritation and often leads to eye infections (*see* CONJUNCTIVITIS, p.570). In severe cases, corneal ulcers (p.571) may develop. Dry eye affects more women than men and is more common over the age of 35. The condition may be linked to autoimmune disorders, such as Sjögren's syndrome (p.463), in which the body attacks its own tissues.

Your doctor will prescribe artificial tears to restore moisture to the eye. He or she may also investigate and treat an underlying cause. Sometimes, surgery may be performed to plug the channel through which the tears normally drain.

(WWW) ONLINE SITES: p.1031

Xerophthalmia

Dryness of the eye due to a dietary deficiency of vitamin A

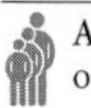 AGE More common in children but can occur at any age

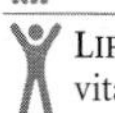 LIFESTYLE Caused by a diet low in vitamin A

 GENDER GENETICS Not significant factors

Xerophthalmia, which occurs mainly in developing countries, means dryness of the eye. The condition is caused by a dietary deficiency of vitamin A (*see* NUTRITIONAL DEFICIENCIES, p.630).

Left untreated, xerophthalmia leads to chronic (long-term) infection and the transparent cornea at the front of the eye may soften and perforate. Infection may then spread inside the eye and blindness (p.591) may result. Artificial tears may relieve dryness, but the main treatment is large doses of vitamin A.

VISION DISORDERS

Disorders of vision are very common; most people have a visual problem at some time in their lives. The most common disorders of vision are shortsightedness (myopia) and longsightedness (hyperopia), which are types of refractive (focusing) errors. Most refractive errors can be corrected by aids, such as glasses or contact lenses, or cured by surgical techniques.

The opening articles in this section discuss refractive errors and show how variations in the size and shape of the eye may lead to distortions of vision. Tests and treatments for refractive errors are also described. However, special tests for children's vision are covered separately (*see* VISION TESTS IN CHILDREN, p.857). Presbyopia, the deterioration of vision that occurs with aging, is covered next.

The following articles describe colour blindness, a condition that is more common in men, and serious visual problems, including double vision and partial or total blindness.

Disorders that affect the structure of the eye, including glaucoma, are covered elsewhere (*see* EYE DISORDERS, pp.570–582), as are blindness at birth (*see* CONGENITAL BLINDNESS, p.856) and two disorders that mainly affect children: crossed eyes (*see* STRABISMUS, p.857) and abnormal vision in an eye that is otherwise structurally normal (*see* AMBLYOPIA, p.858).

KEY ANATOMY

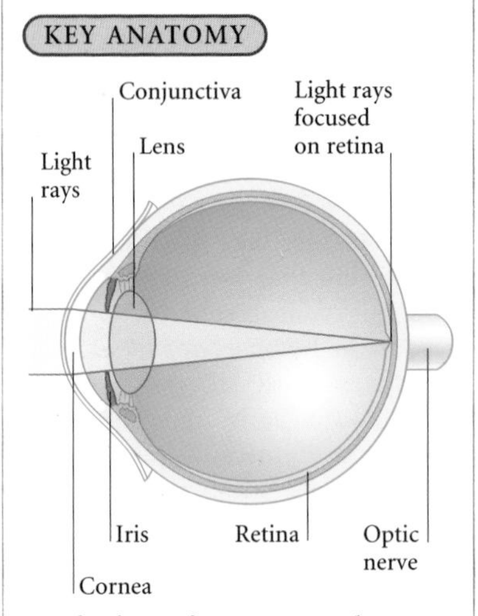

For further information on the structure and function of the eye, *see* pp.566–569.

Myopia

Inability to see distant objects clearly, commonly known as shortsightedness

 AGE Usually becomes apparent around puberty

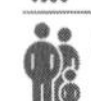 GENETICS Sometimes runs in families

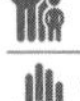 GENDER LIFESTYLE Not significant factors

To enable us to see clearly, light rays need to be focused by the transparent cornea at the front of the eye and by the eye's lens so that they form a sharp image on the retina, the light-sensitive membrane at the back of the eye. In people who have myopia (shortsightedness), the eyeball is long relative to the combined focusing power of the cornea and the lens. Light rays from distant objects are therefore bent too much and are focused in front of the retina, resulting in blurred vision. Myopia is a very common condition that sometimes runs in families and can usually be corrected.

WHAT ARE THE SYMPTOMS?

The symptoms of myopia often become apparent around puberty, but the condition may begin to develop a few years before. The earlier myopia starts, the more severe it is likely to become. However, the condition usually stabilizes in early adulthood when growth stops. The main symptoms are:

- Increasing difficulty in seeing objects clearly from a distance.
- In children, deteriorating schoolwork as a result of not seeing clearly.

If you are seriously myopic, you are more susceptible to eye disorders such as retinal detachment (p.578), chronic glaucoma (p.576), and macular degeneration (p.580). All of these disorders can badly damage eyesight. If you have problems seeing distant objects clearly, you should visit your optician.

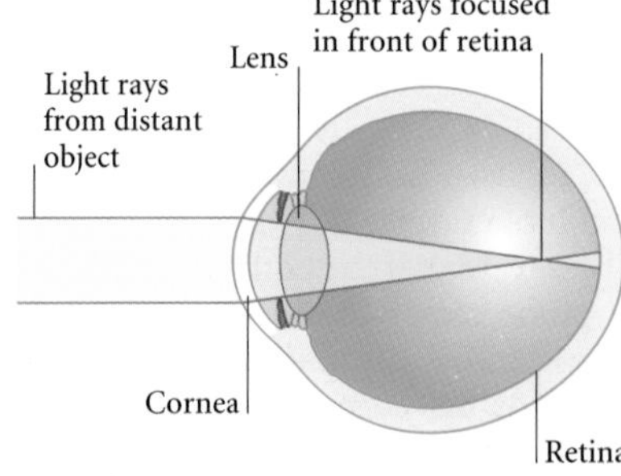

Myopia

In myopia, the eyeball is too long relative to the focusing power of the cornea and lens. Light from distant objects is focused in front of the retina and the image is blurred.

WHAT MIGHT BE DONE?

The optician will carry out vision tests (opposite page) to check for myopia. Myopia can be corrected with concave-lensed glasses or, for older children and adults, contact lenses (*see* GLASSES AND CONTACT LENSES, p.588). In mild cases, the cornea's shape can be altered by surgery to correct vision (*see* SURGERY FOR REFRACTIVE ERRORS, p.589).

(WWW) ONLINE SITES: p.1031

Hypermetropia

Inability to see close objects clearly, commonly known as longsightedness

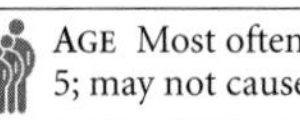 AGE Most often detected at about the age of 5; may not cause problems until middle age

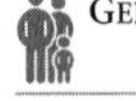 GENETICS Sometimes runs in families

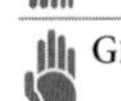 GENDER LIFESTYLE Not significant factors

The transparent cornea and the lens act together to focus light rays and create a clear image on the light-sensitive retina at the back of the eye. Hypermetropia (longsightedness) occurs if the eyeball is short relative to the combined focusing power of the cornea and lens. When the image falls behind the retina, it causes blurred vision that is

TEST VISION TESTS

You should have your vision tested every 2 years, especially if you are over the age of 40. The most common tests assess the acuity (sharpness) of your distance vision and your ability to focus on near objects. The tests also show which corrective lenses, if any, you need. Additional tests for specific eye disorders, such as glaucoma (p.575), may be performed, depending on your age and medical history.

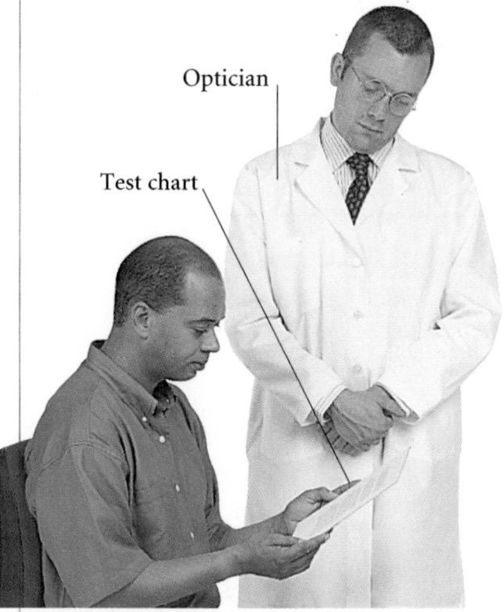

Near-vision test
Wearing your usual glasses or contact lenses, if you use them, you will be asked to read very small print on a chart held at normal reading distance. This test checks your ability to focus on near objects.

Phoropter
This device can hold different lenses in front of each eye, allowing the eyes to be tested separately

Adjustable arm
The position of the trial frame is adjusted to your height

Snellen chart
The acuity of your distance vision is tested separately for each eye. The test involves noting how far down a Snellen chart you can read letters of decreasing sizes.

Having a vision test
Lenses in the phoropter are changed until you can accurately read the letters near the bottom of the Snellen chart. This enables the optician to make the appropriate prescription for your corrective lenses.

often worse when viewing near objects. Young people with hypermetropia often see distant objects very clearly because the lens is flexible and changes focus easily, but with age, focusing ability lessens and distant vision is also affected.

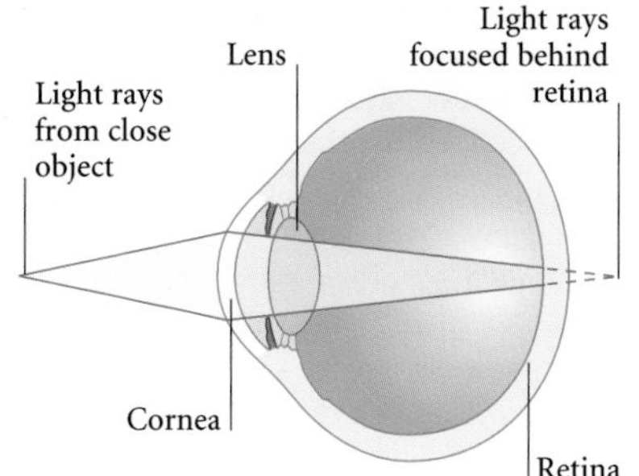

Hypermetropia
In hypermetropia, the eye is too short relative to the focusing power of the cornea and lens. Light rays are focused behind the retina and the image is blurred.

WHAT ARE THE SYMPTOMS?

Mild or moderate hypermetropia will probably not affect vision in young people because they can compensate by focusing the lens, but, the more severe the condition, the earlier in life symptoms may appear. Symptoms of severe hypermetropia, which may be apparent from infancy, can include:

- Lack of interest in small objects.
- Difficulty with reading or following picture stories.

If the eyes are not equally affected by hypermetropia, they may be unable to focus together on the same object. Without early treatment, young children may develop crossed eyes (*see* STRABISMUS, p.857) and may eventually lose vision in one eye (*see* AMBLYOPIA, p.858). You should take your child to the doctor immediately if you notice any of the symptoms described here.

If you have trouble seeing near objects clearly or have difficulty in reading or doing other close work, you should visit your optician for vision tests (above). These problems may indicate that you have presbyopia (p.589), which develops earlier in people with hypermetropia than in most people.

WHAT MIGHT BE DONE?

Your optician will check your visual acuity and the level of detail you can see, and then assess the severity of hypermetropia. Although the condition is sometimes detected in children during routine vision testing at school, all children who have a family history of severe hypermetropia should be tested before the age of 3 because early treatment is important.

Hypermetropia can be corrected with contact lenses or glasses that have

TREATMENT GLASSES AND CONTACT LENSES

Most refractive errors can be corrected by wearing glasses or, for older children and adults, contact lenses. Glasses are suitable for most refractive errors, are comfortable to wear, and do not cause complications. Contact lenses are also available for many refractive errors, but they are most effective for myopia (p.586) and hypermetropia (p.586). All contact lenses require careful cleaning to reduce the chance of an infection of the transparent cornea over which they are placed.

HOW LENSES WORK

Glasses and contact lenses correct refractive errors in the eye by altering the angle of light rays before the rays reach the surface of the cornea, the transparent front part of the eye. The cornea at the front of the eye and the lens can then focus the rays correctly on the retina. Concave lenses make the light rays diverge (bend apart) and convex lenses make the light rays converge (bend together).

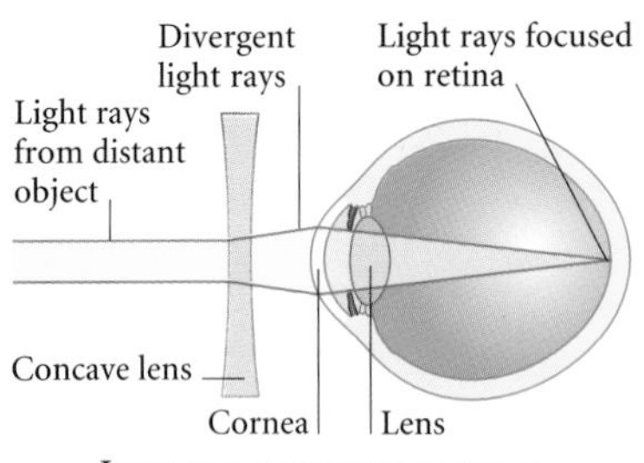

LENS TO CORRECT MYOPIA

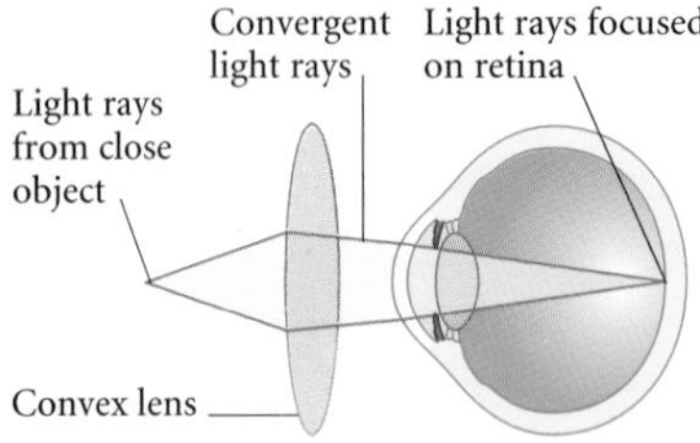

LENS TO CORRECT HYPERMETROPIA

Myopia and hypermetropia
Myopia is corrected by concave lenses, which make light rays diverge and focus on the retina, not in front of it. Hypermetropia requires a convex lens to make light rays converge, focusing them on the retina and not behind it.

CONTACT LENSES

Three types of contact lenses are available: rigid, gas-permeable, and soft. Soft lenses are the most widely used and rigid the least. Some soft lenses are worn only once or for a few days. Nondisposable lenses should be disinfected daily unless worn for an extended period (not usually recommended). If an eye becomes red or painful, you should stop wearing your lenses and consult your optician immediately.

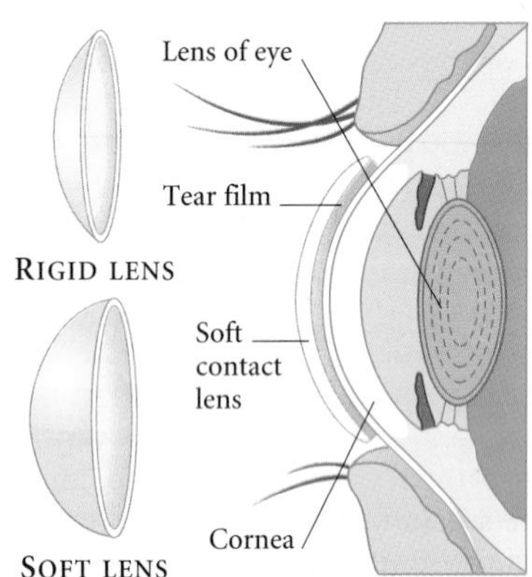

Rigid and soft lenses
A contact lens floats on the tear film on the front of the eye. Soft lenses cover the whole cornea; rigid and gas-permeable lenses cover only the central part of the cornea.

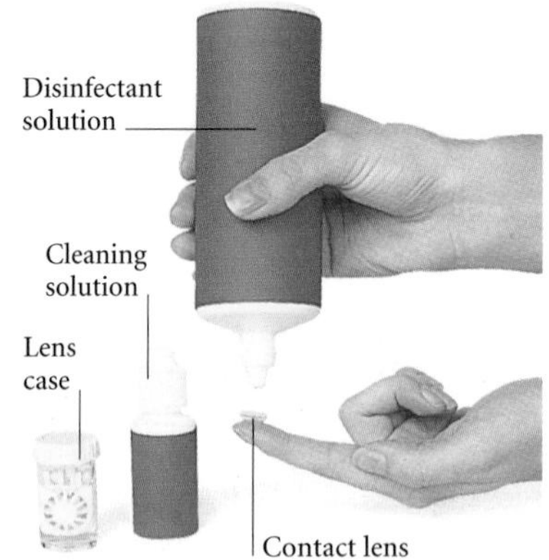

Contact lens care
Good lens hygiene prevents eye infections. Nondisposable lenses must be carefully cleaned before and after use and soaked overnight in disinfectant solution.

convex lenses (*see* GLASSES AND CONTACT LENSES, left). The focusing power of the eye decreases gradually with age, and your prescription may need to be updated regularly. People who have hypermetropia may be helped by laser treatment that increases the focusing power of the cornea (*see* SURGERY FOR REFRACTIVE ERRORS, opposite page).

Hypermetropia does not cause complications, but people who have the condition are more prone to acute glaucoma (p.575), a condition that must be treated promptly. Regular tests for glaucoma (*see* COMMON SCREENING TESTS, p.44) are therefore especially important.

(WWW) ONLINE SITES: p.1031

Astigmatism

Distorted vision caused by an uneven curvature of the transparent cornea at the front of the eye

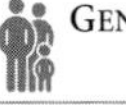
GENETICS Sometimes runs in families

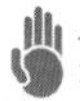
AGE GENDER LIFESTYLE Not significant factors

In people with astigmatism, the transparent cornea at the front of the eye is unevenly curved and refracts (bends) the light rays striking different parts of it to differing degrees. The lens is then unable to bring all the rays into focus on the light-sensitive retina at the back of the eye, and vision becomes blurred. Astigmatism can run in families and often occurs in combination with myopia (p.586) or hypermetropia (p.586).

WHAT ARE THE CAUSES?

The most common form of astigmatism is present from birth and is due to a slight buckling of the cornea in both eyes. Instead of being round like a football, the cornea is shaped like a rugby ball, with a steep curvature in one direction and a shallow curvature in the other. This type may worsen slowly with age. Less often, astigmatism is due to an eye disorder such as keratoconus (p.572) or an eye injury that causes a corneal ulcer (p.571) to develop.

WHAT ARE THE SYMPTOMS?

The majority of people have a slight degree of astigmatism. If you are only slightly affected, you probably will not notice much wrong with your vision.

TREATMENT SURGERY FOR REFRACTIVE ERRORS

Surgery can be used to correct some refractive errors permanently. The main techniques are: laser-assisted in-situ keratomileusis (LASIK), photorefractive keratectomy (PRK), and radial keratotomy (RK). LASIK, in which the cornea is reshaped by a laser, causes the least scarring and is becoming more widely used. In PRK, areas of the cornea are shaved away by laser, and mild corneal scarring may result. RK, in which the cornea is flattened by scalpel cuts, can weaken the cornea.

LASIK treatment of myopia
After a flap has been created, a laser beam, guided by computer, removes part of the cornea. The flap is then replaced. The reshaped cornea is flatter, and light rays are focused to form a sharp image. The LASIK technique leaves very little scarring.

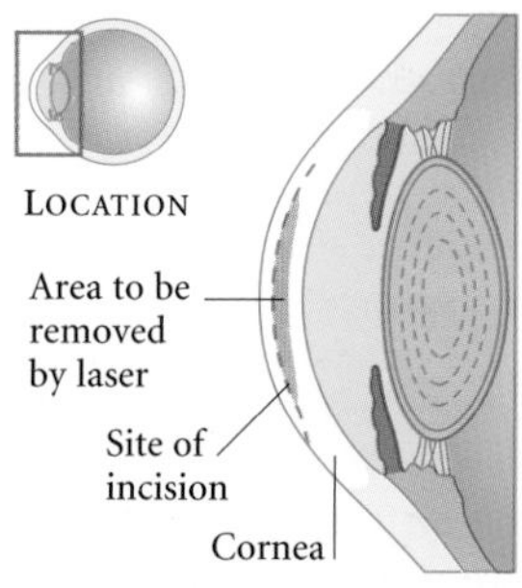

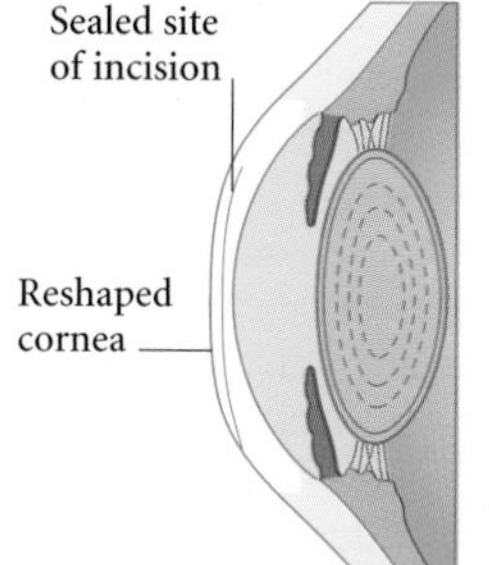

More severe astigmatism, however, may lead to significant visual problems.

Astigmatism can affect vision in a number of different ways. Symptoms may include the following:

- Blurring of small print, causing difficulty in reading.
- Inability to see both near and distant objects clearly.

If you are experiencing difficulty in seeing objects clearly at any distance, it is important to visit your optician as soon as possible to have a vision test (p.587).

WHAT IS THE TREATMENT?

In people with astigmatism, vision can usually be corrected by glasses that have special lenses that compensate for the unevenly shaped cornea. Rigid contact lenses are also effective because they smooth out the surface of the cornea. Conventional soft contact lenses mould to the shape of the cornea and can normally correct only mild astigmatism. However, soft contact lenses known as toric lenses, which are designed to correct the condition, are also available.

In some people, astigmatism may be corrected permanently by laser treatment that alters the shape of the cornea, leaving only minimal scarring (*see* SURGERY FOR REFRACTIVE ERRORS, above). This type of surgery is rarely used in the UK but it is more common in some other countries.

WWW ONLINE SITES: p.1031

Presbyopia

Gradual age-associated loss of the eye's ability to focus on near objects

AGE Generally develops over the age of 40

GENDER GENETICS LIFESTYLE Not significant factors

After about the age of 40, almost everyone starts to notice increased difficulty in reading small print because of the development of presbyopia. A person with normal vision is able to see close objects clearly because the elastic lens of the eye changes shape, becoming thicker and more curved when focusing on near objects. The thicker lens brings light rays from close objects into sharp focus on the light-sensitive retina at the back of the eye in a process known as accommodation. As we age, the lens becomes less elastic and the power of accommodation is reduced. Eventually, light rays from near objects can no longer be focused on the retina and the objects we see appear blurred.

WHAT ARE THE SYMPTOMS?

Since presbyopia develops very slowly, most people are unaware of the initial stages of this condition. However, the symptoms usually become noticeable between the ages of 40 and 50. Longsighted people (*see* HYPERMETROPIA, p.586) may have noticeable symptoms from an earlier age. Common symptoms of presbyopia include:

- The need to hold newspapers and books at arm's length so that you can read them.
- Increased difficulty in focusing on near objects in poor light.
- If you are shortsighted (*see* MYOPIA, p.586), the need to take off your glasses to see near objects clearly.

If you develop any of these problems, consult your optician.

WHAT IS THE TREATMENT?

Presbyopia can be corrected by wearing glasses with convex (outward-curved) lenses, which bring light rays from near objects into focus on the retina. If you are longsighted, shortsighted, or have astigmatism (opposite page), you may be prescribed glasses with a different power in different parts of the lens. For example, bifocals have an upper lens to correct distance vision and a lower lens to correct presbyopia. Progressive lenses that gradually alter the focusing power from top to bottom are also available. Presbyopia can sometimes be corrected with contact lenses, but glasses may still be necessary for reading.

Presbyopia tends to worsen with age, and you will probably need to have your lens prescription updated every few years. You should see your optician regularly in order to have vision tests. The condition eventually stabilizes at about the age of 60 by which time little natural focusing power is left. By this stage most of the focusing work is done by glasses instead of the eye.

WWW ONLINE SITES: p.1031

Double vision

Seeing two separate images of a single object instead of one

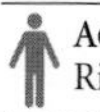
AGE GENDER GENETICS LIFESTYLE Risk factors depend on the cause

People with double vision see two images of a single object. The images are separate but often clearly focused. This disorder can have a number of causes, and usually disappears when one eye is closed. You should consult your doctor immediately if you start to experience double vision because it may indicate that you have a serious underlying disorder.

WHAT ARE THE CAUSES?

The most common cause of double vision is weakness or paralysis of one or more of the muscles that control the movements of one eye. The movement of the affected eye is impaired, causing crossed eyes (*see* STRABISMUS, p.857). Two different views of the same object are received by the visual system and the brain cannot combine them. Tilting or turning the head may briefly correct the problem. However, not all types of crossed eyes cause double vision.

Many serious conditions that affect the brain and nervous system may cause impaired eye movements, leading to double vision. Potential causes include multiple sclerosis (p.541), head injuries (p.521), brain tumours (p.530), and bulging of an artery inside the head due to a weakness in the vessel wall (called an aneurysm). In older people, impaired eye movement resulting in double vision may be linked with diabetes mellitus (p.687) and, rarely, with atherosclerosis (p.402) and high blood pressure (*see* HYPERTENSION, p.403).

Very rarely, double vision can also occur as a result of a tumour or blood clot behind one of the eyes, causing the movement of that eye to be affected.

HOW IS IT DIAGNOSED?

Your doctor may ask you to shut one eye at a time to see whether the double vision disappears. He or she may also ask you to describe the double images, or ask if they appear side by side or one on top of the other or whether one of the images appears to be tilted. Your doctor will probably observe the movements of your eyes closely in order to establish whether any of the eye muscles are weak or paralysed. He or she may also carry out special vision tests to identify weak eye movement.

If double vision has come on suddenly, or if no obvious cause can be found, urgent CT scanning (p.247) or MRI (p.248) may be carried out to check for any abnormality in the eye sockets or brain that might be affecting the alignment of the eyes. You may also have a neurological examination.

WHAT IS THE TREATMENT?

Treatment of double vision is aimed at the underlying cause. A serious disorder such as an aneurysm may need hospital treatment. Double vision due to diabetes mellitus usually disappears over time. If it does not, you may be advised to wear a patch over one eye to eliminate the second image. Surgery to adjust the eye muscles helps if double vision has been present for some time.

(WWW) ONLINE SITES: p.1031, p.1035

(TEST) VISUAL FIELD TEST

Visual field testing (perimetry) is used to check the whole area that each eye can see (the visual field). The development of blank sections in the visual field may be caused by various underlying disorders (*see* VISUAL FIELD DEFECTS, right). Many eye disorders cause characteristic visual field defects that can develop without being noticed. Testing allows early detection and treatment.

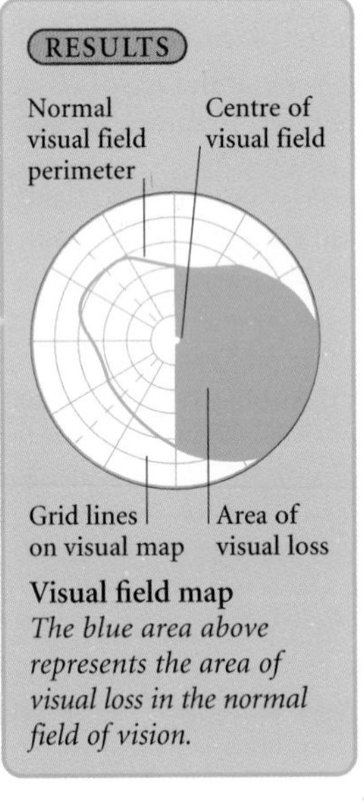

Visual field map
The blue area above represents the area of visual loss in the normal field of vision.

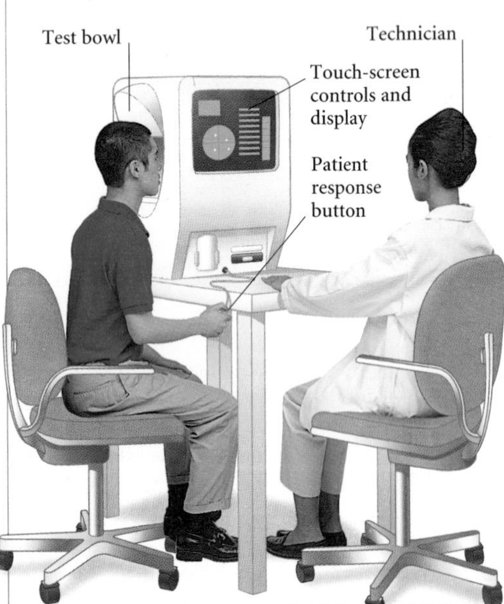

Visual field test
One eye is covered while you look at a central target inside the test bowl. When you see lights flashing in different parts of your visual field, you press a response button.

Visual field defects

Loss of part of the normal area of vision in one or both eyes

AGE GENDER GENETICS LIFESTYLE
Risk factors depend on the cause

Visual field defects take different forms, ranging from loss of areas at the outer edges of vision (peripheral vision) or small blind spots to loss of most of the area that you normally see (the visual field). If you notice a loss of vision, you should seek urgent medical advice because visual field defects sometimes indicate a serious underlying disorder. Regular vision tests (p.587) are important because visual field defects may develop slowly without being noticed.

WHAT ARE THE CAUSES?

Visual field defects may be caused by damage to the light-sensitive retina at the back of the eye; the optic nerve, along which nerve signals are carried from the retina to the brain; or the parts of the brain involved with vision.

Several eye disorders cause characteristic patterns of visual field loss. For example, a gradual increase in fluid pressure in the eye (*see* CHRONIC GLAUCOMA, p.576) can damage nerve fibres in the retina, causing loss of peripheral vision. If glaucoma is left untreated, only a narrow area of central vision will remain (tunnel vision). Inflammation of the optic nerve (*see* OPTIC NEURITIS, p.581) can cause various visual field defects, and a pituitary tumour (p.676) often causes loss of the outer half of the visual field in each eye. Brain damage due to a stroke (p.532) or tumour (*see* BRAIN TUMOUR, p.530) may result in loss of the right or left half of the visual field in both eyes. Migraine (p.518) can cause temporary visual field defects.

What are the symptoms?

Visual field defects usually appear gradually and often remain unnoticed. In other cases, depending on the type of defect, symptoms may include:

- Bumping into objects on one side.
- Missing whole sections of text while you are reading.
- Being able to see only straight ahead (tunnel vision).

The majority of visual field defects can be detected during routine vision tests. However, you should see your doctor immediately if you notice a change in your normal field of vision.

What might be done?

Your doctor may carry out a visual field test (opposite page) to assess the pattern and extent of the defect.

The treatment for the defect depends on the underlying cause. For example, if you have chronic glaucoma, you will be given drugs to reduce the pressure in the eye (*see* DRUGS FOR GLAUCOMA, p.920). Existing defects are usually permanent, but treatment of the underlying condition may prevent further deterioration. Many people who have a visual field defect become used to it, but it may affect their lifestyle or choice of occupation. For example, if you have tunnel vision, you should not drive.

(WWW) ONLINE SITES: p.1031

Eyestrain

Temporary discomfort or aching in or around the eyes

 AGE GENDER GENETICS LIFESTYLE Not significant factors

Eyestrain is neither a medical term nor a diagnosis. In contrast to widespread belief, you cannot damage or strain your eyes by using them under difficult conditions, such as reading small print in poor light or wearing glasses of the wrong strength. Although aching and discomfort are commonly attributed to eyestrain, they are often headaches that are caused by tension or tiredness of the muscles around the eye as a result of frowning or squinting.

The symptoms normally attributed to eyestrain do not require treatment and normally disappear on their own, but, if the problem worsens or persists, you should consult your doctor.

Colour blindness

Below-normal ability to distinguish between colours

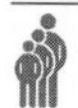 AGE Usually present from birth

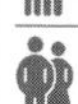 GENDER More common in males

GENETICS Usually due to an abnormal gene inherited from the mother

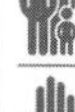 LIFESTYLE Not a significant factor

Colour blindness is the reduced ability to tell certain colours apart. It is due to a defect in the cones, the specialized cells in the light-sensitive retina at the back of the eye. There are three types of cone cell, each of which is sensitive to blue, green, or red light. If one or more type of cell is faulty, colour blindness results. The condition is usually inherited.

What are the types?

The most common type of colour blindness, red–green colour blindness, affects far more males than females, and may take one of two forms. In one form, people are unable to distinguish between pale reds, greens, oranges, and browns. The other form makes shades of red appear dull and indistinct. Red–green colour blindness is caused by an abnormal gene carried on the X chromosome. It mainly affects men because women have a second X chromosome that usually masks the effect of the gene (*see* GENE DISORDERS, p.271). However, women may pass the abnormal gene to their children.

Another, much rarer, type of colour blindness makes it difficult to distinguish between blues and yellows. This form of the condition can be inherited, but because it is not linked to the X chromosome, it affects both females and males in equal numbers. Macular degeneration (p.580) and other eye disorders may cause colour blindness. The toxic effects of some drugs, including chloroquine (*see* ANTIMALARIAL DRUGS, p.888), may also cause colour blindness.

What might be done?

Colour blindness is usually noticed during routine vision testing in childhood (*see* VISION TESTS IN CHILDREN, p.857). It may also be detected during medical tests for jobs requiring normal colour vision, such as flying aeroplanes. The test checks your ability to see numbers in patterns of coloured dots.

Colour blindness is rarely a serious problem. Inherited forms are untreatable, but, if the condition is caused by eye disorders or drugs, the underlying cause can sometimes be treated.

(WWW) ONLINE SITES: p.1031

Blindness

Severe to total loss of vision that cannot be rectified by corrective lenses

 AGE GENDER GENETICS LIFESTYLE Risk factors depend on the cause

Complete or almost complete loss of sight, usually termed blindness, affects at least 40 million people worldwide. Although most of those affected are in developing countries, about 190,000 people in the UK are registered as blind, and many more are visually handicapped. The risk of becoming blind increases with age, but the condition can be present from birth (*see* CONGENITAL BLINDNESS, p.856).

What are the causes?

Blindness may be caused by disorders of the eyes, the nerves that connect the eyes to the brain, or the areas of the brain that process visual information.

In developed countries, blindness is most often caused by a damaged retina due to diabetic retinopathy (p.579) or macular degeneration (p.580), raised fluid pressure in the eye due to glaucoma (p.575), or clouding of the lens due to cataracts (p.573). Cataracts are also a common cause in developing countries, together with the eye infection trachoma (p.572) and vitamin A deficiency (*see* XEROPHTHALMIA, p.585).

What might be done?

Early diagnosis can help some underlying disorders that cause blindness to be treated to preserve vision. For example, if you have glaucoma, you will be given drugs to reduce the pressure in the eye (*see* DRUGS FOR GLAUCOMA, p.920).

If you are registered as blind or visually handicapped, you may be eligible for certain benefits and services. Visual aids, such as magnifying glasses, can make some daily tasks easier.

(WWW) ONLINE SITES: p.1031

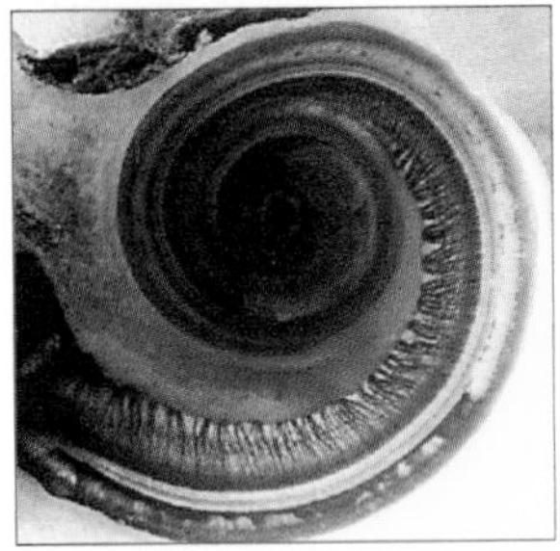

The cochlea in the inner ear
Resembling the shell of a snail, the cochlea is a coiled tubular structure in the inner part of the ear. The central duct of the cochlea contains the spiral organ of Corti, the receptor for hearing.

EARS, HEARING, AND BALANCE

OUR EARS PROVIDE US with two vital but very different senses: hearing and balance. Sound detected by the ears provides essential information about our external surroundings and allows us to communicate in highly sophisticated ways, such as through speech and music. In addition, our ears contribute to our sense of balance, the largely unconscious understanding of the body's orientation in space that allows us to maintain an upright posture and move without falling over.

The ear contains separate organs of hearing and balance, which detect sound from the world around us and internal information about our posture and movement. Sensory structures inside our ears convert the different forms of information into nerve impulses, which travel along nerves to various parts of the brain where the information is analysed. Our ability to interpret sounds and use information about balance develops during infancy and childhood.

THE QUALITIES OF SOUND

Sound is actually a vibration of the molecules in the air all around us. The pitch of a noise (how "high" or "low" it sounds) is determined by a property of sound waves called the frequency. Frequency is the number of vibrations per second and is measured in units called hertz (Hz). The higher the frequency, the higher the pitch.

The intensity or loudness of a sound depends on the power of the sound waves and is measured in units called decibels (dB). For every 10 dB increase in power, our ears hear double the loudness, so noises at 90 dB sound twice as loud as those at only 80 dB. Conversation is typically about 60 dB, and sound from nearby traffic is usually about 80 dB. Even brief exposure to noises over 120 dB can damage our hearing.

We all vary in the acuteness of our hearing (how loud a sound has to be for us to hear it) and in our ability to analyse complex sounds such as music. The human ear can normally detect sounds with frequencies between about 30 Hz and 20,000 Hz, but our ability to hear high-frequency sounds tends to decline with age. Animals such as bats and dogs can hear sounds with frequencies much higher than the normal human range.

BALANCE AND MOVEMENT

The structures of the inner ear that are concerned with balance have two functions: awareness of the head's orientation – where it is in space – and detection of the head's rotation and movement in all directions. The brain combines information from the ears with that from position sensors in the muscles, tendons, and joints and visual information from the eyes. Taken together, this information enables us to move in many different ways without losing our balance.

(STRUCTURE) CONNECTING PASSAGEWAYS

Although the ears may appear to be isolated structures, they are directly linked to the nose and throat. The visible part of the ear, the pinna, is connected to the ear canal, which ends at the eardrum. Beyond this membrane lies the middle ear, an air-filled space connected to the back of the nasal cavity and to the throat by a channel called the eustachian tube. This tube ensures that the air pressure is the same on both sides of the eardrum. The structures of the inner ear lie deep within the skull and contain the sensory organs for sound and balance.

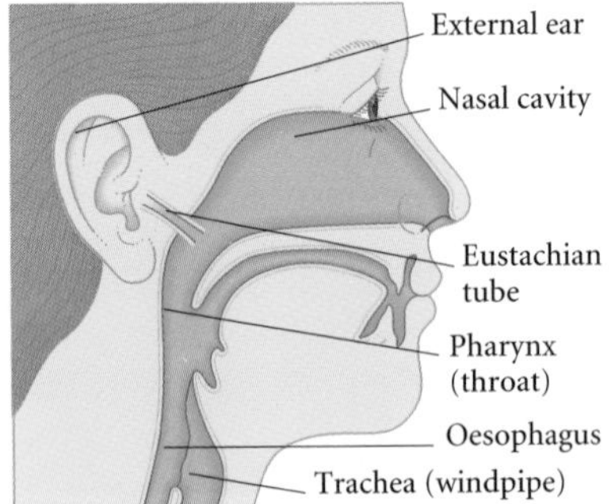

Link between the ear, nose, and throat
The eustachian tube connects the ear to the nasal cavity and throat and maintains equal air pressure on both sides of the eardrum.

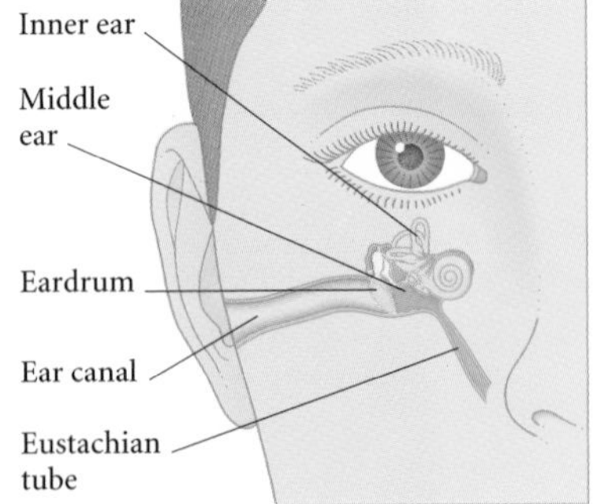

Internal components of the ear
The ear canal runs from the external ear to the middle and inner ear, which are situated inside the skull.

STRUCTURE COMPONENTS OF THE EAR

The ear is made up of the outer, middle, and inner ear. The outer ear consists of the visible pinna and the ear canal. This air-filled tube ends at the eardrum, which vibrates in response to sound. Beyond the eardrum lies the middle ear, also filled with air, which contains three tiny bones called the auditory ossicles – the malleus, incus, and stapes. These bones transmit vibrations from the eardrum to the membrane of the oval window, which separates the middle ear from the inner ear. In the fluid-filled inner ear is the cochlea, which contains the sensory receptor for hearing together with other structures that detect movement and balance.

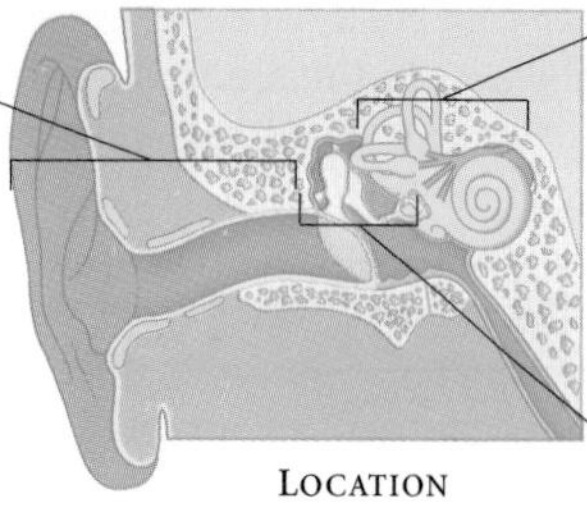

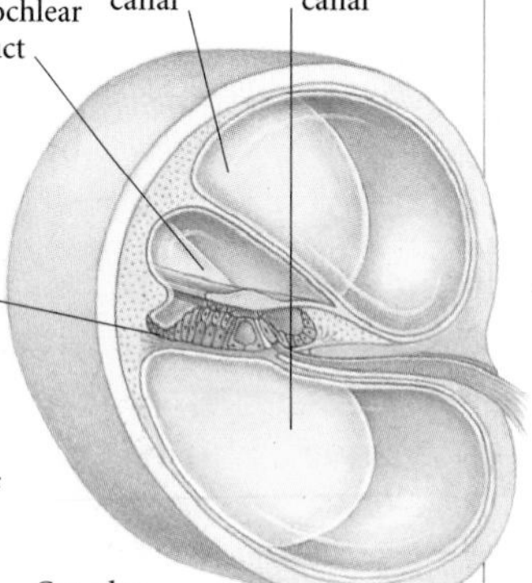

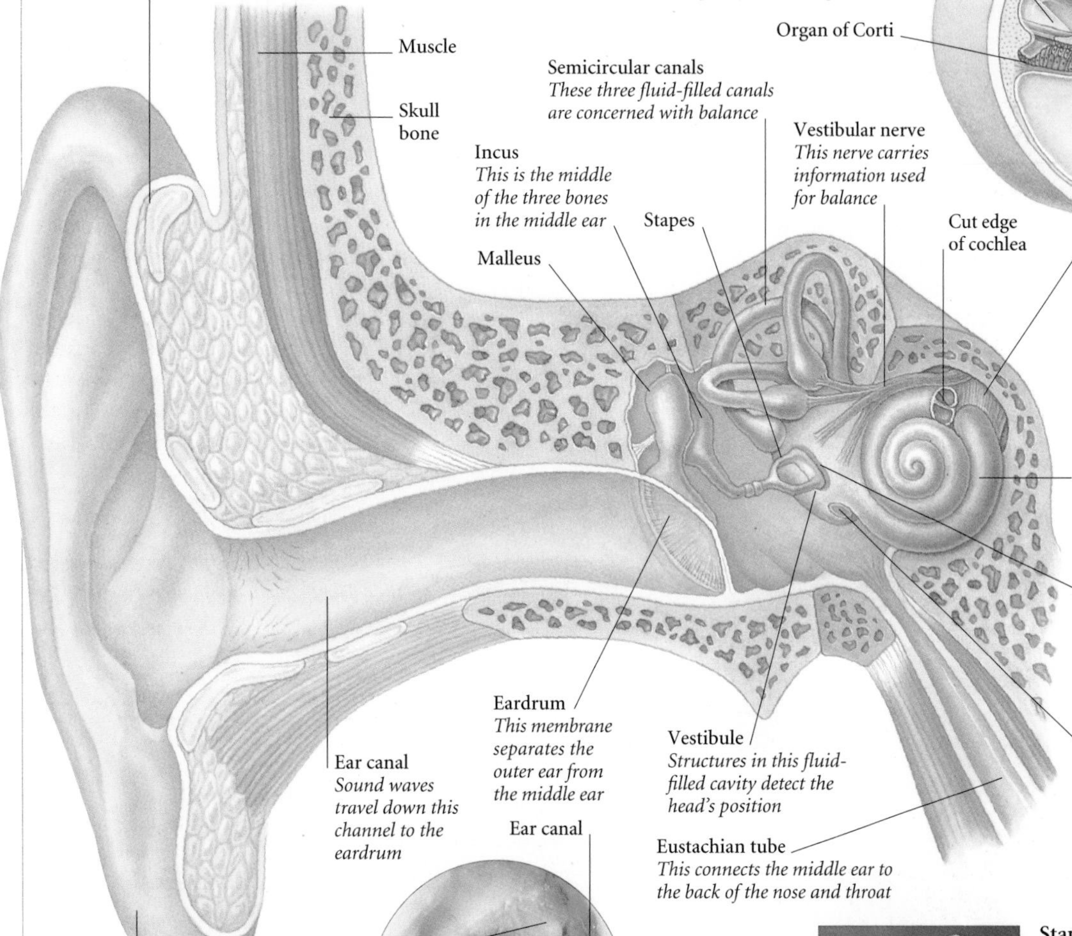

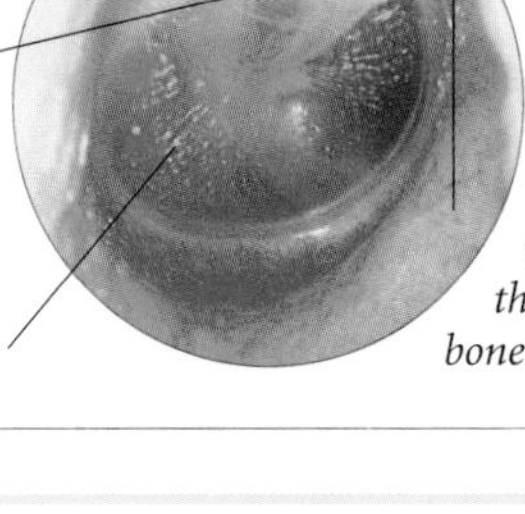

Eardrum
Sound causes this membrane to vibrate. These vibrations pass to the malleus, a tiny bone in the middle ear.

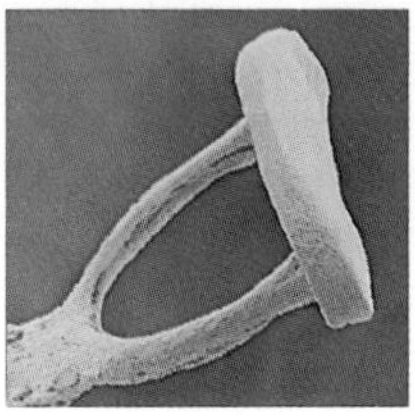

Stapes
This stirrup-shaped bone is one of the three tiny bones in the middle ear. It is the smallest bone in the body.

STRUCTURE AND FUNCTION THE MECHANISM OF HEARING

Our ability to hear depends on a complex series of events that occur in the ear. Sound waves in the air are transmitted as vibrations through a series of structures to the receptor for hearing, the organ of Corti in the inner ear. Inside the organ of Corti, these physical vibrations are detected by sensory hair cells, which respond by producing electrical signals. Nerves carry these signals to the brain, where they are interpreted. Sounds of different frequencies stimulate hair cells in different parts of the organ of Corti, allowing us to perceive the subtleties of sounds such as speech and music.

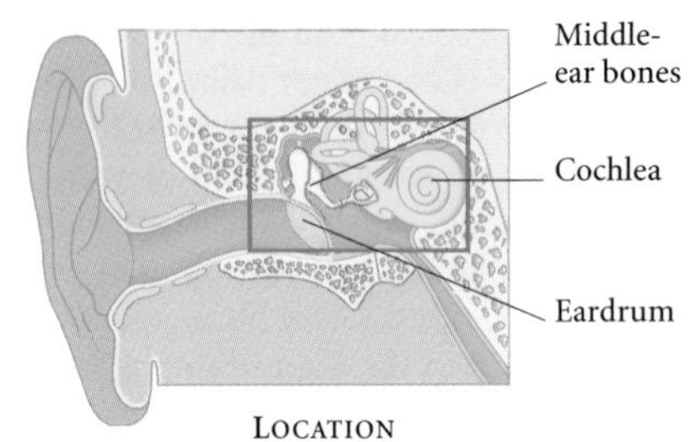

LOCATION

Malleus
This bone is attached to the eardrum and transmits vibrations to a bone called the incus

Incus

Path of incoming vibration

Oval window

Stapes

Vestibular canal
Vibrations of the oval window membrane pass to the fluid in this duct, then to the vestibular membrane

Cochlear duct
The fluid in this duct transmits vibrations to the basilar membrane

Basilar membrane
Vibration of this membrane stimulates the sensory hair cells in the organ of Corti

Cochlear nerve
This carries auditory information from the ear to the brain

Direction of sound wave

Ear canal

Vestibular membrane
Vibrations of this membrane are transmitted to the fluid in the cochlear duct

Eardrum
This thin membrane vibrates in response to sound waves that enter the ear

Round window
This membrane transmits fluid vibrations in the tympanic canal back to the middle ear

Eustachian tube
This tube controls air pressure in the middle ear

Tympanic canal
Residual vibrations pass along the fluid in this duct

Nerve fibres
These join to form the cochlear nerve

Hair cells

Path of weak residual vibrations

Organ of Corti
This receptor for hearing rests on the basilar membrane and contains sensory hair cells

Tectorial membrane
The hair cells of the organ of Corti move against this membrane, producing electrical signals

Direction of nerve impulse
Impulses from the organ of Corti travel along nerve fibres to the cochlear nerve

Hair cell

Sensory hairs

Cochlear nerve

Hair cells in the organ of Corti
This highly magnified cross section shows hair cells in the organ of Corti. The electrical signals produced by these cells travel along the cochlear nerve to the brain.

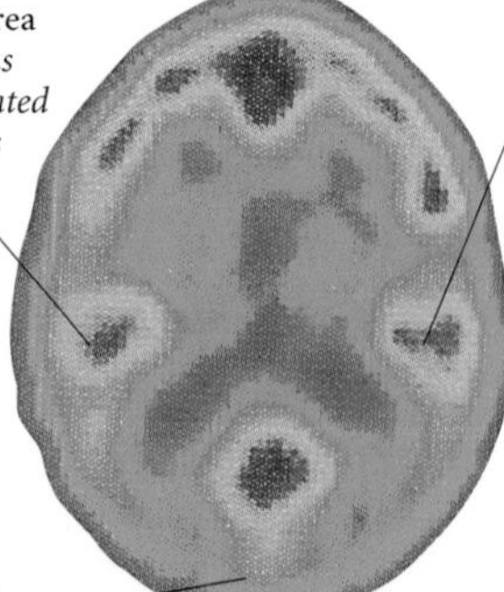

Language area
This area has been stimulated by the words of a song

Music area
This area has been stimulated by music

Back of brain

Brain during auditory stimulation
Sound is processed in auditory areas on both sides of the brain, but speech is interpreted mainly on the left side. This PET scan was taken while the subject was listening to a song, stimulating activity on both sides of the brain.

STRUCTURE AND FUNCTION THE SENSE OF BALANCE

The ability to stand upright and move without falling over depends on our sense of balance. Structures in the inner ear, known as the vestibular apparatus, contribute to balance by detecting the position and movements of the head. The vestibular apparatus is composed of three semicircular canals and the two-chambered vestibule.

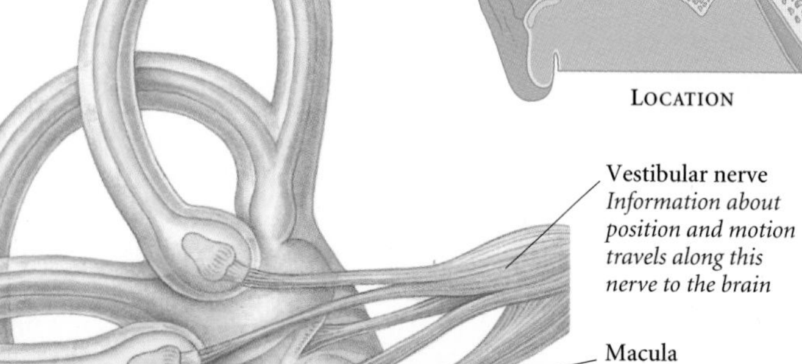

THE ROLE OF HAIR CELLS

The head's movements are detected by hair cells found in structures called cristae in the semicircular canals and in two structures called maculae in the vestibule.

Semicircular canal
The three semicircular canals lie at right angles to each other. When the head turns, fluid in the canals moves, giving information about the speed and direction of motion

Vestibular nerve
Information about position and motion travels along this nerve to the brain

Macula
This sensory area contains hair cells that detect the position of the head

Crista
Sensory hair cells in the cristae are embedded in gelatinous caps called cupulae

Vestibule
The two chambers of the fluid-filled vestibule each contain a sensory structure called a macula

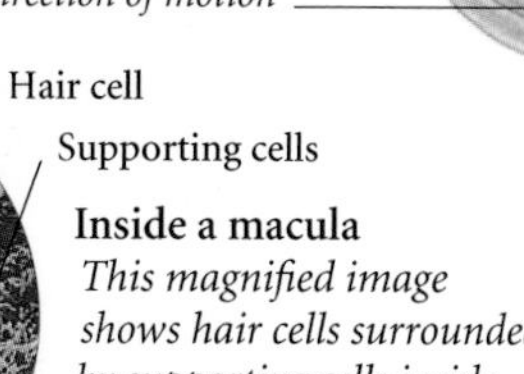

Inside a macula
This magnified image shows hair cells surrounded by supporting cells inside a macula. When the hairs move, the hair cells send electrical impulses to the brain.

LINEAR MOVEMENT AND STATIC POSITION

The two maculae within the vestibule of the inner ear sense linear movements – for example, when travelling by car or using a lift – and the orientation of the head relative to gravity. Detecting the head's position in relation to gravity helps us, for example, to know instantly which way is up when we dive into deep water.

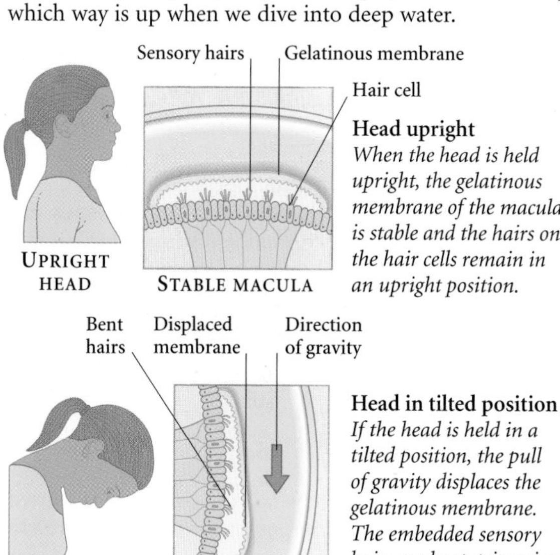

Head upright
When the head is held upright, the gelatinous membrane of the macula is stable and the hairs on the hair cells remain in an upright position.

Head in tilted position
If the head is held in a tilted position, the pull of gravity displaces the gelatinous membrane. The embedded sensory hairs are bent, triggering the hair cells to produce electrical signals.

ROTATIONAL MOVEMENT

Rotational movements of the head are detected by the cristae in the fluid-filled semicircular canals. The three semicircular canals are at right angles to each other, so head rotation in any direction is detected by at least one canal. The information is used both to maintain balance and to keep vision stable when the head moves.

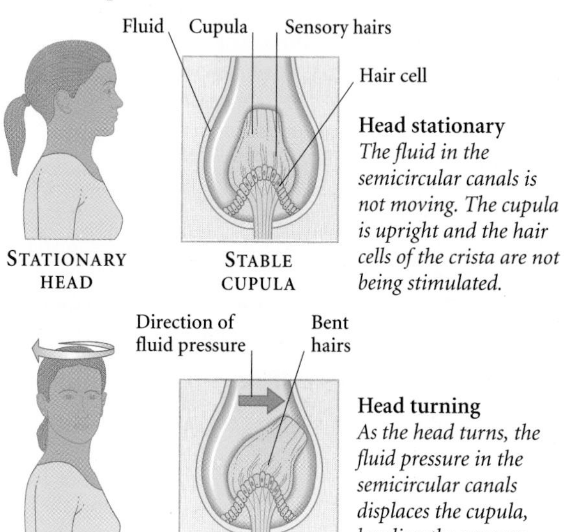

Head stationary
The fluid in the semicircular canals is not moving. The cupula is upright and the hair cells of the crista are not being stimulated.

Head turning
As the head turns, the fluid pressure in the semicircular canals displaces the cupula, bending the sensory hairs, which create electrical impulses.

OUTER- AND MIDDLE-EAR DISORDERS

The outer ear consists of the visible part, called the pinna, which is composed of skin and cartilage, and the ear canal, the channel that leads to the eardrum. Behind the eardrum is the air-filled middle ear, which contains three tiny, delicate bones. The middle ear is directly linked to the respiratory system by the eustachian tube, the passage connecting the ear to the nose and throat.

This section covers disorders of the visible parts of the ear and of the ear canal, followed by conditions that affect the eardrum and middle ear. Outer- and middle-ear disorders have a number of causes, including injury, infections, obstruction, damage from atmospheric pressure changes, and inherited disease. The symptoms of these disorders include irritation, discomfort, pain, and, in some cases, partial hearing loss.

Most outer- and middle- ear problems are more easily treatable than those affecting the inner ear and are less likely to lead to permanent loss of hearing. Most causes of hearing loss are covered elsewhere (*see* HEARING AND INNER-EAR DISORDERS, pp.599–605), as are disorders of the middle ear that particularly affect children (*see* ACUTE OTITIS MEDIA IN CHILDREN, p.860, and CHRONIC SECRETORY OTITIS MEDIA, p.860).

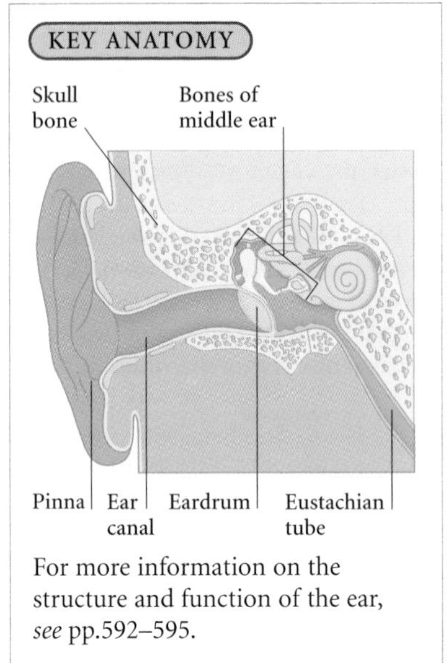

For more information on the structure and function of the ear, *see* pp.592–595.

Outer-ear injury

Damage to the visible part of the ear, sometimes leading to deformity

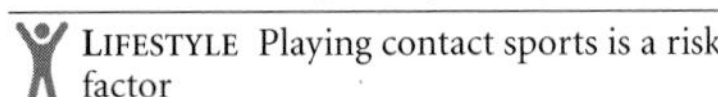

LIFESTYLE Playing contact sports is a risk factor

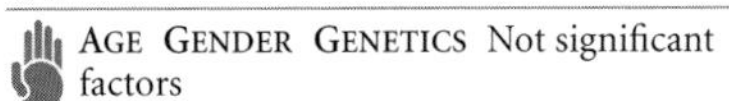

AGE GENDER GENETICS Not significant factors

If the visible part of the outer ear is injured, blood may collect between the skin of the ear and its underlying cartilage, leading to pain and swelling. The collected blood (haematoma) may cut off the supply of blood to the cartilage, which may break down and be gradually replaced by scar tissue. Severe or repeated injury may result in a "cauliflower ear", a deformity that sometimes occurs in boxers and other athletes.

You can reduce the discomfort of an injured ear by applying an ice pack. If the ear is severely swollen, you should consult your doctor. He or she may drain a haematoma under a local anaesthetic or apply a pressure bandage to reduce swelling. Plastic surgery may be necessary to correct a deformity.

When playing contact sports, make sure you wear headgear to protect your ears (*see* EXERCISING SAFELY, p.59).

(WWW) ONLINE SITES: p.1031, p.1036

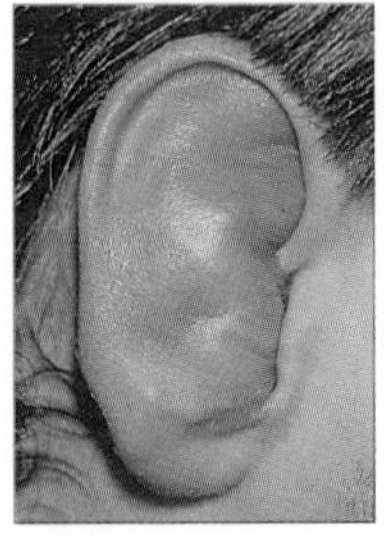

Outer-ear injury *The visible part of this ear is swollen and distorted due to a large collection of blood under the skin. The injury was caused by a blow to the ear.*

Otitis externa

Inflammation of the ear canal, commonly known as "swimmer's ear"

LIFESTYLE Swimming or wearing a hearing aid or earplugs are risk factors

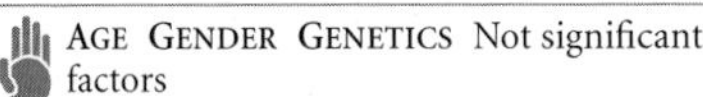

AGE GENDER GENETICS Not significant factors

In otitis externa, the ear canal becomes inflamed, usually because of bacterial, viral, or fungal infection. Otitis externa often develops after swimming because persistent moisture within the ear canal increases the risk of infection. The condition can also affect people who work in a hot and humid environment or who wear a hearing aid or earplugs. Scratching the ear with a cotton swab or fingernail is another cause of otitis externa. Less commonly, the infection occurs as a reaction to chemicals such as those in eardrops or hair dye.

WHAT ARE THE SYMPTOMS?

The symptoms of otitis externa usually appear over 1–2 days and may include:

- Itching and/or pain within the ear canal at the affected site.
- Discharge of pus from the ear.

If pus blocks the canal, see your doctor rather than trying to remove it yourself.

WHAT MIGHT BE DONE?

Your doctor will examine your ear with an otoscope (*see* OTOSCOPY, opposite page). If there is pus present, indicating infection, he or she may take a swab to identify the organism responsible. The ear canal may also be cleaned out using a suction device. Depending on the type of infection present, your doctor may prescribe eardrops that contain an antibiotic or antifungal and/or a corticosteroid (*see* DRUGS ACTING ON THE EAR, p.921). An oral painkiller (p.912) may also be given to relieve discomfort.

If you have a severe bacterial infection, your doctor may prescribe oral antibiotics (p.885). Most viral infections are treated solely with painkillers. However, if the condition is caused by the herpes virus, you may be prescribed an oral antiviral drug (p.886), sometimes with a corticosteroid (p.930). The disorder usually clears up in a few days.

(WWW) ONLINE SITES: p.1031, p.1033

Wax blockage

Blockage of the ear canal by earwax, often causing a feeling of fullness and irritation in the ear

AGE GENDER GENETICS LIFESTYLE
Not significant factors

Earwax, produced by glands in the ear canal, cleans and moistens the canal. Usually, wax is produced in small quantities and emerges naturally from the ear. However, if the canal becomes blocked with wax, it causes a feeling of fullness and discomfort and sometimes hearing loss. A common cause of wax blockage is insertion of a cotton swab or finger into the canal in an attempt to remove the wax. This action usually pushes the wax deeper into the canal. Excessive secretion of wax may also lead to blockage.

Wax blockage can be treated with over-the-counter eardrops, which usually dissolve the earwax in about 4–10 days. If the ear remains blocked, you should consult your doctor. He or she will probably use a viewing instrument to inspect the ear canal (*see* OTOSCOPY, right). You may have the wax removed with a probe or suction device, or the ear may be gently flushed out with warm water from a syringe. Wax blockage sometimes recurs after treatment.

(WWW) ONLINE SITES: p.1031

Otitis media

Inflammation of the middle ear, usually as a result of a bacterial or viral infection

AGE More common in children but can occur at any age

GENDER GENETICS LIFESTYLE
Not significant factors

In otitis media, tissues lining the middle ear are inflamed, and pus and fluid accumulate in the middle ear, causing pain and partial hearing loss. The condition occurs when a viral infection, such as a common cold (p.288) or influenza (p.289), or a bacterial infection spreads from the throat to the middle ear. The infection may cause a ruptured eardrum (right). Otitis media is common in children. This is because their eustachian tubes, which connect the ear to the back of the nose and throat and ventilate the middle ear, are immature and easily blocked by large structures, such as adenoids (*see* ACUTE OTITIS MEDIA IN CHILDREN, p.860). Sometimes, a sticky fluid persistently collects in the middle ear, impairing hearing (*see* CHRONIC SECRETORY OTITIS MEDIA, p.860).

WHAT ARE THE SYMPTOMS?

The symptoms of otitis media often develop over a few hours and include:

- Pain in the ear, which may be severe.
- Partial hearing loss.
- Fever.

If the eardrum ruptures, there may be a bloodstained discharge from the ear and a decrease in pain. Untreated otitis media may become a chronic infection with a constant discharge of pus from the ear. Rarely, the infection results in a cholesteatoma, a collection of skin cells and debris, in the middle ear. This complication may damage the middle ear and rarely the inner ear, causing permanent loss of hearing.

WHAT MIGHT BE DONE?

Your doctor will examine your ear with an otoscope (*see* OTOSCOPY, below) to check if your eardrum is inflamed and to see if there is pus in the middle ear. You may be prescribed oral antibiotics (p.885) and may be given painkillers (p.912). In most cases, the pain subsides in a few days, but mild hearing loss may sometimes persist for a week or two. If a cholesteatoma has developed, it is usually necessary for it to be removed by surgery.

(WWW) ONLINE SITES: p.1031, p.1033

Ruptured eardrum

A tear or hole in the membrane between the outer and middle ear

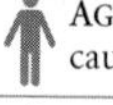
AGE LIFESTYLE Risk factors depend on the cause

GENDER GENETICS Not significant factors

Rupture of the eardrum most commonly results from an acute bacterial infection of the middle ear (*see* OTITIS MEDIA, left). Pus or other fluid produced by the infection builds up inside the middle ear and eventually bursts through the eardrum. Less commonly, a rupture occurs when an object, such as a cotton swab or hairpin, is poked into the ear. In some cases, the eardrum suddenly ruptures because there is an imbalance between the pressures inside the middle ear and the outer ear. Such an imbalance of pressure in different parts of the ear may occur after a blow to the ear, an explosion, a head injury (p.521), or when flying or diving (*see* BAROTRAUMA, p.598).

WHAT ARE THE SYMPTOMS?

The symptoms usually last for only a few hours and may include:

- Sudden, sometimes intense pain in the affected ear.
- Bloodstained discharge from the ear.
- Partial hearing loss.

If you suspect that you have a ruptured eardrum, keep the affected ear dry and consult your doctor as soon as possible.

(TEST) OTOSCOPY

The ear canal and eardrum can be examined directly by using an otoscope, a viewing instrument that illuminates and magnifies the inside of the ear. Otoscopy is used to diagnose disorders such as otitis media and ruptured eardrum.

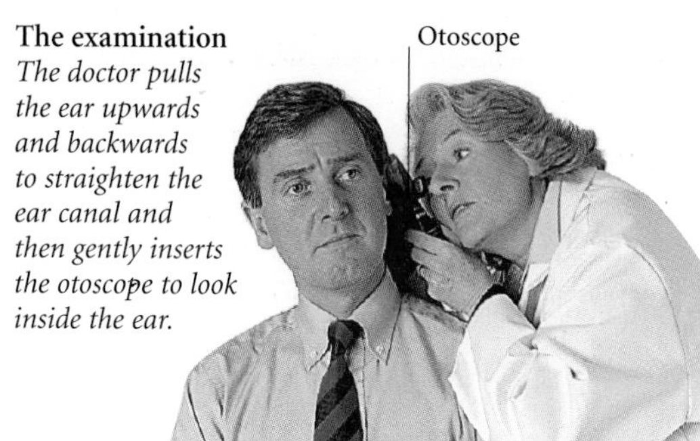

The examination
The doctor pulls the ear upwards and backwards to straighten the ear canal and then gently inserts the otoscope to look inside the ear.

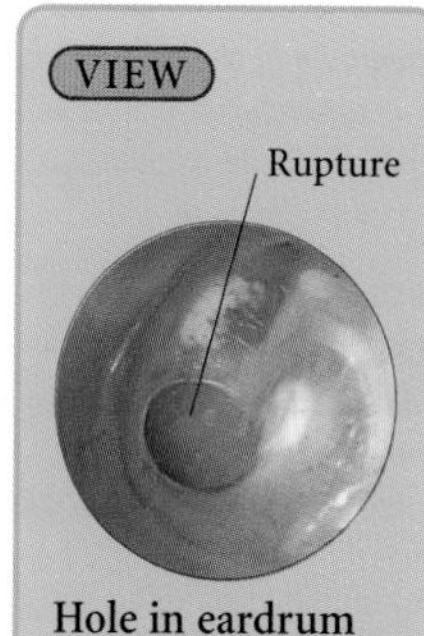

Hole in eardrum
This eardrum has ruptured as a result of a long-standing bacterial infection of the middle ear.

WHAT MIGHT BE DONE?

Your doctor may inspect your ear (*see* OTOSCOPY, p.597). A ruptured eardrum usually heals within a month. Infection can be treated with antibiotics (p.885). Rarely, ruptures caused by an infection need to be repaired with a tissue graft.

(WWW) ONLINE SITES: p.1031, p.1036

Barotrauma

Damage or pain, mainly affecting the middle ear, caused by pressure changes

LIFESTYLE Air travel and diving are risk factors

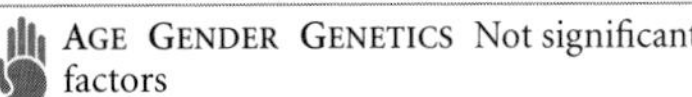

AGE GENDER GENETICS Not significant factors

If the pressure on the outer side of the eardrum exceeds the pressure on the inner side, the middle ear may become damaged or painful, a condition called barotrauma. Changes in outside pressure are common when flying or diving and may cause pain or a feeling of fullness in the ears. If you swallow or hold your nose and exhale with your mouth closed, the eustachian tubes, which connect the ears to the nose and throat will usually open, allowing air into the middle ear and equalizing the pressure. If insufficient air enters the middle ear, barotrauma occurs. The condition is more likely if the eustachian tubes are blocked as a result of a cold or ear infection (*see* OTITIS MEDIA, p.597).

Small pressure changes may cause pain and temporary ringing or buzzing in the ears (*see* TINNITUS, p.602). An extreme pressure imbalance may lead to a ruptured eardrum (p.597), bleeding into the middle ear, or damage to the inner ear, which may result in hearing loss and vertigo (p.603).

If symptoms do not clear up in a few hours, see your doctor. If you have a cold or ear infection, avoid flying or diving. If you must fly, use a decongestant (p.909) beforehand to clear the eustachian tubes.

(WWW) ONLINE SITES: p.1031, p.1036.

(TREATMENT) STAPEDOTOMY

This operation is carried out to treat otosclerosis (right), a disorder in which the stapes bone in the middle ear becomes immobilized by bony overgrowth, causing hearing loss. Under local or general anaesthesia, parts of the stapes are removed and replaced by a prosthesis. Stapedotomy is usually successful, but there is a small risk that hearing may deteriorate further.

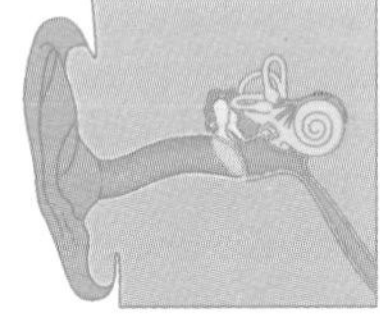

LOCATION

Before surgery
The stapes has become immobilized due to bony overgrowth around its base, so that sound vibrations cannot travel to the inner ear. During the operation, the body of the stapes bone is removed and a hole is drilled in the bony area around the base.

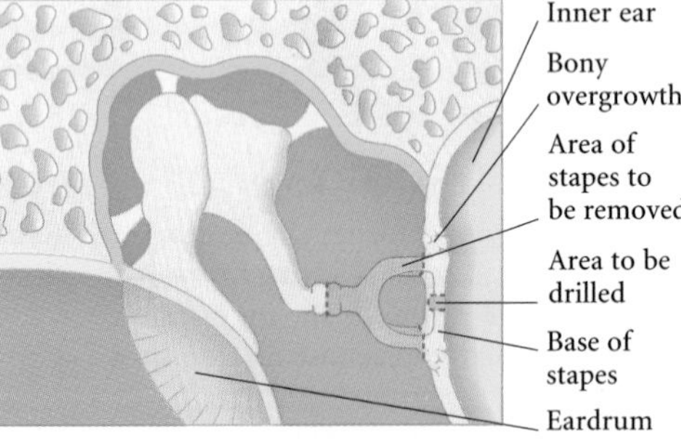

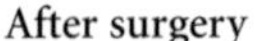

After surgery
The body of the stapes is replaced by a prosthetic piston. The piston is able to move freely in and out of the hole in the bony area, transmitting vibrations to the inner ear.

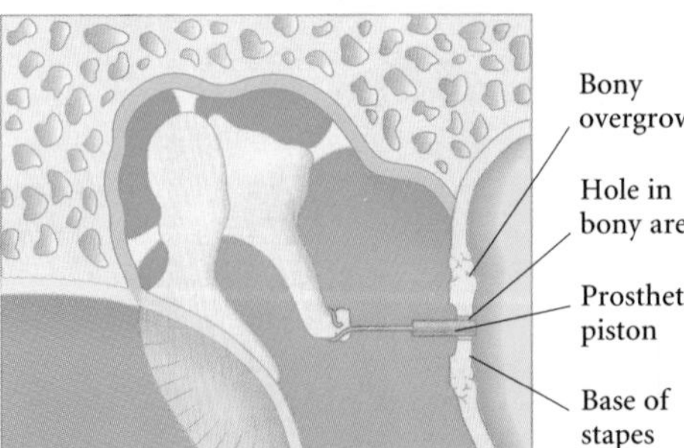

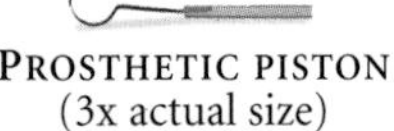

PROSTHETIC PISTON
(3x actual size)

Otosclerosis

Abnormal growth of bone between the middle and inner ear, often leading to hearing loss

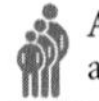

AGE Symptoms usually develop between the ages of 20 and 30

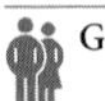

GENDER Twice as common in females

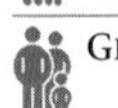

GENETICS Often runs in families

LIFESTYLE Not a significant factor

Otosclerosis is a condition in which, for unknown reasons, bone begins to overgrow around the base of the stapes, the innermost of the three tiny bones in the middle ear. The stapes gradually becomes immobilized, preventing the transmission of sound vibrations to the inner ear and causing progressive loss of hearing. Usually both ears are affected, although not always equally. As the disease progresses, nerve damage may occur in the inner ear.

Although otosclerosis affects about 1 in 12 people, the condition does not usually cause symptoms. If symptoms do develop, they usually first appear between the ages of 20 and 30. The disorder is twice as common in women as it is in men and often progresses more quickly during pregnancy. In 6 out of 10 people with otosclerosis, the condition runs in the family.

WHAT ARE THE SYMPTOMS?

The symptoms of otosclerosis develop gradually and may include:

- Hearing loss in which sounds are muffled but may appear to be clearer if there is background noise.
- Ringing or buzzing noises in the ears (*see* TINNITUS, p.602).

In severe cases, dizziness and imbalance (*see* VERTIGO, p.603) may also develop.

WHAT MIGHT BE DONE?

Your doctor will probably be able to diagnose otosclerosis from the results of hearing tests (p.600) and from your family history. There is no drug treatment that halts the progression of the disease, but you will be offered a choice between using a hearing aid (p.601) and having surgery to replace the immobilized stapes (*see* STAPEDOTOMY, left).

(WWW) ONLINE SITES: p.1032

HEARING AND INNER-EAR DISORDERS

Disorders of hearing are very common and, in severe cases, they may interfere with communication, causing significant disability. In some cases, hearing loss is due to a disorder of the ear canal or the middle ear, but inner-ear disorders can also cause hearing problems. The inner ear also contains the vestibular apparatus, which helps to maintain the sense of balance. Inner-ear disorders may therefore lead to other symptoms such as dizziness.

This section starts by discussing all types of hearing loss from partial loss of hearing to total deafness. Hearing defects that are due to disorders of the inner ear, including noise-induced hearing loss and tinnitus (various sounds heard in one or both ears in the absence of an external source), are then covered in greater detail.

Problems in other parts of the ear that may cause hearing loss or deafness are covered elsewhere in the book (*see* OUTER- AND MIDDLE-EAR DISORDERS, pp.596–598), as is hearing loss or deafness that is present from birth (*see* CONGENITAL DEAFNESS, p.859).

Inner-ear disorders do not only affect hearing; if the vestibular apparatus is disturbed, the sense of balance may be disrupted. Three common inner-ear disorders that affect balance – motion sickness, labyrinthitis, and Ménière's disease – are described in this section. All of these disorders may cause symptoms such as dizziness and nausea. Ménière's disease can also lead to hearing loss. The final article in this section discusses acoustic neuroma, a rare, noncancerous tumour affecting the vestibulocochlear nerve, which connects the inner ear to the brain.

KEY ANATOMY

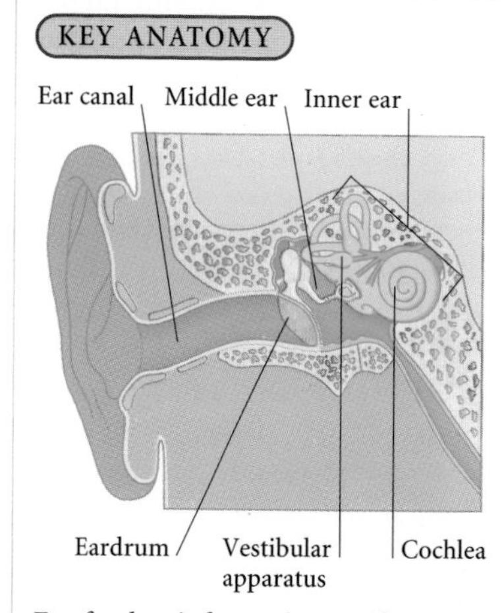

For further information on the structure and function of the ear, *see* pp.592–595.

Hearing loss

Partial or total loss of hearing in one or both ears

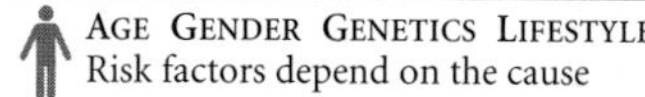

Partial or total hearing impairment can severely restrict social interaction, leading to isolation and depression (p.554). Hearing loss may result from disease or injury, and most people experience deterioration of hearing with age (*see* PRESBYACUSIS, p.601). Hearing defects may also be present from birth; about 2 in every 1,000 babies are born with some degree of hearing impairment (*see* CONGENITAL DEAFNESS, p.859).

WHAT ARE THE TYPES?

There are two different types of hearing loss: conductive and sensorineural. Conductive hearing loss is caused by a failure of the outer or middle ear to transmit sound to the inner ear. This type of hearing loss is often temporary. Sensorineural hearing loss may be caused by disorders of the cochlea, which is the part of the inner ear that detects sound, or the vestibulocochlear nerve, which connects the inner ear to the brain. Sensorineural hearing loss is usually permanent.

CONDUCTIVE HEARING LOSS The most common cause of conductive hearing loss in children is chronic secretory otitis media (p.860), in which the middle ear fills with fluid following an infection. In adults, conductive hearing loss is often due to blockage of the ear canal (*see* WAX BLOCKAGE, p.597). It can also result from a ruptured eardrum (p.597) or sudden changes in air pressure (*see* BAROTRAUMA, p.598). In rare cases, conductive hearing loss is due to otosclerosis (p.598), a condition in which one of the three very small bones in the middle ear becomes immobilized and unable to transmit sound.

SENSORINEURAL HEARING LOSS This type of hearing loss is commonly due to deterioration of the cochlea with age. Most people over the age of 70 have a degree of sensorineural deafness. The condition may also result from damage to the cochlea by excessive noise (*see* NOISE-INDUCED HEARING LOSS, p.601) or by the inner-ear disorder Ménière's disease (p.604). Rarely, sensorineural hearing loss is caused by a tumour that affects the vestibulocochlear nerve (*see* ACOUSTIC NEUROMA, p.605).

WHAT MIGHT BE DONE?

Your doctor will examine your ear with a viewing instrument called an otoscope (*see* OTOSCOPY, p.597). Hearing tests (p.600) may then be performed to establish whether the hearing loss is conductive or sensorineural and also to assess the degree of loss. If a tumour of the vestibulocochlear nerve is suspected, your doctor may arrange for examination of the nerve using MRI (p.248).

If you have conductive hearing loss, treatment of the underlying cause may restore your hearing to near normal. Sensorineural hearing loss is often permanent, although a hearing aid (p.601) may be helpful. In cases of profound sensorineural deafness, a cochlear implant (p.603), in which electrodes are surgically implanted in the cochlea, may allow hearing of sounds such as speech.

(WWW) ONLINE SITES: p.1032

(TEST) HEARING TESTS

Your doctor may recommend hearing tests if you have difficulty hearing speech or if you work in a noisy environment. He or she may perform preliminary tests in the surgery and may refer you to a hearing specialist for others. Some tests determine the type of hearing loss, while others assess how well you can hear sounds of varying frequency and volume. Children should be tested regularly, especially if they are late in beginning to talk (*see* HEARING TESTS IN CHILDREN, p.859).

PRELIMINARY TESTS

A tuning fork is used to distinguish conductive hearing loss, resulting from a disorder of the outer or middle ear, from sensorineural loss, which is caused by a disorder of the inner ear or of the nerves that transmit hearing to the brain.

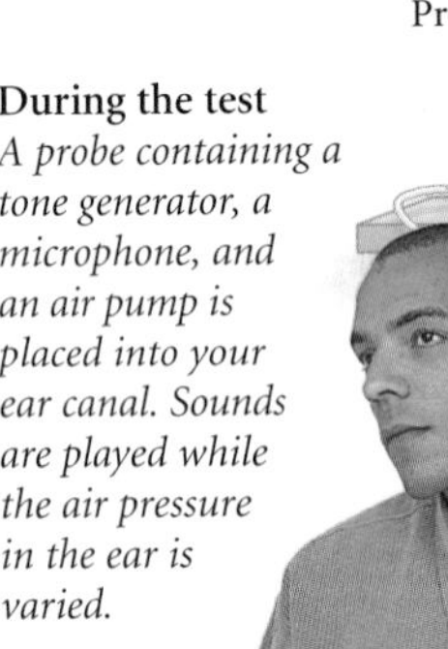

Weber test
A vibrating tuning fork is held against your forehead. If you have conductive hearing loss, the sound will seem louder in the more affected ear. In sensorineural loss, it is louder in the less affected ear.

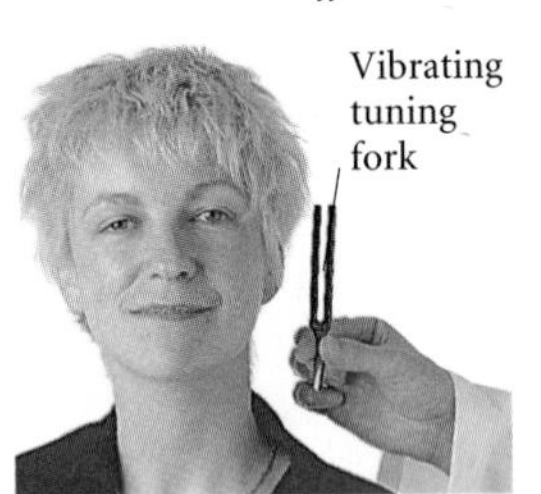

Rinne test
A vibrating tuning fork is held near your ear and then against a bone behind the ear. If it sounds louder in the second position, you have conductive hearing loss. If it is louder in the first position, either the ear is healthy or the hearing loss is sensorineural.

TYMPANOMETRY

Detailed information about the movements of the eardrum and bones of the middle ear in response to sound can be obtained by tympanometry. The test is used to establish the cause of conductive hearing loss and is often used in children because it does not rely on responses from the person being tested.

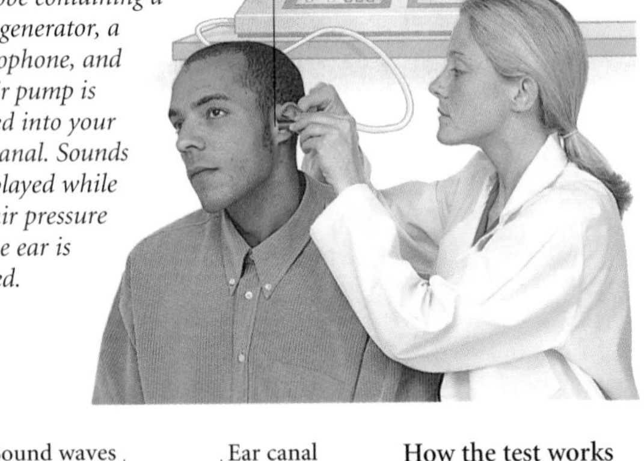

During the test
A probe containing a tone generator, a microphone, and an air pump is placed into your ear canal. Sounds are played while the air pressure in the ear is varied.

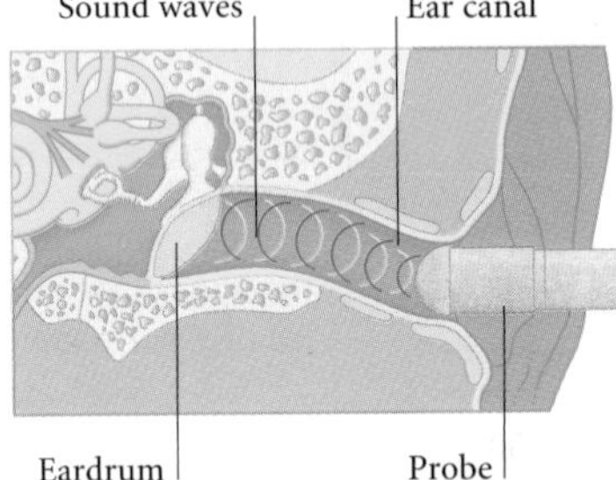

How the test works
The sounds bounce off the eardrum and are picked up by a microphone. The pattern of reflected sound varies at different air pressures and shows whether the eardrum is moving normally.

AUDIOMETRY

This test measures how loud a sound has to be for you to hear it. Sounds of varying frequency are transmitted to one ear at a time through headphones. For each frequency, the volume is increased until you hear it, and the results are recorded. The test is repeated with a speaker held against a bone behind the ear.

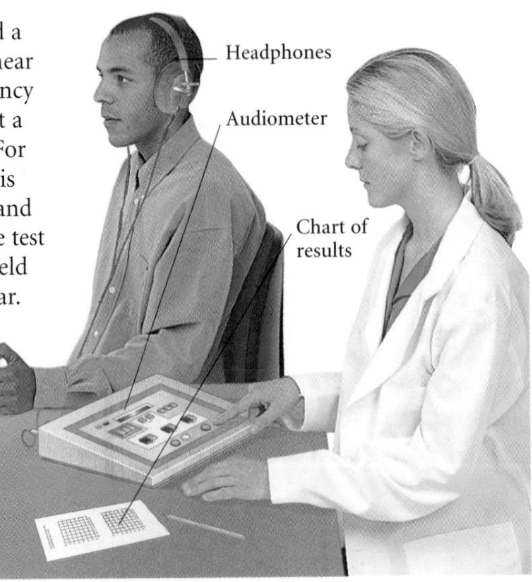

During the test
You will be asked to press a button when you hear a sound in either ear. The softest sound that you can hear at each frequency will be recorded.

(RESULTS)

HEARING LOSS (dB): -20, 0, 20, 40, 60, 80, 100
FREQUENCY (hertz): 125, 250, 500, 1000, 2000, 4000, 8000
Left ear
Right ear

Audiometry trace
This trace is from a person with normal hearing in the left ear and sensorineural hearing loss in the right. At higher frequencies, the right ear can detect sound only if the sound level is much higher than normal.

TREATMENT HEARING AIDS

Hearing aids amplify sounds, improving hearing in people with most types of hearing loss. These devices have a tiny microphone, amplifier, and speaker, all powered by batteries. The range of sounds amplified by a hearing aid is tailored to the individual's pattern of hearing loss.

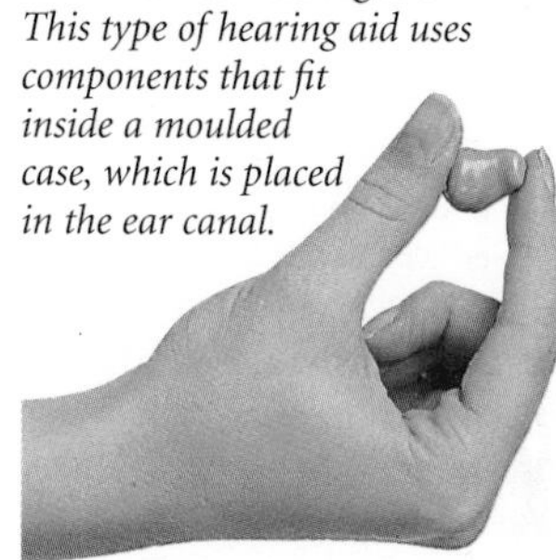

In-the-canal hearing aid
This type of hearing aid uses components that fit inside a moulded case, which is placed in the ear canal.

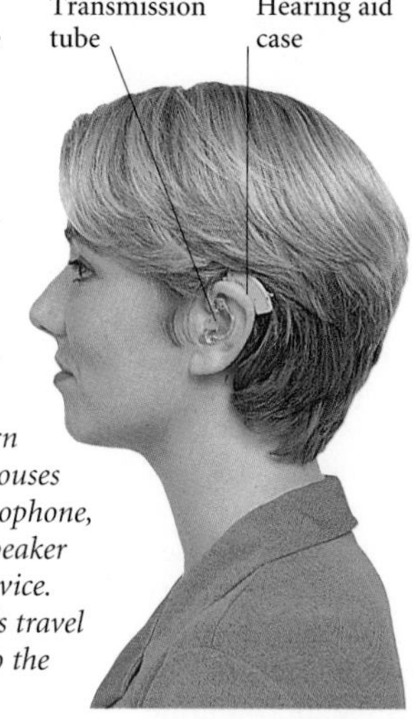

Behind-the-ear hearing aid
A small case worn behind the ear houses the battery, microphone, amplifier, and speaker of this type of device. Amplified sounds travel along a tube into the ear canal.

Presbyacusis

Gradual loss of hearing that develops as a natural part of aging

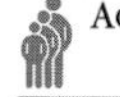 AGE More common over the age of 50

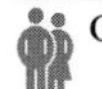 GENDER More common in males

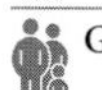 GENETICS Sometimes runs in families

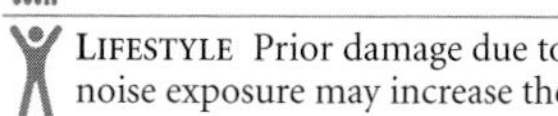 LIFESTYLE Prior damage due to excessive noise exposure may increase the severity

Many people over the age of 50 notice that they find it hard to hear quiet or high-pitched sounds and conversation is sometimes difficult to understand, particularly when there is background noise, such as music. Over a period of years, sounds of all pitches may become increasingly difficult to hear. This progressive decline in hearing is known as presbyacusis and is a common feature of the normal process of aging.

Presbyacusis occurs in about 1 in 5 people aged 50–60, 1 in 3 people aged 60–70, and half of all people over 70. The condition is more common and severe in men and may run in families.

WHAT ARE THE CAUSES?

The body's sensory receptor for hearing, located in the cochlea in the inner ear, is lined with sensory hair cells. Presbyacusis occurs when these sensory hair cells degenerate and die with age. The condition is occasionally more severe in people whose hearing has already been damaged by exposure to excessive levels of noise (*see* NOISE-INDUCED HEARING LOSS, right).

WHAT ARE THE SYMPTOMS?

The symptoms of presbyacusis develop gradually, often over a number of years, and may include:

- Loss of hearing, initially of high-pitched sounds and gradually of lower pitches.
- Difficulty in hearing speech, especially with noise in the background.
- Loss of sound clarity, so that even loud speech is difficult to understand.

Both ears are usually affected, although not always equally. The severity and progression of hearing loss vary from person to person. Severe hearing loss sometimes leads to feelings of isolation, loneliness, and depression (p.554).

WHAT MIGHT BE DONE?

Your doctor will examine your ears with a viewing instrument called an otoscope (*see* OTOSCOPY, p.597). He or she may also arrange for various hearing tests to determine the type and degree of hearing loss (*see* HEARING TESTS, opposite page). There is no cure for presbyacusis. However, a hearing aid (above) may greatly improve your ability to hear and communicate, although it may take a while for you to adjust to using one at first.

WWW ONLINE SITES: p.1032

Noise-induced hearing loss

Hearing loss caused by prolonged exposure to excessive noise or by brief exposure to intensely loud noise

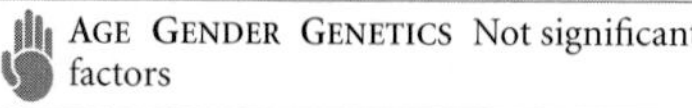 LIFESTYLE A noisy workplace and using a portable stereo are risk factors

AGE GENDER GENETICS Not significant factors

Persistent exposure to extremely loud noise or a single intensely loud sound can both damage the delicate sensory hair cells that line the receptor for hearing within the inner ear. Temporary or permanent hearing loss may result.

Your risk of noise-induced hearing loss is increased if there is excessive noise in your workplace, if you listen to loud music, or if you regularly attend rock concerts. A single excessively loud noise, such as an explosion, may cause immediate hearing loss and can also lead to a ruptured eardrum (p.597).

A few simple steps, such as using earplugs, can reduce your risk of noise-induced hearing loss (*see* PROTECTING YOUR HEARING, p.602).

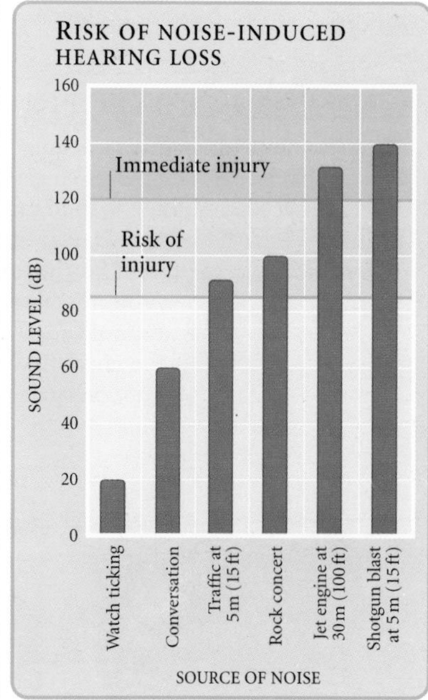

Noise levels and damage to hearing
The intensity of sound is measured in decibels (dB). A 10-dB increase doubles the loudness, so that 90 dB sounds twice as loud as 80 dB. As shown in this graph, noises above 85 dB can damage hearing.

WHAT ARE THE SYMPTOMS?

Exposure to very loud noises can cause immediate symptoms. These usually affect both ears and may include:

- Loss of hearing, particularly of high-pitched sounds.
- Ringing or buzzing sounds in the ears (*see* TINNITUS, right).
- Pain in the ears following intensely loud noises.

Immediate symptoms of noise-induced hearing loss are almost always temporary, and hearing returns to normal after a few hours or days. However, permanent hearing loss may occur as a result of either a single, loud noise or repeated exposure to excessive noise.

If your symptoms persist, or if you work in a noisy environment or regularly listen to loud music and notice a change in your hearing, you should consult your doctor.

WHAT MIGHT BE DONE?

Your doctor may perform hearing tests (p.600) and may arrange for further tests to assess the pattern of any hearing loss. Noise-induced hearing loss cannot be cured, although using a hearing aid (p.601) may make understanding conversation and communication easier.

(WWW) ONLINE SITES: p.1032, p.1036

Tinnitus

Sounds heard in one or both ears in the absence of external noise

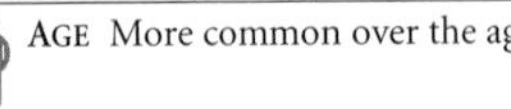
AGE More common over the age of 60

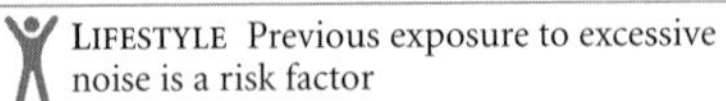
LIFESTYLE Previous exposure to excessive noise is a risk factor

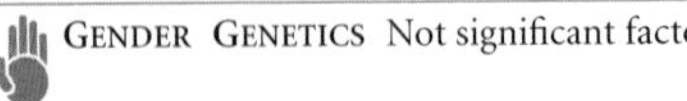
GENDER GENETICS Not significant factors

People with tinnitus hear sounds that originate within the ear itself. These sounds may include ringing, buzzing, whistling, roaring, or hissing noises in the ears. These sounds may vary in intensity and pulse in time with the heartbeat, but they are usually continuous. For some people, the episodes of tinnitus are brief, but for others it is a permanent condition.

In many cases, tinnitus is associated with hearing loss, and your risk of developing tinnitus is increased if you have previously been exposed to loud noises. The condition is more common in older people and affects approximately 3 in 10 people over the age of 60.

Most people with tinnitus are only aware of the sounds when they listen carefully, but for others the condition may be intrusive and lead to difficulties in concentrating or in getting to sleep (*see* INSOMNIA, p.554). In these cases, tinnitus may lead to depression (p.554) and anxiety disorders (p.551).

WHAT ARE THE CAUSES?

Tinnitus may occur for no apparent reason, but it is often associated with certain ear disorders, such as Ménière's disease (p.604), presbyacusis (p.601), or noise-induced hearing loss (p.601).

In some cases, tinnitus can be the result of a deficiency of the blood pigment that carries oxygen (*see* ANAEMIA, p.446) or an overactive thyroid gland (*see* HYPERTHYROIDISM, p.679). Other causes of tinnitus include head injuries (p.521) and treatment with various drugs, such as aspirin (*see* PAINKILLERS, p.912) and certain antibiotics (p.885). Tinnitus that affects one ear only may be a symptom of a tumour affecting the vestibulocochlear nerve, which carries information from the inner ear to the brain (*see* ACOUSTIC NEUROMA, p.605).

If you develop tinnitus, particularly if it affects one ear only, you should consult your doctor.

WHAT MIGHT BE DONE?

Your doctor will examine your ear with a viewing instrument called an otoscope (*see* OTOSCOPY, p.597) and may arrange for hearing tests (p.600). He or she may also arrange for other tests to look for an underlying disorder. These tests may include a blood test for anaemia, as well as CT scanning (p.247) or MRI (p.248) to rule out a tumour.

If an underlying cause is found and successfully treated, the tinnitus may improve. If tinnitus persists, your doctor may recommend a device called a masker. This device, worn in or behind the ear like a hearing aid, produces sounds that distract you from the tinnitus. If tinnitus accompanies hearing loss, a hearing aid (p.601) may provide relief by increasing your awareness of background noise while masking the internal sounds. Many people with tinnitus find that background noise, such as playing music, reduces their awareness of the sounds in their ears.

If tinnitus is particularly distressing or leads to depression or anxiety, counselling (p.971), self-help groups, or relaxation exercises (p.75) may help.

(WWW) ONLINE SITES: p.1032

(SELF-HELP) PROTECTING YOUR HEARING

Excessive noise can damage the inner ear and lead to hearing loss. If possible, you should avoid exposure to loud noise. For example, do not listen to loud music, especially on a portable stereo. If exposure is unavoidable in your work, always take steps to prevent hearing loss by using ear protectors or earplugs. You should also have regular tests to check that your hearing is not being damaged.

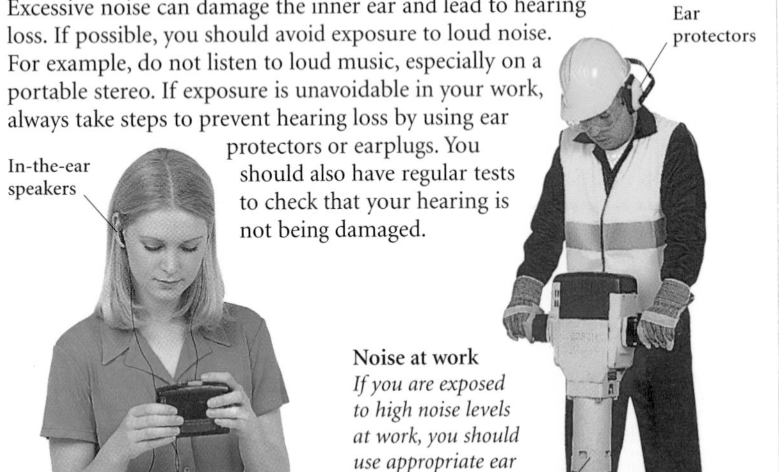

Using a portable stereo
When listening to music on a portable stereo, you should still be able to hear conversation.

Noise at work
If you are exposed to high noise levels at work, you should use appropriate ear protection to prevent noise-induced hearing loss.

TREATMENT COCHLEAR IMPLANTS

A cochlear implant is used to treat profoundly deaf people who are not helped by hearing aids. The device consists of tiny electrodes surgically implanted in the cochlea deep in the inner ear and a receiver that is embedded in the skull just behind and above the ear. A microphone, sound processor, and transmitter are worn externally. A cochlear implant does not restore normal hearing, but it enables patterns of sound to be detected. Combined with lip-reading, it may enable speech to be understood.

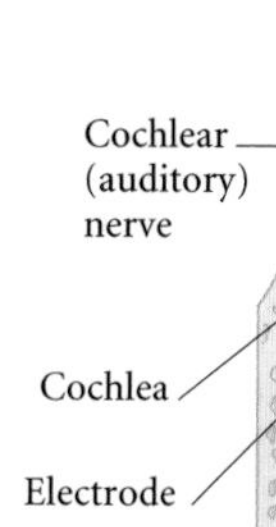

External components
The microphone detects sounds and converts them into electrical signals, which travel to the sound processor. Selected signals are relayed back to the transmitter behind the ear and then transmitted to the implanted components of the cochlear implant.

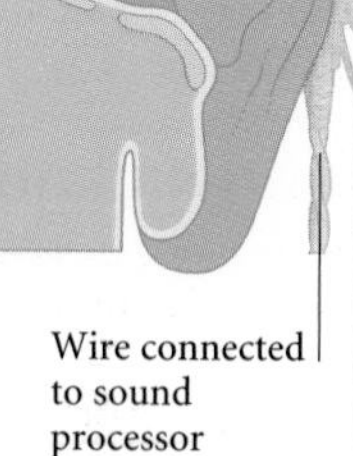

Inside the ear
Signals from the transmitter are detected by the implanted receiver and travel along a wire to the cochlea. Implanted electrodes are activated by the signals and stimulate the cochlear nerve to send impulses to the brain.

Vertigo

A false sensation of movement often combined with nausea and vomiting

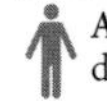
AGE GENETICS LIFESTYLE Risk factors depend on the cause

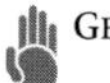
GENDER Not a significant factor

People with vertigo feel as if they or their surroundings are moving. These false sensations are often accompanied by a feeling of spinning and may be associated with nausea and, sometimes, severe vomiting. Vertigo may result from disturbance affecting the organs of balance in the inner ear (the vestibular apparatus), the nerve that connects the inner ear to the brain, or the areas of the brain concerned with balance. Rarely, it is a sign of a serious underlying condition and needs urgent medical attention.

Vertigo often develops suddenly and may last from a few minutes to several days, occurring either intermittently or constantly. The condition can be very distressing and, in severe cases, may make it impossible to walk or even to stand. In most cases, vertigo disappears on its own or following treatment of the underlying disorder.

WHAT ARE THE CAUSES?

Vertigo is often associated with arthritis in the neck (*see* CERVICAL SPONDYLOSIS, p.376), a disorder that mainly affects older people. In this condition, vertigo occurs when the head is turned or tilted, thereby compressing blood vessels that supply the parts of the brain involved with balance.

Another common cause of vertigo is an infection of the vestibular apparatus (*see* LABYRINTHITIS, p.604). The infection usually begins as a viral infection of the respiratory tract, such as a common cold (p.288) or influenza (p.289) or, less frequently, a bacterial infection of the middle ear (*see* OTITIS MEDIA, p.597). This type of vertigo usually starts suddenly and lasts for 1–2 weeks.

Recurrent vertigo combined with hearing loss and sounds in one or both ears (*see* TINNITUS, opposite page) may due to the inner-ear disorder Ménière's disease (p.604). Vertigo may also be a side effect of certain antibiotics (p.885), due to excessive alcohol consumption, or be a symptom of food poisoning (p.629) or heatstroke (*see* HEAT EXHAUSTION AND HEATSTROKE, p.322).

Vertigo is sometimes caused by calcified material moving around in the inner ear and causing dizziness when the head is moved. This condition often improves over a few weeks or months.

Rare causes of vertigo include a tumour affecting the nerve connecting the inner ear to the brain (*see* ACOUSTIC NEUROMA, p.605), a stroke (p.532), a head injury (p.521), or multiple sclerosis (p.541). These serious conditions may also cause other symptoms, such as speech or vision problems or weakness in a limb. If vertigo is accompanied by symptoms of this type, you should seek immediate medical attention.

WHAT CAN I DO?

You may relieve vertigo by lying still and avoiding sudden movement. If you have been vomiting, take small sips of water every 10 minutes to avoid dehydration until the symptoms subside.

If the vertigo persists for more than a few minutes, or if it becomes recurrent, you should consult your doctor.

WHAT MIGHT BE DONE?

Your doctor may examine your ears, eye movements, and nervous system to look for a cause. Tests may include a caloric test, in which air at different temperatures is blown into the ear to check the function of the vestibular apparatus. A neck X-ray (p.244) may be done to look for cervical spondylosis. If you also have tinnitus, you may have CT scanning (p.247) or MRI (p.248) to rule out a tumour pressing on the brain.

Your doctor may recommend drugs to relieve the symptoms of vertigo (*see* ANTIEMETIC DRUGS, p.922, and ANTIHISTAMINES, p.906). If vertigo is a side effect of an antibiotic, you may be given an alternative drug. Other treatment will be aimed at the underlying cause. For example, vertigo caused by a bacterial infection of the vestibular apparatus may be treated with antibiotics.

(WWW) ONLINE SITES: p.1035

Motion sickness

A range of symptoms, generally including nausea, caused by motion during travel by road, sea, or air

AGE Can occur at any age; most common in children aged 3–12

GENDER GENETICS LIFESTYLE Not significant factors

Most people experience some degree of motion sickness at some time in their lives. The condition is especially common in children. Motion sickness occurs when the brain receives messages from the organs of balance in the inner ear and from the eyes that conflict with one another. For example, when you travel in a car, the inner ear senses the motion, but, if you look at the interior of the car, the eyes may perceive it as stationary. The conflicting messages that the brain receives may lead to a feeling of nausea.

WHAT ARE THE SYMPTOMS?

In its mildest form, motion sickness may produce only a feeling of uneasiness. However, the initial symptoms of motion sickness usually include:

- Nausea.
- Headache and dizziness.
- Lethargy and tiredness.

If the motion continues after the onset of symptoms, the initial symptoms typically get worse and other symptoms, such as pale skin, excessive sweating, yawning, hyperventilation (abnormally deep or rapid breathing), and vomiting may occur. Poor ventilation in the vehicle may make the symptoms worse.

WHAT CAN I DO?

Before travelling, you should eat only small amounts and not drink alcohol. When travelling, you should try to sit in a cool, well-ventilated position and avoid reading or looking at nearby objects. Instead, try to look at the horizon or a distant object in the direction of travel. Drivers have to maintain their focus on the road ahead and so are usually unaffected by motion sickness.

There are many drugs, both over-the-counter and prescription, available to prevent or treat motion sickness (*see* ANTIEMETIC DRUGS, p.922, and ANTIHISTAMINES, p.906). To prevent symptoms, the medication should be taken before travelling, but, if you are driving, you should avoid certain drugs that may cause drowsiness. Many of these drugs can also increase the effects of alcohol.

Motion sickness remedies based on ginger plant stems, which have been shown to be effective in preventing nausea in controlled research trials, are available in health-food stores.

(WWW) ONLINE SITES: p.1037

Labyrinthitis

Inflammation of the labyrinth of the inner ear, which contains the organs of balance and the receptor for hearing

AGE GENDER GENETICS LIFESTYLE Not significant factors

The labyrinth of the inner ear consists of the vestibular apparatus, which is composed of the organs of balance, and the cochlea, which contains the receptor for hearing. Inflammation of the labyrinth, known as labyrinthitis, can therefore affect both balance and hearing. Labyrinthitis can be mild, but more often it is extremely unpleasant. The condition is not painful and rarely has serious consequences.

WHAT ARE THE CAUSES?

The most common cause of labyrinthitis is a viral infection. Viral labyrinthitis may develop as a result of a viral infection of the upper respiratory tract, such as a common cold (p.288) or influenza (p.289). Less commonly, labyrinthitis is due to a bacterial infection, usually a complication of a middle-ear infection (*see* OTITIS MEDIA, p.597) or, rarely, an infection elsewhere in the body.

WHAT ARE THE SYMPTOMS?

The symptoms of labyrinthitis usually develop rapidly and are most severe in the first 24 hours. They may include:

- Dizziness and a loss of balance (*see* VERTIGO, p.603).
- Nausea and vomiting.
- Ringing and buzzing noises in the ears (*see* TINNITUS, p.602).

The symptoms may gradually decrease as the brain compensates for the disturbance to the vestibular apparatus, but you should consult your doctor immediately if you develop symptoms of labyrinthitis. Left untreated, bacterial infection of the labyrinth may cause severe damage to the cochlea, possibly leading to permanent hearing loss, or it may spread to the membranes covering the brain, causing meningitis (p.527).

WHAT MIGHT BE DONE?

Labyrinthitis can be diagnosed from your symptoms. Your doctor may prescribe an antiemetic drug (p.922) to ease the nausea. He or she may also advise you to lie in a darkened room with your eyes closed. Viral labyrinthitis often clears up without specific treatment, but, if you have bacterial labyrinthitis, your doctor will prescribe antibiotics (p.885). It may take several weeks to recover completely from labyrinthitis.

(WWW) ONLINE SITES: p.1030

Ménière's disease

A disorder of the inner ear causing sudden episodes of severe dizziness, nausea, and hearing loss

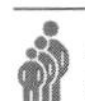
AGE Most common between the ages of 20 and 60

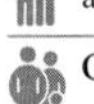
GENETICS Sometimes runs in families

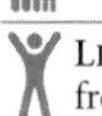
LIFESTYLE A high-salt diet may increase the frequency of attacks

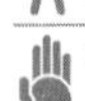
GENDER Not a significant factor

Ménière's disease is a rare disorder in which the amount of fluid in the inner ear increases intermittently. The raised pressure in the inner ear disturbs the organs of hearing and balance, causing sudden attacks of distorted hearing and dizziness so severe that the affected person may fall to the ground.

Usually only one ear is affected, but both ears can become involved. The condition is most common in people aged between 20 and 60 years and sometimes runs in families. The underlying cause of Ménière's disease is unknown, but a high-salt diet may increase the frequency of attacks. The disorder may lead to permanent hearing loss.

WHAT ARE THE SYMPTOMS?

Attacks of Ménière's disease occur suddenly and may last from a few minutes to several days before gradually subsiding. The symptoms may include:

- Sudden, severe dizziness and loss of balance (*see* VERTIGO, p.603).
- Nausea and vomiting.
- Abnormal, jerky eye movements.
- Ringing or buzzing noises in the affected ear (*see* TINNITUS, p.602).
- Loss of hearing, particularly of low-pitched sounds.
- Feeling of pressure or pain in the affected ear.

The time between attacks of Ménière's disease ranges from a few days to years. Tinnitus may be constant or occur only during an attack. Between attacks, vertigo and nausea cease and hearing may improve. With repeated attacks, hearing often deteriorates progressively.

HOW IS IT DIAGNOSED?

Your doctor may arrange for hearing tests (p.600) to assess your hearing loss. He or she may also arrange for a caloric test, in which air at different temperatures is blown into the ears to check the functioning of the organs of balance. A tumour affecting the nerve that connects the ear to the brain (*see* ACOUSTIC NEUROMA, right) may occasionally produce symptoms that resemble those of Ménière's disease. Your doctor may arrange for you to have tests such as CT scanning (p.247) or MRI (p.248) to rule out the possibility of a tumour.

WHAT IS THE TREATMENT?

You may be prescribed drugs to relieve nausea (*see* ANTIEMETIC DRUGS, p.922). Your doctor may also recommend an antihistamine (p.906) to give further relief from nausea and vertigo and to reduce the frequency of the episodes. In addition, sedative drugs such as diazepam may be prescribed to relieve vertigo (*see* ANTIANXIETY DRUGS, p.916). Sometimes, diuretic drugs (p.902) are used to help prevent further attacks.

There are steps you can take to help yourself if you have Ménière's disease. During an attack, lie still with your eyes closed and avoid noise, perhaps by wearing earplugs. Between attacks, try to avoid stress. Relaxation techniques and a low-salt diet may also be helpful.

Despite treatment, some people with Ménière's disease have repeated attacks of, severe, disabling vertigo. For these people, the doctor may recommend surgery to cut the nerve between part of the inner ear and the brain. The operation cures the vertigo and may prevent loss of hearing in the treated ear.

WHAT IS THE PROGNOSIS?

The symptoms of Ménière's disease are usually improved with medication. The frequency and severity of the episodes tend to decrease over a period of years. However, hearing usually worsens progressively with each successive attack, and permanent hearing loss may result. If the deafness becomes total, the other symptoms usually disappear.

(WWW) ONLINE SITES: p.1030

Acoustic neuroma

A noncancerous tumour affecting the vestibulocochlear (acoustic) nerve, which connects the ear to the brain

 AGE Most common between the ages of 40 and 60

 GENETICS One type runs in families

 GENDER LIFESTYLE Not significant factors

An acoustic neuroma is a rare tumour affecting the vestibulocochlear (acoustic) nerve, which carries auditory and balance information from part of the inner ear to the brain. The tumour usually affects the vestibulocochlear nerve on one side of the head only, but it may affect both nerves. The tumour is noncancerous but can cause severe nerve and brain damage. If detected early, it can be removed by surgery.

The cause of acoustic neuroma is unknown but, if the tumour affects both acoustic nerves, it may be associated with neurofibromatosis (p.827), an inherited condition in which multiple tumours grow from the sheaths around nerves. Acoustic neuroma is most common between the ages of 40 and 60.

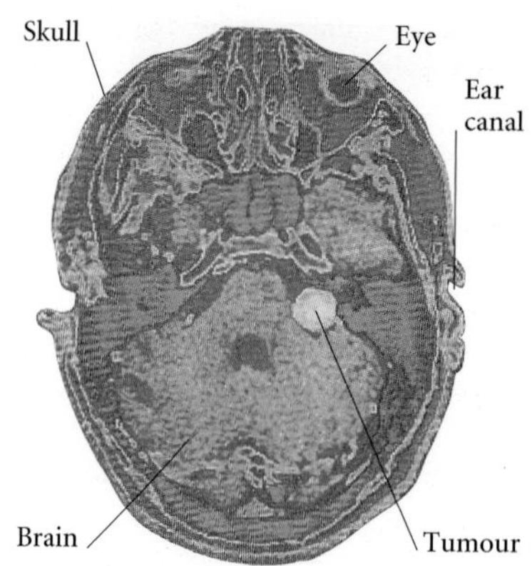

Acoustic neuroma

This MRI scan of the head shows an acoustic neuroma, a tumour of the nerve that connects the ear to the brain.

WHAT ARE THE SYMPTOMS?

The symptoms of an acoustic neuroma usually develop slowly, almost always affect only one ear, and may include:

- Progressive hearing loss.
- Ringing or buzzing noises in the ear (*see* TINNITUS, p.602).
- Headache and pain in the ear.
- Dizziness and a loss of balance (*see* VERTIGO, p.603).

An acoustic neuroma is slow-growing, but as it enlarges it may press on part of the brain, causing lack of coordination of body movements. The tumour may also compress the nerves that supply the face, causing weakness of the facial muscles (*see* FACIAL PALSY, p.548) and pain. Left untreated, a neuroma may cause permanent nerve damage.

WHAT MIGHT BE DONE?

If you have symptoms of an acoustic neuroma, your doctor may arrange for imaging tests such as MRI (p.248) to look for a tumour and hearing tests (p.600) to check for hearing loss.

An acoustic neuroma can usually be removed by surgery, and the earlier this treatment is carried out, the better the outcome. Many of the symptoms disappear with surgery, and, if the tumour is small, hearing may be restored in the affected ear. However, removal of a large tumour may damage the vestibulocochlear or facial nerves. If these nerves are damaged, there may be permanent hearing loss in the affected ear, combined with numbness, weakness, or paralysis of part of the face.

(WWW) ONLINE SITES: p.1032

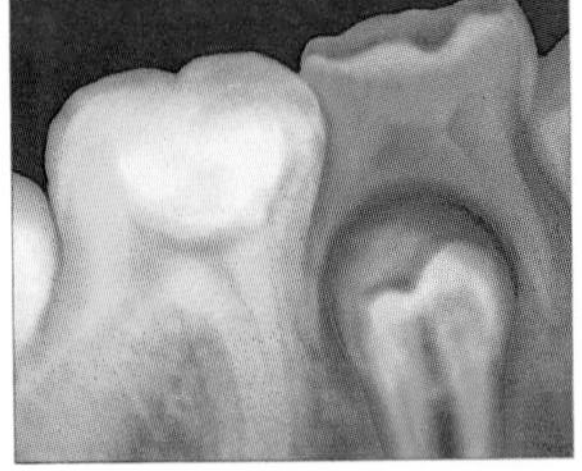

Tooth eruption
In this colour-enhanced X-ray of a child's lower jaw, a secondary tooth that has not yet erupted can be seen below a primary tooth.

TEETH AND GUMS

THE PRIMARY FUNCTION OF TEETH is to break down food ready for digestion. Teeth also help us to pronounce sounds clearly and give the face shape and definition. Each of us grows two sets of teeth in a lifetime, the second set gradually replacing the first during childhood. The gums help to keep the teeth firmly in the jaw and protect their roots from decay. Teeth and gums are vulnerable to the build-up of plaque (a sticky mixture of bacteria, saliva, and food particles), which causes decay and gum disease.

At the beginning of the 20th century, it was common for people to have lost all of their secondary (adult) teeth by the age of 60 as a result of tooth decay and gum disease. Today, because of the advances that have been made in dental health care, improvements in nutrition, and widespread fluoridation of water, many people keep their secondary teeth for life.

THE STRUCTURE OF THE TEETH

The part of the tooth that protrudes from the gum is called the crown; the part beneath the gumline is called the root. The crown is covered with a protective layer of enamel, the hardest substance in the body. Enamel is composed of rod-shaped calcium salt crystals and cannot renew itself. As a result, the enamel may eventually become worn down from abrasion, or it may be damaged by acid present in food and drinks or produced by bacteria in plaque. If the enamel is worn through, a cavity is formed. This can be repaired with a dental filling.

Beneath the enamel layer lies the dentine, a hard ivory-like substance that surrounds the pulp cavity. This central cavity contains nerves and blood vessels that extend through tiny channels into the dentine, making the dentine sensitive to heat, cold, and pain.

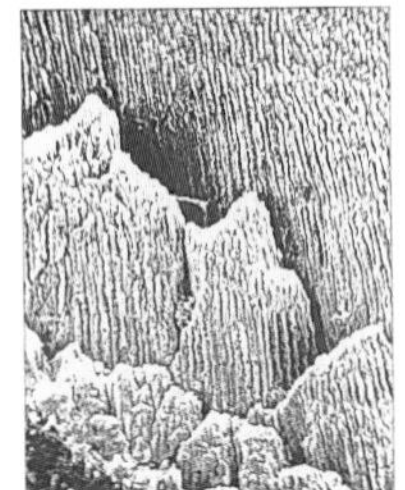

Tooth enamel
This magnified image of tooth enamel shows the many tiny, rod-shaped calcium crystals that lie at right angles to the surface of the tooth.

About two-thirds of a tooth is made up of the root, buried below the gumline in a deep socket in the jaw. Each root is attached to the jawbone by a periodontal ligament, which cushions the root in its socket while the teeth are grinding down food.

Teeth have various shapes and sizes to enable them to hold, cut, tear, and chew food efficiently. For example, to enable teeth to grind down food effectively, the contoured chewing surfaces of the upper and lower back teeth meet and are similar in shape. The actions of the teeth are controlled by the upper and lower jaws, which are able to clamp the teeth together with great force – up to 500 kg/sq. cm (7,000 lb/sq. in) – with the help of four powerful sets of muscles.

STRUCTURE DEVELOPMENT OF TEETH

Our first set of 20 teeth appears between the ages of 6 months and 3 years. These teeth are known as primary, deciduous, or milk teeth. As the jaw grows, a set of 32 secondary (adult or permanent) teeth appears between the ages of 6 and 21. As the secondary teeth erupt, they displace the primary teeth, which usually fall out by the age of 13. In some cases, the third molars, also known as wisdom teeth, never erupt.

Patterns of eruption
The primary and secondary teeth usually erupt in a specific order (as indicated here by the numbers in parentheses).

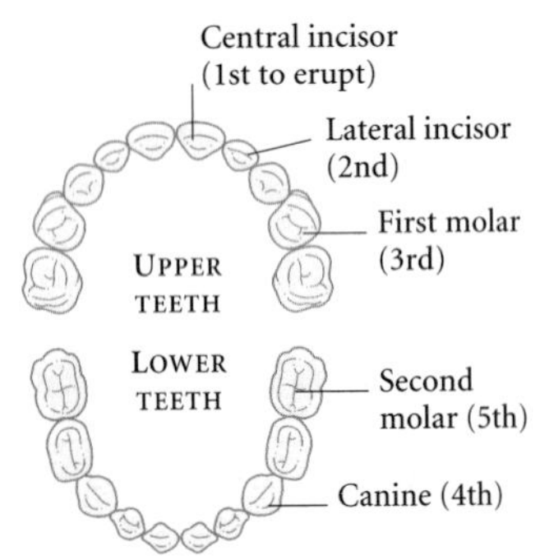

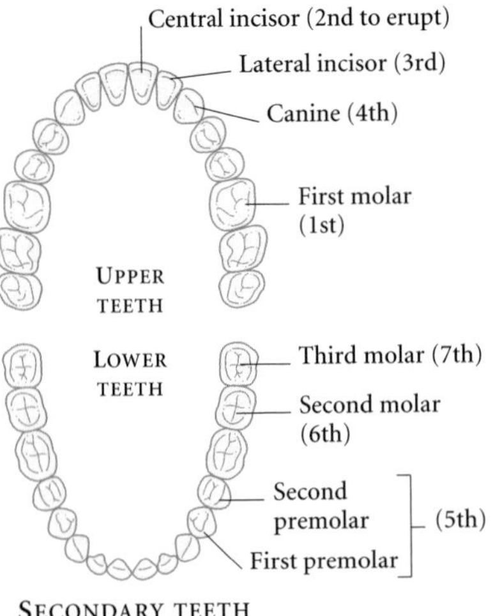

THE ROLE OF THE GUMS

The bone and periodontal ligaments that support the teeth in the jaw are covered by a layer of protective tissue known as the gums or gingiva. Healthy gums are pink or brown and firm. They form a tight seal around the neck of the tooth, preventing food particles and plaque from invading underlying tissues and the root of the tooth.

(STRUCTURE) TEETH AND GUMS

Teeth vary in shape and size but have an identical structure. Each tooth consists of a hard shell that surrounds a cavity of soft tissue, known as pulp. The crown (the exposed part of the shell) is coated in a tough layer of enamel, beneath which is a layer of a yellowish substance similar to ivory, called dentine. The dentine and pulp form long, pointed roots that extend into the jawbone and are covered by a layer of firm, fleshy tissue called the gums.

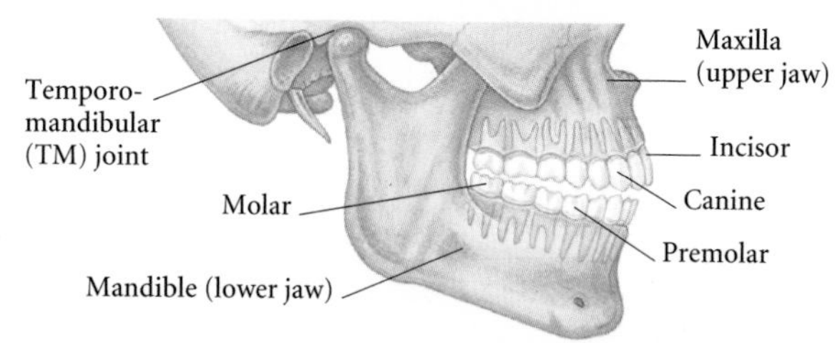

SIDE VIEW OF THE JAWS AND TEETH

Crown
The crown is the part of the tooth exposed above the gumline

Neck
The part of the tooth that narrows slightly at the gumline is called the neck

Root
The root is the long pointed part of the tooth embedded in the jawbone; incisors and canines have one root, premolars one or two, and molars three or four

Incisor
The sharp chisel-like incisors, situated at the front of the mouth, cut and hold food.

Canine
Canines are longer and more pointed than incisors; they are used for tearing food.

Premolar
Premolars have two prominences (cusps) on their biting surfaces and are used for grinding food.

Molar
Molars, the largest teeth, are used for grinding. They have four or five cusps on their chewing surfaces.

Enamel
The crown is coated in enamel, an insensitive, nonliving substance

Dentine
Dentine is a tough, ivory-like material supplied with blood and nerves from the pulp tissue

Gum (gingiva)
This layer of protective tissue fits tightly around the base of the crown and covers the roots of the tooth

Pulp
At the centre of a tooth lies the soft pulp tissue, containing nerves and blood vessels

Periodontal ligament
This tissue joins the tooth to the jawbone and gums

Cementum
This layer of hard tissue covers the roots and anchors the fibres of the periodontal ligament

Jawbone
Deep sockets in the jawbone encase the roots of the tooth

Nerve
Nerves supply the periodontal ligament, pulp, gums, and jaw

Blood vessel
These blood vessels supply nutrients to the pulp tissue, bone, and gums

(FUNCTION) USING THE JAWS

The actions of biting and chewing require the lower jaw to move in all directions. This range of movement is made possible by the temporomandibular joint, a complex but exceptionally flexible type of hinge joint that attaches the lower jaw to the skull.

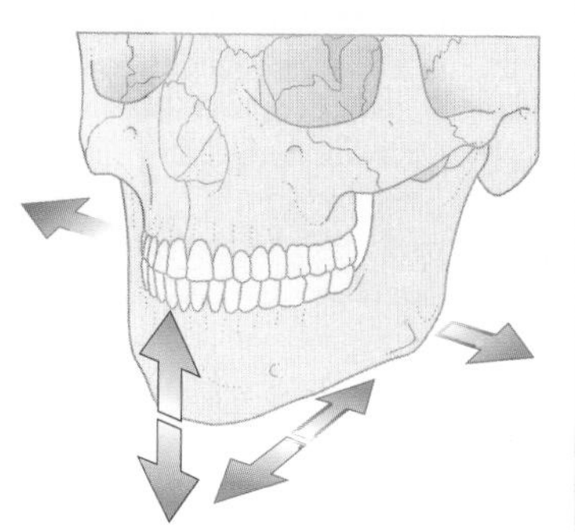

Moving the lower jaw
The lower jaw moves in six directions, side to side, up and down, and backwards and forwards. This mobility is essential for biting off and chewing food.

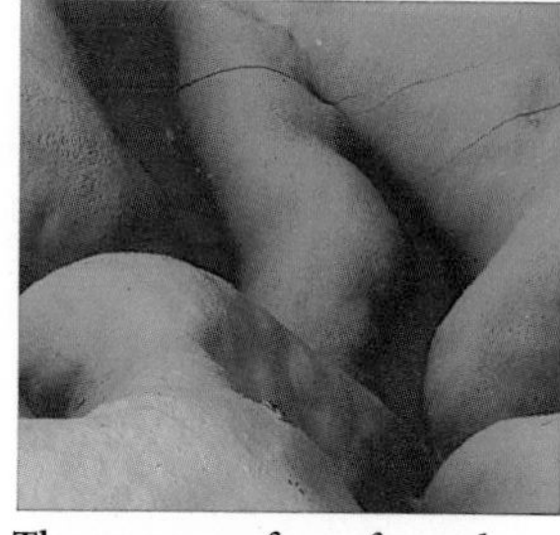

The upper surface of a molar
This magnified image shows the normal undulations on the chewing surface of a molar tooth.

DISORDERS OF THE TEETH

Teeth are necessary for chopping food into small pieces to make digestion easier. Each person has two sets of teeth: the primary teeth, which emerge in infancy, and the secondary teeth, which gradually replace the primary teeth in late childhood. Both sets are protected from damage and decay by a hard coating of enamel and by the gums, which cover the roots.

Good oral hygiene is essential because without regular brushing and flossing of the teeth and gums, tooth decay or gum disease may develop. Improved oral hygiene and the addition of fluoride to water in many parts of the world in order to harden teeth have made tooth decay far less common today than it was several decades ago.

The first articles in this section deal with tooth disorders that are usually caused by neglect of oral hygiene, such as toothache and tooth decay. If left untreated, tooth decay may spread to the central parts of the teeth and cause pulpitis. Pus may eventually build up at the root of a tooth due to infection, resulting in a dental abscess. Poor oral hygiene can also cause teeth to become discoloured. Malocclusion caused by teeth that have grown unevenly or become overcrowded is covered next. Sometimes teeth are missing or are broken or lost due to injury. Problems of the temporomandibular joint are covered in the last article of this section. Teething (p.819) in babies is discussed in the children's section.

KEY ANATOMY

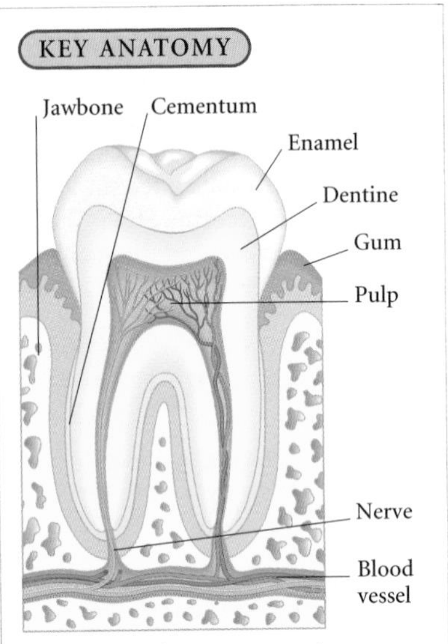

For more information on the structure and function of teeth, *see* pp.606–607.

Toothache

Pain or discomfort in one or more teeth or in the gums

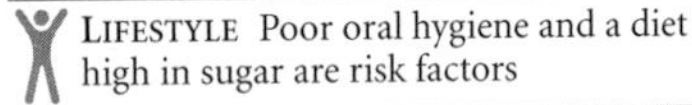
LIFESTYLE Poor oral hygiene and a diet high in sugar are risk factors

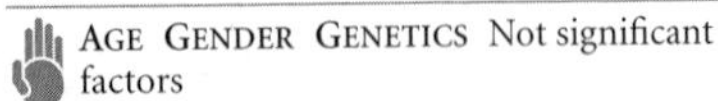
AGE GENDER GENETICS Not significant factors

Pain in one or more teeth is usually a symptom of an underlying problem with the teeth or gums. Depending on the cause, the pain may range from a dull ache to a severe throbbing sensation. Toothache may last only a few minutes or it may be continuous.

WHAT ARE THE CAUSES?

A sharp pain triggered by biting or consuming hot, cold, or sweet foods and drinks may be a symptom of the early stages of tooth decay (*see* DENTAL CARIES, opposite page). A fractured tooth (p.614), receding gums (p.619), or advanced gum disease (*see* PERIODONTITIS, p.618) may also result in toothache. A dull pain in the teeth while chewing may be due to inflammation of the gums (*see* GINGIVITIS, p.617) following a build-up of plaque (a deposit of food particles, saliva, and bacteria). Pain may also be caused by food trapped between the teeth.

A continuous, severe, throbbing pain is usually the result of advanced tooth decay (*see* PULPITIS, p.611), in which the pulp, the central part of the tooth containing the nerves and blood vessels, becomes inflamed. If the pain changes so that the tooth becomes tender to touch, it may be a sign that pulpitis has developed into a dental abscess (p.611) at the root, with infection and death of the pulp tissues. The infection may spread to surrounding tissues and be accompanied by facial swelling and, occasionally, fever. The lymph nodes in the neck may also become enlarged and tender.

Pain and tenderness at the back of the mouth may be due to emerging wisdom teeth. The gums may be particularly painful if the wisdom teeth only partially emerge or grow in the wrong direction (*see* IMPACTED TEETH, p.613).

In some cases, toothache occurs as a result of a disorder elsewhere in the body, such as sinusitis (p.475), an ear infection (*see* OTITIS MEDIA, p.597), or a problem in the joint between the jaw and the skull (*see* TEMPOROMANDIBULAR JOINT DISORDER, p.616).

WHAT CAN I DO?

If you have toothache, you should consult your dentist as soon as possible. If you have a fever and/or a swollen face in addition to toothache, you should see a dentist immediately.

Painkillers (p.912), such as aspirin and paracetamol, can help to relieve toothache while you are waiting for an appointment. Rinsing out your mouth with warm salt water may also help. However, the only permanent remedy for toothache is for the affected tooth to be treated by a dentist.

WHAT MIGHT BE DONE?

Your dentist will ask you about your symptoms and examine your teeth and gums. He or she may also take X-rays of your mouth to look for decay.

If toothache is caused by decay, your dentist will remove the decayed areas and may put in an ordinary filling to stop the pain and prevent further decay (*see* TOOTH FILLING, p.611). If you have gingivitis, your dentist will probably remove the plaque by scaling the teeth. He or she may also prescribe antibiotics (p.885) for an infection. If tooth decay is advanced and you have pulpitis or a dental abscess, you may need root canal treatment (p.612), in which the soft pulp tissues within the tooth are taken out. The cavity is sterilized to clear up the infection, and the root canals and decayed area are filled permanently. A tooth that is very badly damaged or decayed may need to be extracted. Likewise, painful, impacted wisdom teeth may need to be extracted. If your toothache is due to a condition such as sinusitis or an ear infection, you may need to consult your doctor for the necessary treatment.

To prevent toothache, you should brush and floss your teeth and gums regularly (*see* CARING FOR YOUR TEETH AND GUMS, p.610). You should also have regular dental checkups (below).

WWW ONLINE SITES: p.1030

Dental caries

Progressive decay of one or more teeth, causing cavities to form

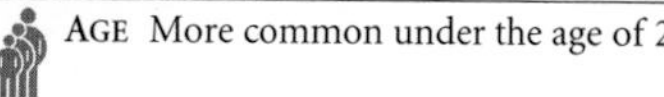
AGE More common under the age of 25

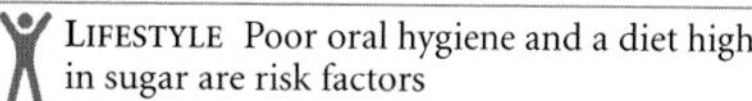
LIFESTYLE Poor oral hygiene and a diet high in sugar are risk factors

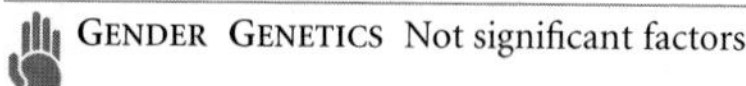
GENDER GENETICS Not significant factors

Gradual, progressive decay of a tooth is known as dental caries. This condition usually starts as a small cavity in the enamel (the hard, protective outer covering of a tooth). If left untreated, the decay eventually penetrates the outer layer of enamel and attacks the dentine, the softer material that makes up the bulk of a tooth. As the tooth decay progresses, the pulp (the living core of the tooth that contains the nerves and blood vessels) may be affected (*see* PULPITIS, p.611). If the pulp is exposed to decay and becomes infected, it may die.

Most people develop dental caries at some time in their lives. In younger age groups, tooth decay most often occurs on the chewing surfaces of the upper and lower teeth and on the surfaces where the teeth touch each other. In older people, tooth decay is more common at the gum margins where the teeth meet the gums.

In developed countries, the number of teeth lost as a result of dental caries has fallen considerably in recent years, particularly among children. This fall is

TEST DENTAL CHECKUP

In order to keep your teeth and gums healthy, you should consult your dentist at least once every 6 months for a checkup. He or she will examine your teeth for signs of decay and your gums for evidence of gum disease. If you have not been to the dentist for some time, you may have X-rays to look for evidence of decay between the back teeth and under existing fillings. Your dentist may also clean and polish your teeth and will advise you on good oral hygiene.

LOOKING AT THE TEETH AND GUMS

Your teeth and gums will be examined for signs of disease while you lie in a dental chair under a bright light. Your dentist will also check that all the teeth are present and aligned correctly and that teeth still emerging are not likely to become impacted.

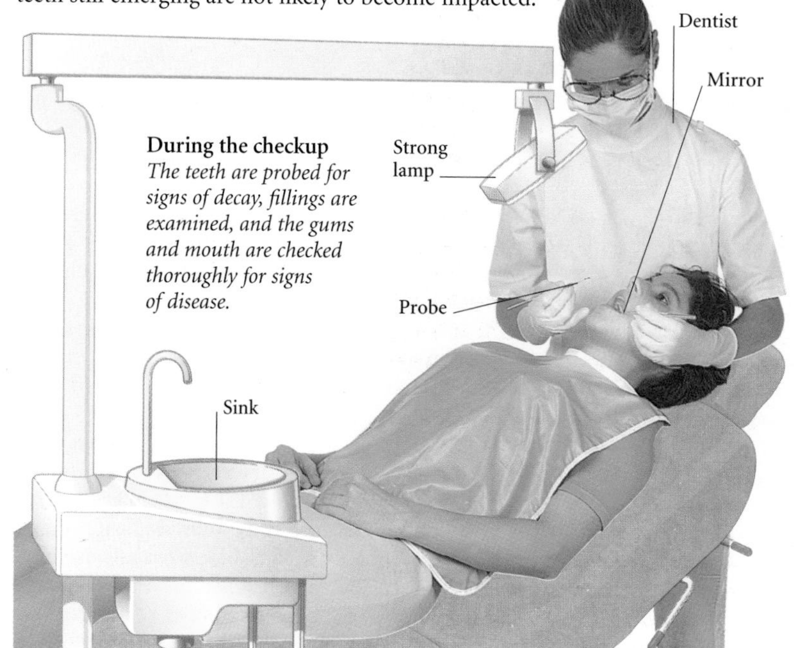

During the checkup
The teeth are probed for signs of decay, fillings are examined, and the gums and mouth are checked thoroughly for signs of disease.

BITE-WING X-RAY

A bite-wing X-ray is used to look for decay. The X-ray film is held between the teeth while the X-ray machine is placed near your cheek. An X-ray may be taken on both sides of the face.

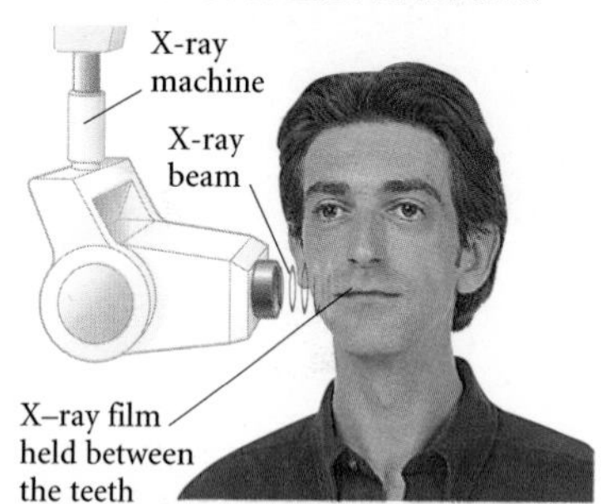

Having an X-ray
The X-ray film is placed in the cheek and held between the teeth using the wing attached to the film. An X-ray is taken.

RESULTS

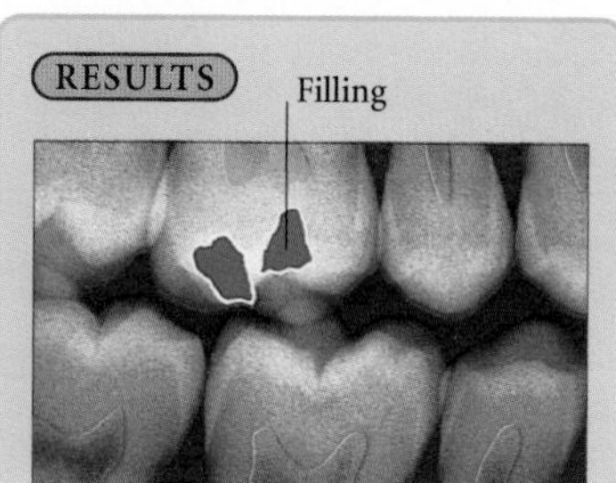

Bite-wing X-ray
This colour-enhanced X-ray shows two fillings in an upper molar tooth. No decay is present.

SELF-HELP CARING FOR YOUR TEETH AND GUMS

Daily care of your teeth is as important as having regular dental checkups. If you adopt a simple routine of regular brushing and flossing, you can prevent food particles and bacteria from building up on the surface of your teeth and reduce the risk of tooth decay and gum disease. If you cannot clean your teeth between meals, chewing sugar-free gum may help. You should avoid sugary foods and drinks, which contribute to tooth decay. If your water does not contain fluoride, which helps to strengthen teeth, consult your dentist about whether to use fluoride tablets or drops.

BRUSHING YOUR TEETH

Your teeth need brushing at least twice a day for 5 minutes and, if possible, after every meal. Use a small-headed, soft toothbrush and fluoride toothpaste. Make sure that you clean all the surfaces of all your teeth, especially where they meet the gum. You should replace your toothbrush every 2–3 months.

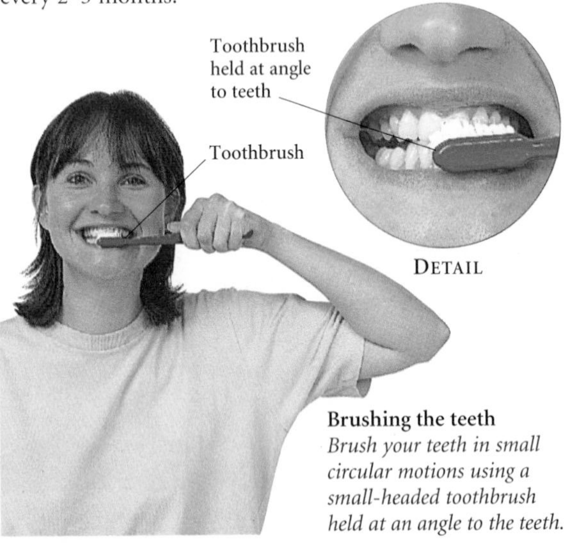

Brushing the teeth
Brush your teeth in small circular motions using a small-headed toothbrush held at an angle to the teeth.

CLEANING BETWEEN TEETH

Dental floss or dental tape is used to clean between the teeth and remove food particles and bacteria from areas between the teeth that cannot be reached easily with a toothbrush. Toothpicks and small interdental brushes may also be used. You should clean between each tooth in turn in a regular pattern so that no teeth are missed.

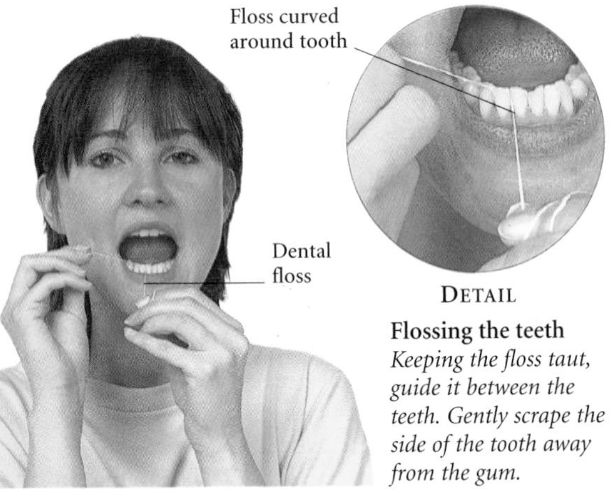

Flossing the teeth
Keeping the floss taut, guide it between the teeth. Gently scrape the side of the tooth away from the gum.

FOOD AND DRINK

You should avoid consuming foods and drinks that have a high sugar content, such as desserts and colas, particularly if you cannot clean your teeth immediately. If you cannot brush soon after eating sugary foods, chew sugar-free gum.

Sugarless snacks
Snacking on foods such as nuts, celery, carrots, and cheese is better for your teeth than eating sugary foods.

partly due to the addition of fluoride to drinking water in some areas and to the widespread use of fluoride toothpaste, both of which help to harden the teeth, making them more resistant to decay.

WHAT ARE THE CAUSES?

Tooth decay is usually caused by a build-up of plaque (a deposit of food particles, saliva, and bacteria) on the surface of the teeth. The bacteria in plaque break down the sugar in food to produce an acid that erodes the tooth enamel. If sugary foods are eaten often and the teeth are not cleaned thoroughly soon afterwards, a cavity is eventually likely to form.

The condition is especially common in children, adolescents, and young adults because they are more likely to have a diet high in sugar and fail to clean their teeth regularly. Babies who frequently fall asleep with a bottle of juice in their mouth may also develop severe caries, especially in the front teeth.

WHAT ARE THE SYMPTOMS?

There may be no signs of dental caries in the early stages, but the symptoms develop gradually as the decay progresses and may include:

- Toothache, which may be constant or sharp and stabbing and triggered by hot, cold, or sweet foods or drinks.
- Persistent, throbbing pain in the jaw and occasionally in the ear and face, which may be worse when chewing.
- Bad breath.

Pain in a tooth can take several forms. It may be persistent, recurrent, or set off by extremes of hot or cold or pressure on the tooth. You should see your dentist as soon as possible after the pain first appears and make an immediate appointment if the pain ends abruptly because this may indicate that the nerves and blood vessels have died. Delaying a visit to your dentist may result in the spread of infection, and an abscess may eventually form (*see* DENTAL ABSCESS, opposite page).

WHAT MIGHT BE DONE?

Your dentist will examine your teeth with a probe and a mirror to look for areas of tooth decay. An X-ray may also be taken to look for decay that may be developing beneath the surface of the teeth (*see* DENTAL CHECKUP, p.609).

If you have superficial dental caries restricted to the surface of the enamel, your dentist may only apply fluoride to the affected area and advise you to be more careful about oral hygiene.

If tooth decay has penetrated further into the enamel or if it has affected the dentine, your dentist will probably need to fill the affected tooth (*see* TOOTH FILLING, right). An injection of a local anaesthetic is often used to numb the tooth and nearby gum to prevent you from feeling pain. When the area is numb, the decayed parts of the tooth are drilled out, and the cavity is cleaned and filled to prevent further decay. If you have pulpitis and the pulp cannot be saved, you may need to have root canal treatment (p.612).

CAN IT BE PREVENTED?

Your teeth and gums should be brushed and flossed regularly to keep them clean (*see* CARING FOR YOUR TEETH AND GUMS, opposite page). You can also help to prevent dental caries from developing by avoiding sweet foods and drinks.

(WWW) ONLINE SITES: p.1030

Pulpitis

Inflammation of the pulp, the living core of a tooth

LIFESTYLE Poor oral hygiene and a diet high in sugar are risk factors

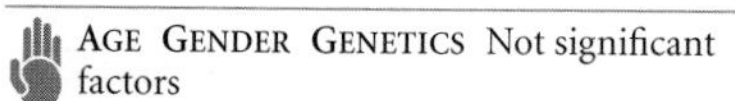

AGE GENDER GENETICS Not significant factors

The soft central part (the pulp) of a tooth contains the blood vessels and nerves. If tooth decay (*see* DENTAL CARIES, p.609) becomes advanced, it will gradually progress to invade the pulp and cause pulpitis. Pulpitis may also develop if the pulp becomes exposed in a fractured tooth (p.614). Some people grind their teeth during sleep, which may inflame the pulp.

There are two varieties of pulpitis: reversible and irreversible. In reversible pulpitis, the decay has not affected the entire pulp, and the remaining tissue with its nerves and blood vessels can be saved. Left untreated, reversible pulpitis may eventually become irreversible, in which the decay is so severe that the remaining pulp, nerves, and vessels die and have to be removed. Eventually, the tooth may become discoloured (*see* DISCOLOURED TEETH, p.612).

The principal symptom of pulpitis is toothache. If it only occurs while eating or drinking, pulpitis is likely to be reversible. In irreversible pulpitis, pain tends to be more constant until the tissues in the pulp die. You may also notice pain if you tap the tooth with a finger. Left untreated, an abscess may form (*see* DENTAL ABSCESS, right).

WHAT MIGHT BE DONE?

Your dentist will examine your teeth and may take an X-ray to look for decay (*see* DENTAL CHECKUP, p.609). He or she will probably treat reversible pulpitis by removing the decayed area and filling the tooth to prevent further damage (*see* TOOTH FILLING, below). If the pulpitis is irreversible, you will probably need root canal treatment (p.612), in which the pulp is removed and the root canals are filled. It is unlikely that the tooth will be extracted.

(WWW) ONLINE SITES: p.1030

Dental abscess

A pus-filled sac that develops in or around the root of a tooth

LIFESTYLE Poor oral hygiene and a diet high in sugar are risk factors

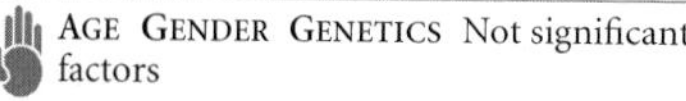

AGE GENDER GENETICS Not significant factors

An accumulation of pus in or around the root of a tooth is known as a dental abscess. An abscess usually develops as a complication of dental caries (p.609), which gradually destroys the layer of enamel on the outside of the tooth and the inner dentine, allowing bacteria to invade the soft central core, or pulp, of the tooth (*see* PULPITIS, left). Eventually, a dental abscess may form. The pulp may also become infected if a tooth is damaged by a blow to the mouth (*see* FRACTURED TOOTH, p.614).

An abscess may also form as a result of certain types of gum disease (*see* PERIODONTITIS, p.618). Periodontitis is usually caused by a build-up of dental plaque (a deposit including food particles, saliva, and bacteria) in a pocket that forms between a tooth and gum.

A dental abscess can be extremely painful and may cause the tooth that is affected to loosen in its socket.

TREATMENT TOOTH FILLING

Teeth are usually filled because of tooth decay. White fillings are often used in front teeth and amalgam (a mixture of silver, tin, and mercury) in back teeth. A local anaesthetic may be used to make the tooth and gum numb. When they are numb, the decayed area of the tooth is drilled away and the hole is shaped to secure the filling. The filling is then pushed into the tooth as a soft paste that will harden within a few hours.

Before treatment
Tooth decay has penetrated the hard enamel covering of the tooth and invaded the dentine, the softer material that makes up the bulk of the tooth.

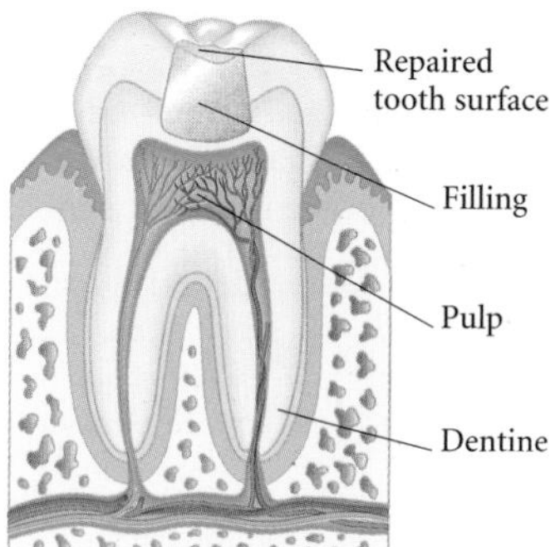

After treatment
The decayed area of the tooth has been drilled out and the hole carefully shaped to hold a filling. The filling has been put in to prevent further tooth decay.

WHAT ARE THE SYMPTOMS?

The main symptoms of a dental abscess develop gradually and may include:

- Severe pain on touching the affected tooth and on biting or chewing.
- Loosening of the affected tooth.
- Red, tender swelling of the gum over the root of the tooth.
- Release of pus into the mouth.

If the abscess is not treated, the infection may make a channel from the tooth to the surface of the gum, and a painful swelling, known as a gumboil, may form. If the gumboil bursts, foul-tasting pus is released into the mouth and the pain decreases. In some cases, the channel may persist, leading to a chronic (long-standing) abscess that discharges pus periodically.

If the infection spreads to the surrounding tissues, the face may become swollen and painful, and a fever may also develop. If you suspect that you have a dental abscess, you should consult your dentist as soon as possible.

WHAT CAN I DO?

If there is a delay before you are able to see your dentist, taking painkillers (p.912), such as paracetamol, may be helpful in the meantime. Rinsing your mouth with warm salt water may also help to relieve the pain and encourage a gumboil to burst. If a gumboil does burst, you should wash away the pus thoroughly with more warm salt water.

WHAT MIGHT THE DENTIST DO?

Your dentist will ask you about your symptoms and examine your teeth and gums. He or she may take an X-ray of your mouth to confirm the diagnosis (*see* DENTAL CHECKUP, p.609).

If the abscess has been caused by decay, your dentist may try to save the tooth. Under a local anaesthetic, a hole is drilled through the top of the tooth to release the pus and relieve the pain. If there is a gumboil, a small cut may be made in the boil to drain the pus. The cavity is then cleaned with an antiseptic solution. A small tube may be left in place for a few days to allow any remaining pus to drain, and you will probably be given a course of antibiotics (p.885). Once the infection has cleared up, you will probably need root canal treatment (above). If it is not possible to save the tooth, it will be extracted.

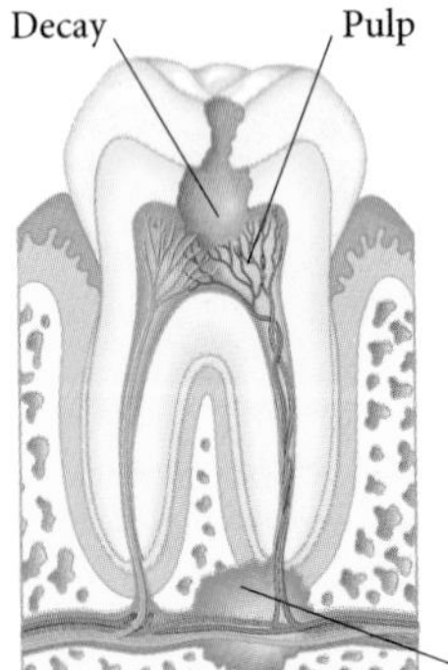

Dental abscess
Tooth decay and infection has spread through the tooth, and pus has gathered at the root of the tooth. If not treated, the tooth will have to be extracted.

In order to treat an abscess caused by gum disease, your dentist may use a probe to scrape out the plaque from the pocket between the affected tooth and gum. Afterwards, the pocket is washed out with an antiseptic solution. In a severe case, the tooth over the abscess may need to be extracted.

WHAT IS THE PROGNOSIS?

Treatment is usually successful, but a small area of infection may persist and further treatment may be required.

To help to prevent the formation of a dental abscess, you should brush and floss your teeth carefully (*see* CARING FOR YOUR TEETH AND GUMS, p.610).

(WWW) ONLINE SITES: p.1030

(TREATMENT) ROOT CANAL TREATMENT

Sometimes, decay invades the pulp, the centre of the tooth, and root canal treatment may be performed. The pulp is removed, as well as the nerves and blood vessels, and an antiseptic solution is used to sterilize the cavity. If infection within the tooth is severe, a temporary filling may be inserted for a few days before the cavity is sterilized again. The root canals and the decayed area of the tooth are then filled.

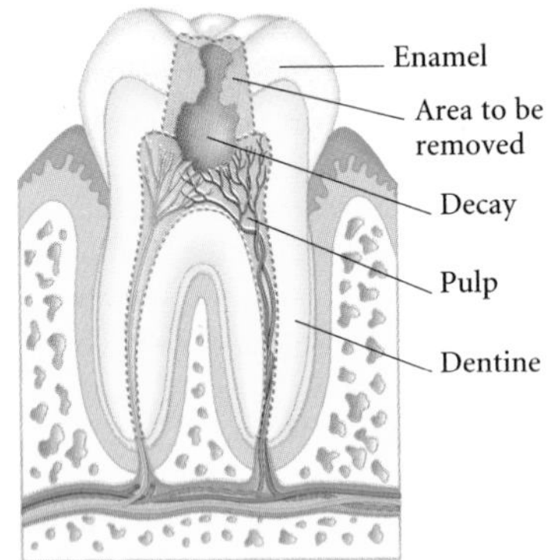

Before treatment
Tooth decay has penetrated the enamel and the dentine and has reached the pulp, the core of the tooth that contains the blood vessels and nerves.

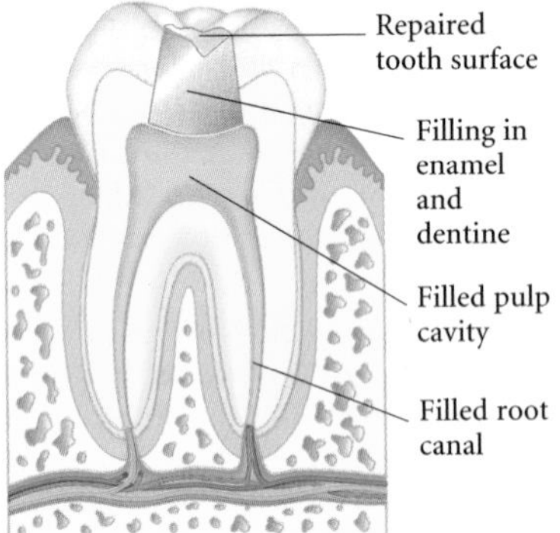

After treatment
The decayed area of the tooth and pulp have been removed, and the pulp cavity has been sterilized. The decayed area, pulp cavity, and root canals have been filled.

Discoloured teeth

Abnormal colouring of the teeth, which may be due to a number of factors

AGE More common with increasing age

LIFESTYLE Poor oral hygiene, using tobacco, and drinking coffee and tea are risk factors

GENDER GENETICS Not significant factors

Tooth colour varies among individuals, and secondary teeth are usually darker than primary teeth. Teeth also normally darken slightly with age. However, abnormal discoloration sometimes occurs because of changes within the teeth.

WHAT ARE THE CAUSES?

A common cause of discoloration is the build-up of dental plaque (a deposit of food particles, saliva, and bacteria) on the surface of the teeth. Plaque-stained teeth are often yellowish-brown, but children's teeth may be black or green. Regularly drinking tea and coffee and using tobacco may also stain the surface of the teeth, as may some liquid medicines that contain iron.

Teeth may also become discoloured if children are given certain drugs while

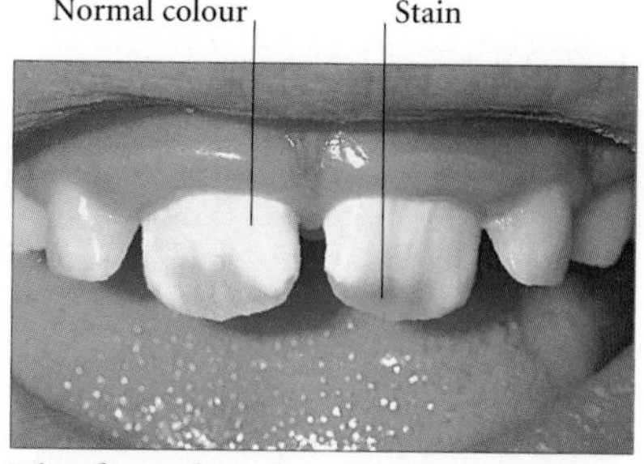

Discoloured teeth
The brown areas of discoloration on this child's two front teeth have been caused by excess amounts of fluoride. This condition is called fluorosis.

their secondary teeth are developing. For example, if tetracycline (*see* ANTIBIOTICS, p.885) is given to babies or children under the age of 10, it may cause a yellow discoloration of the secondary teeth. If the drug is given to a pregnant woman, her baby's teeth may be discoloured when they emerge.

Fluorosis, in which the teeth develop a mottled colour, is due to an excess of natural fluoride in the water in some parts of the world. However, where fluoride is added to the water to reduce tooth decay, the concentration is too low to cause fluorosis. Fluorosis may also develop if children are given too high a dose of fluoride drops or pills.

A tooth may become darker than normal following irreversible pulpitis (*see* PULPITIS, p.611), when the soft centre, or the pulp, of the tooth dies. Root canal treatment (opposite page) may cause a tooth to darken if the material used to fill the tooth is dark in colour.

WHAT MIGHT BE DONE?

Staining on the surface of the teeth is routinely removed by scaling and polishing of teeth by your dentist or oral hygienist. If staining is severe, the teeth can be bleached. If a single tooth is discoloured as a result of a condition such as pulpitis or following root canal treatment, a porcelain or plastic veneer may be bonded to the front of the tooth, or the top of the tooth can be replaced by a crown (*see* CROWNS AND REPLACEMENT TEETH, p.615).

Most discoloration of teeth can be prevented by brushing and flossing the teeth and gums regularly (*see* CARING FOR YOUR TEETH AND GUMS, p.610).

WWW ONLINE SITES: p.1030

Impacted teeth

Failure of teeth to emerge completely from the gum and grow into their normal position, usually due to lack of room

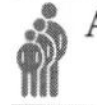
AGE More common under the age of 25

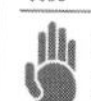
GENDER GENETICS LIFESTYLE Not significant factors

Teeth usually become impacted when there is not enough room in the mouth for them to grow into their correct positions. Impacted teeth may remain entirely buried in the jawbone, with few or no symptoms, or only partly erupt through the gum. Impaction may also occur if a tooth starts to grow in the wrong direction and pushes against other teeth or the jawbone.

Wisdom teeth are the most likely to become impacted, followed by the upper canines. These teeth emerge at a later stage of life than other teeth, and often there is insufficient room in the mouth for them to erupt normally. Impacted teeth most frequently occur in adolescents and young adults when the teeth are still emerging.

Impacted teeth may cause pain and inflammation. A partly erupted tooth may be covered by a flap of gum under which plaque (a sticky deposit of food particles, saliva, and bacteria) accumulates, leading to inflammation of the gum and gradual decay of the tooth (*see* DENTAL CARIES, p.609).

WHAT MIGHT BE DONE?

Your dentist will check at each visit (*see* DENTAL CHECKUP, p.609) whether any emerging teeth are likely to become impacted. He or she may also take X-rays

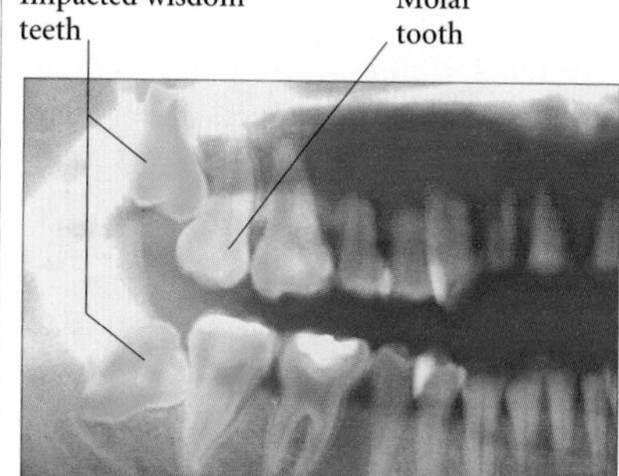

Impacted teeth
This colour-enhanced X-ray shows two wisdom teeth that have impacted on the roots of adjacent molars.

to look at unerupted teeth. One or more teeth may be extracted to allow room for other teeth to come through. You may also need orthodontic treatment (p.614) to straighten the teeth.

Wisdom teeth that appear likely to become impacted are often extracted to avoid complications. If canines are impacted, they may be fully exposed by removing gum tissue. An orthodontic device is then applied to guide the teeth into position.

WWW ONLINE SITES: p.1030

Malocclusion

Unsatisfactory contact between the upper and lower teeth

AGE Most common between the ages of 6 and 14

GENETICS Often runs in families

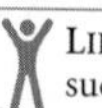
LIFESTYLE Poor oral hygiene and thumb sucking beyond the age of 6 are risk factors

GENDER Not a significant factor

Ideally, the upper front teeth should slightly overlap the lower front teeth and the molars should meet evenly. However, perfect teeth are rare and most people have some teeth that are out of position. Imperfections are not usually a pressing problem unless appearance is adversely affected or biting and chewing are impaired.

Malocclusion may occur when the teeth are crooked because they are crowded and overlap each other or when the upper front teeth protrude too far in front of the lower front teeth. Less commonly, the lower teeth protrude in front of the upper front teeth. Sometimes, the back teeth prevent the front teeth from meeting properly, a condition known as an open bite.

WHAT ARE THE CAUSES?

Malocclusion often runs in families and usually develops in childhood when the teeth and jaws are growing. The condition is usually caused by a discrepancy between the number and size of the teeth and the growth of the jaws. In children, protrusion of the front teeth may also be caused by thumb sucking beyond about the age of 6.

If the primary teeth are lost early (before the ages of 9 or 10) because of

(TREATMENT) ORTHODONTIC TREATMENT

Orthodontics is the correction of crowded or unevenly spaced teeth. Orthodontic treatment is usually performed on older children and adolescents while their teeth are still developing, although adults can also benefit. Casts of the teeth are taken before an orthodontic appliance, or brace, is applied either to move or straighten the teeth gradually. In some cases, it is necessary to extract one or more teeth in order to make room for others. The treatment usually takes several months or years to complete and necessitates regular visits to the orthodontist for checkups.

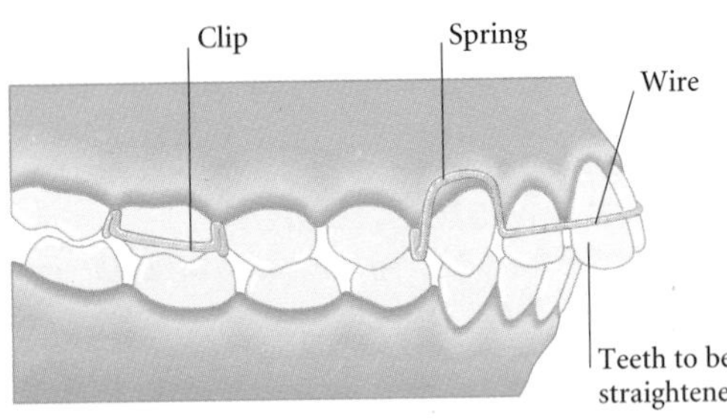

Removable appliances
Removable braces consist of a plastic plate, which fits into the roof of the mouth and clips into place. Springs and wires exert pressure on the teeth. To increase the amount of pressure, the brace may be connected to a headcap that is worn while sleeping.

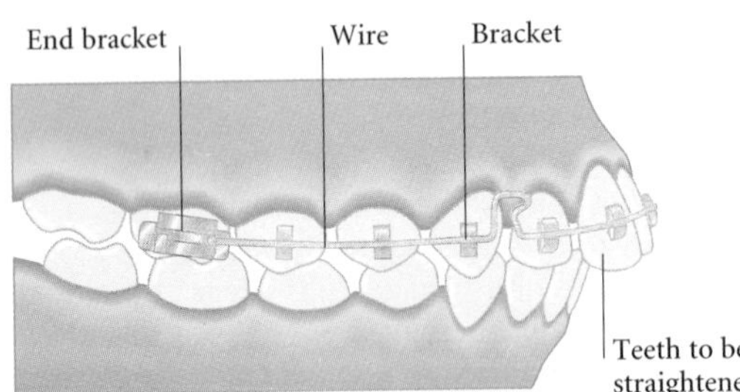

Fixed appliances
Fixed braces consist of wires and springs carried by brackets that are fixed to the teeth with dental adhesive. These braces can exert greater pressure than removable appliances and produce more complex movements of the teeth.

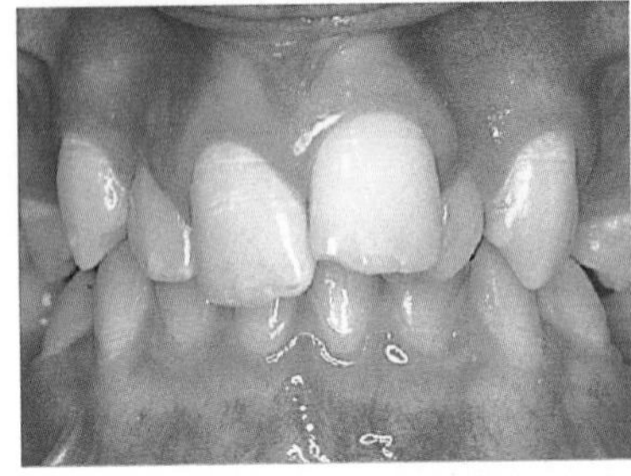

BEFORE TREATMENT

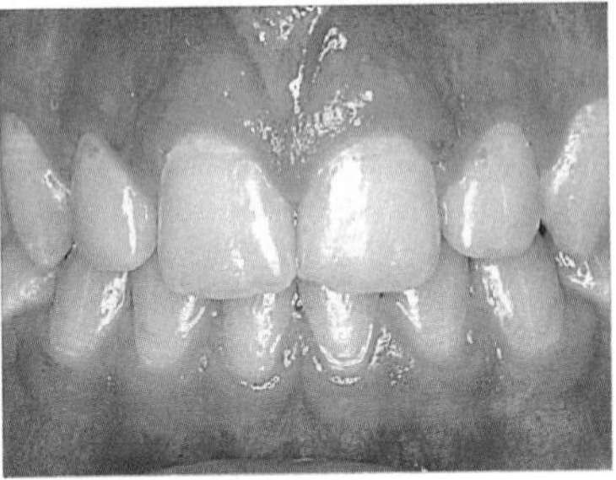

AFTER TREATMENT

Orthodontic treatment
These two photographs show a set of teeth before and after orthodontic treatment. The irregular teeth have been brought into line by the treatment.

decay (*see* DENTAL CARIES, p.609), the secondary molars that are already in position may move forwards to take up some of the space meant for the new front teeth. The new teeth then become crowded and misaligned.

WHAT ARE THE SYMPTOMS?

From about the age of 6, the symptoms develop gradually and may include:

- Out-of-line, crowded, or abnormally spaced teeth.
- Excessive protrusion of the upper teeth in front of the lower, or a protruding lower jaw.
- Front teeth that do not meet.

Some children have mild symptoms, but these are often temporary and tend to result from a growth spurt.

Speech and chewing are affected in severe cases of malocclusion. An abnormal bite may be painful and may also affect the appearance, particularly the lower-jaw profile. Arthritis may develop in the temporomandibular joint (*see* TEMPOROMANDIBULAR JOINT DISORDER, p.616) in rare cases.

WHAT MIGHT BE DONE?

The dentist will look for malocclusion as part of a dental checkup (p.609). If found, a specialist dentist called an orthodontist may take casts of the teeth to study the bite in detail. The orthodontist may also take X-rays, especially if some of the teeth have not erupted.

Treatment is usually necessary only if malocclusion is severe and is causing difficulties when eating and speaking or affecting appearance. If the teeth are overcrowded, some of them may be extracted. Rough or irregular teeth are often reshaped or capped. If required, the teeth may then be aligned using an orthodontic appliance (*see* ORTHODONTIC TREATMENT, above). Surgery is necessary only in rare cases.

It is best to treat malocclusion during childhood, when the teeth and jaw bones are still developing. However, if malocclusion is caused by a severe mismatch in the size of the jaws and teeth, surgery may be needed and treatment may be delayed until adulthood.

(WWW) ONLINE SITES: p.1030

Fractured tooth

A tooth that is cracked, chipped, or broken, often as a result of a blow to the mouth

- AGE More common under the age of 30
- GENDER More common in males
- LIFESTYLE Playing contact sports is a risk factor
- GENETICS Not a significant factor

A hard blow to the mouth is the most common cause of a fractured tooth. Young men are more likely to damage their teeth in this way because they are more likely to participate in contact sports. Protruding front teeth or teeth weakened by heavy filling are particularly susceptible to fracture.

The enamel, the hard outer covering of the crown, is most often damaged, but this does not usually produce any symptoms. Sensitivity to heat or cold and pain when biting may occur if the dentine beneath the enamel is affected.

Pain and bleeding may indicate that the pulp, containing the nerves and blood vessels, has been damaged. You should consult your dentist within 24 hours if the damaged tooth feels sensitive or is bleeding because the pulp may become infected (*see* PULPITIS, p.611), and a dental abscess (p.611) may form at the root. While waiting for an appointment, soft dental wax can be placed over a damaged tooth to protect it.

WHAT MIGHT BE DONE?

Treatment depends on the severity of the damage. Chipped enamel may only be treated for cosmetic reasons. A large fracture may be filled (*see* TOOTH FILLING, p.611) or a crown may be fitted (*see* CROWNS AND REPLACEMENT TEETH, right). A tooth with an extensive fracture may be splinted to neighbouring teeth for 1–2 weeks. If the pulp is infected or has died, you may need root canal treatment (p.612). Severely damaged teeth may have to be extracted.

(WWW) ONLINE SITES: p.1030, p.1032

Missing teeth

The lack of one or more secondary, or adult, teeth

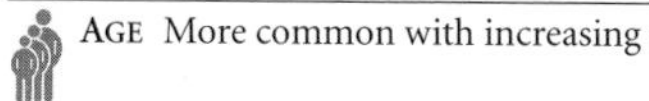
AGE More common with increasing age

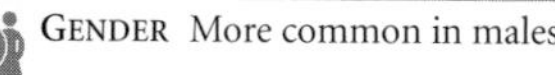
GENDER More common in males

GENETICS In some cases, the cause is inherited

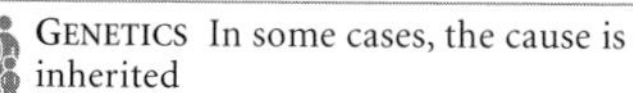
LIFESTYLE Poor oral hygiene and playing contact sports are risk factors

Total absence of many or all of the secondary teeth is very rare. Failure of one or more teeth to develop is more common. Of all the teeth, the wisdom teeth are most likely to be absent, which may be an advantage as it reduces the risk of impaction (*see* IMPACTED TEETH, p.613). The emergence of some teeth may be delayed by the effects of chemotherapy (p.280) and radiotherapy (p.281) and in people with Down's syndrome (p.821) or those with certain other genetic conditions. A delay may also be due to impaction caused by overcrowding.

Teeth may be lost due to injury (*see* AVULSED TOOTH, p.616) or following tooth decay caused by neglect of oral hygiene (*see* DENTAL CARIES, p.609). The risk of tooth loss is higher in men

(TREATMENT) CROWNS AND REPLACEMENT TEETH

If a tooth is damaged but the root and main body of the tooth are healthy, a new biting surface, known as a crown, may be attached. The crown is often coloured to match the surrounding natural teeth. If a tooth is lost or extracted, it may be replaced by an artificial tooth. There are several methods for replacing missing teeth. The method used depends on the circumstances as well as the number of teeth that have been lost.

CROWNS

Up to two or three visits to your dentist may be necessary for a crown to be fitted. White porcelain is usually used for crowns at the front of the mouth. Crowns at the back of the mouth are often made of porcelain bonded to a gold or a gold–platinum alloy.

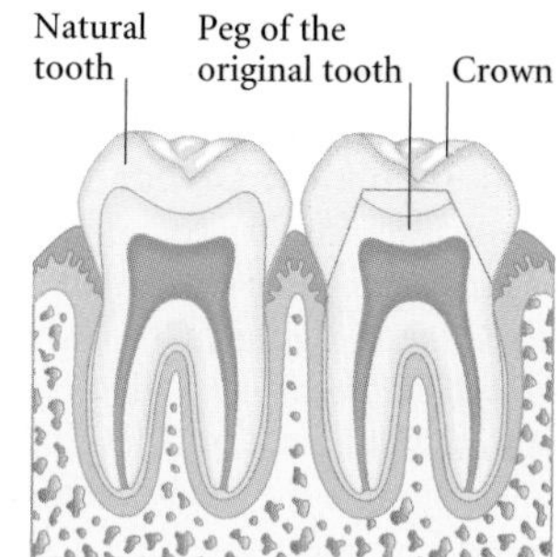

Fitting a crown
The tooth is shaped into a peg and an impression of the peg is taken. A temporary crown is made to fit over the peg while a permanent crown is made. The permanent crown is then cemented into place.

REPLACEMENT TEETH

If one or more teeth have to be extracted, or if they are lost, they can be replaced by one of three different types of artificial teeth: a bridge, a dental implant, or dentures. Bridges and dental implants are permanent and fixed and are used to replace only one or two teeth at a time. Dentures can be removed and are used when many teeth need to be replaced.

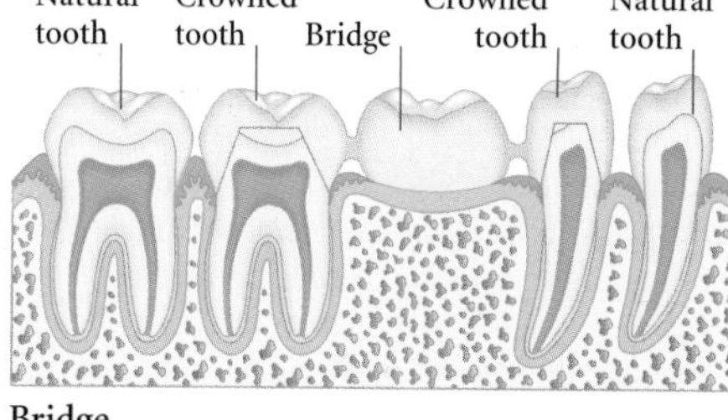

Bridge
A bridge is a permanent fixture used to replace one or two teeth. The teeth on either side of the gap are crowned to support the artificial tooth (bridge).

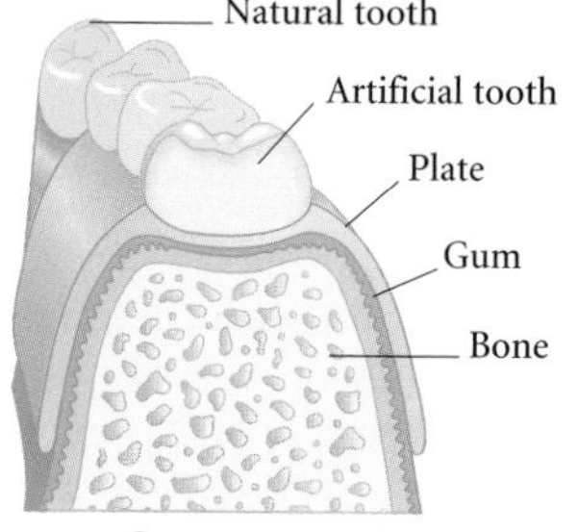

SECTION ACROSS DENTURE

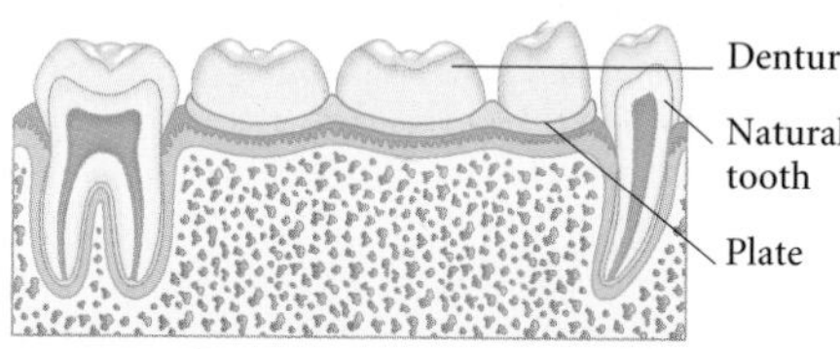

SECTION ALONG DENTURE

Dentures
A denture can be removed and may replace any number of teeth. Dentures have a metal or plastic baseplate and stay in place by resting on the gum ridges or by clasps that fit the natural teeth.

Implants
An implant is a permanent method of replacing a single tooth. A hole is drilled in the jaw at the site of the missing tooth, and an implant, usually titanium, is placed into the hole. The implant must heal for 4–6 months before an artificial tooth is attached to the top of the implant.

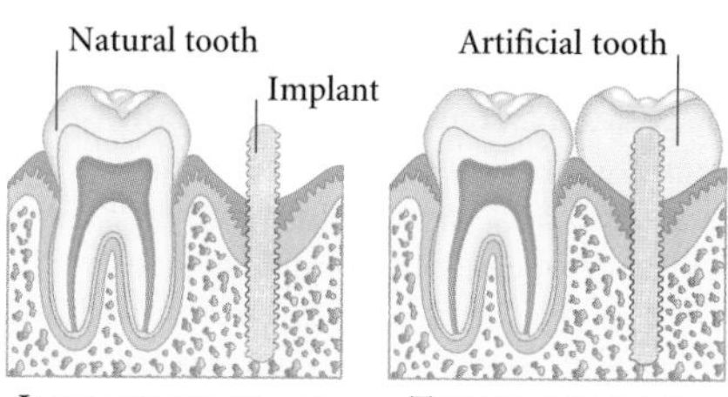

IMPLANT IN PLACE

TOOTH IN PLACE

because they play more contact sports such as boxing and rugby. If the secondary (adult) teeth are not present, adjacent teeth tend to grow into the remaining spaces, which may cause uneven teeth or malocclusion (p.613).

WHAT MIGHT BE DONE?

The dentist will check a child's teeth during each checkup to make sure that all the teeth emerge. If one or more teeth are missing, he or she may take bite-wing X-rays to see if the teeth are absent or still in the jaw (*see* DENTAL CHECKUP, p.609). If you lose a tooth, you should consult a dentist or go to an accident and emergency department at once.

Treatment depends on how many and which teeth are affected. If the teeth are held back or delayed by overcrowding, one or two teeth may be removed to make room for the others. A brace may be needed to move teeth into place or keep them locked in position until the missing teeth have emerged and have become established (*see* ORTHODONTIC TREATMENT, p.614). Teeth that have been lost can sometimes be reattached. If a tooth has failed to develop or one or more teeth have been lost, the missing tooth or teeth may be replaced (*see* CROWNS AND REPLACEMENT TEETH, p.615). Missing wisdom teeth are not replaced.

(WWW) ONLINE SITES: p.1030

Avulsed tooth

A tooth that has been partly or completely knocked out of its socket as a result of a powerful impact to the jaw

AGE More common in children

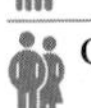
GENDER More common in males

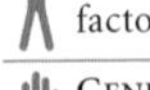
LIFESTYLE Playing contact sports is a risk factor

GENETICS Not a significant factor

Although teeth are commonly lost in childhood accidents, an avulsed tooth is really a problem only if a secondary (adult) tooth is lost because primary (baby) teeth are eventually replaced by secondary teeth. Avulsed teeth are much more common in men because they play more contact sports. The front teeth are most often involved.

If you have a tooth that is dislodged or knocked out, you should consult a dentist or visit an accident and emergency department immediately. If your tooth has been completely knocked out, you should put it back into the socket if possible. Alternatively, put the tooth in a glass of milk or salt water, or wrap it in a clean, damp cloth. In 9 out of 10 cases, a tooth will reattach itself to the jaw if it is replaced in the socket within 30 minutes of being knocked out.

WHAT MIGHT BE DONE?

The dentist will replace the tooth and splint it to other teeth to immobilize it for 10–14 days. Complete avulsion usually kills the pulp (containing nerves and blood vessels), in which case you may need root canal treatment (p.612) when the tooth has been replaced.

If you have lost a tooth and may have inhaled it, a chest X-ray (p.490) may be taken to ensure that the tooth is not lodged in your airways or lungs. A lost or damaged tooth may have to be replaced with an artificial tooth (*see* CROWNS AND REPLACEMENT TEETH, p.615).

(WWW) ONLINE SITES: p.1030, p.1032

Temporomandibular joint disorder

Problems in the joint between the jaw and skull, causing headaches or pain in the face

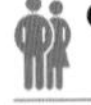
GENDER Much more common in females

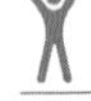
LIFESTYLE Stress may be a risk factor

AGE GENETICS Not significant factors

The temporomandibular joint connects the mandible (lower jawbone) to the part of the skull known as the temporal bone. The joint allows the lower jaw to move in all directions so that the teeth can be used to bite off and chew food efficiently. In temporomandibular joint disorder, the joint and the muscles and ligaments that control the joint do not work together properly, causing pain. The condition is three times more common in women than in men.

Temporomandibular joint disorder is most commonly caused by spasm of the chewing muscles, often as a result of clenching the jaw or grinding the teeth. Clenching the jaw and grinding the teeth may be increased by stress. A poor bite (*see* MALOCCLUSION, p.613) places stress on the muscles and may also result in temporomandibular joint disorder, as may an injury to the head, jaw, or neck that causes displacement of the joint. In rare cases, arthritis (p.374) is a cause of the condition.

WHAT ARE THE SYMPTOMS?

If you have temporomandibular joint disorder, you may notice one or more of the following symptoms:

- Headaches.
- Tenderness in the jaw muscles.
- Aching pain in the face.
- Severe pain near the ears.

In some cases, pain is caused by chewing or by opening the mouth too widely when yawning. There may be difficulty in opening the mouth, locking of the jaw, and clicking noises from the joint as the mouth is opened or closed.

WHAT MIGHT BE DONE?

Your dentist may take a panoramic X-ray of your mouth and jaws. He or she may also arrange for you to have special X-rays or an MRI (p.248) of the joint.

Treatment is aimed at eliminating muscle spasm and tension and relieving the pain. There are several self-help measures that you can take, including applying a warm, wet towel to the face, massaging the facial muscles, eating only soft foods, and using a device that fits over the teeth at night to prevent you from clenching or grinding your teeth. Taking a painkiller (p.912), such as aspirin or paracetamol, may also help. If tension of the muscles used for chewing is severe, your doctor may prescribe a muscle relaxant drug (p.896). If stress is a major factor, you may find relaxation exercises (p.75) helpful.

If your bite needs to be adjusted, your dentist may recommend wearing a fixed or removable orthodontic appliance for a specified period of time (*see* ORTHODONTIC TREATMENT, p.614).

WHAT IS THE PROGNOSIS?

In about 3 in 4 people, the symptoms improve within 3 months of treatment. However, in some cases, if symptoms do not improve, surgery may be needed to repair the temporomandibular joint.

(WWW) ONLINE SITES: p.1030, p.1032

GUM DISORDERS

The gums form a layer of protective tissue that surrounds the base of each tooth and covers part of the jawbones. Healthy gum forms a tight seal around the crown of a tooth and protects the sensitive tissues below from bacterial invasion. If the gums are damaged, the teeth may become unsupported and loose. Most gum disorders can be prevented by good oral hygiene.

Most adults have some degree of gum disease which, if left untreated, may eventually lead to loss of teeth. Good oral hygiene is essential to help to prevent gum disorders. During regular dental checkups, most dentists and oral hygienists provide information on the correct way to brush and floss teeth and on general mouth care.

The first topics covered here are gum disorders such as gingivitis and periodontitis, which may be caused by poor oral hygiene. Inadequate teeth cleaning leads to a build-up of plaque (a deposit of food particles, saliva, and bacteria) on the surfaces of the teeth. If the plaque is not removed, it causes the gums to become inflamed. In more serious cases, the teeth may be affected and loosen or come out, either because the periodontal tissues are inflamed and detach from the teeth or because the gums recede, exposing the roots and leading to tooth decay. The final article in this section discusses a condition called dry socket, in which a tooth socket becomes inflamed after the tooth has been extracted.

KEY ANATOMY

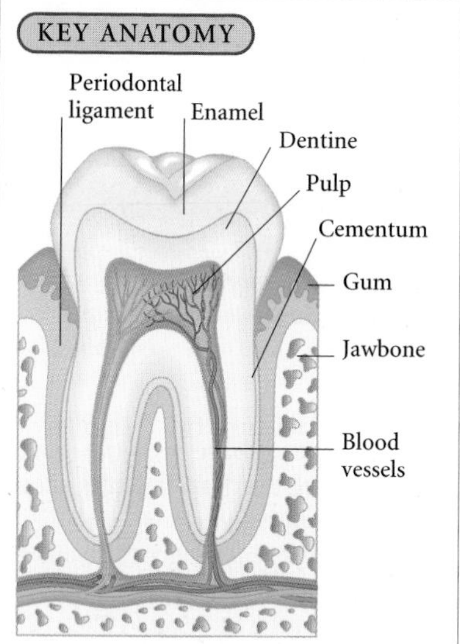

For more information on the structure and function of the gums, *see* pp.606–607.

Gingivitis

Inflammation of the gums, usually caused by poor oral hygiene

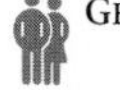 GENDER More common in females

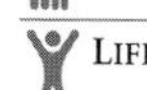 LIFESTYLE Poor oral hygiene is a risk factor

 AGE GENETICS Not significant factors

Mild gingivitis, also known as gum disease, is a very common disorder and occurs in about 9 in 10 adults. Healthy gums are pink or brown and firm. In gingivitis, the gums become purple-red, soft, and shiny. They also bleed easily, especially when the teeth are brushed. The condition is usually caused by a build-up of plaque (a deposit of food particles, saliva, and bacteria) where the gum meets the base of the tooth.

Gingivitis can be made worse by taking certain drugs, such as phenytoin (*see* ANTICONVULSANT DRUGS, p.914), immunosuppressants (p.906), and some antihypertensives (p.897). These drugs may cause overgrowth of the gums, making the removal of dental plaque difficult. Certain contraceptive drugs can also make symptoms worse. Pregnant women are more susceptible to gingivitis because of dramatic changes in hormone levels during pregnancy.

If gingivitis develops suddenly, it is known as acute necrotizing ulcerative gingivitis (ANUG) or "trench mouth". ANUG usually occurs in teenagers and young adults. The condition sometimes develops from chronic gingivitis and is caused by an abnormal growth of the bacteria that normally exist harmlessly within the mouth. ANUG is more common in people who are under stress or run down and in people with AIDS (*see* HIV INFECTION AND AIDS, p.297).

WHAT ARE THE SYMPTOMS?

The symptoms of gingivitis develop gradually and usually include:

- Purple-red, soft, shiny, swollen gums.
- Gums that bleed easily when the teeth are brushed.

If gingivitis is not treated, the gum eventually pulls away from the tooth, and a pocket develops between the tooth and the gum in which more plaque can form. Bacteria in the plaque may cause the inflammation to spread. Eventually, chronic periodontitis (p.618) or receding gums (p.619) may develop. In severe cases, one or more teeth may be lost.

Symptoms of ANUG usually develop over 1–2 days and may include:

- Bright red gums that are covered with a greyish deposit.
- Crater-like ulcers on the gums.
- Gums that bleed easily.
- Bad breath and a metallic taste in the mouth.
- Pain in the gums.

As ANUG progresses, the lymph glands in the neck may become enlarged, and a fever may develop.

WHAT IS THE TREATMENT?

If you have gingivitis, your dentist will probably scale your teeth to remove the plaque and calculus (hardened plaque). The procedure involves using an ultrasonic scaler to remove the calculus and scraping away at resistant areas with a hand tool. The teeth are then polished. Regular follow-up visits may be needed to monitor the condition of your gums. Your dentist may also recommend that you use a mouthwash that contains hydrogen peroxide, which helps to prevent plaque from building up.

If you have ANUG, your dentist will clean carefully around all the teeth. He or she will also prescribe antibiotics (p.885) and an antiseptic mouthwash.

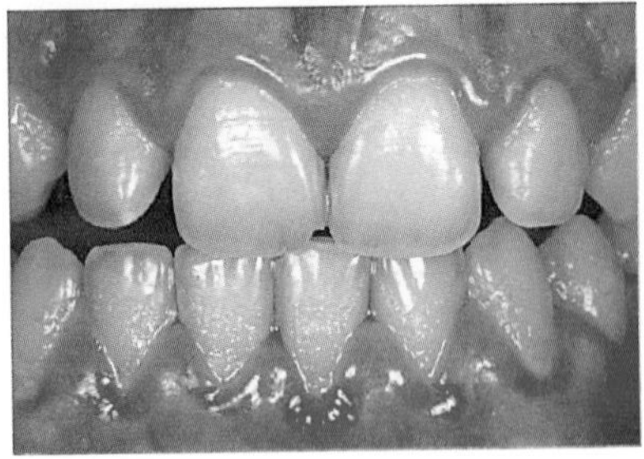

Gingivitis
In gingivitis, the gums become inflamed and soft due to a build-up of plaque on the teeth. The gums also bleed easily.

Painkillers (p.912) may be prescribed. Once your teeth have been thoroughly scaled and cleaned, your gums should gradually return to normal.

You can prevent gingivitis by adopting good oral hygiene (*see* CARING FOR YOUR TEETH AND GUMS, p.610).

(WWW) ONLINE SITES: p.1030

Periodontitis

Inflammation of the tissues that support the teeth

 AGE More common over the age of 55

 GENETICS In rare cases, the cause is inherited

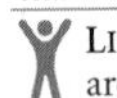 LIFESTYLE Poor oral hygiene and smoking are risk factors

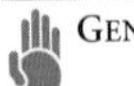 GENDER Not a significant factor

Periodontitis affects many people over the age of 55 and is a major cause of tooth loss. In this condition, the periodontal tissues that secure teeth in their sockets become inflamed, and the teeth become loose and, eventually, may fall out. The damage from periodontitis is irreversible, but further inflammation can be prevented with treatment and by improving oral hygiene (*see* CARING FOR YOUR TEETH AND GUMS, p.610). There is evidence that if periodontal disease is left untreated, it may predispose to cardiovascular disease.

WHAT ARE THE CAUSES?

The most common form of periodontitis is chronic adult periodontitis. This condition often develops as a complication of gingivitis (p.617), in which the gums are inflamed, usually due to poor oral hygiene and/or smoking. If toothbrushing is neglected, plaque (a deposit of food particles, saliva, and bacteria) and calculus (hardened plaque) build up on the teeth. As a result of this build-up, the gums become inflamed and pull away from the teeth, leaving pockets in which more plaque can collect. As gingivitis develops, bacteria in the plaque attack the periodontal tissues, causing them to become inflamed and detach from the teeth. The inflammation also results in the loss of bone supporting the teeth, and teeth may fall out.

Periapical periodontitis is another form of periodontitis and is caused by tooth decay (*see* DENTAL CARIES, p.609), usually due to poor oral hygiene. If tooth decay is left untreated, the hard enamel that covers the tooth and the dentine underneath will eventually be destroyed, allowing bacteria into the pulp (central part) of the tooth (*see* PULPITIS, p.611).

Some rare genetic forms of the disorder, such as juvenile periodontitis, occur in children or young adults and are particularly severe.

WHAT ARE THE SYMPTOMS?

In the early stages of periodontitis, there may be no symptoms. Symptoms of chronic periodontitis may include:

- Red, soft, shiny gums that bleed easily and may recede (*see* RECEDING GUMS, opposite page).
- Bad breath and an unpleasant taste.
- Toothache when hot, cold, or sweet foods or drinks are consumed.

In the late stages of chronic periodontitis, there may be loosening of the teeth.

The symptoms of periapical periodontitis may include:

- Toothache in a specific area, especially when biting.
- Loosening of a tooth.
- Swelling of the jaw.

In some cases, a dental abscess (p.611) forms. If any of these symptoms occur, consult your dentist promptly.

WHAT MIGHT BE DONE?

Your dentist will examine your teeth and gums and check the depth of the pockets between them using a special probe. He or she may also take dental X-rays (*see* DENTAL CHECKUP, p.609) to check how much of the bony support around the teeth has been lost.

Chronic periodontitis is treated by removing plaque and calculus from the teeth in a procedure known as scaling. In some cases, a gingivectomy (surgical trimming of the gums) may also be performed to reduce the size of the pockets between the gums and teeth. The diseased lining of the pockets may be removed to allow healthy tissue to attach itself to the teeth.

After surgery, you will probably be prescribed an antiseptic mouthwash, which you should use regularly. If the periodontitis is severe, your dentist may prescribe a course of antibiotics (p.885), or an antibiotic paste or pellet may be pushed into the deep pockets between the teeth and gums. Loose teeth may be fixed to other teeth in order to prevent them from falling out.

Periapical periodontitis is treated by removing the bacteria from the tooth and carrying out root canal treatment (p.612). A tooth that cannot be saved may need to be extracted.

After treatment, your dentist will advise that you brush and floss your teeth at least twice a day to prevent further build-up of plaque and calculus. If you smoke, giving up will help to prevent further inflammation.

WHAT IS THE PROGNOSIS?

If you have chronic periodontitis, better oral hygiene and giving up smoking should help to prevent the gums from receding further and teeth becoming loose. It may also reduce the risk of complications. Periapical periodontitis may need root canal treatment. About 1 in 10 people with periodontitis has a rapidly progressive form of the condition, leading to loss of teeth around the age of 50.

(WWW) ONLINE SITES: p.1030

Inflamed gum
Receding gum

Periodontitis
The gums and tissues securing the teeth have become inflamed, and the gums have receded, leaving the teeth unsupported. The condition is known as periodontitis.

Receding gums

Withdrawal of the gums from around the teeth, exposing part of the roots

 AGE Usually develops after the age of 55

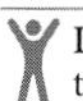 LIFESTYLE Poor oral hygiene and abrasive tooth-brushing are risk factors

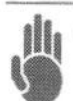 GENDER GENETICS Not significant factors

Healthy gums form a tight seal around the tooth where the crown of the tooth meets the root. If the gums recede, the root of the tooth becomes exposed, causing the attachment between the tooth and the socket to weaken. Eventually, the tooth may become loose and, in severe cases, may have to be extracted by the dentist.

If the roots are exposed, the teeth may be sensitive to hot, cold, or sweet substances. Since the roots are softer than the enamel on the crown of the tooth, they are also more susceptible to decay (*see* DENTAL CARIES, p.609).

WHAT ARE THE CAUSES?

Severely receding gums are usually a symptom of long-term gingivitis (p.617) or periodontitis (opposite page). These disorders are usually a result of poor oral hygiene, which results in a build-up of plaque (a deposit of food particles, saliva, and bacteria) and calculus (hardened plaque) between the base of the teeth and the gums.

The gums will eventually become inflamed and recede, exposing the roots of the teeth. Vigorous, abrasive tooth-brushing along the margins of the gums, particularly in a horizontal direction with a hard toothbrush, may also cause the gums to recede.

WHAT MIGHT BE DONE?

If you have receding gums, improving your oral hygiene (*see* CARING FOR YOUR TEETH AND GUMS, p.610) and giving up smoking, should prevent any further recession of the gums.

Your dentist will probably use a procedure known as scaling to remove the plaque and calculus from your teeth. Scaling should help to prevent your gums from receding further. He or she will also advise you on your tooth-brushing and flossing techniques to avoid further damage to the exposed roots. Your dentist may suggest that you use a desensitizing toothpaste or fluoride mouthwash, which will also reduce the risk of decay. If your teeth are very sensitive, the dentist may treat them with a desensitizing varnish or an adhesive filling material. Very rarely, grafting procedures, which help to cover the exposed surfaces of roots, are used. If severely receding gums cause any teeth to become loose, these loose teeth can sometimes be fixed to teeth that are more firmly anchored in the jawbone.

(WWW) ONLINE SITES: p.1030

Gingival hyperplasia

Enlargement and swelling of the gums due to various causes

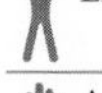 LIFESTYLE Poor oral hygiene is a risk factor

AGE GENDER GENETICS Not significant factors

The gums most commonly enlarge and swell, a condition known as gingival hyperplasia, as a result of the gum disease gingivitis (p.617). This condition is usually the result of poor oral hygiene, which allows plaque (a deposit of food particles, saliva, and bacteria) and calculus (hardened plaque) to build up where the gums meet the teeth. The gums become inflamed and bleed easily, especially when the teeth are brushed.

Gingival hyperplasia can also be a side effect of certain drugs, such as antihypertensives (p.897), anticonvulsants (p.914), and some immunosuppressants (p.906). The condition may occur during pregnancy due to certain hormonal changes. Less common causes include acute leukaemia (p.454) and scurvy, in which there is a deficiency of vitamin C.

To treat gingival hyperplasia, your dentist will probably scale your teeth to remove the plaque and advise you to brush and floss regularly (*see* CARING FOR YOUR TEETH AND GUMS, p.610). In some cases, excess gum tissue may be removed. If gingival hyperplasia is due to drugs, alternatives will be given. An underlying disorder, such as acute leukaemia, will be treated if possible, and the condition of your gums should then improve. Gingival hyperplasia due to pregnancy should clear up after the birth as hormone levels return to normal.

(WWW) ONLINE SITES: p.1030

Dry socket

Inflammation of a tooth socket that will not heal after extraction of the tooth

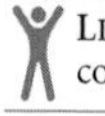 LIFESTYLE Smoking and taking oral contraceptives are risk factors

 AGE GENDER GENETICS Not significant factors

After a tooth is extracted, the tooth socket fills with blood. The blood clots and provides the framework for healing the socket. If the clot is washed away for some reason, such as by overvigorous rinsing, or if the clot becomes infected, the bony lining of the socket can become inflamed, a condition that is known as "dry socket" or post-extraction alveolitis. Dry socket occurs after about 1 in 25 tooth extractions and is more common following a difficult extraction of a molar tooth from the lower jaw. The condition occurs more frequently in people who smoke and in women taking oral contraceptives.

The symptoms of dry socket may include a severe, throbbing pain that commonly radiates to the ear 2–4 days after extraction of the tooth, a bad taste in the mouth, and bad breath. The tooth socket may only partly heal, and occasionally small pieces of bone may come out of the tooth socket.

WHAT MIGHT BE DONE?

Your dentist may prescribe antibiotics (p.885) after extracting a tooth to help to prevent the tooth socket from becoming infected. If after a few days the socket is not healing or you are still feeling pain, make an appointment to see your dentist as soon as possible. While waiting for an appointment, you can relieve symptoms with over-the-counter painkillers (p.912), such as paracetamol.

To treat dry socket, your dentist may initially wash out the tooth socket with warm salt water or a dilute antiseptic solution. He or she will then pack the socket with antiseptic paste. This treatment is repeated every 2–3 days until the tooth socket begins to heal. Your dentist may also suggest that you use hot saltwater mouthwashes at home to help to reduce the inflammation. The socket should start to heal within a few days, and healing should be complete within a few weeks.

(WWW) ONLINE SITES: p.1030

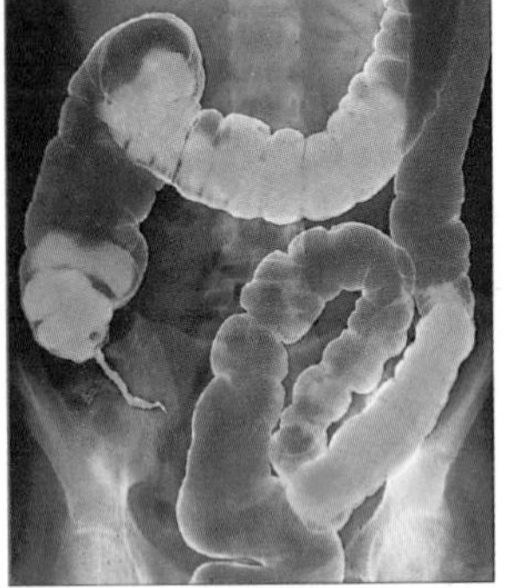

Colon
The colon, a looped tube about 1.3 m (4 ft) long, is the main component of the large intestine.

DIGESTIVE SYSTEM

THE DIGESTIVE SYSTEM breaks down food into simple components that the body's cells can absorb and eliminates remaining waste. Food is propelled by muscular contractions through the digestive tract, the long tube that runs from the mouth to the anus. Digestion begins in the mouth, where saliva moistens and dissolves the food and the chewing action of the teeth and tongue breaks up large particles. The process of digestion is completed when nutrients (the useful parts of food) have been absorbed into the bloodstream and waste has passed out of the anus. The body uses nutrients for energy, growth, and tissue repair.

The digestive system consists of a long, convoluted, muscular tube or tract, which extends from the mouth to the anus, and a number of other digestive organs. These associated organs include the salivary glands, liver, and pancreas. The digestive tract is made up of a series of hollow organs, which includes the stomach and the small and large intestines.

The functions of the digestive system are to ingest food, break it down, extract the useful components, or nutrients, and dispose of the remaining waste as faeces. Food can take many hours to pass through the tract. However, the oesophagus and stomach enable us to swallow a large amount of food quickly and digest it at leisure. In an average person's lifetime, the digestive system processes 30,000 kg (66,000 lb) of food. The digestive system can process a variety of diets, from a typical meat-based Western diet to a Japanese diet consisting mainly of rice and fish.

FOOD BREAKDOWN

Most food molecules are too large to pass through cell membranes and must be broken down before they can be absorbed. Organs of the digestive system secrete juices containing enzymes (proteins that speed up chemical reactions) and acids that help to convert large molecules into small, absorbable units. Chewing physically breaks down food into small particles, exposing a large surface area to the action of enzymes. In the stomach, food is churned with digestive juices to make chyme, a semi-liquid mixture.

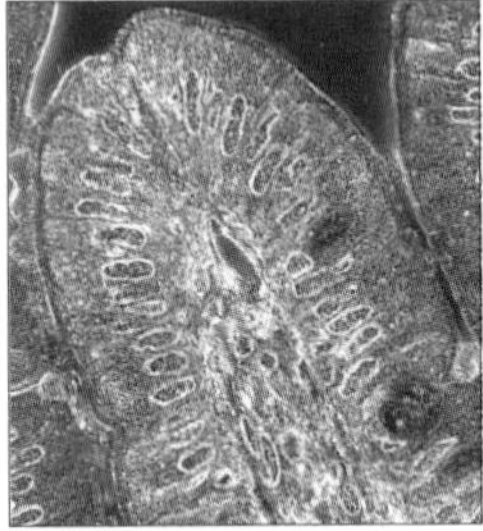

Villus
A villus is one of many, tiny, finger-like projections lining the small intestine.

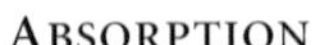

ABSORPTION

By the time food reaches the end of the small intestine, most large nutrient molecules have been broken down into smaller molecules. These are absorbed into the blood through tiny pores in the villi, the fronds that project from the intestinal wall. The blood carries nutrients to the liver, then to the body's cells. Indigestible matter passes into the large intestine, where some water is absorbed before the remainder is expelled from the anus as faeces.

REGULATING DIGESTION

The nervous and hormonal systems work together to ensure that digestive juices are secreted at the right time in different parts of the digestive tract. For example, when food enters the stomach or intestines, local glands release hormones that activate the production of digestive juices. These systems also control the action of the muscular walls of the digestive tract.

PROCESS HUNGER AND APPETITE

How much and how often we eat is determined by both hunger and appetite. When the body needs food or at times of day when it expects a routine meal, the nervous and hormonal systems cause the stomach to contract, resulting in hunger pangs. Appetite is a pleasurable sensation caused by the production of digestive juices in the mouth and stomach.

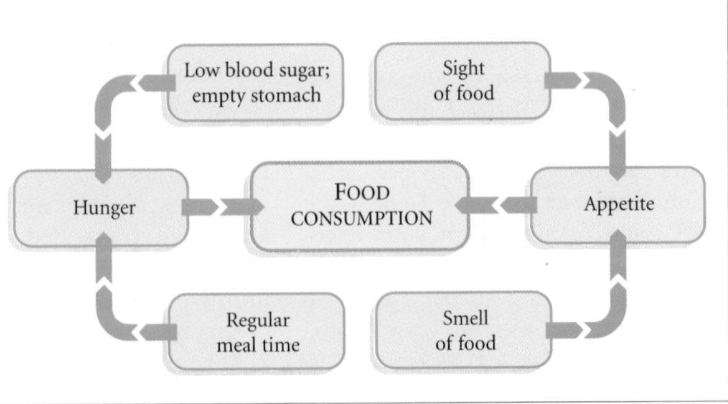

Stimulating hunger and appetite
Hunger is stimulated by the body's need for food or by the routine of meal times. The anticipation of food stimulates the appetite. Both sensations trigger a desire to eat.

STRUCTURE AND FUNCTION

THE DIGESTIVE SYSTEM

The digestive system consists of the digestive tract and its associated organs. The digestive tract is a tube about 7 m (24 ft) long through which food passes while it is broken down. The tract consists of the mouth and pharynx (throat), oesophagus, stomach, the small and large intestines, and the anus. The associated digestive organs include three pairs of salivary glands, the liver, the pancreas, and the gallbladder.

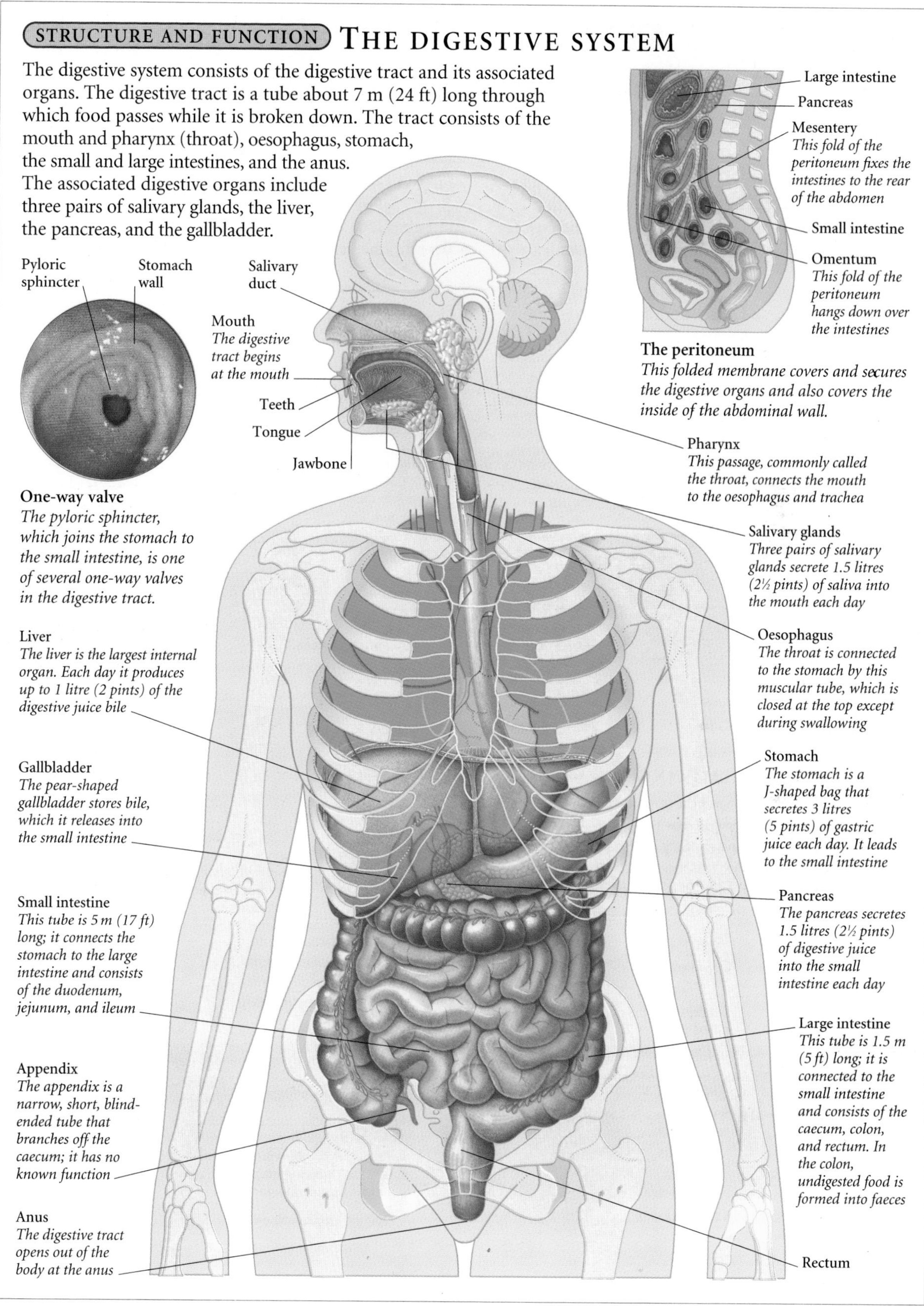

STRUCTURE AND FUNCTION

THE DIGESTIVE TRACT

The digestive tract is a series of hollow organs – the mouth, oesophagus, stomach, small and large intestines, and anus – connected to form a long tube. The tract has muscular walls that rhythmically propel food along the tube (*see* PERISTALSIS, opposite page), breaking it down and mixing it with digestive juices. Muscular activity is controlled by a network of nerves that covers the tract. Several muscular valves control the passage of food and prevent it from moving backwards.

MOUTH

The tongue, teeth, and saliva work together to start digestion and aid swallowing. Teeth chop and grind food, increasing the surface area over which digestive enzymes in saliva can act. Saliva also softens food so that the tongue can mould it into a bolus, or ball, for swallowing.

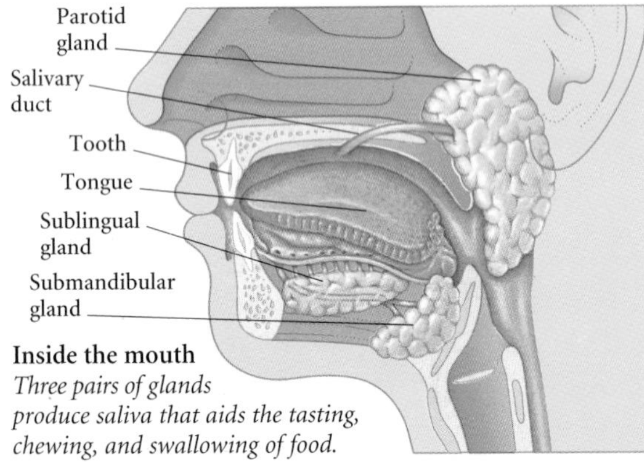

Inside the mouth
Three pairs of glands produce saliva that aids the tasting, chewing, and swallowing of food.

FUNCTION

SWALLOWING

Swallowing begins when you push a bolus (ball of food) towards the oesophagus with your tongue. This action triggers two involuntary events: the soft palate, the back of the roof of the mouth, closes off the nasal cavity, and the epiglottis, a flap of cartilage, tilts downwards to seal the trachea (windpipe).

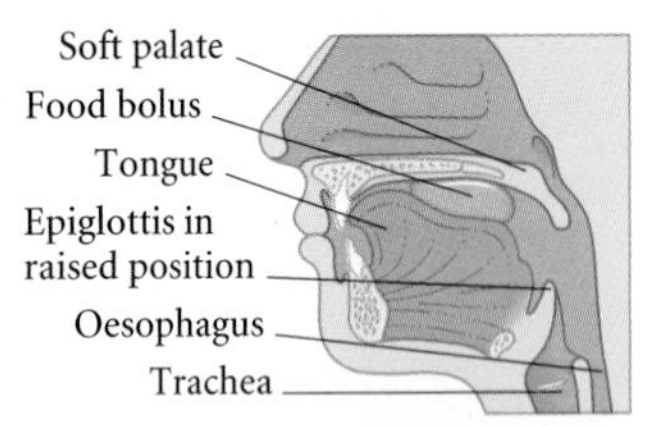

1 *In their normal positions, the soft palate and the epiglottis allow air to pass from the nasal cavity into the trachea.*

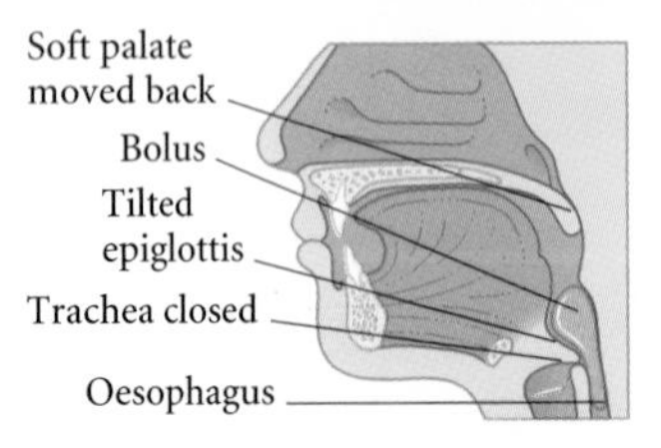

2 *While swallowing, the epiglottis tilts to seal the trachea, the soft palate lifts to close off the nasal cavity, and the bolus enters the oesophagus.*

OESOPHAGUS AND STOMACH

The throat opens into the oesophagus, a muscular tube that propels food to the stomach. In the stomach, solid food spends up to 5 hours being churned to a pulp and mixed with gastric juice to form chyme before being squirted into the small intestine. Liquids pass from the mouth to the intestine in a matter of minutes.

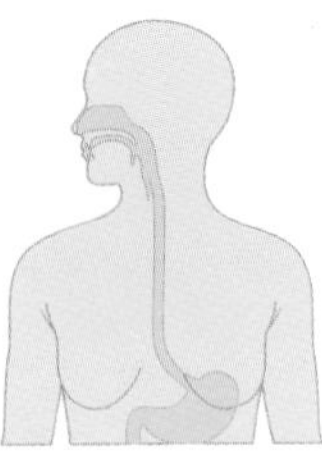

LOCATION

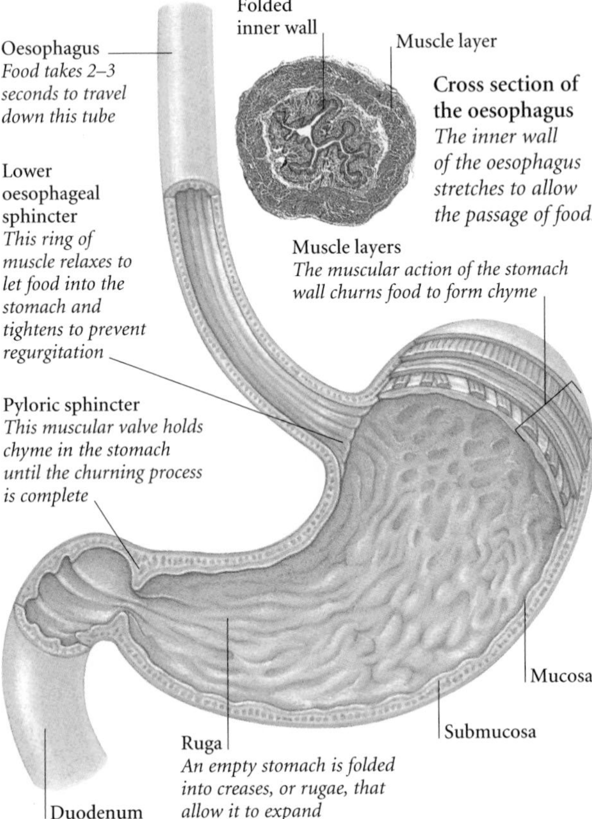

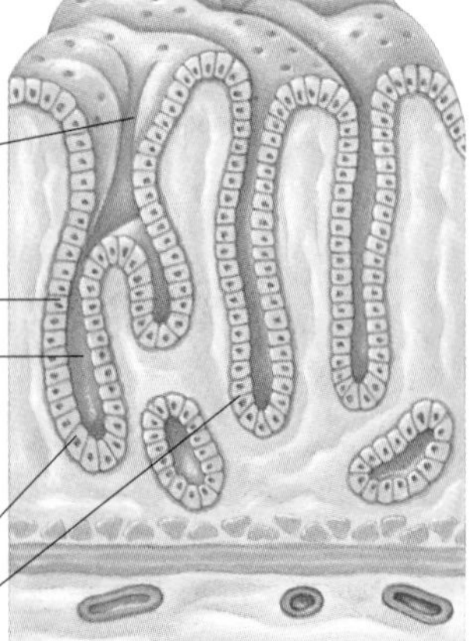

Section of the stomach lining
The stomach is lined by mucosa, which secretes mucus to prevent the stomach from digesting itself.

SMALL AND LARGE INTESTINES

At about 6.5 m (22 ft) in length, the intestines form the longest part of the digestive tract. In the small intestine, which consists of the duodenum, jejunum, and ileum, food mixes with digestive juices, and nutrients and water are absorbed into the blood. In the large intestine, which is divided into the caecum, colon, and rectum, faeces are formed before passing out of the anus.

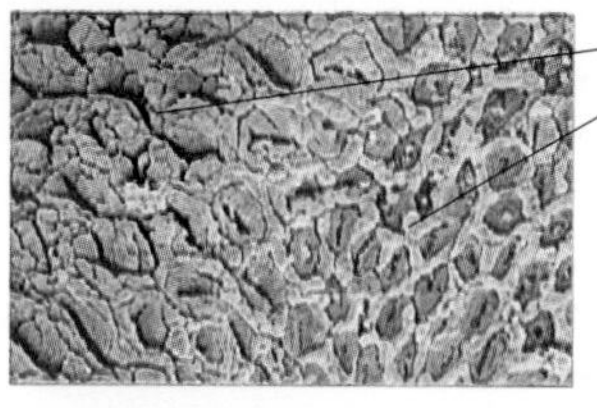

Intestinal junction
The small intestine has a folded lining to absorb nutrients; the lining of the large intestine is flatter.

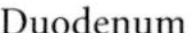

Cross section of the large intestine
The large intestine wall has a wider diameter and less developed muscle layers than the small intestine.

CROSS SECTION OF SMALL INTESTINE

CROSS SECTION OF THE SMALL INTESTINE LINING

Villi of the small intestine
The mucosa, the inner layer of the small intestine, has millions of finger-like fronds called villi covered in smaller fronds called microvilli. These fronds provide a surface area the size of a tennis court for nutrient absorption.

FUNCTION PERISTALSIS

Food is propelled along the digestive tract by a sequence of muscular contractions called peristalsis. The muscular wall behind a piece of food squeezes to push it forwards into the next part of the tract, where the muscle is relaxed. Other types of muscular action churn food in the stomach and form faeces in the colon.

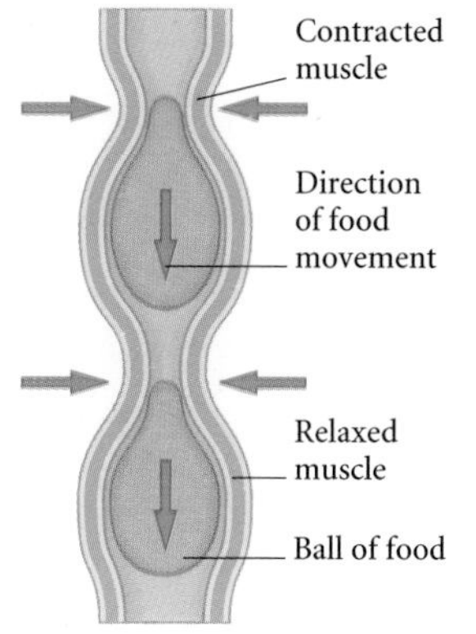

The peristaltic wave
The muscular action of the digestive tract moves food continuously in an action known as a "peristaltic wave".

(STRUCTURE) LIVER, GALLBLADDER, AND PANCREAS

The liver, gallbladder, and pancreas all take part in the process of digestion by secreting digestive juices that break down food molecules. The liver produces a greenish digestive juice called bile, which is stored in the sac-like gallbladder. The pancreas produces a powerful digestive fluid known as pancreatic juice. When food enters the duodenum from the stomach, the duodenal lining releases hormones that stimulate the gallbladder and pancreas to release their juices.

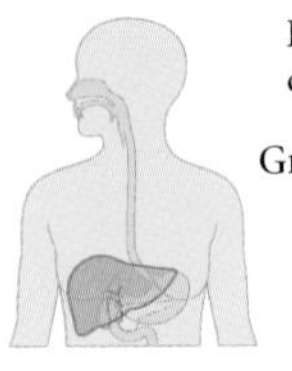

LOCATION

Pancreatic cell

Granule

Cell nucleus

Pancreatic enzymes
This magnified view shows granules that contain enzymes in pancreatic cells.

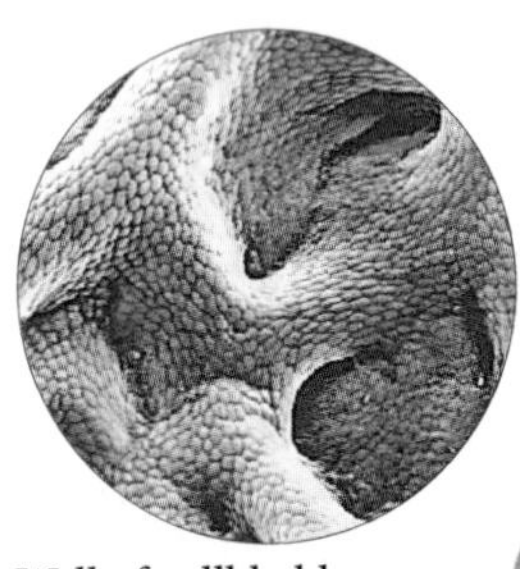

Wall of gallbladder
The heavily folded inner wall of the gallbladder can be seen in this highly magnified image.

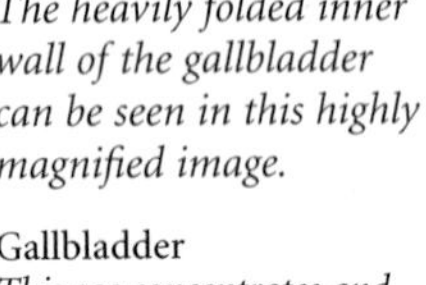

Liver
The liver manufactures, stores, and breaks down substances as required by the body

Inferior vena cava
Blood that has been processed by the liver is carried to the heart by this vein

Hepatic veins
These veins drain blood from the liver

Oesophagus

Stomach

Gallbladder
This sac concentrates and stores bile, a digestive fluid made by the liver from waste products of the blood

Pancreas
The pancreas secretes enzymes and mucus that neutralize stomach acid

Central vein

Lobule

Pancreatic duct
This duct carries pancreatic juice into the duodenum

Cystic duct
This carries bile from the gallbladder to the common bile duct

Hepatic artery
This artery carries oxygenated blood from the heart to the liver

Cross section of liver lobules
The liver consists of thousands of lobules, tiny blood-processing units each 1 mm (1/25 in) wide.

Duodenum
When food enters this tube, the pancreas and gallbladder release digestive juices

Common bile duct
This carries bile from the liver and gallbladder to the duodenum

Portal vein
This vein carries nutrient-rich blood from the small intestine to the liver

LIVER FUNCTION

The liver is the body's chemical factory, converting molecules into simpler or more complex forms as the body requires. For example, nutrients are modified in the liver, then stored there or distributed throughout the body; toxins such as alcohol are broken down into less harmful substances. The liver also produces the digestive juice bile.

Inside a liver lobule
Branches of the portal vein, hepatic artery, and bile duct surround each lobule. A central vein carries blood to the heart.

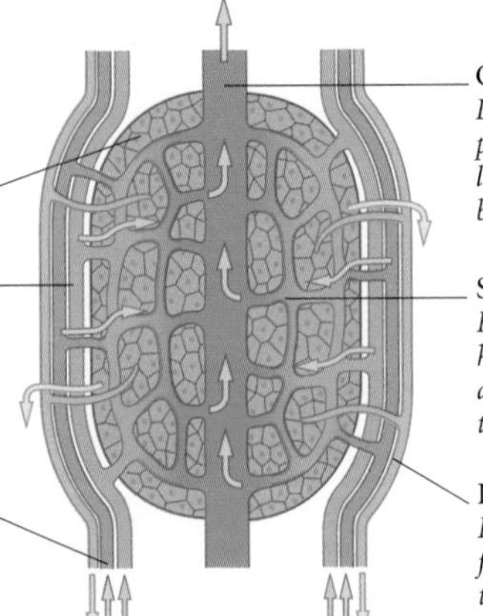

Lobule
Each lobule contains specialized cells that perform all of the liver's chemical functions

Branch of portal vein
Nutrient-filled blood from the small intestine enters each lobule through six small veins

Branch of hepatic artery
Oxygenated blood from the heart reaches each lobule through six small arteries

Central vein
Deoxygenated and processed blood from the lobule collects in this vein before returning to the heart

Sinusoids
Blood is processed by hepatocytes as it passes along these channels to the centre of the lobule

Branch of bile duct
Bile made by liver cells flows into tiny channels that converge to form the common bile duct

PROCESS CHEMICAL BREAKDOWN

Food consists mainly of water and the three main types of nutrient – protein, carbohydrate, and fat – that the body needs to survive. Before these nutrients can be used, their large molecules must be broken down in the digestive system into units small enough for the body to absorb. Absorption occurs in the small intestine (the duodenum, jejunum, and ileum) and the colon. Vitamins and minerals, which are also essential nutrients, consist of molecules tiny enough for the body to absorb without breaking them down first.

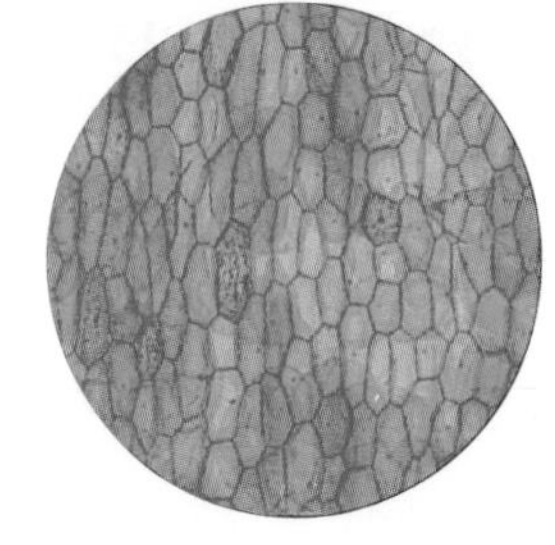

Indigestible fibre
This magnified view shows cells of fibre, an indigestible plant material that is a vital part of the diet. Fibre adds bulk to faeces and helps them to retain some water, making them easier to expel.

In the mouth
Enzymes in saliva begin to break down starch, a type of carbohydrate, into simple sugars

Liver (site of bile production)

Salivary glands

Oesophagus

In the stomach
Gastric juice secreted by glands in the stomach wall contains acid and enzymes. The acid kills bacteria in food; enzymes help to break down protein into amino acids. Special cells secrete mucus, which prevents the stomach from digesting itself

Gallbladder (site of bile storage)

Pancreas

Transfer of pancreatic juice and bile into the duodenum

In the duodenum
Bile breaks down fat particles into smaller droplets; pancreatic juice contains enzymes that convert fats into fatty acids and glycerol and sodium bicarbonate to neutralize stomach acid

In the jejunum
Pancreatic enzymes and enzymes produced by the jejunum wall complete the breakdown of carbohydrate, protein, and fat

Nutrient transfer to liver
Absorbed nutrients flow in the bloodstream to the liver, where they are processed and either stored or distributed to other parts of the body. Some fats pass along lymph vessels before entering the bloodstream

In the ileum
The main function of the ileum is to absorb nutrients; bile is also absorbed here and returned to the liver through blood vessels

In the colon
The absorption of water from waste matter to form faeces, which consist mainly of fibre, is completed in the colon. Bacteria in the colon produce some vitamins that are then absorbed

In the rectum
Faeces formed in the colon collect in the rectum before being excreted

Anus

DIGESTIVE ENZYMES

Food molecules are too large to pass through the walls of the digestive tract into the blood and lymph vessels and must be broken down into smaller molecules. Digestive enzymes help to break down proteins into amino acids, fats into fatty acids and glycerol, and starch (a complex carbohydrate) into simple sugars.

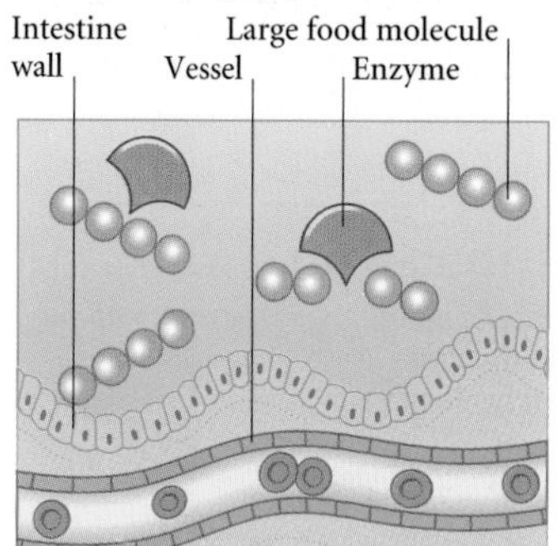

1 *A particular enzyme combines with a large food molecule, such as a protein. The enzyme breaks down the large molecule into two or more smaller molecules.*

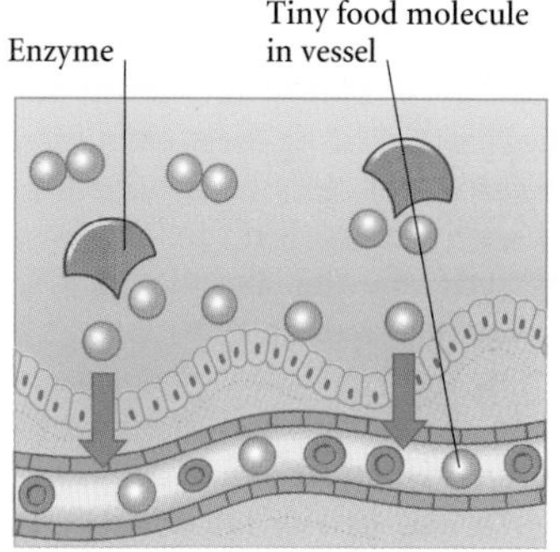

2 *The tiny molecules separate from the enzyme and are able to pass through the wall of the digestive tract into the bloodstream. The enzyme molecule remains unchanged.*

GENERAL DIGESTIVE AND NUTRITIONAL PROBLEMS

Most common digestive problems cause short-term symptoms, such as indigestion, diarrhoea, and constipation. However, long-term symptoms affecting the digestive system sometimes reflect a more serious underlying disorder.

The first part of this section looks at indigestion, the upper abdominal discomfort that most people feel at some time. Occasionally, as is described in the second article, discomfort may be more vague and persist without an identifiable cause, in which case it is known as nonulcer dyspepsia.

The next articles cover diarrhoea and constipation. These problems often clear up on their own. If they persist, you should seek medical advice because there may be an underlying disorder that needs treatment. Diarrhoea may be a result of gastroenteritis or food poisoning, both of which can be serious in elderly people and young children.

Bleeding from the digestive tract can indicate a serious disorder and is discussed in the next article. New techniques developed in the last 25 years have enabled most cases of digestive tract bleeding to be diagnosed and treated without the need for surgery.

The final articles look at nutritional deficiencies, which are rare in the UK, and obesity, a condition that affects about a fifth of the UK population.

KEY ANATOMY

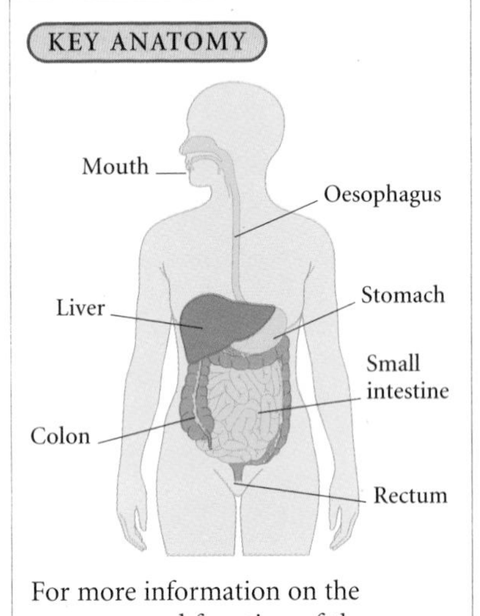

For more information on the structure and function of the digestive system, *see* pp.620–625.

Indigestion

Pain or discomfort in the upper abdomen, usually after eating, that may have a variety of causes

 AGE More common in adults

 LIFESTYLE Stress, being overweight, smoking, and certain dietary habits are risk factors

 GENDER GENETICS Not significant factors

Most people have had a few episodes of upper abdominal discomfort related to eating, usually called indigestion. The condition is more common in adults. Smoking and being overweight increase the risk. Most cases are not serious.

Usually, indigestion follows a meal, especially one that includes rich, fatty, or heavily spiced food. Overeating, consuming too much alcohol or coffee, and eating too quickly can also cause discomfort, as can stress and drugs such as aspirin that irritate the digestive tract. If indigestion persists or becomes more severe, or if you start to vomit, lose your appetite, or lose weight, you should consult your doctor. These symptoms may be a sign of a more serious condition such as gastro-oesophageal reflux (p.636), a peptic ulcer (p.640), or, in rare cases, stomach cancer (p.642).

Antacids (p.923) can usually relieve mild indigestion. There are also some self-help measures that you can follow to avoid future attacks (*see* PREVENTING INDIGESTION, opposite page).

(WWW) ONLINE SITES: p.1030

Nonulcer dyspepsia

Pain or discomfort in the upper abdomen that is not associated with a structural abnormality

 AGE More common in adults

 GENDER More common in males

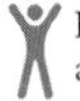 LIFESTYLE Stress, being overweight, smoking, and certain dietary habits are risk factors

 GENETICS Not a significant factor

Nonulcer dyspepsia describes recurrent and persistent indigestion (left) that occurs without an identifiable cause or abnormality of the digestive tract. The condition is more common in adults, especially men, and may be made worse by stress, being overweight, smoking, and a diet high in rich, fatty foods.

The symptoms may include pain in the upper abdomen, often made worse by eating, and nausea, particularly in the morning. People who have nonulcer dyspepsia often experience these symptoms several times a week for months. If you have such symptoms, you should consult your doctor because they could be a sign of a more serious underlying disorder, such as a peptic ulcer (p.640) or stomach cancer (p.642).

WHAT MIGHT BE DONE?

Your doctor will probably arrange for tests to exclude other disorders. For example, a blood test may be carried out to check for infection of the stomach lining with the bacterium *H. pylori* (*see* HELICOBACTER PYLORI INFECTION, p.639). In addition, upper digestive tract endoscopy (p.641) or contrast X-rays (p.245) may be carried out to look for abnormalities in the digestive tract. If no underlying disorder is found, you will be diagnosed with nonulcer dyspepsia.

There are measures that you can try to reduce the frequency or severity of symptoms (*see* PREVENTING INDIGESTION, opposite page). If these measures do not resolve the problem, your doctor may prescribe a drug to neutralize

SELF-HELP **PREVENTING INDIGESTION**

Some measures can be taken to prevent or reduce the frequency of episodes of indigestion. You may find some of the following helpful:

- Eat small portions of food at regular intervals without rushing or overfilling your stomach.
- Avoid eating in the 3 hours before going to bed to allow your body enough time to digest food.
- Reduce or eliminate your intake of alcohol, coffee, and tea.
- Avoid rich, fatty foods such as butter and fried foods.
- Keep a food diary to help identify foods that cause indigestion.
- Learn to overcome stress, which can often trigger episodes of indigestion (*see* RELAXATION EXERCISES, p.75).
- Try to lose excess weight and avoid tight-fitting clothing.
- If possible, avoid medicines that irritate the digestive tract, such as aspirin and other nonsteroidal anti-inflammatory drugs (p.894).

or reduce stomach acid production (*see* ANTACIDS, p.923, and ULCER-HEALING DRUGS, p.923). You may also be given drugs that help the stomach to empty more effectively, such as metoclopramide (*see* ANTISPASMODIC DRUGS AND MOTILITY STIMULANTS, p.926).

WWW ONLINE SITES: p.1030

Diarrhoea

The passage of loose or watery stools and/or an increase in the frequency of bowel movements

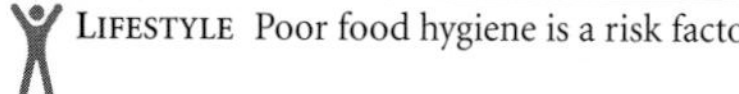

LIFESTYLE Poor food hygiene is a risk factor

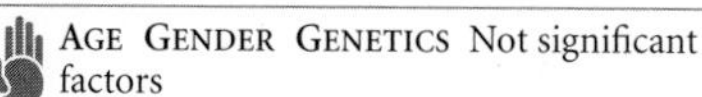

AGE GENDER GENETICS Not significant factors

Diarrhoea is the production of stools that are more watery, more frequent, or greater in volume than is normal for a particular individual. Although it is not a disease in itself, diarrhoea may be a symptom of an underlying disorder.

In some cases, diarrhoea is accompanied by abdominal pain, bloating, loss of appetite, and vomiting. Severe diarrhoea can also lead to dehydration that may be life-threatening, particularly in babies (*see* VOMITING AND DIARRHOEA, p.864) and elderly people.

Short bouts of diarrhoea, especially if they are associated with vomiting, are often due to gastroenteritis (p.628) or food poisoning (p.629). Diarrhoea that lasts more than 3–4 weeks usually indicates that there is an intestinal disorder and requires medical attention.

WHAT ARE THE CAUSES?

Diarrhoea that starts abruptly in a person who is otherwise healthy is often caused by contaminated food or water and may last a few hours to 10 days. This sort of diarrhoea often occurs during travel in a developing country, where food hygiene and sanitation may be poor. Diarrhoea can also be caused by a viral infection that is spread by close personal contact. For example, infectious gastroenteritis is a common cause of diarrhoea in babies and young children.

People with reduced immunity, such as those with AIDS (*see* HIV INFECTION AND AIDS, p.297), are more susceptible to infectious gastroenteritis, which also tends to be more severe in these people. People taking drugs such as antibiotics (p.885) may develop sudden diarrhoea if the drugs disturb the normal balance of bacteria in the colon.

Persistent diarrhoea may result from long-standing inflammation of the intestine due to disorders such as ulcerative colitis (p.659) or Crohn's disease (p.658) or some conditions in which the small intestine is unable to absorb nutrients (*see* MALABSORPTION, p.656). Lactose intolerance (p.657), a disorder in which lactose (a natural sugar present in milk) cannot be broken down and absorbed, can also cause diarrhoea.

Infections with protozoal parasites, such as giardiasis (p.307) and amoebiasis (p.306), can cause persistent diarrhoea. Irritable bowel syndrome (p.655) may produce abnormal contractions of the intestine, which result in alternating episodes of diarrhoea and constipation.

WHAT MIGHT BE DONE?

In most cases, diarrhoea clears up after a day or two. Other symptoms that can accompany diarrhoea, such as headache, weakness, and lethargy, are most often caused by dehydration. The symptoms of dehydration disappear as soon as lost fluids and salts are replaced (*see* PREVENTING DEHYDRATION, below).

If your diarrhoea lasts longer than 3–4 days, you should consult your doctor, who may request a sample of faeces to look for evidence of either infection or unabsorbed nutrients. If the diarrhoea persists for more than 3–4 weeks or if there is blood in the faeces, your doctor will probably arrange for you to have investigations, such as contrast X-rays (p.245) of the intestines, sigmoidoscopy, or colonoscopy (p.661).

Specific treatments given for diarrhoea depend on the underlying cause. If you need to relieve your diarrhoea quickly, your doctor may prescribe an antidiarrhoeal drug (p.924), such as loperamide. However, antidiarrhoeal drugs should be avoided if your diarrhoea is due to an infection because they may prolong the infection. Antibiotics are only needed to treat persistent diarrhoea that has a known bacterial cause.

WWW ONLINE SITES: p.1030, p.1033

SELF-HELP **PREVENTING DEHYDRATION**

For normal body functioning, the body's water and salt content must be kept at a constant level. During an attack of diarrhoea or vomiting, the body can become dehydrated due to loss of large amounts of fluids and salts. Babies, children, and elderly people are particularly vulnerable to dehydration, which can be reversed or prevented by following these simple measures:

- Drink plenty of fluids every 1–2 hours, while symptoms last. Choose fluids such as dilute orange juice, weak sweet tea, or rehydration solution, which is available over the counter as a powder that you reconstitute.
- Do not give children milk because it may perpetuate the diarrhoea. However, if a breast-feeding baby is affected, continue to breast-feed and give the baby additional fluids.
- Stay out of the sun and try to keep yourself cool in order to prevent further loss of body fluids in sweat.

Constipation

Difficult and infrequent passage of small, hard stools

AGE Most common in children and elderly people

GENDER More common in females

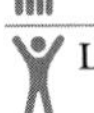
LIFESTYLE A low-fibre diet is a risk factor

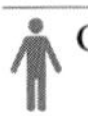
GENETICS Risk factors depend on the cause

If your stools are small and hard or if you have to strain to pass them, you are probably constipated. How frequently you pass stools is less important because healthy people have bowel movements at widely differing intervals. Usual intervals range from three times a day to three times a week. Most people tend to have a regular routine, and bowels usually function best if they are allowed to follow a consistent pattern.

Bouts of constipation are common and usually harmless, but occasionally they may indicate an underlying disorder. You should consult your doctor if you have recently developed constipation that is severe or lasts more than 2 weeks, particularly if it first occurs after the age of 50 or if blood is present in the faeces. Persistent constipation may lead to faecal impaction, in which hard faeces remain in the rectum. Liquid faeces may leak around the partial obstruction, resulting in diarrhoea (p.627).

WHAT ARE THE CAUSES?

A diet that is low in fibre and fluids is the most common cause of constipation. Drinking too much alcohol or drinks containing caffeine, which may lead to dehydration, can also make faeces hard and difficult to pass. Other factors that decrease the frequency of bowel movements are taking too little exercise and long periods of immobility. Several disorders, such as the metabolic disorder hypothyroidism (p.680) and depression (p.554), may also lead to constipation. In addition, the condition is associated with disorders of the large intestine, such as diverticular disease (p.663).

People recovering from abdominal surgery and people with anal disorders, such as haemorrhoids (p.668) or an anal fissure (p.669), may find it painful to defaecate and then develop constipation. Certain drugs, including some antidepressants (p.916) and antacids (p.923) containing aluminium and calcium carbonate, may cause constipation.

Poor toilet training in infants (*see* CONSTIPATION IN CHILDREN, p.865) and increasing immobility in elderly people make constipation much more common in these age groups. For unknown reasons, it is more common in women.

WHAT MIGHT BE DONE?

If constipation is associated with your lifestyle, there are several measures you can take to relieve it and prevent recurrence (*see* PREVENTING CONSTIPATION, below). If constipation persists despite taking these measures, you should consult your doctor, who will perform tests to look for an underlying cause. He or she will probably first examine your abdomen and check your rectum by inserting a gloved finger. You may be asked to give a faecal sample, which will be examined for the presence of blood (*see* FAECAL OCCULT BLOOD TEST, p.233).

If a cause is not found, you may have your large intestine examined with a viewing instrument (*see* COLONOSCOPY, p.661) or have contrast X-rays (p.245) of your intestines to reveal abnormalities. If your doctor finds an underlying cause, its treatment should relieve constipation. Your doctor will prescribe an alternative drug if a particular drug is the cause of constipation.

You may have an enema, in which liquid is passed through a tube into the rectum to stimulate bowel movements. This treatment should be followed by a change in diet to include more fibre.

Constipation linked to a painful anal disorder may be relieved with a soothing ointment or suppositories.

(WWW) ONLINE SITES: p.1030, p.1035

SELF-HELP PREVENTING CONSTIPATION

There are some simple steps you can take to prevent or reduce the severity of constipation:

- Increase your daily fibre intake. Fibre-rich foods include bran, wholemeal bread, cereals, fruit, leafy vegetables, potato skins, beans, and dried peas.
- Reduce your intake of highly refined and processed foods, such as cheese and white bread.
- Increase your daily fluid intake, but avoid drinks containing caffeine or alcohol.
- Do not use stimulant laxatives (p.924) persistently because the colon may eventually be unable to function without them.
- Do not ignore the urge to defaecate. The longer that faeces remain in the colon, the drier and harder they become.
- Try to achieve a regular routine in which you go to the toilet at the same time of day.

Gastroenteritis

Inflammation of the lining of the stomach and intestines, usually due to infection

AGE Most common in babies and children but can occur at any age

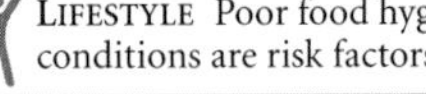
LIFESTYLE Poor food hygiene or unsanitary conditions are risk factors

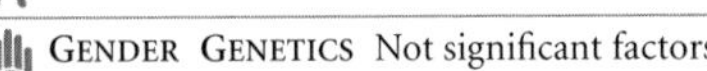
GENDER GENETICS Not significant factors

Gastroenteritis usually starts suddenly, with symptoms of vomiting, diarrhoea (p.627), and fever. Outbreaks commonly occur within families and among people who are in close contact, such as schoolchildren. Most people recover from the disorder without problems, but gastroenteritis may be serious in elderly people and very young children (*see* VOMITING AND DIARRHOEA, p.864) because there is a risk of dehydration. In developing countries, gastroenteritis is a common cause of death in these age groups.

WHAT ARE THE CAUSES?

Gastroenteritis is usually due to a viral or bacterial infection that inflames the lining of the stomach and intestines. The infection may be acquired from contaminated food or water (*see* FOOD POISONING, opposite page), or it may be spread among people who are in close contact, especially if hygiene is poor.

Viral gastroenteritis is often caused by rotaviruses or astroviruses, particularly in young children, and by the Norwalk virus in older children and adults. Most people acquire immunity to these viruses by the time they are adults. Bacterial causes of gastroenteritis include salmonella and *Escherichia coli*.

What are the symptoms?

The symptoms of gastroenteritis often develop rapidly over 1–2 hours and may vary in severity. They include:

- Nausea and vomiting.
- Cramping abdominal pain.
- Fever, often with headache.
- Diarrhoea.

In some people, vomiting or diarrhoea may lead to dehydration. Babies and elderly people are much more susceptible to the effects of dehydration, which are often difficult to recognize. Babies may become listless and cry feebly, and an elderly person may become confused. Consult your doctor promptly if you are not able to keep fluids down or have not passed urine for over 6 hours, especially if you have a long-term illness, such as diabetes mellitus (p.687) or kidney disease. Without appropriate treatment, dehydration may be life-threatening.

What might be done?

A mild attack of gastroenteritis usually clears up without treatment, but you should follow self-help measures and drink plenty of fluids every few hours (*see* PREVENTING DEHYDRATION, p.627). Over-the-counter antidiarrhoeal drugs (p.924) are useful if you need to relieve your symptoms quickly. However, these treatments are best avoided because they may prolong gastroenteritis by retaining the infective organism inside the gastrointestinal tract.

If your symptoms are severe or prolonged, you should consult your doctor. You may be asked to provide a sample of faeces, which will be tested for infection. Antibiotics (p.885) are rarely given unless a bacterial infection is identified. Severe dehydration requires emergency treatment in hospital to replace fluids and salts intravenously.

What is the prognosis?

Most people recover rapidly from gastroenteritis with no long-lasting effects. Occasionally, short-term damage to the intestine may reduce its ability to digest lactose, the natural sugar present in milk (*see* LACTOSE INTOLERANCE, p.657). This disorder occurs particularly in infants and often results in diarrhoea that can persist for days or weeks. In rare cases, gastroenteritis may trigger irritable bowel syndrome (p.655).

(WWW) ONLINE SITES: p.1030, p.1033

Food poisoning

Sudden illness caused by consuming food or drink contaminated by a toxin or infectious organism

LIFESTYLE Poor food hygiene is a risk factor

AGE GENDER GENETICS Not significant factors

Food poisoning is the term used to describe a sudden illness that is caused by consuming food or drink that may taste normal but is contaminated with a toxin or infectious organism.

The diagnosis of food poisoning is easily made if a group of people all develop the same symptoms, usually vomiting and diarrhoea, after they have consumed the same food or drink. The symptoms may start hours or days after consuming the food or drink.

Usually, the symptoms are confined to the gastrointestinal tract. However, some food poisoning may cause more widespread symptoms. For example, the *Clostridium botulinum* bacterium causes muscle weakness and paralysis (*see* BOTULISM, p.301), and listeriosis (p.301) may cause flu-like symptoms and lead to meningitis (p.527).

Food poisoning is becoming increasingly common, and there are more than 10 million cases every year in the UK. However, it can usually be avoided by careful preparation, storage, and cooking of food (*see* FOOD HYGIENE, p.79).

What are the causes?

Most cases of food poisoning result from contamination of food or water by bacteria, viruses, or, less commonly, protozoal parasites. Poor food hygiene can enable microorganisms to multiply. In some cases of bacterial food poisoning, it is not the presence of the bacteria themselves that cause poisoning but the effect of toxins produced by the bacteria.

If infectious organisms are ingested with the food, they can multiply in the digestive tract. If the food poisoning is caused by bacterial toxins, they may be produced in the food before it is eaten.

Most types of food poisoning cause diarrhoea and/or vomiting, often with abdominal pain. The severity of symptoms, the speed at which they develop, and the duration of the illness depend on the cause of food poisoning.

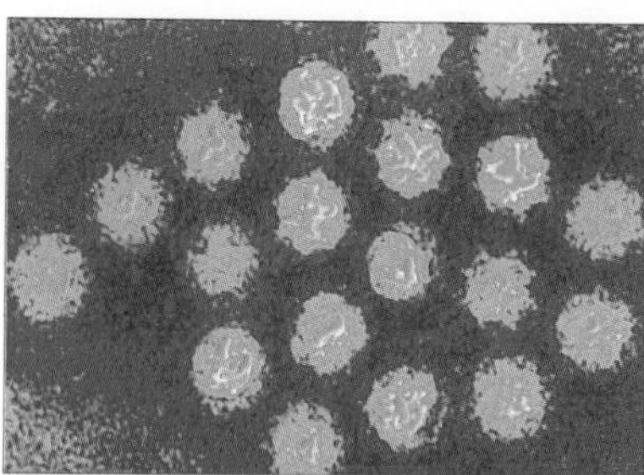

Norwalk virus
This magnified image shows particles of Norwalk virus, which often contaminates shellfish and causes food poisoning.

STAPHYLOCOCCI BACTERIA A number of foods, such as poultry, eggs, pâté, and previously prepared sandwiches can be infected by staphylococci bacteria. These bacteria produce toxins that are ingested with food. The toxins usually produce diarrhoea and/or vomiting within 4 hours. In most cases, symptoms clear up within 24 hours.

ESCHERICHIA COLI BACTERIA Certain types of *E. coli* can contaminate meat and water and produce toxins of varying potency. Types of *E. coli* are usually responsible for causing traveller's diarrhoea, which is usually mild. However, some types of *E. coli* may cause a severe illness because they produce a potent type of toxin that can damage blood cells and lead to kidney failure (p.705).

SALMONELLA BACTERIA Up to half a million people develop the disease salmonellosis every year in the UK from eating eggs or poultry that are infected with salmonella bacteria. It typically causes symptoms such as vomiting, mild fever, and severe diarrhoea that may be bloodstained. The symptoms usually begin 12–72 hours after eating the contaminated food and last for 1–3 days.

CAMPYLOBACTER BACTERIA These bacteria are one of the most common causes of diarrhoea. They may contaminate meat and more rarely water or unpasteurized milk. Symptoms usually develop about 2–5 days after eating contaminated food and may include severe, watery diarrhoea. The diarrhoea may contain blood and/or mucus. In most cases, the symptoms subside within 2–3 days, but bacteria may be present in faeces for up to 5 weeks after infection.

OTHER INFECTIONS Viral infections can be contracted from contaminated food or water. Shellfish are a common source of infection, especially with the Norwalk virus. Symptoms often start suddenly after contaminated food has been eaten, but recovery is usually rapid. Protozoal infections that may be contracted from contaminated food or water include cryptosporidiosis (p.307), amoebiasis (p.306), and giardiasis (p.307). Cryptosporidiosis may cause symptoms such as vomiting and loose, watery diarrhoea to develop about a week after contaminated substances have been consumed. Symptoms of amoebiasis may include watery, often bloody, diarrhoea persisting for several days or weeks. In giardiasis, there may be diarrhoea, bloating, and flatulence that often last more than a week.

NONINFECTIOUS CAUSES In some cases, food poisoning may be caused by poisonous mushrooms or contamination of fruit or vegetables with high concentrations of pesticides. Symptoms may include vomiting and diarrhoea.

WHAT MIGHT BE DONE?

Usually, symptoms disappear without treatment. If your symptoms are mild, use self-help measures to prevent dehydration (*see* PREVENTING DEHYDRATION, p.627). If the symptoms are severe or last more than 3–4 days, consult your doctor. If an elderly person or child is affected, you should consult a doctor immediately. Keep a sample of any remaining food in addition to the faeces, which can be tested for the presence of infectious microorganisms. If the cause is noninfectious, such as poisonous mushrooms, you may need to be treated urgently to eliminate the poison from the body.

Treatment of food poisoning is usually aimed at preventing dehydration. In severe cases, fluids and salts may be administered intravenously in hospital. Antibiotics (p.885) are given only if specific bacteria have been identified. People usually recover rapidly from a bout of food poisoning and rarely experience long-lasting consequences.

In rare cases, there is a risk of septicaemia (p.299) if bacteria spread into the bloodstream. Both dehydration and septicaemia can lead to shock (p.414), a condition that may be fatal.

(WWW) ONLINE SITES: p.1030, p.1033

Bleeding from the digestive tract

Loss of blood from the lining of the digestive tract, sometimes resulting in bloodstained faeces or vomit

AGE GENDER GENETICS LIFESTYLE
Risk factors depend on the cause

Bleeding can occur in any part of the digestive tract and should always be investigated because there may be a serious underlying cause. In some cases, only small amounts of blood are lost over a long period of time and go unnoticed. In other cases, severe, sudden bleeding from the digestive tract may result in blood being vomited or passed out of the anus in the faeces. You should seek medical help if you notice any bleeding.

WHAT ARE THE CAUSES?

The causes of bleeding in the digestive tract include inflammation of or damage to the tract's lining and tumours.

Bleeding from the upper tract, which includes the oesophagus, stomach, and duodenum, may occur if stomach acid damages the lining of these organs. This is a common complication of gastro-oesophageal reflux (p.636) and peptic ulcers (p.640). Severe bleeding is sometimes due to enlargement of veins in the oesophagus, which may be a complication of chronic liver diseases (*see* PORTAL HYPERTENSION AND VARICES, p.648).

Most cases of bleeding from the lower digestive tract, which includes the colon, rectum, and anus, are due to minor disorders, such as haemorrhoids (p.668) or anal fissure (p.669) caused by straining to defaecate. However, bleeding may be a sign of colorectal cancer (p.665). Diverticular disease (p.663) and other disorders of the colon can also lead to the presence of blood in the faeces.

WHAT ARE THE SYMPTOMS?

The symptoms vary according to the site and severity of the bleeding. If it is mild, blood loss may go unnoticed, but it may eventually cause symptoms of iron-deficiency anaemia (p.447), such as pale skin and shortness of breath. Severe bleeding from the oesophagus, stomach, or duodenum may cause:

- Vomit containing bright red blood or resembling coffee grounds.
- Light-headedness.
- Black, tarry stools.

If there is a heavy loss of blood from the lower part of the tract, there will probably be visible blood in the stools. When there is severe blood loss from any part of the tract, shock (p.414) may develop. Shock causes symptoms that include fainting, sweating, and confusion and requires immediate hospital treatment.

WHAT MIGHT BE DONE?

Minor bleeding may be detected only during an investigation for anaemia or screening to detect colorectal cancer. If the bleeding is severe, you may need intravenous fluids and a blood transfusion (p.447) to replace lost blood. You will be examined to detect the location of the bleeding, usually by endoscopy through the mouth (*see* UPPER DIGESTIVE TRACT ENDOSCOPY, p.641) or anus (*see* COLONOSCOPY, p.661).

Treatment for bleeding depends on the underlying cause. For example, peptic ulcers are treated with antibiotics (p.885) and ulcer-healing drugs (p.923), but colorectal cancer requires surgery. It may be possible to stop the bleeding by a treatment such as laser surgery (*see* LASER TREATMENT, p.951), which is carried out during endoscopy. If the cause of the bleeding is identified and treated early, treatment is usually successful.

(WWW) ONLINE SITES: p.1030

Nutritional deficiencies

Deficiencies of one or more nutrients essential for normal body function

AGE More common in children

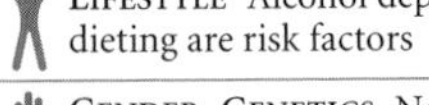
LIFESTYLE Alcohol dependence and extreme dieting are risk factors

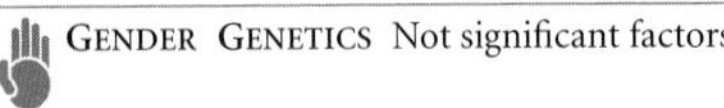
GENDER GENETICS Not significant factors

Nutritional deficiencies occur when the body lacks essential elements that are obtained from food. In developing countries, such deficiencies are usually the result of poverty and insufficient food supplies. In the UK, nutritional deficiencies are due mainly to disorders that limit the body's intake or absorption of nutrients or to self-imposed dietary restrictions. Deficiencies may be noticed when nutritional needs increase, such as in growth spurts in childhood.

WHAT ARE THE TYPES?

There are two main types of nutritional deficiency: a general deficiency of calories and all nutrients; and deficiency of specific nutrients. A general deficiency may be the result of poor eating because of severe illness or surgery. It may also be due to extreme dieting or deliberate starvation, as occurs in the eating disorder anorexia nervosa (p.562). Some people may neglect their diet because of other psychological problems, such as alcohol dependence (p.564). A general deficiency of nutrients may also result from poor absorption of food in the small intestine (*see* MALABSORPTION, p.656). Symptoms of a general deficiency may include weight loss, muscle weakness, and tiredness.

Specific nutritional deficiencies may occur if people limit their diets because of certain beliefs. In some cases, malabsorption causes deficiency of a specific nutrient. For example, the bowel disorder Crohn's disease (p.658) can affect the last section of the small intestine, through which vitamin B_{12} is absorbed. Specific nutritional deficiencies result in a variety of disorders. These include iron-deficiency anaemia (p.447) and the bone disorders osteomalacia and rickets (p.370), which are caused by a lack of calcium or vitamin D.

WHAT MIGHT BE DONE?

If your doctor suspects that you have a nutritional deficiency, he or she will weigh you and make a full assessment of your diet. You may also have blood tests to look for anaemia and to measure levels of specific nutrients. Investigations, such as contrast X-rays (p.245) of the gastrointestinal tract, may be carried out to check for underlying disorders.

If the deficiency is severe, you will be admitted to hospital and given nutrients using a tube passed through the nose into the stomach or through a drip directly into the bloodstream.

If the deficiency is a result of a treatable physical problem, it should resolve with treatment. Changing your diet should resolve the problem if poor eating is the cause. Psychological problems will also require treatment. In some cases, such as Crohn's disease, long-term vitamin and mineral supplements (pp.927–929) may be required.

(WWW) ONLINE SITES: p.1031, p.1035

Obesity

A condition in which there is an accumulation of excess body fat

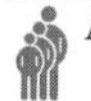
AGE More common with increasing age

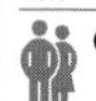
GENDER More common in females

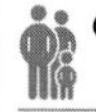
GENETICS Sometimes runs in families

LIFESTYLE Overeating and a sedentary lifestyle are risk factors

A person is considered obese if he or she weighs at least 20 per cent more than the maximum healthy weight for his or her height (*see* ARE YOU A HEALTHY WEIGHT?, p.53). About 1 in 5 people in the UK are obese, and the condition is becoming increasingly common.

Obesity can cause many health problems due to the strain it puts on organs and joints. For example, back pain, painful hips and knees, and shortness of breath are common problems. Obesity increases the risk of some widespread and potentially fatal disorders, such as coronary artery disease (p.405), stroke (p.532), and high blood pressure (*see* HYPERTENSION, p.403). Obesity may also lead to psychological problems, including depression (p.554).

WHAT ARE THE CAUSES?

Obesity occurs when food taken into the body provides more energy than is used. The main causes of obesity are overeating and a sedentary lifestyle. Obesity may run in families as a result of learned eating habits in addition to inherited factors. In rare cases, obesity may be a symptom of a hormonal disorder, such as hypothyroidism (p.680). Some drugs, particularly corticosteroids (p.930), can also lead to obesity. Occasionally, obesity may be a result of an underlying psychological problem.

ARE THERE COMPLICATIONS?

Obesity increases the risk of various long-term problems. For example, obese people are more likely to have high blood cholesterol levels (*see* HYPERCHOLESTEROLAEMIA, p.691). High cholesterol in turn increases the risk of atherosclerosis (p.402), in which fatty deposits build up on the inner linings of the arteries. Atherosclerosis may contribute to high blood pressure and coronary artery disease. Arterial thrombosis and embolism (p.431), which is blockage of a blood vessel by a blood clot, occurs more frequently in obese people. Obese adults are at greater risk of gallstones (p.651) and are more likely to develop diabetes mellitus (p.687). Certain cancers, such as breast cancer (p.759) and cancer of the uterus (p.748), are also more common in obese people.

Excess weight puts strain on joints. Osteoarthritis (p.374), especially in the hips and knees, is common in obese people. Sleep apnoea (p.477), a respiratory disorder, is also linked to obesity.

WHAT MIGHT BE DONE?

Your doctor will probably measure your weight and height and discuss your diet with you (*see* A HEALTHY DIET, p.48) and will probably also ask you how much exercise you take (*see* EXERCISE AND HEALTH, pp.55–61). Tests may be performed to measure blood sugar levels (to look for diabetes) and cholesterol levels (*see* BLOOD CHOLESTEROL TESTS, p.231). Rarely, you may have blood tests to check for a hormonal disorder.

Obesity is most commonly treated by a weight-reduction diet and increased exercise. Calorie intake per day is usually reduced to 500–1,000 calories less than the average requirement for a person of your age, sex, and height (*see* CONTROLLING YOUR WEIGHT, p.53). This type of eating plan is designed to produce slow, sustainable weight loss. The diet may be formulated by your doctor or a dietitian, although you may also choose to join a self-help group. Moderate, regular exercise is essential in losing weight.

Appetite suppressant drugs are available but few are recommended because of the side effects. However, newer treatments with fewer side effects, such as drugs that control the appetite by affecting neurotransmitters in the brain, may soon be available. Drugs that reduce fat absorption from the digestive tract, such as orlistat, may also help. Rarely, surgery is used to treat obesity. The stomach may be stapled to reduce its size so that you feel full after only a small meal.

Changes in diet and lifestyle need to be maintained throughout life. Support from your family, doctor, and a self-help group should help you to follow your weight-loss plan successfully.

(WWW) ONLINE SITES: p.1031, p.1035

DISORDERS OF THE MOUTH, TONGUE, AND OESOPHAGUS

Digestion begins in the mouth, where food is chewed by the teeth and mixed by the tongue with saliva secreted by the salivary glands. Swallowing forces the food into the oesophagus, where it progresses to the stomach by coordinated muscle contractions. The mouth, tongue, and oesophagus are constantly exposed to irritants and infection from food and airborne particles.

The first half of this section deals with disorders of the mouth and tongue. These conditions range from mouth ulcers, which are common and relatively mild, to the serious disease mouth cancer. Also included are disorders that involve inflammation, such as glossitis (inflammation of the tongue), and disorders that cause white patches in the mouth, such as oral leukoplakia.

Two disorders affecting the salivary glands are described next. Salivary gland stones are painful but can usually be removed successfully. The majority of salivary gland tumours are not cancerous, and their outlook is generally good, but they may recur.

The last part of the section covers disorders of the oesophagus, the most common being gastro-oesophageal reflux; cancer of the oesophagus, which is much rarer, is also described.

For disorders specifically affecting the teeth and gums, *see* pp.606–619.

KEY ANATOMY

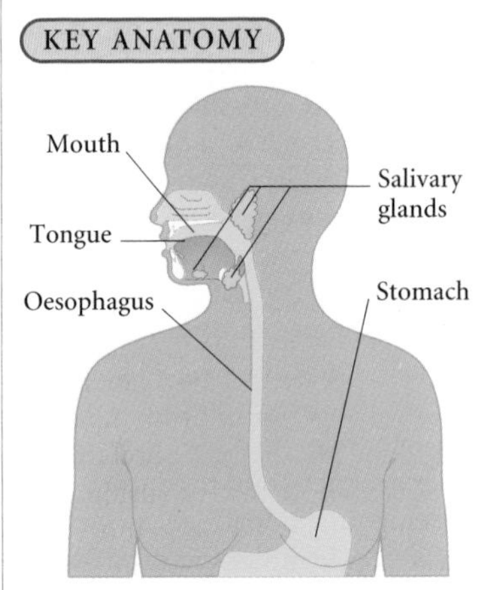

For more information concerning the structure and function of the mouth, tongue, and oesophagus, *see* pp.620–625.

Mouth ulcers

Painful sores in the lining of the mouth, also called aphthous ulcers or canker sores

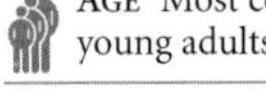
AGE Most common in adolescents and young adults

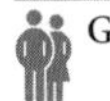
GENDER Slightly more common in females

GENETICS Sometimes run in families

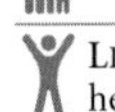
LIFESTYLE Stress, illness, and poor general health are risk factors

Mouth ulcers are shallow, grey-white pits with a red border. They can cause pain, particularly when you are chewing spicy, hot, or acidic food. Mouth ulcers are extremely common and may occur singly or in clusters anywhere in the mouth. They may recur several times a year, but they usually disappear without treatment within 2 weeks.

The cause of mouth ulcers is not known, but the ulcers tend to occur in people who are run down or ill and before menstruation in women. Mouth ulcers are often stress-related. Injuries to the lining of the mouth caused by ill-fitting dentures, a roughened tooth, or careless tooth-brushing can also result in the development of mouth ulcers.

Occasionally, recurrent mouth ulcers are due to anaemia (p.446), a deficiency of either vitamin B_{12} or folic acid, or an intestinal disorder such as Crohn's disease (p.658) or coeliac disease (p.658). In rare cases, they are due to the autoimmune disorder Behçet's syndrome (p.465).

Ulcers may also occur as a result of specific infections, such as herpes simplex infections (p.291). Rarely, an ulcer that enlarges slowly and does not heal may be mouth cancer (p.634).

Mouth ulcers usually heal without treatment. If you are prone to them, avoid possible irritants, such as spicy foods, and use a saltwater mouthwash. Over-the-counter treatments containing a corticosteroid to reduce inflammation or an anaesthetic are available in paste, lozenge, and gel form. The most suitable type depends on the site of the ulcer.

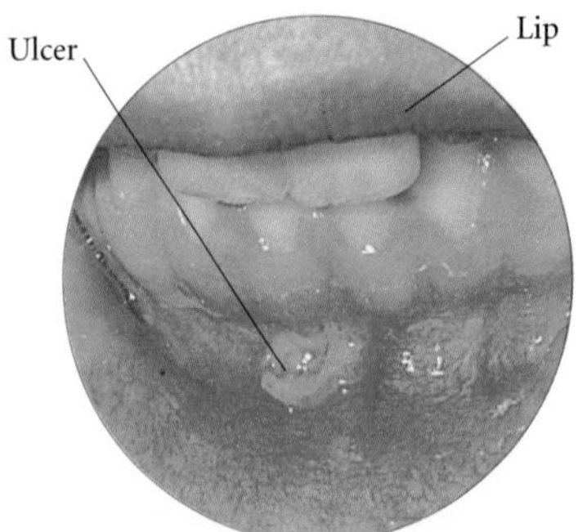

Mouth ulcer
The typical grey-white pit of a mouth ulcer has developed inside the lower lip of the mouth shown above.

Consult a doctor or dentist about a mouth ulcer that does not heal within 3 weeks. He or she may carry out tests to look for an underlying cause.

(WWW) ONLINE SITES: p.1030, p.1033

Stomatitis

Inflammation of the lining of the mouth that may be mild or severe

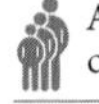
AGE May occur at any age but most common in children and elderly people

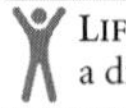
LIFESTYLE Poor oral hygiene, smoking, and a diet deficient in iron are risk factors

GENDER GENETICS Not significant factors

Stomatitis is a general inflammation of the lining of the mouth including the tongue. The disorder is usually caused by an infection. If the inflammation affects the tongue, it is called glossitis (opposite page); if it affects the gums, it is called gingivitis (p.617). Mouth ulcers (left) are another form of stomatitis.

Whichever part of the mouth is affected, stomatitis is usually a short-lived condition and, although it may be painful, it does not usually cause serious problems.

WHAT ARE THE CAUSES?

The most common causes of stomatitis are infections with viruses, bacteria, or fungi and eating a poor diet. Smoking may also cause the condition.

Viral stomatitis is mainly caused by the herpes simplex virus (*see* HERPES SIMPLEX INFECTIONS, p.291) and the coxsackie virus. Viral stomatitis occurs most commonly in childhood.

Bacterial stomatitis, particularly gingivitis, usually results from neglected dental problems and poor oral hygiene, such as ineffective tooth-brushing. Oral bacterial infections are also more likely when saliva production is reduced, such as in Sjögren's syndrome (p.463).

Stomatitis may also result from the fungal infection candidiasis (p.309), in which a fungus that is normally present in the mouth grows excessively and causes inflammation. Candidiasis occurs most commonly in infants, elderly people, those who wear dentures, and pregnant women. People with reduced immunity, such as those with diabetes mellitus (p.687) and people with AIDS (*see* HIV INFECTION AND AIDS, p.297), are also susceptible to candidiasis. The infection may also occur in people who are being treated with antibiotics (p.885) and in people who use inhaled corticosteroids to treat asthma (*see* CORTICOSTEROIDS FOR RESPIRATORY DISEASE, p.911) and fail to rinse their mouth thoroughly afterwards.

The most common deficiency that causes stomatitis is a shortage of iron, which also leads to anaemia (*see* IRON-DEFICIENCY ANAEMIA, p.447). Deficiency of vitamin B_{12} or folic acid in the diet may also cause stomatitis.

WHAT ARE THE SYMPTOMS?

The symptoms of stomatitis may range from mild to severe and include:

- Sore mouth.
- Bad breath.
- In some cases, mouth ulcers.

In gingivitis, the gums may be sore and swollen and may bleed during tooth-brushing. Chronic gingivitis and poor oral hygiene may lead to teeth loosening and eventually falling out.

WHAT MIGHT BE DONE?

If your doctor cannot make a diagnosis from your symptoms immediately, a swab may be taken from the affected area of the mouth and sent to a laboratory for testing. If stomatitis is due to infection, antibiotics or antifungal drugs (p.889) may be prescribed. Most viral infections clear up spontaneously, and treatment is usually aimed at relieving symptoms such as pain. Antiviral drugs (p.886) may also be prescribed.

To relieve the symptoms, you should keep your mouth clean by using salt-water mouthwashes regularly. If eating and drinking are particularly painful, your doctor may prescribe a pain-relieving mouthwash or gel containing a local anaesthetic to apply to the inside of your mouth just before meals. If children are unable to drink, they may be admitted to hospital to be given fluids intravenously to rehydrate them.

Gingivitis can be prevented by good oral hygiene (*see* CARING FOR YOUR TEETH AND GUMS, p.610). Once it has developed, more extensive treatment by your dentist or dental hygienist may be necessary to control the progression of the condition.

WWW ONLINE SITES: p.1029, p.1033

Glossitis

Inflammation of the tongue, making it smooth, red, and swollen

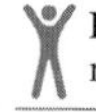 LIFESTYLE Alcohol abuse and smoking are risk factors

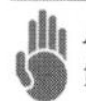 AGE GENDER GENETICS Not significant factors

Glossitis (inflammation of the tongue) is usually a temporary condition that heals quickly with treatment. The most common cause of glossitis is an injury to the tongue, which can be due to ill-fitting dentures, roughened teeth, or scalding liquids. Smoking, eating spicy foods, and excessive alcohol intake may cause mild irritation and inflame the tongue. Glossitis may also be the primary symptom of a fungal infection such as candidiasis (p.309) or a viral infection such as herpes simplex infection (p.291). In some cases, the tongue becomes inflamed as a result of a deficiency of iron, vitamin B_{12}, or folic acid in the diet. Rarely, some people find that particular oral hygiene products,

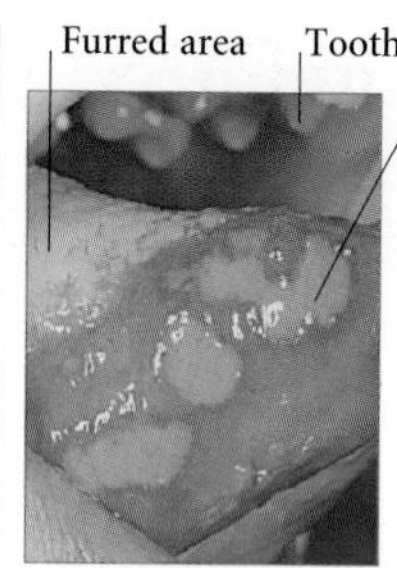

Glossitis
This tongue has inflammation (glossitis), along with thick furring and ulceration, as a result of herpes simplex infection.

such as mouthwashes, breath fresheners, and toothpastes, cause an allergic reaction in the mouth, which leads to inflammation of the tongue.

WHAT ARE THE SYMPTOMS?

In many cases, the symptoms of glossitis develop gradually. With time, the tongue may become:

- Painful, swollen, and tender.
- Smooth and red.
- Furred.
- Dotted with multiple small ulcers.
- Cracked.

In cases of glossitis caused by damage from scalding liquids, a viral infection, or an allergic reaction, the symptoms often develop rapidly. Swallowing and speaking may become painful. Other symptoms may also be present in addition to a swollen tongue, depending on the cause. For example, you may have ulcers on your tongue if you have a herpes simplex infection, or if you have candidiasis, you may have sore patches that are creamy-yellow or white.

WHAT MIGHT BE DONE?

Your doctor may take swabs from the tongue to identify an infection. A blood sample may also be taken to look for mineral or vitamin deficiencies.

Whatever the cause, you can relieve the discomfort by rinsing your mouth regularly with a salt solution and antiseptic or pain-relieving mouthwashes. It should also help if you stop smoking and avoid acidic and spicy foods that exacerbate the soreness. In many cases, the symptoms clear up without a cause being identified. However, if a clear diagnosis is made, specific treatment for the infection is usually effective. For example, if your condition is caused by candidiasis, your doctor may prescribe an antifungal drug (p.889), such as miconazole in an oral gel form.

WWW ONLINE SITES: p.1030, p.1033

Oral lichen planus

White patches in the mouth, sometimes associated with an itchy skin rash

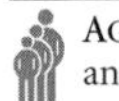 AGE Most common between the ages of 30 and 60

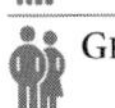 GENDER More common in females

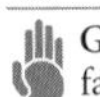 GENETICS LIFESTYLE Not significant factors

Oral lichen planus is a rare condition in which small, white patches develop on the inside of the cheeks and sometimes elsewhere in the mouth. The patches often have a lacy pattern. In most people these white patches are painless, but sometimes they develop into persistent ulcers that can be very painful.

Oral lichen planus usually occurs in episodes that may last months or even years and frequently recurs after treatment. The condition occurs most often in people between the ages of 30 and 60 and affects more women than men. A small number of people who have oral lichen planus may also develop the general skin condition lichen planus (p.336), in which an itchy rash appears on the skin, most commonly on the inner surfaces of the wrists.

WHAT ARE THE CAUSES?

Often no cause can be found, but oral lichen planus may be due to an abnormal immune response and may occur with other immune disorders, such as systemic lupus erythematosus (p.461). Oral lichen planus is sometimes due to an adverse reaction to amalgam tooth fillings or particular drugs, including gold-based antirheumatic drugs (p.895) and some of the drugs used to treat diabetes mellitus (p.687). Stress sometimes triggers the symptoms.

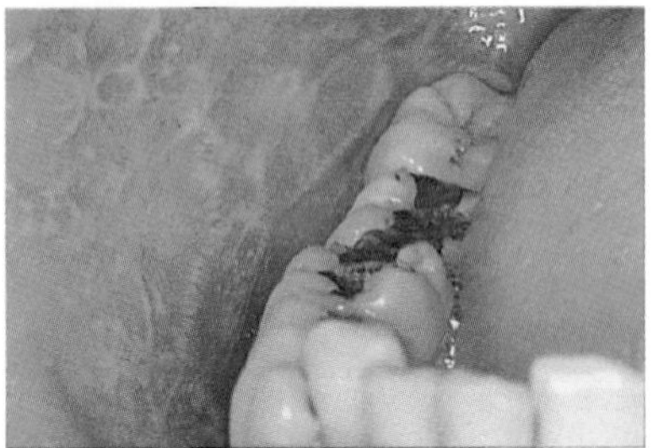

Oral lichen planus
The distinctive lacy pattern of oral lichen planus can be seen clearly here on the lining of the inside of the cheek.

WHAT MIGHT BE DONE?

If you have white patches in your mouth that last longer than 3 weeks, you should consult your doctor or dentist. It may be possible to make a diagnosis from your symptoms, but to confirm the diagnosis and exclude other disorders, a sample of tissue from the affected area may be taken under local anaesthesia and examined microscopically.

If the symptoms are only mild, no treatment may be necessary. However, a topical corticosteroid in an oral paste may be given to relieve pain. Oral lichen planus sometimes disappears spontaneously after several years.

(WWW) ONLINE SITES: p.1030, p.1033

Oral leukoplakia

Small, thickened, white patches on the lining of the mouth or tongue

 AGE Nearly always occurs over the age of 40

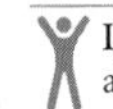 LIFESTYLE Smoking, chewing tobacco, and alcohol abuse are risk factors

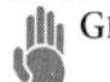 GENDER GENETICS Not significant factors

In oral leukoplakia, thickened white patches develop on the lining of the mouth or on the tongue. The patches develop slowly and painlessly, starting most often on the sides of the tongue. Unlike the white patches in the mouth caused by oral thrush (*see* CANDIDIASIS, p.309), leukoplakia patches cannot be scraped off. Sometimes, these patches harden, causing the surface to crack.

WHAT ARE THE CAUSES?

Occasionally, the condition is caused by repeated mild damage to one area of the mouth, such as by a roughened tooth, but often the cause is unknown. If there is no obvious cause, there is a 1 in 20 chance that the patch may become cancerous (*see* MOUTH CANCER, right). The risk of cancer is higher if the patch is on the floor of the mouth or is ulcerated. Oral leukoplakia is much more common in smokers and people who chew tobacco. The risk of the condition is increased further if people drink excessive amounts of alcohol. The disorder nearly always occurs in people over 40.

A form of leukoplakia known as hairy leukoplakia affects people with reduced immunity, especially people with AIDS (*see* HIV INFECTION AND AIDS, p.297). White patches occur on the sides of the tongue and have a rough or corrugated surface. Hairy leukoplakia does not usually become cancerous.

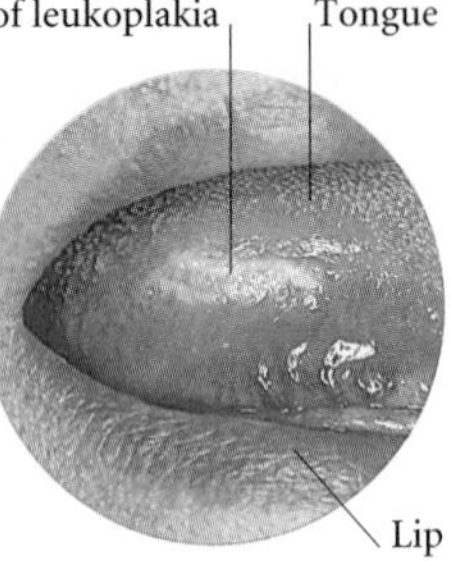

Leukoplakia
The thickened white patches of oral leukoplakia usually develop on the side of the tongue. The patches often harden and crack.

WHAT MIGHT BE DONE?

An obvious cause for the patches, such as damage from dentures, can be treated, and the patches may then disappear. If no cause is found or the condition persists, your doctor or dentist may take a tissue sample from your mouth to exclude mouth cancer. Persistent patches may be removed by surgery or laser treatment (p.951). Even with treatment, oral leukoplakia may recur and needs to be monitored regularly.

(WWW) ONLINE SITES: p.1030

Mouth cancer

Cancerous tumour of the lips, tongue, or lining of the mouth

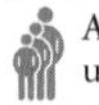 AGE Most common over the age of 60; rare under the age of 40

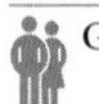 GENDER Twice as common in males

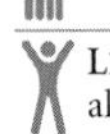 LIFESTYLE Smoking, chewing tobacco, alcohol abuse, and excessive exposure to sunlight are risk factors

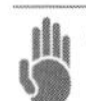 GENETICS Not a significant factor

About half of all cancerous tumours of the mouth occur on either the tongue or the lower lip. The gums, inside of the cheeks, floor of the mouth, and palate are less commonly affected.

In developed countries, mouth cancer accounts for around 2–4 per cent of all new cases of cancer. In developing countries such as India, where people chew tobacco, betel leaves, and nuts, mouth cancer is much more common. Worldwide, the disease is twice as common in men as it is in women, although the incidence is beginning to increase in women. Mouth cancer occurs most commonly in people over the age of 60 and is rare in those under the age of 40. The outlook for lip cancer is good. The outcome is generally poorer for other forms of mouth cancer but is improved with early diagnosis.

What are the causes?

In half of all people with mouth cancer, the tumour develops from oral leukoplakia (opposite page), a condition in which thickened white patches appear on the lining of the mouth or on the tongue. The main factor that encourages the growth of leukoplakia and mouth tumours is smoking, particularly pipes and cigars, and chewing tobacco. The risk of mouth cancer is increased further when tobacco use is combined with excessive alcohol consumption.

Diet may also play a part, particularly if the diet is deficient in vitamins A, C, and E and in iron. In addition, lip cancer is strongly associated with repeated unprotected exposure to strong sunlight.

What are the symptoms?

If you have mouth cancer, you may experience the following symptoms:

- An ulcer that enlarges slowly and fails to heal, occurring on the lining of the mouth or on the tongue.
- A swelling that develops anywhere inside the mouth or on the lips.

Left untreated, mouth cancer usually spreads from the mouth to nearby tissues, the lymph nodes in the neck, and from there to other parts of the body.

How is it diagnosed?

Cancerous tumours in the mouth are often detected early by a dentist during a checkup. If your doctor suspects that a lump or nonhealing ulcer is a tumour, a small sample of tissue may be taken for examination. If cancer is found, further tests will establish how far it has spread (*see* STAGING CANCER, p.279).

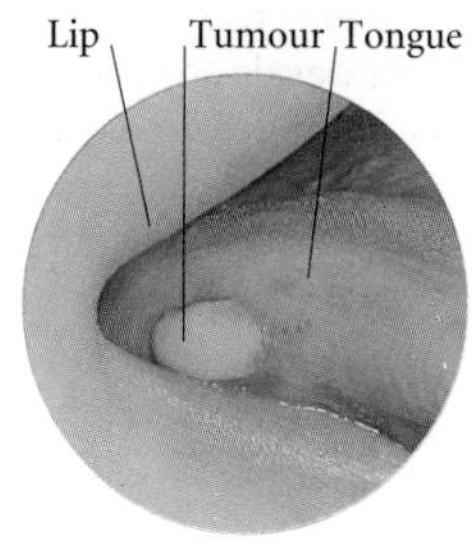

Mouth cancer
A cancerous tumour can be seen here in the form of a small, white lump that has developed on the right side of the tongue.

What is the treatment?

A small cancerous tumour that is discovered early may be removed surgically or by laser treatment (p.951). In about 8 in 10 people, surgery is successful and the cancer does not recur following removal of the tumour. If the tumour is large, it will be removed surgically, and plastic surgery (p.952) may be necessary to restore a more normal facial appearance. Following surgery, radiotherapy (p.281) may be carried out to ensure that all cancerous cells have been destroyed and the cancer does not recur.

What is the prognosis?

Tumours that are found early and are in an easily accessible part of the mouth can usually be treated successfully. The outlook is best for lip cancer, which is the most accessible site. For cancers within the mouth, less than half of the affected people survive for 5 years.

(WWW) ONLINE SITES: p.1028

Salivary gland stones

Stones that form in the ducts of the salivary glands

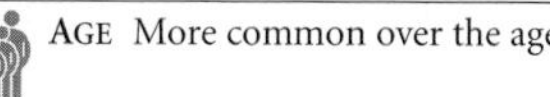
AGE More common over the age of 40

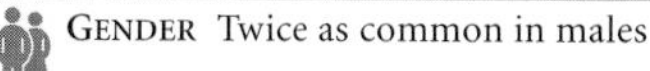
GENDER Twice as common in males

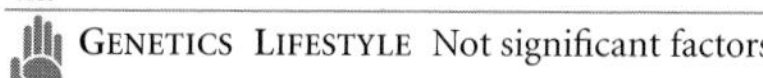
GENETICS LIFESTYLE Not significant factors

There are three pairs of salivary glands in the mouth, and sometimes the salivary ducts (tubes through which saliva enters the mouth) become blocked by stones. The stones are composed of calcium salts and vary in size. They either partially or, rarely, completely block the duct. The salivary gland then becomes swollen and feels painful during eating because saliva cannot escape from the gland into the mouth. In most cases, no cause can be found. Stones are twice as common in men and occur most often in people over the age of 40.

What are the symptoms?

In most cases, the symptoms of salivary gland stones include:

- A visible swelling on the outside of the mouth or the sensation of a lump inside the mouth.
- Pain during or after a meal due to a build-up of saliva behind the stone.

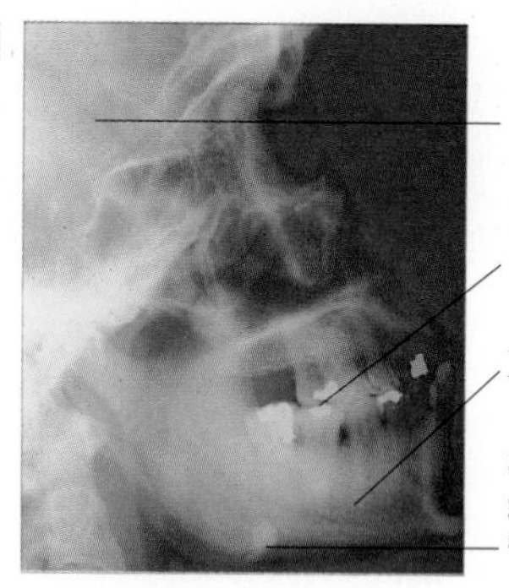

Salivary gland stone
In this X-ray, a salivary gland stone shows up as a white mass. The stone is blocking the duct of the gland beneath the jaw bone.

A blocked salivary duct is liable to become infected, causing the swelling to become red and inflamed with possible leakage of pus into the mouth.

What might be done?

To confirm the presence of a salivary gland stone, you may have imaging tests, such as X-rays (p.244) or CT scanning (p.247). If the location is unclear, you may have a test called a sialogram, in which a dye is injected directly into the blocked duct and an X-ray of the area is taken. The doctor may be able to tease out the stone using his or her fingers. Failing this, the stone can be removed surgically or by lithotripsy, in which ultrasound is used to break up stones so that they can be flushed out. Salivary gland stones may recur after treatment.

(WWW) ONLINE SITES: p.1030

Salivary gland tumours

Noncancerous or cancerous tumours in the salivary glands

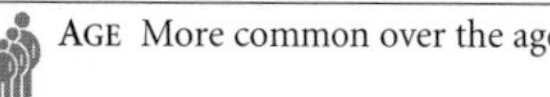
AGE More common over the age of 45

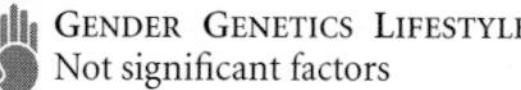
GENDER GENETICS LIFESTYLE Not significant factors

Tumours that affect the salivary glands are rare, particularly in people under the age of 45. Three-quarters of the tumours occur in one of the two parotid salivary glands that lie behind the angles of the jaw. Only about 1 in 5 salivary gland tumours is cancerous.

The symptoms of a salivary gland tumour depend on whether or not it is a cancerous tumour, but in all cases there is a lump that may be felt either

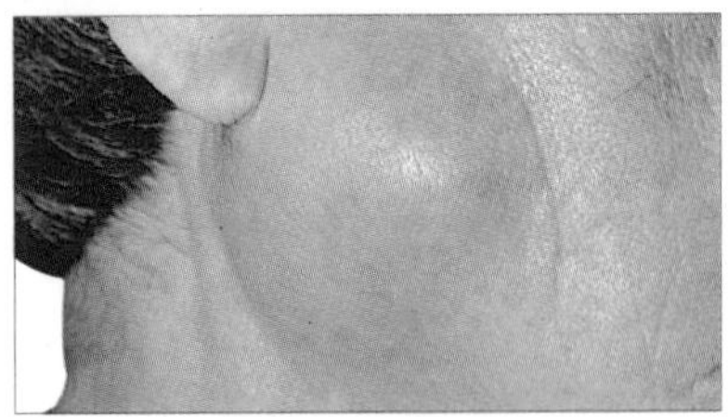

Salivary gland tumour
This swelling close to the ear and over the angle of the jawbone is caused by a noncancerous tumour of a salivary gland.

protruding inside the mouth or on the face. Noncancerous tumours are usually painless, rubbery in consistency, and mobile when touched. These benign tumours usually grow slowly.

Cancerous tumours of the salivary gland usually grow quickly, feel hard, and are sometimes painful. The facial nerve, which passes through the gland, may be affected as the cancer develops, leading to paralysis of part of the face (*see* FACIAL PALSY, p.548). If the tumour is left untreated, the cancer may spread to nearby lymph nodes in the neck and from there to other parts of the body, such as the chest and liver.

WHAT IS THE TREATMENT?

Treatment for a noncancerous tumour of the parotid gland is an operation to remove the affected part of the gland. This is a very delicate procedure and there is a risk that the facial nerve may be damaged. If damage does occur, the mouth may droop as a result. The nerve sometimes recovers, but in other cases the damage may be permanent.

If a tumour is cancerous, all of the affected gland is removed. If the tumour has spread to the lymph nodes in the neck, these nodes may also need to be removed. After surgery, it may be necessary to perform radiotherapy (p.281) to destroy remaining cancerous cells.

WHAT IS THE PROGNOSIS?

Noncancerous tumours can usually be treated but may recur. Untreated, up to 1 in 10 become cancerous within 20 years.

Most people with cancerous tumours survive for more than 5 years after diagnosis. However, the earlier the diagnosis and treatment, the greater the chance of a cure. If the disease spreads beyond the salivary glands, it may be fatal.

(WWW) ONLINE SITES: p.1028, p.1030

Gastro-oesophageal reflux

Regurgitation of acidic stomach juices into the oesophagus, causing pain in the upper abdomen and chest

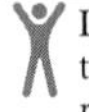
LIFESTYLE Obesity, a high-fat diet, drinking too much coffee or alcohol, and smoking are risk factors

AGE GENDER GENETICS Not significant factors

Gastro-oesophageal reflux (GOR), usually known as acid reflux, is probably the most common cause of attacks of indigestion (p.626). The discomfort is due to acidic juices from the stomach flowing back up into the oesophagus (the tube leading from the throat to the stomach). The lining of the oesophagus is not adequately protected against the harmful effects of stomach acid, which causes inflammation and a burning pain known as heartburn.

Attacks of GOR are usually brief and relatively mild but if they are persistent, the lining of the oesophagus may be permanently damaged or scarred. In some cases, GOR causes bleeding from the digestive tract (p.630).

(SELF-HELP) MANAGING GASTRO-OESOPHAGEAL REFLUX

The following steps will either relieve the symptoms of gastro-oesophageal reflux (GOR) or prevent them from recurring:

- Take antacids (p.923) to help neutralize stomach acids.
- Avoid spicy, acidic, tomato-based foods and high-fat foods such as chocolate and cream.
- Avoid alcohol, colas, and coffee.
- Stop smoking.
- Lose excess weight.
- Eat smaller amounts of food to avoid overfilling the stomach and do not eat late at night.
- After eating, do not exercise or lie down since both may lead to food being regurgitated.
- Raise the head of your bed or sleep on extra pillows so that your head is higher than your feet during the night.

WHAT ARE THE CAUSES?

The stomach contents are kept from entering the oesophagus by a double-action valve mechanism. One part of this mechanism is the muscular ring at the lower end of the oesophagus, known as the lower oesophageal sphincter. The other part is the effect of the diaphragm muscle on the oesophagus as the tube passes through a narrow opening in the muscle, called the hiatus. These mechanisms provide an effective one-way valve.

GOR may develop as a result of several factors acting together to make the valve leak. These factors include poor muscle tone in the sphincter; increased abdominal pressure due to pregnancy; obesity; or a weakness in the hiatus that allows part of the stomach to slide into the chest (a hiatus hernia). Many people develop mild attacks of GOR after eating certain foods or drinks, especially pickles, fried or fatty meals, carbonated soft drinks, alcohol, or coffee. Smoking may also worsen symptoms.

WHAT ARE THE SYMPTOMS?

Some of the symptoms of GOR are most noticeable immediately after eating a large meal or when a person bends over. The main symptoms include:

- Burning pain or discomfort in the chest behind the breastbone, known as heartburn.
- Acidic taste in the mouth due to regurgitation of acidic fluid into the throat or mouth.
- Persistent cough.
- Belching.
- Blood in the vomit or faeces.

GOR that persists for many years can cause scarring in the oesophagus, which eventually may become severe enough to cause a stricture (narrowing). A stricture can make swallowing difficult and may lead to weight loss. Long-term GOR can lead to a condition called Barrett's oesophagus, in which part of the lining of the oesophagus is replaced by the stomach lining. People with Barrett's oesophagus are at increased risk of cancer of the oesophagus (p.638).

If you have recently developed pain in the centre of your chest that seems unrelated to eating or drinking, you should seek immediate medical help because the far more serious condition angina (p.407) is sometimes mistaken for the pain of severe heartburn.

TEST BARIUM SWALLOW

A barium swallow is a test used to visualize the oesophagus, the tube that connects the mouth to the stomach. The test can detect disorders or abnormalities of the oesophagus, such as narrowing or tumours. A barium solution is used because it shows up on X-rays, which are taken continuously to monitor the flow of the solution. The barium may cause temporary constipation.

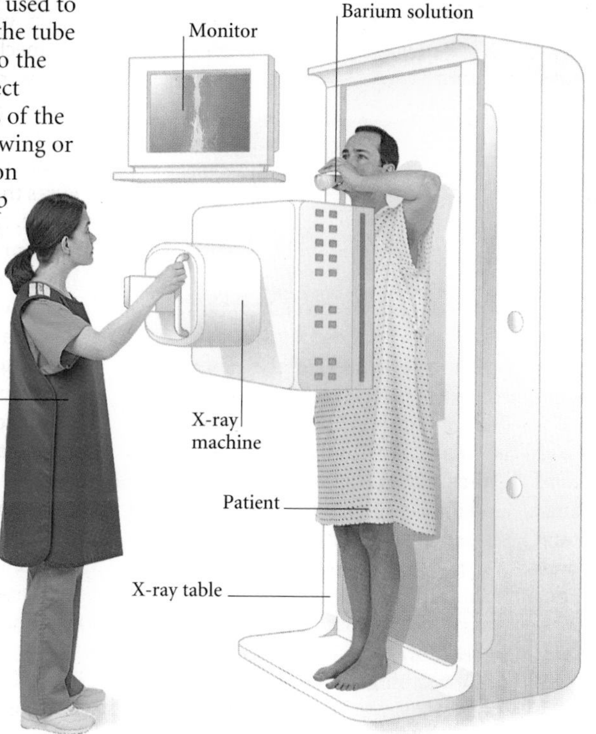

Radiographer
The radiographer ensures that you are comfortable and then positions the X-ray machine

During the procedure
While standing in front of the X-ray machine, you are asked to swallow a barium solution as a series of X-rays is taken. The procedure takes about 15 minutes to complete.

RESULTS

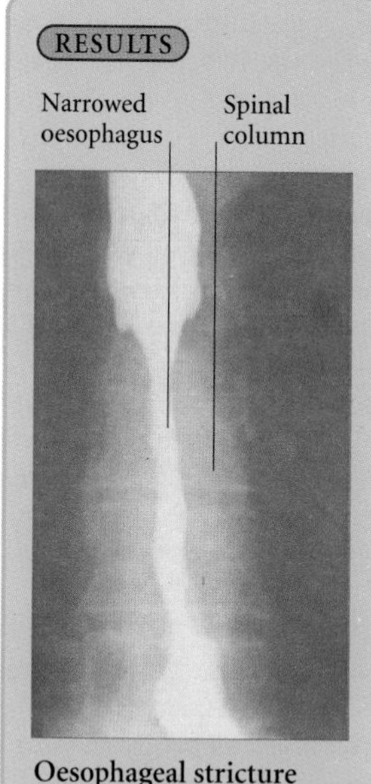

Oesophageal stricture
This contrast X-ray shows a narrowed area called a stricture in the lower section of the oesophagus.

WHAT MIGHT BE DONE?

Self-help measures can relieve many symptoms of heartburn (*see* MANAGING GASTRO-OESOPHAGEAL REFLUX, opposite page). However, if your heartburn is troublesome and persistent, consult your doctor about the problem.

The doctor may arrange for contrast X-rays that can show any abnormalities in the oesophagus (*see* BARIUM SWALLOW, above). You may also undergo endoscopy (p.255), in which a flexible viewing tube is used to examine the lining of the oesophagus. During this procedure, a small sample of tissue may be removed from the oesophagus for examination under a microscope.

If self-help measures do not relieve your symptoms, your doctor may prescribe a drug that reduces the stomach's acid production (*see* ULCER-HEALING DRUGS, p.923). The rate at which the stomach is emptied may be increased by a drug such as metoclopramide (*see* ANTISPASMODIC DRUGS AND MOTILITY STIMULANTS, p.926), making heartburn less likely. In most cases, the symptoms of GOR disappear with treatment. If they do not, you may need surgery to return the stomach to its normal position and tighten the lower oesophageal sphincter muscle. The procedure may be carried out by endoscopic surgery (p.948), in which an endoscope and surgical instruments are manipulated through tiny incisions in the abdomen.

WWW ONLINE SITES: p.1030

Achalasia

Difficulty in swallowing due to a muscle disorder of the oesophagus

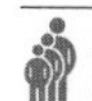 AGE Most common between the ages of 20 and 40; rare in childhood

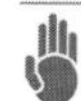 GENDER GENETICS LIFESTYLE Not significant factors

In people with achalasia, the passage of food and drink into the stomach from the oesophagus is delayed or prevented. The problem is mainly caused by failure of the lower oesophageal sphincter (the ring of muscle at the lower end of the oesophagus) to relax normally and allow food to pass into the stomach during swallowing. Achalasia may also be caused by poor muscle coordination in the oesophagus. The condition causes the lower part of the oesophagus to be progressively distorted and widened over months or years, and makes swallowing increasingly difficult. Achalasia most commonly occurs in people between the ages of 20 and 40.

WHAT ARE THE SYMPTOMS?

Symptoms of achalasia usually develop slowly and include the following:

- Difficulty in swallowing.
- Chest pain or a feeling of discomfort behind the breastbone, which may be related to eating.
- Regurgitating undigested food during meals or some hours afterwards, especially at night.
- Eventually, weight loss.

If achalasia is left untreated, there is a slightly increased risk of developing cancer of the oesophagus (p.638).

HOW IS IT DIAGNOSED?

If your doctor suspects that you have achalasia, a chest X-ray (p.490) may be arranged to look for the typical widening and distortion of the oesophagus. The diagnosis may be apparent from a barium swallow (above), in which the action of muscles in the oesophagus can be observed. Your doctor may look down your oesophagus using a flexible viewing instrument called an endoscope (*see* ENDOSCOPY, p.255) to confirm the diagnosis and eliminate other possible disorders, such as cancer of the oesophagus. Oesophageal manometry may be arranged, in which a flexible tube is passed down the oesophagus in order to measure pressures. Normally, the procedure shows changing pressures as a result of the alternate contractions and relaxations of the muscles that propel the food towards the stomach. In achalasia, these pressure changes are absent, and the overall pressure is high due to incomplete muscle relaxation.

WHAT IS THE TREATMENT?

Several different effective treatments are available for achalasia. The choice of treatment depends on your age and general health in addition to the severity and duration of your symptoms.

The simplest treatment is for your doctor to prescribe drugs called calcium channel blockers (p.900), which temporarily relax the lower oesophageal sphincter muscle. However, for longer-term relief, the treatment most often used is to pass a small balloon down to the oesophageal sphincter. Once the balloon is in place, it is inflated with either air or water to stretch the sphincter and is then removed. This procedure is successful in at least half of all people with the disorder. However, for a few people, it may have to be repeated over periods varying from 6 months to several years.

An alternative treatment is the injection of botulin toxin into the sphincter. In small doses, this toxin paralyses the affected muscles, causing them to relax and allow food and liquids to pass. This effect typically lasts a little over a year and may need to be repeated.

If none of these methods is successful, endoscopic surgery (p.948) may be performed using instruments passed down an endoscope. Some of the muscle at the lower end of the oesophagus may be cut to allow food to pass into the stomach. In about 1 in 10 cases, this procedure leads to the stomach contents flowing back up the oesophagus, a condition that will also need treatment (*see* GASTRO-OESOPHAGEAL REFLUX, p.636).

WWW ONLINE SITES: p.1030

Cancer of the oesophagus

Cancerous tumour in the tissue of the oesophagus

AGE Most common between the ages of 60 and 70; rare before the age of 50

GENDER About 2–3 times more common in males

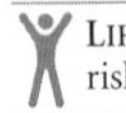
LIFESTYLE Smoking and alcohol abuse are risk factors

GENETICS Not a significant factor

In the UK, cancer of the oesophagus accounts for more than 1 in 50 of all new cases of cancer. It is much more common in countries such as Iran and parts of China. The disease is more than twice as common in men than in women and occurs most frequently in people between the ages of 60 and 70. Death rates from cancer of the oesophagus are relatively high because the tumour is often present for some time before it begins to cause symptoms. As a result, the cancer has often spread to other parts of the body by the time medical help is sought.

WHAT ARE THE CAUSES?

The exact cause of cancer of the oesophagus is unknown, but factors known to increase the risk of developing it include smoking and excessive alcohol consumption. In China, fungal toxins in food are thought to be responsible for the high rate of the cancer. People who have particular disorders of the oesophagus, such as gastro-oesophageal reflux (p.636), achalasia (p.637), and Barrett's oesophagus (in which the lining of the stomach replaces part of the oesophageal lining), are at increased risk of developing cancer of the oesophagus. People with long-term oesophageal diseases should have regular endoscopy (p.255) to look for early evidence of cancerous growths.

Tumour

Wall of oesophagus

Oesophageal cancer
This endoscopic view shows a cancerous tumour on the lining of the oesophagus.

WHAT ARE THE SYMPTOMS?

Early in the disease, there are often no symptoms. When they begin to develop, they do so slowly over weeks or months as the oesophagus becomes obstructed. The symptoms may include:

- Pain and difficulty in swallowing solid foods, particularly bread and meat.
- Difficulty in swallowing liquids.
- Regurgitation of recently eaten food.
- Cough as a result of food spilling into the lungs.
- Loss of appetite and weight loss.

If the tumour spreads and involves the trachea, there may also be shortness of breath and blood in the sputum.

HOW IS IT DIAGNOSED?

Your doctor may arrange for a tissue sample to be taken during endoscopy, which involves passing a flexible viewing tube into the oesophagus (see UPPER DIGESTIVE TRACT ENDOSCOPY, p.641). A barium swallow (p.637) may be performed to detect an obstruction in the oesophagus. Once the diagnosis has been confirmed, tests such as CT scanning (p.247) of the chest or of the abdomen may be carried out to determine if the tumour has spread beyond its original site (*see* STAGING CANCER, p. 279).

WHAT IS THE TREATMENT?

The treatment depends on whether the cancer is limited to the oesophagus or has spread to the structures around it. A localized cancer can be removed, but the operation is a major procedure and only a small proportion of affected people are diagnosed early enough to make attempting surgery worthwhile.

If the cancer has already spread or if general health is not good enough for major surgery, treatment is given to relieve the symptoms. Insertion of a rigid tube into the oesophagus in the narrowed area can relieve swallowing difficulties (*see* PALLIATIVE SURGERY FOR CANCER, p. 282). Additional treatment may involve radiotherapy (p.281) and chemotherapy (p.280).

WHAT IS THE PROGNOSIS?

About 1 in 4 people in whom curative surgery is attempted survive for more than 5 years. However, people for whom curative surgery is not an option usually survive for less than a year.

WWW ONLINE SITES: p.1028, p.1030

DISORDERS OF THE STOMACH AND DUODENUM

The stomach and the duodenum (the first part of the intestine) are exposed to many potentially damaging substances, including acid produced by the stomach to aid food digestion, alcohol, and irritative foods such as spices. The stomach and duodenum have a natural defence mechanism that protects against damage, but sometimes this mechanism fails, leading to disease.

The first article in this section covers infection with the *Helicobacter pylori* bacterium, which was only discovered in the early 1980s. It is now estimated that about half the world's population is infected with *H. pylori*. In most cases, there are no symptoms. However, *H. pylori* is known to be associated with the disorders of the stomach and duodenum discussed in this section: gastritis, which is inflammation of the lining of the stomach; peptic ulcer, which is an area of the stomach lining or the duodenum that has been eroded by acidic digestive juices; and stomach cancer. Both gastritis and peptic ulcer are common disorders of the digestive system that affect thousands of people in the UK every year. However, if either of these disorders occurs with *H. pylori* infection, it can usually be treated successfully with drugs. The final article covers stomach cancer, which is now rare in many developed countries. General problems that may involve the stomach or another part of the upper digestive tract are covered elsewhere (*see* INDIGESTION, p.626; NONULCER DYSPEPSIA, p.626; and GASTRO-OESOPHAGEAL REFLUX, p.636).

KEY ANATOMY

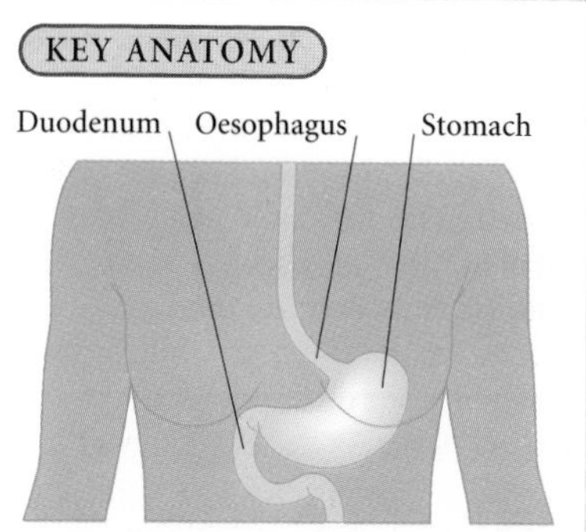

For further information about the structure and function of the stomach and duodenum, *see* pp.620–625.

Helicobacter pylori infection

A common bacterial infection, which may lead to inflammation or ulceration in the upper digestive tract

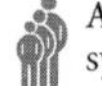 AGE Often contracted in childhood, but symptoms usually develop in adulthood

 GENDER More common in males

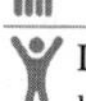 LIFESTYLE Living in overcrowded, unsanitary conditions is a risk factor

 GENETICS Not a significant factor

The *Helicobacter pylori* bacterium was discovered in the early 1980s. Research since then has shown that about half of the world's population is infected. The infection is usually contracted during childhood and, in most cases, causes no symptoms. However, in some people, *H. pylori* infection may lead to the development of gastritis (p.640), in which the stomach lining becomes inflamed, or to a peptic ulcer (p.640), in which an area of the lining of the stomach or the duodenum is eroded by the action of the acidic digestive juices.

The *H. pylori* bacterium can lead to peptic ulcers or gastritis when it damages the mucous layer of the stomach or duodenum. The mucus usually protects the lining of the stomach and the duodenum from acidic digestive juices, and the lining may become inflamed or eroded in areas where the mucous layer is damaged. Long-term infection with *H. pylori* may also increase the risk of developing stomach cancer (p.642).

The exact way in which *H. pylori* is transmitted is unknown. It is believed that the bacterium may be carried in faeces and saliva and is most readily passed on by close contact with others, especially among people living in overcrowded, unsanitary conditions. The infection is more common in males.

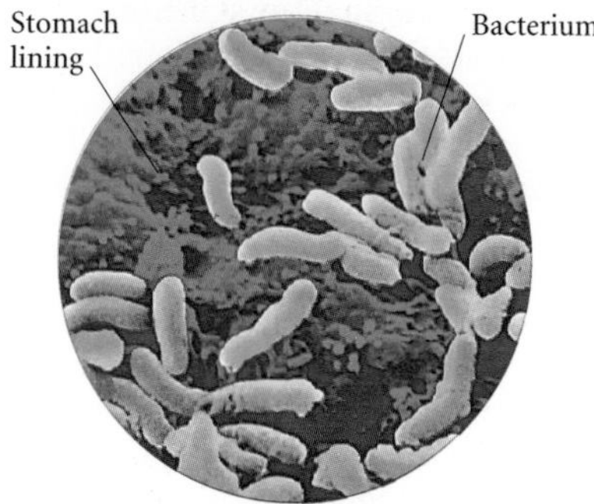

Helicobacter pylori
A number of Helicobacter pylori *bacteria can be seen in this magnified view of the mucous lining of the stomach.*

HOW IS IT DIAGNOSED?

If you have discomfort or pain in the upper abdomen, your doctor may suspect that you have gastritis or a peptic ulcer. He or she may arrange for tests to check for *H. pylori* infection. One of these tests may be a blood test to check for the presence of antibodies against *H. pylori* (*see* TESTS FOR ANTIGENS AND ANTIBODIES, p.235). A positive result confirms that you have had the infection at some time. Alternatively, you may be given a breath test. This test involves first drinking a substance that is normally broken down by *H. pylori*. If the bacteria are present, the substance is changed into a chemical that can be detected with a breathalyser. You may also have an upper digestive tract endoscopy (p.641), in which the stomach or duodenum is examined with a flexible viewing tube. At the same time, a small piece of the lining may be taken for examination under a microscope.

What is the treatment?

Treatment for *H. pylori* is given only if the infection has led to a disorder such as gastritis or a peptic ulcer. Your doctor will prescribe a combination of antibiotics (p.885) to treat the infection and other drugs to suppress the production of stomach acid (*see* ULCER-HEALING DRUGS, p.923). In about 9 in 10 cases, *H. pylori* infection can be successfully treated. The infection may recur in a small number of cases.

(WWW) ONLINE SITES: p.1030

Gastritis

Inflammation of the stomach lining, which may be caused by irritation or infection

AGE More common over the age of 50; rare in children

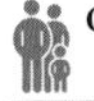
GENETICS Sometimes runs in families

LIFESTYLE Alcohol abuse and smoking are risk factors

GENDER Not a significant factor

Gastritis, which is inflammation of the stomach lining, is a common disorder. More than half of the population over the age of 50 have gastritis, although in some cases there are no symptoms. The disorder may be acute and have a sudden onset, but it is more frequently chronic, developing gradually over months or years. The symptoms commonly include discomfort in the upper abdomen. The inflammation may be complicated by bleeding from the stomach.

Some types of gastritis run in families. However, in the 1980s, *Helicobacter pylori* infection (p.639) was found to be a major cause of chronic gastritis. This discovery has led to effective treatment for many people with the disorder.

What are the causes?

Acute gastritis may occur when the stomach lining is damaged by drinking an excessive amount of alcohol or by taking aspirin or another nonsteroidal anti-inflammatory drug (p.894), such as ibuprofen. Acute gastritis can also develop after serious illness, such as blood poisoning (*see* SEPTICAEMIA, p.299).

Chronic gastritis is often caused by infection with *H. pylori* bacteria, which are found in the stomach lining of about half of the population. The bacterium damages the mucous layer that protects the stomach lining from digestive juices, allowing acid to attack the lining. Chronic gastritis may also occur in Crohn's disease (p.658), a disorder which may cause digestive tract inflammation. Long-term use of alcohol, tobacco, and nonsteroidal anti-inflammatory drugs (p.894), such as aspirin, may also lead to chronic gastritis.

One type of chronic gastritis, known as atrophic or autoimmune gastritis, is caused by an abnormal reaction of the immune system in which the body produces antibodies that attack the tissues of the stomach lining.

What are the symptoms?

Chronic gastritis often does not cause any symptoms, but it may gradually result in damage to the stomach lining that will eventually produce symptoms similar to those of acute gastritis. The onset of symptoms in acute gastritis is much faster and the symptoms are more severe. The symptoms of both types of gastritis may include:

- Discomfort or pain in the stomach area, often after eating.
- Nausea and vomiting.
- Loss of appetite.

Bleeding from the stomach lining may go unnoticed until it gives rise to iron-deficiency anaemia (p.447), which causes tiredness and pale skin. If the bleeding is severe, you may vomit blood or pass black, tarry stools (*see* BLEEDING FROM THE DIGESTIVE TRACT, p.630).

Atrophic gastritis is usually painless, and the only symptoms may be those of pernicious anaemia due to a deficiency of vitamin B_{12}. Atrophic gastritis damages the stomach so that it cannot make intrinsic factor, a substance essential for the absorption of this vitamin. People with chronic gastritis, especially atrophic gastritis, also have an increased risk of developing stomach cancer (p.642).

What can I do?

The symptoms of mild gastritis can be treated with over-the-counter antacids (p.923), which neutralize the acid in the stomach. You may also find that your symptoms are relieved by eating small, regular meals, reducing alcohol intake, and giving up smoking. If symptoms persist or are severe or you are losing weight, consult your doctor.

What might be done?

Your doctor will ask you about your smoking, drinking, and dietary habits, and your use of medications. You may be given a blood or breath test to look for *H. pylori* infection. You may also have a blood test for anaemia to see if there has been bleeding from the stomach lining. Your doctor may arrange for you to have endoscopy (*see* UPPER DIGESTIVE TRACT ENDOSCOPY, opposite page) to examine the stomach lining.

If *H. pylori* infection is confirmed, a combination of antibiotics (p.885) and ulcer-healing drugs (p.923) may be prescribed. If you have gastritis and need to take aspirin or another nonsteroidal anti-inflammatory drug for a period of time, you may also be advised to take a drug called misoprostol. This drug reduces the production of stomach acid and helps to protect the stomach lining.

Gastritis usually improves if lifestyle changes, such as reducing intake of alcohol, are made. If chronic gastritis is caused by *H. pylori* infection, complete recovery usually follows treatment with antibiotics and ulcer-healing drugs. However, infection sometimes recurs, requiring further treatment.

(WWW) ONLINE SITES: p.1030

Peptic ulcer

An eroded area of the tissue lining the stomach or the duodenum, the first part of the small intestine

AGE Stomach ulcers are more common over the age of 50; duodenal ulcers are most common between the ages of 20 and 45

GENDER Duodenal ulcers are more common in males

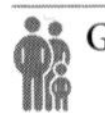
GENETICS Sometimes runs in families

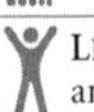
LIFESTYLE Stress, excess alcohol, smoking, and unsanitary conditions are risk factors

The lining of the stomach and duodenum normally has a barrier of mucus to protect it from the effects of acidic digestive juices. If this barrier is damaged, the acid may cause inflammation and erosion of the lining. The resulting eroded areas are known as peptic ulcers, of which there are two types: duodenal ulcers and gastric (stomach) ulcers. Duodenal ulcers are more common than gastric ulcers and usually occur in people aged 20 to 45, particularly men.

Gastric ulcers are more common in people over the age of 50. Peptic ulcers are common, and it is estimated that about 1 in 10 people in the UK develops an ulcer at some time.

WHAT ARE THE CAUSES?

Peptic ulcers are most commonly associated with *Helicobacter pylori* infection (p.639). This bacterium is thought to be transmitted most easily in unsanitary living conditions and releases substances that reduce the effectiveness of the mucous layer. Acidic digestive juices are then able to erode the lining of the stomach or the duodenum, which allows peptic ulcers to develop.

Peptic ulcers may sometimes result from the long-term use of nonsteroidal anti-inflammatory drugs (p.894), such as ibuprofen or aspirin, that damage the lining of the stomach. Other factors that may lead to peptic ulcers include smoking and consumption of alcohol and possibly caffeine. In some people, there is a strong family history of peptic ulcers, suggesting that a genetic factor may be involved in their development. Psychological stress is no longer believed to be one of the primary causes of peptic ulcers, but it may play a part in making an existing ulcer worse.

WHAT ARE THE SYMPTOMS?

Many people with a peptic ulcer do not experience symptoms or dismiss their discomfort as indigestion (p.626). Those with persistent symptoms may notice:

- Pain or discomfort that is felt in the upper abdomen.
- Loss of appetite and weight loss.
- A feeling of fullness in the abdomen.
- Nausea and sometimes vomiting.

Pain is often present for several weeks and then disappears for months or even years. The pain from a duodenal ulcer can be worse before meals when the stomach is empty. This pain may be quickly relieved by eating but usually recurs a few hours afterwards. By contrast, pain caused by a gastric ulcer is often aggravated by food.

ARE THERE COMPLICATIONS?

The most common complication of a peptic ulcer is bleeding as the ulcer becomes deeper and erodes into nearby blood vessels (*see* BLEEDING FROM THE DIGESTIVE TRACT, p.630). Minor bleeding from the digestive tract may cause no symptoms apart from those of iron-deficiency anaemia (p.447), such as pale skin, tiredness, and faintness. Bleeding from the digestive tract may lead to vomiting of blood. Alternatively, blood may pass through the digestive tract, resulting in black, tarry stools. In some cases, an ulcer perforates all the layers of the stomach or duodenum, allowing gastric juices to enter the abdomen and causing severe pain (*see* PERITONITIS, p.665). Bleeding from the digestive tract and perforation of the stomach or the duodenum may be life-threatening and require immediate medical attention.

In rare cases, stomach ulcers may result in narrowing of the stomach outlet into the duodenum, which prevents the stomach from emptying fully. Symptoms may then include bloating after meals, vomiting undigested food hours after eating, and weight loss.

WHAT MIGHT BE DONE?

If your doctor suspects that you have a peptic ulcer, he or she may arrange an endoscopy (*see* UPPER DIGESTIVE TRACT ENDOSCOPY, below) to view the stomach and duodenum. During endoscopy, a sample of the stomach lining may be taken to look for evidence of *H. pylori* infection and exclude stomach cancer (p.642), which may cause similar symptoms. Your doctor may also arrange for you to have blood tests to detect antibodies against the *H. pylori* bacterium and to check for evidence of anaemia.

TEST AND TREATMENT UPPER DIGESTIVE TRACT ENDOSCOPY

This technique involves passing a flexible viewing tube through the mouth to examine the oesophagus, stomach, and duodenum (the first part of the small intestine) to look for disorders such as peptic ulcers. Diathermy (a heat treatment) or laser therapy can be performed or injections of drugs given to stop any bleeding.

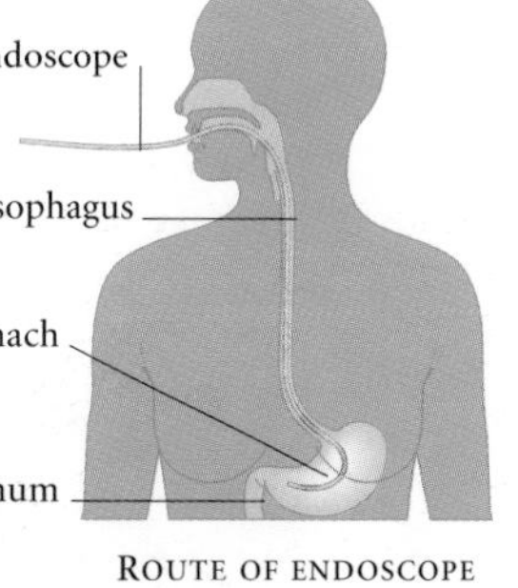

ROUTE OF ENDOSCOPE

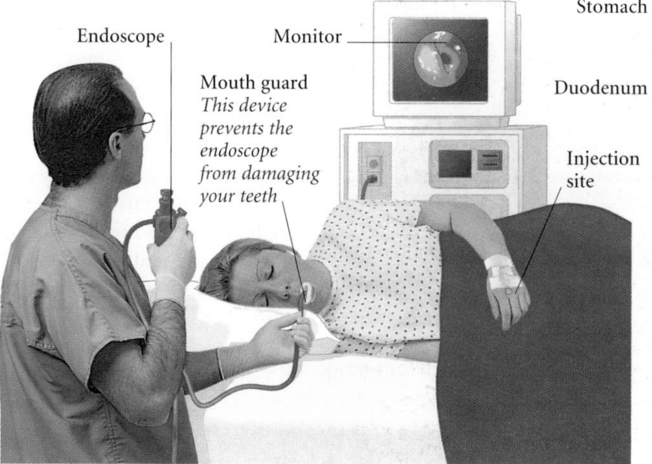

During the procedure
You may have a local anaesthetic spray to numb the back of your throat and/or intravenous sedation. You then swallow the endoscope, through which the doctor views your upper digestive tract. The procedure usually takes about 15 minutes.

VIEW

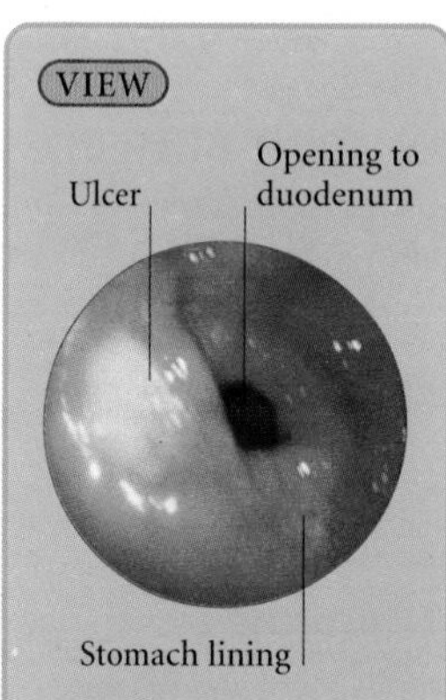

Gastric ulcer
In this view through an endoscope, a gastric ulcer is clearly visible in the mucous membrane lining the stomach. Close by is the opening from the stomach into the duodenum.

Treatment of a peptic ulcer is designed to heal the ulcer and to prevent it from recurring. You will be advised to make some lifestyle changes, such as giving up smoking and drinking less alcohol.

If *H. pylori* is found, a combination of antibiotics (p.885) and ulcer-healing drugs (p.923) will usually be prescribed. Ulcer-healing drugs are usually given to maximize the chance of healing even if tests for *H. pylori* prove negative.

If long-term treatment with aspirin or another nonsteroidal anti-inflammatory drug is the cause, your doctor may prescribe an alternative or an additional drug, such as misoprostol, to protect the lining of the stomach and duodenum.

A bleeding or perforated ulcer is an emergency requiring urgent admission to hospital. If the blood loss is severe, a blood transfusion (p.447) may be necessary. Endoscopy may be used to view the stomach lining; during this, bleeding blood vessels may be treated with diathermy, a technique that uses heat to seal them. Alternatively, an injection of drugs may be given to stop bleeding. If bleeding is severe or the ulcer is perforated, surgery is usually necessary.

With treatment, about 19 in 20 peptic ulcers disappear completely within a few months. However, the ulcer may recur if lifestyle changes are not made or if there is reinfection with *H. pylori*.

(WWW) ONLINE SITES: p.1030

Stomach cancer

A cancerous tumour in the lining of the stomach wall

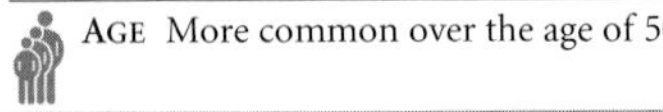
AGE More common over the age of 50

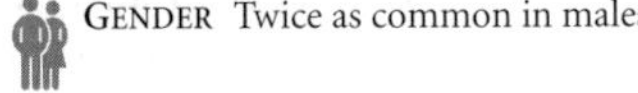
GENDER Twice as common in males

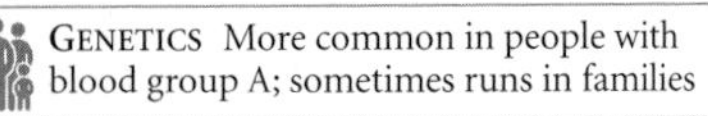
GENETICS More common in people with blood group A; sometimes runs in families

LIFESTYLE Certain foods, smoking, and a high alcohol intake are risk factors

Worldwide, stomach cancer is the second most common cancer after lung cancer. Stomach cancer is a particular problem in Japan and China, possibly because of dietary factors. However, in most other countries the disease has become less common, perhaps because diets now contain less smoked and salted foods. There are about 6,000 new cases of stomach cancer each year in the UK. Few cases occur before the age of 50, but the incidence then increases with age. Stomach cancer is twice as common in males. It is also more common in people of blood group A and can run in families, suggesting a genetic factor.

In most cases, stomach cancer develops in the stomach lining. The cancer may spread rapidly to other parts of the body. Early diagnosis is rare because the symptoms are usually mild, and by the time people seek medical help, the cancer has often spread.

What are the causes?

The causes of stomach cancer are not fully understood, but there are a number of factors. Chronic gastritis due to infection with the *H. pylori* bacterium (*see* HELICOBACTER PYLORI INFECTION, p.639) increases the risk of stomach cancer. Certain diets may increase the risk, such as a diet with a high intake of salt, pickled and smoked foods, and a low intake of fresh fruit and green vegetables. Smoking and a high alcohol intake are also risk factors.

What are the symptoms?

The early symptoms of stomach cancer are mild and vague, and many people ignore them. They may include:

- Discomfort in the upper abdomen.
- Pain in the stomach after eating.
- Loss of appetite and weight loss.
- Nausea and vomiting.

In many people, iron-deficiency anaemia (p.447) develops due to minor bleeding from the stomach lining. Later on, swelling may be felt in the upper abdomen.

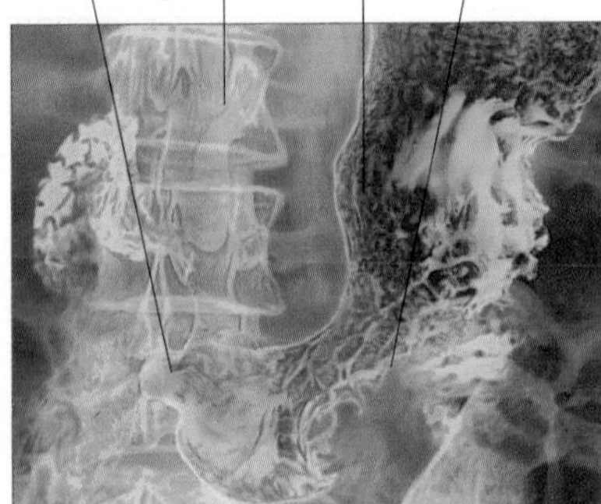

Cancer in the lower stomach
In this X-ray, barium has been used to outline the stomach. The lining of the stomach has an irregular area where there is a large tumour.

How is it diagnosed?

Your doctor may arrange for you to have upper digestive tract endoscopy (p.641), in which a thin, flexible viewing tube is used to examine the lining of the stomach. Samples of tissue are taken from abnormal areas of the stomach lining during the procedure and tested to look for the presence of cancerous cells. You may also have a barium meal (*see* CONTRAST X-RAYS, p.245), in which a liquid barium mixture is swallowed to show the stomach clearly on an X-ray. The doctor may arrange blood tests for anaemia, which may show that there has been bleeding from the stomach lining.

If a diagnosis of stomach cancer is confirmed, further investigations, such as CT scanning (p.247) and blood tests, may be performed to check whether the cancer has spread to other organs (*see* STAGING CANCER, p.279).

What is the treatment?

The only effective treatment for stomach cancer is early surgery to remove the tumour. However, this option is suitable in only about 2 in 10 cases; in the rest the cancer has already spread too widely to be operable. The operation involves the removal of part or all of the stomach. The surrounding lymph nodes are also removed since they are possible sites of cancer spread. In some cases in which the cancer has spread to other parts of the body, surgery may help to improve life expectancy, but in other cases the operation is carried out to relieve the symptoms rather than to attempt a definitive cure. Radiotherapy (p.281) and chemotherapy (p.280) are used to slow the progress of the disease and to relieve pain. Strong painkillers (p.912) can be given to help to relieve severe discomfort.

What is the prognosis?

If detected and treated early, stomach cancer has a good cure rate. Some countries in which stomach cancer is common, such as Japan, have efficient screening programmes to detect the cancer early. In these countries, about 8 in 10 people have surgery and are alive 5 years after diagnosis. However, the outlook worldwide is generally poor, with only about 2 in 10 affected people surviving for 5 years after diagnosis.

(WWW) ONLINE SITES: p.1028, p.1030

DISORDERS OF THE LIVER, GALLBLADDER, AND PANCREAS

One of the main functions of the liver and pancreas is to aid food digestion. The liver makes the digestive fluid bile, which is stored in the gallbladder. The pancreas makes digestive enzymes. These organs have other vital functions. The liver uses digestion products to make new substances such as proteins and fats, and the pancreas produces hormones that control the level of glucose in the blood.

The yellow discoloration of the skin and eyes known as jaundice is a sign of liver disease but also has other causes, which are discussed in the first article in this section. The next two articles cover hepatitis due to viral infection, which is the most common cause of liver disease worldwide, as well as other forms of hepatitis. Excessive alcohol consumption is the main cause of liver disease in Western countries; three articles deal with alcoholic liver disease and its complications – cirrhosis and portal hypertension and varices. Liver cancer is then described; the first type, which originates in the liver, is less common in Western countries than cancer that spreads from other organs to the liver (liver metastases). Liver failure, which may be fatal unless treated with liver transplantation, is also discussed.

Gallstones do not usually cause symptoms and may not need to be treated, as explained in the next articles, but can lead to inflammation of the gallbladder, called cholecystitis. Articles on the inflammatory conditions, acute and chronic pancreatitis follow, and the final article covers pancreatic cancer, which is increasingly common in Western countries.

KEY ANATOMY

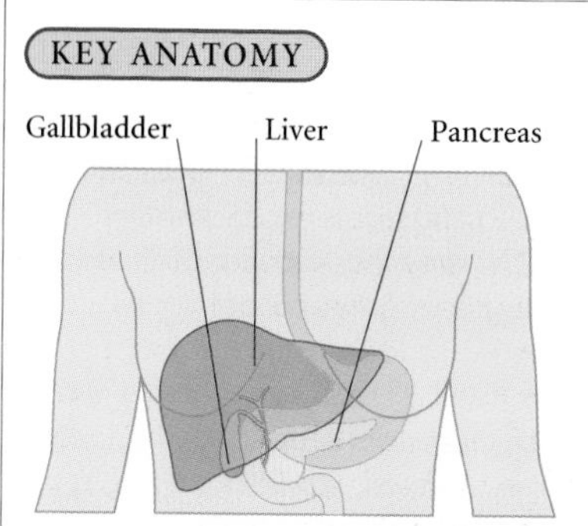

For information on the structure and function of the liver, gallbladder, and pancreas, *see* pp.620–625.

Jaundice

Yellow discoloration of the skin and the whites of the eyes

AGE GENDER GENETICS LIFESTYLE
Risk factors depend on the cause

Jaundice, a yellow discoloration of the skin and the whites of the eyes, is a symptom of many disorders of the liver, gallbladder, or pancreas. It may also be caused by some blood disorders. Jaundice results from excessively high blood levels of the pigment bilirubin, a breakdown product of red blood cells. Bilirubin is processed by the liver and then excreted as a component of the digestive fluid bile.

Jaundice always requires investigation because the underlying disorder may be serious. A few days after birth, many babies develop a form of jaundice that is usually harmless and disappears quickly (*see* NEONATAL JAUNDICE, p.817).

WHAT ARE THE CAUSES?

Levels of bilirubin in the blood can increase if the amount of bilirubin produced is too great for the liver to process. Damaged liver cells or obstruction of the bile ducts, which carry bile from the liver to the gallbladder and small intestine, can also lead to high levels of bilirubin in the blood.

EXCESS RED BLOOD CELL BREAKDOWN In a healthy person, red blood cells have a lifespan of about 120 days, after which they are removed from the blood and broken down by the spleen to produce bilirubin. The bilirubin then passes to the liver. If the number of red blood cells being broken down is above normal, the liver cannot process the large amounts of bilirubin produced. This condition is known as haemolytic jaundice and may be caused by disorders such as haemolytic anaemia (p.450), in which the lifespan of red blood cells is shorter than normal. It may be accompanied by other symptoms, such as tiredness.

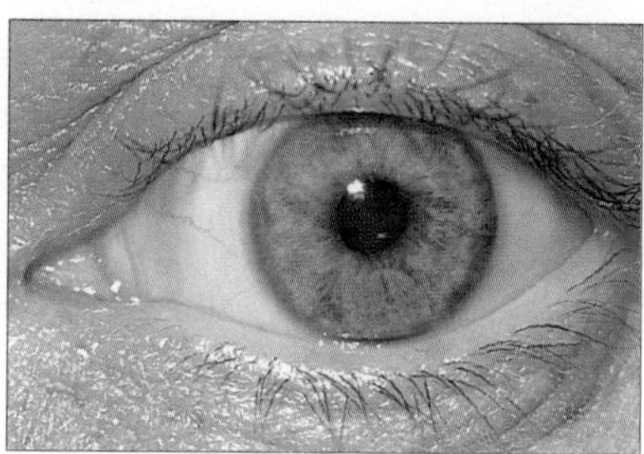

Jaundice
The skin and the white of the eye have become yellow. These symptoms, known as jaundice, can occur as a result of many disorders, including liver disease.

LIVER CELL DAMAGE If the liver cells are damaged, the liver is less able to process bilirubin. Possible causes of damage include infection (*see* ACUTE HEPATITIS, p.644, and CHRONIC HEPATITIS, p.645), alcohol abuse (*see* ALCOHOL-RELATED LIVER DISEASE, p.646), and an adverse reaction to some drugs. Jaundice that is due to liver cell damage is sometimes accompanied by nausea, vomiting, and abdominal pain and swelling.

BILE DUCT OBSTRUCTION An obstruction in the bile ducts, the channels through which bile leaves the liver, may result in jaundice. Obstruction may be due to disorders such as pancreatic cancer (p.654) or gallstones (p.651). If bile ducts are blocked, bile builds up in the liver, and bilirubin is forced back into the blood. This type of jaundice may be accompanied by itching, dark-coloured urine, and paler than normal faeces.

WHAT MIGHT BE DONE?

Your doctor may arrange blood tests to assess liver function and to look for signs of excess red blood cell destruction, viral hepatitis, or other disorders affecting the liver. To look for evidence of inflammation or obstruction, your doctor may use imaging techniques such as CT scanning (p.247) or MRI (p.248) or techniques such as ERCP (p.653) and ultrasound scanning (p.250), which may be carried out using an endoscope. A sample of liver tissue may be taken and examined for underlying liver disease (*see* LIVER BIOPSY, p.647).

If the underlying cause of jaundice can be treated, jaundice will disappear. If the cause is not curable, as in the case of pancreatic cancer, treatment may be given to relieve symptoms associated with jaundice, such as itching.

(WWW) ONLINE SITES: p.1034

Acute hepatitis

Sudden, short-term inflammation of the liver due to a variety of causes

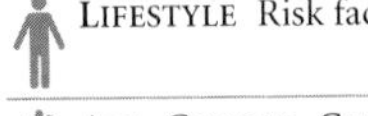

LIFESTYLE Risk factors depend on the cause

AGE GENDER GENETICS Not significant factors

Short-term inflammation of the liver is known as acute hepatitis. The condition has various causes and has a sudden onset. Most people with acute hepatitis recover within a month or two, but in some cases inflammation of the liver persists for many months or even years (*see* CHRONIC HEPATITIS, opposite page) or progresses to liver failure (p.650).

WHAT ARE THE CAUSES?

Worldwide, the most common cause of acute hepatitis is infection with any one of the several types of hepatitis viruses. Until the late 1980s, there were only two known hepatitis viruses, hepatitis A and B. Additional hepatitis viruses have now been identified, including hepatitis C, D, and E. Other hepatitis viruses are almost certainly yet to be discovered. The known viruses can all cause acute hepatitis, and they have many features in common, although the way in which they are transmitted and their long-term effects may differ. Infections with some types of bacteria, other nonhepatitis viruses, and some parasites can also lead to acute hepatitis. In addition, the condition may be caused by noninfectious agents, such as some drugs and toxins, including alcohol (*see* ALCOHOL-RELATED LIVER DISEASE, p.646).

HEPATITIS A VIRUS The hepatitis A virus is common in southern and eastern Europe and some parts of Africa and Asia, but it is much less common in the UK. However, many cases are not reported because the virus often produces no symptoms or symptoms are so mild that the infection passes unrecognized. The virus can be detected in the urine and faeces of infected people, and it can be transmitted to other people in contaminated food or water.

HEPATITIS B VIRUS It is estimated that each year 1 million people in Europe become infected with hepatitis B, and about 1 in 1,000 people in the UK carry the virus at any one time. The virus is spread by contact with an infected person's body fluids. For example, the virus can be spread by sexual intercourse or sharing contaminated needles for taking drugs intravenously. In developing countries, hepatitis B infection is most commonly transmitted from mother to baby at birth. Before blood banks routinely screened blood for the hepatitis B virus, as they do now, blood transfusions were a source of infection, and a number of people with haemophilia (*see* HAEMOPHILIA AND CHRISTMAS DISEASE, p.452) contracted hepatitis.

HEPATITIS C VIRUS About 3 per cent of people worldwide have been infected with the hepatitis C virus. The virus is most commonly transmitted by contact with an infected person's blood, often by sharing contaminated needles used for taking drugs intravenously. All of the blood used for transfusions in the UK is now routinely screened for the hepatitis C virus. Hepatitis C infection can also be spread through sexual intercourse.

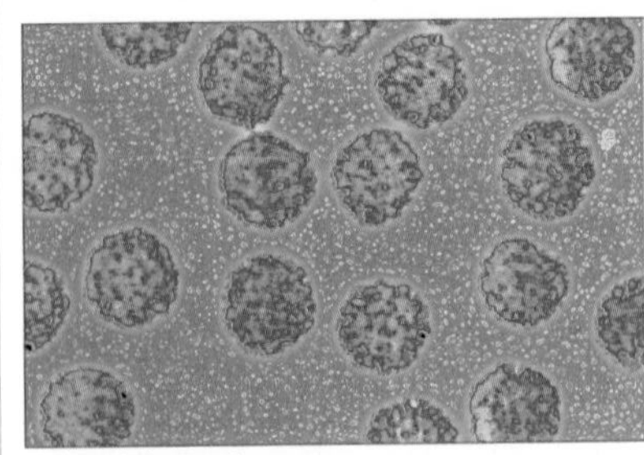

Hepatitis B viruses
This highly magnified image shows spherical hepatitis B viruses. Infection with these viruses is one of the many causes of the liver disorder acute hepatitis.

HEPATITIS D AND E VIRUSES Infection with hepatitis D occurs only in people who already have hepatitis B infection. It is spread by contact with infected body fluids. The hepatitis E virus is a rare cause of hepatitis in the developed world. The virus is excreted in the faeces of infected people and is spread in much the same way as the hepatitis A virus.

OTHER INFECTIOUS CAUSES Acute hepatitis may also be caused by other viral infections, such as cytomegalovirus (*see* CYTOMEGALOVIRUS INFECTION, p.292) and the Epstein–Barr virus, the cause of infectious mononucleosis (p.291). Some bacterial infections, such as leptospirosis (p.302) and Legionnaires' disease, can cause acute hepatitis. Parasitic infections that may lead to acute hepatitis include infection with plasmodium organisms, the cause of malaria (p.305).

NONINFECTIOUS CAUSES In developed countries, excessive alcohol intake is one of the most common causes of acute hepatitis. The disease can also be caused by other toxins, such as those found in poisonous fungi. Certain drugs, such as the anaesthetic gas halothane (*see* GENERAL ANAESTHETICS, p.914), some anticonvulsants (p.914), and an overdose of paracetamol (*see* PAINKILLERS, p.912), may cause acute hepatitis. Occasionally, the condition occurs in pregnancy, although the cause is not fully understood.

WHAT ARE THE SYMPTOMS?

Some people infected with a hepatitis virus have no symptoms or symptoms are so mild that they are not recognized. In other cases, the disorder may be life-threatening. If hepatitis is due to a viral infection, the time from infection to the appearance of symptoms can vary from up to 6 weeks for hepatitis A to 6 months for hepatitis B. Some people who have no symptoms may become carriers of the virus. If symptoms do develop, they may initially include:

- Tiredness and a feeling of ill health.
- Poor appetite.

- Nausea and vomiting.
- Fever.
- Discomfort in the upper right side of the abdomen.

In some cases, several days after the initial symptoms develop, the whites of the eyes and the skin take on a yellow tinge, a condition known as jaundice (p.643). Often, the initial symptoms improve once jaundice appears. At this time, the faeces may become paler than usual, and widespread itching may be present. Acute hepatitis caused by the hepatitis B virus may also cause joint pains.

Severe acute hepatitis may result in liver failure, causing mental confusion, seizures, and sometimes coma (p.522). Liver failure is relatively common following an overdose with the painkiller paracetamol but is less common with some types of hepatitis, such as those due to the hepatitis A virus.

How is it diagnosed?

If your doctor suspects that you have hepatitis, he or she may arrange for you to have blood tests to evaluate your liver function and to look for possible causes of your symptoms. Blood tests will probably be repeated in order to help monitor your recovery. If the diagnosis is unclear, you may undergo ultrasound scanning (p.250) and may need to have a liver biopsy (p.647), in which a small piece of liver is removed and examined under a microscope.

What is the treatment?

There is no specific treatment for most cases of acute hepatitis, and people are usually advised to rest. Consult your doctor before taking any medicines, such as painkillers, because there is a risk of side effects. If you have viral hepatitis, you will need to take precautions to prevent the spread of the disease, including practising safe sex (p.68).

You should avoid drinking alcohol during the illness and for a minimum of 3 months after you have recovered. However, if the cause was alcohol-related, you will be advised to give up drinking alcohol permanently.

What is the prognosis?

Most people with acute hepatitis feel better after 4–6 weeks and recover by 3 months. However, for some people with hepatitis C, recovery is followed by a series of relapses over the course of several months. About 3 in 4 people with hepatitis C and 1 in 20 with hepatitis B and D develop chronic hepatitis. People with acute hepatitis caused by an infection other than the hepatitis viruses usually recover completely once the infection has cleared up. Recovery from acute hepatitis that has been caused by excessive alcohol consumption, drugs, or other toxins depends on the extent of the resulting damage to the liver. The substance that caused acute hepatitis must be avoided in the future.

In the rare cases in which hepatitis progresses to liver failure, a liver transplant (p.650) may be necessary.

Can it be prevented?

Infection with hepatitis A and E may be prevented by maintaining good personal hygiene. The risk of being infected with hepatitis B, C, and D can be reduced by practising safe sex and by not sharing needles or other objects that might be contaminated with body fluids infected with the virus. Infection with one of the hepatitis viruses provides future immunity against that virus but not against any of the other types of hepatitis virus.

Immunizations that protect people against the hepatitis A and B viruses are given to those at particular risk of contracting the infection, such as travellers (*see* TRAVEL IMMUNIZATIONS, p.86).

In order to avoid the transmission of hepatitis through blood transfusions, blood banks routinely screen all blood for the presence of the hepatitis B and hepatitis C viruses.

(WWW) ONLINE SITES: p.1033, p.1034

Chronic hepatitis

Inflammation of the liver, due to a variety of causes, that lasts more than 6 months

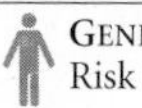
GENDER GENETICS LIFESTYLE Risk factors depend on the cause

AGE Not a significant factor

Chronic hepatitis is inflammation of the liver that lasts for at least 6 months. Sometimes, the condition persists for many years. Although chronic hepatitis is often mild with no symptoms, it can slowly damage the liver, causing cirrhosis (p.647), in which healthy liver tissue is replaced by fibrous scar tissue. Eventually, liver failure (p.650) may develop. People who are affected with chronic hepatitis and cirrhosis have a higher than normal risk of developing liver cancer (p.649).

What are the causes?

Chronic hepatitis can have a number of causes, including a viral infection, an autoimmune reaction in which the body's immune system attacks liver cells, certain drugs, alcohol abuse, and some metabolic disorders.

Some of the hepatitis viruses that cause acute hepatitis (opposite page) are more likely than others to cause persistent inflammation. The virus that most commonly causes chronic inflammation is the hepatitis C virus. Less commonly, the hepatitis B and D viruses are responsible. Infections with the hepatitis A and E viruses never become chronic. Some people may be unaware that they have had a previous episode of acute viral hepatitis until long-term symptoms of chronic hepatitis appear.

The underlying cause of autoimmune chronic hepatitis is still not known, but the condition is more common among women than it is in men.

Some drugs, such as isoniazid (*see* ANTITUBERCULOUS DRUGS, p.886) may cause chronic hepatitis. The condition can also result from regular excessive alcohol consumption (*see* ALCOHOL-RELATED LIVER DISEASE, p.646).

In addition, chronic hepatitis can be due to rare metabolic diseases in which liver inflammation is caused by excess amounts of certain minerals that accumulate in the body. For example, in the inherited disorder haemochromatosis (p.692) there are abnormally high levels of iron in the blood and tissues.

What are the symptoms?

In some cases, chronic hepatitis causes no symptoms. If symptoms do develop, they are usually mild but can vary in severity. They may include:

- Loss of appetite and weight loss.
- Tiredness.
- Yellowing of the skin and whites of the eyes (*see* JAUNDICE, p.643).
- Swelling of the abdomen.
- Abdominal discomfort.

If cirrhosis develops due to persistent inflammation, there may be increased blood pressure in the blood vessels that connect the digestive tract to the liver. This pressure may lead to bleeding into the digestive tract (*see* PORTAL HYPERTENSION AND VARICES, p.648). In some cases, cirrhosis can result in liver failure, which may be fatal.

WHAT MIGHT BE DONE?

Your doctor will give you a physical examination and arrange for blood tests to evaluate your liver function and to look for causes of your symptoms. To confirm the diagnosis, he or she may use an imaging technique such as ultrasound scanning (p.250). A liver biopsy (opposite page), in which a small piece of liver is taken for microscopic examination, may be used to determine the nature and severity of liver damage.

Chronic hepatitis caused by infection with the hepatitis B or C viruses may respond to treatment with particular antiviral drugs (p.886), such as interferon alfa (*see* INTERFERON DRUGS, p.907). These drugs are usually taken as long-term courses to prevent hepatitis from recurring. They can cause significant side effects, and monitoring is needed.

People with chronic hepatitis caused by an autoimmune reaction are usually treated indefinitely with corticosteroids (p.930), which may be combined with immunosuppressant drugs (p.906). If the liver has been damaged by a drug, it should recover slowly as long as the drug is stopped. If chronic hepatitis is due to a metabolic disorder, treatment of that underlying disorder may slow the progress of liver damage.

WHAT IS THE PROGNOSIS?

The outlook depends on the cause of the hepatitis. Chronic viral hepatitis usually progresses slowly, and it may take years before problems such as cirrhosis and liver failure develop. People with chronic hepatitis are at increased risk of developing liver cancer, particularly if hepatitis is due to infection with the hepatitis B or C virus.

Without treatment, approximately 1 in 2 people who have autoimmune chronic hepatitis develop liver failure after 5 years. Hepatitis due to a metabolic disorder tends to get progressively worse, often ending in liver failure. In the case of liver failure, a liver transplant (p.650) may be considered.

(WWW) ONLINE SITES: p.1034

Alcohol-related liver disease

Short-term or progressive liver damage due to excessive alcohol consumption

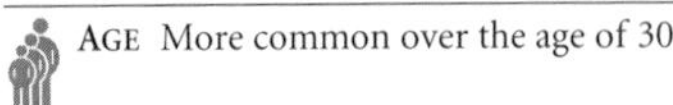
AGE More common over the age of 30

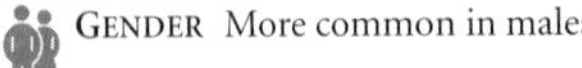
GENDER More common in males

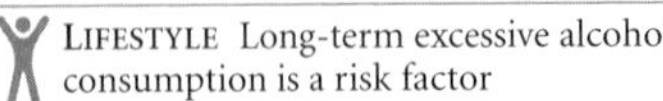
LIFESTYLE Long-term excessive alcohol consumption is a risk factor

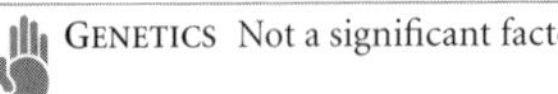
GENETICS Not a significant factor

The most common cause of severe long-term liver disease in developed countries is excessive alcohol consumption (*see* ALCOHOL AND HEALTH, p.62, and ALCOHOL DEPENDENCE, p.564). More men than women have alcohol-related liver disease because more men drink heavily. However, women are more susceptible to liver damage from alcohol because of differences in the way that men and women metabolize alcohol. For both men and women, regular excessive alcohol consumption is more likely to damage the liver than sporadic heavy drinking. The longer excessive alcohol consumption continues, the greater the likelihood of liver disease developing. Long-term alcohol-related liver disease is known to increase the risk of liver cancer (p.649).

WHAT ARE THE TYPES?

Alcohol may cause three types of liver disease: fatty liver, alcoholic hepatitis, and cirrhosis (opposite page). Typically, these conditions occur in sequence, but this is not always the case. Over a period of several years, most heavy drinkers develop a fatty liver, in which fat globules develop within liver cells. If alcohol consumption continues, hepatitis (inflammation of the liver) develops. With continued drinking, cirrhosis develops. In this condition, liver cells that are damaged by alcohol are replaced by fibrous scar tissue. If cirrhosis has developed, liver damage is irreversible. It is not known why some heavy drinkers go on to develop hepatitis or cirrhosis while others do not.

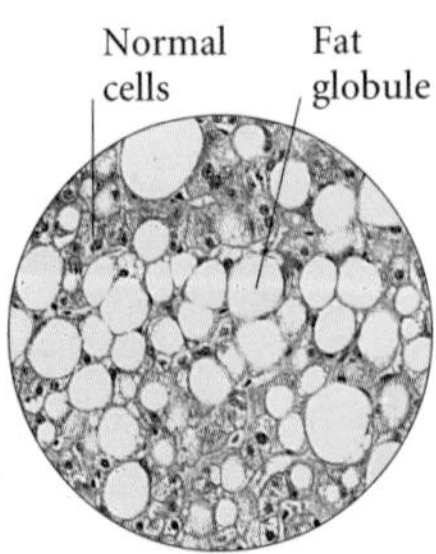

Fatty liver *Excessive alcohol consumption can damage the liver, causing fat globules to form in liver cells, as seen in this magnified view.*

WHAT ARE THE SYMPTOMS?

In many cases, fatty liver does not cause symptoms and often remains undiagnosed. However, in about 1 in 3 affected people, the liver becomes enlarged, which may lead to discomfort in the right upper abdomen.

Alcoholic hepatitis may also produce no symptoms at first, but after about 10 years of heavy drinking in men and sooner in women, the first symptoms usually develop. These may include:

- Nausea and occasional vomiting.
- Discomfort in the upper right side of the abdomen.
- Weight loss.
- Fever.
- Yellowing of the skin and the whites of the eyes (*see* JAUNDICE, p.643).
- Swollen abdomen.

Cirrhosis often causes no symptoms for a number of years or only mild symptoms, including:

- Poor appetite and weight loss.
- Nausea.
- Muscle wasting.

In some cases, severe cirrhosis may lead to a serious condition in which there is bleeding into the digestive tract from abnormal blood vessels that develop in the wall of the oesophagus (*see* PORTAL HYPERTENSION AND VARICES, p.648). Severe alcoholic hepatitis and cirrhosis can lead to liver failure (p.650), which may result in coma (p.522) and death.

HOW IS IT DIAGNOSED?

A history of heavy alcohol consumption is essential for the diagnosis of alcohol-related liver disease. It is important that you are honest and tell your doctor exactly how much you drink. However, many people who drink heavily are reluctant to do this.

Your doctor may arrange for blood tests to evaluate your liver function. You may also have a liver biopsy (opposite page), a procedure in which a hollow needle is inserted into the liver to obtain a sample of liver tissue. The sample is then examined under a microscope to look for cell abnormalities.

TEST LIVER BIOPSY

In a liver biopsy, a sample of tissue is removed from the liver to diagnose a variety of disorders, including cirrhosis, hepatitis, and cancer. This procedure is performed in hospital under local anaesthesia and the sample is sent to a laboratory for microscopic examination. You will need to remain in bed for up to 6 hours afterwards, lying on your right side at first to prevent bleeding. The biopsy site may be tender for a few days.

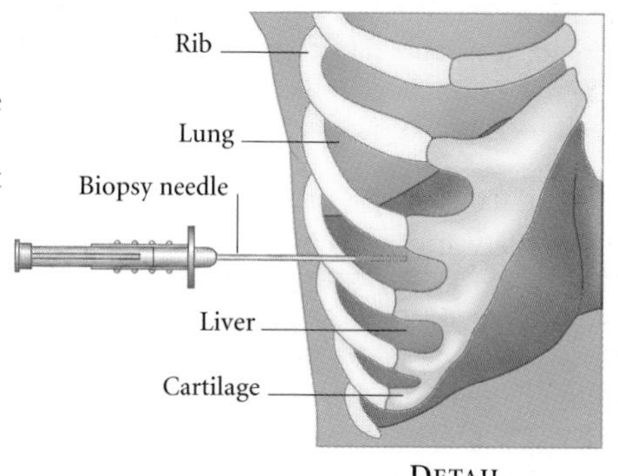

DETAIL

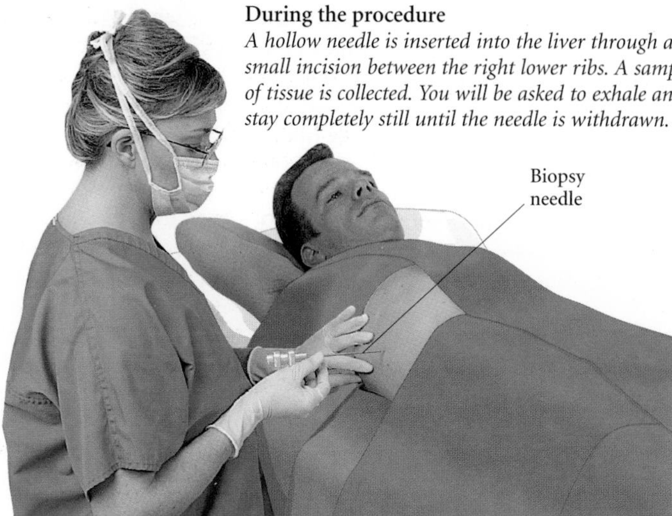

During the procedure
A hollow needle is inserted into the liver through a small incision between the right lower ribs. A sample of tissue is collected. You will be asked to exhale and stay completely still until the needle is withdrawn.

RESULTS

Cirrhosis
This magnified view of a sample of liver tissue shows normal liver cells surrounded by bands of fibrous scar tissue. Such an appearance is typical of the damage caused by cirrhosis.

Normal cells
Fibrous tissue

WHAT IS THE TREATMENT?

People with alcohol-related liver disease must stop drinking permanently. Many people need professional help to achieve this. If drinking continues, the disease will probably progress and may be fatal. If drinking stops, the outlook is likely to improve.

Fatty liver often disappears after 3–6 months of abstinence from alcohol. Some people with alcoholic hepatitis who stop drinking recover completely. However, in most cases damage to the liver is irreversible, and the condition progresses to cirrhosis. Severe alcoholic cirrhosis can cause a number of serious complications, which in some cases may be fatal. About half of all people who have cirrhosis die from liver failure within 5 years. More than 1 in 10 people who have cirrhosis go on to develop liver cancer. People who have alcohol-related liver disease but have no other serious health problems and have managed to stop drinking may be candidates for a liver transplant (p.650).

Many of the symptoms and some of the complications of alcohol-related liver disease can be treated successfully. For example, swelling of the abdomen as a result of fluid accumulating in the abdominal cavity can be reduced by diuretic drugs (p.902) and by following a diet that is low in salt. Nausea and vomiting can frequently be relieved by antiemetic drugs (p.922).

WWW ONLINE SITES: p.1026, p.1034

Cirrhosis

Irreversible scarring of the liver, occurring in the late stages of various liver disorders

 AGE More common over the age of 40

 GENDER More common in males

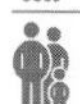 GENETICS In some cases, the underlying cause is inherited

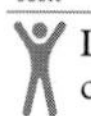 LIFESTYLE Long-term excessive alcohol consumption is a risk factor

In cirrhosis, normal liver tissue is destroyed and replaced by fibrous scar tissue. The condition may be caused by several different disorders, including viral infections and excessive alcohol consumption. The liver damage is irreversible and prevents the liver from functioning properly. Some people with cirrhosis may feel well for years despite having severe liver damage. However, with time they may develop complications, such as liver failure (p.650) and liver cancer (p.649).

In developed countries, cirrhosis is the third most common cause of death in people aged between 45 and 65, after coronary artery disease and cancer. Cirrhosis is much more common in men than in women in the UK and accounts for about 3,000 deaths a year.

WHAT ARE THE CAUSES?

There are various causes of cirrhosis. Worldwide, the most common cause is infection with a hepatitis virus, particularly the hepatitis B and C viruses (*see* CHRONIC HEPATITIS, p.645). However, in developed countries, cirrhosis is most frequently caused by excessive alcohol consumption (*see* ALCOHOL-RELATED LIVER DISEASE, opposite page). Another cause is the autoimmune disorder primary biliary cirrhosis, which is more common in women than in men. Bile, a liquid produced by the liver to aid digestion, normally leaves the liver through the bile ducts. In primary biliary cirrhosis, the bile ducts become inflamed, blocking the flow of bile from the liver.

This causes bile to build up, damaging the liver tissue. Cirrhosis may also be caused by sclerosing cholangitis, a condition in which the bile ducts inside the liver become inflamed. The cause of this condition is not known, although it can be associated with some inflammatory bowel diseases, such as ulcerative colitis (p.659) and Crohn's disease (p.658). Cirrhosis may also develop after bile duct surgery or as a result of a blockage of the bile ducts by gallstones (p.651). In addition, certain inherited disorders, such as haemochromatosis (p.692), may cause cirrhosis to develop.

What are the symptoms?

Often, cirrhosis produces no symptoms and is detected during a routine examination for another condition. If there are symptoms, they may include:

- Poor appetite and weight loss.
- Nausea.
- Yellowing of the skin and the whites of the eyes (*see* Jaundice, p.643).

After some time, life-threatening complications may develop. For example, cirrhosis can lead to high blood pressure in veins in the oesophagus, which causes them to be fragile and to bleed easily (*see* Portal hypertension and varices, right). Malnutrition may also develop from being unable to absorb fats and certain vitamins. Eventually, cirrhosis can lead to liver cancer or liver failure. The symptoms of liver failure include a swollen, fluid-filled abdomen and visible spider-like blood vessels in the skin, known as spider naevi. A failing liver may also result in abnormal bleeding and easy bruising. This is as a result of reduced production of blood clotting factors in the liver.

What might be done?

If your doctor suspects that you have cirrhosis from your symptoms, he or she will take blood samples to assess liver function and look for hepatitis viruses. You may also have ultrasound scanning (p.250), CT scanning (p.247), or MRI (p.248) to assess the liver. To confirm the diagnosis, you may have a liver biopsy (p.647), in which a small sample of tissue is removed from your liver for microscopic examination.

Damage to the liver caused by cirrhosis is always irreversible. However, if the underlying cause can be treated, further deterioration may be prevented. Whatever the cause of the cirrhosis, you should not drink alcohol. Nutritional deficiencies can be corrected by taking supplements and altering your diet. If the condition worsens but you are otherwise in good health, you may be suitable for a liver transplant (p.650).

What is the prognosis?

The outlook for cirrhosis is extremely variable and depends on the degree of liver damage, whether complications have developed, and whether further damage can be prevented. If the condition is mild, people may live for many years. About 7 in 10 people survive for more than a year after a liver transplant.

(WWW) ONLINE SITES: p.1026, p.1034

Portal hypertension and varices

Elevated pressure in the vein carrying blood to the liver, leading to distended veins, particularly in the oesophagus

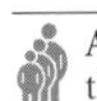 Age More common in adults, especially those over the age of 40

 Gender More common in males

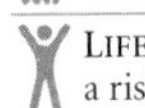 Lifestyle Excessive alcohol consumption is a risk factor

 Genetics Not a significant factor

In a liver damaged by disease, normal blood flow may become blocked. This obstruction leads to portal hypertension, in which the pressure is increased inside the portal vein, a large vein that carries blood from the digestive tract to the liver. The high pressure forces blood through other smaller veins in the digestive tract. These veins become distended and fragile (like varicose veins in the legs), and are known as varices.

In most cases, varices develop at the lower end of the oesophagus. They are prone to rupture, and heavy bleeding from them can be life-threatening. In some cases, varices develop in other areas of the body, such as in the skin over the abdomen and in the rectum.

Portal hypertension occurs mainly in adults and is more common in men. The condition is often associated with excessive consumption of alcohol (*see* Alcohol and health, p.62).

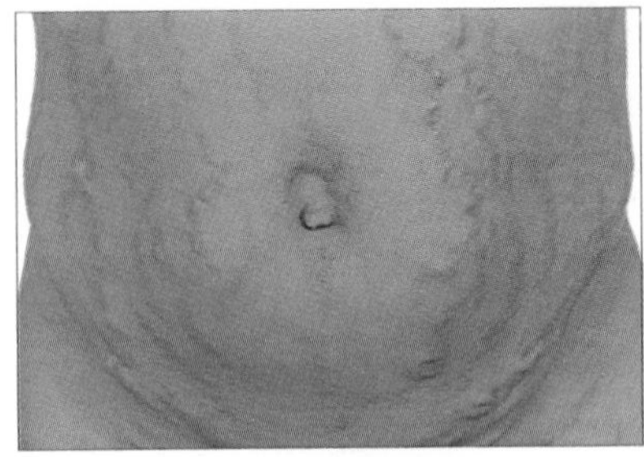

Effect of portal hypertension
Increased pressure in the portal vein, which carries blood from the digestive tract to the liver, can cause distended veins in the skin over the abdomen, as shown here.

What are the causes?

In Western countries, about 8 in 10 cases of portal hypertension are associated with cirrhosis (p.647), which is often due to chronic hepatitis (p.645) or long-term alcohol abuse (*see* Alcohol-related liver disease, p.646). A blood clot blocking the portal vein, schistosomiasis (p.312), and in rare cases congenital liver disorders may also cause portal hypertension.

What are the symptoms?

Portal hypertension is usually undetected until complications develop. If symptoms develop, they may include:

- Swollen abdomen due to accumulation of fluid.
- Visible swelling of the veins in the skin over the abdomen, sometimes around the navel.

In about 1 in 3 people with varices in the oesophagus, the veins eventually rupture. The bleeding is usually sudden and massive and leads to vomiting of blood and later passage of black, tarry faeces that contain partly digested blood (*see* Bleeding from the digestive tract, p.630). Loss of large volumes of blood can result in shock (p.414). If not treated immediately, shock may cause damage to internal organs and lead to disorders such as acute kidney failure (p.706) and liver failure (p.650).

What might be done?

Your doctor will check for signs of portal hypertension if you have chronic hepatitis. Ultrasound scanning (p.250) or CT scanning (p.247) may be done to detect enlarged veins, or endoscopy may be used to visualize them (*see* Upper digestive tract endoscopy, p.641).

Usually, once portal hypertension has developed, liver damage is irreversible. However, beta-blocker drugs (p.898) may be prescribed to lower pressure in the portal vein and decrease the risk of bleeding from varices.

Ruptured varices require urgent treatment in hospital with intravenous fluids and a blood transfusion (p.447) to replace lost blood. The source of internal bleeding will be investigated using endoscopy. If possible, the varices will be injected through the endoscope with a chemical that causes the blood vessel to close and therefore stops bleeding. The drug vasopressin may also be given to help to reduce bleeding.

If these measures do not stop the bleeding, a tube encircled by a deflated balloon may be passed through the mouth into the oesophagus. The balloon is inflated to compress the varices and is left in place until bleeding stops. In some cases, a procedure is carried out to allow blood from the digestive tract to bypass the liver. This may involve using X-rays to view and direct the insertion of a tube that connects the portal vein directly to the hepatic vein, through which blood normally leaves the liver.

WHAT IS THE PROGNOSIS?

The outlook depends on whether or not varices develop and bleed and also on the severity of bleeding. About 7 in 10 people survive ruptured varices, but in over half of them bleeding will recur.

(WWW) ONLINE SITES: p.1026, p.1034

Liver cancer

A cancerous tumour that originates in the cells of the liver

AGE More common with increasing age

GENDER Up to four times more common in males

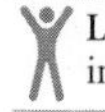
LIFESTYLE Excess alcohol consumption and intravenous drug abuse are risk factors

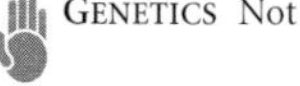
GENETICS Not a significant factor

Worldwide, liver cancer is one of the most common forms of cancer, with over 500,000 cases in 1997. However, in developed countries, the disease is less common, and most cases occur following long-standing cirrhosis (p.647) due to long-term alcohol abuse. In developing countries, liver cancer is closely linked with viral hepatitis, especially that due to the hepatitis B and C viruses (*see* CHRONIC HEPATITIS, p.645), which account for about 7 in 10 cases of liver cancer. People with haemochromatosis (p.692), a condition in which excess iron builds up in the liver, are also at high risk of developing liver cancer.

Another cause of liver cancer is contamination of food by carcinogens (cancer-causing agents) such as aflatoxin, a toxin produced by a fungus that grows on stored grain and peanuts. Occasionally, liver cancer results from infection with a form of liver fluke (a parasitic worm) that is common in the Far East or exposure to certain chemicals in the workplace.

WHAT ARE THE SYMPTOMS?

People with liver cancer may experience the following symptoms:

- Weight loss and fever.
- Pain in the upper right side of the abdomen.
- Yellowing of the skin and the whites of the eyes (*see* JAUNDICE, p.643).

As the disease progresses, the abdomen may become swollen because of an accumulation of fluid.

WHAT MIGHT BE DONE?

Your doctor may suspect liver cancer from your symptoms if you already have cirrhosis. You may have blood tests to look for signs of cancer and to assess liver function. Imaging tests, such as ultrasound scanning (p.250) or MRI (p.248), may be performed to confirm the diagnosis. You may also have a liver biopsy (p.647), in which a piece of tissue is removed and tested for cancer cells.

Surgery offers the only chance of a cure. A liver transplant (p.650) may be considered but is rarely done because in many cases the cancer is likely to recur. More commonly, the aim is to slow the progress of the disease with treatments that include chemotherapy (p.280) and blocking the blood supply to the tumour, causing it to shrink.

WHAT IS THE PROGNOSIS?

The outlook for people who have liver cancer is poor. Many people do not respond to treatment and survive less than a year after diagnosis.

(WWW) ONLINE SITES: p.1026, p.1028, p.1034

Liver metastases

Cancerous tumours in the liver that have spread from other parts of the body

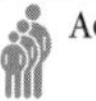
AGE More common with increasing age

GENDER GENETICS LIFESTYLE Not significant factors

Metastases are cancerous tumours in the liver that originate from cancers elsewhere in the body, commonly those of the lung, breast, colon, pancreas, and stomach. Other types of cancer, such as leukaemia (p.453) and lymphoma (p.459), may also spread to the liver. Liver metastases form when cancerous cells separate from the original cancer, circulate in the blood, and settle in the liver, where they multiply. Several metastases of varying size may develop.

In developed countries, liver metastases occur more commonly than liver cancer (left). The disease is more common in elderly people.

WHAT ARE THE SYMPTOMS?

People may already have symptoms due to the original cancer, but sometimes this cancer is not apparent. The symptoms of liver metastases may be the only warning of illness. They include:

- Weight loss.
- Reduced appetite.
- Fever.
- Pain in the upper right side of the abdomen.
- Yellowing of the skin and the whites of the eyes (*see* JAUNDICE, p.643).

As the disease progresses, the abdomen may become swollen due to enlargement of the liver or fluid accumulation.

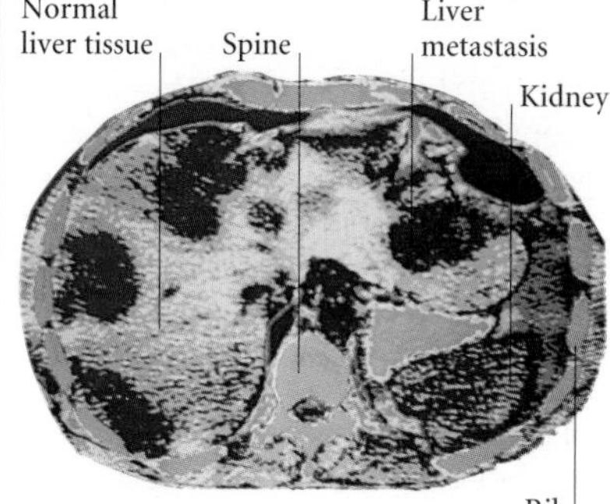

Liver metastases
The dark areas in the liver shown in this CT scan are metastases, which are cancerous tumours that have spread from a cancer elsewhere in the body.

WHAT MIGHT BE DONE?

Anyone who has cancer will have tests, such as ultrasound scanning (p.250), CT scanning (p.247), or MRI (p.248), to find out if the liver is affected. To confirm the diagnosis, a piece of liver tissue may be removed for microscopic examination (*see* LIVER BIOPSY, p.647). Most treatment aims to maintain liver function and relieve symptoms. You may be offered painkillers (p.912) for pain and chemotherapy (p.280) or radiotherapy (p.281) to reduce the size of the metastases. Surgery may be considered if there is a solitary metastasis.

WHAT IS THE PROGNOSIS?

The outlook is poor for most people with liver metastases because by this stage the cancer is usually advanced. Few people survive longer than a year.

(WWW) ONLINE SITES: p.1028, p.1034

(TREATMENT) LIVER TRANSPLANT

This procedure involves the transfer of a healthy liver, usually from a recently deceased donor, into a person with liver disease. Sometimes, part of a liver is donated by a living relative. The donor and recipient must have the same blood type. After the transplant, the recipient is monitored in an intensive care unit for a few days and remains in hospital for up to 4 weeks. Transplants are successful in 9 out of 10 children and 7 out of 10 adults. If the new liver fails, further transplants may be possible.

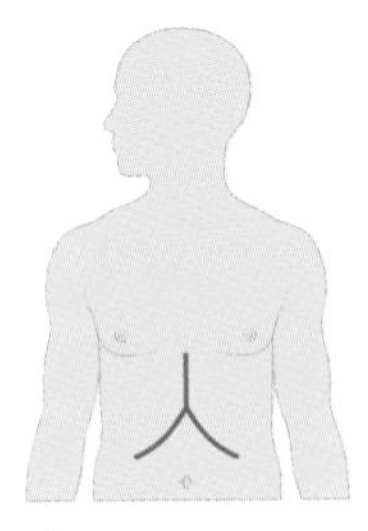

SITE OF INCISION

Transplanted gallbladder
Transplanted liver
Recipient's aorta
Bile duct
Donor's blood vessels
Recipient's blood vessels

The procedure
The liver, gallbladder, and portions of the connected blood and bile vessels are removed. The donor organs and vessels are connected to the recipient's vessels.

Liver failure

Severe impairment of liver function, occurring either suddenly or at the final stages of chronic liver disease

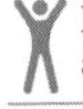 LIFESTYLE Excessive alcohol consumption is a risk factor

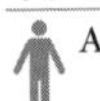 AGE Risk factors depend on the cause

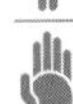 GENDER GENETICS Not significant factors

The liver performs many vital functions, such as the breakdown of toxins in the blood. Liver failure allows toxin levels to rise, affecting the brain and other organs. In acute liver failure, the liver may fail suddenly. In chronic liver failure, it may fail over months or years.

Acute liver failure may be due to a disorder such as acute viral hepatitis (*see* ACUTE HEPATITIS, p.644) or damage from drugs, such as an overdose of paracetamol. Chronic liver failure is usually due to an underlying disorder such as alcohol-related liver disease (p.646) or chronic hepatitis (p.645).

WHAT ARE THE SYMPTOMS?

The symptoms of acute liver failure can develop over several hours or days and are caused by the effect of toxins on the brain. They may include:

- Poor memory.
- Confusion and agitation.
- Drowsiness.

As acute liver failure progresses, other major organs, including the kidneys and the lungs, may gradually begin to fail. The condition may eventually lead to coma (p.522) and death.

Chronic liver failure may produce no symptoms for several months or even years. When the symptoms do begin to appear, they usually develop gradually and may include:

- Yellowing of the skin and whites of the eyes (*see* JAUNDICE, p.643).
- Itching.
- Easy bruising and bleeding.
- Swollen abdomen.
- Abnormally shaped fingernails.
- Numerous small, spider-like blood vessels in the skin, called spider naevi.
- Redness of the palms of the hands.

Spider naevi
In people with liver failure, numerous spider-like blood vessels known as spider naevi may appear on the skin, particularly in the chest area.

- Thickened tissue in the palms of the hands (*see* DUPUYTREN'S CONTRACTURE, p.390).
- In men, enlargement of the breasts and shrunken testes.

Bleeding into the digestive tract may occur from enlarged blood vessels that form in the wall of the oesophagus (*see* PORTAL HYPERTENSION AND VARICES, p.648). Sometimes, chronic liver failure deteriorates suddenly and causes the symptoms of acute liver failure.

WHAT MIGHT BE DONE?

Acute liver failure or chronic liver failure that has deteriorated suddenly requires immediate hospital care, often in an intensive care unit (p.958). Antibiotics (p.885) may be given to reduce the numbers of intestinal bacteria. These bacteria produce toxins that accumulate in the blood and adversely affect the brain and other organs.

If you have chronic liver failure, your doctor will arrange for blood tests to determine the extent of damage to the liver. You may need to follow a diet that is low in protein to reduce the work of the liver. Your doctor may also advise you to reduce the salt in your diet and may prescribe diuretic drugs (p.902) to reduce swelling of the abdomen. You should stop drinking alcohol immediately and permanently. There is no treatment that can repair the damage that has already occurred to the liver.

What is the prognosis?

Most people who have severe liver failure need a liver transplant (opposite page) to survive. Fewer than 1 in 10 people survive acute liver failure without having a transplant. In those who do survive, the liver often recovers completely, provided that it was previously undamaged. In chronic liver failure, the outlook depends to a large extent on the underlying cause. Many people with chronic liver failure lead normal lives for many years.

(WWW) ONLINE SITES: p.1026, p.1034

Gallstones

Stones of various sizes and content that form in the gallbladder

AGE More common over the age of 40; rare in childhood

GENDER Twice as common in females

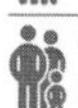
GENETICS Sometimes run in families; more common in people of Asian and white European origin

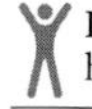
LIFESTYLE Being overweight and eating a high-fat diet are risk factors

Gallstones occur in about 1 in 10 people over the age of 40, with twice as many women as men being affected. The stones usually occur in the gallbladder, and, in most cases, do not cause symptoms. Gallstones are formed from bile, a liquid that aids digestion and is produced by the liver and then stored in the gallbladder. Bile is made up mainly of the fatty substance cholesterol, pigments, and various salts. A change in the composition of bile may trigger stone formation. Most gallstones are a mixture of cholesterol and pigments. In about 1 in 5 cases, stones consist of cholesterol only, and in about 1 in 20 cases, stones consist of pigment only. Often, there are many stones, and some can reach the size of a golf ball. Gallstones may run in families, and they are more common in people of Asian and white European origin, for reasons that are unclear.

What are the causes?

There is often no obvious cause for gallstones. However, cholesterol stones are more common in people who are very overweight (*see* OBESITY, p.631) and the risk of stones forming may also be greater than normal in people who have a high-fat diet.

Pigment stones may form if there is excessive destruction of red blood cells, as in the disorders haemolytic anaemia (p.450) and sickle-cell disease (p.448). Insufficient emptying of the gallbladder caused by narrowed bile ducts may also increase the risk of gallstones.

What are the symptoms?

Gallstones often cause no symptoms. However, symptoms may occur if one or more stones block the cystic duct (the exit tube from the gallbladder) or the common bile duct (the main bile duct from the liver to the duodenum). A stone that partially or completely blocks the flow of bile will cause attacks known as biliary colic, which cause symptoms that may include:

- Mild to severe upper abdominal pain.
- Nausea and vomiting.

Episodes are normally brief and typically occur following a fatty meal, which causes the gallbladder to contract.

Are there complications?

Stones that remain lodged in the bile ducts block the drainage of bile. This can cause severe inflammation or infection of the gallbladder (*see* CHOLECYSTITIS, p.652) and bile ducts. Blocked bile ducts may also cause jaundice (p.643), in which the skin and whites of the eyes become yellow. In addition to jaundice, blockage of the common bile duct may cause inflammation of the pancreas (*see* ACUTE PANCREATITIS, p.652).

Gallstones
A gallbladder full of gallstones is visible in this colour-enhanced X-ray. In some people, gallstones are detected only when an X-ray is taken for another purpose.

How are they diagnosed?

Most people only become aware that they have gallstones by chance when an unrelated condition is being investigated. However, if your doctor suspects from your symptoms that you have gallstones, you may have blood tests to check your red blood cell count and cholesterol levels (*see* BLOOD CHOLESTEROL TESTS, p.231). You may also have imaging tests, such as ultrasound scanning (p.250). If a bile duct is found to be blocked, the exact position of the gallstones may be located using a specialized imaging procedure called ERCP (p.653), in which an endoscope is used to inject a specialized dye into the bile ducts prior to X-rays being taken.

What is the treatment?

Gallstones that do not cause symptoms need no treatment. If you have mild or infrequent symptoms, adopting a diet that is low in fat may prevent further discomfort. However, if your symptoms are persistent or become worse, you may have your gallbladder removed by conventional surgery or by minimal access surgery (*see* HAVING MINIMALLY INVASIVE SURGERY, p.949). Removal of the gallbladder usually cures the problem. However, in very rare cases, the stones re-form in the bile duct and may need to be removed by open surgery or during ERCP. The absence of a gallbladder does not usually cause any health problems, and the bile simply drains continuously through a duct directly into the intestines.

Drugs are available that dissolve gallstones made of pure cholesterol, but it may take months or years for the stones to dissolve completely. Occasionally, you may be treated with ultrasonic shock waves (*see* LITHOTRIPSY, p.702), which shatter the stones into tiny pieces so that they pass painlessly into the small intestine and are excreted in the faeces. Use of drugs or ultrasonic shock waves avoids the need for surgery. However, because the gallbladder is still present there is an ongoing risk that further gallstones will form.

(WWW) ONLINE SITES: p.1030, p.1035

Cholecystitis

Inflammation of the gallbladder, usually associated with gallstones blocking the flow of the digestive fluid bile

AGE More common over the age of 40; rare in childhood

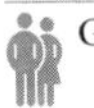
GENDER Twice as common in females

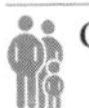
GENETICS Sometimes runs in families

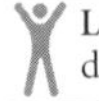
LIFESTYLE Being overweight and a high-fat diet are risk factors

Cholecystitis is inflammation of the gallbladder wall. It usually occurs when the outlet from the gallbladder, through which the digestive liquid bile is normally released, becomes blocked by a gallstone (p.651). Bile becomes trapped in the gallbladder, causing inflammation of its walls. A bacterial infection may then develop in the stagnant bile. In rare cases, cholecystitis occurs when there are no gallstones present.

Anyone with gallstones is at risk of developing cholecystitis. Gallstones are more common in people over 40 and in women and sometimes run in families. Gallstones are associated with obesity (p.631), a high-fat diet, and blood disorders, such as sickle-cell disease (p.448).

What are the symptoms?

The symptoms of cholecystitis can vary in severity. They usually develop over a period of hours and may include:

- Constant pain in the right side of the abdomen, just below the ribcage.
- Pain in the right shoulder.
- Nausea and vomiting.
- Fever and chills.

Sometimes, jaundice (p.643), causing yellowing of the skin and the whites of the eyes, may develop. Symptoms often improve over a few days and disappear after about a week. However, in some cases symptoms become progressively worse and need urgent treatment.

Rarely, bacterial infection may cause the gallbladder to perforate. This allows irritant bile to leak into the abdomen, resulting in peritonitis (p.665), a serious condition in which the peritoneum (the membrane lining the wall of the abdomen) becomes inflamed. Cholecystitis may also be accompanied by acute pancreatitis (right), in which there is sudden inflammation of the pancreas.

What might be done?

Your doctor may suspect cholecystitis from your symptoms and after a physical examination. If so, he or she may arrange for you to have ultrasound scanning (p.250) or ERCP (opposite page) to confirm the diagnosis and to indicate the position of any gallstones.

What is the treatment?

If your symptoms are mild, you may be treated at home with antibiotics (p.885) and painkillers (p.912). If your symptoms are severe, you will need treatment in hospital with intravenous fluids, painkillers, and antibiotics. You may have a tube passed into your nose and down to your stomach to remove the contents by suction. This procedure stops digestive juices from entering the duodenum, which would cause the gallbladder to contract.

Although cholecystitis often subsides after treatment with antibiotics, surgery to remove the gallbladder is usually recommended to prevent the condition from recurring. Surgery is always necessary if complications arise, such as perforation of the gallbladder.

What is the prognosis?

Removal of the gallbladder, at the time cholecystitis occurs or some weeks later, prevents recurrences of the disorder. Absence of the gallbladder has no long-term ill effects on the digestive system.

(WWW) ONLINE SITES: p.1034, p.1035

Acute pancreatitis

Sudden inflammation of the pancreas due to damage from its own enzymes

AGE Almost exclusively affects adults

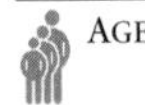
LIFESTYLE Excessive alcohol consumption is a risk factor

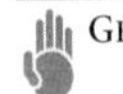
GENDER GENETICS Not significant factors

In acute pancreatitis, the pancreas suddenly becomes inflamed, causing severe abdominal pain. The condition is serious and can be life-threatening if left untreated. The main function of the pancreas is to secrete a fluid containing enzymes that aid digestion. In addition, the pancreas secretes the hormones insulin and glucagon, which control the level of sugar in the blood.

What are the causes?

Often, the cause of acute pancreatitis is unclear. If there is a cause, it may be a gallstone (p.651) blocking the common bile duct (the duct that transports bile from the liver to the duodenum). The gallstone obstructs the flow of digestive juices from the pancreas so that enzymes in these juices leak into the pancreatic tissue and cause severe inflammation.

Excessive alcohol consumption over a long period can also cause the disorder. However, it is not fully understood how alcohol causes inflammation of the pancreas. Typically, an attack of acute pancreatitis occurs 12–24 hours after a heavy bout of drinking.

Certain drugs such as immunosuppressants (p.906) and thiazide diuretics (p.902) can cause pancreatitis. Less common causes include viral infection of the pancreas and high levels of fatty substances in the blood (*see* INHERITED HYPERLIPIDAEMIAS, p.692).

What are the symptoms?

Acute pancreatitis causes a range of symptoms that occur suddenly and may be severe. These symptoms may include:

- Severe upper abdominal pain, often spreading to the back and made worse by movement.
- Nausea and vomiting.
- Bruised appearance of the skin around the abdomen.
- Fever.

In severe cases, inflammation affects the whole abdomen, making it rigid and increasing the pain (*see* PERITONITIS, p.665). There is also a risk of shock (p.414), a potentially fatal condition in which blood pressure falls extremely low.

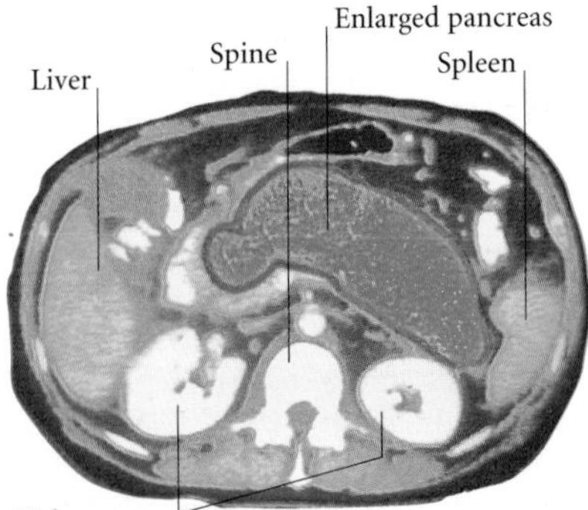

Acute pancreatitis
The enlarged pancreas seen in this CT scan through the abdomen is due to the inflammatory disorder acute pancreatitis.

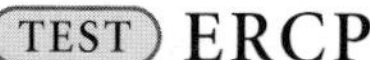

ERCP

Endoscopic retrograde cholangiopancreatography (ERCP) is a procedure used to look for blockages or other abnormalities in the bile ducts and pancreatic duct. Contrast dye is injected into the ducts using an endoscope passed through the mouth into the duodenum. The doctor's view down the endoscope can also be seen on a monitor. The flow of the dye is followed on X-ray images shown on a second monitor. ERCP is done in hospital under sedation and takes up to 1 hour.

Endoscope
Site of injection
X-ray machine
X-ray beam
X-ray monitor
ERCP monitor

During the procedure
The endoscope is passed painlessly down the throat into the duodenum, and dye is injected into the ducts.

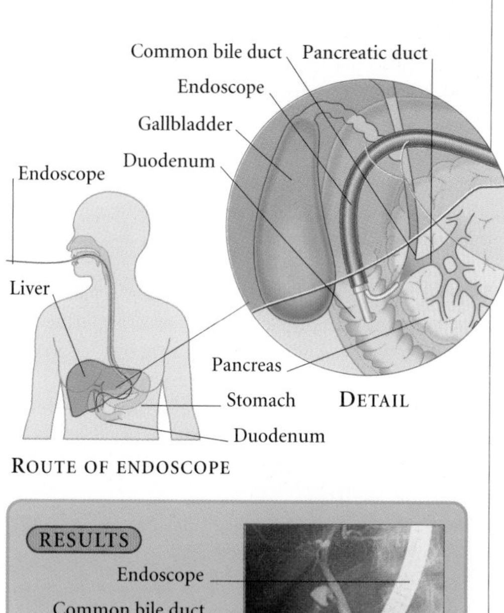

ROUTE OF ENDOSCOPE

RESULTS

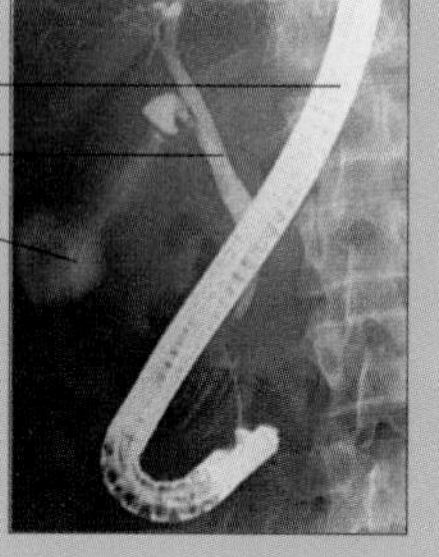

Contrast X-ray
The common bile duct and gallbladder, made visible by a dye injected through the endoscope, appear normal.

How is it diagnosed?

If your doctor suspects that you have acute pancreatitis, he or she may arrange for blood tests to detect pancreatic enzymes that have leaked directly into the blood. You may need imaging tests, such as CT scanning (p.247), ultrasound scanning (p.250), or MRI (p.248), to look for a blockage of the common bile duct by gallstones. The imaging tests may also reveal enlargement of the pancreas due to inflammation.

What is the treatment?

If you have acute pancreatitis, you will probably be admitted to hospital. If the condition is severe, you may need continuous monitoring in an intensive care unit (p.958). Your stomach will be kept empty to prevent the pancreas from being stimulated to produce more enzymes. A tube will be passed through your nose into your stomach to remove its contents by suction, and you will be given fluids intravenously. If imaging tests have detected a gallstone, ERCP (above) may be performed to locate the stone more precisely and remove it. In rare cases, damaged pancreatic tissue becomes infected and may need to be drained surgically. If the pancreatitis was caused by gallstones, it may be advisable to have your gallbladder removed once you have recovered.

What is the prognosis?

About 9 in 10 people survive an attack of acute pancreatitis, but the gland may be damaged so that it is unable to produce adequate amounts of enzymes. You may then need to take enzyme supplements. Severe damage to the hormone-secreting areas of the pancreas may affect the production of insulin and lead to diabetes mellitus (p.687). Treatment with insulin will then be necessary to control your blood sugar levels. A single attack of acute pancreatitis may not cause permanent damage, and long-term treatment is needed only if the condition recurs. If your gallbladder is removed because of stones, there should be no long-term ill effects.

WWW ONLINE SITES: p.1026, p.1030

Chronic pancreatitis

Long-term inflammation of the pancreas, leading to progressive loss of function

AGE Most common between the ages of 35 and 45

LIFESTYLE Excessive alcohol consumption is a risk factor

GENDER GENETICS Not significant factors

Chronic pancreatitis is a progressive disorder in which the pancreas is persistently inflamed. One of the functions of the pancreas is to secrete a fluid containing digestive enzymes that is added to the intestinal contents. The pancreas also forms the hormones insulin and glucagon, which are released into the bloodstream to control blood sugar levels. In chronic pancreatitis, normal pancreatic tissue becomes damaged and is replaced by scar tissue, gradually impairing pancreatic function. The condition is usually painful and may lead to complications. Damage to the pancreas is usually irreversible.

What are the causes?

Chronic pancreatitis most commonly results from long-term alcohol abuse. Less commonly, the condition may be caused by haemochromatosis (p.692), an inherited disorder in which excessive levels of iron accumulate in the tissues of organs such as the pancreas. In some cases, the cause of chronic pancreatitis is unclear.

What are the symptoms?

Symptoms usually develop over several years and vary in severity depending on the extent of damage to the pancreas. Most people do not experience symptoms during the early stages, but, as the disease progresses, they may develop symptoms such as:

- Persistent upper abdominal pain, often radiating to the back.
- Nausea and vomiting.
- Loss of appetite.

Complications result mainly from the reduced production of enzymes and hormones. A reduced level of pancreatic enzymes causes malabsorption (p.655), which may lead to greasy, bulky stools, vitamin deficiencies, and weight loss. Diabetes mellitus (p.687) may result if the production of insulin is reduced.

How is it diagnosed?

There is no simple test to diagnose chronic pancreatitis. Your doctor may arrange for X-rays (p.244), ultrasound scanning (p.250), or MRI (p.248) to look for calcium deposits in the pancreas, which are an indication that the pancreas has been inflamed. Other tests may include ERCP (p.653), in which a tube-like instrument called an endoscope is used to inject a contrast dye into the pancreatic duct to look for abnormalities. You may also have ultrasound scanning, which may be done through an endoscope, to look for gallstones. In addition, you may have blood tests to determine blood sugar levels.

What is the treatment?

Your doctor will probably advise you to avoid alcohol and fatty foods. You may need drugs to replace the hormones and enzymes that should be produced by the pancreas. Enzymes in tablet or powder form can be taken with each meal to aid digestion. Regular injections of insulin may also be necessary to control blood sugar levels and will probably be needed for life. If pain is severe, strong opiate painkillers (p.912) are given. In some cases, pain may be relieved by a nerve block. In this procedure, an injection is used to destroy the nerves that carry pain sensations from the pancreas to the spinal cord.

What is the prognosis?

The symptoms of chronic pancreatitis may recede over time, but in some cases the disorder worsens and symptoms become more severe. People who have chronic pancreatitis are more likely to develop pancreatic cancer (below).

(WWW) ONLINE SITES: p.1026

Pancreatic cancer

A cancerous tumour of the pancreas that may cause no symptoms in its early stages

 **Age** More common over the age of 50

 **Gender** Almost twice as common in males

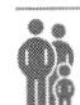 **Genetics** More common in black people

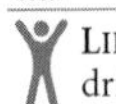 **Lifestyle** Smoking, a high-fat diet, and drinking alcohol to excess are risk factors

Pancreatic cancer is a relatively rare disorder; it is diagnosed in about 7,000 people each year in the UK. However, the disease, which mainly affects people over the age of 50, is becoming more common in the UK as life expectancy increases. Cancer of the pancreas occurs almost twice as frequently in men as in women and the disease is slightly more common in black people. This form of cancer is almost always fatal and is one of the 10 most common causes of death from cancer in the UK.

People with pancreatic cancer usually have few symptoms until the disorder reaches an advanced stage and often not until it has spread to other parts of the body, typically to the lymph nodes in the abdomen and the liver.

Little is known about the causes of pancreatic cancer, but it has been linked with diet, in particular with fatty foods and high alcohol consumption. A higher incidence of the cancer in certain ethnic groups indicates that genetic factors may be involved. The risk of the disease is greater in people who smoke and in those with chronic pancreatitis (p.653).

What are the symptoms?

Symptoms often develop gradually over a few months and may include:

- Pain in the upper abdomen that radiates to the back.
- Loss of weight.
- Reduced appetite.

Many pancreatic tumours cause obstruction of the bile ducts, through which the digestive liquid bile leaves the liver. Such blockage leads to jaundice (p.643), in which the skin and whites of the eyes turn yellow. Jaundice may be accompanied by itching, dark-coloured urine, and paler than normal faeces.

How is it diagnosed?

Imaging techniques, such as ultrasound scanning (p.250), CT scanning (p.247), or MRI (p.248), are normally used to diagnose pancreatic cancer. In addition, specialized imaging procedures such as ERCP (p.653) and ultrasound scanning through an endoscope may be used to look for abnormalities in the bile and pancreatic ducts. To confirm the diagnosis, a sample of pancreatic tissue may be taken for microscopic examination.

What is the treatment?

Surgery to remove part or all of the pancreas offers the only chance of cure. However, the cancer has usually spread by the time it is diagnosed. In such cases, surgery to relieve symptoms may be possible. For example, if the bile duct is obstructed by a tumour, a rigid tube known as a stent may be inserted to keep the duct open. This procedure is usually carried out during ERCP and helps to reduce jaundice. Treatment such as chemotherapy (p.280) and radiotherapy (p.281) may be used to slow the progress of the disease.

Pain can often be relieved with painkillers (p.912). If the pain is severe, it may be treated by a nerve block, a procedure using an injection of a chemical to inactivate the nerves supplying the pancreas.

What is the prognosis?

In many cases, pancreatic cancer is not diagnosed until it is far advanced, at which time the outlook is poor. Fewer than 1 in 50 people survive more than 5 years. Even with surgery, only 1 in 10 people survive more than 5 years. Most people survive for less than a year.

(WWW) ONLINE SITES: p.1028, p.1030

DISORDERS OF THE INTESTINES, RECTUM, AND ANUS

The intestines, rectum, and anus are exposed to infectious agents and toxins in food, and disorders resulting from these factors are common. Disorders may also be linked to diet, but in many other cases the cause is unknown. Many problems cause changes in the consistency of faeces and in the frequency of bowel movements.

The first article in this section covers irritable bowel syndrome, an extremely common disorder affecting about 2 in 10 people. Disorders that affect the body's ability to absorb nutrients from food, such as malabsorption and lactose intolerance are described next. Two subsequent articles deal with the inflammatory bowel disorders Crohn's disease and ulcerative colitis. Digestive disorders that can affect the movement of the intestinal contents, such as hernias, are then discussed. The section also covers appendicitis and colorectal cancer, a common cause of death due to cancer in the UK. Disorders of the rectum and anus are described last.

Articles on diarrhoea (p.627) and constipation (p.628) can be found in the section that deals with general digestive and nutritional problems. Intestinal infections (*see* INFECTIONS AND INFESTATIONS, pp.284–313) and intestinal disorders in children (*see* INFANCY AND CHILDHOOD, pp.862–865) are also covered elsewhere in the book.

KEY ANATOMY

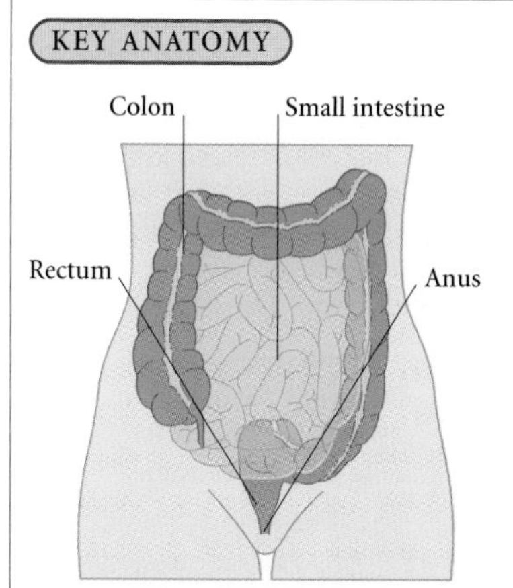

For further information on the structure and function of the intestines, rectum, and anus, *see* pp.620–625.

Irritable bowel syndrome

A combination of intermittent abdominal pain, constipation, and/or diarrhoea

 AGE Most commonly develops between the ages of 20 and 30

 GENDER Twice as common in females

 GENETICS Sometimes runs in families

 LIFESTYLE Stress and certain foods may make symptoms worse

Irritable bowel syndrome accounts for more referrals to gastroenterologists than any other disorder, although many affected people never consult a doctor. The condition most often develops in people between the ages of 20 and 30 and is twice as common in women as in men. As many as 2 in 10 people have symptoms of irritable bowel syndrome at some time in their lives. The symptoms, which include abdominal pain, constipation, and/or diarrhoea, tend to be intermittent but typically persist for many years. Although irritable bowel syndrome can be distressing, it does not lead to serious complications.

WHAT ARE THE CAUSES?

The precise cause of irritable bowel syndrome is unknown. It may result from abnormal contractions of the muscles in the intestinal walls. An increased sensitivity to certain foods, such as fruit, sorbitol (an artificial sweetener), and fat, may also contribute. The disorder sometimes develops after a gastrointestinal infection (*see* GASTROENTERITIS, p.628). The problem can run in families, which suggests that genetic factors are involved. Stress, anxiety, and depression are associated with the syndrome and can make symptoms worse.

WHAT ARE THE SYMPTOMS?

The symptoms are typically intermittent but usually recur for many years and often persist into old age. They vary widely among people and with each episode. The main symptoms include:

- Abdominal bloating combined with excessive quantities of wind.
- Abdominal pain, often on the lower left side, that may be relieved by defaecation or passing wind.
- Diarrhoea, which may be most severe on waking and sometimes alternates with bouts of constipation that may produce "rabbit pellet" stools.
- Feeling that the bowel has not been emptied completely.
- Passage of mucus during defaecation.
- Nausea and vomiting.
- Feeling of fullness and difficulty in finishing meals.

Many people have symptoms unrelated to the digestive tract, such as tiredness, headache, back pain, and an increased urge to pass urine. In women, sexual intercourse may be painful, and symptoms may be worse before menstrual periods.

You should consult your doctor if the symptoms are severe, persistent, or recurrent or if you have unexpectedly lost weight. If you are over 40 when the symptoms first develop, you should seek medical advice so that serious disorders with similar symptoms, such as colorectal cancer (p.665), can be ruled out.

HOW IS IT DIAGNOSED?

There is no single test to diagnose irritable bowel syndrome. Instead, your doctor will want to make sure that you have no other serious condition. The type and number of tests used to investigate the disorder depend on your age.

If your symptoms suggest that you may have an inflammatory bowel disorder such as Crohn's disease (p.658) or

SELF-HELP LIVING WITH IRRITABLE BOWEL SYNDROME

Some people learn to control the symptoms of irritable bowel syndrome by making dietary and lifestyle changes. The symptoms may improve if you follow a diet that is high in fibre and low in fat (*see* DIET AND HEALTH, p.48). You may need to try several different approaches before finding one that helps you. Try the following:

- Keep a food diary. Try to eliminate any food or drink that seems to bring on an attack of irritable bowel syndrome.
- Avoid large meals; spicy, fried, fatty foods; and milk products.
- If constipation is a problem, try gradually increasing your fibre intake. If bloating and diarrhoea are particular problems, reduce your fibre intake.
- Cut out or reduce your intake of tea, coffee, milk, cola, and beer.
- Eat at regular times.
- Stop smoking.
- Try relaxation exercises (p.75) to alleviate stress, which is often a contributing factor.

if you are over the age of 40, your doctor will probably want to investigate your symptoms further. You may have a blood test to check for inflammation, which can indicate the presence of Crohn's disease. If the result is positive or if your doctor suspects a colorectal tumour, you will probably have a contrast X-ray (p.245) of the intestines or undergo a colonoscopy (p.661). You may also have tests to exclude food intolerance (opposite page) and lactose intolerance (opposite page), which cause symptoms similar to those of irritable bowel syndrome.

WHAT IS THE TREATMENT?

Although the symptoms can be distressing, irritable bowel syndrome is not a serious condition. You should usually be able to control your symptoms with a combination of a change in diet and relaxation techniques (*see* LIVING WITH IRRITABLE BOWEL SYNDROME, above). However, if symptoms are troublesome enough to interfere with daily routines, you should consult your doctor for advice on treatment. You may be given antispasmodic drugs to relax the contractions of the digestive tract and help to relieve abdominal pain (*see* ANTISPASMODIC DRUGS AND MOTILITY STIMULANTS, p.926). Your doctor may also prescribe antidiarrhoeal drugs (p.924) to help to alleviate diarrhoea, especially if you have diarrhoea on waking. If you regularly have problems with constipation, bulk-forming agents (*see* LAXATIVES, p.924) may help.

If you have psychological symptoms such as anxiety in addition to irritable bowel syndrome, you should ask your doctor to refer you to a therapist for advice on how to control anxiety.

Irritable bowel syndrome tends to be a long-term disorder, often lasting into old age. However, attacks usually become less frequent and severe with time.

WWW ONLINE SITES: p.1030

Malabsorption

Impaired absorption of nutrients from the small intestine

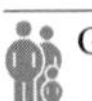 GENETICS Sometimes runs in families

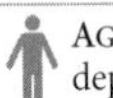 AGE GENDER LIFESTYLE Risk factors depend on the cause

Malabsorption occurs when the small intestine cannot absorb nutrients from food passing through it. The disorder may cause various symptoms, including diarrhoea and weight loss. If malabsorption is left untreated, certain nutritional deficiencies (p.630) can develop, which may lead to further problems, such as anaemia (p.446) or nerve damage (*see* NUTRITIONAL NEUROPATHIES, p.545).

WHAT ARE THE CAUSES?

Malabsorption is due to disorders that result in inadequate breakdown of food during digestion, damage to the lining of the small intestine, or impairment of motility, which is the ability of the muscular intestinal walls to contract.

In some cases, the small intestine cannot break down food because digestive enzymes or juices are missing or in short supply. For example, disorders affecting the pancreas, the organ that produces digestive juices, may prevent the breakdown of food. Such disorders include chronic pancreatitis (p.653) and cystic fibrosis (p.824). Sometimes, there is a problem in breaking down a specific nutrient. For example, people with lactose intolerance (p.657) lack an enzyme in the intestine needed to break down the sugar lactose from milk.

Damage to the lining of the intestine may result from inflammation due to disorders such as coeliac disease (p.658) and Crohn's disease (p.658) and certain infections, such as giardiasis (p.307). As a result, nutrients are unable to cross the lining and pass into the bloodstream. In the autoimmune disorder scleroderma (p.462), changes in the structure of the intestinal walls affect motility and lead to malabsorption of nutrients. Diabetes mellitus (p.687) may cause abnormal motility and malabsorption by damaging the nerves that supply the muscles in the intestinal walls.

WHAT ARE THE SYMPTOMS?

The most common symptoms of malabsorption include:

- Bulky, pale, foul-smelling diarrhoea.
- Flatulence and abdominal bloating.
- Weight loss.
- Abdominal pain with cramps.
- Tiredness and weakness.

Left untreated, malabsorption can lead to deficiencies in vitamin B_{12} and iron, which may result in anaemia, the symptoms of which include pale skin and shortness of breath. A deficiency of vitamin B_{12} can also affect the spinal cord and peripheral nerves, causing numbness and tingling in the hands and feet.

HOW IS IT DIAGNOSED?

Your doctor may arrange for a variety of blood tests to look for anaemia, vitamin deficiencies, and other signs of malabsorption. If the doctor suspects that your pancreas is damaged, he or she will probably arrange for additional tests to assess its function. A test may be carried out to confirm the enzyme deficiency that causes lactose intolerance.

Further tests may be carried out to check for other disorders of the small intestine. You may have a blood test to look for the antibodies that are present in coeliac disease. A special X-ray in which barium is used to highlight the inside of the small intestine (*see* CONTRAST X-RAYS, p.245) may be carried out to look for damage to the digestive tract caused by Crohn's disease. You may also require an endoscopy (p.255) to obtain a sample of intestinal tissue for microscopic analysis.

WHAT IS THE TREATMENT?

If possible, the underlying cause of the malabsorption is treated. Coeliac disease is usually treated with a special diet, and Crohn's disease usually responds to corticosteroids (p.930) or sulfasalazine (*see* AMINOSALICYLATE DRUGS, p.924). If the cause of malabsorption is giardiasis, antiprotozoal drugs (p.888) will be prescribed. Specific nutritional deficiencies can be corrected by taking vitamin and mineral supplements (*see* VITAMINS, p.927, and MINERALS, p.929).

If you are severely malnourished, you may need treatment in hospital, where you will be given intravenous nutrients or special liquid food supplements.

Most disorders that lead to malabsorption can be treated effectively, and the majority of affected people recover fully from the condition.

(WWW) ONLINE SITES: p.1030, p.1035

Food intolerance

Symptoms that are related to eating a specific food

 AGE GENDER GENETICS LIFESTYLE Not significant factors

If you develop troublesome symptoms such as stomach-ache each time you eat a particular food, you may have food intolerance. The cause of food intolerance is usually unknown, although in some cases there is a definite abnormality, such as an enzyme deficiency (*see* LACTOSE INTOLERANCE, right). The condition is different from a food allergy (p.467), in which the immune system reacts inappropriately to a specific food.

WHAT ARE THE SYMPTOMS?

The symptoms of food intolerance vary among individuals. Symptoms are usually related to a particular type of food, such as milk or wheat flour. They may occur within minutes or hours of eating and include the following:

- Nausea and vomiting.
- Abdominal pain.
- Diarrhoea.

Some people develop other symptoms, such as aching muscles or headaches.

WHAT MIGHT BE DONE?

In most cases of food intolerance, the diagnosis is based on your symptoms. Tests will then be performed to confirm the diagnosis. In some cases, endoscopy (*see* UPPER DIGESTIVE TRACT ENDOSCOPY, p.641) is carried out to examine the digestive tract and to look for evidence of an intestinal disorder such as coeliac disease (p.658). During the procedure, a small piece of tissue may be taken from the intestinal wall for microscopic examination. Levels of fat and certain sugars in a sample of faeces may also be measured. Higher than normal levels may indicate a food intolerance.

Often, the only way to diagnose food intolerance is to exclude the suspect food from your diet for a time to see if your symptoms improve. The food is later reintroduced, and you are monitored to see if your symptoms worsen. An exclusion diet, especially one for a child, should be undertaken only under the supervision of a doctor and a dietitian because restricted diets can cause vitamin and mineral deficiencies.

Once the cause of your intolerance has been identified, you should avoid eating foods that aggravate the problem. You will probably need to consult a dietitian, who will advise you on a diet that provides all the nutrients you need.

(WWW) ONLINE SITES: p.1030, p.1035

Lactose intolerance

An inability to digest lactose, the natural sugar found in milk

 AGE Most commonly develops from adolescence onwards

 GENETICS More common in certain ethnic groups

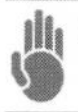 GENDER LIFESTYLE Not significant factors

A person who is lactose intolerant is unable to digest lactose, a natural sugar found in milk and dairy products. As a result, the lactose remains undigested in the intestines. In an affected person, even small amounts of lactose can cause abdominal pain and diarrhoea. Lactose intolerance usually develops in adolescence or adulthood, and only rarely affects babies. Worldwide, about 8 in 10 people of African, Native American, Asian, and Jewish origin develop an inability to digest lactose in the diet.

WHAT ARE THE CAUSES?

Normally, the enzyme lactase breaks down lactose in the intestines to form the sugars glucose and galactose, which are easily absorbed through the intestinal wall. If this enzyme is absent, the unabsorbed lactose ferments in the large intestine and produces painful symptoms. Although high levels of lactase are present at birth, in many ethnic groups the levels can drop with increasing age, becoming very low by adolescence so that milk can no longer be digested.

In children and babies, lactose intolerance sometimes develops temporarily following an attack of gastroenteritis (p.628) that causes short-term damage to the lining of the intestine.

WHAT ARE THE SYMPTOMS?

The symptoms of lactose intolerance usually develop a few hours after eating or drinking products containing milk. They may include the following:

- Abdominal bloating and cramping.
- Diarrhoea.
- Vomiting.

The severity of the symptoms depends on the degree of lactase deficiency. One person may experience symptoms only after drinking several glasses of milk, but another may feel discomfort after consuming only a small amount of a dairy product. The symptoms are often initially mild but can become more severe with each subsequent episode.

WHAT MIGHT BE DONE?

Your doctor may be able to diagnose lactose intolerance from your symptoms. He or she will probably ask you to keep a diary of all the foods you eat and the symptoms that occur. You may then have a specialized test to confirm lactose intolerance. Alternatively, your doctor may ask you to eliminate all dairy products from your diet for a few days. If your symptoms improve but return when dairy products are reintroduced into your diet, the diagnosis of lactose intolerance is confirmed.

Lactose intolerance is usually permanent in adults. However, the symptoms can be completely relieved by eliminating lactose from the diet. It is important to remember that you should avoid all dairy products, such as milk, yogurt, cheese, cream, and butter. Milk products that have been specially treated by having the lactose broken down are available over the counter. In addition, your doctor may suggest lactase supplements in the form of liquid or capsules. In babies whose lactose intolerance is caused by gastroenteritis, milk may be gradually introduced into the diet after a few weeks as the intestine recovers.

(WWW) ONLINE SITES: p.1030, p.1035

Coeliac disease

Malabsorption due to the intestine being damaged by a reaction to gluten, a protein found in many foods

AGE Usually occurs in the first year of life but can occur at any age

GENDER More common in females

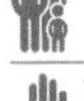
GENETICS Sometimes runs in families

LIFESTYLE Not a significant factor

Coeliac disease, commonly called sprue, is a condition caused by the protein gluten, which is found in wheat, rye, barley, and to some extent in oats. In people with the disease, the lining of the small intestine is damaged so that food cannot be properly absorbed (*see* MALABSORPTION, p.655). The exact mechanism of damage is uncertain, but it seems to be due to an abnormal immune response in which antibodies against gluten are produced. The resulting malabsorption leads to a deficiency of many nutrients, including vitamins and minerals that are vital for good health. Coeliac disease can run in families, which suggests that genetic factors are involved.

In the UK, coeliac disease affects about 1 in 1,000 people. The condition is very rare in Africa and Asia.

WHAT ARE THE SYMPTOMS?

In babies, the symptoms of coeliac disease first appear soon after cereals are introduced into the diet, usually at 3 or 4 months. In adults, the symptoms usually develop gradually and include:

- Bulky, loose, foul-smelling faeces that look greasy.
- Abdominal bloating and flatulence.
- Weight loss.
- Weakness and tiredness.
- Sometimes, a persistent, itchy rash on the knees, buttocks, elbows, and shoulders (*see* BLISTERING DISEASES, p.336).

In babies and children, the following symptoms may also occur:

- Diarrhoea.
- Failure to grow or gain weight.
- Muscle wasting, especially around the buttocks.

Vitamin and mineral deficiencies may lead to disorders such as iron-deficiency anaemia (p.447) and osteomalacia (*see* OSTEOMALACIA AND RICKETS, p.370), which is due to a lack of vitamin D and calcium. Untreated, coeliac disease may increase the risk of cancers, particularly cancer of the small intestine.

HOW IS IT DIAGNOSED?

Your doctor may suspect coeliac disease from your symptoms, especially if you have the characteristic rash described above. A blood test for antibodies may help to confirm the diagnosis. The doctor may suspect the condition in a baby if symptoms developed soon after solid foods were introduced.

Diagnosis involves removing a small sample of tissue from the lining of the small intestine. This procedure is performed using an endoscope inserted through the mouth (*see* UPPER DIGESTIVE TRACT ENDOSCOPY, p.641). When the tissue is examined under a microscope, the intestinal lining appears flattened. You may also have blood tests to look for evidence of anaemia.

WHAT IS THE TREATMENT?

Coeliac disease is treated by removing gluten from your diet. The recommended diet can be complicated, and it is advisable to see a dietitian for guidance.

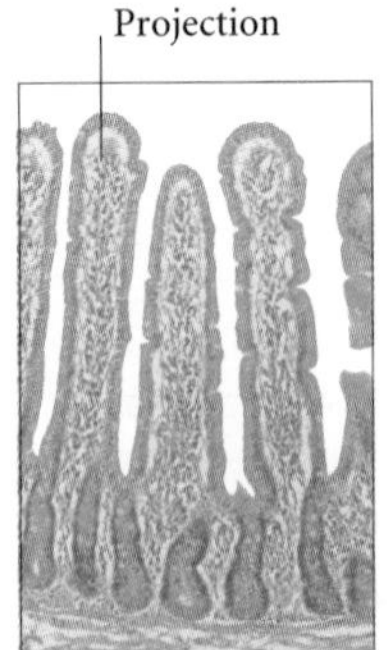

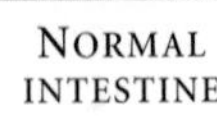

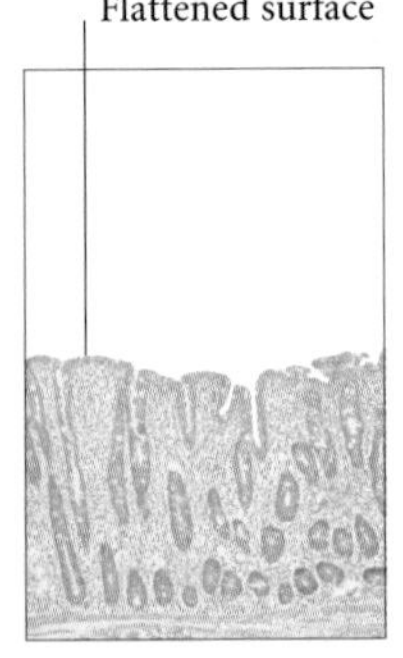

Intestine in coeliac disease

These magnified sections of small intestine show the effects of coeliac disease. The finger-like projections that normally absorb nutrients are flattened in coeliac disease.

You should avoid foods that contain wheat, rye, and barley. Of the cereals, only rice, corn, and possibly oats are suitable. It is not advisable to eat mustard, pasta, salad dressing, and some margarines because they contain wheat or wheat extracts, and you should avoid drinking beer. Initially, you may also need to take supplements of vitamins (p.927) and minerals (p.929).

Removing gluten from the diet usually produces a substantial and rapid improvement, and eventually the symptoms may totally disappear. However, coeliac disease is a long-term disorder and may reappear if gluten is reintroduced. Since coeliac disease sometimes runs in families, relatives of an affected person may be screened for the disorder by having a blood test to check for antibodies produced in the disease.

(WWW) ONLINE SITES: p.1030

Crohn's disease

A long-term inflammatory disease that can affect any part of the digestive tract

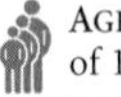
AGE Onset most common between the ages of 15 and 30

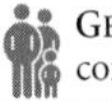
GENETICS Sometimes runs in families; more common in certain ethnic groups

LIFESTYLE Smoking is a risk factor

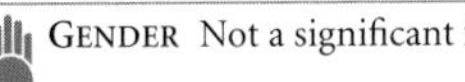
GENDER Not a significant factor

Crohn's disease is a long-term illness that usually begins in early adulthood and may cause serious ill health throughout life. Areas of the digestive tract become inflamed, causing a range of symptoms such as diarrhoea, abdominal pain, and weight loss. The disorder can occur in any part of the digestive tract from the mouth to the anus. However, the parts most frequently affected are the ileum (the last part of the small intestine) and the colon (the major part of the large intestine). Inflammation often occurs in more than one part of the digestive tract, with unaffected or mildly affected areas between the inflamed areas.

Crohn's disease is a relatively uncommon disorder; 30,000–40,000 people are affected in the UK. In Europe and North America, the condition most commonly affects white people, especially those of Jewish origin, and the onset of symptoms usually occurs between the ages of

15 and 30. Crohn's disease tends to recur despite treatment, and in the majority of cases the condition is lifelong.

The exact cause of Crohn's disease is unknown. Genetic factors are likely to contribute since about 1 in 10 affected people has one or more relatives with Crohn's disease or another inflammatory bowel disorder. Smoking may also play a part; smokers are three times more likely to develop Crohn's disease.

WHAT ARE THE SYMPTOMS?

The symptoms of Crohn's disease vary between individuals. The disorder usually recurs at intervals throughout life. Episodes may be severe, lasting weeks or several months, before settling down to periods when symptoms are mild or absent. The symptoms include:

- Diarrhoea.
- Abdominal pain.
- Fever.
- Weight loss.
- General feeling of ill health.

If the colon is affected, symptoms may also include the following:

- Diarrhoea, often containing blood.
- Rectal bleeding.

About 1 in 10 people also develops other disorders associated with Crohn's disease. These other conditions may occur even in mild cases of Crohn's disease and include arthritis (*see* ANKYLOSING SPONDYLITIS, p.378), eye disorders (*see* UVEITIS, p.574), kidney stones (p.701), gallstones (p.651), and a rash (*see* ERYTHEMA NODOSUM, p.348).

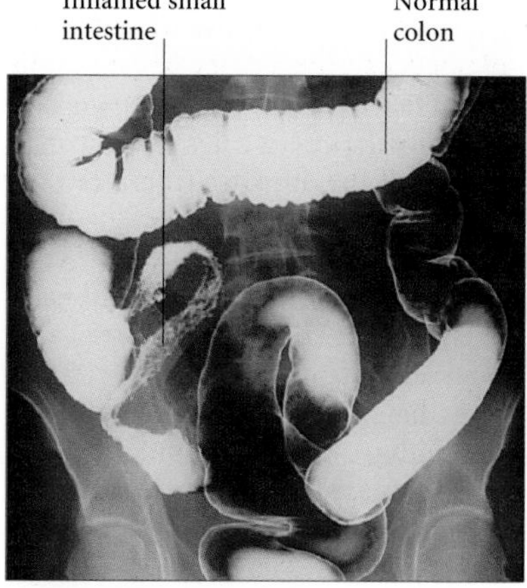

Crohn's disease
This contrast X-ray shows a normal colon and also shows a section of small intestine that has become inflamed and ulcerated as a result of Crohn's disease.

ARE THERE COMPLICATIONS?

Complications of Crohn's disease may include pus-filled cavities near the anus (*see* ANAL ABSCESS, p.669). These cavities can develop into abnormal passages between the anal canal and the skin around the anus, called anal fistulas.

Intestinal obstruction (p.663) caused by thickening of the intestinal walls is a fairly common complication of Crohn's disease. Damage to the small intestine may prevent the absorption of nutrients (*see* MALABSORPTION, p.655) and thus lead to anaemia (p.446) or vitamin deficiencies. Inflammation of the colon over a long period of time may also be associated with an increased risk of developing colorectal cancer (p.665).

HOW IS IT DIAGNOSED?

If your doctor suspects that you have Crohn's disease, he or she may arrange for a colonoscopy (p.661), in which the intestine is examined and tissue samples are taken from affected areas for microscopic examination. If the small intestine is affected, you may have a contrast X-ray (p.245) of the intestine, known as a small bowel enema study, to look for abnormalities.

Blood tests may be done to check for anaemia and to assess how severely the intestine is inflamed. If your doctor suspects that you have gallstones or kidney stones, you may have imaging tests.

WHAT IS THE TREATMENT?

Mild attacks of Crohn's disease can often be treated with antidiarrhoeal drugs (p.924) and painkillers (p.912). For an acute attack, your doctor may prescribe oral corticosteroids (p.930). As soon as symptoms subside, the dosage will be reduced to avoid the risk of side effects. If your symptoms are very severe, you may need hospital treatment with intravenous corticosteroids. In all cases, once the dosage of corticosteroids has been reduced, your doctor may recommend oral sulfasalazine or mesalazine (*see* AMINOSALICYLATE DRUGS, p.924) to prevent recurrent attacks. He or she may also give you an immunosuppressant drug (p.906), such as azathioprine.

You may need dietary supplements, such as extra protein and vitamins (p.927), to counteract malabsorption. During severe attacks, nutrients may have to be given intravenously.

Many people who have Crohn's disease need surgery at some stage. The procedure involves removing the diseased area of the intestine and rejoining the healthy ends (*see* COLECTOMY, p.665). However, surgery is not usually performed until it is absolutely necessary because further affected regions may develop in the remaining intestine.

WHAT IS THE PROGNOSIS?

Crohn's disease is a recurrent disorder. Most affected people learn to live reasonably normal lives, but 7 in 10 people eventually need surgery. Complications and repeated surgery can occasionally reduce life expectancy. Crohn's disease may increase the risk of colorectal cancer, and, for this reason, your doctor may advise you to have regular check-ups that include colonoscopy.

(WWW) ONLINE SITES: p.1030

Ulcerative colitis

Long-term, intermittent inflammation and ulceration of the rectum and colon

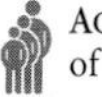 AGE Onset most common between the ages of 15 and 35

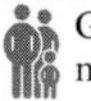 GENETICS Sometimes runs in families; more common in white people and in certain other ethnic groups

 LIFESTYLE More common in nonsmokers and ex-smokers

 GENDER Not a significant factor

Ulcerative colitis is a long-term, intermittent inflammatory disorder that most commonly develops in young adults. The disorder causes ulceration of the rectum and the colon (the major part of the large intestine). It may either affect the rectum alone (*see* PROCTITIS, p.667) or extend from the rectum further up the colon. In some cases, the disorder involves the entire colon.

Ulcerative colitis affects about 1 in 1,000 people. It occurs most frequently in white people, particularly those of Jewish descent. Smoking may give some protection against the disease.

WHAT IS THE CAUSE?

The exact cause of ulcerative colitis is unknown. However, there is some evidence that genetic factors are involved, since about 1 in 10 people with ulcerative colitis has a close relative who has

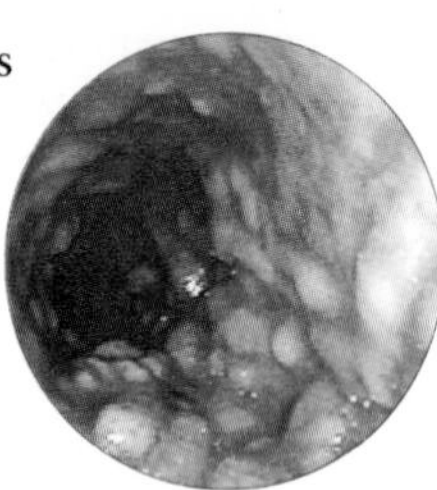
Ulcerative colitis
This endoscopic view of a colon affected by ulcerative colitis shows extensive ulceration of the intestinal lining.

the disease. There may also be a family history of intestinal diseases, such as Crohn's disease (p.658), and of allergic disorders, such as eczema (p.333).

WHAT ARE THE SYMPTOMS?

The symptoms of ulcerative colitis are often intermittent, and there may be several months or years in which there are few or no symptoms. In a mild episode, symptoms often develop over a few days and may include the following:

- Diarrhoea, sometimes with blood and mucus in the stool.
- Abdominal pain.
- Tiredness.
- Loss of appetite.

In a severe attack, the symptoms may begin suddenly, developing over just a few hours. Symptoms may include:

- Severe bouts of diarrhoea, at least six times a day.
- Passage of blood and mucus from the anus.
- Pain and swelling in the abdomen.
- Fever.
- Weight loss.

People with ulcerative colitis often have other associated disorders. These include pain in the joints and in the spine (*see* ARTHRITIS, p.374, and ANKYLOSING SPONDYLITIS, p.378), inflammation in the eye (*see* UVEITIS, p.574), and the skin condition erythema nodosum (p.348).

ARE THERE COMPLICATIONS?

A severe, sudden attack of ulcerative colitis may lead to toxic megacolon. In this condition, the colon becomes inflamed and greatly distended. As a result, the wall of the colon can perforate, allowing intestinal contents containing bacteria to leak into the abdominal cavity. This leakage can cause peritonitis (p.665), a potentially fatal disorder.

People with ulcerative colitis are also at greater risk of developing colorectal cancer (p.665). The risk is increased further if the ulcerative colitis is severe and began at an early age.

HOW IS IT DIAGNOSED?

If your symptoms are fairly mild, your doctor will probably ask you for a faecal sample, which will be tested to exclude the possibility of an infection. You may also have a colonoscopy (opposite page), during which a small sample of tissue may be removed from the lining of the rectum or the colon for microscopic examination. Sometimes, a specialized contrast X-ray (p.245) called a barium enema, which detects abnormalities in the intestinal lining, may be performed. You may also have blood tests to look for anaemia (p.446) and to assess the extent of inflammation of the colon.

WHAT IS THE TREATMENT?

Ulcerative colitis is usually treated with drugs, but surgery may be necessary if you are experiencing frequent severe attacks or if complications develop.

DRUGS Your doctor may prescribe the anti-inflammatory drug sulfasalazine (*see* AMINOSALICYLATE DRUGS, p.924) to prevent attacks of ulcerative colitis or treat mild episodes. Alternatively, you may be given mesalazine, which has fewer side effects. If the inflammation is confined to the rectum or the lower part of the colon, your doctor may prescribe aminosalicylate drugs for you to self-administer in the form of an enema or suppositories. If the ulcerative colitis has spread further up the colon, you will be given the drugs to take orally.

If you have severe, sudden attacks of the disorder, your doctor will probably prescribe corticosteroids (p.930) to be taken orally or as an enema. Long-term use of corticosteroids may cause side effects, such as weight gain and a moon-shaped face. For this reason, the doctor will reduce the dose once your symptoms have started to subside and stop the treatment as soon as possible.

SURGERY Surgical treatment is usually necessary for people who experience persistent symptoms despite treatment with drugs. It may also be recommended for people who have a sudden, severe attack that does not respond to medical treatment and that may lead to toxic megacolon. In addition, surgery may be advisable for people with an increased risk of colorectal cancer. Surgery usually involves the removal of the diseased colon and rectum (*see* COLECTOMY, p.665) and creation of a stoma, which is an artificial opening in the abdominal wall through which the small intestine can expel faeces (*see* COLOSTOMY, p.666). A newer procedure called a pouch operation is suitable for some people. In this procedure, part of the small intestine is used to create a pouch that connects the small intestine to the anus. This operation avoids the need for a stoma, but the pouch may become inflamed and the frequency of bowel movements often increases.

WHAT IS THE PROGNOSIS?

Some people have only one attack of ulcerative colitis, but most have recurring episodes. About 1 in 5 people needs to have surgery. Colorectal cancer is the greatest long-term risk, and it eventually develops in about 1 in 6 people whose entire rectum and colon have been affected for 25 years or more. If you have long-standing, extensive ulcerative colitis but have not had surgery, you will need regular colonoscopy to detect early signs of colorectal cancer.

(WWW) ONLINE SITES: p.1030

Polyps in the colon

Noncancerous growths in the large intestine that often do not produce symptoms

 AGE More common over the age of 60, but some forms develop in childhood

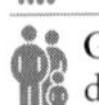 GENETICS In some cases, the condition is due to an abnormal gene

 GENDER LIFESTYLE Not significant factors

Polyps in the colon are very common in developed countries, where at least 1 in 3 people over the age of 60 may be affected. However, most people are unaware that they have polyps because they often do not cause symptoms.

Polyps are slow-developing growths that protrude inwards from the lining of the large intestine. Some are small and spherical and are attached directly to the intestinal wall; others are over 2.5 cm (1 in) long and attached to the wall by a stalk. Polyps can occur either singly or in groups. Growths larger than 1 cm (½ in) in diameter may become cancerous (*see* COLORECTAL CANCER, p.665) and must be treated early.

TEST AND TREATMENT COLONOSCOPY

In colonoscopy, a flexible tube called a colonoscope is used to view the colon to look for disorders such as polyps. The day before a colonoscopy, you will be given laxatives. You may also be given sedatives before the procedure, which takes 15–60 minutes and is usually painless. Attachments on the colonoscope can be used to take tissue samples or perform certain treatments. A similar viewing technique called sigmoidoscopy is used to examine the rectum and lower part of the colon.

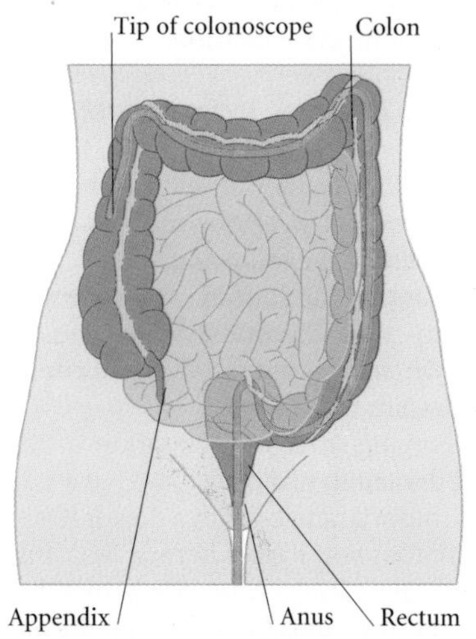

During the procedure
The colonoscope is passed through the anus and rectum into the colon. Once the tube is inside, you will not feel it moving.

VIEW

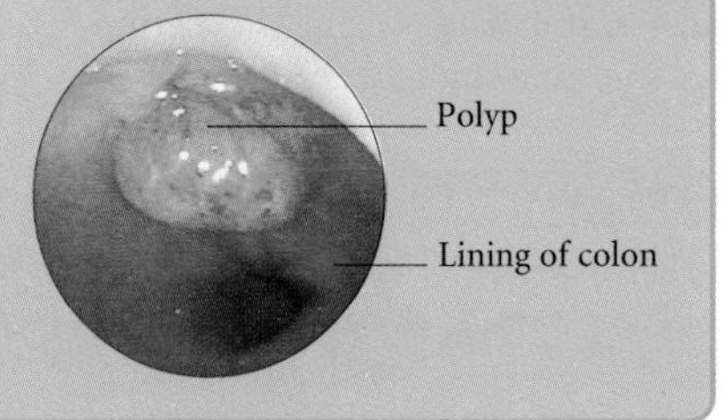

Intestinal polyp
An intestinal polyp attached to the wall of the colon can be seen in this view through a colonoscope. Small polyps can often be painlessly removed during the colonoscopy.

WHAT ARE THE CAUSES?

In most cases, the cause of the condition is not known. Rarely, polyps result from an inherited condition such as familial adenomatous polyposis (FAP). This condition, in which hundreds of polyps cover the lining of the large intestine, is due to an abnormal gene inherited in an autosomal dominant manner (*see* GENE DISORDERS, p.271).

WHAT ARE THE SYMPTOMS?

In most cases, intestinal polyps do not cause symptoms. However, if symptoms do occur, they may include:

- Diarrhoea.
- Blood in the faeces or bleeding from the anus, sometimes with mucus.

In some cases, anaemia (p.446) develops due to blood loss, causing tiredness and shortness of breath. In rare cases, a polyp protrudes through the anus.

WHAT MIGHT BE DONE?

In many people who do not have symptoms, polyps may be detected during routine screening for colorectal cancer or by investigations that are performed for other reasons. If you do have symptoms, your doctor may arrange for a colonoscopy (above) to examine the lining of the intestine. Most polyps can be removed painlessly during the colonoscopy, but occasionally surgery may be necessary to remove larger growths. Polyps that have been removed will be examined under a microscope to look for precancerous cells. If you are found to have precancerous polyps, you may need a colonoscopy every 3–5 years to check for new growths.

If you have FAP, the polyps will be too numerous to be removed individually. There is a high risk of colorectal cancer associated with FAP, and for this reason you will probably be advised to have your colon completely removed (*see* COLECTOMY, p.665). If you have a close relative with FAP, you may be offered regular screening using colonoscopy to look for polyps (p.660). In some cases, testing for the abnormal gene may be carried out (*see* TESTS FOR ABNORMAL GENES, p.239). If no polyps have developed by the time you reach the age of 40, they are unlikely to occur.

WHAT IS THE PROGNOSIS?

Polyps that do not cause any symptoms may never be diagnosed. Those polyps that do cause symptoms can almost always be treated successfully. In such cases, further polyps may develop. However, with treatment the condition can be controlled and the risk of colorectal cancer kept to a minimum.

(WWW) ONLINE SITES: p.1028, p.1030

Hernias

Protrusions of part of an organ, usually the intestine, through a weakened muscle

LIFESTYLE Obesity and lifting heavy weights may be risk factors

AGE GENDER Risk factors depend on the type

GENETICS Not a significant factor

Hernias, commonly called "ruptures", most often occur at sites in the abdomen where there is a weakness in the muscles. If pressure in the abdomen is increased due to activities such as lifting heavy weights, persistent coughing, or straining at defaecation, the muscles of the abdomen become stretched at the weak point. A visible bulge can then develop, which may contain fatty tissue or part of the intestine. Abdominal hernias are frequently found in men who have manual jobs.

An abdominal hernia usually disappears when you lie flat, but sometimes a section of intestine becomes trapped inside the bulge. If the trapped portion of intestine becomes twisted, its blood supply may be cut off. This is known as a strangulated hernia and causes severe

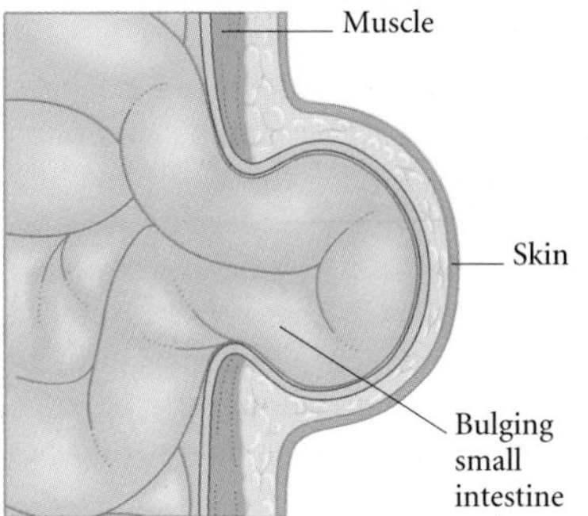

How a hernia develops
Part of the small intestine pushes through a weak area of muscle in the abdominal wall, causing a noticeable bulge to appear on the surface of the body.

pain and vomiting. Immediate surgery is essential to prevent the intestine from becoming gangrenous.

Occasionally, hernias occur in other areas. Hiatus hernias develop when part of the stomach protrudes into the chest cavity through a weakened area in the diaphragm (the sheet of muscle that lies beneath the lungs and is involved in breathing) and may be accompanied by gastro-oesophageal reflux (p.636).

WHAT ARE THE TYPES?

Hernias are classified according to the site where they occur in the body. Some types occur more often in men; others are more frequently found in women.

INGUINAL HERNIA This type of hernia occurs when a portion of the intestine pushes through into the inguinal canal, which is a weak spot in the abdominal muscle wall. The hernia causes a visible bulge in the groin or scrotum. These hernias usually affect men, but sometimes occur in women.

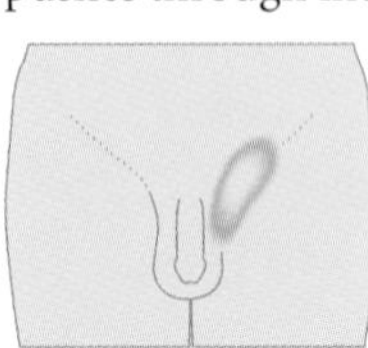

FEMORAL HERNIA This type of hernia occurs in the part of the groin where the femoral vein and artery pass from the lower abdomen to the thigh. Women who are overweight or who have had several pregnancies are at increased risk of these hernias because their abdominal muscles are weakened.

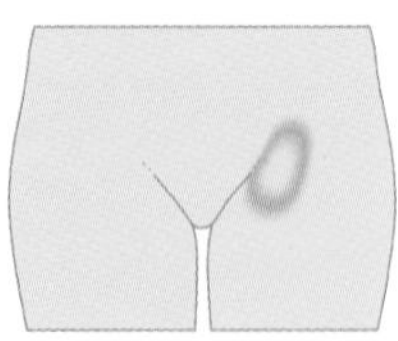

UMBILICAL HERNIA Babies may be born with an umbilical hernia, which develops behind the navel due to a weakness in the abdominal wall. Hernias that develop near the navel are known as paraumbilical hernias and are most common in women who are overweight or have had several pregnancies.

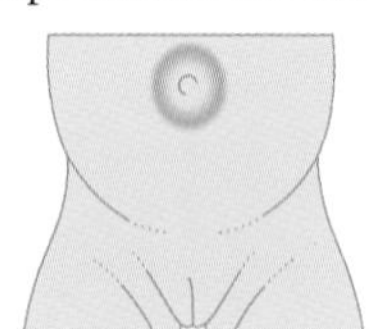

OTHER TYPES OF HERNIA Epigastric hernias develop in the midline between the navel and the breastbone and are three times more common in men. Incisional hernias may develop after abdominal surgery if there is weakness around the scar. Risk factors include being overweight and having several operations through the same incision.

WHAT ARE THE SYMPTOMS?

The symptoms may come on suddenly, but more often they develop over a period of several weeks or months. They may include the following:

- A lump in the abdomen or groin; the lump may disappear when you lie down and reappear when you cough or strain to defaecate.
- Dragging or aching sensation in the abdomen or groin.

It is important to consult a doctor if you think that you have a hernia. Seek immediate medical advice for a hernia that cannot be pushed back through the abdominal wall or one in which the skin is tender or inflamed because these symptoms suggest a strangulated hernia.

WHAT MIGHT BE DONE?

Your doctor may be able to feel a hernia by examining your abdomen or groin. Even small hernias eventually need to be repaired (*see* HERNIA REPAIR, below) because, if they are left untreated, they may become strangulated. The type of operation depends largely on the size of the hernia and on your age and general health. Some procedures are done under local anaesthetic as day surgery. Umbilical hernias in babies can usually be left untreated since they tend to disappear naturally by the age of 5 years.

Surgery is usually effective. However, there is a risk that the hernia will recur in the same place or elsewhere. After a hernia repair, you may be advised to avoid strenuous activity for a few weeks. You can help to prevent a recurrence by losing excess weight, taking gentle exercise, and avoiding constipation.

(WWW) ONLINE SITES: p.1028, p.1030

(TREATMENT) HERNIA REPAIR

A hernia repair is a simple operation, often performed as day surgery. A local or general anaesthetic will be given depending on the size and location of the hernia. The procedure may be done either as open surgery, in which a 3–5 cm (1–2 in) incision is made over the hernia, or by endoscopic surgery (p.948). In both types of operation, the contents of the hernia are eased back into place and the weakened muscle is repaired. After the operation, the area is likely to be painful at first, but you will be given painkillers for relief. You can resume most normal activities within 7 days, but you should avoid lifting heavy objects for up to 3 months.

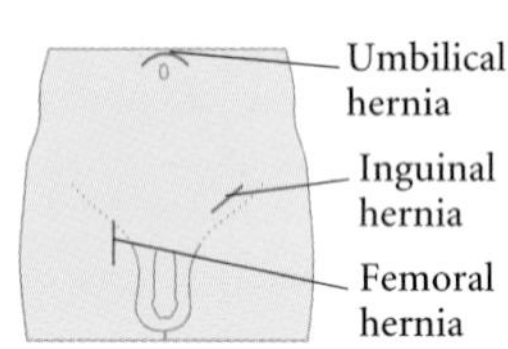

SITES OF INCISIONS

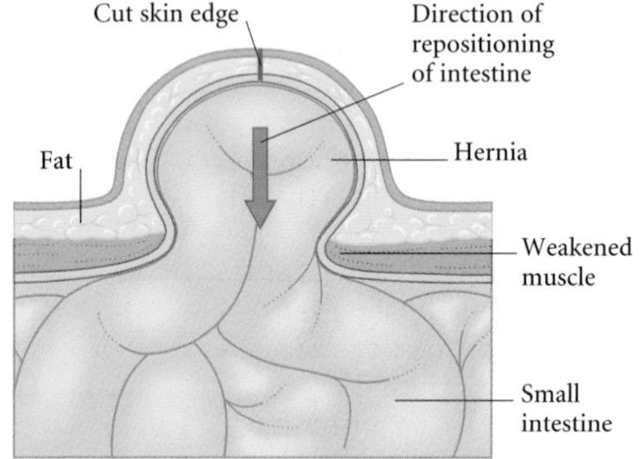

1 An incision is made through the layers of skin and fat to uncover the hernia. The intestine is then gently pushed back into the abdominal cavity.

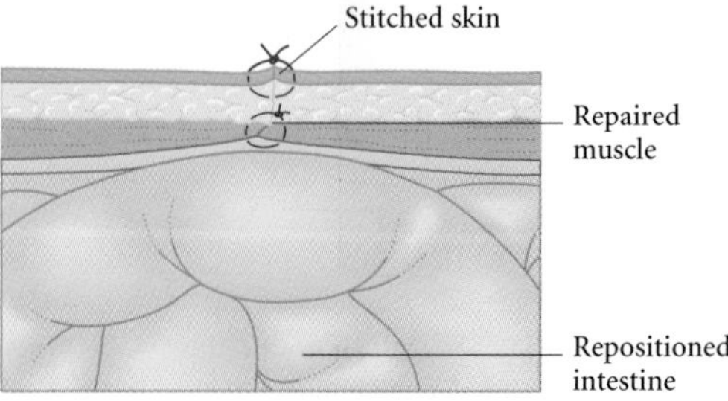

2 Once the hernia has been repositioned, the weakened area is repaired, usually by suturing the muscle. However, in some cases, a repair may have to be reinforced with a piece of synthetic mesh placed over the abdominal muscle.

Intestinal obstruction

Failure of partly digested material to move through the intestine due to a blockage or paralysis of the intestinal muscles

AGE GENDER GENETICS LIFESTYLE Risk factors depend on the cause

In intestinal obstruction, a section of the intestine is partially or totally blocked (mechanical obstruction) or the muscles in the intestinal walls stop contracting (functional obstruction). In both circumstances, the intestinal contents are unable to move along the digestive tract normally. Left untreated, the condition can be life-threatening.

What are the causes?

Many disorders can cause mechanical obstruction. For example, the intestine may be blocked by a tumour inside it or by external compression from a growth in another organ. Obstruction may also be due to narrowing of the intestine as a result of inflammation, which occurs in Crohn's disease (p.658). In addition, an obstruction can be the result of a strangulated hernia, in which a small part of the intestine protrudes through a weakened area in the muscles of the abdominal wall and becomes trapped (*see* HERNIAS, p.661). After abdominal surgery, scar tissue can form between loops of intestine and cause an obstruction months or even years later.

Functional obstruction, in which the intestinal muscles fail to contract properly, may be a complication of certain disorders, such as the serious abdominal inflammation peritonitis (p.665), or it may follow major surgery.

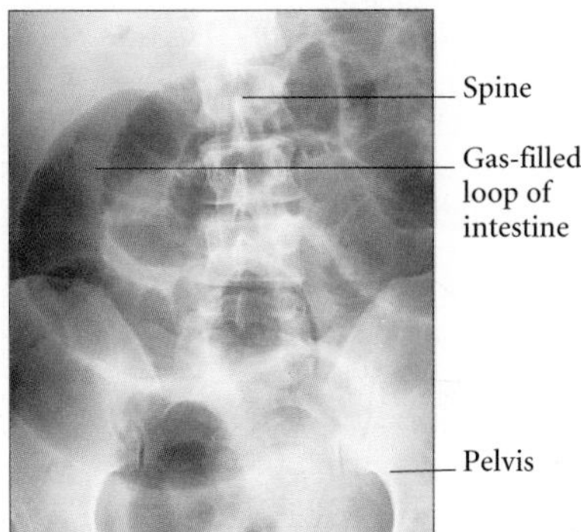

Intestinal obstruction
This abdominal X-ray shows enlarged loops of gas-filled intestine due to an obstruction in the colon.

What are the symptoms?

The symptoms of intestinal obstruction may appear suddenly or develop gradually depending on the cause. In all cases, symptoms may include:

- Vomiting fluid that may be greenish-yellow, or brown with a faecal odour.
- Severe constipation.
- Abdominal bloating.
- Pain, usually occurring in waves that may later become continuous.
- Total absence of flatulence, implying a complete intestinal obstruction.

Repeated vomiting may cause dehydration due to fluid loss. The intestinal wall may tear due to increased pressure and leak its bacteria-rich contents into the abdomen, causing peritonitis.

What might be done?

If your doctor suspects that you have an obstruction in the intestine, you will be admitted to hospital immediately. You will have abdominal X-rays (p.244) to confirm the diagnosis and determine the nature and position of the obstruction. A tube may be inserted through your nose and down into your stomach to remove digestive juices and prevent vomiting. You will probably be given intravenous fluids to prevent further dehydration. Surgery is often needed to relieve an obstruction. If the cause is Crohn's disease or peritonitis, treating the inflammation may relieve the condition. If a blockage occurs after major surgery, the intestinal wall usually starts to contract normally after a few days.

(WWW) ONLINE SITES: p.1030

Diverticular disease

The presence of small pouches known as diverticula in the wall of the colon

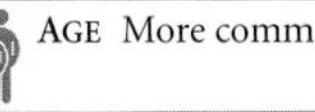

AGE More common over the age of 50

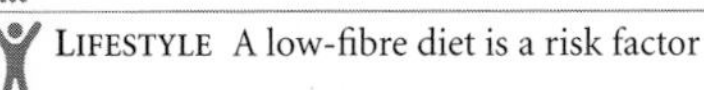

LIFESTYLE A low-fibre diet is a risk factor

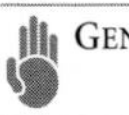

GENDER GENETICS Not significant factors

In diverticular disease, pea- or grape-sized pouches (diverticula) protrude from the wall of the large intestine, usually from the part of the colon closest to the rectum. The pouches form when parts of the wall of the intestine bulge outwards through weakened areas, often close to an artery. In many cases, the

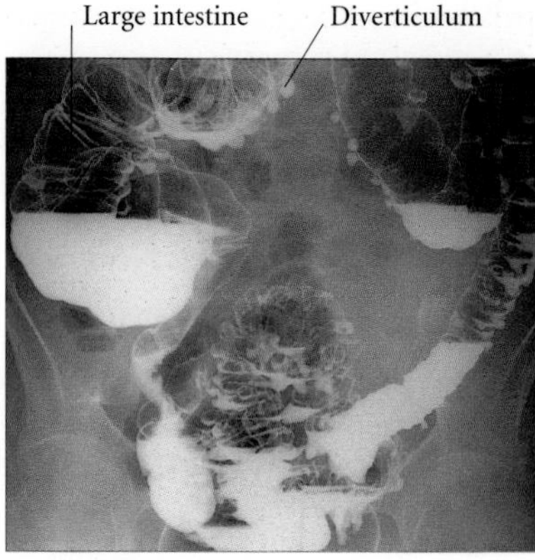

Diverticular disease
In this special X-ray, a contrast dye shows small pouches (diverticula) protruding from the wall of the large intestine.

bulging of the intestinal wall is associated with persistent constipation (p.628) and occurs when the pressure inside the intestine increases as the person strains to defaecate. Sometimes, one or more pouches become inflamed, a condition known as diverticulitis.

About 1 in 3 people between the ages of 50 and 60 has diverticular disease, and the disorder becomes increasingly common after the age of 60. However, most affected people have no symptoms. The disease is strongly associated with a low-fibre diet, which can lead to constipation. The disease is very rare in developing countries, where fibre comprises a large part of the diet.

What are the symptoms?

More than three-quarters of all people with diverticular disease are unaware of the condition because they have no symptoms. If symptoms are present, they may include the following:

- Episodes of abdominal pain, especially in the lower left abdomen, that are relieved by a bowel movement or a release of intestinal wind.
- Intermittent episodes of constipation and diarrhoea.
- Occasional bright red bleeding from the rectum, which may be painless.

Diverticular disease is sometimes difficult to distinguish from irritable bowel syndrome (p.656), which has similar symptoms. If diverticulitis develops, the symptoms may become worse and be accompanied by:

- Severe lower abdominal pain and tenderness in the abdomen.

- Fever.
- Nausea and vomiting.

If you notice any change in your bowel habits or you have rectal bleeding, you should consult your doctor immediately because these symptoms may indicate a more serious underlying disease, such as colorectal cancer (p.665).

ARE THERE COMPLICATIONS?

If an inflamed diverticulum bursts, faeces and bacteria can spill into the abdominal cavity. As a result, an abscess may form next to the colon or peritonitis (opposite page), an inflammation of the membrane that lines the abdominal cavity, may develop. Peritonitis is a potentially life-threatening condition.

An abnormal channel called a fistula may develop between a diverticulum and the bladder, resulting in pain, a more frequent urge to pass urine, or recurrent bladder infections (*see* CYSTITIS, p.709). In some women, a fistula may develop between a diverticulum and the vagina, causing faecal material to be discharged through the vagina. An inflamed diverticulum may also cause intestinal obstruction (p.663).

HOW IS IT DIAGNOSED?

If your doctor suspects that you have diverticular disease, he or she may arrange for you to have a contrast X-ray (p.245) in which a barium enema is used to highlight the shape of the intestines. If your symptoms include rectal bleeding, a colonoscopy (p.661) may be carried out to examine the colon and exclude colorectal cancer. Sometimes, diverticular disease is found during an investigation for another disease.

If your symptoms develop suddenly, you may be admitted to hospital for investigative tests. You may have X-rays and a colonoscopy. In addition, CT scanning (p.247) or ultrasound scanning (p.250) may be performed.

WHAT IS THE TREATMENT?

Often, a high-fibre diet with plenty of fluids is the only treatment needed for diverticular disease, together with antispasmodic drugs (*see* ANTISPASMODIC DRUGS AND MOTILITY STIMULANTS, p.926) if you have abdominal pain.

If you develop severe diverticulitis, you will be admitted to hospital and given intravenous fluids and antibiotics (p.885) to treat bacterial infection. These measures produce improvements in most cases, and no further treatment is needed. However, surgery is sometimes necessary if you have severe rectal bleeding or if an abscess or a fistula develops. Anyone who has two or three attacks of diverticulitis within a few years is also likely to need surgery. The most common operation is a partial colectomy (p.665), in which the diseased part of the colon is removed and the healthy ends of the intestine are rejoined. At the same time, a temporary colostomy (p.666) may be performed.

WHAT IS THE PROGNOSIS?

The outlook for diverticular disease is generally good. If a high-fibre diet is adopted early enough, the condition is unlikely to progress. Among people with diverticulitis, 2 in 3 have only one attack, but in other people it recurs and surgery may be needed. About 2 in 10 people who experience bleeding will have a recurrence within the next few months to a year unless the problem is treated surgically.

(WWW) ONLINE SITES: p.1030

Appendicitis

Inflammation of the appendix, leading to severe abdominal pain

 AGE More common under the age of 40, especially among adolescents

 GENDER Slightly more common in males

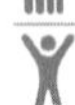 LIFESTYLE A low-fibre diet is a risk factor

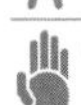 GENETICS Not a significant factor

Appendicitis is inflammation affecting the appendix, the small, blind-ended tube attached to the first section of the large intestine. The disorder is common, especially among adolescents, affecting about 1 in 500 people every year in the UK. Appendicitis is a common cause of sudden, severe pain in the abdomen, and removal of the appendix is one of the most commonly performed emergency operations. The disorder occurs most commonly in developed countries where the typical diet is low in fibre.

In most cases of appendicitis, no cause is detected, but in some instances the inflammation is the result of a blockage inside the appendix. Blockages sometimes occur when a lump of faecal material passes from the large intestine into the appendix and becomes lodged there. The closed end of the appendix beyond the obstruction then becomes infected with bacteria and inflamed.

WHAT ARE THE SYMPTOMS?

Symptoms differ from one person to another. The early symptoms usually develop over a few hours and include:

- Sudden onset of intermittent pain that is first felt in the upper abdomen or around the navel.
- Nausea, with or without vomiting.

Less often, there may be:

- Diarrhoea.
- Mild fever.
- Loss of appetite.
- Frequent passing of urine.

After a few hours, the pain shifts to the lower right abdomen. If treatment is delayed, the appendix may rupture, and intestinal matter containing a high concentration of bacteria can leak into the abdomen. The result may be peritonitis (opposite page), a potentially serious condition in which the membrane that lines the abdominal cavity becomes inflamed. If the appendix ruptures, the pain becomes widespread and severe.

WHAT MIGHT BE DONE?

Your doctor will first ask you about the development of your symptoms. He or she will then examine your abdomen and may also insert a gloved finger into the rectum to determine whether there is tenderness in the area around the appendix. You may also have a blood test to measure the white blood cell count. An elevated white cell count may be a sign of inflammation. If your doctor suspects that you have appendicitis, you will be admitted to hospital immediately, where imaging with ultrasound scanning (p.250) or CT scanning (p.247) may confirm the diagnosis.

The usual treatment is removal of the appendix by minimally invasive surgery (*see* ENDOSCOPIC SURGERY, p.948) or by conventional open surgery. The operation is relatively simple and is performed under general anaesthesia. There are usually no long-term adverse effects following either type of operation, and recovery normally takes only 3–4 days.

(WWW) ONLINE SITES: p.1030

Peritonitis

Inflammation of the peritoneum, the membranous lining of the abdomen

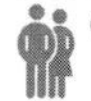
GENDER More common in males

AGE GENETICS LIFESTYLE Not significant factors

Inflammation of the peritoneum, the membrane that surrounds the organs in the abdomen and lines the abdominal cavity, is called peritonitis. The condition is more common in men. It usually occurs as a complication of another abdominal disorder, such as appendicitis (opposite page). Severe peritonitis may be fatal if not treated rapidly.

What are the causes?

The most common cause of peritonitis is a bacterial infection that has spread from elsewhere in the abdomen. For example, bacteria from the intestine may escape into the abdominal cavity if the intestine is perforated. Possible causes of a perforation include a severe flare-up of a long-term inflammatory disorder, such as ulcerative colitis (p.659); intestinal obstruction (p.663); a wound such as a stab injury (p.319); or surgery.

A less common cause of peritonitis is irritation of the peritoneum. For example, stomach acid may leak out into the abdominal cavity and cause irritation if a peptic ulcer (p.640) perforates the wall of the stomach or the duodenum (the first part of the small intestine). Peritonitis may also develop if bile leaks out from an inflamed gallbladder (*see* CHOLECYSTITIS, p.652). Occasionally, the condition is caused by leakage of digestive enzymes into the abdominal cavity as a result of acute pancreatitis (p.652).

What are the symptoms?

The symptoms of peritonitis usually develop rapidly. They may include:

- Severe, constant abdominal pain.
- Fever.
- Abdominal swelling.
- Nausea and vomiting.

In severe cases, dehydration and shock (p.414) may also occur. Rarely, after an attack of peritonitis, adhesions may develop, in which bands of scar tissue grow between loops of intestine, causing the loops to stick together. Adhesions may cause abdominal pain months after the attack of peritonitis. Another complication may be intestinal obstruction.

If you believe that you may have peritonitis, you should seek medical attention without delay.

What might be done?

It is important that peritonitis is diagnosed and treated as soon as possible. If your doctor suspects that you have peritonitis, he or she will have you admitted to hospital immediately. In hospital, a doctor will examine your abdomen to check for pain or tenderness and you will have X-rays (p.244) of the abdomen. In addition, you may need a procedure called a laparoscopy (p.742), in which the abdominal cavity is examined for abnormalities.

If peritonitis is the result of a bacterial infection, you will be given antibiotics (p.885). You may also need intravenous fluids to treat dehydration and shock. Your doctor will treat the underlying cause of the peritonitis. For example, a perforated peptic ulcer will be repaired or a ruptured appendix removed.

If peritonitis is treated immediately, recovery is usually rapid and long-term problems, such as adhesions, are rare.

(WWW) ONLINE SITES: p.1030

Colorectal cancer

A cancerous tumour of the lining of the colon or rectum

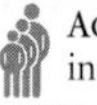
AGE Rare under the age of 40; becomes increasingly common over the age of 40

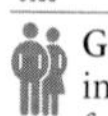
GENDER Rectal cancer is more common in males; colon cancer is more common in females

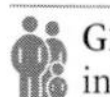
GENETICS In some cases, the condition is inherited

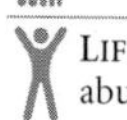
LIFESTYLE A high-fat, low-fibre diet, alcohol abuse, and obesity are risk factors

Colorectal cancer is one of the most common cancers in the UK and is the second leading cause of cancer death. However, it is one of the few cancers that can be detected early by screening people who are at risk (*see* SCREENING, p.42, and COLONOSCOPY, p.661), and when it is detected early enough, it can be treated successfully by surgery.

Colorectal cancer is rare under 40 and most often occurs in people over 60. Rectal cancer tends to be more common in men, while colon cancer is more common in women. Cancer can occur anywhere in the colon or rectum, but about 6 in 10 tumours develop in the part of the colon nearest the rectum.

(TREATMENT) Colectomy

A colectomy is an operation in which part or all of the large intestine (the colon and the rectum) is removed under general anaesthesia. It is usually performed to treat inflammatory conditions, such as Crohn's disease, or cancer of the colon. In most cases, the cut ends of the large intestine are rejoined once the diseased section has been removed, but sometimes a colostomy (p.666) is needed. You will have to stay in hospital for at least a week after the operation, depending on the extent of the surgery.

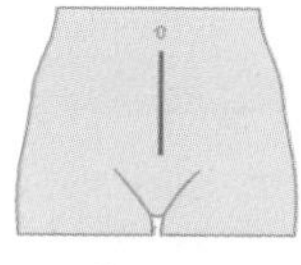

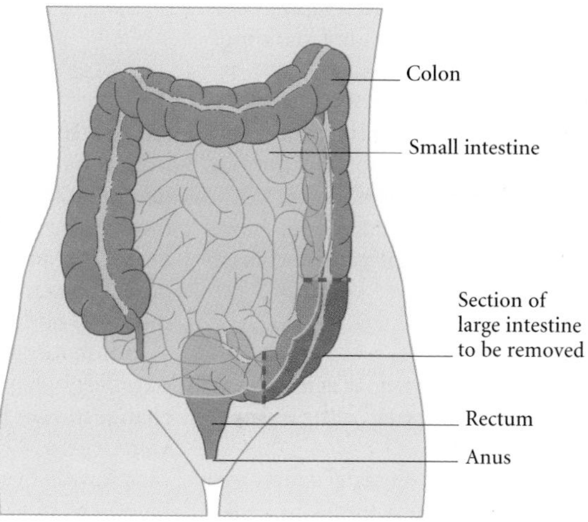

Partial colectomy
During the procedure, the abnormal section of the colon is cut out, and the healthy ends of the remaining intestine are joined together. A colostomy is performed only in a minority of partial colectomies.

WHAT ARE THE CAUSES?

In less affluent countries, where people traditionally live on a high-fibre diet consisting mainly of cereals, fruit, and vegetables, colorectal cancer is rare. However, a typical Western diet, which tends to be high in meat and animal fats and low in fibre, seems to increase the risk of developing colorectal cancer. It is not known how fibre in the diet reduces the risk of the disorder. A possible explanation is that dietary fibre shortens the time that it takes for waste matter to pass through the intestines. As a result, potentially cancer-causing substances (known as carcinogens) in food are expelled from the body at a faster rate. Other lifestyle factors, such as excessive alcohol consumption, obesity, and lack of exercise, may also contribute to the risk of developing colorectal cancer. The reasons for this increased risk are also unknown.

About 1 in 8 cases of colorectal cancer is hereditary. Most of these cases are caused by inheritance of an abnormal gene. People who have this gene are at increased risk of developing a form of the cancer known as hereditary non-polyposis colorectal cancer (HNPCC). Rarely, colorectal cancer may be caused by the inherited disorder familial adenomatous polyposis (FAP), in which polyps (growths of tissue) form inside the large intestine (*see* POLYPS IN THE COLON, p.660). In FAP, there is a 9 in 10 chance that some of the polyps will become cancerous over time.

Inflammatory disorders affecting the large intestine, such as ulcerative colitis (p.659) or Crohn's disease (p.658), can also increase the risk of developing colorectal cancer if they are long-standing.

TREATMENT COLOSTOMY

In a colostomy, part of the colon is cut and the edges are attached to the skin of the abdomen to form an artificial opening called a stoma. Faeces are expelled through the stoma into a disposable bag. A colostomy is performed following a colectomy (p.665) and may be either temporary or permanent. If part of the colon has been removed, a temporary colostomy may be carried out to allow the rejoined ends to heal without faeces passing through the site. A permanent colostomy is needed when the rectum and anus are removed with part of the colon.

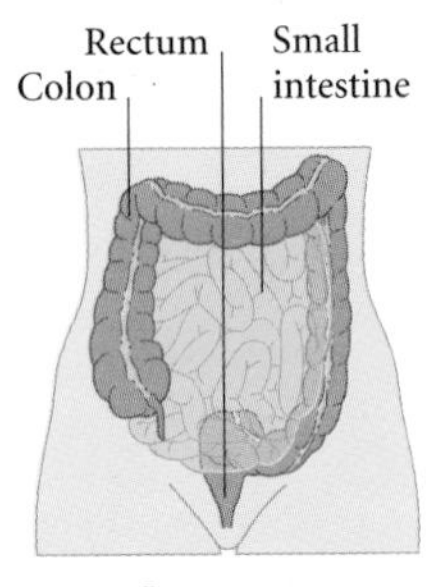

LOCATION

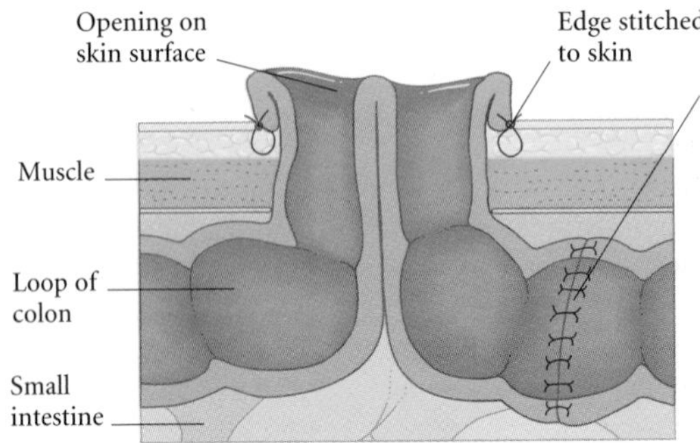

Temporary colostomy
An incision is made in a loop of colon and the edges of the loop are stitched to the skin surface. When the colectomy site has healed, the incision in the colon is closed and the colon is then returned under the skin.

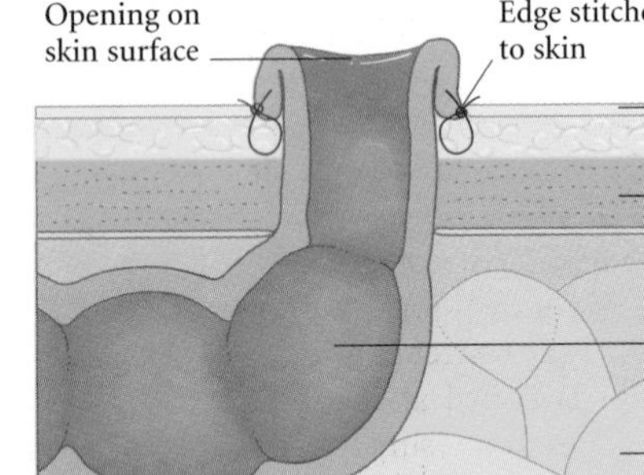

Permanent colostomy
The cut end of the colon is passed through the abdominal wall. The edges are then stitched to the skin surface to create a permanent opening. Normal defaecation is no longer possible.

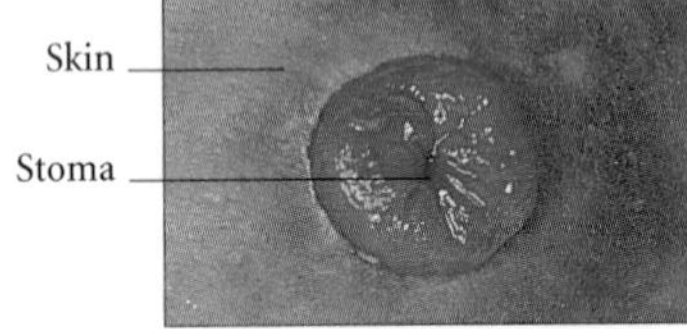

Permanent stoma
An artificial opening (stoma) can be seen on the surface of the abdomen. Faeces discharged from the intestine are collected in a disposable bag fitted over the stoma.

WHAT ARE THE SYMPTOMS?

The symptoms of colorectal cancer vary depending on the site of the tumour. They may include the following:

- Changes in the frequency of bowel movements or in the general consistency of the faeces.
- Abdominal pain.
- Blood in the faeces.
- Rectal discomfort or a sensation of incomplete emptying of the rectum.
- Loss of appetite.

The symptoms of colorectal cancer may be mistaken for the symptoms of a less serious disorder, such as haemorrhoids (p.668). If there is heavy loss of blood from the rectum, iron-deficiency anaemia (p.447) may result. This condition produces symptoms such as pale skin, headaches, and tiredness. As the tumour grows bigger, it may eventually cause intestinal obstruction (p.663).

You should consult your doctor without delay if you notice an obvious change in your bowel habits or blood in your faeces. Left untreated, colorectal cancer will eventually spread via the bloodstream to the lymph nodes, liver, and other organs in the body.

HOW IS IT DIAGNOSED?

Often, colorectal cancer is diagnosed during screening before symptoms have developed. If you do have symptoms, your doctor may feel your abdomen to detect swelling and carry out a rectal examination, in which a gloved finger is inserted into the rectum to feel for a tumour. A stool sample is tested for the presence of blood (*see* FAECAL OCCULT BLOOD TEST, p.233) and a blood sample is tested for evidence of anaemia.

The rectum may be examined visually with a viewing instrument inserted through the anus. Your doctor may also arrange for a colonoscopy, in which a flexible viewing instrument is used to examine the entire colon. A biopsy, in which a sample of intestinal tissue is removed for microscopic examination, may be performed during the procedure. You may also have a contrast X-ray (p.245) in which a barium enema is used to detect an abnormality of the rectum or colon. If a cancerous tumour is detected, you will probably need to have CT scanning (p.247) to see if the cancer has spread to the lymph nodes in the abdomen or to the liver.

In the UK, an annual faecal occult blood test is being considered for everyone over the age of 50. People who have a family history of colorectal cancer may wish to consult their doctor about the possibility of screening for the disorder.

What is the treatment?

Treatment of colorectal cancer depends on the site of the tumour. In most cases of early cancer, the affected part of the intestine can be removed and the cut ends rejoined (*see* Colectomy, p.665). In a few cases, if most of the rectum has been removed, a permanent colostomy (opposite page) may be necessary. In this procedure, an opening is created on the surface of the abdomen for the discharge of faeces. If the cancer cannot be cured, treatment is aimed at relieving the symptoms. For example, surgery may be done to remove a tumour obstructing the bowel. If cancer has spread to other parts of the body, chemotherapy (p.280), radiotherapy (p.281), or both may be necessary to treat the disease.

About 9 in 10 people treated at an early stage live at least 5 years free from cancer. Surgical removal of affected tissue at a more advanced stage of the disease gives the person a 3 in 4 chance of living 5 years free from cancer. If the cancer has spread, the outlook is poor.

(WWW) ONLINE SITES: p.1028, p.1030

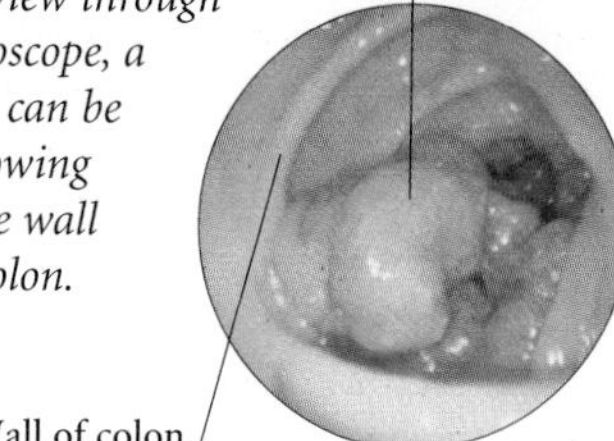

Colorectal cancer
In this view through a colonoscope, a tumour can be seen growing from the wall of the colon.

Proctitis

Inflammation of the rectum, most often due to ulcerative colitis

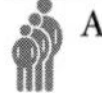 Age Rare in childhood

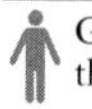 Gender Lifestyle Risk factors depend on the cause

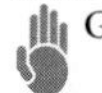 Genetics Not a significant factor

In proctitis, the lining of the anus and the rectum becomes inflamed. The disorder most commonly develops as part of ulcerative colitis (p.659), a condition that can either be restricted to the rectum or be a more widespread disease that also affects the colon.

Proctitis may also result from an infection of the lining of the rectum. Unprotected anal sex increases the risk of contracting a sexually transmitted infection (STI), such as herpes simplex infection (p.291) or gonorrhoea (p.764). Because anal sex may also lead to proctitis by causing physical injury to the rectum, the disorder is more common in homosexual men. Other causes of proctitis include the gastrointestinal infection amoebic dysentery (*see* Amoebiasis, p.306) and radiotherapy (p.281) used to treat cancers close to the rectum, such as prostate cancer (p.726).

What are the symptoms?

In most cases, the symptoms of proctitis include the following:

- Blood, mucus, or pus in the faeces.
- Discomfort and pain in the anus and rectum that becomes more severe with a bowel movement.
- Diarrhoea or constipation.
- An increased urge to defaecate.

Inflammation due to an STI may be accompanied by fever and pelvic pain. If the rectum is inflamed, there may also be an increased risk of acquiring or transmitting STIs, such as HIV infection (*see* HIV infection and AIDS, p.297), through unprotected anal sex.

In some cases, proctitis is complicated by the presence of an anal fissure (p.669) or an anal abscess (p.669).

How is it diagnosed?

Your doctor may ask for a stool sample or take a rectal swab to look for infection. He or she may also examine your rectum by using a viewing instrument called a proctoscope to determine the extent of the inflammation. A small sample of rectal tissue may be taken for examination under a microscope.

What is the treatment?

Treatment of proctitis depends on the cause. However, pain and inflammation, whatever the cause, may be eased with painkillers (p.912) and drugs to soften the faeces (*see* Laxatives, p.924). If the cause is ulcerative colitis, sulfasalazine (*see* Aminosalicylate drugs, p.924) or corticosteroids (p.930) are generally used to reduce inflammation.

Antibiotics (p.885) are usually given to treat a bacterial STI. Topical corticosteroids (p.892) can be used to reduce rectal inflammation caused by injury. Avoiding anal intercourse will help to speed up the healing process. Antibiotics may be given to treat amoebic dysentery, while proctitis due to radiotherapy is often treated with corticosteroids. Treatment is usually successful.

(WWW) ONLINE SITES: p.1030

Rectal prolapse

Protrusion of the lining of the rectum outside the anus

 Age Most common in young children and in elderly people

 Gender More common in males

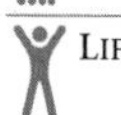 Lifestyle A low-fibre diet is a risk factor

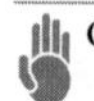 Genetics Not a significant factor

Rectal prolapse is an uncommon condition in which the lining of the rectum protrudes through the anus. It is usually associated with a low-fibre diet and constipation (p.628). The condition is more common in males and in elderly people and may be a recurrent problem in people who have weak pelvic floor muscles. In addition, rectal prolapse may sometimes occur temporarily in very young children during toilet training.

What are the symptoms?

If you have a rectal prolapse, you may experience symptoms after straining to defaecate. These include:

- Bleeding and discharge of mucus from the anus.
- Pain or discomfort on defaecation.

- The sensation of a lump protruding from the anus.

If the prolapse is large, there may also be some faecal incontinence.

What might be done?

Your doctor may examine the prolapse with a gloved finger and gently push the rectum back into place. Further treatment is used to relieve the underlying cause, such as a high-fibre diet to relieve constipation. If the prolapse recurs and you have persistent constipation, your doctor may arrange for tests, such as colonoscopy (p.661) or contrast X-rays (p.245), to look for an underlying disease, such as colorectal cancer (p.665).

In children, rectal prolapse will usually disappear when measures are taken to prevent constipation. Elderly people may require surgery to fix the rectum in position permanently.

(WWW) ONLINE SITES: p.1028, p.1030

Haemorrhoids

Swollen veins inside the rectum and around the anus, also known as piles

 AGE More common in adults

 GENDER More common in females during pregnancy and after childbirth

 LIFESTYLE Being overweight and a low-fibre diet are risk factors

 GENETICS Not a significant factor

Haemorrhoids are a common problem, affecting up to half of all people at some time in their lives. In this disorder, veins in the soft tissues around the anus and inside the lower part of the rectum become swollen. Swellings around the anus are called external haemorrhoids, and those within the rectum are called internal haemorrhoids. Internal haemorrhoids that protrude outside the anus are called prolapsing haemorrhoids.

Haemorrhoids often cause bleeding, itching, and discomfort. However, these symptoms are usually intermittent, and the condition is not in itself serious.

What are the causes?

Haemorrhoids most often result from constipation, when a person strains to pass stools. Straining in this way increases the pressure inside the abdomen, which in turn causes blood vessels around the rectum to swell. Constipation is often due to a low-fibre diet. Excess weight also exerts pressure on blood vessels and thus increases the risk of haemorrhoids. During pregnancy, the growing fetus has the same effect, frequently resulting in haemorrhoids.

What are the symptoms?

The symptoms of haemorrhoids commonly develop following constipation. They may include:

- Fresh blood on toilet paper or in the toilet after a bowel movement.
- Increasing discomfort on defaecation.
- Discharge of mucus from the anus, sometimes leading to itching.
- Visible swellings around the anus.
- Feeling that the bowels have not been fully emptied.

A prolapsing haemorrhoid may protrude through the anus after a bowel movement and may then retract or can be pushed back inside with a finger. In some cases, a blood clot (thrombus) may form within a prolapsing haemorrhoid, causing severe pain and a visible, tender, blue, grape-sized swelling.

If you have bleeding from the anus, you should consult your doctor without delay, especially if you are over 40, since it may indicate a more serious disorder, such as colorectal cancer (p.665).

What might be done?

Your doctor will probably examine your rectum by inserting a gloved finger into it, and, if there has been bleeding that suggests a serious underlying disease, may arrange for colonoscopy (p.661).

Small haemorrhoids do not usually need treatment. Haemorrhoids due to pregnancy usually disappear soon after the birth. A high-fibre diet helps to prevent constipation, and laxatives (p.924) may help to ease defaecation. Over-the-counter topical corticosteroids (p.892) and corticosteroid suppositories can reduce swelling and itching, and anaesthetic sprays may relieve pain. If these measures are not effective within a few days, you should consult your doctor, who may consider surgery.

Small internal haemorrhoids may be treated by sclerotherapy, in which the affected area is injected with a solution that causes the veins to shrink. Alternatively, the doctor may place a band around the base of an internal haemorrhoid, causing it to shrink and fall off (*see* BANDING HAEMORRHOIDS, below).

Persistent, painful, bleeding haemorrhoids can be destroyed by electrical, laser, or infrared heat treatment or be removed surgically. Treatment is usually successful, but they may recur.

(WWW) ONLINE SITES: p.1030

(TREATMENT) Banding haemorrhoids

Large or prolapsing haemorrhoids can be successfully treated by using a procedure called banding, in which a rubber band is placed around the base of the haemorrhoid. As a result, the haemorrhoid gradually shrinks over a period of several days and eventually drops off. Before the procedure, you may need a laxative to ensure that the rectum is empty. The procedure can be carried out in a doctor's surgery and is usually painless. The treated area may be sore for a few days afterwards.

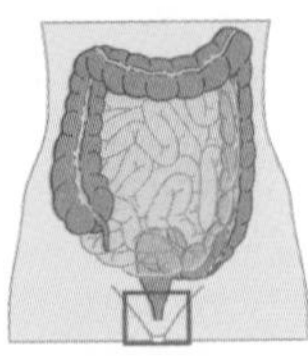
LOCATION

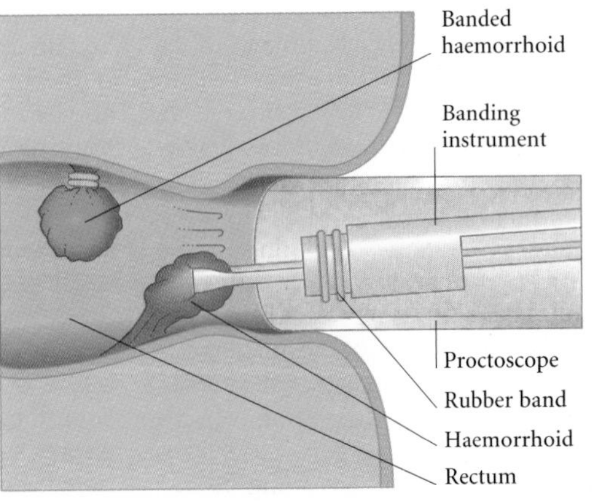

During the procedure
Using a short tube called a proctoscope, the doctor first grasps the haemorrhoid with forceps and then attaches a rubber band around the base using a banding instrument.

Anal abscess

An infected, pus-filled cavity in the anal or rectal area

 GENDER More common in males

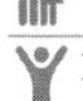 LIFESTYLE Anal sex is a risk factor

 AGE GENETICS Not significant factors

An anal abscess is a pus-filled cavity that develops when bacteria enter a mucus-secreting gland in the anus or rectum and multiply. The abscess may be deep within the rectum or close to the anus.

Inflammatory disorders of the colon, such as Crohn's disease (p.658), can be associated with anal abscesses. Anal sex also increases the risk.

You should consult a doctor if you have swelling or redness in the anal area or have a throbbing pain that worsens with defaecation. If the infection spreads from the anal area, you may also have a fever and feel generally unwell.

An anal abscess is usually diagnosed by a physical examination. Treatment involves draining the abscess through an incision under local anaesthesia. Drainage of deep or large abscesses may need a general anaesthetic. You may be given oral antibiotics (p.885) and advised to soak the affected area in warm water three or four times a day. An abscess may take several weeks to heal.

(WWW) ONLINE SITES: p.1030

Anal fissure

A tear in the lining of the anus that is usually a result of constipation

 LIFESTYLE A low-fibre diet is a risk factor

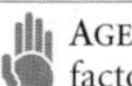 AGE GENDER GENETICS Not significant factors

The most common cause of an anal fissure is the passage of a large, hard stool due to constipation (p.628). This type of stool can tear the anal lining so that subsequent defaecation is extremely painful. You may also notice bright red blood on your faeces or the toilet paper.

Your doctor will diagnose an anal fissure during an examination of the anus. In some cases, the doctor views the anal lining using a viewing instrument called an anuscope.

Self-help measures to relieve constipation, such as using laxatives (p.924) and eating a high-fibre diet, may help the anal fissure to heal. However, further episodes of constipation may cause the fissure to recur. Persistent or recurrent anal fissures may eventually require surgery to loosen or stretch the ring of muscle around the anus.

(WWW) ONLINE SITES: p.1030

Anal itching

Irritation in or, more commonly, around the anus

 AGE GENDER LIFESTYLE Risk factors depend on the cause

GENETICS Not a significant factor

Anal itching (pruritus ani) is rarely a serious condition, although it may be embarrassing and hard to treat. Itching may be either localized around the anus or part of a generalized itching disorder (*see* ITCHING, p.339). It may be worse in older people because their skin is drier, less elastic, and more easily irritated.

Localized anal itching may be caused by poor personal hygiene, haemorrhoids (opposite page), or threadworm infestation (p.310). Generalized itching around the anal area may be a symptom of a skin disease, such as psoriasis (p.332) or eczema (p.333), or be due to an allergic reaction to a substance such as detergent or soap.

WHAT MIGHT BE DONE?

There are several measures you can take to relieve anal itching. It is important to keep the anal area clean by washing and drying carefully after a bowel movement. Avoid using soaps that irritate the skin, and try not to scratch because it will worsen the itching. A warm bath or shower before bed may soothe night-time itching. Loose underclothes made of natural fibres are less likely than synthetic materials to cause irritation. An over-the-counter cream containing a topical corticosteroid (p.892) may give relief. Itching that lasts for longer than 3 days should be assessed by a doctor.

Your doctor may examine your anus and arrange for tests to look for causes that require treatment. For example, haemorrhoids may need to be removed.

(WWW) ONLINE SITES: p.1030, p.1036

Anal cancer

Cancer of the anus or anal canal, which may cause pain and bleeding

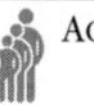 AGE More common with increasing age

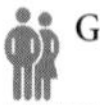 GENDER More common in males

 GENETICS LIFESTYLE Not significant factors

Cancer of the anus or the anal canal (the passage from the rectum to outside the body) is very rare. Although the cause is not known, there may be a link between anal cancer and human papillomaviruses, which cause genital warts (p.768) and are also associated with cancer of the cervix (p.750).

WHAT ARE THE SYMPTOMS?

The symptoms of anal cancer usually develop gradually and include:

- Bleeding from the anus.
- Itching or discomfort in the anal area.
- Frequent desire to defaecate.
- A lump in or near the anus.

If you have any of these symptoms, you should consult your doctor to determine the cause. Left untreated, anal cancer may spread to nearby tissues and eventually to other parts of the body.

WHAT MIGHT BE DONE?

Your doctor will first examine the anus and then insert a gloved finger into the rectum to feel for lumps. Under local anaesthesia, your doctor may remove a sample of tissue from the anal canal for examination under a microscope.

If anal cancer is diagnosed, you will need further tests to detect whether the cancer has spread. These tests include blood tests and CT scanning (p.247) or MRI (p.248) of the abdomen and pelvis.

The usual treatment is chemotherapy (p.280) with radiotherapy (p.281). In about 2 in 3 people, this treatment causes the tumour to shrink so that surgery is not needed. In most people, treatment is curative. However, in rare cases, surgery is necessary to remove the anus and part of the rectum.

If the cancer has already spread to other parts of the body, the outlook is poor. However, surgery in combination with radiotherapy may relieve the symptoms and prolong life.

(WWW) ONLINE SITES: p.1028, p.1030

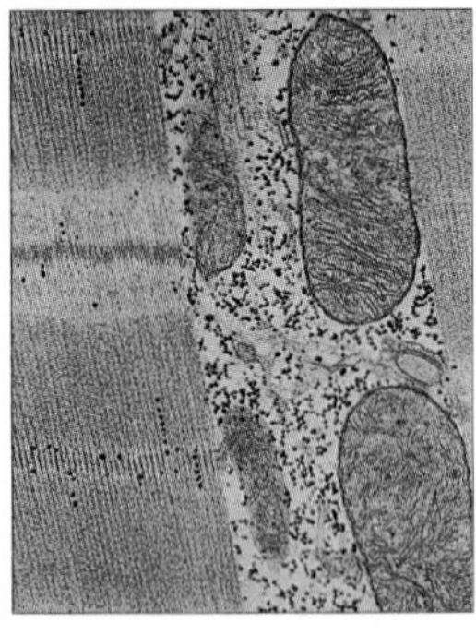
Glycogen in muscles
Glycogen stores, which break down into glucose to supply energy, appear as black dots in this view of muscle cells.

HORMONES AND METABOLISM

THE WORD HORMONE is derived from a Greek term meaning "to excite" or "to spur on". Hormones are chemical messengers that alter the activity of or "excite" targeted cells. They are produced in various specialized glands and cells throughout the body and are transported in the bloodstream to their specific sites of action. Hormones regulate many important body processes and functions, including growth, reproduction, and metabolism, the collective term for all the chemical reactions that occur in the body.

Hormones are produced by a number of different glands and cells that are described collectively as the endocrine system. The major endocrine glands – the pituitary, thyroid, parathyroid, and adrenal glands and the pancreas, ovaries, and testes – are all primarily dedicated to the production of various hormones. However, other organs in the body with major functions of their own also contain cells that produce hormones. For example, the main function of the kidneys is to filter the blood, but they also contain endocrine cells that secrete hormones.

Hormones are transported in the bloodstream to their target tissues, which may then be stimulated to produce other hormones in a chain reaction. For example, the pituitary gland produces thyroid-stimulating hormone (TSH), which travels to the thyroid gland where it stimulates the production of thyroid hormones.

Hormones also regulate the balance of certain substances in the blood.If there is too much or too little of a substance, a feedback mechanism restores the correct levels. The pituitary, a pea-sized gland regulated by a part of the brain called the hypothalamus, has overall control of most hormone production.

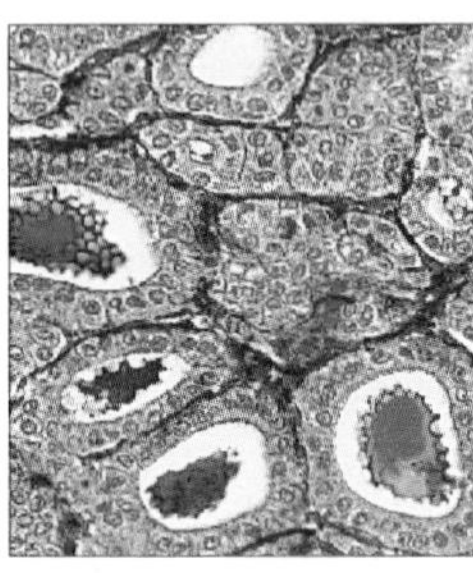
Thyroid gland tissue
This image shows hormone-secreting cells in the thyroid gland. The red areas are stores of hormones.

Some hormones work on cells throughout the body. For example, certain thyroid hormones influence metabolic rate. Others have specific target cells, such as the hormone vasopressin, which acts on specific cells in the kidneys to regulate urine concentration.

When we are under stress or excited, the two adrenal glands increase production of hormones that affect our blood pressure, circulation, and breathing, creating the heightened states that form part of our "fight or flight" response to danger.

Throughout life, hormone levels rise and fall. For example, during puberty sex hormones rise sharply, and in women levels fall after the menopause.

PROCESS FEEDBACK MECHANISM

Hormone secretion is regulated by feedback mechanisms in order to maintain correct levels of substances in the blood. For example, a drop in the calcium level in the bloodstream stimulates an increase in the secretion of parathyroid hormone (PTH), which acts on various parts of the body to raise calcium levels. When calcium reaches the normal level, PTH secretion decreases.

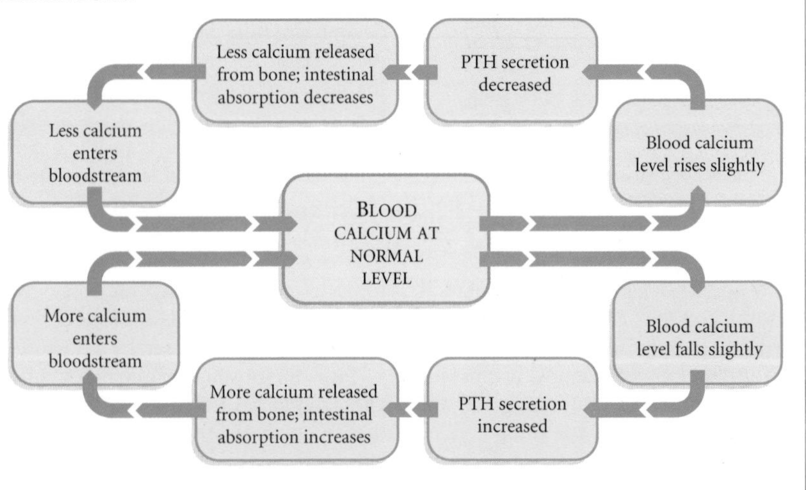

Maintaining blood calcium levels
The parathyroid glands detect fluctuations in calcium levels in the blood and secrete appropriate amounts of parathyroid hormone (PTH) to correct them.

STRUCTURE AND FUNCTION HORMONE-SECRETING GLANDS AND CELLS

Most endocrine cells are grouped together in organs, such as the pituitary, thyroid, and adrenal glands, whose only purpose is to produce hormones. However, hormone-secreting cells are also present in many other tissues that have a different primary function. For example, the kidneys secrete hormones that stimulate red blood cell production, although their main role is to filter the blood. New chemical substances that act as hormones are still being discovered and their specific roles in the body clarified.

Pituitary gland
The pituitary gland secretes many hormones. Some of these act on other glands, stimulating them to produce their own hormones, while others act directly on target tissues and organs

Thymus
This gland is part of the immune system but also produces hormones that control the production of a group of white blood cells called T cells

Adrenal gland
The two adrenal glands produce hormones that control metabolism and hormones involved in the body's responses to stress

Kidney
The main role of the kidneys is to filter blood, but they also produce erythropoietin, which stimulates red blood cell production

Duodenum
The duodenum secretes hormones that act on other digestive organs, such as the gallbladder

Intestines
Endocrine cells in the lining of the intestines release several hormones that are involved in digestion

Ovary
The two ovaries produce progesterone and oestrogen, two hormones involved in the menstrual cycle. Oestrogen also plays a part in the development of female secondary sexual characteristics

Placenta
During pregnancy, the placenta, which forms in the uterus, produces certain hormones that are essential for fetal development

Hypothalamus
Although not strictly part of the endocrine system, the hypothalamus acts as the link between the nervous system and the endocrine system. It produces hormones called releasing factors that control the pituitary gland

Pineal gland
This gland produces the hormone melatonin, which controls body rhythms, such as sleeping and waking, and may also play a role in sexual development

Parathyroid gland
The four parathyroid glands are embedded in the back of the thyroid gland. They produce parathyroid hormone, which helps to regulate calcium levels in the blood

Thyroid gland
This gland produces hormones that have important roles in many aspects of metabolism, including energy use

Heart
During physical exertion, the heart muscle produces natriuretic hormone, which helps to control blood pressure

Stomach
Endocrine cells in the lining of the stomach secrete the hormone gastrin, which stimulates the secretion of acid to aid digestion

Pancreas
The pancreas secretes many different hormones. The most important of these are insulin and glucagon, which control glucose levels in the bloodstream

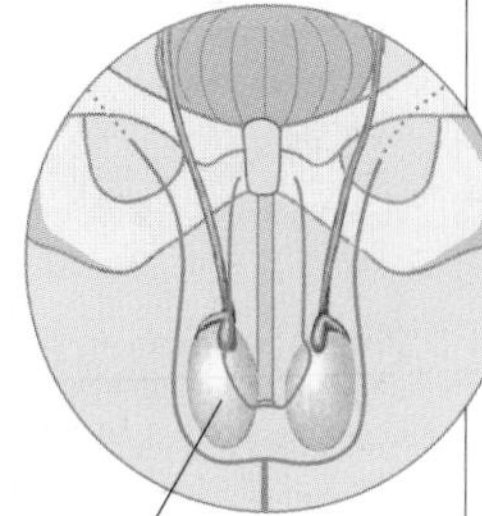

Testis
The two testes produce male sex hormones (mainly testosterone). These hormones stimulate sperm production and the development of male secondary sexual characteristics

STRUCTURE AND FUNCTION

PITUITARY GLAND

The pituitary gland controls the activities of many other endocrine glands and hormone-producing cells around the body. The pituitary gland has two parts, the anterior and posterior lobes, which are under the control of a part of the brain known as the hypothalamus. The hypothalamus secretes releasing hormones that pass through the circulation to the pituitary's anterior lobe, where they trigger the production of hormones that control other glands. Nerve cells in the hypothalamus secrete two hormones that pass down nerve fibres to be stored in the posterior lobe until they are needed.

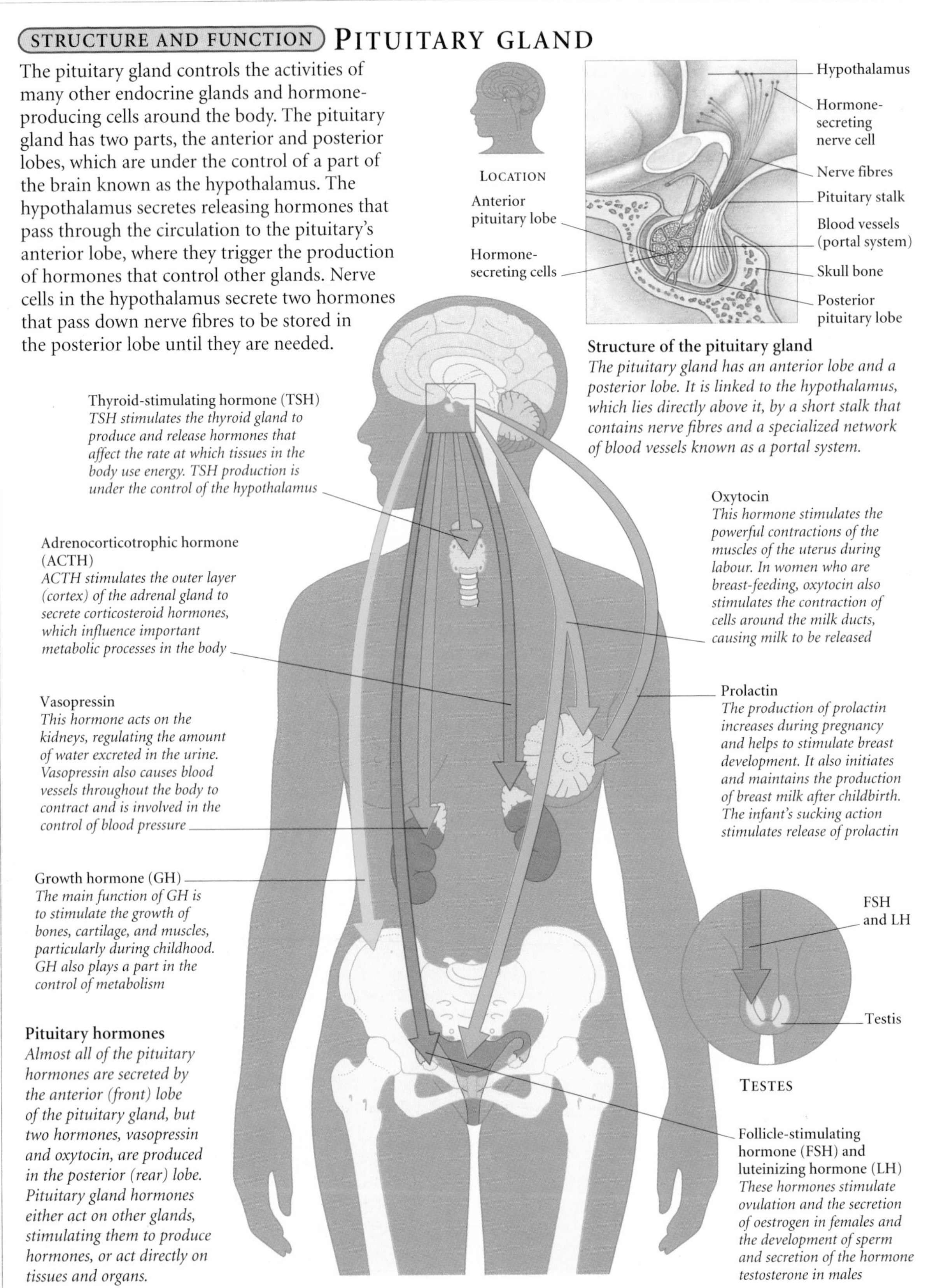

Structure of the pituitary gland
The pituitary gland has an anterior lobe and a posterior lobe. It is linked to the hypothalamus, which lies directly above it, by a short stalk that contains nerve fibres and a specialized network of blood vessels known as a portal system.

Pituitary hormones
Almost all of the pituitary hormones are secreted by the anterior (front) lobe of the pituitary gland, but two hormones, vasopressin and oxytocin, are produced in the posterior (rear) lobe. Pituitary gland hormones either act on other glands, stimulating them to produce hormones, or act directly on tissues and organs.

STRUCTURE AND FUNCTION THYROID AND PARATHYROID GLANDS

The thyroid and parathyroid glands are situated close to each other in the front of the neck. The thyroid gland produces the hormone thyroxine (T_4) and its more active form, T_3, which act on body cells to regulate metabolism (the chemical reactions continually occurring in the body). Some thyroid cells secrete the hormone calcitonin, which lowers calcium in the blood. The parathyroid glands produce parathyroid hormone (PTH), the main regulator of calcium.

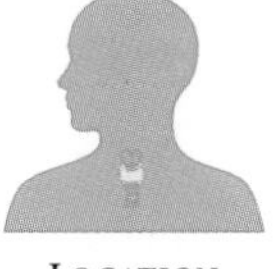

Structure of the thyroid and parathyroid glands
The thyroid gland is wrapped around the front of the trachea. The four parathyroid glands are at the back of the thyroid gland.

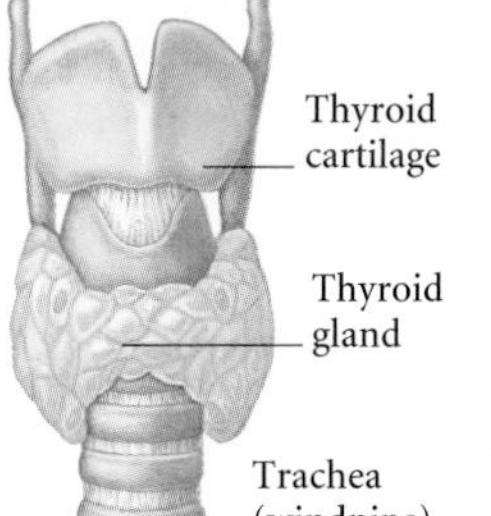

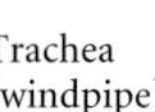

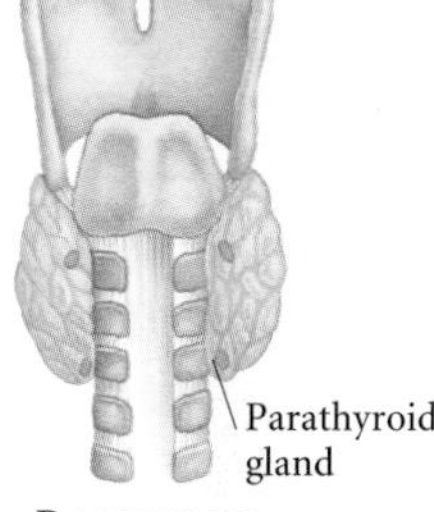

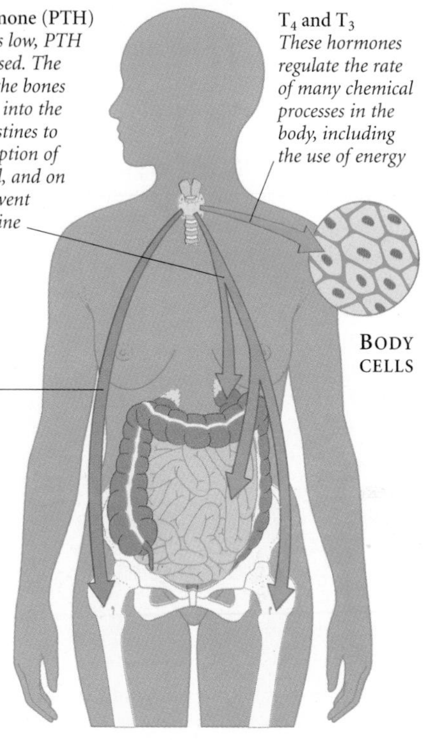

Thyroid and parathyroid hormones
Iodine from the diet is used to make the hormones T_4 and T_3. These hormones are produced by the thyroid gland and regulate body metabolism. Parathyroid hormone (PTH) and, to a lesser extent, calcitonin regulate levels of calcium and phosphate.

STRUCTURE AND FUNCTION ADRENAL GLANDS

Each adrenal gland has two parts. The cortex (outer layer) is controlled by the pituitary gland and produces several corticosteroid hormones, the most important of which affect metabolism and blood pressure. The cortex also secretes small amounts of male sex hormones (androgens). The medulla (core) influences the autonomic nervous system by releasing the hormones epinephrine (adrenaline) and norepinephrine (noradrenaline), which increase heart activity and blood flow in response to excitement or stress.

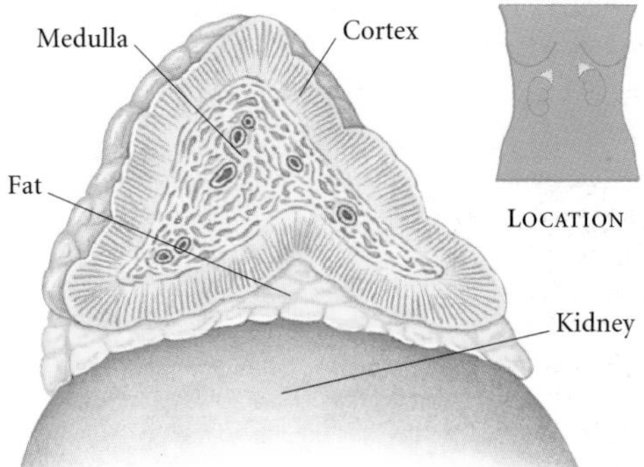

Structure of the adrenal gland
The adrenal glands rest on pads of fat above the kidneys. Each gland has an outer cortex, which makes up 90 per cent of its weight, and an inner medulla.

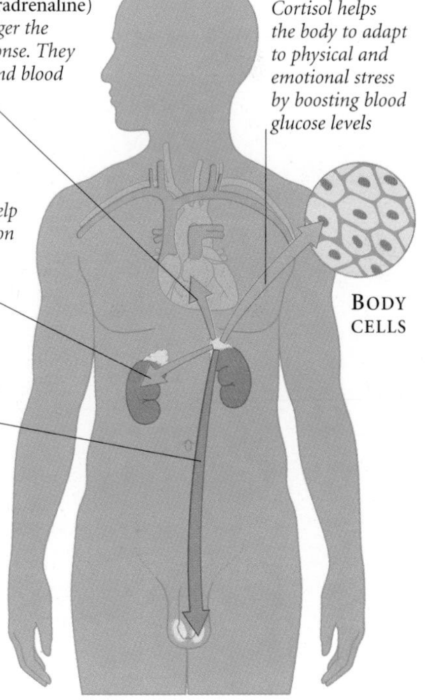

Adrenal hormones
The corticosteroid hormones cortisol and aldosterone and small amounts of male sex hormones are secreted by the cortex. The medulla secretes epinephrine (adrenaline) and norepinephrine (noradrenaline).

STRUCTURE AND FUNCTION

PANCREAS

The pancreas has two functions. It plays a major role in digestion, releasing enzymes that break down fat, starch, and proteins through the pancreatic ducts into the intestine. It also contains clusters of cells, called islets of Langerhans, that secrete hormones directly into the bloodstream. These cells secrete insulin and glucagon, two hormones that regulate glucose levels in the body, and other digestive hormones.

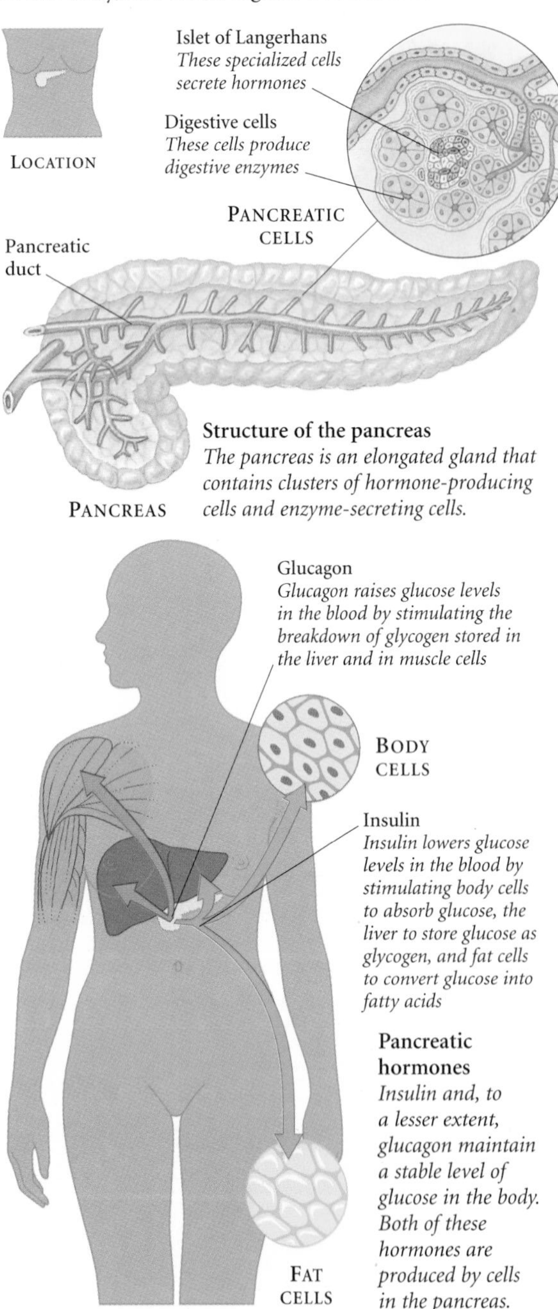

Structure of the pancreas
The pancreas is an elongated gland that contains clusters of hormone-producing cells and enzyme-secreting cells.

Pancreatic hormones
Insulin and, to a lesser extent, glucagon maintain a stable level of glucose in the body. Both of these hormones are produced by cells in the pancreas.

PROCESS

METABOLISM

Thousands of chemical reactions and conversions take place continuously in body cells to keep the body alive and healthy and to generate energy. Metabolism is the collective term for all these chemical processes. The raw materials for metabolic processes are obtained from nutrients in food, which are broken down into simple molecules during digestion. These molecules are either recycled and built up into new complex molecules that can be used to repair or make new cells (anabolism) or are further broken down to release energy (catabolism).

ANABOLISM AND CATABOLISM

In anabolic processes, body cells are built up and repaired, or complex substances are constructed out of simpler ones. In catabolic processes, complex molecules are broken down into simple molecules, such as glucose and amino acids, and these simple molecules are broken down to supply the cells with energy and materials for renewing cell structures.

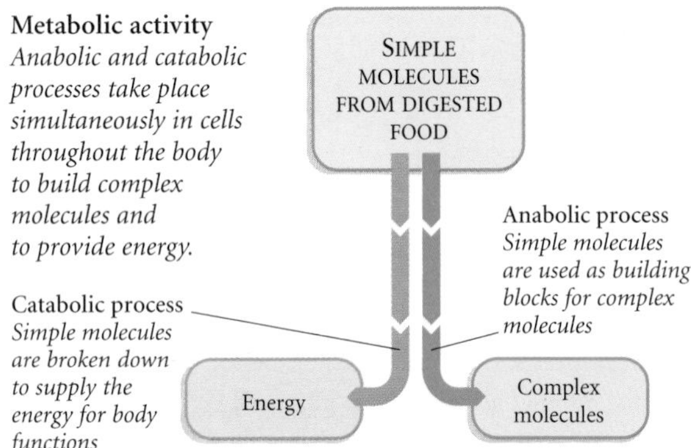

Metabolic activity
Anabolic and catabolic processes take place simultaneously in cells throughout the body to build complex molecules and to provide energy.

BASAL METABOLIC RATE

The amount of energy a person uses for essential functions, such as maintaining body heat, breathing, and heart rate, is called the basal metabolic rate (BMR). BMR decreases naturally with age, but it is raised in the short term by factors such as illness, pregnancy, breast-feeding, and menstruation. All forms of exercise increase the body's use of energy above the BMR.

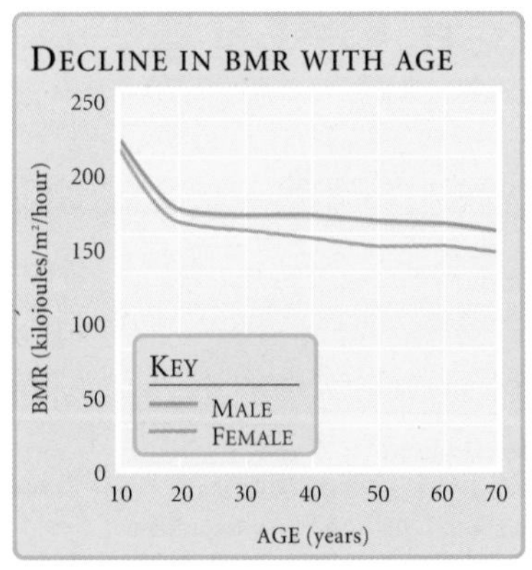

Basal metabolic rate (BMR)
After about the age of 10, basal metabolic rate decreases with age and tends to be lower in females than in males. BMR is measured at rest and is often expressed as kilojoules used per square metre of body surface per hour (1 kilojoule equals about 4 kilocalories).

How the body uses food

Every living body cell depends on essential nutrients in food. Carbohydrates, proteins, and fats are converted into glucose, amino acids, and fatty acids respectively during digestion. These molecules enter the lymphatic system and the bloodstream and are converted into a usable form (metabolized) in the liver and in all body cells. Glucose is used to produce energy, as are fatty acids when glucose is in short supply. Amino acids are used to build the complex proteins needed to make and repair cells.

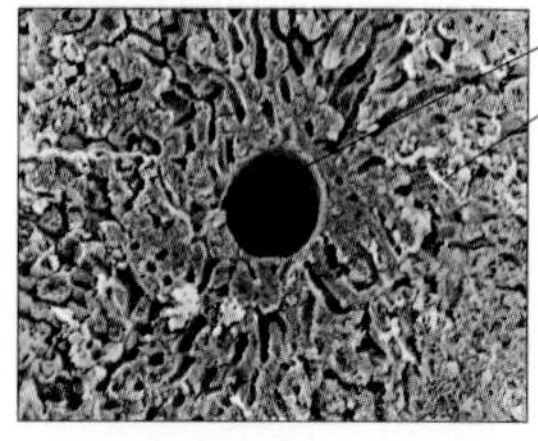

Liver tissue
The liver has a rich blood supply. This magnified view of liver tissue shows a blood vessel surrounded by large liver cells (hepatocytes).

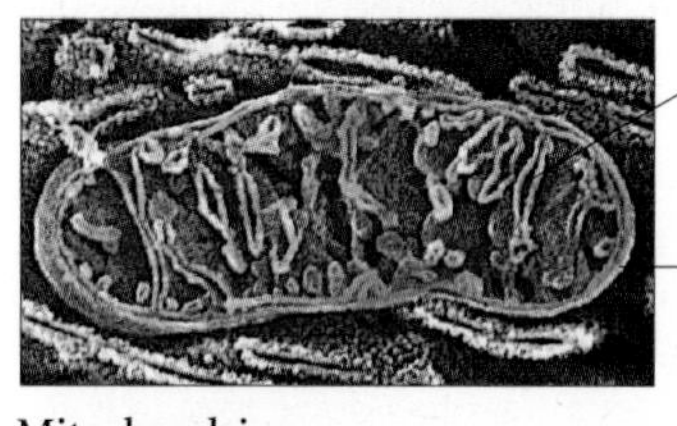

Mitochondrion
Each body cell contains many mitochondria. This magnified image of a mitochondrion, the cell "powerhouse", shows the folds (cristae) where energy-producing reactions take place.

Digestion
During digestion, complex carbohydrates are converted into simple sugars, such as glucose; fats and oils are broken down into fatty acids and glycerol; and proteins are broken down into amino acids. The bloodstream transports these nutrients to the liver, the body's major metabolic site, and then to all body cells.

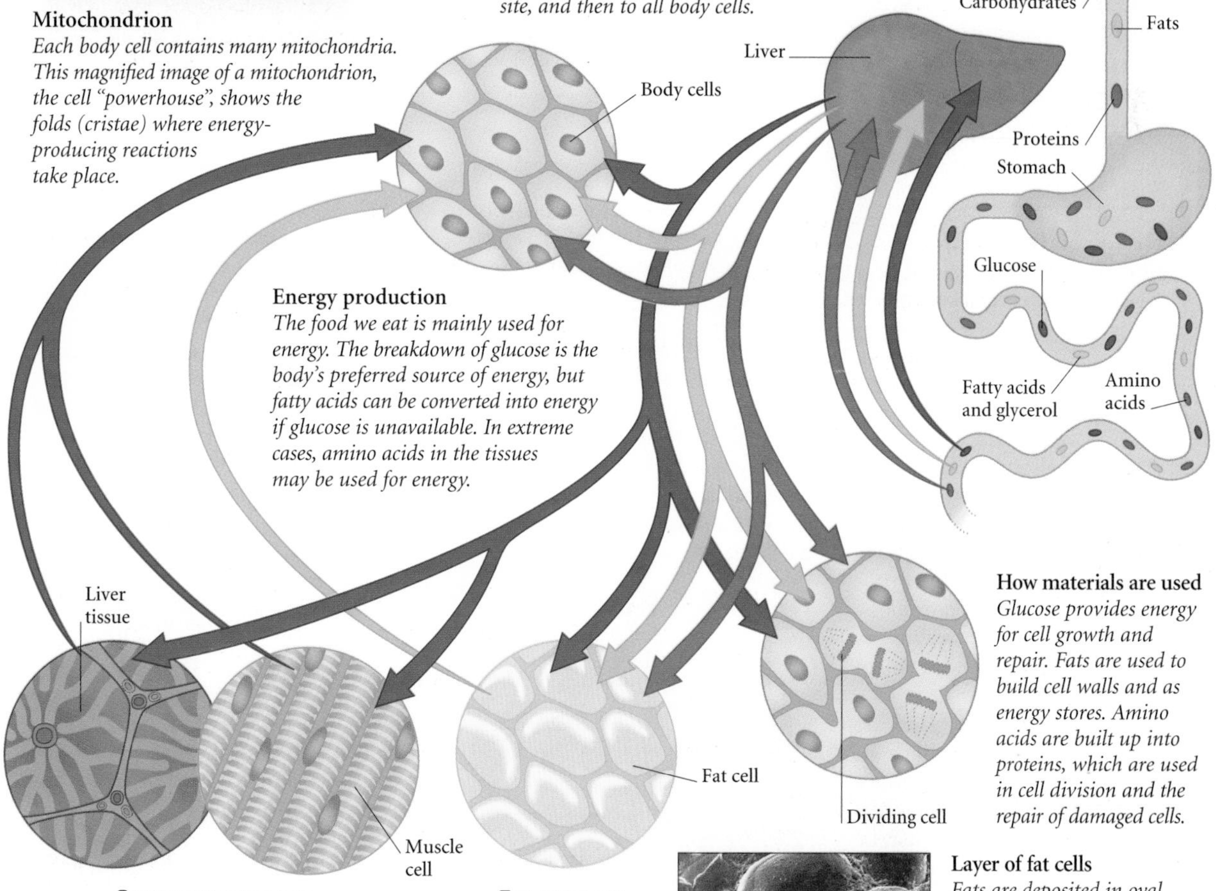

Carbohydrates
Fats
Liver
Body cells
Proteins
Stomach
Glucose
Fatty acids and glycerol
Amino acids

Energy production
The food we eat is mainly used for energy. The breakdown of glucose is the body's preferred source of energy, but fatty acids can be converted into energy if glucose is unavailable. In extreme cases, amino acids in the tissues may be used for energy.

Liver tissue
Muscle cell
Fat cell
Dividing cell

GLYCOGEN STORAGE
FAT STORAGE

How materials are used
Glucose provides energy for cell growth and repair. Fats are used to build cell walls and as energy stores. Amino acids are built up into proteins, which are used in cell division and the repair of damaged cells.

Storage of materials
Surplus glucose is stored in the liver and muscle cells as glycogen. This substance can be broken down into glucose and used for instant energy. Excess fats are stored as fatty acids in fat cells. Excess amino acids cannot be stored, but they can be converted into fatty acids for storage in fat cells. If glycogen stores are full, excess glucose is also converted into fatty acids for storage.

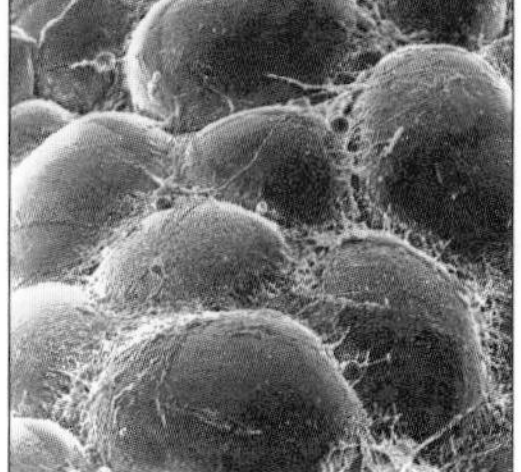

Layer of fat cells
Fats are deposited in oval storage cells known as fat cells or adipocytes. These cells form a layer, which varies in thickness, beneath the skin to insulate the body. A thin layer of adipose tissue surrounds the heart, kidneys, and other delicate internal organs.

PITUITARY GLAND DISORDERS

The pituitary gland is a small gland at the base of the brain that produces a large number of the hormones controlling growth, sexual development, and water balance. The gland also produces hormones that control many other hormone-secreting glands, such as the thyroid gland. Most pituitary disorders are caused by tumours that alter the output of particular pituitary hormones.

This section opens with a discussion of various tumours of the pituitary gland. Some types cause underproduction of particular hormones, and others cause overproduction. The abnormal hormone levels can have adverse effects elsewhere in the body; these effects are discussed in the articles that follow.

Particular pituitary hormones affect other hormone-secreting glands in the body; a pituitary disorder may thus lead to a disorder in another gland (*see* THYROID AND PARATHYROID GLAND DISORDERS, pp.679–683, and ADRENAL GLAND DISORDERS, pp.684–686). Sex hormone disorders that may be caused by a problem with the pituitary gland are discussed elsewhere (*see* MALE HORMONAL DISORDERS, pp.728–729, and MENSTRUAL, MENOPAUSAL, AND HORMONAL PROBLEMS, pp.734–740), as are growth abnormalities in children that result from pituitary disorders (*see* GROWTH DISORDERS, p.869).

KEY ANATOMY

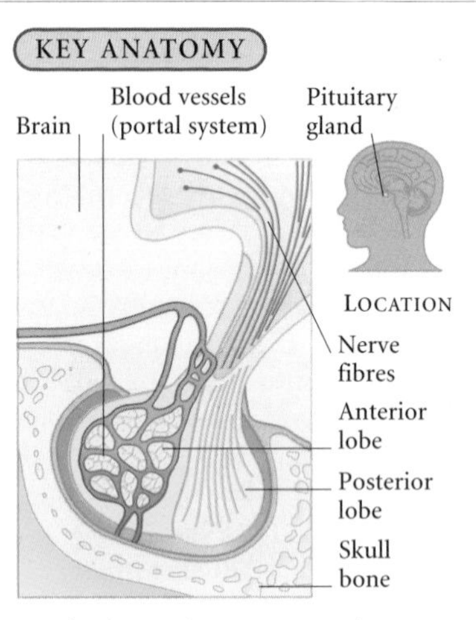

For further information on the structure and function of the pituitary gland, *see* pp.670–675.

Pituitary tumours

Abnormal growths in the pituitary gland, which may cause hormonal disturbances

AGE GENDER GENETICS LIFESTYLE
Risk factors depend on the type

The pituitary gland, located at the base of the brain, secretes hormones that either have a direct effect on the body or affect other hormone-secreting glands. For this reason, an abnormality in the pituitary gland may affect several body systems. Some pituitary tumours produce excessive amounts of hormones; others do not produce hormones themselves but can disrupt the production of hormones from adjacent cells.

Tumours of the pituitary gland are rare. Usually, tumours occur in the front part of the gland and are noncancerous. The cause of most pituitary tumours is not known, although rarely they may be associated with the inherited disorder multiple endocrine neoplasia (p.683).

WHAT ARE THE TYPES?

Nearly half of all hormone-secreting pituitary tumours make excess prolactin. Increased levels of prolactin may lead to infertility in women and to impotence in men (*see* PROLACTINOMA, opposite page). Some pituitary tumours secrete growth hormone, causing enlargement of certain parts of the body (*see* ACROMEGALY, opposite page). Others secrete hormones that overstimulate the adrenal glands, causing changes in body chemistry and physical appearance (*see* CUSHING'S SYNDROME, p.684).

As it grows, any pituitary tumour may press against the optic nerves, which lie above the gland. Such compression may cause headaches and loss of part of the field of vision (*see* VISUAL FIELD DEFECTS, p.590). Growing pituitary tumours may also damage surrounding cells, thereby reducing secretion of one or more pituitary hormones (*see* HYPOPITUITARISM, p.678). Reduced secretion of thyroid-stimulating hormone (TSH) may cause hypothyroidism (p.680). A tumour that presses on the posterior part of the pituitary gland may reduce secretion of vasopressin, which controls water balance (*see* DIABETES INSIPIDUS, p.678).

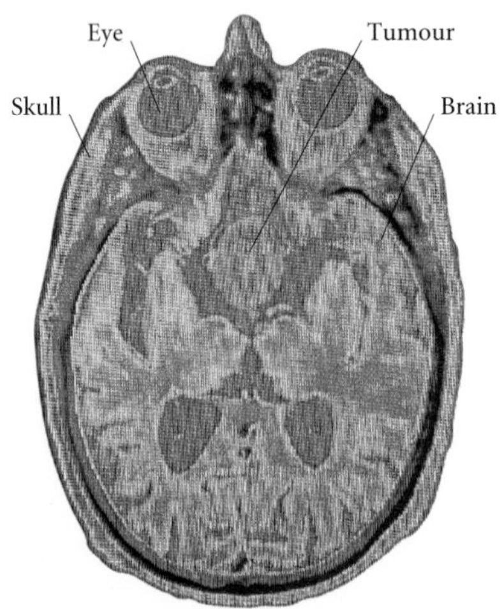

Pituitary tumour
This MRI scan of the head reveals a large pituitary tumour, which may affect vision and produce headaches.

WHAT MIGHT BE DONE?

You may have several blood tests to look for abnormal levels of pituitary hormones. You may also have MRI (p.248) or CT scanning (p.247) to look for a tumour and a visual field test (p.590) to check for blind areas. In some instances, a pituitary tumour is discovered during tests for another disorder. In this case, the tumour may be monitored without treatment unless symptoms develop.

Some tumours are treated with drugs (*see* PITUITARY DRUGS, p.934). Others must be removed surgically. If it is not possible to remove the whole tumour, radiotherapy (p.281) may be given to prevent further growth of abnormal tissue. These treatments can result in hypopituitarism, which may need hormone replacement for life.

(WWW) ONLINE SITES: p.1028, p.1033

Prolactinoma

A pituitary tumour causing excess secretion of prolactin, a hormone that influences fertility and breast milk production

GENDER More common in females

AGE GENETICS LIFESTYLE Not significant factors

A prolactinoma is a noncancerous type of pituitary tumour. The tumour causes an excess of the hormone prolactin, which is essential for breast development and milk production in women. Although women's prolactin levels normally increase during pregnancy, an excessive level of the hormone can have adverse effects in both men and women. Prolactinomas occur more frequently in women. The cause is unknown.

WHAT ARE THE SYMPTOMS?

A prolactinoma usually develops over a period of several years, and the symptoms appear gradually. Symptoms that affect only women include:

- Irregular or absent menstrual periods (*see* AMENORRHOEA, p.735).
- Infertility.

Some symptoms of prolactinoma affect only men, and these include:

- Impotence.
- Breast enlargement.

There are some symptoms that affect both sexes, and these include:

- Leakage of fluid from the nipples.
- Reduced interest in sex.

An untreated tumour may grow large enough to put pressure on surrounding areas of the brain. The pressure may cause headaches, loss of the normal field of vision (*see* VISUAL FIELD DEFECTS, p.590), or hypopituitarism (p.678).

WHAT MIGHT BE DONE?

If your doctor suspects that you have a prolactinoma, he or she will initially want to know if you could be pregnant or taking drugs, such as certain antipsychotics (p.917), that raise levels of prolactin and are not related to the presence of a prolactinoma. You will probably have a blood test to measure hormone levels. If the prolactin level is high, you may have imaging tests such as CT scanning (p.247) or MRI (p.248) to look for a pituitary tumour. If a tumour is found, drugs may be given to reduce production of prolactin (*see* PITUITARY DRUGS, p.934). If treatment with drugs is unsuccessful, surgery or radiotherapy (p.281) may be necessary to remove or destroy the tumour.

WHAT IS THE PROGNOSIS?

Drug treatment is successful in more than 3 in 4 cases. In the others, surgery or radiotherapy is usually effective. Less commonly, the tumour may recur and treatment may need to be repeated.

If a woman becomes pregnant after treatment for a prolactinoma, she will be monitored carefully because the tumour may recur as a result of the hormonal changes. Drugs to lower prolactin levels are discontinued during pregnancy.

(WWW) ONLINE SITES: p.1033

Acromegaly

Excessive growth of parts of the body due to overproduction of growth hormone by the pituitary gland

AGE May occur at any age

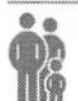
GENETICS Occasionally runs in families

GENDER LIFESTYLE Not significant factors

Acromegaly is a rare condition that results from overproduction of growth hormone by the pituitary gland. Overproduction of growth hormone causes certain bones, particularly those in the face, hands, and feet, to enlarge. Soft tissues, such as the tongue, also become enlarged. Acromegaly may occur at any age. If excess growth hormone is produced during childhood, the condition causes exaggerated bone growth resulting in excessive height, and is called gigantism (*see* GROWTH DISORDERS, p.869).

Acromegaly is usually caused by a pituitary tumour (opposite page). In rare cases, acromegaly occurs as part of multiple endocrine neoplasia (p.683), an inherited disorder in which tumours develop in several of the endocrine glands around the body.

WHAT ARE THE SYMPTOMS?

If acromegaly develops in adulthood, the resulting physical changes occur almost imperceptibly over a period of years. Sometimes, the condition is detected by comparing old photographs with more recent ones. The following symptoms may become noticeable:

- Changes in the shape of the face, such as enlargement of the jaw.
- Enlargement of the hands or feet, resulting in a larger glove or shoe size.
- Deepening of the voice.
- Enlargement of the tongue.
- Tingling in the hands and feet.
- Excessive sweating.
- Increased growth of coarse body hair.

A growing pituitary tumour may press on the brain, causing headaches and loss of the normal field of vision (*see* VISUAL FIELD DEFECTS, p.590) in addition to the symptoms of acromegaly. If not treated, acromegaly may cause serious disorders, such as diabetes mellitus (p.687) and enlargement of the heart (*see* DILATED CARDIOMYOPATHY, p.427), which may lead to chronic heart failure (p.413).

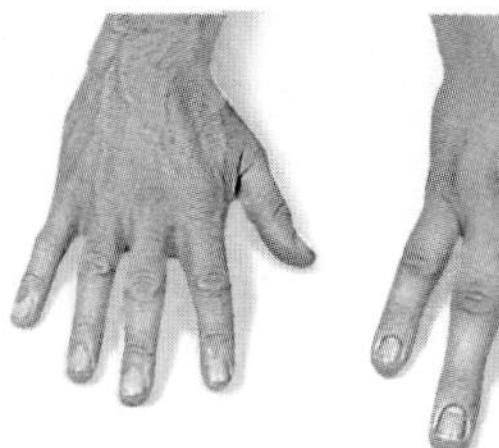
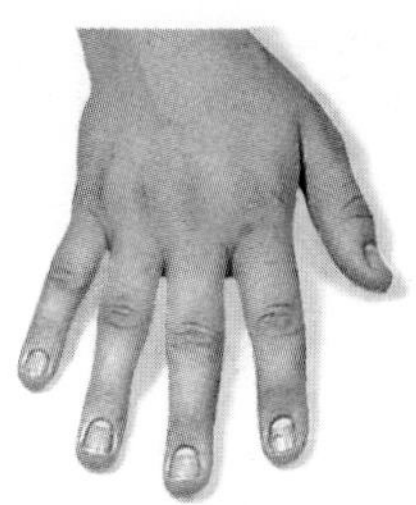

Enlarged hand in acromegaly
Acromegaly can lead to enlarged hands, as shown in this comparison between the hand of an affected man and that of an unaffected man of similar build.

WHAT MIGHT BE DONE?

Your doctor may arrange for you to have several blood tests. If these tests reveal high growth hormone levels, you may also undergo imaging procedures, such as MRI (p.248) or CT scanning (p.247), to look for a pituitary tumour.

Small pituitary tumours can usually be removed completely by surgery. If a tumour is large or cannot be removed entirely, radiotherapy (p.281) may be necessary to destroy the remaining tumour cells, or drugs may be given to reduce the production of growth hormone (*see* PITUITARY DRUGS, p.934).

Treatment is usually effective and prevents life-threatening complications from developing. Soft tissues will gradually decrease in size. However, changes in the size of bones cannot be reversed.

(WWW) ONLINE SITES: p.1033

Hypopituitarism

Insufficient production of some or all of the pituitary hormones

AGE GENDER GENETICS LIFESTYLE
Not significant factors

Hypopituitarism is a rare condition in which the pituitary gland secretes inadequate amounts of one or more of its hormones. In some cases, the disorder is progressive, ultimately causing underproduction of all pituitary hormones.

Hypopituitarism is usually caused by a pituitary tumour that damages normal tissue in the gland as it grows. The disorder may also be due to other factors that damage the pituitary gland or the hypothalamus, the part of the brain directly above the pituitary gland. Such factors include surgery or radiotherapy (p.281) to treat a pituitary tumour or other head or neck tumour, head injury (p.521), or heavy blood loss that deprives the gland of oxygen.

WHAT ARE THE SYMPTOMS?

The symptoms may appear suddenly but more commonly develop gradually and can go unrecognized for months or years. They may include:

- Loss of interest in sex.
- Lack of menstrual periods in women.
- Loss of facial hair and shrinking of the testes in men.
- Loss of underarm and pubic hair.
- Dizziness, nausea, and vomiting.
- Paleness of the skin.
- Tiredness, constipation, weight gain, and intolerance to cold.

Left untreated, hypopituitarism can lead to coma and be fatal. This is because the body is unable to increase the output of hormones needed to respond to physical stresses such as injury or infection.

WHAT MIGHT BE DONE?

If your doctor suspects that you have hypopituitarism, he or she will probably arrange for blood tests to check your hormone levels. You may also need to undergo tests in hospital to determine hormone production in response to various chemical stimulants, and you may have MRI (p.248) or CT scanning (p.247) to look for a pituitary tumour.

If a tumour is detected, you may have surgery to remove it, followed by radiotherapy to prevent a recurrence. Hypopituitarism can be treated with lifelong hormone-replacement drugs. These drugs do not usually replace pituitary hormones; they replace hormones, such as thyroid hormones and corticosteroids, that are produced by other glands stimulated by the pituitary.

You may need additional doses of corticosteroid drugs (p.930) if you become injured or ill. It is important for you to carry identification that provides information about the drugs you need in case a medical emergency arises.

(WWW) ONLINE SITES: p.1033

Diabetes insipidus

Inadequate production of, or resistance to the effects of, the pituitary hormone involved in controlling water balance

AGE GENDER GENETICS LIFESTYLE
Risk factors depend on the type

Diabetes insipidus is a rare condition in which the kidneys produce large volumes of dilute urine. The condition is not related to diabetes mellitus (p.687), although both conditions cause thirst and excessive passing of urine.

In diabetes insipidus, the body lacks or cannot fully respond to the hormone vasopressin. This hormone is produced by the hypothalamus, the part of the brain directly above the pituitary gland. However, vasopressin is stored in and secreted by the pituitary gland, which is why it is usually considered a pituitary hormone. The role of vasopressin is to maintain the water balance of the body by controlling urine production.

WHAT ARE THE TYPES?

Diabetes insipidus occurs in two forms: the more common form, called cranial diabetes insipidus, and a form known as nephrogenic diabetes insipidus.

Cranial diabetes insipidus is due to the reduced secretion of vasopressin. Possible causes of this condition include a pituitary tumour (p.676), a tumour near the hypothalamus, surgery, radiotherapy (p.281), or head injuries (p.521). In some cases, the cause is not known.

In nephrogenic diabetes insipidus, the kidneys fail to respond to normal levels of vasopressin. In some cases, the condition is present from birth and is permanent. In these cases, it is more common in males because it is due to an inherited recessive gene carried on the X chromosome (*see* GENE DISORDERS, p.271). The condition may also be due to chronic kidney failure (p.706) or to kidney damage resulting from the use of drugs such as certain antibiotics (p.885) or lithium, a mood-stabilizing drug (p.918). In such cases, the condition may be reversible.

WHAT ARE THE SYMPTOMS?

Symptoms of both forms of diabetes insipidus usually develop over days or weeks, but they may appear suddenly if the pituitary gland has been damaged. Symptoms may include:

- Passing excessive amounts of urine.
- Insatiable thirst.
- Disturbed sleep due to the need to pass urine frequently.

If water lost from the body is not replaced, dehydration will occur. Severe dehydration may need immediate hospital treatment with intravenous fluids.

WHAT MIGHT BE DONE?

If your doctor suspects that you have diabetes insipidus, he or she may measure your urine volume over a 24-hour period. Also, urine output is measured after you have been deprived of fluids for several hours. If you have diabetes insipidus, you will continue to produce a large volume of urine. Your response to synthetic vasopressin is then measured. If vasopressin lowers your urine output, you probably have cranial diabetes insipidus; if output remains high, you probably have the nephrogenic form. If a tumour is suspected as the cause of the cranial form, you may also undergo imaging tests, such as MRI (p.248).

Cranial diabetes insipidus is most commonly treated with synthetic vasopressin (*see* PITUITARY DRUGS, p.934). If there is an underlying cause, such as a pituitary tumour, this will be treated.

Nephrogenic diabetes insipidus that is inherited is usually treated with a low-sodium diet and thiazide diuretics (p.902), which paradoxically reduce urine volume. Treatment must be continued for life. Nephrogenic diabetes due to kidney damage may clear up as the kidneys recover; otherwise, drug treatment is needed. If you have diabetes insipidus, carry identification to alert others to the fact in an emergency.

(WWW) ONLINE SITES: p.1033

THYROID AND PARATHYROID GLAND DISORDERS

The thyroid and parathyroid glands are situated in the neck, where they produce and secrete hormones into the bloodstream. There are two types of thyroid hormone, both of which help to control the rate of metabolism (the chemical reactions constantly occurring in the body). The four small parathyroid glands produce a hormone that controls calcium levels in the blood.

Thyroid disorders are common, but their onset is often gradual and they may not be detected or diagnosed for months or even years. Low levels of thyroid hormones at birth can prevent normal development of the brain and, for this reason, a thyroid function test is one of the first tests to be performed on a newborn baby (*see* SCREENING FOR METABOLIC DISORDERS, p.867). Over- and underactivity of the thyroid gland are the most common thyroid disorders and are discussed first. Swellings and growths are covered next, followed by disorders in which there is over- or underproduction of hormones by the parathyroid gland.

The last article describes multiple endocrine neoplasia, a group of rare inherited disorders in which tumours develop in several endocrine glands, including the thyroid and parathyroid.

KEY ANATOMY

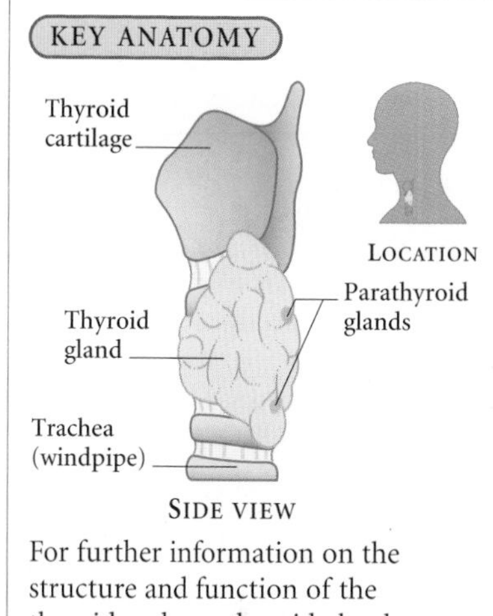

For further information on the structure and function of the thyroid and parathyroid glands, *see* pp.670–675.

Hyperthyroidism

Overproduction of thyroid hormones, causing many body functions to speed up

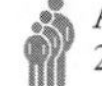 AGE Most common between the ages of 20 and 50

 GENDER More common in females

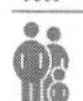 GENETICS Sometimes runs in families

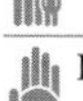 LIFESTYLE Not a significant factor

When the thyroid gland produces an excess of hormones, many of the body's functions are stimulated by these hormones and speed up. This condition is known as hyperthyroidism and is one of the most common hormonal disorders. Hyperthyroidism is 7–10 times more common in women and usually develops between the ages of 20 and 50.

About 3 in 4 cases of the condition are due to Graves' disease, an autoimmune disorder in which the immune system produces antibodies that attack the thyroid gland, resulting in overproduction of thyroid hormones. Graves' disease tends to run in families and is thought to have a genetic basis. In rare cases, hyperthyroidism may be associated with other autoimmune disorders, in particular the skin disorder vitiligo (p.342) and pernicious anaemia, a disorder of the blood (*see* MEGALOBLASTIC ANAEMIA, p.448). In some cases, thyroid nodules (p.681) that secrete hormones may be the cause of hyperthyroidism. Inflammation of the thyroid gland (*see* THYROIDITIS, p.681) may temporarily produce symptoms of hyperthyroidism.

WHAT ARE THE SYMPTOMS?

In most cases, symptoms of hyperthyroidism develop gradually over several weeks and may include:

- Weight loss despite increased appetite and food consumption.
- Rapid heartbeat, which is sometimes also irregular.
- Tremor (persistent trembling) affecting the hands.
- Warm, moist skin as a result of excessive sweating.
- Intolerance to heat.
- Anxiety and insomnia.
- Frequent bowel movements.
- Swelling in the neck caused by an enlarged thyroid (*see* GOITRE, p.680).
- Muscle weakness.
- In women, irregular menstruation.

People with hyperthyroidism caused by Graves' disease may also have bulging eyes (*see* EXOPHTHALMOS, p.582).

HOW IS IT DIAGNOSED?

If your doctor suspects that you have hyperthyroidism, he or she may arrange for a blood test to check for abnormally high levels of thyroid hormones and for antibodies that can attack the thyroid gland. Your doctor will also feel around your neck for lumps caused by general enlargement of the gland. If swelling is detected in this area, radionuclide scanning (p.251) may be used to identify the cause of the hyperthyroidism.

WHAT IS THE TREATMENT?

Symptoms of hyperthyroidism can initially be relieved by beta-blocker drugs (p.898), which reduce tremor and anxiety but do not affect thyroid hormone levels. There are three main treatments aimed at reducing the production of thyroid hormones. The most common is antithyroid drugs (*see* DRUGS FOR HYPERTHYROIDISM, p.932), which are used when hyperthyroidism is due to Graves' disease and work by suppressing production of thyroid hormones. These drugs need to be taken daily for 12–18 months, after which the thyroid gland often functions normally. Radioactive iodine may be the most effective treatment for hormone-secreting thyroid nodules. Treatment involves taking a capsule of radioactive iodine orally. The radioactive iodine is absorbed by the body and accumulates in the thyroid gland, destroying part of it. Surgical removal of part of the thyroid gland is an alternative treatment.

WHAT IS THE PROGNOSIS?

Many people recover fully following treatment. However, hyperthyroidism may recur, particularly in people who have Graves' disease. If the treatment involves surgery or radioactive iodine, the remaining part of the thyroid may not be able to produce sufficient hormones (*see* HYPOTHYROIDISM, below). It is therefore important for thyroid hormone levels to be monitored regularly after treatment so that hormone supplements can be given if needed.

(WWW) ONLINE SITES: p.1033

Hypothyroidism

Underproduction of thyroid hormones, causing many body functions to slow down

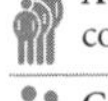
AGE May be present from birth but most common over the age of 40

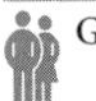
GENDER More common in females

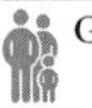
GENETICS Sometimes runs in families

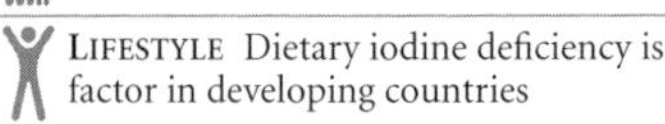
LIFESTYLE Dietary iodine deficiency is a risk factor in developing countries

In hypothyroidism, the thyroid gland does not produce enough thyroid hormones. These hormones are important in metabolism (the chemical reactions constantly occurring in the body). A deficiency causes many of the body's functions to slow down. The condition may be present from birth, in which case treatment is begun before symptoms appear, but it is more common in people over the age of 40, particularly women.

WHAT ARE THE CAUSES?

Hypothyroidism that is present from birth has no known cause. In adults, a common cause of hypothyroidism is thyroiditis (opposite page). The most common type of thyroiditis that leads to hypothyroidism is an autoimmune disorder known as Hashimoto's thyroiditis, which tends to run in families. In Hashimoto's thyroiditis, the body produces antibodies that attack the thyroid gland, damaging it permanently. Other forms of thyroiditis may lead to temporary or permanent hypothyroidism. Treatments for an overactive thyroid gland that involve radioactive iodine or surgery (*see* HYPERTHYROIDISM, p.679) can lead to permanent hypothyroidism.

Rarely, hypothyroidism is due to an underproduction of thyroid-stimulating hormone (TSH) by the pituitary gland, often as the result of a pituitary tumour (p.676). TSH stimulates the thyroid gland to secrete its own hormones.

Insufficient dietary iodine, essential for the production of thyroid hormones, can also cause hypothyroidism.

WHAT ARE THE SYMPTOMS?

The symptoms of hypothyroidism vary in severity and usually develop slowly over months or years. They may include:

- Extreme tiredness.
- Weight gain.
- Constipation.
- Hoarseness of the voice.
- Intolerance to cold.
- Swelling of the face, puffy eyes, and dry, thickened skin.
- Generalized hair thinning.
- In women, heavy menstrual periods.

Some people with hypothyroidism develop a swelling in the neck due to an enlarged thyroid (*see* GOITRE, right).

WHAT MIGHT BE DONE?

Blood tests to measure the levels of thyroid hormones and antibodies that act against the thyroid gland are used to diagnose hypothyroidism. In the UK, all newborns are tested for hypothyroidism shortly after birth (*see* SCREENING FOR METABOLIC DISORDERS, p.867).

Babies with an underactive thyroid are treated promptly with synthetic thyroid hormones, which need to be taken for life (*see* DRUGS FOR HYPOTHYROIDISM, p.932). Lifelong hormone treatment may also be needed if permanent hypothyroidism is diagnosed in adulthood, in which case symptoms should improve about 3 weeks after starting treatment. Hormone treatment must be monitored regularly to ensure that the correct dose is maintained. If hypothyroidism is the result of a pituitary disorder, this will need to be investigated and treated.

Temporary hypothyroidism does not usually need to be treated. Supplements can be taken to correct iodine deficiency.

(WWW) ONLINE SITES: p.1033

Goitre

A swelling in the neck due to enlargement of the thyroid gland

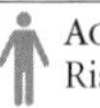
AGE GENDER GENETICS LIFESTYLE
Risk factors depend on the cause

If the thyroid gland becomes enlarged, it causes a swelling to appear in the neck. This swelling is known as a goitre. A goitre can range in size from a barely noticeable lump to a swelling the size of a grapefruit. In rare cases, a very large goitre may press against the oesophagus and trachea (windpipe) in the neck, which can cause difficulty in swallowing and breathing.

WHAT ARE THE CAUSES?

The thyroid gland may enlarge without any disturbance of its function at certain times, particularly at puberty and during pregnancy. Disorders that may be associated with goitre include hyperthyroidism (p.679), hypothyroidism (left), thyroid nodules (opposite page), and certain types of thyroiditis (opposite page). Goitre is a known side effect of drugs such as lithium (*see* MOOD-STABILIZING DRUGS, p.918), which is used to treat bipolar affective disorder (p.557). Iodine deficiency may also be a cause of goitre, although this is extremely rare in developed countries. Rarely, goitre is due to thyroid cancer (opposite page).

WHAT MIGHT BE DONE?

Your doctor will examine your neck to assess the size and shape of the thyroid gland. A sample of your blood may be taken to measure your thyroid hormone levels, and ultrasound scanning (p.250) may be carried out to look at the thyroid.

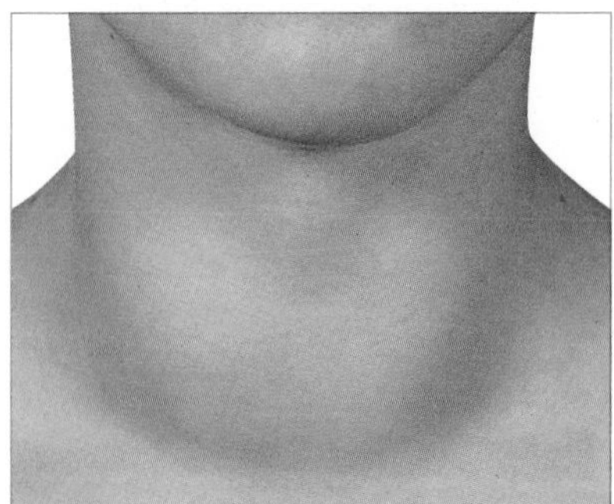

Goitre
This swelling in the neck, called a goitre, is due to enlargement of the thyroid gland. Most goitres are painless.

Needle aspiration of the thyroid gland (p.682) may be performed to provide a more precise diagnosis.

Treatment with surgery, radioactive iodine, or antithyroid drugs (*see* DRUGS FOR HYPERTHYROIDISM, p.932) is sometimes successful in shrinking a goitre in people with hyperthyroidism. Surgery may also be necessary if breathing or swallowing is obstructed or if thyroid cancer is suspected. A small goitre that has no effect on thyroid function may not need treatment and may decrease in size or disappear completely with time.

(WWW) ONLINE SITES: p.1033

Thyroiditis

Inflammation of the thyroid gland, causing permanent or temporary damage

 AGE More common in adults; rare in children

 GENDER GENETICS Risk factors depend on the type

 LIFESTYLE Not a significant factor

Inflammation of the thyroid gland is known as thyroiditis. This disorder can disrupt thyroid activity, causing underactivity (*see* HYPOTHYROIDISM, opposite page) or overactivity (*see* HYPERTHYROIDISM, p.679) of the thyroid gland. The under- or overproduction of thyroid hormones that results is usually temporary, but it can be permanent.

WHAT ARE THE TYPES?

Thyroiditis may take a number of different forms, depending on its cause. The three most common types of thyroiditis are described below.

HASHIMOTO'S THYROIDITIS The most common type of thyroid inflammation is Hashimoto's thyroiditis, an autoimmune disorder in which antibodies are produced that attack the thyroid gland. It often causes thyroid underactivity (*see* HYPOTHYROIDISM, opposite page) and sometimes swelling in the neck due to enlargement of the gland (*see* GOITRE, opposite page). Hashimoto's thyroiditis is eight times more common in women and sometimes runs in families. It may occur with other autoimmune disorders, such as the skin disorder vitiligo (p.342) or pernicious anaemia of the blood (*see* MEGALOBLASTIC ANAEMIA, p.448).

VIRAL THYROIDITIS This form of thyroiditis can sometimes be mistaken for a throat infection because it causes pain on swallowing. There may also be pain in the jaws or ears, fever, and weight loss. Viral thyroiditis can cause overactivity followed by underactivity of the gland.

POSTPARTUM THYROIDITIS About 1 in 10 women develops postpartum thyroiditis within a few months of giving birth. It is thought that this condition results from certain changes that occur in a woman's immune system during pregnancy. Symptoms are uncommon but may include those associated with hyperthyroidism followed by those of hypothyroidism. Postpartum thyroiditis usually clears up after a few months but may recur after future pregnancies.

WHAT MIGHT BE DONE?

Your doctor may arrange for a blood test to check your thyroid hormone levels and look for specific antibodies that attack the thyroid gland. Radionuclide scanning (p.251) may also be necessary to assess the level of thyroid activity.

If you have Hashimoto's thyroiditis, you will usually need lifelong treatment with synthetic thyroid hormones (*see* DRUGS FOR HYPOTHYROIDISM, p.932). In severe cases of viral thyroiditis, corticosteroids (p.930) or aspirin may be used to relieve the inflammation. Postpartum thyroiditis is usually temporary.

(WWW) ONLINE SITES: p.1033

Thyroid nodules

Growths that develop in the thyroid gland, which are usually noncancerous

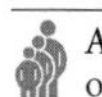 AGE Most common between the ages of 40 and 60

 GENDER More common in females

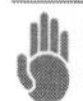 GENETICS LIFESTYLE Not significant factors

Thyroid nodules are abnormal growths that develop in the thyroid gland. They are generally small and occur as single or multiple solid lumps or cysts. Some nodules produce excess thyroid hormones (*see* HYPERTHYROIDISM, p.679). All types of thyroid nodule are most common in people between the ages of 40 and 60 and are three times more common in women than in men.

WHAT ARE THE SYMPTOMS?

Nodules may cause no symptoms, but some people may develop the following:

- Lump or swelling in the neck.
- Difficulty in swallowing or breathing.

If nodules cause hyperthyroidism, additional symptoms may develop, such as rapid heartbeat and loss of weight.

WHAT MIGHT BE DONE?

Imaging of the thyroid gland with ultrasound scanning (p.250) or radionuclide scanning (p.251) may be necessary to diagnose a thyroid nodule. Needle aspiration of the thyroid gland (p.682) may be carried out to establish whether a nodule is a solid lump or a cyst or if it is cancerous. If the nodule is cancerous, further investigation and treatment are necessary (*see* THYROID CANCER, below).

Noncancerous thyroid nodules that do not cause symptoms may not require treatment but should be monitored on a regular basis. Radioactive iodine will be used to treat a nodule that secretes excess thyroid hormones (*see* DRUGS FOR HYPERTHYROIDISM, p.932).

(WWW) ONLINE SITES: p.1033

Thyroid cancer

An uncommon, cancerous tumour occurring in the thyroid gland

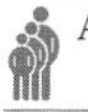 AGE More common over the age of 40

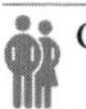 GENDER More common in females

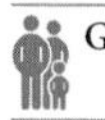 GENETICS Risk factor depends on the type

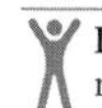 LIFESTYLE Previous exposure of the neck to radiation is a risk factor

Abnormal growths in the thyroid gland can sometimes be cancerous. Thyroid cancer is rare, accounting for only 1 in 100 of all cancers, but it is twice as common in women as men. The condition generally occurs in people who are over the age of 40, and evidence suggests that previous exposure of the neck area to radiation increases the risk. The cure rates of most types of thyroid cancer are among the highest of all cancers.

WHAT ARE THE TYPES?

There are three main types of thyroid cancer, each arising from different cell types in the gland: papillary, follicular, and medullary. About 7 in 10 thyroid

TEST NEEDLE ASPIRATION OF THE THYROID GLAND

Needle aspiration of the thyroid gland is used to determine the cause of a lump and, if the lump is a cyst, to drain it. During the procedure, cells are removed from the abnormal area using a fine hollow needle attached to a syringe. Ultrasound guidance may be used if a lump is inaccessible. The sample is then examined in a laboratory for cancerous cells. This procedure is safe and almost painless and can be carried out in an outpatient clinic.

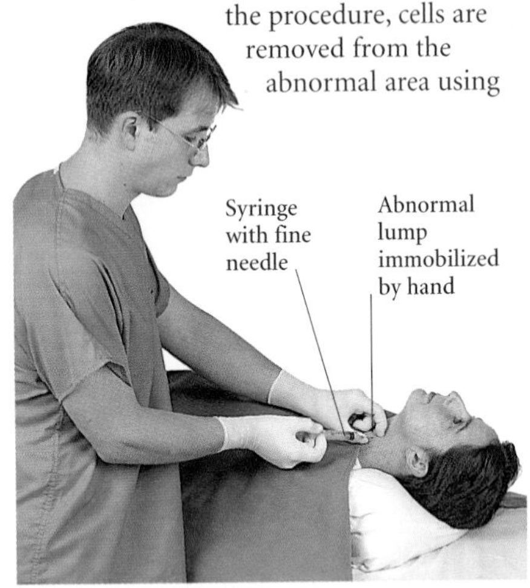

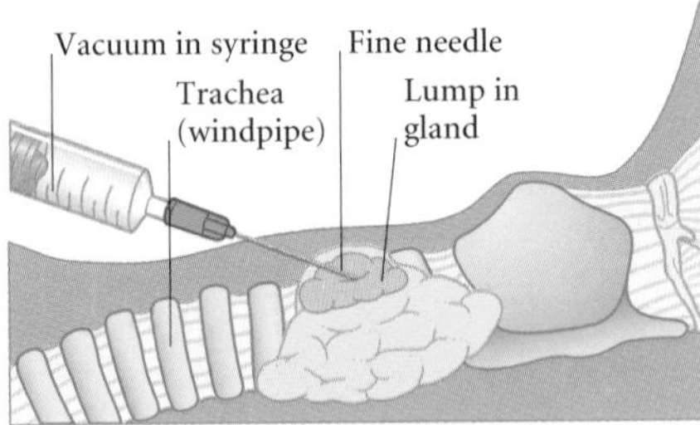

Taking a sample
A pillow is placed under your neck to raise the thyroid area. The doctor withdraws cells from the abnormal area using a syringe with a fine needle.

RESULTS

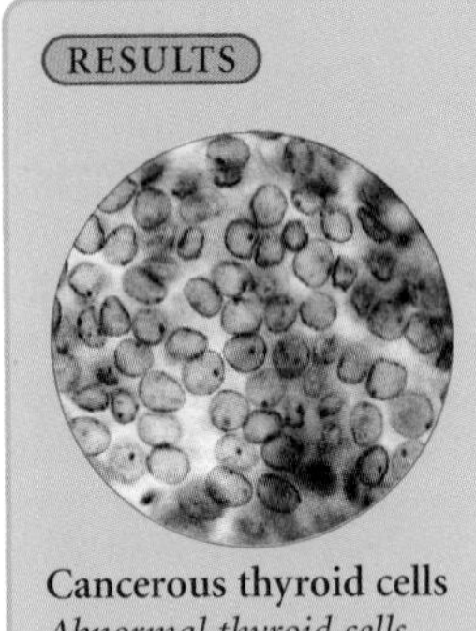

Cancerous thyroid cells
Abnormal thyroid cells obtained using needle aspiration are viewed through a microscope in the laboratory by a specialist. These cells, taken from an abnormal lump, are cancerous.

cancers are papillary, and this type of thyroid cancer spreads most often to the lymph nodes. Exposure to radiation increases the risk of developing papillary cancer. Follicular thyroid cancer is less common and may spread to the lungs or the bones. Medullary cancer of the thyroid is rare and is usually associated with multiple endocrine neoplasia (opposite page), an inherited condition.

WHAT ARE THE SYMPTOMS?

The symptoms depend on the type of thyroid cancer, but they often include:

- Painless, hard lump in the neck.
- Difficulty swallowing.
- Hoarseness.

The first symptom of papillary thyroid cancer may be a lump in the side of the neck due to enlarged lymph nodes.

WHAT MIGHT BE DONE?

If you develop a lump in your neck, your doctor will examine you and may arrange for a blood test to measure thyroid hormone levels. The thyroid gland may be imaged using ultrasound scanning (p.250) or radionuclide scanning (p.251). Needle aspiration of the thyroid gland (above) may be carried out to remove cells from the lump so that they can then be tested for cancer.

Thyroid cancer is usually treated by surgical removal of the whole thyroid gland. Further treatment often involves an oral dose of radioactive iodine. The radioactive iodine accumulates in the remaining thyroid tissue and destroys any cancer cells that may still be present. After treatment, you will need to take thyroid hormone drugs for the rest of your life (*see* DRUGS FOR HYPOTHYROIDISM, p.932). If thyroid cancer is diagnosed and treated early, the survival rate after 5 years is as high as 95 per cent.

(WWW) ONLINE SITES: p.1028, p.1033

Hyperparathyroidism

Overproduction of parathyroid hormone, which may lead to a high level of calcium in the blood

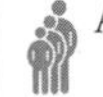
AGE More common over the age of 50

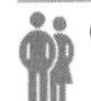
GENDER More common in females

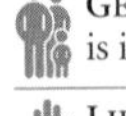
GENETICS In some cases, the condition is inherited

LIFESTYLE Not a significant factor

Parathyroid hormone (PTH), which is produced by four pea-sized parathyroid glands embedded in the thyroid tissue, helps to regulate the body's calcium levels. Overproduction of PTH is called hyperparathyroidism and leads to high calcium levels in the blood. The condition rarely develops before the age of 50 and is much more common in women.

WHAT ARE THE CAUSES?

The most common cause of hyperparathyroidism is a tumour in one or more of the four parathyroid glands. In some cases, development of parathyroid tumours is associated with the inherited disorder multiple endocrine neoplasia (opposite page), in which tumours form in several endocrine glands. Parathyroid tumours are rarely cancerous.

The parathyroid glands may become enlarged and overproduce PTH in an attempt to compensate for disorders that cause a low level of calcium in the blood, such as chronic kidney failure (p.706). In these cases, the condition is called secondary hyperparathyroidism.

WHAT ARE THE SYMPTOMS?

A slightly raised level of calcium in the blood due to hyperparathyroidism may not cause obvious symptoms. However, people with a very high calcium level may develop the following symptoms:

- Abdominal pain.
- Nausea and vomiting.
- Constipation.
- Increased thirst and passing of urine.
- Depression.

An abnormally high level of calcium in the blood may also lead to dehydration, confusion, and unconsciousness, and it can be life-threatening. Serious complications of hyperparathyroidism include the formation of kidney stones (p.701), due to a build-up of calcium, and bone fractures (p.392), resulting from calcium gradually leaking out of the bone into the bloodstream.

WHAT MIGHT BE DONE?

If you develop the symptoms of hyperparathyroidism, your doctor is likely to arrange for you to have blood tests to assess your kidney function and check for raised levels of calcium and PTH. If you have not experienced symptoms, hyperparathyroidism is usually detected by chance during a routine checkup. Sometimes, the condition is diagnosed during investigations to look for the cause of kidney stones.

You may not require treatment if the level of calcium in your blood is only slightly raised; however, your blood calcium level and kidney function will need to be monitored annually. If your calcium levels are very high, you will be given fluids and drugs intravenously in hospital to lower blood calcium.

If a parathyroid tumour is accompanied by high blood calcium levels, the affected parathyroid gland will be removed surgically. You may need calcium supplements immediately after surgery, but body calcium levels usually return to normal after a few days. The underlying disorder causing secondary hyperparathyroidism will be treated if possible; alternatively, some of the parathyroid glands may be removed surgically.

(WWW) ONLINE SITES: p.1033

Hypoparathyroidism

Underproduction of parathyroid hormone, which may lead to a low level of calcium in the blood

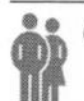 GENDER More common in females

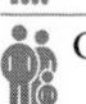 GENETICS Sometimes runs in families

 AGE LIFESTYLE Not significant factors

Hypoparathyroidism occurs when the parathyroid glands, which are embedded in the thyroid tissue, produce an inadequate amount of parathyroid hormone (PTH). PTH regulates the amount of calcium in the body. A lack of PTH results in an abnormally low level of calcium in the blood and may lead to the development of disorders of the muscles and nerves, which need calcium in order to function properly. In rare cases, hypoparathyroidism is present from birth. It is twice as common in women as men and sometimes runs in families.

Muscular spasm
A muscular spasm has caused this hand to turn inwards, the fingers to bend, and the thumb to turn across the palm. This spasm, due to low calcium levels, is a symptom of hypoparathyroidism.

WHAT ARE THE CAUSES?

Damage to the parathyroid glands during surgery on the thyroid gland is the most common cause of hypoparathyroidism. In this case, the disorder tends to develop suddenly. In rare cases, hypoparathyroidism is associated with autoimmune disorders, in which the body attacks its own tissues.

WHAT ARE THE SYMPTOMS?

If hypoparathyroidism develops after thyroid surgery, symptoms appear within a few hours. In other cases, symptoms develop gradually and are usually less severe. In either case, symptoms are due to low calcium levels and include:

- Tetany (muscular spasm) in the feet, the hands, and sometimes the throat.
- Tingling and numbness in the hands, the feet, and around the mouth.
- Seizures.

If the condition is left untreated, long-term complications, such as cataracts (p.573), may develop.

WHAT MIGHT BE DONE?

If your doctor suspects hypoparathyroidism from your symptoms, he or she will probably arrange for blood tests to measure the levels of PTH and calcium.

If the symptoms are severe, you may require emergency hospital treatment, including intravenous injections of calcium to relieve muscle spasms. Lifelong treatment with dietary supplements of calcium (*see* MINERALS, p.929) and vitamin D (*see* VITAMINS, p.927) may be necessary, as well as regular blood tests to monitor your blood calcium level.

(WWW) ONLINE SITES: p.1033

Multiple endocrine neoplasia

A rare inherited disorder in which tumours develop in several of the endocrine glands

 GENETICS Due to an abnormal gene inherited from one parent

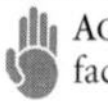 AGE GENDER LIFESTYLE Not significant factors

In the rare disorder known as multiple endocrine neoplasia (MEN), tumours form in several of the endocrine glands around the body. The condition exists in many forms, each caused by a different abnormal gene. In each case, this abnormal gene is inherited in an autosomal dominant manner, which means that the condition can be inherited from just one parent (*see* GENE DISORDERS, p.271). Each child of an affected person has a 1 in 2 chance of inheriting the abnormal MEN gene, and the condition can appear at any age.

Tumours may develop in several endocrine glands at the same time or at different times over a period of years. In the most common type of the disorder, known as MEN 1, tumours develop in the pancreas, parathyroid glands, and pituitary gland (*see* PITUITARY TUMOURS, p.676). Less commonly, a variant known as MEN 2 causes tumours to develop in the adrenal glands (*see* PHAEOCHROMOCYTOMA, p.686) and the thyroid gland. Thyroid tumours may be cancerous (*see* THYROID CANCER, p.681), but tumours that develop in other endocrine glands are usually noncancerous. The affected glands may produce excess hormones.

WHAT MIGHT BE DONE?

If your doctor detects an abnormality in one gland, he or she may arrange for you to have blood tests to check the function of the other endocrine glands. If MEN is diagnosed, your family may be offered screening tests (*see* TESTS FOR ABNORMAL GENES, p.239). Members with the abnormal gene can be monitored to detect tumours at an early stage.

Tumours are usually removed surgically. After treatment, you will probably be monitored periodically to check for endocrine abnormalities. If endocrine tumours are diagnosed early, they can usually be treated successfully.

(WWW) ONLINE SITES: p.1032, p.1033

Adrenal gland disorders

There are two adrenal glands, one situated above each kidney. Hormones produced by the adrenal glands are vital in controlling body chemistry. If adrenal hormone levels become imbalanced, the effects tend to be widespread throughout the body and are often serious, even life-threatening. However, these disorders are rare.

KEY ANATOMY

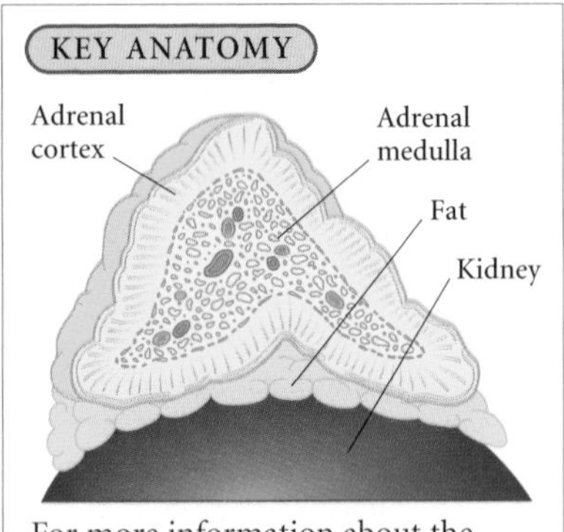

For more information about the structure and function of the adrenal glands, *see* pp.670–675.

Adrenal gland disorders may involve either the over- or underproduction of adrenal hormones. This section first discusses disorders in which adrenal hormones are overproduced. The overproduction of adrenal hormones is most commonly due to the presence of an adrenal tumour. These tumours are usually noncancerous and can often be removed by means of surgery.

The final article discusses Addison's disease, a disorder in which the adrenal gland underproduces hormones. The lack of adrenal hormones is frequently caused by an autoimmune disorder that damages the gland. Addison's disease can be treated successfully with synthetic hormones.

Adrenal disorders are sometimes caused by changes in the levels of hormones that are produced by the pituitary gland (*see* PITUITARY GLAND DISORDERS, pp.676–678). There is also an extremely rare adrenal disorder that is caused by a genetic defect (*see* CONGENITAL ADRENAL HYPERPLASIA, p.866). Disorders that are due to the abnormal production of sex hormones by the adrenal glands are described elsewhere in the book (*see* MALE HORMONAL DISORDERS, pp.728–729, and MENSTRUAL, MENOPAUSAL, AND HORMONAL PROBLEMS, pp.734–740).

Adrenal tumours

Tumours in the adrenal glands, usually noncancerous, that may produce excess adrenal hormones

AGE GENDER GENETICS LIFESTYLE
Risk factors depend on the type

Tumours of the adrenal glands are rare, and in 9 out of 10 cases they are noncancerous. In almost all cases, tumours occur in only one adrenal gland, and their effects depend on which part of the gland is affected. Most adrenal tumours secrete excessive amounts of one or more of the adrenal hormones, which can upset metabolism (the chemical reactions constantly occurring in the body) and water balance and may alter the body's response to physical stress such as injury.

What are the types?

Adrenal tumours can develop in either the cortex (outer layer) or the medulla (centre) of the adrenal gland.

Adrenal tumours in the cortex may secrete corticosteroids, aldosterone, or androgens (male sex hormones). Overproduction of corticosteroids leads to changes in physical appearance as well as in body chemistry (*see* CUSHING'S SYNDROME, right) and may cause serious complications. An excess of the hormone aldosterone, a condition known as hyperaldosteronism (opposite page), disturbs the body's salt and water balance and is a rare cause of high blood pressure (*see* HYPERTENSION, p.403). A high level of androgens in women may lead to the development of male characteristics (*see* VIRILIZATION, p.740); in males, an excess often goes unnoticed.

Tumours that develop in the adrenal medulla are known as phaeochromocytomas (p.686). These tumours produce large amounts of either or both of the hormones epinephrine (adrenaline) and norepinephrine (noradrenaline), excessive levels of which cause sweating, high blood pressure, and palpitations.

What might be done?

Adrenal tumours are usually diagnosed by detecting abnormal levels of adrenal hormones in the blood. Imaging tests, such as MRI (p.248) and CT scanning (p.247), may also be carried out to look for abnormalities in the adrenal glands.

Most adrenal tumours can be treated by surgical removal. In the rare cases in which an adrenal tumour is found to be cancerous, treatment with chemotherapy (p.280) may also be necessary.

(WWW) ONLINE SITES: p.1028, p.1033

Cushing's syndrome

Changes in body chemistry and physical appearance caused by excessive amounts of corticosteroid hormones

GENDER More common in females

AGE GENETICS LIFESTYLE
Not significant factors

Corticosteroid hormones are involved in the regulation of metabolism (the chemical reactions that continually occur in the body) and play a part in the control of salt and water balance and blood pressure. In Cushing's syndrome, an excess of corticosteroids causes disruption of these control mechanisms. The distribution of fat around the body and the growth of body hair are affected, resulting in significant changes in physical appearance. Depression and other psychological problems may also develop. Cushing's syndrome is more common in women than in men.

What are the causes?

The most common cause of Cushing's syndrome is long-term treatment with oral corticosteroid drugs (p.930), such as prednisolone, which are used to treat rheumatoid arthritis (p.377) and other inflammatory conditions. These drugs mimic the effects of natural corticosteroids produced by the adrenal glands. Less commonly, Cushing's syndrome is due to the overproduction of corticosteroids by the adrenal glands. This may be caused by a hormone-secreting tumour in one of the adrenal glands (*see* ADRENAL TUMOURS, opposite page) or by a tumour in the pituitary gland (*see* PITUITARY TUMOURS, p.676) that produces the hormone ACTH, which stimulates the adrenal glands.

Some cancers, such as primary lung cancer (p.503), produce hormones that mimic pituitary hormones and may cause Cushing's syndrome as a result.

WHAT ARE THE SYMPTOMS?

The symptoms of Cushing's syndrome appear gradually and become increasingly obvious over a period of weeks or months. Any of the following may occur:

- Changes in the appearance of the face, which may become red and rounded.
- Weight gain concentrated around the chest and abdomen.
- Excessive growth of facial or body hair (more noticeable in women).
- In women, irregular menstruation. Eventually, menstruation may stop.
- Reddish-purple stretch marks on the abdomen, thighs, and arms.
- Small pads of fat between the shoulder blades at the base of the neck.
- Difficulty climbing stairs, associated with muscle wasting and weakness of the legs. Arms may also be affected.
- Tendency to bruise easily, especially on the limbs.
- Acne (p.340).
- Lack or loss of sexual drive; men may become impotent.
- Depression and mood swings.

If the condition is left untreated, it may eventually lead to complications such as high blood pressure (*see* HYPERTENSION, p.403), thinning of the bones (*see* OSTEOPOROSIS, p.368), diabetes mellitus (p.687), and chronic heart failure (p.413).

HOW IS IT DIAGNOSED?

If you have been taking large doses of corticosteroid drugs, your doctor will probably be able to diagnose Cushing's syndrome from your symptoms. Otherwise, tests on blood or urine may be carried out to look for raised levels of natural corticosteroids. Abnormally high

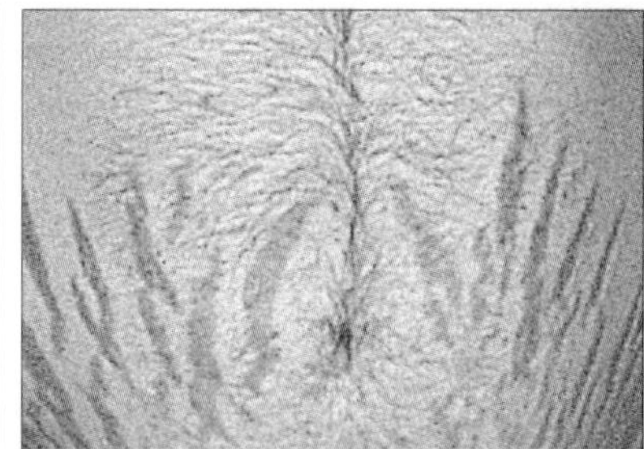

Stretch marks in Cushing's syndrome
Large, reddish-purple stretch marks on the trunk, especially the abdomen, are often seen in people with Cushing's syndrome.

levels of corticosteroids may indicate that you have an adrenal tumour or that your adrenal glands are overstimulated.

Once the diagnosis is confirmed, the cause will be investigated. You may have tests in hospital to distinguish between raised hormone levels that may be due to a pituitary tumour and those possibly due to an adrenal tumour. MRI (p.248) or CT scanning (p.247) of the adrenal glands may be carried out.

WHAT IS THE TREATMENT?

The treatment of Cushing's syndrome depends on the underlying cause. If you are on a long-term course of corticosteroid drugs, your doctor may reduce your dosage or, if possible, discontinue the treatment. However, you should not stop taking corticosteroid drugs without first consulting your doctor.

If the cause is a tumour in one of the adrenal glands, your doctor may initially prescribe drugs to lower corticosteroid levels. After that, it may be necessary to have the affected adrenal gland surgically removed.

If the adrenal glands have been overstimulated by a pituitary tumour, the tumour may be surgically removed. In most cases, the surgery is successful but radiotherapy (p.281) or drug treatment are sometimes necessary to destroy any remaining abnormal cells.

You may need to take small doses of corticosteroid drugs for several months after surgery until your adrenal gland or glands adapt and produce normal amounts of hormones. The symptoms of Cushing's syndrome should then improve gradually. In rare cases, if both adrenal glands are removed, you will need corticosteroid drugs for life.

(WWW) ONLINE SITES: p.1033

Hyperaldosteronism

Changes in body chemistry caused by an excess of the hormone aldosterone

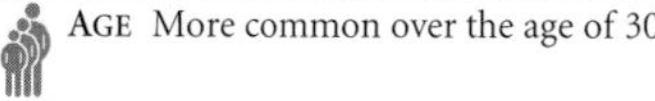
AGE More common over the age of 30

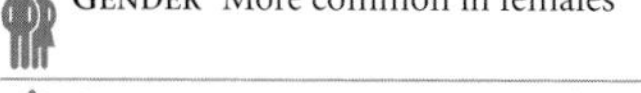
GENDER More common in females

GENETICS LIFESTYLE Not significant factors

Aldosterone is a hormone that is produced by the outer layers of the adrenal glands and acts on the kidneys to regulate salt balance and blood pressure. Overproduction of aldosterone by one or both adrenal glands is called hyperaldosteronism and leads to a high level of salt in the body and loss of the mineral potassium in the urine. High salt levels cause high blood pressure (*see* HYPERTENSION, p.403), but fewer than 1 in 100 people with high blood pressure have hyperaldosteronism.

Hyperaldosteronism is usually due to a noncancerous tumour in the adrenal cortex. It may also result from other conditions, such as chronic heart failure (p.413), cirrhosis (p.647), and nephrotic syndrome (p.700). Hyperaldosteronism due to an adrenal tumour is more common after the age of 30 and in women.

WHAT ARE THE SYMPTOMS?

Hyperaldosteronism does not always produce noticeable symptoms, but if symptoms of the condition do develop, they may include:

- Muscle weakness and cramps.
- Frequent passage of large amounts of urine, accompanied by thirst.

Normal adrenal gland
Spine
Adrenal tumour
Kidney

Aldosterone-producing tumour
This vertical CT scan through the upper abdomen shows an adrenal tumour. Such tumours may cause hyperaldosteronism.

Hyperaldosteronism also leads to high blood pressure, which rarely produces noticeable symptoms but may be detected during a routine health checkup.

WHAT MIGHT BE DONE?

Your doctor may arrange blood tests to measure salt, potassium, and aldosterone levels and CT scanning (p.247) to look for a tumour. If a tumour is found, the adrenal gland may be surgically removed. Treatment may include drugs to block the action of excess aldosterone and drugs to control blood pressure (*see* ANTIHYPERTENSIVE DRUGS, p.897).

(WWW) ONLINE SITES: p.1033

Phaeochromocytoma

A tumour in the centre of the adrenal gland that produces an excess of certain adrenal hormones

AGE Most common between the ages of 30 and 60 but may occur at any age

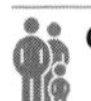
GENETICS Sometimes runs in families

GENDER LIFESTYLE Not significant factors

A phaeochromocytoma is a tumour that develops in the medulla (centre) of one of the adrenal glands. Phaeochromocytomas produce excessive amounts of the hormones epinephrine (adrenaline) and norepinephrine (noradrenaline), which are normally produced by the adrenal glands to prepare the body for action or physical stress. Phaeochromocytomas are rare. Only 1 in 10 is cancerous. Such tumours may develop as part of multiple endocrine neoplasia (p.683), an inherited condition in which tumours occur in several hormone-secreting glands.

WHAT ARE THE SYMPTOMS?

Exercise, emotion, or even a change in body position can trigger the tumour to release hormones into the blood. When this happens, you may experience the following symptoms:

- Palpitations (awareness of an abnormally fast or irregular heartbeat).
- Pale, cold skin and profuse sweating.
- Nausea and vomiting.
- Feelings of intense anxiety.
- Headache.

Raised levels of epinephrine and norepinephrine also lead to a rise in blood pressure (*see* HYPERTENSION, p.403).

WHAT MIGHT BE DONE?

If your doctor suspects a phaeochromocytoma, he or she may ask you to collect your urine over a 24-hour period so that tests can be performed on it. Chemicals in the urine provide information about levels of epinephrine and norepinephrine in your body. If the levels of these hormones are higher than normal, you will probably have MRI (p.248) or CT scanning (p.247) to look for a tumour.

Initially, drug treatment is used to lower your blood pressure. The tumour is then removed surgically. People who have had a noncancerous phaeochromocytoma removed usually make a full recovery. However, cancerous tumours are more likely to recur.

(WWW) ONLINE SITES: p.1028, p.1033

Addison's disease

Insufficient levels of corticosteroid hormones in the blood, causing changes in body chemistry

GENDER Twice as common in females

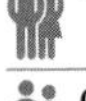
GENETICS Sometimes runs in families

AGE LIFESTYLE Not significant factors

Corticosteroids are adrenal hormones involved in metabolism (the chemical reactions constantly occurring in the body). They also help to control blood pressure and salt and water balance in the body. In the rare disorder Addison's disease, underproduction of corticosteroids leads to changes in body chemistry. The condition is twice as common in women and sometimes runs in families.

The usual cause of Addison's disease is damage to an adrenal gland by an autoimmune disorder (p.461), in which the body attacks its own tissues. Less common causes of the disorder include HIV infection and AIDS (p.297), tuberculosis (p.491), growth of cancer cells in the adrenal glands, lack of stimulation from the pituitary gland (*see* HYPOPITUITARISM, p.678), and sudden, severe low blood pressure (*see* SHOCK, p.414).

Corticosteroid secretion is also suppressed if you take corticosteroid drugs (p.930) long term for another disorder. If you suddenly stop treatment, undergo surgery, or become ill, levels of natural corticosteroids will be too low.

WHAT ARE THE SYMPTOMS?

The symptoms of Addison's disease appear gradually but become increasingly obvious over a period of several weeks or months. You may develop:

- Vague feeling of ill health.
- Tiredness and weakness.
- Gradual loss of appetite.
- Weight loss.
- Skin pigmentation similar to suntan, especially in the creases of the palms and on knuckles, elbows, and knees.

People with Addison's disease usually develop low blood pressure (*see* HYPOTENSION, p.414). If you develop a serious illness or sustain an injury, corticosteroid levels may be too low for your body's needs, and this may result in a condition called an Addisonian crisis. In such a crisis, excessive loss of salt and water results in dehydration, extreme weakness, abdominal pain, vomiting, and confusion. Left untreated, a crisis may lead to coma (p.522) and death.

HOW IS IT DIAGNOSED?

The diagnosis will be obvious if you have suddenly stopped taking corticosteroid drugs. Otherwise, if your doctor suspects Addison's disease, you may have a blood test to measure salt and potassium levels. Further tests may include blood tests to check levels of corticosteroids or to assess your response to an injection of a substance that normally stimulates the adrenal glands.

WHAT IS THE TREATMENT?

Any underlying conditions will be treated if possible. In addition, people with Addison's disease usually need long-term treatment with oral corticosteroid drugs (p.930).

The dose of corticosteroid drugs will need to be increased in times of illness or stress. If you develop an infection while taking corticosteroid drugs long term, you should double the dose and consult your doctor. If you are vomiting or unable to take the drugs orally, you will need an injection of corticosteroids. Corticosteroid injections are also needed as emergency treatment in an Addisonian crisis along with intravenous fluids and glucose. If you are taking corticosteroid drugs long term for any reason, you should carry a card or wear a tag with this information.

(WWW) ONLINE SITES: p.1033

METABOLIC DISORDERS

The chemical processes that take place in the body are known collectively as metabolism. These processes are largely controlled by hormones, and either overproduction or underproduction of a particular hormone can have wide-ranging effects on the body's internal chemistry. Metabolic disorders can also be caused by underlying conditions affecting major organs that regulate metabolism, such as the liver and the kidneys.

One important group of metabolic disorders is due to faulty or blocked chemical pathways, which cause the build-up of a chemical that is usually eliminated from the body. As the chemical accumulates, it may damage organs such as the brain and the liver. Many of these disorders, such as haemochromatosis, are due to genetic defects, some of which tend to run in families. If you have a close relative with one of these disorders, you may be at increased risk of developing the metabolic disorder yourself (*see* GENE DISORDERS, p.271).

Most metabolic disorders can be diagnosed using blood or urine tests to measure levels of hormones or other specific chemicals. If the disorders are recognized early, they can sometimes be treated by a change in diet or the replacement of missing hormones or other chemicals. The sooner treatment is started, the better the prospects are for avoiding permanent damage.

The opening article in this section describes diabetes mellitus, the most common metabolic disorder. The next discusses hypoglycaemia, a condition sometimes associated with treatment for diabetes. The final articles cover disorders, including amyloidosis, in which abnormal levels of particular chemicals collect in the body.

Certain metabolic disorders are also disorders of particular endocrine (hormone-secreting) glands and are described elsewhere (*see* PITUITARY GLAND DISORDERS, pp.676–678; THYROID AND PARATHYROID GLAND DISORDERS, pp.679–683; and ADRENAL GLAND DISORDERS, pp.684–686).

Diabetes mellitus

Inability of the body to use glucose for energy due to inadequate amounts of or loss of sensitivity to the hormone insulin

GENETICS Sometimes runs in families

AGE GENDER LIFESTYLE
Risk factors depend on the type

Diabetes mellitus is one of the most common long-term diseases occurring in the UK, affecting more than 3 in 100 people. In this disorder, either the pancreas produces insufficient amounts of the hormone insulin or body cells become resistant to the hormone's effects.

Normally, insulin is produced by the pancreas and enables the body's cells to absorb the sugar glucose (their main energy source) from the blood. In diabetes mellitus, the cells have to use other sources of energy, leading to a build-up of toxic by-products in the body. Unused glucose accumulates in the blood and urine, causing symptoms such as excessive passing of urine and thirst.

Treatment is designed to control glucose levels in the blood. Among people treated for diabetes mellitus, 1 in 10 depends on self-administered injections of insulin for life. The rest require a carefully managed diet and often oral drugs. These measures enable most affected people to lead normal lives. However, in many cases, complications eventually develop, although their onset may be delayed by treatment. Complications include problems with the eyes, kidneys, cardiovascular system, and nervous system. Diabetes mellitus also weakens the immune system and thus increases susceptibility to infections such as cystitis (p.709). The condition is usually permanent, and there is no known cure.

WHAT ARE THE TYPES?

There are two main forms of diabetes mellitus, which are designated as type 1 and type 2 diabetes.

TYPE 1 DIABETES This form of diabetes occurs when the pancreas produces far too little insulin or produces none at all. The disorder usually develops suddenly in childhood or adolescence. Although dietary measures are also important, it must be treated with insulin injections. About 350,000 people in the UK have this type of diabetes.

TYPE 2 DIABETES Type 2 is by far the most common form of diabetes, affecting about 3 million people in the UK. In this condition, the pancreas continues to secrete insulin, but the cells of the body become resistant to its effects. This form of diabetes mainly affects people over the age of 40 and is more common in people who are overweight. The condition develops slowly and often goes unnoticed for many years. In the initial stages, dietary measures may be sufficient to control the condition, but oral drugs and sometimes insulin injections become necessary as it progresses.

Diabetes mellitus can sometimes develop during pregnancy (*see* DIABETES DEVELOPING IN PREGNANCY, p.788). This condition is called gestational diabetes and may require treatment with insulin to maintain the health of the mother and baby. Gestational diabetes usually disappears after childbirth; however, women who have had it are at increased risk of developing type 2 diabetes in later life.

WHAT ARE THE CAUSES?

Type 1 diabetes is usually caused by an abnormal reaction in which the immune system destroys insulin-secreting cells in the pancreas. The cause of this reaction is unknown, but it may be triggered by a viral infection. In some cases, destruction of insulin-secreting tissues occurs following inflammation of the pancreas (*see* ACUTE PANCREATITIS, p.652).

Genetics may also play a role, but the pattern of inheritance is complicated. A

SELF-HELP INJECTING INSULIN

If you need regular injections of insulin, you will be shown how to inject yourself. You can use a syringe and needle, but many people prefer insulin pens, which are easier to use and more discreet. Insulin can be injected into any fatty area, such as the upper arms, abdomen, or thighs. Insert the needle quickly into a pinch of skin and then inject the insulin slowly. You should try not to use exactly the same site each time for the injection.

Dose selector dial
Turn the dial to select the dose in units

Insulin cartridge
Each cartridge is prefilled with insulin

Dosage window

Needle

Push button
Press this button to release the insulin

Insulin scale
The scale shows how many units are left

Insulin pen
This device for carrying and delivering insulin holds an insulin cartridge and has a dial that lets you set the required dose. Disposable needles attach to one end.

Learning to inject
From an early age, children who have diabetes can be taught how to inject themselves.

Injection site
For children, the thigh is often an easy site for injection

child of a person with type 1 diabetes is at greater risk of developing the same type of diabetes, but most affected children do not have a parent with diabetes.

The causes of type 2 diabetes are less well understood, but genetics and obesity are important factors. About 1 in 3 affected people has a relative with the same type of diabetes. Type 2 diabetes is a major health problem in affluent societies and a growing problem in some developing countries. As food intake increases, more people become overweight and the prevalence of the condition rises.

In people who are predisposed to diabetes, the condition can be triggered by corticosteroid drugs (p.930) or by excessively high levels of natural corticosteroid hormones (*see* CUSHING'S SYNDROME, p.684), which act against insulin.

WHAT ARE THE SYMPTOMS?

Although some of the symptoms of both forms of diabetes mellitus are similar, type 1 diabetes tends to develop more quickly and become more severe. The symptoms of type 2 may not be obvious and may go unnoticed until a routine medical checkup. The main symptoms of both forms may include:

- Excessive passing of urine.
- Thirst and a dry mouth.
- Insufficient sleep because of the need to pass urine at night.
- Lack of energy.
- Blurred vision.

Type 1 diabetes may also cause weight loss. In some people, the first sign of the disorder is ketoacidosis, a condition in which toxic chemicals called ketones build up in the blood. These chemicals are produced when the tissues of the body are unable to absorb glucose from the bloodstream, due to inadequate production of insulin, and have to use fats for energy. Ketoacidosis can also occur in people with type 1 diabetes who are taking insulin if they miss several doses or if they develop another illness (because any form of illness increases the body's requirement for insulin). The symptoms of ketoacidosis may include:

- Nausea and vomiting, sometimes with abdominal pain.
- Deep breathing.
- Acetone smell to the breath (like nail-polish remover).
- Confusion.

The development of these symptoms is a medical emergency because they can lead to severe dehydration and coma (p.522) if they are not treated urgently. Emergency treatment for ketoacidosis includes intravenous infusion of fluids to correct dehydration and restore the chemical balance of the blood, and injections of insulin to enable body cells to absorb glucose from the blood.

ARE THERE COMPLICATIONS?

Diabetes mellitus may give rise to both short-term and long-term complications. Short-term problems are usually easy to treat, but long-term complications are more difficult to control and can lead to premature death.

SHORT-TERM COMPLICATIONS Poorly controlled or untreated type 1 diabetes may lead to ketoacidosis, the symptoms of which are described at left.

A common complication of insulin treatment for either type of diabetes is hypoglycaemia (p.691), in which blood sugar falls to abnormally low levels. Hypoglycaemia is often caused by an imbalance between food intake and the dose of insulin. The disorder is more common in people with type 1 diabetes but may also affect people with type 2 diabetes who take sulphonylurea drugs or insulin (*see* DRUGS FOR DIABETES MELLITUS, p.931). If left untreated, it can cause unconsciousness and seizures.

LONG-TERM COMPLICATIONS Certain long-standing problems pose the main health threat to people with diabetes and may eventually affect even people whose diabetes is well controlled. Close control of blood sugar reduces the risk of developing these problems, and early recognition of complications helps in their control. For these reasons, all affected people should see their doctor at least four times a year (*see* LIVING WITH DIABETES, p.690). Type 2 diabetes is often not diagnosed until years after its onset. As a result, complications may be evident at the time of initial diagnosis.

People who have diabetes are at increased risk of cardiovascular disorders (*see* DIABETIC VASCULAR DISEASE, p.432). Large blood vessels may be damaged by atherosclerosis (p.402), which is a major cause of coronary artery disease (p.405) and stroke (p.532). Raised amounts of cholesterol in the blood (*see* HYPERCHOLESTEROLAEMIA, p.691), which accelerate the development of atherosclerosis, are more common in people who have diabetes. Diabetes is also associated with hypertension (p.403), another risk factor for cardiovascular disease.

Other long-term complications result from damage to the small blood vessels throughout the body. Damage to blood vessels in the light-sensitive retina at the back of the eye may cause diabetic retinopathy (p.579). Diabetes also increases the risk of developing cataracts (p.573). People with diabetes mellitus should have their eyes examined yearly in an organized screening programme.

If diabetes affects blood vessels that supply nerves, it may cause nerve damage (*see* DIABETIC NEUROPATHY, p.545). There may be a gradual loss of sensation, starting at the hands and feet and sometimes gradually extending up the limbs. Symptoms may also include dizziness upon standing and impotence (p.770) in men. Loss of feeling, combined with poor circulation, makes the legs more susceptible to ulcers (*see* LEG ULCERS, p.350) and gangrene (p.435).

Damage to small blood vessels in the kidneys (*see* DIABETIC KIDNEY DISEASE, p.705) may lead to chronic kidney failure (p.706) or end-stage kidney failure (p.708), which requires lifelong dialysis (p.707) or a kidney transplant (p.708).

HOW IS IT DIAGNOSED?

Your doctor will first ask you to provide a urine sample, which will be tested for glucose. The diagnosis is confirmed by a blood test to check for a high glucose level. If the level is borderline, you may undergo another blood test after fasting overnight. Your blood may also be tested for glycosylated haemoglobin, an altered form of the pigment in red blood cells, which increases in concentration when the blood glucose level has been high for several weeks or months.

WHAT IS THE TREATMENT?

For anyone with diabetes mellitus, the aim of treatment is to maintain the level of glucose in the blood within the normal range without marked fluctuations. This aim may be achieved with dietary measures, a combination of diet and insulin injections, or diet and pills that lower blood glucose levels. Treatment is usually lifelong, and you will have to take responsibility for the daily adjustment of your diet and medication.

TYPE 1 DIABETES This form of diabetes mellitus is always treated with injections of insulin. Treatment with oral drugs alone is ineffective. Insulin is available in various forms, including short-acting, long-acting, and combinations of both (*see* DRUGS FOR DIABETES MELLITUS, p.931). Treatment regimens need to be individually tailored, and they may include combinations of insulin and oral drugs. Your doctor will talk to you about your needs and arrange for you to learn how to inject yourself (*see* INJECTING INSULIN, opposite page). You will also have to control your diet and monitor your blood glucose as described below. If the diabetes is difficult to control, you may be given an insulin pump, which dispenses insulin through a catheter that is inserted into your skin.

The only way to cure type 1 diabetes is by having a pancreas transplant, but this surgery is not routinely offered because the body may reject the new organ and because lifelong treatment with immunosuppressant drugs (p.906) is needed afterwards. However, in some cases, a pancreas transplant is given at the same time as a kidney transplant. A method is currently being devised to transplant insulin-secreting cells isolated from a normal pancreas, but this technique is still at an experimental stage.

TYPE 2 DIABETES Many people with this form of diabetes can control their blood glucose levels by taking exercise regularly and by following a healthy diet to maintain ideal weight.

You should follow general guidelines for a healthy diet (*see* DIET AND HEALTH, pp.48–54) and seek advice from a dietitian if necessary. You should try to keep fat intake low, and obtain energy from complex carbohydrates (such as bread and rice) to minimize fluctuations in the blood glucose level. Your diet should have a fixed calorie content. The proportions of protein, carbohydrate, and fat must be consistent to keep a balance between food intake and medication.

TEST MONITORING YOUR BLOOD GLUCOSE

You can monitor your blood glucose level using a digital meter. The method of use varies, depending on the type of meter, but usually involves applying a drop of blood to a test strip impregnated with a chemical that reacts with glucose. Checking your blood glucose at least once a day or as often as your doctor recommends allows you to monitor your treatment to confirm that it is effective and to alter it as necessary.

Pricking device

1 Before starting, wash your hands thoroughly and dry them. Once your hands are clean, obtain a drop of blood by using a spring-loaded pricking device on the fingertip.

Drop of blood

Target area of test strip

2 Cover the chemically impregnated target area of the test strip with the drop of blood. Wait for 1 minute (or as long as is recommended by the instructions that come with the meter).

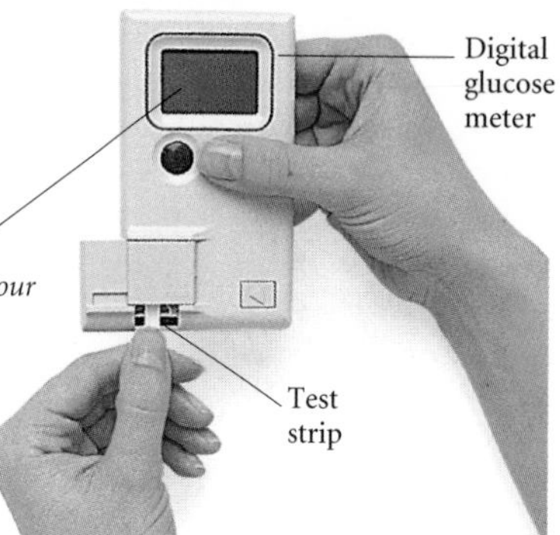

3 Finally, wipe or wash the excess blood from the strip and insert the strip into the digital glucose meter. The meter analyses the blood and gives an almost instant reading of the glucose level.

SELF-HELP LIVING WITH DIABETES

People with diabetes mellitus can lead normal lives, and they can continue to exercise and to eat most foods. However, it is very important to eat a healthy diet, maintain fitness, and, if necessary, lose weight. Following a healthy lifestyle helps to minimize the risk of developing complications over time, including heart disease, circulatory problems, and kidney failure.

A HEALTHY DIET

For some people with diabetes, a healthy diet and weight loss are enough to keep blood glucose levels normal. Your diet should be high in complex carbohydrates, such as rice, pasta, and cereals, and low in fats, particularly fats of animal origin.

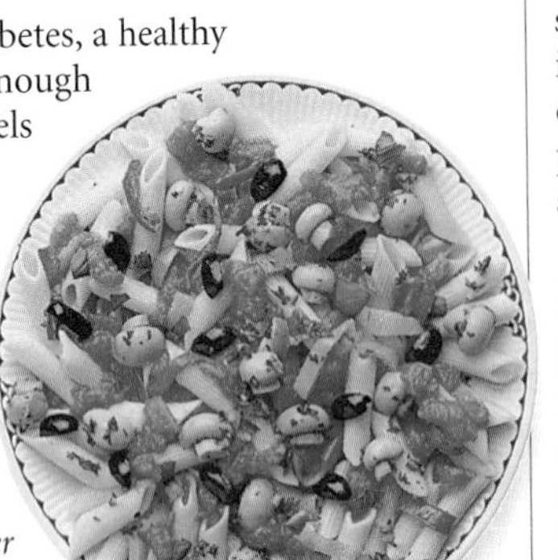

Complex carbohydrates
Rice, pasta, cereals, and other complex carbohydrates are the basis of a healthy diet.

DRINKING AND SMOKING

Alcohol in moderation is safe for most people, but in excess it may lower blood glucose levels. In addition, it is high in calories and may cause weight gain. Smoking is very harmful because it greatly increases the risk of long-term complications, such as heart disease and stroke.

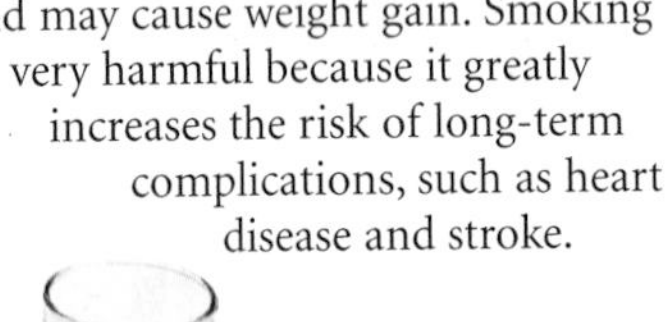

Cigarettes and alcohol
If you have diabetes and smoke, you should stop. If you drink alcohol, you can continue to do so, but you should make sure that you drink in moderation.

SPECIAL CARE FOR YOUR FEET

Diabetes can increase the risk of skin infections and ulcers on the feet. You can reduce the risk by wearing shoes that fit comfortably, visiting a chiropodist regularly, not walking barefoot, and cutting your toenails straight across. You should inspect and clean your feet daily and consult your doctor promptly if you develop a sore on your foot.

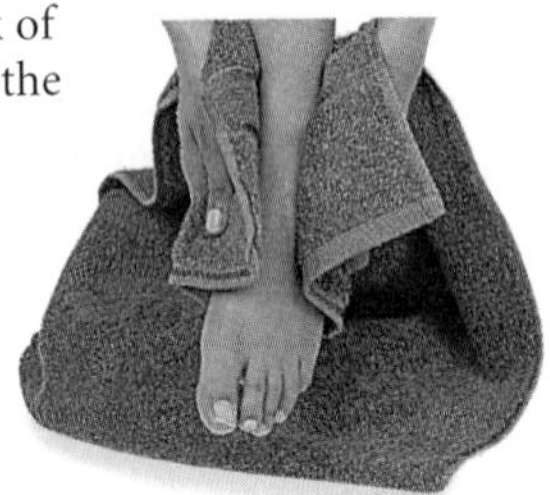

Foot care
Wash and dry your feet carefully. If the skin is dry, use a moisturizer every day.

EXERCISE AND SPORTS

Regular exercise makes you feel healthier, reduces the risk of heart disease, stroke, and high blood pressure, and can help if you need to lose weight. If you have type 1 diabetes, you may need to monitor your blood glucose before, during, and after exercise to check how the activity affects your requirements for both insulin and food.

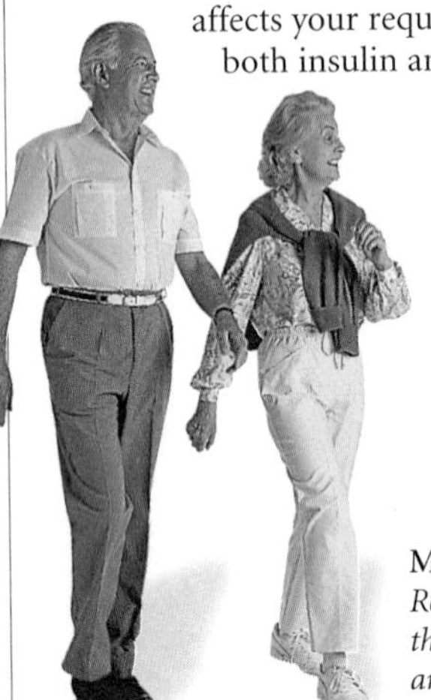

Strenuous exercise
Blood glucose levels usually drop during strenuous exercise. You may need to adjust your dose of insulin or eat more before strenuous activity.

Moderate exercise
Regular moderate exercise reduces the chance of developing coronary artery disease and may improve the control of your diabetes.

YOUR MEDICAL CHECKUP

If you have diabetes, you should have a checkup every 6 months. This will be carried out either by your GP or by a doctor at a hospital diabetes clinic. During the checkup, you will be given a full physical examination, including blood pressure measurement, an assessment of your nervous system, and an eye examination. A sample of your urine will also be tested to check for kidney disease.

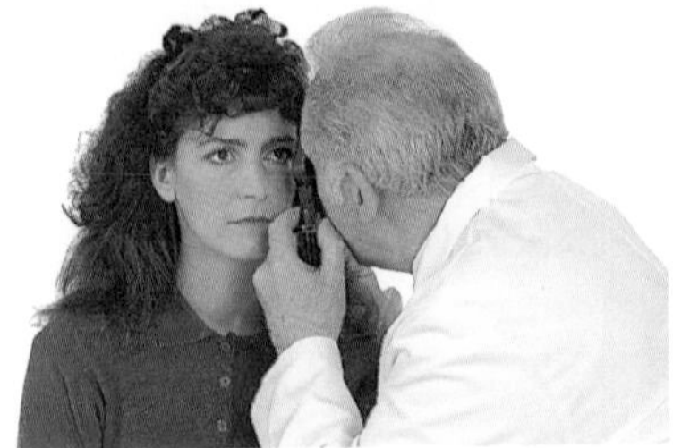

Eye examination
Inspection of the retina (the light-sensitive membrane at the back of the eye) can detect retinal damage caused by diabetes.

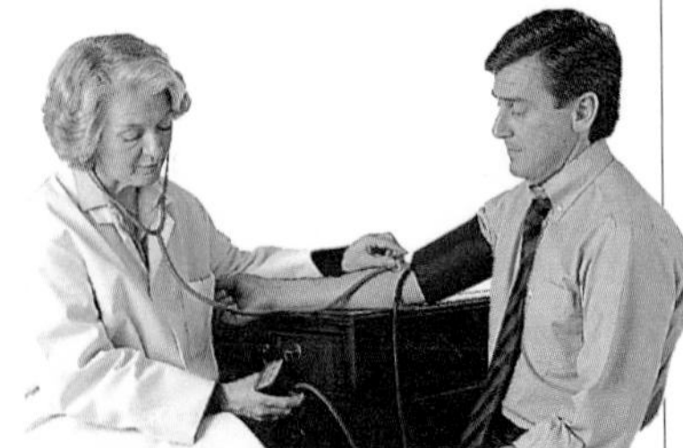

Blood pressure measurement
People with diabetes mellitus have an increased risk of high blood pressure, and regular monitoring is important.

You must also check your blood glucose regularly (*see* MONITORING YOUR BLOOD GLUCOSE, p.689). If the glucose level is higher or lower than recommended, you may need to alter your diet or adjust your insulin or drug dose with the help of your doctor. Effective monitoring is particularly important if you develop another illness, such as influenza (p.289), and in situations such as taking strenuous exercise or planning to eat a larger meal than usual.

When dietary measures are not sufficient to control your blood sugar, one or more drugs may be prescribed (*see* DRUGS FOR DIABETES MELLITUS, p.931). You are likely to begin with oral drugs, such as sulphonylureas, which stimulate the pancreas to release more insulin, and metformin, which helps the body tissues to absorb glucose and is often used to treat diabetes in people who are overweight. If oral drugs are ineffective, you may need to have insulin injections.

WHAT IS THE PROGNOSIS?

Diabetes mellitus is not a curable disease, but advances in monitoring blood glucose levels, combined with a healthy lifestyle, have made it easier to control, allowing people who have the condition to lead a relatively normal life. Children who develop diabetes quickly learn to manage their disease and can participate in sports and lead full social lives.

(WWW) ONLINE SITES: p.1030

Hypoglycaemia

An abnormally low level of glucose in the blood, depriving body cells of glucose

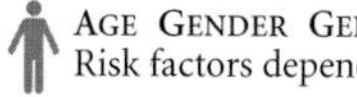
AGE GENDER GENETICS LIFESTYLE
Risk factors depend on the cause

In hypoglycaemia, the body's cells are deprived of glucose, which is their main source of energy. Symptoms of the condition include sweating, nausea, hunger, and anxiety. Hypoglycaemia is usually temporary, and it occurs most often as a side effect of insulin treatment for type 1 diabetes (*see* DIABETES MELLITUS, p.687). It is less common in people who have type 2 diabetes and is rare in those who do not have diabetes. Vague feelings of faintness or nausea that some people attribute to hypoglycaemia are in fact usually due to other disorders, tiredness, or stress (p.74).

WHAT ARE THE CAUSES?

In people who have type 1 diabetes, hypoglycaemia is usually due to a dose of insulin that is excessive in relation to food intake and that lowers glucose levels in the blood too much. People taking insulin must balance their insulin dosage with food intake, which raises blood glucose levels, and physical activity, which lowers blood glucose. If the balance is disturbed and the glucose level falls, hypoglycaemia may result.

Hypoglycaemia in people with type 2 diabetes and impaired kidney function may be due to the gradual build-up of glucose-lowering drugs in the blood (*see* DRUGS FOR DIABETES MELLITUS, p.931).

The rare cases occurring in people without diabetes are usually due to serious medical problems. Such problems include severe liver disease, adrenal failure, or very rarely an insulin-secreting tumour of the pancreas. In babies, especially in newborns, hypoglycaemia may develop because the liver does not yet contain sufficient stores of glucose.

WHAT ARE THE SYMPTOMS?

When blood glucose levels become low, the symptoms of hypoglycaemia develop rapidly. Some people may get warning signs of an attack, which may include:

- Sweating, nausea, hunger, and anxiety.
- Rapid, forceful heartbeat.

If blood glucose continues to fall, further symptoms may develop, including:

- Confusion.
- Slurred speech and unsteady movements, similar to drunkenness.
- Seizures (particularly in children).

Unconsciousness may result. If not treated promptly, the condition may cause permanent brain damage or death.

WHAT IS THE TREATMENT?

If you have diabetes mellitus and experience the above symptoms, take food or drink that contains sugar immediately. Always carry sweets or biscuits with you and wear an information tag to inform people that you have diabetes. If you develop hypoglycaemia and lose consciousness, you will need an immediate injection of glucagon, a hormone that restores consciousness by raising blood glucose levels. If the treatment fails or is not available, you will need emergency treatment with intravenous glucose.

(WWW) ONLINE SITES: p.1030, p.1032

Hypercholesterolaemia

Raised levels of cholesterol in the blood, which increase the risk of developing cardiovascular disease

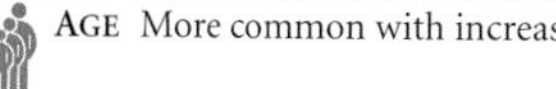
AGE More common with increasing age

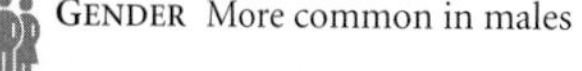
GENDER More common in males

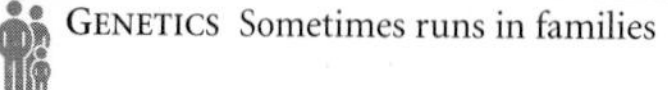
GENETICS Sometimes runs in families

LIFESTYLE A diet high in saturated fats, obesity, and lack of exercise are risk factors

More than 1.5 million people in the UK have a very high level of cholesterol in their blood, and many more have a level that is high enough to increase their risk of illness. Raised cholesterol levels are associated with increased risk of coronary artery disease (p.405) and stroke (p.532) due to atherosclerosis (p.402).

Cholesterol is a substance known as a lipid. It is used in the manufacture of cell walls and in the production of bile acids (which aid the digestion of fat) and hormones. Most of the body's supply of cholesterol is produced in the liver, but some cholesterol is derived from food, particularly from eggs, meat, and shellfish. The level of cholesterol in the body can be affected by diet (*see* DIET AND HEALTH, p.48) and other lifestyle factors.

Cholesterol is carried in the bloodstream in the form of lipid–protein molecules known as lipoproteins. There are two main types of these molecules: low-density lipoproteins (called LDLs) and high-density lipoproteins (known as HDLs). LDLs carry larger amounts of cholesterol than HDLs and deposit the cholesterol around the body. A high level of LDLs in the blood increases the risk of arterial disease. The reason is that excess LDLs form fatty deposits on the walls of arteries. As these deposits grow, they restrict blood flow and can cause the formation of clots that block the vessels. HDLs pick up free molecules of cholesterol and return them to the liver to be broken down. A high level of HDLs in the blood thus protects against arterial disease.

WHAT ARE THE CAUSES?

Cholesterol level is determined by a combination of genetic and lifestyle factors, including diet, weight, and exercise. A high cholesterol level is associated with a diet that is high in fats, particularly saturated fats (*see* CHOOSING HEALTHY FATS, p.50). Being overweight and lack of exercise also lead to high cholesterol levels. Although hypercholesterolaemia often runs in families, some people have one of the specific inherited disorders known as inherited hyperlipidaemias (right), which affect lipid metabolism in the body and are associated with extremely high levels of cholesterol.

A high cholesterol level does not usually cause symptoms until it leads to the development of another disorder, such as coronary artery disease.

HOW IS IT DIAGNOSED?

Regular screening tests to measure the level of cholesterol in the blood (*see* COMMON SCREENING TESTS, p.44) are recommended from early adult life for people who have a family history of raised cholesterol levels, heart disease, or stroke. Cholesterol testing may also be offered as part of a general health checkup. Hypercholesterolaemia is frequently first diagnosed as a result of a routine screening test.

The optimal range of cholesterol for a middle-aged person is 3–5.2 mmol/L (115–200 mg/dL). If the total cholesterol level exceeds 5.2 mmol/L (200 mg/dL), your doctor may carry out a further blood test to check your levels of LDL and HDL cholesterol.

WHAT IS THE TREATMENT?

Whether or not you require treatment depends on how high your blood cholesterol level is and whether other risk factors for coronary artery disease, such as high blood pressure (*see* HYPERTENSION, p.403) or smoking, are present. Even if your cholesterol level falls within the normal range, you may be given treatment to lower blood cholesterol if you are already known to have heart disease or atherosclerosis.

If you are found to have an excessively high level of cholesterol in your blood, your doctor may initially advise you about changes in diet and exercise habits that should lower the level. However, if these measures fail to lower your cholesterol level sufficiently, your doctor may prescribe drugs, which you will need to take for the rest of your life (*see* LIPID-LOWERING DRUGS, p.935).

(WWW) ONLINE SITES: p.1032, p.1035

Inherited hyperlipidaemias

Inherited conditions in which the blood contains abnormally high levels of cholesterol and/or triglycerides

AGE Present from birth but usually become apparent in early adulthood

GENETICS Due to an abnormal gene inherited from one or both parents

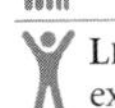
LIFESTYLE A diet high in fats and lack of exercise aggravate the conditions

GENDER Not a significant factor

Many people have an elevated level of cholesterol in their blood (*see* HYPERCHOLESTEROLAEMIA, p.691). In some of these people, blood levels of cholesterol and of lipids called triglycerides are high due to specific genetic disorders called hyperlipidaemias. These disorders create high levels of lipoproteins (lipid–protein molecules in the blood), and they tend to produce symptoms earlier in adulthood than other hypercholesterolaemias. Raised blood levels of lipids (especially cholesterol) increase the risk of complications of atherosclerosis (p.402), such as coronary artery disease (p.405).

There are several different forms of inherited hyperlipidaemias. The most common affects about 1 in 500 people of European descent, who inherit one copy of an abnormal gene. Affected people have a cholesterol level two or three times higher than normal. There is a one in a million risk that people will inherit the abnormal gene from both parents. If two copies of the gene are inherited, the cholesterol level is six to eight times higher than normal. Affected people have a high probability of a heart attack (*see* MYOCARDIAL INFARCTION, p.410), which may occur even in childhood.

WHAT ARE THE SYMPTOMS?

Extremely high cholesterol levels associated with inherited hyperlipidaemias may cause some of the following symptoms, which develop gradually over a period of several years:

- Yellow swellings under the skin (xanthomas) on the back of the hands.
- Swellings on the tendons around the ankle and wrist joints.
- Yellow swellings on the skin of the eyelids (xanthelasmas).
- White ring around the iris (the coloured part of the eye).

Raised triglyceride levels do not usually produce any symptoms but do increase the risk of acute pancreatitis (p.652).

Men with these disorders can develop symptoms of coronary artery disease, such as chest pain (*see* ANGINA, p.407), in their 20s or 30s. In women, oestrogen usually gives protection from these problems until after the menopause.

WHAT MIGHT BE DONE?

There is no cure for inherited hyperlipidaemias, but symptoms can be treated with a combination of exercise, a diet that is low in cholesterol and saturated fats (*see* CHOOSING HEALTHY FATS, p.50), and lipid-lowering drugs (p.935). The outlook varies, but early treatment can reduce the risk of having a heart attack. Relatives of an affected person may be offered screening for the disorder.

(WWW) ONLINE SITES: p.1032, p.1035

Haemochromatosis

An inherited disorder affecting body chemistry, in which iron is deposited in body tissues, causing damage to them

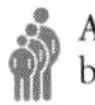
AGE Present from birth but does not usually become apparent until the age of 40

GENDER Much more common in males

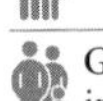
GENETICS Due to an abnormal gene inherited from both parents

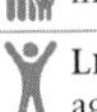
LIFESTYLE Excessive alcohol intake aggravates the condition

In haemochromatosis, the level of iron in the blood is too high. Excess iron gradually accumulates in the liver, pancreas, and heart. The build-up of iron causes damage to these organs. Haemochromatosis is an inherited condition. Men are much more likely to develop the symptoms of haemochromatosis than women because women regularly lose iron from the body when menstruating.

WHAT ARE THE CAUSES?

Haemochromatosis is the result of an abnormal gene that causes the body to absorb too much iron from food. The gene is inherited in an autosomal recessive manner; a person must inherit one abnormal gene from each parent for symptoms to develop (*see* GENE DISORDERS, p.271). If both parents are carriers (people who have just one abnormal gene instead of a pair), there is a 1 in 4 chance of their children having the disease. Carriers do not develop symptoms.

WHAT ARE THE SYMPTOMS?

The symptoms develop gradually and usually do not appear until after the age of 40. Initial symptoms may include:

- Weakness and lack of energy.
- Abdominal pain.
- Shrinking of the testes in men and loss of interest in sex.
- Pain or stiffness in the joints, particularly in the hands.
- Bronzing of the skin.

Symptoms occur earlier in people who drink excessive alcohol because alcohol increases the amount of iron that is absorbed by the intestines.

As the disease progresses, damage to organs can lead to chronic heart failure (p.413), diabetes mellitus (p.687), cirrhosis (p.647), and liver cancer (p.649).

HOW IS IT DIAGNOSED?

Haemochromatosis is diagnosed by testing blood for an abnormally high iron level. CT scanning (p.247) or ultrasound scanning (p.250) may be used to look for liver damage. A liver biopsy (p.647), in which a small sample of the liver is removed and examined under a microscope, may also be carried out to check for the presence of iron deposits in the liver. Members of an affected person's family may want to consider screening (p.42) for the condition.

WHAT IS THE TREATMENT?

Treatment is aimed at removing some of the excess iron from the body. About 500 ml (1 pint) of blood is removed each week until the iron levels are normal. Thereafter, blood needs to be removed less often. If you have haemochromatosis, avoid alcohol and iron-rich foods. You may also need treatment for complications such as diabetes mellitus.

WHAT IS THE PROGNOSIS?

Early treatment, before liver damage has occurred, can prevent the disease from reducing life expectancy. If severe organ damage has occurred, haemochromatosis is potentially fatal. In rare cases, a heart transplant (p.427) or liver transplant (p.650) may be necessary.

WWW ONLINE SITES: p.1032

Amyloidosis

A group of disorders in which abnormal proteins accumulate in internal organs

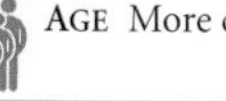
AGE More common in elderly people

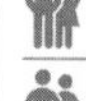
GENDER Twice as common in males

GENETICS In some cases the condition is inherited

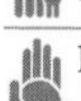
LIFESTYLE Not a significant factor

The various rare conditions known as amyloidosis develop when deposits of abnormal proteins, called amyloid, collect in organs and interfere with their function. There are various forms of amyloidosis, each of which is caused by a different type of amyloid. The condition mainly affects elderly people and is twice as common in men as in women.

Amyloidosis may be due to an abnormal gene or have no apparent cause; in these cases it is called primary amyloidosis. More commonly, it occurs as a complication of another disorder and is therefore called secondary amyloidosis. Disorders associated with the condition include inflammatory disorders such as rheumatoid arthritis (p.377), long-term infections, and the bone marrow cancer multiple myeloma (p.456).

WHAT ARE THE SYMPTOMS?

Often, there are no symptoms in the early stages of amyloidosis. Over months or years, various symptoms develop, depending on which organs and tissues are affected. Diseased organs such as the kidneys, heart, liver, and nerves often become enlarged and cannot function properly. Resulting complications may include chronic kidney failure (p.706), chronic heart failure (p.413), chronic liver failure (p.650), or nerve damage (*see* PERIPHERAL NEUROPATHIES, p.543).

WHAT MIGHT BE DONE?

Amyloidosis is diagnosed by examining a tissue sample from an affected organ under a microscope to detect deposits of protein. In cases of secondary amyloidosis, treating the underlying disorder may halt or even reverse the condition. However, amyloidosis that is associated with multiple myeloma tends to progress rapidly, and the outlook is poor. For primary amyloidosis, immunosuppressant drugs (p.906) or drugs that are more commonly used in the treatment of cancer (*see* ANTICANCER DRUGS, p.907) may be prescribed. If amyloidosis has already caused the failure of an organ, a transplant may be a treatment option, but the replacement organ could also be affected if the disease is not controlled.

WWW ONLINE SITES: p.1033

Porphyria

A set of rare disorders in which chemicals called porphyrins accumulate in tissues

GENETICS Some types are inherited

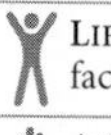
LIFESTYLE Excessive alcohol intake is a risk factor

AGE GENDER Not significant factors

As the body makes haemoglobin, the red pigment in blood, it produces chemicals called porphyrins. Normally, porphyrins are turned into haemoglobin, but in porphyria this change is blocked and they build up in the body. There are several forms of porphyria. Most forms are due to abnormal genes. The most common is inherited in an autosomal dominant manner (*see* GENE DISORDERS, p.271). Some forms are associated with sunlight exposure, liver disease, excessive alcohol use, or AIDS (*see* HIV INFECTION AND AIDS, p.297). In susceptible people, porphyria may be a side effect of some drugs.

WHAT ARE THE SYMPTOMS?

Each type of porphyria causes different symptoms. In some, the symptoms are persistent; in others, they are intermittent and triggered by sunlight, alcohol, or drugs. Symptoms may include:

- Dark, purplish urine.
- Rashes or blisters in areas that are exposed to sunlight.
- Abdominal pain.
- Pain or weakness in the arms or legs.

Severe intermittent porphyria can cause psychiatric problems such as delusions.

WHAT MIGHT BE DONE?

Porphyria is diagnosed by testing blood, faeces, or urine for porphyrins. There is no cure, but avoiding triggers may reduce the frequency of attacks. In some forms, intravenous glucose may help to prevent attacks or limit their severity.

WWW ONLINE SITES: p.1032

URINARY SYSTEM

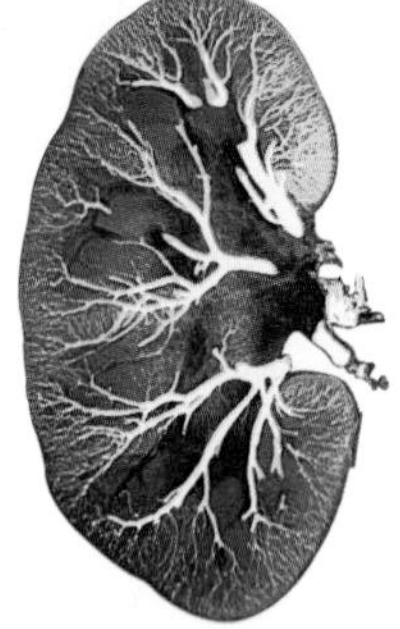

Rich blood supply
Numerous blood vessels supply the kidney with blood.

THE URINARY SYSTEM, also known as the urinary tract, acts as a filtering unit for the body's blood, excreting waste products and excess water as urine. The system consists of a pair of kidneys; the bladder; the ureters, which connect each kidney to the bladder; and the urethra, through which urine leaves the body. As the urinary system filters the blood, it regulates body water levels and maintains the balance of body fluids. The kidneys also produce hormones, one of which helps to control blood pressure. Every day the body's entire volume of blood passes through the kidneys over 300 times – a flow of about 1,700 litres (375 gallons).

Every action of our daily lives, from eating and breathing to walking and running, is made possible by chemical reactions in our body cells. Wastes produced as a result of these reactions collect in the blood. In order for us to remain healthy, these wastes must be filtered out and excreted. This is the main function of the urinary system.

The kidneys are connected to the aorta, the body's main artery that runs directly from the heart. When the body is at rest, the kidneys receive about a quarter of the blood pumped by the heart. Filtered blood is returned to the heart through the inferior vena cava, the largest vein in the body.

BLOOD FILTRATION

Each kidney contains about 1 million nephrons, mini-filtering units that consist of a knot of capillaries called the glomerulus and a long, thin tube called the renal tubule. Pores in the glomerulus allow only some of the molecules in the blood to pass through, depending on their size and shape. For example, red blood cells and proteins are much too large to pass through these pores and do not enter the filtered fluid. Smaller molecules pass into the renal tubule, where useful substances, such as glucose, are reabsorbed into the bloodstream. The fluid remaining in the tubule, called urine, is a mixture of wastes, such as urea, and other substances that are not required by the body, such as excess water and salts.

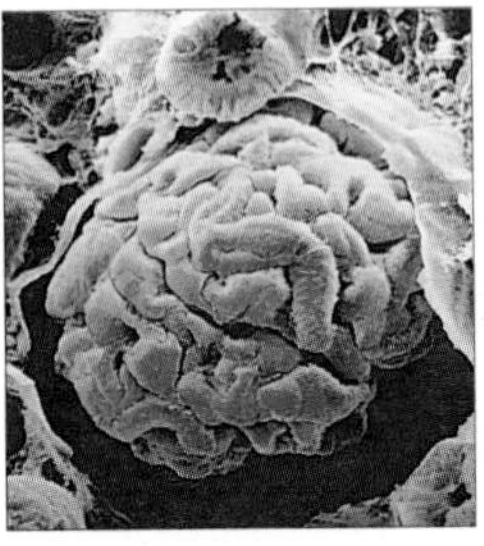

A glomerulus
This knot of capillaries is the glomerulus, which filters blood in the kidney.

This constant filtration of blood not only removes harmful wastes from the body but also helps to regulate water levels. If, for example, you drink more water than is needed for the body's requirements, the excess is excreted in urine. However, if you need to conserve water, the kidneys make the urine more concentrated and excrete as little water as possible. Furthermore, if your blood becomes too acidic or too alkaline, the kidneys change the urine's acidity level to restore the correct balance.

HORMONE PRODUCTION

The kidneys produce a number of hormones, each with different roles. Their functions include stimulating the formation of blood cells and controlling blood pressure by helping to regulate blood flow through arteries.

STRUCTURE SEXUAL DIFFERENCES

The lower urinary tract is different in males and females. The urethra from the male bladder passes through the prostate gland, carrying either urine or semen to the opening at the tip of the penis. The female bladder sits under the uterus, and the urethra carries urine to the opening in the front of the vagina. In both sexes, the passing of urine is partly controlled by muscles in the neck of the bladder.

Length of the urethra
The male urethra is usually about 20 cm (8 in) long. In females, the urethra is about 4 cm (1½ in) long.

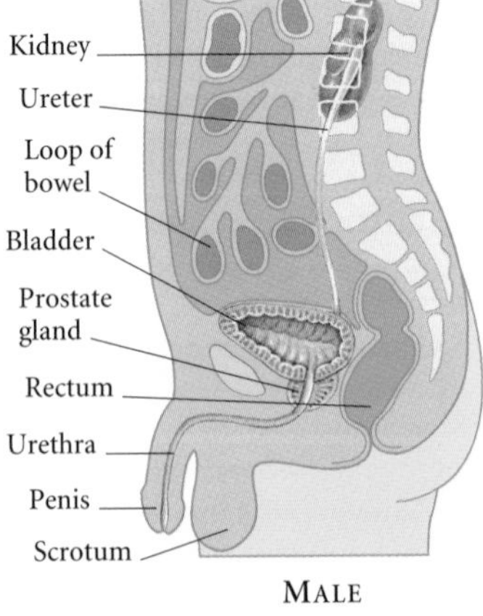

MALE

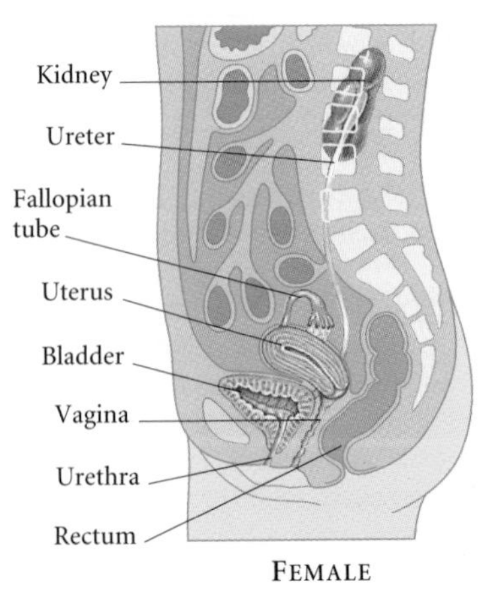

FEMALE

STRUCTURE URINARY SYSTEM

The urinary system consists of two kidneys, each linked by a ureter to the bladder, and a urethra, which connects the bladder to the outside of the body. The kidneys lie at the back of the abdomen, on either side of the spine. They are reddish-brown, bean-shaped organs, about 10–12.5 cm (4–5 in) long and 5–7.5 cm (2–3 in) wide. The ureters are thin, muscular tubes about 25–30 cm (10–12 in) long, and the bladder is a hollow, muscular organ located in the pelvis. The bladder's lower opening is surrounded by muscle that helps to control the release of urine through the urethra.

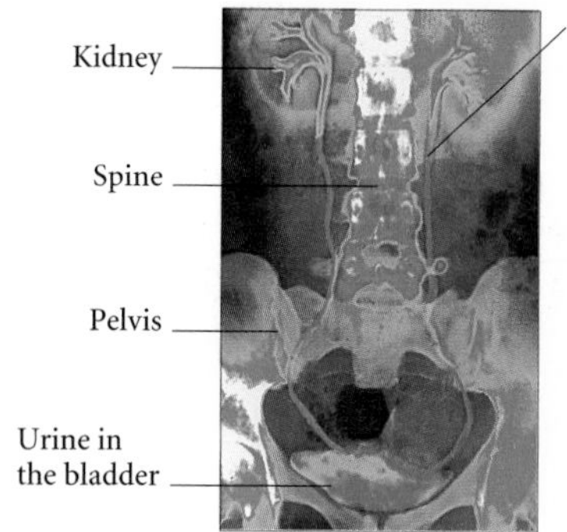

X-ray of urinary system
This specialized X-ray, known as an intravenous urogram (IVU), is used to highlight structures of the urinary system. The image clearly shows part of the kidneys; the ureters lying at either side of the spine; and the bladder. No abnormalities are seen.

Inferior vena cava
Blood from the lower part of the body returns to the heart in this vein

Adrenal gland (whole)
One adrenal gland sits on top of each kidney and secretes hormones

Kidney (whole)
The kidney on the right side of the body is slightly lower than the left one

Renal artery
Branching directly from the aorta, this artery supplies the kidney with blood

Renal vein
This vein takes blood from the kidney to the inferior vena cava

Peritoneum
This membrane, shown in part here, lines the abdomen and covers the surface of the bladder

Opening of ureter
This opening acts like a valve to stop urine flowing back up the ureter

Bladder outlet
Muscles at the bladder neck control the outflow of urine

Prostate gland
In males, the urethra passes through the prostate gland

Male urethra
The male urethra runs from the bladder to the tip of the penis

Adrenal gland (cross section)

Aorta
This artery carries blood from the heart to the rest of the body

Kidney (cross section)

Renal pelvis
This area is the drainage system of the kidney

Cortex of the kidney

Medulla of the kidney

Ureter
One ureter leads from each kidney and carries urine to the bladder

Bladder
Urine collects in the bladder, which has a thick, muscular wall

Ureter

Urethra

Bladder

Female lower urinary tract
The female urethra is shorter than the male urethra, and sits slightly lower in the pelvis.

STRUCTURE THE KIDNEY

The kidney has three regions: the cortex, the medulla, and the renal pelvis. The outer layer, the cortex, contains filtering units called nephrons, each consisting of a glomerulus and a renal tubule. The middle layer, the medulla, consists of cone-shaped groups of urine-collecting ducts. The inner region, the renal pelvis, branches into cavities called major and minor calyces. Each minor calyx gathers urine from the medulla; the urine is then collected in major calyces and funnelled into the ureter.

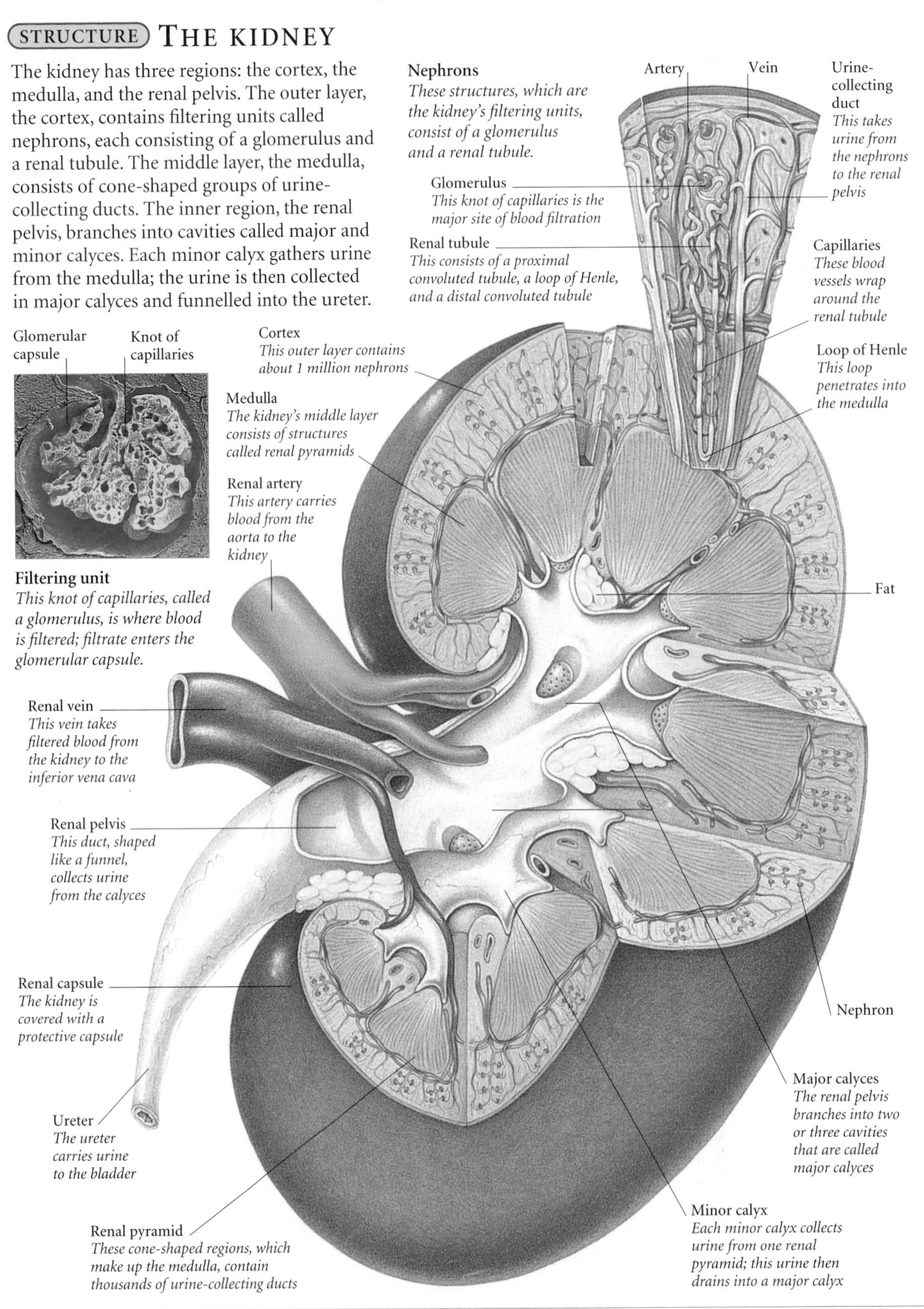

FUNCTION URINE FORMATION AND EXCRETION

Urine is composed of unwanted substances that have been filtered from the blood by nephrons, the functional units of the kidneys. The urine formed in the kidneys passes through the ureters and is temporarily stored in the bladder. From here it is emptied, normally under voluntary control, through the urethra. A healthy adult excretes 0.5–2 litres (1–4 pints) of urine each day.

HOW A NEPHRON MAKES URINE

Blood entering the nephron is filtered through a cluster of capillaries called the glomerulus. The filtrate then enters the renal tubule, along which a complex process of secretion and reabsorption occurs. Useful substances such as glucose are reabsorbed; the acidity of the blood is regulated; and water levels are adjusted. The resulting fluid is called urine.

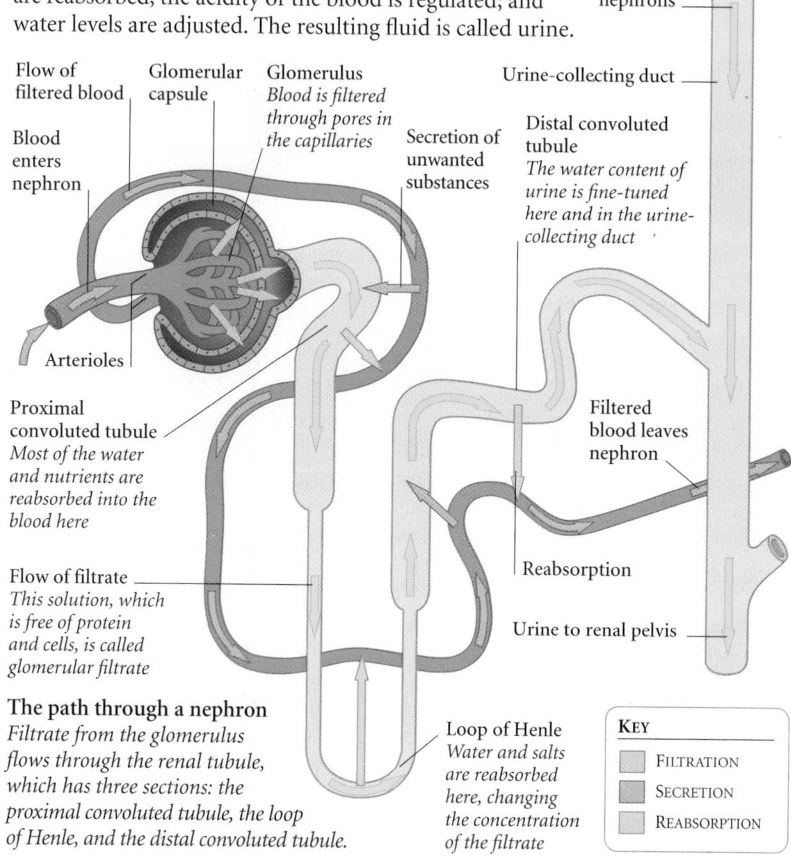

The path through a nephron
Filtrate from the glomerulus flows through the renal tubule, which has three sections: the proximal convoluted tubule, the loop of Henle, and the distal convoluted tubule.

WHAT IS URINE MADE OF?

Urine consists of a mixture of waste products and other substances. The mixture is balanced so that the body's internal environment remains constant. The water content of urine depends on whether there is too much or too little water in the body.

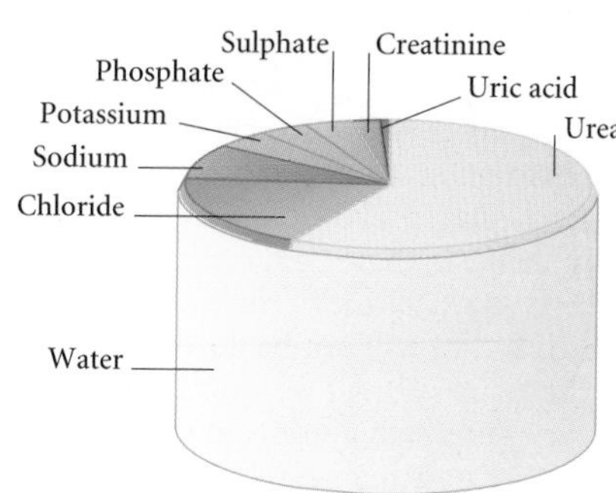

Mainly water
Urine is about 95 per cent water. The remainder includes wastes and other substances not needed by the body.

HOW URINATION IS CONTROLLED

When the bladder is full, nerves in the bladder wall send signals to the spinal cord. Signals are then sent back to the bladder, making it contract and expel urine. In older children and adults, the timing of urination can be regulated because this process is controlled by the brain. Infants lack this control, and the bladder empties when full.

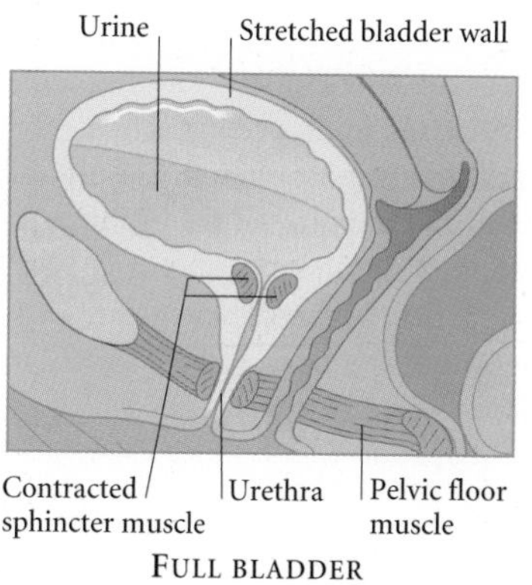

FULL BLADDER

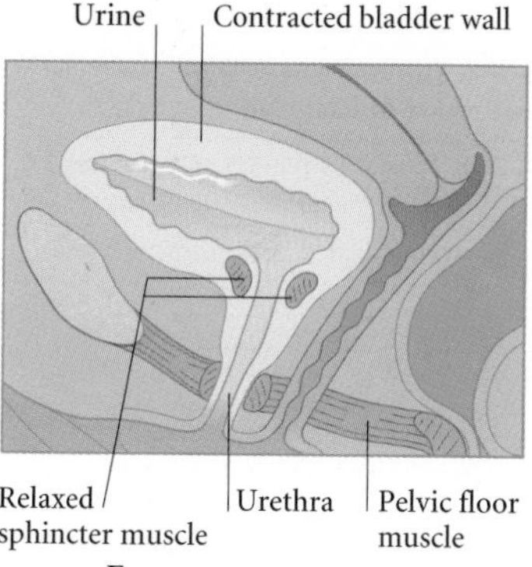

EMPTYING BLADDER

Emptying the bladder
To empty the bladder, muscles in the bladder wall contract and the sphincter muscles relax, forcing urine out of the bladder and down the urethra.

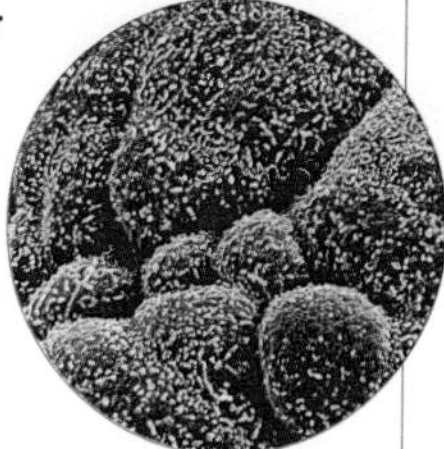

Inside the bladder
This highly magnified view shows the folds in the lining of the bladder wall. The folds in the wall stretch out as the bladder fills.

Kidney disorders

The kidneys keep the body's chemistry in balance by removing waste products and excess water. They also regulate blood pressure and stimulate red blood cell production. Although the body can stay healthy with only a single kidney, it is important that kidney disorders are treated promptly because some disorders progress rapidly, often affecting both kidneys.

The first article in this section covers pyelonephritis, a common disorder in which kidney tissue becomes inflamed, usually due to a bacterial infection. Glomerulonephritis, which develops when inflammation damages the glomeruli (the kidneys' filtering units), is discussed in the second article. This condition is most often the result of an abnormal response of the immune system rather than infection.

The next articles discuss stones and cysts in the kidneys. Kidney stones are often treated by a technique called lithotripsy, in which shock waves are used to pulverize the stones. Cysts are usually harmless, but multiple cysts resulting from a genetic disorder may cause kidney failure. The final articles cover cancer of the kidneys and kidney failure. The latter disorder may occur suddenly, especially if it results from a reduction in the blood flow to the kidneys, but more often it develops gradually due to a long-term disease such as diabetes mellitus. Kidney infections in children and the rare kidney cancer called Wilms' tumour (p.872) are discussed in the section on infancy and childhood (pp.870–872).

KEY ANATOMY

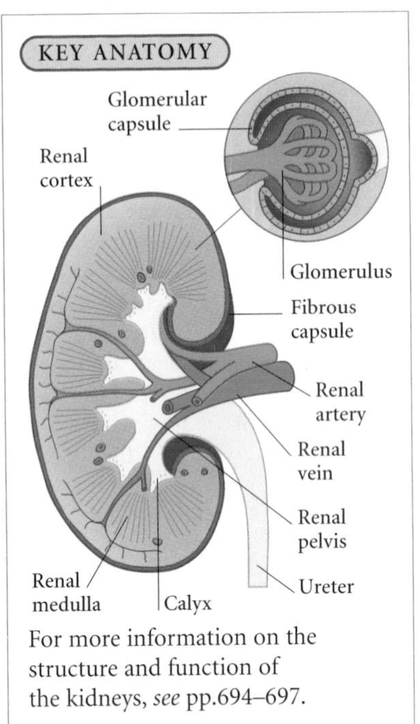

For more information on the structure and function of the kidneys, *see* pp.694–697.

Pyelonephritis

Inflammation of one or both kidneys, usually due to bacterial infection

AGE Most common between the ages of 16 and 45

GENDER Much more common in females

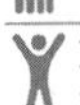
LIFESTYLE May be related to sexual activity in females

GENETICS In some cases, the cause is inherited from one parent

Pyelonephritis is one of the most common kidney disorders, particularly in young and middle-aged adults. In this condition, one or both of the kidneys become inflamed, usually as a result of a bacterial infection. In adults, pyelonephritis causes intense pain around the kidneys. The condition can usually be promptly diagnosed and treated and, for this reason, rarely leads to long-term damage to the kidneys. However, the symptoms of pyelonephritis may be less obvious in children. As a result, it may go unnoticed and lead to serious kidney damage (*see* URINARY TRACT INFECTIONS IN CHILDREN, p.871), possibly resulting in kidney failure in later life.

What are the causes?

Pyelonephritis may be caused by bacteria entering the urinary tract through the urethra (the passage from the bladder to the outside of the body). Often the bacteria migrate from an infection in the bladder (*see* CYSTITIS, p.709). Urinary infections, and therefore pyelonephritis, are much more common in females because the female urethra is shorter than that of the male, and its opening is nearer the anus. Bacteria from the anal area may enter the urethra during sex or if the area is wiped from back to front after a bowel movement. People with diabetes mellitus (p.687) are more likely to have urinary infections, partly because glucose in the urine may encourage bacterial growth.

In both sexes, pyelonephritis is more likely to develop if there is a physical obstruction anywhere in the urinary tract that prevents the normal flow of urine. In these circumstances, if bacteria have already contaminated the urine, they will not be flushed through the urinary tract as normal. Instead, they multiply in the stagnant urine. An obstruction may result from pressure on parts of the urinary tract. Possible causes of blockage include the expanding uterus in pregnant women or an enlarged prostate gland (p.725) in men. Normal urine flow may also be obstructed by bladder tumours (p.715) or kidney stones (p.701). In addition, kidney stones may harbour bacteria and can therefore predispose affected people to infection in the urinary tract. All of these conditions are likely to lead to recurrent episodes of pyelonephritis.

Bacteria may also enter the bladder during bladder catheterization (p.713), a procedure in which a tube is passed up the urethra into the bladder to drain urine. In addition, bacteria may be carried in the bloodstream from elsewhere in the body to the kidneys.

What are the symptoms?

The symptoms of pyelonephritis may appear suddenly, often over a period of a few hours, and include:

- Intense pain that begins in the back just above the waist and then moves to the side and groin.
- Fever over 38°C (100°F), resulting in shivering and headache.
- Painful, frequent passing of urine.
- Cloudy, blood-stained urine.

- Foul-smelling urine.
- Nausea and vomiting.

If you develop these symptoms, consult your doctor immediately.

HOW IS IT DIAGNOSED?

If your doctor suspects pyelonephritis, he or she will probably examine a sample of your urine to find out whether it contains bacteria. If there is evidence of infection, the urine sample will be sent for laboratory analysis to establish which type of bacterium has caused the infection. Men and children may need further tests to detect an underlying cause after a single episode of the disorder. Pyelonephritis is more common in women. For this reason, further tests are carried out for women only if they have recurrent episodes, or if the doctor suspects an underlying cause.

Further investigations may include a blood test to assess the function of the kidneys. Imaging procedures, such as ultrasound scanning (p.250), CT scanning (p.247), or intravenous urography (below), may also be carried out to check for signs of kidney damage or a disorder such as kidney stones.

WHAT IS THE TREATMENT?

Pyelonephritis is usually treated with a short course of oral antibiotics (p.885), and symptoms often improve within 2 days of treatment. When the course of antibiotics is finished, further urine tests may be carried out to confirm that the infection has cleared up. However, if you are vomiting, in pain, or seriously ill, you may be admitted to hospital and given intravenous fluids and antibiotics.

If you experience repeated episodes of pyelonephritis, you may be advised to take low-dose antibiotics for a period of 6 months to 2 years to reduce the frequency of the attacks. If you have an underlying disorder, such as kidney stones, this may also need to be treated.

WHAT IS THE PROGNOSIS?

In most cases, prompt treatment of pyelonephritis is effective, and the condition causes no permanent damage to the kidneys. However, rarely, frequent episodes of pyelonephritis may lead to scarring of the kidneys and result in irreversible damage (*see* END-STAGE KIDNEY FAILURE, p.708).

(WWW) ONLINE SITES: p.1037

Glomerulonephritis

Inflammation of the glomeruli, the tiny filtering units of the kidney

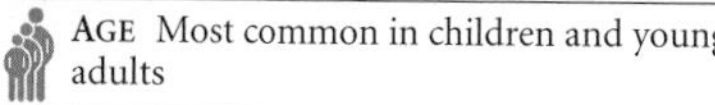
AGE Most common in children and young adults

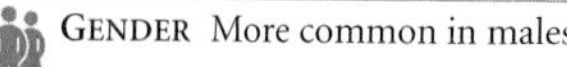
GENDER More common in males

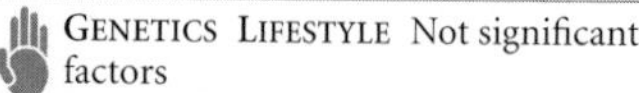
GENETICS LIFESTYLE Not significant factors

Glomerulonephritis is an uncommon disorder in which many of the tiny filtering units of the kidneys, known as glomeruli, become inflamed. As a result, the kidneys are unable to carry out their usual function of removing waste products and excess water from the body efficiently. In addition, blood cells and protein molecules, which normally remain in the blood, leak through the glomeruli into the urine.

Glomerulonephritis can be a short-term (acute) or long-standing (chronic) disorder. An episode with a sudden onset is usually followed by complete recovery, but in severe cases damage to the glomeruli may be permanent. Chronic glomerulonephritis sometimes

TEST INTRAVENOUS UROGRAPHY

Intravenous urography (IVU) is a procedure used to give a clear X-ray picture of the urinary tract. The procedure involves intravenous injection of a contrast medium (a substance that shows up on X-rays) into the arm. The contrast medium is carried in the blood to the urinary system, where it passes through the kidneys, ureters, and bladder to be excreted in the urine. X-rays taken at intervals show outlines of the kidneys, ureters, and bladder. IVU detects abnormalities, such as tumours and obstructions, and signs of kidney disease.

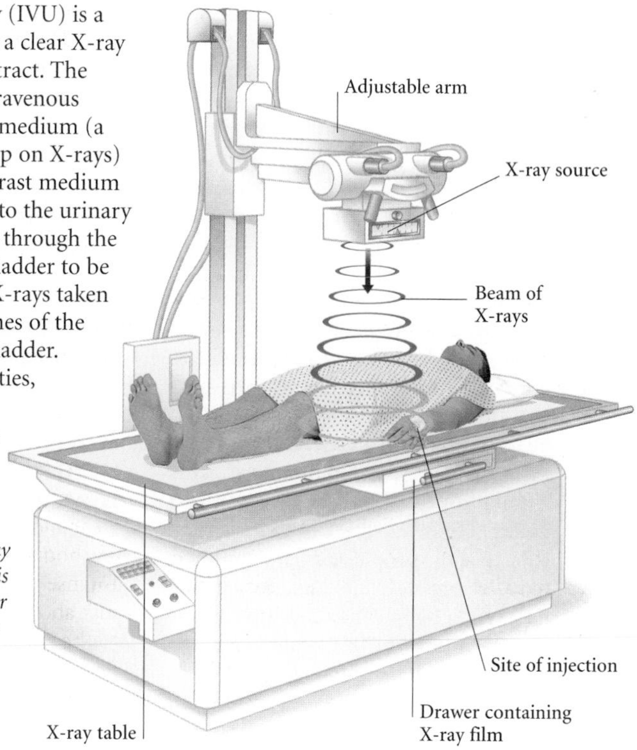

Undergoing urography
While you are on the X-ray table, a contrast medium is injected into a vein in your arm. You may feel a slight flushing sensation as this is done. X-rays are then taken at intervals over a 30-minute period.

RESULTS

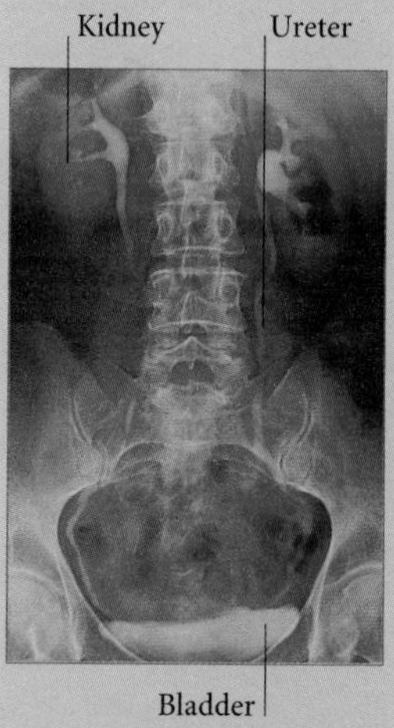

Normal urinary tract
This X-ray was taken 15 minutes after a contrast medium had been injected into the bloodstream. The kidneys, ureters, and bladder are clearly outlined.

develops after an acute attack. Progressive kidney damage then occurs over several months or years as a result of continual inflammation. Most people who develop glomerulonephritis have no previous history of kidney disease.

Although glomerulonephritis affects both kidneys, not all of the glomeruli are affected to the same degree.

WHAT ARE THE CAUSES?

Acute glomerulonephritis sometimes occurs as a complication of certain infectious diseases. The antibodies that are produced by the immune system to fight the infection attack the glomeruli in the kidneys, causing inflammation and damage. The most common cause of acute glomerulonephritis, especially in children, is a bacterial throat infection, such as a streptococcal infection. Occasionally, acute glomerulonephritis develops after a viral infection, such as infectious mononucleosis (p.291). In developing countries, the disorder may occur as a result of parasitic diseases, such as malaria (p.305).

Chronic glomerulonephritis is usually caused by an abnormal reaction of the immune system, in which certain antibodies of the immunoglobulin A type are deposited in the kidney tissues. However, chronic glomerulonephritis may also be associated with an autoimmune disorder that affects many organs in the body, such as systemic lupus erythematosus (p.461).

WHAT ARE THE SYMPTOMS?

In acute glomerulonephritis, symptoms develop rapidly over a few days. In contrast, the initial symptoms of chronic glomerulonephritis develop slowly and may only become apparent when the kidneys have already been severely damaged. The symptoms of both forms of the disorder may include:

- Frequent passing of urine.
- Frothy or cloudy urine.
- Blood in the urine.
- Puffiness of the face, with swelling around the eyes in the morning.
- Swollen feet and legs in the evening.
- Shortness of breath.
- Loss of appetite.

A serious complication of glomerulonephritis is high blood pressure (*see* HYPERTENSION, p.403), which may result in further damage to the kidneys.

HOW IS IT DIAGNOSED?

In the initial stages of chronic glomerulonephritis there may be no symptoms, and the condition may only be diagnosed during routine screening tests or investigations for another disorder. If you do develop symptoms of acute or chronic glomerulonephritis, the doctor may test a urine sample to detect blood and protein. Further urine tests and a blood test may be necessary to assess kidney function. In addition, your doctor may arrange for imaging tests to assess the size of your kidneys because the kidneys are likely to become larger in cases of acute glomerulonephritis and to shrink in chronic glomerulonephritis. The imaging tests usually include X-rays (p.244) or ultrasound scanning (p.250), and intravenous urography (p.699), a form of X-ray in which the urinary tract is highlighted with a contrast dye. However, the use of this dye is avoided in people with suspected serious kidney problems. A kidney biopsy (opposite page) may also be needed to determine the extent of kidney damage.

WHAT IS THE TREATMENT?

Treatment depends on the severity and, if known, the cause of the disorder. Some cases are so mild that they do not need treatment and are simply monitored. However, if the disorder follows a bacterial infection, antibiotics (p.885) and sometimes corticosteroids (p.930) may be prescribed. Glomerulonephritis due to an autoimmune disorder can usually be treated with immunosuppressants (p.906) and corticosteroids. If the condition is accompanied by high blood pressure, this will be treated at the same time. For chronic glomerulonephritis, a low-salt diet with reduced fluid intake may be recommended to prevent fluid retention in body tissues.

WHAT IS THE PROGNOSIS?

In most cases, the symptoms of acute glomerulonephritis disappear after 6–8 weeks. However, the outlook is variable. In some people, kidney function is reduced but does not deteriorate further. Other people may develop chronic kidney failure (p.706), which can lead to end-stage kidney failure (p.708), an irreversible loss of kidney function that may be fatal if not treated promptly.

(WWW) ONLINE SITES: p.1037

Nephrotic syndrome

A group of symptoms resulting from kidney damage that causes loss of protein into the urine and swelling of body tissues

 AGE Most common in young children but can affect people of any age

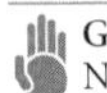 GENDER LIFESTYLE GENETICS Not significant factors

The urine of a healthy person does not normally contain protein because the molecules are too large to pass across the glomeruli (the blood-filtering units in the kidneys). However, if the delicate glomeruli are damaged, large amounts of protein can leak into the urine from the blood. Eventually, this leakage results in low protein levels in the blood, an accumulation of fluid in body tissues, and widespread swelling.

WHAT ARE THE CAUSES?

Nephrotic syndrome can be due to various kidney diseases, most commonly glomerulonephritis (p.699) and diabetic kidney disease (p.705). It may also be a complication of infection elsewhere in the body, such as hepatitis B (*see* ACUTE HEPATITIS, p.644). Rarely, it can be due to amyloidosis (p.693), in which an abnormal protein collects in organs. Other possible causes include reactions to drugs and chemicals, as well as certain autoimmune disorders (in which the body attacks its own tissues), such as systemic lupus erythematosus (p.461).

WHAT ARE THE SYMPTOMS?

The symptoms of nephrotic syndrome appear gradually over days or weeks and worsen as more and more protein is lost. You may notice:

- Frothy urine.
- Decreased urine production.
- Puffiness of the face, with swelling around the eyes in the morning.
- Swollen feet and legs in the evening.
- Shortness of breath.
- Loss of appetite and weight loss.
- Swelling of the abdomen.

If you develop these symptoms, you should see a doctor immediately.

WHAT MIGHT BE DONE?

If your doctor suspects that you have nephrotic syndrome, he or she will first test your urine for the presence of protein. The doctor may also ask you to collect the urine that you produce over a 24-hour period so that daily protein loss can be measured. You may have blood tests to measure your protein levels and assess kidney function. In some cases, a kidney biopsy (right) is carried out to find the cause of the condition.

Your doctor may prescribe diuretics (p.902) to help to remove excess fluid from your body and may recommend a low-salt diet to prevent further fluid retention. If symptoms are severe, you may need treatment in hospital where you will be given diuretics and protein-rich intravenous fluids. You may also be given corticosteroids (p.930) and immunosuppressants (p.906). If possible, the underlying disorder will be treated.

What is the prognosis?

The outlook for someone with nephrotic syndrome depends on the extent of the kidney damage. Children usually respond well to corticosteroids and often make a full recovery, but adults may experience recurrent episodes. In the most severe cases, chronic kidney failure (p.706) and eventually end-stage kidney failure (p.708), an irreversible loss of kidney function, may develop.

(WWW) ONLINE SITES: p.1037

(TEST) Kidney biopsy

A kidney biopsy is used to identify the nature and extent of kidney damage. The biopsy may be carried out as an outpatient procedure, or you may have to stay in hospital overnight. During the biopsy, a small piece of kidney tissue is removed. This tissue is then sent to a laboratory for microscopic examination. After the biopsy, you will be advised to rest for about 2 hours to minimize the risk of bleeding from the kidney.

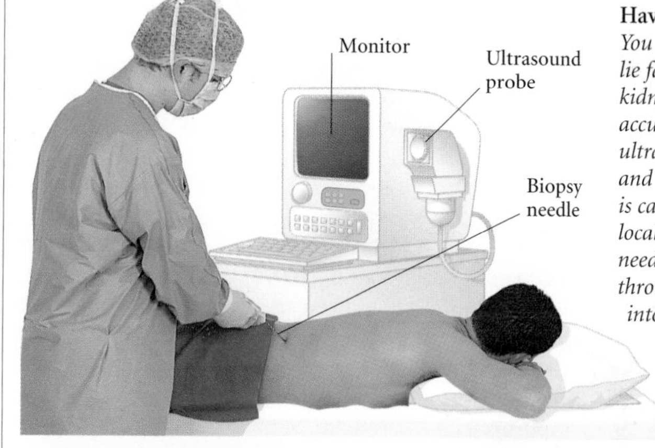

Having a biopsy
You will be asked to lie face down. The kidney is first located accurately using ultrasound scanning and then the biopsy is carried out. Under local anaesthesia, a needle is inserted through your skin into the kidney to remove a sliver of tissue.

(RESULTS)

Normal kidney tissue
This highly magnified view shows healthy kidney tissue. Several of the filtering units of the kidney, known as glomeruli, and the kidney tubules that lead from them are clearly visible.

Glomerulus
Kidney tubule
Glomerular capsule

Kidney stones

Crystal deposits of varying sizes that form in the kidney

AGE Most common between the ages of 30 and 50

GENDER More common in males

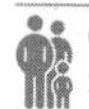
GENETICS In some cases, the cause is inherited

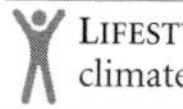
LIFESTYLE Certain diets and living in a hot climate are risk factors

Normally, the waste products of the body's chemical processes pass out of the kidneys in the urine. Kidney stones occur when the urine is saturated with waste products that are able to crystallize into stone-like structures, or when the chemicals that normally inhibit this crystallization process are not present. Kidney stones can take years to form.

If the stones are small, they may become dislodged from the kidney and move through the urinary tract, eventually passing out of the body in the urine. Larger stones stay in the kidney but may occasionally move into the ureter (the tube that takes urine from the kidney to the bladder). If a stone becomes lodged in the ureter, it can cause severe pain. A large stone in the kidney is not usually painful, but it can increase the risk of urinary infection.

What are the causes?

The risk of stones forming in the kidneys is greatest when there is a high concentration of dissolved substances in the urine. Inadequate intake of fluid increases the risk of kidney stones. When there is too little water in the body, the kidneys conserve water by forming less urine, and as a result the urine they produce is highly concentrated. People who live in hot climates may be susceptible to kidney stones if they do not drink enough to replace the fluid lost through perspiration.

Different types of kidney stone can form, depending on the waste products that crystallize out of the urine. Most are made of calcium salts. These stones may be associated with a diet containing foods rich in calcium or a substance called oxalic acid. They may also develop if your body produces too much parathyroid hormone (*see* HYPERPARATHYROIDISM, p.682), a process causing high levels of calcium to build up in the bloodstream. A small percentage of stones contain uric acid and may occur in people who have gout (p.380).

Kidney stones may also result from a long-standing urinary tract infection. In such cases, the stones can grow into a staghorn shape and fill the central cavity of the kidney. Rarely, they are formed from cystine, a substance present in abnormally high levels in people who have the inherited disorder cystinuria. Kidney stones are also associated with some drugs, such as indinavir, which is used to treat HIV infection (*see* DRUGS FOR HIV INFECTION AND AIDS, p.887).

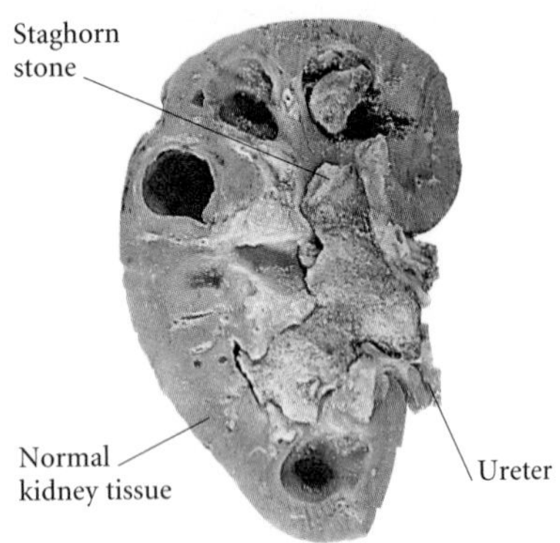

Staghorn kidney stone
Named for its shape, this staghorn kidney stone has enlarged over many years to fill the entire centre of the kidney.

WHAT ARE THE SYMPTOMS?

Very small kidney stones may pass unnoticed in the urine. Larger stones or small fragments of stones that pass into the ureter may cause painful spasms of the ureter wall. The symptoms usually appear suddenly and may include:

- Excruciating pain that starts in the back, spreads to the abdomen and groin, and may be felt in the genitals.
- Frequent, painful passing of urine.
- Nausea and vomiting.
- Blood in the urine.

If a kidney stone is passed in the urine, the pain will subside rapidly. However, if a stone lodges in a ureter, it may cause a build-up of urine, which will then result in swelling of the kidney (*see* HYDRONEPHROSIS, opposite page).

HOW IS IT DIAGNOSED?

If your doctor suspects that you have kidney stones, he or she will take a specimen of urine to look for blood, crystals, and evidence of an underlying infection. Stones that have been passed in the urine may be collected and analysed so that their composition can be determined. An ordinary X-ray (p.244) may be used to look for calcium stones; other types of kidney stone can be detected by taking specialized X-rays of the urinary tract (*see* INTRAVENOUS UROGRAPHY, p.699). You may also have a blood test to assess kidney function by measuring the levels of calcium, uric acid, and other substances in your blood. You may be asked to collect your urine for 24 hours for chemical analysis. These tests enable the doctor to determine the presence and composition of kidney stones still in the urinary tract.

WHAT IS THE TREATMENT?

If the stones are small and remain in the kidney, you may simply be advised to rest, take painkillers (p.912) to relieve discomfort, and drink plenty of fluids to help to flush the stones into the urine. In some cases, kidney stones that have become lodged in the lower part of the ureter can be removed during cystoscopy (p.715). In this procedure, a viewing tube is passed into the ureter through the urethra and bladder. Forceps are then passed through the tube to crush or remove the stone.

If a stone moves into the ureter, it usually causes severe pain that can last for several hours. You may need to go to hospital for strong painkillers. You may also be given intravenous fluids to increase the volume of urine and help to flush the stone out of the ureter. The most frequently used treatment for kidney stones is lithotripsy (below), in which shock waves are used to break the stones into powder that can be passed easily in the urine. Surgical removal of kidney stones is needed only if they are very large. Rarely, a staghorn stone is so large that the entire kidney must be surgically removed.

The underlying cause needs to be treated to prevent the kidney stones from recurring. Your doctor will probably advise you to drink at least 2–3 litres (4–6 pints) of fluids every day and to avoid foods that may encourage the formation of stones (*see* PREVENTING KIDNEY STONES, opposite page).

TREATMENT LITHOTRIPSY

Lithotripsy is a procedure that is usually carried out in hospital. It uses high-energy shock waves to disintegrate stones in the kidneys, ureters, or bladder. The fragmented stones will then be passed in the urine, avoiding the need for surgery. Painkillers are given before the procedure since there may be some discomfort; children are usually given a general anaesthetic. For a few days after lithotripsy, you may have blood in your urine, and the treated area will feel bruised and tender. However, serious complications are uncommon.

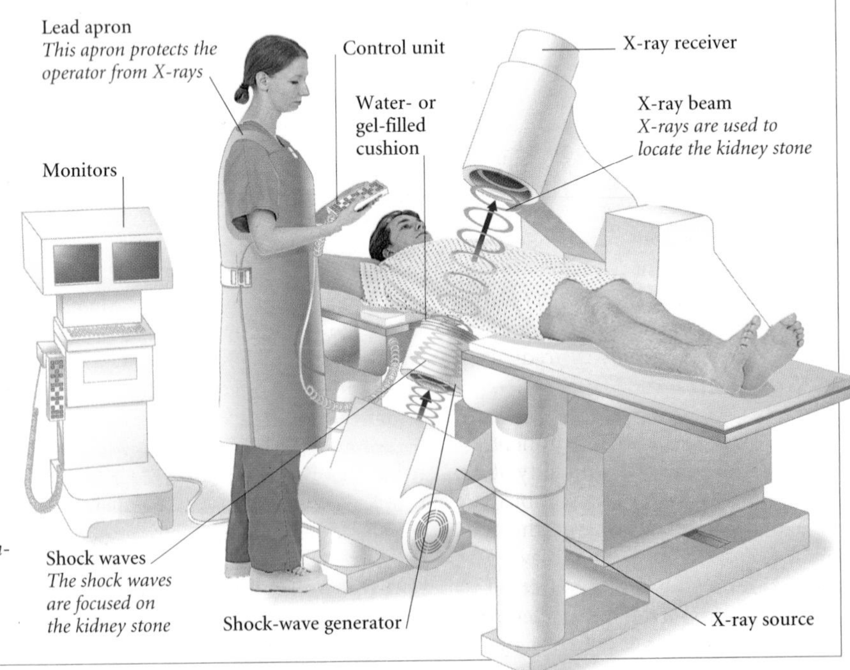

Undergoing lithotripsy
The stone is located using X-rays. A machine called a lithotripter focuses high-energy ultrasonic shock waves on to the stone through a water- or gel-filled cushion placed under the back.

SELF-HELP PREVENTING KIDNEY STONES

If you have kidney stones, these dietary precautions may help prevent their recurrence:

- Drink 2–3 litres (4–6 pints) of fluids daily.
- Drink fluids before going to bed to ensure that urine production continues overnight.
- Drink more fluids in hot weather, after strenuous exercise, or if you have a fever.
- Ask your doctor or dietitian if you should alter your diet to reduce your calcium intake. If you drink bottled water, check the calcium content.
- To prevent oxalate stones, avoid rhubarb, spinach, and asparagus.

WHAT IS THE PROGNOSIS?

More than half the people treated for a kidney stone develop another within about 7 years. However, the self-help measures above may reduce the risk of recurrence. Kidney stones rarely cause permanent damage to the kidneys.

WWW ONLINE SITES: p.1037

Hydronephrosis

Swelling of the kidney due to a blockage of the urinary tract

AGE Most common in very young children and elderly people

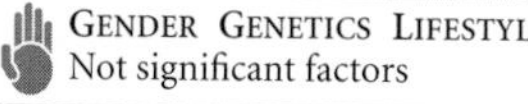
GENDER GENETICS LIFESTYLE Not significant factors

In hydronephrosis, a blockage in the urinary tract prevents urine from flowing normally through the system. As a result, the kidney becomes swollen with urine and pressure builds up within it, preventing normal function. The condition can affect one or both kidneys and may occur suddenly or gradually.

WHAT ARE THE CAUSES?

The blockage that causes hydronephrosis may be due to an abnormality of the urinary tract that is present at birth or to narrowing of the ureter (the tube that takes urine from the kidney). This narrowing may develop as a result of pressure from outside the ureter, such as that caused by a tumour or by the enlargement of the uterus during pregnancy. Hydronephrosis may also occur if a ureter is blocked by a kidney stone (p.701) moving towards the bladder.

In addition, the disorder can be due to blockage of the urethra (the passage that leads from the bladder to outside the body). A blocked urethra is usually due to a urethral stricture (p.714) or an enlarged prostate gland (p.725).

WHAT ARE THE SYMPTOMS?

If hydronephrosis results from a sudden obstruction in the urinary tract, the following symptoms may develop:

- Severe pain in the abdomen.
- Acute lower back pain.
- Nausea and vomiting.

However, hydronephrosis that develops gradually over a long period of time does not usually produce the symptoms listed above. In these cases, chronic kidney failure (p.706) may be the first sign that the condition exists.

People with hydronephrosis have an increased risk of urinary tract infection because bacteria are likely to multiply in urine that is not flowing freely.

HOW IS IT DIAGNOSED?

If your doctor suspects that you have hydronephrosis, he or she may arrange for blood tests and urine tests to find out how well your kidneys are functioning. The doctor may also arrange for imaging tests, including ultrasound scanning (p.250) and intravenous urography (p.699). These tests will enable the blockage in your urinary tract to be located and the cause of the obstruction determined. In some instances, hydronephrosis is detected only when another disorder, such as an enlarged prostate gland, is being investigated.

WHAT IS THE TREATMENT?

Initially, the aim of treatment is to prevent permanent damage to the kidney by relieving the pressure that has built up inside it as soon as possible. If there is a blockage in the urethra, a tube will be inserted into the bladder to drain the urine (*see* BLADDER CATHETERIZATION, p.713). If the blockage is higher in the urinary tract, a tube may be inserted directly into the affected kidney to drain the urine. Once the pressure in the kidney has been relieved, your doctor can treat the cause of the blockage.

Hydronephrosis that is associated with pregnancy is usually mild and does not require treatment. The condition should improve spontaneously after the birth.

WHAT IS THE PROGNOSIS?

If hydronephrosis is detected early, the affected kidney tissue normally recovers once the cause has been treated. However, in rare cases, hydronephrosis may lead to permanent kidney damage, and chronic kidney failure may develop if both kidneys are affected.

WWW ONLINE SITES: p.1037

Kidney cyst

A fluid-filled swelling within the cortex, the outer part of the kidney

AGE More common over the age of 50

GENDER GENETICS LIFESTYLE Not significant factors

Kidney cysts form in the cortex (outer layer) of the kidney. They often occur singly, but three or four may develop. Kidney cysts are very common; up to half of all people over the age of 50 have at least one cyst, often without realizing it. The cause is not known.

Unlike the multiple cysts that occur in polycystic kidney disease (p.704), kidney cysts do not affect kidney function and are usually harmless. In most cases, they cause no symptoms. Rarely, a kidney cyst may become large enough to cause back pain, or it may bleed, causing blood to appear in the urine.

WHAT MIGHT BE DONE?

A kidney cyst is often detected by chance during ultrasound scanning (p.250), CT scanning (p.247), or intravenous urography (p.699) performed to investigate another condition. In some cases, a fluid sample may be taken from the cyst through a hollow needle to be examined for cancerous cells. This procedure is carried out under local anaesthesia and uses ultrasound to locate the cyst.

A simple kidney cyst does not usually require treatment unless symptoms develop. However, if the cyst becomes painful, you may be sent to hospital to have fluid removed from it using a needle and syringe. Alternatively, the cyst can be removed surgically.

WWW ONLINE SITES: p.1037

Polycystic kidney disease

An inherited disorder in which multiple fluid-filled cysts gradually replace the tissue in both kidneys

AGE Juvenile form usually evident at birth; adult form usually apparent by the age of 45

GENETICS Due to an abnormal gene inherited from one or both parents

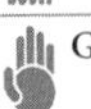
GENDER LIFESTYLE Not significant factors

Polycystic kidney disease is an inherited condition in which the kidneys have a honeycomb appearance as a result of the presence of numerous fluid-filled cysts. The cysts gradually replace normal tissue so that the kidneys become larger and progressively less able to function until eventually they fail completely (*see* END-STAGE KIDNEY FAILURE, p.708). Polycystic kidney disease is not the same as simple kidney cysts (p.703), which are generally harmless.

Polycystic kidneys may affect adults or, rarely, infants. Adult polycystic kidney disease does not usually become apparent until about the age of 45, although symptoms can appear as early as the age of 20. In children, the condition is known as juvenile polycystic kidney disease and is sometimes fatal.

What are the causes?

Polycystic kidney disease is caused by an abnormal gene. In the adult form, the gene is inherited in an autosomal dominant manner, and as a result the disease can be inherited from just one parent (*see* GENE DISORDERS, p.271). Each child of such a parent has a 1 in 2 chance of developing the disorder in adulthood. The juvenile form is inherited in an autosomal recessive way; both parents must pass the faulty gene to the child for the disorder to develop. When both parents have one copy each of the faulty gene, each child has a 1 in 4 chance of developing the disorder.

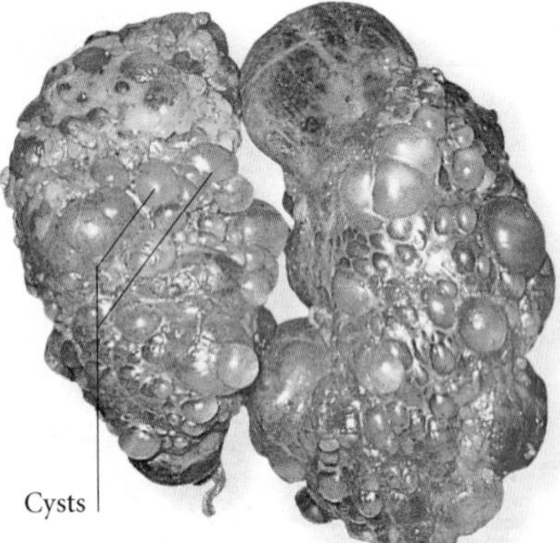

Polycystic kidneys
Multiple fluid-filled cysts have replaced the normal tissue in both of these kidneys. As a result, the kidneys have become very large and irregularly shaped.

Can it be prevented?

The gene responsible for polycystic kidneys in adults has been identified, and genetic counselling (p.272) is available for people who have a family history of the disease. If both parents are aware that they carry the gene that is responsible for the juvenile form, they will also need counselling. Otherwise, it is possible to check the kidneys of a fetus for signs of the disorder using ultrasound scanning (*see* ULTRASOUND SCANNING IN PREGNANCY, p.793). If an ultrasound scan reveals polycystic kidneys in the fetus, the parents can discuss the options available with the doctor.

What are the symptoms?

The symptoms of adult polycystic kidney disease may not appear for many years. The main symptoms are:

- Vague discomfort in the abdomen or aching in the lower back.
- Episodes of severe and sudden pain in the abdomen or lower back.
- Blood in the urine.

A baby with juvenile polycystic disease will have a very swollen abdomen due to enlargement of the kidneys.

In adults, as the disease progresses, high blood pressure (*see* HYPERTENSION, p.403) may develop, which can lead to further kidney damage. Occasionally, one or more of the kidney cysts become infected, resulting in pain and fever. Sometimes, cysts develop in other organs, such as the pancreas and liver.

If you have abdominal pain and notice blood in your urine, you should consult your doctor as soon as possible.

What might be done?

In many people, adult polycystic kidney disease is first discovered during a routine physical examination. It may also be detected when family members are screened because a relative already has polycystic kidney disease. Blood and urine tests may be performed to assess kidney function, and ultrasound scanning (p.250) or CT scanning (p.247) may be carried out to confirm the diagnosis. Healthy children of people with polycystic kidney disease are advised to have periodic ultrasound scans to check for the development of the disorder.

If it has not been detected in the fetus, juvenile polycystic kidney disease may be obvious at birth because the baby will have a very swollen abdomen. Doctors can then confirm the diagnosis by using ultrasound scanning to look for enlarged kidneys with cysts.

There is no effective way to prevent the cysts forming, but careful control of high blood pressure may slow the rate of the kidney damage. If the fluid in the cysts is infected, antibiotics (p.885) may be prescribed. If end-stage kidney failure occurs, dialysis (p.707) or a kidney transplant (p.708) will be needed.

What is the prognosis?

The progression of polycystic kidney disease in adults varies considerably. However, the outlook tends to be similar for affected members of the same family. About 7 in 10 of the people who have polycystic kidney disease develop kidney failure by the age of 65.

In a child who has juvenile polycystic kidney disease, the kidneys will fail, and eventually the child will need dialysis or a kidney transplant. Some affected infants may die at only a few months of age due to kidney failure.

(WWW) ONLINE SITES: p.1032, p.1037

Kidney cancer

Cancerous tumours that either originate in the kidney or have spread from a cancer elsewhere in the body

AGE GENDER GENETICS LIFESTYLE Risk factors depend on the cause

In most cases of kidney cancer, a tumour develops within the kidney tissue itself. Rarely, cancer may spread to the kidney from other organs in the body.

There are three main types of kidney cancer. The most common type, adenocarcinoma, develops from the cells that make up the main body of the kidneys. A second, rare form, known as transitional cell carcinoma, develops from

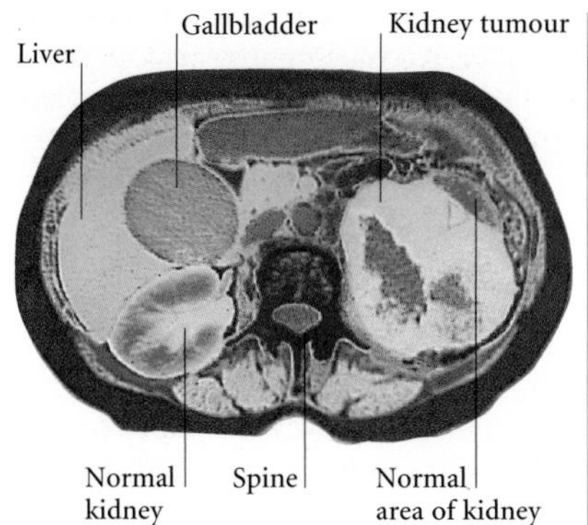

Kidney cancer
This CT scan through the abdomen shows a large kidney tumour that has grown to replace most of the normal kidney tissue.

the cells that line the urine-collecting system within the kidney, bladder, and ureters (the tubes that carry urine from the kidneys to the bladder). This form is more common in people who smoke, because tobacco contains carcinogens (cancer-inducing substances), and in people who have been exposed to other carcinogens, such as chemical dyes, even many years previously. A third type, called Wilms' tumour (p.872), is usually either present at birth or develops during the first 5 years of life.

What are the symptoms?

There are often no symptoms in the early stages of kidney cancer. If symptoms do develop, they may include:

- Painful, frequent passing of urine.
- Blood in the urine.
- Pain in the back or sides.
- Weight loss.

If you notice blood in your urine (indicated by a red, pink, or smoky colour), consult your doctor immediately.

What might be done?

If your doctor suspects kidney cancer, he or she may image the kidneys using ultrasound scanning (p.250), CT scanning (p.247), or intravenous urography (p.699). An affected kidney will be surgically removed. (The other kidney can usually compensate.) If the cancer has spread, you may need chemotherapy (p.280). A form of the natural hormone progesterone (*see* Sex hormones and related drugs, p.933) and cancer treatments such as aldesleukin (*see* Anticancer drugs, p.907) have been successful in treating some cases.

About 7 in 10 people who have a kidney tumour removed survive for more than 5 years, even if the tumour was large. If the cancer has spread to other organs before it is diagnosed, the chance of survival decreases. However, treatments such as radiotherapy (p.281) may slow the spread of cancer and relieve pain.

(WWW) ONLINE SITES: p.1028, p.1037

Diabetic kidney disease

Damage to the filtering units of the kidneys that occurs in people who have diabetes mellitus

Age Usually occurs in adults who have had diabetes mellitus for many years

Genetics Diabetes mellitus sometimes runs in families

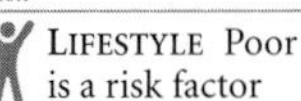
Lifestyle Poor control of diabetes mellitus is a risk factor

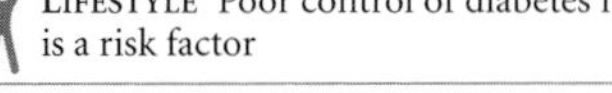

Gender Not a significant factor

Long-term diabetes mellitus (p.687) may result in damage to various organs in the body. Kidney damage caused by diabetes mellitus is known as diabetic kidney disease. The disorder develops in about 4 in 10 of the people who have had diabetes for over 15 years.

Diabetes mellitus affects small blood vessels in the glomeruli (the filtering units of the kidney). Damage to these vessels causes protein to leak into the urine and reduces the kidneys' ability to remove wastes and excess water from the body. Symptoms do not usually appear until kidney damage is severe, and they may then include vomiting, drowsiness, and shortness of breath (*see* Chronic kidney failure, p.706). Many people with long-term diabetes mellitus also have high blood pressure (*see* Hypertension, p.403), which may cause further damage to the kidneys.

What might be done?

People who have diabetes mellitus are monitored regularly by their doctor so that complications such as kidney damage can be detected at an early stage. The doctor may look for the first signs of diabetic kidney disease by arranging for urine tests to detect protein, and blood tests may also be performed to check how well the kidneys are functioning. Once the condition has been diagnosed, the primary aim of treatment is to slow the progression of the disease to kidney failure. Control of blood glucose levels and blood pressure can help to prevent deterioration of kidney function. However, even if diabetes is under control, diabetic kidney disease can still lead to damage. Drugs known as ACE inhibitors (p.900) can be effective in treating kidney disease due to diabetes mellitus but, nevertheless, the outcome may be end-stage kidney failure (p.708). If this occurs, there is a complete loss of function in both kidneys.

End-stage kidney failure due to diabetic kidney disease can usually be treated with dialysis (p.707) or a kidney transplant (p.708). It is sometimes possible to combine a kidney transplant with a transplant of the pancreas, treating both kidney failure and diabetes mellitus at the same time. However, the surgery involved is complex and is only carried out in certain specialist centres.

(WWW) ONLINE SITES: p.1030, p.1037

Kidney failure

Loss of the normal function of both kidneys due to a variety of causes

Age Gender Genetics Lifestyle Risk factors depend on the cause

In kidney failure, the kidneys cease to function normally, and waste products and excess water build up in the body, disrupting the chemical balance of the blood. The condition may take one of three forms: acute kidney failure (p.706), chronic kidney failure (p.706), or end-stage kidney failure (p.708).

Acute kidney failure is a sudden, drastic loss of kidney function that can be fatal if not treated rapidly. Chronic kidney failure is a gradual reduction in function of the kidneys over months or years. Some people have the condition for years without knowing it. End-stage kidney failure is a permanent and almost total loss of kidney function and is the last stage of chronic kidney failure. Left untreated, the condition is fatal.

Treatment for kidney failure involves first reversing or slowing the damage, then restoring the chemical balance of the blood and treating the underlying disorder. Methods of treatment for kidney failure may include drugs, dialysis (p.707), or a kidney transplant (p.708).

(WWW) ONLINE SITES: p.1037

Acute kidney failure

Sudden loss of the function of both kidneys, which is potentially life-threatening

AGE GENDER GENETICS LIFESTYLE Risk factors depend on the cause

Acute kidney failure occurs when both kidneys suddenly cease their normal function of filtering waste products and excess water from the blood into the urine. The waste substances build up to dangerous levels in the body, and the chemical balance of the blood is upset. The condition is life-threatening and requires immediate hospital treatment.

WHAT ARE THE CAUSES?

The kidneys will stop working properly if their blood supply is greatly reduced. This reduction may be due to a fall in blood pressure associated with shock (*see* HYPOTENSION, p.414), such as after severe bleeding, serious infection, or a heart attack (*see* MYOCARDIAL INFARCTION, p.410). Kidney failure may also result from damage by disorders such as glomerulonephritis (p.699), by toxic chemicals, or by drugs. Another cause may be a blockage in the urinary tract that causes both kidneys to swell with urine (*see* HYDRONEPHROSIS, p.703).

WHAT ARE THE SYMPTOMS?

The symptoms of acute kidney failure may appear rapidly, sometimes over a period of hours, and include:

- Greatly reduced urine volume.
- Nausea and vomiting.
- Drowsiness and headache.
- Back pain.

If you develop these symptoms, you should call your doctor immediately. Without treatment, acute kidney failure may be fatal within a few days.

HOW IS IT DIAGNOSED?

If your doctor suspects acute kidney failure, he or she will have you admitted to hospital for emergency treatment and tests to find the cause. In some cases, there may be an obvious cause, such as severe bleeding. In other cases, ultrasound scanning (p.250) or CT scanning (p.247) may be performed to look for a blockage of the urinary tract. A kidney biopsy (p.701) may also be performed to examine kidney tissue.

WHAT IS THE TREATMENT?

If you have acute kidney failure, you will need immediate treatment for the disorder and any associated conditions. You will probably be treated in an intensive care unit (p.958). You may have to undergo dialysis (opposite page) for a short time so that the excess fluid and waste products can be removed from your bloodstream while the doctors investigate the cause of the kidney failure. If you have lost a large amount of blood, you may need to have a blood transfusion (p.447) to restore your normal blood volume. If an underlying disorder is diagnosed, treatment with drugs may be necessary. Finally, if there is a blockage anywhere in your urinary tract, you may need to undergo surgery to have the obstruction removed.

WHAT IS THE PROGNOSIS?

If your kidneys have not already been damaged irreversibly, there is a good chance that you will make a complete recovery, which may take up to 6 weeks. However, in some cases, the resulting damage is not completely reversible, and in this situation chronic kidney failure (below) may develop. If chronic kidney failure eventually progresses to end-stage kidney failure (p.708), in which there is a permanent and almost total loss of kidney function, you will need treatment that involves long-term dialysis or a kidney transplant (p.708) to restore normal kidney function.

(WWW) ONLINE SITES: p.1037

Chronic kidney failure

Gradual and progressive loss of function in both kidneys

AGE Some causes are increasingly common with age

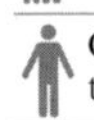
GENDER GENETICS Risk factors depend on the cause

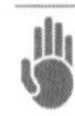
LIFESTYLE Not a significant factor

In chronic kidney failure, progressive damage gradually reduces the ability of the kidneys to remove excess water and wastes from the blood for excretion as urine. As a result, waste substances start to build up in the body and cause problems. In many cases, kidney function is reduced by over 60 per cent before the build-up begins; by this time, often after months or even years, the kidneys may be irreversibly damaged. Dialysis (opposite page) or a kidney transplant (p.708) may therefore become necessary.

WHAT ARE THE CAUSES?

Chronic kidney failure can be due to disorders that progressively damage kidney tissue, such as polycystic kidney disease (p.704) or glomerulonephritis (p.699). The condition may also be the result of generalized disorders, such as diabetes mellitus (p.687) or high blood pressure (*see* HYPERTENSION, p.403). People who have sickle-cell disease (p.448) are at risk of developing chronic kidney failure if abnormal blood cells block the small vessels that supply the kidneys. Chronic kidney failure can also follow prolonged blockage of the urinary tract, such as that caused by an enlarged prostate gland (p.725).

WHAT ARE THE SYMPTOMS?

The initial symptoms of chronic kidney failure appear gradually over weeks or months and are often vague, such as weakness and loss of appetite. Obvious symptoms may then develop, including:

- Frequent passing of urine, particularly during the night.
- Pale, itchy, and easily bruised skin.
- Shortness of breath.
- Persistent hiccups.
- Nausea and vomiting.
- Muscular twitching.
- Pins and needles.
- Cramps in the legs.

The condition is associated with a number of complications, such as high blood pressure, which may be an effect as well as a cause of kidney failure; bone thinning (*see* OSTEOPOROSIS, p.368); and anaemia (p.446), in which the oxygen-carrying capacity of the blood is reduced. Disturbance in blood chemistry caused by kidney failure may lead to conditions such as hyperparathyroidism (p.682).

HOW IS IT DIAGNOSED?

If you have symptoms of chronic kidney failure, your doctor will probably arrange for tests of your blood and urine to detect abnormally high waste levels. You may also have ultrasound scanning (p.250), radionuclide scanning (p.251), or CT scanning (p.247) to assess the size of the kidneys; abnormally small kidneys are often a sign of

TREATMENT DIALYSIS

Dialysis is used to treat kidney failure by replacing the functions of the kidneys, which filter out wastes and excess water from the blood. It can be a temporary treatment for acute kidney failure (opposite page) or a long-term measure used in end-stage kidney failure (p.708). There are two forms: peritoneal dialysis, in which the peritoneal membrane in the abdomen is used as a filter; and haemodialysis, in which a kidney machine filters the blood.

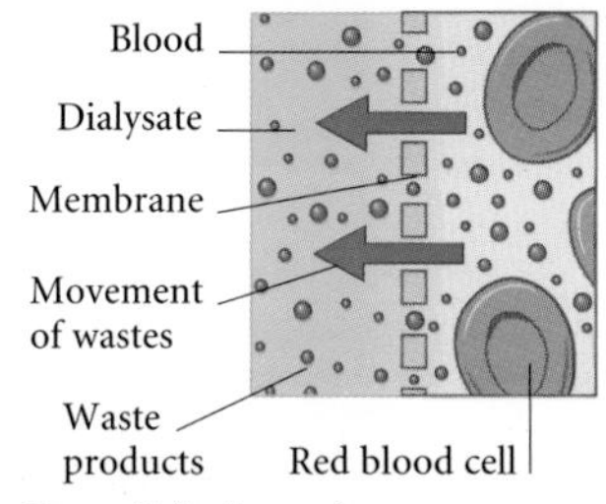

How dialysis works
During dialysis, excess water and waste products from the blood pass across a membrane into a solution (the dialysate), which is then discarded.

PERITONEAL DIALYSIS

In peritoneal dialysis, the peritoneum, the membrane that surrounds the abdominal organs, is used instead of the kidneys to filter the blood. A procedure called an exchange is carried out four times a day at home. During an exchange, dialysis fluid that was infused into the abdomen 4–6 hours earlier is drained out of the peritoneum through a catheter in the abdominal wall. The fluid is replaced with fresh solution, then the equipment is disconnected and you can carry out normal activities. Between exchanges, wastes and excess water pass continually from the peritoneal blood vessels into the dialysis fluid.

Fresh dialysate
The bag of fresh dialysate is slowly emptied into the peritoneal cavity

Dialysate tubing

Undergoing peritoneal dialysis
In peritoneal dialysis, dialysis fluid is changed at regular intervals and is continually present in the abdomen. Once a fluid exchange has taken place, the bags and tubing are detached, and you can move freely.

Bag of used dialysate
Used dialysate drains out of the body and collects in this bag before fresh fluid is allowed to flow in

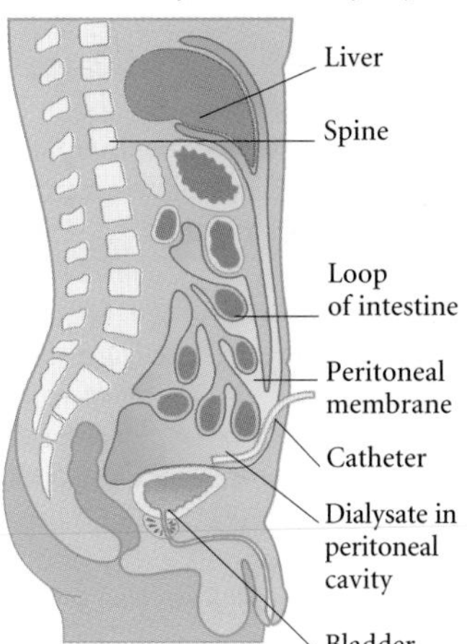

Using the peritoneum as a filter
The abdominal organs are covered by the peritoneal membrane, which is rich in blood vessels. In peritoneal dialysis, waste products and water pass from the blood across the membrane and into dialysate fluid in the abdomen.

HAEMODIALYSIS

In haemodialysis, blood is pumped by a kidney machine through a filter attached to the side of the machine. Inside the filter, blood flows on one side of a membrane and dialysis fluid flows on the other. Waste products and water pass from the blood across the membrane and into the dialysate fluid, and the filtered blood returns to the body. Each treatment takes 3–4 hours and is usually repeated three times a week.

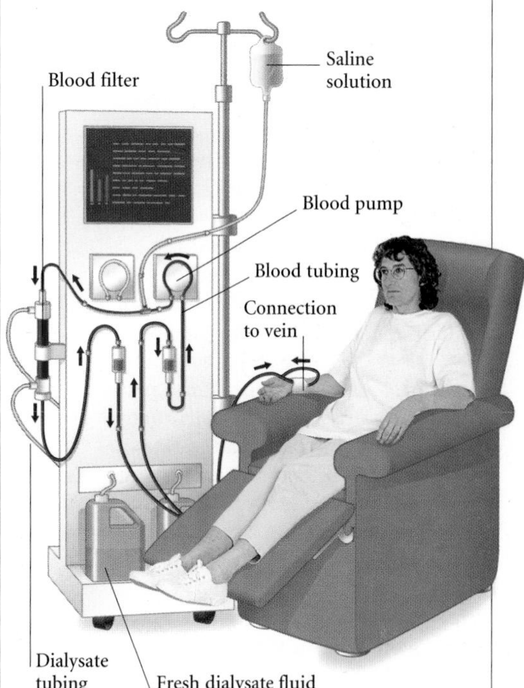

Undergoing haemodialysis
During haemodialysis, you are attached to the kidney machine for several hours while waste products and water are removed from your blood. Haemodialysis is usually carried out in outpatient dialysis centres, but some people are able to treat themselves at home.

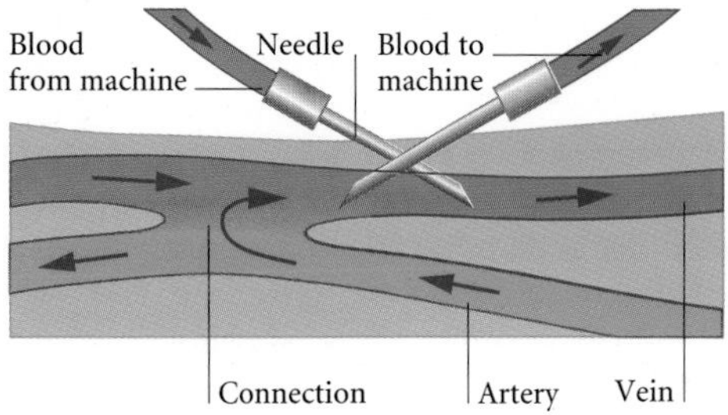

Access to the bloodstream
Dialysis requires fast blood flow. A vein and an artery near the skin surface are surgically joined so that the vein carries blood at high pressure. This vein can then be used for access to the circulatory system.

chronic kidney failure. In addition, you may need to undergo a kidney biopsy (p.701), a procedure in which a small piece of kidney tissue is removed and examined under a microscope to determine the nature of kidney damage.

What is the treatment?

Treatment is directed at the underlying cause. Corticosteroids (p.930) may be used to treat some forms of glomerulonephritis. Drugs for high blood pressure (*see* Antihypertensive drugs, p.897) may also be given, whether the condition is a cause or a result of chronic kidney failure. If there is an obstruction in the urinary tract, you will probably need surgery to relieve it. In addition, your doctor will monitor the progress of the disease and the effectiveness of your treatment with regular checkups.

What is the prognosis?

The outlook for chronic kidney failure depends on the cause and severity of the kidney damage. If your doctor is able to treat the cause and prevent further damage to your kidneys, you may not need dialysis. However, in many cases, treatment only slows the rate of deterioration. After several months or even years, chronic kidney failure may develop into end-stage kidney failure (below), in which the damage is irreversible. At this stage, dialysis or a kidney transplant operation is required.

(WWW) ONLINE SITES: p.1037

TREATMENT Kidney transplant

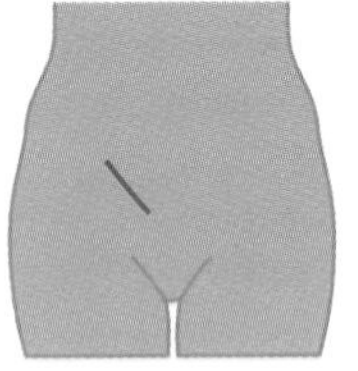

End-stage kidney failure may be treated with a kidney transplant, which can take over the function of both diseased kidneys. An organ may be donated by a living relative or spouse or by someone who has consented to the use of his or her organs after death. The new kidney is sited in the pelvis and the diseased ones are usually left in place. A kidney transplant avoids the need for dialysis and often allows a return to a normal lifestyle.

Site of incision

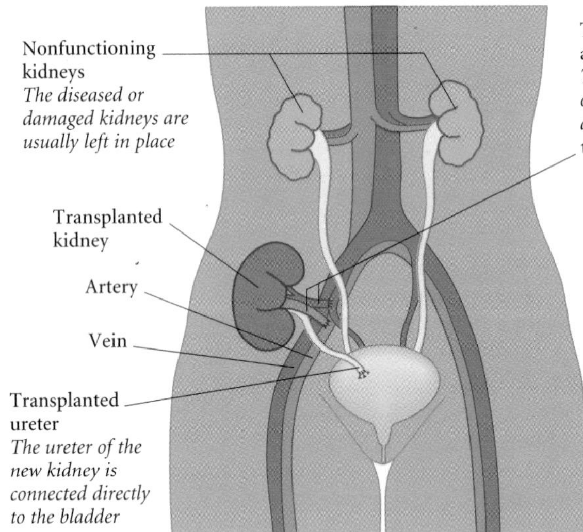

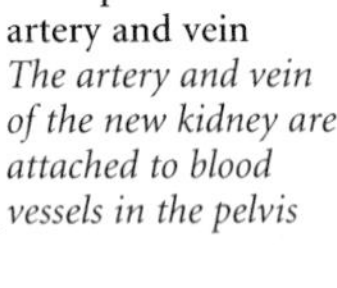

The operation
The new kidney is placed in the pelvis through an incision in the abdomen. The kidney is carefully positioned so that it can be connected easily to a nearby vein and artery and to the bladder.

End-stage kidney failure

Irreversible loss of the function of both kidneys, which is often life-threatening

Age Gender Genetics Lifestyle
Risk factors depend on the cause

In end-stage kidney failure, the kidneys have permanently lost over 90 per cent of their normal function. They are therefore unable to filter waste products and excess water out of the blood for excretion as urine. End-stage kidney failure usually progresses from chronic kidney failure (p.706). If prompt action is not taken to replace the function of the failed kidneys with dialysis (p.707) or a kidney transplant (above), the condition is inevitably fatal.

What are the symptoms?

The main symptoms of end-stage kidney failure usually include:

- Greatly reduced volume of urine.
- Swelling of the face, the limbs, and the abdomen.
- Severe lethargy.
- Weight loss.
- Headache and vomiting.
- Furred tongue.
- Very itchy skin.

Many people who have end-stage kidney failure also have breath that smells like ammonia, an odour similar to that of household bleach.

How is it diagnosed?

If your doctor suspects end-stage kidney failure, he or she will first arrange for urine tests and blood tests to detect abnormal levels of waste products in these body fluids. If the cause of kidney failure has not already been identified, you may also have to undergo imaging procedures such as ultrasound scanning (p.250), CT scanning (p.247), or radionuclide scanning (p.251) to detect abnormalities in your kidneys.

What is the treatment?

Kidney dialysis, the usual treatment for end-stage kidney failure, takes over the function of filtering harmful waste products from the blood and controlling the water balance of the body. However, long-term dialysis may lead to complications such as gradual weakening of the bones (*see* Osteoporosis, p.368). Anaemia (p.446), in which the oxygen-carrying capacity of the blood is reduced, may develop due to a lack of the hormone erythropoietin, which is made in the kidneys and stimulates red blood cell production. However, anaemia is easily treated by injections of erythropoietin.

A kidney transplant offers the best hope of returning to a normal lifestyle. The main drawback of a transplant is that you will need to take immunosuppressants (p.906) for the rest of your life to prevent your immune system from rejecting the donor organ. Occasionally, a second transplant is needed if the first kidney stops functioning. If you do not have a kidney transplant, you will need dialysis for the rest of your life.

(WWW) ONLINE SITES: p.1037

DISORDERS OF THE BLADDER AND URETHRA

Urinary disorders are very common. The symptoms may include an increased need to empty the bladder, urinary leakage, blood in the urine, and pain during and after urination. These symptoms can often disrupt daily routine. However, most disorders of the bladder and urethra (the passage from the bladder to the outside of the body) are curable or at least controllable by treatment.

The first article in this section deals with cystitis, a condition in which the bladder becomes inflamed. Cystitis is often due to infection by bacteria from the skin around the anus. Women are particularly susceptible to the disorder because the female urethra is short and close to the anus, allowing bacteria to enter easily. In men, bladder infections are often related to an obstruction due to an enlarged prostate gland.

The next three articles cover urinary incontinence, which is the inability to control bladder function. There are several types of incontinence, all of which are more common in women and in older people of both sexes.

Structural disorders are covered in the next articles; they include stones that form in the bladder and strictures that narrow the urethra, making the passing of urine difficult.

The last article in this section covers bladder tumours, which are often first indicated by the presence of blood in the urine. Early diagnosis usually leads to successful treatment.

Sexually transmitted infections that affect the male urethra are discussed elsewhere (*see* SEXUALLY TRANSMITTED INFECTIONS, pp.764–768). Urinary tract problems that occur in children are covered in the section on infancy and childhood (pp.870–872).

KEY ANATOMY

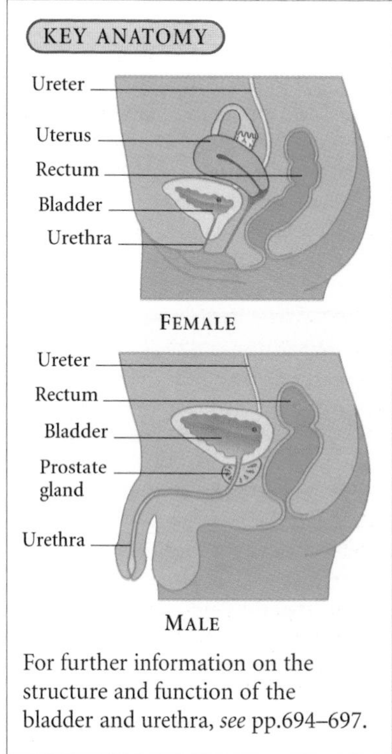

For further information on the structure and function of the bladder and urethra, *see* pp.694–697.

Cystitis

Inflammation of the bladder lining, causing painful, frequent passing of urine

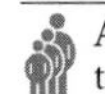 AGE Rare in children; more common in teenage girls and women of all ages

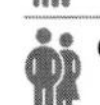 GENDER Much more common in females

 LIFESTYLE For some women, sexual intercourse may bring on an episode

 GENETICS Not a significant factor

In cystitis, the lining of the bladder becomes inflamed, resulting in a frequent need to pass urine and pain when passing urine. In most cases, the condition is due to a bacterial infection.

Cystitis affects women much more commonly than men. About half of all women have at least one attack of bacterial cystitis in their lifetime, and some women have recurrent attacks. In men, cystitis is rare and is usually associated with a disorder of the urinary tract. In children, cystitis can be the result of an anatomical or structural problem and can damage the kidneys (*see* URINARY TRACT INFECTIONS IN CHILDREN, p.871).

WHAT ARE THE TYPES?

There are several types of cystitis. The most common form is bacterial cystitis, which is often caused by *Escherichia coli*, a bacterium that normally lives in the intestines. Cystitis usually occurs when bacteria from the anal or vaginal areas enter the bladder through the urethra (the tube from the bladder to the outside of the body), often during sex or when the anus is wiped after a bowel movement. Women are at much greater risk of infection than men because the female urethra is shorter than that of the male and the opening is nearer the anus. The risk of bacterial cystitis is increased if the bladder cannot be emptied fully. Incomplete emptying causes urine to be retained in the bladder, and bacteria can multiply in the trapped urine. Postmenopausal women are especially prone to bacterial cystitis because they have reduced levels of the hormone oestrogen, which leaves their urethral lining vulnerable. Women who use a diaphragm and spermicide for contraception are at increased risk because a diaphragm, which has to stay in place for several hours, can prevent complete bladder emptying, and spermicide may encourage the growth of bacteria in the vagina. People with diabetes mellitus (p.687) are also susceptible for several reasons: there may be glucose in their urine, which encourages the growth of bacteria; they may have reduced immunity to infection; or they may have nerve damage that prevents the bladder from emptying completely. Other disorders that prevent complete bladder emptying include an enlarged prostate gland (p.725) and urethral stricture (p.714), in which the urethra is narrowed.

Interstitial cystitis is a rare, long-term inflammation of the lining and tissues of the bladder that may lead to ulceration. The cause is unknown.

In radiation cystitis, the lining of the bladder is damaged as a result of radiotherapy (p.281) to treat prostate cancer (p.726), bladder tumours (p.715), or cancer of the cervix (p.750).

Some women have repeated bouts of painful, frequent urination but with no bacteria in the urine. These symptoms are known as urethral syndrome. Minor bruising following sexual intercourse is sometimes a factor, particularly in postmenopausal women whose genital tissues may be thin and easily damaged.

WHAT ARE THE SYMPTOMS?

The main symptoms of all types of cystitis are the same and include:

- Burning pain when passing urine.
- Frequent and urgent need to urinate, with little urine passed each time.
- A feeling of incomplete emptying of the bladder.

If the cause of the cystitis is a bacterial infection, you may also notice:

- Pain in the lower abdominal region and sometimes in the lower back.
- Fever and chills.

A bladder infection can spread upwards to a kidney, causing severe pain in the back (*see* PYELONEPHRITIS, p.698). In some severe cases of cystitis, complete or partial loss of control over bladder function can occur as a result of irritation of the muscle in the bladder wall (*see* URGE INCONTINENCE, p.712).

SELF-HELP PREVENTING BACTERIAL CYSTITIS

If you have had bacterial cystitis, the following measures can help you to avoid further attacks:

- Drink 2–3 litres (4–6 pints) of fluids each day. Drink even more in hot weather.
- Empty your bladder frequently and completely.
- Be careful about hygiene. After a bowel movement, wipe yourself from front to back to prevent bacteria around the anus from entering the urethra.
- Wash your genital area before sexual intercourse. Make sure your partner washes, too.
- Pass urine shortly after having sexual intercourse.
- Use unperfumed toiletries and avoid vaginal deodorants.
- Do not use a diaphragm or spermicide for contraception.

WHAT MIGHT BE DONE?

If you develop the symptoms of cystitis, arrange to see your doctor. You may be able to relieve symptoms by drinking ½ litre (about 1 pint) of fluid every hour for 4 hours. Drinking cranberry juice can relieve the burning sensation when passing urine, and painkillers (p.912) may ease discomfort. Self-help measures (*see* PREVENTING BACTERIAL CYSTITIS, left) may prevent a recurrence.

Your doctor will arrange for urine tests to detect any evidence of infection. While awaiting the results, he or she may prescribe antibiotics (p.885). Almost all attacks of bacterial cystitis are cured by a single course of antibiotics. Recurrent attacks in women or a single episode in men need further investigation, usually involving urodynamic studies (p.711) and ultrasound scanning (p.250) of the urinary tract and sometimes cystoscopy (p.715), in which a viewing instrument is used to look for underlying conditions. If there is no evidence of a disorder but the cystitis still recurs, your doctor may prescribe a long course of low-dose antibiotics. Women may be given a single high dose of antibiotics to be taken after intercourse or at the first sign of symptoms.

If urine tests show no infection but you have recurrent attacks of pain and a frequent urge to pass urine, your doctor may suspect urethral syndrome and will probably refer you to a specialist. To relieve symptoms, you may have urethral dilation, a procedure to widen the urethra that can be carried out during cystoscopy. Some postmenopausal women find that oestrogen-containing creams help to relieve symptoms.

If the attacks continue, you may have interstitial cystitis. Your doctor may arrange for cystoscopy to view the bladder, and a sample of tissue may be taken. If you have interstitial cystitis, your doctor may suggest a procedure in which the bladder is stretched by filling it with water. This procedure, which is carried out under general anaesthesia, often relieves the symptoms of cystitis.

(WWW) ONLINE SITES: p.1037

Urinary incontinence

Complete or partial loss of voluntary control over bladder function

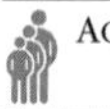
AGE More common with increasing age

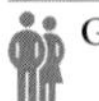
GENDER More common in females

GENETICS LIFESTYLE Risk factors depend on the type

Normally, muscles in the bladder wall push the urine out of the bladder, while muscles in the neck of the bladder and urethra (the tube from the bladder to the outside of the body) control the opening and closing of the bladder outlet. Any disorder affecting these muscles or their nerve supply can result in a partial or complete loss of bladder control.

Urinary incontinence becomes more common with increasing age. The condition is more common in women than in men. It sometimes accompanies dementia (p.535) or stroke (p.532).

WHAT ARE THE TYPES?

There are four main types of incontinence: stress, urge, overflow, and total. The symptoms and treatment are different for each type.

The most common type of incontinence is stress incontinence (opposite page), in which small amounts of urine are expelled involuntarily.

People who have urge incontinence (p.712) feel an unexpected and urgent need to pass urine due to an involuntary contraction of the bladder, resulting in the uncontrollable and sudden passage of large amounts of urine.

In overflow incontinence, the bladder cannot empty because of a blockage at the bladder neck or in the urethra or because of a weak bladder muscle. The volume of urine then builds up in the bladder, causing an intermittent dribble. Urine outflow is usually obstructed by a urethral stricture (p.714) or, in men, by an enlarged prostate gland (p.725) constricting the urethra. A weak bladder muscle may be due to an obstruction, diabetes mellitus (p.687), pelvic surgery, or a nervous system disorder such as spina bifida (*see* NEURAL TUBE DEFECTS, p.844) or multiple sclerosis (p.541).

In total incontinence, there is no bladder control. The condition usually results from a nervous system disorder

TEST URODYNAMIC STUDIES

Urodynamic studies are carried out to investigate problems with bladder control, including incontinence and restricted urine flow. In these studies, probes are inserted into the bladder and rectum or vagina to monitor pressure changes while the bladder is being filled through a catheter and emptied. In some cases, the bladder is filled with a contrast medium (a dye that shows up on X-rays), which enables the doctor to view the shape of the bladder on an X-ray monitor. You will be asked to cough as the bladder fills, which may cause leakage of urine if you have stress incontinence.

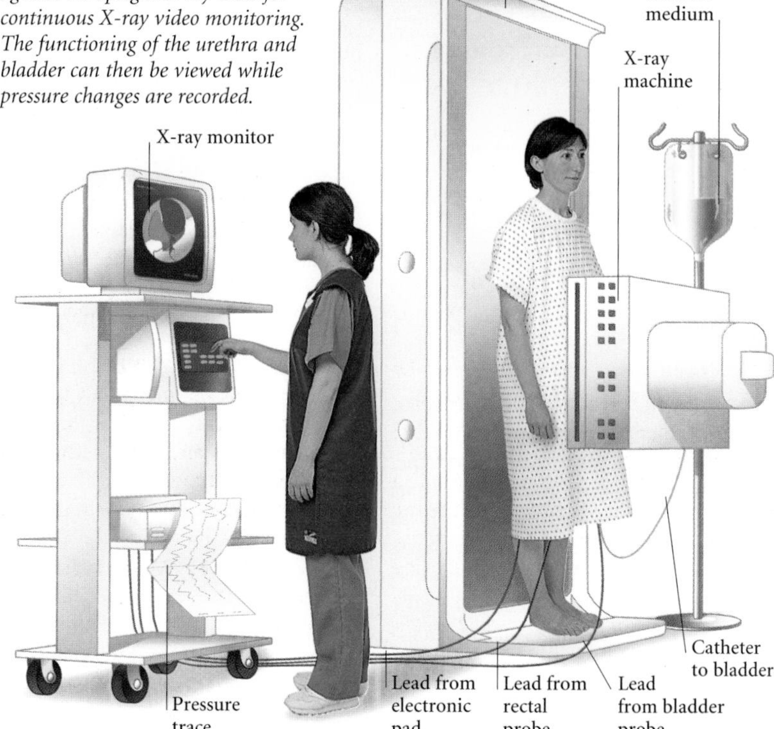

X-ray monitoring
During the procedure, you stand against an upright X-ray table for continuous X-ray video monitoring. The functioning of the urethra and bladder can then be viewed while pressure changes are recorded.

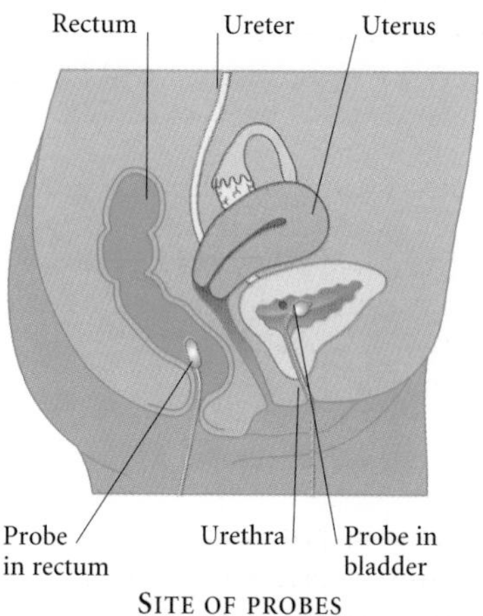

SITE OF PROBES

RESULTS

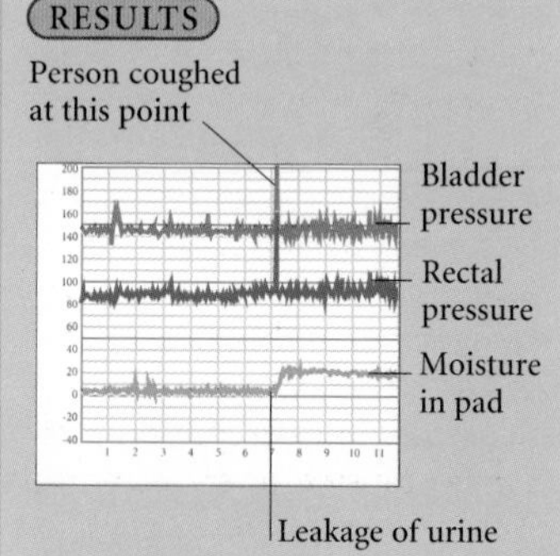

Pressure tracing
As the bladder filled, the person was asked to cough. This action increased pressure in and around the bladder, causing a leakage of urine on to an electronic absorbent pad. This result is typical of stress incontinence.

such as dementia or spinal injury (p.524). Surgery to treat pelvic cancers can also cause incontinence by damaging nerves that supply the bladder.

WHAT MIGHT BE DONE?

Urodynamic studies (above) can determine the type of incontinence. Pads to absorb urine can be worn to protect clothes. Pelvic floor exercises (p.712) and physiotherapy (p.961) may help to improve bladder muscle tone. Incontinence due to incomplete bladder emptying can be relieved by intermittent self-catheterization to drain the urine or permanent bladder catheterization (p.713) if the person is disabled.

WWW ONLINE SITES: p.1037

Stress incontinence

Involuntary loss of urine during exertion, coughing, or sneezing

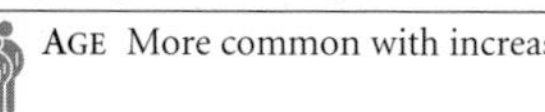
AGE More common with increasing age

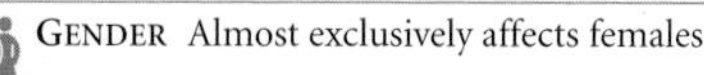
GENDER Almost exclusively affects females

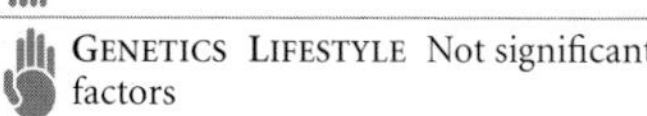
GENETICS LIFESTYLE Not significant factors

Stress incontinence results from weakness of the urethra (the tube from the bladder to the outside of the body) and pelvic floor muscles. These muscles support the bladder and help to control the opening and closing of the bladder outlet when passing urine. Weakness of the muscles allows the bladder neck to drop. Involuntary loss of urine occurs when pressure in the abdomen is increased.

In mild stress incontinence, a small amount of urine leaks out of the bladder during strenuous activities, such as running. In severe cases, urine escapes during activities such as coughing or lifting. Stress incontinence is the most common type of incontinence and mostly affects women.

The disorder commonly occurs during and after pregnancy; after surgery in the pelvic area; during the menopause, when a reduced level of the hormone oestrogen causes the pelvic muscles to lose elasticity; and with increasing age. Stress incontinence may also be linked

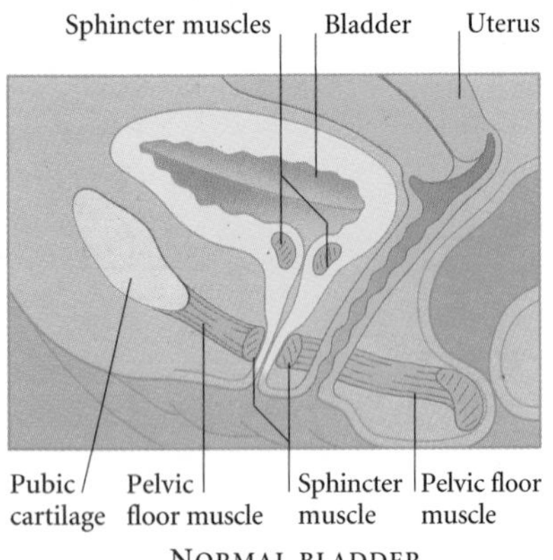

NORMAL BLADDER

Dropped bladder neck
Uterus
Pubic cartilage
Sagging muscles

INCONTINENT BLADDER

Cause of stress incontinence
In stress incontinence, the muscles in the pelvic floor cannot support the bladder. The bladder neck drops, and the sphincter muscles become unable to keep it closed.

to a prolapse of the uterus and vagina (p.747), rectal prolapse (p.667), or a prolapsed bladder. The condition is more likely to develop if you have a persistent cough. Rarely, men develop stress incontinence after prostate surgery.

How is it diagnosed?

Your doctor may diagnose stress incontinence after asking about your fluid intake, how often you pass urine, the amount of urine you pass, and when you leak urine. He or she will perform a pelvic examination to check your pelvic floor muscles and find out if you have a prolapsed uterus. The doctor may refer you to hospital for urodynamic studies (p.711) to assess your bladder function.

What is the treatment?

Strengthening the pelvic floor muscles with pelvic floor exercises (right) is an effective form of self-help treatment for stress incontinence, whatever the cause. If the condition occurs after childbirth, muscle tone will gradually return, but pelvic floor exercises may speed recovery. Postmenopausal women may be advised to have hormone replacement therapy (p.937) to counteract loss of muscle tone in the pelvic floor. If you are overweight, your doctor may recommend a diet to help you to lose weight (*see* CONTROLLING YOUR WEIGHT, p.53). In severe cases, surgery to reposition the bladder and improve its support may be needed to restore near-normal bladder control.

(WWW) ONLINE SITES: p.1037

Urge incontinence

Repeated episodes of involuntary loss of urine preceded by a sudden, urgent need to empty the bladder

 AGE More common with increasing age

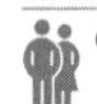 GENDER More common in females

 GENETICS LIFESTYLE Not significant factors

A person with urge incontinence feels a sudden, urgent need to pass urine that is followed by involuntary loss of urine. This condition varies in severity. At its mildest, the person is usually able to reach a toilet before the bladder starts to empty. However, if the condition is severe, it can be impossible to stop the flow of urine voluntarily once the bladder has begun to empty.

What are the causes?

Urge incontinence is most commonly caused by irritability of the muscle that forms the bladder wall. When irritated, the muscle contracts involuntarily and empties the bladder. Bladder irritability can due to infection or inflammation of the bladder lining (*see* CYSTITIS, p.709). Incontinence in women, especially after the menopause, may be caused by weak muscles in the bladder neck and pelvic floor or by gynaecological disorders, such as a prolapsed uterus (*see* PROLAPSE OF THE UTERUS AND VAGINA, p.747).

Urge incontinence can also be due to disorders such as bladder stones (p.714). Other causes are disorders that affect the nervous system, such as stroke (p.532), multiple sclerosis (p.541), or spinal injury (p.524). Some cases are thought to be linked with anxiety disorders (p.551).

What might be done?

You will be asked to keep a record of how often you need to pass urine, the amount of urine passed, and how much fluid you drink. You may also need to provide a urine sample to be checked for infection. Your doctor will examine you to look for an underlying disorder and may refer you to hospital for further investigations.

Any underlying cause of urge incontinence should be treated first. If no underlying disorder is found, there are several self-help measures that you can try. For example, you can learn to control your bladder function by extending the intervals between the times when you pass urine. Pelvic floor exercises (below) strengthen the muscles that control the bladder outlet. If you smoke, you should try to stop since smoking is known to irritate the bladder. It is also advisable to avoid drinks containing caffeine and alcohol. In addition, you may be given an anticholinergic drug such as oxybutynin in order to reduce the irritability of the bladder wall (*see* DRUGS ACTING ON THE BLADDER, p.926).

(WWW) ONLINE SITES: p.1037

SELF-HELP PELVIC FLOOR EXERCISES

Exercises can be used to help to strengthen the pelvic floor muscles. These muscles support the bladder, uterus, and rectum. If performed regularly, pelvic floor exercises can help in both the treatment and prevention of incontinence.

You can perform pelvic floor exercises sitting, standing, or lying down. Do the exercises as often as you can, ideally for 5 minutes every hour throughout the day.

In order to identify the pelvic floor muscles, imagine that you are passing urine and have to stop suddenly midstream. The muscles that you feel tighten around your vagina, urethra, and rectum are the pelvic floor muscles. To strengthen these muscles, practise the following exercises:

- Contract the pelvic floor muscles and hold them for 10 seconds.
- Relax the muscles slowly.
- Repeat 5 to 10 times, as often as you can.

Urinary retention

Inability to empty the bladder completely or at all

AGE More common over the age of 50

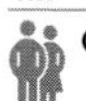
GENDER More common in males

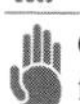
GENETICS LIFESTYLE Not significant factors

Urinary retention may be either acute or chronic. In acute retention, the bladder cannot be emptied at all despite a desperate urge to do so, and a sudden and painful build-up of urine occurs. In chronic retention, some urine can be passed with difficulty, but the bladder cannot be emptied completely, and as a result a gradual and painless build-up of urine occurs. Both forms of urinary retention are more common in men.

What are the causes?

Anything that exerts pressure on the urethra (the tube from the bladder to the outside of the body) can restrict the flow of urine, causing acute or chronic urinary retention. The most common cause in men is an enlarged prostate gland (p.725). Sometimes, the flow of urine is restricted by a narrowed urethra (*see* URETHRAL STRICTURE, p.714) or by a tightened foreskin of the penis (*see* PHIMOSIS, p.721). In women, retention may occur during early pregnancy due to pressure by the enlarging uterus on the urethra, but it may disappear later as the uterus rises up into the abdomen. In both sexes, urinary retention may be caused by constipation because faeces in the rectum can press on the urethra. Rarely, the flow of urine from the bladder is restricted by conditions in which the neck of the bladder is obstructed, such as bladder stones (p.714) and bladder tumours (p.715).

Damage to the nerves supplying the bladder muscles can also cause urinary retention. Damage may occur in disorders such as multiple sclerosis (p.541) and diabetes mellitus (p.687), or it may be caused by spinal injury (p.524).

In some cases, chronic urinary retention can become acute because of a sudden increase in the amount of urine produced, which can be triggered by diuretic drugs (p.902), cold weather, or alcohol consumption. In other cases, acute urinary retention is a side effect of antidepressant drugs (p.916), drugs for Parkinson's disease (*see* PARKINSON'S DISEASE AND PARKINSONISM, p.539), or cold and flu remedies (p.910).

What are the symptoms?

Symptoms of acute urinary retention develop over a few hours and include:

- Abdominal pain.
- A distressing and painful urge to pass urine without being able to do so.

In contrast to acute retention, chronic retention is unlikely to cause any pain, although the condition can be uncomfortable. The symptoms tend to develop more slowly and include:

- A frequent urge to pass urine.
- Swelling of the abdomen.
- Difficulty starting to pass urine.
- A weak flow of urine that ends in a dribble. In some cases, there may be involuntarily dribbling of urine between visits to the toilet.

Urinary retention can cause kidney damage if urine cannot drain from the kidneys (*see* HYDRONEPHROSIS, p.703).

What might be done?

If you have acute urinary retention, you will probably need to have your bladder emptied in hospital (*see* BLADDER CATHETERIZATION, below). You will have a rectal or pelvic examination and may later have special tests (*see* URODYNAMIC STUDIES, p.711, and CYSTOSCOPY, p.715) to identify the underlying cause.

Chronic urinary retention may be suspected if a routine medical examination reveals that you have an enlarged bladder. Diagnostic tests are the same as those for acute retention. The cause of the retention is treated if possible, and, in most cases, bladder function returns to normal. If the condition results from nerve damage, permanent or intermittent catheterization to drain the urine may be necessary. You may be taught how to catheterize yourself.

Urinary retention that occurs during pregnancy usually disappears when the uterus enlarges and moves up and out of the pelvis into the abdominal area, relieving pressure on the urethra.

(WWW) ONLINE SITES: p.1037

TREATMENT BLADDER CATHETERIZATION

In this procedure, a catheter is inserted into the bladder through the urethra (urethral catheterization) or through an incision in the abdomen (suprapubic catheterization). The catheter allows urine to drain out of the body if passing urine is not possible, if a person is incontinent, or if urine flow needs to be measured for diagnostic reasons. The catheter is held in place by a small, water-filled balloon and may be removed after urine has been drained or left in permanently. Some people may be taught to insert a catheter themselves several times a day to drain urine.

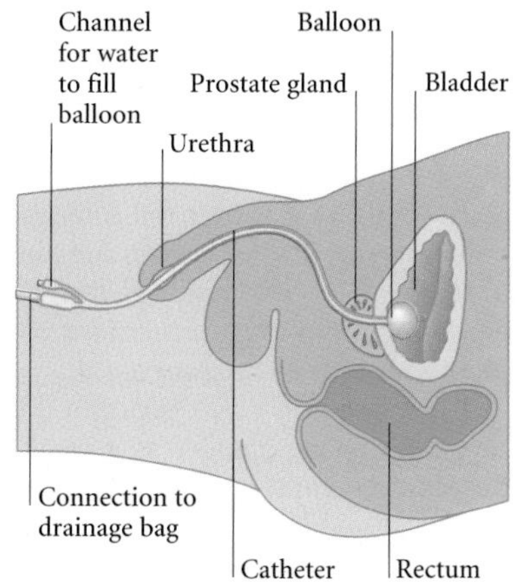

Urethral catheterization
The catheter is inserted along the urethra and into the bladder. Urine passes down the catheter into a drainage bag attached to a stand or worn around the thigh.

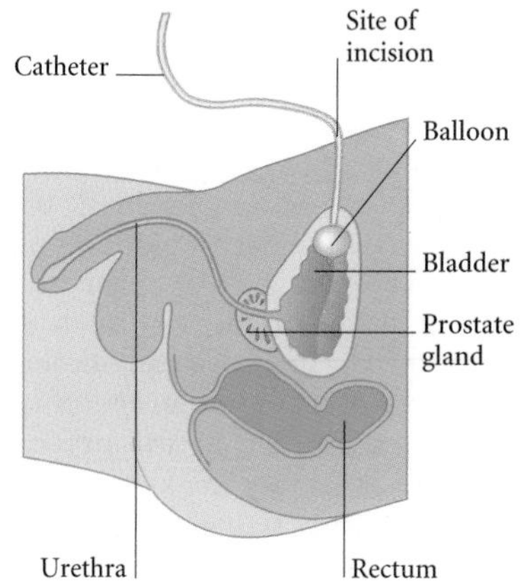

Suprapubic catheterization
This catheterization is used for long-term drainage if the urethra is blocked. The catheter enters the bladder via an incision in the abdomen. Urine is collected in a bag.

Urethral stricture

Abnormal narrowing of part of the urethra, the passage from the bladder to the outside of the body

 AGE Can affect adults of any age but most common over the age of 50

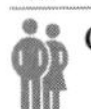 GENDER Almost exclusively affects males

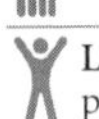 LIFESTYLE Unprotected sex with multiple partners is a risk factor

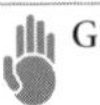 GENETICS Not a significant factor

In urethral stricture, scar tissue forms within the wall of the urethra, causing narrowing of the urethra and difficulty passing urine. In developed countries, scar tissue usually results from damage to the area during certain medical procedures, such as bladder catheterization (p.713), cystoscopy (opposite page), or prostatectomy (p.725). Scarring from these procedures usually affects people over 50 years old. Worldwide, the most common causes of scarring are persistent urethral inflammation as a result of sexually transmitted infections, such as gonorrhoea (p.764) or nongonococcal urethritis (p.765), and accidental injury to the genital area, such as a fracture of the pelvis. Such conditions are usually more common in young adults.

WHAT ARE THE SYMPTOMS?

The symptoms of a stricture gradually get worse over time and may include:

- Difficulty passing urine.
- Poor flow of urine.
- Dribbling after passing urine.
- The sensation that the bladder has been only partly emptied.
- Frequent need to pass urine.

An untreated stricture may block the flow of urine from the bladder, causing urinary retention (p.713). Incomplete emptying of the bladder can result in cystitis (p.709). In a few cases, incomplete emptying may cause an abnormal build-up of pressure in the urinary tract that can damage the kidneys (*see* HYDRONEPHROSIS, p.703).

WHAT MIGHT BE DONE?

Your doctor will carry out a physical examination to find out if your bladder is enlarged. He or she may then arrange for specialized X-rays of the urinary tract to establish whether your bladder empties completely when you pass urine and to look for bladder abnormalities. A stricture may be suspected if X-rays reveal slow bladder emptying and an abnormally large volume of retained urine. Further studies (*see* URODYNAMIC STUDIES, p.711) may show whether or not a stricture exists, and cystoscopy and imaging may be used to locate it.

If a stricture is detected, treatment depends on its location and factors such as the age of the affected person. The simplest treatment is urethral dilation (widening). Under local anaesthesia, a slim, flexible instrument is passed into the urethra to stretch the narrowed area gently. The procedure is repeated weekly over several months.

For more serious strictures, the scar tissue may be removed surgically during cystoscopy. If there is substantial scarring, the narrowed section may be removed and the urethra reconstructed using plastic surgery techniques.

(WWW) ONLINE SITES: p.1037

Bladder stones

Ball-like masses of variable size, made of chemical deposits, that gradually form within the bladder

 AGE Can affect adults of any age but much more common over the age of 45

 GENDER More common in males

 GENETICS LIFESTYLE Not significant factors

Stones can form in the bladder if waste products in the urine crystallize. About 8 in 10 stones consist of calcium, which comes from excess salts in the urine. Most are between 2 mm ($^1/_{16}$ in) and 2 cm ($^3/_4$ in) in diameter, but some grow much larger. Bladder stones are about three times more common in men than in women and are much more common in people over 45 years old.

The condition may develop if urine stagnates in the bladder as a result of incomplete emptying (*see* URINARY RETENTION, p.713). It is also more likely to develop in people who have recurrent or persistent urinary tract infections (*see* CYSTITIS, p.709). Certain metabolic disorders, such as gout (p.380), can also give rise to increased levels of waste products in the urine and encourage the formation of bladder stones.

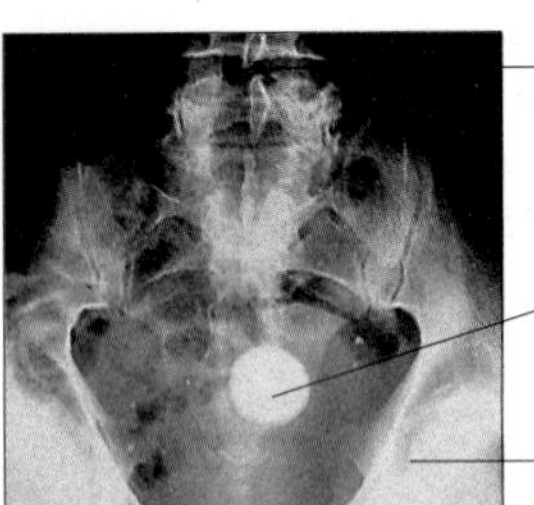

Bladder stone
A large bladder stone can be seen in this X-ray. Stones, especially of this size, can make passing urine painful and difficult.

WHAT ARE THE SYMPTOMS?

A small bladder stone may not cause any symptoms. However, as a stone increases in size, it may start to irritate the bladder lining, causing some or all of the following symptoms:

- Pain and difficulty passing urine.
- Frequent and sometimes urgent need to pass urine.
- Blood in the urine.

If you develop any of these symptoms, you should consult your doctor without delay. Left untreated, a stone may irritate the muscles in the bladder wall and cause urge incontinence (p.712). A stone that blocks the bladder outlet can cause urinary retention or cystitis, which may be intensely painful.

WHAT MIGHT BE DONE?

If bladder stones are suspected, you will be referred to hospital for tests such as an abdominal X-ray (p.244) or specialized X-rays of your urinary tract (*see* INTRAVENOUS UROGRAPHY, p.699). You may also have samples of your blood and urine analysed to look for signs of infection and rule out an underlying metabolic disorder, such as gout. In addition, cystoscopy (opposite page) may be carried out to examine the lining of your bladder.

Bladder stones can usually be broken into fragments and washed out during cystoscopy. Alternatively, a form of ultrasound (*see* LITHOTRIPSY, p.702) is used to pulverize the stones, which are washed out in the urine soon after the procedure. If the stones are very large, surgery may be needed to remove them.

Bladder stones often recur. About 3 in 5 of the people successfully treated for bladder stones develop the condition again within 7 years.

(WWW) ONLINE SITES: p.1037

Bladder tumours

Cancerous growths that develop in the lining of the bladder

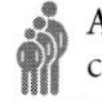
AGE Rare under the age of 50; more common with increasing age

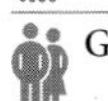
GENDER More common in males

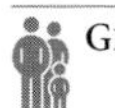
GENETICS May be a significant factor

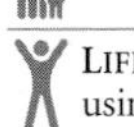
LIFESTYLE Smoking and some occupations using chemicals are risk factors

Tumours in the bladder are all treated as cancerous. Most of these tumours begin as superficial, wart-like growths, called papillomas, which grow from the lining of the bladder and project into the bladder cavity. Bladder tumours are about three times more common in men than in women.

What are the causes?

More than half of all bladder tumours develop in people who smoke. About 1 in 6 tumours occurs in people who are employed in the rubber-manufacturing industry or work with industrial dyes or solvents. These people are susceptible to tumours since they handle carcinogens (cancer-causing substances), which are absorbed by the body and excreted in the urine. Carcinogens therefore come into contact with the bladder lining, where they can trigger the growth of abnormal tissue. The underlying cause of bladder tumours is unknown, but the possibility that they may be inherited is currently under investigation.

In tropical regions, a common cause of bladder tumours is the parasitic infestation schistosomiasis (p.312).

What are the symptoms?

Bladder tumours initially do not cause symptoms, but the following symptoms may develop over time:

- Blood in the urine.
- Dull ache in the lower abdomen.
- Difficulty passing urine.

If urine flow is restricted, urine may stagnate, leading to infections in the urinary tract (*see* CYSTITIS, p.709). Large tumours may block the bladder outlet, causing urinary retention (p.713). Left untreated, the cancer may spread to nearby areas. Cancerous cells can also break away from the tumour and travel in the blood to other parts of the body.

TEST AND TREATMENT — Cystoscopy

During cystoscopy, a thin, hollow viewing tube, known as a cystoscope, is inserted into the urethra and then into the bladder to look for tumours and other abnormalities affecting the urethra and bladder. The cystoscope may be rigid or flexible. Instruments to take tissue samples or destroy or remove tumours and stones can be inserted through the cystoscope. The procedure may be carried out under local or general anaesthesia.

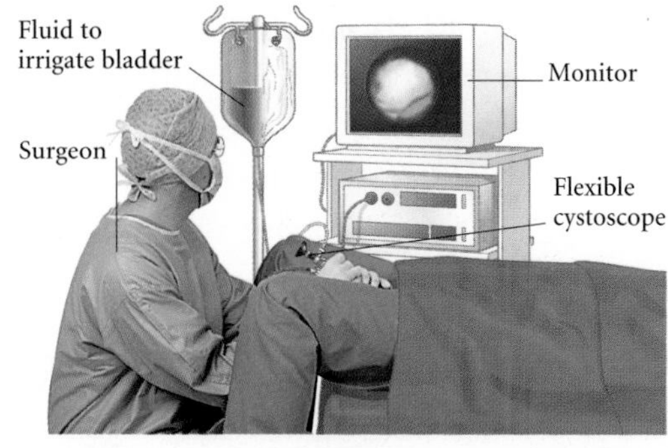

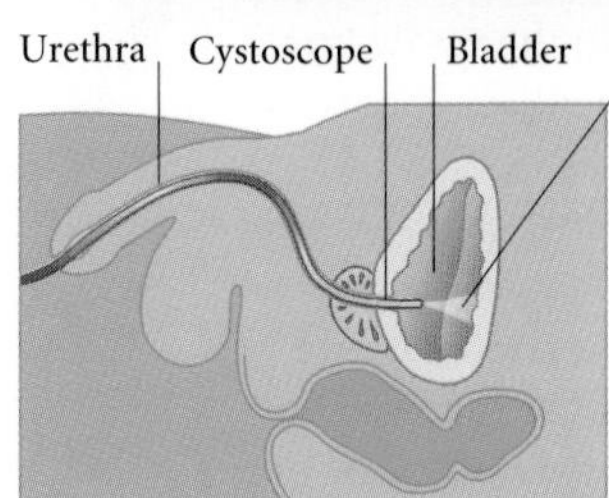

During the procedure
An illuminated and magnified view of part of the bladder lining is transmitted from the cystoscope to a monitor.

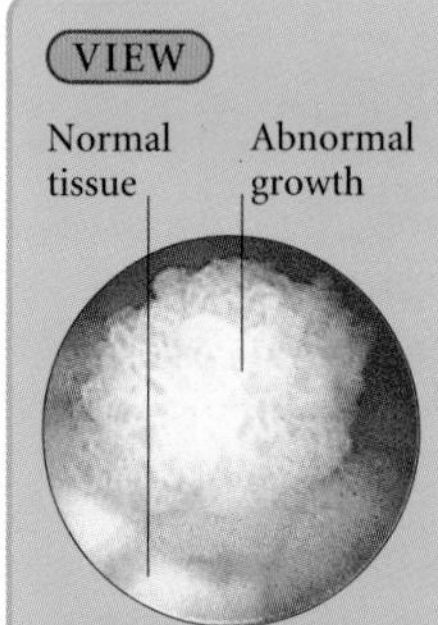

Bladder lining
This magnified view through a cystoscope shows a growth in the lining of the bladder. Samples taken from such a growth will be analysed under a microscope to look for cancerous cells.

What might be done?

Your doctor will have a urine sample tested in the laboratory for blood and cancerous cells. Ultrasound scanning (p.250), intravenous urography (p.699), CT scanning (p.247), or MRI (p.248) may be used to image the bladder and reveal abnormalities. Your doctor will also arrange for you to have cystoscopy (above), in which a viewing instrument is used to examine the bladder lining. If a tumour is found, surgical instruments are inserted through the cystoscope to take a tissue sample, remove the tumour, or destroy it by heat treatment. Tumours may also be treated by drugs that are delivered directly into the bladder through a catheter.

If a tumour is large or has spread deep into the tissues of the bladder, abdominal surgery may be necessary to remove the tumour along with part or all of the bladder. If the whole bladder must be removed, urine will be diverted through an opening on the skin in the abdominal area by way of a passage constructed from a piece of intestine. Radiotherapy (p.281) and chemotherapy (p.280) may be used for tumours that would be difficult to treat with cystoscopy or surgery or where a person is too ill or frail for surgery.

What is the prognosis?

Bladder tumours that have been diagnosed at an early stage can usually be treated successfully. However, lifelong monitoring will be necessary because further bladder tumours may develop. Regular checkups should ensure that, if more papillomas develop, they can be treated before they have the chance to become more serious.

If you smoke, giving up will greatly reduce your risk of developing a bladder tumour. Once you have had a tumour treated, giving up smoking will reduce the risk of recurrence. If you work with high-risk chemicals or have done so in the past, you should see your doctor for regular checkups because tumours can develop many years after exposure to carcinogenic chemicals.

(WWW) ONLINE SITES: p.1028, p.1037

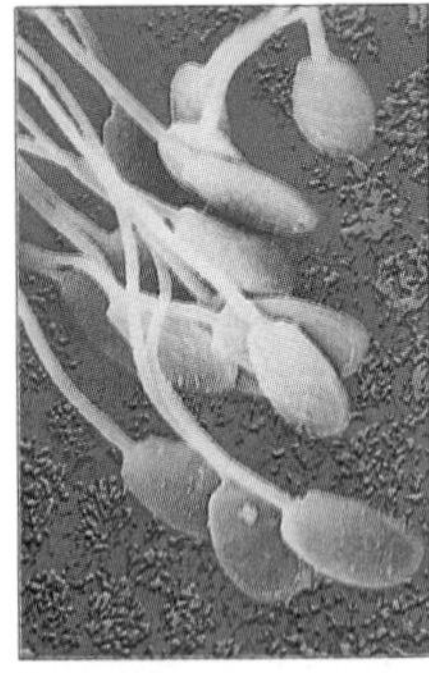

Sperm
Each sperm has a long tail that enables it to swim inside the female reproductive tract.

MALE REPRODUCTIVE SYSTEM

MEN REACH THEIR SEXUAL PEAK between the ages of 16 and 18, shortly after puberty. Since they are able to produce sperm continuously from puberty onwards, men remain fertile for a longer period than women; some men can become fathers at the age of 70 or older. Sperm are produced in the testes, and, during sexual intercourse, the penis delivers them into the female reproductive system. The male reproductive system also manufactures sex hormones that are essential for sperm production and for sexual development during puberty.

The male reproductive system begins to develop before a male baby is even born. The only visible parts of the male reproductive system are the penis and the scrotum, but inside the body there is a complicated network of ducts, glands, and other tissues that work together to make the production and transport of sperm possible.

SPERM PRODUCTION

Once puberty is reached, sperm are manufactured continuously in the two testes at a rate of about 125 million each day. Since sperm production is not efficient at body temperature, the testes are kept cool by being suspended outside the body in a sac of skin called the scrotum. Mature sperm leave each testis through an epididymis, a long coiled tube that lies above and behind each testis. The sperm are stored in the epididymis and mature there before going to the vas deferens, the tube that connects an epididymis to an ejaculatory duct. During sexual activity, each vas deferens contracts and pushes sperm towards the urethra (the tube that connects the bladder to the outside of the body). The sperm are ejaculated during sexual activity or are reabsorbed into the body. Some dribble through the upper end of the vas deferens into the urethra and are later washed away in the urine.

The sperm are carried in a fluid consisting of secretions from various glands. Most of these secretions are produced by glands called seminal vesicles as the sperm leave the vas deferens. Fluid is also added by the prostate gland. In addition to acting as a vehicle for the sperm to help them to swim, the fluid provides nutrients that keep the sperm healthy. Together, these secretions and sperm form semen, containing about 50 million sperm per millilitre.

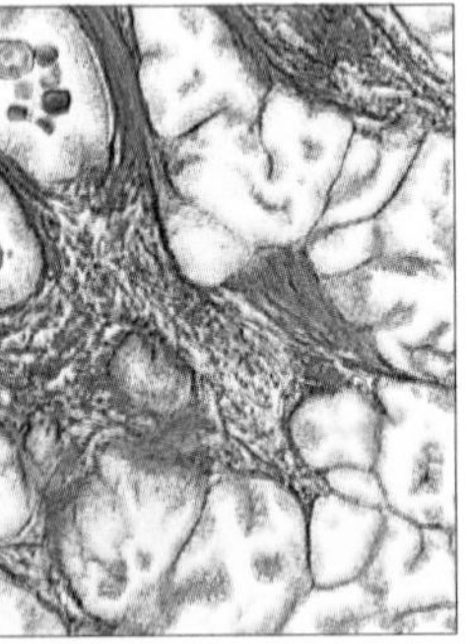

Prostate gland
The prostate gland secretes a milky fluid that helps the sperm to swim.

In order for reproduction to take place, sperm must enter the female reproductive system (*see* SEX AND REPRODUCTION, pp.762–763). During arousal, the penis becomes enlarged and firm. Muscular contractions at the base of the penis then force sperm through the male urethra and into the vagina during male orgasm.

MALE HORMONES

The principal male sex hormone, testosterone, is produced throughout life. Testosterone plays an important part in the development of the genitals and other male sexual characteristics. During puberty, there is a dramatic increase in the level of testosterone. This increase triggers the growth of the genitals and the development of secondary male sexual characteristics, such as body and facial hair, deepening of the voice, and muscle development.

PROCESS PUBERTY

Puberty is the process of sexual development. In boys, puberty usually occurs between the ages of 12 and 15 and lasts 3–4 years. Hormones secreted by the pituitary gland cause levels of the male sex hormone testosterone to rise, stimulating changes such as genital growth and the development of secondary sexual characteristics.

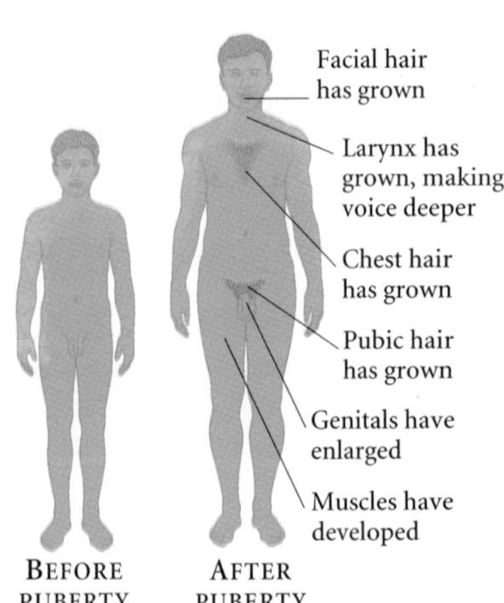

Physical development
During puberty, the penis, scrotum, and testes enlarge, and pubic hair grows. Hair also appears on the face and other parts of the body. Rapid growth occurs, the muscles develop, and the voice deepens.

STRUCTURE MALE REPRODUCTIVE SYSTEM

The male genitals consist of the penis, scrotum, and the two testes, which are suspended in the scrotum. Above and behind each testis is an epididymis, a coiled tube that leads to another tube called the vas deferens. The upper end of each vas deferens is joined by a duct draining from a gland called the seminal vesicle. This duct and a vas deferens together form an ejaculatory duct. The two ejaculatory ducts then join the urethra where it is surrounded by the prostate gland, and the urethra passes through the penis to the outside.

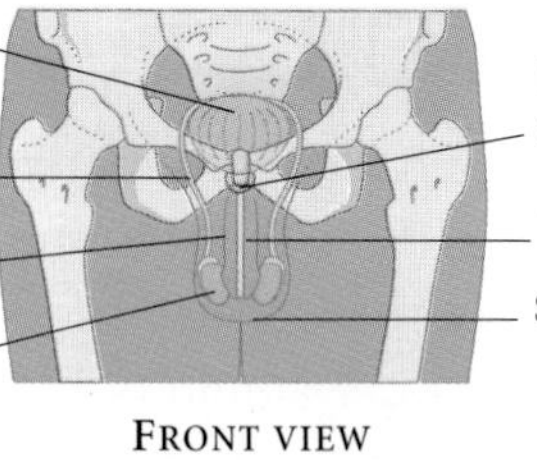

FRONT VIEW

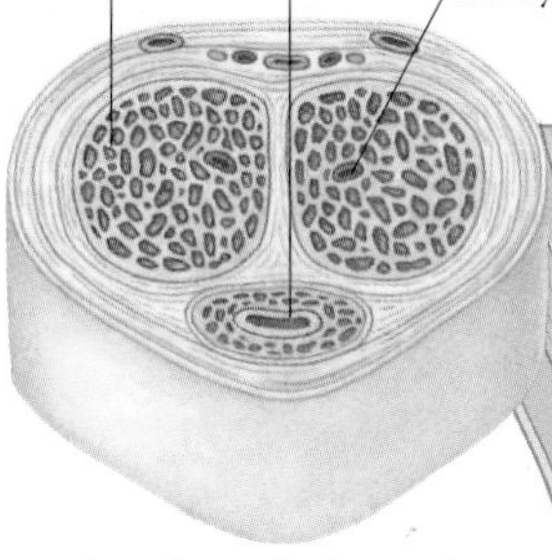

Section through the penis
The penis contains three columns of spongy tissue and many blood vessels.

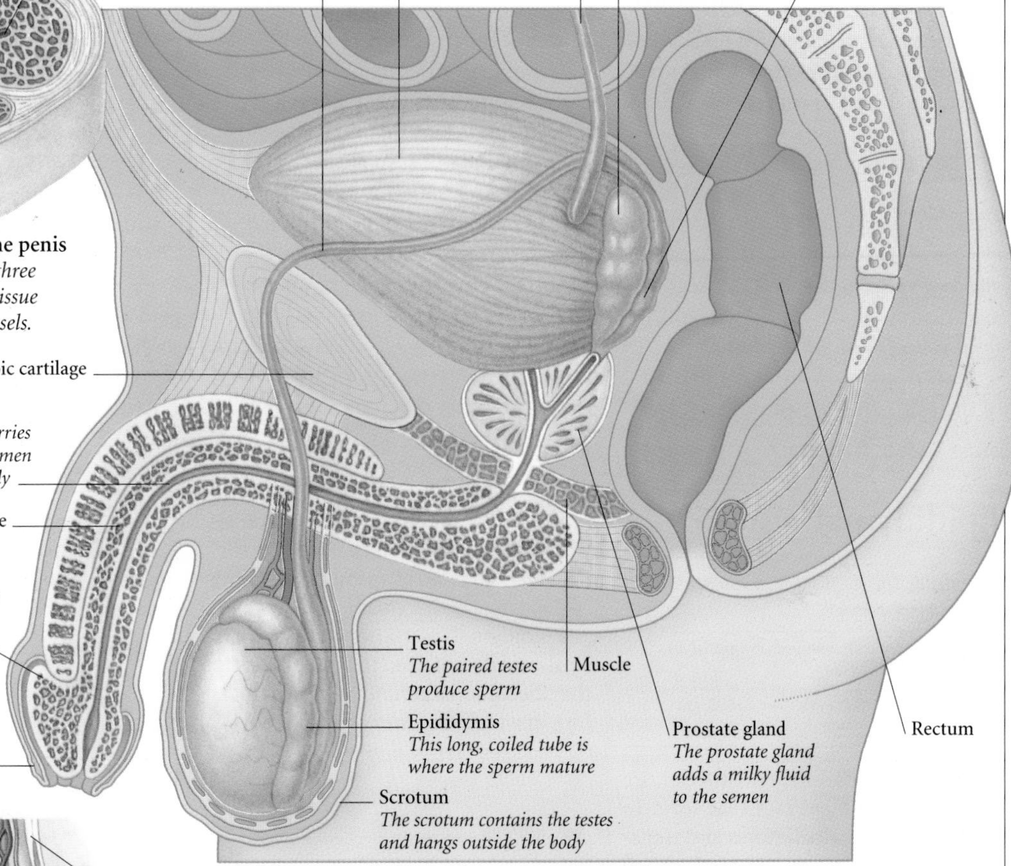

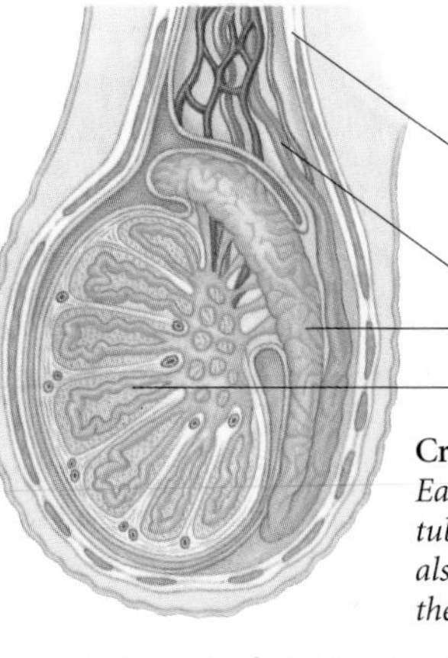

Cross section of the testis
Each testis is packed with seminiferous tubules, which make sperm. The testes also contain Leydig cells that manufacture the sex hormone testosterone.

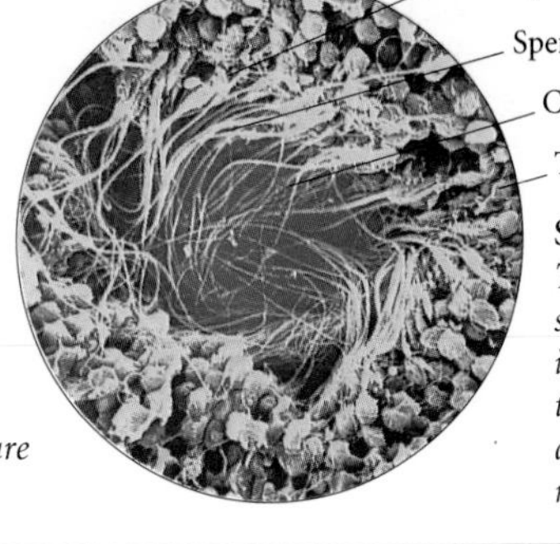

Sperm production
This magnified image shows maturing sperm in a seminiferous tubule. The tails of developing sperm are near the centre.

DISORDERS OF THE TESTES, SCROTUM, AND PENIS

Most of the male reproductive system – the penis, scrotum, and testes – is outside the abdomen. Consequently, symptoms of disorders in these structures are usually obvious at an early stage. Such symptoms should not be ignored out of embarrassment since most genital disorders can be cured by prompt treatment.

In this section, disorders that affect the epididymis (the coiled tube that carries sperm away from each testis) and the testes are described first. These disorders range from epididymal cysts, which are harmless collections of fluid, to cancer of the testis.

The next articles discuss disorders of the scrotum, the sac in which the testes are suspended. These disorders are usually not serious and include varicose veins in the scrotum, known as varicocele, and hydrocele, in which fluid collects around the testis.

Disorders caused by inflammation of the penis and foreskin are covered next, followed by two disorders of erectile function of the penis. The final article in this section discusses cancer of the penis, a very rare but distressing disorder that, if diagnosed early, responds well to treatment.

Skin conditions that may affect the penis and scrotum are discussed elsewhere (*see* SKIN, HAIR, AND NAILS, pp.328–361), as are male hormonal disorders (pp.728–729) including abnormal puberty, sexual problems (pp.769–773) such as impotence, infertility (pp.774–777), and sexually transmitted infections (pp.764–768). Conditions that develop in the male genitals during childhood are covered in disorders of the urinary and reproductive systems (*see* INFANCY AND CHILDHOOD, pp.870–872).

KEY ANATOMY

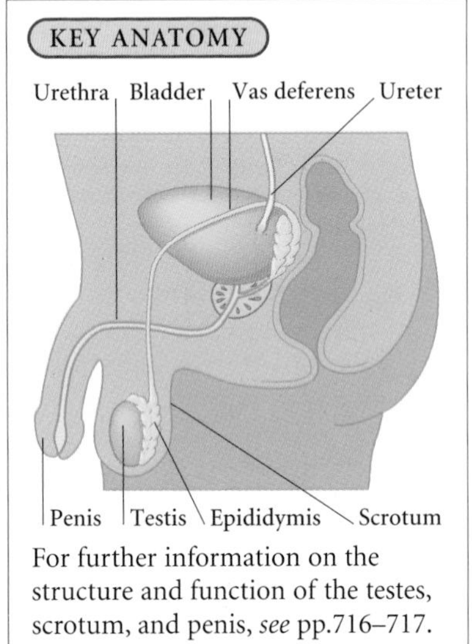

For further information on the structure and function of the testes, scrotum, and penis, *see* pp.716–717.

Epididymal cysts

Swellings in the epididymis, the coiled tube inside the scrotum that stores and transports sperm

 AGE More common over the age of 40

 GENETICS LIFESTYLE Not significant factors

Epididymal cysts, or spermatoceles, are harmless fluid-filled sacs that form in the epididymis, which stores and transports sperm away from the testis. Small epididymal cysts are common, particularly in men over the age of 40. The cysts develop slowly and are usually painless.

In many cases, there are multiple cysts, which can be felt as distinct, painless swellings like a tiny bunch of grapes on top of and behind the testis. The epididymal tubes in both testes may be affected by cysts at the same time.

If you detect a swelling on one or both sides of your scrotum, you should consult your doctor to rule out a serious condition, such as cancer of the testis (opposite page). He or she will probably be able to make a diagnosis from a physical examination, but further tests such as ultrasound scanning (p.250) may be necessary.

Epididymal cysts normally remain small and do not need treatment. Rarely, they become large and cause discomfort, in which case they can be removed.

(WWW) ONLINE SITES: p.1034

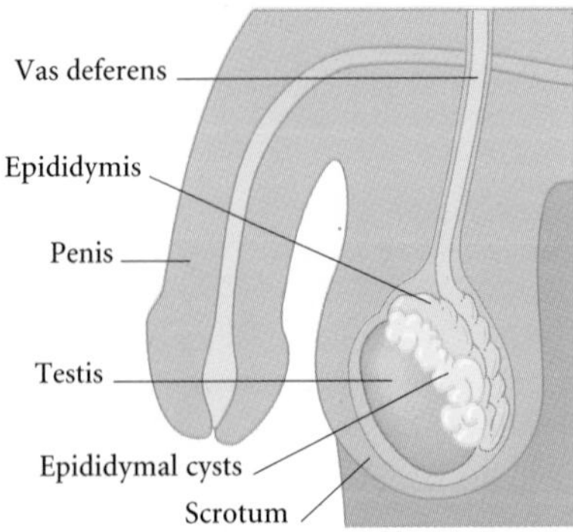

Epididymal cysts
Fluid-filled cysts that develop next to the testis in the epididymis are known as epididymal cysts and are usually painless.

Epididymo-orchitis

Inflammation of the epididymis, the coiled tube inside the scrotum that stores and transports sperm, and of the testis

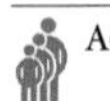 AGE Rare before puberty

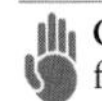 GENETICS LIFESTYLE Not significant factors

Infection of the testis and epididymis (the coiled tube that stores and transports sperm away from the testis) can lead to inflammation called epididymo-orchitis. This condition usually causes painful swelling of one testis and may be accompanied by fever.

WHAT ARE THE CAUSES?

Epididymo-orchitis is usually caused by bacteria that have travelled from the urinary tract along the spermatic duct (vas deferens) to the epididymis. In men under 35 years of age, a common cause of the condition is a sexually transmitted infection (STI), such as nongonococcal urethritis (p.765). In older men, a urinary tract infection, prostatitis (p.724), or recently having had a catheter inserted to drain urine (*see* BLADDER CATHETERIZATION, p.713) are possible causes. In rare cases, an infection that is transmitted through the bloodstream, such as tuberculosis (p.491), leads to the development of epididymo-orchitis.

In boys and young men, the most common cause of the condition used to be inflammation due to mumps (p.293), but this has become less common since the introduction of immunization.

WHAT ARE THE SYMPTOMS?

The symptoms of epididymo-orchitis usually develop over a period of several hours and may include:

- Swelling, redness, and tenderness of the scrotum on the affected side.
- In severe cases, extreme pain in the scrotum, with fever and chills.

You may also have some symptoms of the underlying disorder, such as painful and frequent passage of urine in the case of a urinary tract infection.

The symptoms of epididymo-orchitis are similar to those of a more serious condition called torsion of the testis (right). For this reason, you should consult your doctor immediately if you have any of the symptoms listed above.

WHAT MIGHT BE DONE?

Your doctor will ask you to provide a urine sample to be tested for infection. If the doctor suspects an STI, he or she will take a swab from your urethra (the tube from the bladder to the outside of the body) to check for infection. If the diagnosis is unclear, you will need to go to hospital as an emergency for tests to rule out torsion of the testis. In some cases, exploratory surgery is necessary.

Your doctor will probably prescribe antibiotics (p.885) unless the inflammation is caused by infection with the mumps virus, in which case antibiotics are ineffective. You may be advised to rest in bed and drink plenty of fluids. Taking painkillers (p.912) may help to ease the discomfort, and using an ice pack may reduce the swelling and pain in the scrotum. An athletic support can be worn to support the scrotum.

Pain is usually relieved in 1–2 days, but the swelling of the scrotum may take several weeks to subside.

(WWW) ONLINE SITES: p.1034

Torsion of the testis

Twisting of the testis within the scrotum, causing severe pain

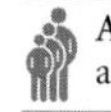
AGE Most common between the ages of 12 and 18 but can occur at any age

GENETICS LIFESTYLE Not significant factors

Each testis is suspended in the scrotum on a spermatic cord. The spermatic duct (vas deferens) and the blood vessels that supply the testis are contained in the spermatic cord. If the spermatic cord becomes twisted, the flow of blood to the testis is restricted, causing severe pain in the scrotum.

Torsion of the testis usually affects only one of the two testes. It sometimes occurs after strenuous activity but may develop for no apparent reason, even during sleep. Torsion of the testis most commonly occurs during adolescence, but it can develop at any age. The condition is potentially serious; torsion may result in permanent damage to the testis if not treated immediately.

WHAT ARE THE SYMPTOMS?

Symptoms of torsion of the testis usually appear suddenly. They may include:

- Sudden pain in the scrotum that tends to increase in severity.
- Pain in the groin and lower abdomen.
- Redness and extreme tenderness of the scrotum on the affected side.

The severity of the pain can cause nausea and vomiting. If you develop any of these symptoms, you should seek medical advice urgently.

WHAT MIGHT BE DONE?

Your doctor may arrange for ultrasound scanning (p.250) of the scrotum to exclude other disorders that cause similar symptoms, such as epididymo-orchitis (opposite page). If you have torsion of the testis, an operation is carried out to untwist the spermatic cord. Both testes are then anchored in the scrotum with stitches to prevent a recurrence of the condition. If this operation is performed promptly, the testis is usually undamaged. However, if a testis is irreversibly damaged, it will be removed.

Occasionally, the spermatic cord will untwist spontaneously. If your symptoms disappear, you should still consult your doctor because they may recur.

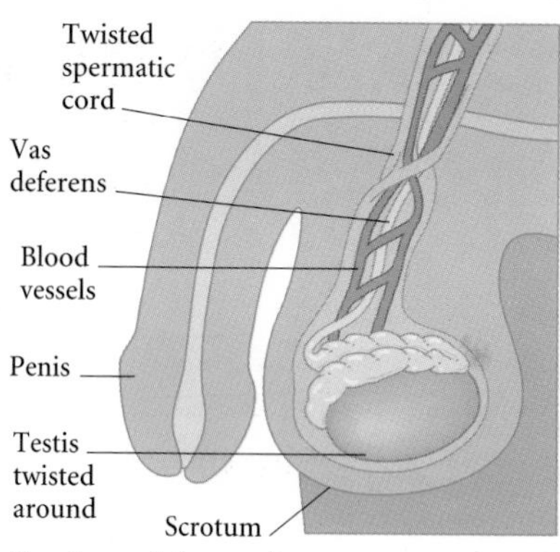

Torsion of the testis

In torsion of the testis, the spermatic cord, from which the testis hangs in the scrotum, becomes twisted, which restricts the flow of blood to and from the testis.

WHAT IS THE PROGNOSIS?

The testis is usually undamaged if the spermatic cord is untwisted within 6 hours. Removal of one testis does not normally affect fertility because the remaining one is able to produce sufficient sperm. A testis can be replaced by an artificial implant for cosmetic reasons.

(WWW) ONLINE SITES: p.1034

Cancer of the testis

A cancerous tumour that develops within a testis

AGE Most common between the ages of 20 and 40

GENETICS Sometimes runs in families

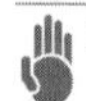
LIFESTYLE Not a significant factor

Although cancer of the testis is a rare condition, it is one of the most common forms of cancer diagnosed in men between the ages of 20 and 40. It is also one of the most easily cured cancers if discovered at an early stage. However, cancer of the testis may spread to the lymph nodes and eventually to other parts of the body if left untreated, and it may ultimately be fatal. The condition usually affects only one testis.

Most testicular tumours develop in the sperm-producing cells of the testis. There are four types of tumour: seminoma, embryonal carcinoma, teratoma, and choriocarcinoma. Seminomas are the most common type of testicular tumour, and they are usually found in men between the ages of 35 and 45.

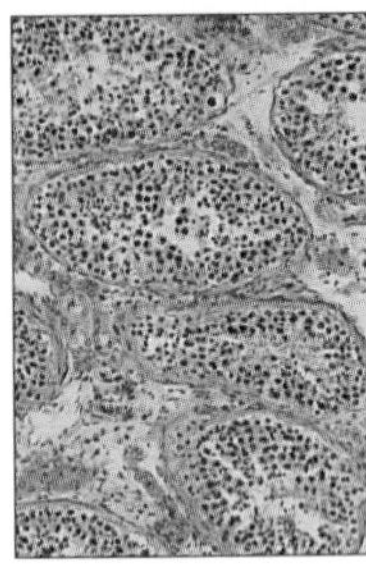
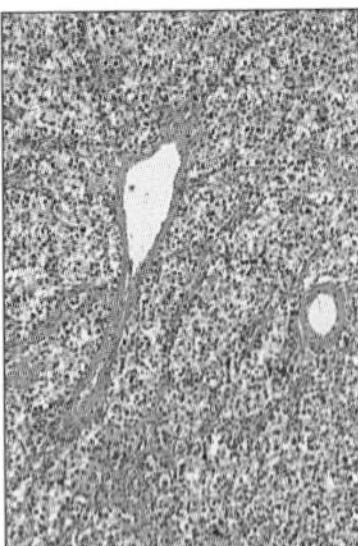

NORMAL ABNORMAL

Cancer of the testis
These tissue samples from testes compare normal tissue structures in a healthy testis with the disordered tissue structures that are found in a cancerous testis.

WHAT ARE THE CAUSES?
The causes of cancer of the testis are not known, but certain factors increase the risk, such as having a family history of the condition or having had an undescended testis (p.870), a condition in which a testis fails to descend into the scrotum before birth.

WHAT ARE THE SYMPTOMS?
You may not notice the symptoms unless you examine your testes regularly (*see* EXAMINING YOUR TESTES, below). The symptoms may include:

- Hard, painless lump in the affected testis.
- Change in the usual size and texture of the testis.
- Dull ache in the scrotum.
- Rarely, a sudden, sharp pain in the affected testis.

In some cases, fluid may accumulate in the scrotum (*see* HYDROCELE, opposite page). If you find any changes, consult your doctor immediately.

HOW IS IT DIAGNOSED?
Your doctor will examine the affected testis and may arrange for you to have ultrasound scanning (p.250) of the testes. A special blood test may also be arranged to look for cancer (*see* TUMOUR MARKER TESTS, p.233). If a tumour is found, further blood tests, CT scanning (p.247), and MRI (p.248) will be performed to determine whether the cancer has spread to other parts of the body.

WHAT IS THE TREATMENT?
If cancer of the testis is diagnosed, the affected testis will have to be surgically removed. If the cancer has not spread beyond the testis, no further treatment may be needed. However, even after the testis has been removed, blood tests to check tumour marker levels are usually carried out every 6 months to make sure that the cancer has not spread.

If the cancer has spread to tissues in other parts of the body, you may need to have further treatment, which may include surgery, radiotherapy (p.281), and chemotherapy (p.280). If the cancer has spread to the lymph nodes in the abdomen, surgery may be required to remove the affected nodes. Of the four types of testicular tumour, seminomas are the most easily treated by surgery and radiotherapy.

WHAT IS THE PROGNOSIS?
The outlook depends on the type of cancer and the stage at which it is diagnosed. Cancer of the testis has a very high cure rate. About 4 in 10 testicular cancers are seminomas, which have a survival rate of more than 9 in 10, but, if the cancer has spread to other tissues, this rate drops to 8 in 10.

Surgical removal of a testis is not likely to affect sexual function or fertility if they were normal before surgery. However, both chemotherapy and radiotherapy reduce sperm production, and fertility may be temporarily or permanently affected by these treatments. For this reason, some men choose to have semen containing normal sperm frozen before treatment is started.

(WWW) ONLINE SITES: p.1028, p.1034

SELF-HELP EXAMINING YOUR TESTES

Cancer of the testis is one of the most easily treated cancers if it is diagnosed at an early stage. For this reason, all men should examine their testes regularly to check for lumps or swellings. An early cancerous tumour can usually be felt as a hard lump embedded in the surface of the testis. This lump is not usually tender when pressed. Soft swellings in the testis may be harmless cysts, and painful swellings are often due to infection. You should also check for changes in the skin of the scrotum. If you detect any change in the normal appearance or texture of your testes or scrotum, consult your doctor immediately.

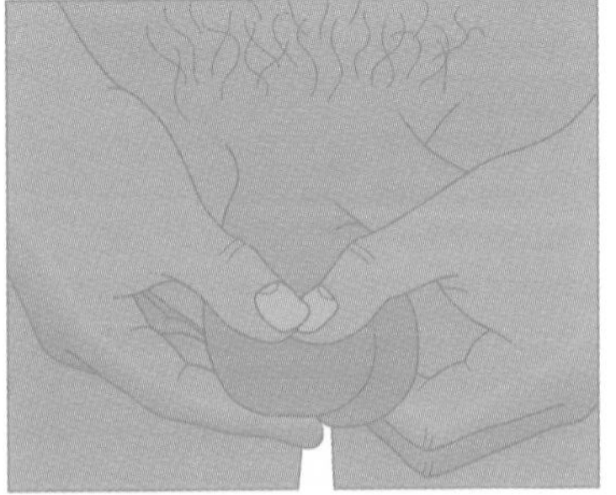

How to examine your testes
After a bath or shower, when the scrotum is relaxed, carefully feel across the entire surface of each testis by rolling each one slowly between fingers and thumb. Check for lumps or swellings and be thorough.

Varicocele

A collection of varicose veins in the scrotum

AGE GENETICS LIFESTYLE Not significant factors

A varicocele is a knot of dilated veins in the scrotum. The condition is caused by leaking valves in the testicular veins, which drain blood away from the testes, and it affects as many as 1 in 6 men. There is usually no identifiable reason for the leakage of these valves, but, in rare cases, a varicocele can result from pressure on a vein, usually in the pelvis, which prevents blood draining efficiently from the testis. This pressure may be due to a tumour in a kidney. Varicoceles most commonly occur on the left-hand side of the scrotum.

If you develop a varicocele, you may notice some swelling of your scrotum and a dragging, aching discomfort. The affected side of your scrotum may hang lower than normal, and the swelling may feel like a bag of worms.

WHAT MIGHT BE DONE?
Your doctor will probably be able to make a diagnosis by examining your scrotum while you are standing up and again while you are lying on your back. If the swelling is caused by a varicocele, it should disappear when you lie down because the veins will empty.

Small, painless varicoceles do not need to be treated because they usually cause no other symptoms and often disappear. Wearing an athletic support or close-fitting underwear can relieve mild discomfort. If the varicocele is due to a kidney tumour, all or part of the kidney will be removed surgically.

A varicocele may reduce your fertility, but sexual performance should not be affected. If tests reveal that you have a low sperm count or if you have persistent discomfort, surgery may be needed to divide and tie off the swollen veins. Varicoceles sometimes recur.

(WWW) ONLINE SITES: p.1034

Hydrocele

An abnormal accumulation of fluid between the double-layered membrane that surrounds the testis

 AGE Most common in infants and the elderly

 GENETICS LIFESTYLE Not significant factors

The double-layered membrane that surrounds each testis normally contains a small amount of fluid. If an excessive amount of fluid accumulates within this membrane, a swelling called a hydrocele will result. This condition is most common in infant boys and elderly men. In most cases, there is no apparent cause, but hydroceles have been linked to infection, inflammation, or injury to the testis. Rarely, a hydrocele that develops in adulthood is due to the presence of a tumour in the testis (*see* CANCER OF THE TESTIS, p.719).

A hydrocele usually develops as a visible swelling in the scrotum. There may be a heavy, dragging sensation in the scrotum due to its increased size, but the swelling is not normally painful.

WHAT MIGHT BE DONE?

If you think you may have a hydrocele, you should consult your doctor. He or she will first try to identify a hydrocele by holding a torch against the affected area of your scrotum. If the swelling is due to excess fluid, light will shine through the swelling. Your doctor may also arrange for you to have ultrasound scanning (p.250) of the scrotum to confirm the diagnosis and to exclude an underlying testicular disorder such as a tumour.

Hydroceles that develop in infants often subside by the age of 6 months without requiring treatment. However, in all cases, if a hydrocele becomes very large, uncomfortable, or painful, it is usually treated by a minor operation in which the sac of testicular membrane containing the excess fluid is removed.

If the hydrocele is associated with an infection, an antibiotic (p.885) may be prescribed. If a tumour is found in the testis, you will be referred for further tests and treatment.

(WWW) ONLINE SITES: p.1034

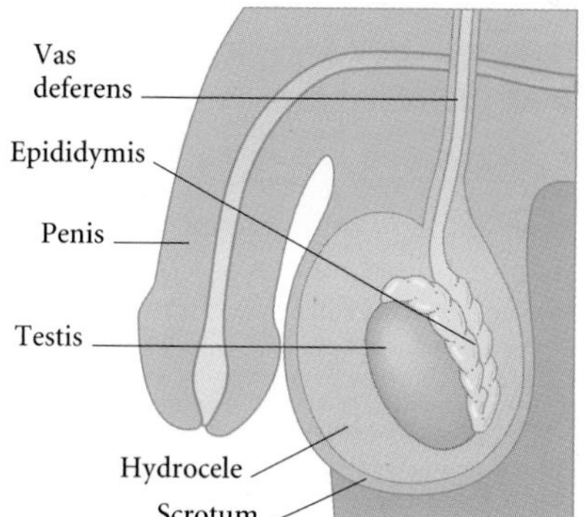

Hydrocele
If fluid accumulates in the double-layered membrane enclosing the testis, it forms a swelling in the scrotum called a hydrocele.

Phimosis

A foreskin that is tight or has a very small opening at the tip, preventing it from being retracted over the head of the penis

 AGE More common in children but may occur at any age

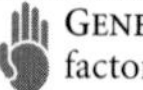 GENETICS LIFESTYLE Not significant factors

In phimosis, the foreskin is too tight or the opening at its tip is too narrow, so that it cannot be retracted (pulled back) over the head of the penis (the glans). Phimosis may make it difficult to clean the head of the penis thoroughly and, as a result, infections may occur under the foreskin (*see* BALANITIS, p.722). In some cases, the condition also interferes with the normal flow of urine.

WHAT ARE THE CAUSES?

In most cases, phimosis is present at birth or becomes apparent during childhood, although it can occur at any age.

By the time a boy is 12 months old, it is usually possible to retract the foreskin. If it is not possible to pull a boy's foreskin back over the glans by the age of 5, he has phimosis and probably needs

(TREATMENT) VASECTOMY

Vasectomy is a method of male sterilization. Counselling is given to make sure the man and his partner do not wish to have children in the future. The procedure has no effect on sex drive or ejaculation, but the semen no longer carries sperm, which are reabsorbed in each testis. Additional contraception is needed until 12–16 weeks later, when semen is tested to ensure sperm are no longer present.

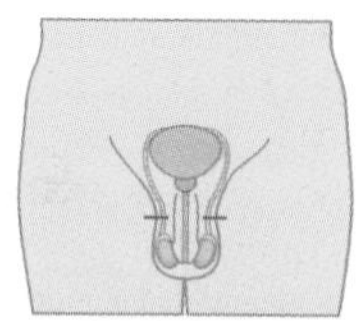

SITES OF INCISIONS

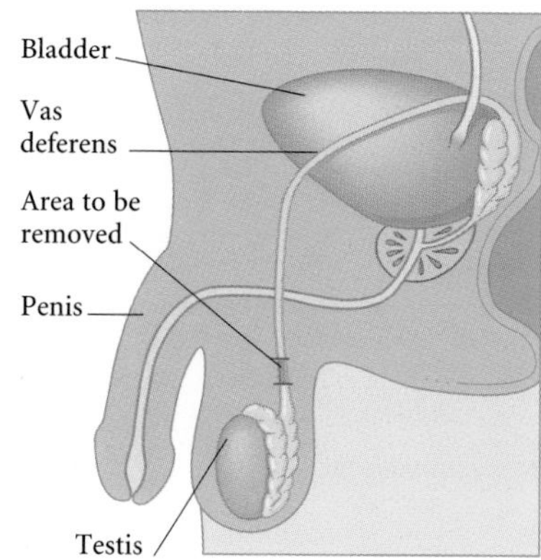

The procedure
A small section of each vas deferens (spermatic duct) is removed through small incisions on either side of the scrotum.

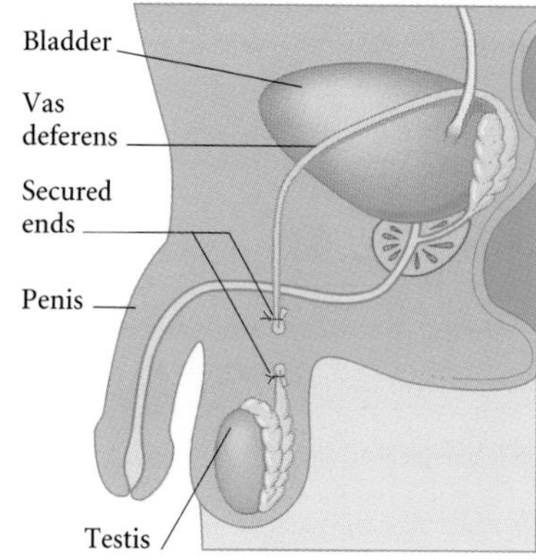

After the procedure
The open ends of the vas deferens have been turned back and secured with a stitch to prevent them from rejoining.

treatment. The cause of the condition in babies and young children is unknown, but in older children and adults, it may result from scarring of the penile tissue due to recurrent episodes of balanitis.

What are the symptoms?

The only symptom of phimosis may be an inability to pull back the foreskin, but this may be accompanied by:

- Weak urinary stream.
- Gradual ballooning of the foreskin when passing urine.
- Painful erection.

If bacteria become trapped behind the foreskin, balanitis and recurrent urinary tract infections may occur.

A complication of phimosis called paraphimosis may occur. In this condition, it is not possible for a foreskin that has been retracted to be rolled forwards again. The condition needs immediate medical attention because it constricts the flow of blood to the head of the penis, causing the area to become swollen and extremely painful.

What might be done?

Boys under the age of 5 will probably not need treatment because the condition is likely to improve by itself. If the condition has resulted in a urinary tract infection or difficulty passing urine, or if it occurs in adolescent boys or men, the doctor will probably recommend that surgical removal of the foreskin (*see* Circumcision, below) is carried out.

Paraphimosis needs immediate treatment. The doctor may ease the foreskin forwards by applying an ice pack to the penis, then gently squeezing the head. Alternatively, the doctor may make a small incision in the foreskin to enable it to be pulled forwards. Circumcision is often required to prevent recurrence.

(WWW) ONLINE SITES: p.1028, p.1034

Balanitis

Inflammation of the head of the penis and foreskin

 Age More common in children

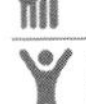 Lifestyle Not being circumcised is a risk factor

 Genetics Not a significant factor

In balanitis, the head of the penis (the glans) and foreskin become itchy, sore, and inflamed. In addition, there may be a discharge, and a rash may develop.

The disorder can be caused by a bacterial infection, a fungal infection such as thrush (*see* Candidiasis, p.309), or an allergic reaction. It may also be due to a sexually transmitted infection (STI), such as the protozoal infection trichomoniasis (p.767). A tighter than normal foreskin (*see* Phimosis, p.721) may increase the risk of infection by preventing effective cleaning of the glans.

Men with diabetes mellitus (p.687) are more susceptible to the condition because their urine contains high levels of glucose, which can encourage the growth of microorganisms. This leads to infection and inflammation at the opening of the urethra (the tube leading from the bladder to the outside of the body). Excessive use of antibiotics (p.885) can increase the risk of a fungal infection by temporarily lowering the body's natural defences. Children are especially vulnerable to balanitis.

The condition may also occur as a result of sensitivity of the penis to certain chemicals, such as those found in some condoms, contraceptive creams, detergents, and washing powders.

What might be done?

If the head of your penis or your foreskin is inflamed, you should consult your doctor. He or she will examine the area and probably take a swab to look for evidence of infection. The doctor will also test your urine to check for glucose.

The treatment of balanitis depends on the cause. For example, if you have a bacterial infection, antibiotics may be prescribed, and, if the infection is due to a tight foreskin, circumcision (below) may be carried out to prevent balanitis from recurring. If the condition is the result of a sexually transmitted infection, your partner should be checked for evidence of infection and treated if necessary to prevent the condition from recurring (*see* Preventing STIs, p.765). If the cause seems to be sensitivity to a

(TREATMENT) Circumcision

Circumcision is the surgical removal of the foreskin, the skin covering the head of the penis (the glans). This procedure is sometimes carried out in infancy for religious reasons. In the past, circumcision was often performed routinely in childhood in the belief that it would improve hygiene, but this practice is no longer recommended. In older boys and men, circumcision may be necessary if the foreskin becomes too tight to be pulled back fully (*see* Phimosis, p.721). When the operation is carried out in infancy, only local anaesthesia is required, but boys and men are usually given a general anaesthetic before undergoing surgery.

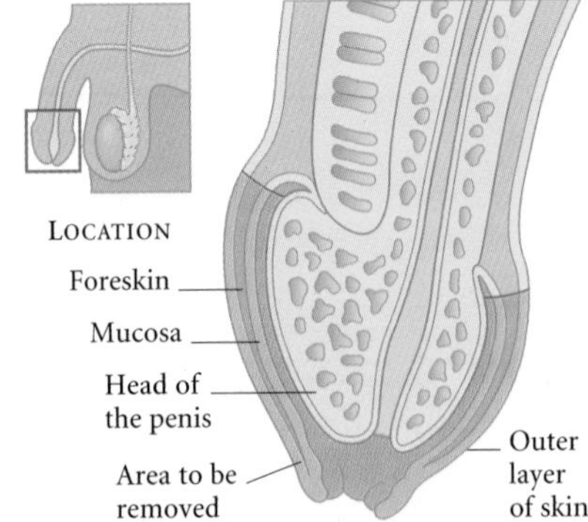

The operation
The foreskin, which covers the head of the penis, consists of an inner layer of mucosa and an outer layer of skin. During the operation, both layers are removed.

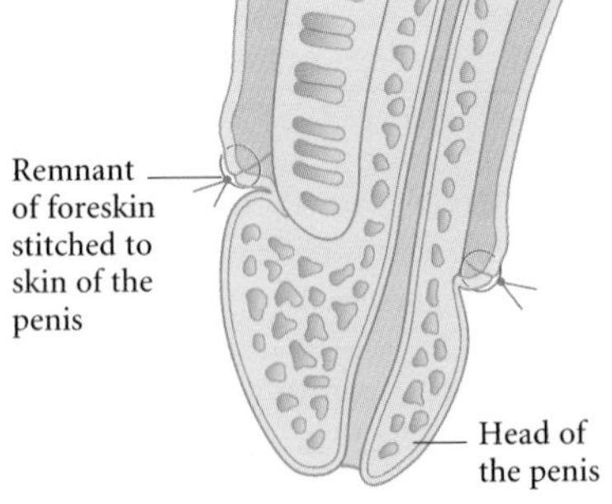

After the operation
The remnant of the foreskin has been stitched to the skin just behind the head of the penis, leaving the head of the penis uncovered. These stitches either dissolve or fall out after a few days.

chemical, the irritant should be identified, if possible, so that you can avoid it.

The inflamed area should be kept clean, dry, and free of irritants. Most cases of balanitis clear up rapidly once the cause has been found and treated.

(WWW) ONLINE SITES: p.1028, p.1034

Priapism

Prolonged, painful erection of the penis, which may not be related to sexual desire

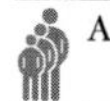
AGE More common in young adults

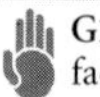
GENETICS LIFESTYLE Not significant factors

Priapism is a persistent erection of the penis occurring for 4 hours or longer, with or without any sexual arousal. The condition is usually painful, and it requires urgent treatment in hospital to avoid permanent damage to the erectile tissues of the penis.

Priapism develops if blood cannot drain away from the spongy tissues of the erect penis. Causes of the condition include damage to the nerves that control the supply of blood to the penis; disorders of the blood, including sickle-cell disease (p.448), leukaemia (p.453), and polycythaemia (p.457); and, in some instances, prolonged sexual intercourse. Priapism may also occur as a side effect of treatment with certain antipsychotic drugs (p.917). Drug treatments for impotence (p.770), whether they are taken orally, such as the erectile dysfunction medication sildenafil, or injected into the penis, may rarely result in priapism.

What might be done?

If you develop a painful and very prolonged erection, particularly one that is not a result of sexual arousal, you must consult your doctor or go to your nearest accident and emergency department immediately. In most cases of priapism, blood can be drained from the erectile tissues of the penis by using a needle and syringe, which produces immediate relief of symptoms.

If priapism is a result of an underlying disorder, further treatment will depend on the cause. In all cases, there is a risk of permanent damage, and full erection of the penis may be adversely affected in the future.

(WWW) ONLINE SITES: p.1034

Peyronie's disease

Scarring of the erectile tissue of the penis, causing it to bend at an angle when erect

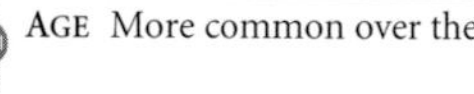
AGE More common over the age of 40

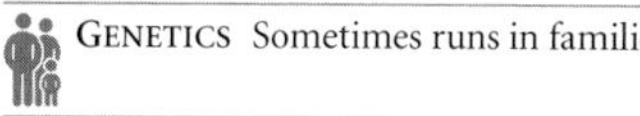
GENETICS Sometimes runs in families

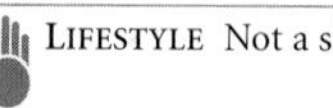
LIFESTYLE Not a significant factor

In Peyronie's disease, the fibrous tissue of the penis becomes thickened, causing it to bend during erection. The penis may bend so much that sexual intercourse is difficult and painful. Peyronie's disease occurs in about 1 in 100 men, most commonly in those over 40.

In many cases, there is no apparent cause for the condition, but previous damage to the penis may be a risk factor. Peyronie's disease is also associated with Dupuytren's contracture (p.390), a condition in which the fibrous tissue in the palm of the hand becomes thick and shortened, causing the fingers to bend inwards. Peyronie's disease sometimes runs in families, suggesting that a genetic factor is involved.

What are the symptoms?

The symptoms of Peyronie's disease develop gradually and may include:

- Curvature of the penis to one side during an erection.
- Pain in the penis on erection.
- Thickened area within the penis that can usually be felt as a firm nodule when the penis is flaccid.

Eventually, the thickened region of the penis may extend to include parts of the erectile tissue. In this case, the condition may lead to impotence (p.770).

What is the treatment?

Peyronie's disease sometimes improves without any treatment. In some mild cases, in which painless intercourse is still possible, no treatment is necessary. However, in other cases, the condition becomes worse if left untreated.

If the condition is severe, the penis may be straightened by a surgical procedure. If Peyronie's disease has led to impotence, a permanent implant may be surgically inserted into the penis under general anaesthesia to correct the deformity and restore erectile function.

(WWW) ONLINE SITES: p.1034

Cancer of the penis

A rare, cancerous tumour that usually occurs on the head of the penis

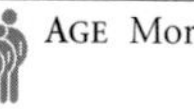
AGE More common over the age of 40

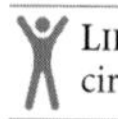
LIFESTYLE Smoking and not being circumcised are risk factors

GENETICS Not a significant factor

Cancer of the penis is a rare disorder that almost exclusively occurs in uncircumcised men, particularly those in whom the foreskin does not retract (*see* PHIMOSIS, p.721). It is more common in men over the age of 40. Infection with the human papillomavirus, which causes genital warts (p.768), is thought to increase the risk of developing the cancer. Smoking also seems to be a risk factor.

The tumour usually develops on the head of the penis (the glans). It appears as a wart-like growth or flat, painless sore that may be hidden by the foreskin. Sometimes, the growth may bleed or produce an unpleasant-smelling discharge. The cancer usually grows slowly, but, if left untreated, it may eventually spread to the lymph nodes in the groin.

A sore area on the penis should be examined by a doctor immediately.

What might be done?

Your doctor will carry out a physical examination and may take a swab to check for infections that can produce similar symptoms. He or she may also arrange for a biopsy (*see* SKIN BIOPSY, p.344), in which a sample of the growth is removed to be examined under the microscope for evidence of cancer.

If it is detected early, a tumour on the penis can often be treated successfully with surgery, radiotherapy (p.281), or a combination of both. Surgery involves either partial or complete amputation of the penis. In some cases, penile reconstruction may be possible following amputation. Radiotherapy may be recommended as the first choice treatment because it offers the chance of curing the cancer without loss of the penis.

The outlook depends on how far the disease has advanced before diagnosis and treatment. More than 8 in 10 men who have received treatment for penile tumours survive for 5 years or more.

(WWW) ONLINE SITES: p.1028, p.1034

PROSTATE DISORDERS

The prostate gland is a firm, round organ about the size of a chestnut. It surrounds the upper part of the urethra (the tube through which urine is emptied from the bladder) and lies underneath the bladder and directly in front of the rectum. The secretions that are produced by the prostate gland are added to semen, the fluid that contains sperm.

Disorders affecting the prostate gland are very common, particularly in men over the age of 30. Prostatitis, in which the prostate gland is inflamed, is the first disorder discussed in this section. Enlargement of the prostate gland is covered next. Some degree of prostate enlargement occurs in most men over the age of 50 and is often viewed as a natural part of aging. The final article covers prostate cancer. In many cases, prostate cancer is not life-threatening, and in older men it may not require treatment because the tumour is often slow-growing and does not affect life expectancy. However, prostate cancer in younger men may spread to other parts of the body more quickly and can be life-threatening. Current research is therefore aimed at developing tests to detect prostate cancer before symptoms start to appear. However, although these tests can help to identify prostate cancer in its early stages, they cannot identify which cancers are more likely to spread and require early treatment.

KEY ANATOMY

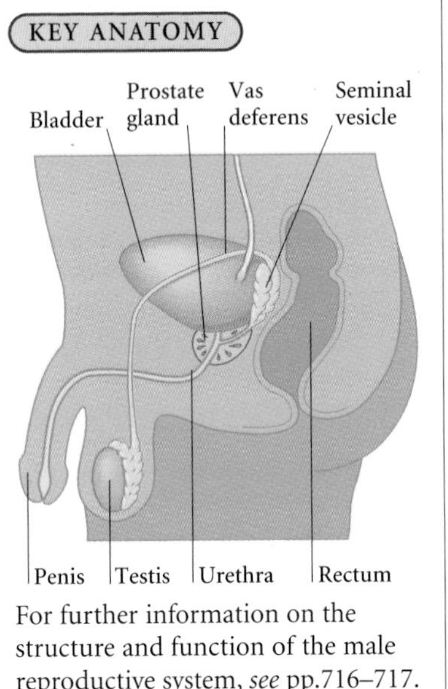

For further information on the structure and function of the male reproductive system, *see* pp.716–717.

Prostatitis

Inflammation of the prostate gland, sometimes due to infection

AGE Most common between the ages of 30 and 50

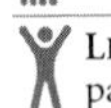
LIFESTYLE Unprotected sex with multiple partners is a risk factor

GENETICS Not a significant factor

Inflammation of the prostate gland, known as prostatitis, may be acute or chronic. Acute prostatitis is uncommon and tends to produce sudden, severe symptoms that clear up rapidly with treatment. By contrast, chronic prostatitis usually causes mild but persistent symptoms and can be difficult to treat. Both types are most common in sexually active men aged between 30 and 50.

WHAT ARE THE CAUSES?

In most cases of acute or chronic prostatitis, an exact cause of the disorder cannot be determined. However, both forms of the condition can be the result of bacterial infection that spreads from the urinary tract to the prostate gland. Inflammation of the prostate gland may also develop in association with sexually transmitted infections (pp.764–768).

WHAT ARE THE SYMPTOMS?

The symptoms of acute prostatitis develop suddenly and are usually severe. They may include the following:

- Fever and chills.
- Pain around the base of the penis.
- Lower back pain.
- Pain during bowel movements.
- Frequent, urgent, and painful passing of urine.

Acute prostatitis sometimes causes urinary retention (p.713), painful swelling behind the testes, or the formation of an abscess in the prostate gland.

Chronic prostatitis may not produce symptoms. If symptoms do occur, they develop gradually and may include:

- Pain and tenderness at the base of the penis and in the testes, groin, pelvis, or back.
- Pain on ejaculation.
- Blood in the semen.
- Frequent, painful passing of urine.

If you suspect that you have either acute or chronic prostatitis, you should consult your doctor immediately.

HOW IS IT DIAGNOSED?

Your doctor will perform a digital rectal examination, in which a finger is inserted into the rectum to feel the prostate. The doctor may also ask you to provide a urine sample and may obtain a sample of prostate gland secretions by massaging the prostate through the rectum and collecting secretions from the urethra. Both the urine sample and the prostate gland secretions will then be tested for the presence of infectious organisms. Ultrasound scanning (p.250) may also be carried out to check for an abscess and to rule out prostate cancer (p.726).

WHAT IS THE TREATMENT?

If a bacterial infection is found, antibiotics (p.885) will be prescribed. It may take several months for the infection to clear up completely. In the meantime, your doctor may recommend painkillers (p.912) and give you drugs that soften the stools (*see* LAXATIVES, p.924) to make bowel movements more comfortable. If your symptoms are severe, your doctor may advise bed rest. Prostatitis that is not caused by a bacterial infection may be treated with painkillers and drugs to relax the muscle at the exit of the bladder (*see* DRUGS FOR PROSTATE DISORDERS, p.938). To help to relieve the symptoms of chronic prostatitis, you may need repeated massage of the prostate gland.

Although most affected men recover fully, both types of prostatitis can recur.

(WWW) ONLINE SITES: p.1034, p.1036

Enlarged prostate gland

Noncancerous enlargement of the prostate gland, causing difficulty in passing urine

 AGE Rare before the age of 40; increasingly common after the age of 50

 GENETICS LIFESTYLE Not significant factors

In most men over the age of 50, the prostate gland has become enlarged to some degree. Such prostate enlargement is termed benign prostatic hyperplasia. The condition is noncancerous and is not associated with prostate cancer (p.726). Minor prostate enlargement is considered a natural part of the aging process. The cause of the condition is unknown.

What are the symptoms?

As the prostate gland grows larger, it constricts and distorts the urethra (the tube from the bladder to the outside of the body). At first, this enlargement does not cause any symptoms. However, if the prostate gland continues to enlarge,

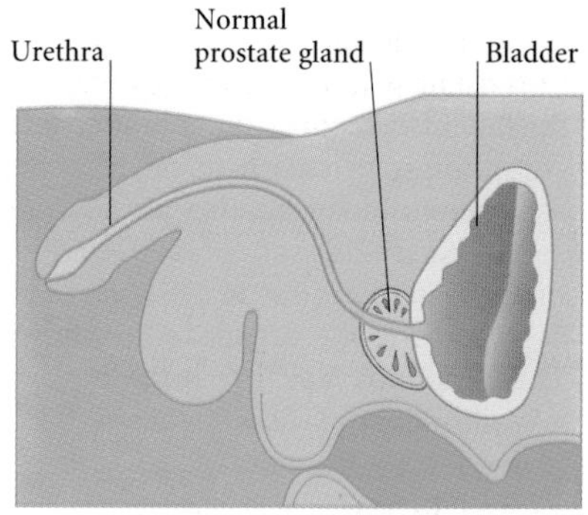

NORMAL PROSTATE

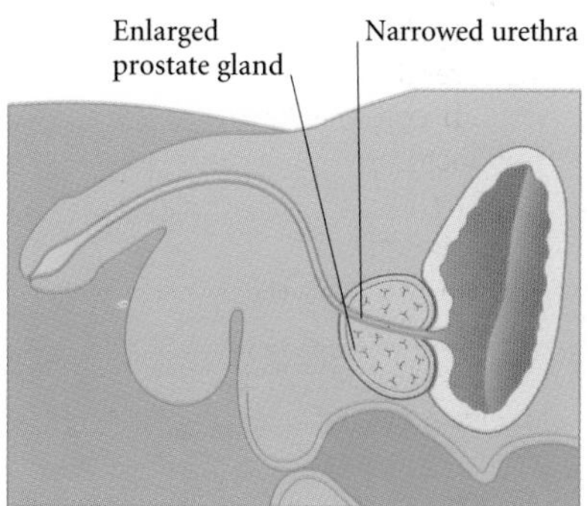

ENLARGED PROSTATE

Prostate enlargement

The prostate encircles the upper part of the urethra. An enlarged prostate may constrict the urethra, making it difficult to pass urine, and indent the base of the bladder, preventing it from emptying completely.

(TREATMENT) Partial prostatectomy

There are several operations to treat an enlarged prostate gland. The most common is a partial or transurethral prostatectomy, in which only part of the gland is removed. The operation is performed under general or spinal anaesthesia and requires a hospital stay of about 3 days. Since the rest of the gland will continue to enlarge, symptoms may recur and further surgery may be necessary later. About 8 in 10 men are infertile after this type of surgery because sperm pass into the bladder on ejaculation, but orgasm is normal. In a minority of cases, partial prostatectomy results in impotence.

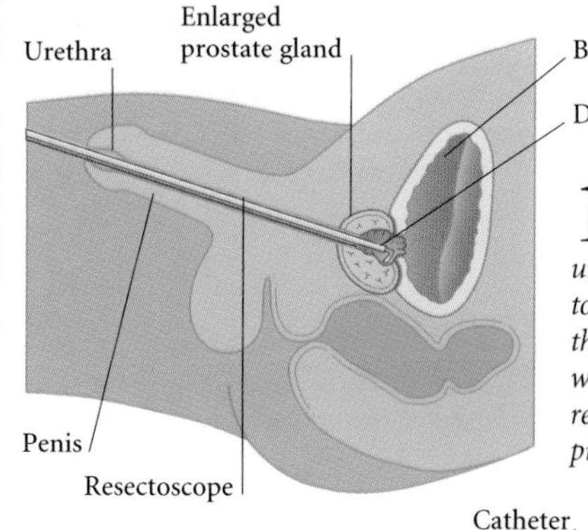

1 A specialized viewing instrument called a resectoscope is passed along the urethra (the tube leading from the bladder to the outside of the body) until it reaches the prostate. A heated wire (diathermy wire) is then introduced through the resectoscope and used to cut away excess prostate tissue, thus widening the urethra.

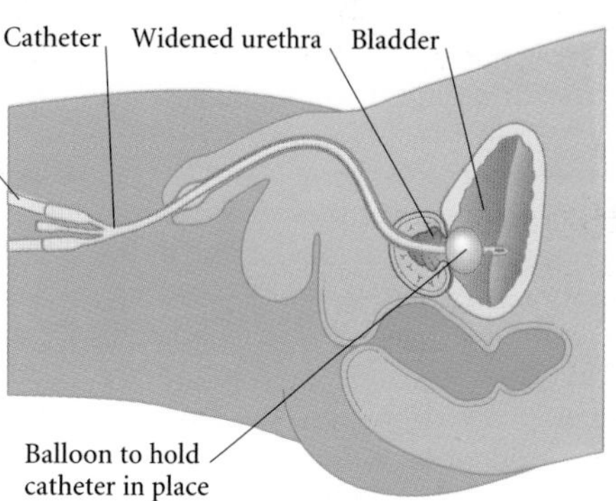

2 After surgery, the diathermy wire and the resectoscope are withdrawn. A catheter is passed along the urethra into the bladder to drain urine. An irrigation system is attached to the catheter to wash out prostate tissue and to stop blood clots from forming. The catheter is left in place for 2–3 days.

it may cause difficulty in passing urine, resulting in the following symptoms:

- Frequent need to pass urine, during the day and night.
- Delay in starting to pass urine, especially at night or if the bladder is full.
- Weak, intermittent flow of urine.
- Dribbling at the end of urine flow.
- Feeling that the bladder has not completely emptied.

These symptoms may be worsened by cold weather; drinking large volumes of fluids (especially alcohol); taking drugs that increase urine production, such as diuretics (p.902); or taking drugs that may cause urinary retention, such as antispasmodics (*see* ANTISPASMODICS AND MOTILITY STIMULANTS, p.926).

If the bladder does not empty completely, it may enlarge and make the abdomen swell visibly. Urine may collect in the bladder and stagnate. If the condition is left untreated, the urinary tract may become infected (*see* CYSTITIS, p.709) and there is an increased risk of bladder stones (p.714). Rarely, retained urine can produce a build-up of backward pressure from the bladder to the kidneys, leading to kidney damage (*see* HYDRONEPHROSIS, p.703), and kidney failure (p.706) may occur. Occasionally, an enlarged prostate gland may suddenly block the outflow of urine completely (*see* URINARY RETENTION, p.713), causing rapidly increasing pain. This problem requires emergency treatment.

How is it diagnosed?

Your doctor will perform a digital rectal examination, in which a finger is inserted into the rectum to feel the prostate. The doctor may also arrange for blood tests to assess kidney function and rule out prostate cancer and urine tests to look for evidence of infection. Urine flow may also be assessed (*see* URODYNAMIC STUDIES, p.711). Ultrasound scanning (p.250) may be carried out to measure the amount of urine left in your bladder after passing urine and check that your kidneys are not abnormally enlarged.

WHAT IS THE TREATMENT?

The choice of treatment depends on factors such as age, general health, the degree of the prostate enlargement, and whether the obstruction of urine flow is having harmful effects on the bladder and kidneys. Treatment may affect sexual function, and you should discuss the available treatments with your doctor.

If your symptoms are mild, your doctor may simply advise you not to drink fluids in the evening so that urinary frequency is decreased at night. If the symptoms persist, drugs, surgery, or catheterization may be necessary.

Alpha blockers are commonly used to treat prostate enlargement and can relieve the symptoms in some cases (*see* DRUGS FOR PROSTATE DISORDERS, p.938). If your symptoms are more severe, your doctor may suggest prostate surgery to remove part of the gland through the urethra (*see* PARTIAL PROSTATECTOMY, p.725). Only tissue that is obstructing urine flow is removed. Rarely, if the prostate is very enlarged and the excess tissue cannot be removed through the urethra, most of the gland is removed through an abdominal incision. This procedure may result in infertility. It may also cause impotence (p.770), especially in older men. Laser surgery and shrinkage of the prostate using microwaves are alternative treatments that are currently being developed.

If surgery is not advisable due to old age or poor health, a catheter may be left in permanently to drain the urine (*see* BLADDER CATHETERIZATION, p.713).

WHAT IS THE PROGNOSIS?

The outlook varies greatly. Mild cases may be improved with drug treatment, but surgery is more effective for severe cases. About 1 in 7 men needs a second partial prostatectomy after 8–10 years.

(WWW) ONLINE SITES: p.1034, p.1036

Prostate cancer

A cancerous tumour arising from the glandular tissue of the prostate gland

 AGE Rare under the age of 40; increasingly common over the age of 65

 GENETICS Sometimes runs in families; more common in certain ethnic groups

 LIFESTYLE Not a significant factor

Prostate cancer is the most commonly diagnosed male cancer in the UK, affecting about 1 in 12 men at some time in their lives. The disorder is more common in northern Europeans and black men, but it is rare in men from Asian countries. The number of cases of prostate cancer identified in the UK has been rising since the 1970s, not only in elderly men, in whom it is most common, but also in men in their 40s and 50s. This increased identification of the cancer in recent years has been largely due to a new screening test that measures the level of a protein called prostate-specific antigen, secreted by the prostate gland. Although prostate cancer is the cause of about 10,000 deaths each year in the UK, many tumours grow slowly, especially in elderly men, and may never cause symptoms. Treatment is more likely to be necessary in younger men.

WHAT ARE THE CAUSES?

The exact cause of prostate cancer is not known, although the male sex hormone testosterone, produced by the testes, has been found to influence the growth and spread of the tumour. In about 1 in 10 cases, the cancer is partly due to an inherited abnormal gene. In these cases, it is more likely to occur before the age of 60. Although there has been concern that having had a vasectomy (p.721) increases the risk of prostate cancer, there is no firm evidence to support this view.

WHAT ARE THE SYMPTOMS?

Prostate cancer may not produce any symptoms, particularly in elderly men. If symptoms do occur, they are likely to develop when the tumour starts to constrict the urethra (the tube leading from the bladder to the outside of the body). The symptoms may then include:

- Weak urinary stream or inability to pass urine normally.

(TEST) PROSTATE GLAND BIOPSY

A prostate gland biopsy is used to diagnose prostate cancer. In the most common type of biopsy, an ultrasound probe is inserted into the rectum in order to visualize the prostate. A hollow needle attached to the probe is gently pushed through the rectal wall and into the prostate several times, removing pieces of tissue for examination. After the biopsy, urine and semen may contain blood for a few days.

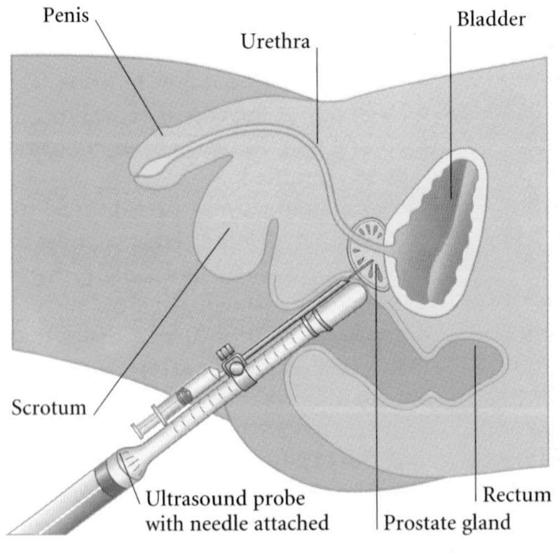

The procedure
A slight pricking sensation may be felt as each biopsy sample is taken, but anaesthesia is usually not required.

(RESULTS)

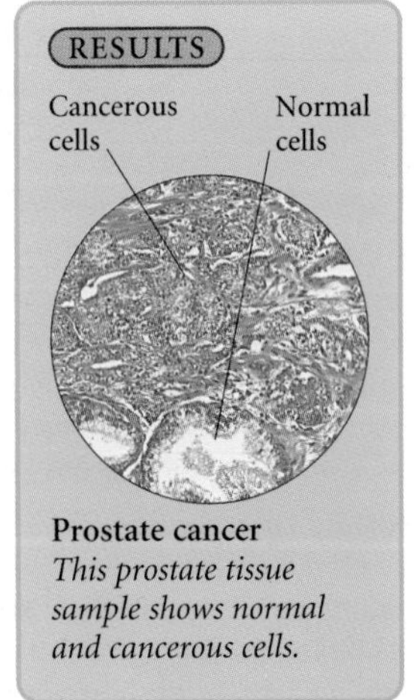

Prostate cancer
This prostate tissue sample shows normal and cancerous cells.

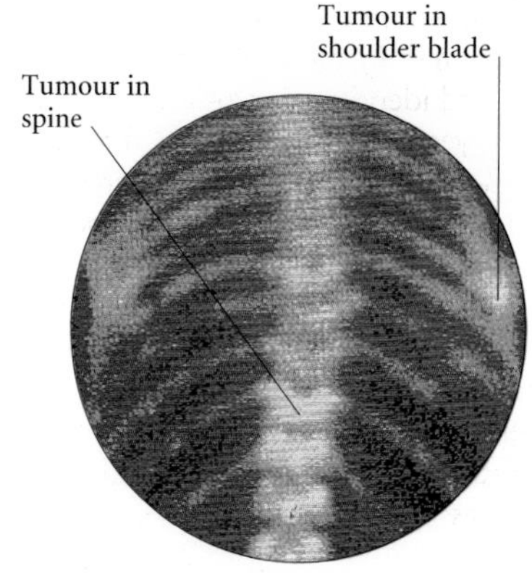

Metastatic cancer
This radionuclide bone scan of the chest shows "hot spots" in the spine and in the shoulder blade due to the spread of a cancer that originated in the prostate gland.

- Frequent urge to pass urine, especially during the night.
- Rarely, blood in the urine.

In some men, the initial symptoms of prostate cancer are due to the metastasis (spreading) of the cancer to other parts of the body, most commonly the bones, lymph nodes, and lungs. In these cases, the symptoms may include back pain, enlarged lymph nodes, shortness of breath, and significant weight loss.

How is it diagnosed?

If you develop the symptoms of prostate cancer or if the disorder runs in your family, you should consult your doctor. The doctor will perform a digital rectal examination, in which a finger is inserted into the rectum to feel the prostate gland. He or she may also arrange for a blood test to measure your prostate-specific antigen levels.

You may be referred to hospital to have a type of ultrasound scanning in which a probe is inserted into the rectum to visualize the prostate gland. This procedure enables the doctor to assess the size of the gland and to look for any abnormalities. During scanning, a prostate gland biopsy (opposite page) may also be carried out. In this procedure, some cells are removed from areas of the gland that appear abnormal and are examined under a microscope. If prostate cancer is diagnosed, you may need imaging tests, such as MRI (p.248) and radionuclide scanning (p.251), to check whether the prostate cancer has spread to other parts of the body.

What is the treatment?

The choice of treatment for prostate cancer depends on age, general health, and whether the cancer has spread to other parts of the body. If the cancer is confined to the prostate and your health is otherwise good, your doctor may recommend that the entire prostate gland be surgically removed, along with some of the surrounding tissues (*see* Radical prostatectomy, below). Alternatively, radiotherapy (p.281) may be given. This form of therapy involves either having a radioactive implant or radioactive seeds placed in the prostate gland or undergoing external radiotherapy over several weeks. In elderly men in whom the cancer is confined to a small area of the prostate gland, no immediate treatment may be required, but the course of the disease will be closely monitored.

If the cancer has spread beyond the prostate, a cure may not be possible. However, progress of the disease can be slowed significantly with hormone therapy. In this treatment, drugs that block the release or actions of testosterone are given to suppress the effects of the hormone on the cancer (*see* Drugs for prostate disorders, p.938). In some cases, part of both of the testes may be surgically removed to stop the production of testosterone. Rarely, treatments that block the actions or production of testosterone result in impotence (p.770) and loss of interest in sex.

What is the prognosis?

A diagnosis of cancer of the prostate gland does not necessarily mean that the cancer will cause symptoms or be life-threatening. Sometimes the best policy, especially in elderly men, is to defer treatment and begin regular checkups to monitor the disease. Men with certain types of small tumour do not need treatment and are likely to live for several years with no symptoms before dying from some other cause. For men who have had surgery for a tumour confined to the prostate gland, the outlook is good, with more than 9 out of 10 men surviving for 5 years after diagnosis. Unfortunately, surgery may result in impotence and urinary incontinence.

Cancer that has spread beyond the prostate gland is unlikely to be cured completely, but hormone therapy often controls the symptoms for many years.

(WWW) ONLINE SITES: p.1034, p.1036

(Treatment) Radical prostatectomy

A radical prostatectomy may be done to treat prostate cancer if the cancer has not spread beyond the gland. The procedure is performed under general anaesthesia and usually requires a hospital stay of about 3–5 days. The operation completely removes the cancer in most men, but afterwards about 1 in 2 men will be impotent, and some will have a degree of urinary incontinence.

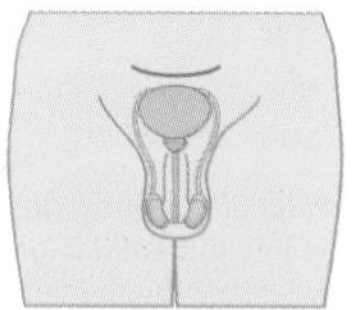

Site of incision

The procedure
The tumour is removed, together with the entire prostate gland, the seminal vesicles, and the neck of the bladder.

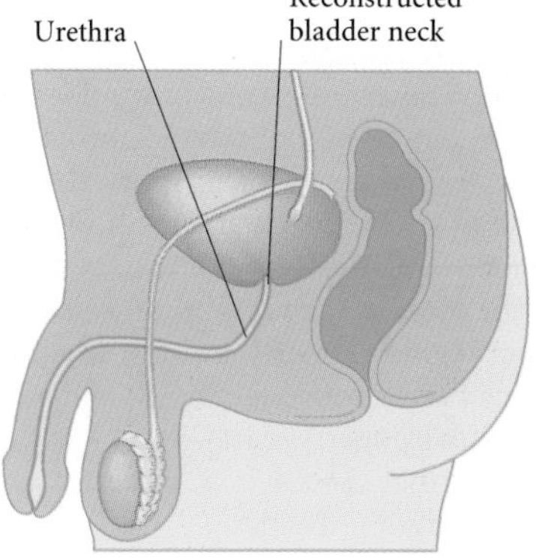

After the procedure
The bladder neck has been reconstructed and rejoined to the urethra (the tube from the bladder to the outside of the body).

MALE HORMONAL DISORDERS

The most important male sex hormone is testosterone, which influences sperm production, fertility, and sex drive. Male sex hormones also promote the development of secondary sexual characteristics at puberty. Over- or underproduction of male sex hormones may be due to a variety of factors, including inherited disorders, long-term illnesses, tumours, or lifestyle factors.

Male sex hormones, or androgens, are produced mainly by the testes but also by the adrenal glands. The production of male sex hormones is controlled by hormones secreted by the pituitary gland. In turn, the pituitary gland is under the control of a part of the brain called the hypothalamus.

The changes that occur at puberty are controlled by the sex hormones. This section starts by discussing early or late onset of puberty in boys, which may be a symptom of under- or overproduction of male sex hormones.

Hypogonadism, in which male sex hormones are underproduced, is covered next. In boys, this condition can suppress sexual development; in men, hypogonadism lowers sperm production and fertility. The final article discusses gynaecomastia, a common disorder causing breast enlargement that temporarily affects nearly half of all boys during puberty.

Male hormonal disorders may lead to sexual problems (pp.769–773) and can sometimes be a cause of infertility (*see* MALE INFERTILITY, p.777).

KEY ANATOMY

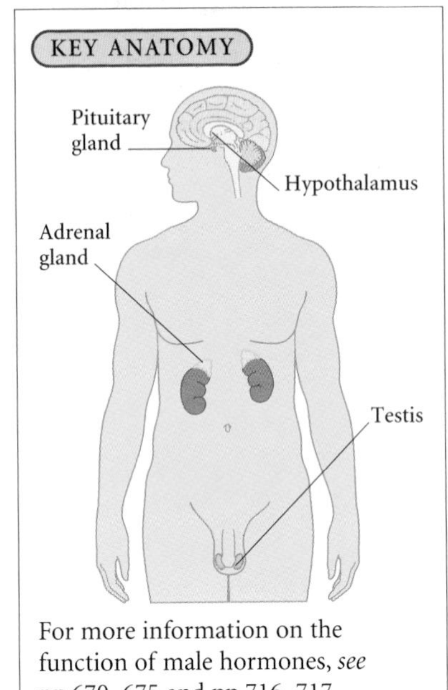

For more information on the function of male hormones, *see* pp.670–675 and pp.716–717.

Abnormal puberty in males

Very early or late onset of puberty, usually due to a hormonal imbalance

 AGE Occurs before or after the normal age range for puberty

 GENETICS Sometimes runs in families; rarely due to a chromosomal abnormality

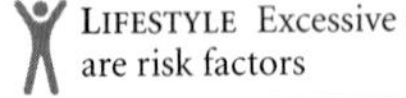 LIFESTYLE Excessive exercise and a poor diet are risk factors

The natural process of sexual development and maturation that takes place over several years is known as puberty (p.716). In boys, puberty is normally characterized by a growth spurt; deepening of the voice; enlargement of the genitals; and the development of hair on the face, in the armpits, and in the pubic region. Puberty in boys usually begins between the ages of 10 and 15. Abnormal puberty starts either earlier than normal (precocious puberty) or later (delayed puberty).

Precocious puberty is rare and is usually an indication of an underlying hormonal disorder. Delayed puberty is more common and less likely to indicate a serious underlying condition.

WHAT ARE THE CAUSES?

In boys, puberty is controlled by male sex hormones produced by the testes and adrenal glands. The production of these hormones is controlled by hormones from the pituitary gland and from the hypothalamus (the part of the brain that regulates the pituitary gland). Disorders in these organs may lead to abnormal early or late puberty.

Precocious puberty is caused by the overproduction of male sex hormones in a young boy. For example, congenital adrenal hyperplasia (p.866), in which the adrenal glands produce excessive amounts of male sex hormones, may lead to precocious puberty.

Boys in whom puberty is delayed are usually just late developers, a tendency that often runs in families. However, delayed puberty may also be caused by the underproduction of male sex hormones. Rarely, there is a more serious underlying cause, such as a brain tumour pressing on the hypothalamus or pituitary gland, or a chromosome disorder, such as Klinefelter's syndrome (p.822), in which the sex organs do not develop normally. Some long-term illnesses, such as Crohn's disease (p.658), kidney failure (p.705), cystic fibrosis (p.824), and diabetes mellitus (p.687), can also cause delayed puberty and growth. Certain lifestyle factors such as excessive exercise and an inadequate diet may delay the onset of puberty. Rarely, a pituitary tumour (p.676) may lead to either precocious or delayed puberty.

WHAT MIGHT BE DONE?

Early or late puberty should be investigated by a doctor, who will carry out a physical examination to see if puberty has started or how far it has progressed. A blood test may also be performed to measure hormone levels and to check for a chromosomal abnormality. X-rays (p.244) of the wrist and hand may be used to assess bone maturity, and ultrasound scanning (p.250) of the testes or adrenal glands may also be carried out to look for abnormalities. If a pituitary tumour is suspected, MRI (p.248) or CT scanning (p.247) may be performed.

If tests identify an underlying cause, it will be treated. For example, precocious puberty may be treated with drugs that block the production of male sex hormones or inhibit their action. These drugs may be given in the form of injections, implants under the skin, or nasal sprays. If delayed puberty runs in the family, no treatment may be needed. In many other cases, puberty is induced by giving injections of testosterone or a drug that stimulates the production of testosterone (*see* SEX HORMONES AND RELATED DRUGS, p.933). Some boys benefit from counselling for psychological problems caused by abnormal puberty.

Abnormal puberty is often treatable, but lifelong treatment may be needed. Future fertility depends on the cause.

(WWW) ONLINE SITES: p.1028, p.1033, p.1034

Hypogonadism in males

Underactivity of the testes, resulting in low levels of the sex hormone testosterone and impaired production of sperm

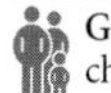 GENETICS Sometimes caused by a chromosomal abnormality

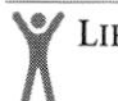 LIFESTYLE Alcohol abuse is a risk factor

 AGE Not a significant factor

Reduced activity of the testes, known as hypogonadism, results in the underproduction of the male sex hormone testosterone and impaired sperm production. In boys who have not reached puberty, growth is often slowed, and sexual development may be delayed. Hypogonadism is uncommon.

Abnormal development of the testes due to a chromosome disorder, such as Klinefelter's syndrome (p.822), may cause hypogonadism, as may failure of the pituitary gland to produce sufficient hormones, which may be the result of a pituitary tumour (p.676). There are also a number of disorders that may cause damage to the testes and lead to hypogonadism, such as torsion of the testis (p.719) and mumps (p.293). Excessive consumption of alcohol, chemotherapy (p.280), and radiotherapy (p.281) can also cause hypogonadism.

WHAT ARE THE SYMPTOMS?

If hypogonadism occurs after puberty, the only effect may be infertility (*see* MALE INFERTILITY, p.777) due to the reduced production of sperm. However, some of the following symptoms may also be evident:

- Impotence.
- Reduction in the size of the genitals.
- Lowered sex drive.
- Reduced growth of facial, underarm, and pubic hair.
- Reduced muscle strength.

When hypogonadism develops before adolescence, it may result in late onset of puberty (*see* ABNORMAL PUBERTY IN MALES, opposite page).

WHAT MIGHT BE DONE?

The doctor will carry out a physical examination to determine whether the genitals and secondary sexual characteristics have developed normally. A blood test may be done to measure the levels of testosterone and other hormones and to look for a chromosomal abnormality.

Treatment is aimed at the underlying cause. For example, synthetic male hormones (*see* SEX HORMONES AND RELATED DRUGS, p.933) may be used to treat disorders of the testes. If underactivity of the pituitary gland is the cause, pituitary hormones may be given (*see* PITUITARY DRUGS, p.934). A pituitary tumour may be removed surgically. In boys, hormone treatment stimulates puberty, including growth and sexual development; in men, it encourages growth of facial hair, muscle strength, potency, and sex drive. Side effects of treatment with hormones may include temporary breast development (*see* GYNAECOMASTIA, below) and acne.

If the genitals are normal, treatment may improve sexual potency and fertility; if hypogonadism is due to a testicular disorder, fertility is rarely achieved.

(WWW) ONLINE SITES: p.1032, p.1033, p.1034

Gynaecomastia

Noncancerous enlargement of one or both breasts in males

 AGE Most common in newborn babies and adolescents

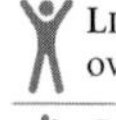 LIFESTYLE Alcohol abuse and being overweight are risk factors in adults

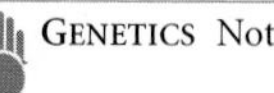 GENETICS Not a significant factor

All males produce small amounts of the female sex hormone oestrogen. If too much oestrogen is produced, breast enlargement, called gynaecomastia, occurs. One or both breasts may be affected. The condition is common in newborn boys and affects 1 in 2 male adolescents. It is usually temporary in both of these age groups. Older men can also be affected.

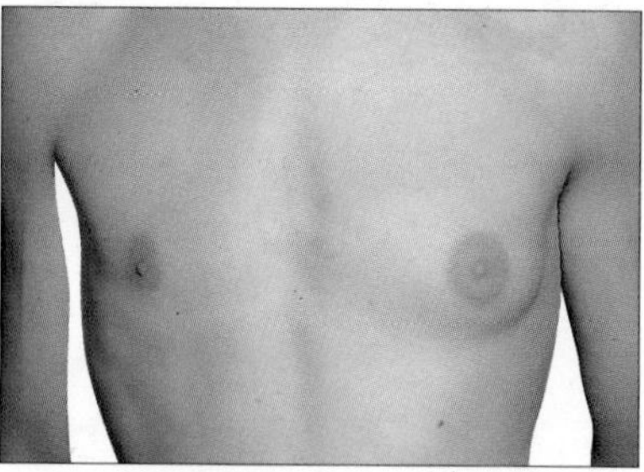

Gynaecomastia
An excess of the female sex hormone oestrogen in the blood may cause one or both male breasts to enlarge, as seen here.

WHAT ARE THE CAUSES?

Gynaecomastia in the newborn occurs when the fetus has been exposed to the mother's oestrogen within the uterus. Increased levels of oestrogen, resulting in breast enlargement, are also common during puberty. In adults, alcohol abuse and being overweight are the most common causes of gynaecomastia.

Drugs that affect levels of female sex hormones, such as spironolactone (*see* DIURETIC DRUGS, p.902) and corticosteroids (p.930), may lead to enlargement of the breasts. Some drugs for prostate cancer (*see* DRUGS FOR PROSTATE DISORDERS, p.938) may have the same effect.

WHAT ARE THE SYMPTOMS?

The symptoms of gynaecomastia may include the following:

- Tender and swollen breast or breasts.
- Firm or rubbery button of tissue that can be felt underneath the nipple.
- Discharge from the nipple.

One breast may enlarge more than the other. The symptoms listed here should always be investigated because they are similar to those of breast cancer (p.759).

WHAT MIGHT BE DONE?

Newborn boys do not need treatment, and gynaecomastia usually disappears within a few weeks. In most adolescents, the condition disappears in less than 18 months without any treatment. In older men, the doctor will ask about lifestyle factors and carry out a physical examination. He or she may arrange for tests to measure hormone levels and to look for evidence of breast cancer. The treatment and outlook depend on the underlying cause, but, if gynaecomastia persists, the excess tissue may be removed surgically.

(WWW) ONLINE SITES: p.1032, p.1033, p.1034

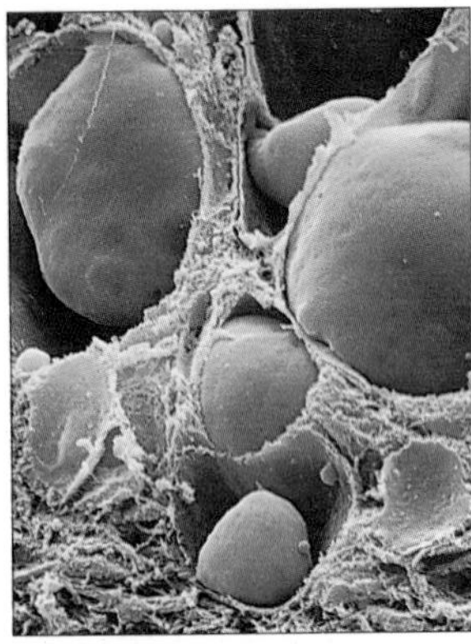

Developing egg follicles
A woman's eggs mature in fluid-filled follicles in the ovaries. This magnified image shows follicles at various stages of development.

FEMALE REPRODUCTIVE SYSTEM

THE CENTRAL ROLE of the female reproductive system is carried out by the ovaries, which produce sex cells, called ova or eggs, containing genetic material. When an egg fuses with a male sex cell, called a sperm, it has the potential to develop into a fetus. The ovaries also secrete sex hormones that control sexual development and the menstrual cycle. The breasts play a part in sexual arousal and produce milk after childbirth.

The only visible parts of the female reproductive system are the tissues that make up the vulva. The labia are folds of skin that protect the entrance to the vagina, which is lined with cells that produce a slightly acidic fluid to prevent infection. The vagina leads from the outside of the body to the uterus, the thick-walled organ in which a fetus develops. Two fallopian tubes lead from the uterus to the two ovaries, where eggs are stored.

FEMALE FERTILITY

Newborn girls have a supply of about 150,000 immature eggs, which are present in their ovaries before birth. The eggs are stored in the ovaries and do not begin to mature until a rise in the levels of female sex hormones at puberty triggers the start of monthly menstrual cycles.

Once a month, an egg matures for 14 days in its follicle and is released from the ovary into the fallopian tube in a process called ovulation. The egg survives for 24 hours after ovulation and can only be fertilized by a sperm during this time. It takes about 5–6 days for the egg, fertilized or not, to pass along the tube to the uterus. If fertilized, the egg eventually implants in the lining of the uterus, which becomes thicker after ovulation, ready for an egg to implant. The egg then grows into an embryo. If not fertilized, the egg passes out of the vagina, along with the uterine lining. This blood loss is called menstruation.

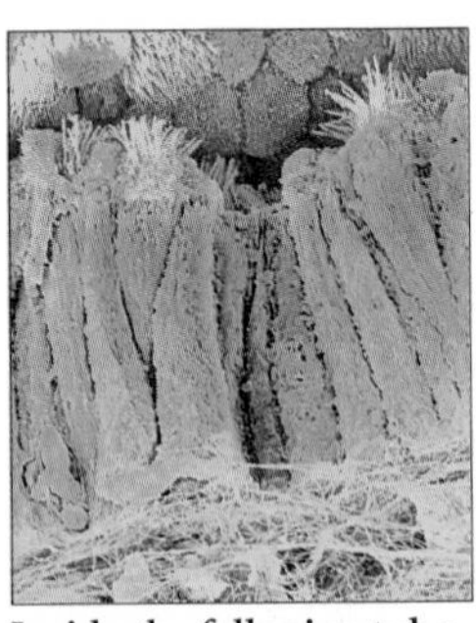

Inside the fallopian tube
Hair-like projections (cilia) in the fallopian tube propel the egg towards the uterus.

The cycle of egg maturation, ovulation, and menstrual bleeding occurs at intervals of, on average, 28 days during a woman's reproductive life. At the menopause, which usually occurs between the ages of 45 and 55, eggs stop maturing and are no longer released by the ovaries. Menstruation stops, and the reproductive phase of a woman's life comes to an end.

(PROCESS) PUBERTY

Puberty is the period during which visible sexual characteristics develop and sexual organs mature. In girls, puberty usually starts between the ages of 10 and 14 and lasts for about 3–4 years. Puberty can occur up to 2 years earlier in black people, and girls tend to enter puberty about 1–2 years before boys.

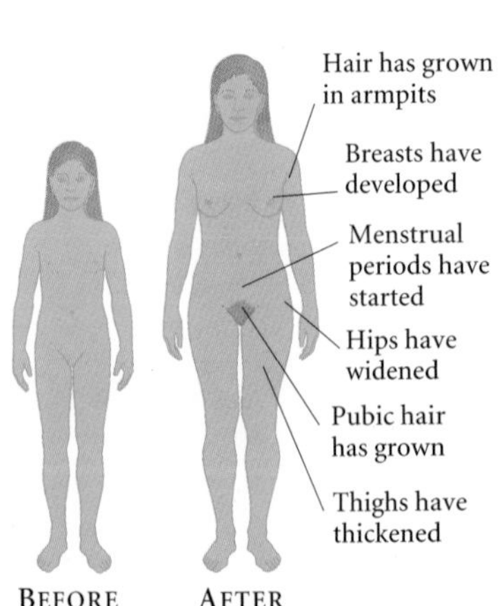

Physical development
During puberty, the breasts start to develop, pubic hair grows, and there is a rapid increase in height. The hips also widen, hair grows in the armpits, and menstruation begins.

FEMALE HORMONES

The ovaries produce the hormones oestrogen and progesterone, but secretion of these is controlled by follicle-stimulating hormone and luteinizing hormone, which are produced in the pituitary gland, a tiny structure just below the brain. Sex hormones control sexual development at puberty, the menstrual cycle, and fertility. Oestrogen also stimulates the fat distribution that results in a woman's rounded shape. Changes in hormone levels during the menstrual cycle and at menopause may affect mood and behaviour.

(STRUCTURE) FEMALE REPRODUCTIVE SYSTEM

The internal organs of the female reproductive system are all located in the lower third of the abdomen. The ovaries store and release eggs, which pass along the fallopian tubes into the uterus. The vagina connects the uterus to the outside of the body. The visible external organs are collectively known as the vulva and consist of the sexually sensitive clitoris surrounded by folds of skin called the labia, which protect the entrances to the vagina and the urethra. Just inside the entrance to the vagina lie the two Bartholin's glands, which secrete a fluid for lubrication during sexual intercourse.

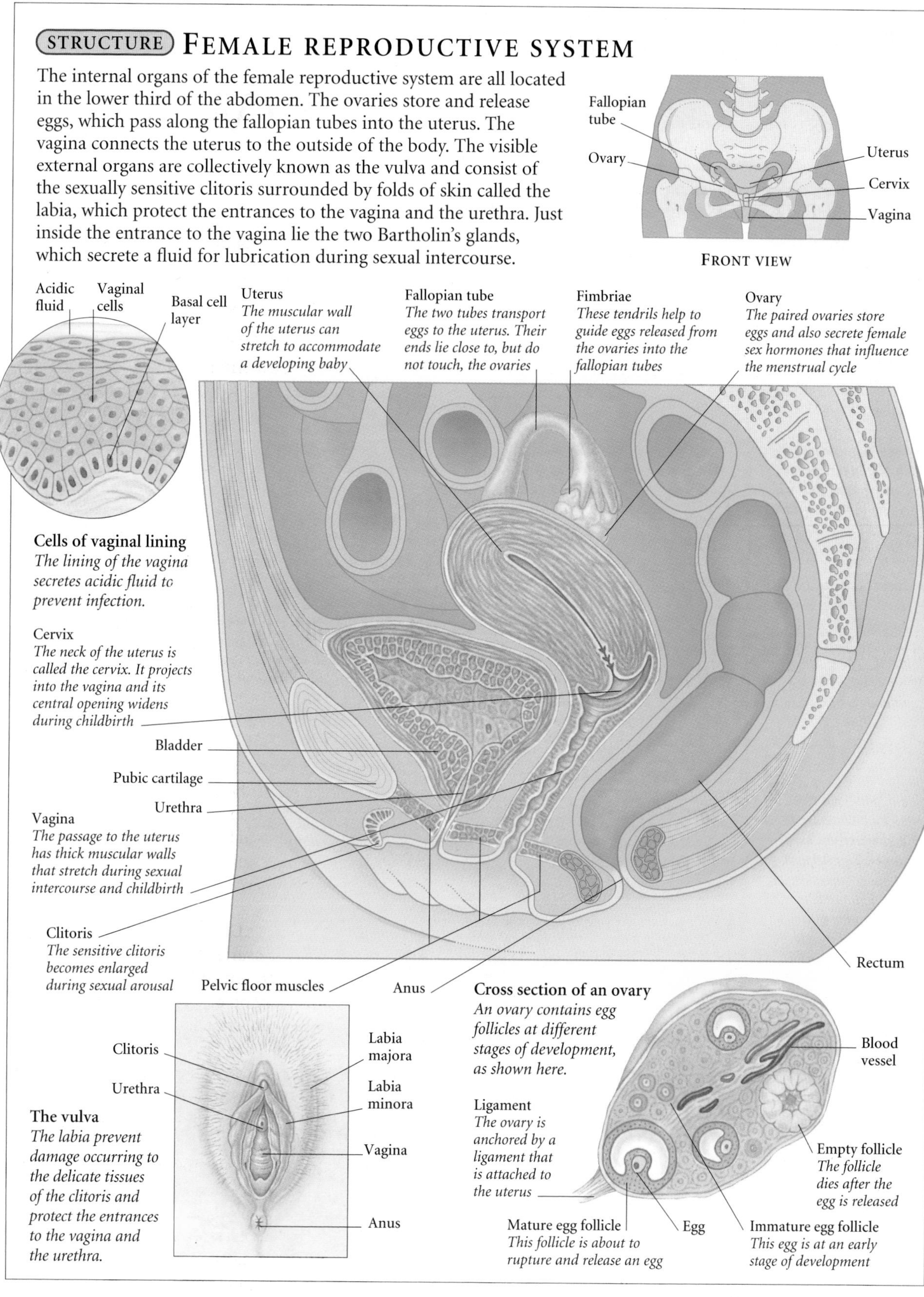

PROCESS MENSTRUAL CYCLE

Each month between puberty and the menopause, a woman's body goes through the menstrual cycle in preparation for conception and pregnancy. A mature egg is released, and the lining of the uterus (the endometrium) becomes thicker, ready for a fertilized egg to implant. If the egg is not fertilized, it passes out of the body during menstruation. The menstrual cycle lasts 28 days on average but may not be the same length every month and varies from woman to woman. The cycle is regulated by a complex interaction between four sex hormones. Follicle-stimulating hormone (FSH) and luteinizing hormone (LH) are produced in the pituitary gland, and oestrogen and progesterone are secreted by the ovaries.

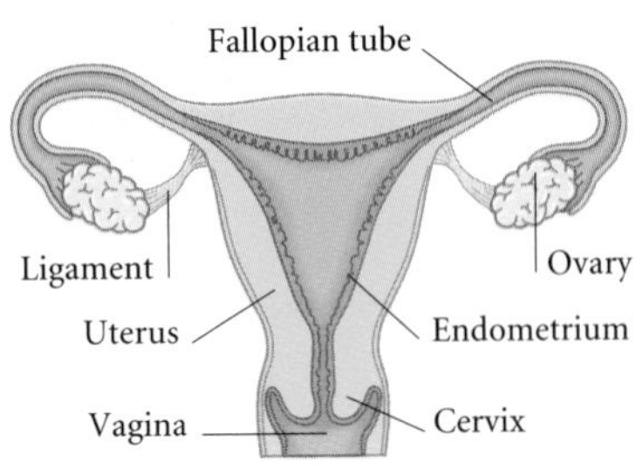

FEMALE REPRODUCTIVE SYSTEM

Hormones
Once a month, FSH causes an egg to mature and LH triggers its release. Just before ovulation, oestrogen levels peak. A rise in progesterone causes the lining of the uterus to thicken.

Inside the ovary
The cycle begins with an egg developing inside a follicle in the ovary. The mature egg is released into the fallopian tube, leaving the empty follicle, called the corpus luteum, in the ovary.

Endometrium
Hormones cause the endometrium to double in thickness, to about 6 mm (¼ in). If fertilization does not occur, some of the endometrial cells are shed as menstrual blood, together with the unfertilized egg.

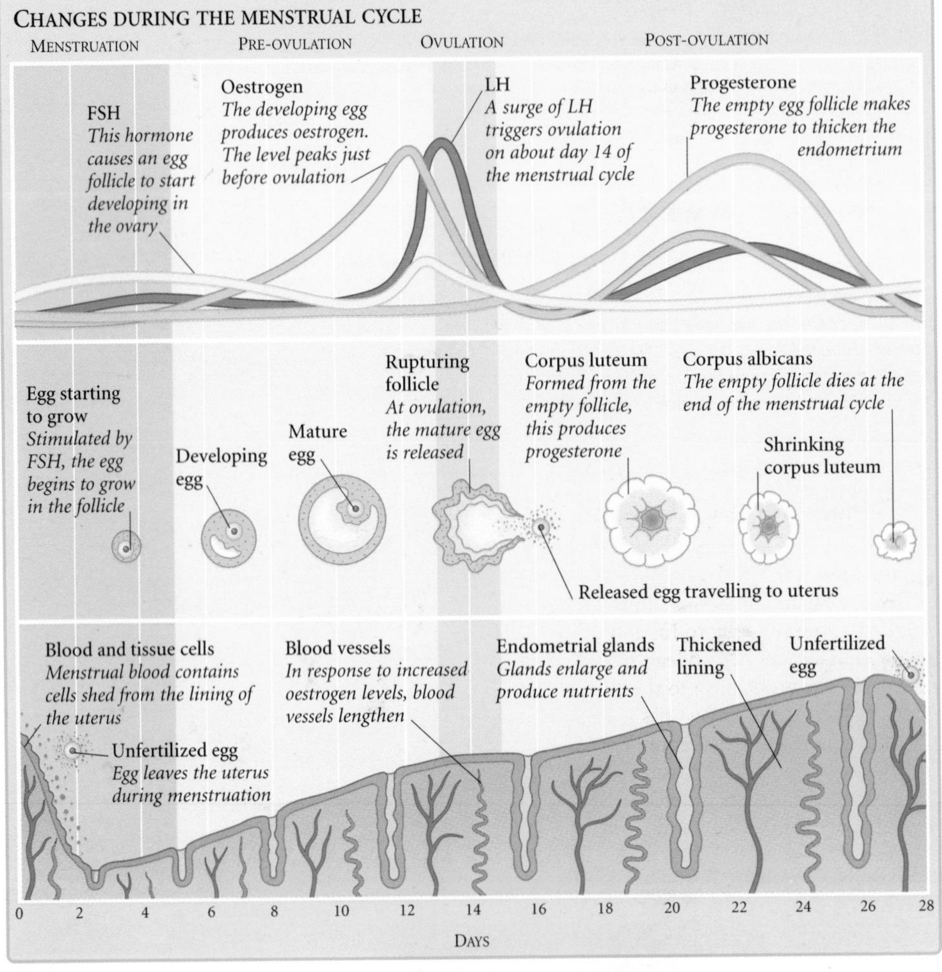

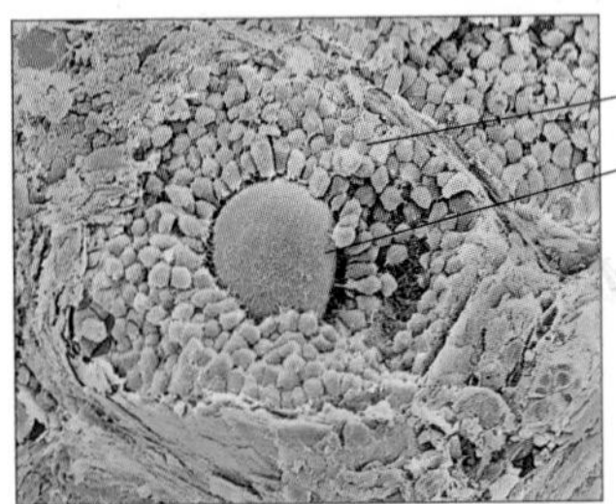

Developing follicle
By absorbing nutrients from cells inside the follicle, an immature egg is able to develop and grow to maturity.

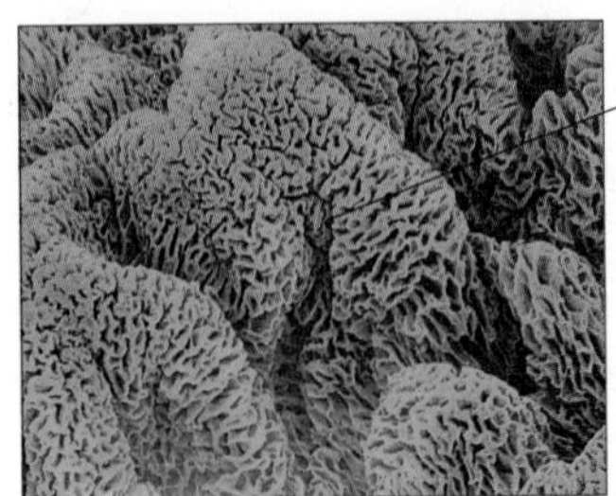

Endometrium
After ovulation, the thickened endometrium tissue looks spongy and is ready to receive the fertilized egg.

FUNCTION CHANGES DURING THE MENOPAUSE

The menopause occurs between the ages of 45 and 55, when a woman's ovaries stop responding to follicle-stimulating hormone (FSH) and produce less of the female sex hormones oestrogen and progesterone. This drop in hormone levels brings an end to ovulation and menstruation. In the years just before and after the menopause, hormone changes produce physical symptoms such as mood swings, hot flushes, vaginal dryness, and night sweats. The menopause may also cause long-term physical changes, such as osteoporosis.

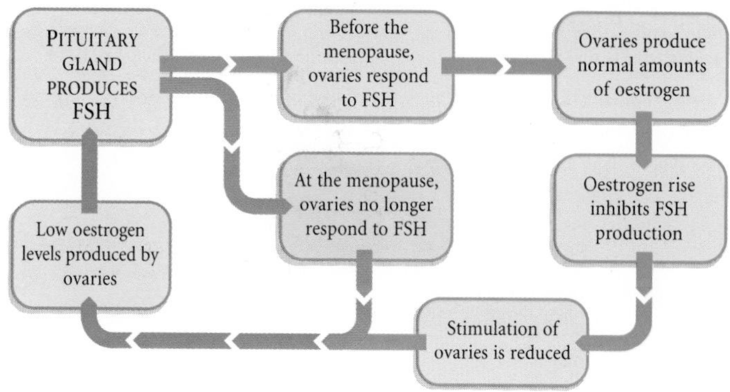

Hormone cycle
At the menopause, the ovaries no longer respond to FSH and produce little oestrogen. The pituitary gland reacts by increasing its production of FSH. The raised levels of FSH cause symptoms such as hot flushes.

KEY
- BEFORE THE MENOPAUSE
- AT THE MENOPAUSE

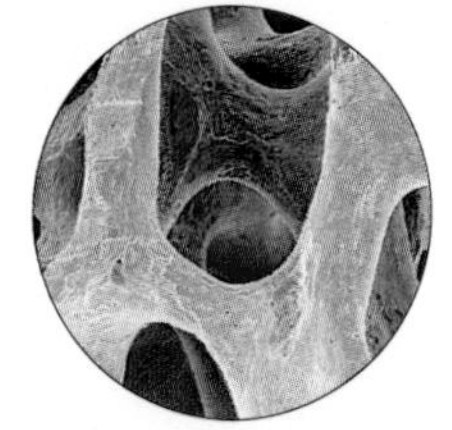
BEFORE THE MENOPAUSE

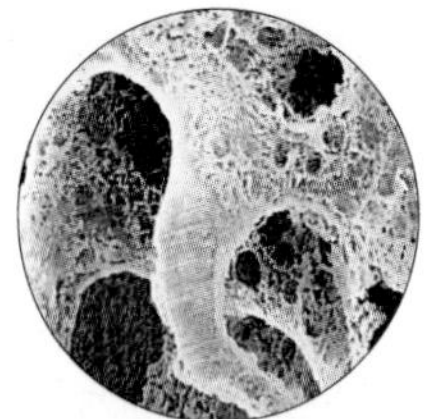
AFTER THE MENOPAUSE

Osteoporosis in bone tissue
Oestrogen is needed to give bones strength. After the menopause, when oestrogen levels are low, osteoporosis can develop. Bones lose density and may become thin and brittle, as shown in the microscopic image above.

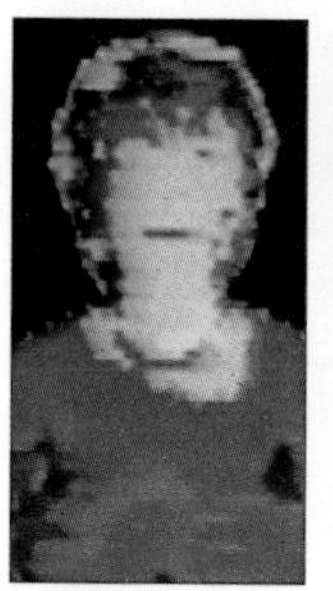

NORMAL HOT FLUSH

Hot flushes
These thermal images show increased skin temperature in a hot flush caused by high FSH levels.

FUNCTION ROLE OF THE BREASTS

Breasts have a role in sexual arousal, but their main function is to produce and deliver milk to a newborn baby. Hormonal changes in late pregnancy stimulate the production of milk in glands called lobules, which lead to ducts that converge and then open on to the surface of the nipple. The remaining breast tissue is mostly fat, with a small amount of connective tissue that helps to support the breasts. The variety in size and shape of breasts is determined by genetic factors, fat content, and muscle tone.

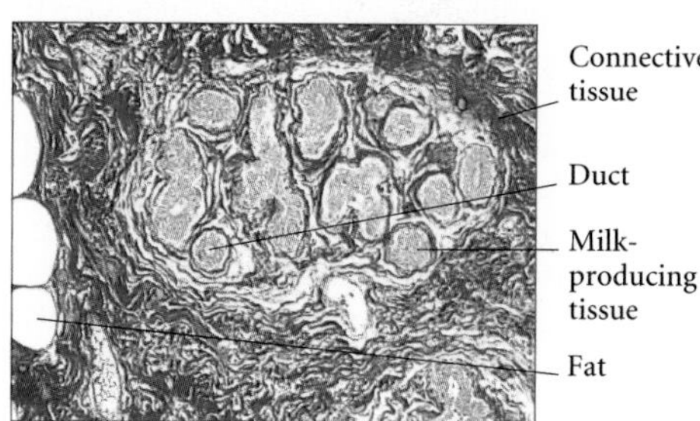

Breast tissue
A milk-producing lobule of the breast and the drainage ducts leading from it are shown here. Each lobule is surrounded by fat and connective tissue.

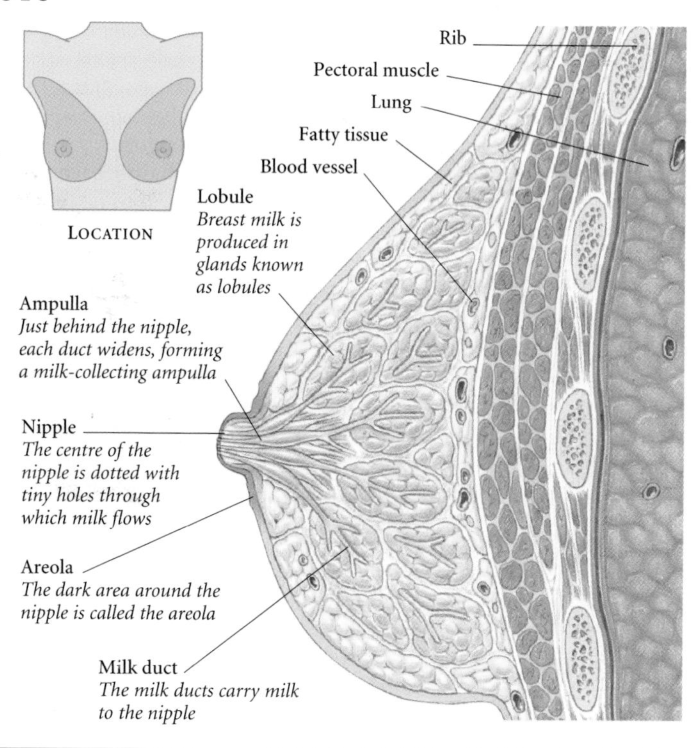

MENSTRUAL, MENOPAUSAL, AND HORMONAL PROBLEMS

Menstruation usually starts at puberty and ceases at the menopause. These two stages in a woman's life are determined by the levels of female sex hormones in the body. The menstrual cycle itself is also governed by a combination of hormones, all of which are produced at varying levels throughout the cycle. Many conditions or disorders upset the balance of these hormones.

This section begins by discussing some common menstrual disorders. Several of these disorders are still not fully understood, but advances in diagnostic techniques have made investigation easier, and modern surgical methods have improved treatment. The articles that follow discuss health problems associated with the menopause and other disorders caused by an imbalance of the sex hormones. The widespread use of hormonal treatment has helped to relieve many of these disorders.

Related disorders that affect the female reproductive system are dealt with in other sections (*see* DISORDERS OF THE FEMALE REPRODUCTIVE ORGANS, pp.741–753, and SEX AND REPRODUCTION, pp.762–777), as are disorders involving hormones other than the sex hormones (*see* HORMONES AND METABOLISM, pp.670–693).

KEY ANATOMY

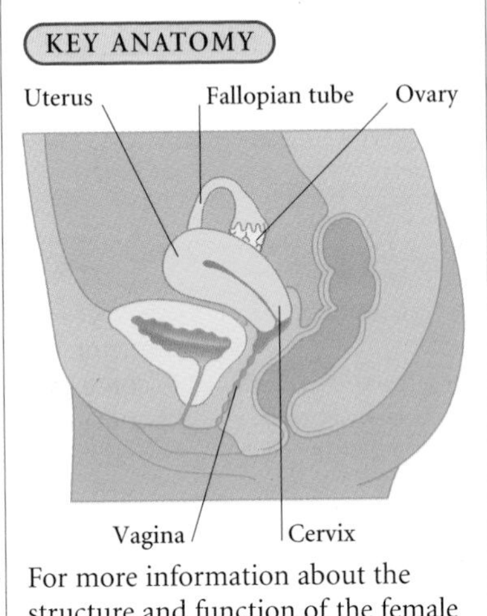

For more information about the structure and function of the female reproductive system, *see* pp.730–733.

Irregular periods

A menstrual cycle that has wide variations in the length of time between periods

 AGE Most common just after puberty and just before the menopause

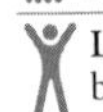 LIFESTYLE Stress, excessive exercise, and being underweight are all risk factors

 GENETICS Not a significant factor

Periods start at puberty and continue until the menopause. The average menstrual cycle lasts 28 days, but periods may occur as often as every 24 days or as infrequently as every 35 days. After puberty, most women develop a regular menstrual cycle with a relatively consistent length of time between periods. In some women, however, periods remain irregular. Menstrual bleeding normally lasts between 2 and 7 days, with the average length of bleeding being 5 days.

WHAT ARE THE CAUSES?

Variations in the length of the menstrual cycle are usually the result of a temporary hormonal imbalance. Fluctuations in hormone levels during puberty mean that periods are often irregular when they first start, and wide variations in a woman's normal pattern of bleeding are common in the first few months following childbirth and with the approach of the menopause.

Hormonal imbalances at other times may be caused by factors such as stress, depression, and severe or long-term illness. Excessive exercise and extreme loss of weight (*see* ANOREXIA NERVOSA, p.562) are also common causes of hormonal disturbance that can cause menstruation to become irregular.

Occasionally, irregular menstruation may be a symptom of a disorder of the ovaries or of the uterus. For example, polycystic ovary syndrome (p.744), in which there is an imbalance of the sex hormones, or endometriosis (p.742), in which fragments of the tissue that normally lines the uterus are displaced and become attached to other organs in the pelvis, may disrupt periods.

In some cases, an unsuspected pregnancy produces irregular bleeding that could easily be mistaken for a period. A single, late, heavy period may be due to a miscarriage (p.791). If you have a late period that is accompanied by severe abdominal pain, you should seek medical attention urgently because it may be due to an ectopic pregnancy (p.790). In some cases, the cause of irregular menstruation is unknown.

WHAT MIGHT BE DONE?

Irregular periods due to the normal hormonal changes that follow puberty or childbirth usually become more regular with time. In women who are approaching the menopause, irregular periods will eventually cease altogether. In all these cases, treatment is not usually necessary. However, if the problem persists and interferes with a woman's lifestyle, drugs may be given to regulate menstruation. These drugs include oral contraceptives for younger women and hormone replacement therapy (p.937) for women near the menopause. Irregular menstruation that is due to extreme weight loss, excessive exercise, stress, or depression should become more regular once these problems have been overcome.

If there is no obvious cause for your irregular periods and no apparent pattern to menstrual bleeding, your doctor may arrange for you to have tests to look for an underlying disorder. These may include a pregnancy test, blood tests to measure hormone levels, and ultrasound scanning (p.250) of the pelvic region to look at the ovaries and uterus. If an underlying disorder is discovered, treatment of that disorder should regulate periods in most cases.

(WWW) ONLINE SITES: p.1037

Amenorrhoea

The absence of menstruation for at least 3 months in women who would otherwise be having periods

AGE Occurs between puberty and the menopause

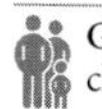
GENETICS In some cases, due to a chromosomal abnormality

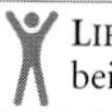
LIFESTYLE Stress, excessive exercise, and being underweight are all risk factors

There are two types of amenorrhoea: primary and secondary. If a girl has not started to menstruate by the age of 16, she is said to have primary amenorrhoea. Once menstruation has become established during puberty, it is normal for periods to stop during pregnancy, for a few months following childbirth, while breast-feeding, temporarily after ceasing to take oral contraceptive pills, and permanently at the menopause. If menstruation stops at any other time for at least 3 months, the condition is known as secondary amenorrhoea.

What are the causes?

Amenorrhoea is often caused by a disturbance in the female sex hormones, which may be brought on by factors such as stress or depression. Excessive exercise and extreme or sudden weight loss (*see* ANOREXIA NERVOSA, p.562) may also lead to such hormonal disturbances and are common causes of amenorrhoea in athletes, gymnasts, and ballet dancers. Hormonal changes may lead to primary or secondary amenorrhoea, depending on when they occur.

Primary amenorrhoea is a characteristic feature of delayed puberty (*see* ABNORMAL PUBERTY IN FEMALES, p.739) and may be caused by a chromosomal abnormality. The failure of menstruation to start at puberty may also be due to a condition in which the hymen (the thin membrane over the vagina) has no opening, and menstrual blood cannot leave the body. In rare cases, the uterus is absent from birth, and therefore no menstruation can occur.

Secondary amenorrhoea may be due to a pituitary gland disorder, such as a pituitary tumour (*see* PROLACTINOMA, p.677). Some women have a premature menopause, in which periods cease before the age of 35. Other possible causes include disorders of the ovaries, such as polycystic ovary syndrome (p.744), and treatments such as radiotherapy (p.281) and chemotherapy (p.280), which can result in damage to the ovaries.

What might be done?

Treatment is not needed if amenorrhoea lasts for only a few months after stopping oral contraceptive pills or occurs during pregnancy or breast-feeding. Menstruation normally resumes within a few months of giving birth if you are not breast-feeding or within a month of stopping breast-feeding. After the menopause, amenorrhoea will be permanent.

Amenorrhoea that occurs at any other time should be investigated. Your doctor will examine you and may perform a pregnancy test. You may also need to have blood tests to measure hormone levels, ultrasound scanning (p.250) of the ovaries and uterus, and CT scanning (p.247) of the pituitary gland.

Treatment of the underlying disorder induces menstruation in most cases. If the cause cannot be treated, hormonal treatment may be used to start menstruation. If periods are absent due to stress, weight loss, or excessive exercise, they should occur if the problem is overcome.

(WWW) ONLINE SITES: p.1037

Menorrhagia

Menstrual bleeding that is heavier than normal

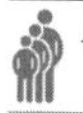
AGE More common over the age of 40

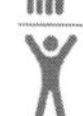
LIFESTYLE Being overweight is a risk factor

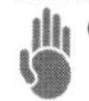
GENETICS Not a significant factor

Some women have heavier periods than others. However, if menstrual bleeding lasts for longer than 7 days, cannot be controlled by sanitary towels or tampons, or includes large blood clots, it is classed as menorrhagia. In some cases, this condition may be associated with a dragging pain in the lower abdomen. Menstruation may also be irregular (*see* IRREGULAR PERIODS, opposite page). Severe menstrual bleeding may lead to iron-deficiency anaemia (p.447), causing light-headedness and tiredness. About 1 in 20 women has menorrhagia regularly. The condition is more common in women approaching the menopause.

What are the causes?

Heavy or prolonged menstrual bleeding can be a symptom of various disorders of the uterus, such as fibroids (p.745), uterine polyps (p.746), or cancer of the uterus (p.748). Menorrhagia is also a well-known side effect of using an intrauterine contraceptive device (IUD). A single heavy period that is late may be a miscarriage (p.791). Menorrhagia may also be caused by a hormonal disorder, such as hypothyroidism (p.680). The condition occurs more commonly in women who are overweight.

Sometimes, the cause is not clear. If your periods have always been heavy, there is probably no need for concern. However, you should consult your doctor if the problem affects your lifestyle.

How is it diagnosed?

Your doctor will examine you and may arrange for blood tests to measure your hormone levels and to look for signs of anaemia. Further investigations, such as ultrasound scanning (p.250) to look for fibroids or polyps in the uterus, may be necessary. You may also have a hysteroscopy (p.745), in which a viewing instrument is passed through the cervix to examine the uterus. A small sample of the endometrium (the lining of the uterus) may be taken for analysis (*see* ENDOMETRIAL SAMPLING, p.738).

What is the treatment?

Treatment depends on the cause, your age, and the severity of the bleeding. Any underlying disorder will be treated. If no cause is found, drugs may initially be given to reduce blood loss. You may want to consider changing your method of contraception if you use an IUD. If you are overweight, losing weight may help.

If initial treatments do not help or if menorrhagia is severe, you may require laser surgery to remove the endometrium (*see* LASER TREATMENT, p.951) or an operation to remove the uterus (*see* HYSTERECTOMY, p.747). These procedures are irreversible and are only offered to women who do not want to have children in the future. Laser removal of the endometrium is a minor procedure, but it carries a small risk that problems will recur if any endometrial tissue remains. A hysterectomy is a major operation but ensures that menorrhagia will not recur.

(WWW) ONLINE SITES: p.1037

Dysmenorrhoea

Lower abdominal pain and discomfort experienced just before or during menstruation

 GENETICS Sometimes runs in families

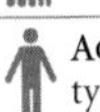 AGE LIFESTYLE Risk factors depend on the type

Up to three-quarters of women have period pain, also known as dysmenorrhoea, at some time. In about a fifth of these women, the pain is severe and can seriously disrupt normal activities. Pain is usually experienced in the 24 hours before menstruation or over the first 1 or 2 days of the period.

WHAT ARE THE TYPES?

There are two types of dysmenorrhoea: primary, which has no obvious cause; and secondary, which is the result of a disorder of the reproductive organs.

PRIMARY DYSMENORRHOEA This form of dysmenorrhoea usually appears in the early teens and is associated with the hormones involved in the monthly release of eggs from the ovaries. Periods often become painful about 1–2 years after the start of menstruation, when ovulation begins. A rise in the level of hormone-like substances called prostaglandins in the body occurs some days after ovulation and makes the muscles of the uterus contract. This contraction interferes with the blood supply to the uterus and causes period pain. This type of menstrual pain tends to lessen after the age of 25, often disappearing by the age of 30, and it usually becomes less severe after childbirth, probably because the blood supply to the uterus increases.

Women with close female relatives who have had primary dysmenorrhoea are more likely to develop it, suggesting that genetic factors are involved.

SECONDARY DYSMENORRHOEA Painful periods in women who have not experienced menstrual pain before or have only had mild pain is called secondary dysmenorrhoea. This type of period pain usually affects women between the ages of 20 and 40. The cause is often endometriosis (p.742), in which fragments of the tissue that normally lines the uterus become attached to other organs in the pelvis, or a disorder of the uterus, such as fibroids (p.745). A persistent infection of the reproductive organs (*see* PELVIC INFLAMMATORY DISEASE, p.741) and use of an intrauterine contraceptive device (IUD) may also cause painful periods.

WHAT ARE THE SYMPTOMS?

The symptoms of dysmenorrhoea begin either just before or at the start of menstruation and are worst when bleeding is heaviest. The pain may be described as either or both of the following:

- Cramping lower abdominal pain that comes in waves, radiating to the lower back and down the legs.
- Dragging pain in the pelvis.

This pain may be accompanied by any of the symptoms of premenstrual syndrome (right), such as headache.

WHAT CAN I DO?

Taking certain over-the-counter painkillers (p.912), such as ibuprofen, may help to alleviate the discomfort. Relaxing in a hot bath and applying a source of heat, such as a hot-water bottle, to your abdomen may also provide pain relief. However, consult your doctor if you are experiencing period pain for the first time or if the pain becomes severe.

WHAT MIGHT THE DOCTOR DO?

Your doctor will probably examine you, especially if you have secondary dysmenorrhoea. Various tests may be carried out, including a cervical swab to look for infection, ultrasound scanning (p.250) of the lower abdomen, or examination of the uterus with an instrument called a hysteroscope (*see* HYSTEROSCOPY, p.745).

Treatment depends on the type of dysmenorrhoea. If you have primary dysmenorrhoea, your doctor may prescribe a nonsteroidal anti-inflammatory drug (p.894) or an antispasmodic drug (*see* ANTISPASMODIC DRUGS AND MOTILITY STIMULANTS, p.926) to reduce cramping pain. In some cases, your doctor may prescribe oral contraceptive pills, which relieve period pain by preventing ovulation and can also decrease menstrual blood loss. Once ovulation has been suppressed, primary dysmenorrhoea should improve, but the pain may recur at any time if you stop treatment. Secondary dysmenorrhoea usually disappears once the underlying condition is treated.

(WWW) ONLINE SITES: p.1037

Premenstrual syndrome

Varying symptoms that may affect women in the days leading up to menstruation

 AGE Usually develops in late adolescence; may occur in all menstruating females

 GENETICS Sometimes runs in families

 LIFESTYLE Stress and certain foods may aggravate symptoms

As many as 1 in 3 women experiences symptoms of premenstrual syndrome (PMS) as her period approaches. In up to 1 in 20 women, these symptoms may be severe enough to disrupt activities.

The cause of PMS is disputed, but it is thought that the symptoms are triggered by the action of the female sex hormones oestrogen and progesterone before menstruation. Stress may make the symptoms worse, as may excessive consumption of chocolate and caffeine-containing drinks, such as coffee and cola. A women is more likely to have

(SELF-HELP) PREVENTING PREMENSTRUAL SYNDROME

The following self-help measures may help either to prevent or to relieve premenstrual syndrome. If these measures do not help and you have persistent symptoms, visit your doctor for advice.

- Relax as much as possible and try to avoid stress.
- Try taking up a light, relaxing exercise, such as yoga.
- Take warm baths.
- Eat little and often, making sure your diet includes plenty of carbohydrates and fibre.
- Try to reduce your salt intake.
- Avoid eating excessive amounts of chocolate.
- Avoid drinks containing large amounts of caffeine, such as coffee, tea, and cola.
- A vitamin B_6 supplement may be helpful, although very high doses can be harmful.
- Evening primrose oil capsules are often effective, especially in relieving breast tenderness.

severe symptoms of PMS if close relatives have experienced similar problems, although no specific genetic factors have as yet been identified.

WHAT ARE THE SYMPTOMS?

The symptoms of PMS vary between women, and some women find that the symptoms also differ from month to month. Symptoms may appear just a few hours before a period begins, but they can start up to 14 days beforehand. In most affected women, the symptoms disappear by the time menstruation has finished or a few days afterwards. The symptoms of PMS may include:

- Tenderness or generalized lumpiness of the breasts.
- A feeling of bloating caused by the retention of fluid.
- Mood changes, including feelings of tension, irritability, depression, anxiety, and tiredness.
- Difficulty concentrating and making everyday decisions.
- Headaches, including migraine.
- Backache and muscle stiffness.
- Disruption of normal sleep patterns.
- Unusual food cravings.

Less commonly, nausea, vomiting, cold sweats, dizziness, and hot flushes may also be experienced.

WHAT MIGHT BE DONE?

The diagnosis of PMS is usually easily made from the timing of your symptoms. Your doctor may ask you to keep a record of symptoms to confirm that they are related to menstruation.

There are a number of self-help measures you can take to try to prevent PMS (*see* PREVENTING PREMENSTRUAL SYNDROME, opposite page). If these are not effective or your symptoms are severe, you should seek medical advice. Certain painkillers (p.912), such as ibuprofen, can help to relieve headaches and muscle stiffness. If you experience mood swings, your doctor may prescribe antidepressant drugs (p.916), which may be more effective if taken throughout the menstrual cycle. Diuretic drugs (p.902) may help to relieve fluid retention. Your doctor may also prescribe treatment with the hormone progesterone (*see* SEX HORMONES AND RELATED DRUGS, p.933). No treatment is consistently successful, but the symptoms can usually be relieved.

(WWW) ONLINE SITES: p.1037

Abnormal vaginal bleeding

Vaginal bleeding that is not related to menstruation

AGE LIFESTYLE Risk factors depend on the cause

GENETICS Not a significant factor

Normally, vaginal bleeding occurs only during a period. Bleeding that occurs outside menstruation is abnormal. In women under the age of 35, abnormal vaginal bleeding is often the result of starting oral contraceptives. Abnormal bleeding caused by a disorder of the reproductive organs is more common in women over this age.

WHAT ARE THE CAUSES?

Light bleeding between periods, known as spotting, is common in the first few menstrual cycles after starting oral contraceptives or changing to a different type of pill. Spotting is usually brought on by the body adjusting to changes in hormone levels, but this type of bleeding is also associated with using an intrauterine contraceptive device (IUD).

Abnormal bleeding, especially within a few hours of sexual intercourse, may indicate a disorder of the cervix, such as cervical erosion (p.749) or cancer of the cervix (p.750). In older women, sex may damage the walls of the vagina, which become thinner and more fragile after the menopause, causing bleeding.

Abnormal vaginal bleeding that is not associated with sexual intercourse or contraception may be caused by a disorder such as endometriosis (p.742) or uterine polyps (p.746). Loss of blood from the uterus can also occur in early pregnancy and could indicate a miscarriage (p.791). Various disorders of the female reproductive organs may cause postmenopausal bleeding (p.738), such as cancer of the uterus (p.748).

If you notice abnormal bleeding, you should see your doctor immediately so that the cause can be investigated.

WHAT MIGHT BE DONE?

Your doctor may be able to make a diagnosis based on the timing of the bleeding and a physical examination. You may also need to have tests, such as a cervical smear test (p.749) to check for disorders of the cervix, ultrasound scanning (p.250) to look at the uterus, or endoscopy to view the inside of the uterus (*see* HYSTEROSCOPY, p.745).

The treatment for abnormal vaginal bleeding depends on the cause. Spotting caused by oral contraceptives may be prevented by changing the dose or type of pill. Hormone treatments can be used to restore the elasticity of fragile vaginal walls in older women. Surgery may be required to treat more serious underlying disorders. In most cases, abnormal vaginal bleeding disappears once the cause has been successfully treated.

(WWW) ONLINE SITES: p.1037

Menopausal problems

Symptoms associated with the normal changes that take place in a woman's body as her period of fertility ends

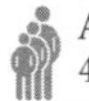
AGE Most common between the ages of 45 and 55

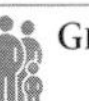
GENETICS Sometimes runs in families

LIFESTYLE Smoking may lower the age at which the menopause occurs

The menopause, the time at which a woman stops menstruating, is a normal consequence of the aging process. More than 8 in 10 women feel well throughout the menopause or experience only mild symptoms, but some women have severe problems that affect their lifestyle.

The onset of the menopause usually occurs between the ages of 45 and 55, although some women develop symptoms before or after this time. Smoking can lower the age at which the menopause takes place. A woman is generally considered to be menopausal if she has not had a period for at least 6 months and there is no other underlying cause. The tendency to have either an early or a late menopause can run in families.

WHAT ARE THE CAUSES?

As women age, their ovaries gradually become less active and produce smaller amounts of the sex hormone oestrogen. The menopause occurs as a result of this reduction in oestrogen levels. As levels of oestrogen in the body decline, the pituitary gland begins to secrete more follicle-stimulating hormone (FSH) to try to stimulate the ovaries. Most of the symptoms associated with the menopause are a consequence of the reduced levels of oestrogen or increased levels of FSH. These tend to be more severe when the menopause takes place prematurely or abruptly. A sudden menopause can be brought about by surgical removal of the ovaries or anticancer treatments that can damage the ovaries, such as chemotherapy (p.280) and radiotherapy (p.281).

WHAT ARE THE SYMPTOMS?

Menopausal symptoms may begin up to 5 years before menstruation finally stops and usually last for a year or two. Many women find that one of the first signs of the menopause is irregularity in their menstrual cycle. Menstrual bleeding may also become heavier (*see* MENORRHAGIA, p.735). Increased levels of FSH in the body cause many of the other common symptoms that can occur during the menopause. These include:

- Hot flushes, in which the head, chest, and arms become red and feel hot, lasting from a couple of minutes to as long as an hour.
- Heavy sweating, which is often especially troublesome at night.
- Feelings of anxiety, panic, or depression, which may be made worse if the menopause coincides with a stressful life event such as the departure of adult children from the home.

The longer-term effects of a decline in oestrogen levels include:

- Drying of the skin, which encourages the formation of wrinkles.
- Vaginal dryness and discomfort during sexual intercourse as a result of thinning of the lining of the vagina.
- Urinary infections that occur due to thinning of the lining of the urethra (the passage leading from the bladder to the outside of the body).

The decline in oestrogen levels following the menopause may also increase your risk of developing certain long-term conditions, such as coronary artery disease (p.405) and age-related thinning of the bones (*see* OSTEOPOROSIS, p.368).

WHAT MIGHT BE DONE?

Hormone replacement therapy (p.937), commonly known as HRT, may help to relieve many of the symptoms that occur at the menopause by boosting the level of oestrogen in the body and reducing the production of FSH. Your doctor may prescribe HRT as pills, implants under the skin, or skin patches. To achieve maximum benefit, HRT is usually given for at least 5 years. However, long-term use may carry certain risks, which you should discuss with your doctor.

Alternative treatments are available in the form of oestrogen creams, which help to control vaginal dryness and discomfort, and the drug clonidine, which can be used to relieve hot flushes. Some women find complementary therapies, such as homeopathy (p.974), helpful.

The process of the menopause normally lasts between 1 and 5 years, after which symptoms usually disappear.

(WWW) ONLINE SITES: p.1037

Postmenopausal bleeding

Bleeding from the uterus occurring at least 6 months after menstruation has stopped

AGE Occurs after the menopause

GENETICS LIFESTYLE Not significant factors

Menstrual bleeding should cease at the menopause. Postmenopausal bleeding is normal only with certain forms of hormone replacement therapy (p.937) that cause withdrawal bleeding once a month. Other postmenopausal bleeding may be a sign of a serious disorder, such as cancer of the reproductive tract, and should be investigated by a doctor. Postmenopausal bleeding may range from light spotting to a heavier flow of blood and is usually painless.

WHAT ARE THE CAUSES?

Postmenopausal bleeding can be a symptom of several disorders of the vulva, vagina, cervix, and uterus. The most common and least serious cause of such bleeding is atrophic vaginitis, in which the vagina becomes inflamed due to low levels of oestrogen after the menopause (*see* VULVOVAGINITIS, p.752).

Postmenopausal bleeding could be caused by a disorder of the cervix, such as cervical erosion (p.749) or cancer of the cervix (p.750). In these disorders, bleeding from the cervix may be more

(TEST) ENDOMETRIAL SAMPLING

During endometrial sampling a small sample of tissue is removed from the endometrium (the lining of the uterus) to investigate symptoms such as heavy vaginal bleeding and to rule out cancer of the uterus. The sample is examined under a microscope for abnormalities. The procedure may be slightly uncomfortable but usually lasts for only a few minutes and does not require anaesthesia.

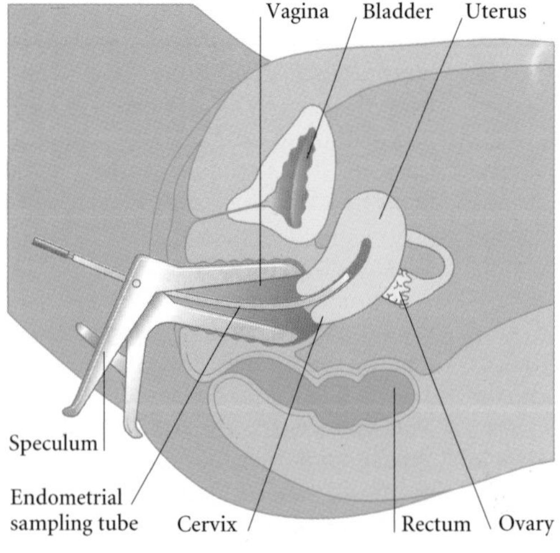

During the procedure
An instrument called a speculum is used to hold the vagina open while a thin, flexible tube is inserted into the uterus. A small sample of tissue is then drawn into the tube by vacuum suction.

(RESULTS)

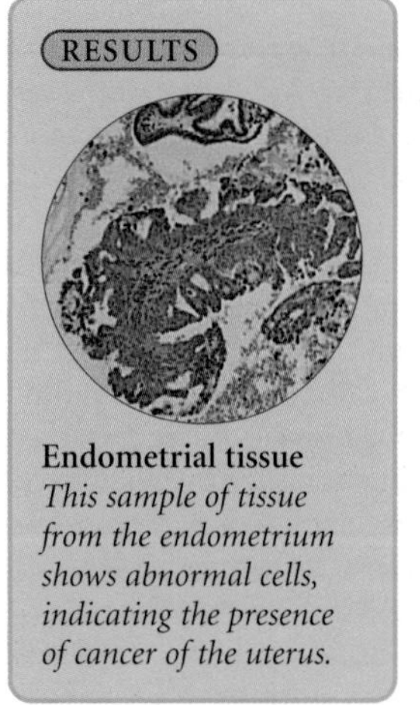

Endometrial tissue
This sample of tissue from the endometrium shows abnormal cells, indicating the presence of cancer of the uterus.

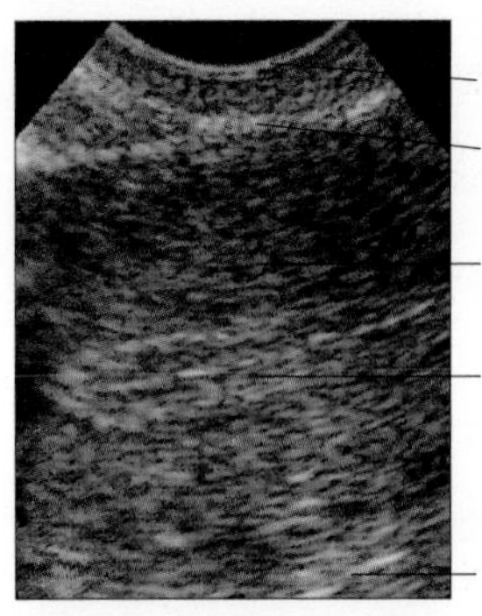

Thickened endometrium
This ultrasound scan of the uterus shows that the endometrium (the lining of the uterus) is thickened. This may be a cause of postmenopausal bleeding.

likely to occur after sexual intercourse. Postmenopausal bleeding may also be the result of a thickened endometrium (the lining of the uterus) or cancerous or noncancerous growths in the uterus (*see* CANCER OF THE UTERUS, p.748, and UTERINE POLYPS, p.746). Cancer of the vulva and vagina (p.753) may also lead to postmenopausal bleeding, although both of these disorders are very rare.

WHAT MIGHT BE DONE?

Your doctor will examine the vagina and cervix to look for abnormalities. If abnormal areas are seen in the vagina, a small sample of tissue may be taken for examination under a microscope. Your doctor may also perform a cervical smear test (p.749) to check for abnormal cells in the cervix. In some cases, a sample of endometrial tissue may be taken for analysis (*see* ENDOMETRIAL SAMPLING, opposite page).

Ultrasound scanning (p.250) may be carried out to image the uterus and to measure the thickness of the lining. The inside of your uterus may also be examined (*see* HYSTEROSCOPY, p.745).

The treatment for postmenopausal bleeding varies depending on the underlying cause. Oestrogen creams that are applied to the vagina may be prescribed to relieve atrophic vaginitis. Surgery may be necessary to remove cancerous growths. Surgery may also be carried out to treat disorders of the cervix and uterus, such as cervical polyps or a thickened endometrium. Postmenopausal bleeding should cease once the underlying disorder has been treated.

(WWW) ONLINE SITES: p.1037

Hypogonadism in females

Underactivity, developmental failure, or absence of the ovaries, leading to low levels of female sex hormones

 GENETICS Sometimes due to a chromosomal abnormality

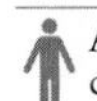 AGE LIFESTYLE Risk factors depend on the cause

Female sex hormones control sexual development and the menstrual cycle. Underactivity of the ovaries, known as hypogonadism, leads to low levels of these hormones in the body. A decline in hormone levels occurs naturally during the menopause, but at other times it may indicate an underlying disorder. Hypogonadism may cause distressing symptoms but is often treatable.

WHAT ARE THE TYPES?

There are two types of hypogonadism: primary and secondary. Either type can occur at any age. Primary hypogonadism is often caused by a disorder or failure of the ovaries, which may result from a chromosomal abnormality such as Turner's syndrome (p.823). It may also be caused by the surgical removal of the ovaries. In most cases, primary hypogonadism occurs as a natural consequence of the menopause.

Secondary hypogonadism is caused by an abnormality of the pituitary gland or of the hypothalamus (a part of the brain) that leads to underproduction of the hormones that stimulate the ovaries to function. This abnormality may be due to a disorder such as a pituitary tumour (p.676) or, rarely, to damage to the pituitary gland or the hypothalamus as a result of a head injury (p.521) or an infection such as viral encephalitis (p.528). Sometimes, it results from excessive exercise or sudden weight loss.

WHAT ARE THE SYMPTOMS?

The symptoms depend on the age at which hypogonadism develops and the amount of sex hormones produced. If the onset occurs before puberty, hypogonadism causes abnormal puberty in females (right). If the onset occurs after puberty, symptoms may include:

- Reduced or absent menstruation (*see* AMENORRHOEA, p.735).
- Reduced fertility.
- Hot flushes, excessive sweating, and anxiety, together with other symptoms associated with the menopause (*see* MENOPAUSAL PROBLEMS, p.737).
- Rarely, the pubic hair may recede and the breasts may become smaller.

There may also be other symptoms, depending on the underlying cause.

WHAT MIGHT BE DONE?

Your doctor may arrange for you to have blood tests to measure your hormone levels. You may also have CT scanning (p.247) of the brain to look for a pituitary abnormality or ultrasound scanning (p.250) of the ovaries.

The treatment depends on the cause. For example, a pituitary tumour may be removed by surgery. If the condition is due to weight loss, gaining weight may help. In some cases, hormone treatment may be prescribed to induce puberty. Hormone replacement therapy (p.937) may be recommended for menopausal women to help to relieve symptoms of the menopause and protect against diseases associated with low levels of sex hormones, such as osteoporosis (p.368) and coronary artery disease (p.405).

(WWW) ONLINE SITES: p.1032, p.1033, p.1037

Abnormal puberty in females

Very early or late start of puberty, usually due to a hormonal imbalance

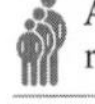 AGE Occurs before or after the normal age range for puberty

LIFESTYLE Excessive exercise and weight loss are risk factors

GENETICS In some cases, due to a chromosomal abnormality

Puberty is the period during which sexual development occurs (*see* PUBERTY, p.730). In girls, puberty is characterized by a growth spurt, hair growth in the armpits and pubic region, the development of the breasts and reproductive organs, and the onset of menstruation. Although there is some variation in the age of onset of puberty, girls tend to start this process between the ages of 10 and 14. Puberty may be considered abnormal if it starts either earlier than normal (precocious) or later (delayed). Early puberty occurs if a girl develops breasts before the age of 8 or if menstruation starts before the age of 10. In extreme cases, puberty may begin at the age of 4. Puberty is delayed if menstruation has not started by the age of 16 (*see* AMENORRHOEA, p.735) or breast development is absent at the age of 14.

Early puberty is rare and may be due to a hormone disorder. Delayed puberty is more common. Although there may be an underlying cause of delayed puberty, many girls who have not menstruated by the age of 16 are simply late developers, a tendency that often runs in families.

Abnormal puberty can be disturbing for a girl and her family because physical and sexual development will not coincide with that of her peers. Medical advice should be sought as soon as abnormal puberty is suspected.

WHAT ARE THE CAUSES?

Puberty in girls is controlled by female sex hormones produced by the ovaries. The production of these hormones is controlled by hormones from the pituitary gland in the brain and from the hypothalamus (the part of the brain that regulates the pituitary gland). Disorders of any of these organs may lead to an abnormally early or late puberty.

Early puberty may be due to a disorder that causes a premature rise in sex hormones. For example, an ovarian cyst (p.743) developing in childhood may produce sex hormones, causing early sexual development. A tumour of the hypothalamus or damage to the pituitary gland as the result of head injury (p.521) or an infection such as meningitis (p.527) may also cause early puberty.

Delayed puberty may be caused by certain chromosome disorders, such as Turner's syndrome (p.823), or less commonly by a pituitary tumour (p.676). Excessive weight loss or exercise may create a temporary hormonal imbalance that can lead to delayed puberty.

In many cases of abnormal puberty, no underlying cause is found.

WHAT MIGHT BE DONE?

The doctor will carry out an examination to determine whether puberty has started or how far it has progressed. A blood sample may be taken to measure hormone levels or check for a chromosomal abnormality. The doctor may also arrange for MRI (p.248) or CT scanning (p.247) of the brain to look for a pituitary tumour, or ultrasound scanning (p.250) of the ovaries to check for cysts.

If there is an underlying condition, it will be treated. For example, an ovarian cyst will be surgically removed. Hormonal treatment may be prescribed to suspend precocious puberty or to promote sexual development if puberty is delayed. In some cases, delayed puberty is associated with infertility (*see* FEMALE INFERTILITY, p.775), and further evaluation and treatment may be required in the future if a woman who has had a delayed puberty wants to have children.

Sometimes, puberty is simply late, and treatment is not necessary. Gaining weight and reducing strenuous activity may help if delayed puberty has been caused by weight loss or exercise.

(WWW) ONLINE SITES: p.1028, p.1037

Virilization

Development of male characteristics in a female due to a hormonal imbalance

 AGE May be present at birth but usually develops later in life

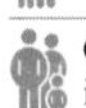 GENETICS In some cases, the cause is inherited

 LIFESTYLE Not a significant factor

Normally, low levels of male sex hormones are present in females and are produced by the adrenal glands and the ovaries. However, if the production of these hormones increases significantly, various male characteristics begin to develop, a condition called virilization.

Virilization most commonly occurs in adulthood, causing symptoms such as deepening of the voice, excessive hair growth on the face and body known as hirsutism, and thinning of the hair on the temples and crown. These symptoms often cause psychological distress. Rarely, the condition is present at birth. If present at birth, virilization is usually due to a genetic disorder that causes abnormal hormone levels (*see* CONGENITAL ADRENAL HYPERPLASIA, p.866).

WHAT ARE THE CAUSES?

When virilization develops later in life, the possible causes include abnormalities of the ovaries, such as certain types of ovarian cysts (p.743), cancer of the ovary (p.744), and polycystic ovary syndrome (p.744). Hormone levels can also be increased by adrenal tumours (p.684) and the use of certain male hormone supplements by athletes.

WHAT ARE THE SYMPTOMS?

Symptoms appear gradually as male sex hormone levels rise. They include:

- Excessive growth of hair on the face and body.
- Less regular or absent menstruation (*see* AMENORRHOEA, p.735).
- Reduction in breast size or in rare cases failure of the breasts to develop.
- Enlargement of the clitoris.
- Irreversible enlargement of the larynx (Adam's apple), causing the voice to become deeper.
- Thinning of the hair around the temples and crown (*see* MALE-PATTERN BALDNESS, p.359).

The hormonal imbalance may lead to increased muscular development, producing a male body shape.

WHAT MIGHT BE DONE?

Your doctor will examine you and may arrange tests to determine the cause of your symptoms. These tests include blood tests to measure hormone levels, MRI (p.248) or CT scanning (p.247) to look for an adrenal tumour, and ultrasound scanning (p.250) to check the ovaries. Treatment of the cause, such as removal of a tumour, should reverse some of the changes. If no cause is found, oral contraceptives may be given to suppress hormone production by the ovaries and reduce male sex hormone levels. You may be given advice on how to manage excessive hair, perhaps by using electrolysis or waxing. Counselling (p.971) is often helpful.

(WWW) ONLINE SITES: p.1032, p.1033, p.1037

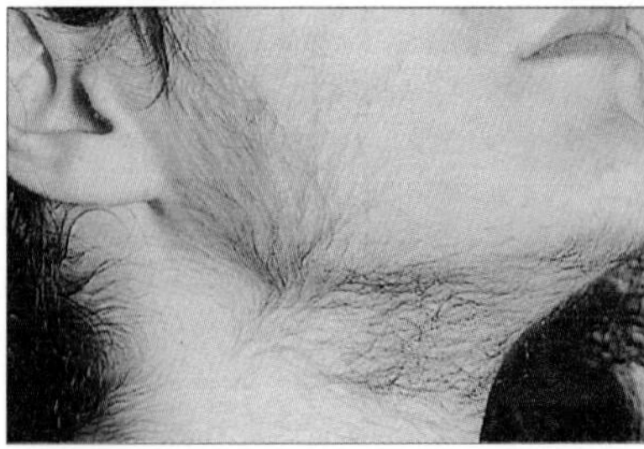

Excessive facial hair
This young woman has excessive facial hair (hirsutism), a common symptom of virilization, a condition caused by the excess production of male sex hormones.

DISORDERS OF THE FEMALE REPRODUCTIVE ORGANS

The female reproductive organs are the ovaries, fallopian tubes, uterus, cervix, vagina, and vulva. Since the combined primary function of these organs is reproduction, disorders affecting them can result in infertility and should be treated as soon as possible, particularly if children are planned. Such disorders may be caused by infections, physical damage, or hormonal imbalances.

The first two articles in this section discuss pelvic inflammatory disease and endometriosis, disorders that may affect more than one female reproductive organ. The next articles discuss disorders of the ovaries, uterus, and cervix. Disorders affecting the vagina and vulva are covered last.

Many disorders affecting the female reproductive organs are common, and most women develop one or more of them at some time. However, many of these disorders are easily treated.

Disorders affecting menstruation, the menopause, or sexual development are covered in other sections (*see* MENSTRUAL, MENOPAUSAL, AND HORMONAL PROBLEMS, pp.734–740), as are sexual disorders of both sexes (*see* SEXUALLY TRANSMITTED INFECTIONS, pp.764–768, INFERTILITY, pp.774–777, and SEXUAL PROBLEMS, pp.769–773).

KEY ANATOMY

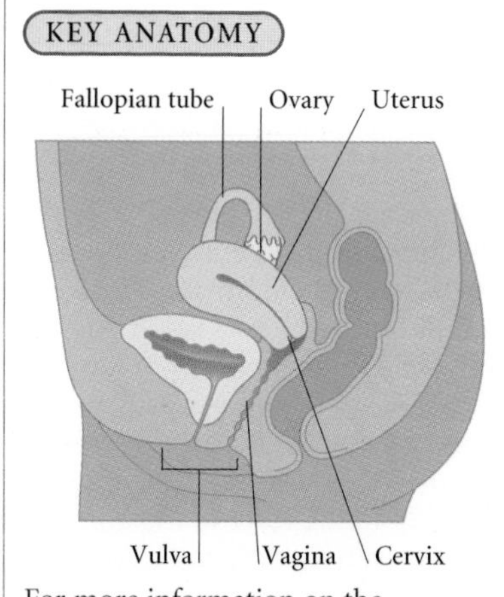

For more information on the structure and function of the female reproductive organs, *see* pp.730–733.

Pelvic inflammatory disease

Inflammation of the female reproductive organs, most often due to a sexually transmitted infection

 AGE Most common between the ages of 15 and 24; rare before puberty

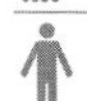 LIFESTYLE Risk factors depend on the cause

 GENETICS Not a significant factor

Pelvic inflammatory disease (PID) is a common cause of pain in the pelvic region in women. In this condition, some of the female reproductive organs become inflamed, usually as a result of an infection. Young and sexually active women are most likely to be affected. PID may have no obvious symptoms, and some women are unaware that they have had the condition until, years later, they are investigated for infertility (*see* FEMALE INFERTILITY, p.775).

PID is usually caused by a sexually transmitted infection (STI), such as gonorrhoea (p.764) or chlamydial infection (p.765). PID may also be caused by an infection developing after a termination of pregnancy (p.789) or after childbirth. In rare cases, tuberculosis (p.491) can develop in the pelvis.

The infection spreads upwards from the vagina to the uterus and fallopian tubes. The ovaries may also be affected. An intra-uterine contraceptive device (IUD) makes this spread of infection more likely. If you think you may have an infection, tests will usually be performed so that you can be treated before PID develops. When PID is discovered during investigations for infertility, the original cause may remain unknown.

WHAT ARE THE SYMPTOMS?

PID may have no obvious symptoms, especially when caused by chlamydia. If there are symptoms, they may include:

- Pain in the pelvic region.
- Fever.
- An abnormal vaginal discharge.
- Heavy or prolonged periods (*see* MENORRHAGIA, p.735).
- Pain during sexual intercourse.
- Tiredness.

If PID develops suddenly, you may have severe pain, nausea, and vomiting, and urgent hospital attention is required.

If the condition is not treated, the fallopian tubes may be damaged. The infection may also spread to other organs in the pelvis and the abdomen.

WHAT MIGHT BE DONE?

If your doctor suspects that you have PID, he or she will carry out a pelvic examination. Swabs may be taken from both the cervix and the vagina to identify the organisms causing the infection. Ultrasound scanning (p.250) of the pelvis may also be performed. If you have severe symptoms, you will be admitted to hospital, and a laparoscopy (p.742) may be performed to view the abdominal and pelvic cavities.

Your doctor will probably prescribe antibiotics (p.885), which will be given intravenously if you are in hospital. You may also be given painkillers (p.912).

You should not have sexual intercourse until your recovery is complete. Your sexual partner should have tests to look for sexually transmitted infections and should be treated if necessary to prevent a reinfection (*see* PREVENTING STIs, p.765). If you use an IUD, you may be advised to change to a different method of contraception.

If PID is detected and treated early, you should make a complete recovery. If PID is not treated, damage to the fallopian tubes can increase the risk of having an ectopic pregnancy (p.790) or may lead to infertility.

(WWW) ONLINE SITES: p.1033, p.1037

Endometriosis

A condition in which endometrial tissue, which normally lines the uterus, becomes attached to other organs in the abdomen

AGE Most common between the ages of 30 and 45

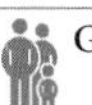
GENETICS Sometimes runs in families

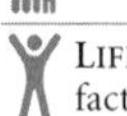
LIFESTYLE Not having had children is a risk factor

The lining of the uterus, known as the endometrium, is normally shed once a month during menstruation and then regrows. In endometriosis, some pieces of the lining become attached to organs in the pelvic cavity, such as the ovaries and the lower intestine. The misplaced pieces of lining react to the hormones of the menstrual cycle and bleed during periods. The blood cannot leave the body through the vagina and causes irritation of the surrounding tissues, leading to pain in the abdomen and eventually scarring. Irritation of the ovaries may lead to painful cysts.

Endometriosis is a common condition, affecting as many as 1 in 5 women of childbearing age. Women who do not have children until they are in their 30s and those who remain childless are more likely to develop the condition. Severe endometriosis can often cause problems with fertility (*see* FEMALE INFERTILITY, p.775).

The exact cause of endometriosis is not known, but there are many theories. One theory is that fragments of endometrium shed during menstruation do not leave the body in the usual way through the vagina. Instead, they travel along the fallopian tubes, from where they may pass into the pelvic cavity and become attached to the surfaces of nearby organs.

WHAT ARE THE SYMPTOMS?

Endometriosis may not produce symptoms. If symptoms do develop, their severity varies from woman to woman. Symptoms may also vary depending on which organs are affected by the condition. They may include:

- Pain in the lower abdomen, which usually becomes more severe just before and during menstrual periods (*see* DYSMENORRHOEA, p.736).
- Irregular periods or very heavy menstrual bleeding.
- Pain during sexual intercourse.
- Lower abdominal pain on urination.

If the endometrium grows on the lower intestine, you may develop diarrhoea or constipation, pain during bowel movements, and, in rare cases, bleeding from the rectum during menstruation.

WHAT MIGHT BE DONE?

In women who do not have symptoms, endometriosis may only be suspected following investigations for infertility. To help make a diagnosis, your doctor will carry out a pelvic examination. The diagnosis may be confirmed with a laparoscopy (left), in which the organs in the pelvic and abdominal cavities are examined using a viewing instrument.

There are many different treatments for endometriosis, and the one chosen depends on your age, which organs are affected, the severity of symptoms, and whether you wish to have children in the future. You may be offered hormonal or surgical treatment. In mild cases, treatment may not be necessary.

If your symptoms are troublesome, your doctor may prescribe one of several different hormonal treatments that stop menstruation for several months. These drugs may include the synthetic hormone gonadorelin, gonadorelin analogues, and danazol (*see* SEX HORMONES AND RELATED DRUGS, p.933), all of which suppress production of the female sex hormone oestrogen and have the effect of stopping menstruation. Alternatively, you may be given the combined oral contraceptive pill. This treatment is usually given for approximately 6–12 months, during

TEST AND TREATMENT LAPAROSCOPY

During laparoscopy, a rigid viewing instrument called a laparoscope is used to view the inside of the pelvis and the abdomen through small abdominal incisions. Laparoscopy may be used to look for disorders of the female reproductive organs, such as endometriosis, and to investigate other abdominal disorders, such as appendicitis. Some types of surgery, such as female sterilization (opposite page), may also be carried out during the procedure. Laparoscopy is always performed under general anaesthesia. Recovery is faster than after normal surgery due to the smaller incisions.

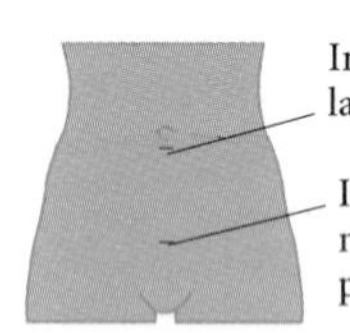

SITES OF INCISIONS

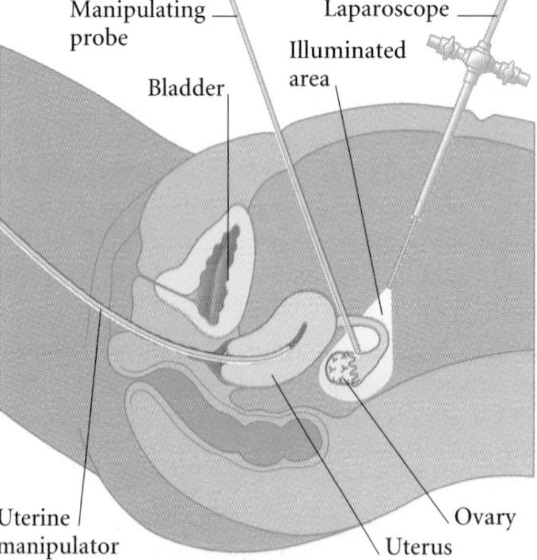

The procedure
The laparoscope and a tool to manipulate the internal organs are inserted through incisions. Gas is pumped through the laparoscope so that the organs separate and can be seen clearly. In women, a second tool may be inserted through the vagina.

VIEW

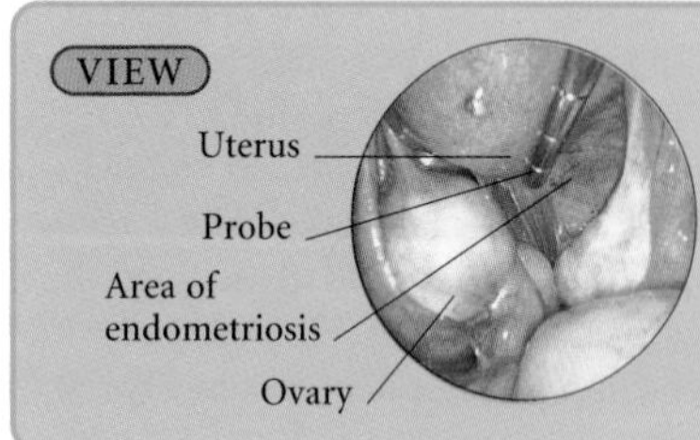

Endometriosis
This view through a laparoscope shows areas of endometriosis on the lining of the pelvic cavity next to the uterus. The tip of a manipulating probe and one of the ovaries can also be seen.

TREATMENT FEMALE STERILIZATION

Sterilization, by a method known as tubal ligation, is a permanent means of contraception for women who do not want any more children or for whom pregnancy would be harmful. The operation can be performed through two small incisions in the abdomen (laparoscopic sterilization) or a single incision in the pubic area (minilaparotomy). The operation seals the fallopian tubes, usually by using clips or by cutting and tying them, so that sperm cannot travel through the tubes to fertilize eggs.

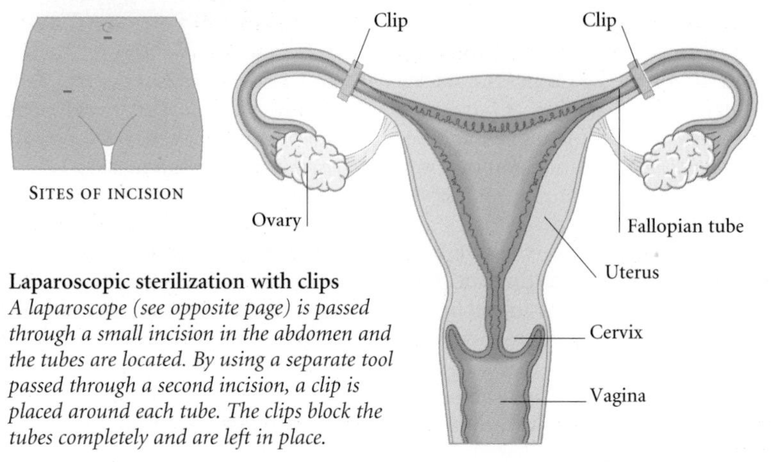

Laparoscopic sterilization with clips
A laparoscope (see opposite page) is passed through a small incision in the abdomen and the tubes are located. By using a separate tool passed through a second incision, a clip is placed around each tube. The clips block the tubes completely and are left in place.

which time the endometriosis should improve. If the condition does recur, it is usually milder than before.

Small fragments of endometrial tissue that do not respond to a period of hormonal treatment may be destroyed by laser surgery during a laparoscopy. However, endometriosis sometimes recurs after this treatment, and further operations may be necessary.

If you have severe endometriosis and you do not plan to have children or have gone through the menopause, your doctor may recommend that you have a hysterectomy (p.747) to remove the uterus. Both ovaries will also be removed, together with other areas that are affected by endometriosis. If the ovaries are removed before you have reached the menopause naturally, you will develop menopausal symptoms. To alleviate these symptoms, your doctor will probably recommend hormone replacement therapy (p.937).

WHAT IS THE PROGNOSIS?

Although treatment is usually successful, endometriosis may recur until the menopause occurs and the menstrual cycle ends. Endometriosis is unlikely to recur if the ovaries are removed.

WWW ONLINE SITES: p.1037

Ovarian cysts

Fluid-filled swellings that grow on or in one or both ovaries

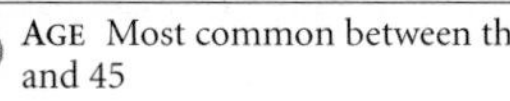
AGE Most common between the ages of 30 and 45

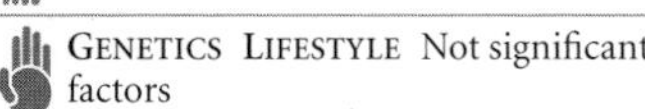
GENETICS LIFESTYLE Not significant factors

Ovarian cysts are fluid-filled sacs that grow on or in the ovaries. Most ovarian cysts are noncancerous and not harmful, but a cyst may sometimes become cancerous (*see* CANCER OF THE OVARY, p.744). Cancerous cysts are more likely to develop in women over the age of 40.

WHAT ARE THE TYPES?

There are many types of ovarian cyst. The most common type is a follicular cyst, in which one of the follicles, where eggs develop, grows and fills with fluid. This type of ovarian cyst may grow to 5 cm (2 in) in diameter and usually occurs singly. Multiple small cysts that develop in the ovaries are thought to be caused by a hormonal disorder, and this condition is known as polycystic ovary syndrome (p.744).

Less commonly, cysts may form in the corpus luteum, the yellow tissue that develops from a follicle after the release of an egg. These cysts fill with blood and can grow to 3 cm ($1\frac{1}{4}$ in).

A dermoid cyst is a cyst that contains cells that are normally found elsewhere in the body, such as skin and hair cells. A cystadenoma is a cyst that grows from one type of cell in the ovary. In rare cases, a single cystadenoma can fill the entire abdominal cavity.

WHAT ARE THE SYMPTOMS?

Most ovarian cysts do not cause symptoms, but when there are symptoms, they may include:

- Discomfort in the abdomen.
- Pain during sexual intercourse.
- Irregular periods, which sometimes have heavy blood loss.
- Postmenopausal bleeding (p.738).

Large cysts can put pressure on the bladder, leading to urinary retention (p.713) or a frequent need to pass urine.

ARE THERE COMPLICATIONS?

If an ovarian cyst ruptures or becomes twisted, severe abdominal pain, nausea, and fever may develop. Cysts may grow so large that the abdomen is distended. In rare cases, a cyst producing the sex hormone oestrogen may develop before puberty, which leads to early sexual development (*see* ABNORMAL PUBERTY IN FEMALES, p.739). Some ovarian cysts produce male sex hormones, which can cause the development of male characteristics, such as growth of facial hair (*see* VIRILIZATION, p.740).

WHAT MIGHT BE DONE?

Sometimes, ovarian cysts are only discovered when a pelvic examination is carried out during a routine checkup. If you have symptoms of a cyst, your doctor will perform a pelvic examination.

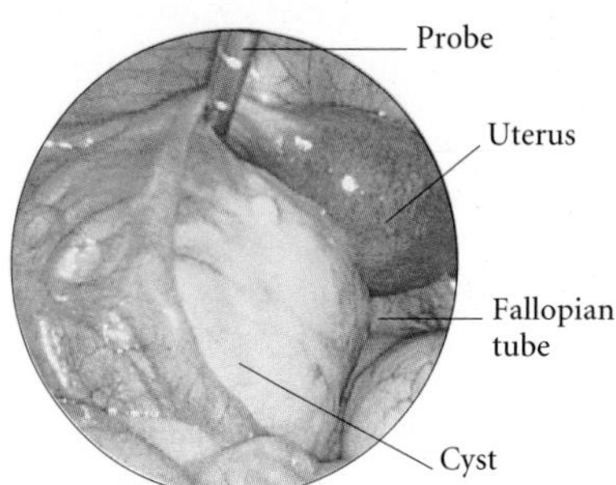

Ovarian cyst
This view through a laparoscope shows a large ovarian cyst next to the uterus. Most ovarian cysts are noncancerous.

You may also be sent for ultrasound scanning (p.250) or for a laparoscopy (p.742) to confirm the diagnosis and determine the size and position of the cyst. You may also have blood tests to see if a cyst is cancerous.

Ovarian cysts may disappear without treatment, although the size of a cyst may be monitored with regular ultrasound scans. Large or persistent cysts may be drained or removed. If there is a chance that the cyst is cancerous, it will be removed, leaving the ovary and fallopian tube if possible. Ovarian cysts may recur if the ovary is not removed.

(WWW) ONLINE SITES: p.1037

Polycystic ovary syndrome

Multiple, small, fluid-filled cysts in the ovaries, which may be caused by a sex hormone imbalance

 AGE Affects females of childbearing age

 GENETICS Sometimes runs in families

 LIFESTYLE Not a significant factor

In polycystic ovary syndrome, both of the ovaries become enlarged with multiple, fluid-filled cysts. The condition is thought to be caused by an imbalance of sex hormones, sometimes by a relative excess of luteinizing hormone, produced by the pituitary gland, and of the male sex hormone testosterone. This imbalance may prevent ovulation (egg release), thus reducing fertility (*see* FEMALE INFERTILITY, p.775), and sometimes leads to the excessive growth of body hair (*see* VIRILIZATION, p.740).

This syndrome is the most common female reproductive disorder, affecting about 1 in 20 women of childbearing age in the UK. The condition sometimes runs in families.

WHAT ARE THE SYMPTOMS?

The symptoms of polycystic ovary syndrome are variable. The condition may go unnoticed until a woman is tested for infertility. Symptoms include:

- Infrequent or absent periods (*see* AMENORRHOEA, p.735).
- Obesity.
- Excessive hair growth.

Women with polycystic ovary syndrome have an increased risk of developing resistance to the action of the hormone insulin and this resistance may lead to diabetes mellitus (p.687). Women who are affected by the condition are also more likely to develop hypertension (p.403), coronary artery disease (p.405), and myocardial infarction (p.410).

WHAT MIGHT BE DONE?

If your doctor suspects that you have polycystic ovary syndrome, he or she will take blood samples to measure your levels of sex hormones and see if you have an imbalance. You may also have ultrasound scanning (p.250) to look for ovarian cysts.

Treatment depends on the severity of your symptoms and whether you want to conceive. Infertility can be treated with drugs, such as clomiphene (*see* DRUGS FOR INFERTILITY, p.936). If you do not want to have children, abnormal periods can be treated with a combined oral contraceptive pill.

To treat insulin resistance and reduce your risk of developing diabetes mellitus, your doctor may prescribe drugs such as metformin (*see* DRUGS FOR DIABETES MELLITUS, p.931), which may also help to make your periods more regular and aid weight loss. Excess hair can be removed by electrolysis.

(WWW) ONLINE SITES: p.1037

Cancer of the ovary

A cancerous tumour that can develop in one or both ovaries

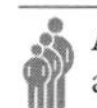 AGE Most common between the ages of 50 and 70; rare under the age of 40

GENETICS Sometimes runs in families

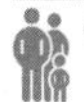 LIFESTYLE Not having had children is a risk factor

Cancer of the ovary is the fifth most common type of cancer in women and causes about 4,300 deaths each year in the UK, more than any other cancer of the reproductive tract. This high death rate is usually explained by the fact that symptoms do not develop until late in the progress of the disease, which delays the diagnosis and treatment.

The cause of cancer of the ovary is not known, but the tumour sometimes develops from an ovarian cyst (p.743).

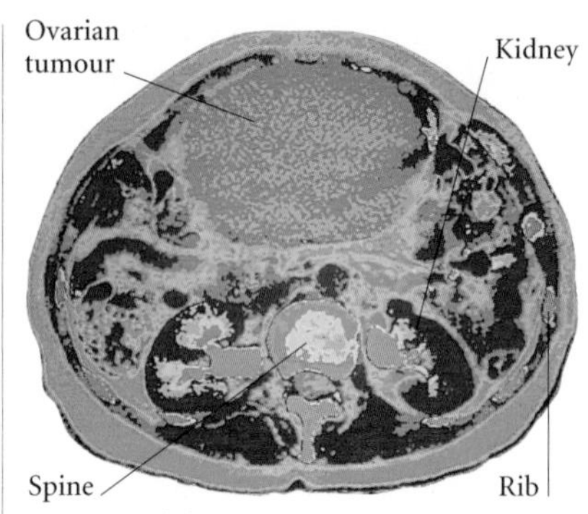

Cancer of the ovary
Most of the abdominal cavity seen in this colour-enhanced CT scan is filled by a large cancerous ovarian tumour.

There seem to be hormonal and genetic risk factors for developing the disease. Women who have never had children or have had a late menopause are more likely to develop cancer of the ovary. Women with a close relative who developed ovarian cancer before the age of 50 are also at greater risk.

WHAT ARE THE SYMPTOMS?

Ovarian cancer rarely produces symptoms in the early stages, although there may be symptoms similar to those of an ovarian cyst, such as irregular periods. In most cases, symptoms occur only if the cancer has spread to other organs and may include:

- Pain in the lower abdomen.
- Swelling in the abdomen caused by excess fluid.
- Frequent need to pass urine.
- Rarely, abnormal vaginal bleeding.

There may also be general symptoms of cancer, such as loss of weight, nausea, and vomiting. Left untreated, the cancer may spread to other organs in the body, such as the liver or lungs.

HOW IS IT DIAGNOSED?

If a close relative has had cancer of the ovary, you should consult your doctor about screening for this type of cancer. Screening may detect cancerous changes before symptoms develop and allows treatment to be given in the early stages of the disease. You may be offered ultrasound scanning (p.250) through the vagina to look for a tumour or blood tests to look for a specific protein that is produced by this cancer. Otherwise, if your doctor suspects cancer of the ovary, he or she will examine your abdomen for the presence of swellings or lumps. You may have an ultrasound scan of your ovaries and a laparoscopy (p.742). Other tests that may be carried out include a chest X-ray (p.490) and CT scanning (p.247) of the lungs or liver to see if the disease has spread.

WHAT IS THE TREATMENT?

If cancer of the ovary is diagnosed in a woman who wishes to have children, usually only the affected ovary and fallopian tube are removed. If the cancer has spread to other parts of the reproductive tract or the woman does not wish to have children, a total hysterectomy may be performed, in which the uterus and both the fallopian tubes and ovaries are removed. Surgery is followed by chemotherapy (p.280) to kill any remaining cancer cells. If the cancer has spread to other organs in the body, radiotherapy (p.281) may also be given. After treatment, blood tests and physical examinations are carried out regularly to check for recurrence.

WHAT IS THE PROGNOSIS?

A complete recovery from cancer of the ovary is possible only if the condition is diagnosed and treated while in the early stages. However, the disease has spread in up to 3 in 4 women by the time of diagnosis. In these women, chemotherapy can prevent further spread of the cancer, sometimes for years, but it can rarely eliminate the cancer completely.

(WWW) ONLINE SITES: p.1028, p.1037

Fibroids

Common, noncancerous tumours that grow slowly within the muscular wall of the uterus

AGE Most common between the ages of 35 and 55

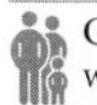
GENETICS More common in black women

LIFESTYLE Not a significant factor

Fibroids are abnormal growths in the uterus that consist of muscular and fibrous tissue. Fibroids are found in up to 1 in 3 women of childbearing age in the UK and are more common in black women. Fibroids occur singly or in groups and may be as small as a pea or as big as a grapefruit. Small fibroids may not cause problems, but larger ones may affect menstruation or fertility (*see* FEMALE INFERTILITY, p.775).

WHAT IS THE CAUSE?

The cause of fibroids is unknown, but they are thought to be related to an abnormal response by the uterus to the female sex hormone oestrogen. Fibroids do not occur before puberty, when the ovaries begin to increase oestrogen production, and they usually stop growing after the menopause. They also increase in size at times when there are increased levels of oestrogen in the body, such as during pregnancy and when taking the combined contraceptive pill or hormone replacement therapy (p.937).

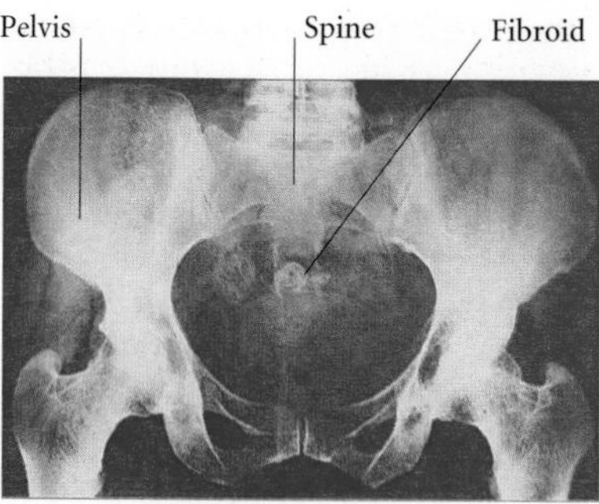

Fibroid in the uterus
A noncancerous tumour, known as a fibroid, can be seen within the wall of the uterus in this X-ray of the pelvis.

WHAT ARE THE SYMPTOMS?

Most small fibroids do not cause symptoms, but the common symptoms of larger fibroids include:

- Prolonged menstrual bleeding.
- Abdominal pain during periods (*see* DYSMENORRHOEA, p.736).
- Heavy bleeding during periods (*see* MENORRHAGIA, p.735).

Heavy blood loss may lead to anaemia (p.446), causing pale skin and tiredness. Large fibroids may distort the uterus, which can often result in infertility or in recurrent miscarriages (p.791). During pregnancy, a large fibroid may cause the fetus to lie in an abnormal position (*see* ABNORMAL PRESENTATION, p.800). Fibroids may also press on the bladder, causing a need to pass urine often, or on the rectum, causing back pain. Rarely, a fibroid may become twisted, resulting in sudden pain in the lower abdomen.

(TEST AND TREATMENT) HYSTEROSCOPY

A hysteroscope is an instrument used to see inside the uterus and fallopian tubes. Hysteroscopy is used to diagnose disorders such as uterine polyps and can be performed under general or local anaesthesia in an outpatient clinic. Minor surgery, such as the removal of fibroids, may also be carried out through the hysteroscope. The procedure usually lasts 15 minutes or less.

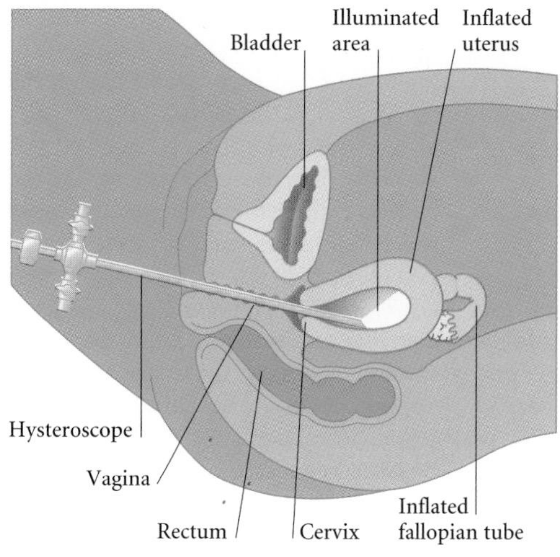

The procedure
After the hysteroscope is inserted down the vagina, the uterus and fallopian tubes are filled with gas passed through the hysteroscope. This allows them to be seen easily. Light provides a clear view.

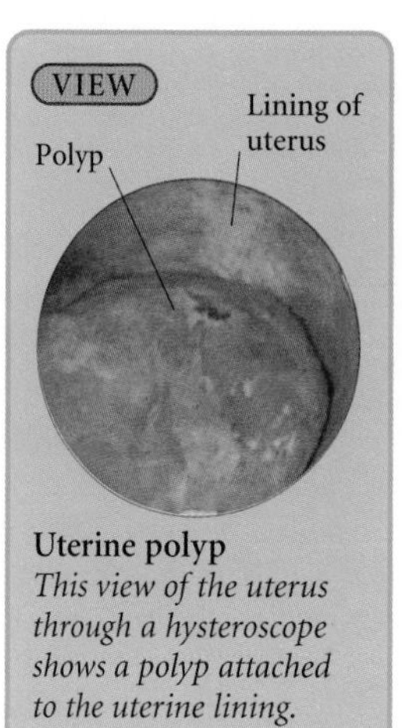

Uterine polyp
This view of the uterus through a hysteroscope shows a polyp attached to the uterine lining.

How are they diagnosed?

The doctor will perform a pelvic examination. You may also have ultrasound scanning (p.250) of the uterus or a hysteroscopy (p.745), in which a viewing instrument is inserted into the uterus through the cervix. A sample of the fibroid will be removed during the hysteroscopy to check that the growth is not cancerous. Sometimes, fibroids show up on X-rays (p.244) that are taken for other reasons.

What is the treatment?

Small fibroids often do not need treatment but should be checked regularly by your doctor to make sure that they have not grown. If treatment is necessary, fibroids may be removed during a hysteroscopy if they are on an inner wall. Rarely, fibroids are treated using an injection of a substance that blocks the blood vessels supplying them, causing the fibroids to shrink.

Large fibroids can be removed via an incision in the abdomen. Before having the surgery, you may be prescribed hormones that suppress the production of oestrogen so that the fibroids shrink. If you have persistent, large fibroids and do not want children, you may consider having a hysterectomy (opposite page).

Removal of fibroids usually results in regained fertility, but in about 1 in 10 women fibroids recur. Fibroids usually start to shrink after the menopause, when oestrogen levels in the body fall.

(WWW) ONLINE SITES: p.1037

Uterine polyps

Noncancerous growths that develop in the uterus or the cervix

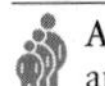
AGE Most common between the ages of 30 and 50

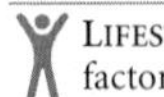
LIFESTYLE Not having had children is a risk factor

GENETICS Not a significant factor

Uterine polyps are painless growths that are attached to the cervix or to the inside of the uterus. The polyps may occur singly or in groups and vary in length up to about 3 cm (1 in). Polyps are usually harmless, but they may become cancerous in rare cases. Uterine polyps are common, especially in premenopausal women over the age of 30.

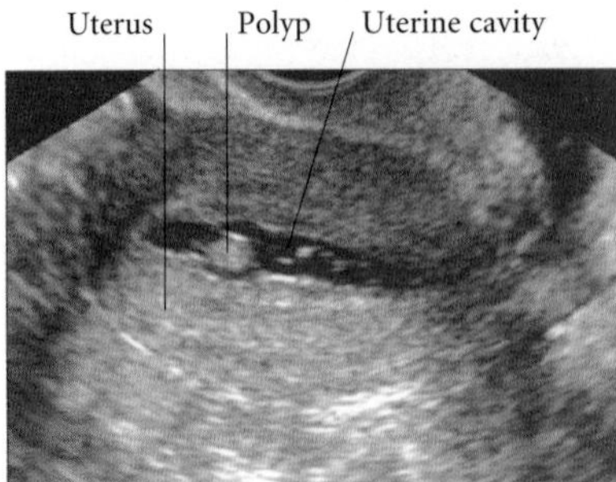

Uterine polyp
This ultrasound scan of the pelvis shows a single polyp in the uterine cavity that has grown from the lining of the uterus.

The reason why uterine polyps form is unknown, but they may develop on the cervix if it is already affected by a cervical erosion (p.749), in which the cells on the surface of the cervix are more delicate than usual. Polyps also sometimes form on the cervix following an infection of the area. Women who have not had children are more likely to develop uterine polyps.

Symptoms of uterine polyps include a watery, bloodstained discharge from the vagina and bleeding after sexual intercourse, between periods, or after the menopause. Such bleeding may also be a sign of a more serious disorder, such as cancer of the cervix (p.750).

What might be done?

Your doctor will usually be able to see polyps on the cervix by looking at the cervix while holding your vagina open with an instrument called a speculum. If polyps in the uterus are suspected, further investigations will be arranged, such as ultrasound scanning (p.250) or hysteroscopy (p.745), in which a viewing instrument is inserted through the cervix to view the inside of the uterus.

Treatment of polyps is usually quick and easy. Polyps on the cervix may be removed surgically during examination through the speculum, and uterine polyps can be removed during a hysteroscopy. Mild pain and slight vaginal bleeding are likely for a few days after surgery. Samples of tissue from the polyps are examined under a microscope to make sure that there are no cancerous cells. Uterine polyps may recur after treatment, and then further surgery is usually required.

(WWW) ONLINE SITES: p.1037

Retroverted uterus

A usually harmless condition in which the uterus is tilted backwards

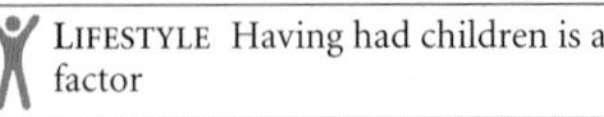
LIFESTYLE Having had children is a risk factor

AGE GENETICS Not significant factors

The uterus is normally inclined upwards and forwards. In about 1 in 10 women the uterus is tilted backwards, lying close to the rectum. This condition is known as a retroverted uterus and is a harmless variation of the normal position. There is often no cause for the condition, although it may occur after childbirth or because an ovarian cyst (p.743) pushes the uterus backwards.

A retroverted uterus usually causes no symptoms and does not affect fertility, pregnancy, or childbirth. However, you may feel pain during sexual intercourse or have low backache, especially during menstrual periods.

What might be done?

Your doctor may be able to feel that the uterus is retroverted during a pelvic examination. If an underlying disorder is thought to be causing the condition, laparoscopy (p.742) may be carried out to view the pelvis and abdominal cavity. Mild painkillers (p.912) may relieve backache, and pain during intercourse may be relieved through trying a different sexual position. If there is an underlying cause, such as a cyst, this may be treated, allowing the uterus to return to its normal position.

(WWW) ONLINE SITES: p.1037

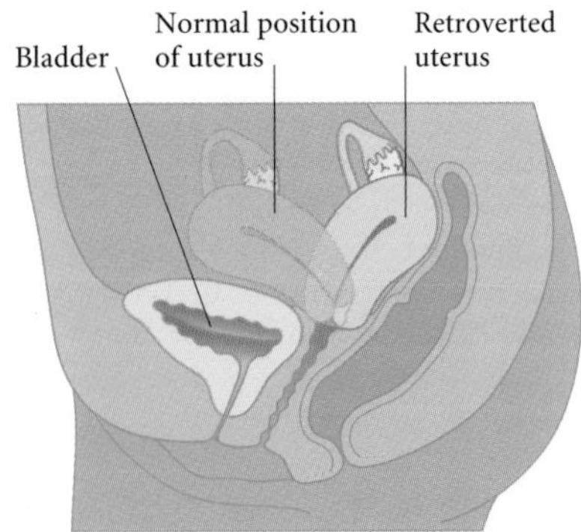

Retroverted uterus
The uterus usually tilts forwards, resting close to and just above the bladder. A retroverted uterus tilts backwards so that it lies close to the rectum.

Prolapse of the uterus and vagina

Downwards displacement of the uterus and/or wall of the vagina

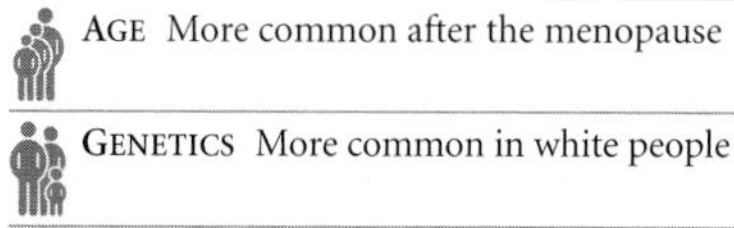

AGE More common after the menopause

GENETICS More common in white people

LIFESTYLE Being overweight and having had children are risk factors

The uterus and vagina are held in place by ligaments and muscles in the pelvis. If these supporting structures become weakened or stretched, often as a result of childbirth, the uterus and/or vaginal walls may be displaced. Prolapse usually occurs only after the menopause, when low levels of the hormone oestrogen lead to weakening of the ligaments. The risk of prolapse is increased by conditions that put extra pressure on the muscles and ligaments in the pelvis, such as obesity, a persistent cough, or straining during bowel movements. For reasons that are unknown, prolapse is more common in white people.

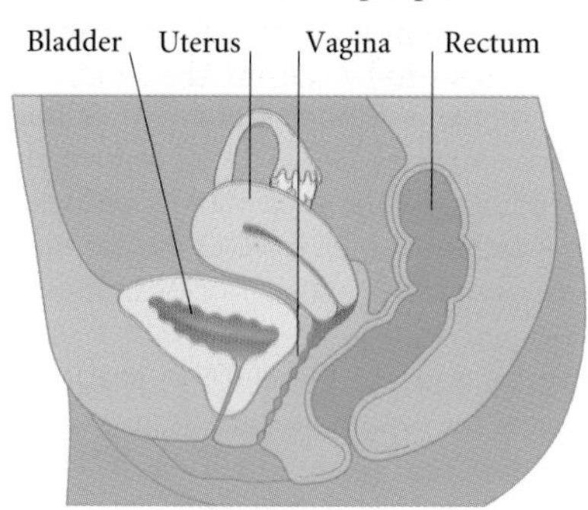

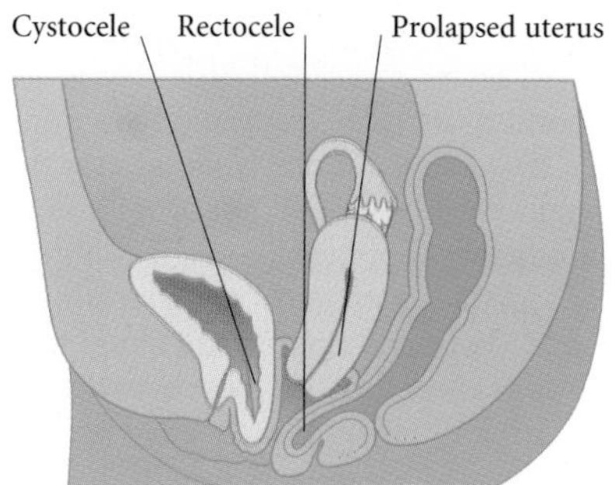

Prolapse of the uterus and vagina
In this prolapse, the uterus is displaced, the bladder bulges into the front vaginal wall (cystocele), and the rectum bulges into the back vaginal wall (rectocele).

TREATMENT HYSTERECTOMY

A hysterectomy is an operation in which the uterus and the cervix are removed to treat conditions such as endometriosis or cancer of the uterus. Occasionally, the ovaries and fallopian tubes are also removed. The operation is carried out through an incision in the abdomen or through the vagina and is done under a general anaesthetic. The upper end of the vagina is then stitched. Afterwards, you may have vaginal bleeding and some pain. You will need to stay in hospital for 4–6 days. Recovery may take about 6 weeks, depending on your health.

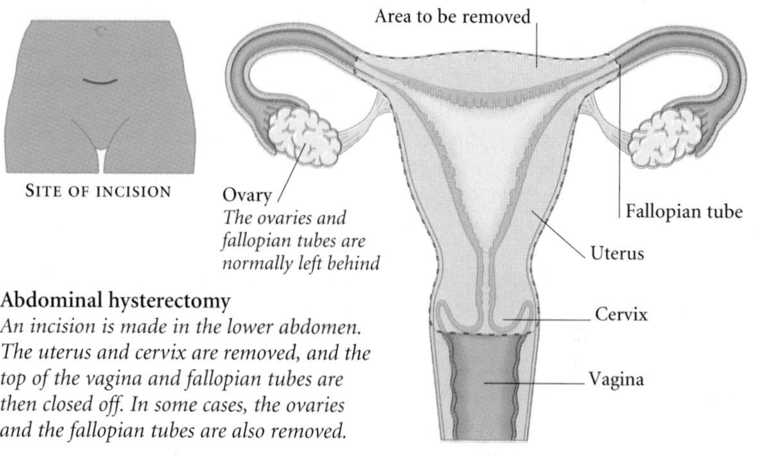

Abdominal hysterectomy
An incision is made in the lower abdomen. The uterus and cervix are removed, and the top of the vagina and fallopian tubes are then closed off. In some cases, the ovaries and the fallopian tubes are also removed.

WHAT ARE THE TYPES?

In uterine prolapse, the uterus moves down into the vagina. The amount of movement ranges from slight displacement into the vagina to projection of the uterus outside the vulva.

There are two main types of vaginal prolapse: cystocele and rectocele. In a cystocele, the bladder presses inwards against the weak front vaginal wall. In a rectocele, the rectum bulges against the weakened back vaginal wall. Both types of vaginal prolapse may occur together with or without uterine prolapse.

WHAT ARE THE SYMPTOMS?

The symptoms of any type of uterine or vaginal prolapse may include:

- A feeling of fullness in the vagina.
- A lump protruding into or even out of the vagina.
- A dragging sensation or mild pain in the lower back.
- Difficulty passing urine or stools.
- Passing urine more frequently.

A cystocele can cause leakage of urine when laughing or coughing (*see* STRESS INCONTINENCE, p.711). It also increases the risk of an infection in the bladder (*see* CYSTITIS, p.709) because the bladder may not empty properly.

WHAT MIGHT BE DONE?

Your doctor may be able to see that you have a prolapse by looking at the position of the uterus and the walls of the vagina while using a speculum to hold the vagina open. He or she may ask you to cough or strain so that the prolapse can be assessed. A sample of urine may also be taken to check for infection.

Pelvic floor exercises (p.712), which strengthen the supporting muscles, can help to treat a mild prolapse. Practising the exercises before and after childbirth can help to prevent a prolapse.

If you are past the menopause and have a mild prolapse, your doctor may prescribe oestrogen hormones, either orally or as a cream that you can apply to the vaginal wall (*see* SEX HORMONES AND RELATED DRUGS, p.933). Oestrogen helps to strengthen the supporting tissues. A plastic device, known as a ring pessary, is also sometimes inserted into the vagina to help to keep the uterus in place. Surgical techniques may also be used. For example, if a uterine prolapse is severe and you do not want to have children in the future, your doctor may recommend a hysterectomy (above) to completely remove the uterus.

(WWW) ONLINE SITES: p.1037

Cancer of the uterus

A cancerous tumour that grows in the lining of the uterus

 AGE Most common between the ages of 55 and 65

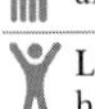 LIFESTYLE Being overweight and not having had children are risk factors

 GENETICS Not a significant factor

Cancer of the uterus is one of the most common cancers of the female reproductive organs in the UK, with about 3,500 new cases diagnosed each year. Most uterine cancers develop in the endometrium (the lining of the uterus). More rarely, cancer occurs in the muscular wall of the uterus.

WHAT ARE THE CAUSES?

The causes of cancer of the uterus are unclear. The disorder is more common in women aged 55–65 and in those who have or have previously had abnormally high levels of the female sex hormone oestrogen. Raised oestrogen levels may be caused by being overweight and by certain disorders, such as polycystic ovary syndrome (p.744). The disorder is also more likely in women who have had a late menopause (after the age of 52) or who have not had children.

WHAT ARE THE SYMPTOMS?

The symptoms of cancer of the uterus vary depending on whether it develops before or after the menopause. These symptoms may include:

- In premenopausal women, heavier than normal periods (*see* MENORRHAGIA, p.735) or bleeding between periods or after sexual intercourse.
- In postmenopausal women, vaginal bleeding that may vary from spotting to heavier bleeding.

Left untreated, cancer of the uterus may spread to the fallopian tubes and the ovaries and to other organs, including the lungs and sometimes the liver.

HOW IS IT DIAGNOSED?

If your doctor suspects cancer from your symptoms, he or she will perform a pelvic examination. During the examination, a small sample of tissue may be taken from the endometrium to check for the presence of cancerous cells (*see* ENDOMETRIAL SAMPLING, p.738). Your doctor may also arrange for ultrasound scanning (p.250), using a probe inserted into the vagina to measure the thickness of the lining of the uterus. A thicker than normal lining may indicate cancer of the uterus.

If these tests are not conclusive, a hysteroscopy (p.745) may be needed to remove a larger amount of tissue from the uterus. Samples of the endometrial tissue are then microscopically examined for cancerous cells. During the hysteroscopy, your doctor is also able to directly view the endometrium to check for any obvious abnormalities.

If cancer of the uterus is diagnosed, tests will be carried out to see if the cancer has spread. For example, you may have a chest X-ray (p.490) or MRI (p.248) of the chest to view the lungs. You may also have blood tests to assess the function of the liver.

WHAT IS THE TREATMENT?

The treatment for cancer of the uterus depends on the stage at which the cancer is diagnosed and whether or not it has spread elsewhere in the body.

In most women, the tumour can be treated by a hysterectomy (p.747), in which the uterus is surgically removed. Usually, the ovaries and the fallopian tubes are removed at the same time. In addition, samples from nearby pelvic lymph nodes are usually taken and examined under a microscope to see if the disease has spread and to check whether further treatment is required. Surgery may be followed by radiotherapy (p.281) to destroy any cancer cells that remain in the body.

If cancerous cells are found in the lymph nodes, you will be treated with chemotherapy (p.280) and the female hormone progesterone (*see* SEX HORMONES AND RELATED DRUGS, p.933), which slows down the growth of cancer cells. After treatment, you will have regular tests to look for signs of cancerous changes in samples of cells taken from the top of the vagina.

The outlook for cancer of the uterus depends on whether the tumour is treated at an early stage before the condition has spread to other parts of the body. About 4 in 5 women who are treated when the cancer is at an early stage survive for 5 years or longer.

(WWW) ONLINE SITES: p.1028, p.1037

Choriocarcinoma

A cancerous tumour that develops from the placenta after a pregnancy

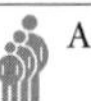 AGE Affects females of childbearing age

 GENETICS LIFESTYLE Not significant factors

A choriocarcinoma is a rare cancerous tumour that occurs in 1 in every 20,000 pregnancies. The tumour develops from the placental tissue and usually arises from a noncancerous placental tumour called a hydatidiform mole (*see* MOLAR PREGNANCY, p.790). A choriocarcinoma may also occur after an ectopic pregnancy (p.790) or rarely after childbirth or termination of pregnancy (p.789) if some placental cells remain. Occasionally, the tumour may not develop until months or even years after pregnancy. The main symptom is persistent vaginal bleeding. If left untreated, the tumour grows quickly, and the disease spreads first to the walls of the uterus and then to other organs such as the liver.

WHAT MIGHT BE DONE?

Choriocarcinoma is usually diagnosed by blood or urine tests to measure levels of the hormone human chorionic gonadotropin (HCG). HCG is normally produced by the placenta in pregnancy, but extremely high levels of the hormone are associated with a choriocarcinoma. Women who have had a molar pregnancy, and are therefore at particular risk of the disease, are usually given regular tests to measure the levels of HCG. Women who have had persistent bleeding after childbirth, a termination, or an ectopic pregnancy may also have their HCG levels checked. If HCG levels are found to be high, ultrasound scanning (p.250) using a probe inserted into the vagina will be carried out to look for a tumour. If choriocarcinoma is confirmed, further tests, such as CT scanning (p.247) of the abdomen and blood tests to assess liver function, may be arranged to check whether the disease has spread.

Choriocarcinoma is usually treated with chemotherapy (p.280), whether or not the disease has spread to other organs. Rarely, a hysterectomy (p.747) may be necessary. Most women recover completely following treatment.

(WWW) ONLINE SITES: p.1028, p.1035, p.1037

Cervical erosion

Extension of cells that normally line the inside of the cervical canal on to the surface of the cervix

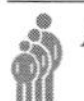
AGE More common after puberty

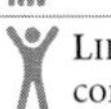
LIFESTYLE Long-term use of oral contraceptives is a risk factor

GENETICS Not a significant factor

In cervical erosion, the layer of delicate cells that line the cervical canal extend on to the outer surface of the cervix, which is usually covered with stronger tissue. The term cervical erosion is misleading because there is no actual loss of cervical tissue. Instead, since the cervix is covered with delicate tissue, it is more easily damaged than normal and has a tendency to bleed.

In many cases, there is no obvious reason for cervical erosion, but the disorder often occurs in association with long-term use of oral contraceptives or after the cervix has been stretched during childbirth. In many cases, cervical erosion does not result in any obvious symptoms. However, a few women may notice increased vaginal discharge and bleeding between menstrual periods or after sexual intercourse.

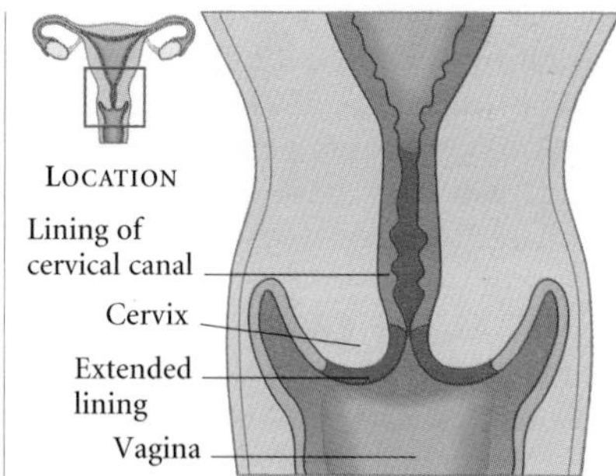

Cervical erosion
In cervical erosion, the delicate cells that line the inside of the cervical canal extend on to the surface of the cervix.

WHAT MIGHT BE DONE?

Cervical erosion is often detected by a routine cervical smear test (below). Treatment is usually not necessary, but if troublesome symptoms develop, the abnormal cells can be destroyed using a freezing technique called cryotherapy. The cells can also be treated with an electrical current, a technique known as diathermy, or by laser surgery (p.951). Following treatment, you may have a discharge for 2–3 weeks, and you will be advised to avoid sexual intercourse during this period. The cells of the cervix return to normal after treatment and the disorder does not usually recur.

(WWW) ONLINE SITES: p.1037

Cervical dysplasia

Changes in the surface cells of the cervix that may become cancerous

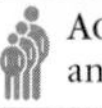
AGE Most common between the ages of 25 and 35

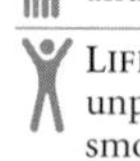
LIFESTYLE Unprotected sex at an early age, unprotected sex with multiple partners, and smoking are risk factors

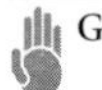
GENETICS Not a significant factor

In some women, the cells of the cervix gradually change from normal to cancerous. The condition between these two extremes, when the cells are abnormal and have the potential to become cancerous, is known as cervical dysplasia. There are three grades of dysplasia: mild, moderate, and severe. Mild dysplasia may return to a normal state, but severe dysplasia may progress to cancer of the cervix (p.750) if not treated.

Many developed countries, including the UK, have established screening programmes that check for cervical dysplasia using the cervical smear test (below). Regular testing, which helps to ensure that cervical dysplasia is diagnosed and treated before the abnormal cells become cancerous, has led to a dramatic fall in the total number of cases of cancer of the cervix.

(TEST) CERVICAL SMEAR TEST

A cervical smear test is a painless procedure used to detect abnormal cells on the cervix. Cells are collected from the cervix using a spatula or brush and are sent away to be examined under a microscope. Women in the UK are offered a smear test every 5 years from the start of sexual activity onwards. More frequent tests may be necessary if abnormal cells are detected. Early treatment of some cervical abnormalities helps to prevent the development of cancer of the cervix (*see* TREATING CERVICAL DYSPLASIA, p.751).

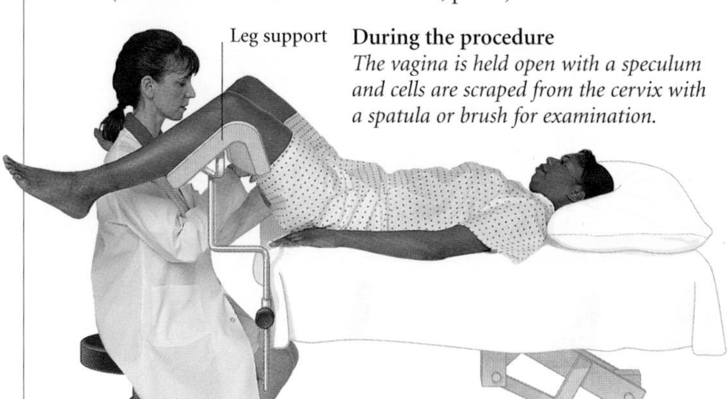

During the procedure
The vagina is held open with a speculum and cells are scraped from the cervix with a spatula or brush for examination.

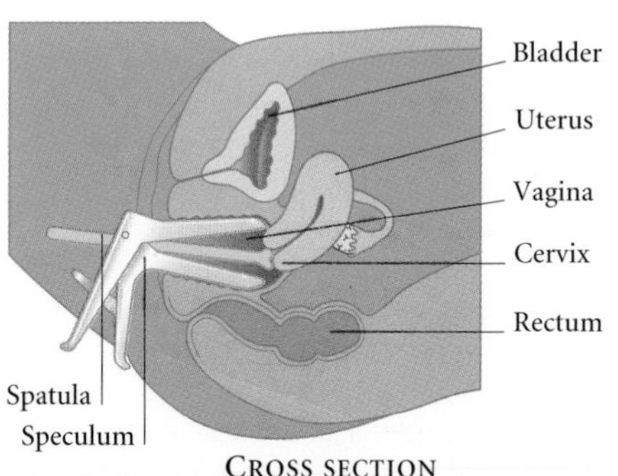

CROSS SECTION

(RESULTS)

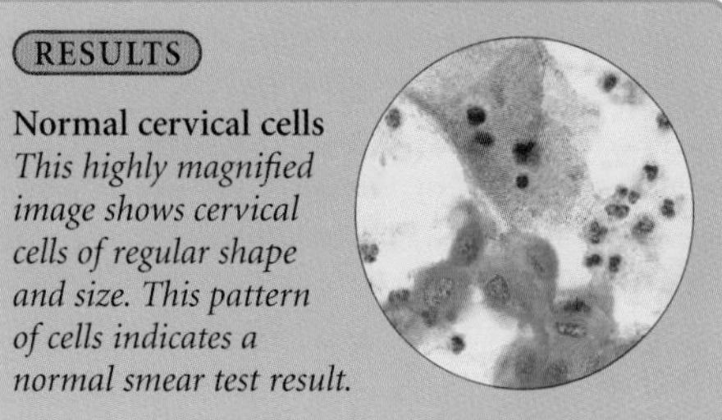

Normal cervical cells
This highly magnified image shows cervical cells of regular shape and size. This pattern of cells indicates a normal smear test result.

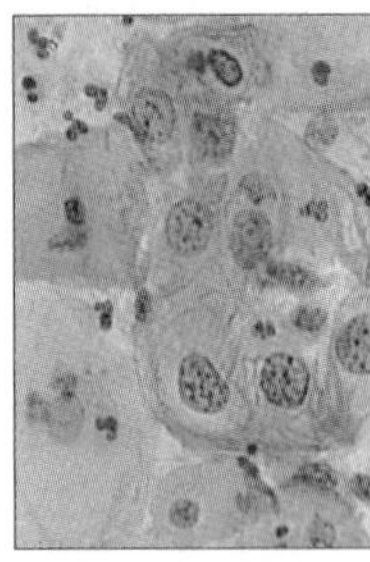

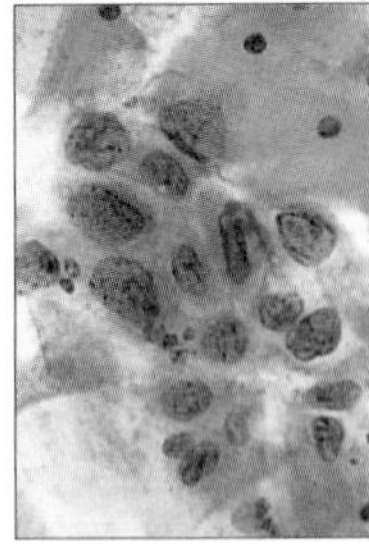

MILD DYSPLASIA SEVERE DYSPLASIA

Cervical dysplasia
These highly magnified images of cells taken from the cervix illustrate the degree of cell distortion that is present in mild and severe cervical dysplasia.

WHAT ARE THE CAUSES?

The exact cause of cervical dysplasia is not known, but a number of different risk factors have been identified. For example, the risk of developing cervical dysplasia appears to be slightly higher after exposure to some types of human papillomavirus (HPV). Other risk factors for the development of cervical dysplasia include unprotected sex at an early age, unprotected sex with many partners, and a pregnancy before the age of 20. Exactly how these risk factors are connected to cervical dysplasia is unknown. Smoking also increases the risk of developing the condition.

HOW IS IT DIAGNOSED?

Cervical dysplasia does not produce symptoms. Normally, the condition is only diagnosed after a cervical smear test, during which a sample of cells is taken from the cervix and sent for microscopic examination. If you are found to have abnormal cells, your doctor may arrange for you to have a colposcopy (right), in which the cervix is viewed through a magnifying instrument to examine abnormal-looking areas. A small sample of tissue may be removed from the cervix for examination under the microscope.

WHAT IS THE TREATMENT?

If you are diagnosed with cervical dysplasia, the treatment depends on the degree of abnormality of the cells. Mild dysplasia may not require treatment because the abnormal cells revert to normal in up to 2 in 5 cases. However, the disorder will be monitored with smear tests every 6 months. If cervical dysplasia persists or worsens, treatment to destroy or remove the abnormal cells will be needed (*see* TREATING CERVICAL DYSPLASIA, opposite page). After treatment, you may have a bloodstained discharge for a few weeks.

WHAT IS THE PROGNOSIS?

In many cases of cervical dysplasia, the cells of the cervix return to normal after treatment. However, your condition will be monitored for the next few years to ensure that no further abnormalities develop. About 3 months after treatment, you will have a smear test and colposcopy, followed by regular smear tests at 6 months and then yearly until your doctor advises otherwise. The risk of cancer of the cervix is higher in cases of severe cervical dysplasia.

(WWW) ONLINE SITES: p.1037

Cancer of the cervix

A cancerous growth occurring in the lower end of the cervix

 AGE Most common between the ages of 45 and 65

 LIFESTYLE Unprotected sex at an early age, unprotected sex with multiple partners, and smoking are risk factors

 GENETICS Not a significant factor

Cancer of the cervix is one of the most common cancers affecting women. In the UK, there are over 4,000 new cases each year. However, it is one of the few cancers that can be prevented by regular screening (p.42) before symptoms appear. Cancer of the cervix usually develops slowly. In the precancerous stage, cervical cells gradually change

TEST AND TREATMENT COLPOSCOPY

A colposcope is a binocular viewing instrument used to magnify the cervix for examination. Colposcopy is often performed after an abnormal cervical smear test (p.749) to look for signs of cervical dysplasia. During the procedure, which is painless and lasts for 15–30 minutes, your doctor may paint solutions on to the cervix to highlight abnormal areas. A sample of cervical tissue may also be taken, or abnormal areas of the cervix may be treated (*see* TREATING CERVICAL DYSPLASIA, opposite page).

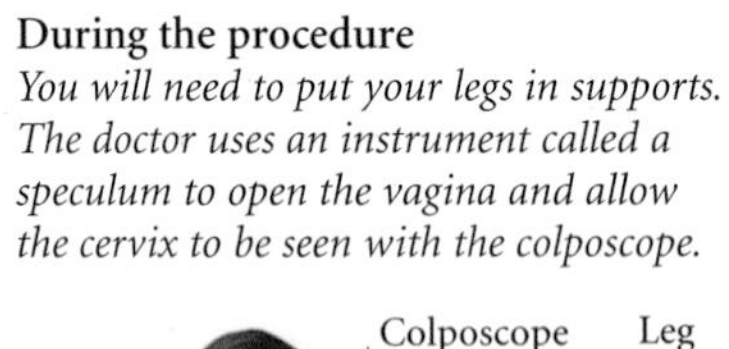

During the procedure
You will need to put your legs in supports. The doctor uses an instrument called a speculum to open the vagina and allow the cervix to be seen with the colposcope.

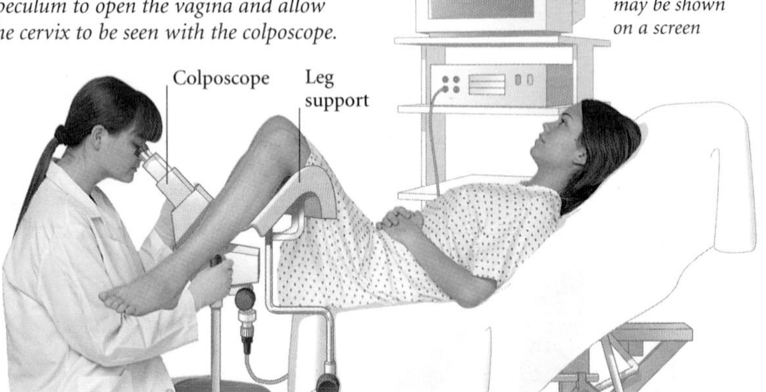

VIEW

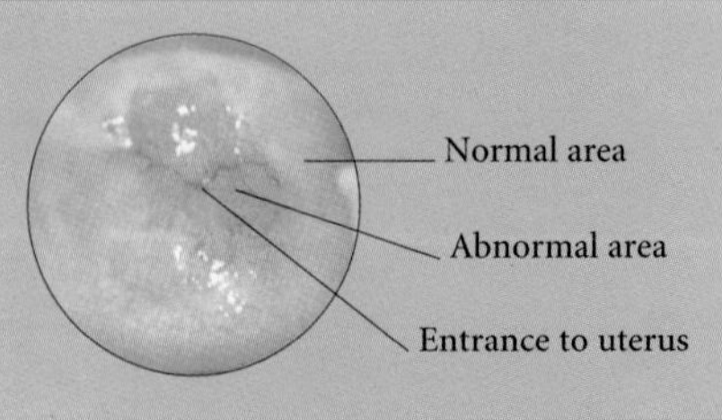

View of the cervix
Normal and abnormal areas of tissue can be seen on this cervix. The abnormal area close to the centre of the cervix proved to be due to moderate cervical dysplasia.

TREATMENT — TREATING CERVICAL DYSPLASIA

Treatment of cervical dysplasia varies depending on the severity of the condition. In mild or moderate cases, the abnormal cells may be destroyed by laser treatment (p.951) or by freezing tissue using a probe. Alternatively, cells may be surgically removed. In severe cases, a cone-shaped area is removed. All treatment is carried out through the vagina. You may have a discharge for a few weeks afterwards.

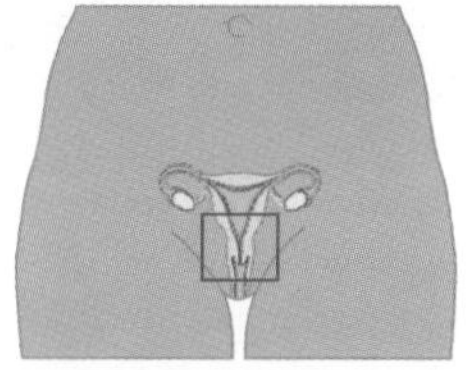

LOCATION

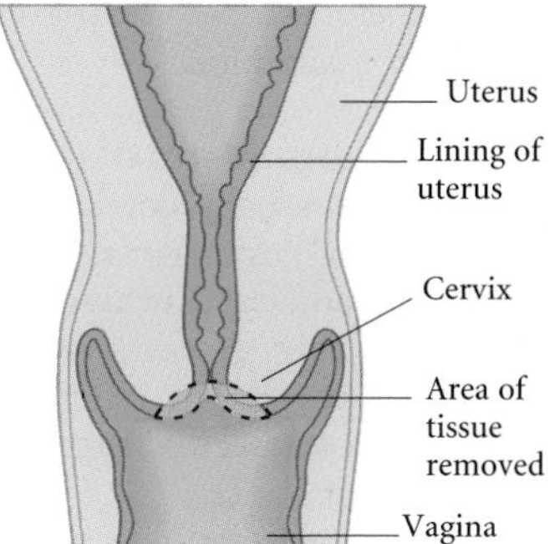

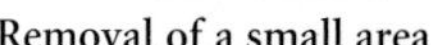

Removal of a small area
In mild to moderate cervical dysplasia, a small area of tissue containing abnormal cells may be removed from the cervix. Treatment is carried out under local anaesthesia and takes 5–10 minutes.

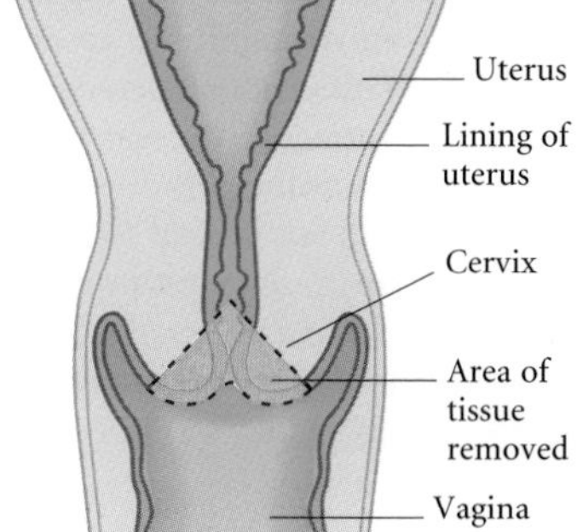

Cone biopsy
In severe cervical dysplasia, in which the abnormal cells are extremely distorted, a larger cone-shaped section of the cervix is removed, often under general anaesthesia, and the wound is left to heal.

from being mildly to extremely abnormal, a condition known as cervical dysplasia (p.749). These changes can be detected using a cervical smear test (p.749), allowing treatment to be carried out before cancer develops.

WHAT ARE THE CAUSES?

The cause of cancer of the cervix is not clear, but there is evidence that changes in cells in the cervix are associated with some types of human papillomavirus (HPV). The virus is transmitted through unprotected sexual intercourse, and the risk of cervical cancer is increased if you have unprotected sex from an early age or with many partners. Smoking is also a risk factor for cervical cancer. Women who have reduced immunity or who are taking immunosuppressant drugs (p.906) are at increased risk of developing cancer of the cervix.

WHAT ARE THE SYMPTOMS?

Cancer of the cervix does not always cause symptoms. However, in some women, there may be some abnormal vaginal bleeding, especially after sexual intercourse. As the cancer progresses, further symptoms may include:

- A watery, bloodstained, and offensive-smelling vaginal discharge.
- Pelvic pain.
- Pain during intercourse.

Left untreated, cancer of the cervix may spread to the uterus and then to the lymph glands in the pelvis. Eventually, cancer may spread to other parts of the body, such as the liver and lungs.

HOW IS IT DIAGNOSED?

If your doctor suspects that you have cancer of the cervix from your symptoms, he or she may perform a smear test. If the test shows abnormal cells, your doctor may arrange for you to have a colposcopy (opposite page), in which the cervix is viewed through a magnifying instrument and checked for abnormal areas. A sample of tissue will probably be taken from the cervix during the procedure and later examined under a microscope for evidence of cancerous cells.

If cancer of the cervix is diagnosed, you may have further tests to see if the condition has spread to other parts of the body. These tests may include a chest X-ray (p.490) or MRI (p.248) of the chest to look at the lungs and blood tests and CT scanning (p.247) of the abdomen to assess liver function.

WHAT IS THE TREATMENT?

The treatment for cancer of the cervix depends on the stage of the disease and your individual circumstances.

If the cancer is confined to the cervix and you plan to have children, it may be possible to remove only the affected area of the cervix. More often, a hysterectomy (p.747) to remove the cervix and the uterus will be performed. If the disease has spread to the uterus, it may be necessary to remove the uterus as well as the fallopian tubes, the ovaries, the top of the vagina, and the nearby lymph nodes. In women who are premenopausal, the ovaries are left if possible because they produce sex hormones and removing them causes premature menopause. If the cancer has spread to other organs in the body, radiotherapy (p.281), and sometimes chemotherapy (p.280), may be needed.

WHAT IS THE PROGNOSIS?

If cancer of the cervix is diagnosed and treated early, almost all women recover completely. However, if the disease has spread beyond the cervix, the disease is fatal in 2 out of 5 women.

Routine smear tests and the early treatment of abnormal cervical cells have greatly reduced the incidence of cancer of the cervix in the developed world. In addition to having regular smear tests, it is advisable to try to reduce the risks of cervical cancer by not smoking and by using barrier methods of contraception (p.69).

(WWW) ONLINE SITES: p.1028, p.1037

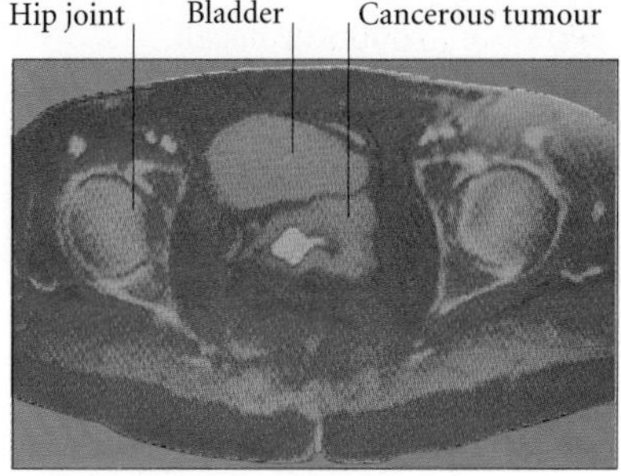

Cancer of the cervix
This colour-enhanced MRI through the pelvis shows a large cancerous tumour of the cervix lying just behind the bladder.

Vulvovaginitis

Inflammation of the vulva and vagina, causing itching and soreness

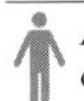 AGE LIFESTYLE Risk factors depend on the cause

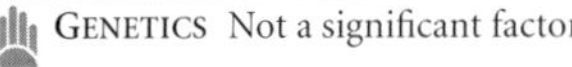 GENETICS Not a significant factor

Vulvovaginitis is a very common disorder affecting most women at some time during their life. In this condition, the vulva and the vagina become inflamed, itchy, and sore. There may also be pain during sexual intercourse and a discharge from the vagina. The condition can also affect children.

WHAT ARE THE CAUSES?

Most cases of vulvovaginitis are caused by an infection, either with the fungus *Candida albicans*, which causes vaginal thrush (right), or with the protozoan *Trichomonas vaginalis*, which is the cause of the sexually transmitted infection trichomoniasis (p.767). Women with diabetes mellitus (p.687) have an increased risk of fungal vulvovaginitis. Overgrowth of the harmless bacteria that normally live in the vagina (*see* BACTERIAL VAGINOSIS, opposite page) may also lead to vulvovaginitis.

In some cases, the condition may be caused by irritation from perfumed bath products, detergents, deodorants, or contraceptive creams. Following the menopause, the disorder may develop as the vaginal tissues become thinner, drier, and more susceptible to irritation. These changes in the tissues of the vagina occur when levels of oestrogen fall. In rare cases, vulvovaginitis may be the result of cancerous changes in the cells that line the surface of the vulva or the vagina (*see* CANCER OF THE VULVA AND VAGINA, opposite page).

In children, the cause of the disorder is often unclear. In some cases, a foreign body in the vagina or, rarely, sexual abuse may be the cause.

WHAT MIGHT BE DONE?

Your doctor will take a swab from the inflamed area to look for an infection and to identify the causative organism. If you have repeated episodes of fungal vulvovaginitis, your urine may also be tested for glucose to exclude diabetes mellitus. If cancerous changes are suspected, a tissue sample will be taken and examined for abnormal cells.

Treatment of vulvovaginitis depends on the cause of the inflammation. If you have bacterial vaginosis, you will be prescribed antibiotics (p.885); if necessary, your sexual partner should also be treated to avoid reinfecting you. Hormone replacement therapy (p.937) or topical creams that contain oestrogen can relieve vulvovaginitis that is caused by low levels of oestrogen following the menopause. If vulvovaginitis is caused by a particular bath product, detergent, deodorant, or contraceptive cream, you should change to another product.

Your doctor will advise you to avoid sexual intercourse until your symptoms have cleared up. Most affected people recover completely after treatment, but the condition may recur.

(WWW) ONLINE SITES: p.1037

Vaginal thrush

Inflammation of the vagina caused by infection with the candida fungus

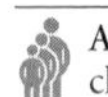 AGE Most common in females of childbearing age

 LIFESTYLE Stress may trigger the condition

 GENETICS Not a significant factor

Vaginal thrush affects many women at some point in their adult lives, most commonly at some time during the childbearing years, and can recur regularly. The condition develops when a fungus called *Candida albicans*, which can occur naturally in the vagina, grows more rapidly than usual. Vaginal thrush is not serious, but it may cause unpleasant itching of the vulva and vagina and a discharge. Candida infections may occur in other areas, such as the mouth (*see* ORAL THRUSH, p.862).

WHAT ARE THE CAUSES?

The candida fungus is found in the vagina of about 1 in 5 women and does not usually cause disease. The growth of the fungus is suppressed by both the immune system and harmless bacteria that normally live in the vagina. If these bacteria are destroyed by antibiotics or spermicides, the fungus can multiply, which may lead to symptoms. Harmless bacteria in the vagina may also be destroyed as a result of changes in levels of female sex hormones. Such changes may occur during pregnancy or before periods or may be due to drugs that affect female sex hormone levels, such as the oral contraceptive pill. Vaginal thrush may also develop after having sexual intercourse with a partner who has a candida infection.

Women who have diabetes mellitus (p.687) are more susceptible to vaginal thrush. Sometimes, stress can trigger an episode of the condition.

WHAT ARE THE SYMPTOMS?

The symptoms usually develop gradually over several days and may include:

- Intense irritation and itching of the vagina and vulva (*see* VULVOVAGINITIS, left).
- Thick, white vaginal discharge that is cheesy in appearance.

Left untreated, vulvovaginitis may lead to redness and eventually cracking of the delicate skin of the vulva.

WHAT CAN I DO?

If you are confident that your symptoms are due to vaginal thrush because you have had the condition before, you can treat yourself with over-the-counter

SELF-HELP PREVENTING VAGINAL THRUSH

If you often have vaginal thrush, the following self-help measures may help to prevent further episodes of infection:

- Wash the vaginal area with water only. Try to avoid using bath additives, perfumed soaps, or vaginal deodorants or douches.
- Avoid spermicidal creams, lubricants, and latex condoms if you find they irritate the vagina.
- Avoid scented sanitary towels or tampons, change tampons frequently, and use sanitary towels instead of tampons as often as possible.
- Keep your external genital area clean, dry, and cool. Wear cotton underwear and loose-fitting clothes if possible.
- If thrush seems to be triggered by stress, try to avoid stressful situations whenever possible.

drugs. Antifungal drugs (p.889) are readily available and include vaginal pessaries and creams or pills.

It is advisable not to have sexual intercourse for the next few days until your symptoms have cleared up. Your sexual partner should also be treated in order to avoid reinfection.

If you get vaginal thrush regularly, some simple measures can be taken to avoid the condition (*see* PREVENTING VAGINAL THRUSH, opposite page). If you are not sure about the cause of your symptoms or if treatment with over-the-counter preparations does not help, you should consult your doctor.

WHAT MIGHT THE DOCTOR DO?

Your doctor may diagnose thrush from the vaginal discharge. He or she will perform a pelvic examination and may take a swab from your vagina for examination. If vaginal thrush is diagnosed, your doctor may advise you on self-help measures or prescribe a stronger antifungal drug. Although treatment for vaginal thrush is usually successful, the condition tends to recur.

(WWW) ONLINE SITES: p.1037

Bacterial vaginosis

Bacterial infection of the vagina that sometimes causes an abnormal discharge

 AGE Can affect sexually active females of any age

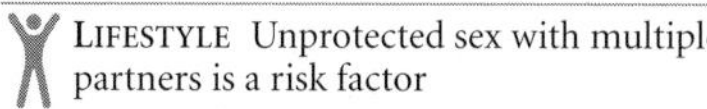 LIFESTYLE Unprotected sex with multiple partners is a risk factor

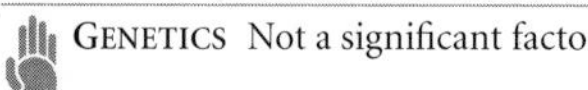 GENETICS Not a significant factor

Bacterial vaginosis is caused by excessive growth of some of the bacteria that normally live in the vagina, particularly *Gardnerella vaginalis* and *Mycoplasma hominis*. As a result, the natural balance of these organisms in the vagina is altered. The reason for this is unknown, but the condition is more common in sexually active women and often, but not always, occurs in association with sexually transmitted infections. Vaginal infections can also be caused by an excessive growth of the candida fungus (*see* VAGINAL THRUSH, opposite page) and the protozoan *Trichomonas vaginalis* (*see* TRICHOMONIASIS, p.767).

Bacterial vaginosis often causes no symptoms. However, some women may have a greyish-white vaginal discharge with a fishy or musty odour and vaginal or vulval itching. Rarely, the disorder leads to pelvic inflammatory disease (p.741), in which some of the reproductive organs become inflamed.

WHAT MIGHT BE DONE?

Your doctor may be able to diagnose bacterial vaginosis from your symptoms. Swabs of any discharge may be taken and tested to confirm the diagnosis. Vaginosis is usually treated with antibiotics (p.885), either orally or as pessaries inserted in the vagina. Sexual partners should also be checked for infection and treated if necessary. Vaginosis usually clears up completely within 2 days of starting treatment, but the condition does tend to recur.

(WWW) ONLINE SITES: p.1037

Bartholinitis

Infection of one or both Bartholin's glands, located in the vulva, and/or of their ducts

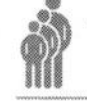 AGE More common after puberty

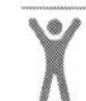 LIFESTYLE Poor hygiene and unprotected sex with multiple partners are risk factors

 GENETICS Not a significant factor

Bartholin's glands are two pea-sized glands with ducts that open into the vulva. The glands produce a fluid that lubricates the genital area during sexual intercourse. In bartholinitis, one or both of the glands and/or their ducts become infected. In some cases, the disorder is caused by bacteria from faeces entering the glands as a result of poor hygiene. A sexually transmitted infection may also cause the condition. The condition causes swelling in the surrounding tissues and a painful abscess may develop. One or both ducts may also become blocked, causing a painless swelling called a Bartholin's cyst.

Your doctor will prescribe antibiotics (p.885) to treat bartholinitis, and the disorder should clear up within a few days. Painkillers (p.912) may help to relieve discomfort. An abscess may be drained under local anaesthesia. Bartholin's cysts are not usually removed unless they are very large or cause discomfort. Bartholinitis may recur.

(WWW) ONLINE SITES: p.1037

Cancer of the vulva and vagina

Cancerous growths occurring on the vulva or in the vagina

 AGE More common over the age of 60

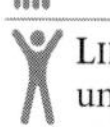 LIFESTYLE Unprotected sex at an early age, unprotected sex with multiple partners, and smoking are risk factors

 GENETICS Not a significant factor

Cancers of the vulva and vagina are rare and usually affect women over the age of 60. They account for about 1 in 20 cancers of the female reproductive organs. Although these cancers do not usually occur together, they may both be associated with certain types of the human papillomavirus (HPV), which is sexually transmitted. Smoking may also be a risk factor. If not treated, these cancers may spread to the pelvic lymph nodes and to other parts of the body.

Cancer of the vulva may cause vulval itching, but often the first symptom is a hard lump or ulcer on the vulva. If the ulcer is not treated, it may produce an offensive, bloody discharge. Cancer of the vagina often causes no symptoms until the tumour is at an advanced stage, although bleeding and pain may occur after sexual intercourse. If you develop any of these symptoms, you should consult your doctor at once.

WHAT MIGHT BE DONE?

Your doctor may make a diagnosis of cancer of the vulva or vagina from your symptoms. A sample of tissue may also be removed from the affected area and examined to look for cancerous cells.

Cancer of the vulva is usually treated surgically by removing the affected area. The nearby lymph nodes are also usually removed and examined to see if the disease has spread and if further treatment is necessary. Cancer of the vagina is usually treated with radiotherapy (p.281). However, it may also be necessary to remove part of the vagina and the nearby lymph nodes.

The outlook for both these cancers depends on whether they have spread. If they are diagnosed and treated early, there is often a full recovery.

(WWW) ONLINE SITES: p.1028, p.1037

BREAST DISORDERS

The breasts consist of fatty tissue that gives them their size and shape, lobules that secrete milk after childbirth, and milk ducts that carry the milk to the nipple during breast-feeding. The nipples are sensitive to touch and play a role in sexual arousal. Most disorders of the breasts are not serious, although breast cancer is becoming increasingly common in developed countries.

Throughout life, the breasts change size and shape in response to varying levels of female sex hormones. The breasts usually enlarge during puberty, before periods, and during pregnancy and breast-feeding. This enlargement can be associated with breast pain and generalized lumpiness.

This section opens with an overview of the causes of breast lumps, both normal and abnormal. Many women associate a breast lump with breast cancer, but in fact most lumps are noncancerous. Two common causes of noncancerous lumps in the breasts, fibroadenomas and breast cysts, are discussed next in this section.

The following articles cover breast pain, abnormalities in breast size, and problems that affect the nipples. The final article deals with breast cancer. Since early diagnosis of this disease significantly improves the chances of long-term survival, this section includes information about screening for breast cancer and how to examine your breasts so that abnormalities are detected as soon as possible.

KEY ANATOMY

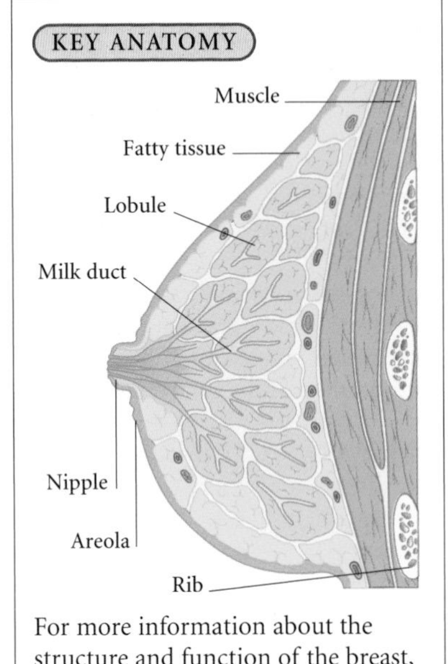

For more information about the structure and function of the breast, *see* pp.730–733.

Breast lumps

Any masses or swellings that can be felt in the breast tissue

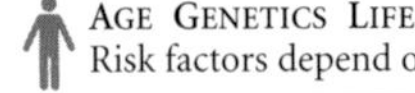

AGE GENETICS LIFESTYLE
Risk factors depend on the cause

Breast lumps are a common problem. Many women notice generalized breast lumpiness, especially when the breasts enlarge during puberty and pregnancy and before menstruation. This generalized lumpiness is usually a variation in normal breast development and does not increase the risk of breast cancer. A single, discrete breast lump may cause concern, but in fact only 1 in 10 breast lumps is due to cancer.

WHAT ARE THE CAUSES?

Generalized lumpiness in the breasts, often with associated breast tenderness, is thought to be related to the hormonal changes that occur during the menstrual cycle. The lumpiness usually becomes worse just before a period, and this worsening may be due to oversensitivity of the breast tissue to female sex hormones at this time.

A discrete lump is often a fibroadenoma (right). This noncancerous lump is caused by overgrowth of one or more breast lobules (the structures that produce milk). Breast cysts (opposite page) are fluid-filled sacs in the breast tissue. One or more cysts may be present, and both breasts may be affected. Occasionally, a breast lump is caused by an infection that has developed into an abscess. A breast abscess may develop if mastitis (p.809), which is most common in women who are breast-feeding, is not treated. An abscess may be associated with inflammation and localized pain. A lump in the breast may also be a symptom of breast cancer (p.759).

WHAT MIGHT BE DONE?

You should check your breasts regularly (*see* BREAST SELF-EXAMINATION, opposite page), so that you become familiar with their normal appearance and texture. Consult your doctor if you notice a new lump or a change in an existing lump. He or she will probably refer you to a breast clinic, where you may have ultrasound scanning (p.250) or mammography (p.759). The doctor at the clinic may also take a tissue sample from the lump (*see* ASPIRATION OF A BREAST LUMP, p.756) to look for cancerous cells. Many noncancerous breast lumps do not need treatment. Generalized breast lumpiness tends to decrease after the menopause, but the condition may continue if you take hormone replacement therapy (p.937). However, breast cysts usually need to be drained. Modern screening techniques and treatments mean that breast cancer can often be diagnosed early and treated successfully. If a breast tumour is found, further treatment will be planned.

(WWW) ONLINE SITES: p.1037

Fibroadenoma

A firm, round, noncancerous growth in the breast tissue

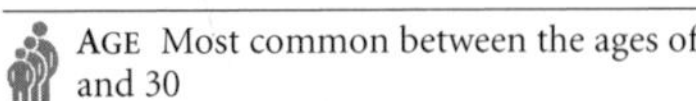

AGE Most common between the ages of 15 and 30

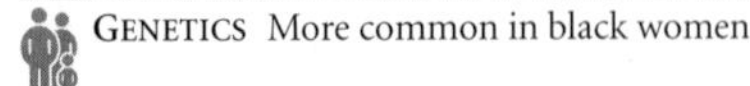

GENETICS More common in black women

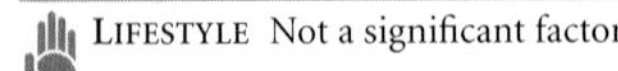

LIFESTYLE Not a significant factor

A fibroadenoma is an overgrowth of a breast lobule (the part of the breast that produces milk) and surrounding connective tissue. Although the cause of this condition is not fully understood, the development of a fibroadenoma is thought to be linked to the sensitivity of

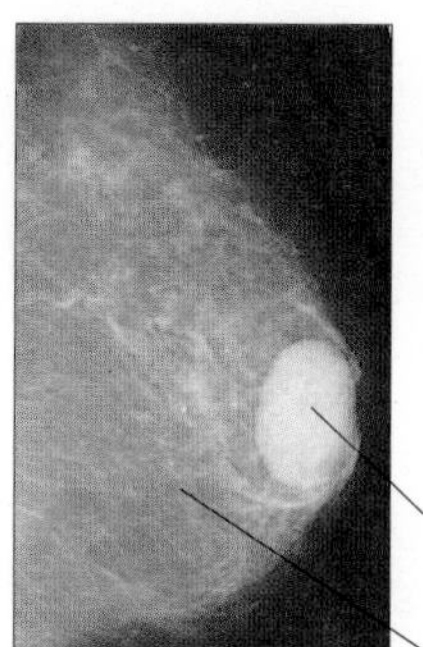

Fibroadenoma
A fibroadenoma can be seen in the breast tissue in this colour-enhanced mammogram (breast X-ray).

breast tissue to female sex hormones. The lumps tend to grow more quickly during pregnancy, probably because of the increased levels of female sex hormones. Fibroadenomas appear more commonly in women aged between 15 and 30 and in black women.

A fibroadenoma is usually painless. These lumps can develop in any part of the breast, but they are most commonly found in the upper, outer part and are usually about 1–5 cm (½–2 in) in size. There is often more than one lump, and sometimes both breasts are affected. In some women, multiple fibroadenomas develop together with a generalized thickening of the breast tissue.

It is important to carry out a regular breast self-examination (right) to look for any changes in the appearance or texture of your breasts. Fibroadenomas are harmless, but, if you find a lump in your breast, you should consult your doctor so that the possibility of breast cancer (p.759) can be ruled out.

What might be done?

Your doctor will probably refer you to a breast clinic, where you may have mammography (p.759) or ultrasound scanning (p.250) of the breast tissue. A sample of cells may be removed from the lump (*see* Aspiration of a breast lump, p.756) to be examined microscopically for cancerous cells.

Small fibroadenomas do not usually need treatment. About 1 in 3 fibroadenomas becomes smaller or disappears completely within 2 years. If you are worried about the fibroadenoma, or if it grows larger, surgical removal may be recommended. After removal, the lump will be examined under a microscope for the presence of cancerous cells. In most cases, fibroadenomas do not recur after treatment.

(WWW) ONLINE SITES: p.1037

Breast cyst

A firm, round, fluid-filled swelling within the breast tissue

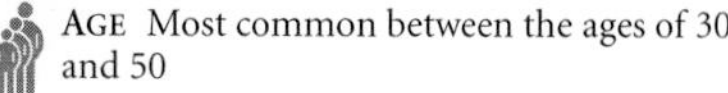
AGE Most common between the ages of 30 and 50

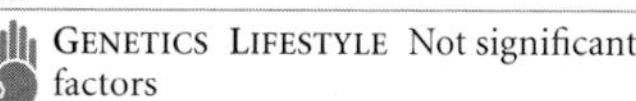
GENETICS LIFESTYLE Not significant factors

A breast cyst is a firm, round lump in the breast tissue that forms when a lobule (the part of the breast that produces milk) fills with fluid. The development of cysts is influenced by levels of female sex hormones. Breast cysts most often affect women aged 30–50, particularly those approaching the menopause.

A cyst may be felt just under the skin or may occur deeper within the breast tissue. The lump is usually not painful.

Breast cysts may occur singly, but in about half of all cases there is more than one cyst, and both breasts may be affected. Some women also have generalized lumpiness of the breast tissue.

You should always consult your doctor if you detect a lump during breast self-examination (below) so that the possibility of breast cancer (p.759) can be ruled out. In rare cases, cancerous cells may be found in the wall of a cyst.

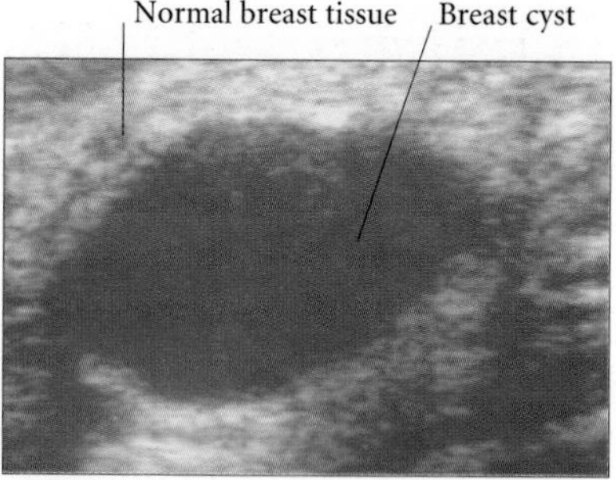

Breast cyst
This ultrasound scan of a breast shows a fluid-filled breast cyst, visible as a dark area within the breast tissue.

What might be done?

If your doctor suspects a cyst, he or she may refer you to a clinic, where you may have breast X-rays (*see* Mammography, p.759) or ultrasound scanning (p.250).

The usual treatment for breast cysts is to drain them of fluid (*see* Aspiration of a breast lump, p.756). The fluid will be examined for cancerous cells only if it is bloodstained. Cysts usually disappear after aspiration but may recur and require further drainage. If a cyst recurs several times or contains bloodstained fluid, it will be removed surgically.

(WWW) ONLINE SITES: p.1037

(SELF-HELP) Breast self-examination

Regular examination of your breasts helps you to become familiar with their normal feel and appearance so that you will notice if a change occurs. The best time to examine your breasts is just after your period. If you detect a new lump, changes in a long-standing lump, a change in nipple shape, or a change in the skin overlying the breast, you should consult your doctor. In many cases, breast lumps are harmless, but they are sometimes caused by a cancerous tumour.

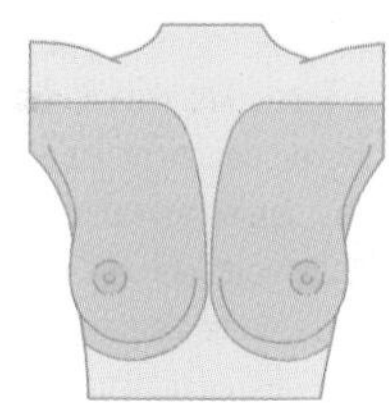

Area to be examined

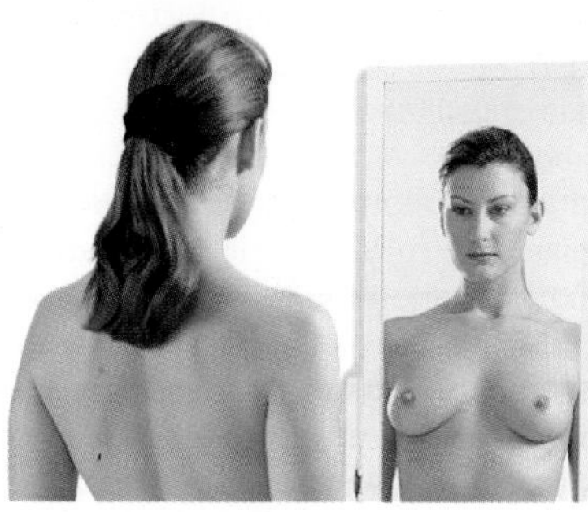

1 *Look at the appearance of your breasts in a mirror. Look closely for dimpled skin and any changes to your nipples or to the size and shape of your breasts.*

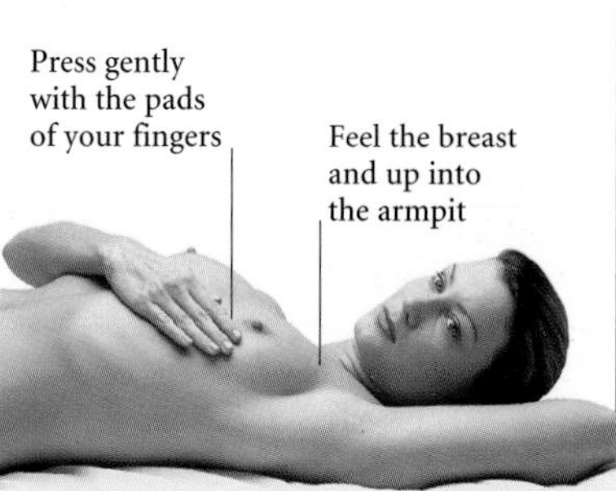

2 *With one arm behind your head, gently but firmly press the breast with small circular movements. Feel around the entire breast, armpit area, and nipple.*

TEST AND TREATMENT ASPIRATION OF A BREAST LUMP

Aspiration of a breast lump is used as a diagnostic procedure to detect breast cancer and also as a treatment for fluid-filled breast cysts. If aspiration confirms that a breast lump is solid tissue, a sample of cells is withdrawn and examined under a microscope for evidence of cancer. If the lump is a cyst, the fluid will be drained and the lump may disappear. Aspiration may be uncomfortable but usually takes less than a minute.

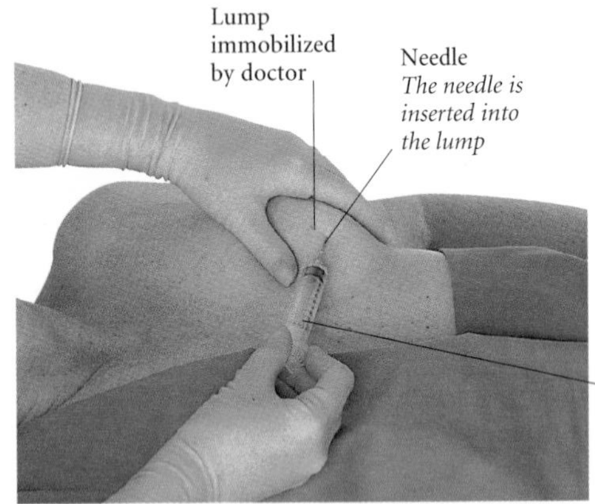

During the procedure
The doctor immobilizes the breast lump with one hand and inserts a needle attached to a syringe into the lump. Cells or fluid are then withdrawn through the needle for analysis.

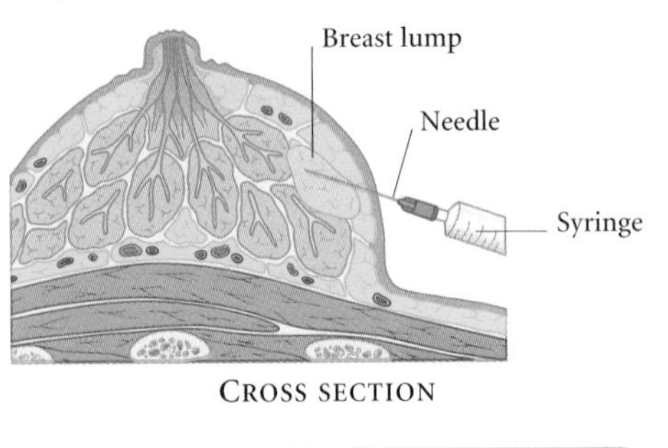

CROSS SECTION

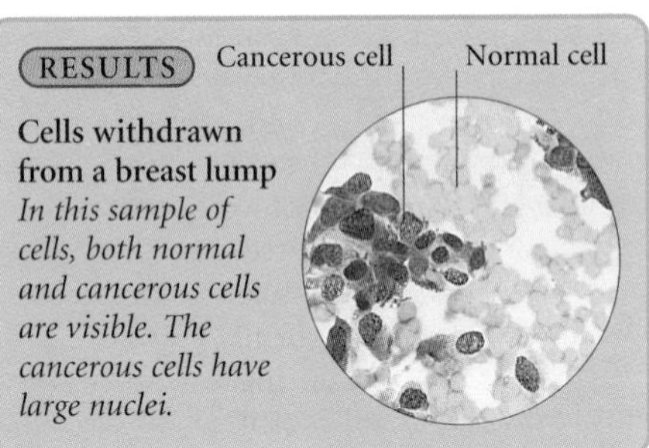

Cells withdrawn from a breast lump
In this sample of cells, both normal and cancerous cells are visible. The cancerous cells have large nuclei.

Breast pain

Pain or discomfort usually affecting one or both breasts

AGE Most common between the ages of 15 and 50

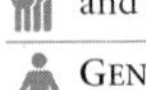
GENETICS LIFESTYLE Risk factors depend on the cause

Breast pain is an extremely common problem. In most women, the pain is cyclical, varying in severity in response to the hormonal changes of the menstrual cycle. This cyclical pain is usually most severe before periods and tends to affect both breasts.

Cyclical breast pain affects as many as 1 in 2 women and is commonly a long-term problem. Women who experience cyclical breast pain frequently also have generalized breast lumpiness, which tends to become worse before a period. The pain may be aggravated by stress and by caffeine in certain drinks.

In some women, breast pain is not related to menstruation. One cause of noncyclical breast pain is muscle strain. Rarely, pain is caused by a breast cyst (p.755) or breast cancer (p.759). Breast pain may also be due to a short-term problem, such as inflammation of the breast tissue caused by an infection (*see* MASTITIS, p.809) or engorgement of the breasts with milk after childbirth (*see* BREAST ENGORGEMENT, p.808). Sometimes, the cause of breast pain is not known. If you have large breasts, you are more likely to suffer from both cyclical and noncyclical breast pain.

WHAT MIGHT THE DOCTOR DO?

Your doctor will ask you about your breast pain to see if there is a pattern. He or she will examine your breasts to look for an underlying cause, such as a breast cyst, or any tender areas in the surrounding muscles. If it is apparent from the consultation and examination that you do not have an underlying disorder, your doctor may ask you to keep a record of when you experience breast pain to help to confirm that the pain is cyclical. If your doctor suspects that an underlying disorder may be causing the pain, he or she will probably refer you to a breast clinic for mammography (p.759) or ultrasound scanning (p.250) to look for any abnormalities in the breast tissue.

Mild cyclical pain does not normally require treatment. However, in about 1 in 10 women, the pain is so severe that it can interfere with everyday life. Taking large doses of evening primrose oil may reduce the response of the breast tissue to female sex hormones. However, if this treatment is ineffective or the pain is severe, your doctor may prescribe danazol, a drug that reduces the effects of female sex hormones acting on the breast (*see* SEX HORMONES AND RELATED DRUGS, p.933). Although this drug is effective in relieving pain, it can sometimes have side effects such as acne and weight gain. Cyclical breast pain tends to diminish following the menopause. If you are taking hormone replacement therapy (p.937), the pain may continue after the menopause, but it often improves after a few months.

If your breast pain is noncyclical, the cause will be treated if necessary. Cysts are usually drained (*see* ASPIRATION OF A BREAST LUMP, above), and antibiotics (p.885) can be used to treat infection. Nonsteroidal anti-inflammatory drugs (p.894) may help to relieve muscle pain.

WHAT CAN I DO?

Breast pain may be eased by wearing a bra that supports your breasts properly. If your breasts are heavy and the pain is severe, you may need to wear a bra at night. Cyclical pain may be relieved by cutting down on caffeine, practising relaxation exercises (p.75) to help to control stress, and trying to lose weight to reduce the size of the breasts. Some women find that taking vitamin E supplements is also helpful, but this effect has not been scientifically proven.

(WWW) ONLINE SITES: p.1037

Abnormality of breast size

Abnormally large, small, or asymmetrical breasts

AGE Develops during puberty

GENETICS LIFESTYLE Not significant factors

There is considerable variation in breast size among women. A slight asymmetry in the size of the breasts in an individual woman is also common. However, having abnormally large, small, or asymmetrical breasts can lead to emotional distress and, in the case of very large breasts, may cause pain (*see* BREAST PAIN, opposite page) and discomfort.

Breasts that grow abnormally large often develop rapidly during puberty and are thought to be the result of oversensitivity of the breast tissue to the female sex hormone oestrogen. Large breasts may lead to pain in the back, shoulders, and neck, and in some cases a skin infection may develop under the breast. Women who have abnormally large breasts may experience discomfort when running or playing sports and have difficulty in finding clothes that fit.

In some women, the breasts develop to only a very small size. A woman who has very small breasts may find her appearance unfeminine. However, having small breasts does not cause any physical problems and does not affect a woman's ability to breast-feed.

Occasionally, there is a marked difference in size between the two breasts because one breast develops more than the other at puberty. This asymmetry may cause embarrassment and anxiety.

WHAT MIGHT BE DONE?

Women with large breasts can benefit from a well-fitting, supportive bra. You may also find that wearing a bra at night makes you feel more comfortable. If this does not relieve your discomfort or distress, you may wish to consider the possibility of a surgical operation to permanently reduce the size of your breasts (*see* BREAST REDUCTION, below).

Women with small breasts may find that a padded bra improves their body shape under clothes. The only permanent way to enlarge small breasts is by surgically inserting an implant behind the breast tissue. The most frequently used implants are filled with a silicone gel. In the past, leakage of the gel sometimes occurred, but improved materials have made such problems rare.

Some women who experience distress as a result of having abnormally large, small, or asymmetrical breasts may find counselling (p.971) of benefit.

(WWW) ONLINE SITES: p.1037

(TREATMENT) BREAST REDUCTION

Breast reduction operations relieve the discomfort of very large, heavy breasts. The procedure takes place under general anaesthesia and involves a short hospital stay. During the operation, some skin and breast tissue are removed, and the breast is reshaped. The nipple and areola (the dark area around the nipple) may be moved up and made smaller. After surgery, your breasts will be smaller and firmer. The scarring is usually minimal and is mostly hidden under the breast. However, sensation in the nipple will be reduced, and breast-feeding will not be possible.

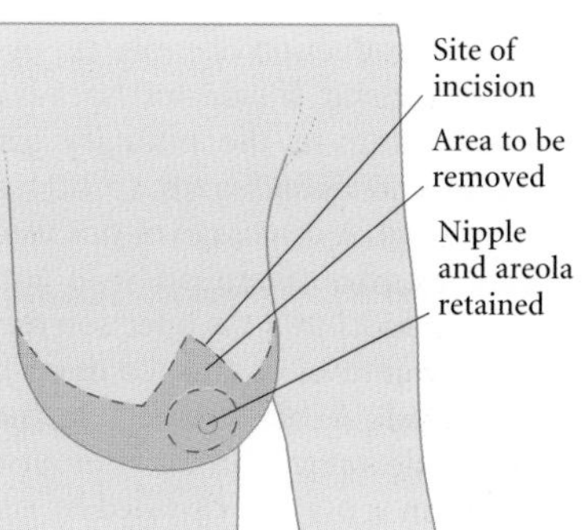

1 *A substantial area of skin and tissue is removed from the lower part of the breast. The nipple and areola are retained, along with the blood vessels and some of the nerves that supply the area.*

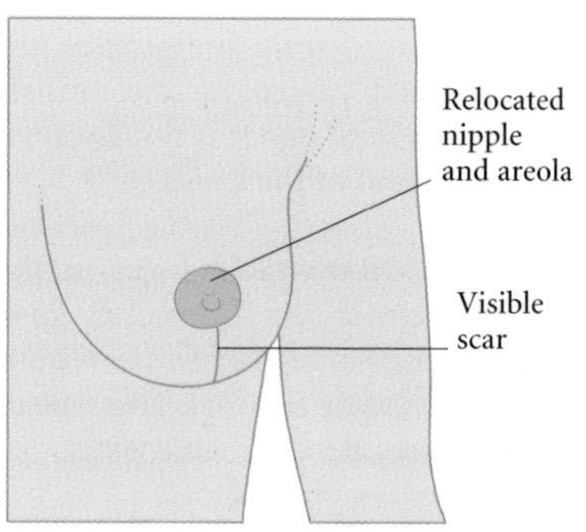

2 *The nipple and areola are repositioned higher up, and the V-shaped part of the incision is sewn together below it. The remaining skin edges are rejoined under the breast and are not visible.*

Abnormal nipples

Change in the appearance of a nipple or the area around it (areola)

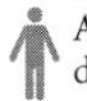
AGE GENETICS LIFESTYLE Risk factors depend on the cause

There are two main types of nipple abnormality: retraction into the breast (nipple inversion) and disorders affecting the skin on or around the nipple. Although these abnormalities are most often caused by minor problems that are easily treatable, any changes in the condition of the nipples should receive medical attention because, in rare cases, they may indicate breast cancer (p.759).

WHAT ARE THE CAUSES?

Inversion of the nipples may occur during puberty if the breasts do not develop properly. This type of inversion is usually harmless, although it may later make breast-feeding difficult. Nipple inversion may also occur as a result of inflammation of the milk ducts behind the nipple. This condition most often affects nonpregnant women who smoke. Changes in the structure of the breasts as they age may cause the nipple to be drawn into the breast in older women. Less commonly, nipple inversion that develops in adulthood may be due to breast cancer.

Many women develop fine cracks and tender areas on their nipples during the first few weeks of breast-feeding (*see* CRACKED NIPPLES, p.808). These cracks are most often the result of the baby not taking the whole nipple into his or her mouth properly when feeding. Leaving the nipples wet after a feed can also cause them to become sore and cracked. Cracked nipples often cause stabbing or burning pain as the baby starts or stops feeding and may become infected, causing inflammation of the breast tissue (*see* MASTITIS, p.809).

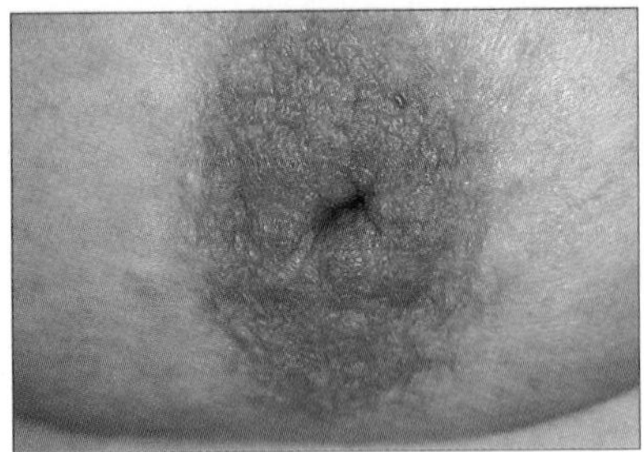

Inverted nipple
This nipple has become drawn into the breast (inverted), which may be due to shortening of the milk ducts with age.

Dry, flaky patches of skin that occur on or around both nipples may be due to eczema (p.333). Eczema is usually itchy and tends to occur in several sites on the body. However, occasionally, skin changes on the nipples that resemble eczema are in fact caused by Paget's disease of the breast, a rare form of cancer that originates in the milk ducts. Unlike eczema, Paget's disease rarely develops on both nipples and does not heal. This type of breast cancer often causes soreness and bleeding from the nipple and is often associated with a breast lump.

WHAT MIGHT BE DONE?

Your doctor will examine your breasts, paying particular attention to your nipples. If nipple inversion has occurred in adulthood but is not related to breast-feeding, your doctor may refer you to a breast clinic, where you may have ultrasound scanning (p.250) or mammography (opposite page) to look for breast abnormalities. If a breast lump is found, cells or fluid may be taken from it using a needle and syringe (*see* ASPIRATION OF A BREAST LUMP, p.756) and examined for cancerous cells. If you have a persistent rash on or around a nipple, a skin sample may be taken and tested for cancerous cells.

Occasionally, it is possible to correct nipple inversion that has been present since puberty by gently drawing the nipples out between your thumb and forefinger every day for several weeks. Suction devices, such as nipple shells, which are temporarily worn in your bra, can also help to draw out the nipple.

If your nipples have become cracked, washing and drying them carefully and applying a moisturizer may help. Make sure that you wash the moisturizer off before breast-feeding. You should also avoid plastic-lined breast pads, which may become damp and encourage infection. Infection is usually treated with antibiotics (p.885), and eczema can be improved by hydrocortisone cream (*see* TOPICAL CORTICOSTEROIDS, p.892).

If cancer of the breast is discovered, you will be referred for treatment, and additional tests, including blood tests and X-rays (p.244), may be performed to find out if the cancer has spread to other parts of the body. If Paget's disease is diagnosed, the affected skin will be removed along with surrounding tissue. If a lump is found, treatment can include surgery, radiotherapy (p.281), or chemotherapy (p.280).

(WWW) ONLINE SITES: p.1037

Nipple discharge

Discharge of fluid from one or both nipples

AGE GENETICS LIFESTYLE Risk factors depend on the cause

It is normal for women to release milk from their nipples during late pregnancy and while breast-feeding. At any other time, a nipple discharge may be due to hormonal changes in the menstrual cycle or a symptom of a minor disorder. However, because the condition may be a sign of a more serious disorder, such as breast cancer (opposite page), you should see your doctor if you notice an unusual discharge.

WHAT ARE THE CAUSES?

The main causes of nipple discharge are hormonal changes, infection within the breast, or, more rarely, a breast tumour. Fluid discharged from the nipples can vary considerably in colour and consistency, and its appearance is not always a good indication of the cause.

HORMONAL CHANGES Changes in the levels of female sex hormones may produce a discharge, usually from both nipples, just before a period. This type of discharge may be clear and watery or yellow, green, or blue-black.

A watery, milky discharge in women who are not pregnant or breast-feeding is known as galactorrhoea. This is usually due to overproduction of prolactin from the pituitary gland. The condition may be due to a noncancerous tumour of the pituitary gland, called a prolactinoma (p.677), or more rarely be an effect of a hormonal disorder such as hyperthyroidism (p.679). Some drugs, such as antipsychotics (p.917), cause galactorrhoea as a side effect.

BREAST INFECTION In breast-feeding women, blocked milk ducts may become infected and produce a discharge of pus from the nipples (*see* MASTITIS, p.809). In nonbreast-feeding women, smoking may cause inflammation of the milk ducts, producing a pus-containing nipple discharge. This is most common in women under 40.

BREAST TUMOURS A profuse, watery discharge from the nipple may be associated with a cancerous breast tumour. A bloodstained discharge may also be a symptom of cancer, although, more commonly, this type of discharge is the result of a noncancerous tumour forming within a duct.

WHAT MIGHT BE DONE?

Your doctor will carry out a physical examination of your breasts. He or she may take a sample of the discharge to be examined for evidence of infection or cancerous cells. X-rays of the breast (*see* MAMMOGRAPHY, opposite page) and ultrasound scanning (p.250) may be performed. A blood sample may be taken to measure hormone levels.

In most cases, a discharge caused by normal hormonal functions is harmless and does not need treatment. Galactorrhoea can often be treated successfully using the drug cabergoline (*see* PITUITARY DRUGS, p.934), which reduces production of prolactin by the pituitary gland. If galactorrhoea is due to a tumour in the pituitary gland, surgery and radiotherapy (p.281) may be required. A discharge of pus usually clears up after treatment with antibiotics (p.885), but if the infection recurs, surgical removal of affected ducts may be needed. A bloodstained discharge caused by a noncancerous tumour of a milk duct is normally treated by surgical removal of the duct.

If initial tests reveal that your nipple discharge has been caused by a cancerous growth in the breast, you will be referred for further tests and treatment.

(WWW) ONLINE SITES: p.1037

Breast cancer

A cancerous growth that originates in the breast

AGE Risk increases with age

GENETICS In some cases, due to an abnormal gene

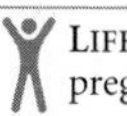
LIFESTYLE Obesity and delaying or avoiding pregnancy are risk factors

Breast cancer is one of the most common cancers affecting women. In the UK, about 32,500 women develop cancer of the breast each year. The disease can also occur in men, although cancer of the male breast accounts for less than 1 in 100 breast cancer cases.

The risk of breast cancer increases with age, doubling every 10 years. The disease is most commonly diagnosed in women over the age of 50. Only a very few women under the age of 30 develop breast cancer. The number of cases diagnosed each year in Europe and North America is increasing slightly. However, there has been a small drop in the number of deaths from breast cancer in recent years, and only about a fifth of cases are fatal. This reduction is due to improved treatment and the increased use of mammography (below) to screen for cancer, which means that tumours can be detected early, when they often respond well to treatment. Screening may reduce the number of breast cancer deaths in women over the age of 50 by up to 4 in 10. In the UK, women between the ages of 50 and 64 are offered a mammogram every 3 years.

A tumour may first develop in the breast lobules (the structures that produce milk). A tumour that originates in the milk ducts may lead to Paget's disease of the breast (*see* ABNORMAL NIPPLES, p.757). Tumours may spread to other organs, such as the lungs or the liver, before being detected.

WHAT ARE THE CAUSES?

The underlying cause of most breast cancers is unclear. However, some risk factors have been identified, many of which suggest that the female hormone oestrogen is an important factor in the development of the disease. Women who have their first period before the age of 11 or who have a late menopause seem to be at increased risk of developing breast cancer, probably because they are exposed to high levels of oestrogen for longer. The number of menstrual cycles before a first pregnancy also has some influence on the risk of breast cancer. A woman who never has children is more than twice as likely to develop breast cancer as a woman who has her first child before the age of 20. Breast-feeding is thought to have an additional protective effect.

Obesity slightly increases the risk of breast cancer because excess body fat causes an increase in oestrogen levels.

TEST MAMMOGRAPHY

A mammogram is an X-ray of the breast and is used to screen for signs of breast cancer and to investigate lumps. Mammograms can show precancerous cells as well as tumours but may not detect every case of breast cancer. For this reason, it is important to examine your breasts regularly. You should have routine mammograms from the age of 50 because the risk of developing breast cancer increases with age. The procedure is slightly uncomfortable but lasts only a few seconds. Two pictures are taken of each breast.

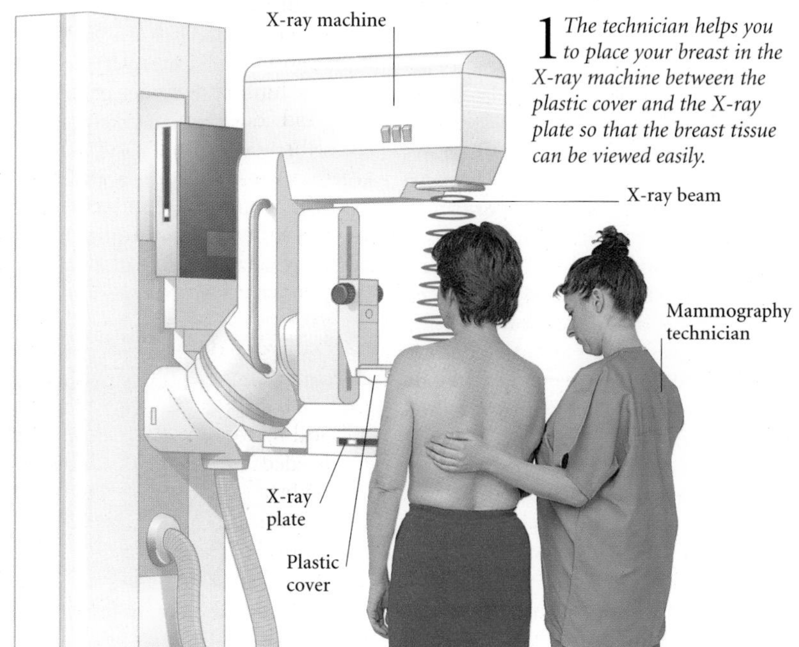

1 The technician helps you to place your breast in the X-ray machine between the plastic cover and the X-ray plate so that the breast tissue can be viewed easily.

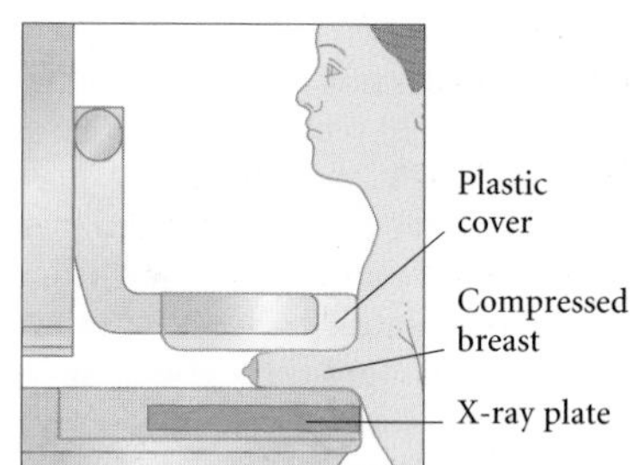

2 The breast is firmly compressed between the plastic cover and the X-ray plate. X-rays pass down through the breast and on to the X-ray plate.

RESULTS

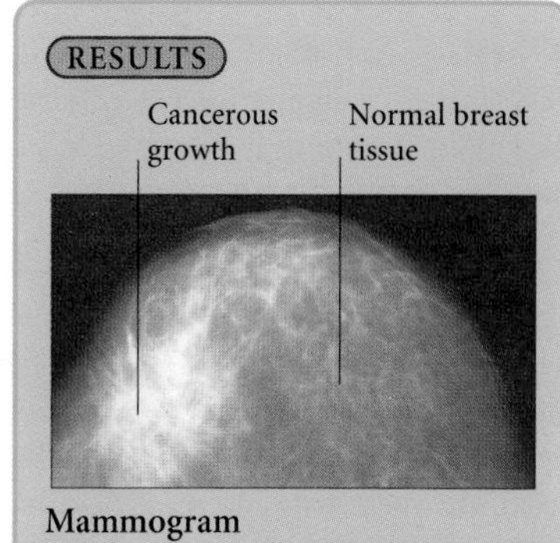

Mammogram
In this X-ray image, a tumour is visible within the breast. The tumour is denser than normal breast tissue and appears opaque on the X-ray.

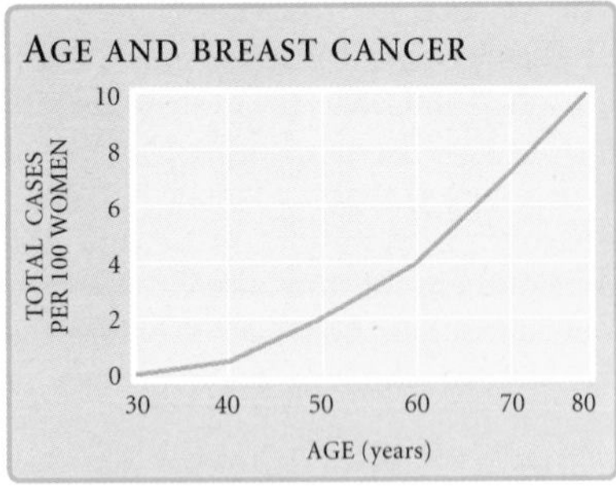

Lifetime risk of breast cancer
This graph shows that of all women who are alive at the age of 80, approximately 1 in 10 will have developed breast cancer at some time in her life.

Artificial oestrogen in some medications may also influence susceptibility to breast cancer. Many cancerous tumours are oestrogen-sensitive, and oestrogen encourages them to grow once they have formed. Combined oral contraceptive pills slightly increase the risk of developing breast cancer, although only while they are being taken. Hormone replacement therapy (p.937) in postmenopausal women is associated with a small increase in risk, but this is significant only after 10 years of treatment.

About 1 in 20 cases of breast cancer is linked to an abnormal gene, and several of these genes have now been identified. Breast cancer with a genetic basis most commonly affects women in their 30s and 40s and may also affect men. If you have a close relative who had breast cancer before the age of 40, you may carry an abnormal gene. Genetic testing is not widely available in the UK, but you may be given additional screening. If close relatives have had breast cancer after the age of 40, you will have only a slightly increased risk. Often, there is no family history.

Noncancerous breast lumps do not increase the risk of breast cancer.

What are the symptoms?

It is very unusual for breast cancer to produce symptoms in its early stages. When symptoms do occur, they usually affect only one breast and may include:

- A lump in the breast, which is usually painless and may be situated deep in the breast or just under the skin.
- Dimpling of the skin in the area of the lump, or swelling of the skin with an "orange peel" appearance.
- Inversion of the nipple.
- A bloodstained nipple discharge.

In Paget's disease, the only symptom may be a patch of dry, flaky skin on the nipple. Although these symptoms most often result from noncancerous conditions, you should consult your doctor if you notice a change in the appearance or texture of your breasts. If breast cancer is not treated, it can spread to the lymph nodes in the armpit and then to other organs, such as the lungs, liver, or bones, causing additional symptoms.

How is it diagnosed?

You should check your breasts regularly (*see* BREAST SELF-EXAMINATION, p.755) to look for lumps and other abnormalities. Screening using mammography enables tumours to be detected before any symptoms have appeared. Although this procedure is reliable, it may not detect every case, and it is therefore important that you continue to examine your breasts regularly even after a normal mammogram.

If you visit your doctor because you have noticed a lump or other abnormality of your breast, he or she will carry out a breast examination and check for signs of spread to the lymph nodes in the armpit. If he or she finds a lump or other evidence of breast cancer, you will be referred to hospital, where mammography or ultrasound scanning (p.250) may be carried out. A sample of cells from the lump may be removed using a needle and syringe (*see* ASPIRATION OF A BREAST LUMP, p.756) and examined for cancerous cells.

If the diagnosis of cancer is confirmed, further tests will be performed to find out whether the cancer is sensitive to oestrogen and if it has spread. Certain blood tests provide a measure of liver function and indicate whether the cancer has spread to the liver. Chest X-rays (p.490) may be arranged to look for evidence of spread to the lungs, and a bone scan (*see* RADIONUCLIDE SCANNING, p.251) may be carried out to see if the bones have been affected.

What is the treatment?

The extent of the cancerous growth within the breast, whether it has spread to other parts of the body, and whether it is oestrogen-sensitive are the main considerations when deciding on the most appropriate course of treatment. Once a full assessment has been made, your doctor will discuss your treatment options with you. Treatment of breast cancer may include surgery, radiotherapy, chemotherapy, hormone therapy, or, most frequently, a combination of these. Counselling may help you to come to terms with cancer, and some complementary therapies can be used to promote a sense of well-being.

SURGERY Surgery is normally the first stage of breast cancer treatment. There are many possible types of operation used to treat breast cancer (*see* SURGERY FOR BREAST CANCER, opposite page).

If the tumour is small, a lumpectomy may be performed, in which the tumour and a small area of surrounding tissue are removed. A larger tumour is treated by a quadrantectomy, in which about a quarter of the breast tissue is removed.

In some cases, all of the tissue from the affected breast is surgically removed in a procedure known as a mastectomy. Some women choose to have a mastectomy because they want to make sure that all of the tumour has been removed. However, medical studies have shown that this operation is not necessary for most single, small tumours.

During surgery, a number of lymph nodes from the armpit on the same side as the affected breast may be removed. These lymph nodes are examined to look for signs of cancer. If the lymph nodes are found to be free of cancerous cells, the cancer is unlikely to have spread from the tumour site.

Surgery will affect the appearance of your breast. If one breast looks smaller after surgery, you may want to have the other breast reduced to the same size (*see* BREAST REDUCTION, p.757). After a

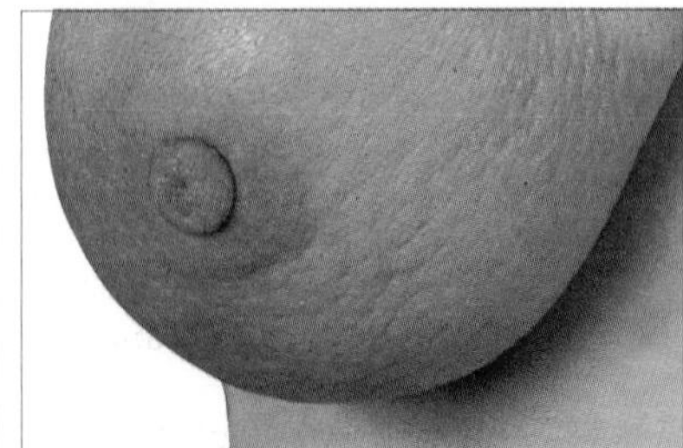

Appearance of the skin in breast cancer
A cancerous growth in this breast has caused the skin to become swollen with fluid, giving an "orange peel" appearance.

mastectomy, some women have a breast reconstruction. This operation can either be performed at the same time as the mastectomy or at a later date.

RADIOTHERAPY Treatment with radiotherapy (p.281) is given to almost all women after lumpectomy, regardless of the size of the tumour. It may also be used after mastectomy if a large tumour is removed or if the cancer has spread to the lymph nodes. Treatment usually begins 1 month after surgery and is given 5 days a week for about 6 weeks. The aim is to destroy any cancer cells that may remain after surgery.

DRUG TREATMENTS Tumours that are oestrogen-sensitive usually respond to drugs that block the action of oestrogen, whereas chemotherapy (p.280) is often effective for all types of tumour.

Tamoxifen (*see* SEX HORMONES AND RELATED DRUGS, p.933) inhibits the effects of oestrogen so that the tumour becomes smaller or does not grow as quickly. Tamoxifen is usually taken for at least 5 years. The drug has also been found effective in preventing breast cancer in women at increased risk.

Chemotherapy involves using combinations of drugs that destroy rapidly dividing cancerous cells. Treatment is usually given at intervals of 3–4 weeks over a period of 4–6 months. In most cases, chemotherapy is used in addition to surgery. These drugs can also kill normal cells, such as those in the lining of the mouth. Hair loss and mouth ulcers are common side effects.

COMPLEMENTARY THERAPIES Women with breast cancer may choose to complement conventional treatments with other therapies, such as relaxation exercises (p.75), meditation, homeopathy (p.974), or acupuncture (p.973). These therapies should not be regarded as alternatives to conventional treatment. If you are considering using complementary therapies, you should consult your doctor. Counselling (p.971) may also be helpful in coping with cancer.

TREATMENT SURGERY FOR BREAST CANCER

The aim of breast cancer surgery is to remove all cancerous tissue. The procedure varies depending on the size and position of the tumour. Two operations are described here: lumpectomy, which is commonly used to treat small tumours; and mastectomy, sometimes used to treat larger or multiple tumours. Usually, the surgeon also removes some lymph nodes from the armpit. These are checked to see whether the cancer has spread.

LUMPECTOMY

In a lumpectomy, the small area of breast tissue containing the tumour is removed, along with a small number of lymph nodes from the armpit. This procedure takes place under general anaesthesia. After the operation, the shape of the breast remains essentially unchanged.

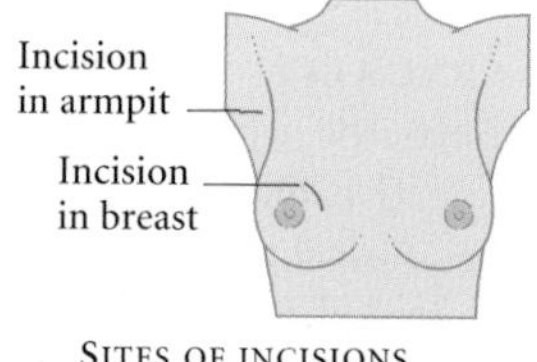

SITES OF INCISIONS

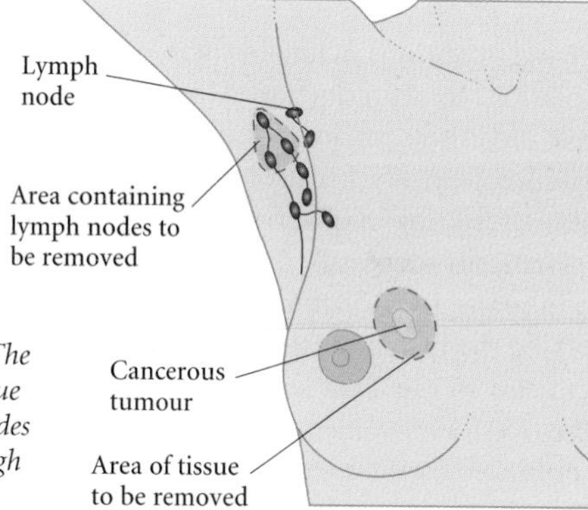

During the procedure
An incision is made in the breast. The tumour and some surrounding tissue are removed. Some of the lymph nodes from the armpit are removed through a separate incision.

MASTECTOMY

In a mastectomy, the whole breast is removed. This operation is used to treat large or multiple cancerous breast tumours. The procedure takes place under general anaesthesia, and you will need to stay in hospital for several days. You may choose to have plastic surgery to reconstruct your breast at the same time as you have the mastectomy or at a later time.

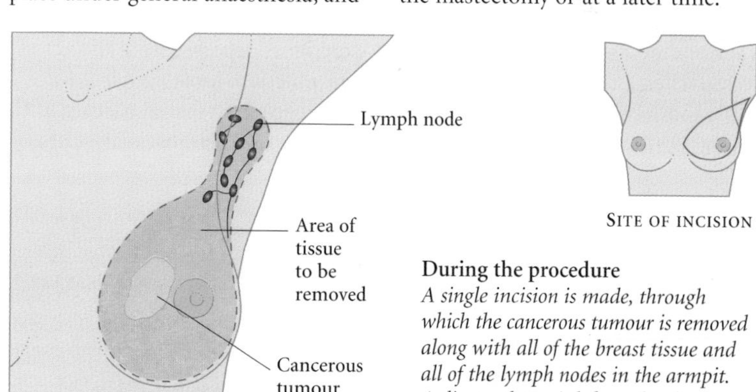

SITE OF INCISION

During the procedure
A single incision is made, through which the cancerous tumour is removed along with all of the breast tissue and all of the lymph nodes in the armpit. A diagonal scar is left on the chest.

WHAT IS THE PROGNOSIS?

If breast cancer is diagnosed before it has spread to other body organs, treatment is more likely to be successful and the cancer is less likely to recur after treatment. Combining drug treatment with surgery has been found to improve the chances of long-term survival.

Following treatment, you will have follow-up examinations with your doctor and regular mammograms to check for recurrence of the disease. About 1 in 4 women treated for breast cancer has a recurrence within 5 years. Cancer may recur close to the site of the original tumour or in a different area. Any recurrence requires further treatment.

About 7 in 10 women who receive treatment for breast cancer in its early stages survive for 10 years or more.

(WWW) ONLINE SITES: p.1028

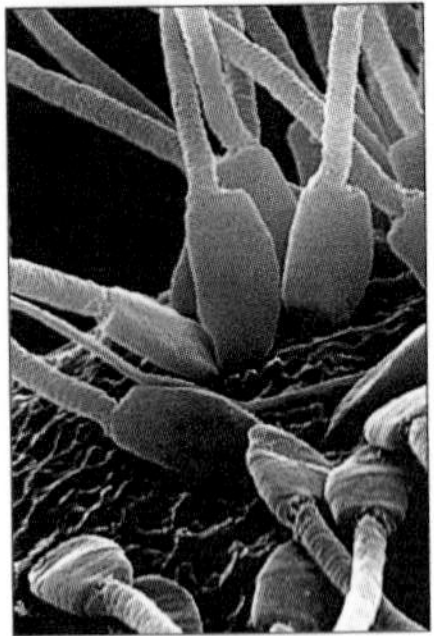

Sperm meet egg
Many sperm attempt to penetrate the surface of an egg to fertilize it.

SEX AND REPRODUCTION

IN BIOLOGICAL TERMS, the urge to reproduce is one of the strongest basic drives. Producing a new generation to ensure the continuation of the species fulfils one of the primary functions of the human body. However, in humans, sexual intercourse is not only the means by which males and females reproduce but also an outlet for emotional expression. A sexual relationship can therefore play an important role in creating and maintaining the bond between partners.

All living organisms maintain their populations by reproduction. Most simple organisms, such as bacteria, reproduce asexually, usually by cell division, resulting in offspring that are genetically identical.

In humans, reproduction is sexual, involving the fusion of two cells: a sperm and an egg. Eggs are produced by the ovaries in women, and sperm are produced by the testes in men. These cells are normally brought into contact through sexual intercourse. If a sperm succeeds in fertilizing an egg, DNA (genetic material) from each parent combines to create a unique individual.

Sexual reproduction results in an infinite variety of offspring. The only exceptions are identical twins, which develop when a fertilized egg divides equally to produce two individuals with the same genetic make-up.

HUMAN SEXUALITY

In many animals, the urge to reproduce is largely instinctive, but, in humans, many social and psychological factors also significantly influence sexuality and reproduction. Changing social attitudes towards sexual behaviour in the last few decades have enabled both men and women to express their sexual needs more freely to each other.

Sex drive varies widely between individuals of both sexes and ranges from a complete lack of sexual interest to very powerful urges. The ease with which sexual arousal can be achieved also varies between individuals.

Human beings are probably unique among animals in seeking to engage in sexual intercourse as a pleasurable experience separate from the act of reproduction. Most people have a preference for a sexual partner of the opposite sex (heterosexual). Others have a preference for members of the same sex (homosexual), and some individuals experience attraction to members of either sex (bisexual).

FERTILITY

Reproduction depends on an egg being fertilized and embedding in the uterus of the woman. Sexual behaviour and fertility affect the likelihood that these events will occur. If a fertile man and a woman at the fertile stage of her menstrual cycle have sex without contraception, a sperm has about a 1 in 5 chance of fertilizing an egg.

With medical advances, the process of reproduction can increasingly be controlled. Couples can choose to prevent conception by using a form of contraception. On the other hand, if a couple is unable to conceive naturally, conception can be assisted in a number of ways.

FUNCTION SEXUAL RESPONSE

Sexual thoughts, the sight of a partner's body, and foreplay all contribute to sexual arousal. Excitement makes breathing quicken, heart rate increase, and blood pressure rise. In a male, the penis becomes firm and erect. In a female, the labia and clitoris swell, the vagina lengthens and becomes lubricated, and the breasts enlarge. The time taken for sexual arousal varies between men and women.

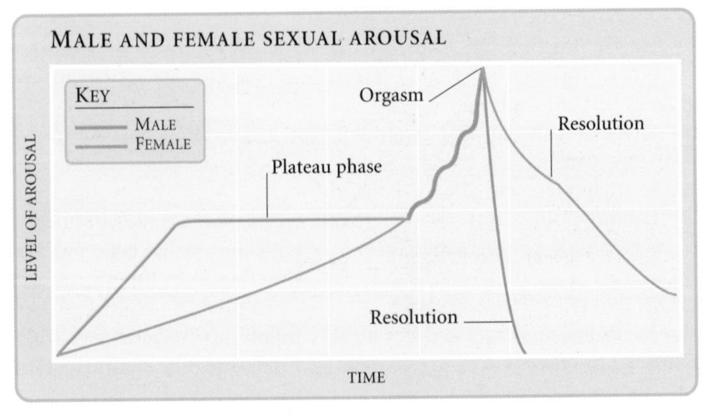

Phases of sexual arousal
In men, sexual excitement rises rapidly to reach a plateau; in women, arousal is more gradual. In both sexes, arousal peaks at orgasm, which may not occur simultaneously, and wanes in the resolution phase.

FUNCTION SEXUAL INTERCOURSE

When a couple is sexually aroused (*see* SEXUAL RESPONSE, opposite page), the man's penis becomes erect and the woman's vagina is lubricated. During sexual intercourse, also called coitus, the penis is inserted into the vagina and the man begins thrusting pelvic movements. At orgasm, which the partners may experience simultaneously or at different times, intense, pleasurable sensations spread throughout the body. The woman's vaginal walls contract rhythmically and the man ejaculates, releasing sperm.

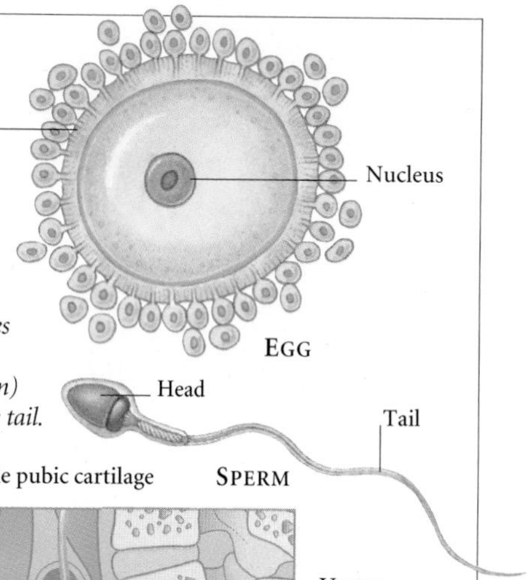

Protective layer
Nucleus
EGG
Head
Tail
SPERM

Egg and sperm
The egg is about 0.1 mm ($\frac{1}{250}$ in) in diameter. The sperm (not shown to scale) is 20 times smaller – about 0.005 mm ($\frac{1}{5000}$ in) long, including the tail.

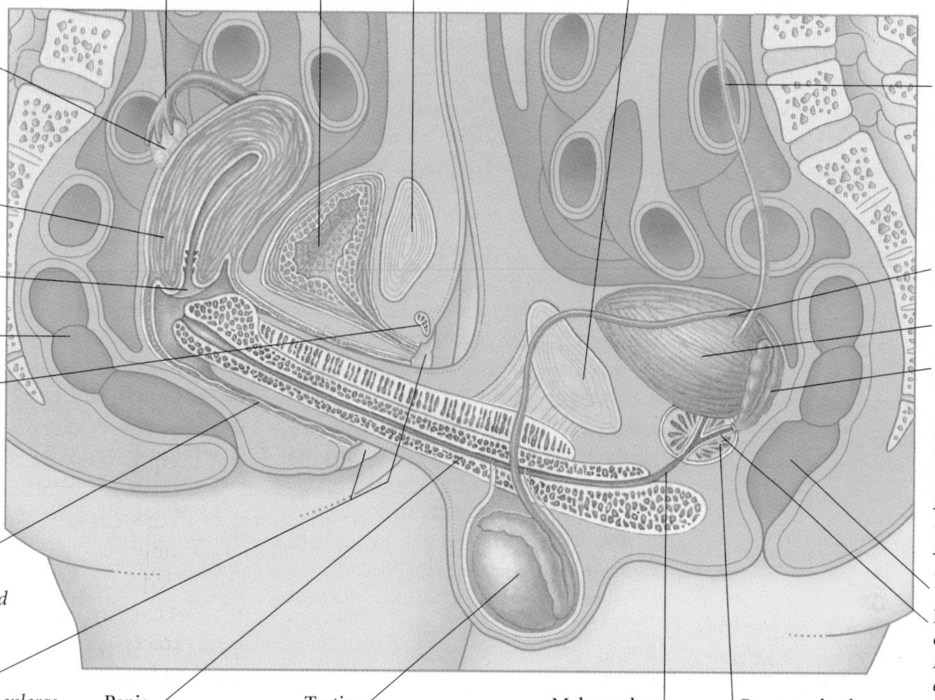

Fallopian tube
Female bladder
Female pubic cartilage
Male pubic cartilage
Ovary
Uterus
The uterus lifts to extend the vagina
Cervix
Rectum
Clitoris
The clitoris becomes enlarged and more prominent
Vagina
The vagina expands and moistens
Labia
The labia enlarge as they become engorged with blood
Penis
The penis stiffens to enter the vagina
Testis
The testes draw closer to the body during intercourse
Male urethra
Semen is ejaculated through this tube
Prostate gland
This gland adds secretions to the semen
Ureter
Vas deferens
Sperm is carried from each testis to ejaculatory ducts by these tubes
Male bladder
Seminal vesicles
These glands, one on either side of the bladder, add fluid to the sperm to form semen
Rectum
Ejaculatory duct
Each of these ducts joins the vas deferens to the urethra

Ovary
Direction of sperm
Fallopian tube
Uterus
Cervix
Vagina
Penis

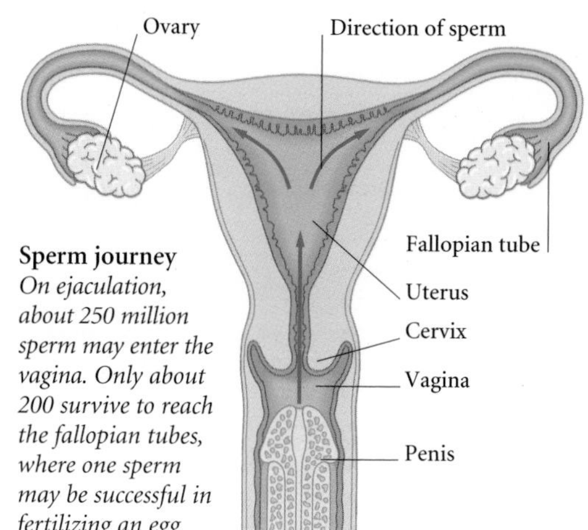

Sperm journey
On ejaculation, about 250 million sperm may enter the vagina. Only about 200 survive to reach the fallopian tubes, where one sperm may be successful in fertilizing an egg.

FUNCTION FERTILIZATION

Fertilization takes place in one of the fallopian tubes. Many sperm reach the egg and try to penetrate its outer covering. If a sperm succeeds, its head enters the egg and its tail is then shed. A membrane then rapidly forms around the egg, creating a barrier to prevent other sperm from entering. Fertilization occurs when the head of the sperm fuses with the nucleus of the egg.

Sperm
Egg

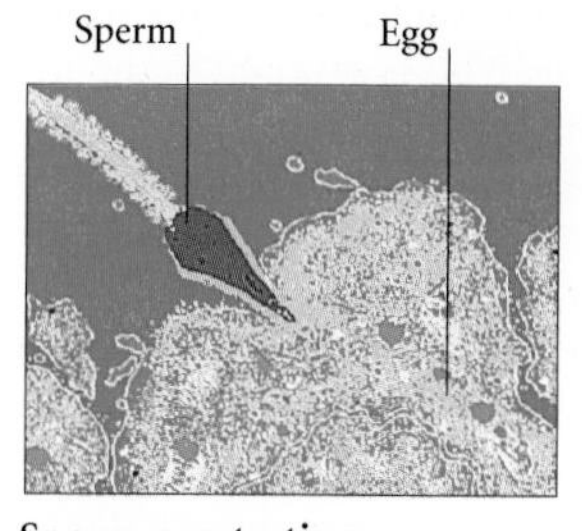

Sperm penetrating egg
The head of the sperm pushes through the egg's outer coating in order to reach the nucleus.

SEXUALLY TRANSMITTED INFECTIONS

Sexually transmitted infections (STIs) are infections that are passed primarily from person to person during sexual activity. Many people delay seeking medical help for STIs because of embarrassment, but early diagnosis often prevents complications. Most STIs can be treated successfully with modern drugs.

The diseases covered in this section are grouped according to the type of organism that causes them. The first few articles discuss bacterial infections such as gonorrhea. The protozoal infection trichomoniasis is then described, and the following articles deal with viral infections, such as genital warts. The final article looks at parasitic infestation with pubic lice.

Early treatment of STIs is essential because some, such as chlamydial infection, may cause infertility. Sexually active people who frequently change their partners should have routine tests because some STIs may not cause symptoms, and many people are unaware that they have an STI. Syphilis, a progressive and once fatal disease, can now usually be fully cured if it is treated when it is first detected. STIs such as genital herpes and genital warts can often recur. Some types of genital wart virus increase the risk of cancer of the cervix. Pregnant women with an STI must carefully follow their recommended treatment because STIs can pass to the baby during pregnancy or in the birth canal during childbirth.

HIV infection and AIDS (p.297) and certain forms of hepatitis (pp.644–645) are viral infections that can also be transmitted by sexual contact.

The risk of contracting STIs can be reduced by using the safe sex practices, covered here and in detail elsewhere (*see* SEX AND HEALTH, pp.67–71).

Gonorrhoea

A bacterial infection that causes genital inflammation and discharge

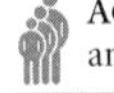 AGE Can affect sexually active people of any age

 GENDER More frequent in males

 LIFESTYLE Unprotected sex with multiple partners is a risk factor

 GENETICS Not a significant factor

The bacterium *Neisseria gonorrhoeae* (gonococcus), which causes gonorrhoea, can be transmitted by various forms of sexual contact, including vaginal, oral, and anal sex. The infection is usually confined to the site where the bacteria enter the body, such as the vagina or the mouth, but can spread through the bloodstream to other parts of the body. A baby who is exposed to the infection in the birth canal during delivery may develop neonatal ophthalmia, a severe eye infection that can cause blindness (*see* CONJUNCTIVITIS, p.570).

The incidence of gonorrhoea is decreasing, partly due to the practice of safe sex (p.68). By the end of the 20th century, there were about 12,000 cases of gonorrhoea each year in the UK. Nongonococcal urethritis (opposite page), genital herpes (p.767), and chlamydial pelvic infection (opposite page) are all more prevalent diseases.

WHAT ARE THE SYMPTOMS?

Gonorrhoea often causes no symptoms. If symptoms occur, they usually appear 1–14 days after sex with an infected person. In men, they may include:

- Discharge of pus from the penis.
- Pain on passing urine.

Without treatment, the symptoms may start to disappear after about 2 weeks, but the person remains infectious.

About 1 in 5 infected women has symptoms, which may include:

- Yellowish-green discharge of pus from the vagina.
- Pain on passing urine.
- Lower abdominal pain.
- Irregular vaginal bleeding.

In both sexes, if gonorrhoea occurs as a result of anal intercourse, the anus and the rectum may become inflamed (*see* PROCTITIS, p.667), but usually there are no symptoms. If the infection has been transmitted during oral sex, the first symptom may be a sore throat.

ARE THERE COMPLICATIONS?

Gonorrhoea in men can lead to inflammation of the testes and epididymides (the tubes that carry sperm from the testes), a condition called epididymo-orchitis (p.718). Gonorrhoea may also result in inflammation of the prostate gland (*see* PROSTATITIS, p.724) or of the bladder (*see* CYSTITIS, p.709). Rarely, the disorder results in urethral stricture (p.714), scarring and blockage of the urethra (the tube from the bladder) that causes difficulty in passing urine.

In women, the infection may spread from the vagina to the fallopian tubes and cause pelvic inflammatory disease (p.741). Left untreated, the disorder increases the risk of ectopic pregnancy (p.790) and can make women infertile (*see* FEMALE INFERTILITY, p.775).

Occasionally, gonorrhoea spreads in the bloodstream, causing fever, rash, and, rarely, infection of the joints (*see* SEPTIC ARTHRITIS, p.381).

WHAT MIGHT BE DONE?

If you suspect that you or your partner has gonorrhoea, go to a clinic specializing in STIs or to your doctor. To confirm the diagnosis, a swab will be taken from areas that are likely to be infected and

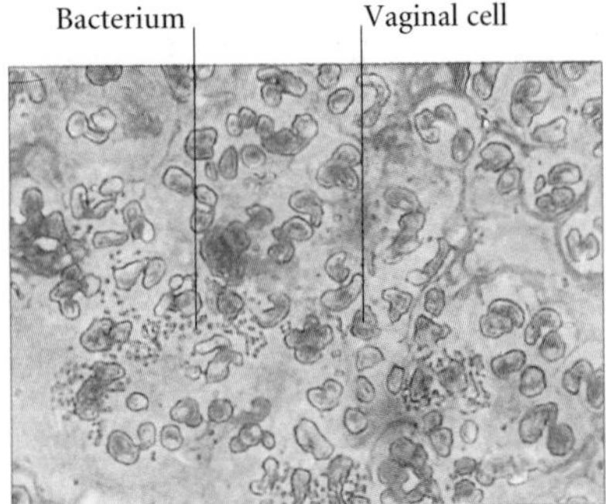

Cells infected by gonorrhoea bacteria
The vaginal cells in this image have been infected by Neisseria gonorrhoeae, *the bacterium that causes gonorrhoea.*

tested for the bacteria. You will also have tests for other STIs, such as chlamydial infection. Gonorrhoea is treated with antibiotics (p.885) and usually clears up in 3–4 days. If bacteria have spread throughout the body, treatment with intravenous antibiotics in hospital is necessary. All sexual partners should be tested and offered treatment.

CAN IT BE PREVENTED?

You can take steps to reduce your risk of contracting gonorrhoea (*see* PREVENTING STIs, right). If you are infected, avoid sex until you and your partner have finished treatment and your doctor says that you are free of infection.

(WWW) ONLINE SITES: p.1036

Nongonococcal urethritis

Inflammation of the urethra in men that may be caused by several different organisms

 AGE Can affect sexually active males of any age

 GENDER Affects men. Women can carry the infection

 LIFESTYLE Unprotected sex with multiple partners is a risk factor

 GENETICS Not a significant factor

Inflammation of the male urethra (the tube leading from the bladder to the tip of the penis) that is not due to the bacterium causing gonorrhoea (opposite page) is known as nongonococcal urethritis (NGU). Worldwide, NGU is one of the most common sexually transmitted infections (STIs) in men.

WHAT ARE THE CAUSES?

Nearly half of all cases of NGU are due to a bacterium, *Chlamydia trachomatis*, which can also infect the female reproductive organs (*see* CHLAMYDIAL PELVIC INFECTION, right). NGU can also be due to another bacterium, *Ureaplasma urealyticum;* the protozoan *Trichomonas vaginalis*, which also causes trichomoniasis (p.767); and the fungus *Candida albicans*, which can cause candidiasis (p.309). The viruses that cause genital warts (p.768) and genital herpes (p.767) can result in NGU if they affect the urethra. Often, no cause is found.

WHAT ARE THE SYMPTOMS?

About 1–6 weeks after you have become infected with NGU, the following group of symptoms may develop:

- Pain on passing urine, especially the first time in the morning.
- Discharge from the penis.
- Redness and soreness at the opening of the urethra.

If you have any of these symptoms, you should go to a clinic specializing in STIs or consult your doctor.

ARE THERE COMPLICATIONS?

Various complications may result from NGU, including inflammation of the prostate gland (*see* PROSTATITIS, p.724), which causes pain around the rectum and anus, in the genitals, and on ejaculation. Occasionally, the testes and the epididymides (the tubes carrying sperm from the testes) become inflamed (*see* EPIDIDYMO-ORCHITIS, p.718). The infection may trigger an immune response that causes inflammation of the joints (*see* REACTIVE ARTHRITIS, p.379).

WHAT MIGHT BE DONE?

Your doctor will take a swab from your urethra, together with a urine sample, to check for the presence of an infectious organism that could cause NGU. Tests for other STIs will probably be carried out at the same time.

Depending on the organism found, your doctor may then prescribe antibiotics (p.885), antifungal drugs (p.889), or antiviral drugs (p.886). With treatment, NGU usually clears up in about a week; however, it sometimes returns, and treatment may need to be repeated. You can also be reinfected if your sexual partner has the disease. Sexual partners must be tested and treated even if they have no symptoms because in women the infection causes pelvic inflammation, which can lead to infertility (*see* FEMALE INFERTILITY, p.775).

CAN IT BE PREVENTED?

The risk of contracting NGU can be reduced by following safe sex measures (*see* PREVENTING STIs, right). To avoid spreading the infection, it is important that you do not have sexual contact until you and your partner have finished your treatment and your doctor confirms that you are no longer infected.

(WWW) ONLINE SITES: p.1036

SELF-HELP

PREVENTING STIs

There are several safe sex measures that you can follow to reduce the risk of acquiring an STI:

- Avoid sex with multiple partners.
- In a new sexual relationship, you or your partner should use a condom and a spermicide containing nonoxinol "9", which may have an antiviral effect.
- If you use lubricants, use water-based types; oil-based lubricants damage the rubber in condoms.
- Avoid sexual activity that may split a condom or sex that causes breaks in the skin or the tissues of the vagina or anus.

If you suspect that you or your partner has an STI, you should both consult an STI clinic or a doctor. Complete your course of treatment and avoid sexual contact until your doctor confirms that you are free of infection (*see* SEX AND HEALTH, pp.67–71).

Chlamydial pelvic infection

An infection of the genital tract in women that is usually symptomless

 AGE Affects sexually active women of any age

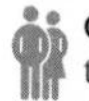 GENDER Affects women. Men can carry the infection

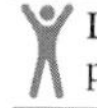 LIFESTYLE Unprotected sex with multiple partners is a risk factor

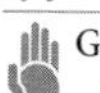 GENETICS Not a significant factor

The bacterium *Chlamydia trachomatis* causes a common sexually transmitted infection (STI). In women, the infection can cause serious inflammation of the reproductive organs. In men, it is the most common cause of nongonococcal urethritis (left). A baby exposed to infection during delivery may develop the eye disorder conjunctivitis (p.570).

WHAT ARE THE SYMPTOMS?

Most women are symptom-free, but if symptoms do occur, they may include:

- Abnormal vaginal discharge.
- Frequent urge to pass urine.

- Pain in the lower abdomen.
- Pain on deep penetration during sex.

Left untreated, chlamydial infection can spread from the cervix to the fallopian tubes (*see* PELVIC INFLAMMATORY DISEASE, p.741), and is a common cause of infertility in women. The infection sometimes triggers an immune response that leads to a form of arthritis (*see* REACTIVE ARTHRITIS, p.379).

WHAT MIGHT BE DONE?

Infection with chlamydia may not be suspected until symptoms develop or a partner is tested for an STI. The disorder may also be suspected during investigations for infertility, which can be a complication of untreated chlamydial infection. For this reason, screening is important for sexually active women at high risk, including those who have been treated previously for an STI or who have multiple partners.

If you think that you or your partner has a chlamydial infection you should go to a clinic that specializes in STIs or consult your own doctor. In women, diagnosis is confirmed by taking a swab from the cervix. Tests for other STIs may be performed at the same time.

Treatment for the infection is with antibiotics (p.885). Even if they are free of symptoms, sexual partners should be tested and treated.

CAN IT BE PREVENTED?

You can reduce your risk of contracting chlamydial infection by following safe sex measures (*see* PREVENTING STIs, p.765). You and your partner should abstain from sexual contact until treatment has been completed.

(WWW) ONLINE SITES: p.1036

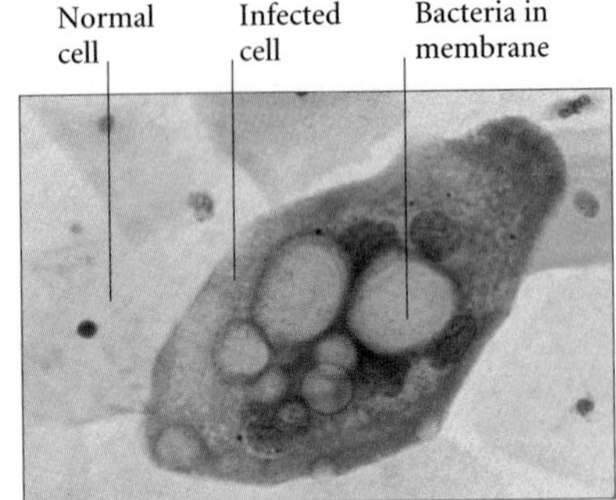

Cervical cell infected by chlamydia
The magnified view of a cervical specimen shows an infected cell in which chlamydia bacteria are enclosed within a membrane.

Syphilis

A bacterial infection initially affecting the genitals that, left untreated, can damage other parts of the body years later

AGE Can affect sexually active people of any age

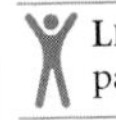
LIFESTYLE Unprotected sex with multiple partners is a risk factor

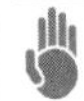
GENDER GENETICS Not significant factors

Syphilis is caused by the bacterium *Treponema pallidum*. This organism enters the body through the mucous membranes of the genital area or the skin. Left untreated, the disease may be fatal.

Syphilis was once a widespread disease throughout the world but became less common with the introduction of the antibiotic penicillin in the 1940s. Today, the disease rarely progresses to its most advanced stage. A rise in incidence in homosexual men in the 1960s and 70s was reversed by safe sex practices to combat HIV infection in the 1980s. Incidence is now very low.

A pregnant woman with syphilis can pass the disease to the fetus, causing it to develop congenital syphilis (*see* CONGENITAL INFECTIONS, p.817). However, screening during pregnancy has now made congenital syphilis very rare.

WHAT ARE THE SYMPTOMS?

The symptoms of syphilis develop in three stages. The primary and secondary stages are infectious for up to 2 years. The tertiary stage is not infectious.

PRIMARY STAGE Within 1–12 weeks of contact with an infected person, the following symptoms may develop:

- Hard, painless, and highly infectious sore known as a chancre. The chancre usually appears on the penis or vulva but may occur in the mouth or rectum as a result of oral or anal sex.
- Painless enlargement of the lymph nodes in the groin or neck.

The chancre may go unnoticed and disappears after 1–6 weeks.

SECONDARY STAGE About 6–24 weeks after the appearance of the chancre, the following symptoms develop:

- Nonitchy, infectious rash over the whole body, including the palms of the hands and soles of the feet.

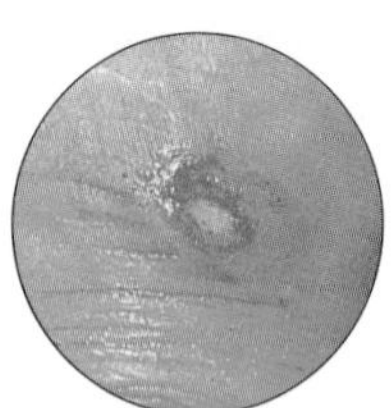

Chancre on penis
In primary stage syphilis, a hard, painless sore, called a chancre, appears. It usually develops on the genitals.

- Thickened, grey or pink, moist, wartlike patches in the skin folds of the genitals and anus.
- In rare cases, patchy hair loss.
- Fever and tiredness.
- Headaches and muscle pain.

After 4–12 weeks, these symptoms disappear, and the disease then enters a symptomless stage of indefinite length.

TERTIARY STAGE Some people remain without further symptoms for the rest of their lives. However, if treatment is not given, tertiary syphilis may develop 10–20 years after the initial infection. The symptoms vary and may include changes in personality; mental illness; meningitis (p.527); tabes dorsalis (destruction of the spinal cord), which causes weakness and difficulty in walking; and aortic aneurysm (p.430).

WHAT MIGHT BE DONE?

If you think you or your partner has syphilis go to a clinic specializing in STIs or consult your doctor. In the primary stage, you may have a swab of the chancre taken for microscopic examination. Diagnosis of both primary and secondary syphilis may be confirmed by a blood test. At the same time you will probably be tested for other STIs. If tertiary syphilis is suspected, a lumbar puncture (p.527) may be carried out to look for antibodies to the bacterium in the cerebrospinal fluid.

Syphilis is treated with injections of antibiotics (p.885). In the primary or secondary stages, treatment usually results in complete recovery. Damage due to tertiary syphilis may be permanent.

CAN IT BE PREVENTED?

The risk of contracting syphilis is reduced by taking safe sex measures (*see* PREVENTING STIs, p.765). If you have the disease, or your partner has it, avoid sexual contact until you have both finished your treatment and your doctor confirms that you are free of infection.

(WWW) ONLINE SITES: p.1036

Trichomoniasis

A genital tract infection that may cause a vaginal discharge in women but is usually symptomless in men

AGE Can affect sexually active people of any age

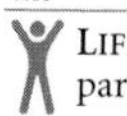
LIFESTYLE Unprotected sex with multiple partners is a risk factor

GENDER GENETICS Not significant factors

Trichomoniasis is an infection caused by the protozoan *Trichomonas vaginalis.* In women, this infection may cause vulvovaginitis (p.752), inflammation in and around the vagina, which may lead to a profuse vaginal discharge and to cystitis (p.709). In men, the infection may cause mild inflammation of the urethra (the tube from the bladder to the outside of the body) and occasionally results in nongonococcal urethritis (p.765). In most cases, trichomoniasis is a sexually transmitted infection, but an infected pregnant woman may pass the infection to her baby during birth (*see* CONGENITAL INFECTIONS, p.817).

WHAT ARE THE SYMPTOMS?

Some women have no symptoms, and the infection may only be detected on a routine smear test (p.749). If symptoms do occur, they may include:

- Profuse, yellow, frothy, and offensive-smelling discharge from the vagina.
- Painful inflammation of the vagina.
- Itching and soreness of the vulva (the skin around the vagina).
- Burning sensation on passing urine.
- Discomfort during intercourse.

Men, usually have no symptoms, but if present, they may include:

- Discomfort on passing urine.
- Discharge from the penis.

If you or your partner develop any of these symptoms, go to a clinic specializing in STIs or consult your doctor.

WHAT MIGHT BE DONE?

Swabs will be taken from infected areas and tested for the presence of the protozoan. You will probably be tested for other STIs at the same time. If you have trichomoniasis, you will be prescribed antibiotics (p.885). Sexual partners, and babies who are born to infected mothers, should also be tested and treated, even if they have no symptoms.

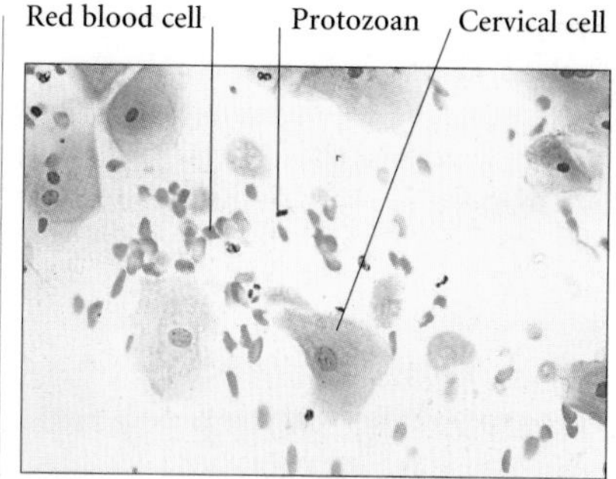

Trichomoniasis protozoan
This magnified image of cells from the cervix shows the presence of Trichomonas vaginalis, *the protozoan responsible for causing trichomoniasis.*

CAN IT BE PREVENTED?

You can reduce your risk of contracting trichomoniasis by practising safe sex (*see* PREVENTING STIs, p.765). If you or your partner have been infected, you should avoid spreading the infection further by abstaining from sexual contact until you have both finished your course of drug treatment and your doctor has confirmed that the infection has cleared up completely.

(WWW) ONLINE SITES: p.1036

Genital herpes

A viral infection that causes painful blisters on and around the genitals that can recur

AGE Can affect sexually active people of any age

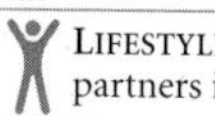
LIFESTYLE Unprotected sex with multiple partners is a risk factor

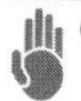
GENDER GENETICS Not significant factors

Genital herpes is caused by the herpes simplex virus, of which there are two forms, known as type 1 (HSV-1) and type 2 (HSV-2). Genital herpes is usually due to type 2; type 1 mainly causes blisters around the mouth (*see* COLD SORE, p.354). However, HSV-1 can be transmitted from the mouth to the genitals during oral sex, producing genital herpes. In the UK, there are 15,000 new cases of genital herpes each year.

The disease can recur, especially in the first few years after the initial attack. In women, it tends to recur 5–12 days before a period and to clear up in a few days. Subsequent attacks are milder, but still infectious. A pregnant woman with genital herpes should inform her midwife of the fact because, very rarely, the infection causes serious illness in a baby exposed to it during birth (*see* CONGENITAL INFECTIONS, p.817).

WHAT ARE THE SYMPTOMS?

The first attack of genital herpes is usually the most severe and occurs within 5 days of contact with an infected person. The symptoms may include:

- Painful, fluid-filled blisters on the genitals. Blisters may occur on the thighs and buttocks and, rarely, in the mouth or rectum due to oral or anal sex.
- Tingling, burning, soreness, and redness of the affected area.
- Enlarged and painful lymph nodes in the groin.
- Pain on passing urine.
- Headache, fever, and muscle aches.
- In women, vaginal discharge.

After 10–21 days the symptoms usually disappear. There may be further milder attacks, often affecting the same areas.

WHAT MIGHT BE DONE?

If you suspect genital herpes in yourself or your partner go to a clinic specializing in STIs or consult your doctor. A diagnosis will probably be made from your symptoms and a physical examination. Swabs of the blisters may be taken to test for the virus. You may also have tests for other STIs. Partners need to attend for a checkup even if they have no obvious symptoms.

Genital herpes cannot be cured. Your doctor may prescribe aciclovir or another antiviral drug (p.886) during an attack. If aciclovir is taken early, it usually reduces the severity of symptoms.

WHAT IS THE PROGNOSIS?

About 2 in 10 infected people have only one attack. However, the virus remains in the body, and some people have recurrent attacks a few times a year for several years. Symptoms are usually less severe in subsequent attacks and the time between attacks increases.

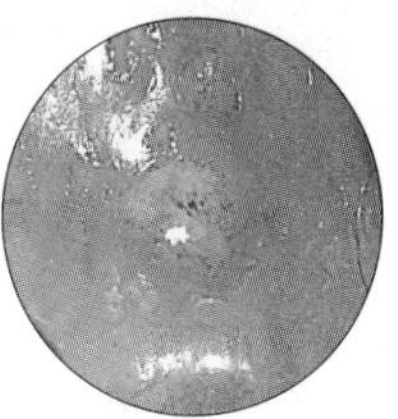

Genital herpes
The fluid-filled blisters shown in this close-up of a penis are caused by the genital herpes virus.

CAN IT BE PREVENTED?

The risk of contracting genital herpes can be reduced by practising safe sex (*see* PREVENTING STIs, p.765). However, a condom may not always provide total protection since areas of skin around the genitals may have blisters or be less obviously infected. The virus can be passed on even if no blisters are present. If you have an attack, avoid sex until the symptoms have gone.

If you have repeated attacks, your doctor may prescribe preventive treatment with an antiviral drug to reduce the risk of a recurrence. Treatment is rarely needed for more than a year.

A pregnant woman who has a genital herpes attack close to delivery may need a caesarean section to prevent the infection passing to the baby.

(WWW) ONLINE SITES: p.1033, p.1036

Genital warts

Fleshy, painless growths on and around the genitals caused by a virus

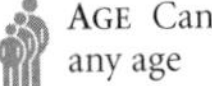 AGE Can affect sexually active people of any age

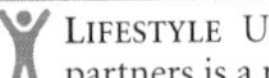 LIFESTYLE Unprotected sex with multiple partners is a risk factor

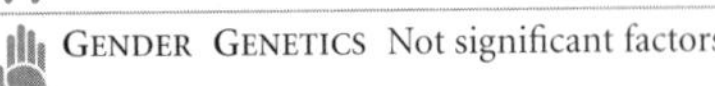 GENDER GENETICS Not significant factors

Genital warts are skin growths caused by the human papillomavirus (HPV). In the UK, genital warts is one of the most prevalent sexually transmitted infections (STIs). At the end of the 20th century, there were about 60,000 cases each year. The disorder is reported more often by men than by women, probably because warts are more visible on the penis. An infected person can transmit the virus to sexual partners even if he or she has no symptoms.

The warts appear from a few weeks to as long as 20 months after infection. They are usually soft with a rough surface and are painless. A few may have a hard surface. Genital warts become larger rapidly, and in some instances the growths cluster together in one area.

In men, warts may occur on the shaft of the penis, on the foreskin, on the glans (head of the penis), or around the anus. In women, warts may appear on the vulva (the external part of the female genitals) or develop inside the vagina, on the cervix, and around the anus. The warts may also occur in the rectum due to infection through anal intercourse. If a pregnant woman has genital warts, she should make sure that her midwife is aware of the fact because there is a very small risk of passing the infection to the baby during delivery.

WHAT MIGHT BE DONE?

If you or your partner has genital warts, or if you have been exposed to infection, you should or go to a clinic that specializes in STIs or consult your doctor. Diagnosis is based on a physical examination. Tests may also be performed to check for other STIs.

There are several ways of treating genital warts. You may be prescribed a cream containing imiquimod or podophyllin for use on external genital areas and applied directly to the warts. The treatment is repeated until the warts have gone. Other techniques include cryotherapy, in which the warts are destroyed by freezing; electrocautery, which burns them off; laser treatment; surgical removal; or injecting each wart with interferon drugs (p.907), proteins that stimulate the body's immunity to the virus. Warts may recur, but in most cases the body's immune system controls them eventually.

Some types of HPV that occur in the cervix have been associated with cancer of the cervix (p.750). If HPV is identified on a cervical smear test (p.749), close monitoring, follow-up tests, and treatment will be given. However, these are not the same types of HPV that cause genital warts, and no link has been established between genital warts and cancer of the cervix.

CAN IT BE PREVENTED?

You can reduce your risk of contracting genital warts by practising safe sex (*see* PREVENTING STIs, p.765). People are often advised to avoid sexual contact when warts are visible. However, warts can be acquired from someone who is a carrier of the virus but has no symptoms, so there is a risk of becoming infected from any new partner. To prevent short-term recurrence of warts, condoms should be used for 12 weeks after treatment has finished, but condoms may not give total protection since they may not cover all affected areas.

(WWW) ONLINE SITES: p.1036

Pubic lice

Infestation of pubic hair by a type of small wingless parasite causing irritation

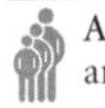 AGE Can affect sexually active people of any age

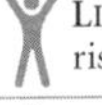 LIFESTYLE Sex with multiple partners is a risk factor

GENDER GENETICS Not significant factors

Pubic lice, often called "crabs", are usually spread by sexual contact. The lice live in pubic hair, where they feed on blood and lay eggs called nits. About 10,000 cases of infestation with pubic lice are treated in STI clinics in the UK each year. The most common symptom is itching in the pubic area and around the anus, especially at night. Some people have no symptoms and only realize that they are infested when they see the nits or the tiny insects. Normal washing does not remove the nits since they are firmly stuck to the hair.

If you think that you or your partner has pubic lice, you should consult your doctor or go to a clinic specializing in sexually transmitted infections (STIs).

WHAT MIGHT BE DONE?

Your doctor will probably prescribe a preparation containing lindane or permethrin to apply to affected areas (*see* PREPARATIONS FOR SKIN INFECTIONS AND INFESTATIONS, p.892). A second application is needed about 10 days after the first to destroy freshly hatched lice.

To prevent the spread of lice, sexual partners should be checked and treated if necessary. The clothing and sheets used by an infested person should be machine-washed in hot water.

(WWW) ONLINE SITES: p.1036

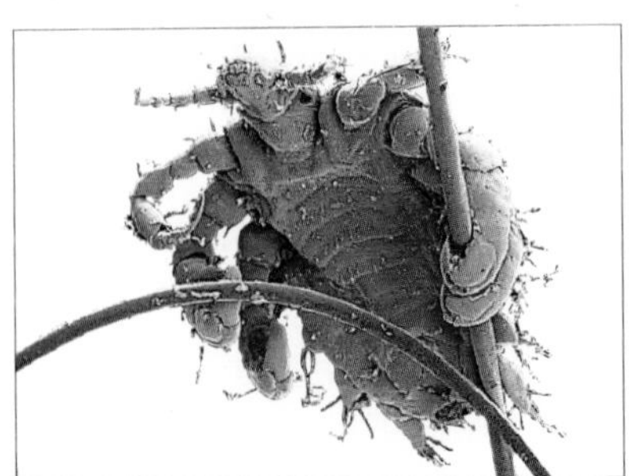

Pubic louse

This highly magnified image shows a pubic louse attached to a human hair. Lice are about 2 mm ($^1/_{12}$ in) in width.

SEXUAL PROBLEMS

Most men and women experience a sexual problem at some time in their lives. Some problems, such as decreased sex drive and pain during intercourse, may be experienced by either partner, while others, such as impotence and vaginismus, are specific to men or women. Sexual problems have many causes, including physical and psychological disorders and certain drug treatments.

The most common sexual problem that affects both sexes is decreased sex drive. This is often a natural response to changing hormone levels, although there are many other causes. Other common problems include failure of orgasm in women, and, in men, impotence and premature ejaculation, which affect most men at some time.

A sexual problem may begin with an underlying physical cause, but anxiety about sexual performance can often develop and compound the original problem. Sometimes, a sexual problem experienced by one partner may be caused by the response or behaviour of the other partner. For these reasons, doctors and sex therapists generally prefer to involve both partners in discussions and therapy sessions to promote mutual understanding and appreciation. This is particularly important when the recommended treatment involves exercises to be practised at home by both partners.

A variety of treatments is currently available, and there are many doctors and therapists who specialize in treating sexual problems. Sources of specialized help include urologists, gynaecologists, sex therapists, and counsellors. For some problems, assistance from a psychiatrist or psychologist may be helpful. Treatments for sexual problems have a high success rate.

Decreased sex drive

A temporary or long-term reduction of interest in sex

AGE More common with increasing age

GENETICS In rare cases, due to an extra chromosome

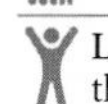
LIFESTYLE Physical and mental stress and the use of certain drugs may be risk factors

GENDER Not a significant factor

Someone whose sex drive has decreased loses interest in sex, does not fantasize about sex, and feels little or no pleasure during sexual activity. It is common for a person to experience a temporary loss of sex drive, or libido, at some point in his or her life. However, a long-term decrease in a person's sex drive may become a problem if it causes distress either to the individual concerned or to his or her sexual partner.

Sex drive is partly controlled by sex hormones, which decrease gradually as you grow older. As a result, sex drive also declines naturally with age. However, men and women have different patterns of sexual desire. Sex drive is most intense in young men in their teens and 20s, whereas most women reach their sexual peak later in life, often not until their 30s. Different people have different levels of sex drive and activity. For this reason, a decrease in your sex drive should be judged only in comparison with your own normal sex drive and activity, not in comparison with the claims of other people.

WHAT ARE THE CAUSES?

Many women experience a temporary decline in sex drive after childbirth or gynaecological surgery, and sometimes during pregnancy. Menopausal women may also be affected both because of fluctuations in the levels of their sex hormones and because of their emotional responses to the menopause. Many women experience regular fluctuations in sexual desire that reflect the normal changes in hormone levels that occur during the menstrual cycle.

A number of psychological problems may trigger a loss of interest in sex in either men or women. Such problems may include anxiety disorders (p.551), depression (p.554), stress (p.74), and general problems with the relationship.

A reduction in sex drive may be a side effect of certain drugs, including some contraceptive pills; some types of antidepressant drug (p.916); and certain antihypertensive drugs (p.897), such as beta-blockers (p.898). Heavy drinking may also decrease sex drive.

Other possible causes include illness and tiredness as well as a few rare genetic disorders, such as Klinefelter's syndrome (p.822), which affects only males and results in low levels of sex hormones.

WHAT CAN I DO?

You may be able to identify the reason for your loss of sex drive. If you suspect that stress or heavy drinking may be the cause, try changing your lifestyle. If you think that the cause is an underlying problem in your relationship, it may help to discuss the issue with your partner (*see* COMMUNICATING YOUR SEXUAL NEEDS, p.770). If you cannot improve the situation, consult your doctor.

WHAT MIGHT THE DOCTOR DO?

Your doctor will discuss your lifestyle and relationship with you to determine which factors are contributing to the problem. If your doctor suspects that your decreased sex drive is the result of a physical condition, he or she may examine you and arrange for tests to look for a disorder. For example, blood tests may be used to check for abnormally low hormone levels in men. If your decreased sex drive is a side effect of a particular drug, your doctor may give you a different medication. The doctor may also suggest changes in your lifestyle, such as reducing stress or cutting down on alcohol intake. If the cause seems to be psychological, your doctor may recommend that you and your partner have sex therapy (p.773).

Most people who consult a doctor about a decrease in their sex drive can be treated successfully.

(WWW) ONLINE SITES: p.1034, p.1036, p.1037

Failure of orgasm

Inability to reach the peak of sexual excitement

 AGE Can affect sexually active people of any age

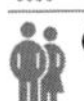 GENDER Common in females; rare in males

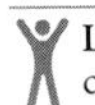 LIFESTYLE Stress, alcohol, and the use of certain drugs are risk factors

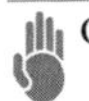 GENETICS Not a significant factor

Failure to reach orgasm, the peak of sexual excitement, is called anorgasmia. The causes are usually psychological. Anorgasmia is the most frequently reported sexual problem in women and affects up to half of all women at some time in their lives. Fewer than 1 in 10 men report failure to reach orgasm.

WHAT ARE THE CAUSES?

Psychological factors that can inhibit orgasm include anxiety about sexual performance, fear of pregnancy, a previous unpleasant sexual experience, physical or mental abuse during childhood, and sexual inhibitions as a result of a strict upbringing regarding sex.

Poor sexual technique on the part of one or both partners may lead to failure of orgasm. Most often, insufficient time is allowed for the woman to become fully aroused. Poor sexual technique is common between new partners who know little about each other's sexual responses. The problem may also be due to inexperience or a lack of communication between partners.

Some long-term disorders that result in damage to nerves, including diabetes mellitus (p.687), may lead to failure of orgasm. Certain drugs, such as particular antidepressants (p.916) and some antihypertensive drugs (p.897), including beta-blockers (p.898), can cause a decreased sex drive (p.769) that may result in anorgasmia. Heavy drinking may also cause failure of orgasm.

WHAT MIGHT BE DONE?

If you or your partner repeatedly fail to reach orgasm, it is important to discuss the matter together (*see* COMMUNICATING YOUR SEXUAL NEEDS, right). Your doctor should be consulted if the situation does not improve. If the problem is psychological or due to poor sexual technique, you will probably be referred to a sex therapist (*see* SEX THERAPY, p.773). If the problem is caused by drug treatment, the doctor may change your medication. However, if you have nerve damage, the problem is usually permanent and cannot be treated.

Sex therapy is effective in most cases, but, if you or your partner have deep-rooted problems such as difficulties due to abuse in childhood, some form of psychological therapy (pp.968–971) may be needed. Failure of orgasm can be treated successfully in many people.

(WWW) ONLINE SITES: p.1034, p.1036, p.1037

Impotence

Inability to achieve or sustain an erection, also known as erectile dysfunction

 AGE More common with increasing age

 LIFESTYLE Smoking, alcohol, stress, and the use of certain drugs are risk factors

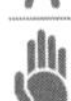 GENETICS Not a significant factor

Most men experience temporary difficulty in achieving or maintaining an erection at some time in their lives. Such occasional impotence is normal. Persistent, long-term difficulty in achieving an erection may indicate a physical cause and should prompt you to seek medical advice. Impotence over a long period often results in distress for both the individual and his partner. Despite this, only 1 in 10 men who has the condition seeks medical advice.

WHAT ARE THE CAUSES?

Impotence can be due to a physical or a psychological disorder and in many cases may be a combination of the two. Anxiety disorders (p.551) and depression (p.554) can lead to impotence, and may themselves be a reflection of stress in a man's life, a relationship difficulty, or fear of sexual failure. Impotence may also be a side effect of drugs, such as antidepressants (p.916) and antihypertensives (p.897). The risk of impotence can be increased by factors such as tiredness, heavy drinking, and smoking.

The condition is more common in middle-aged and elderly men and often has a physical cause. The most common cause is a vascular disease, such as atherosclerosis (p.402), that reduces the blood supply to the penis. Impotence can also result if the nerves supplying the penis are damaged due to surgery, such as operations on the prostate gland (*see* PARTIAL PROSTATECTOMY, p.725, and RADICAL PROSTATECTOMY, p.727), or to long-term conditions such as multiple sclerosis (p.541) or diabetes mellitus (p.687). Rarely, impotence is due to low levels of the sex hormone testosterone.

Episodes of sudden and intermittent impotence usually have a psychological cause. Impotence that develops gradually and is persistent or progressive is primarily due to physical causes.

WHAT MIGHT BE DONE?

If you have persistent problems with impotence, you should consult your doctor. He or she will ask if you have full morning erections. If you do, it is more likely that your impotence has a psychological cause. Your doctor will also ask about your lifestyle and about any medication that you use to see if there are factors contributing to your problem that can be altered.

The doctor may give you a physical examination. He or she may take a blood sample to check for diabetes mellitus

(SELF-HELP)

COMMUNICATING YOUR SEXUAL NEEDS

Many people feel that the sexual side of their relationship could be better. The key to improving your sex life is communication with your partner and mutual understanding. Bear the following points in mind when you discuss your problems with your partner:

- Think carefully about your words and timing to avoid sounding hostile or critical.
- Talk about the positive aspects of your sex life.
- Suggest things that you would like to do or would like to spend more time on; watch your partner's reaction carefully.
- Keep your comments open and your suggestions positive.
- Listen to what your partner says.
- Create an action plan together, and include the points that you would both like to work on.

and to measure your testosterone level. You may also be referred to a specialist for Doppler ultrasound scanning (p.432) to assess the blood flow to your penis.

If the blood vessels to the penis are narrowed due to atherosclerosis, surgery may restore normal blood flow and allow you to achieve an erection. Your doctor may change your medication if drug treatment is a likely cause. If you have diabetes, your doctor should make sure that it is well controlled to prevent further nerve damage.

In addition, if your doctor suspects that an aspect of your lifestyle is causing your impotence, he or she may suggest changes that you can make, such as reducing stress or your alcohol intake.

If the impotence appears to have a psychological basis or if you have difficulties in your relationship, your doctor may suggest that you and your partner consult a sex therapist or a counsellor (*see* SEX THERAPY, p.773).

In cases where the underlying cause cannot be treated, a range of drug treatments and physical aids is available.

DRUG TREATMENTS The oral medication sildenafil has proved an effective treatment for impotence in many men. The drug relaxes the muscles of the penis and the walls of the arteries that supply blood to the penis. More blood then flows into the penis, making erection easier. In the UK, the prescription of sildenafil through the NHS is limited to certain specified conditions. Since there is a risk of serious side effects in some men, you should not obtain the drug from nonmedical sources and not take sildenafil without first having a medical assessment.

The drug alprostadil may also help you to achieve an erection. This drug can be inserted into the urethra (the tube through which urine and semen leave the body). Alternatively, the drug is injected directly into the penis. However, alprostadil can sometimes have serious side effects. For the small number of men with low testosterone levels, testosterone injections may be effective.

PHYSICAL TREATMENTS There are many physical aids that can help you to achieve and maintain an erection. The vacuum constriction device consists of a plastic cylinder that is fitted over the penis. A hand-held pump is used to create a vacuum in the cylinder, causing the penis to fill with blood and become erect. The cylinder is then removed and the erection is maintained by a special rubber band fitted on the base of the penis.

An alternative is a penile prosthesis, which is surgically implanted into the penis. One type consists of paired rods that enable the position of the penis to be adjusted manually. However, once the rods are implanted, the size of the penis cannot be altered. Another device is the inflatable penile implant, which consists of paired cylinders and a small pump. The pump can be triggered to inflate the cylinders, which then hold the penis erect. When not in use, this implant enables the erection to subside.

The outlook for impotence is good. In many men, the cause can be treated. If the cause is not treatable, drugs and physical aids are usually effective.

(WWW) ONLINE SITES: p.1034, p.1036

Premature ejaculation

Release of seminal fluid from the penis that occurs before or immediately after penetration and with minimal stimulation

 AGE Most common in young, sexually inexperienced males

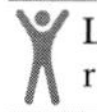 LIFESTYLE Early sexual encounters in rushed conditions may be a risk factor

 GENETICS Not a significant factor

Premature ejaculation is a very common sexual problem, particularly for young men. Ejaculation is considered to be premature when semen is released from the penis before or very shortly after penetration and with minimal sexual stimulation. Most sex therapists agree that the experience of premature ejaculation is part of the normal sexual learning curve; inexperienced men, particularly if they are young, often ejaculate prematurely. The problem may also occur in experienced men when they have intercourse after a long period of abstinence from sex.

Recurrent premature ejaculation can be a frustrating problem. Repeated episodes may make a man anxious about his performance and possibly result in impotence (opposite page). If premature ejaculation does occur repeatedly, medical advice should be sought.

WHAT ARE THE CAUSES?

The causes of premature ejaculation are usually psychological. Problems may include anxiety about performance or result from early sexual experiences in which there was a fear of being discovered. Some men cannot recognize the physical sensations that they experience immediately before they ejaculate and therefore cannot control the timing of their orgasm. Premature ejaculation is more common during the early stages of a sexual relationship, when the partners may lack confidence and may be nervous about their performance.

Rarely, premature ejaculation may be caused by a physical disorder such as inflammation of the prostate gland (*see* PROSTATITIS, p.724) or may result from damage to the spinal cord.

WHAT MIGHT BE DONE?

If you experience recurrent problems with premature ejaculation, you should discuss the matter with your doctor. You will have an examination to look for a physical cause, and any underlying disorder will be treated.

(SELF-HELP) SQUEEZE TECHNIQUE

The squeeze technique can be used to prevent premature ejaculation. Just before ejaculation, the shaft of the penis is firmly squeezed between the thumb and forefinger. The squeezing causes the erection to be partially lost, thus preventing ejaculation. Repeated regularly, the exercise can dramatically improve control of ejaculation.

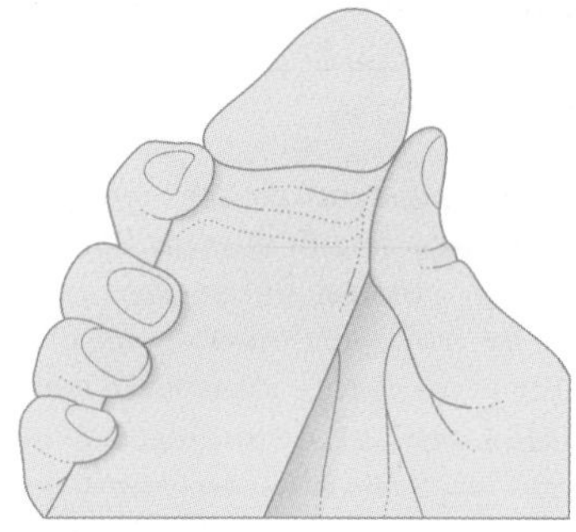

Applying pressure
The thumb and forefinger are used to apply pressure just behind the head of the penis, on the upper and lower sides. This pressure prevents ejaculation.

If premature ejaculation does not have a physical cause, treatment of the disorder is aimed at teaching you how to recognize and control sexual arousal. Your doctor will probably recommend that you see a sex therapist, who can teach you exercises for managing arousal (*see* SEX THERAPY, opposite page).

Exercises may include the start/stop technique, in which the man's penis is stimulated by his partner. When the man feels that he is close to ejaculation, he asks his partner to stop stimulating him. After a few minutes, stimulation is resumed by his partner and then stopped again. When the stop/start exercise is repeated many times over a period of weeks, it can help men to achieve better control. The squeeze technique (p.771) can be used together with the start/stop technique or used separately.

Some antidepressant drugs (p.916), such as sertraline, have the side effect of delaying ejaculation. They may be prescribed as a short-term measure to treat premature ejaculation because delaying ejaculation can boost confidence and assist in solving the problem.

The outlook is excellent: most men who seek help vastly improve their control over the timing of ejaculation.

(WWW) ONLINE SITES: p.1034, p.1036

Painful intercourse in men

Pain experienced in the genital area during sexual intercourse

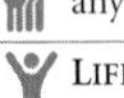
AGE Can affect sexually active males of any age

LIFESTYLE Unprotected sex is a risk factor

GENETICS Not a significant factor

Painful sexual intercourse, known as dyspareunia, is rare in men. The cause is usually physical, but in some cases it may be psychological. Pain occurring in the penis during intercourse may be accompanied by a burning sensation both during and after ejaculation.

WHAT ARE THE CAUSES?

The most common cause of painful sexual intercourse in men is an infection of the genitals, the prostate gland, or the urethra (the tube through which urine and semen pass out of the body). These infections, which include genital herpes (p.767) and nongonococcal urethritis (p.765), are often transmitted through unprotected sexual intercourse. Friction on the penis during sexual intercourse can aggravate the pain of an infection. Other causes of pain during intercourse may include inflammation of the head of the penis (*see* BALANITIS, p.722) and persistent inflammation of the prostate gland (*see* PROSTATITIS, p.724), which may result in pain on ejaculation. Dyspareunia may also be due to Peyronie's disease (p.723), a condition in which the shape of the penis is abnormal when erect. A tight foreskin is another possible cause of painful intercourse (*see* PHIMOSIS, p.721).

In some instances, discomfort during penetration results from skin irritation caused by an allergic reaction to a particular brand of condom or spermicide. Less commonly, sharp pain during penetration can be caused by threads of an intrauterine contraceptive device that protrude from the woman's cervix (*see* USING CONTRACEPTIVES, p.70). Rarely, there may be a psychological reason, such as sexual abuse in childhood.

WHAT MIGHT BE DONE?

If you think that the pain is due to an allergy to condoms or spermicide, try changing to another brand. If the pain persists, consult your doctor. The doctor will examine you and may take a swab from the tip of the penis to test for infection. If you have an infection, the doctor may prescribe antibiotics (p.885) for both you and your partner so that you do not reinfect each other, or may refer you to a clinic that specializes in sexually transmitted infections.

Any disorder that interferes with the erection of the penis may require surgery if it is causing pain. If your partner has an intrauterine contraceptive device that causes you discomfort, her doctor may trim its threads so that they do not protrude as far through the cervix.

If no physical cause is found, your doctor may refer you to a sex therapist, who will help you to work through any psychological problems together with your partner (*see* SEX THERAPY, opposite page). Painful sexual intercourse in men can usually be treated successfully.

(WWW) ONLINE SITES: p.1034, p.1036

Painful intercourse in women

Pain experienced in the genital area or the lower abdomen during sexual intercourse

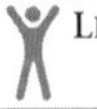
AGE Can affect sexually active females of any age

LIFESTYLE Unprotected sex is a risk factor

GENETICS Not a significant factor

Many women experience painful sexual intercourse, known as dyspareunia, at some point in their lives. The pain may be superficial, in the vulva or vagina, or deep in the pelvis. It may have either a psychological or a physical cause.

WHAT ARE THE CAUSES?

For many women, superficial pain during sexual intercourse may be caused by psychological factors, such as anxiety disorders (p.551), guilt, or fear of sexual penetration. These factors can also result in vaginismus (opposite page).

There are many physical causes of superficial pain during intercourse. A fairly common cause is vaginal dryness. This problem may result from insufficient sexual arousal before penetration. It may also be a side effect of certain drugs, such as some antidepressants (p.916), or be due to hormonal changes after childbirth or the menopause (*see* MENOPAUSAL PROBLEMS, p.737). Many women find intercourse painful for some time after giving birth, especially if they had a vaginal tear. Pain during a woman's first sexual experience is common, particularly if the hymen is intact.

Superficial pain during intercourse may also be caused by infections of the urinary tract or the genitals, including cystitis (p.709), trichomoniasis (p.767), and vaginal thrush (p.752). In rare cases, an abnormally shaped vagina may make sexual intercourse painful.

Pain that is felt deep within the pelvis during intercourse may be due to a disorder of the pelvic cavity or of the pelvic organs, such as pelvic inflammatory disease (p.741), fibroids (p.745), or endometriosis (p.742). Another possible cause of pain may be an intrauterine contraceptive device that is incorrectly positioned in the uterus (*see* USING CONTRACEPTIVES, p.70).

Despite common belief, a large penis does not make sex painful, although certain positions can cause pain in the vagina and vulva or deep in the pelvis.

WHAT CAN I DO?

If you think your pain is due to vaginal dryness caused by lack of arousal, you may need to talk to your partner about spending more time on foreplay (*see* COMMUNICATING YOUR SEXUAL NEEDS, p.770). Alternatively, you may find it helpful to use a lubricant, particularly after childbirth and during and after the menopause. If certain sexual positions cause discomfort, try other ones.

WHAT MIGHT THE DOCTOR DO?

If you consult your doctor, he or she may take swabs from your vagina and cervix to test for infection and may arrange for ultrasound scanning (p.250) and CT scanning (p.247) of the pelvis to look for abnormalities. If pain is due to an underlying disorder, the disorder will be treated if possible. If the pain is due to vaginal dryness caused by a drug, your doctor may prescribe an alternative. If no physical cause is found, your doctor may refer you for sex therapy (right) with your partner. In most cases, the pain ceases following treatment.

(WWW) ONLINE SITES: p.1036, p.1037

Vaginismus

Spasm of the muscles around the entrance to the vagina, making sexual intercourse painful or impossible

AGE Can affect sexually active females of any age

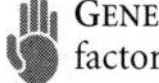
GENETICS LIFESTYLE Not significant factors

In vaginismus, the pelvic floor muscles go into painful involuntary spasm and reduce the size of the vaginal opening. As a result, sexual intercourse may be very painful and vaginal penetration can often be impossible. The condition varies in severity for different women. Some women are affected by vaginismus to such an extent that they cannot insert even a finger or a tampon into the vagina and may need an anaesthetic for a vaginal examination. Other women may be able to tolerate a vaginal examination by a doctor or nurse but cannot tolerate sexual intercourse.

WHAT ARE THE CAUSES?

Vaginismus is usually psychological in origin and often occurs in women who fear that penetration may be painful. This fear may result from a previous traumatic sexual experience, such as a rape or sexual abuse in childhood. Another cause of vaginismus may be the fear of pregnancy. Anxiety or guilt concerning sex may also be a contributing factor to this condition.

Certain physical disorders can also lead to vaginismus. Inflammation of the vagina (*see* VULVOVAGINITIS, p.752) may make intercourse painful and lead to vaginismus. Some women develop the condition because they expect that sex will be painful after childbirth or that they will experience sexual difficulties during or after the menopause (*see* MENOPAUSAL PROBLEMS, p.737).

WHAT MIGHT BE DONE?

Your doctor will examine you gently to look for any physical problem that could make penetration painful or difficult. If there is an underlying physical cause, he or she will treat it. If the problem is psychological, you may need some form of psychological therapy (pp.968–971) or, alternatively, you may be referred to a sex therapist (*see* SEX THERAPY, below). The sex therapist will explain that the vaginal wall is elastic and may teach you relaxation exercises. He or she may then show you how a small dilator can be inserted into the vagina. By practising this technique and gradually using larger dilators, you should lose your fear that penetration will be painful. Treatment for vaginismus is successful in about 9 out of 10 women.

(WWW) ONLINE SITES: p.1036, p.1037

(TREATMENT) SEX THERAPY

Sex therapy is often helpful when a sexual problem has a psychological basis rather than a physical cause. The type of therapy used depends on your problem but often involves discussions with a sex therapist. To overcome particular problems, the therapist may set exercises for you to practise at home, either by yourself or with your partner.

DISCUSSION SESSIONS

Discussing sexual problems with a trained sex therapist or counsellor can often help a couple to analyse and understand their relationship and sexual needs more clearly. It is important that both partners attend the therapy sessions. Each visit lasts about 1 hour, and several sessions may be necessary.

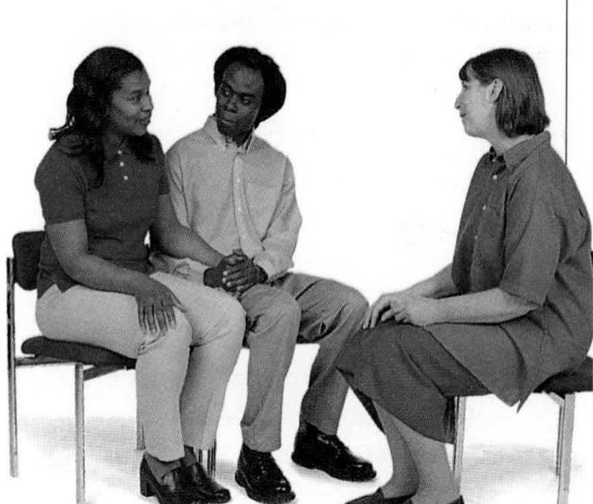

Counselling
Talking with a counsellor can help you to understand your relationship and deal with sexual problems.

EXERCISES

A sex therapist may assign you exercises to practise at home to improve the way in which you and your partner communicate. Exercises may include techniques such as sensate focus. This technique involves experiencing your partner simply through touch and is helpful for problems stemming from anxiety about performance.

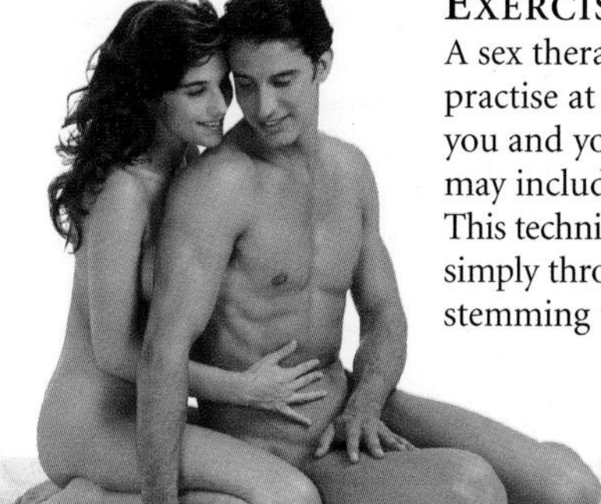

Sensate focus technique
This technique involves discovering pleasure in your own body and that of your partner by means of touch rather than sexual intercourse.

INFERTILITY

Infertility affects 1 in 10 couples who want children. Fertility declines in both sexes after the ages of 25–30, and because more and more couples are delaying starting a family until their 30s, infertility is becoming more common in the developed world. If conception has not occurred after a year of unprotected, regular sex, one or both partners may have a fertility problem.

For every 10 couples who try to have a child, 8 conceive within a year and 9 conceive within 2 years. The remainder may have fertility problems. Some problems may be temporary or can be treated medically, but certain problems can prevent a couple from ever having children. Infertility can also affect people who have children already.

It is important that both partners visit the doctor together if they are worried about an inability to conceive. In about half of all couples who have difficulty conceiving, the problem lies with the female partner, and in about a third of couples it lies with the male partner. However, in some couples, no cause can be found.

In this section, the first article covers the advice that a doctor might give to a couple who are having difficulties in conceiving. The following two articles describe specific infertility problems in women and in men. Each article describes the tests that a doctor may carry out to identify fertility disorders and discusses how specific problems may be treated. Other conditions that can lead to infertility are covered elsewhere in the book. Such conditions include polycystic ovary syndrome (p.744) and endometriosis (p.742) in women, and varicocele (p.720) and hypogonadism in men (p.729).

In many couples, the cause of infertility can be identified and treated. If a specific cause cannot be found or is untreatable, assisted conception may be advised. This section discusses the techniques in current use, including recent sophisticated developments.

Problems conceiving

When pregnancy does not result after a couple have had regular, unprotected sex for more than a year

AGE GENDER GENETICS LIFESTYLE
Risk factors depend on the cause

The average time taken by a couple who are trying to conceive is 6 months, and 8 in 10 couples will be successful within a year. It is very common for a couple to feel anxious if pregnancy does not occur in the first few months, but most young couples are advised to continue trying for a year before seeking medical help. Older couples may decide to ask for medical help earlier because fertility in both sexes declines with age. Women over the age of 35 may find it particularly difficult to conceive.

WHAT MIGHT BE DONE?

If you are having problems conceiving, you and your partner should consult a doctor together. The doctor will ask about your sex life and whether you are having any specific difficulties with sexual intercourse (*see* SEXUAL PROBLEMS, pp.769–773). He or she will also check whether you have been having sexual intercourse around the middle of the woman's menstrual cycle, when conception is most likely to take place.

Your doctor will take a medical history from both of you because previous illnesses or operations may be relevant. You will be asked how often you drink alcohol and how much, whether you smoke, and if you use any prescribed or recreational drugs. You may also be given a physical examination that includes your genitals.

If you are both relatively young and there is no obvious problem, your doctor may give you advice about measures that you can take to improve your likelihood of conceiving (*see* MAXIMIZING YOUR CHANCE OF CONCEPTION, right) and suggest that you keep trying. If you have not had preconception counselling for advice on a healthy pregnancy, the doctor may discuss your health, diet, and lifestyle with you.

If your doctor suspects there may be a problem preventing conception or if the female partner is over 35, you may be referred to a specialist for a series of tests (*see* FEMALE INFERTILITY, opposite page, and MALE INFERTILITY, p.777).

WHAT IS THE PROGNOSIS?

For most couples, it is only a matter of time before they conceive, and 9 in 10 couples are successful within 2 years.

If a problem is detected, the treatment and outlook will depend on the cause. Assisted conception (p.776) or artificial insemination (opposite page) may be suitable for some couples if no cause is discovered or if the problem cannot be treated successfully.

(WWW) ONLINE SITES: p.1033

SELF-HELP MAXIMIZING YOUR CHANCE OF CONCEPTION

The overall health of both partners has an important effect on fertility. You may find that following the self-help measures below improves your chance of conception:

- Make sure your weight is in or near the normal range (*see* ARE YOU A HEALTHY WEIGHT?, p.53).
- Eat a healthy diet.
- Do not smoke.
- Cut down on alcohol, which is known to reduce the sperm count and can damage the fetus if pregnancy occurs.
- Have sex every day at the woman's most fertile time, in the middle of the menstrual cycle.
- Try not to worry, because stress can lower your fertility. Learn relaxation exercises (p.75) to lower your stress levels.
- Men should avoid taking hot baths or using saunas.

Female infertility

Inability of a woman to conceive with a partner of normal fertility

AGE Increases with age; most common over the age of 35

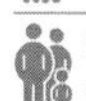
GENETICS In rare cases, may be due to a chromosomal abnormality

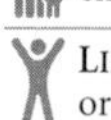
LIFESTYLE Stress, excessive exercise, and low or excess body weight are risk factors

About half of all couples who experience difficulties conceiving do so as a result of female infertility. Fertility in women decreases with age and is generally lower after the age of 35, making conception more difficult.

For conception to occur, all of the following steps must take place: ovulation (the production and release of a mature egg by an ovary), fertilization of the egg by a sperm, transport of the fertilized egg along the fallopian tube to the uterus, and implantation of the fertilized egg in the lining of the uterus. If any stage does not occur or is interrupted, conception cannot take place.

WHAT ARE THE CAUSES?

There are a number of fertility problems in females that may affect one or more of the processes required for conception. The problems can develop at different stages of conception.

PROBLEMS WITH OVULATION A common cause of female infertility is failure of the ovaries to release a mature egg during each monthly cycle. Ovulation is controlled by a complex interaction of hormones produced by the hypothalamus (an area of the brain), the pituitary and thyroid glands, and the ovaries. A common and treatable cause of female infertility is polycystic ovary syndrome (p.744), which may cause a hormonal imbalance that prevents ovulation from taking place. Disorders of the thyroid gland, such as hypothyroidism (p.680), may also lead to a hormonal imbalance that can affect the frequency of ovulation. Pituitary gland disorders, such as prolactinoma (p.677), a noncancerous tumour, may cause a similar imbalance. Ovulation does not always occur in some women for reasons that are unclear. In some cases, women who have been using oral contraceptives for a number of years may take time to re-establish a normal hormonal cycle after discontinuing them. Excessive exercise, stress, and obesity or low body weight may affect hormone levels and cause temporary infertility.

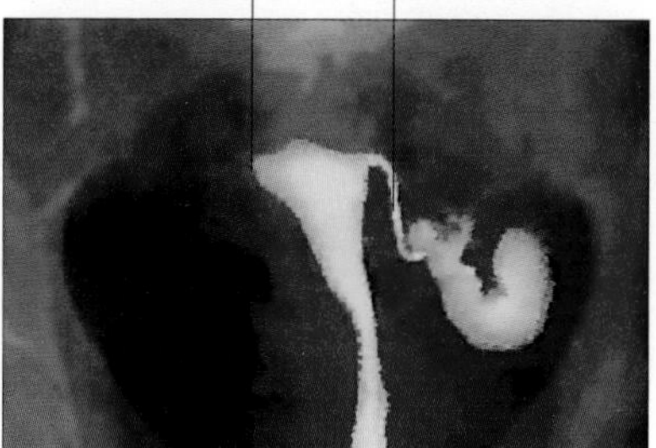

Damaged fallopian tubes
In this X-ray, a contrast dye has been used to show the female reproductive organs. One fallopian tube is blocked and is not visible; the other is narrowed and distorted.

Premature menopause also results in a failure to ovulate. It can occur for no apparent reason or may be the result of pelvic surgery, chemotherapy (p.280), or radiotherapy (p.281). In rare cases, the ovaries do not develop normally due to a chromosomal abnormality, such as Turner's syndrome (p.823).

PROBLEMS WITH EGG TRANSPORT AND FERTILIZATION The passage of the egg from the ovary to the uterus may be impeded by damage to one of the fallopian tubes. This damage may be due to pelvic infection (*see* PELVIC INFLAMMATORY DISEASE, p.741), which may in turn result from a sexually transmitted infection such as chlamydial infection (p.765). Such disorders may exist with no symptoms and may be detected only if you have difficulty conceiving.

Endometriosis (p.742), a condition that can lead to the formation of scar tissue and cysts within the pelvis, may also damage the fallopian tubes, preventing the passage of an egg.

In some women, the egg cannot be fertilized because the mucus produced naturally by the cervix contains antibodies that destroy the partner's sperm before they reach the egg.

PROBLEMS WITH IMPLANTATION If the lining of the uterus has been damaged by an infection, such as gonorrhoea (p.764), the implantation of a fertilized egg may not be possible. Hormonal problems may also result in the uterine lining not being adequately prepared for successful implantation. Noncancerous tumours that distort the uterus (*see* FIBROIDS, p.745) and, rarely, structural abnormalities present from birth may make it impossible for a fertilized egg to embed itself in the uterine lining.

(TREATMENT) ARTIFICIAL INSEMINATION

Artificial insemination is a simple procedure to introduce sperm into a woman's vagina or uterus. Sperm from the woman's partner or from a donor is drawn into a syringe and injected into the top of the vagina or through the cervix into the uterus. The procedure is painless and takes only minutes, and the woman can go home after half an hour of rest.

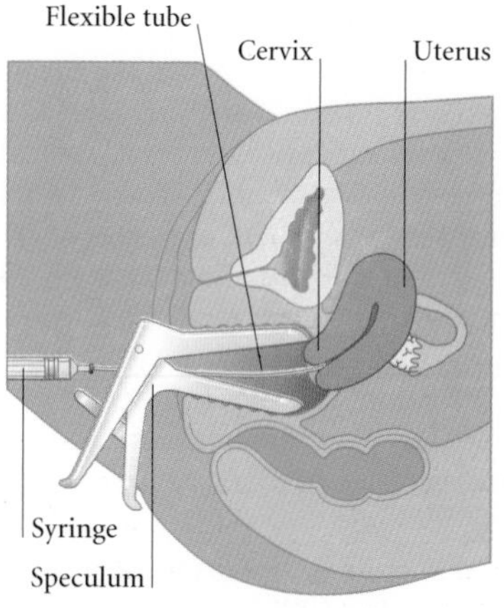

Artificial insemination
The vagina is held open by a speculum so that sperm can be injected into the top of the vagina or into the uterus.

WHAT MIGHT BE DONE?

Your doctor will ask you about your general state of health, your lifestyle, your medical and menstrual history, and your sex life before recommending particular tests and treatments.

Most causes of female infertility can now be identified through testing. You can find out if and when you ovulate by using an ovulation prediction kit, available over the counter, or by recording your body temperature daily (*see* USING CONTRACEPTIVES, p.70). If your doctor suspects that you are not ovulating regularly, you may have repeated blood tests during your menstrual cycle to assess the level of the hormone progesterone, which normally rises after ovulation. Repeated ultrasound scanning (p.250) of the ovaries during the cycle may also be carried out to check if and when ovulation occurs. In addition, a tissue sample may be taken from the uterus and examined for abnormalities (*see* ENDOMETRIAL SAMPLING, p.738).

If tests show that you are not ovulating, you may need further blood tests to check the levels of certain hormones, including thyroid hormones, and drugs may be prescribed to stimulate ovulation (*see* DRUGS FOR INFERTILITY, p.936). However, if you are ovulating, the next step is to find out whether your partner is producing sufficient normal sperm by analysing two or more semen samples (*see* SEMEN ANALYSIS, opposite page).

If you are ovulating normally and your partner's sperm are healthy, your doctor will check if there is a problem preventing the egg and sperm from meeting. For example, you and your partner may be asked to have sex during the time that you are ovulating so that a sample of your cervical mucus (collected within a few hours of intercourse) can be tested for antibodies to sperm. If antibodies are found, there are several methods of treatment. Corticosteroids (p.930) may be prescribed to suppress the production of antibodies, or your partner's semen may be injected directly into your uterus to avoid contact with the mucus (*see* ARTIFICIAL INSEMINATION, p.775). If these steps are not successful, your doctor may recommend assisted conception (right).

If the cause of the infertility has still not been found, your doctor may arrange for further investigations to look for a blockage in the fallopian tubes or an abnormality of the uterus. One such test is laparoscopy (p.742), in which an endoscope containing a camera is inserted through a small incision in the abdomen. Another test is hysterosalpingography, in which a dye is injected through the cervix and X-rays are taken as the dye enters the reproductive organs. The treatment depends on the problem. For example, a blockage of the fallopian tube may be corrected by microsurgery (p.950), and endometriosis may be treated with drugs (*see* SEX HORMONES AND RELATED DRUGS, p.933).

TREATMENT ASSISTED CONCEPTION

Infertility treatments that involve mixing eggs and sperm outside the body include in-vitro fertilization (IVF), gamete intrafallopian transfer (GIFT), and zygote intrafallopian transfer (ZIFT). IVF is also used to treat some genetic disorders because the embryo can be tested for abnormalities before implantation.

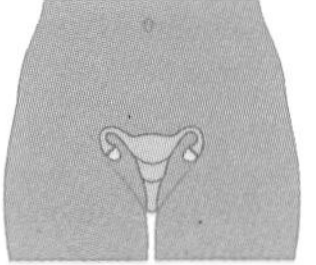

LOCATION

IN-VITRO FERTILIZATION

IVF may be performed if the cause of infertility cannot be determined or treated or if there is a blockage in a fallopian tube. Successful pregnancies occur in about 15 per cent of IVF attempts.

1 *Drugs are given to stimulate several eggs to mature in the ovaries. Under ultrasound guidance, the eggs are collected with a needle inserted through the vaginal wall.*

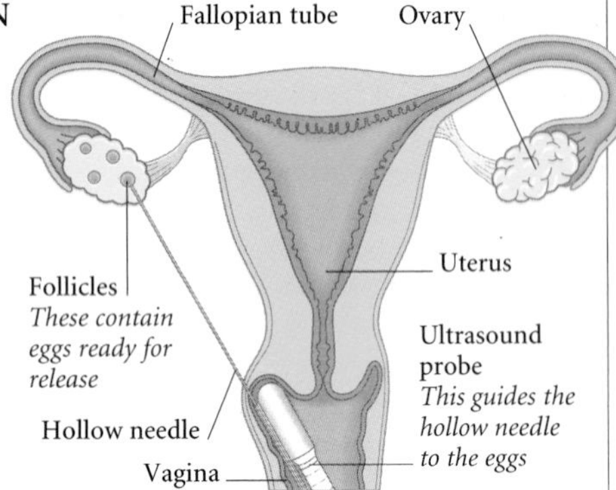

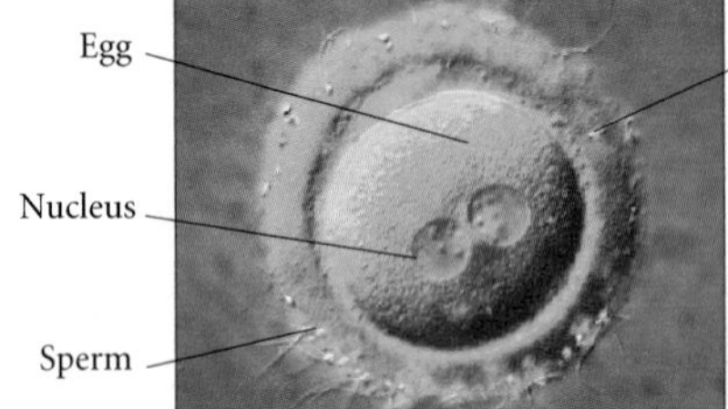

2 *A sperm sample, provided by the woman's partner, is combined with the collected eggs and the mixture is incubated for 48 hours at normal body temperature (37°C or 98.6°F) to allow fertilization to take place.*

3 *The fertilized eggs are introduced into the woman's uterus. Up to three eggs are injected through a thin tube that is fixed to a syringe and passed through the cervix. This procedure takes around 20 minutes. If one or more fertilized eggs implant, conception occurs.*

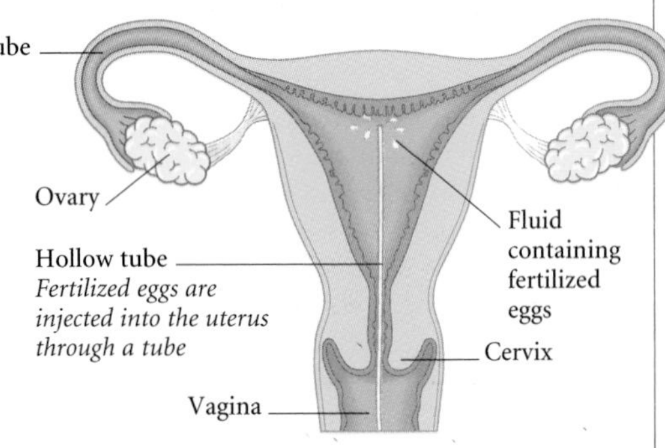

OTHER METHODS

The techniques GIFT and ZIFT may help couples who have unexplained infertility. In each method, eggs are collected as in IVF but are returned to the fallopian tube rather than the uterus. The success rate for both methods is 25–30 per cent.

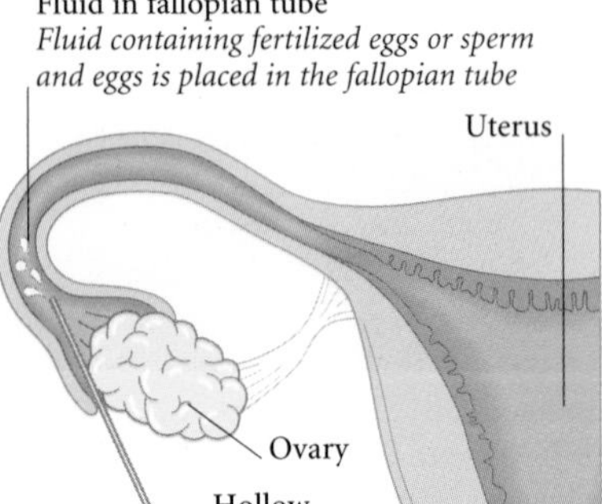

GIFT and ZIFT replacement methods
In GIFT, eggs are mixed with sperm and then returned to the fallopian tube before fertilization. In ZIFT, the eggs are fertilized and returned to the fallopian tube.

What is the prognosis?

Treatments for female infertility have greatly increased the chance of pregnancy. Success rates vary, depending on the cause of the infertility and the type of treatment. Fertility drugs stimulate ovulation in 1 in 3 women, but there is a risk of multiple pregnancy. Microsurgery to clear obstructed fallopian tubes can be successful but increases the risk of ectopic pregnancy (p.790). Success rates for assisted conception methods range from 15 to 30 per cent for each individual treatment.

(WWW) ONLINE SITES: p.1033

Male infertility

Inability of a man to produce or deliver sufficient numbers of healthy sperm to achieve fertilization

GENETICS In rare cases, may be due to a chromosomal abnormality

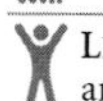
LIFESTYLE Smoking and drinking alcohol are risk factors

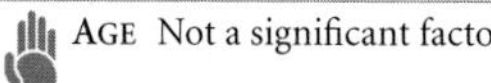
AGE Not a significant factor

In about 1 in 3 couples who have difficulty conceiving, the problem results from male infertility. In men, fertility depends partly on the production of enough normal sperm to make it likely that one of them will fertilize an egg and partly on the ability to deliver the sperm into the vagina during sexual intercourse. If either of these processes is faulty, infertility may result.

What are the causes?

Unlike the causes of female infertility, which are more easily identifiable, the cause of infertility can be difficult to determine in some men. A cause is discovered in only 1 in 3 men investigated.

PROBLEMS WITH SPERM PRODUCTION A low sperm count or the production of abnormal sperm may have various causes. One is a rise in the temperature of the testes. Normally, the testes are about 2°C (4°F) cooler than the rest of the body. Any factors that raise their temperature can reduce the sperm count.

Aspects of your lifestyle that may impair sperm production include smoking, drinking alcohol, using certain medications and recreational drugs, and wearing tight clothing.

Sperm production can be adversely affected by certain long-term illnesses, such as chronic kidney failure (p.706), and by some infections that occur after puberty, such as mumps (p.293). Conditions affecting the urethra, such as hypospadias (p.870), or the scrotum, such as a varicocele (p.720), may also reduce fertility. In addition, fertility problems may occur if the testes are damaged by medical procedures including surgery, chemotherapy (p.280), or radiotherapy (p.281) for disorders such as cancer of the testis (p.719).

Low sperm production may also be due to a hormonal deficiency. Insufficient production of the sex hormone testosterone by the testes (*see* HYPOGONADISM IN MALES, p.729) can cause a low sperm count. Since the pituitary gland controls testosterone secretion, pituitary disorders, such as a tumour (*see* PROLACTINOMA, p.677), may also lead to reduced sperm production. Rarely, low testosterone levels are due to a chromosomal abnormality such as Klinefelter's syndrome (p.822). The most common cause of a low sperm count is idiopathic oligospermia, in which there is a reduced sperm count for no identifiable reason. There is no effective treatment for this condition.

PROBLEMS WITH SPERM DELIVERY A number of factors may prevent sperm from reaching the vagina. The most easily identifiable is impotence (p.770), the inability to achieve or maintain an erection. Other factors include damage to the epididymides and vas deferens (tubes that transport sperm). Damage is often due to a sexually transmitted infection such as gonorrhoea (p.764). It may also be caused by retrograde ejaculation, in which semen flows back into the bladder when the bladder neck does not close properly. This condition can occur following prostate surgery (*see* PARTIAL PROSTATECTOMY, p.725, and RADICAL PROSTATECTOMY, p.727).

What might be done?

Your doctor will ask about your health, medical history, and sex life and give you a physical examination, including an examination of your genitals. You may also need to provide semen samples (*see* SEMEN ANALYSIS, right). If your sperm count is low or your sperm are abnormal, you may have further investigations such as blood tests to check your hormone levels.

Low testosterone levels can be treated with injections of hormones (*see* SEX HORMONES AND RELATED DRUGS, p.933). Artificial insemination (p.775) may be used in cases of impotence or retrograde ejaculation; for the latter, the sperm may be taken from urine. Damage to the epididymides or vas deferens can be treated by microsurgery (p.950). If you produce only a few healthy sperm, a sample may be taken from an epididymis or testis by microsurgery. A process called intracytoplasmic sperm injection (ICSI) may then be used to fertilize an egg with a single sperm.

What is the prognosis?

If the infertility is treatable, the chance of regaining fertility is high. Artificial insemination gives a 10–15 per cent chance of conceiving in one menstrual cycle, and the treatment usually works within 6 months. Each attempt at assisted conception (opposite page) or ICSI is successful in 15–30 per cent of cases, depending on the technique.

(WWW) ONLINE SITES: p.1033

(TEST) Semen analysis

Microscopic examination of several samples of a man's semen is carried out to investigate male infertility. If there are too few sperm or if many are deformed or dead, fertility will be reduced. An abnormally small volume of semen may also indicate that there is a fertility problem.

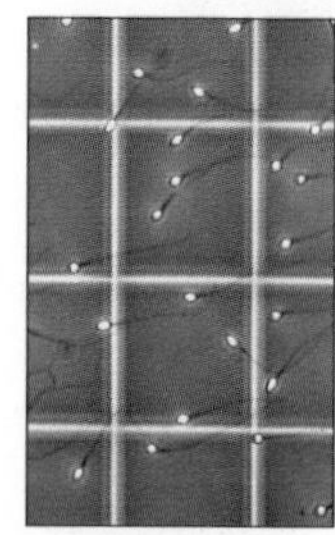
NORMAL SPERM COUNT

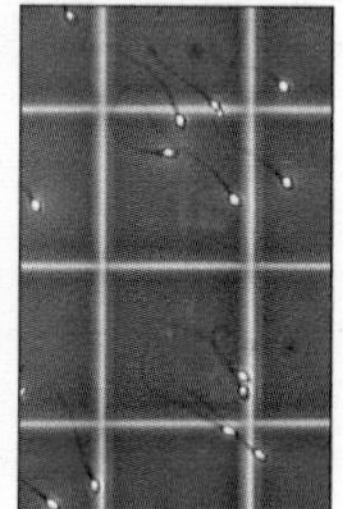
LOW SPERM COUNT

The sperm count

Each millilitre of normal semen contains at least 50 million sperm, most of which are healthy. If the sperm count is low, there are fewer than 20 million sperm.

Pregnancy and Childbirth

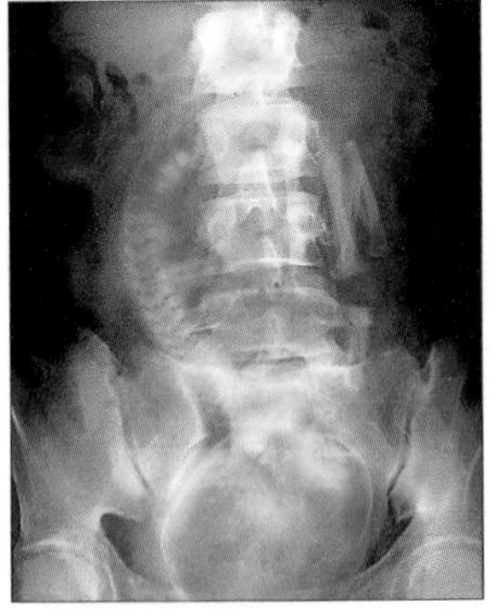

A fully grown fetus
This X-ray shows the skeleton of a fetus at full term. Its head is low in the mother's pelvis.

From the moment of conception, when an egg is fertilized, to the moment of birth, complex changes take place within a pregnant woman's body. Genetic material from the father and the mother fuses together, eventually forming a new, genetically distinct individual. During this time, the mother provides a nourishing and protective environment in which the fetus can develop. When the baby is born, he or she is able to survive outside the mother's body and begin a separate existence.

About a week after fertilization, the egg embeds itself securely in the lining of the uterus, at which stage it is known as an embryo. Only 8 weeks later, the embryo is recognizable as a human being and has developed all its vital organs, including the heart and brain. From this stage onwards, it is called a fetus. Between 8 and 12 weeks, the fetus grows rapidly, and its weight increases by up to 15 times. By the time the baby is born, it weighs just over 3 kg (7 lb) on average.

The pregnant woman

Changes in the mother's hormone levels control the physical changes necessary for a healthy pregnancy and for birth. First, menstruation ceases, and then the ligaments and joints in the mother's pelvis begin to soften and become more flexible in preparation for the birth of the baby. In addition, the mother's breasts enlarge as their milk-producing glands increase in number, ready for breast-feeding the newborn baby.

Each new pregnancy runs a slightly different course. Many prospective mothers feel well throughout their pregnancies. Others experience uncomfortable symptoms such as nausea, vomiting, heartburn, indigestion, and tiredness. These are a result of the biological changes, such as pressure of the fetus on surrounding organs and hormone changes, occurring in the body as the fetus grows. Such symptoms develop at particular stages during the pregnancy.

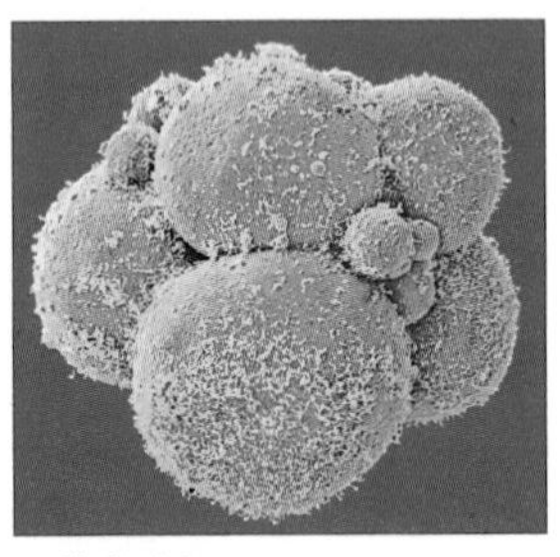

Cell division
In the days after fertilization, the egg has divided to form a cluster of cells called a morula.

The baby's birth

After about 36 weeks, the fetus is fully formed and is able to survive outside its mother's body. Around the 40th week, a change in the mother's hormones triggers the first of the three stages of labour. After the baby is born, the mother begins to produce nourishing breast milk, and her body gradually returns to its state before pregnancy.

(Process) From egg to embryo

Pregnancy begins when an egg is fertilized by a sperm. This event takes place in the outer third of one of the fallopian tubes, when a single sperm meets and fuses with an egg following sexual intercourse. Within 2 days of fertilization, the egg starts its journey towards the uterus, propelled by the muscular action of the fallopian tube. As the egg travels, its cells gradually divide to form a cluster of cells called a morula. After 5–7 days, the morula arrives in the uterus and then embeds securely in the uterine lining. From this moment onwards, the pregnancy is properly established, and the morula is known as an embryo.

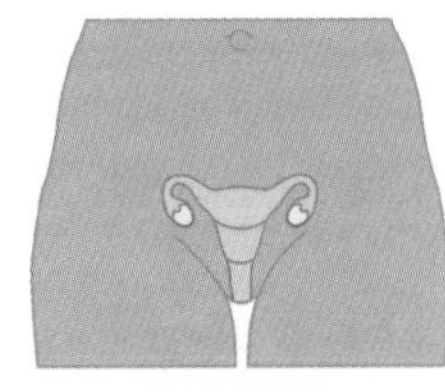

Location

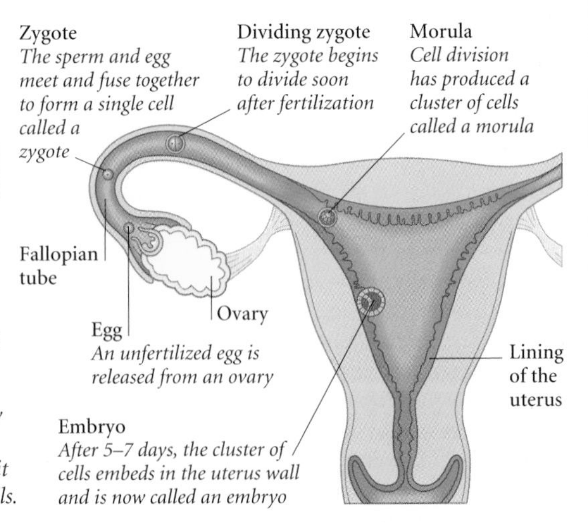

The beginning of life
After fertilization, the egg begins to move along the fallopian tube, its cells doubling in number every 12 hours. By the time the egg arrives in the uterus, it consists of hundreds of cells.

(STRUCTURE AND FUNCTION) PREGNANCY

Inside the uterus, the fetus is surrounded by a protective, fluid-filled bag known as the amniotic sac. Nourishment is provided through the placenta, an organ attached to the wall of the uterus and connected to the fetus by the umbilical cord. As the fetus grows, the uterus increases in size and weight and gradually expands into the mother's abdomen. Many of the mother's organs, such as the bladder and the intestines, are pushed out of their normal positions by the enlarging uterus. By the end of pregnancy, the fetus is usually tightly curled up with its head pointing downwards towards the mother's pelvis.

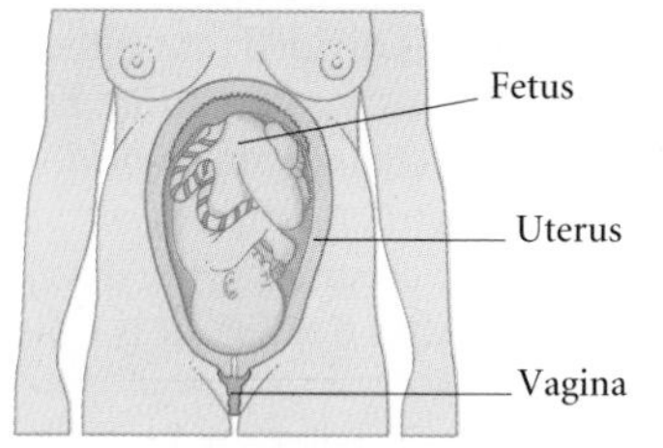

LOCATION

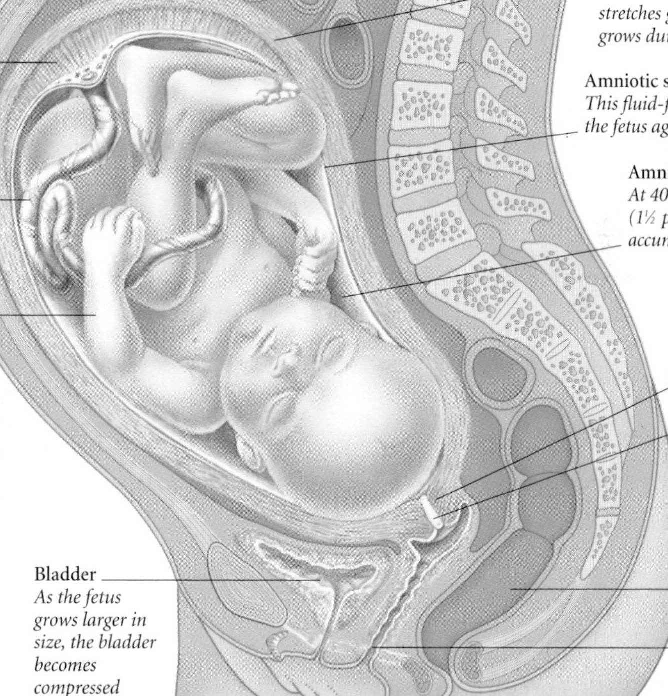

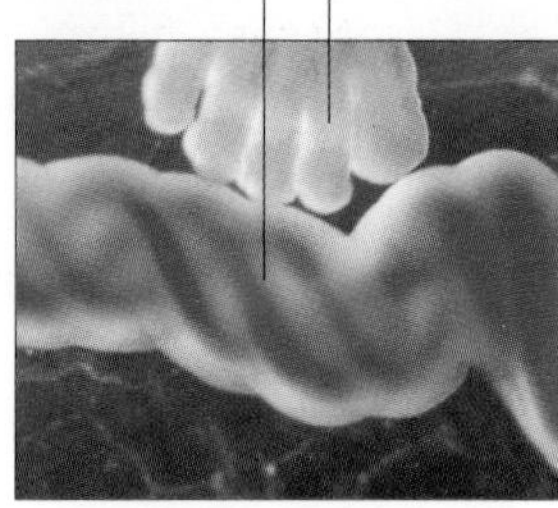

Nourishing the fetus
The umbilical cord provides a link to the placenta and the mother's nourishing blood supply.

(PROCESS) MULTIPLE PREGNANCY

Most multiple pregnancies produce twins; birth of three or more babies is rare. The majority of twins are nonidentical and develop when two eggs are released from an ovary and are fertilized by two separate sperm. These twins may or may not be the same sex. Less commonly, fertilization of a single egg takes place as normal, but the fertilized cell divides to form two identical, same-sex embryos.

Twins in the uterus
Nonidentical twins develop in their own amniotic sacs and have their own separate placentas. Identical twins may share an amniotic sac or a placenta, or both. Twins can lie in any position in the uterus.

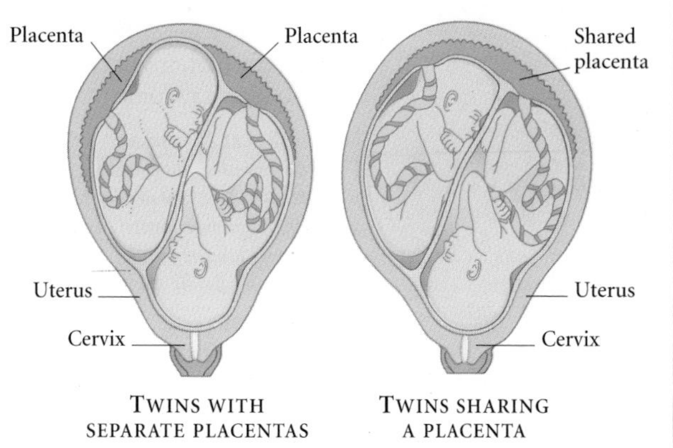

TWINS WITH SEPARATE PLACENTAS

TWINS SHARING A PLACENTA

PROCESS STAGES OF PREGNANCY

Pregnancy is divided into three stages, or trimesters, each about 3 months in duration. Each trimester brings about significant changes in the mother's body and progressive development and growth of the baby. During the first 8 weeks of pregnancy, the developing baby is called an embryo. After 8 weeks, it is called a fetus.

Embryo at 4 weeks
At 1 month old, the embryo has bulges on either side of its head where the eyes are beginning to form.

Developing eye
Developing arm
Placental blood vessel

FIRST TRIMESTER (WEEKS 1–12)

There are few visible changes in the mother's body during this trimester. However, her heart rate increases by about 8 beats per minute to increase the blood circulation. Most of the growing fetus's major organs, such as the heart and the brain, become fully developed during the first 3 months.

The mother at 12 weeks
At 12 weeks, the mother's waistline is only slightly thickened. The breasts are tender and the areola, the area around the nipple, becomes darker in colour.

Nipple
Lobule (milk-producing gland)
Stomach
Slightly thickened waistline
Intestine
Uterus
Fetus
Bladder

From embryo to fetus
The first trimester is crucial in the baby's development; 8 weeks after fertilization, the embryo has developed most of its organs and is now called a fetus. During the third month, it more than doubles in length.

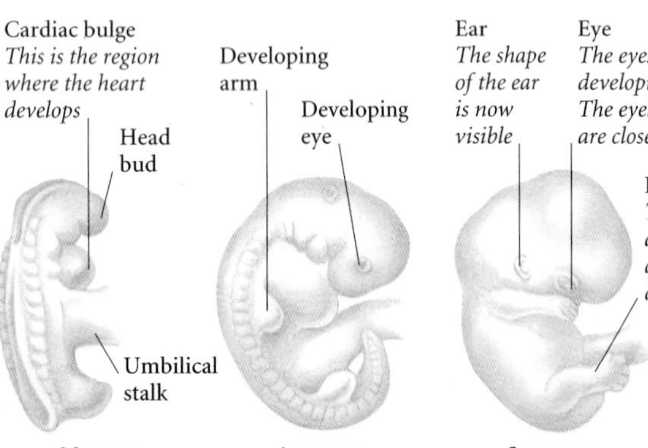

Arm
The fetus can now move its limbs
Face
All the facial features are fully formed
Umbilical cord

12 WEEKS
6 cm (2½ in) long

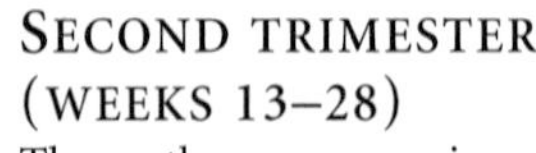

SECOND TRIMESTER (WEEKS 13–28)

The mother may experience backache as she copes with the growing weight of the fetus. Her appetite tends to increase. The fetus starts moving at 18–20 weeks, producing sensations of fluttering in the mother's abdomen.

The mother at 24 weeks
The mother's abdomen swells as the fetus grows. There may be discharge from the nipples, caused by enlarging lobules (milk-producing glands) in the breasts.

Enlarging uterus
Fetus

The fetus
The fetus grows in size and accumulates a layer of fat, and its internal organs become more complex. Its sense of hearing is now developed.

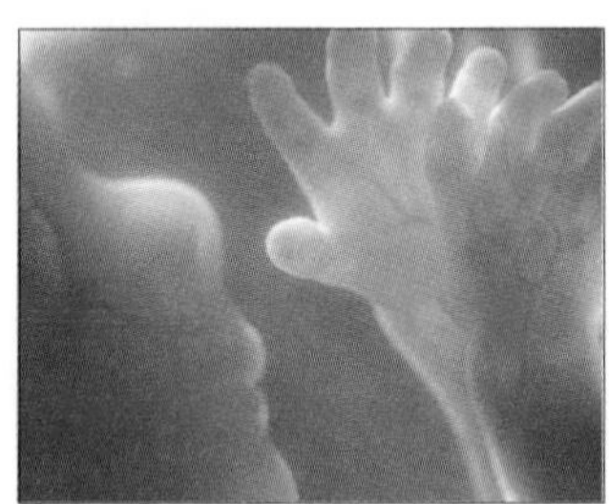

Fetus at 20 weeks
At this stage, the hands are well developed and the fetus is able to flex its fingers. The fetus now has recognizable features and the profile of the face shows the forehead, nose, lips, and chin.

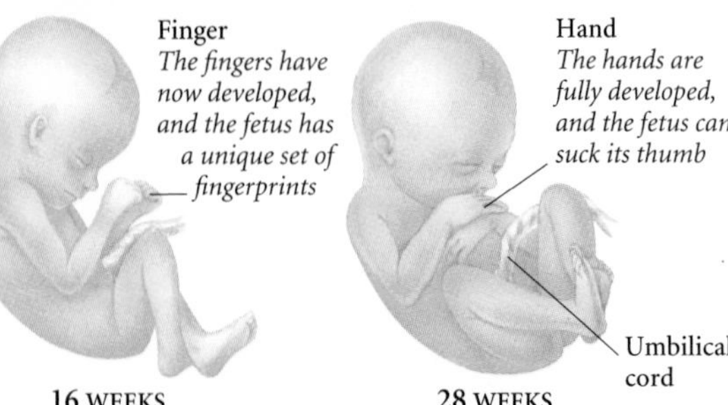

THIRD TRIMESTER (WEEKS 29–40)

During the third trimester, the mother rapidly gains weight as the fetus undergoes a growth spurt. The top of the uterus is high in the abdomen, almost to the level of the breastbone. This can cause slight shortness of breath due to compression of the mother's lungs.

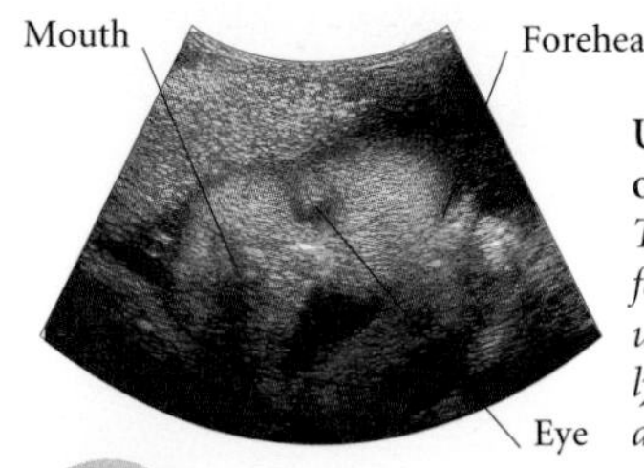

Ultrasound scan of the fetus
The face of a fully grown fetus is clearly visible on this ultrasound scan. The head is lying sideways and the eyes and lips are closed.

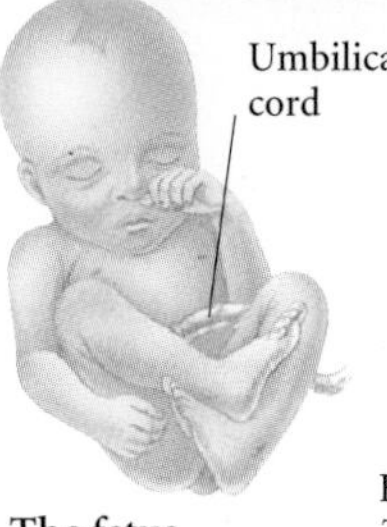

The fetus at 36 weeks
The fetus is now fully formed, weighs about 3 kg (6½ lb), and is about 50 cm (20 in) in length.

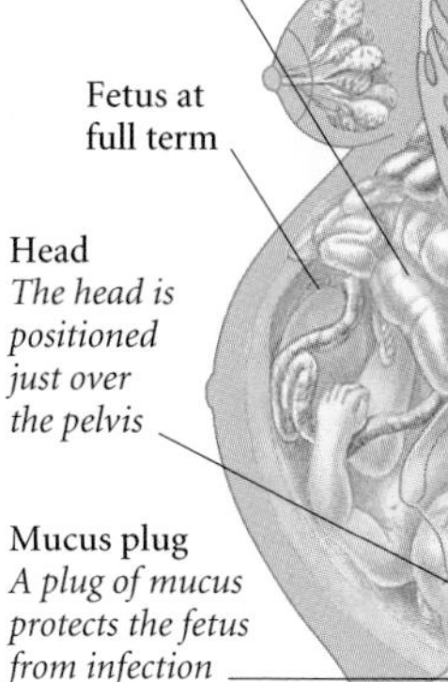

The mother at 36 weeks
The growing uterus presses on the intestines. The stomach may also be compressed, causing heartburn.

PROCESS ENGAGEMENT

A few weeks before labour begins, the head of the fetus moves down to sit snugly in the pelvis. The head is then said to be engaged. In women who have given birth before, this process may not occur until labour begins.

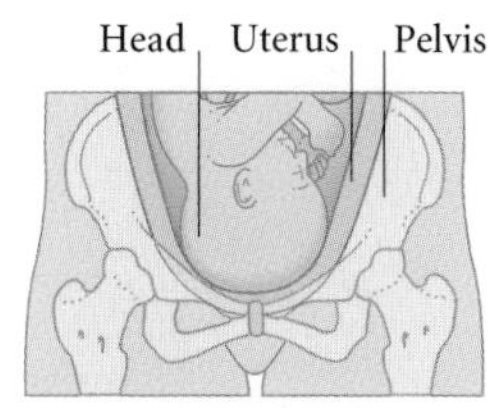

BEFORE ENGAGEMENT

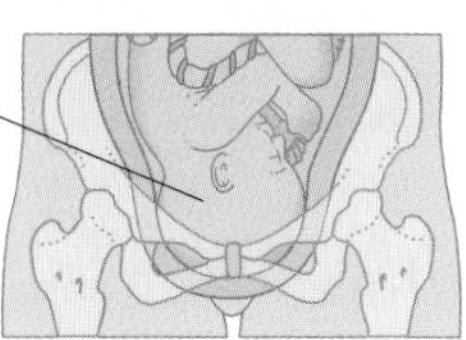

AFTER ENGAGEMENT

Fetus at 40 weeks
In preparation for the birth, the fetus drops lower in the mother's abdomen so that its head sits low in her pelvic cavity.

PROCESS NOURISHING THE FETUS

The fetus is dependent on the mother for nourishment and oxygen. These substances are transferred from the mother's blood to the fetus's blood inside the placenta, an organ attached to the uterus and connected to the fetus by the umbilical cord. About 600 ml (1.1 pints) of maternal blood passes through the placenta every single minute, carrying a continuous supply of nutrients.

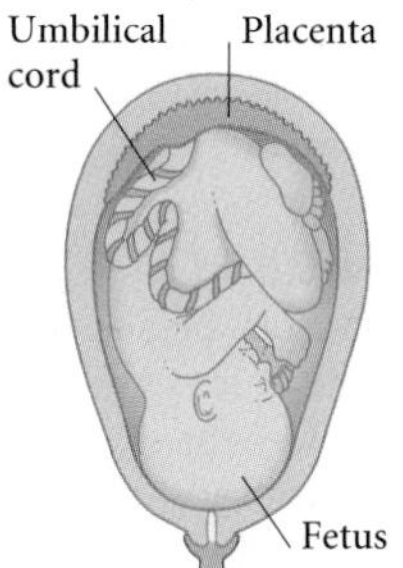

LOCATION

Maternal artery
This artery circulates blood, which contains oxygen and nutrients for the fetus, around the chorionic villi

Chorionic villus
Tiny projections, called villi, form from a thin membrane called the chorion and contain the fetal blood vessels

Flow of oxygen and nutrients

Wall of uterus

Maternal vein
This vein carries waste products away from the fetus

Lining of uterus (endometrium)

Flow of wastes

Pool of mother's blood

Umbilical vein
Blood, oxygen, and nutrients pass to the fetus from this vein

Umbilical artery
This artery carries waste products away from the fetus

Amniotic fluid

Umbilical cord

Blood vessels of the placenta
Inside the placenta, various substances are exchanged between the mother's blood and that of the fetus through a thin membrane called the chorion. Oxygen, nutrients, and antibodies pass from the mother's blood to the fetus's blood, and waste products pass in the opposite direction.

Lining of the uterus
The placenta is firmly attached to the uterine lining

Fetal blood vessel
The blood vessels of the fetus are surrounded by the mother's blood

Placental tissue
This magnified image of a section of placenta shows tissue from both the mother and the fetus. In the placenta, their blood circulations do not mix but are in very close proximity.

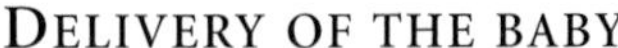

PROCESS CHILDBIRTH

The process of childbirth, known as labour, begins at about the 40th week of pregnancy. There are three distinct stages of labour: first, the contractions in the uterus and the widening of the cervix; second, the birth of the baby; and finally, the delivery of the placenta. The length of each stage varies between women and often depends on the number of previous pregnancies.

THE FIRST SIGNS OF LABOUR

Labour begins when contractions start. The passing of the mucus plug from the cervix occurs up to 10 days before the start of contractions. The amniotic sac that surrounds the baby ruptures either shortly before or at any time during the first stage of labour. The first stage of labour lasts on average 6–12 hours.

1 The passing of the mucus plug from the cervix is known as the show. It is a sign that labour is soon to start, but it goes unnoticed by many women.

Fetus

Uterus

Amniotic fluid

Mucus plug
This bloodstained plug leaves the cervix up to 10 days before labour begins

Pelvis

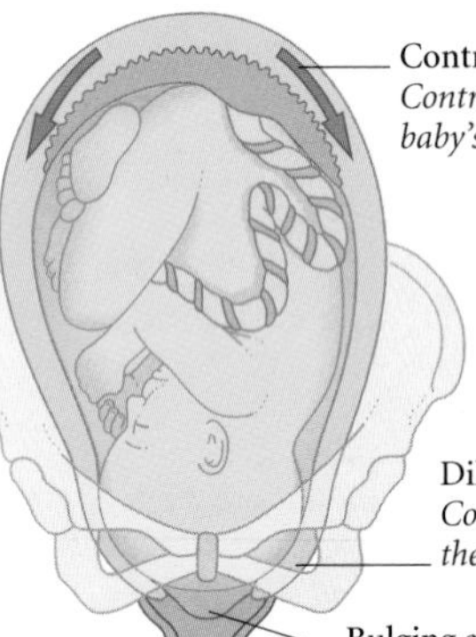

2 Contractions begin at any time in the few days following the show. With each contraction, the uterine muscles shorten and thicken.

Contracting uterus
The uterus continues to contract, pushing the baby down

Dilated cervix
The cervix has a diameter of about 10 cm (4 in) when fully dilated

3 The contractions gradually become stronger and more regular. By this stage, the amniotic sac has usually burst.

DELIVERY OF THE BABY

During the second stage of labour, the baby travels from the uterus down the vagina and is born. This stage is much quicker than the first stage and usually lasts 1–2 hours. The cervix is fully dilated, and the uterine contractions are very strong and usually painful. The baby's head presses down on the pelvic floor, which causes the mother to have an overwhelming urge to push down. Once the baby's head is visible at the vaginal opening, the birth is imminent.

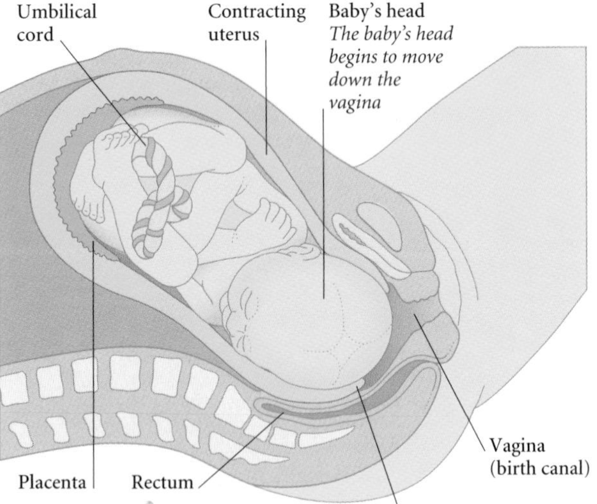

1 As the mother starts to push, the baby turns towards the mother's back and begins to move out of the uterus, with its head bent on to its chest. The vagina, or birth canal, stretches as the baby descends.

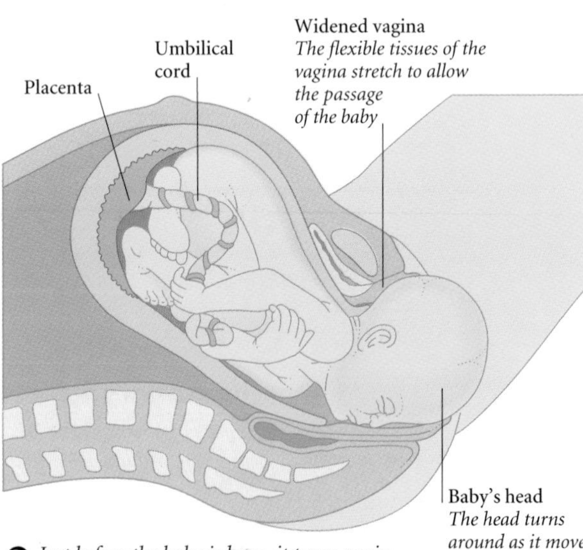

2 Just before the baby is born, it turns again. The head rotates so that it can negotiate the bend in the vagina. The baby is usually facing the mother's anus as it leaves the vagina.

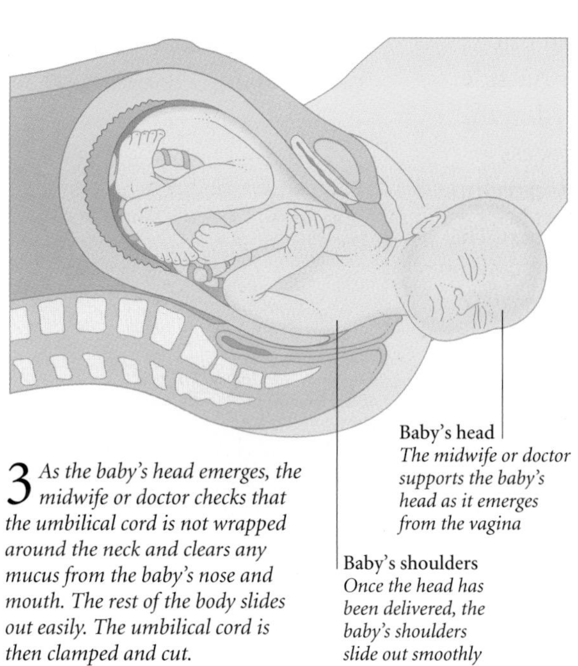

3 *As the baby's head emerges, the midwife or doctor checks that the umbilical cord is not wrapped around the neck and clears any mucus from the baby's nose and mouth. The rest of the body slides out easily. The umbilical cord is then clamped and cut.*

Delivery of the placenta

During the third stage of labour, the placenta is expelled from the uterus. The placenta peels away from the lining of the uterus and is gently pushed through the vagina and out of the body. Often, the mother is injected with a drug that helps the muscles of the uterus to contract and so stop any bleeding from the site where the placenta was attached.

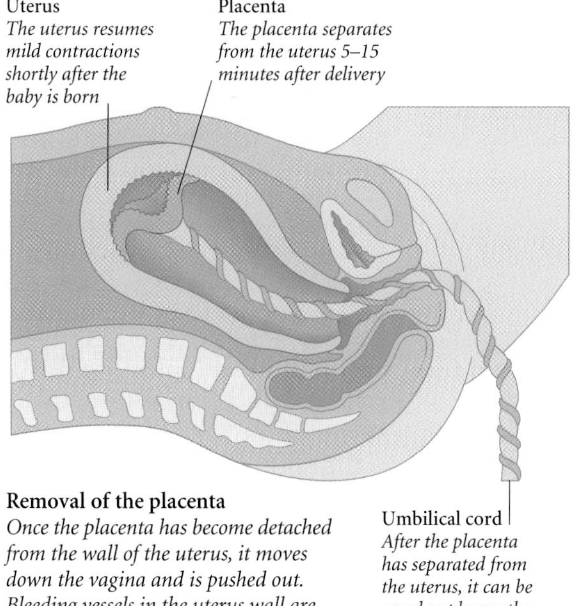

Removal of the placenta
Once the placenta has become detached from the wall of the uterus, it moves down the vagina and is pushed out. Bleeding vessels in the uterus wall are sealed as the uterine muscles contract.

PROCESS After the birth

After birth, the mother's breasts produce colostrum, a fluid rich in nutrients and antibodies, before milk production begins. The mother's uterus, cervix, vagina, and abdomen, which enlarged during pregnancy, begin to return to their normal sizes.

Preparing for lactation

During pregnancy, the lobules (milk-producing glands), which are dormant in nonpregnant women, gradually become able to produce milk in preparation for nourishing the newborn baby. At the same time, they increase in number so that enough milk is produced.

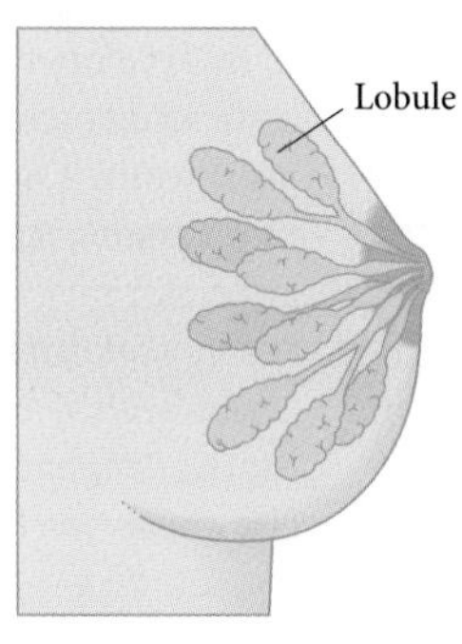

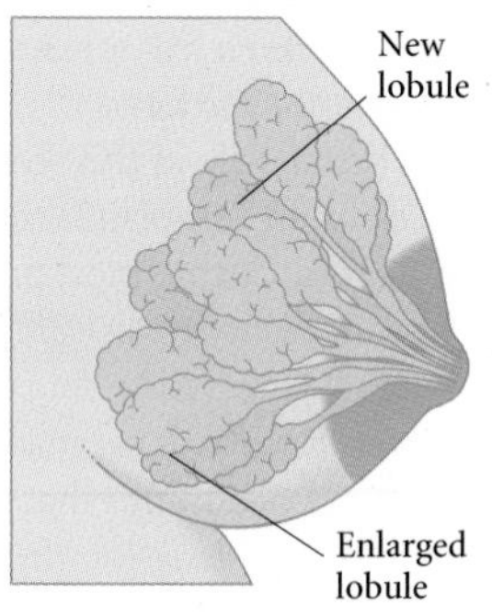

Changes in the breasts
The number of lobules (milk-producing glands) in the breasts increases during pregnancy. After 3 months, they are able to produce colostrum, and after the baby is born, they can produce around 1 litre (2 pints) of milk each day.

The uterus returns to normal

The uterus begins to shrink immediately after birth and continues to decrease in size for the next 6–8 weeks, helped by hormones circulating in the mother's body. There may be some mild pains as the uterus shrinks, but these usually disappear a few weeks after delivery.

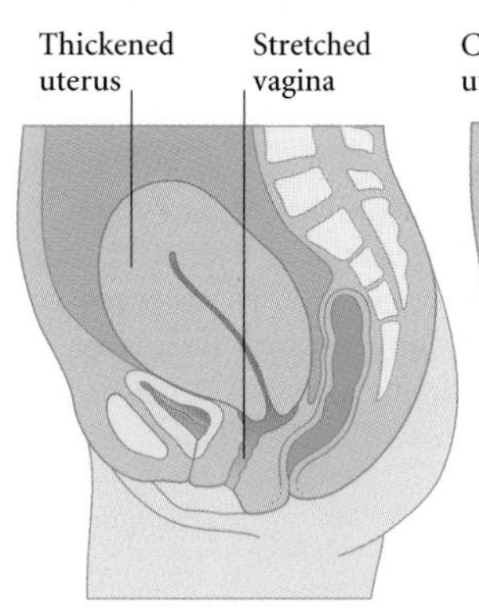

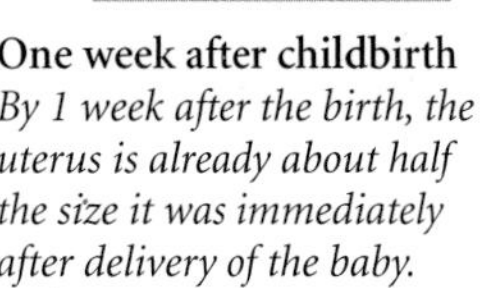

One week after childbirth
By 1 week after the birth, the uterus is already about half the size it was immediately after delivery of the baby.

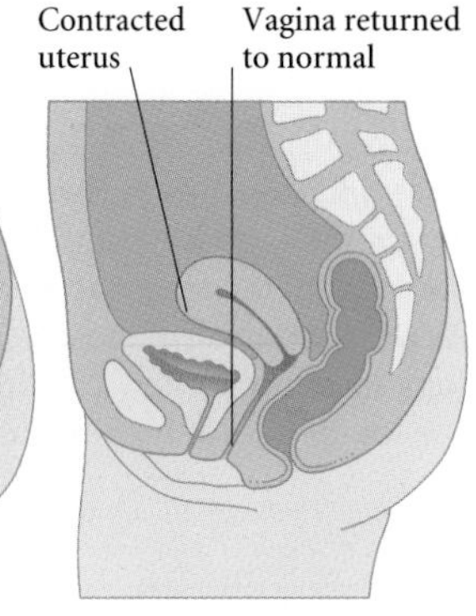

Six weeks after childbirth
After 6 weeks, the uterus has contracted, although not quite to its original size, and returned to its usual position.

PROBLEMS IN PREGNANCY

Pregnancy normally lasts about 40 weeks from conception to delivery of the baby. During this time, a single fertilized cell develops into a fully grown fetus that is able to survive outside the uterus. For the fetus to develop, it must be protected in the uterus and nourished by the mother. Although this process usually progresses smoothly, sometimes problems may develop.

Problems during pregnancy may affect the mother, the fetus, or both. Many of the most common disorders are mild and short-lived, but others may be severe or even life-threatening to the mother or the fetus.

The first article in this section deals with common complaints that occur at some time during most pregnancies. These complaints are usually minor and can often be relieved by simple self-help measures. High-risk pregnancies and pre-existing conditions that should be taken into consideration when planning a pregnancy are discussed next. The remaining articles in this section cover various problems that may occur at different stages of pregnancy.

In developed countries, pregnancy is no longer a major health risk for most women. In some cases, problems in pregnancy can be averted by good antenatal care and a healthy lifestyle before and during pregnancy. Advice about healthy eating and exercise during pregnancy can be found elsewhere (*see* HEALTH IN PREGNANCY AND AFTER CHILDBIRTH, p.33).

KEY ANATOMY

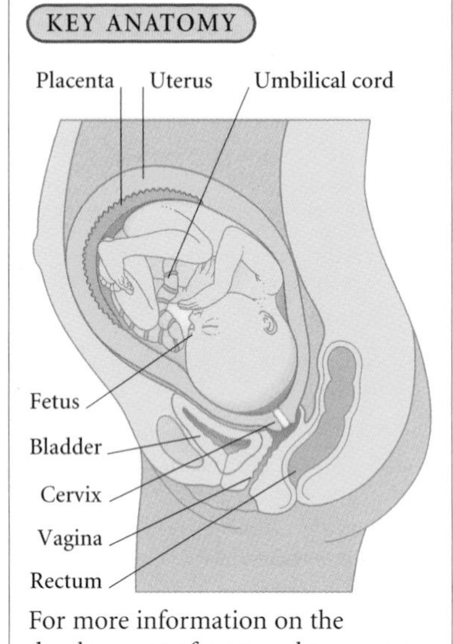

For more information on the development of a normal pregnancy, *see* pp.778–783.

Common complaints of normal pregnancy

Minor problems commonly experienced during pregnancy

AGE GENETICS LIFESTYLE Not significant factors

Most of the common complaints that occur during pregnancy are not serious and are a result of the normal changes in the body that take place as the pregnancy progresses. Some problems are caused by changes in the levels of sex hormones in the mother, others by the weight and pressure of the developing fetus on the organs around the uterus. Although many pregnant women experience some or all of these complaints, others have only a few problems, and some feel even healthier than usual.

WHAT ARE THE SYMPTOMS?

Some symptoms that occur in pregnancy are due to the hormonal changes taking place in the body. They often develop early and may include:

- Breast tenderness.
- Nausea, often with vomiting (known as morning sickness).
- Constipation (p.628).
- Heartburn (*see* GASTRO-OESOPHAGEAL REFLUX, p.636).
- Skin changes, such as increased pigmentation and dryness.

The weight and pressure of the growing fetus and its surrounding fluid may also cause symptoms. These usually develop later in pregnancy than those due to hormonal changes and may include:

- An increased urge to pass urine.
- Increased constipation, which sometimes leads to haemorrhoids (p.668).
- Swollen ankles.
- Varicose veins (p.438).
- Stretch marks (p.349).
- Backache.
- Sciatica (p.546).
- Shortness of breath.
- Difficulty sleeping due to discomfort.

You may also feel very tired, feel faint on occasion, and have headaches.

It is normal to have several different symptoms during pregnancy and often to have more than one problem at a time. If you are worried about a specific symptom, you should obtain medical advice. You should also speak to your doctor if you are having problems with severe vomiting and cannot keep any food or fluids down (*see* HYPEREMESIS, p.789). If you find it painful to pass urine or your urine appears cloudy, you should consult your doctor to make sure that you do not have a urinary tract infection, such as cystitis (p.709).

WHAT CAN I DO?

There is little that you can do to relieve some of the symptoms associated with pregnancy, such as breast tenderness. However, some other complaints may be eased by various self-help measures (*see* COPING WITH PREGNANCY, opposite page). For example, you may be able to relieve morning sickness by eating before you get out of bed. Eating frequent, small snacks throughout the day rather than a few larger meals and sleeping propped up by several pillows may help to reduce nausea and heartburn. If heartburn is severe, you may be prescribed drugs to help to reduce stomach acidity (*see* ANTACIDS, p.923).

It is important that you check with your doctor before you take any over-the-counter drugs because there are several common medications, such as laxatives and painkillers, that can harm a developing baby and should not be taken at any time during pregnancy.

(WWW) ONLINE SITES: p.1035

SELF-HELP COPING WITH PREGNANCY

It is normal to experience a variety of complaints during pregnancy. These are usually caused by hormonal changes within the body and by the increasing weight of the fetus. Although such complaints may cause discomfort, they are usually not serious. Many symptoms can be relieved by self-help measures, but you should consult your pharmacist or doctor before using any drugs and see your doctor if symptoms are severe.

DIGESTIVE COMPLAINTS

A healthy diet is important throughout pregnancy. It not only provides the fetus with the correct nutrients for growth but also helps to prevent you having digestive problems associated with pregnancy, such as nausea, heartburn, and constipation. Avoid spicy foods because they can cause heartburn, and always have something plain available to eat in case you feel hungry.

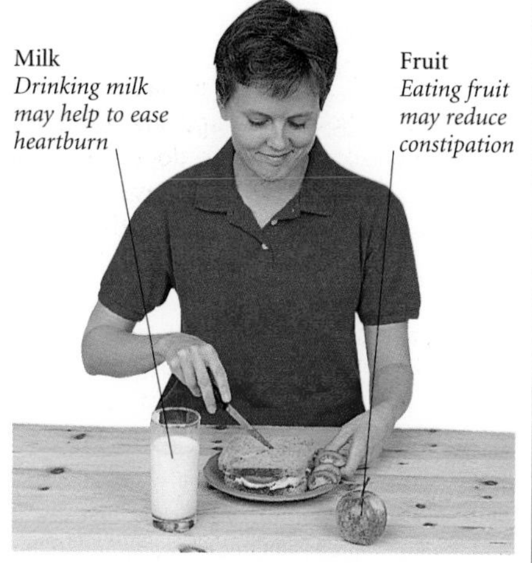

Eating during pregnancy
Small, frequent meals may help to reduce nausea, and milky drinks may ease heartburn. Plenty of fruit, vegetables, and other fibre-rich foods in your diet should help to reduce constipation.

CIRCULATORY COMPLAINTS

Increased pressure on the blood vessels in the pelvis may lead to varicose veins, swollen ankles, and feeling faint in late pregnancy. To relieve symptoms, avoid standing still for long periods of time and sit or lie down whenever you feel faint. Support tights may help to relieve varicose veins.

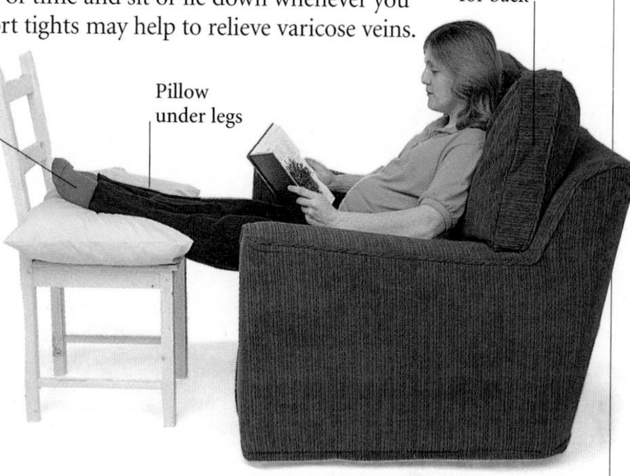

Sitting comfortably
Try to rest and put your feet up whenever possible. Support your back and always try to elevate your feet above the level of your hips.

BACKACHE AND SCIATICA

Backache is an increasingly common problem as pregnancy progresses, and poor posture may place pressure on the sciatic nerve, causing a shooting pain from the buttock down one leg (sciatica). Both of these problems may be eased by adopting good posture when standing, using a chair with good back support, sleeping on a firm mattress, and wearing flat shoes.

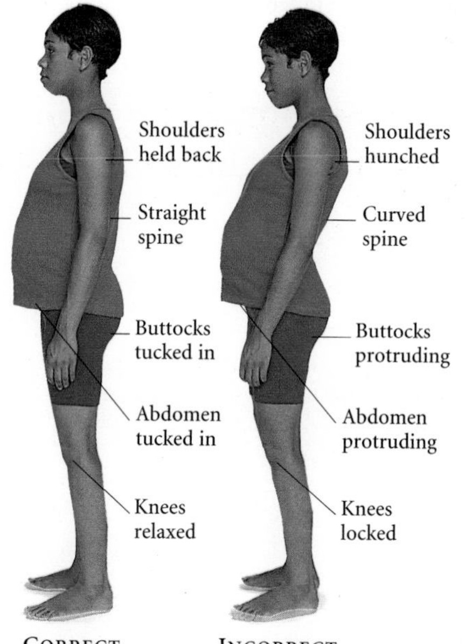

Standing correctly
Stand with your feet apart and your weight equally balanced on each foot. Hold your back straight and your shoulders back. Tuck in your buttocks and abdomen and relax your knees.

TIREDNESS AND DIFFICULTY SLEEPING

You will probably feel tired from early pregnancy onwards. As your pregnancy progresses and your abdomen enlarges, you may also find it more difficult to get into a comfortable position in which to sleep. Before going to bed, try to relax, have a warm bath and a milky drink, and watch television, listen to the radio, or read until you feel sleepy.

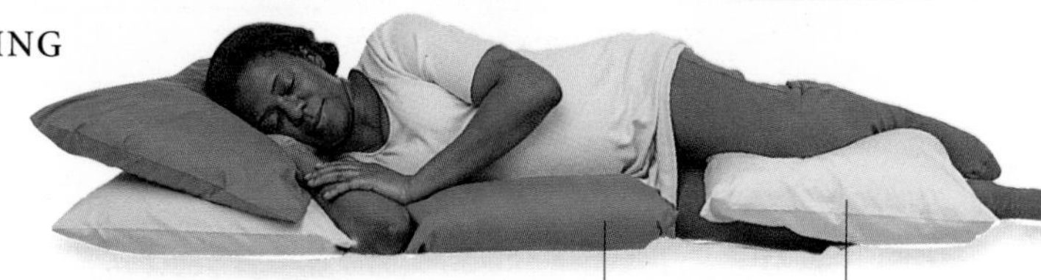

Sleeping comfortably
Try to sleep on your side, with a pillow between your legs. You may feel more comfortable if you place another pillow under your abdomen.

High-risk pregnancy

A pregnancy with a higher than average risk for the mother or the fetus

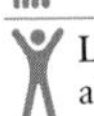
AGE Most common under the age of 15 or over the age of 35

LIFESTYLE Smoking and alcohol or drug abuse during pregnancy are risk factors

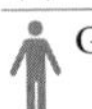
GENETICS Risk factors depend on the cause

For the majority of women, pregnancy progresses well except for some minor problems, such as tiredness and swollen ankles (*see* COMMON COMPLAINTS OF NORMAL PREGNANCY, p.784). However, pregnancy is not without risks. Although the risk of death for both mother and fetus is low, it increases in certain situations. Some women are at higher risk of developing problems in pregnancy, and one of the functions of routine antenatal care (below) is to identify these women so that they can be monitored and receive additional treatment if needed.

WHAT ARE THE RISK FACTORS?

There are many different risk factors that may lead to a high-risk pregnancy. Women under the age of 15 or over the age of 35 are more likely to have problems, as are women with a small build. Other risk factors in pregnancy include certain lifestyle factors, such as smoking; a history of problems in previous pregnancies; and pre-existing illnesses.

AGE Women under the age of 15 who become pregnant are at increased risk of going into labour before the end of the pregnancy (*see* PREMATURE LABOUR, p.798). They are also at risk of certain complications during pregnancy, such as pre-eclampsia and eclampsia (p.794) in which blood pressure is high.

Women over the age of 35 are more likely to have pre-existing disorders, such as noncancerous tumours in the uterus (*see* FIBROIDS, p.745) or diabetes mellitus (p.687). They are also at greater risk of developing pre-eclampsia or diabetes while pregnant (*see* DIABETES DEVELOPING IN PREGNANCY, p.788), which may place the pregnancy at risk. There is also an increased likelihood of the fetus having a chromosomal abnormality, such as Down's syndrome (p.821), if the mother is over the age of 35.

PHYSICAL FACTORS Women who have a small build and a small pelvis are at greater risk of a delayed first stage of labour (p.801), particularly if they are carrying a large baby who cannot easily fit through the pelvis.

Women who weigh less than 47.5 kg (105 lb) before pregnancy are more likely to have small babies. Conversely, women who are overweight are at increased risk of developing diabetes mellitus during pregnancy, which increases their risk of having a large baby. Overweight women are also at greater risk of high blood pressure (*see* HYPERTENSION, p.403).

LIFESTYLE FACTORS Having a poor diet, smoking, and abusing alcohol or drugs during pregnancy all increase the risk of problems occurring, including miscarriage (p.791), premature labour, and intra-uterine growth retardation (p.796).

PROBLEMS IN PREVIOUS PREGNANCIES Any problems in a previous pregnancy, such as a premature labour or stillbirth (p.805), tend to increase the risk for the current pregnancy. A woman who had a small baby in a previous pregnancy will be more likely to have another baby who is underweight.

PRE-EXISTING ILLNESSES Any disorder that is already present (*see* PRE-EXISTING DISEASES IN PREGNANCY, p.788), such as diabetes mellitus, epilepsy (p.524), or high blood pressure, may lead to

(TEST) ROUTINE ANTENATAL CARE

Antenatal care is essential to make sure that a pregnancy is progressing well. Regular antenatal visits include urine and blood tests and one or more ultrasound scans of the developing fetus. Occasionally, antenatal genetic tests (opposite page) may also be carried out to look for a gene or chromosome disorder in the fetus.

Routine tests

Antenatal care usually starts at about 11 weeks into the pregnancy. Follow-up occurs monthly at first; every 2 weeks from 28 to 36 weeks; and then every week after 36 weeks.

WHEN DONE	TYPE OF TEST	REASON FOR TEST
First visit	Medical history and examination	To look for pre-existing risk factors, such as long-term illnesses
	Urine tests	To check the urine for glucose, which may indicate diabetes developing in pregnancy (p.788), and for protein, which may indicate pre-existing kidney disease
	Blood tests	To determine blood type and look for anaemia (p.446), antibodies to rubella (p.294), and certain infectious diseases, such as hepatitis B and, after discussion, HIV infection (p.297)
	Weight and blood pressure	To provide initial measurements against which later ones are compared
Between 11 and 20 weeks	Ultrasound scans (one or more)	To check the age of the fetus and look for fetal abnormalities (*see* ULTRASOUND SCANNING IN PREGNANCY, p.793)
Follow-up visits at regular intervals from 11 weeks to delivery	Weight and examination	To assess the growth of the fetus and to see which way it is lying in the uterus
	Urine tests	To detect diabetes or pre-eclampsia (*see* PRE-ECLAMPSIA AND ECLAMPSIA, p.794)
	Blood pressure	To detect developing pre-eclampsia
	Blood tests (at some visits only)	To look for anaemia and, in combination with ultrasound scanning, to assess the risk of fetal abnormalities, such as neural tube defects (p.844) or Down's syndrome (p.821). A test to screen for diabetes mellitus in the mother may also be necessary

(TEST) ANTENATAL GENETIC TESTS

You may be offered blood tests and/or ultrasound scanning to determine whether you are at increased risk of having a baby with a genetic disorder. Ultrasound can detect thickening of the tissues at the back of the neck of the fetus (nuchal translucency) and absence of the nasal bone, which indicate a risk of a genetic disorder such as Down's syndrome. If tests suggest a disorder, you may be offered chorionic villus sampling or amniocentesis.

CHORIONIC VILLUS SAMPLING

Chorionic villus sampling is usually carried out between weeks 8 and 11 of pregnancy. Tissue from the edge of the placenta (chorionic villi) is taken and then analysed to look for a chromosomal or genetic abnormality. The risk of miscarriage is increased slightly by having this test.

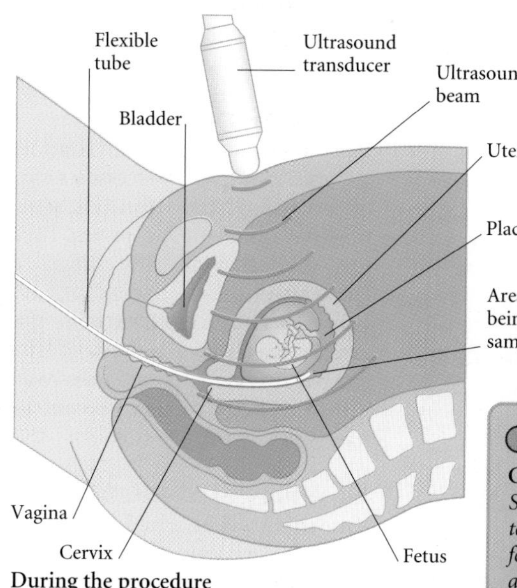

During the procedure
A small sample of the placenta is taken either by inserting a needle through the abdominal wall or, as shown here, using a flexible tube that is passed through the cervix. Ultrasound is used to guide the tube, and the sample is removed using gentle suction.

AMNIOCENTESIS

Amniocentesis is usually carried out between weeks 14 and 18 of pregnancy. A small sample of the amniotic fluid surrounding the fetus is removed and analysed for genetic abnormalities. The procedure is associated with a very small risk of miscarriage (about 1 in 200 women).

During the procedure
Ultrasound is used to guide a needle into the sac containing the fetus and the amniotic fluid. A small sample of fluid is then withdrawn using a syringe. A slight pricking sensation may be felt.

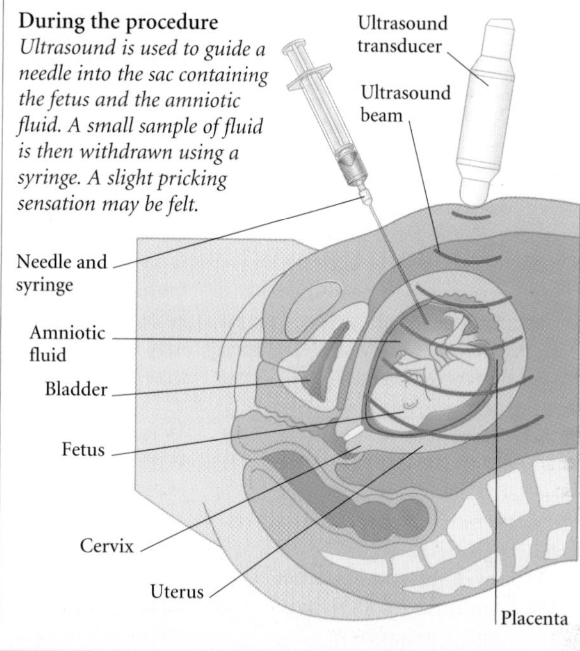

(RESULTS)

Chromosome analysis
Samples from genetic tests are analysed to look for a chromosomal abnormality. This test result shows one extra chromosome number 21, indicating Down's syndrome in the fetus.

1 2 3 4 5
6 7 8 9 10 11 12
13 14 15 16 17 18
19 20 21 22 XX

Normal chromosome pair
Extra chromosome

certain problems for both mother and fetus. Changes to the mother's current medication and additional monitoring of mother and fetus may be necessary before and during pregnancy.

WHAT MIGHT BE DONE?

At your first antenatal visit, your doctor or midwife will examine you and ask you questions to determine whether or not you are at increased risk. If you are, you will need additional monitoring and possibly specialized treatment during your pregnancy or labour.

If you have a high-risk pregnancy, you will probably need more frequent antenatal visits than usual to make sure that the pregnancy is progressing normally. You may also be offered additional tests if you are at increased risk of having a baby with a gene or chromosome disorder (*see* ANTENATAL GENETIC TESTS, above). Frequent blood tests may be needed to monitor any pre-existing diseases, and additional ultrasound scans may be required to monitor the development and growth of the fetus (*see* ULTRASOUND SCANNING IN PREGNANCY, p.793). You may be supervised by several doctors, including specialists, who will work together to maximize your chances of a successful pregnancy.

WHAT IS THE PROGNOSIS?

With careful monitoring and appropriate delivery techniques, the majority of problems in pregnancy can be treated successfully. Although complications are still more likely to occur in a high-risk pregnancy, modern treatments have significantly improved the outlook.

(WWW) ONLINE SITES: p.1035

Pre-existing diseases in pregnancy

Long-term pre-existing diseases that could affect the progress of pregnancy or the health of the fetus

AGE More common over the age of 35

GENETICS LIFESTYLE Not significant factors

If a woman who becomes pregnant has a long-term medical condition, she may need specialist care throughout pregnancy and labour. Pre-existing disorders that could adversely affect pregnancy or the health of the fetus are more common in women over the age of 35.

Long-term pre-existing disorders and their treatment may affect the progress of the pregnancy. For example, women who have diabetes mellitus (p.687) are more prone to problems such as cystitis (p.709) or premature labour (p.798), particularly if the diabetes is not well controlled. Changes in hormone levels during pregnancy can have adverse effects on diabetes, which often worsens. However, in some women who have mild asthma (p.483), symptoms improve during pregnancy.

The fetus may also be affected by pre-existing diseases in the mother. For example, a mother who has high blood pressure (*see* HYPERTENSION, p.403) is at an increased risk of having a smaller than average baby (*see* INTRA-UTERINE GROWTH RETARDATION, p.796). A baby who is born to a mother with diabetes mellitus may have low blood sugar levels immediately after birth.

If you have a long-term condition, you should consult your doctor before becoming pregnant. Your condition, and that of your fetus, will need monitoring throughout pregnancy and your doctor will work with your obstetrician to ensure you remain healthy.

WHAT MIGHT BE DONE?

If you have a long-term disorder, your doctor will review your condition before you become pregnant to make sure that it is as well controlled as possible.

Your usual treatment may need to be altered while you are pregnant because some drugs can affect the fetus. For example, if you normally take tablets to control your diabetes mellitus, you will have to change to insulin injections (*see* DRUGS FOR DIABETES MELLITUS, p.931). The dose of some treatments may need to be altered, and additional measures may be required. For example, women who have epilepsy (p.524) and are taking anticonvulsant drugs (p.914) will usually be prescribed a higher than normal dose of folic acid to reduce the risk of their medication causing neural tube defects (p.844) in the fetus.

You may have antenatal checkups at more frequent intervals than usual, and your doctor may refer you to an obstetrician specializing in your condition. You may have additional tests, including ultrasound scanning (*see* ULTRASOUND SCANNING IN PREGNANCY, p.793). Extra monitoring may be necessary during labour, and after the delivery, your baby may be given a series of tests to ensure that he or she is healthy.

WHAT IS THE PROGNOSIS?

With monitoring and treatment, pre-existing conditions in pregnancy can be controlled, and they usually carry little risk for the mother or the fetus. Changes in the condition that have occurred as a result of the pregnancy are normally reversed soon after delivery.

(WWW) ONLINE SITES: p.1035

Diabetes developing in pregnancy

Inability of the tissues to absorb glucose from the bloodstream during pregnancy due to a lack of the hormone insulin

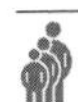
AGE More common over the age of 30

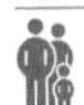
GENETICS A family history of diabetes mellitus is a risk factor

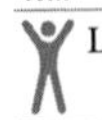
LIFESTYLE Being overweight is a risk factor

During the course of pregnancy, up to 1 in 50 women temporarily develops diabetes mellitus (p.687). The condition is called gestational diabetes. Normally, the hormone insulin, which is produced by the pancreas, enables body cells to absorb glucose from the bloodstream. During pregnancy, additional hormones, which have an anti-insulin effect, are produced by the placenta. If the body does not produce enough insulin to counter this effect, the result is high levels of glucose in the blood and gestational diabetes.

Diabetes developing in pregnancy is more common in women over the age of 30, women who are overweight, and those who have a family history of diabetes mellitus. Gestational diabetes can usually be controlled by a special diet.

In most cases, gestational diabetes disappears after the birth of the baby, but about 1 in 3 women who has had gestational diabetes develops permanent type 2 diabetes mellitus, often within 5 years of pregnancy.

WHAT ARE THE SYMPTOMS?

Many women with gestational diabetes do not develop symptoms. Others may develop symptoms that include:

- Tiredness.
- Increased thirst and appetite.
- Passing large amounts of urine.

If gestational diabetes is not controlled, the fetus may gain an excessive amount of weight and have difficulty passing through the mother's pelvis. Labour may then be particularly difficult (*see* DELAYED FIRST STAGE OF LABOUR, p.801). Babies born to mothers with gestational diabetes are also at risk of having low blood sugar levels at birth. Women whose diabetes cannot be controlled have a greater risk of a stillbirth (p.805).

HOW IS IT DIAGNOSED?

Your urine will be tested for glucose at each antenatal visit. If glucose is found, your doctor may arrange for a glucose tolerance test, in which you are given a sugar solution to drink and a sample of blood is tested. If your blood shows higher glucose levels than would normally be anticipated, the diagnosis is confirmed. Your doctor may also suggest that you have this test if you had an unexplained stillbirth in the past, you have given birth to a larger than average baby, or if diabetes mellitus runs in your family. This test may be performed routinely during weeks 24–28 of pregnancy.

WHAT IS THE TREATMENT?

If you have gestational diabetes, your doctor will recommend that you follow a modified diet that contains less sugar than normal and greater amounts of fibre and starchy carbohydrates. Some women also need insulin injections.

You will need to have a blood test at least once every 2 weeks to check your blood sugar levels. You may also be advised to test your blood sugar levels at home (*see* MONITORING YOUR BLOOD GLUCOSE, p.689) and check your urine daily for glucose. More frequent antenatal visits than usual may be necessary, and you may also need to have extra ultrasound scanning (*see* ULTRASOUND SCANNING IN PREGNANCY, p.793).

For most women with gestational diabetes, pregnancy progresses safely to about 40 weeks, and vaginal delivery is possible. However, if diabetes becomes difficult to control, early induction of labour (p.797) may be necessary. If the fetus is very large, the doctor may carry out a caesarean section (p.802) to avoid a difficult vaginal delivery.

After delivery, your blood sugar levels and those of your baby will be monitored. If the baby's blood sugar level is low, he or she may need to be admitted to a special care baby unit (p.959) for treatment. Since you may be at risk of developing permanent diabetes mellitus after pregnancy, you will be given a glucose tolerance test at your 6-week postnatal checkup.

WHAT IS THE PROGNOSIS?

Usually, glucose levels return to normal soon after delivery of the baby, and you should be able to resume your normal diet. If you were having insulin injections, they can be stopped. However, you are likely to develop diabetes during future pregnancies.

(WWW) ONLINE SITES: p.1030, p.1035

Hyperemesis

Severe vomiting associated with early pregnancy

LIFESTYLE Stress may aggravate the condition

AGE GENETICS Not significant factors

In hyperemesis, vomiting in early pregnancy is so severe that no food or fluids can be kept down. Hyperemesis is more severe than common morning sickness (*see* COMMON COMPLAINTS OF NORMAL PREGNANCY, p.784), in which nausea and vomiting during early pregnancy are usually not serious and can often be relieved by a few simple measures. When morning sickness occurs in pregnancy, the mother continues to gain weight steadily. In contrast, a mother who has hyperemesis will lose weight. Excessive vomiting eventually leads to dehydration, which, in turn, decreases urine volume and causes an imbalance of chemicals in the blood. Allowed to continue without treatment, dehydration may become life-threatening for both the mother and the fetus.

The cause of hyperemesis is usually not known, although it is thought that very high amounts of human chorionic gonadotropin (HCG), a hormone that is produced in pregnancy, may contribute to excessive vomiting in the mother. High levels of HCG occur if more than one fetus is present (*see* MULTIPLE PREGNANCY AND ITS PROBLEMS, p.792) or, less commonly, if a tumour develops from part of the placenta (*see* MOLAR PREGNANCY, p.790). Psychological factors, such as emotional stress, may aggravate the condition in some cases.

WHAT MIGHT BE DONE?

If you are unable to keep any food or fluids down, you need to be admitted to hospital. You may have blood tests to assess the degree of dehydration. You may also have ultrasound scanning (*see* ULTRASOUND SCANNING IN PREGNANCY, p.793) to investigate the possibility of a multiple or molar pregnancy.

Usually, dehydration is treated with intravenous fluids. You may be given drugs that help to stop the vomiting (*see* ANTIEMETIC DRUGS, p.922) and possibly sedatives to help you to relax.

Once the vomiting has been treated, you should be able to start eating small quantities of plain food and gradually build up to a normal diet. However, vomiting often recurs, and further hospital stays may be necessary to prevent dehydration. Hyperemesis usually subsides after the 14th week of pregnancy, although the condition is likely to recur in subsequent pregnancies.

(WWW) ONLINE SITES: p.1035

(TREATMENT) TERMINATION OF PREGNANCY

A termination of pregnancy may be carried out if the pregnancy threatens the woman's physical or emotional health or if tests show a severe fetal disorder. All types of termination cause some abdominal pain for a few hours and a brown discharge for several days. Sexual intercourse should be avoided for 2 weeks.

Methods of termination

There are several different methods of termination, depending on the stage of the pregnancy. Most terminations are carried out using suction between 6 and 14 weeks.

WHEN DONE	WHERE DONE	PROCEDURE USED
Before 7 weeks	At a clinic. Two visits of several hours each are required	This method of termination uses the drug mifepristone, which causes the placenta to detach from the uterus. This drug is taken orally under supervision, and monitoring is carried out for at least 2 hours. 36–48 hours later, a prostaglandin pessary is placed in the vagina in order to encourage the uterus to contract and expel the contents. Monitoring is carried out for a further 6–8 hours.
At 6–14 weeks	At a clinic or hospital. No overnight stay is required	A suction device is inserted through the cervix and into the uterus under either general or local anaesthesia. A vaginal pessary may be given first to soften the cervix. The contents of the uterus are then removed
After 14 weeks	In the hospital. An overnight stay is required	A prostaglandin drug is given to stimulate uterine contractions, which expel the contents. The drug may be given as an intravenous infusion, a vaginal pessary, or an injection through the abdomen into the uterus. Pain relief (*see* PAINKILLERS, p.912) and mild sedatives may be needed

Molar pregnancy

A rare condition in which part of the placenta develops into a tumour

AGE More common over the age of 35

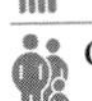
GENETICS More common in Asian women

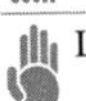
LIFESTYLE Not a significant factor

In about 1 in 2,000 pregnancies, part of the placenta develops into a hydatidiform mole, a tumour that looks similar to a small bunch of grapes. Although a hydatidiform mole is noncancerous, in a few cases it develops into a cancerous tumour (*see* CHORIOCARCINOMA, p.748). A hormone called human chorionic gonadotropin (HCG), which is normally produced by the placenta in pregnancy, is present in very high levels in molar pregnancy. In most molar pregnancies, the tumour prevents a fetus from developing. If a fetus does develop, it will be abnormal and die before birth. Placental cells left after a miscarriage or pregnancy can develop into a hydatidiform mole.

In about 1 in 10 molar pregnancies, a hydatidiform mole invades the wall of the uterus. In about 3 in 100 cases, a hydatidiform mole becomes cancerous, and the cancer may spread. Molar pregnancy occurs more often in women over the age of 35 and is more common in Asian women. The cause is unknown.

WHAT ARE THE SYMPTOMS?

A hydatidiform mole exaggerates some of the symptoms of a normal, healthy pregnancy, such as tiredness, and it may also produce the following:

- Bleeding from the vagina and passing material that looks like grapes.
- Extreme nausea and vomiting (*see* HYPEREMESIS, p.789).

A hydatidiform mole grows faster than a normal fetus, making the uterus larger than normal for the stage of pregnancy. If the pregnancy progresses, additional problems, including pre-eclampsia (*see* PRE-ECLAMPSIA AND ECLAMPSIA, p.794) and anaemia (p.446), may develop.

WHAT MIGHT BE DONE?

If you are experiencing severe nausea and vomiting or if your uterus appears much larger than normal for the stage of your pregnancy, your doctor may suspect a molar pregnancy. He or she will arrange for an ultrasound scan (*see* ULTRASOUND SCANNING IN PREGNANCY, p.793) to look for signs of a molar pregnancy, and your blood will be tested to measure levels of HCG. If a hydatidiform mole is diagnosed, the abnormal tissue will be removed from the uterus under general anaesthesia.

WHAT IS THE PROGNOSIS?

A molar pregnancy will never result in the birth of a fetus. Most women recover fully and need no further treatment once the molar pregnancy has been removed. However, a choriocarcinoma sometimes develops and further treatment, such as chemotherapy (p.280), is required.

Women who have had a molar pregnancy should have regular urine tests for at least 2 years to measure HCG levels and ensure that any cancerous changes are detected early. It is advisable not to conceive for at least 1 year after treatment for a hydatidiform mole because the risk of choriocarcinoma is greatest during this time and a pregnancy will interfere with HCG monitoring. In up to 3 in 100 subsequent pregnancies, a hydatidiform mole recurs.

(WWW) ONLINE SITES: p.1035

Ectopic pregnancy

A pregnancy that develops outside the uterus, usually in a fallopian tube

AGE Most common between the ages of 20 and 29

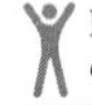
LIFESTYLE Use of an intra-uterine contraceptive device is a risk factor

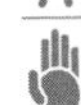
GENETICS Not a significant factor

About 1 in 100 pregnancies is ectopic. In an ectopic pregnancy, a fertilized egg becomes implanted in tissues outside the uterus instead of in the uterine lining. The egg then begins to develop into an embryo. In most ectopic pregnancies, the fertilized egg lodges inside one of the two fallopian tubes. Rarely, the egg implants in the cervix, in one of the ovaries, or in the abdominal cavity. The embryo is not able to grow normally in an ectopic pregnancy and only rarely survives.

If the placenta develops inside a fallopian tube and the embryo grows, the fallopian tube will eventually rupture, causing life-threatening bleeding into the mother's abdominal cavity. Ectopic pregnancies need to be removed surgically as soon as possible after detection because of the risk to the mother.

WHAT ARE THE CAUSES?

Ectopic pregnancy is more common in women aged between 20 and 29, but the cause is not always known. However, previous damage to one of the fallopian tubes may obstruct the passage of a fertilized egg along the tube to the uterus. The egg then implants in the wall of the tube instead of in the uterus. This prior damage may have been caused by an unsuccessful or a reversed sterilization procedure (*see* FEMALE STERILIZATION, p.743) or a fallopian tube infection (*see* PELVIC INFLAMMATORY DISEASE, p.741). Ectopic pregnancies are also more common in women using an intra-uterine contraceptive device (*see* CONTRACEPTION, p.69), partly because these devices increase the risk of a pelvic infection in women who are regularly exposed to sexually transmitted infections (p.764).

WHAT ARE THE SYMPTOMS?

An ectopic pregnancy usually produces symptoms in the first 6–7 weeks, sometimes even before the woman realizes she is pregnant. However, most women who have an ectopic pregnancy will have missed a menstrual period by the time symptoms appear. The symptoms of an ectopic pregnancy may include:

- Pain that is low down on one side of the abdomen.
- Irregular vaginal bleeding that may be confused with menstruation.

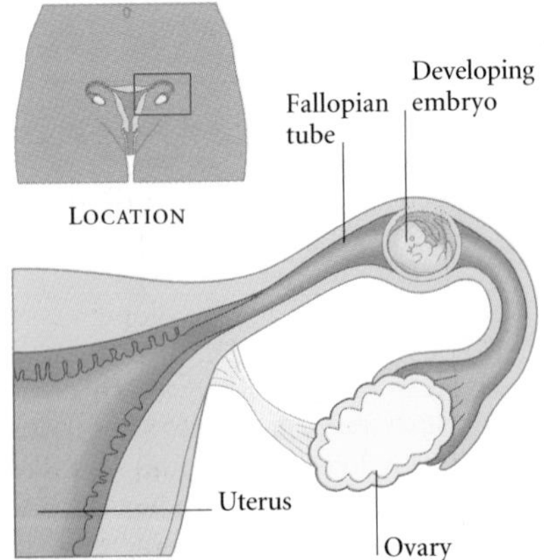

Ectopic pregnancy
In most ectopic pregnancies, the fertilized egg implants in a fallopian tube and starts to develop there, rather than in the uterus.

If the ectopic pregnancy is not detected and a fallopian tube ruptures, further symptoms may develop that include:

- Sudden, severe pain that gradually spreads throughout the abdomen.
- Shoulder pain (referred pain due to overlapping nerve pathways).

Sudden internal bleeding follows the rupture of the fallopian tube and may cause shock (p.414). If you are in shock, you may sweat profusely and feel faint. It is important to see your doctor at once if you have abdominal pain or vaginal bleeding and might be pregnant. If you experience severe pain or shock, call an ambulance immediately.

WHAT MIGHT BE DONE?

If you are not sure whether or not you are pregnant, a pregnancy test will be performed. If the test is positive, your doctor may arrange for you to have an ultrasound scan using a probe in your vagina to find out the position of the embryo. You may also have a blood test to measure blood levels of human chorionic gonadotropin (HCG), a hormone that is produced in lower amounts than normal in ectopic pregnancies. To confirm the diagnosis, an examination of the inside of the abdominal cavity may be performed under general anaesthesia (*see* LAPAROSCOPY, p.742).

If an ectopic pregnancy is confirmed, the embryo and surrounding tissue are usually surgically removed. A damaged fallopian tube will be repaired if possible, but, if it is badly damaged, the tube may be removed to prevent another ectopic pregnancy from occurring at the same site. If an ectopic pregnancy is diagnosed early, it may be treated with the drug methotrexate rather than by surgery.

WHAT IS THE PROGNOSIS?

Although approximately 1 in 10 women will have a further ectopic pregnancy, most affected women can have normal pregnancies even if one fallopian tube has been removed. If both tubes have been damaged, in-vitro fertilization (*see* ASSISTED CONCEPTION, p.776) may help a woman to become pregnant.

In subsequent pregnancies, an ultrasound scan (*see* ULTRASOUND SCANNING IN PREGNANCY, p.793) may be carried out at an early stage to check that the fetus is developing in the uterus.

WWW ONLINE SITES: p.1035

Vaginal bleeding in pregnancy

Bleeding from the vagina at any time during pregnancy

AGE GENETICS LIFESTYLE Not significant factors

If you experience vaginal bleeding in pregnancy, you should seek immediate advice from your doctor. If you develop heavy bleeding, particularly late in pregnancy, you should call an ambulance. Severe bleeding may be life-threatening for both you and your baby, so it is vital that you receive emergency care.

WHAT ARE THE CAUSES?

The causes of vaginal bleeding in pregnancy vary, depending on the stage of the pregnancy. Some common conditions can cause bleeding at any stage. These include noncancerous growths on the cervix (*see* UTERINE POLYPS, p.746) and cervical erosion (p.749), in which cells on the inner lining of the cervix extend on to its surface.

BLEEDING BEFORE 14 WEEKS Bleeding in early pregnancy can be caused by a miscarriage (right) and may be accompanied by cramping, period-like pain. Light to heavy bleeding accompanied by severe pain at 6–7 weeks may be due to a pregnancy outside the uterus (*see* ECTOPIC PREGNANCY, opposite page).

Rarely, light, painless vaginal bleeding called spotting persists during the first 14 weeks of pregnancy. In most of these cases, the pregnancy continues.

BLEEDING AT 14–24 WEEKS After week 14 of pregnancy, bleeding may be due to a late miscarriage, the causes of which can include a weak cervix (*see* CERVICAL INCOMPETENCE, p.794). Bleeding due to miscarriage at this stage may be painful.

BLEEDING AFTER 24 WEEKS After the 24th week of pregnancy, painful, light to heavy vaginal bleeding is most often caused by placental abruption (p.799), in which the placenta becomes partially separated from the wall of the uterus. Painless vaginal bleeding after 24 weeks may be due to placenta praevia (p.798), in which the placenta covers some or all of the opening of the cervix.

WHAT MIGHT BE DONE?

A manual examination is rarely carried out, particularly if you are in late pregnancy, because the examination could damage the placenta if it is lying low in the uterus. Using a speculum to hold the vagina open, your doctor will examine your cervix to look for the cause of the bleeding. You may also have ultrasound scanning (*see* ULTRASOUND SCANNING IN PREGNANCY, p.793). If you are in the advanced stages of pregnancy, the fetus's heartbeat may be monitored (*see* FETAL MONITORING, p.803).

Treatment depends on the cause and extent of the bleeding and the stage of your pregnancy. If you have light to moderate bleeding in early pregnancy, your doctor may suggest that you rest in bed. Most of these pregnancies continue normally. However, surgery may be necessary in some cases of miscarriage or if the cause of the bleeding is found to be an ectopic pregnancy. If you have heavy vaginal bleeding later in your pregnancy, your baby may have to be delivered by an emergency caesarean section (p.802). If you have lost a large amount of blood, you may need to have a blood transfusion (p.447).

WWW ONLINE SITES: p.1036

Miscarriage

The spontaneous end of a pregnancy before week 24, also known as a spontaneous abortion

AGE Most common under the age of 16 and over the age of 35

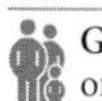

GENETICS In some cases, due to a genetic or chromosomal abnormality in the fetus

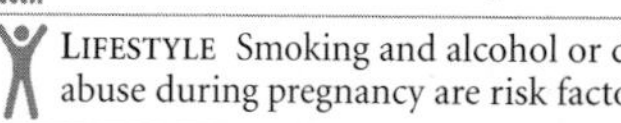

LIFESTYLE Smoking and alcohol or drug abuse during pregnancy are risk factors

More than 1 in 4 of all pregnancies end in miscarriage, the loss of a fetus before the 24th week of pregnancy. Most miscarriages occur in the first 14 weeks of pregnancy, and some occur so early that the woman may not be aware that she is pregnant. Generally, women who miscarry have abnormal vaginal bleeding and abdominal cramps.

WHAT ARE THE CAUSES?

About 3 in 5 miscarriages in the first 14 weeks of pregnancy are caused by a genetic disorder or an abnormality in the fetus. An early miscarriage may also result from lower than normal levels of the hormone progesterone. Early miscarriage is more common in multiple pregnancies (*see* MULTIPLE PREGNANCY AND ITS PROBLEMS, right).

Later miscarriages (between weeks 14 and 24) may be due to a weak cervix (*see* CERVICAL INCOMPETENCE, p.794) or to a severe infection in the mother. An abnormally shaped uterus or noncancerous tumours in the wall of the uterus (*see* FIBROIDS, p.745) may also cause a late miscarriage. Smoking and alcohol or drug abuse in pregnancy are also risk factors. Women who have diabetes mellitus (p.687) are at increased risk of a late miscarriage.

Any of the above factors may cause recurrent miscarriages. Generally, miscarriage is more common in women under the age of 16 or over 35. It is a commonly held belief that stress or minor injuries may lead to miscarriage, but there is no evidence to support this.

WHAT ARE THE TYPES?

A miscarriage can be classified into one of several different types: threatened, inevitable, and missed miscarriage.

In a threatened miscarriage, the fetus is alive and the cervix remains closed. There is some vaginal bleeding, which is usually painless, but the pregnancy often continues for its full term of about 40 weeks. However, sometimes a threatened miscarriage develops into an inevitable miscarriage.

In an inevitable miscarriage, the fetus is usually dead and the cervix is open. An inevitable miscarriage is frequently painful because the uterus contracts to expel the fetus. Pain varies from mild, menstrual period-type pains to severe pain, and there may be heavy vaginal bleeding with clots. An inevitable miscarriage may be either complete (all the contents of the uterus are expelled) or incomplete (some contents remain in the uterus after the miscarriage).

In a missed miscarriage, the fetus is dead, but there is usually no bleeding or pain. The uterus does not contract, and the cervix is closed with the fetus still inside. Although pregnancy symptoms, such as nausea, come to an end, a missed miscarriage is often not detected until a routine ultrasound scan is carried out (*see* ULTRASOUND SCANNING IN PREGNANCY, opposite page).

You should consult your doctor if you have vaginal bleeding or pain in pregnancy. If bleeding or pain is severe, call an ambulance immediately.

HOW IS IT DIAGNOSED?

Your doctor will examine your cervix using a speculum. If your cervix is closed, an ultrasound scan will be performed and, if the fetus is alive, the pregnancy often continues. However, if the cervix is open, miscarriage is usually inevitable. An ultrasound scan will be carried out to check that all the contents of the uterus have been expelled.

HOW MIGHT THE DOCTOR TREAT IT?

If you have a threatened miscarriage, your doctor will probably suggest that you rest for a few days until the bleeding has stopped and any identifiable cause, such as an infection, is treated. In the event of an inevitable miscarriage, your treatment will depend on whether the miscarriage is complete or incomplete. Normally, no further medical treatment is needed for a complete miscarriage, although you may be given painkillers (p.912) if necessary. If a miscarriage was incomplete, you may need to be admitted to hospital so that any tissue left behind in the uterus can be removed surgically. This procedure is also used for an early missed miscarriage. The doctor may also prescribe antibiotics (p.885) to prevent an infection developing. If a missed miscarriage occurs in later pregnancy, you may require induction of labour (p.797).

WHAT CAN I DO?

The loss of a baby is always distressing, and you should take time to grieve and talk about your feelings. You may want to discuss your concerns about future pregnancies with your doctor. If you want to become pregnant again, it is best to wait several months to give yourself time to recover from your loss.

WHAT IS THE PROGNOSIS?

Most women who have a miscarriage do not have problems with subsequent pregnancies. Some women have recurrent miscarriages, but with specialist investigation and treatment they may eventually have a successful pregnancy.

(WWW) ONLINE SITES: p.1029, p.1035

Multiple pregnancy and its problems

The presence of more than one fetus in the uterus and the problems that may arise

 AGE Multiple pregnancy more common over the age of 30

 GENETICS Multiple pregnancy sometimes runs in families

 LIFESTYLE Not a significant factor

Multiple pregnancy occurs when more than one fetus develops in the uterus. Although most multiple pregnancies progress smoothly, the risk of problems is increased for both mother and fetuses.

Nonidentical fetuses may develop if two or more eggs are fertilized at the same time, whereas two or more identical fetuses may develop if an egg splits after fertilization. Fetuses may share a placenta or each fetus may have its own.

In the UK, twins occur naturally in about 15 in 1,000 births and triplets occur in about 1 in 2,000 births. Natural pregnancies of more than three fetuses are extremely rare, but there has been a dramatic increase in multiple pregnancies as a result of fertility treatment.

You are more likely to have nonidentical twins if you are over the age of 30 or if there are multiple births in your family history on your mother's side. However, these factors do not increase your chance of having identical twins.

WHAT ARE THE CAUSES OF MULTIPLE PREGNANCY?

Multiple pregnancies may occur naturally, but 2 in 3 pregnancies with three or more fetuses result from infertility treatments (*see* ASSISTED CONCEPTION,

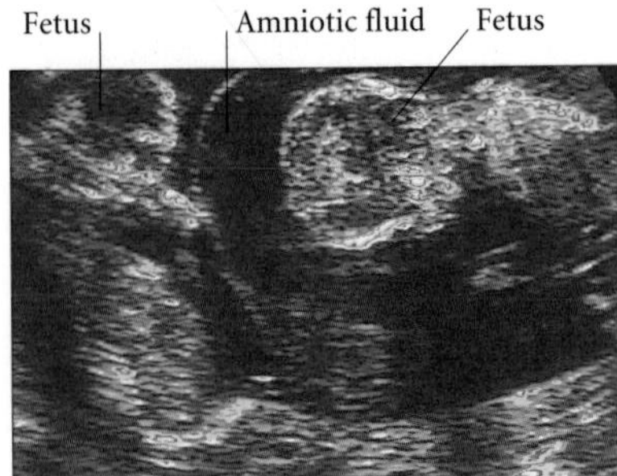

Twins in the uterus
Two fetuses, each in its own sac of fluid, can be seen lying at right angles to each other in this colour-enhanced ultrasound scan.

p.776). This is because drugs for infertility (p.936) stimulate the ovaries to release more than one egg each month, and more than one egg is inserted into the uterus during in-vitro fertilization.

What are the problems?

The common problems associated with normal pregnancy (*see* Common complaints of normal pregnancy, p.784) are sometimes more severe in a multiple pregnancy. This is partly due to the increased size of the uterus and partly because the placenta or placentas produce a higher level of hormones.

Women who are carrying more than one fetus are more likely to have certain problems, such as high blood pressure during pregnancy (*see* Pre-eclampsia and eclampsia, p.794). Such women are also more likely to develop excessive vomiting during early pregnancy (*see* Hyperemesis, p.789), have greater than normal amounts of fluid surrounding the fetus (*see* Polyhydramnios, p.795), and have a low-lying placenta or placentas (*see* Placenta praevia, p.798). Iron-deficiency anaemia (p.447) is also more likely because the mother must supply iron to more than one fetus.

A multiple pregnancy is more likely to result in a miscarriage (p.791) or in premature labour (p.798). The fetuses in a multiple pregnancy are often smaller than single babies, and there is a greater risk of one baby not being in the normal position for labour (*see* Abnormal presentation, p.800). Since there may be more than one placenta, bleeding after the delivery may be heavy (*see* Postpartum haemorrhage, p.806).

What might be done?

Your doctor may suspect a multiple pregnancy if your abdomen is larger than would be expected for the stage of the pregnancy. The diagnosis is usually confirmed by ultrasound scanning (*see* Ultrasound scanning in pregnancy, below). You may be monitored with ultrasound scans every month, possibly with Doppler ultrasound scanning every 2 weeks to check that each fetus is receiving adequate blood. Some hospitals have multiple pregnancy clinics.

Additional treatment may be needed if problems develop. For example, you may be prescribed iron supplements to treat anaemia. You should rest often, especially after the 28th week, to help to reduce the risk of a premature labour. Multiple fetuses are usually delivered in hospital because of the risks of a difficult or premature labour. Twins may be delivered vaginally if the first baby is in the head-down position. A caesarean section (p.802) is usually necessary for the delivery of three or more babies.

Since the babies are often premature and small, they may need to be looked after in a special care baby unit (p.959).

(WWW) ONLINE SITES: p.1035

(TEST) Ultrasound scanning in pregnancy

Ultrasound scanning uses sound waves to produce an image of the internal organs. The procedure is routinely used during pregnancy to assess the health of the fetus, determine the fetus's age, and measure fetal growth. Scanning may also be used to investigate problems, such as vaginal bleeding, and diagnose fetal abnormalities. For example, the procedure may identify neural tube defects and can sometimes detect heart disease. A scan takes about 20–30 minutes and is painless and safe. Doppler scanning may be used to measure blood flow to the fetus.

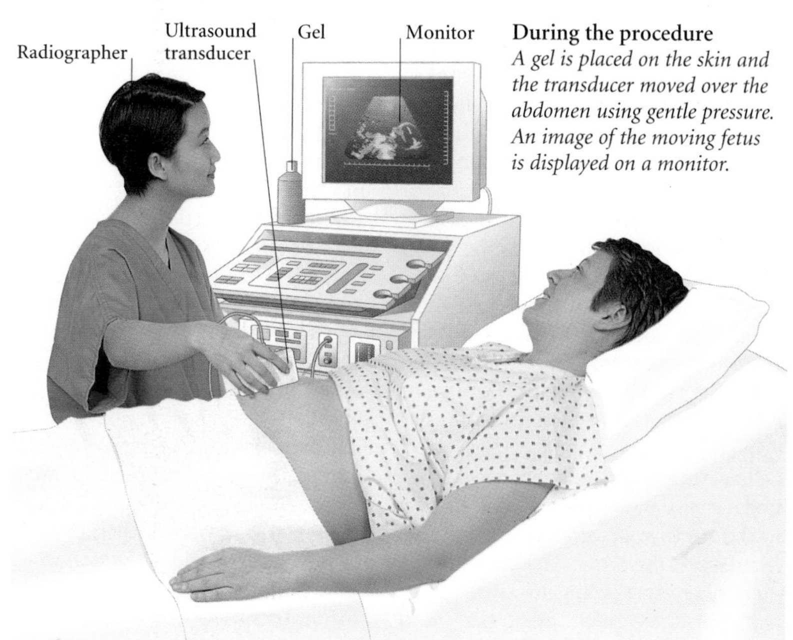

During the procedure
A gel is placed on the skin and the transducer moved over the abdomen using gentle pressure. An image of the moving fetus is displayed on a monitor.

(RESULTS)

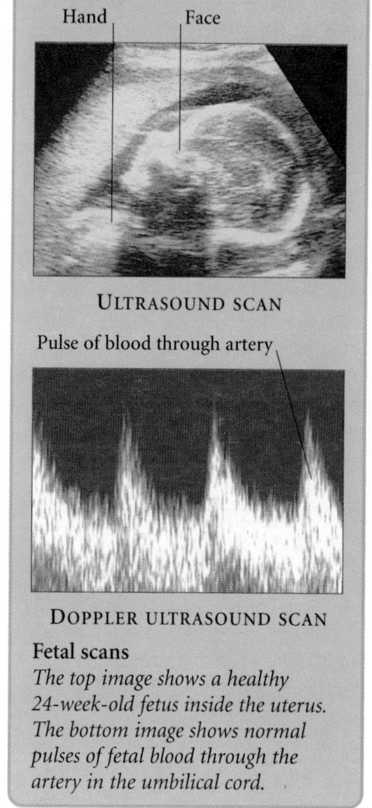

Ultrasound scan

Doppler ultrasound scan

Fetal scans
The top image shows a healthy 24-week-old fetus inside the uterus. The bottom image shows normal pulses of fetal blood through the artery in the umbilical cord.

Cervical incompetence

Weakness of the cervix, which may result in a late miscarriage

AGE GENETICS LIFESTYLE Not significant factors

The cervix normally stays closed until labour begins. However, if the cervix has become weak, a condition known as cervical incompetence, the weight of the growing fetus and its surrounding amniotic fluid may cause the cervix to open early, resulting in a miscarriage (p.791). Cervical incompetence is the cause of about 1 in 4 miscarriages after the 14th week of pregnancy.

The cervix may be weakened by previous surgery, such as a cone biopsy (*see* TREATING CERVICAL DYSPLASIA, p.751), or by any procedure that involves artificial opening of the cervix. For example, a woman who has had more than three terminations of pregnancy (p.789) at an early stage is more likely to develop cervical incompetence.

Often there are no symptoms of cervical incompetence before miscarriage occurs. At this stage, the mother may feel pressure in the lower abdomen or a "lump" in the vagina.

WHAT MIGHT BE DONE?

If you have had a previous miscarriage after the 14th week of pregnancy, your doctor may arrange for you to have ultrasound scanning (p.250) to check for cervical incompetence. The scan is performed through the vagina to measure the thickness of the cervix and may be carried out at an early stage in your next pregnancy or when you are planning a pregnancy. If you are at high risk of cervical incompetence, possibly due to previous surgery on the cervix, you may also be investigated for cervical incompetence before or early in pregnancy.

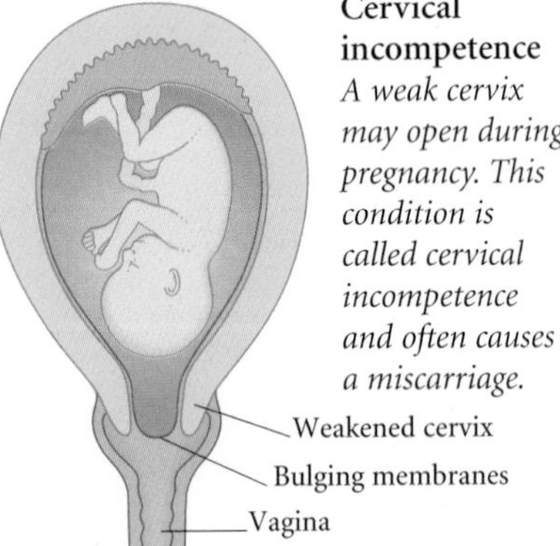

Cervical incompetence
A weak cervix may open during pregnancy. This condition is called cervical incompetence and often causes a miscarriage.

If the cervix is weak, a stitch can be inserted in it to hold it closed. The procedure is carried out under general or epidural anaesthesia between weeks 12 and 16 of pregnancy. The stitch is usually removed at 37 weeks, before the beginning of labour. If labour starts while the stitch is still in place, it will be removed immediately to prevent the cervix from becoming torn. If the stitch fails to prevent a miscarriage, another pregnancy may be successful if a stitch is inserted higher in the cervix, sometimes during an abdominal operation.

Cervical incompetence is likely to recur in subsequent pregnancies, so the cervix may need to be stitched each time to prevent miscarriage.

(WWW) ONLINE SITES: p.1035

Pre-eclampsia and eclampsia

High blood pressure, fluid retention, and protein in the urine in pregnancy, which may lead to seizures and coma

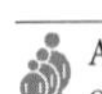
AGE Most common under the age of 19 or over the age of 35

GENETICS Sometimes runs in families

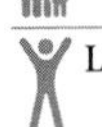
LIFESTYLE Being overweight is a risk factor

Pre-eclampsia, also called pre-eclamptic toxaemia, develops in about 1–2 out of 20 pregnancies, most often in the second half of pregnancy. The condition is a combination of high blood pressure with excessive fluid retention and/or protein in the urine. Mild pre-eclampsia is common in the last weeks of pregnancy and is usually easy to treat. Severe pre-eclampsia may threaten the life of the mother and/or the fetus. If it is left untreated, severe pre-eclampsia may lead to a potentially fatal disorder known as eclampsia that causes seizures and may bring on a coma (p.522).

The cause of pre-eclampsia is not yet understood, but it may be due in part to the mother developing an immune reaction to the fetus. The condition is most likely to develop in a first pregnancy, a subsequent pregnancy with a new father, or a multiple pregnancy. Pre-eclampsia can run in families and is most common in women under the age of 19 or over 35. There is also an increased risk of pre-eclampsia in overweight women and in women who have chronic kidney disease, diabetes mellitus (p.687), or pre-existing high blood pressure (*see* HYPERTENSION, p.403).

WHAT ARE THE SYMPTOMS?

Initially, pre-eclampsia may produce no symptoms. As the condition progresses, the symptoms tend to develop gradually, but occasionally the onset is rapid. Symptoms may include:

- Swollen feet, ankles, and hands and excessive weight gain due to retention of fluid.
- Headaches.
- Visual disturbances, such as blurred vision and seeing flashing lights.
- Vomiting.
- Upper abdominal pain.

You should consult your doctor immediately if you develop any of the above symptoms during pregnancy. Without immediate hospital treatment, the condition may worsen rapidly.

HOW IS IT DIAGNOSED?

Your doctor will examine you for evidence of pre-eclampsia at every antenatal checkup. He or she will examine you for signs of fluid retention, take your blood pressure, and test your urine for protein. If your doctor suspects pre-eclampsia, he or she may also arrange for various blood tests, including tests to check your kidney function.

WHAT IS THE TREATMENT?

Treatment for pre-eclampsia depends on the stage of your pregnancy and the severity of your symptoms. If you have mild to moderate pre-eclampsia and are less than 36 weeks pregnant, you will probably be advised to rest at home. Your blood pressure will be taken frequently to check that it is not raised. In some women, monitoring in hospital and bed rest may be needed.

If pre-eclampsia becomes severe and the fetus is mature enough to survive an early delivery, induction of labour (p.797) or a caesarean section (p.802) may be recommended. Before an early delivery, you may have injections of corticosteroids to help the lungs of the fetus to mature. In rare cases, severe pre-eclampsia that develops before the

24th week requires a termination of pregnancy (p.789) to save the mother.

Regardless of the severity, if you have pre-eclampsia later than 36 weeks into your pregnancy, your doctor is likely to recommend that labour be induced at once or that a caesarean section be performed to deliver the baby.

If eclampsia develops, you may be given antihypertensive drugs (p.897) to lower your blood pressure and intravenous anticonvulsant drugs (p.914) to stop seizures. Delivery by emergency caesarean section is then performed.

WHAT IS THE PROGNOSIS?

If pre-eclampsia is treated before it becomes severe, the outlook is usually good. If eclampsia develops, the lives of the mother and fetus are at risk. High blood pressure usually returns to normal within about 1 week of delivery, but there is an increased risk of the mother developing high blood pressure in later life. About 1 in 10 affected women has pre-eclampsia in a future pregnancy.

(WWW) ONLINE SITES: p.1035

Polyhydramnios

An excessive amount of amniotic fluid surrounding the fetus in the uterus

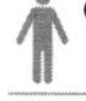
GENETICS Risk factors depend on the cause

AGE LIFESTYLE Not significant factors

Normally, the amount of amniotic fluid surrounding the fetus does not exceed 1.5 litres (3 pints). In polyhydramnios, more than 2 litres (4 pints) of amniotic fluid build up, causing abdominal discomfort or pain in the mother.

Excess fluid makes it easier for the fetus to move around in the uterus. For this reason, the fetus may not lie in the normal head-down position at the end of pregnancy (*see* ABNORMAL PRESENTATION, p.800). Excessive amounts of fluid also increase the likelihood of a premature labour (p.798) or of premature rupture of membranes (p.797).

WHAT ARE THE TYPES?

There are two types of polyhydramnios: chronic, in which the amniotic fluid accumulates slowly over several weeks; and acute, in which the amniotic fluid accumulates over a few days.

Chronic polyhydramnios is the more common form. It develops from about week 32 of pregnancy and causes gradually worsening abdominal discomfort. Breathing difficulties, indigestion, and retention of fluid also sometimes occur. In many women, no cause is found for chronic polyhydramnios. However, the condition occurs more often in mothers who have pre-existing diabetes mellitus (p.687) and in women carrying more than one fetus (*see* MULTIPLE PREGNANCY AND ITS PROBLEMS, p.792). The disorder is more likely if the fetus has a developmental defect, such as spina bifida (*see* NEURAL TUBE DEFECTS, p.844).

The acute form of polyhydramnios develops from 22 weeks and is typically associated with an identical twin pregnancy. The symptoms are similar but more severe than those of chronic polyhydramnios. Frequently, there is severe abdominal pain, nausea, and vomiting.

WHAT MIGHT BE DONE?

Your doctor may suspect that you have polyhydramnios if your abdomen is larger than would be expected for the stage of your pregnancy. You will probably undergo ultrasound scanning (*see* ULTRASOUND SCANNING IN PREGNANCY, p.793) to confirm the diagnosis and to look for fetal abnormalities. You may also need a blood test to check whether you have diabetes mellitus.

Usually, chronic cases can be treated by bed rest. If troublesome symptoms occur late in pregnancy, induction of labour (p.797) may be recommended.

If you have acute polyhydramnios, your doctor may recommend induction of labour if the fetus or fetuses are mature enough. If the fetus is immature, you may be given corticosteroid injections to help the lungs of the fetus mature so that it can be delivered early. Abdominal pain may be relieved temporarily by removing some of the amniotic fluid from the uterus using a needle inserted into the abdomen. If required, the procedure can be repeated.

If you have diabetes mellitus, polyhydramnios may recur in subsequent pregnancies. However, careful control of your diabetes should reduce this risk. If you have polyhydramnios due to other causes, you are not at increased risk in future pregnancies.

(WWW) ONLINE SITES: p.1035

Rhesus incompatibility

A mismatch between the Rh blood group of a pregnant woman and that of her fetus

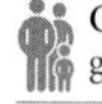
GENETICS Due to incompatibility of genetically determined blood groups

AGE LIFESTYLE Not significant factors

One of the systems for classifying blood is the Rhesus (Rh) group. This system classifies blood according to the presence or absence of certain proteins on the surface of red blood cells. About 17 in 20 people in the UK have Rh proteins on the surface of their red blood cells and are Rh positive. The remaining 3 in 20 people do not have these proteins and are therefore Rh negative.

Rh incompatibility occurs when a mother is Rh negative and her fetus is Rh positive. The situation rarely causes problems in a first pregnancy. However, the mother may develop antibodies if stray blood cells from the baby enter her circulation. These antibodies may attack red blood cells in an Rh-positive fetus in a future pregnancy. The destruction of fetal blood cells may result in severe anaemia (p.446) in the fetus and in anaemia and yellowing of the skin and whites of the eyes (*see* NEONATAL JAUNDICE, p.817) in the newborn baby.

Women who are Rh negative now routinely have preventive treatment at 28 and 34 weeks of pregnancy, and fewer than 1 in 100 women develop problems in future pregnancies.

WHAT IS THE CAUSE?

Blood groups are inherited from both parents. A baby who is Rh positive can be born to an Rh-negative mother only if the baby's father is Rh positive. The circulatory systems of the mother and the fetus are separate, and the red blood cells do not usually cross from one to the other. However, there are circumstances in which stray red blood cells from the fetus can enter the mother's circulation. The fetus's blood cells may leak into the mother's system during delivery, miscarriage (p.791), or termination of pregnancy (p.789). There is also a risk of blood mixing when an amniocentesis test is carried out (*see* ANTENATAL GENETIC TESTS, p.787) or after a placental abruption (p.799), in which part or all of the placenta detaches from the uterus before delivery. The mother's immune system reacts by producing antibodies to destroy the fetal red blood cells in her circulation. In future pregnancies in which the fetus is Rh positive, these antibodies cross the placenta and destroy fetal red blood cells. Untreated, these effects become increasingly severe in each subsequent Rh-incompatible pregnancy.

WHAT ARE THE EFFECTS?

The mother remains well and is usually unaware that there is a problem. The effects on the fetus depend on the level of antibodies present and when in the pregnancy they are produced.

The fetus may develop swelling and progressive anaemia, in which destruction of the red blood cells leads to low levels of oxygen-carrying pigment in the blood. Rarely, a severely anaemic fetus develops acute heart failure (p.412) and may die in the uterus (*see* STILLBIRTH, p.805). After an Rh-incompatible pregnancy, a baby may be born with severe anaemia. Jaundice in the newborn baby occurs due to build-up of bilirubin, a pigment produced from the destruction of fetal red blood cells. Rarely, severe jaundice may cause brain damage.

WHAT MIGHT BE DONE?

If Rh antibodies develop, treatment depends on the amount of antibodies and their effect on the fetus. A sample of the fluid in the uterus is tested for evidence of high bilirubin in the fetus. Additional ultrasound scanning (*see* ULTRASOUND SCANNING IN PREGNANCY, p.793) may be used to check whether the fetus is swollen. If antibody levels are low, the pregnancy may continue until labour is induced at 38 weeks (*see* INDUCTION OF LABOUR, opposite page); if levels are high, labour may be induced earlier. A fetus that is too immature for delivery may have a blood transfusion of Rh-negative blood into the umbilical cord or abdominal cavity. After birth, the baby may need more transfusions and treatment for jaundice.

CAN PROBLEMS BE PREVENTED?

All women are tested at their first antenatal visit to determine their Rh blood group. If you are Rh negative, you will have a blood test at about 28 weeks to see if you have developed antibodies. You will also be given an injection of antibodies against Rh-positive blood at about week 28 and soon after the birth to destroy any fetal red blood cells in your blood. This prevents you from developing antibodies that might react against future Rh-positive fetuses. You may also have this injection after a miscarriage or other procedure that causes fetal and maternal blood to mix. With this treatment, you are very unlikely to develop antibodies that will cause problems in the future.

(WWW) ONLINE SITES: p.1035

Intra-uterine growth retardation

Failure of the fetus to grow properly in the uterus so that it is smaller than expected throughout the pregnancy

AGE Most common under the age of 17 or over the age of 34

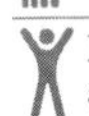
LIFESTYLE Smoking, alcohol or drug abuse, and an inadequate diet during pregnancy are risk factors

GENETICS Risk factors depend on the cause

Intra-uterine growth retardation affects about 1 in 20 babies and occurs when a fetus fails to put on sufficient weight during pregnancy. On average, a baby weighs just over 3 kg (7 lb) at full term. A baby who has growth retardation weighs less than 2.5 kg (5½ lb) at full term and is usually thinner than average rather than shorter in length. Underweight, thin babies are more commonly born to mothers who are under the age of 17 or over the age of 34.

WHAT ARE THE CAUSES?

Poor fetal growth is usually caused by lack of nourishment, which may be due to a disorder in the mother or a factor in her lifestyle. The condition may also be caused by a problem with the placenta or a fetal abnormality.

Maternal disorders that may affect the function of the placenta and lead to malnourishment of the fetus include pre-eclampsia (*see* PRE-ECLAMPSIA AND ECLAMPSIA, p.794), in which high blood pressure and other symptoms develop during pregnancy, chronic high blood pressure (*see* HYPERTENSION, p.403), or pre-existing kidney failure (p.705). Poor fetal growth can also be caused by a serious infection in the mother, such as rubella (p.294). In addtion, several factors in the mother's lifestyle are thought to be linked to intra-uterine growth retardation. Smoking, abusing alcohol or drugs, and eating an inadequate diet may all affect levels of nutrients passing across the placenta to nourish the fetus.

In addition, there are problems with the placenta itself that may lead to fetal malnourishment. For example, part of the placenta may separate from the wall of the uterus (*see* PLACENTAL ABRUPTION, p.799). Rarely, an inherited or a chromosomal abnormality in the fetus, such as Down's syndrome (p.821), leads to intra-uterine growth retardation.

WHAT MIGHT BE DONE?

You will probably have no symptoms, but your doctor may be concerned if measurements of your abdomen during pregnancy show that your uterus is not increasing in size at the normal rate. You will have regular ultrasound scans to monitor the rate of growth of the fetus and may be given scans that measure blood flow through the umbilical cord to the fetus (*see* ULTRASOUND SCANNING IN PREGNANCY, p.793).

If intra-uterine growth retardation is diagnosed, you may need to be admitted to hospital for bed rest. You will be treated for any underlying condition, if possible. For example, you may be given drugs to treat high blood pressure. If your diet is inadequate, you may be offered dietary advice. The fetus's heartbeat will probably be monitored twice daily. If the fetus continues to grow slowly, it may be delivered early, either by induction of labour (opposite page) or by caesarean section (p.802).

WHAT IS THE PROGNOSIS?

After they are born, small babies may initially need to be monitored and cared for in a special care baby unit (p.959) because they tend to be more susceptible to problems such as infections, low blood glucose, and low body temperature (hypothermia). Most small babies gain weight rapidly and reach a normal size. Having a small baby slightly increases the risk of your next baby also being small. However, each new baby tends to be larger than the last.

(WWW) ONLINE SITES: p.1035

Premature rupture of membranes

Rupture of the membrane sac surrounding the fetus that is not closely followed by labour or that occurs before labour is due

LIFESTYLE Smoking is thought to be a risk factor

AGE GENETICS Not significant factors

The fetus is protected in the uterus inside a fluid-filled bag called the amniotic sac. The membranes that form this sac normally rupture during or just before the start of labour, but in about 1 in 14 women they rupture early.

It is not known exactly what causes the membranes to break early, although smoking during pregnancy appears to increase the risk. In some pregnancies, premature rupture of the membranes may be due to an infection that spreads upwards to the uterus from the vagina.

Rupture of the membranes causes the amniotic fluid to leak from the vagina. The amount of fluid lost varies from a light trickle to a heavy gush. If your membranes break at night, you may wake in a pool of liquid, which can easily be mistaken for urine. If you think that your membranes may have broken, you should contact your doctor.

Are there complications?

If labour does not commence within a few hours of the membranes rupturing, there is a risk of the uterus or the fetus becoming infected. There is also a possibility of a cord prolapse, in which the umbilical cord drops into the cervix or vagina. If this occurs, the blood supply to the fetus may be reduced, depriving it of oxygen (*see* FETAL DISTRESS, p.804). In women who have not yet reached week 37 of pregnancy, rupture of the membranes may lead to premature labour (p.798). In this event, the risk to the fetus of an early delivery must be balanced against the risk of an infection developing if labour is stopped.

What might be done?

You may need to be admitted to hospital and monitored for evidence of an infection. Your doctor will feel your abdomen and examine you internally using a speculum to hold the vagina open. He or she will also take your temperature because a fever may indicate an infection. Your doctor may also take a vaginal swab and arrange for blood tests to look for signs of an infection. If there is an infection, you will be treated with antibiotics (p.885). The heart rate of the fetus may be monitored (*see* FETAL MONITORING, p.803) to look for indications of fetal distress. If you are at least 37 weeks into your pregnancy, labour usually begins within 24 hours of the rupture of the membranes. Labour will be induced (*see* INDUCTION OF LABOUR, below) if it fails to start.

If you are 36 weeks pregnant or the fetus is mature enough for delivery, labour may be induced; otherwise, you may be kept in hospital and monitored for signs of infection. If you are less than 34 weeks pregnant, you may be given injections of corticosteroids to help the fetus's lungs mature.

After birth, the baby may need to be monitored in a special care baby unit (p.959), but most babies are healthy and have no ill effects from early delivery.

(WWW) ONLINE SITES: p.1035

(TREATMENT) Induction of labour

If a pregnancy continues beyond 42 weeks or if the health of the mother or fetus is at risk, labour may need to be artificially induced. Various methods are used depending on the stage of labour: a pessary may be inserted into the vagina to encourage the cervix to open, the membranes containing the fetus may be ruptured, or a hormone may be given intravenously to stimulate uterine contractions. In some cases, all three methods need to be used. The last two methods may also be used to speed up labour if it is delayed.

Closed cervix

Pessary

Insertion of a pessary
If the cervix is closed, a prostaglandin pessary is placed at the top of the vagina to soften the cervix, which then thins and begins to open.

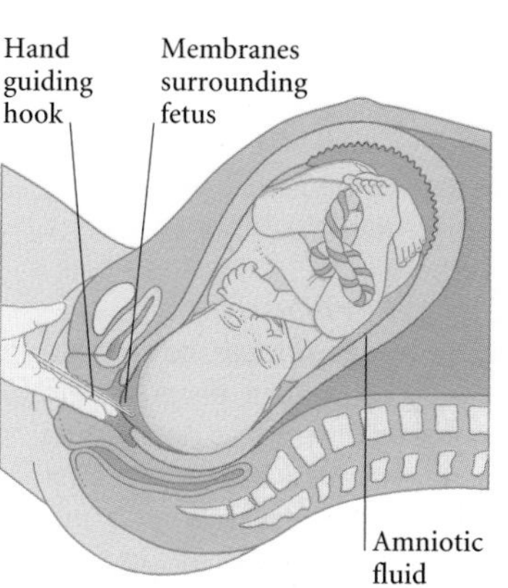

Rupture of membranes
If the cervix is already open, a small hook may be used to rupture the membranes that contain the fetus and its surrounding amniotic fluid.

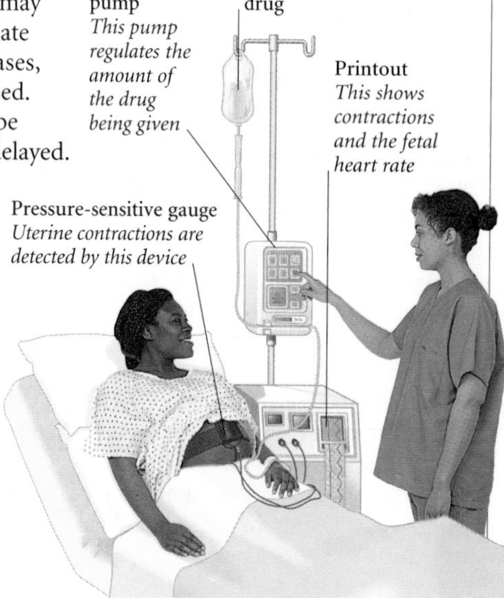

Stimulating uterine contractions
If the cervix is open and the membranes have ruptured, a drug may be given intravenously to encourage the uterus to contract. The contractions and the fetal heart rate will be monitored.

Premature labour

The onset of labour before the 37th week of pregnancy

AGE Most common under the age of 17 or over the age of 35

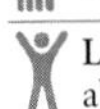
LIFESTYLE Smoking and alcohol or drug abuse during pregnancy are risk factors

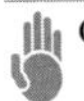
GENETICS Not a significant factor

The normal duration of pregnancy is about 40 weeks. Labour that starts before 37 weeks is considered premature. Premature labour involves few extra risks for the mother, but premature babies often have problems because of their small size and immaturity (*see* PROBLEMS OF THE PREMATURE BABY, p.816).

If premature labour is diagnosed early, there is a chance that it can be stopped and that the pregnancy will continue. If labour cannot be stopped completely, it may be delayed for a day or two so that corticosteroids (p.930) can be given to help the fetus to mature. Premature labour occurs in approximately 1 in every 10 births and is more common in very young mothers and those who are over the age of 35.

What are the causes?

Often, the cause of premature labour is not known, but triggering factors can sometimes be identified.

A multiple pregnancy often results in premature labour, possibly because the uterus is stretched (*see* MULTIPLE PREGNANCY AND ITS PROBLEMS, p.792). An excessive amount of fluid around the fetus (*see* POLYHYDRAMNIOS, p.795) has the same effect. An infection of the urinary tract (*see* CYSTITIS, p.709) or of the vagina (*see* BACTERIAL VAGINOSIS, p.753) may also act as a trigger.

Factors that increase the risk of premature labour include smoking and alcohol or drug abuse during pregnancy, heavy work, stress, a previous premature labour, and long-term disorders such as diabetes mellitus (p.687).

What are the symptoms?

The symptoms of premature labour may be mistaken initially for the backache and painless contractions that commonly occur in late pregnancy. They include:

- Intermittent pain in the lower back.
- Tightenings felt in the abdomen that become regular painful contractions.
- A discharge of blood and mucus from the vagina.

If you think you are going into premature labour, you should contact your doctor immediately. The earlier premature labour is diagnosed, the greater the chances of stopping it. You may be admitted to hospital and transferred to a special care baby unit (p.959) in case it is impossible to stop labour and you deliver your baby early.

What might be done?

Your doctor will examine you to make sure that you are in labour and to assess how far it has advanced. The uterine contractions and the heartbeat of the fetus will be monitored regularly (*see* FETAL MONITORING, p.803). Tests may also be carried out to try to find the cause of the premature labour.

If the fetus is not mature enough to be delivered safely, your doctor may try to stop labour by giving you an intravenous infusion of drugs (*see* DRUGS FOR LABOUR, p.938) that sometimes stop the muscles of the uterus from contracting. You should rest completely during treatment because movement encourages uterine contractions.

If your labour cannot be stopped, the doctor may try to postpone it for a couple of days so that you can be given two injections of corticosteroid drugs, which help the lungs of the fetus to mature. This procedure reduces the risk of breathing problems in the baby after delivery. The fetus will be monitored for signs of fetal distress (p.804). In many cases, a carefully monitored vaginal delivery is possible, but, if there are risk factors such as a multiple pregnancy, it may be necessary to carry out a caesarean section (p.802).

What is the prognosis?

In many cases, labour can be stopped and the pregnancy then progresses to about 40 weeks. Otherwise, postponing labour for a day or two allows time for corticosteroid drug treatment to improve the fetus's chance of survival. Babies born before 37 weeks may need to be cared for and monitored in a special care baby unit until they are more mature. Premature labour often recurs in subsequent pregnancies.

(WWW) ONLINE SITES: p.1035

Placenta praevia

A condition in which the placenta covers or partially covers the opening of the cervix into the uterus

AGE More common over the age of 35

GENETICS LIFESTYLE Not significant factors

In some pregnancies, the placenta is implanted lower down in the uterus and closer to the cervix than is normal. Although a placenta that is lying low will usually move upwards gradually as the uterus expands, the placenta may remain in this position and cover some or all of the opening of the cervix. This condition, known as placenta praevia, occurs in about 1 in 200 pregnancies and is more common in women over the age of 35. Placenta praevia causes up to 1 in 5 cases of vaginal bleeding that occurs after week 24 of pregnancy.

The severity of this condition is related to how much of the opening of the cervix is covered by the placenta. In marginal placenta praevia, the placenta lies low in the uterus and just reaches the edge of the cervix. When complete placenta praevia occurs, the whole of the cervix is covered. Symptoms caused by the condition vary, and mild cases may cause no adverse effects. In other cases, intermittent light to heavy vaginal bleeding occurs from week 24 of pregnancy onwards. Complete placenta praevia may cause severe bleeding that can be life-threatening to the mother

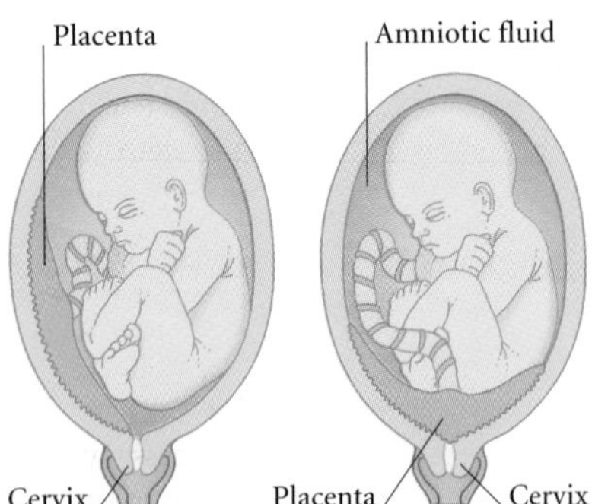

Placenta praevia
In marginal placenta praevia, the placenta implants low in the uterus but only just reaches the opening of the cervix. In complete placenta praevia, the placenta covers the entire opening of the cervix.

and/or fetus. Women who have placenta praevia are at increased risk of developing postpartum haemorrhage (p.806) because the lower part of the uterus may not be able to contract sufficiently to constrict the blood vessels of the uterus and stop bleeding after birth.

WHAT ARE THE CAUSES?

There is an increased risk of placenta praevia in women who have had several pregnancies or if the uterus has been scarred by previous surgery, such as a caesarean section (p.802). The placenta may also develop low in the uterus if there are noncancerous tumours present (*see* FIBROIDS, p.745). The risk of placenta praevia is increased in a multiple pregnancy because there may be more than one placenta or because the placenta may be larger than in a normal pregnancy (*see* MULTIPLE PREGNANCY AND ITS PROBLEMS, p.792).

WHAT MIGHT BE DONE?

Usually, placenta praevia is detected after week 20 by routine ultrasound scanning (*see* ULTRASOUND SCANNING IN PREGNANCY, p.793). If the placenta is lying low, you will be given follow-up scans to monitor its position. The problem may disappear because, in most cases, the placenta moves upwards and away from the cervix by week 32.

If the placenta remains low and you develop vaginal bleeding, you will be admitted to hospital. If you have light bleeding, you may need only bed rest, but if bleeding is heavy, you may need to have an emergency caesarean section and possibly a blood transfusion (p.447) to replace the blood you have lost.

Even if there are no problems, when placenta praevia is complete you will normally be admitted to hospital for monitoring at about the 30th week of pregnancy because of the risk of bleeding. Your baby will then be delivered by caesarean section at 38 weeks. A caesarean section is usually necessary even if there is marginal placenta praevia because of the risk of haemorrhage.

WHAT IS THE PROGNOSIS?

With close monitoring, the pregnancy is usually successful. Placenta praevia may recur in a future pregnancy if an underlying cause cannot be treated.

(WWW) ONLINE SITES: p.1035

Placental abruption

Separation of the placenta from the wall of the uterus before the baby is delivered

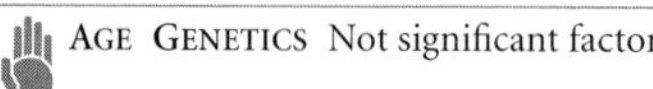

LIFESTYLE Smoking and alcohol or drug abuse during pregnancy are risk factors

AGE GENETICS Not significant factors

The placenta normally separates from the wall of the uterus after the baby has been born. In placental abruption, part or all of the placenta separates from the uterus before the baby has been delivered. The condition occurs in about 1 in 120 pregnancies and is potentially life-threatening, especially for the fetus. Placental abruption is the most common cause of vaginal bleeding in pregnancy after the 28th week.

There are two basic types of placental abruption: revealed and concealed. A revealed placental abruption causes mild to severe vaginal bleeding. In a concealed placental abruption, there is no visible bleeding from the vagina because blood collects between the placenta and the wall of the uterus.

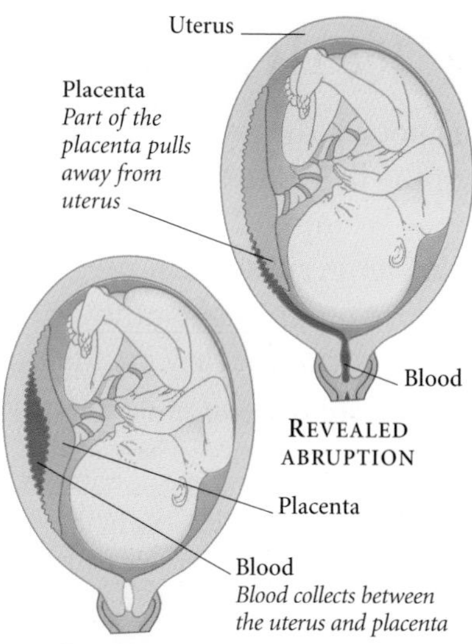

Placental abruption
In a placental abruption, part of the placenta separates from the uterine wall before birth. A revealed abruption causes vaginal bleeding; in a concealed abruption, blood collects behind the placenta.

WHAT ARE THE CAUSES?

The exact cause of placental abruption is not known. However, the condition appears to be more common in women who have long-term high blood pressure (*see* HYPERTENSION, p.403). The risk is also increased if a woman smokes during pregnancy, drinks large amounts of alcohol, and/or abuses drugs. The disorder occurs more often after several previous pregnancies or in women who have had a placental abruption in a previous pregnancy. Abdominal injury sometimes leads to placental abruption.

WHAT ARE THE SYMPTOMS?

Symptoms usually occur suddenly and depend on how much of the placenta has separated from the wall of the uterus. If only a small part of the placenta has pulled away, bleeding may be minor, but a large separation can cause severe haemorrhage. In increasing order of severity, symptoms may include:

- Slight to heavy vaginal bleeding.
- Abdominal cramps or backache.
- Severe, constant abdominal pain.
- Reduced fetal movements.

If you develop vaginal bleeding at any stage of pregnancy, you should consult your doctor immediately. If the bleeding is heavy, it is advisable to call an ambulance without delay because you may need emergency care.

WHAT MIGHT BE DONE?

Your doctor will examine you internally using a speculum, which is an instrument that holds the vagina open. You may also have ultrasound scanning (*see* ULTRASOUND SCANNING IN PREGNANCY, p.793), and the fetal heartbeat will probably be checked. A small separation may be treated by bed rest in hospital, where the fetal heartbeat can be monitored (*see* FETAL MONITORING, p.803).

If bleeding does not stop or restarts, labour may be induced (*see* INDUCTION OF LABOUR, p.797). After a large placental abruption, an emergency caesarean section (p.802) is often needed to save the fetus. You may have a blood transfusion (p.447) if you lose a lot of blood.

The outlook varies depending on the degree of separation. With appropriate treatment, the mother is not usually in danger. If the condition is minor, the pregnancy often progresses, although the fetus may be at risk of intra-uterine growth retardation (p.796). Severe cases may lead to death of the fetus.

(WWW) ONLINE SITES: p.1035

PROBLEMS IN LABOUR

Labour is the process of birth, from the first strong contractions of the uterus to the delivery of the baby and placenta. Labour may last up to 24 hours for a first pregnancy but tends to be shorter in subsequent pregnancies. In most cases, the stages of labour progress smoothly. When problems do occur, they are rarely serious if they are identified and treated promptly.

Improvements in monitoring and more effective pain relief have made labour a safer and much less traumatic experience than it once was. In the past, little relief was available to help mothers cope with the extreme pain of a difficult labour, and complications often threatened the life of the mother or baby, or sometimes both.

The first article in this section looks at abnormal presentation, a condition in which the fetus is not lying in the normal position in the uterus, the easiest position for delivery. Problems that may complicate labour and delivery, usually because the fetus is unable to pass through the mother's pelvis, are covered next.

Two relatively rare conditions are discussed in the final part of this section. Fetal distress arises when the fetus is deprived of sufficient oxygen for its needs. This condition may occur at any stage of pregnancy, but is more common during labour. The final article discusses stillbirth, a rare and distressing situation that occurs when a fetus dies in the womb later than 20 weeks into a pregnancy or, even more rarely, when a baby dies during labour.

KEY ANATOMY

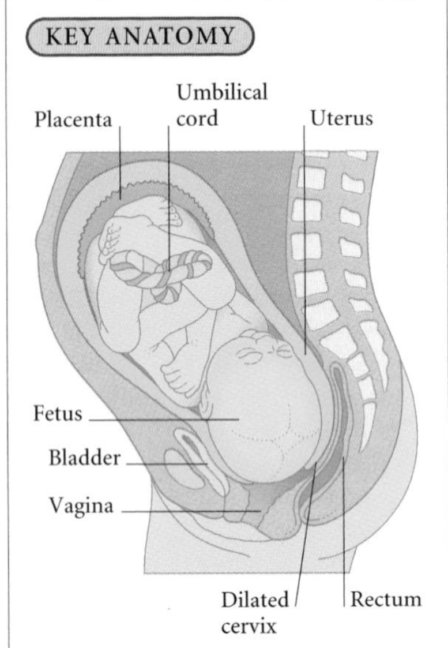

For more information on pregnancy and the stages of childbirth, *see* pp.778–783.

Abnormal presentation

Any deviation from the normal position of the fetus for delivery

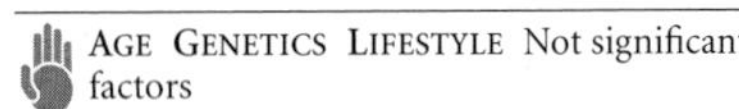

AGE GENETICS LIFESTYLE Not significant factors

In most normal pregnancies, the fetus settles into the mother's pelvic cavity from week 36 onwards, ready for labour and birth. About 8 in 10 fetuses settle head downwards, facing the mother's back, with the chin resting on the chest. In this presentation, the fetus is in the optimum position for birth, and a normal vaginal delivery is usually possible. All other fetal positions are considered to be abnormal presentations and may cause problems during labour.

When a fetus is lying in an abnormal position in the uterus, a vaginal delivery may be possible, but the labour may be prolonged (*see* PROBLEMS DURING DELIVERY, p.802). If the fetus becomes stuck, it may need an assisted delivery (p.805) or caesarean section (p.802).

Most abnormal presentations can be diagnosed before labour begins, and arrangements to deliver the fetus safely can be discussed in advance.

WHAT ARE THE CAUSES?

Abnormal presentation may occur if the fetus is able to move more freely within the uterus than usual, either because the fetus is small and does not fit closely into the pelvis (*see* PREMATURE LABOUR, p.798) or because there is excess amniotic fluid surrounding the fetus (*see* POLYHYDRAMNIOS, p.795). There is also an increased risk of an abnormal presentation when there is more than one fetus in the uterus (*see* MULTIPLE PREGNANCY AND ITS PROBLEMS, p.792).

Occasionally, the fetus cannot settle into the pelvic cavity because of an obstruction, such as the placenta lying low in the uterus (*see* PLACENTA PRAEVIA, p.798) or a noncancerous growth in the uterine wall (*see* FIBROIDS, p.745). An unusually shaped uterus may also contribute to an abnormal presentation.

WHAT ARE THE TYPES?

The most common abnormal presentations are the breech position and the occipitoposterior position. Rarer types include face, compound, brow, and shoulder presentations, named according to the parts of the fetus that are over the dilated cervix at delivery.

BREECH In a breech birth, the fetus presents buttocks first. Many fetuses lie in a breech position before week 32 of pregnancy but most turn by 36 weeks.

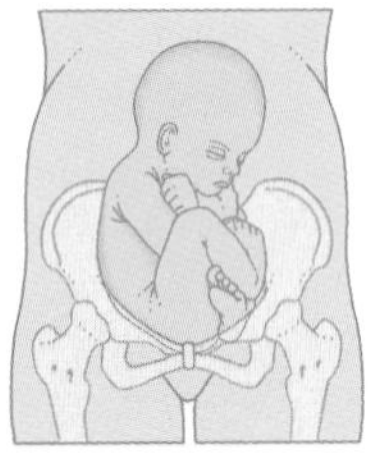

The 3 in 100 that do not turn are in one of three types of breech presentation. A complete breech is one in which the fetus is curled up. In a frank breech, the legs are extended and the feet are close to the face. In a footling breech, one or both feet are positioned over the cervix. Often one twin fetus is a breech.

OCCIPITOPOSTERIOR At the beginning of labour, about 1 in 5 fetuses lies in an occipitoposterior position, head-down but facing the mother's abdomen instead of her back.

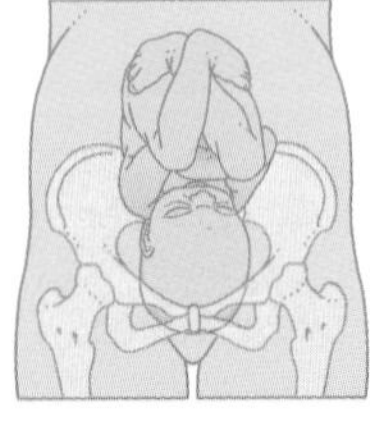

Most fetuses will turn at some stage during labour, but 2 in 100 do not and are still in this presentation when they are delivered.

RARE PRESENTATIONS In a face presentation, the neck of the fetus is bent backwards so that the face is positioned over the cervix. This type of presentation occurs in 1 in every 400 births. In a compound presentation, which occurs in 1 in every 700 births, an arm or leg lies over the cervix in addition to the head or buttocks. In a brow presentation, the fetus's head is bent slightly backwards with the brow over the cervix and occurs in about 1 in every 1,000 births. A shoulder or oblique presentation, in which the fetus lies across the uterus with its shoulder over the cervix, occurs in 1 in every 2,500 births.

ARE THERE COMPLICATIONS?

If the fetus lies in an abnormal position just before delivery, there may be complications that place both the fetus and mother at risk. A fetus in the normal head-down position blocks the cervix and prevents the umbilical cord from passing out of the uterus before the fetus. Some abnormal presentations leave space for the cord to drop through the cervix when the membranes surrounding the fetus rupture. When this occurs, the cord may be compressed by the fetus, or, rarely, its blood vessels may go into spasm because of the drop in temperature outside the uterus. As a result, the fetus may be deprived of oxygen (*see* FETAL DISTRESS, p.804). This may cause brain damage or fetal death. A breech delivery may cause problems if the legs and body of the fetus are able to pass through the cervix when it is not completely dilated, but the head becomes stuck. If, in a footling breech, one foot drops through the cervix, this may prompt the mother to try to push too early. An abnormal presentation may also increase the risk of the cervix or vagina being torn during delivery.

HOW IS IT DIAGNOSED?

Normally, the position of the fetus in the uterus is assessed at each antenatal visit. Your doctor will usually be able to tell if your baby is lying in an abnormal position at the end of your pregnancy. A fetal stethoscope determines where the heartbeat is loudest, and this helps to identify the approximate position of the fetus in the uterus. If your doctor suspects an abnormal presentation, you will be given ultrasound scanning to confirm the position (*see* ULTRASOUND SCANNING IN PREGNANCY, p.793).

WHAT IS THE TREATMENT?

Abnormal presentation is usually diagnosed towards the end of a pregnancy, and, if necessary, a caesarean section is arranged. A vaginal birth may be possible for some breech or occipitoposterior presentations. Sometimes, a mother with a fetus in a breech presentation is offered a procedure to turn the fetus around after week 36 of pregnancy. The doctor attempts to manipulate the fetus into the correct position by pushing gently on the wall of the abdomen. This technique is performed using ultrasound guidance. It is not painful for the mother or fetus, and the mother does not require an anaesthetic.

If the abnormal presentation was due to a structural problem, such as an unusually shaped uterus, there is an increased risk of recurrence in a subsequent pregnancy. However, if the presentation was caused by a condition associated with that particular pregnancy, such as placenta praevia, the risk of recurrence is not increased.

(WWW) ONLINE SITES: p.1035

Delayed first stage of labour

Prolonged or complicated labour in the predelivery stage

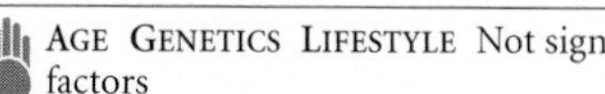

The first stage of labour begins with the onset of regular, strong contractions of the uterus and ends when the cervix is fully dilated. In this period, the cervix widens until it is 10 cm (4 in) in diameter to allow the fetus to pass into the vagina. The average length of the first stage of labour is 6–12 hours, but it can take much longer in a first pregnancy.

(TREATMENT) EPIDURAL ANAESTHESIA IN LABOUR

Epidural anaesthesia is a method of pain relief in labour. The anaesthetic is given through a catheter inserted between two of the vertebrae (bones in the spine) in the lower back. The tip of the catheter is put into the epidural space formed by membranes surrounding the spinal cord. The other end is taped to the shoulder, so that further doses can be given. The anaesthetic numbs nerves from below the waist, including those from the uterus. Intravenous fluids are given, and the baby's heart rate is monitored.

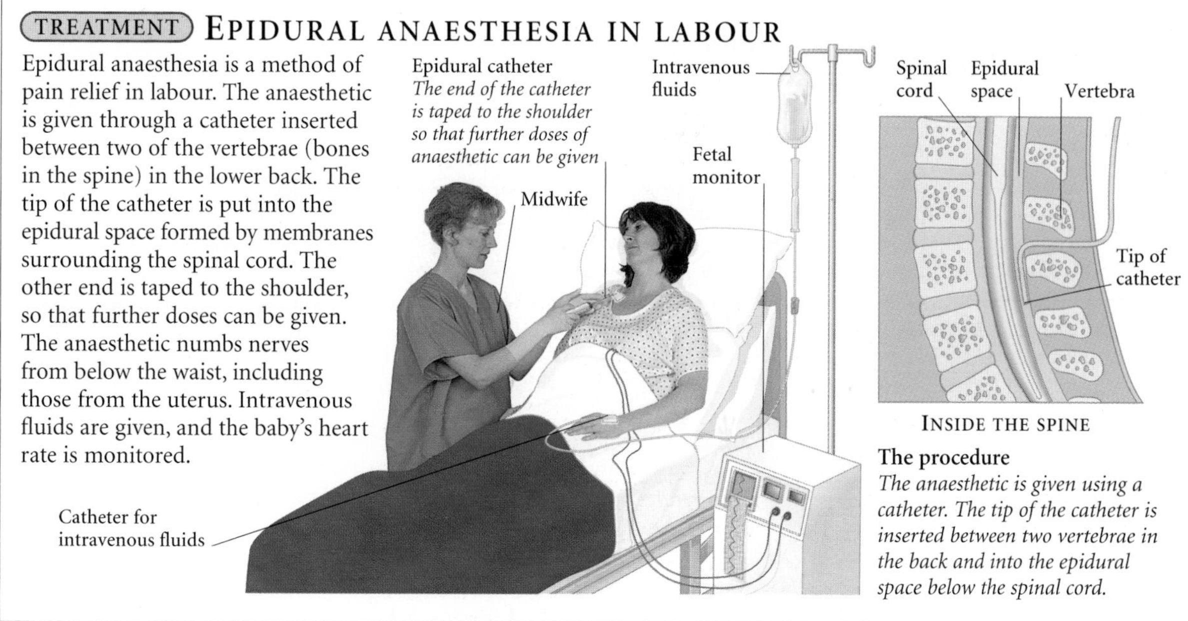

The procedure
The anaesthetic is given using a catheter. The tip of the catheter is inserted between two vertebrae in the back and into the epidural space below the spinal cord.

(TREATMENT) CAESAREAN SECTION

In a caesarean section, the baby is delivered through an incision in the mother's abdomen. The operation is carried out when circumstances make it safer than a vaginal birth for the mother and baby. The delivery is carried out either under general anaesthesia or using an epidural anaesthetic injected into the lower back, which numbs the body below the waist (*see* EPIDURAL ANAESTHESIA IN LABOUR, p.801). An incision is made in the lower abdomen and the baby and placenta are delivered within minutes. The mother stays in hospital for about 4 days afterwards.

During the procedure
A caesarean section may be performed under epidural anaesthesia so that you can remain awake. Your partner can be with you during the operation, and you can hold the baby immediately afterwards.

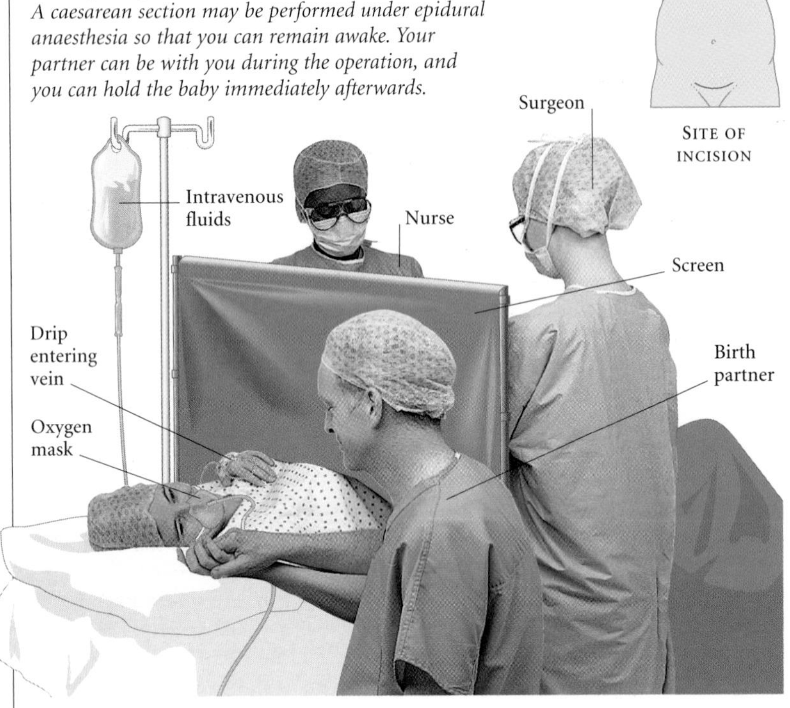

Labour is delayed when the first stage is prolonged and the cervix is not dilating normally. A prolonged labour occurs in about 3 in 10 first births and about 1 in 8 subsequent births.

When it has been recognized that the first stage of labour is not progressing, the problem can usually be treated successfully with modern techniques and monitoring. The mother may become exhausted during a long first stage of labour and this can cause problems during delivery (right). Left untreated, a delay in the first stage may threaten the life of the mother and/or the fetus.

WHAT ARE THE CAUSES?

A delay in the first stage of labour may be due to uterine contractions that are too weak to fully dilate the cervix. In first pregnancies, weak uterine contractions are especially common, and the cervix often takes longer to dilate than normal. Drugs given to relieve pain in labour, such as epidural anaesthesia (*see* EPIDURAL ANAESTHESIA IN LABOUR, p.801), may also weaken contractions.

Sometimes, the cervix fails to dilate because it is scarred from surgery. In some labours, the fetus is in an unusual position and cannot put enough pressure on the cervix to assist dilation (*see* ABNORMAL PRESENTATION, p.800).

WHAT CAN I DO?

If your labour is taking an abnormally long time, try to keep walking around because gentle movement encourages the uterus to contract more effectively, and gravity increases the pressure from the fetus on the cervix. If you cannot get out of bed, try to sit upright. A prolonged labour can be exhausting and may cause dehydration. It is therefore important that you keep your fluid intake up by drinking plenty of water.

WHAT MIGHT THE DOCTOR DO?

At regular intervals during your labour, a nurse will measure your blood pressure and check whether your cervix is dilating. Your contractions and the heart rate of the fetus will be monitored continually (*see* FETAL MONITORING, opposite page). If the fetal heart rate is abnormal, a blood sample may be taken from the fetus's scalp to check for signs of distress. An intravenous drip is used to increase your fluid levels if you are dehydrated. If your uterine contractions cannot dilate the cervix effectively, your doctor may be able to speed up labour by using a number of different methods (*see* INDUCTION OF LABOUR, p.797). If labour is still delayed, you may need to have a caesarean section (left).

WHAT IS THE PROGNOSIS?

With careful monitoring and management, a delayed first stage of labour is unlikely to cause problems.

The chance of having a delayed first stage of labour in future pregnancies depends on the cause. Weak or ineffective uterine contractions are less likely to occur in subsequent pregnancies, and dilation of the cervix is usually quicker. However, if the cervix has been scarred by surgery or damaged by a difficult delivery, a caesarean section may be necessary in future births.

(WWW) ONLINE SITES: p.1035

Problems during delivery

Any problem that prolongs the second stage of labour or prevents normal delivery

AGE GENETICS LIFESTYLE Not significant factors

The delivery of a baby, called the second stage of labour, begins as soon as the mother's cervix has fully dilated to 10 cm (4 in) and ends when the baby is born. About 4 in 10 mothers experience problems during delivery, and the risk is higher for a first pregnancy. With careful management, it may be possible to carry out a normal vaginal delivery,

(TEST) FETAL MONITORING

Fetal monitoring, also known as cardiotocography, is used to detect fetal distress, usually as a result of oxygen deficiency. During labour, changes in the fetal heart rate in response to uterine contractions are recorded. An abnormal heart rate is a sign of fetal distress. If the fetus is distressed, a more accurate reading may be taken using a probe attached to the fetus's head. A blood sample may be taken from the fetus's scalp to check the level of oxygen. Monitoring normally takes place during labour but may also be used to detect problems during pregnancy.

External fetal monitoring
Two devices are strapped to your abdomen: an ultrasound transducer to detect the fetus's heartbeat and a pressure-sensitive gauge to measure your contractions.

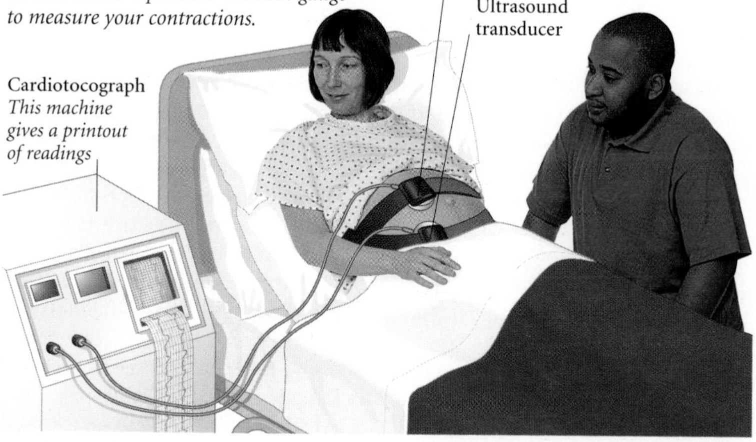

Pressure-sensitive gauge

Ultrasound transducer

Cardiotocograph
This machine gives a printout of readings

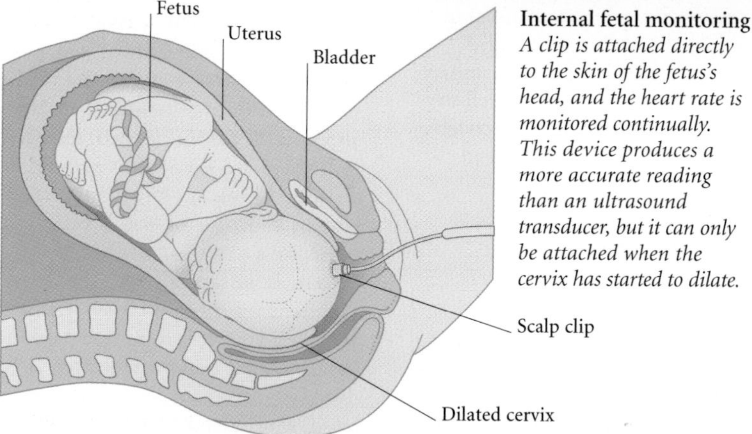

Internal fetal monitoring
A clip is attached directly to the skin of the fetus's head, and the heart rate is monitored continually. This device produces a more accurate reading than an ultrasound transducer, but it can only be attached when the cervix has started to dilate.

(RESULTS)

Cardiotocograph during labour
Readings from the two devices around the mother's abdomen are converted into tracings on a cardiotocograph. The heart rate of a healthy fetus speeds up at the start of a contraction, as the peaks in the graph show, then rapidly returns to a normal level.

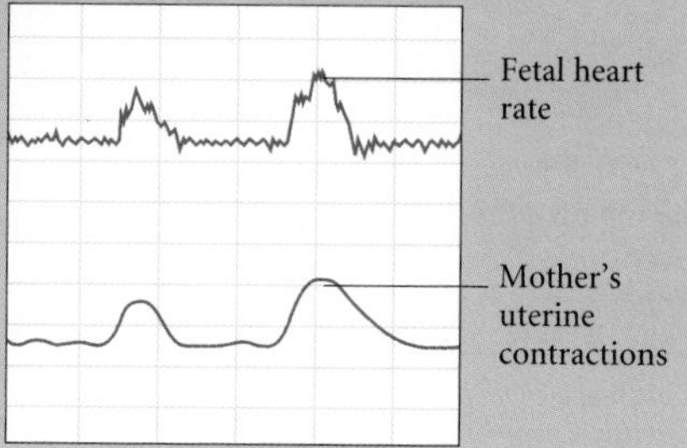

Fetal heart rate

Mother's uterine contractions

but if the second stage of labour is long, and the fetus's oxygen supply becomes low, there is an increased risk of fetal distress (p.804). The doctor may then carry out an assisted delivery (p.805), using vacuum suction or forceps, or a caesarean section (opposite page).

WHAT ARE THE CAUSES?

Any of the problems that cause a delayed first stage of labour (p.801) can prevent a normal delivery. However, even if the first stage has progressed smoothly, a problem may arise at the second stage.

Weak or ineffective uterine contractions may slow down the delivery. Pain relief, such as epidural anaesthesia during labour (p.801), may also affect the strength of contractions. If the mother is exhausted as a result of a long first stage of labour or because of poor general health, contractions may be weak and delivery may be difficult.

There may be a delay in the baby's passage through the cervix and vagina if the baby is not in the normal position (*see* ABNORMAL PRESENTATION, p.800). Normal delivery may also be difficult if the baby cannot pass easily through the pelvis, either because the baby is large or because the mother has a narrow or irregularly shaped pelvis.

Once the baby has reached the vaginal opening, there may be problems in delivery if the surrounding tissues cannot stretch enough to let the head out.

HOW IS IT DIAGNOSED?

When your cervix has dilated fully and the second stage of labour begins, your doctor will monitor the baby's passage through the cervix and into the vagina and will check the heartbeat (*see* FETAL MONITORING, left) for signs of distress. The strength and frequency of uterine contractions are monitored. This information is then used to help determine whether a vaginal delivery is possible.

WHAT IS THE TREATMENT?

If your uterine contractions are too weak, the doctor may give an intravenous drip of oxytocin, a hormone that stimulates strong contractions (*see* INDUCTION OF LABOUR, p.797). When a baby is slow to pass through the cervix and vagina, your doctor may perform an assisted delivery using forceps or vacuum suction. Just before an assisted delivery, an incision, called an episiotomy (right), is usually made in the tissue between the vagina and the anus. This cut eases the baby's passage and prevents the tissues around the vaginal opening from tearing. An episiotomy is also used to help delivery when a mother's vaginal opening is too small for the baby's head to pass through.

A caesarean section will be necessary if the baby cannot pass easily through your pelvis or if an assisted delivery would put either of you at risk.

WHAT IS THE PROGNOSIS?

You may feel disappointed if you need an assisted delivery, a caesarean section, or an episiotomy, but these methods are only used to ensure that your baby is delivered safely. Your ability to have normal vaginal deliveries in the future is not usually affected by any of these procedures. Many women who have a difficult first birth have no problems with subsequent births. However, if there is a physical reason why normal childbirth is difficult for you, such as an abnormally shaped pelvis or one that is too narrow, a caesarean birth will usually be required for future pregnancies.

(WWW) ONLINE SITES: p.1035

Fetal distress

Physical stress experienced by a fetus due to a lack of oxygen

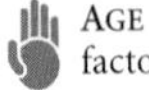
AGE GENETICS LIFESTYLE Not significant factors

Fetal distress develops when there is an insufficient oxygen supply reaching the fetus. Although this condition usually occurs during labour or after week 28 of pregnancy, it can develop at any time. Fetal distress occurs in about 1 in 20 pregnancies, but the fetus is usually delivered before lasting harm occurs. However, left untreated, fetal distress may cause fetal brain damage or death.

WHAT ARE THE CAUSES?

A common cause of fetal distress in pregnancy is a problem with the placenta, the organ that supplies oxygen and nutrients via the umbilical cord to the fetus. The function of the placenta may be affected if the mother develops pre-eclampsia (see PRE-ECLAMPSIA AND ECLAMPSIA, p.794). The oxygen supply to the fetus may also be reduced if part or all of the placenta separates from the uterus during pregnancy (see PLACENTAL ABRUPTION, p.799).

Frequently, the cause of fetal distress during labour is unknown. There may be a placental abruption during labour, or the umbilical cord may become tangled, preventing oxygen from reaching the fetus. Another, less common, cause of fetal distress is cord prolapse. This condition may develop if the fetus is not securely fitted into the mother's pelvis because it is not lying in the normal head-down position facing the mother's back (*see* ABNORMAL PRESENTATION, p.800). An abnormal position may create space for the umbilical cord to drop through the cervix into the vagina. Once it is outside the uterus, the blood vessels in the cord may become compressed or, rarely, may go into spasm. Both of these situations can reduce the oxygen supply to the fetus.

The risk of fetal distress is increased if the fetus is weak or smaller than average (*see* INTRA-UTERINE GROWTH RETARDATION, p.796) or if your labour starts before the 37th week of pregnancy (*see* PREMATURE LABOUR, p.798).

HOW IS IT DIAGNOSED?

If your doctor is concerned that there is a risk of fetal distress during your pregnancy, he or she may decide to refer you for an additional ultrasound scan (*see* ULTRASOUND SCANNING IN PREGNANCY, p.793). This scan enables your doctor to observe fetal movements and also to look at the blood flow in the vessels carrying blood from the placenta to the fetus. Reduced fetal movements may indicate oxygen deficiency. Your doctor may also recommend fetal monitoring (p.803). This monitors the fetus's heart rate, which may be abnormal if the fetus is not getting enough oxygen.

During labour, the fetal heartbeat is continuously monitored, and a sample of blood may be taken from the fetus's scalp to measure blood oxygen levels. The amniotic fluid from the uterus may be examined regularly for signs of staining from fetal faeces (meconium), which are sometimes released from the fetus when it is under stress.

WHAT IS THE TREATMENT?

Treatment for fetal distress depends on the cause, the severity of the distress, whether it occurs before or in labour, and how far labour has progressed.

If there are signs of even mild fetal distress during late pregnancy or early labour, your doctor will probably recommend a caesarean section (p.802). If labour is advanced and the fetus is experiencing only mild levels of distress, an assisted delivery (opposite page) may be a possible option. However, if fetal distress is severe, or there is a cord prolapse, your doctor will probably advise an emergency caesarean section.

WHAT IS THE PROGNOSIS?

If fetal distress is diagnosed and treated promptly, there is a good chance that your baby will be delivered safely and with no permanent harm. However, in some situations – for example, when a baby is premature (*see* PROBLEMS OF THE PREMATURE BABY, p.816) – careful monitoring is needed after birth (*see* SPECIAL CARE BABY UNIT, p.959).

(WWW) ONLINE SITES: p.1035

(TREATMENT) EPISIOTOMY

An episiotomy is an incision made in the perineum (the area of tissue between the vagina and anus) to enlarge the birth opening and prevent a ragged tear. The cut may be used before an assisted delivery or if the perineum fails to stretch sufficiently for the baby's head.

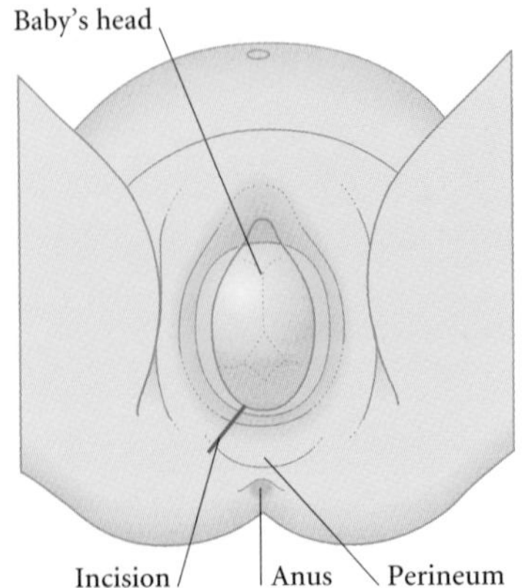

Having an episiotomy
A local anaesthetic is injected into the perineum and a small cut is made during a contraction. The cut is made at an angle to avoid the anus, enabling the baby's head to pass through the vaginal opening more easily.

TREATMENT ASSISTED DELIVERY

When a vaginal delivery does not progress smoothly, a baby may need an assisted delivery. This sometimes occurs if the mother is too exhausted to push the baby out or the baby becomes stuck or distressed. In these circumstances, the doctor may use vacuum suction or forceps to assist the delivery. An episiotomy (opposite page) to enlarge the birth opening is usually carried out just before an assisted delivery. Vacuum suction and forceps procedures are used in about 1 in 10 vaginal births.

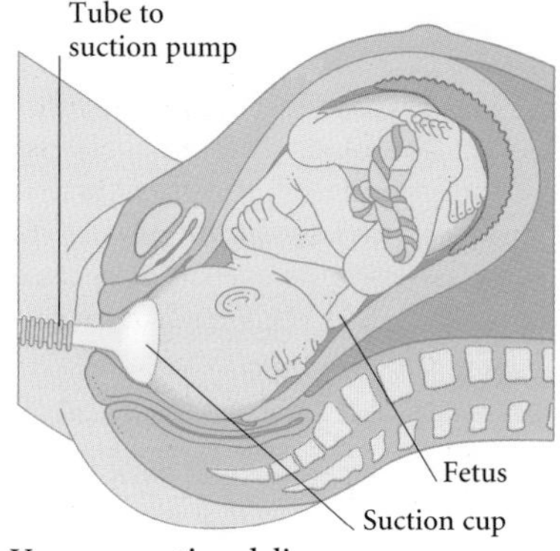

Vacuum suction delivery
A suction cup is placed on the baby's scalp, and the baby is pulled out while the mother pushes. The suction cup leaves a temporary swelling on the baby's head.

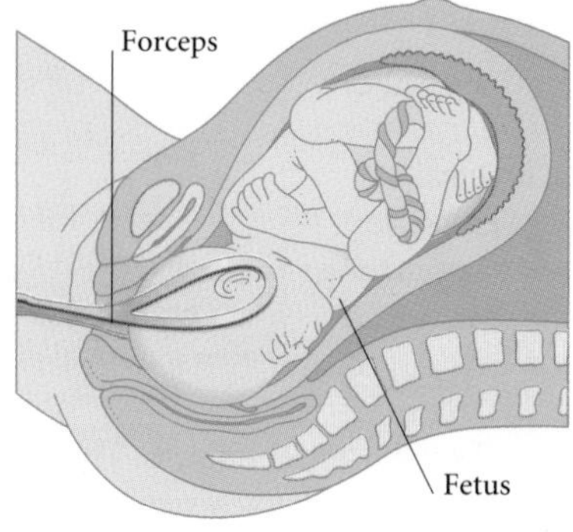

Forceps delivery
Metal forceps are inserted into the vagina and placed on each side of the baby's head. The doctor pulls with the forceps as the mother pushes the baby out.

Stillbirth

The delivery of a dead fetus after week 20 of pregnancy

 AGE More common over the age of 35

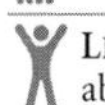 LIFESTYLE Smoking and alcohol or drug abuse during pregnancy are risk factors

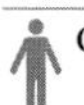 GENETICS Risk factors depend on the cause

The death of a fetus in the uterus or during birth is a very distressing event. Bereaved parents may experience confused feelings of anger, shock, guilt, and inadequacy, in addition to overwhelming grief. Stillbirths are extremely rare. Their incidence has decreased dramatically in developed countries during the past 50 years, and fewer than 6 in 1,000 babies are now stillborn in the UK each year. Stillbirth is slightly more common in mothers over the age of 35.

WHAT ARE THE CAUSES?

Often, the precise cause of fetal death is unknown. The death may be caused by a decrease in the fetus's oxygen supply (*see* FETAL DISTRESS, opposite page) due to a problem with the umbilical cord or the placenta. For example, the umbilical cord may be tangled or knotted, or the placenta may separate from the uterus before the baby is born (*see* PLACENTAL ABRUPTION, p.799). If the mother has very high blood pressure or poorly controlled diabetes mellitus (p.687), the risk of stillbirth is increased.

Stillbirth may also occur if the fetus has a severe genetic disorder or, rarely, if the blood groups of the mother and fetus are not compatible (*see* RHESUS INCOMPATIBILITY, p.795). Certain infectious diseases that pass from the mother to the fetus, such as listeriosis (p.301), may harm the fetus and, if they are severe, may be fatal. Women who smoke or abuse drugs or alcohol are at greater risk of a stillbirth.

WHAT MIGHT BE DONE?

The first sign that a fetus may have died in the uterus is the absence of movement. If, after week 20 of pregnancy, you are aware that fetal movements have decreased or ceased altogether, you should call your doctor without delay. The doctor will listen for the fetal heartbeat and then confirm his or her findings with an ultrasound scan (*see* ULTRASOUND SCANNING IN PREGNANCY, p.793). In most cases, the results of the scan confirm that the fetus is well and the pregnancy is progressing normally. Rarely, if the fetus has died in the uterus and labour has not started, induction of labour (p.797) will be necessary.

If there is no immediate risk to your health, such as an infection, you may be given time to come to terms with the loss of the baby before it is delivered. A caesarean section is not usually used to deliver the baby because of the risks associated with any operation and the small risk of the scar reopening during a subsequent vaginal delivery. In the very rare event of a baby dying during labour, delivery will continue.

Parents are encouraged to see and hold their stillborn baby after the birth as part of the grieving process. After the delivery, the mother and baby undergo tests to determine the cause of death. Before leaving hospital, the mother may be given drugs to inhibit her milk production and provide pain relief.

Your doctor may recommend professional counselling to help you to recover from your loss (*see* LOSS AND BEREAVEMENT, p.76). You should not be afraid to seek support from family and friends. You may also find it helpful to join a self-help group and meet people who have been through a similar experience. Some people may find comfort in a funeral ceremony. About 6 weeks after the birth, your doctor will review the results of tests and the postmortem with you and discuss the cause of the death, if it is known.

WHAT IS THE PROGNOSIS?

After a stillbirth, you may feel strongly that you want to begin another pregnancy straight away. However, it may be better to wait until you are emotionally ready for a new baby and are fully recovered from your pregnancy. If you do decide on another pregnancy, your doctor will ensure that you are given extra care because you will be considered to be at high risk (*see* HIGH-RISK PREGNANCY, p.786). The risk of having a further stillbirth depends on the original cause, if one can be found, but most subsequent pregnancies are successful. As with all grief, the pain of losing a baby lessens with time.

(WWW) ONLINE SITES: p.1029, p.1035

PROBLEMS AFTER CHILDBIRTH

Childbirth is an exhilarating experience for many women, but it can also be difficult and painful. In addition to recovering from physical trauma, the body has to adapt to the abrupt changes in hormone levels after the birth. This hormonal fluctuation, which causes physiological changes, particularly in the breasts in preparation for breast-feeding, often leads to emotional swings.

KEY ANATOMY

Uterus after delivery
Rectum
Cervix
Bladder
Vagina

REPRODUCTIVE ORGANS

Milk duct
Lobule
Nipple
Areola

BREAST

For more information on the physical changes during and after a normal pregnancy, *see* pp.778–783.

Once the baby and the placenta have been delivered, the uterus starts to revert to its size before pregnancy. This process takes about 6 weeks. However, it may take several months for muscle tone to be regained in the abdomen, and any excess weight gained during pregnancy will have to be lost through a careful diet and exercise. The breasts remain enlarged while breast-feeding and only return to their normal size once the baby has been weaned.

The first article covers excessive bleeding occurring immediately after the delivery of the baby or in the first few weeks following childbirth. This condition is now relatively rare due to developments in drug treatment over the past few decades.

Depression, which is covered next, is very common after the birth of a baby. Feelings range from mild baby blues to severe depression that requires hospital treatment. The final articles in this section cover breast disorders that can occur after childbirth, often in association with breast-feeding.

Postpartum haemorrhage

Excessive loss of blood immediately after delivery of a baby or in the first few weeks following childbirth

 AGE More common over the age of 35

 GENETICS LIFESTYLE Not significant factors

Almost all women have some degree of blood loss over the 3 or 4 days after childbirth, and most women have some light vaginal bleeding for up to 4 weeks afterwards. Postpartum haemorrhage is defined as the loss of more than 500 ml (1 pint) of blood after childbirth.

After delivery of the baby, the placenta normally separates from the wall of the uterus and is then expelled from the body through the vagina. The site where the placenta was attached continues to bleed until strong contractions of the uterus constrict the blood vessels in the wall of the uterus and gradually stop the flow of blood. The majority of postpartum haemorrhages, especially if severe, are the result of bleeding from the uterus. However, bleeding may also come from the cervix or the vagina.

Postpartum haemorrhage occurs in about 1 in 50 births, usually immediately after delivery (early postpartum haemorrhage). Only a few women have a late postpartum haemorrhage, in which excessive bleeding occurs more than 24 hours after delivery. Severe postpartum haemorrhage may be life-threatening, but it is now uncommon due to the routine injection of drugs after childbirth to help the uterus to contract.

WHAT ARE THE CAUSES?

In most cases, early postpartum haemorrhage occurs because the uterus is unable to contract sufficiently to constrict the blood vessels in its wall. This may be due to exhaustion of the muscles of the uterus after a prolonged labour, overstretching of the uterus as a result of a multiple pregnancy (*see* MULTIPLE PREGNANCY AND ITS PROBLEMS, p.792), excess amniotic fluid (*see* POLYHYDRAMNIOS, p.795), or a large baby.

Contraction of the uterus may also be impaired by noncancerous growths in the uterus (*see* FIBROIDS, p.745) or if some or all of the placenta remains in the uterus after birth. Occasionally, a general anaesthetic given for a caesarean section (p.802) can impair contractions. Early postpartum haemorrhage may also occur if the placenta has implanted in the lower uterus (*see* PLACENTA PRAEVIA, p.798). In this case, the muscles in the lower uterus may not contract sufficiently to stop bleeding.

Less commonly, a tear in the cervix or vagina during childbirth may cause early postpartum haemorrhage. Such tears are more likely to occur if the baby is born rapidly, is not born head first (*see* ABNORMAL PRESENTATION, p.800), or is delivered with forceps or suction (*see* ASSISTED DELIVERY, p.805).

Late postpartum haemorrhage is usually caused by fragments of the placenta left in the uterus or by an infection.

WHAT ARE THE SYMPTOMS?

The main symptom of early postpartum haemorrhage is excessive loss of bright red blood through the vagina after birth.

A late postpartum haemorrhage may occur between 24 hours and 6 weeks after the birth. Symptoms may include:

- Sudden, heavy vaginal bleeding that is bright red in colour.

- Lower abdominal pain.
- Fever.

Sudden, severe loss of blood may lead to shock (p.414). Postpartum haemorrhage almost always occurs while you are hospitalized. If you are not in hospital and develop severe bleeding through the vagina after giving birth, you should seek medical advice immediately.

How is it diagnosed?

If you are not already in hospital, you will usually be admitted immediately. Your pulse and blood pressure will be monitored to look for any evidence of shock. If an early postpartum haemorrhage has occurred, your doctor will feel your lower abdomen to see if the uterus is contracted. The placenta will be checked to ensure that it is complete. If the uterus appears to be contracted but bleeding continues, your cervix and vagina will be examined. This may be carried out under general anaesthesia or epidural anaesthesia.

If you are having a late postpartum haemorrhage, your doctor may arrange for a special ultrasound scan, using a probe inserted into the vagina, to check for remaining pieces of placenta in the uterus. A vaginal swab may be taken to check for evidence of infection.

What is the treatment?

If an early postpartum haemorrhage is due to poor contraction of the uterus, you may be given an injection to help the uterus to contract. Your doctor may also massage your abdomen. If these measures do not work, further drugs may be given to help the uterus to contract. If the bleeding continues, surgery may be required. In rare cases, a hysterectomy (p.747) may be necessary. Bleeding caused by a retained placenta is treated by manually removing the remaining placenta through the vagina. If the blood loss is due to tears in the cervix or vagina, these will be stitched.

If a late postpartum haemorrhage is the result of an infection, antibiotics (p.885) will be prescribed. If the bleeding continues, surgery may be needed to examine the uterus and remove any remaining fragments of placenta.

Blood lost due to a postpartum haemorrhage may have to be replaced by a blood transfusion (p.447).

(WWW) ONLINE SITES: p.1036

Depression after childbirth

Depressive feelings or psychological disturbances in the first few weeks or months after childbirth

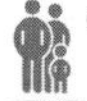 GENETICS Sometimes runs in families

 LIFESTYLE Lack of emotional support and additional stressful life events are risk factors

 AGE Not a significant factor

It is very common for a new mother to feel low or miserable during the first few days or weeks after childbirth. A new baby leads to major changes in lifestyle, and adjustments will need to be made. This mild mood change is commonly known as the "baby blues" and affects up to 8 in 10 women following the birth of a child.

More severe postpartum depression is a relatively common disorder in the first few weeks or months after childbirth and affects about 1 in 10 women. About 1 in 1,000 women develops a serious psychiatric condition known as postpartum psychosis that requires immediate treatment in hospital.

What are the causes?

Baby blues are thought to be caused by the sudden fall in hormone levels (particularly of oestrogen and progesterone) that occurs after a baby is born. These hormonal changes may also cause postpartum depression and possibly also postpartum psychosis.

Women who have suffered from depression (p.554) before are at increased risk of becoming depressed after childbirth. Postpartum depression may run in families. Other factors, such as feelings of isolation and inadequacy and concerns about the new responsibilities of motherhood, can cause stress and contribute to depression. Lack of sleep due to caring for the baby, exhaustion from a long labour, or painful wounds, such as tears in the vagina or scars from a caesarean section, may aggravate the problem. Mothers who have had a difficult labour are more likely to experience postpartum depression. Extra stresses or problems with a partner can make feelings of depression worse. Some women experience anxiety after childbirth, and they may have panic attacks with palpitations and shortness of breath (*see* ANXIETY DISORDERS, p.551). If recurrent panic attacks are untreated, they may lead to postpartum depression.

Although the precise cause of postpartum psychosis is not understood, a previous history of episodes of depression that alternate with episodes of mania (*see* BIPOLAR AFFECTIVE DISORDER, p.557) significantly increases the risk. Women who have close relatives with a medical history of bipolar affective disorder or severe depression are at greater risk of postpartum psychosis.

What are the symptoms?

The symptoms of baby blues start 3–10 days after giving birth. They are often worse by about day 5 and include:

- Dramatic mood swings.
- Weeping.
- Tiredness and irritability.
- Lack of concentration.

Postpartum depression may begin any time in the first 6 months after childbirth. The condition is similar to baby blues but much more severe, and, unlike baby blues, it can interfere with the mother's ability to carry out day-to-day activities. The symptoms include:

- Constantly feeling exhausted.
- Having little interest or no interest at all in the new baby.
- Sense of anticlimax.
- Feeling inadequate and overwhelmed by new responsibilities.
- Difficulty sleeping.
- Loss of appetite.
- Feelings of guilt.

The symptoms of postpartum psychosis usually develop rapidly about 2–3 weeks after childbirth. They often include:

- Insomnia and overactivity.
- Extreme mood swings from depression to mania.
- False beliefs of being disliked and persecuted by people.
- Hallucinations.
- Confusion.

Sometimes, threats of suicide or of harming the baby may be made.

What can I do?

You should try to get as much support as possible from medical staff, friends, and family after childbirth. Make sure you are not left alone until you feel happy caring for your baby, and rest as much as possible. You may also wish to find out about local self-help groups or mother-and-baby groups.

Baby blues do not usually require medical treatment and, with emotional support and time, almost always disappear. If you develop severe depression and find it hard to carry out day-to-day activities and look after your baby, you should consult your doctor.

What might the doctor do?

If postpartum depression is interfering with your life and simple reassurance and support are not helping, your doctor may prescribe antidepressant drugs (p.916) and advise counselling (p.971).

If you have very severe postpartum depression or postpartum psychosis, you will need to be admitted to hospital. The hospital will make sure that your baby can stay with you so that the bond between you can be maintained. To treat severe depression, you may be given a higher dose of antidepressant drugs or a different type of antidepressant drug. Antipsychotic drugs (p.917) are usually prescribed for postpartum psychosis and psychotherapy may be recommended. You will also be offered practical help looking after your baby.

You may not be able to breast-feed while you are taking antidepressant or antipsychotic drugs because of the risk of the drugs passing into your breast milk and harming your baby.

What is the prognosis?

Baby blues usually improve within a few weeks. Postpartum depression is likely to start responding to antidepressant drugs within 2–4 weeks, but full recovery may take up to a year. Antipsychotic drugs are usually helpful for postpartum psychosis within 2–3 months. However, the drugs may need to be taken for several months, and long-term follow-up and support will be given.

Any form of depression may recur after subsequent pregnancies. Women who have an increased risk of developing either postpartum depression or psychosis will be offered extra support during and after future pregnancies. They will also be monitored for signs of depression and may be given hormone patches after birth to counter the sudden fall in their hormone levels.

(WWW) ONLINE SITES: p.1034, p.1035

Breast engorgement

Swollen, painful breasts caused by congestion with milk after childbirth

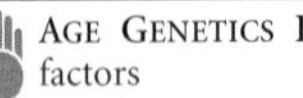

AGE GENETICS LIFESTYLE Not significant factors

All mothers normally produce breast milk after childbirth and develop some degree of breast engorgement before feeding is established and milk production adapts to match the needs of their baby. During engorgement, the breasts become full of milk and may swell to up to twice their normal size. They also become hard, red, and painful.

Breast engorgement may occur if a woman stops breast-feeding or if her baby needs special care in an incubator and she is unable to breast-feed. In these situations, milk accumulates inside the breasts until milk production ceases. In women who are breast-feeding, breast engorgement may develop because the baby is weak and unable to feed properly, so that the initial milk supply exceeds demand. In all cases, the accumulation of excess milk may lead to the development of infection in the breast (*see* MASTITIS, opposite page).

What can I do?

After childbirth, you should wear a firm, supportive bra, whether or not you are going to breast-feed your baby. Local heat treatment may ease discomfort in the breasts, as may taking painkillers (p.912) such as paracetamol. Do not try to express milk if you are not going to breast-feed because this may stimulate further milk production. Your breasts should gradually become less painful after a few days of not breast-feeding. Rarely, you may be prescribed a drug to stop milk production.

If you decide to breast-feed, try to encourage your baby to feed as soon as possible. You can remove some of the excess milk by gently expressing it using your hands or a breast pump. Once your baby is feeding regularly, the production of milk should adapt to match the demands of your baby, and your breasts will become less engorged.

When you stop breast-feeding, cut out feeds one at a time over several days or weeks in order to help prevent your breasts from becoming engorged.

(WWW) ONLINE SITES: p.1035

Cracked nipples

Fine cracks in the nipple caused by breast-feeding

AGE GENETICS LIFESTYLE Not significant factors

During the first few weeks of breast-feeding, fine cracks and raw areas may develop in the skin on and surrounding the nipple. These cause a stabbing or burning pain, usually as the baby starts or stops feeding. Cracked nipples are most often caused by the baby failing to take the whole nipple into his or her mouth properly when feeding. Leaving your nipples wet after each feed may also cause them to become tender and cracked. Occasionally, cracked nipples can become infected and inflamed (*see* MASTITIS, opposite page).

Your doctor or breast-feeding counsellor will advise you on how to feed your baby. You can also take preventive measures to stop cracks forming (*see* AVOIDING CRACKED NIPPLES, opposite page) and to avoid infection.

Cracked nipples normally heal over time as the nipples become tougher and as you become more used to breast-feeding. However, if your nipples are very painful or if discomfort develops after several weeks of successful breast-feeding, you should consult your doctor. If your doctor suspects that an infection is present, he or she will probably prescribe a course of antibiotics (p.885) for you and possibly treatment for your baby if his or her mouth has become infected. This treatment should clear up the infection in a few days.

(WWW) ONLINE SITES: p.1035

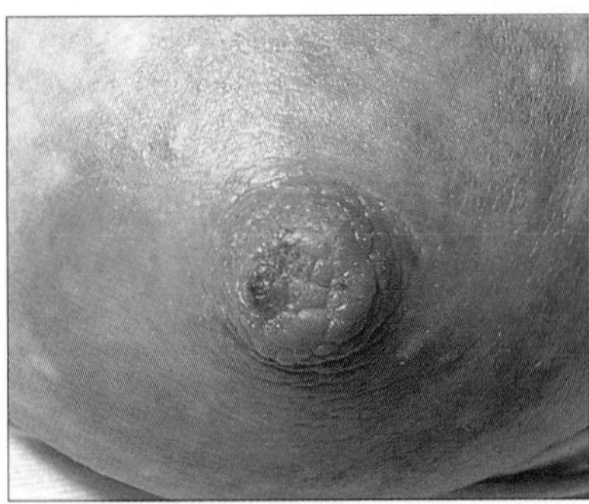

Cracked nipple

Breast-feeding sometimes causes cracks and raw areas on the nipple and surrounding skin, often when the baby is not properly positioned on the nipple during feeding.

SELF-HELP AVOIDING CRACKED NIPPLES

Cracked nipples are usually caused by the baby not taking the nipple into his or her mouth properly. To avoid cracked nipples, make sure that your baby is positioned on your nipple correctly each time you breast-feed. Dry your nipples thoroughly after each feed and avoid plastic-lined breast pads, which may become damp and encourage soreness and infection. Emollient creams can prevent the skin from drying out but should be washed off before breast-feeding.

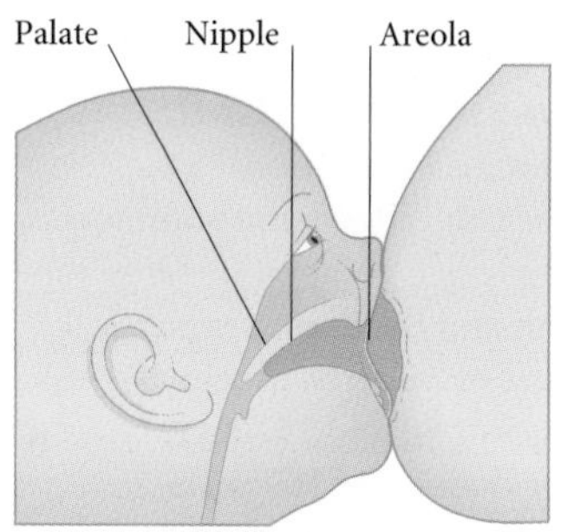

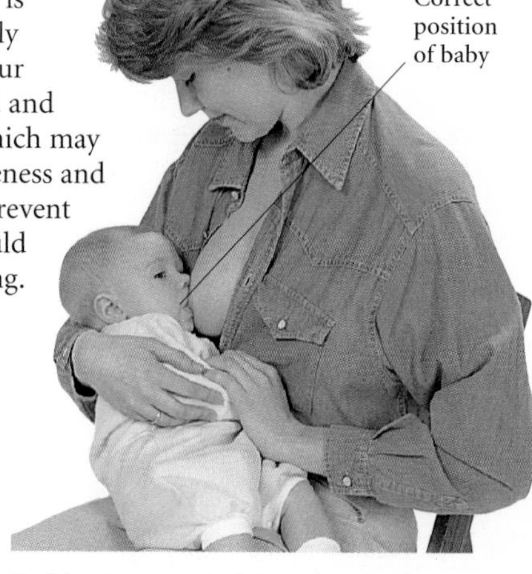

Positioning your baby on the nipple
When breast-feeding, the entire nipple and most of the areola (the darker area around the nipple) should be taken into the baby's mouth to prevent the skin around the nipple becoming cracked.

Mastitis

Painful inflammation of breast tissue in part of one or both breasts

AGE GENETICS LIFESTYLE Not significant factors

Inflammation of one or both breasts is called mastitis. The condition usually occurs in the first 6 weeks of breast-feeding. However, mastitis may develop if breast-feeding is stopped suddenly and the breasts become overfilled with milk (*see* BREAST ENGORGEMENT, opposite page). Mastitis in nonbreast-feeding women is often related to smoking, which causes inflammation of the milk ducts (*see* NIPPLE DISCHARGE, p.758).

Mastitis is caused by infection of a blocked milk duct or an area of the breast that is inadequately drained of milk. The bacterium *Staphylococcus aureus*, which enters the breast through broken skin, most often on the nipple (*see* CRACKED NIPPLES, opposite page). Mastitis affects up to 1 in 10 women who breast-feed. Women breast-feeding for the first time are particularly likely to develop the condition because they may not have learned how to position their baby on the breast.

WHAT ARE THE SYMPTOMS?

Mastitis usually affects only one area of a breast. Symptoms develop gradually over several days and may include:

- Tender, red area that spreads away from the nipple.
- Swelling and pain in the affected area.

A severe, flu-like illness with fever and chills may also develop.

Left untreated, inflammation of the breast gradually becomes worse and a pus-filled cavity, called a breast abscess, may develop, causing a firm lump that is painful to the touch. However, such breast abscesses are now relatively uncommon because antibiotics (p.885) are usually prescribed at the first sign of an infection before a breast abscess has had a chance to develop.

WHAT CAN I DO?

You should keep breast-feeding if you develop mastitis because stopping may cause the breasts to become engorged with milk and encourage an abscess to develop. The infection will not harm your baby because the bacteria in your milk are destroyed by the baby's stomach acid. The regular flow of milk will help to keep the breast well drained and thereby prevent the condition getting worse. Any milk that still remains in the affected breast following breast-feeding should be expressed if possible.

A heat pad or a well-wrapped hot water bottle placed on the affected area of the breast may help to encourage the flow of milk and relieve the pain. Mild painkillers (p.912), such as paracetamol, may be useful. You should try to rest as much as possible and drink plenty of nonalcoholic fluids.

If an abscess develops, you should not breast-feed with the affected breast but should empty the breast of milk by gently using a pump or your hands.

WHAT MIGHT THE DOCTOR DO?

A diagnosis of mastitis is usually obvious from the symptoms, especially if you are currently breast-feeding your baby or if you have recently stopped breast-feeding. Your doctor will examine your breasts and may arrange for a sample of your milk to be sent to a laboratory in order to identify the bacteria that are causing the infection. He or she may also arrange for you to have ultrasound scanning (p.250) to examine any lumps that may be present in the breast. Your doctor will probably prescribe a course of oral antibiotics to treat the infection.

Mastitis usually clears up within 2 or 3 days of beginning treatment with antibiotics. However, if a breast abscess has developed, the pus that has collected may have to be removed from the breast under local anaesthesia using a needle and syringe. This procedure may need to be repeated daily until the abscess has cleared up. Recurrence of the abscess is unlikely.

(WWW) ONLINE SITES: p.1035

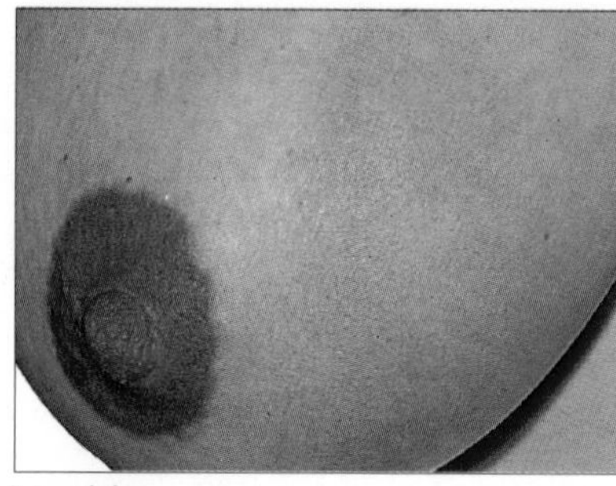

Mastitis
The red triangular area of inflammation radiating away from the nipple indicates mastitis, a condition that may develop in women who are breast-feeding.

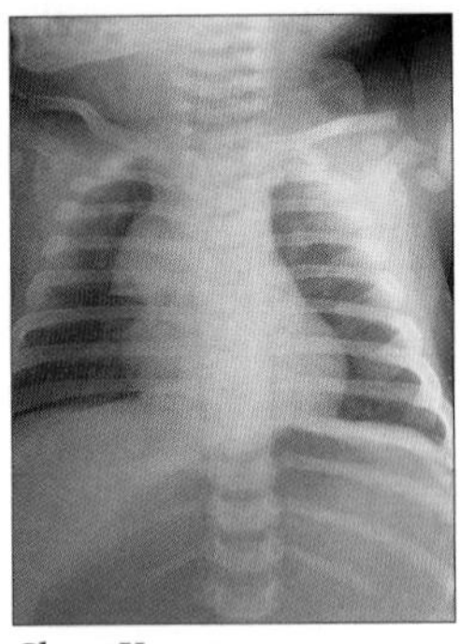

Chest X-ray
This X-ray shows the heart and thymus gland, which is large in newborn babies.

INFANCY AND CHILDHOOD

FROM THE MOMENT OF BIRTH, babies begin a process of adaptation to the world. Over a short space of time, dependent newborns grow and develop physically, mentally, and socially into capable, self-sufficient individuals. In the first year, a baby grows faster than at any time in later life. Within the first five years, children learn basic skills and go on throughout childhood to acquire a wide range of intellectual and physical accomplishments.

Children pass through predictable patterns of growth and development, but each child progresses at a different rate. Physical growth and intellectual development are partly determined by genetic factors, but these processes are also affected by general health and stimulation from the environment.

EARLY GROWTH AND LEARNING

Before babies develop their basic life skills, they have a number of primitive reflexes that help them to survive. They communicate by crying and are born with an instinctive sucking response when offered a nipple.

At first, babies grow fast, and most triple in weight and grow in length by about 25 cm (10 in) during their first year. After the age of 2, children begin a long, slower period of growth, which allows time for complex skills to be learned and perfected.

Both a child's intellectual skills and physical coordination depend on the healthy development of the muscular and nervous systems. The earliest accomplishments for toddlers are fundamental skills such as walking, talking, and feeding themselves. As their independence grows, children recognize themselves as individuals and become more active learners, interacting with their surroundings and developing close relationships. Children learn through imitation and practice. By the age of 12, they have usually acquired sophisticated language and numeracy skills and wide-ranging physical abilities.

TOWARDS ADULTHOOD

Adolescence is the transition period between childhood and adulthood during which children undergo rapid growth and the dramatic physical changes of puberty, usually between the ages of 10 and 15. Puberty occurs earlier than it did 100 years ago, probably because of improvements in nutrition. Reproductive organs mature and secondary sexual characteristics, such as breasts and body hair, appear some time before adolescents have the emotional maturity to cope with adult relationships. They need to adjust to physical changes and new feelings.

At the age of 18, young people are considered adults in most societies, although they continue to mature psychologically for many more years.

STRUCTURE AND FUNCTION — THE HEART BEFORE AND AFTER BIRTH

In the fetus, only a little blood passes through the lungs because the task of adding oxygen to the blood and filtering out waste gases is done by the mother's placenta. Before birth, most blood bypasses the lungs by flowing through two openings in the heart. With a baby's first breath the lungs expand, triggering changes in the circulation so that all blood then flows through the lungs to be oxygenated.

Changes in the heart's circulation
An opening in the fetal heart, the foramen ovale, diverts blood from the right atrium (chamber) to the left, and a duct, the ductus arteriosus, diverts blood into the aorta. The openings close soon after birth.

STRUCTURE AND FUNCTION THE NEWBORN BABY

A full-term newborn baby weighs on average 3.5 kg (7 lb 11 oz), measures 51 cm (20 in) in length, and is well prepared for survival. Many aspects of a newborn's appearance, such as the shape of the skull, are a result of the transition from the uterus to the outside world and are different from those of a fetus or older child. Such differences are normal and usually disappear relatively quickly. Other structures, such as the long bones, are not yet fully formed. The baby also has primitive reflexes, such as a grasp reflex, which are important to survival but disappear with increasing age.

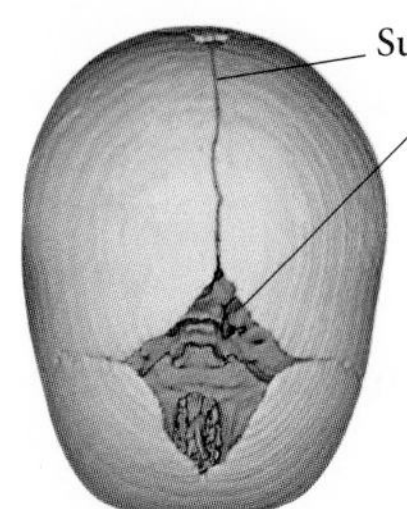

Fontanelles
The bone plates of a baby's skull are separated by fontanelles (soft gaps) and sutures (seams) that allow the plates to move and overlap during childbirth.

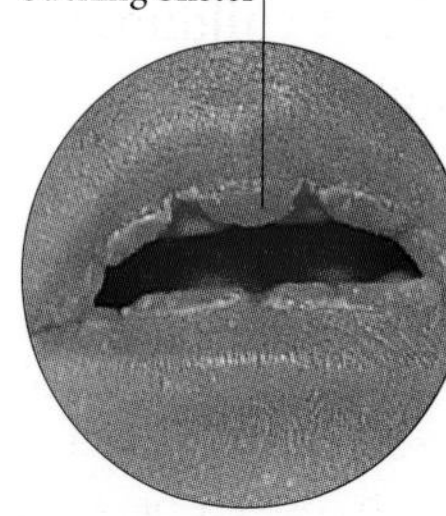

Sucking blister
Blisters, or small white bumps, can be seen on the lips of a newborn baby above. The blisters form as a result of vigorous sucking.

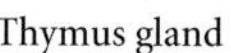

Skull
The baby's skull may look oddly shaped for a few days after birth

Lung
At the first breath, the baby's lungs fill with air, expand, and begin to function

Jaw
At birth, the teeth are fully formed in the jaw, but in most cases they have not yet erupted

Puffy upper lid

Eye
In a newborn baby, the eyelids are puffy and vision is poor even when the eyes are wide open.

Thymus gland
This gland, which forms part of the immune system, is large at birth when the immune system is maturing rapidly

Liver
The liver is large in proportion to the body at birth because it is a major site of blood cell formation in the fetus

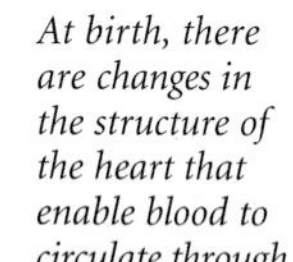

Heart
At birth, there are changes in the structure of the heart that enable blood to circulate through the lungs

Lanugo hair
Premature babies may have downy hair, called lanugo hair, all over the body. This hair disappears after about a month.

Pelvis
At birth, the pelvis is made mostly of cartilage, a connective tissue, which turns into bone during childhood

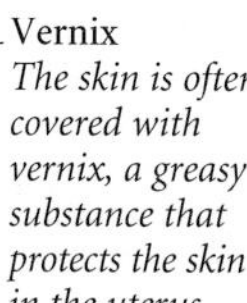

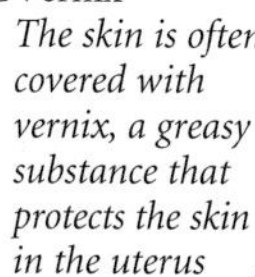

Vernix
The skin is often covered with vernix, a greasy substance that protects the skin in the uterus

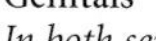

Genitals
In both sexes, the genitals appear large in relation to the rest of the body

Long bone of leg
At birth, only the shafts of the long bones of the legs and arms have hardened. The ends still consist of cartilage

Hand
At birth, the hands are often clenched and the skin is wrinkled. The tips of babies' nails often flake off on their own and do not need cutting.

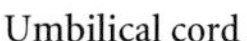

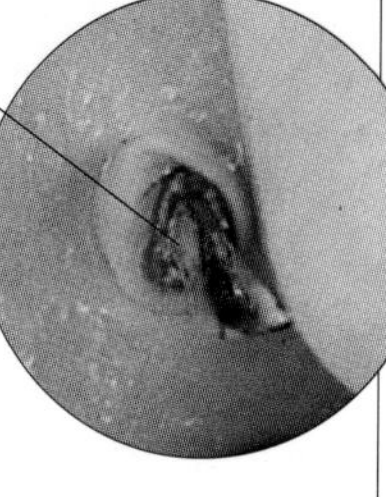

Umbilical cord
The umbilical cord, which is cut at delivery, shrinks and falls off within 10 days to form the navel.

Foot
The foot bones of a newborn are mostly cartilage and are often twisted outwards because of their position in the uterus

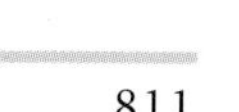

STRUCTURE AND FUNCTION THE DEVELOPING BODY

A child's body grows and changes continuously from birth to adulthood through processes that are largely controlled by hormones. The most dramatic changes take place during infancy, when rapid growth occurs, and during puberty, when the body is approaching sexual maturity. At certain times, some parts of the body develop faster than others, which is why body proportions change throughout childhood. A child's brain is almost fully grown by the age of 6, while the rest of the body remains relatively undeveloped.

CHANGING BODY PROPORTIONS

At birth, a baby's head is as wide as the shoulders and appears large in relation to the rest of the body. The head continues to grow quickly, and by the age of 2, the brain is four-fifths of its adult size. As the child gets older, the rate of growth of the head decreases compared with the rest of the body. Eventually, usually by the age of 18, the proportion of the head with the rest of the body stays the same and growth stops.

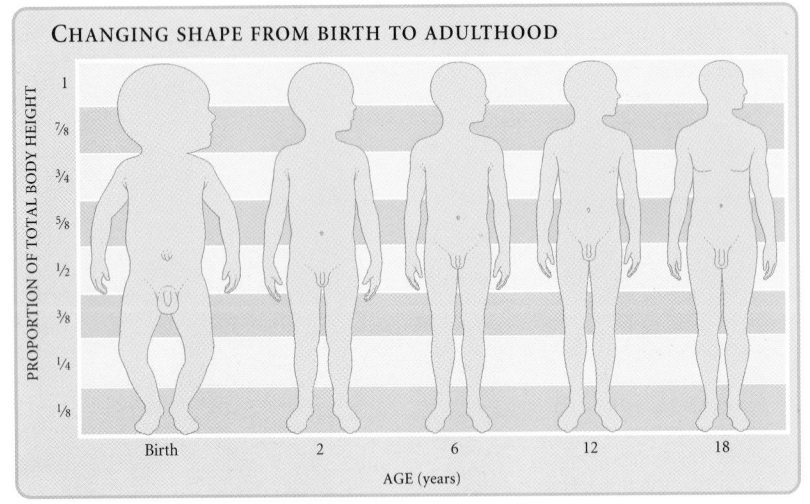

How proportions change
A newborn baby's head makes up about a quarter of total body length, and the legs three-eighths. By 18 years, proportions have changed; the head is an eighth of total body length and the legs a half.

HOW BONES DEVELOP

Hard-bone formation (ossification) commences before birth at sites in the bone shafts known as primary ossification centres. In a newborn baby, only the shafts (diaphyses) are ossified. The ends of these bones (epiphyses) consist of tissue called cartilage, which is gradually replaced by bone that develops from secondary ossification centres. Between the shaft and the ends is a zone called the growth plate, which produces more cartilage to elongate the bones.

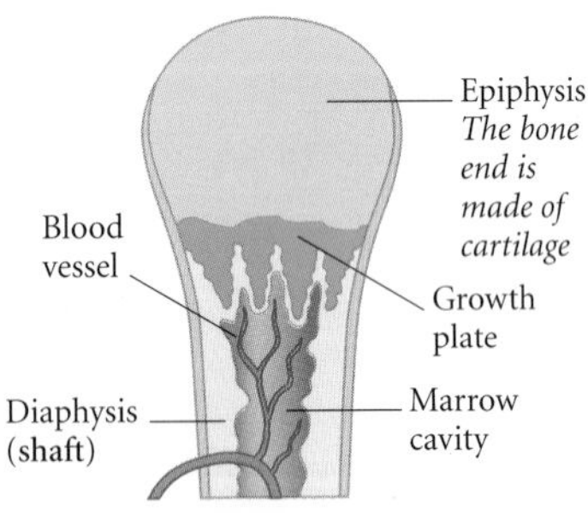

Long bone of a newborn baby
The shaft (diaphysis) is mostly bone, while the ends (epiphyses) are made of cartilage that gradually hardens.

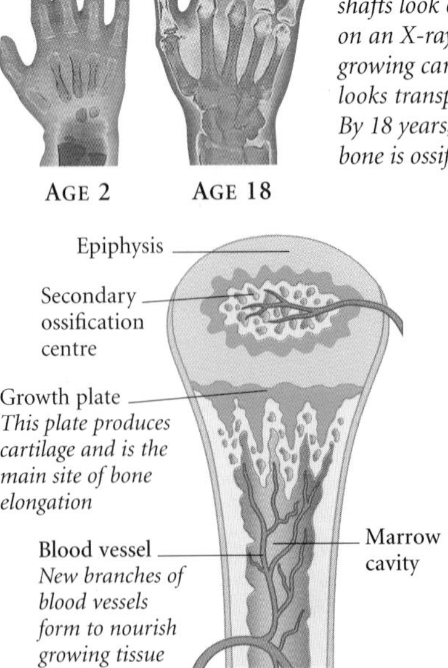

Hand growth
At the age of 2, ossified hand bone shafts look opaque on an X-ray. The growing cartilage looks transparent. By 18 years, all bone is ossified.

Long bone of a child
The epiphyses contain secondary ossification centres from which bone forms. A growth plate near the ends produces new cartilage.

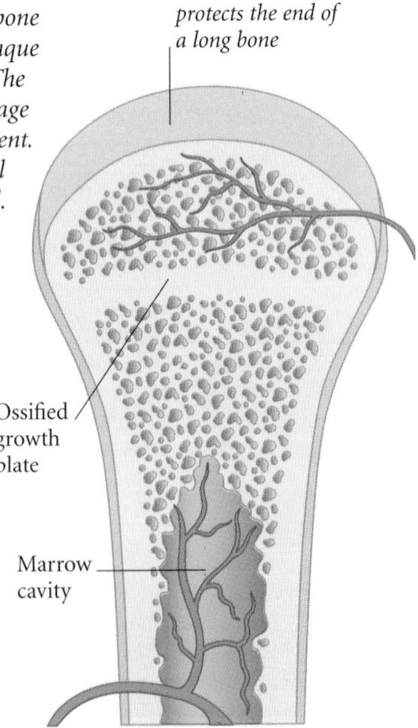

Long bone of an adult
By the age of 18, the shafts, growth plates, and epiphyses have all ossified and fused into continuous bone.

How the skull and brain develop

At birth, a newborn's brain has its full complement of billions of neurons (nerve cells) that transmit and receive messages along axons (nerve fibres). At first, these neural networks are partially developed. In the first 6 years, the networks expand, and the brain grows rapidly to allow new skills to be learned. The skull expands to accommodate this growth. Between the ages of 6 and 18, neural pathways develop at a slower rate.

How the brain and skull grow
During infancy, the part of the skull around the brain (cranium) grows rapidly at the seams (sutures) and soft gaps (fontanelles) between the bone plates. By the age of 6, the brain is almost full size.

Fontanelle (soft gap)

Cranium
The cranium appears large in relation to the immature facial bones

Neural network

Brain

Suture

At birth

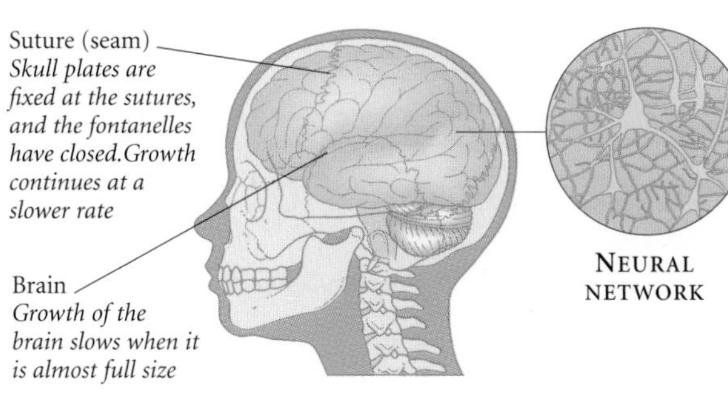

At 6 years

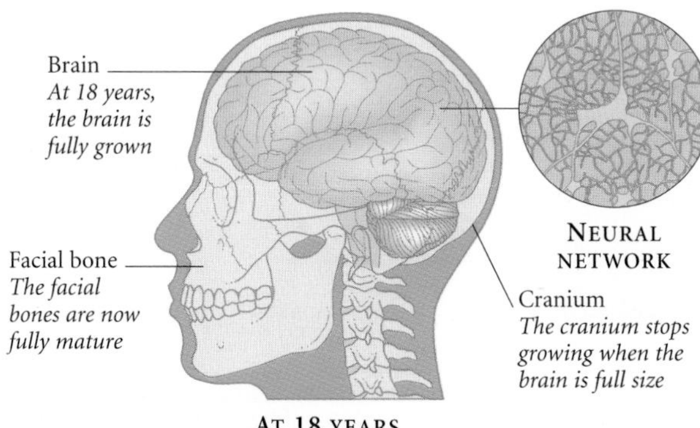

At 18 years

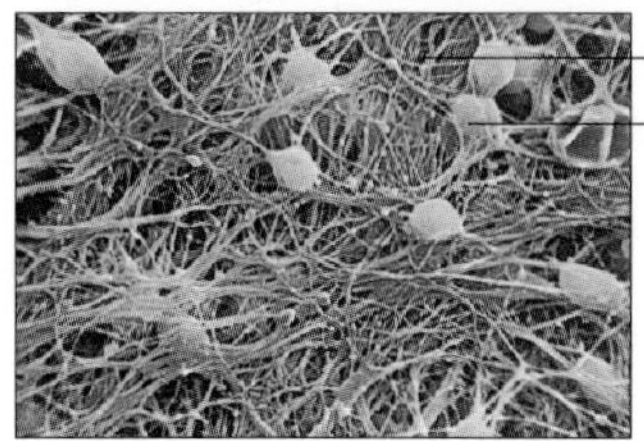

Neural network
This highly magnified view of adult brain tissue shows neurons within a complex network of neural pathways.

How nerves develop

Early in life, most nerve fibres (axons) become wrapped in insulating sheaths made of a fatty substance known as myelin. This insulation speeds up nerve transmission by as much as 100 times and is essential for the body to grow and function normally.

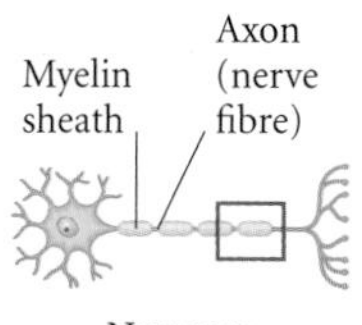

Neuron

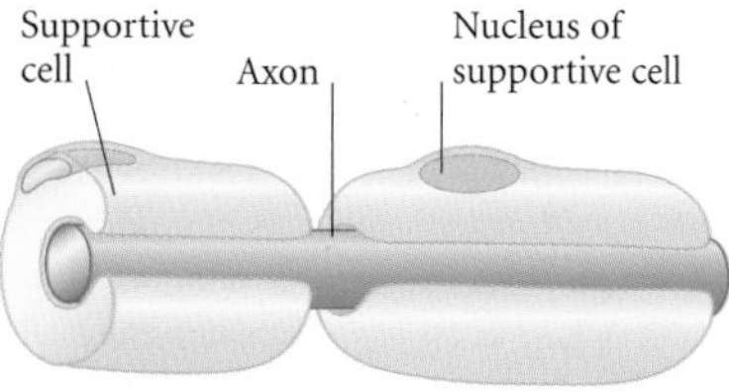

1 *Supportive cells, composed mainly of fatty material known as myelin, wind around an axon to form a protective and insulating sheath.*

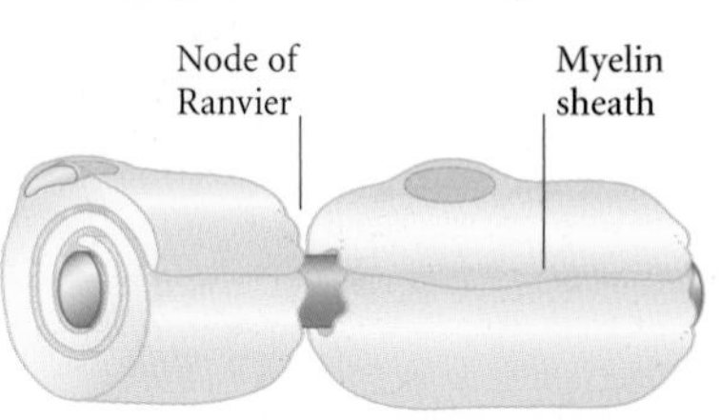

2 *The axon is now wrapped in sections of myelin sheath separated by gaps (nodes of Ranvier). Nerve signals jump from one gap to the next.*

Factors affecting growth

A child's potential maximum growth is determined by genes, but achieving the maximum depends on a number of other factors, such as nutrition and general health. Girls and boys have similar patterns of yearly growth in childhood (below). A growth spurt at puberty is triggered by sex hormones, which also speed up the fusion of growth plates in the bone. Growth is complete by about the age of 18.

Why boys grow taller than girls
In boys, the growth spurt occurs later in puberty than in girls, giving them longer to grow in childhood before their full growth is complete.

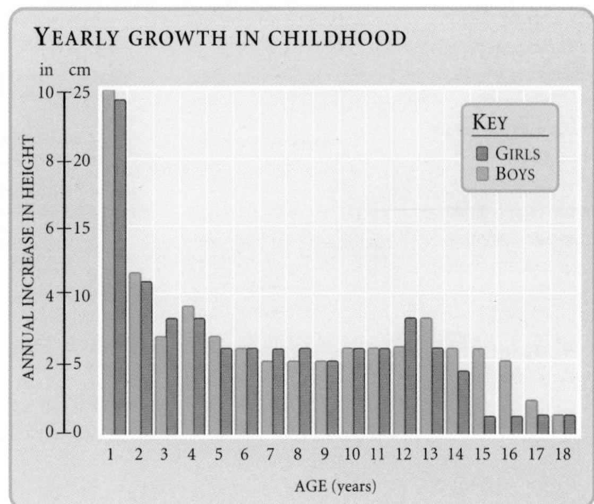

DATA GAINING SKILLS DURING THE FIRST FIVE YEARS

During their first 5 years, children learn the basic skills necessary for their future development. The four main areas are physical skills, manual dexterity, language, and social skills. Although children progress at different rates, developmental milestones occur in a predictable order. This is partly because the ability to learn particular skills depends upon the maturity of the child's nervous system. In addition, for some complex skills, children need to develop a lesser skill first; for example, babies must learn to stand before they can walk.

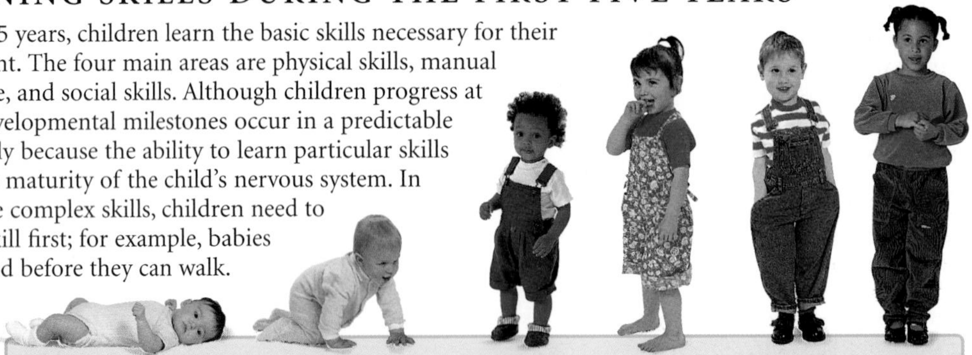

DEVELOPMENTAL MILESTONES

AGE (years): 0, 1, 2, 3, 4, 5

Physical skills
Babies first master control of their body posture and head, then go on to develop physical skills, including standing, crawling, and walking.

Can lift head to 45°
Can walk without help
Can catch a bounced ball
Can roll over
Can stand without help
Can crawl
Can throw a ball
Can balance on one foot for a second
Can stand by hoisting up own weight
Can kick a ball
Can sit unsupported
Can walk up stairs without help
Can bear weight on legs
Can walk holding on to furniture
Can pedal a tricycle
Can hop on one leg

Manual dexterity and vision
Children have to coordinate their movement and vision to perform manipulative tasks, such as picking up objects or drawing.

Holds hands together
Likes to scribble
Can copy a circle
Plays with feet
Can build a tower of four bricks
Passes rattle from hand to hand
Can draw a straight line
Can copy a square
Reaches out for a rattle
Can pick up a small object
Can draw rudimentary likeness of a person
Can grasp object between finger and thumb

Hearing and language
Early on, babies turn towards voices and respond to sounds by cooing. At about 1 year, children speak their first word.

Startled by loud sounds
Can talk in full sentences
Says "dada" and "mama" to parents
Turns towards voice
Can point to parts of the body
Can define seven words
Squeals
Says "dada" and "mama" to anyone
Knows first and last names
Can put two words together
Makes cooing noises
Starts to learn single words
Can name a colour

Social behaviour and play
Self-care begins with basic skills, such as dressing and toilet training. Social skills range from smiling to making the first new friends.

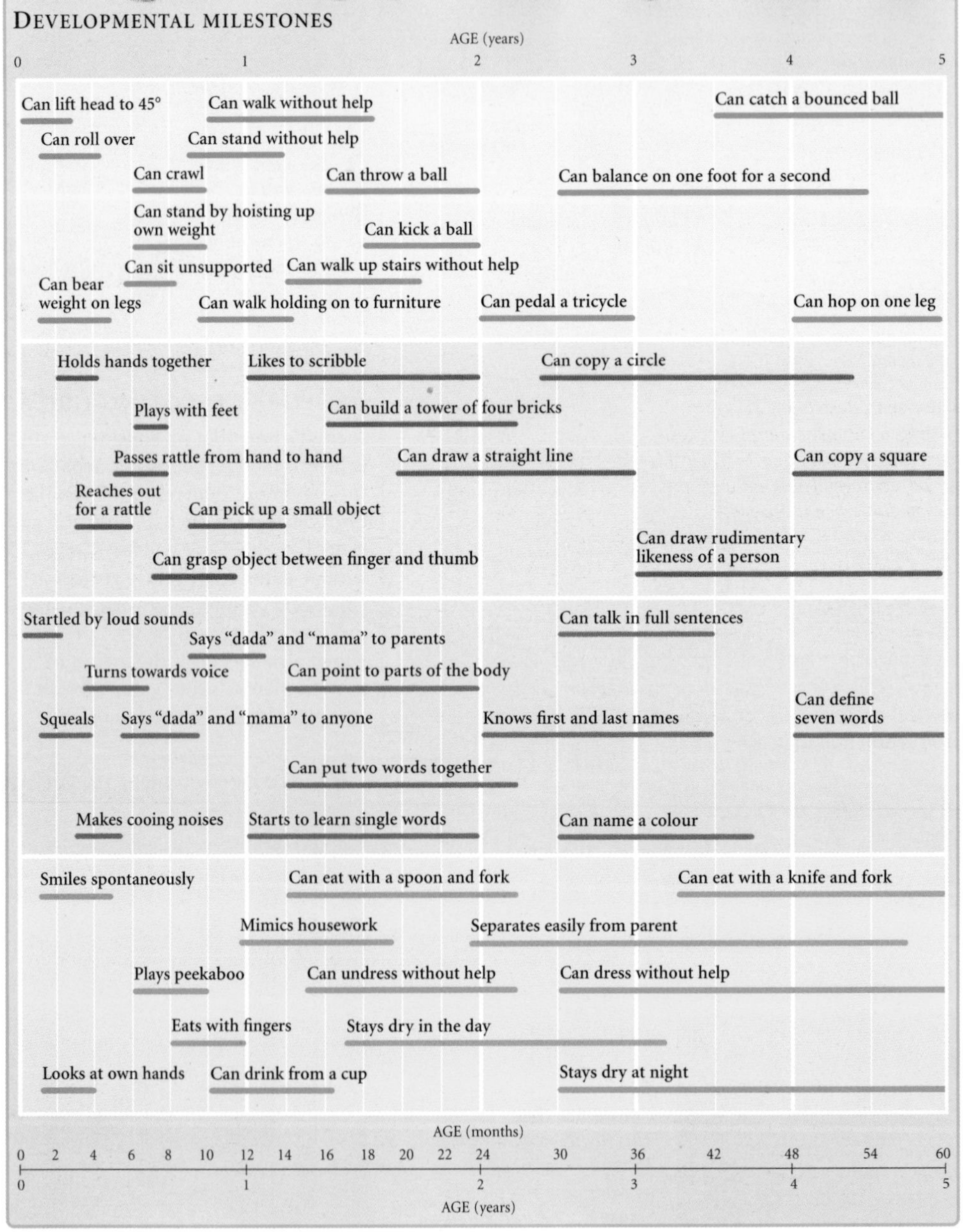

Smiles spontaneously
Can eat with a spoon and fork
Can eat with a knife and fork
Mimics housework
Separates easily from parent
Plays peekaboo
Can undress without help
Can dress without help
Eats with fingers
Stays dry in the day
Looks at own hands
Can drink from a cup
Stays dry at night

AGE (months): 0 2 4 6 8 10 12 14 16 18 20 22 24 30 36 42 48 54 60

AGE (years): 0 1 2 3 4 5

FUNCTION PUBERTY

Puberty is a period of rapid growth and physical change, during which adolescents become sexually mature. The age at which puberty begins and the rate of growth are influenced by genetics, general health, and weight. Puberty begins when the pituitary gland, located at the base of the brain, secretes hormones that stimulate the production of sex hormones. Within about 2 years of the start of puberty, sexual reproduction is possible, but it takes longer for adolescents to become mature enough emotionally for adult relationships.

CHANGES IN GIRLS DURING PUBERTY

In girls, puberty begins between the ages of 10 and 14, when luteinizing hormone (LH) and follicle-stimulating hormone (FSH) stimulate the ovaries to secrete the sex hormones oestrogen and progesterone. These hormones prompt physical changes and, later, stimulate ovulation and menstruation.

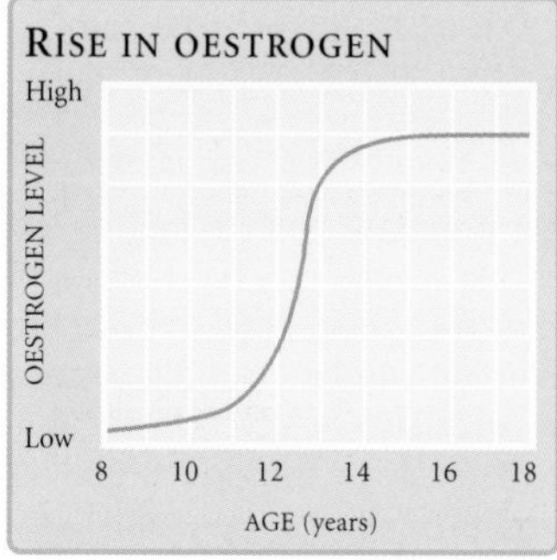

The rise in oestrogen at puberty
Oestrogen levels rise sharply between about the ages of 11 and 14. After this period, oestrogen levels out until the menopause, when it decreases.

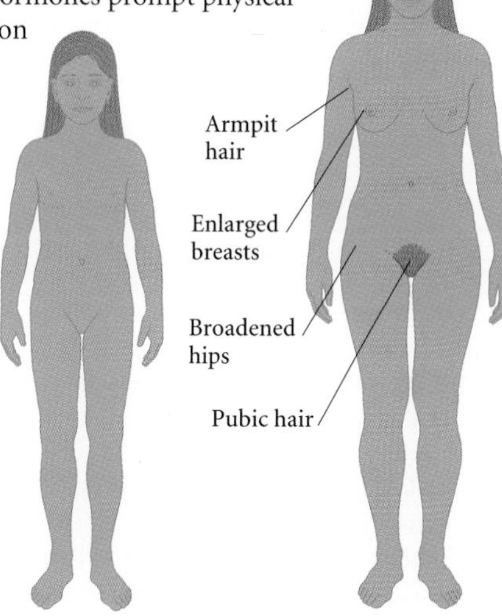

Magnified breast tissue
At puberty, the breasts start to enlarge as they develop the milk glands and ducts that supply milk after a baby is born.

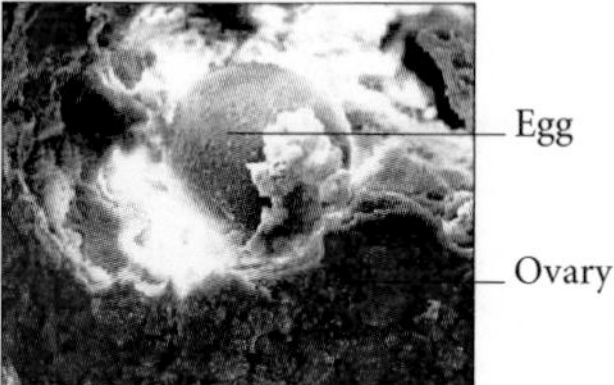

Ovulation
Late in puberty, ovulation begins; every month an egg is released from the ovary (as shown here) and travels to the uterus.

CHANGES IN BOYS DURING PUBERTY

In boys, puberty usually begins between the ages of about 12 and 15, when the pituitary gland starts to secrete the hormones LH and FSH. These hormones stimulate the testes to secrete the male sex hormone testosterone, which prompts physical changes and, later, sperm production and increased sex drive.

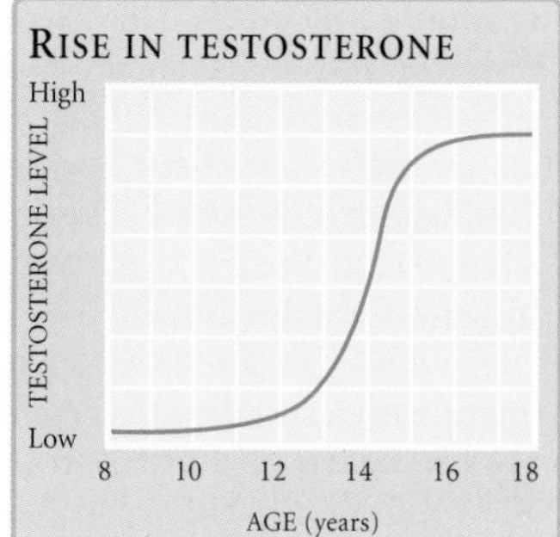

The rise in testosterone at puberty
Testosterone levels rise sharply between about the ages of 13 and 16. After this period, testosterone levels out until old age, when it gradually decreases.

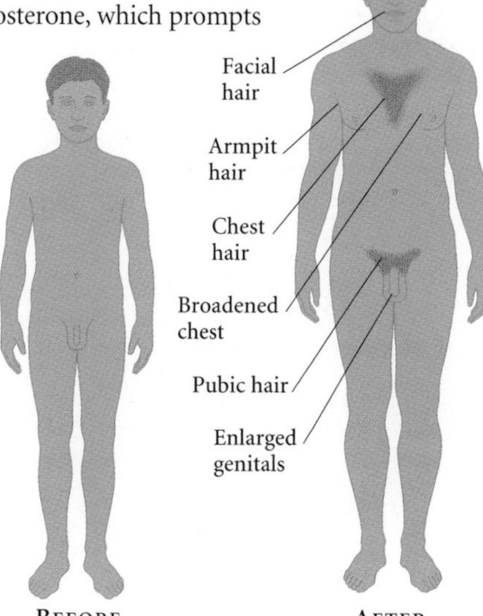

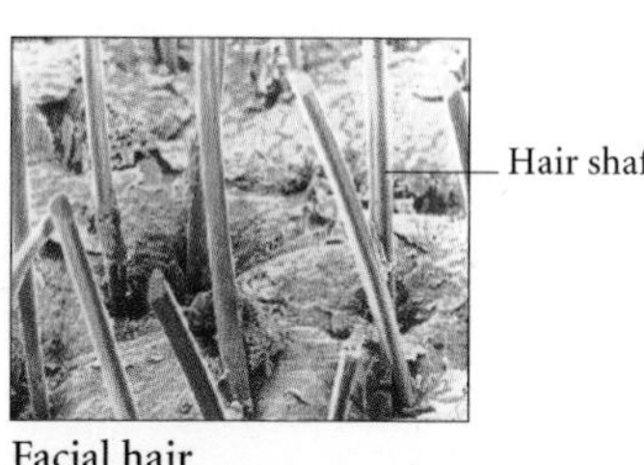

Facial hair
Hair on the face is part of the typical male pattern of hair growth triggered by increasing levels of testosterone.

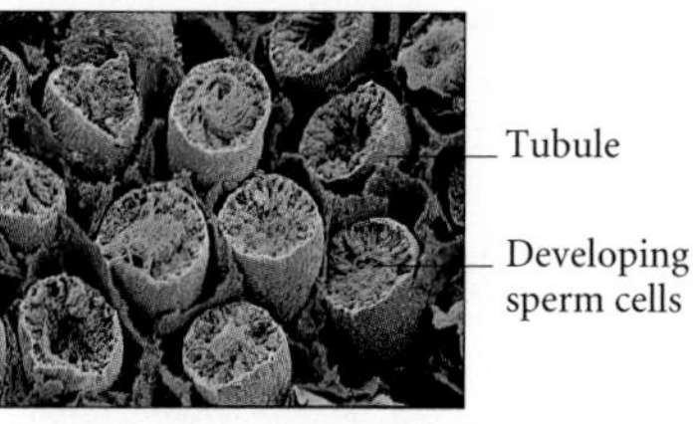

Cross section of testis tissue
In each testis, there are about 1,000 tubules. During puberty, these tubules begin to produce sperm cells.

PROBLEMS IN BABIES

Many problems in babies are associated with their immaturity and adjustment to a new environment. Premature babies are at particular risk of life-threatening conditions, but medical advances have greatly increased the number of babies that survive.

The first article in this section covers problems experienced by premature babies, those born more than 3 weeks before their expected birth date, who may have special problems as a result of their immaturity. The next article discusses congenital infections, which are transmitted from the mother to the fetus either during pregnancy or at birth as the baby passes through the birth canal. Although these infections are rare, they may have serious effects. Neonatal jaundice, which is discussed next, occurs in many newborn babies. In most cases, the jaundice is normal, but rarely there is a serious cause, such as the underdevelopment of the bile ducts in the baby's liver. Problems experienced with sleeping, feeding, crying, colic, and teething are also covered. These minor problems can be stressful for parents but rarely require medical treatment. The section ends with an article on sudden infant death syndrome (SIDS), which is also known as cot death, and advice on how to prevent it. The cause of SIDS is not known, but the incidence of it has decreased since parents have been advised to position babies on their backs to sleep. Other conditions that affect babies from birth are discussed in chromosome and gene disorders (pp.821–827) and endocrine and metabolic disorders (pp.866–869).

Problems of the premature baby

Problems experienced by babies born more than 3 weeks earlier than their expected birth date

AGE Present from birth

GENDER GENETICS LIFESTYLE Not significant factors

Pregnancy usually lasts about 40 weeks. Babies born before 37 weeks of pregnancy (*see* PREMATURE LABOUR, p.798) are called premature, and these babies may have problems because of their small size and immaturity. The severity of these problems will depend on how far the pregnancy has progressed and the baby's weight at birth. With specialist care, babies born as early as 23 weeks now have a chance of survival.

WHAT ARE THE PROBLEMS?

All premature babies lose heat easily because they are smaller than full-term babies and have thin skin and little fat. In addition, respiratory problems may occur because the lungs are immature and may not produce enough surfactant, a chemical that is required for the lungs to function properly. This problem is known as respiratory distress syndrome. Irregular breathing is a common problem due to immaturity of the brain. Premature babies are also particularly vulnerable to injury and infection. The trauma of birth, lack of oxygen, and infection can all affect the developing brain. In very premature babies (born before 28 weeks), tiny blood vessels in the brain may rupture and bleed. There are usually no lasting problems, but specific learning disabilities (p.854) and problems with movement and posture (*see* CEREBRAL PALSY, p.846) may occur.

About 8 in 10 premature babies are affected by neonatal jaundice (opposite page), due to immaturity of the liver. In this condition, there is yellowing of the skin and the whites of the eyes.

WHAT MIGHT BE DONE?

The doctor will assess your baby's condition at birth and start treatment if necessary. A baby who is only a few weeks premature may not need specialist care. However, you will be advised to feed your baby frequently and to make sure that he or she is kept warm.

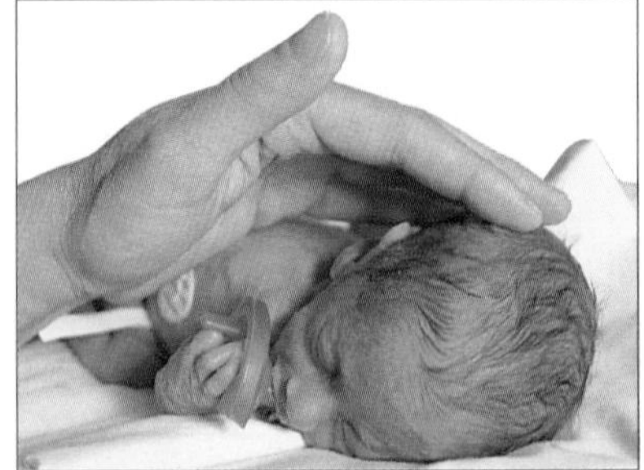

A premature baby
This baby was born prematurely and is smaller than normal. Premature babies need specialist care and monitoring.

Other premature babies may be looked after in a special care baby unit and are placed in an incubator so that their environment can be carefully controlled. They may also be given fluids and fed intravenously or through a tube that is passed through the nose and into the stomach. A premature baby may need to spend several weeks or months in the unit, and parents will be encouraged to take part in the baby's care. Tests may also be performed, such as ultrasound scanning (p.250) of the brain and chest X-rays (p.490), to look for abnormalities that may require treatment.

If your baby has respiratory distress syndrome, mechanical ventilation may be necessary, and surfactant will probably be given directly into the airways to help the lungs to function. A ventilated baby may be given sedatives to make him or her more comfortable. However, the high levels of oxygen that are sometimes needed to treat respiratory difficulties in premature babies have been associated with damage to the retina (the light-sensitive cells at the back of the eye), resulting in visual impairment.

A baby who has jaundice may have treatment with a specific wavelength of fluorescent light (*see* PHOTOTHERAPY, p.818). Antibiotics (p.885) may also be given to treat or prevent infection.

When your baby leaves hospital, the doctor will continue to give you advice and support. Your baby may be given a vision test to look for retinal damage (*see* VISION TESTS IN CHILDREN, p.857) and also a hearing test (*see* HEARING TESTS IN CHILDREN, p.859) to check for hearing loss. Growth and development will be carefully monitored.

WHAT IS THE PROGNOSIS?

The success of treatment depends on how early the baby was born and the weight at birth. About 4 in 10 babies born at 23–24 weeks survive, but they may have long-term problems, such as visual impairment, lung disorders, or cerebral palsy. Most babies born after 30 weeks develop normally with no long-term health problems. Premature babies are more susceptible to sudden infant death syndrome (p.820), thought to be linked with abnormal breathing patterns.

(WWW) ONLINE SITES: p.1035

Congenital infections

Infections contracted before or at birth from the mother

 AGE Present from birth

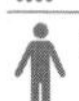 LIFESTYLE Risk factors depend on the cause

 GENDER GENETICS Not significant factors

Most infections contracted by a mother during pregnancy do not affect the fetus, but some cross the placenta and cause harm. These infections are often brief, minor illnesses for the pregnant mother, and she may not even be aware of them. Serious infections such as HIV (*see* HIV INFECTION AND AIDS, p.297) may also be passed on to the fetus.

The effect on the baby depends on the stage of pregnancy at which the infection occurs. In early pregnancy, the development of organs may be disrupted, and a miscarriage (p.791) could occur. Infections in later pregnancy may result in premature labour (p.798) and a baby who is seriously ill at birth. Infections may also be transmitted as the baby passes through the birth canal.

WHAT ARE THE CAUSES?

In the first 3 months of pregnancy, the viral disease rubella (p.294) can lead to fetal heart abnormalities (*see* CONGENITAL HEART DISEASE, p.836) and impaired hearing and vision. Cytomegalovirus (CMV) infection (p.292) and toxoplasmosis (p.307), which is caused by a protozoal parasite found in cats' faeces, may cause miscarriage or malformations of the fetus in early pregnancy. CMV is the leading cause of congenital deafness (p.859) and toxoplasmosis can damage the retina (the light-sensitive cells at the back of the eye). Later in pregnancy, these infections may lead to premature labour, stillbirth (p.805), and serious illness in the newborn baby. Listeriosis (p.301), a bacterial infection that can be contracted from eating soft cheese and pâté, may cause miscarriage or stillbirth.

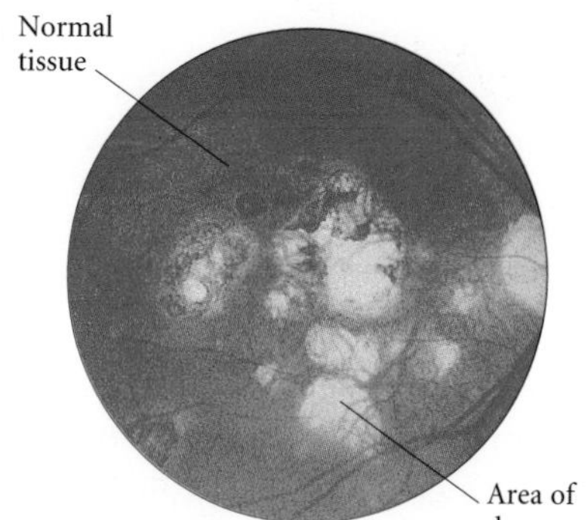

Toxoplasmosis

The pale patches in this view of the retina at the back of a baby's eye indicate the congenital infection toxoplasmosis.

Long-term viral infections that can be passed from mother to fetus include HIV infection and hepatitis B and C (*see* ACUTE HEPATITIS, p.645). The bacterial infection syphilis (p.766) may also be passed on. These infections do not always produce symptoms at birth but can cause serious illness later in life.

Some infections can be transmitted from mother to baby during delivery. Herpes simplex virus (*see* GENITAL HERPES, p.767) and streptococcal bacteria can result in life-threatening infections in the newborn. Other infections such as gonorrhoea (p.764) and chlamydia (*see* CHLAMYDIAL PELVIC INFECTION, p.765) and are less serious.

WHAT MIGHT BE DONE?

If a baby is seriously ill at birth and a congenital infection is suspected, blood and urine samples are taken to identify the infection. Babies are usually nursed in a special care baby unit and treated intravenously with appropriate drugs. Ultrasound scanning (p.250) may be used to image the baby's brain and echocardiography (p.425) may be arranged if there is a heart problem. If the mother is known to be infected with the hepatitis B virus, the baby is given antibodies against the virus. In the UK, newborn babies at high risk are also routinely immunized against hepatitis B infection.

CAN THEY BE PREVENTED?

Women can minimize the risk of contracting many of these infections during pregnancy (*see* HEALTH IN PREGNANCY AND AFTER CHILDBIRTH, p.33). Women can be immunized against rubella before starting a pregnancy. Pregnant women should avoid handling cat litter to prevent toxoplasmosis and should not eat foods linked with listeriosis. Those with HIV infection may be given antiviral drugs to reduce the risk of transmission to the baby. A caesarean section (p.802) is usually advised for women who have HIV infection or active genital herpes.

Mild congenital infections may have no lasting effect on the baby, but severe infections can be life-threatening. Congenital abnormalities may also result in long-term health and learning problems.

(WWW) ONLINE SITES: p.1033, p.1035

Neonatal jaundice

Yellow discoloration of the skin and the whites of the eyes in a newborn baby

 AGE Present from or shortly after birth

 GENETICS Risk factors depend on the cause

 GENDER LIFESTYLE Not significant factors

More than half of all newborn babies develop slight yellowing of the skin in the first week of life, giving them a tanned appearance. This condition is known as neonatal jaundice. In most cases, neonatal jaundice is normal, lasts only a few days, and does not indicate a serious underlying illness.

Neonatal jaundice is caused by high levels of a yellowish-green pigment in the blood known as bilirubin, which is a breakdown product of red blood cells. The liver, which removes bilirubin from the blood, may not be able to process all the bilirubin released by the breakdown of large numbers of red cells after birth. As a result, the level of bilirubin in the blood rises. Breast-feeding may make neonatal jaundice worse, but it can be continued without harming the baby.

Neonatal jaundice may be more severe if it is caused by an underlying condition, for example if the mother and baby have incompatible blood groups because of Rhesus (Rh) incompatibility (p.795). Incompatibility of ABO blood groups is also a common cause of jaundice. Rare conditions that may produce jaundice include congenital infections (p.817) and biliary atresia, in which a baby is born with underdeveloped bile ducts (the tubes that drain bile from the liver).

WHAT ARE THE SYMPTOMS?

In most full-term babies with neonatal jaundice, the skin and the whites of the eyes appear yellow, but there are no other symptoms. However, if bilirubin levels rise, symptoms may include:

- Lethargy.
- Reluctance to feed.

Severe, abnormal jaundice may lead to impaired hearing or brain damage. If the bile ducts are underdeveloped due to biliary atresia, there is a risk of fatal liver damage unless the condition is treated.

WHAT MIGHT BE DONE?

Your baby will probably have a blood test to measure the level of bilirubin and exclude underlying disorders. If biliary atresia is suspected, imaging tests such as ultrasound scanning (p.250) and MRI (p.248) of the liver may be performed. A liver biopsy, in which a small sample of liver tissue is removed for examination, usually confirms the diagnosis.

Most babies with mild jaundice do not require treatment. However, if the level of bilirubin in the blood is high, phototherapy (right) may be necessary, whatever the cause of the jaundice. In phototherapy, bilirubin is converted into a harmless substance that can be excreted. Treatment of Rh incompatibility may involve exchange transfusion, in which a large proportion of the baby's blood is replaced. Biliary atresia is corrected by surgery in the first weeks of the baby's life to prevent liver damage.

Neonatal jaundice does not usually have long-term effects and tends to disappear during the first week of life, or slightly later if the baby is breast-fed. Babies who have had severe jaundice will have a hearing test (*see* HEARING TESTS IN CHILDREN, p.859) and will be monitored for the first few months of life.

(WWW) ONLINE SITES: p.1033

(TREATMENT) PHOTOTHERAPY

In phototherapy, blue fluorescent lights are used in the treatment of neonatal jaundice (p.817), a disorder in which the skin and whites of the eyes become yellow due to high levels of the pigment bilirubin in the blood. In order to maximize exposure, your baby will be undressed and placed under the lights in an incubator to keep him or her warm. You will be allowed to take your baby out of the incubator for feeding, but otherwise he or she will continue phototherapy until blood tests show that bilirubin levels are normal. In most cases, treatment is needed for a few days.

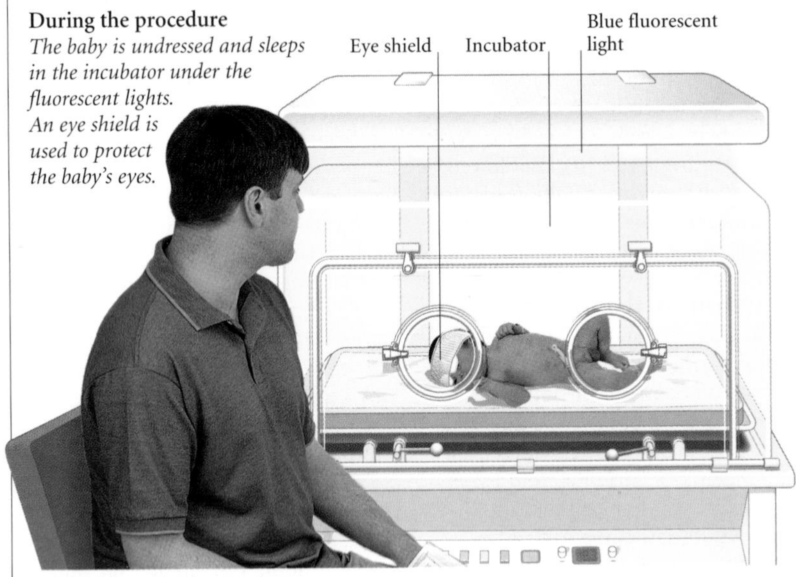

During the procedure
The baby is undressed and sleeps in the incubator under the fluorescent lights. An eye shield is used to protect the baby's eyes.

Sleeping problems in babies

Night-time wakefulness in babies, especially during the first months of life

 AGE More common under the age of 12 months

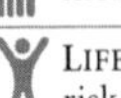 LIFESTYLE An unsettled environment is a risk factor

 GENDER GENETICS Not significant factors

Most newborn babies take time to establish a sleeping pattern that fits in with their parents' sleep and a normal 24-hour day. A baby's sleeping pattern will depend on how frequently he or she needs to feed. Premature babies tend to feed more often than full-term babies and therefore sleep for shorter periods. In older infants, problems may be caused by temperament, an unsettled or stressful environment, or a minor illness such as a common cold (p.288). Some sleeping problems are inevitable with a baby, but they can be stressful for parents.

WHAT CAN I DO?

Although your baby will have an irregular sleeping pattern at first, there are some self-help measures that may be useful. During the day, give your baby plenty of stimulation and try to nap when your baby is asleep. If you are breast-feeding, express milk so that you can share night feeding with your partner. When your baby is about 10 weeks old, you can begin to establish a bedtime routine. Give your baby's last feed in a quiet, darkened room. Check that your baby is comfortable, not hungry, and wearing a clean nappy before putting him or her to bed. Help your baby get to sleep by providing a ticking clock or musical mobile. Do not play with him or her during night-time feeds. If you think your baby's wakefulness may be due to an illness, consult your doctor.

In most babies, night-time wakefulness will improve with time. However, a few may develop sleeping problems later in childhood (*see* SLEEPING PROBLEMS IN CHILDREN, p.851).

(WWW) ONLINE SITES: p.1028

Feeding problems in babies

Feeding difficulties experienced during the first years of life

AGE More common in early infancy

GENDER GENETICS LIFESTYLE
Risk factors depend on the cause

Problems with feeding are common in young babies until a routine is established. These problems are upsetting, particularly for inexperienced parents, but if a baby is gaining weight there is usually no need to worry. However, when a baby who normally feeds well becomes reluctant to feed or vomits, there may be an underlying illness.

WHAT ARE THE CAUSES?

Breast-feeding may not come naturally to mother or baby and takes time to be learned. Problems with bottle-feeding are less common but may be due to the brand of milk or teat size used. A minor illness such as a common cold (p.288) may cause temporary difficulties. Most babies regurgitate some milk after each feed, but in some babies regurgitation is persistent (*see* GASTRO-OESOPHAGEAL REFLUX IN INFANTS, p.863). A few babies vomit forcefully after each feed, which may indicate that the outlet of the stomach is narrowed or blocked (*see* PYLORIC STENOSIS IN INFANTS, p.863).

WHAT MIGHT BE DONE?

If you bottle-feed, you should avoid frequently changing the brands of milk or the teats because such changes may make the problem worse. Wind your baby after a feed and, if he or she tends to vomit, try propping him or her up after feeds. If you are worried, weigh your baby to make sure that he or she is gaining weight. You should seek medical advice if you are still concerned or have problems with breast-feeding.

Your doctor will be able to exclude problems that require treatment, such as gastro-oesophageal reflux or pyloric stenosis, and will give you advice on breast-feeding. Your child may need to have regular weight and measurement checks to assess his or her growth. With time, most feeding problems disappear.

(WWW) ONLINE SITES: p.1028, p.1035

Excessive crying

Prolonged, inconsolable crying in babies that may indicate an underlying illness

AGE More common in early infancy

GENDER GENETICS LIFESTYLE
Not significant factors

Babies let adults know they are hungry or uncomfortable by crying. Prolonged, inconsolable crying, especially at night, is very stressful and tiring for parents. Newborn babies are more likely to cry excessively because they have yet to establish a routine. Regular episodes of crying are called colic (below). Babies also cry more when they are teething (right). However, if the crying is persistent or sounds different from normal, you should consult your doctor because it may indicate that your baby has an infection or disorder.

If your baby is crying but is otherwise well and has been feeding, make sure that you have excluded causes such as wind or a dirty nappy. Holding a crying baby will often soothe him or her, and offering a dummy may help. Many parents find it very stressful if their baby cries for hours on end and feel unable to cope. If you are afraid that you may harm your baby in an attempt to keep him or her quiet, you should put the baby in his or her cot and call someone for support. These feelings are a normal reaction and do not mean that you are a bad parent. Most babies grow out of excessive crying by the age of 6 months.

(WWW) ONLINE SITES: p.1028, p.1035

Colic

Regular episodes of inconsolable crying, usually at the same time every day

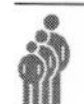
AGE Most common between the ages of 3 weeks and 3 months

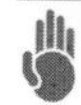
GENDER GENETICS LIFESTYLE
Not significant factors

From the age of about 3 weeks, many babies start to cry vigorously at approximately the same time each day, usually in the evening. This crying sounds different from crying at other times, and the baby may also draw up his or her legs. During these episodes, the baby will usually not respond to any form of comfort, such as feeding or holding, for more than a few minutes. The baby may continue crying for up to 3 hours. Episodes of crying that do not have this regular pattern are not called colic (*see* EXCESSIVE CRYING, left).

Although the baby may appear to be in pain, colic is not due to an illness, and the crying does not cause permanent harm. However, parents may find the condition distressing. The cause of colic is unknown, and it is not thought to be due to abdominal pain or wind, but the crying may be made worse by tiredness or an unsettled environment.

WHAT MIGHT BE DONE?

You should try to arrange your day so that you can comfort your baby when he or she is crying. If you have difficulty coping and require advice and support, consult your doctor or health visitor. You should consult your doctor if your baby develops additional symptoms, such as fever, which may indicate an underlying infection. The doctor will examine your baby and exclude other causes of the crying. Occasionally, he or she may suggest that you try giving your baby an over-the-counter remedy to relieve the colic. However, this treatment is only helpful in some cases. Colic disappears suddenly, on its own, usually when a baby reaches about 3 months of age.

(WWW) ONLINE SITES: p.1035

Teething

Discomfort during early childhood caused by the eruption of the primary teeth

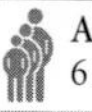
AGE Most common between the ages of 6 months and 3 years

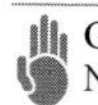
GENDER GENETICS LIFESTYLE
Not significant factors

An infant's first tooth usually appears at about the age of 6 months. Although the primary teeth have usually all erupted by about the age of 3 years, teething is an almost continuous process until the mid-teens, when the primary teeth are completely replaced by secondary teeth.

The eruption of a tooth can be uncomfortable and will probably make your baby irritable and restless. He or she may also be less willing to feed and may sleep poorly at night. Other symptoms include flushed cheeks, dribbling, and red, swollen gums around the site of the new tooth. You may also be able to feel the emerging tooth if you stroke the gum with your finger. Symptoms such as fever, vomiting, or diarrhoea are not due to teething and suggest that an infection may be present. You should take your baby to see the doctor if these symptoms appear.

WHAT CAN I DO?

Babies who are teething often seem to like chewing on a cold, hard object such as a teething ring or a raw carrot. Over-the-counter local anaesthetic gels are available and can be soothing if gently applied to the affected gums. Babies over the age of 3 months can also be given liquid paracetamol to relieve the pain (*see* PAINKILLERS, p.912).

You should avoid using sweet drinks to comfort your baby. Begin to clean his or her teeth with a soft baby toothbrush and fluoride toothpaste as soon as the first tooth appears. Regular brushing will help to prevent decay and establish a routine of good oral hygiene (*see* CARING FOR YOUR TEETH AND GUMS, p.610).

(WWW) ONLINE SITES: p.1028

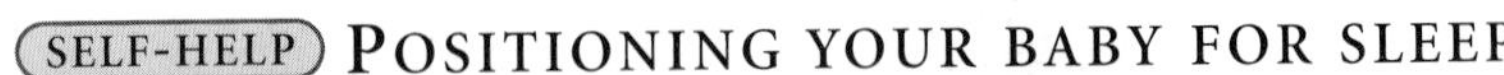

POSITIONING YOUR BABY FOR SLEEP

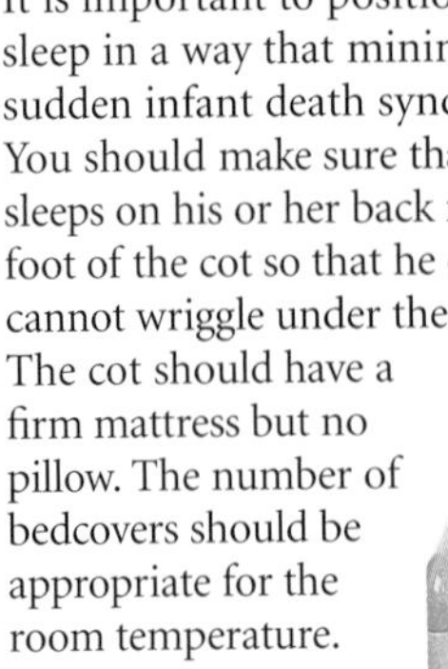

It is important to position your baby for sleep in a way that minimizes the risk of sudden infant death syndrome (SIDS). You should make sure that your baby sleeps on his or her back near the foot of the cot so that he or she cannot wriggle under the bedcovers. The cot should have a firm mattress but no pillow. The number of bedcovers should be appropriate for the room temperature.

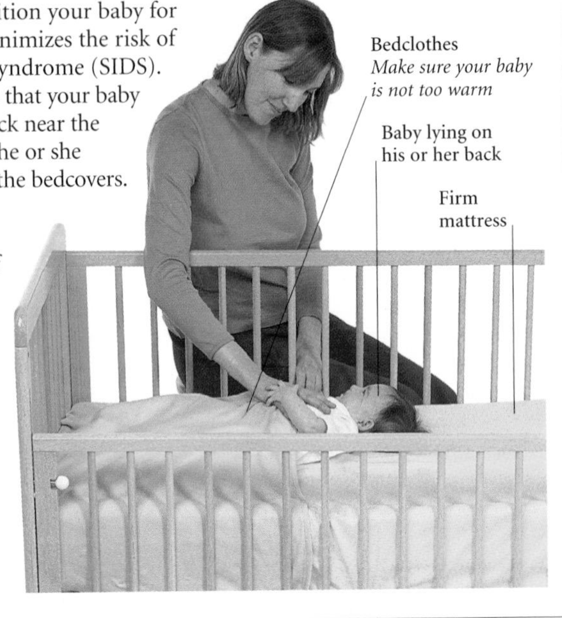

Reducing the risk
Lay your baby down to sleep on his or her back at the foot of the cot, so that his or her face cannot be covered by bedding. Do not overwrap your baby.

Sudden infant death syndrome

The sudden and unexpected death of a baby for which no cause can be found

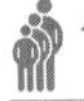 AGE Most common between the ages of 1 and 6 months

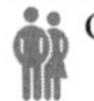 GENDER Slightly more common in boys

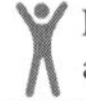 LIFESTYLE Parental smoking and drug abuse are risk factors

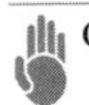 GENETICS Not a significant factor

Sudden infant death syndrome (SIDS), also known as cot death, is devastating for parents of an affected baby. SIDS occurs when healthy babies are put to bed and later found dead for no identifiable reason. In England and Wales, about 60 in 100,000 babies are affected by SIDS each year. The incidence of the condition has been declining steadily since the early 1990s.

WHAT ARE THE CAUSES?

The cause of SIDS is unknown but may be associated with abnormal breathing patterns. Several risk factors have been recognized, such as parental smoking and drug abuse, but in most cases the death is unexplained. Evidence suggests that putting babies to sleep on their fronts and bottle-feeding increase the risk. Babies who are overwrapped, particularly during an illness, can become overheated and may be at increased risk. Parents sometimes report minor symptoms of infection in the hours or days beforehand, but whether these symptoms are significant is not known. The risk of SIDS is slightly higher for siblings of an infant who has died of SIDS and is more common in babies born before 37 weeks (*see* PROBLEMS OF THE PREMATURE BABY, p.816).

WHAT MIGHT BE DONE?

If possible, parents should begin resuscitation immediately after calling for an ambulance (*see* FIRST AID: CARDIOPULMONARY RESUSCITATION FOR INFANTS, p.985). On arrival at hospital, the doctors will attempt to resuscitate the baby, but they are rarely successful. Very occasionally, an infant will be revived, and tests will then be done to try to discover the cause of the condition. The baby will receive follow-up care and monitoring to prevent a recurrence.

The sudden death of a baby is an extremely distressing and shocking event. Bereaved parents will need support from doctors, family, and friends, and they may be offered professional counselling (*see* LOSS AND BEREAVEMENT, p.76). A postmortem examination of the baby is always carried out to exclude other causes of death and to reassure the family that the death could not have been prevented. During this period, everyone concerned may experience intense emotions, including guilt, and relationships can be disrupted. These feelings are quite normal. Many bereaved parents find it helpful to contact a support group that allows them to discuss and share their feelings with other families who have experienced cot death. If the parents decide to have another child, the doctor will provide advice and support and can arrange for special monitoring.

CAN IT BE PREVENTED?

Many parents feel that SIDS is a threat over which they have no control, but there are ways to reduce the risk. All babies should be placed on their backs to sleep, and pillows should not be used until a baby is over one year old (*see* POSITIONING YOUR BABY FOR SLEEP, above). You may feel more confident if you have learned cardiopulmonary resuscitation. Alarms that alert parents if their baby stops breathing are available, but there is no firm evidence to suggest that these devices reduce the risk of SIDS.

(WWW) ONLINE SITES: p.1029

CHROMOSOME AND GENE DISORDERS

The 46 chromosomes in human cells contain about 35,000 pairs of genes, and several thousand rare disorders are directly the result of a defect in a gene or a chromosomal abnormality. Many children affected by such genetic disorders can be identified because their disorders cause a distinctive physical appearance.

This section includes a few examples of chromosome and gene disorders that affect many body systems and become apparent during childhood. The first four articles cover conditions that are caused by an extra or absent chromosome. For example, Down's syndrome is the result of an extra chromosome, and Turner's syndrome, a disorder that affects only girls, is due to an absent chromosome. The articles that follow cover several conditions, including cystic fibrosis, muscular dystrophy, and neurofibromatosis, that are caused by defective genes.

Genetic disorders that mainly affect one part of the body, such as polycystic kidney disease (p.704), are covered in the relevant sections of the book. The principles of chromosome and gene disorders, including how and why they occur and patterns of inheritance, are discussed elsewhere (*see* GENETIC DISORDERS, pp.270–273).

KEY ANATOMY

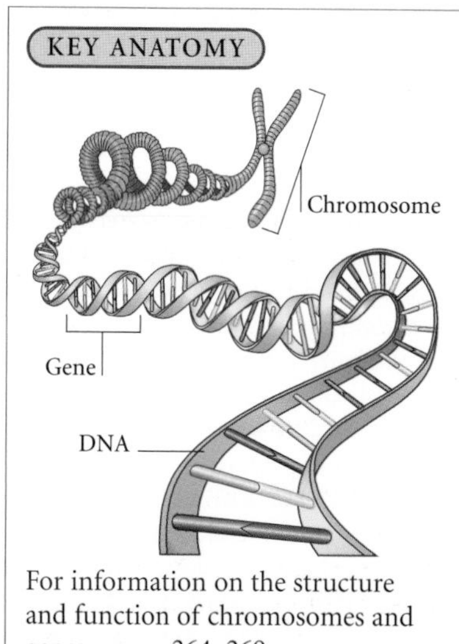

For information on the structure and function of chromosomes and genes, *see* pp.264–269.

Down's syndrome

A chromosome disorder affecting mental development and physical appearance

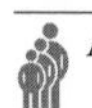 AGE Present at birth

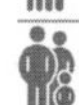 GENETICS Due to an extra chromosome

 GENDER LIFESTYLE Not significant factors

Down's syndrome, also called trisomy 21, is the most common chromosomal abnormality. In the UK, approximately 1 in 650 babies is affected. The condition usually occurs because a baby has three copies of chromosome 21 instead of the normal two copies, giving a total of 47 chromosomes instead of the usual 46. In most cases, the extra chromosome is inherited from the mother due to an abnormality in the egg; less commonly, it is inherited from the father due to a sperm abnormality. Children who have Down's syndrome have a characteristic physical appearance and generalized learning disabilities (p.854).

The risk of a baby having Down's syndrome becomes greater with increasing age of the mother. In women who conceive at the age of 20, there is a risk of 1 in 1,500 that the baby will have the condition. For women aged 40, the risk of Down's syndrome rises to 1 in 100. A woman who has already had an affected child has a slightly increased risk of having other children with the condition in subsequent pregnancies.

WHAT ARE THE SYMPTOMS?

Many of the physical characteristics of Down's syndrome are present at birth and may include:

- Floppy limbs.
- Round face with full cheeks.
- Eyes that slant up at the outer corners with folds of skin covering the inner corners of the eyes.
- Protruding tongue.
- Flattening of the back of the head.
- Excess skin on the back of the neck.
- Short, broad hands that have a single transverse crease on the palm.

Children with Down's syndrome have abnormalities that vary in severity. They are slow in learning to walk and talk, have learning disabilities ranging from mild to severe, and are typically short in stature. However, many affected children are cheerful and affectionate.

ARE THERE COMPLICATIONS?

More than 1 in 3 children with Down's syndrome have an abnormality of the heart (*see* CONGENITAL HEART DISEASE, p.836), usually a hole in the wall (septum) that divides the main chambers of the left and right sides of the heart. Sometimes, abnormalities can occur in the digestive tract, causing the tract to become narrowed or blocked. Affected children are also more likely to have ear infections and an accumulation of fluid in the ear, which may lead to impaired hearing (*see* CHRONIC SECRETORY OTITIS MEDIA, p.860). Problems with vision are also common (*see* CATARACT, p.573). The neck joints may become unstable, which can prevent children with Down's syndrome from taking part in sports. Affected children also have an increased risk of developing cancer of the white blood cells (*see* ACUTE LEUKAEMIA, p.454) and a higher than average risk of having an underactive thyroid gland (*see* HYPOTHYROIDISM, p.680). From about the age of 40, people with Down's syndrome are at increased risk of developing Alzheimer's disease (p.536), a progressive disorder of the brain that results in a gradual decline in mental abilities.

HOW IS IT DIAGNOSED?

An increased risk of Down's syndrome can be determined by tests early in pregnancy (*see* ANTENATAL GENETIC TESTS, p.787). These tests include blood tests and ultrasound scanning. Ultrasound can detect thickening at the back of the neck of the fetus (called nuchal translucency), which indicates an increased risk of Down's syndrome. A definitive diagnosis can only be made by examining the chromosomes from fetal cells obtained at amniocentesis or CVS.

Sometimes, Down's syndrome may not be diagnosed until after the baby is born. The condition is usually recognized by the distinctive appearance of the face. The diagnosis is confirmed by taking a sample of the baby's blood and performing a blood test to look for an extra copy of chromosome 21. Further tests, such as ultrasound scanning of the heart (*see* ECHOCARDIOGRAPHY, p.425) or a contrast X-ray (p.245) of the intestines, called a barium enema, may then be carried out to look for complications.

WHAT IS THE TREATMENT?

In the past, many children with Down's syndrome were given institutional care and lacked the necessary stimulation and support to maximize their mental development. Today, improved facilities mean that it is possible to make the most of their mental capabilities and to treat any physical problems as they arise. In the majority of cases, children are able to remain in their home environment.

Children who have Down's syndrome and their families usually receive medical care and long-term support from a team of professionals. Specialized care may include physiotherapy (p.961) and speech therapy (p.963). Special educational programmes may be adopted to help affected children to develop intellectually as much as possible. In some cases, surgery is necessary to correct abnormalities of the heart or intestine. Parents of affected children may find it helpful to contact a support group.

WHAT IS THE PROGNOSIS?

Most children with Down's syndrome lead happy and fulfilling lives. Although intellectual ability varies widely, affected children are now able to achieve much more because of the improvement in teaching methods and availability of special educational programmes. Some children learn to read and write and may acquire sufficient skills to enable them to work later in life. However, most are unable to live independently and need long-term supervision, provided either by their parents or in a special residential home. Although many survive into middle age, about 1 in 5 children with Down's syndrome dies in childhood, usually as a result of congenital heart disease. Some people who have Down's syndrome live long lives, but of these about 1 in 10 develops Alzheimer's disease from about the age of 50.

(WWW) ONLINE SITES: p.1030

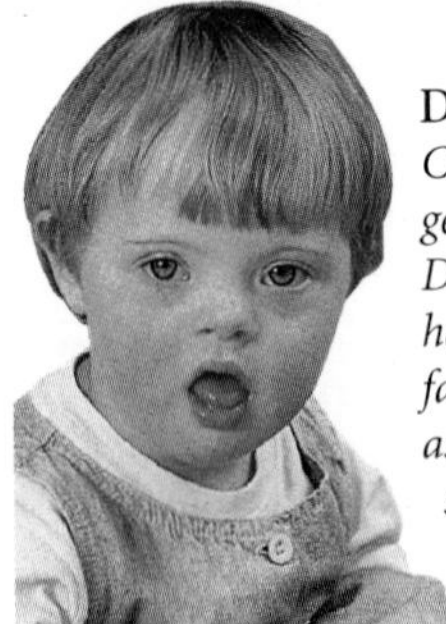

Down's syndrome *Children with the genetic disorder Down's syndrome have characteristic facial features, such as a round face, slanted eyes, and a protruding tongue.*

Fragile X syndrome

A defect in a specific gene on the X chromosome, causing learning difficulties

AGE Present at birth

GENDER Much more common in boys

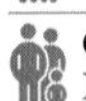
GENETICS Due to an abnormal gene on the X chromosome

LIFESTYLE Not a significant factor

Fragile X syndrome is caused by an abnormality of a specific gene on the X chromosome, one of the two sex chromosomes. This abnormality results in learning difficulties, and the condition is associated with a characteristic physical appearance. In the UK, about 1 in 2,000 boys is affected; the condition is far less common in girls since many women who carry the gene for the condition remain unaffected.

Girls with fragile X syndrome tend to have milder symptoms than affected boys because they have a second copy of the X chromosome that is normal and compensates for the abnormal gene on the other chromosome. However, any woman who carries this gene can pass it on to sons, who would develop more severe symptoms of the disorder.

WHAT ARE THE SYMPTOMS?

The initial symptoms are learning disabilities, which vary from mild to severe and become more obvious as the child grows older (*see* GENERALIZED LEARNING DISABILITIES, p.854). Affected children tend to be taller than normal. Other characteristic physical features of fragile X syndrome often do not appear until puberty and include:

- Large head and a long, thin face with a prominent jaw and large ears.
- In boys, large testes.

Affected children are also susceptible to seizures and behaviour problems (*see* AUTISM SPECTRUM DISORDERS, p.852).

WHAT MIGHT BE DONE?

If your child's doctor suspects fragile X syndrome, he or she will arrange for a blood test to look for the gene abnormality on the X chromosome. Although the condition cannot be treated, affected children may benefit from speech therapy (p.963), specialized teaching, and help from a psychologist for behaviour problems. Some affected children need to take anticonvulsant drugs (p.914) to prevent seizures. Parents of an affected child may wish to join a support group.

Genetic counselling (p.272) is offered to couples who already have a child with fragile X syndrome to assess the risk of having another child with this condition. Antenatal testing can be performed in subsequent pregnancies (*see* ANTENATAL GENETIC TESTS, p.787).

The life expectancy for affected children is normal, but boys usually require lifelong care, either from their parents or in a residential home.

(WWW) ONLINE SITES: p.1032

Klinefelter's syndrome

A chromosomal abnormality in boys, causing tall stature and small genitals

AGE Present at birth

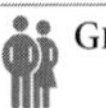
GENDER Affects only boys

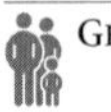
GENETICS Due to an extra chromosome

LIFESTYLE Not a significant factor

Klinefelter's syndrome affects only boys. In the UK, about 1 in every 600 boys has the condition, but it is thought that many cases are never detected. Affected boys have two copies of the X chromosome instead of the usual one. This may lead to insufficient levels of the male sex hormone testosterone and cause infertility and characteristic physical features.

WHAT ARE THE SYMPTOMS?

A boy with Klinefelter's syndrome often appears normal at birth. However, as he reaches puberty, the physical characteristics of the condition become more obvious and include:

- Tall stature.
- Long legs.
- Small penis and testes.

In some cases, breast enlargement also develops (*see* GYNAECOMASTIA, p.729). Most men with Klinefelter's syndrome are infertile because they are unable to produce sperm. A small number of those who have the condition have generalized learning disabilities (p.854).

WHAT MIGHT BE DONE?

Klinefelter's syndrome is often suspected from an affected boy's physical characteristics. The diagnosis is confirmed by a blood test to look for the extra X chromosome. If the condition is diagnosed in childhood, treatment with a testosterone supplement may encourage the development of male characteristics and prevent gynaecomastia. However, if gynaecomastia does occur and causes psychological distress, an operation may be done to reduce breast size. Most boys with Klinefelter's syndrome lead a normal life, although they will not be able to father children. Genetic counselling (p.272) is offered to parents of an affected child who plan to have more children.

(WWW) ONLINE SITES: p.1032

Turner's syndrome

A chromosome disorder in which a girl has only one X chromosome

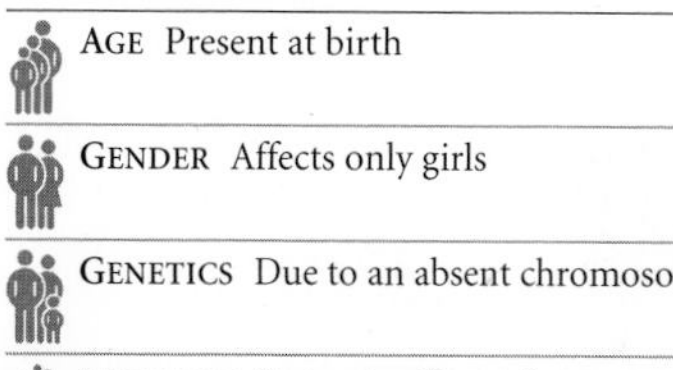

AGE Present at birth

GENDER Affects only girls

GENETICS Due to an absent chromosome

LIFESTYLE Not a significant factor

Normally, girls have two copies of the X sex chromosome. In Turner's syndrome, only one X chromosome is present, giving a total of 45 chromosomes instead of the normal complement of 46. Girls without a second X chromosome have ovaries that do not function normally. As a result, certain hormones that are needed for normal growth and sexual development, such as oestrogen and progesterone, are not produced, leading to infertility. Turner's syndrome affects about 1 in 2,000 girls in the UK.

WHAT ARE THE SYMPTOMS?

Some symptoms of Turner's syndrome may be present at birth and include:

- Puffy hands and feet.
- Small size.
- Broad chest.
- Short, broad neck.
- Prominent ears.

However, in some girls, there may be no symptoms except short stature. In some cases, Turner's syndrome is recognized only when a girl fails to reach puberty at the normal age (*see* ABNORMAL PUBERTY IN FEMALES, p.739). If the condition is recognized and treated before adolescence, a girl is more likely to attain a reasonable height and will develop normal female sexual characteristics, such as breasts, and have menstrual periods.

ARE THERE COMPLICATIONS?

About 1 in 10 girls with Turner's syndrome also has an abnormal narrowing of the aorta, the main artery of the body (*see* CONGENITAL HEART DISEASE, p.836). About 1 in 3 girls with Turner's syndrome has a mild kidney abnormality. Hearing impairment is common and is usually due to a build-up of fluid in the middle ear (*see* CHRONIC SECRETORY OTITIS MEDIA, p.860). Vision problems, including squints, are also common (*see* STRABISMUS, p.857). In later life, other possible complications include infertility (*see* FEMALE INFERTILITY, p.775) and osteoporosis (p.368), in which the bones progressively become thin and brittle.

Girls with Turner's syndrome are of normal intelligence, but some may have minor learning disabilities, especially with respect to mathematics and activities requiring hand–eye coordination. Psychological problems may also arise when a girl becomes aware of her sexual immaturity and short stature.

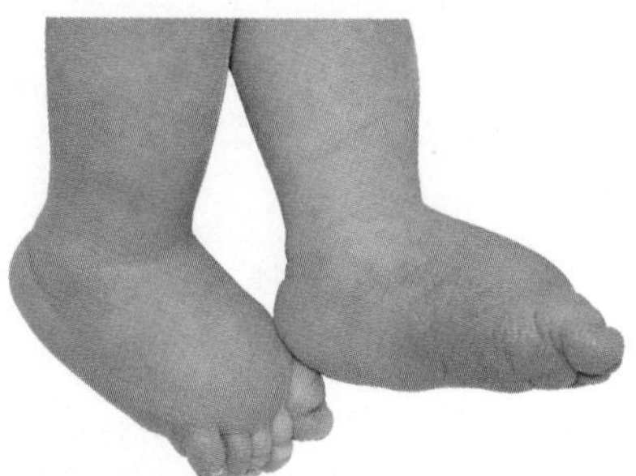

Turner's syndrome
Newborn baby girls with the chromosome disorder Turner's syndrome are sometimes born with temporary puffiness of the feet.

HOW IS IT DIAGNOSED?

Turner's syndrome is often diagnosed in the fetus during routine ultrasound scanning in pregnancy (p.793). Antenatal genetic tests (p.787) can confirm the diagnosis. Most fetuses with severe Turner's syndrome die before birth. If the fetus survives and the condition is suspected in infancy or childhood due to short stature, a blood test will be carried out to analyse the chromosomes. Mild Turner's syndrome may not be suspected until adolescence, when puberty and menstruation do not occur.

WHAT MIGHT BE DONE?

There is no cure for Turner's syndrome, and treatment is aimed at relieving some of the symptoms. Growth hormone and oestrogen may be given to encourage growth, allow normal puberty, and prevent the early onset of osteoporosis. Growth hormone is usually given only until the child reaches the usual age of puberty. Oestrogen is then given from this age and is continued for life.

Other treatments focus on associated complications. The ears will be checked regularly for fluid build-up. Narrowing of the aorta can be corrected surgically if necessary. Women who have Turner's syndrome are unable to conceive naturally, but pregnancy may be possible by using in vitro fertilization (*see* ASSISTED CONCEPTION, p.776).

Genetic counselling (p.272) is usually offered to the parents of a daughter with Turner's syndrome, although the risk of having another affected child is low. Affected individuals and their parents may find it useful to contact a support group.

WHAT IS THE PROGNOSIS?

Although affected girls do not grow to the average height for their age, most should be able to have a normal childhood and eventually to become healthy and independent women. Even serious complications that are associated with Turner's syndrome, such as a narrowed aorta, can now be treated successfully.

(WWW) ONLINE SITES: p.1032

Marfan's syndrome

An inherited condition in which a protein is deficient, resulting in tall stature and defects of the eyes, heart, and arteries

AGE Present at birth

GENETICS Due to an abnormal gene often inherited from one parent

GENDER LIFESTYLE Not significant factors

In Marfan's syndrome, a protein that is a component of the connective tissue between the structures and organs of the body is deficient. The condition most often affects the bones, eyes, heart, and main arteries of the body. Marfan's syndrome is due to an abnormal gene that is inherited in an autosomal dominant manner (*see* GENE DISORDERS, p.271). However, not everyone with this condition is affected to the same extent. In the UK, about 1 in 10,000 children has Marfan's syndrome.

WHAT ARE THE SYMPTOMS?

The symptoms of Marfan's syndrome usually appear at about the age of 10 but may be seen earlier. They may include:

- Very tall stature.
- Long, thin limbs, fingers, and toes.
- Weak joints and ligaments.
- Inward curving of the chest.
- Curvature of the spine.
- Impaired vision.

The risk of complications depends on which tissues are affected and the severity of abnormalities. Most people with Marfan's syndrome are shortsighted (*see* MYOPIA, p.586), and some have other eye defects, such as an incorrectly placed lens. Marfan's syndrome can lead to heart valve disorders (p.421). The aorta, the main artery of the body, may also become weakened and may swell and rupture (*see* AORTIC ANEURYSM, p.430), a condition that is life-threatening.

WHAT MIGHT BE DONE?

Marfan's syndrome is usually diagnosed when the visible features of the condition begin to appear. There is no cure, but an affected child is monitored carefully, and complications are treated as they arise. Many affected children need glasses and should have an eye test once a year. Some people with the condition are given beta-blockers (p.898) to help to prevent weakening of the aorta. In rare cases, affected girls under the age of 10 are given hormone treatment to promote the early onset of puberty and to reduce their growth, preventing excessive height in adulthood. Defects in the heart valves or aorta can be corrected by surgery. Affected individuals may wish to join a support group for advice.

WHAT IS THE PROGNOSIS?

In the past, people with the condition were restricted in their activities and often died before the age of 50. Today, most affected people can lead active lives due to advances in heart surgery, but lifespan may be shortened.

(WWW) ONLINE SITES: p.1032

Cystic fibrosis

An inherited condition that causes body secretions to be thick and abnormal

AGE Present at birth

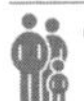
GENETICS Due to an abnormal gene inherited from both parents

GENDER LIFESTYLE Not significant factors

Cystic fibrosis is the most common severe inherited disease among white people of European and North American origin. In the UK, about 1 in 2,500 babies is born with the disorder. Cystic fibrosis is much less common in people of African or Asian descent. The disorder affects all the fluid- and mucus-secreting glands in the body, leading to production of abnormally thick secretions, especially in the lungs and pancreas. As a result, children with cystic fibrosis experience recurrent chest infections and may have difficulty absorbing nutrients from food.

In the past, severe chest infections were a major cause of death in children with cystic fibrosis. Today, with better understanding of the disease and recent advances in treatment, most affected children survive into adulthood.

WHAT ARE THE CAUSES?

Cystic fibrosis is caused by an abnormal gene, which is carried by about 1 in 20 people and inherited in an autosomal recessive manner (*see* GENE DISORDERS, p.271). The abnormal gene occurs on chromosome number 7. Over 350 different mutations (abnormalities) in the gene have now been identified. Of these, the most common is called delta 508, and this is the cause of more than 7 in 10 cases of cystic fibrosis.

WHAT ARE THE SYMPTOMS?

Sometimes, a newborn baby with cystic fibrosis has a swollen abdomen and does not pass meconium (thick, sticky faeces passed by newborn infants) for the first few days following birth. Other symptoms of cystic fibrosis usually develop later in infancy and may include:

- Failure to put on weight or grow at the normal rate.

(TEST) SWEAT TESTING

A sweat test is used to diagnose cystic fibrosis by measuring the levels of salt in sweat. The procedure is painless and is performed in hospital on an outpatient basis. The production of sweat is stimulated for about 3 minutes using two electrodes. The electrodes are then replaced with a pad, which collects the sweat for the next 30 minutes.

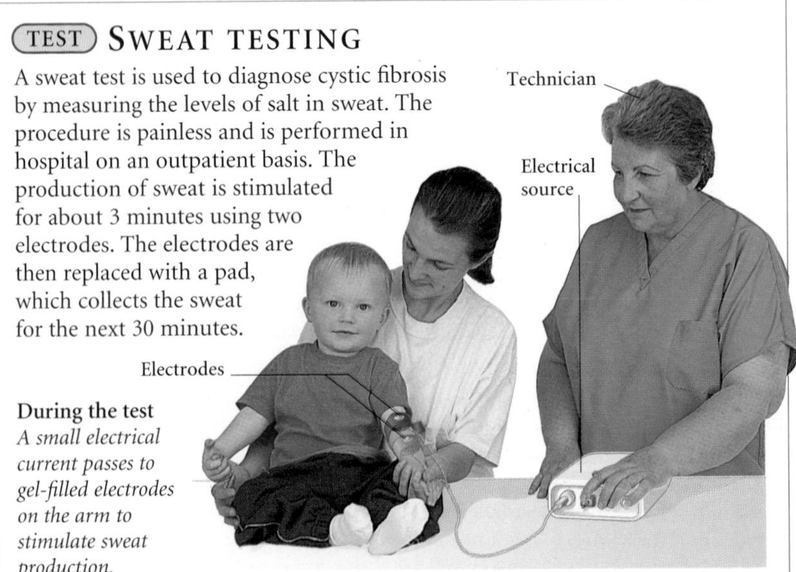

During the test
A small electrical current passes to gel-filled electrodes on the arm to stimulate sweat production.

TREATMENT ANTIBIOTIC DELIVERY SYSTEM

This system enables the easy and regular delivery of intravenous antibiotics and is particularly useful for children with cystic fibrosis (opposite page). Under general anaesthesia, the internal part of the system is placed on the chest wall just under the skin so that it does not interfere with the child's normal activities. A catheter carries the injected antibiotics from the injection site to a vein in the chest just above the heart. The external part of the system is removable.

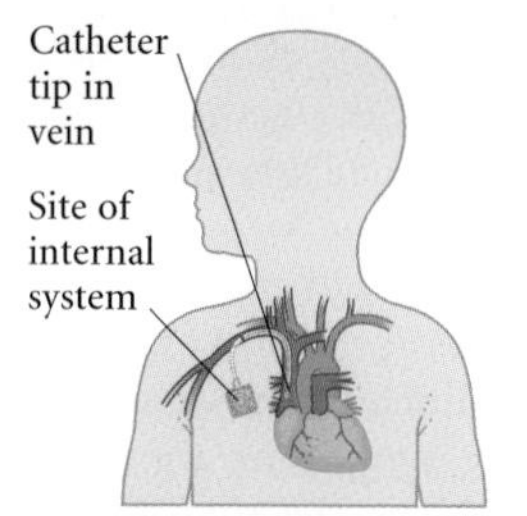

POSITION OF SYSTEM

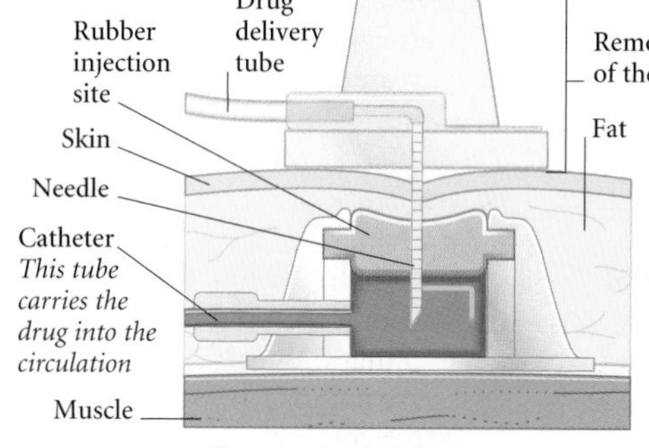

COMPLETE DELIVERY SYSTEM

The injection procedure
The external part of the injection system is positioned over the internal part so that the sterile needle pierces the injection site. Antibiotics are injected into the delivery tube and pass through the catheter into the circulation. Local anaesthetic cream is often used to numb the skin beforehand.

- Pale, greasy faeces that float and have a particularly offensive smell.
- Recurrent chest infections.

In many cases of cystic fibrosis, a constant cough develops, producing large amounts of sticky mucus.

ARE THERE COMPLICATIONS?

As cystic fibrosis progresses, the lung disorder bronchiectasis (p.496) may occur, in which the main airways are abnormally widened. Abscesses may also form in the lungs. Further complications may include liver damage (*see* CIRRHOSIS, p.647) and persistent inflammation of the sinuses (*see* SINUSITIS, p.475). About 1 in 20 children who have cystic fibrosis develop diabetes mellitus (p.687). In all affected children, abnormally high levels of salt are excreted in the sweat, which may lead to dehydration in hot weather.

Children with cystic fibrosis sometimes develop psychological problems as a result of the many difficulties that are associated with lifelong illness. Affected children may be unable to participate in normal childhood and school activities due to continual bad health and may therefore feel isolated.

In later life, almost all males with cystic fibrosis are infertile as a result of a birth defect in which the two vas deferens (the tubes through which sperm are propelled) are absent. About 1 in 5 affected females are infertile because the mucus secretions produced by the reproductive organs are abnormally thick.

HOW IS IT DIAGNOSED?

Some hospitals offer testing for all newborns. An early diagnosis improves the long-term outlook by helping to prevent damage to the lungs in infancy. If the doctor suspects that a child has the condition at birth or later in infancy, a sweat test (opposite page) may be carried out to look for abnormally high levels of salt in the baby's sweat. A sample of blood may also be tested to look for the abnormal gene. If the test result is found to be positive, siblings of the affected child can also be tested.

WHAT IS THE TREATMENT?

Treatment for cystic fibrosis is aimed at slowing the progression of lung disease and maintaining adequate nutrition.

Chest physiotherapy (p.962) is usually performed twice a day to remove secretions from the lungs. Parents and older affected children are often taught how to carry out this procedure at home. If an affected child develops a chest infection, he or she will require immediate treatment with antibiotics (p.885). In addition, long-term use of antibiotics may be necessary to prevent other chest infections from developing. Older children sometimes require regular courses of intravenous antibiotics to eliminate bacteria that become established in the lung secretions. In this case, a permanent catheter may be inserted under general anaesthesia just below the chest wall so that antibiotics can be administered more easily (*see* ANTIBIOTIC DELIVERY SYSTEM, left). Some children with cystic fibrosis can be helped by inhaled drugs that reduce the stickiness of the secretions in the lungs. If the lungs are very severely damaged, it may be necessary to carry out a heart–lung transplant. This operation is always a last resort.

A high-calorie diet helps to ensure that a child with cystic fibrosis grows normally. Most children also need to take pancreatic enzymes and vitamin supplements with every meal.

An affected child and his or her family will be offered psychological support, particularly during adolescence, when long-term illness is especially difficult to cope with. Family members may also find it helpful to join a support group.

CAN IT BE PREVENTED?

Genetic testing means that carriers can be identified and the condition can be detected antenatally. Genetic testing may be offered to adults with a family history of cystic fibrosis and partners of people who have the disease. If these test results are positive, the couple will be offered genetic counselling (p.272). A couple at risk may opt to use assisted conception (p.776), which enables the embryo to be tested for the abnormal gene before it is implanted by in vitro fertilization. Pregnant women may be offered antenatal genetic tests (p.787).

In the future, cystic fibrosis may be treated with gene therapy, in which a normal gene is introduced into relevant tissues to prevent cystic fibrosis from developing. The results of research in this field are promising.

WHAT IS THE PROGNOSIS?

The average life expectancy of a person with cystic fibrosis has increased over the past 30 years. Due to advances in the specialized treatment of cystic fibrosis, most people with the disorder now survive into their third decade.

(WWW) ONLINE SITES: p.1029

Muscular dystrophy

A group of genetic conditions in which muscles become weak and wasted

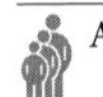 AGE Present at birth

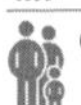 GENETICS Due to an abnormal gene

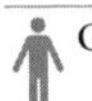 GENDER Risk factors depend on the type

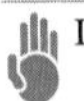 LIFESTYLE Not a significant factor

The two main types of muscular dystrophy almost exclusively affect boys. The most common type is Duchenne muscular dystrophy, which affects about 1 in 3,500 boys in the UK and causes serious disability from early childhood. A second, much rarer type of the disorder is Becker muscular dystrophy, which affects about 1 in 10,000 boys. The onset of Becker muscular dystrophy is slower, and the symptoms tend to start later in childhood. Other rare forms of muscular dystrophy can affect both girls and boys.

What are the causes?

Both Duchenne and Becker muscular dystrophies are caused by an abnormal gene carried on the X chromosome (*see* GENE DISORDERS, p.271). Girls may carry the defective gene, but they do not usually have the disorder because they have two X chromosomes, and the normal X chromosome compensates for the defect in the gene on the other.

Normally, this gene is responsible for the production of a protein called dystrophin, which is necessary for healthy muscles. In Duchenne and Becker muscular dystrophies, the gene is abnormal, resulting in deficiency of the protein and damage to muscle tissue. In Duchenne muscular dystrophy, almost no dystrophin is produced. However, in Becker muscular dystrophy some dystrophin is present, accounting for the difference in severity between the two conditions.

What are the symptoms?

The symptoms of Duchenne muscular dystrophy usually appear around the time a child would begin to walk. Late walking is common; often an affected child does not begin to walk until about 18 months and then will fall more frequently than other children. The more obvious symptoms of the disorder may not appear until the child is between 3 and 5 years old and may include:

- Waddling gait.
- Difficulty climbing stairs.
- Difficulty getting up from the floor. Characteristically, a child will use his hands to "walk up" the thighs.
- Large calf muscles and wasted muscles at the tops of the legs and arms.
- Mild learning disabilities.

The symptoms are progressive, and a child may be unable to walk by the age of 12. The symptoms of Becker muscular dystrophy are similar but usually do not appear until later in childhood or adolescence. This condition progresses more slowly; many of those affected are still able to walk until their 30s or later.

Are there complications?

In Duchenne muscular dystrophy, the heart muscle may become thickened and weakened. The limbs may also become deformed, and abnormal curvature of the spine may develop (*see* SCOLIOSIS, p.371). In the later stages of the disease, a child may have difficulty breathing, and there is an increased risk of chest infections that can be life-threatening.

How is it diagnosed?

If a pregnant woman is known to be a carrier of the disease, she will probably be offered antenatal testing to determine whether the fetus is affected (*see* ANTENATAL GENETIC TESTS, p.787).

In most cases, muscular dystrophy is suspected only when symptoms begin to appear. A blood test to look for the abnormal gene will be carried out to confirm the diagnosis. If the test result is positive, a further blood test may be performed to look for evidence of muscle damage. A muscle biopsy may also be carried out, in which a small piece of muscle tissue is removed under local or general anaesthesia to be examined under the microscope. In addition, tests will be done to find out whether the heart is affected, including a recording of the electrical activity in the heart (*see* ECG, p.406) and ultrasound scanning (*see* ECHOCARDIOGRAPHY, p.425).

What is the treatment?

The treatment for muscular dystrophy is directed at keeping an affected child mobile and active for as long as possible. A team of professionals, including a physiotherapist, a doctor, and a social worker, can provide support for the whole family. Physiotherapy (p.961) is important to keep the limbs supple, and supportive splints may be used. Some children require equipment, such as leg braces or a wheelchair, to aid mobility. If a child develops scoliosis, surgery may be necessary to straighten the spine.

Children with muscular dystrophy and their families usually need a great deal of psychological support. Genetic counselling (p.272) is offered to parents of an affected child who are considering having another child and to sisters of boys affected by the disorder.

Duchenne muscular dystrophy may be fatal before the age of 20. Becker muscular dystrophy has a better outlook; people usually live into their 40s or later.

(WWW) ONLINE SITES: p.1032

Congenital immunodeficiency

Defects of the immune system present from birth, leading to recurrent infection and failure of normal growth

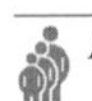 AGE Present at birth

 GENETICS Due to an abnormal gene

 GENDER Risk factors depend on the type

 LIFESTYLE Not a significant factor

In immunodeficiency, the immune system is defective and therefore unable to combat infections effectively. As a result, infections are more frequent and severe and may be life-threatening. A child's growth may also be affected. In children, immunodeficiency is usually caused by an underlying illness (*see* ACQUIRED IMMUNODEFICIENCY, p.460). In rare cases, the condition is inherited and is present at birth, in which case it is called congenital immunodeficiency.

What are the types?

Congenital immunodeficiencies are due to an abnormal gene. This gene is either linked to the X chromosome or inherited in an autosomal recessive manner (*see* GENE DISORDERS, p.271). The type of immunodeficiency depends on which part of the immune system is affected.

The most common type of immunodeficiency is agammaglobulinaemia, a disorder that affects only boys. In this condition, severe bacterial infections, especially of the chest, frequently occur because the production of antibodies is abnormal. Other, less serious, types of immunodeficiency may be caused by failure of the immune system to produce some specific types of antibody.

Chronic granulomatous disease is another type of congenital immunodeficiency. In this disease, the phagocytes, the white blood cells that are responsible for engulfing and killing bacteria and fungi, are unable to function properly. As a consequence, a child who has this disorder may have frequent bacterial and fungal infections, especially of the skin, lungs, and bones.

Severe combined immunodeficiency (SCID) is a disorder in which a child is unable to fight most forms of infection because both the antibodies and the white blood cells are deficient.

WHAT MIGHT BE DONE?

It is possible to screen for congenital immunodeficiency during pregnancy if the fetus is thought to be at risk (*see* ANTENATAL GENETIC TESTS, p.787). More often, congenital immunodeficiency is suspected when a child has persistent unusual infections or fails to grow normally. The doctor may then arrange for blood tests to measure the levels of antibodies and white blood cells and assess the function of the child's immune system. Sometimes, it is possible to detect the abnormal gene by a blood test.

All infections in a child who has a congenital immunodeficiency should be treated as soon as possible. Antibiotics (p.885) will be given if appropriate. If antibodies are deficient, they can be replaced intravenously every few weeks. In some severe types of congenital immunodeficiency, such as SCID, a bone marrow transplant (p.454) may be necessary, and this will be done if a suitable donor can be found. If the transplant is successful, the transplanted bone marrow will start to produce normal white blood cells that can fight infection.

If treatment for congenital immunodeficiencies is started sufficiently early, many children affected with these disorders can lead a normal life and have an average life expectancy.

In the future, treatment of congenital immunodeficiency may include gene therapy. The aim of this new treatment is to correct the genetic defects that affect the function of the immune system.

Genetic tests (pp.238–241) may be offered to relatives of affected people. Genetic counselling (p.272) is offered to couples who are found to have the abnormal gene or who have an affected child and plan to have more children.

(WWW) ONLINE SITES: p.1032, p.1033

Neurofibromatosis

The development of noncancerous tumours along nerve fibres

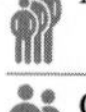 AGE Present at birth

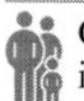 GENETICS Due to an abnormal gene often inherited from one parent

 GENDER LIFESTYLE Not significant factors

Neurofibromatosis is a genetic disorder that causes numerous soft, noncancerous growths, known as neurofibromas, to appear throughout the body. These tumours grow from nerve tissue and develop along nerve pathways. If the condition is severe, it can be disfiguring and may be distressing for the affected child and his or her family.

There are two types of neurofibromatosis. The more common of the two, known as neurofibromatosis 1, affects about 1 in every 2,500 children. The other type, neurofibromatosis 2, is extremely rare, and the symptoms do not usually appear until adulthood. Both types are caused by an abnormal gene that is inherited in an autosomal dominant manner (*see* GENE DISORDERS, p.271). The abnormal gene for neurofibromatosis 1 is located on chromosome 17, and the gene for neurofibromatosis 2 is located on chromosome 22.

WHAT ARE THE SYMPTOMS?

The symptoms of neurofibromatosis 1 usually appear during early childhood. They may include:

- Numerous pale-brown, flat patches with irregular edges, known as café au lait spots, that develop on the skin.
- Soft growths under the skin, which can range in size from hardly noticeable to large and disfiguring.
- Freckles in the armpit and groin areas.

Adults with neurofibromatosis 2 tend to develop tumours in the inner ear, which can affect hearing, but they rarely have tumours on the skin.

ARE THERE COMPLICATIONS?

Complications may occur when growing tumours press on the surrounding organs or nerves. For example, vision may be affected if a tumour develops on the optic nerve, which connects the eye to the brain. Tumours can also cause curvature of the spine (*see* SCOLIOSIS, p.371). Some children with neurofibromatosis may develop epilepsy (p.524) or have learning problems. In rare cases, the tumours become cancerous.

WHAT MIGHT BE DONE?

Neurofibromatosis 1 is normally diagnosed in childhood when the symptoms appear. Neurofibromatosis 2 is usually diagnosed in adulthood. The doctor will arrange for CT scanning (p.247) or MRI (p.248) of the brain to look for tumours, and hearing and vision will be tested.

There is no cure for the disease, and its progression cannot be slowed. Many cases are mild, but long-term care may be needed for severely affected children. Tumours that are large, painful, or disfiguring can often be surgically removed. Complications are usually treated as they arise. For example, a child with learning problems may need special education. Parents of an affected child who want to have more children may be offered genetic counselling (p.272).

In mild cases of neurofibromatosis, life expectancy is normal, but, if tumours are extensive and cancer develops as a complication, lifespan may be reduced.

(WWW) ONLINE SITES: p.1035

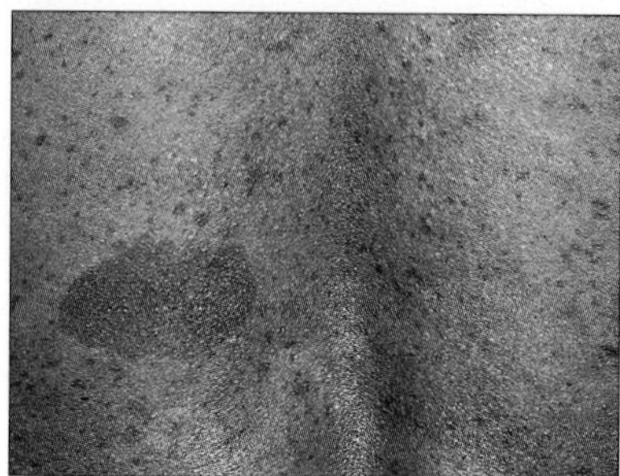

Café au lait spot in neurofibromatosis
This pale-brown, flat patch on the skin is known as a café au lait spot. The development of patches such as this is typical of neurofibromatosis 1.

SKIN AND HAIR DISORDERS

Young skin is sensitive and particularly susceptible to irritation or allergies. Most skin disorders in children are minor, affect only a small area of skin, and disappear as the child grows older. Many skin and hair disorders that affect children can be treated successfully at home with over-the-counter preparations.

Skin and hair disorders that mainly or exclusively affect children include a number of rashes and viral infections. The section begins with disorders that may affect young babies: birthmarks, which are present at birth or develop soon afterwards, and two skin rashes, cradle cap and nappy rash. The next article discusses the more serious rash eczema, which is sometimes caused by an allergy and may persist for many years. Viral infections that cause a rash and affect only young children are also covered. The section concludes with an article on infestation with head lice. Children are especially vulnerable to this problem due to close contact with other children at school.

Skin and hair disorders that affect people of any age are covered either in the main section on skin, hair, and nails (pp.328–361) or, if the disorders are caused by viruses, in the section on viral infections (pp.288–298).

KEY ANATOMY

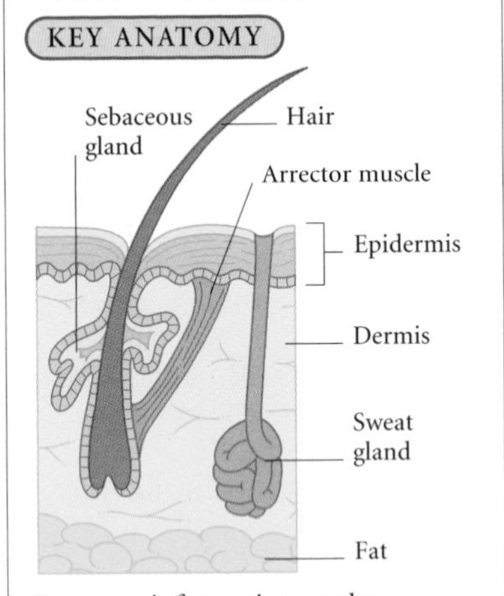

For more information on the structure and function of the skin and hair, *see* pp.328–331.

Birthmarks

Coloured patches of skin that are present at birth or appear soon afterwards

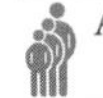 AGE Present at or shortly after birth

 GENETICS Risk factors depend on the type

 GENDER LIFESTYLE Not significant factors

Many babies have patches of coloured skin, known as birthmarks, that may be present at birth or appear during the first weeks of life. Although they can be unsightly and distressing to the parents, most birthmarks are not harmful, and they rarely cause discomfort.

WHAT ARE THE TYPES?

There are two types of birthmark: haemangiomas, which form from the small blood vessels just under the surface of the skin; and pigmented naevi, which form from densely pigmented skin cells.

HAEMANGIOMAS This group of birthmarks includes stork marks, strawberry naevi, and port-wine stains.

Stork marks are very common birthmarks and can occur in up to 5 in 10 babies at birth. A stork mark appears as a flat, pale pink patch, usually between the eyebrows or on the nape of the neck. This type of birthmark usually disappears by the age of 18 months.

Strawberry naevi are common birthmarks, occurring in about 1 in every 50 babies. The naevus appears as a small, flat, red spot at birth. The spot enlarges rapidly and becomes raised during the first year of life but usually disappears completely by the time the child reaches about 5 years of age.

Port-wine stains occur in about 1 in 3,000 babies, and they are usually permanent. The birthmark is visible as an irregularly shaped red patch and may be distressing, particularly if the mark is on the baby's face. In rare cases, a port-wine stain on the face is associated with abnormal blood vessels in the brain that can cause epilepsy (p.524).

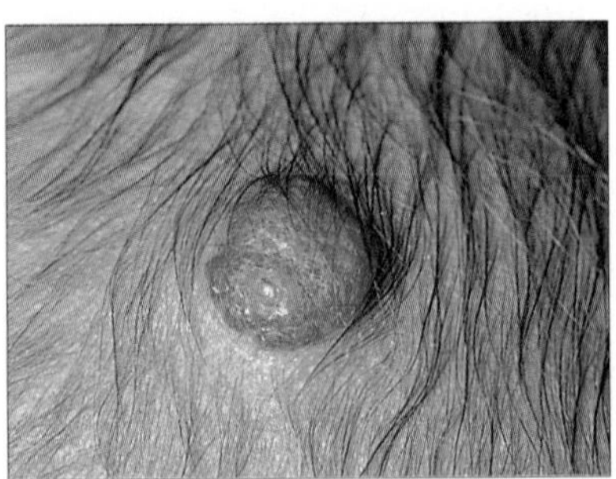

Strawberry naevus on the scalp
This red swelling, known as a strawberry naevus, is a common birthmark that usually disappears by the age of 5.

PIGMENTED NAEVI This group of birthmarks includes Mongolian blue spots and moles. Mongolian blue spots are irregular, bluish areas on the skin. They are commonly seen at birth over the backs and buttocks of black and Asian babies and may be mistaken for bruises. The spots usually disappear by the time the child is 10 years of age.

A mole is a permanent, raised, dark-brown patch on the skin. The presence of a mole at birth is very unusual. In rare cases, such birthmarks may become cancerous in later life.

WHAT MIGHT BE DONE?

Most birthmarks fade as the baby grows. However, a strawberry naevus on the eyelid is usually treated within a few weeks of birth before it can enlarge and affect the baby's vision. Corticosteroids (p.930) may be given orally or injected into the naevus to shrink it, or it may be removed with laser treatment (p.951). Permanent birthmarks, such as port-wine stains, can also be treated with laser surgery, usually during infancy to minimize scarring. All moles should be checked for changes in size, shape, and colour. If moles cause concern, they can be removed by surgery. Treatment for permanent birthmarks usually provides good cosmetic results.

(WWW) ONLINE SITES: p.1028, p.1036

Cradle cap

A thick, scaly rash that appears on the scalp during the first months of life

 AGE Occurs between the ages of 1 month and 1 year

 GENDER GENETICS LIFESTYLE Not significant factors

Babies with cradle cap have reddened skin and thick, yellowish scales on the scalp. Scaly areas may also appear on the baby's forehead and eyebrows and behind the ears. The cause of the condition is unknown. Although cradle cap can be unsightly, it is harmless. Rarely, the rash may become inflamed or infected by bacteria (*see* IMPETIGO, p.351) or fungi (*see* CANDIDIASIS, p.309).

WHAT MIGHT BE DONE?

Cradle cap eventually disappears on its own without any treatment. However, washing your baby's hair and scalp regularly will help to prevent scale build-up. You can also massage baby oil into your baby's scalp at night and then brush out the softened scales in the morning.

You should consult your doctor if these measures are not effective or the rash becomes inflamed or infected. If there is no inflammation or infection, a lotion may be prescribed to dissolve the scales, but such products can cause skin irritation and should be used with care. An infected rash may be treated with topical antibiotics or antifungal drugs (*see* PREPARATIONS FOR SKIN INFECTIONS AND INFESTATIONS, p.892) and an inflamed rash with topical corticosteroids (p.892). The condition should start to improve within a few weeks of treatment but may take longer to disappear.

(WWW) ONLINE SITES: p.1028

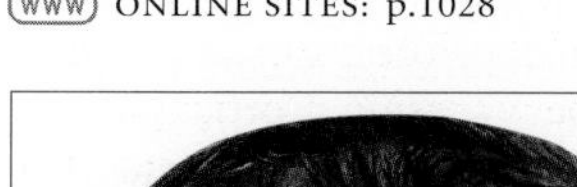

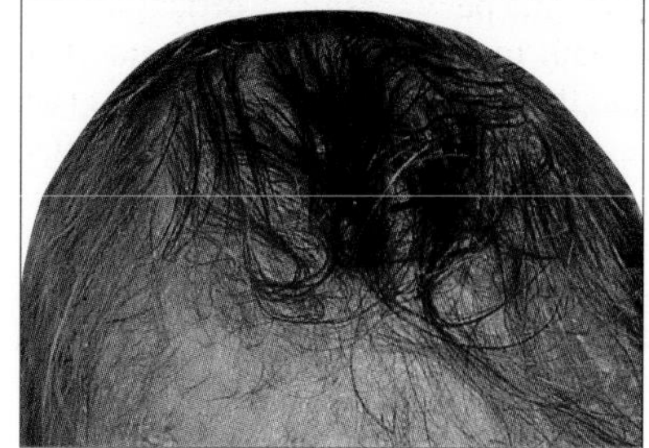

Cradle cap
The reddened skin and thick patches of yellowish scales on top of this baby's head are typical of cradle cap.

Nappy rash

A red rash in the area covered by a nappy, caused by irritation or infection

 AGE May affect babies from birth until they stop wearing nappies

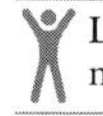 LIFESTYLE Poor hygiene and infrequent nappy changes increase the risk

GENDER GENETICS Not significant factors

Nearly all babies are affected by nappy rash at some time. The rash causes inflammation and soreness in the area of skin covered by a nappy, and the discomfort can make a baby irritable.

WHAT ARE THE CAUSES?

Nappy rash is most commonly caused by urine or faeces irritating the skin. It usually occurs only where the skin and soiled nappy have been in direct contact and does not spread to creases in the baby's skin. The rash is made worse if the baby's nappy is not changed frequently or the nappy area is not cleaned thoroughly. Perfumed skin products and some washing powders used to clean fabric nappies can cause a similar rash.

A fungal infection of the skin such as candidiasis (p.309) or, less commonly, a bacterial infection such as impetigo (p.351) can also cause nappy rash. A rash caused by infection will affect the whole nappy area, including the creases in the baby's skin. Sometimes, a scaly rash similar to cradle cap (left) develops in the baby's nappy area (*see* SEBORRHOEIC DERMATITIS, p.335).

WHAT MIGHT BE DONE?

Your baby's nappy rash will usually clear up within a few days without any medical treatment if you follow the simple self-help measures suggested for managing nappy rash (right).

You should take your baby to the doctor if these self-help measures do not produce an improvement or if you think the nappy rash may be infected. Your baby's doctor will examine the rash and may prescribe topical corticosteroids (p.892) to reduce the inflammation. Oral or topical antibiotics (p.885) may be prescribed to treat a bacterial infection, and topical antifungal drugs may be given to treat candidiasis (*see* PREPARATIONS FOR SKIN INFECTIONS AND INFESTATIONS, p.892).

(SELF-HELP) MANAGING NAPPY RASH

Nappy rash can usually be managed successfully using the measures described below, which also help to prevent recurrence.

- Change your baby's nappies often to prevent skin irritation.
- When changing nappies, clean the nappy area gently with water and allow it to dry thoroughly.
- Use a barrier cream, such as zinc and castor oil cream.
- Avoid perfumed skin products.
- Leave your baby without a nappy as much as possible.
- Wash fabric nappies with a nonbiological washing powder and rinse them thoroughly.
- Use absorbent nappy liners with fabric nappies.

An infected nappy rash should improve with treatment and clear up completely within a week. Nappy rash may recur if preventive self-help measures are not followed regularly throughout the time your child is wearing nappies.

(WWW) ONLINE SITES: p.1028

Eczema in children

Itching and inflammation of the skin, sometimes accompanied by scaling

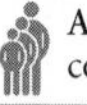 AGE Can occur at any age but most commonly develops under 18 months

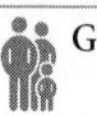 GENETICS Sometimes runs in families

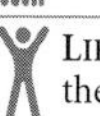 LIFESTYLE Exposure to irritants aggravates the condition

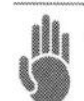 GENDER Not a significant factor

Eczema affects up to 1 in 5 children under school age in the UK. The condition may last for many years but usually disappears in late childhood. A child with eczema has red, inflamed, itchy skin that may make him or her irritable.

WHAT ARE THE CAUSES?

The cause of eczema in children is not fully understood, but an allergic reaction to something in the child's diet or environment is often a factor. Common allergens (substances that provoke an allergic reaction) include cows' milk (*see*

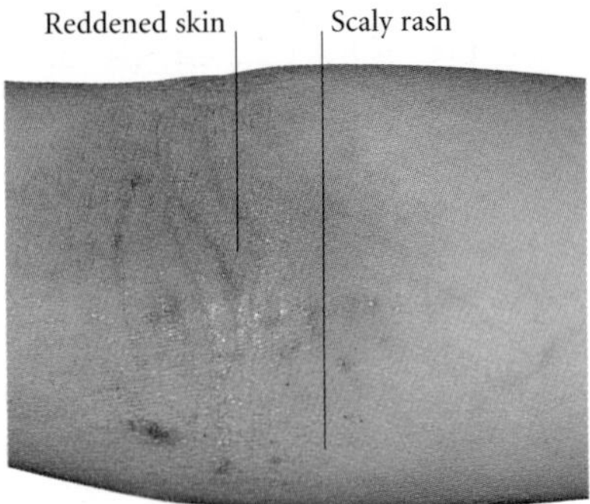

Eczema in children
A red, scaly eczema rash is seen here on the inside of a child's elbow. The inflamed skin is often very itchy and uncomfortable.

COWS' MILK PROTEIN ALLERGY, p.864), soya, wheat, and eggs (*see* FOOD ALLERGY, p.467). Affected children are also susceptible to allergic conditions such as hay fever (*see* ALLERGIC RHINITIS, p.466) and asthma (*see* ASTHMA IN CHILDREN, p.839). Close relatives sometimes have the same allergic disorders, suggesting that a genetic factor is involved.

WHAT ARE THE SYMPTOMS?

The symptoms of eczema vary in severity and usually affect particular areas of the body. Symptoms may include:

- Red, scaly rash.
- Intense itching.
- Gradual thickening of the skin.

In babies, the rash of eczema tends to occur on the face and neck and then on the knees and elbows as the children begin to crawl. In older children, the rash usually appears on the insides of the elbows and wrists and on the backs of the knees. The intense itching causes children to scratch the rash, which may break the skin and lead to bacterial infection. If an infection does occur, the inflammation becomes more severe, and weeping blisters may develop.

A rare but serious complication of eczema is eczema herpeticum, which occurs if a child with eczema is also infected with a type of herpes simplex virus (*see* HERPES SIMPLEX INFECTIONS, p.291). Eczema herpeticum produces a widespread rash with blisters and fever.

HOW IS IT DIAGNOSED?

Your child's doctor will probably diagnose eczema from the inflamed, itchy rash. In some cases, he or she may arrange for a blood test and a skin prick test (p.468) to try to identify a specific food or substance to which your child is allergic. The doctor may also take swabs of the eczema rash to check for signs of bacterial infection.

WHAT IS THE TREATMENT?

Parents play a major part in treating children with eczema, mostly by preventing the affected skin from becoming dry (*see* MANAGING ECZEMA IN CHILDREN, below). Your child's doctor will advise you on day-to-day care and how to moisturize your child's skin with unperfumed emollients, such as bath oils and creams (*see* EMOLLIENTS AND BARRIER PREPARATIONS, p.890). He or she may prescribe a topical corticosteroid (p.892) to reduce inflammation and oral antibiotics (p.885) or antibiotic creams (*see* PREPARATIONS FOR SKIN INFECTIONS AND INFESTATIONS, p.892) if the rash is infected. Your child may also be prescribed an oral antihistamine (p.906) to take at night, which helps to reduce itching and also acts as a sedative.

In very rare cases, a child with severe eczema may be admitted to hospital. Treatment usually consists of applying a corticosteroid cream to the inflamed rash and wrapping the affected areas in bandages soaked in emollient cream.

If your child develops eczema herpeticum, he or she will be admitted to hospital and treated with intravenous antiviral drugs (p.886).

If the cause of eczema is found to be related to something your child eats, elimination of that food from the diet should improve the eczema. However, you should only give your child a special diet under medical supervision. In babies, breast-feeding can help to protect against future food allergies.

Since eczema is a long-term disorder with no reliable cure, you may wish to try alternative treatments such as evening primrose oil or Chinese herbs. These should be discussed with your doctor, who may be able to advise you on reliable sources and caution you against purchasing treatments that may have serious side effects.

> **SELF-HELP MANAGING ECZEMA IN CHILDREN**
>
> Parents play an important role in managing eczema in their children, and the following measures may help to control symptoms and to keep your child comfortable.
>
> - Avoid perfumed skin products.
> - Wash your child with emollient cream instead of soap.
> - Bathe your child at least once a day using moisturizing bath oil.
> - After washing, moisturize your child's skin with a chilled emollient cream.
> - Use prescribed corticosteroid ointments regularly on the affected areas of skin.
> - If your child scratches, make sure his or her fingernails are cut short and he or she wears cotton mittens at night.

WHAT IS THE PROGNOSIS?

Eczema may last throughout childhood. Although there is no reliable cure, the symptoms of the condition can usually be controlled. Eczema usually disappears by adolescence without leaving scars, but in a few cases the rash continues to flare up (*see* ATOPIC ECZEMA, p.334). About half of all affected children develop another allergic disorder later in life.

(WWW) ONLINE SITES: p.1028, p.1036

Roseola infantum

A viral infection that causes a high fever followed by a rash of tiny pink spots

AGE Most common between the ages of 6 months and 2 years

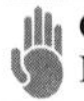
GENDER GENETICS LIFESTYLE Not significant factors

Roseola infantum is a common illness in early childhood that affects about 3 in 10 children in the UK. The infection most commonly occurs in spring and autumn and is caused by strains of the herpes virus that are spread by close contact with other children. One attack of the infection gives lifelong immunity.

WHAT ARE THE SYMPTOMS?

The symptoms of roseola infantum develop in two stages. The first symptoms appear 5–15 days after infection and develop rapidly over a few hours. They include some or all of the following:

- High fever.
- Mild diarrhoea.
- Dry cough.

- Swollen lymph nodes in the neck.
- Earache.

In some children, the high fever causes febrile convulsions (p.849). After about 4 days, the fever subsides and tiny pink spots appear on the face and trunk. This rash usually disappears a few days later.

WHAT MIGHT BE DONE?

Roseola infantum does not require specific treatment, and your child will feel better as soon as his or her temperature drops and the spots appear. You should contact the doctor at once if the self-help measures for bringing down a fever (p.289) are not effective, if a baby under 6 months old is feverish, if your child has a febrile convulsion, or if he or she seems ill even after the fever has been lowered.

(WWW) ONLINE SITES: p.1028, p.1033

Hand, foot, and mouth disease

A common viral infection that causes small blisters in the mouth and blisters on the hands and feet

 AGE More common in children under the age of 4

 GENDER GENETICS LIFESTYLE Not significant factors

Hand, foot, and mouth disease is a common childhood infection that occurs in epidemics during the summer and early autumn. The infection is caused by the coxsackie virus and lasts a few days.

WHAT ARE THE SYMPTOMS?

The symptoms develop 3–5 days after infection and may include:

- Blisters inside the mouth that may develop into painful ulcers.
- Blisters on the hands and feet that typically develop 1–2 days after those in the mouth and disappear spontaneously after 3–4 days.
- Fever.

Children often seem well but may not want to eat if mouth ulcers develop.

WHAT MIGHT BE DONE?

There is no specific treatment for hand, foot, and mouth disease, but self-help measures should relieve the symptoms. You should make sure that your child drinks plenty of fluid, such as chilled milk. However, fruit juices should be avoided because they are acidic and can aggravate mouth ulcers. Liquid paracetamol (*see* PAINKILLERS, p.912) will help in bringing down a fever (p.289) and reduce discomfort. If your child is reluctant to drink, watch for signs of dehydration, such as abnormal drowsiness, and consult your child's doctor immediately if you become concerned.

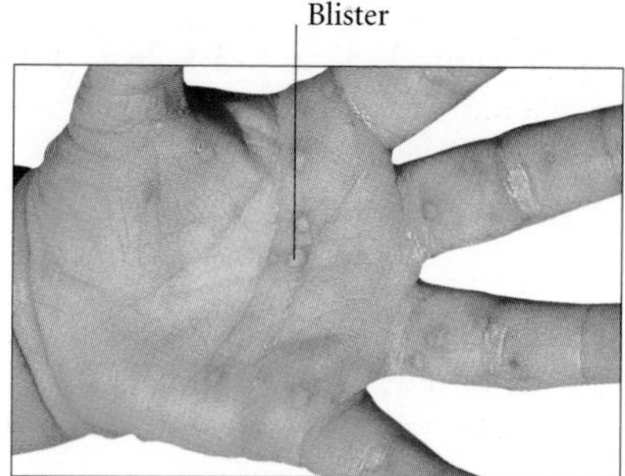

Hand, foot, and mouth disease
The small blisters on this child's hand are characteristic of the viral infection hand, foot, and mouth disease.

You should also consult a doctor if your child has severe symptoms of hand, foot, and mouth infection. Your child's doctor may prescribe a medicated mouthwash to soothe the ulcers and prevent bacterial infection. Blisters clear up in a few days, but ulcers can persist for up to 4 weeks.

(WWW) ONLINE SITES: p.1028, p.1033

Head lice

Infestation of tiny, wingless insects on the scalp that may cause intense itching

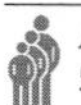 AGE Most common between the ages of 5 and 11

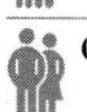 GENDER More common in girls

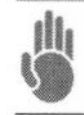 GENETICS LIFESTYLE Not significant factors

Infestation with head lice is common among young schoolchildren, particularly girls, between the ages of 5 and 11 years. These tiny, almost transparent insects are transmitted by close contact and by sharing combs and hats. Head lice prefer clean hair and skin and are not a result of poor hygiene.

The insects live by sucking blood from the scalp and may be seen as they fall off a child's head when the hair is washed or combed. The eggs, known as nits, are visible as tiny white specks attached to the base of the hairs. An infestation of head lice usually causes intense itching, but there may be no other obvious symptoms.

WHAT CAN I DO?

If you think that your child has head lice, check for eggs at the bases of hairs and comb the hair over a piece of white paper to see if adult lice fall out. If head lice are present, you should check the rest of the family for infestation and alert your child's school.

You can normally treat head lice at home using over-the-counter lotions or shampoos containing an insecticide (*see* PREPARATIONS FOR SKIN INFECTIONS AND INFESTATIONS, p.892). You should use the type that is currently recommended because head lice develop resistance to insecticides. If your child is under the age of 2 or has allergies or asthma, discuss treatment with the doctor. To avoid reinfestation, wash bedlinen and combs in very hot water and discourage your child from sharing combs and hats.

(WWW) ONLINE SITES: p.1028

(SELF-HELP) TREATING HEAD LICE

Infestations of head lice can be treated with an over-the-counter lotion or shampoo, and the lice can then be removed with a nit comb. Hair conditioner may make it easier for you to comb out the dead lice and eggs, especially if your child's hair is long, thick, or curly. All combs and towels should be washed in very hot water after use to prevent reinfestation.

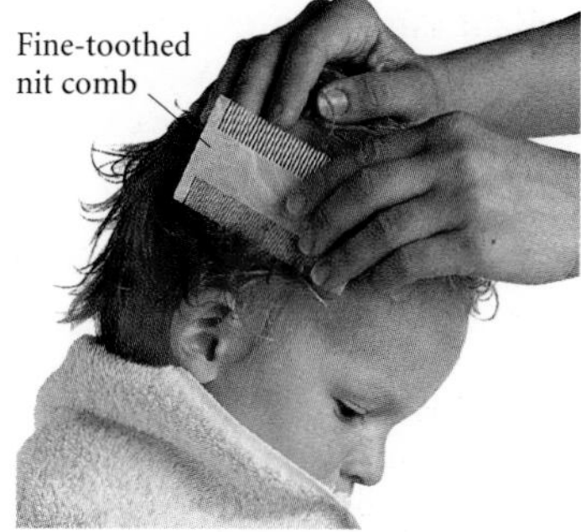

Removing head lice
After applying a recommended lotion or shampoo, carefully comb your child's hair with a fine-toothed nit comb to remove the dead lice and eggs.

MUSCULOSKELETAL DISORDERS

In addition to everyday injuries and fractures, most bone, muscle, and joint problems in children fall into two broad categories: problems that are present at birth and those associated with the changes that occur during the growth spurt of puberty. Early treatment of most of these conditions improves the likelihood of recovery and reduces the risk of complications.

This section begins with articles on three conditions that may be present at birth: congenital hip dysplasia, clubfoot, and achondroplasia, which is caused by an abnormal gene. These are followed by conditions that may develop later in childhood and around puberty. These conditions include two that affect the femur (thighbone), Perthes' disease and slipped femoral epiphysis, and Osgood–Schlatter disease, which causes inflammation of the tibia (shinbone). Minor foot and leg problems, such as flat feet and bow legs, which are often part of normal development, are also covered. The final article discusses the joint disorder juvenile chronic arthritis. Musculoskeletal disorders that affect adults in addition to children are included in the main section on the musculoskeletal system (pp.362–395).

KEY ANATOMY

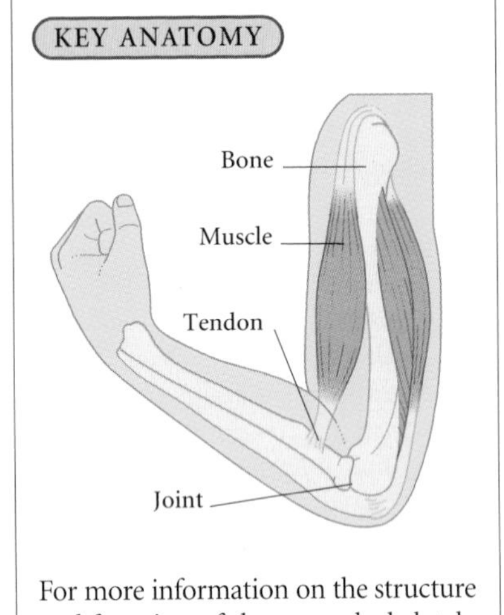

For more information on the structure and function of the musculoskeletal system, *see* pp.362–367.

Congenital hip dysplasia

Problems affecting the hip joint, ranging from mild looseness to dislocation

 AGE Present at birth

 GENDER Six times more common in girls

 GENETICS Sometimes runs in families

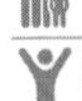 LIFESTYLE Rarely persists in babies who are carried astride the mother's back

Congenital hip dysplasia is a term that covers a range of problems with the hip joint in the newborn. In mild cases, the hip joint moves excessively when manipulated. In moderate cases, the head of the femur (thighbone) slips out of the hip socket when manipulated but can be eased back in. In severe cases, the dislocation is permanent, and the head of the femur lies outside the hip socket.

Mild cases are the result of loose ligaments, but in more severe cases the dislocation is related to abnormal development of the hip socket. Hip dysplasia occurs more often in the left hip and rarely affects both hips. About 1 in 250 babies is affected. Regularly carrying a baby astride the mother's back usually corrects mild dysplasia.

Congenital hip dysplasia is more common in girls and in babies who are born in the breech position. It may also be associated with clubfoot (opposite page).

The cause of hip dysplasia is not fully understood. In about 1 in 5 babies, there is a family history of hip dysplasia, suggesting a genetic factor. The condition may also be due to the effect of maternal hormones that relax the mother's own ligaments in preparation for labour.

WHAT ARE THE SYMPTOMS?

Mild forms of congenital hip dysplasia may have no symptoms. In severe cases, the symptoms may include:

- Asymmetrical creases in the skin on the backs of the baby's legs.
- Inability to turn the affected leg out fully at the hip.
- Shorter appearance of the affected leg.
- Limping when older.

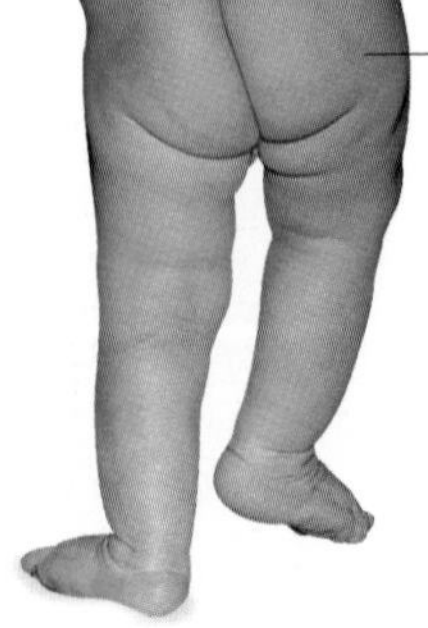

Congenital hip dysplasia
This infant has a dislocated right hip. The right leg appears shorter than the left and cannot be fully straightened.

If congenital hip dysplasia is not corrected early, it may lead to permanent deformity and the early onset of the joint disorder osteoarthritis (p.374).

WHAT MIGHT BE DONE?

The doctor will check your baby's hips for stability and range of movement shortly after birth and then regularly at routine checkups until your child is walking normally. If your doctor suspects congenital hip dysplasia, he or she may arrange ultrasound scanning (p.250) to confirm the diagnosis.

The less severe forms of congenital hip dysplasia often correct themselves during the first 3 weeks of life. However, if the problem persists, prompt treatment is essential because the head of the femur must be positioned correctly if the socket is to develop normally. In a very young baby, the hip joint may be positioned in a harness for 8–12 weeks to hold the head of the femur in the hip. In an older baby, the hip may need holding in a cast for up to 6 months to correct the problem. If treatment is unsuccessful, surgery may be necessary to correct the hip dysplasia.

If congenital hip dysplasia is diagnosed early and treated immediately, most babies develop normal hip joints and there is no permanent damage.

(WWW) ONLINE SITES: p.1028, p.1035

Clubfoot

A condition, also known as talipes, in which a baby is born with one or both feet twisted out of shape or position

 AGE Present at birth

 GENETICS Sometimes runs in families

 GENDER Risk factors depend on the type

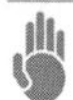 LIFESTYLE Not a significant factor

Babies are often born with their feet in awkward positions (*see* MINOR LEG AND FOOT PROBLEMS, p.834). In severe cases, the defect is known as clubfoot. There are two types of clubfoot: positional clubfoot, in which the twisted foot is flexible and can be manipulated into a normal position, and structural clubfoot, in which the deformity is rigid.

In positional clubfoot, the foot is a normal size but appears twisted, possibly due to compression in the uterus. Most cases are mild and correct themselves. Structural clubfoot occurs in about 1 in 700 babies and is more serious. In this disorder, the foot turns downwards and inwards and is usually abnormally small in size. In about half of these babies, both feet are affected. Structural clubfoot may be related to low levels of fluid in the uterus during pregnancy or may be caused by an underlying condition such as spina bifida (*see* NEURAL TUBE DEFECTS, p.844), and it is sometimes associated with congenital hip dysplasia (opposite page). Structural clubfoot is twice as common in boys and can run in families, suggesting a genetic factor.

WHAT MIGHT BE DONE?

Clubfoot is usually diagnosed during a routine examination after birth. Positional clubfoot may not need treatment, but physiotherapy (p.961) may help to straighten the foot, and a cast may be used to move the foot into position. A normal position can usually be achieved within 3 months. Structural clubfoot requires physiotherapy and a cast for a long period. In 6 out of 10 cases, this treatment is successful. If not, surgery may be needed at the age of 6–9 months. Surgery is usually successful, enabling most children to walk normally.

(WWW) ONLINE SITES: p.1028

Achondroplasia

Defective bone growth due to an abnormal gene, causing short stature

 AGE Present at birth

 GENETICS Due to an abnormal gene

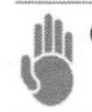 GENDER LIFESTYLE Not significant factors

Achondroplasia causes abnormal body proportions and short stature. The disorder affects the bones of the limbs and base of the skull and prevents normal growth. As a result, although the child's trunk and head grow at a near normal rate, the arms and legs are disproportionately short and the forehead often protrudes. However, the child's intelligence is not usually affected. In the UK, about 2,000 people are affected.

Achondroplasia is caused by an abnormal gene inherited in an autosomal dominant manner (*see* GENE DISORDERS, p.271). Usually, the gene abnormality occurs spontaneously, and there is no family history of the condition. In a few cases, there is a family history of the disorder. People with achondroplasia have a 1 in 2 chance of passing the disorder on to a child, and they may wish to have genetic counselling (p.272) if they are planning a pregnancy.

WHAT ARE THE SYMPTOMS?

Symptoms such as short, bowed legs and a prominent forehead are usually apparent at birth. Other symptoms develop as the baby grows and include:

- Short stature.
- Short, broad hands and feet.
- Forward curve to the lower spine (*see* KYPHOSIS AND LORDOSIS, p.371).
- Waddling gait.

Psychological difficulties may develop when a child starts to realize that other children are different. Rarely, a baby also has hydrocephalus (p.845), in which there is excess fluid around the brain.

WHAT MIGHT BE DONE?

Achondroplasia is sometimes diagnosed during routine ultrasound scanning in pregnancy (p.793) at about 18–20 weeks, but more often the condition is diagnosed at birth. The doctor may arrange for X-rays (p.244) to be taken to confirm the diagnosis, and CT scanning (p.247) or MRI scanning (p.248) may be carried out to look at the baby's head.

There is no cure for achondroplasia, and treatment is rarely needed. The legs can be lengthened slightly by surgery, but many children prefer their natural height. A baby with hydrocephalus may need an operation to drain excess fluid from the brain (*see* SHUNT FOR HYDROCEPHALUS, p.845). Affected children usually have a normal life expectancy, but may have spinal problems as adults.

(WWW) ONLINE SITES: p.1028, p.1032

Perthes' disease

Gradual breaking down and re-forming of the head of the femur (thighbone)

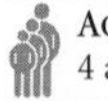 AGE Most common between the ages of 4 and 8

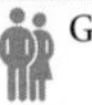 GENDER Five times more common in boys

 GENETICS LIFESTYLE Not significant factors

Perthes' disease is a rare condition in which the head of the femur (thighbone) softens and breaks down, and is gradually replaced by new bone over 18 months to 2 years. The disease causes pain in the hip and sometimes in the knee. An affected child may walk with a limp and have restricted movement of the hip. Perthes' disease occurs mainly in boys between the ages of 4 and 8 and is more severe in older children. The disease affects 1 in 20,000 children. Of these, 1 in 10 has the disease in both hips.

The cause of Perthes' disease is not known. The condition requires treatment, and you should consult your doctor if your child develops a limp or has a painful hip or knee.

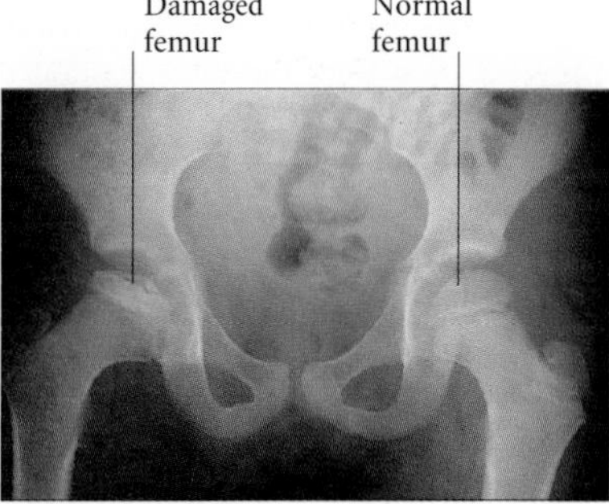

Perthes' disease
The head of the femur (thighbone) seen on the left in this X-ray is flattened compared to the other, as a result of Perthes' disease.

WHAT MIGHT BE DONE?

The doctor will examine your child and will probably arrange for X-rays (p.244) of the hip. MRI scanning (p.248) and radionuclide scanning (p.251) of the hip may also be performed.

Initial treatment is bed rest until the pain subsides. In younger children, bed rest may be sufficient, but sometimes traction is used to place the femur under tension and hold it in the correct position. In more severe cases, casts or braces may be used to protect the hip joint and hold the head of the femur securely in the hip socket while the bone re-forms. Occasionally, surgery is required. Your child's progress will be monitored by X-rays every few months while the head of the femur recovers. He or she will probably have physiotherapy (p.961) to encourage mobility of the joint during healing.

About 3 in 10 of those affected develop the joint condition osteoarthritis (p.374) later in life. In general, a complete recovery is more likely in a child under the age of 8 years.

(WWW) ONLINE SITES: p.1028, p.1035

Slipped femoral epiphysis

Displacement of the head of the femur (thighbone) at the hip joint

AGE Most common in girls aged 11–13 and boys aged 14–16

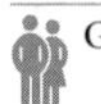
GENDER More common in boys

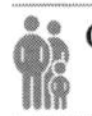
GENETICS Sometimes runs in families

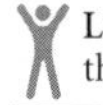
LIFESTYLE Being overweight increases the risk

In children, the epiphysis (the area at the end of a long bone) is separated from the main shaft of the bone by a soft, flexible layer of cartilage where new bone is formed. In the condition known as slipped femoral epiphysis, the epiphysis at the head of the femur (thighbone) becomes displaced. This displacement can happen suddenly as a result of an injury that damages the soft cartilage, or gradually for reasons that are unknown. In about 1 in 5 cases, both hips are affected but usually at different times. Slipped femoral epiphysis occurs in children growing rapidly at puberty. The disorder affects about 3 in 100,000 children in the UK, and overweight children are particularly at risk. Slipped femoral epiphysis can run in families, suggesting a genetic factor.

WHAT ARE THE SYMPTOMS?

Symptoms may appear suddenly but usually develop over several weeks and may include the following:

- Pain in the hip, knee, or thigh.
- Limping with an out-turned foot.
- Restricted hip movement.
- Reluctance and eventually inability to bear weight on the affected leg.

If your child has any of these symptoms, you should contact your doctor within 24 hours.

WHAT MIGHT BE DONE?

If your doctor suspects that the child has slipped femoral epiphysis, he or she will arrange for X-rays (p.244) of the affected hip. If there is displacement, your child will need surgery to fix the epiphysis in place and, sometimes, to strengthen the other hip joint to prevent displacement occurring in both hips. If treated promptly, most children recover completely and the condition is unlikely to recur. Rarely, osteoarthritis (p.374) develops later in life.

(WWW) ONLINE SITES: p.1028, p.1035

Osgood–Schlatter disease

Inflammation of the front of the tibia (shinbone) below the knee

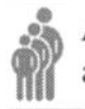
AGE Most common between the ages of 10 and 14

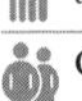
GENDER Much more common in boys

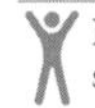
LIFESTYLE Strenuous activity aggravates the symptoms

GENETICS Not a significant factor

In Osgood–Schlatter disease, fragments of cartilage become loose at the front of the tibia (shinbone) just below the knee at the point where a large tendon is attached. The condition is caused by repetitive strong pulls on the tendon that attaches the muscle at the front of the thigh to the tibia. The symptoms include tenderness, swelling, and pain in the affected area and appear slowly over several weeks or months. Physical exercise tends to make the symptoms worse. Osgood–Schlatter disease is most common in boys aged 10–14 who take regular strenuous exercise. The disease usually occurs in only one leg, but in about 1 in 5 cases both legs are affected.

If your doctor suspects that the child has Osgood–Schlatter disease, he or she may arrange for X-rays (p.244) of the affected area to confirm the diagnosis. In most cases, no treatment is required apart from rest and painkillers (p.912) to ease the discomfort. In rare cases, if the condition persists, the affected knee may be immobilized in a cast for 6–8 weeks. Treatment is always successful, and the disorder never recurs in later life. Severely affected children may be advised to avoid strenuous exercise until they are over the age of 14 and the musculoskeletal system has matured.

(WWW) ONLINE SITES: p.1028, p.1035

Minor leg and foot problems

Variations in the position and shape of the feet and legs during childhood

GENETICS Sometimes runs in families

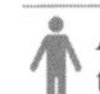
AGE LIFESTYLE Risk factors depend on the type

GENDER Not a significant factor

When a young child stands and walks, the position of the legs or feet may look odd or awkward. Different minor foot problems are common at different ages. However, these problems rarely interfere with walking or require treatment. Specific minor problems with the legs and feet can run in families, suggesting that a genetic factor may be involved.

WHAT ARE THE TYPES?

Minor leg and foot problems include in-toeing and out-toeing, bow legs and knock-knees, and flat feet.

IN-TOEING AND OUT-TOEING The condition known as in-toeing, in which the feet point inwards, is common and occurs at any time from infancy to the age of 8. Out-toeing, in which the feet point away from each other, is less common but may occur from 6 months.

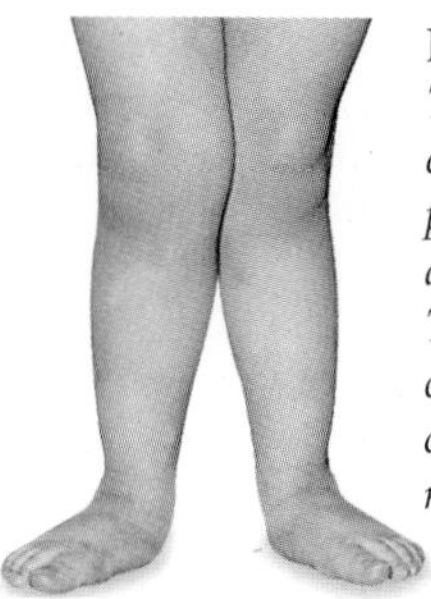

Knock-knees
This child's legs curve inwards, a position known as knock-knees. The condition is common in young children and rarely needs treatment.

BOW LEGS AND KNOCK-KNEES If both tibias (shinbones) curve outwards, a child's knees cannot touch when he or she stands with the feet together. This condition, known as bow legs, is normal until a child is about 3 years of age. Severe bowing is uncommon but may be caused by a deficiency of vitamin D (*see* OSTEOMALACIA AND RICKETS, p.370). In knock-knees, the child's legs curve in at the knees, so that the feet are wide apart even when the knees are touching. Knock-knees is common in children between the ages of 3 and 7 years.

FLAT FEET Most children have flat feet until the arch develops between 2 and 3 years of age. Children also have a pad of fat beneath the foot that accentuates the flat-footed appearance. However, some children have persistent flat feet.

WHAT MIGHT BE DONE?

Your child's legs and feet will be examined regularly during routine medical checkups. However, you should consult your doctor if you are worried by the appearance of your child's legs or feet or if your child has difficulty in walking, has a limp, or complains of pain.

Most children with minor leg and foot problems do not need treatment because walking is rarely affected and the problems disappear naturally as a child grows up. Out-toeing disappears first, usually within a year of a child starting to walk. In-toeing and bow legs have usually disappeared by the age of 3–4 years and knock-knees by the age of 11–12. Persistent flat feet do not often need treatment unless they cause pain.

Your doctor may recommend physiotherapy (p.961) if your child experiences difficulty in walking or the shape of his or her legs is abnormal. Rarely, if your child's legs or feet are seriously affected, he or she may need to have orthopaedic surgery to correct the problem.

Juvenile chronic arthritis

Persistent inflammation of one or more joints that occurs only in childhood

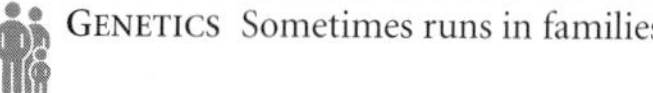
GENETICS Sometimes runs in families

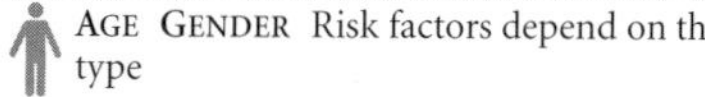
AGE GENDER Risk factors depend on the type

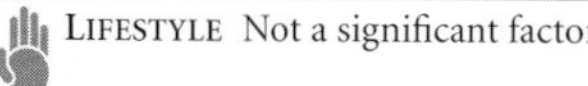
LIFESTYLE Not a significant factor

Children may be affected by the same types of arthritis (p.374) as adults, but juvenile chronic arthritis (JCA) is found only in children. In the UK, about 1 child in 1,000 is affected. The condition is the result of an abnormal response of the body's immune system, leading to inflammation, swelling, and pain in the lining of an affected joint. Although the cause is not known, juvenile chronic arthritis sometimes runs in families, which suggests a genetic factor may be involved. In mild cases, the child is still able to carry out normal activities. In severe cases, there may be joint deformities and reduced mobility.

WHAT ARE THE TYPES?

Juvenile chronic arthritis is divided into three types according to the number of joints affected by the disease and the specific symptoms involved.

POLYARTICULAR ARTHRITIS This type affects more girls than boys and can occur at any age. Symptoms include inflammation, stiffness, and pain in five or more joints. The joints commonly affected include those in the wrists, fingers, knees, and ankles.

PAUCIARTICULAR ARTHRITIS This is the commonest type of JCA and most frequently affects girls under school age. Symptoms include inflammation, stiffness, and pain in four or fewer joints, and girls are at high risk of developing the eye disorder uveitis (p.574). The joints in the knees, ankles, and wrists are commonly involved.

SYSTEMIC ARTHRITIS Also known as Still's disease, this type of JCA affects boys and girls equally. The disorder occurs at any age during childhood but mostly commonly around the age of 2 years. Any number of joints may be affected by pain, swelling, and stiffness. The other symptoms include fever, swollen glands, and a blotchy rash. Some children recover totally, but others develop polyarticular JCA.

WHAT MIGHT BE DONE?

If the doctor suspects that your child has a type of juvenile chronic arthritis, he or she may arrange for X-rays (p.244) of the affected joints and blood tests to look for particular antibodies associated with the condition.

The goal of treatment is to reduce inflammation, minimize damage to the joints, and relieve pain. If your child is mildly affected, he or she may only need to take nonsteroidal anti-inflammatory drugs (p.894) to reduce inflammation and relieve pain. In more severe cases, your child may be prescribed oral corticosteroids (p.930), or he or she may be treated with locally acting corticosteroids (p.895) that are injected into the affected joints. Sometimes, the inflammation can be reduced by using antirheumatic drugs (p.895), such as methotrexate and sulfasalazine.

Other treatments for JCA include physiotherapy (p.961), to help to maintain joint mobility, and occupational therapy (p.962). Splints may be used for support and to help to prevent deformity. Special devices are also available and may help with daily activities such as dressing. If damage to the joints is severe and has caused deformity, joint replacement (p.377) may be necessary.

Juvenile chronic arthritis can clear up within a few years, but severely affected children may be left with deformed joints, and some may have arthritis that persists into in adult life.

(WWW) ONLINE SITES: p.1027, p.1028

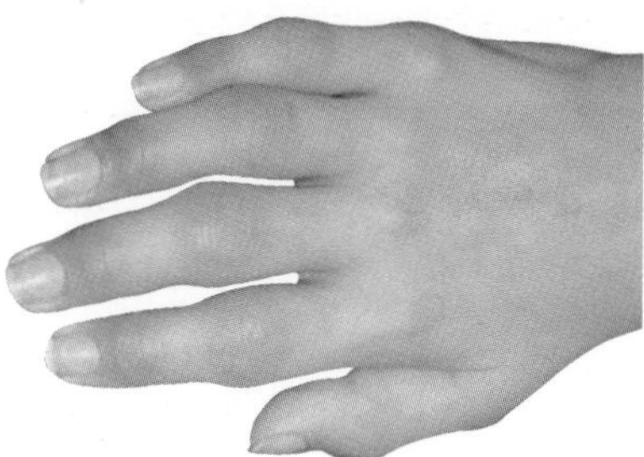

Juvenile chronic arthritis
The joints of this young child's hand are swollen due to the inflammatory disorder polyarticular arthritis.

DISORDERS OF THE CARDIOVASCULAR AND RESPIRATORY SYSTEMS

Disorders of the heart and lungs are relatively common in children. The heart is affected by birth defects more than any other organ, and all children have recurrent bacterial and viral infections of the throat and lungs. Usually these infections are mild and play a role in developing a healthy immune system.

The first articles in this section cover cardiovascular disorders, such as congenital heart disease. Many heart abnormalities correct themselves without medical intervention as a child grows. Many of the more serious heart defects can now be treated successfully because of recent advances in surgical techniques. A rarer disorder that affects the heart in children is Kawasaki disease, which damages the heart and blood vessels. Blood vessels are also damaged in Henoch–Schönlein purpura, which is due to an abnormal response by the immune system. Left untreated, Henoch–Schönlein purpura can eventually cause kidney failure.

The final articles address respiratory disorders, of which asthma is the most common. The incidence of this disorder is increasing for unknown reasons. Respiratory tract infections, such as bronchiolitis, are common in young children. The inflammatory disorder epiglottitis can be dangerous but is now rare in developed countries because of routine immunization of infants against the bacterium responsible for causing the condition, *Haemophilus influenzae* type B.

KEY ANATOMY

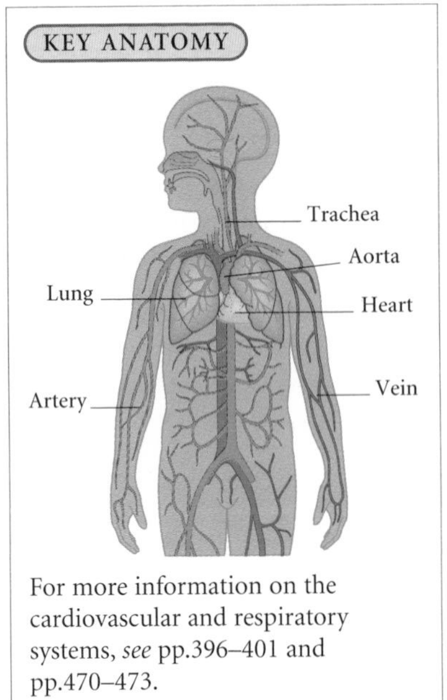

For more information on the cardiovascular and respiratory systems, *see* pp.396–401 and pp.470–473.

Congenital heart disease

One or more defects of the heart that are present at birth

AGE Present at birth

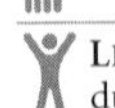
LIFESTYLE Use of certain drugs and alcohol during pregnancy are risk factors

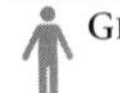
GENETICS Risk factors depend on the type

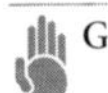
GENDER Not a significant factor

The heart is a complex organ that can develop abnormally in a fetus, leading to defects that affect a baby from birth (congenital heart defects). Congenital heart disease affects about 1 in 100 babies and is one of the most common birth defects. About 2 in 3 of these abnormalities disappear naturally as the baby grows, but more serious defects require complex corrective surgery.

Congenital heart disease commonly causes shortness of breath in affected children, which may inhibit their feeding, growth, and activity.

WHAT ARE THE CAUSES?

In most cases, the cause of congenital heart disease is unknown. However, it can sometimes run in families, suggesting that a genetic factor may be involved. Heart defects at birth may also be associated with genetic disorders, such as Down's syndrome (p.821). Exposure of the fetus to excessive alcohol or drugs such as the anticonvulsant phenytoin increases the risk of congenital heart disease. In early pregnancy, certain infections, such as rubella (p.294), in the mother can lead to fetal heart defects (*see* CONGENITAL INFECTIONS, p.817). More than 1 in 10 babies with congenital heart disease are also found to have a defect elsewhere in the body, commonly in the digestive tract.

WHAT ARE THE TYPES?

Most types of congenital heart disease affect only one part of the heart or one of the major blood vessels, such as the aorta, connected to the heart. Less commonly, several parts of the heart or more than one blood vessel are affected. These multiple heart defects are more serious and can be life-threatening.

SEPTAL DEFECTS The most common type of congenital heart abnormality is a septal defect, also known as a hole in the heart. In this defect, there is a hole in the septum (the inner wall that divides the heart) either between the two lower chambers (ventriculoseptal defect, pictured left) or alternatively between the two upper chambers (atrioseptal defect). In both cases, some oxygen-rich blood passes from the left side to the right side of the heart and is sent back to the lungs instead of going around the body. About 1 in 3 cases of congenital heart disease is due to a ventriculoseptal defect, which is often small and may close naturally. About 1 in 4 cases of congenital heart disease is caused by an atrioseptal defect, which usually produces few symptoms but is likely to require surgical treatment. Both septal defects are common in children with Down's syndrome.

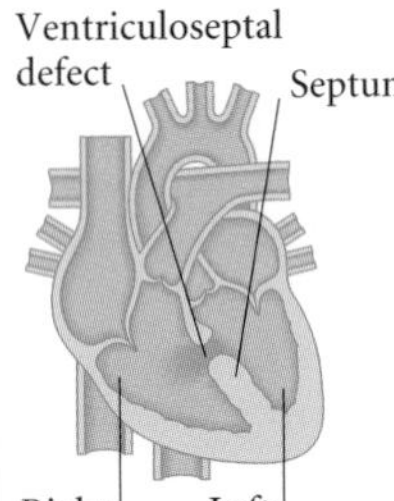

PATENT DUCTUS ARTERIOSUS The ductus arteriosus is a small blood vessel that connects the pulmonary artery to the aorta in the fetus so that blood bypasses the lungs. If this vessel fails to close up soon after birth, normal circulation is prevented. This disorder is often found in premature babies.

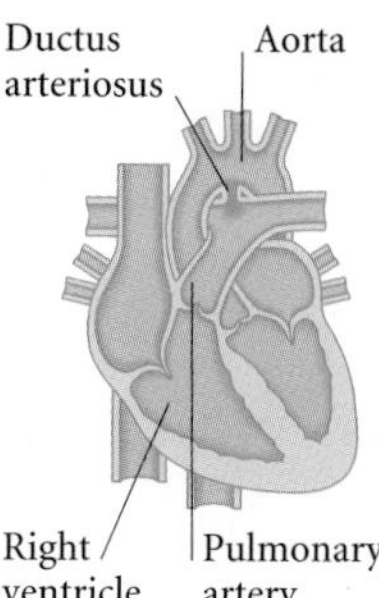

COARCTATION OF THE AORTA In this congenital heart disorder there is a narrowing of an area in the aorta, which restricts the flow of blood to the lower part of the body. As a result, the heart muscle works harder to compensate, and the pressure of blood in the upper part of the body is raised. The disorder requires surgical treatment. Children with coarctation of the aorta may additionally have an abnormality of one or more of the four heart valves.

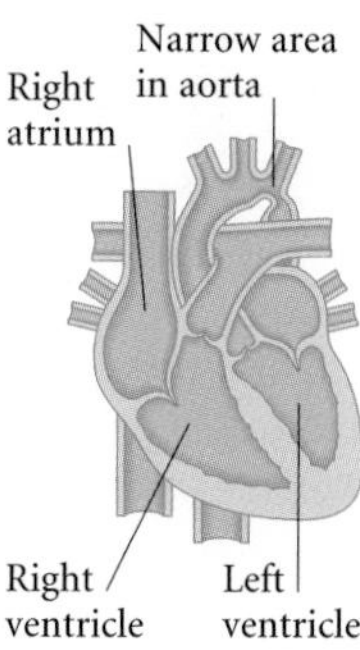

VALVE DEFECTS Any of the four heart valves may develop abnormally. The most common valve disorder is pulmonary stenosis. In this condition, the pulmonary valve, which opens to allow blood to flow from the right ventricle into the pulmonary artery, is narrowed so that blood flow is restricted. Defects of the aortic valve, which opens to allow blood to flow from the left ventricle into the aorta, are less common.

MULTIPLE DEFECTS Sometimes, several heart defects occur together. In addition to placing extra strain on the heart, the defects usually prevent blood from passing through the lungs normally so that blood oxygen levels become very low. Tissues throughout the body may then become oxygen-starved. The most common multiple defect is Fallot's tetralogy, in which four heart abnormalities occur together. These consist of a ventriculoseptal defect, pulmonary stenosis, a displaced aorta, and a thickened right ventricle. Another type of multiple defect is hypoplastic left heart syndrome, in which the chambers and valves on the left side of the heart are underdeveloped. This was once a fatal condition but can now sometimes be treated. A rarer multiple defect involves reversal of the positions of the aorta and the pulmonary artery.

What are the symptoms?

Minor congenital heart defects may not cause symptoms. When symptoms do occur, they vary depending on the severity and type of the heart defect. The symptoms of all types of congenital heart disease may include:

- Shortness of breath, leading to difficulty in feeding.
- Slow weight gain and growth.

Symptoms of severe heart defects may develop suddenly in the first weeks of life. If there are low levels of oxygen in the blood, the tongue and lips may appear bluish in colour. Children with heart defects may be susceptible to chest infections and are at increased risk of infection of the lining of the heart (*see* INFECTIVE ENDOCARDITIS, p.426), especially after surgery or dental treatment. Over a period of several years, congenital heart defects may lead to irreversible damage to the lungs (*see* PULMONARY HYPERTENSION, p.505).

How is it diagnosed?

In some cases, congenital heart disease is diagnosed during routine ultrasound scanning in pregnancy (p.793). Otherwise, defects may be found after birth when symptoms develop or during a routine examination. The doctor may hear a sound (heart murmur) caused by turbulent blood flow while listening to your child's heart. Although many heart murmurs are normal, the doctor is likely to arrange for an ECG (p.406), which monitors the electrical activity of the heart. Your child may also have the imaging technique echocardiography (p.425), which is used to assess the structure and function of the heart.

What is the treatment?

Many heart defects correct themselves or need no treatment. Only about 1 in 3 children requires surgery. Affected children are usually monitored throughout childhood and, if necessary, surgery is performed when the child is older and the operation easier. Rarely, an emergency operation is necessary to save a young baby's life. A heart transplant (p.427) is now a possibility for children who have multiple heart defects. Chest infections need to be treated promptly, and, if the child has dental treatment or surgery, antibiotics (p.885) are necessary to prevent infection of the lining of the heart. Some children will need drugs, such as diuretics (p.902), to control the symptoms of a heart defect.

What is the prognosis?

The outlook depends on the type of heart defect and its severity. Septal defects either close naturally or are corrected surgically. As a result of surgical advances over the last 20 years, even very severe defects can often be corrected, and many severely affected children are leading normal, active lives.

(WWW) ONLINE SITES: p.1027, p.1028, p.1032

Kawasaki disease

A prolonged fever during which the heart and blood vessels may be damaged

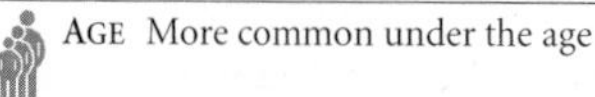
AGE More common under the age of 5

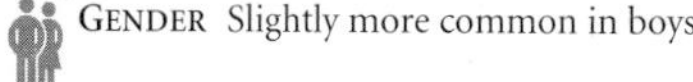
GENDER Slightly more common in boys

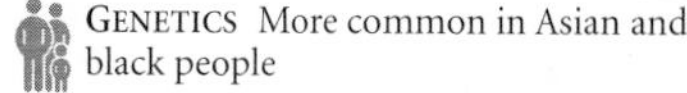
GENETICS More common in Asian and black people

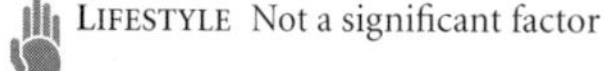
LIFESTYLE Not a significant factor

First observed in Japan in the 1960s, Kawasaki disease is a rare condition in which a prolonged fever is associated with damage to the heart and blood vessels. In the UK, fewer than 1 in every 25,000 children under the age of 5 are affected each year. The disorder is now being diagnosed more often in Western countries, and it occurs more frequently in Asian and black people. Heart damage occurs in about 1 in 5 of all cases of Kawasaki disease. Early diagnosis is very important because the condition can become life-threatening.

The cause of Kawasaki disease is not known, although it is suspected that a viral or bacterial infection may be involved. However, despite a great deal of research, there is as yet no conclusive evidence to confirm this theory.

What are the symptoms?

The first symptoms develop over about 2 weeks and may include:

- Prolonged, constant fever that lasts more than 5 days.
- Sore or itchy, red eyes, possibly associated with a watery discharge (*see* CONJUNCTIVITIS, p.570).
- Cracked, painful, and swollen lips.
- Sore throat.
- Swollen glands in the neck, under the arms, and in the groin.

After about a week of fever, the following symptoms may develop:

- Reddening of the palms of the hands and soles of the feet, usually along with peeling skin on the tips of the fingers and toes.
- Blotchy pink rash over the entire body.

Kawasaki disease may lead to serious complications. For example, balloon-like swellings, called aneurysms, can develop in the walls of the coronary arteries, which supply the heart muscle. Inflammation of the heart muscle (*see* MYOCARDITIS, p.426) may also occur. Kawasaki disease can also damage blood vessels throughout the body.

What might be done?

Diagnosis of Kawasaki disease can be difficult because the symptoms are very similar to those of minor viral infections, such as the common cold. You should consult a doctor if your child develops a fever that cannot be lowered by taking paracetamol and other simple self-help measures (*see* BRINGING DOWN A FEVER, p.289). If Kawasaki disease is suspected, your child will be admitted to hospital immediately because treatment is most effective if started within 10 days of the onset of the disease. Your child will probably have blood tests to look for evidence of Kawasaki disease. The imaging technique echocardiography (p.425) may also be carried out to look for damage to the heart muscle and coronary blood vessels.

If Kawasaki disease is confirmed, the child will probably be given intravenous immunoglobulin. This substance is a blood product containing antibodies that fight infection. Immunoglobulin also reduces the risk of aneurysms and inflammation of the heart muscle in Kawasaki disease for reasons that are not fully understood. High doses of aspirin are usually prescribed until the fever subsides. Lower doses are then continued over a period of several weeks.

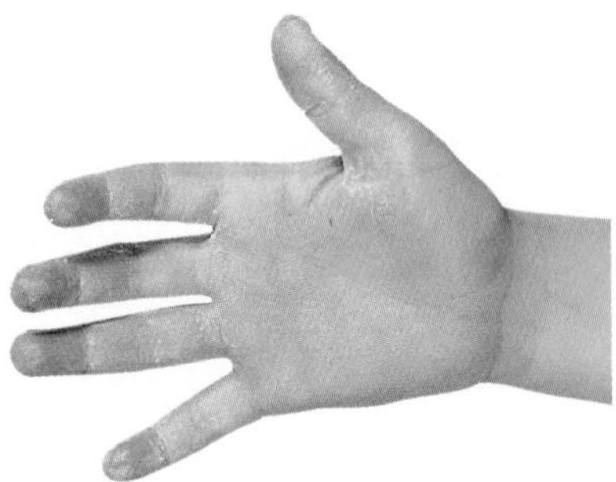

Kawasaki disease
One of the symptoms of the rare disorder Kawasaki disease is reddening of the hands with peeling skin on the tips of the fingers.

What is the prognosis?

Most children who have Kawasaki disease recover completely within 3 weeks but need regular follow-up visits, and possibly echocardiography, over the next few months. Aneurysms and myocarditis, if present, usually disappear over a period of several months. Kawasaki disease is fatal in about 1 in 50 affected children. In children who survive, there is a small risk of developing coronary artery disease (p.405) later in life.

(WWW) ONLINE SITES: p.1028

Henoch–Schönlein purpura

Inflammation of small blood vessels, the kidneys, and joints, caused by an abnormal immune response

 AGE Most common between the ages of 2 and 8

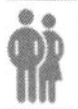 GENDER Twice as common in boys

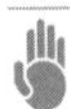 GENETICS LIFESTYLE Not significant factors

In Henoch–Schönlein purpura, small blood vessels are damaged by an abnormal reaction of the immune system, possibly triggered by an infection, such as a common cold (p.288). Antibodies, which are a component of the immune system and normally fight infection, are deposited in the small blood vessels throughout the body, causing them to become inflamed. The inflammation results in blood leaking out of the vessels into the skin, causing a distinctive rash, mainly on the buttocks and the backs of the legs. Bleeding may also occur from the lining of the intestines. The inflammation may also affect the joints and the kidneys.

Henoch–Schönlein purpura is most common in children between the ages of 2 and 8. The disorder occurs more frequently in the winter months and is more common in boys.

What are the symptoms?

The symptoms usually develop over several days and may include:

- A rash of raised, purple lesions that typically appears on the buttocks and legs and sometimes also on the arms.
- Periodic attacks of abdominal pain, often with vomiting and diarrhoea.
- Sometimes, blood in the faeces.
- Painful, swollen joints, most often the knees and ankles.
- Fever.

In about 8 in 10 children with the condition, the kidneys become inflamed, leading to loss of blood and protein in the urine (*see* GLOMERULONEPHRITIS, p.699). The blood is usually present in amounts too small to be seen with the naked eye. If the kidneys are badly affected, they may be damaged permanently, which may result in a rise in blood pressure. If the intestines become inflamed, a rare condition known as intussusception (p.864) may develop, in which part of the intestine "telescopes" in on itself.

How is it diagnosed?

The diagnosis of Henoch–Schönlein purpura is based on the symptoms. Your doctor will probably arrange for a urine test to look for blood or protein, indicating that the kidneys are inflamed. Blood tests will be carried out to assess the function of your child's kidneys and to rule out other possible causes of the symptoms. In some cases, a small sample of kidney tissue may be removed for examination (*see* KIDNEY BIOPSY, p.701).

What is the treatment?

There is no specific treatment for Henoch–Schönlein purpura. Your doctor will probably advise that your child rests in bed and may prescribe painkillers (p.912), such as paracetamol. If the abdominal pain is very severe, he or she may also prescribe corticosteroids (p.930). Joint pain usually disappears

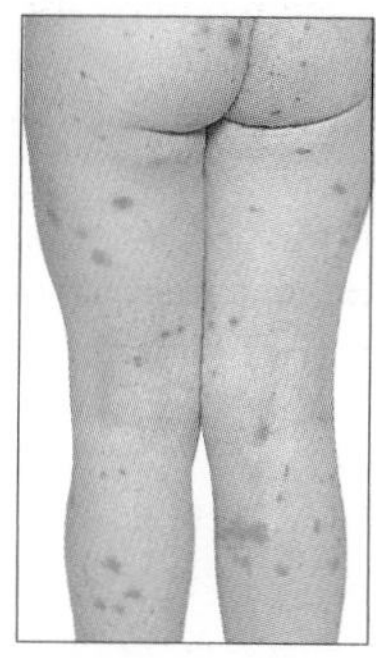

Henoch–Schönlein purpura
The rash of raised purple lesions that has developed over the back of this child's legs and buttocks is one of the symptoms typical of Henoch–Schönlein purpura.

without permanent damage, and the rash should go away without treatment. Symptoms normally take 2–6 weeks to disappear completely. Kidney function is monitored by checking your child's blood pressure and by performing blood tests. Urine tests are carried out for months or even years, until no traces of blood or protein remain in the urine. If the kidneys are severely damaged, the doctor may prescribe immunosuppressants (p.906). Children with kidney damage require long-term follow-up.

WHAT IS THE PROGNOSIS?

Most children with Henoch–Schönlein purpura make a full recovery with no long-term effects. The symptoms may recur over about a year but are rare thereafter. In about 1 in 20 children, there is long-term kidney damage that may lead to kidney failure (p.705).

(WWW) ONLINE SITES: p.1028, p.1033

Asthma in children

Attacks of breathlessness, coughing, and/or wheezing in children due to reversible narrowing of the airways

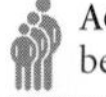
AGE Most common under the age of 6; becomes less common with age

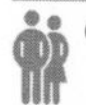
GENDER More common in boys

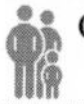
GENETICS Sometimes runs in families

LIFESTYLE Exposure to furry animals, air pollution, and parental smoking are risk factors

In children with asthma, the airways in the lungs tend to narrow temporarily. Narrowing occurs when the linings of the airways become swollen and inflamed and produce excess mucus, which may block the smaller airways.

Asthma affects about 1 in 7 children in the UK and is now the most common long-term respiratory disease in children. The number of children with asthma has risen greatly in recent years. The reason for this is unknown, but allergies and other environmental factors may be involved.

Asthma attacks in children are a common cause of absence from school and admission to hospital. However, between attacks, children can be perfectly well. Severe attacks of asthma are distressing for both children and their parents and can be life-threatening.

WHAT ARE THE CAUSES?

Asthma is more likely to develop in children with a family history of the condition, suggesting that a genetic factor may be involved. Other respiratory disorders, especially those associated with premature birth (*see* PROBLEMS OF THE PREMATURE BABY, p.816), may also increase the risk of developing asthma. Regular exposure to cigarette smoke in the home and pollution from car exhaust and factory fumes may also be risk factors for asthma.

In children under the age of 5, attacks of asthma are usually triggered by a viral infection, such as the common cold (p.288). In older children, asthma attacks are often caused by an allergic reaction to substances such as pollens, moulds, dust mites, and the fur or dander from animals. Exercise, especially outside in cold, dry conditions, may also trigger an asthma attack. In rare cases, certain foods, such as milk, nuts, and eggs, can provoke asthma. In some affected children, emotional stress may make the attacks more severe.

WHAT ARE THE SYMPTOMS?

Symptoms vary in severity from day to day and week to week and with the age of the child. They appear rapidly and may persist for a few hours or longer. Symptoms may include:

- Wheezing.
- Shortness of breath.
- Tightness in the chest.
- Dry cough that may be worse at night and disturb sleep.

Very young children with asthma often have a dry cough at night and no other symptoms. Older children often feel tired due to disturbed sleep and may have difficulty participating in strenuous sports due to shortness of breath. Children with asthma are also predisposed to the allergic disorders eczema (*see* ECZEMA IN CHILDREN, p.829) and hay fever (*see* ALLERGIC RHINITIS, p.466).

A severe asthma attack may cause very rapid breathing, difficulty speaking, and indrawing of the chest wall. If the level of oxygen in the blood is low, a child may develop a bluish tinge to the lips and tongue, a condition known as cyanosis. You should call an ambulance immediately if your child has such an attack, because he or she needs emergency treatment.

Left untreated, severe asthma may impair a child's growth (*see* GROWTH DISORDERS, p.869) and development. Children who have asthma often experience difficulty sleeping, which may lead to tiredness, and in turn to poor performance at school.

(TREATMENT) GIVING INHALED DRUGS TO CHILDREN

The drugs that are used to treat asthma are often inhaled. Devices that administer these drugs are tailored to suit the age of the child (*see* TAKING INHALED ASTHMA DRUGS, p.485). Because babies cannot coordinate their breathing to inhale the drugs, they require special inhalers that incorporate a face mask and a spacer. The spacer retains the drug while the face mask allows the baby to inhale the drug while breathing normally.

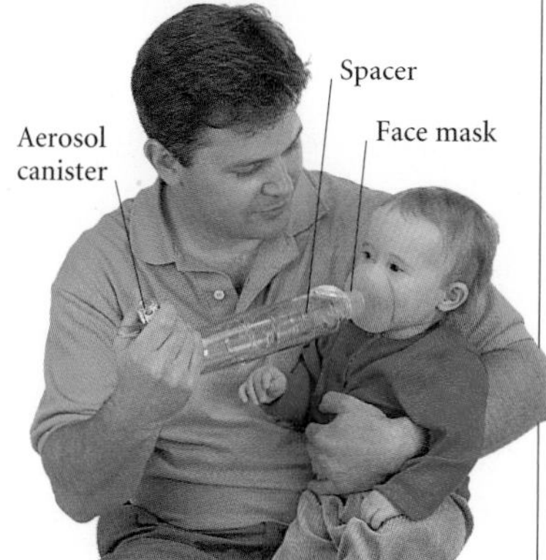

Giving drugs to a young child
A dose of the drug is dispensed from the canister into a spacer, such as the one shown, and the mask is placed over the baby's nose and mouth.

How is it diagnosed?

By the time the doctor sees your child, his or her asthma attack will probably be over. Diagnosis of the condition is therefore often based on a description of your child's symptoms. The doctor will listen to your child's chest with a stethoscope. An older child may be asked to breathe out through a peak flow meter, a special device that measures the child's capacity to exhale (*see* MONITORING YOUR ASTHMA, p.484). To confirm the diagnosis, the doctor may prescribe a trial of a quick-relief drug that opens up the airways in the lungs (*see* BRONCHODILATOR DRUGS, p.910). If your child's symptoms are caused by asthma, they should improve significantly after administration of the drug.

Once the diagnosis has been confirmed, your child may have a skin test to look for specific allergies that may be the trigger factors for his or her asthma attacks (*see* SKIN PRICK TEST, p.468).

What is the treatment?

The aim of treatment for asthma is to enable your child to live as active a life as possible with a minimum of drug treatment. The doctor may give you a detailed plan for managing your child's asthma with advice on when to change treatments and what to do if your child has a sudden attack. It is important that children who have asthma understand their condition and are confident about dealing with their symptoms. Some children will need to take regular peak flow readings at home to monitor their asthma over a period of time. Since the normal peak flow values are determined according to a child's height, growth should also be measured regularly.

ENVIRONMENTAL MEASURES There are many ways in which you can modify your child's environment to minimize contact with factors that may trigger an attack (*see* REDUCING THE RISK OF ASTHMA ATTACKS IN CHILDREN, right).

DRUG TREATMENT The drugs that are used to treat children with asthma fall into two groups: reliever drugs and preventer drugs, which are usually corticosteroids (*see* CORTICOSTEROIDS FOR RESPIRATORY DISEASE, p.911) although sodium cromoglicate and leukotriene antagonists (*see* ANTIALLERGY DRUGS, p.905) may also be used. The reliever drugs act rapidly to open up the airways and relieve wheezing. They usually work within 10 minutes, but their effect lasts for only a few hours. Children who have mild asthma attacks once or twice a week may be prescribed a reliever drug for use when symptoms occur.

Children who have frequent asthma attacks also need to take regular doses of preventer drugs. These drugs take effect slowly over several days and should be taken regularly, even if there are no symptoms of asthma. Preventer drugs reduce inflammation of the airways and prevent the symptoms from occurring. Respiratory corticosteroids are commonly prescribed as preventer drugs, but other drugs, such as sodium cromoglicate, may be given to dampen the allergic response and help to keep the airways open. Leukotriene antagonists are new drugs that may be used in addition to inhaled corticosteroids to treat moderately severe asthma.

Drugs to treat asthma are usually administered with an inhaler. A spacer device attached to an inhaler may be necessary for young children who find an inhaler difficult to use effectively (*see* GIVING INHALED DRUGS TO CHILDREN, p.839). A nebulizer, a device that delivers a drug in aerosol form through a face mask, may be used during a severe asthma attack. It is crucial to learn the correct technique for using inhalers and nebulizers. The doctor or a nurse will show you and your child how to use the devices properly. After a severe asthma attack, oral corticosteroids may be prescribed for your child in addition to the inhaled drugs.

MANAGING AN ASTHMA ATTACK You or your child should always carry a reliever inhaler in case it is needed to treat an asthma attack. An inhaler should also be kept at your child's school and you should ensure that his or her teachers understand its use. If your child's symptoms are not eased by a single dose of a reliever drug, a repeat dose should be taken. If that fails to improve the symptoms, call for an ambulance immediately or take your child to the nearest accident and emergency department. It is important to remain calm and reassure your child. Once in hospital, your child will probably be given oxygen and high doses of reliever drugs through a spacer or with a nebulizer to relieve the symptoms. He or she may need to stay in hospital to recover completely from a severe attack of asthma and may also require a course of oral corticosteroids.

(SELF-HELP) Reducing the risk of asthma attacks in children

Asthma attacks are often triggered by contact with allergy-producing substances, such as cat hair. By adopting simple measures, you can reduce the likelihood of your child having an attack.

- Do not allow people to smoke in the house.
- Do not keep furry animals or birds as pets.
- Dust furniture using a damp cloth and vacuum carpets regularly, if possible when your child is out of the house.
- Do not use fluffy, dust-collecting blankets and make sure pillows and duvets contain artificial fibres and not feathers.
- Enclose mattresses completely in plastic covers.
- If pollen is a problem, keep windows closed, especially while grass is releasing pollen, and use an air purifier.
- Avoid products that have strong odours, such as air fresheners, mothballs, and perfume.

What is the prognosis?

Children with asthma are usually able to lead active lives through careful use of drugs and avoidance of trigger factors, such as animal fur. About half of all children with asthma grow out of the condition by the time they are teenagers. Asthma that persists past the age of 14 is likely to continue into adulthood (*see* ASTHMA, p.483).

Despite the ease with which asthma can be controlled, severe attacks of asthma can cause death. In most cases, fatalities are caused by a delay in getting an affected child to hospital and a lack of understanding about potentially life-threatening symptoms.

(WWW) ONLINE SITES: p.1027, p.1028

Bronchiolitis

Inflammation of the small airways in the lungs caused by a viral infection

AGE Most common under the age of 12 months

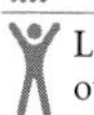
LIFESTYLE Parental smoking and living in overcrowded conditions are risk factors

GENDER GENETICS Not significant factors

Bronchiolitis is a common and usually mild condition that mainly occurs in babies under the age of 12 months. The small airways in the lungs, called bronchioles, become inflamed due to a viral infection and restrict the flow of air in and out of the lungs. In about 9 in 10 cases, the infection is caused by the respiratory syncytial virus, which can be transmitted from person to person in the airborne droplets from coughs and sneezes. By the age of 5, almost all children in the UK have been infected with this virus. Most of those affected only develop the symptoms of a common cold (p.288), but occasionally the infection leads to more severe breathing difficulties. During the cold winter months, bronchiolitis tends to occur in epidemics. The risk of a child having bronchiolitis is increased if his or her family lives in overcrowded conditions, in which a viral infection can spread more quickly among people, or if the child's parents smoke.

What are the symptoms?

Initially, an affected child may have symptoms resembling a common cold, such as a runny nose, fever, and sneezing. However, the following symptoms may develop after 2–3 days:

- Dry cough.
- Rapid breathing.
- Wheezing.
- Feeding difficulties.

If your child is under 1 year old and has these symptoms, you should contact the doctor. Occasionally, babies may experience severe breathing difficulties, especially if they are very young or have an underlying condition such as congenital heart disease (p.836). These babies may develop a blue tinge on the tongue, lips, and skin, a condition called cyanosis. In very small babies who have bronchiolitis, intervals of more than 10 seconds may occur between breaths. You should call for an ambulance immediately if your baby is having difficulty breathing, if his or her tongue, lips, or skin become blue-coloured, or if he or she becomes drowsy at unexpected times because of the extra effort that is needed to breathe.

How is it diagnosed?

The doctor will probably suspect bronchiolitis from the symptoms and by listening to your child's chest with a stethoscope. A chest X-ray (p.490) may be arranged and the doctor may take samples of your child's nasal secretions to look for evidence of infection with the respiratory syncytial virus.

What is the treatment?

If the bronchiolitis is mild, you will probably be able to treat your child at home. The doctor may prescribe inhaled bronchodilators (p.910) to widen the airways and ease breathing. You will probably be advised to give your child liquid paracetamol (*see* PAINKILLERS, p.912) to bring down a fever. You can help to relieve your child's difficulty in breathing by increasing humidity in the bedroom. This can be done by placing a wet towel or a dish of water in the room close to a source of heat, such as a radiator. You should give your child small, frequent drinks and feeds to make sure that he or she is receiving an adequate quantity of fluids, avoiding dehydration, which can be serious.

Children with severe symptoms need to have treatment in hospital, where they may be given an inhaled bronchodilator drug. Intravenous fluids may be administered if the child is unable to feed. Oxygen is usually given, especially if a child is cyanotic. Premature babies and those with problems such as heart disease may be given antiviral drugs (p.886) to treat the infection. These babies may need temporary mechanical ventilation to help them to breathe.

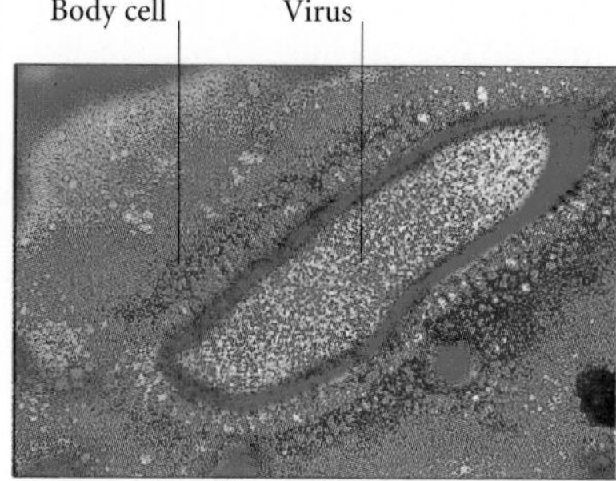

Respiratory syncytial virus
This virus is the most common cause of bronchiolitis, in which small airways in the lungs are inflamed. In some cases, the infection causes severe breathing difficulties.

What is the prognosis?

Mild bronchiolitis usually improves within 5 days and clears up completely in about 10 days. Severe bronchiolitis may require several weeks of hospital treatment but causes no permanent damage. About half of all affected children have recurrent wheezing for a few years following the illness, which worsens if they have a cold.

(WWW) ONLINE SITES: p.1028, p.1033

Croup

Inflammation and narrowing of the main airway (trachea) due to a viral infection

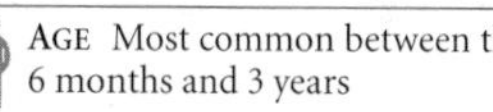
AGE Most common between the ages of 6 months and 3 years

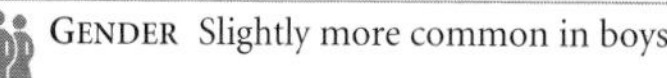
GENDER Slightly more common in boys

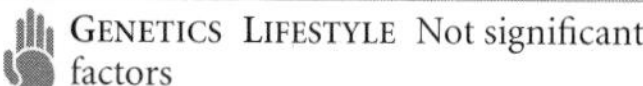
GENETICS LIFESTYLE Not significant factors

Croup is a common disorder that usually affects children between the ages of 6 months and 3 years. During an attack of croup, the airway that leads from the back of the throat to the lungs becomes inflamed because of a viral infection, restricting the flow of air and causing noisy breathing. Although symptoms are usually mild, croup may occasionally cause severe breathing difficulties that require treatment in hospital. Boys appear to be more susceptible to the condition, but the reason for this is not known. Croup occurs more frequently in the autumn and winter months.

What are the symptoms?

Croup usually begins with the symptoms of a common cold, such as a runny nose. About 1–2 days later, the following symptoms may develop:

- Barking cough.
- Harsh, noisy breathing, particularly when inhaling.
- Hoarseness.

In severe cases, breathing may become rapid and difficult. This may cause a lack of oxygen and lead to the development of a bluish colour to the tongue and lips, a condition called cyanosis. If cyanosis develops, you should contact the doctor immediately, and, if he or she is not available, call an ambulance.

What might be done?

The doctor will probably diagnose croup from the symptoms. He or she will assess the severity of your child's condition and may suggest self-help measures to ease your child's breathing. For example, sitting with your child in a steamy bathroom can relieve minor breathing difficulties. You can increase the humidity in your child's room by placing a dish of water near a heat source, such as a radiator. Taking your child outside in the cool night air for a few minutes may also help. The doctor may prescribe an inhaled or oral corticosteroid drug (*see* CORTICOSTEROIDS FOR RESPIRATORY DISEASE, p.911) to reduce inflammation in the airways. If the symptoms are very severe, your child will need to be admitted to hospital. In rare cases, mechanical ventilation may also be necessary.

What is the prognosis?

Most children with croup recover completely within a few days. However, the condition may recur until your child reaches about the age of 5. At this age, the airways are wider and therefore less likely to become severely narrowed by inflammation after an infection.

(WWW) ONLINE SITES: p.1028, p.1031, p.1033

Epiglottitis

Inflammation of the epiglottis, a flap of cartilage that closes over the main airway to the lungs when food is swallowed

AGE Most common between the ages of 1 and 6

GENDER GENETICS LIFESTYLE Not significant factors

In this rare condition, the epiglottis, a flap of tissue behind the tongue that prevents food from entering the airways of the lungs during swallowing, becomes inflamed due to infection. Inflammation causes the epiglottis to swell so that the main airway is partially blocked. The swelling can be so severe that the child is unable to breathe. This situation is life-threatening and needs urgent hospital treatment.

Epiglottitis is caused by infection with the bacterium *Haemophilus influenzae* type B (Hib). Children between 1 and 6 years old are most commonly affected. Epiglottitis is now rare in the UK due to routine immunization (p.45) of babies.

What are the symptoms?

In most cases, the symptoms of epiglottitis develop suddenly over a period of 1–2 hours and may include:

- High fever.
- Severe sore throat.
- Difficulty swallowing.
- Saliva dribbling from the mouth.
- Restlessness and anxiety.
- Rapid, laboured breathing.
- Harsh noise on inhaling.

If there is severe obstruction of the airway, your child may become short of oxygen, possibly causing his or her lips, tongue, and skin to become blue-tinged. If your child develops difficulty swallowing or breathing, you should call for an ambulance without delay because immediate treatment is essential.

What might be done?

Initially, your most important role is to reassure your child and try to keep him or her calm. You should not attempt to examine your child's throat because this may increase distress, resulting in further blockage of the airway. Your child will probably be more comfortable sitting upright with his or her chin jutting out to maintain an unobstructed flow of air into the lungs.

The doctor will probably make a diagnosis from your child's symptoms. Humidified oxygen will need to be given through a mask held near to his or her face. In hospital, your child will probably be taken to the operating theatre and given an inhaled anaesthetic so that a tube can be inserted into the main airway to keep it open. To maintain breathing, your child may need mechanical ventilation. To treat the Hib infection, your child will be given intravenous antibiotics (p.885).

What is the prognosis?

Most children recover in about a week. The tube that keeps the airway open is usually removed after about 2–3 days. There are usually no long-term problems, and the condition does not recur.

(WWW) ONLINE SITES: p.1028, p.1032

Enlarged adenoids

Enlargement of the adenoids, tissue at the back of the nasal cavity that forms part of the body's defence system

AGE Most common under the age of 7

GENDER GENETICS LIFESTYLE Not significant factors

The adenoids, which are located at the back of the nasal cavity, consist of lymphatic tissue that forms part of the body's defences against infection. In some children, particularly those under the age of 7, the adenoids become enlarged, which may lead to difficulties with breathing and speech. This enlargement is sometimes a result of recurrent respiratory infections or can be caused by allergies. In other cases, the cause is unknown. Infected adenoids are sometimes associated with infection of the tonsils (*see* TONSILLITIS, opposite page).

What are the symptoms?

In most children with enlarged adenoids, symptoms are mild and appear gradually. The symptoms may include:

- Breathing through the mouth and snoring during sleep.
- Persistently blocked or runny nose.
- Nasal-sounding voice.

Difficulty in breathing may cause your child to wake frequently during the night, leading to tiredness and inability to concentrate. Enlarged adenoids may cause partial blockage of one or both of the eustachian tubes connecting the throat to the middle ear, causing recurrent middle-ear infections (*see* ACUTE OTITIS MEDIA IN CHILDREN, p.860) or a build-up of fluid in the middle ear that results in deafness (*see* CHRONIC SECRETORY OTITIS MEDIA, p.860). In an older child, obstruction of the flow of nasal secretions may lead to sinusitis (p.475).

What might be done?

The doctor will probably examine your child's throat. If the symptoms are mild, no treatment for enlarged adenoids is required because adenoids shrink naturally with age, and almost always disappear completely before puberty. However, if your child has constantly disrupted sleep, recurrent middle-ear infections, or chronic secretory otitis media, the doctor may advise surgical removal of the adenoids. The tonsils are also sometimes removed at the same time (*see* TONSILLECTOMY AND ADENOIDECTOMY, right). A build-up of fluid in the middle ear may be relieved by inserting a tiny drainage tube called a grommet (p.861) into the eardrum.

The symptoms tend to diminish as a child gets older, and have usually gone by the time adolescence is reached.

WWW ONLINE SITES: p.1028

Tonsillitis

Inflammation of the tonsils, two areas of tissue at the back of the throat that form part of the body's defence system

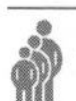 AGE Most common under the age of 8

 GENDER GENETICS LIFESTYLE Not significant factors

The tonsils are two areas of lymphatic tissue at the back of the throat that form an important part of the body's defences against infection. A condition known as tonsillitis develops if the tonsils become inflamed and painful, usually as a result of respiratory infections. The infections may be caused either by viruses, such as those that cause the common cold (p.288), or bacteria, such as streptococci.

In children under the age of 8, tonsillitis is common because the tonsils are exposed to many infections for the first time. Children who have tonsillitis may also have enlarged adenoids (opposite page). Tonsils become smaller with age and therefore tonsillitis occurs far less frequently in adults (*see* PHARYNGITIS AND TONSILLITIS, p.479).

WHAT ARE THE SYMPTOMS?

The symptoms of tonsillitis usually develop over a period of 24–36 hours. Symptoms may include:

- Sore throat and discomfort during swallowing.
- Enlarged and tender lymph nodes in the neck.

Additional symptoms that may be due to a viral infection include:

- Fever.
- Headache.
- Abdominal pain.
- Vomiting and/or diarrhoea.

Babies and children who are too young to talk are unable to tell their parents they have a sore throat, but they may refuse to eat or drink because of the discomfort when swallowing. They may also be lethargic and irritable.

TREATMENT

TONSILLECTOMY AND ADENOIDECTOMY

Surgical removal of the tonsils is performed on children who have recurrent episodes of tonsillitis. Enlarged adenoids may also be removed at the same time if they are causing breathing difficulties and recurrent ear problems. The operation is performed in hospital under general anaesthesia. A child should be able to return home the day after the operation, and he or she should make a full recovery in about 2 weeks.

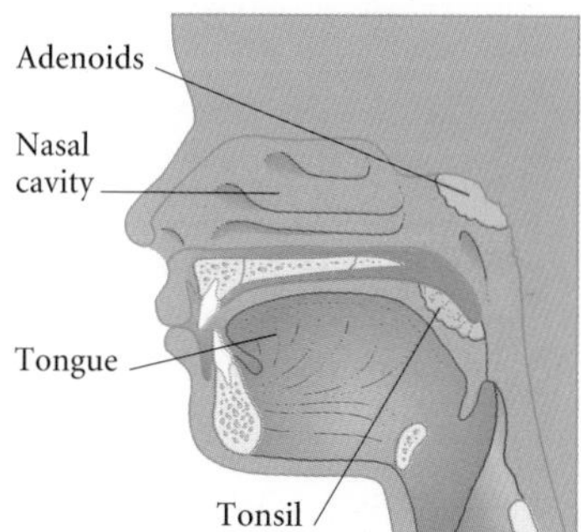

The procedure
Surgical removal of the tonsils and adenoids is performed through the mouth under general anaesthesia.

Tonsillitis which occurs with enlarged adenoids may be associated with a middle-ear infection (*see* ACUTE OTITIS MEDIA IN CHILDREN, p.860). Sometimes, an abscess called quinsy forms next to a tonsil. In young children, the rapid rise in temperature at the start of tonsillitis may cause a convulsion (*see* FEBRILE CONVULSIONS, p.849).

WHAT CAN I DO?

You may be able to make your child more comfortable by practising simple self-help measures at home. To bring down a fever, you can give your child liquid paracetamol (*see* PAINKILLERS, p.912) and sponge him or her down with tepid water (*see* BRINGING DOWN A FEVER, p.289). You should encourage your child to drink small amounts of fluid at regular intervals, particularly if he or she has been vomiting or has diarrhoea. Cold, nonacidic drinks such as milk can help to relieve a sore throat, but older children may prefer ice cream or ice lollies. Older children may also find that sucking throat lozenges or gargling with warm salt water helps to relieve a sore throat.

You should consult the doctor if self-help measures do not bring down body temperature, if your child is taking very little fluid, or if symptoms do not improve in 24 hours.

WHAT MIGHT THE DOCTOR DO?

The doctor will examine your child's throat and may take a swab to test for bacterial infection. He or she may also look inside your child's ears to check for an ear infection (*see* OTOSCOPY, p.597). If the doctor suspects a bacterial throat infection, a course of antibiotics (p.885) will be prescribed.

Most children recover fully from tonsillitis within a few days. However, if your child is not drinking adequate amounts of fluid, he or she may become dehydrated and need to be admitted to hospital for treatment with intravenous fluids and antibiotics. If quinsy has developed, the abscess may need to be surgically drained.

WHAT IS THE PROGNOSIS?

Some children have frequent episodes of tonsillitis, but by the age of 8 these bouts are usually rare. If a child misses school regularly because of tonsillitis, the doctor may recommend surgical removal of the tonsils (*see* TONSILLECTOMY AND ADENOIDECTOMY, left).

WWW ONLINE SITES: p.1028

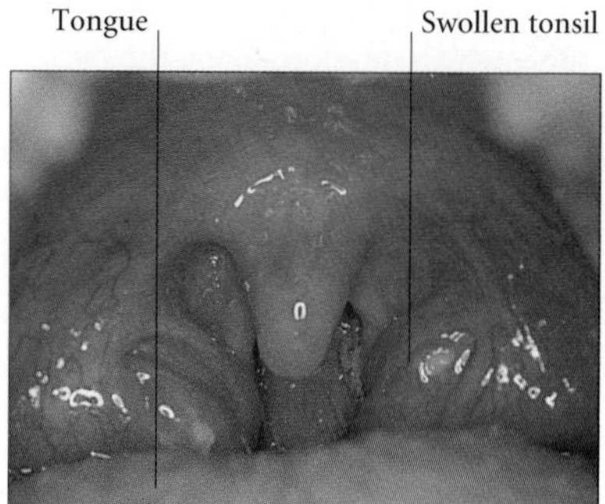

Tonsillitis
These tonsils have become swollen and inflamed as a result of an infection, a condition known as tonsillitis.

DISORDERS OF THE NERVOUS SYSTEM

The nervous system consists of the brain, the spinal cord, and the network of nerves that extends throughout the body. Serious disorders of this system are uncommon in children, although disabling conditions may be present from birth due to defects that occur during pregnancy. The nervous system is sometimes affected by minor disorders and, rarely, by infections and cancers.

Damage to the nervous system, either before birth or in early childhood, can result in varying degrees of physical disability. The first articles in this section describe defects that occur during the development of the spinal cord and brain, causing disorders such as spina bifida and cerebral palsy.

Children are commonly affected by minor disorders of the nervous system, such as headache and migraine, which are described next. Migraine may be more difficult to recognize in young children than in adults because the main symptom is often abdominal pain rather than headache. Further articles discuss serious disorders of great concern to parents, including meningitis, which is a dangerous infection of the coverings of the brain and spinal cord, and Reye's syndrome, an inflammation of the brain and liver. The final articles describe tumours of the brain and of the spinal cord, both of which are rare in children.

Epilepsy (p.524), which usually develops in childhood, is discussed in general nervous system disorders.

KEY ANATOMY

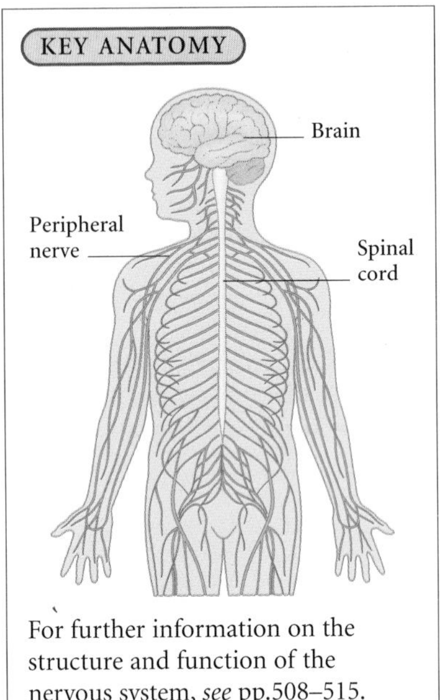

For further information on the structure and function of the nervous system, *see* pp.508–515.

Neural tube defects

Abnormalities of the brain and spinal cord and their protective coverings

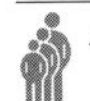 AGE Present from birth

 GENETICS Sometimes run in families

 LIFESTYLE Taking certain drugs during pregnancy is a risk factor

 GENDER Not a significant factor

Neural tube defects occur during pregnancy as a result of abnormalities in the embryo's development. The neural tube, which develops along the back of the embryo by about the third week of pregnancy, later becomes the brain and spinal cord and their coverings. If this tube fails to close completely, defects in any of these body parts can result.

Most commonly, the spinal cord and vertebrae are affected, causing a disorder known as spina bifida. The effects of spina bifida vary from dimpling or a tuft of hair at the base of the spine and a minor abnormality of the vertebrae to complete exposure of part of the spinal cord, known as a myelomeningocele. Rarely, the brain and skull are affected.

Since the discovery in 1992 that folic acid taken during early pregnancy provides protection against neural tube defects, spina bifida is becoming less common. The disorder currently affects only about 1 in 2,500 babies in the UK.

The cause of neural tube defects is not fully understood, but they tend to run in families, which suggests that genetic factors are involved. Certain types of anticonvulsant drug (p.914), such as sodium valproate, are associated with neural tube defects if they are taken during pregnancy.

WHAT ARE THE SYMPTOMS?

The symptoms of a neural tube defect depend upon its severity. Often, there are no obvious symptoms, and spina bifida may be diagnosed only if minor conditions, such as backache, occur in adult life. The symptoms of a severe defect will become apparent at varying stages in childhood; they mainly affect the lower body and include:

- Paralysis or weakness of the legs.
- Absence of sensation in the legs.
- Abnormalities in the functioning of the bladder and bowels.

About 8 in 10 children who have severe spina bifida also have a build-up of fluid within the brain (*see* HYDROCEPHALUS, opposite page). Occasionally, learning difficulties may develop. In some cases, neural tube defects lead to meningitis, a serious infection of the membranes covering the brain and spinal cord (*see* MENINGITIS IN CHILDREN, p.848).

HOW IS IT DIAGNOSED?

Currently, women are routinely offered a blood test at about 16 weeks into pregnancy to allow for early diagnosis of severe neural tube defects. In addition, one or more ultrasound scans (*see* ULTRASOUND SCANNING IN PREGNANCY, p.793) are routinely performed 11–20 weeks into pregnancy to examine the fetus and to detect defects.

After birth, a baby with a neural tube defect will probably have CT scanning (p.247) or MRI (p.248) of the spine to assess the severity of the defect.

WHAT IS THE TREATMENT?

If the defect is minor, no treatment is necessary. However, if a baby has a serious defect, he or she is likely to require surgery in the first few days after birth. If hydrocephalus is present, a drainage tube will probably be inserted to release excess fluid and to prevent further fluid build-up in the cavities of the brain (*see* SHUNT FOR HYDROCEPHALUS, right).

Even with surgery, children born with severe defects will be permanently disabled and need lifelong care. Practical and emotional support will be provided for the whole family. An affected child will often need regular physiotherapy (p.961) to keep as mobile as possible, and some children may need a wheelchair. Training in the regular use of a urinary catheter may be necessary for children who cannot pass urine normally (*see* BLADDER CATHETERIZATION, p.713). Some children may need special teaching. Many families find support through joining a self-help group.

CAN IT BE PREVENTED?

You can reduce the risk of your baby having a neural tube defect by supplementing your daily diet with folic acid while trying to conceive; neural tube defects can occur before you know that you are pregnant. You may also benefit from starting to take folic acid as soon as you know you are pregnant. Your doctor may recommend that you take a slightly higher dose if you already have an affected child. If a close blood relative has a neural tube defect, a couple who are planning a pregnancy may wish to seek genetic counselling (p.272) because their children may be at increased risk of the disorder.

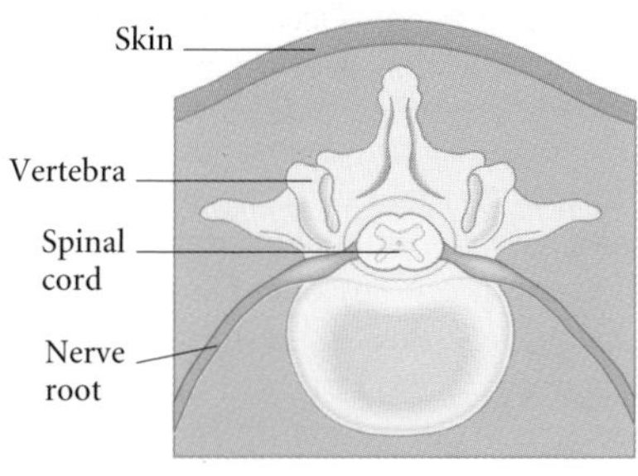

NORMAL VERTEBRA

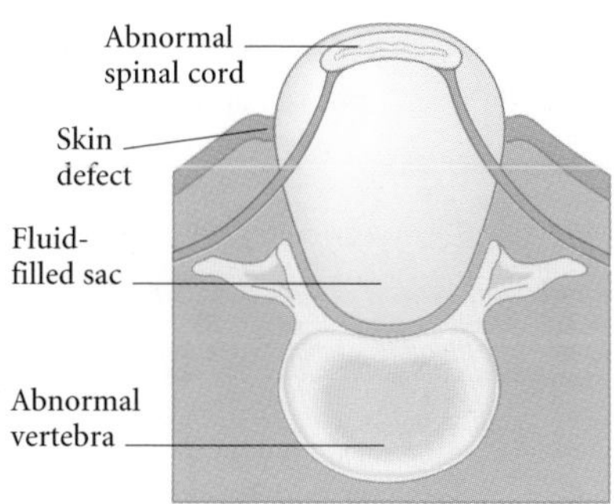

MYELOMENINGOCELE

Neural tube defect

A myelomeningocele, a severe neural tube defect, occurs when the vertebrae are not fully formed. The spinal cord, contained in fluid-filled membranes, bulges outwards through a defect in the skin.

(TREATMENT) SHUNT FOR HYDROCEPHALUS

A shunt is a drainage tube inserted into the brain to treat hydrocephalus, a disorder in which cerebrospinal fluid builds up in the brain cavities. The shunt diverts the excess fluid to another part of the body where it can be absorbed into the bloodstream. The fluid is released through a valve when pressure increases and drains into either the abdominal cavity or, rarely, a chamber in the heart.

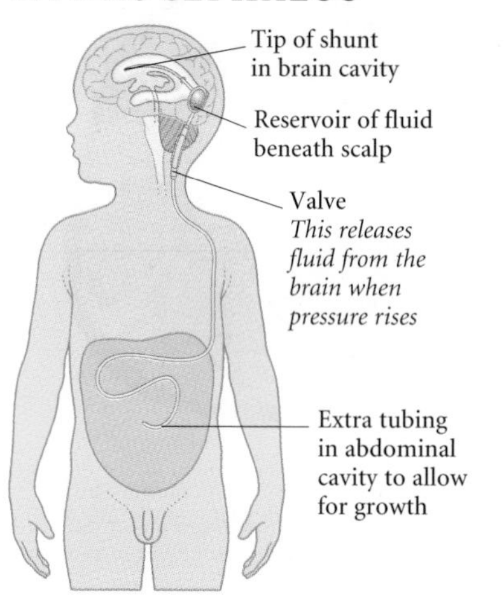

Inserting the shunt

The tip of the shunt is inserted through the skull into the fluid-filled cavity in the brain. The drainage tube is then passed under the skin and ends in the abdomen.

WHAT IS THE PROGNOSIS?

Children with only minor defects have a normal life expectancy. If symptoms affecting posture develop, there may be an increased risk of developing osteoarthritis (p.374). Children with extensive damage to the brain and/or the spinal cord may have a reduced life expectancy.

(WWW) ONLINE SITES: p.1027

Hydrocephalus

An abnormal build-up of fluid within the skull, also known as water on the brain

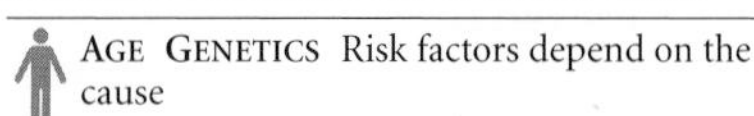
AGE GENETICS Risk factors depend on the cause

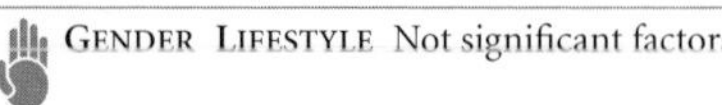
GENDER LIFESTYLE Not significant factors

Hydrocephalus is an uncommon condition that occurs mainly in premature babies or with other disorders present from birth, such as spina bifida (*see* NEURAL TUBE DEFECTS, opposite page).

Cerebrospinal fluid (CSF) is produced in the cavities of the brain and flows around the brain and spinal cord, protecting them from injury. Hydrocephalus develops if CSF builds up in the cavities of the brain, causing them to enlarge. This build-up occurs when the system that drains the CSF away from the brain is damaged or blocked or if excess CSF is produced. In such cases, the resulting increase in pressure in the skull may lead to brain damage.

Hydrocephalus may be caused by a brain defect that is present from birth. The disorder also sometimes develops as a result of meningitis, a serious infection of the membranes covering the brain and spinal cord (*see* MENINGITIS IN CHILDREN, p.848), or a brain tumour (*see* BRAIN AND SPINAL CORD TUMOURS IN CHILDREN, p.850).

WHAT ARE THE SYMPTOMS?

The symptoms vary according to the age of the child, but the following may occur in all affected children:

- Vomiting.
- Drowsiness.
- Reluctance to settle down.

In young babies, the skull bones are not yet fused and are able to separate to some extent to accommodate excess fluid. For this reason, the first signs of hydrocephalus in babies may be an enlarged head that grows too fast and widening of the fontanelles (the soft areas on the top of a baby's skull). In older children with hydrocephalus, the head does not enlarge because the skull bones have fused, and headache due to pressure may be an early symptom.

Left untreated, hydrocephalus may lead to seizures and to cerebral palsy (p.846), in which movement and posture are affected. The disorder may also affect vision and hearing and can result in poor intellectual development.

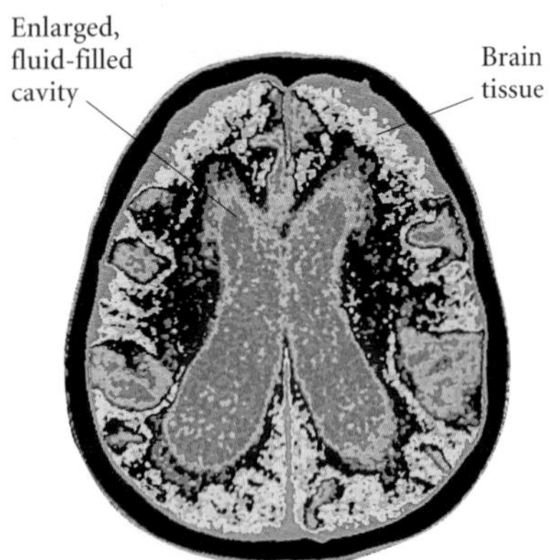

Hydrocephalus
In this CT scan, the small cavities in the centre of the brain have been enlarged by an abnormal build-up of fluid, a condition known as hydrocephalus.

HOW IS IT DIAGNOSED?

Hydrocephalus can sometimes be diagnosed during pregnancy with routine ultrasound scanning (*see* ULTRASOUND SCANNING IN PREGNANCY, p.793).

If the condition is suspected after birth, the doctor will arrange for ultrasound scanning (p.250) or CT scanning (p.247) of the child's head to look for obstructions or other abnormalities.

WHAT IS THE TREATMENT?

A child who has hydrocephalus usually needs surgery. During the operation, a narrow flexible tube, called a shunt, is inserted into a cavity in the brain to drain away the excess fluid (*see* SHUNT FOR HYDROCEPHALUS, p.845). The tube is normally left in place permanently.

In addition, the child may be prescribed drugs that will slow down the production of CSF in the brain. Underlying causes of obstruction, such as a brain tumour, will be treated.

Some children with hydrocephalus are able to lead normal lives if they are given treatment before significant brain damage occurs. However, if the condition is severe or is left untreated, resulting in physical disabilities or difficulties with learning, affected children and their families will need long-term practical and psychological support.

Parents who have a child with hydrocephalus may wish to consider genetic counselling (p.272) because there is an increased risk of the condition occurring in subsequent children.

(WWW) ONLINE SITES: p.1027

Cerebral palsy

Abnormalities of movement and posture caused by damage to the immature brain

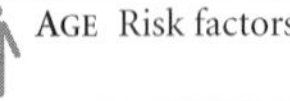

AGE Risk factors depend on the cause

GENDER GENETICS LIFESTYLE Not significant factors

Cerebral palsy is not a specific disease but a general term used to describe a group of disorders affecting movement and posture. These disorders all result from damage to the developing brain either before or during birth or during a child's early years. Children with cerebral palsy lack normal control of limbs and posture, but their intellect is often unaffected. Although the damage to the brain does not progress, the disabilities it causes change as a child grows. Many children have symptoms that are hardly noticeable, but other children may be severely disabled. Cerebral palsy affects about 1 in 500 children born in the UK.

WHAT ARE THE CAUSES?

In many cases of cerebral palsy, there is no obvious cause. However, the fetus can be damaged by an infection, such as rubella or cytomegalovirus, transmitted from the mother during pregnancy (*see* CONGENITAL INFECTIONS, p.817). Cerebral palsy may also result if a baby is deprived of oxygen during a difficult birth (*see* PROBLEMS DURING DELIVERY, p.802). The disorder can develop in premature babies, whose immature brains are often prone to abnormal bleeding (*see* PROBLEMS OF THE PREMATURE BABY, p.816). During early childhood, cerebral palsy can develop after meningitis, an infection of the membranes around the brain (*see* MENINGITIS IN CHILDREN, p.848), or after a head injury (p.521).

WHAT ARE THE SYMPTOMS?

If brain damage has occurred during pregnancy or birth, a newborn baby may be limp and unable to feed properly. Even if the symptoms are vague, such as a reluctance to settle down, parents may suspect that there is a problem from an early age. More commonly, symptoms do not appear until after 6 months of age and may include:

- Weakness or stiffness affecting one or more limbs.
- Reluctance to use a limb.
- Abnormal, uncontrolled movements.
- Delay in achieving normal milestones in development (*see* DEVELOPMENTAL DELAY, p.853).
- Difficulty in swallowing.
- Speech problems.
- Chronic constipation (*see* CONSTIPATION IN CHILDREN, p.865).

Many children have vision disorders, such as squint (*see* STRABISMUS, p.857), and impaired hearing (*see* CONGENITAL DEAFNESS, p.859). About 1 in 4 children has a learning disability (*see* GENERALIZED LEARNING DISABILITIES, p.854).

ARE THERE COMPLICATIONS?

If a child with cerebral palsy has stiff limbs, he or she may experience difficulty in walking and have an abnormal posture. The disorder can also increase the risk of dislocated joints, particularly the hips. Sometimes, children with cerebral palsy develop epilepsy (p.524). Behavioural problems may develop if a child becomes frustrated because of his or her physical disabilities and inability to communicate clearly. Children with severe cerebral palsy are particularly susceptible to chest infections because they cannot cough effectively.

WHAT MIGHT BE DONE?

The diagnosis of cerebral palsy is often difficult to make in a very young child. As a child becomes older, the symptoms become more obvious. Once the condition is suspected, tests such as CT scanning (p.247) or MRI (p.248) may be carried out to identify brain damage.

Once the diagnosis is confirmed, the whole family has to adjust to the lifestyle changes that are often associated

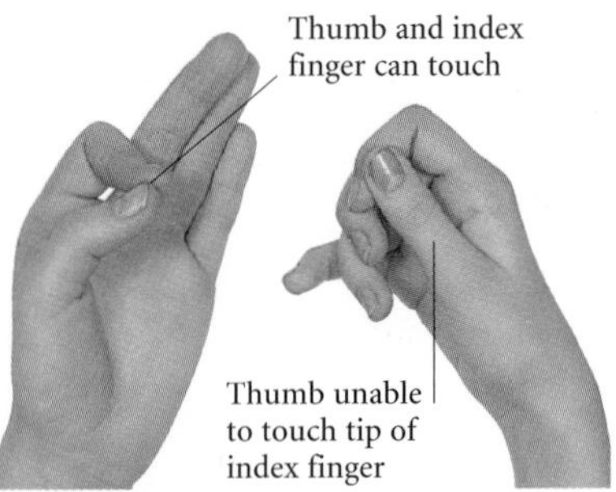

Poor coordination in cerebral palsy
A person with cerebral palsy often cannot coordinate movement in some parts of the body. The right hand shown here has poor coordination but the left hand is normal.

with caring for a child with cerebral palsy. Many affected children have only mild disabilities, requiring some physiotherapy (p.961), but children who have more severe disabilities usually need long-term therapy and specialist support. Emphasis is placed on assessing individual needs and helping a child to achieve his or her maximum potential. Physiotherapy to encourage normal posture plays a major part in the care of an affected child. Parents can encourage a child to play in a way that exercises the muscles and develops coordination.

If a child has only a minor physical disability, he or she may be able to attend a normal school. Children who have more severe disabilities or whose intellectual ability is affected may benefit from special schooling.

Complications and problems associated with cerebral palsy will be treated as necessary. For example, if your child has impaired hearing, he or she may require a hearing aid. Caring for a disabled child at home is stressful, and occasional residential care or residential schools can provide respite.

What is the prognosis?

Children with mild physical disabilities can usually lead active, full, and long lives and often live independently as adults. Severely disabled children, especially those with swallowing difficulties who are more prone to serious chest infections, have a lower life expectancy.

(WWW) ONLINE SITES: p.1028, p.1034

Headache in children

Pain of variable severity affecting the head, sometimes due to an underlying disorder

 AGE More common in school-age children

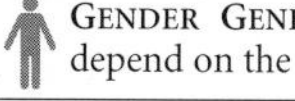 GENDER GENETICS LIFESTYLE Risk factors depend on the cause

Headaches are a common symptom in childhood, and about 9 in 10 children complain of at least one headache a year. Childhood headaches normally cause no more than temporary discomfort, but, if severe or recurrent, they may indicate an underlying condition that requires prompt medical treatment.

Young children, particularly those under the age of 5, are often unable to identify the precise location of pain. They may therefore complain of a headache when the problem is toothache, earache, or even a pain located elsewhere in the body, such as in the abdomen.

What are the causes?

There are many causes of headaches in children, most of which are not serious. In older children especially, the reasons for most headaches are often similar to those in adults (*see* HEADACHE, p.518). However, parents may be understandably worried that their child is suffering from a serious illness such as meningitis, an inflammation of the membranes covering the brain (*see* MENINGITIS IN CHILDREN, p.848), or a brain tumour (*see* BRAIN AND SPINAL CORD TUMOURS IN CHILDREN, p.850). These two disorders account for only a tiny percentage of childhood headaches, but it is important that parents are aware of the main symptoms so that they know when they should seek medical advice (*see* SYMPTOM CHART 10: HEADACHE, p.110).

Short-lived headaches in children are usually caused by a viral infection, such as a common cold (p.288). These infections normally clear up within a few days without needing treatment. Many school-age children suffer from recurrent tension headaches (p.518). In the majority of cases, tension headaches last no longer than 24 hours and may be related to emotional stress either at school or at home. Problems with vision, such as shortsightedness (*see* MYOPIA, p.586), can sometimes result in persistent headaches. By the age of 15, about 1 in 20 children has experienced one or more migraine attacks (*see* MIGRAINE IN CHILDREN, right).

What can I do?

If a severe headache occurs with vomiting or drowsiness, contact your doctor without delay. A child who has lost consciousness after a head injury, however briefly, should be taken to hospital immediately. If the headache is mild, encourage your child to rest and relieve his or her discomfort with paracetamol (*see* PAINKILLERS, p.912).

If you suspect that your child has headaches because of tension, you may be able to help him or her by identifying the particular anxiety. Recurrent headaches that have no obvious cause should be investigated by the doctor.

What might the doctor do?

If the doctor cannot find a cause for concern following a physical examination of your child, further tests are not usually necessary. If the doctor suspects meningitis, he or she will have the child admitted to hospital immediately for treatment. Rarely, your child may need CT scanning (p.247) or MRI (p.248) of the brain to investigate an injury or rule out the presence of a tumour.

If your child is normally well but has regular, persistent headaches, an eye test may be needed to exclude vision problems, and the doctor may refer him or her to an optician.

(WWW) ONLINE SITES: p.1028, p.1032

Migraine in children

Recurring symptoms that may include headache and abdominal pain

 AGE Can occur as early as 2 years of age

 GENDER More common in girls

 GENETICS Sometimes runs in families

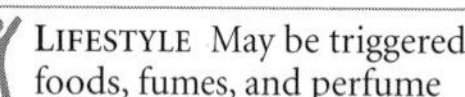 LIFESTYLE May be triggered by certain foods, fumes, and perfume

Migraine is a significant cause of headache in children, particularly girls, and by the age of 15 about 1 in 20 children has experienced an attack. The condition is known to occur in children as young as 2 years of age. However, childhood migraine often differs from that experienced by adults, and the disorder can sometimes be difficult to recognize. In younger children, the symptoms of migraine frequently include recurrent episodes of abdominal pain, and the one-sided headaches and nausea that are typical of the condition in adults (*see* MIGRAINE, p.518) may not occur.

What are the causes?

Why some children develop migraine is not fully understood, but the condition sometimes runs in families, suggesting that genetic factors may be involved. Migraine is thought to be due to changes in the blood flow through the blood vessels inside the skull. There may also be temporary alterations in the levels of chemicals in the brain, which are probably responsible for triggering some of the symptoms elsewhere in the body.

Certain substances are known to trigger attacks of migraine. These include some types of food, commonly chocolate, cheese, citrus fruits, and red wine, and inhaled substances such as perfume, petrol fumes, and tobacco smoke.

WHAT ARE THE SYMPTOMS?

In children under 8 years, the symptoms of migraine may not include headache. Symptoms develop gradually over a few hours, and a child may experience:

- Pain in the centre of the abdomen.
- Pale skin.
- Tiredness.
- Vomiting.

Often, these symptoms persist for several days. If children continue to have attacks of migraine as they grow older, they are likely to have symptoms more similar to those experienced by adults. These symptoms develop over a few hours and may include:

- Visual disturbances, such as seeing flashing lights.
- Headache, typically on one side.
- Nausea and vomiting.
- Dislike of bright lights.

Rarely, a child may experience temporary weakness in one arm or leg.

WHAT MIGHT BE DONE?

The doctor may be able to diagnose migraine from your child's symptoms. Occasionally, he or she may arrange for tests, such as CT scanning (p.247) or MRI (p.248) of the head, or, in young children, ultrasound scanning of the abdomen, to exclude other disorders.

Resting quietly in bed in a darkened room may make your child feel better. Taking painkillers (p.912) will also help to relieve a headache or abdominal pain. If the symptoms are severe, the doctor will probably prescribe specialized drugs (*see* ANTIMIGRAINE DRUGS, p.913). Drugs such as beta-blockers (p.898) may also be prescribed as a long-term treatment to help to prevent continuing attacks of migraine. Your child's diet may also be reviewed by a dietitian to identify foods that may trigger migraine attacks.

With treatment, the symptoms of childhood migraine can usually be controlled. Often, the condition disappears completely as a child becomes older, although in some cases migraine attacks continue throughout adulthood.

(WWW) ONLINE SITES: p.1028, p.1032

Meningitis in children

Inflammation of the membranes that cover the brain and spinal cord, usually caused by a bacterial or viral infection

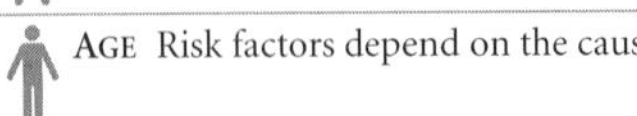

LIFESTYLE Living in close communities is a risk factor

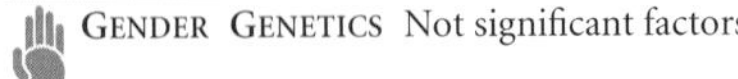

AGE Risk factors depend on the cause

GENDER GENETICS Not significant factors

Meningitis is a serious infection of the meninges (the membranes that cover the brain and spinal cord). Bacterial meningitis is a potentially fatal condition and causes between 150 and 200 deaths each year in the UK. About 8 in 10 cases of bacterial meningitis occur in children under the age of 5, and the disease is a cause of great concern to many parents. Outbreaks of the infection can occur in communities where children are in close contact with one another, such as nurseries and schools.

Meningitis that is caused by a viral infection is a much less severe disorder and is rarely life-threatening.

WHAT ARE THE CAUSES?

Bacterial meningitis in children is most often due to infection with *Neisseria meningitidis* (meningococcus), of which there are several types, or *Streptococcus pneumoniae.* Until recently, another major cause of meningitis was the bacterium *Haemophilus influenza* type b (Hib). In the UK, the introduction of routine immunization (p.45) for Hib and meningococcus type C has made these particular infections uncommon. However, no vaccine is available for meningococcus type B, which is now one of the most common causes of meningitis. A further meningococcal bacterium, type A, is rare in the UK. Tuberculosis (p.491) can also be a cause of bacterial meningitis but this form of the disease is uncommon in children.

Viral meningitis can be caused by a number of different viruses, including those responsible for chickenpox (p.290) and mumps (p.293).

WHAT ARE THE SYMPTOMS?

The symptoms of bacterial and viral meningitis are similar. However, bacterial meningitis tends to develop much more rapidly, and can cause serious illness within a few hours. Unlike adults, young children, especially those under 2 months of age, may not have obvious symptoms, and it is often difficult to distinguish the disease from other less serious infections. Symptoms likely to appear in young children include:

- Fever.
- Drowsiness or restlessness and high-pitched crying.
- Vomiting and/or diarrhoea.
- Reluctance to feed.
- In meningococcal meningitis, a distinctive rash of flat, reddish-purple lesions varying in size from pinheads to large patches that do not fade when pressed (*see* CHECKING A RED RASH, p.129).

Older children may, in addition, have the characteristic symptoms of meningitis in adults, which are:

- Severe headache and an extremely stiff neck, particularly when bending the head forwards.
- Dislike of bright lights.

If bacterial meningitis is left untreated, seizures may occur, followed by loss of consciousness, coma (p.522), and possibly death. Rarely, pus may collect in the brain (*see* BRAIN ABSCESS, p.529).

WHAT MIGHT BE DONE?

A child with meningitis needs urgent hospital treatment, often in an intensive care unit (p.958). When bacterial meningitis is suspected, one or more intravenous antibiotics (p.885) will be given before any tests are carried out. A lumbar puncture (p.527), to remove a sample of fluid from around the spinal cord, will be performed to confirm the diagnosis. The antibiotics will be discontinued if the spinal fluid does not contain bacteria associated with meningitis. The child will be given fluids intravenously to prevent dehydration,

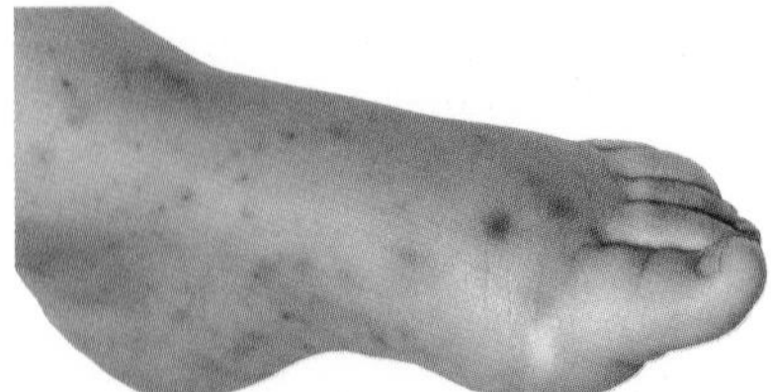

Rash of meningococcal meningitis
This distinctive rash, which can develop anywhere on the body and does not disappear when pressed, is a hallmark of meningococcal meningitis.

and anticonvulsant drugs (p.914) may be prescribed if he or she has seizures.

Close contacts, such as family members and children in the same class as your child, may be given oral antibiotics as a precaution.

WHAT IS THE PROGNOSIS?

Children with viral meningitis usually recover fully in about 2 weeks. Bacterial meningitis proves fatal in about 1 in 20 cases. About 1 in 4 children who recovers has long-term problems such as impaired hearing or epilepsy (p.524).

(WWW) ONLINE SITES: p.1028, p.1033

Febrile convulsions

Seizures caused by a high fever as a result of infection in a part of the body other than the brain

AGE Most common between the ages of 6 months and 5 years

GENDER Slightly more common in boys

GENETICS Sometimes runs in families

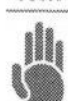
LIFESTYLE Not a significant factor

A febrile convulsion is the most common type of seizure in childhood and may affect as many as 1 in 20 children. The disorder occurs slightly more often in boys. Usually, a febrile convulsion occurs in the first 24 hours of a viral infection, such as a sore throat or common cold (p.288). Sometimes, a seizure may occur in association with a bacterial infection, such as an infection of the ears or upper respiratory tract. The convulsion develops in response to a rapid increase in body temperature that triggers an abnormal burst of electrical activity in the cells of the child's brain.

A febrile convulsion causes jerking body movements and is alarming for parents. However, the disorder is rarely serious, and it does not indicate a brain defect or epilepsy (p.524). Febrile convulsions sometimes run in families.

WHAT ARE THE SYMPTOMS?

Initially, you may notice that your child becomes limp. The symptoms that follow usually include:

- Loss of consciousness.
- Stiffening of the arms and legs and arching of the back.
- Abnormal movements of the limbs.
- Rolling upwards of the eyes.
- A slight pause in breathing, sometimes resulting in bluish skin.

A febrile convulsion usually lasts for about 2–4 minutes and always less than 15 minutes. Your child will probably fall asleep afterwards. If your child has a seizure of any kind, you should contact the doctor immediately. If the convulsion lasts for longer than 5 minutes, call an ambulance at once.

WHAT CAN I DO?

You should not try to restrain a child who is having a febrile convulsion but protect him or her from injury by placing nearby objects out of reach and surrounding the child with pillows or rolled-up towels. After the convulsion is over, sponging the child all over with tepid water helps to bring down a fever, but he or she should not be made too cool (*see* FIRST AID: FEBRILE CONVULSIONS, p.989). When awake enough to be able to swallow, the child should be given a dose of liquid paracetamol (*see* PAINKILLERS, p.912), which also helps to lower body temperature.

WHAT MIGHT THE DOCTOR DO?

The convulsion is usually over by the time the doctor sees your child. He or she will perform a physical examination and make sure that your child's temperature is coming down. The doctor may arrange for your child to be admitted to hospital, particularly if his or her body temperature remains high. A sample of cerebrospinal fluid may be extracted from around the spine (*see* LUMBAR PUNCTURE, p.527) to check that the seizure was not caused by meningitis (*see* MENINGITIS IN CHILDREN, opposite page). Other tests, such as urine tests or throat swabs, may also be performed to look for a bacterial infection.

If your child has a febrile convulsion lasting for longer than a few minutes or has had two or more convulsions, he or she may need to be given anticonvulsant drugs (p.914). The doctor will prescribe antibiotics (p.885) if a bacterial infection is present. Up to 1 in 3 children who have had a febrile convulsion will have another within a year. About 2–6 per cent of affected children will go on to develop epilepsy in later life.

(WWW) ONLINE SITES: p.1028, p.1032, p.1033

Reye's syndrome

A rare illness in which there is sudden inflammation of the brain and liver

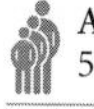
AGE Most common between the ages of 5 and 10

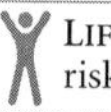
LIFESTYLE Taking aspirin in childhood is a risk factor

GENDER GENETICS Not significant factors

Reye's syndrome is an extremely rare condition, affecting fewer than 1 in 100,000 children each year in the UK. The disorder causes inflammation of the brain (*see* VIRAL ENCEPHALITIS, p.528) and the liver (*see* ACUTE HEPATITIS, p.644) and can be fatal. It almost always occurs in children under the age of 10. The exact cause of Reye's syndrome is not known, but it is thought that in some cases the disorder may be associated with a viral infection, such as chickenpox (p.290). Aspirin is linked to Reye's syndrome and is no longer recommended for children under the age of 12. Exposure to certain insecticides is also believed to trigger Reye's syndrome.

The symptoms develop very rapidly over a few hours and may include vomiting, drowsiness, and seizures. As the disorder progresses, there may be loss of consciousness, coma (p.522), and eventually cessation of breathing.

WHAT MIGHT BE DONE?

If a child is very sick, he or she will be admitted to an intensive care unit (p.958). Tests to confirm the diagnosis include blood tests to assess liver function, a tracing of the electrical activity in the brain (*see* EEG, p.525), and CT scanning (p.247) or MRI (p.248) to look for brain swelling. A sample of the liver may be removed for microscopic examination (*see* LIVER BIOPSY, p.647).

There is no specific cure for Reye's syndrome, but supportive treatment, such as mechanical ventilation, will be given until the condition improves. More than half of all children who have Reye's syndrome recover spontaneously. However, for those who lapse into a deep coma, the outlook is poor, and the condition may be fatal. In some cases, Reye's syndrome leads to long-term developmental problems, such as speech and learning difficulties.

(WWW) ONLINE SITES: p.1028

Brain and spinal cord tumours in children

Abnormal growths in the brain or spinal cord that are usually cancerous

 **AGE** More common under the age of 1

 **GENDER** Slightly more common in boys

 **GENETICS** The underlying cause may be inherited

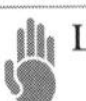 **LIFESTYLE** Not a significant factor

Tumours of the brain and spinal cord are rare in children but still account for almost 1 in 4 cases of all childhood cancers. The disorder is more common in boys and in children under 1 year old. Most of these tumours originate in the nerve cells of the brain or spine or in the cells surrounding the nerves. The tumours are usually cancerous but rarely spread elsewhere. The cause of such tumours is not fully understood, but the risk is increased if a child has the inherited disorder neurofibromatosis (p.827), in which tumours grow along the nerves.

WHAT ARE THE SYMPTOMS?

The symptoms of brain tumours usually develop gradually and at first may be vague, such as failure to gain weight in babies or poor school performance in older children. Tumours are therefore often not diagnosed until they are quite large, when symptoms may include:

- Headache and vomiting, especially in the morning.
- Clumsiness and unsteadiness.
- Abnormal alignment of the eyes (*see* STRABISMUS, p.857).
- Change in personality.

Sometimes, excess fluid builds up in the brain cavities (*see* HYDROCEPHALUS, p.845). If a tumour is in the spinal cord, the symptoms may include:

- Back pain.
- Inability to pass urine.
- Difficulty in walking.

Children with back pain should be seen by a doctor as soon as possible.

WHAT MIGHT BE DONE?

If the doctor is concerned that a child may have a brain or spinal cord tumour, he or she will arrange for imaging tests such as CT scanning (p.247) or MRI (p.248) to look for abnormalities. If a tumour is found, a small piece of tissue may be removed under general anaesthesia for microscopic examination.

Once the diagnosis has been confirmed, surgery is usually carried out to remove the tumour. Radiotherapy (p.281) may also be given, but, because it can affect the normal development of the brain in young children, a reduced dosage is given to children under 3 years of age. In some cases, chemotherapy (p.280) may be used. If there is an accumulation of excess fluid around the brain, a small tube may be inserted to drain the fluid into the abdomen (*see* SHUNT FOR HYDROCEPHALUS, p.845).

If a child has a tumour, a team of professionals will be available to offer his or her whole family psychological support (*see* COUNSELLING, p.971).

WHAT IS THE PROGNOSIS?

Although brain and spinal tumours are serious and often diagnosed late, 1 in 2 children is alive 5 years after diagnosis. The outlook depends on the type of tumour. Some children who survive after treatment may have long-term physical disabilities or learning problems.

(WWW) ONLINE SITES: p.1028

Neuroblastoma

A cancerous tumour that develops from nervous tissue, often in the adrenal gland

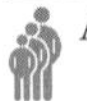 **AGE** More common under the age of 5

 **GENDER** Slightly more common in boys

 **GENETICS** May be due to an abnormal gene

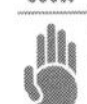 **LIFESTYLE** Not a significant factor

Although rare, neuroblastomas are still the most common cancerous tumours in children under 1 year. The disorder is slightly more common in boys. Most of these tumours originate from nerve tissue that has not developed beyond the embryonic stage. Neuroblastomas may occur in the abdomen or, less commonly, in the chest or pelvic cavity and often spread elsewhere. A third of all neuroblastomas develop in the adrenal glands, above the kidneys. The cause of these tumours is not known, although a genetic factor is thought to be involved.

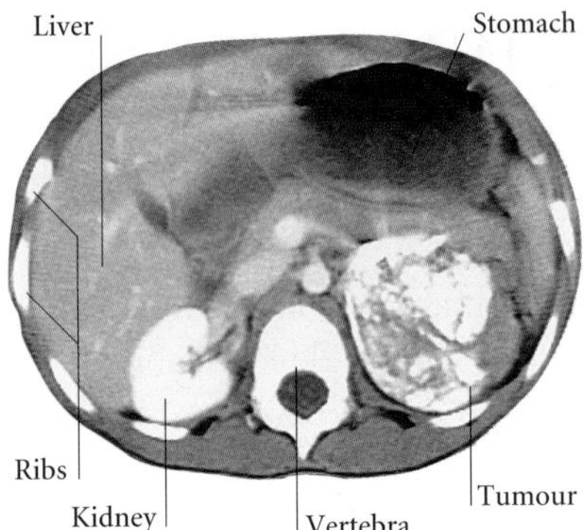

Neuroblastoma

This cross-sectional CT scan of a child's upper abdomen shows a neuroblastoma that has developed from the nervous tissue in one of the adrenal glands.

WHAT ARE THE SYMPTOMS?

The symptoms of neuroblastoma may be present from birth or develop gradually in childhood. They may include:

- Lump in the abdomen.
- Painless, bluish lumps on the skin.
- Tiredness.
- "Dancing" eye movements.

If a neuroblastoma spreads through the body, other symptoms may occur, such as bone pain or, if the lymph nodes are affected, swellings in the neck or armpits. Anaemia (p.446) may result if the cancer spreads to the bone marrow.

WHAT MIGHT BE DONE?

If the doctor suspects a neuroblastoma, he or she may arrange for a urine test to check for substances that indicate the presence of a tumour. The diagnosis is confirmed by a biopsy, in which a tissue sample is removed for examination. MRI (p.248) or radionuclide scanning (p.251) may be needed to find out if the cancer has spread elsewhere. A bone marrow aspiration and biopsy (p.451) may also be performed to look for the spread of cancer to the bones. If possible, the tumour is removed surgically. Chemotherapy (p.280) and radiotherapy (p.281) may also be necessary.

If a tumour has not spread, about 9 in 10 children remain well 5 years after surgery. When a tumour has spread, the outlook is poor, with only about 2 in 10 children surviving more than a year after the diagnosis. In babies under 1 year of age, neuroblastomas may disappear without requiring treatment.

(WWW) ONLINE SITES: p.1028

DEVELOPMENTAL AND PSYCHOLOGICAL DISORDERS

A child's development is a continuous process, marked by identifiable advances in skills and behaviour. The rate at which an individual develops is influenced by many factors, including the family environment and physical health. In some children, psychological disorders may cause developmental delays.

If a child has persistent problems with basic aspects of daily living, such as sleeping, eating, and toilet training, the effects can be very disruptive to the family. The first three articles in this section describe the types of minor behaviour problems that commonly occur in children. These difficulties can often be overcome with simple self-help measures, and most will eventually cease as a child matures. Only rarely do such behaviours indicate underlying psychological problems.

A further article covers the more serious problems that may be caused by autism spectrum disorders, which result in failure to develop normal communication and social skills. Autism, which may be linked to brain abnormalities, is a lifelong condition, but its effects can usually be reduced by appropriate education and therapy.

The next articles describe disorders that may delay children's achievement of certain developmental milestones. These range from generalized learning disabilities, which can affect all areas of development, to specific learning disabilities and speech difficulties in an otherwise normal child.

Attention deficit disorder and conduct disorder are covered in the last two articles. These behavioural disorders tend to have underlying medical, psychiatric, or social causes. Affected children usually respond to skilled guidance and therapy.

Sleeping problems in children

Disturbed sleep at night, which may lead to a disruption of family life

AGE More common under the age of 5

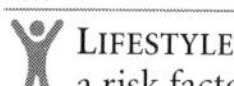
LIFESTYLE A stressful home environment is a risk factor

GENDER GENETICS Not significant factors

Many children sleep through the night by the age of 12 months, but about 1 in 3 children has frequent wakeful nights until the age of 5 or even later. Sleeping problems rarely cause ill health but may disrupt family life and can affect school performance in older children.

Disrupted sleep in children is usually temporary and may occur only because of a lack of or change to daily routine. Sleeping problems may also be related to illnesses, particularly those causing a high temperature, or to anxiety, such as that caused by family quarrels.

WHAT ARE THE TYPES?

Sleeping problems in children take various forms. In toddlers, one of the most common problems is an inability to settle down and go to sleep after being left alone at bedtime. Such restlessness is sometimes caused by anxiety about separation from a parent. Difficulty settling down can also be due to a noisy environment or fear of the dark. The problem may simply be due to bedtime being too early; children vary in the amount of sleep they need.

Most children wake briefly several times during the night without needing attention. However, sudden wakefulness is sometimes caused by nightmares, particularly in children about 5 years of age. Nightmares are commonly triggered by frightening or unusual experiences and, if they occur frequently, may be a sign that a child has a particular worry.

Night terrors are another type of sudden sleep disturbance, which may occur for no apparent reason. During an episode of night terror, a child experiences acute fear and may scream. Although the child seems to be awake, he or she is actually still asleep. If a child wakes from a night terror, he or she usually has little or no memory of the episode. Night terrors usually occur about 2 hours after falling asleep and last only a few minutes. Just before a night terror, a child may appear restless.

Sleepwalking most often occurs in children between the ages of 6 and 12. A sleepwalking child will get out of bed and wander around aimlessly, usually finding his or her own way back to bed.

WHAT MIGHT BE DONE?

Simple measures are often effective in overcoming a sleeping problem. You should try to establish regular routines, with a bath and a story at the same time every night. There is no need to go to a child as soon as he or she cries; often, the crying will stop within a few minutes. If you think that poor sleeping or nightmares are related to an underlying anxiety, such as a frightening television programme or family stress, you should discuss the problem with your child.

If your child has night terrors, it may be possible to wake him or her in the restless period that precedes the terror. Once a terror begins, there is little you can do except stay with the child until the fear recedes. In the case of sleepwalking, try not to wake the child but gently guide him or her back to bed.

You should consult the doctor if your child's sleep problem disrupts the family or if you think that nightmares or night terrors have a particular cause.

In most cases, providing a child with reassurance and introducing a routine will help to establish a normal sleeping pattern within a few weeks. Most children eventually learn to settle down at night and outgrow nightmares, night terrors, or sleepwalking. By the age of 8, few children have sleeping problems.

(WWW) ONLINE SITES: p.1028, p.1036

Eating problems in children

Changes in eating behaviour that may indicate psychological stress

LIFESTYLE A stressful home environment is a risk factor

AGE GENDER Risk factors depend on the type

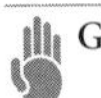
GENETICS Not a significant factor

Eating problems in childhood are very common, affecting about 1 in 10 young children. Usually, the problem is part of growing up and disappears as the child matures. However, persistent problems may be linked to stresses in family life.

WHAT ARE THE TYPES?

Some children appear to eat too little or are fussy about their food. Other children may overeat or have cravings for strange nonfood substances.

Refusing food is often the way in which toddlers try to assert their independence, and the problem is serious only if normal growth or weight gain is affected. Food refusal in older children may be due to emotional distress and, in very severe cases, may be a sign of anorexia nervosa (p.562), particularly in girls. Loss of appetite, which is common during childhood illnesses, is not the same as food refusal, although it may also be caused by anxiety.

Fussy eating habits affect about 1 in 4 children of school age. The fussy child insists on eating only certain foods, but dietary problems rarely occur unless the range of foods is very narrow.

Pica is a craving to eat nonfood substances, such as soil, coal, or chalk. This disorder can sometimes be hazardous. For example, licking or eating certain types of paint can cause severe lead poisoning. Pica usually occurs in children who have other behavioural problems and is possibly associated with a nutritional deficiency, such as a lack of iron.

Overeating commonly leads to obesity. A child may eat for comfort if he or she feels neglected or insecure.

> SELF-HELP
>
> **ENCOURAGING YOUR CHILD TO EAT**
>
> If your child is overly fussy about certain food or refuses to eat, the following hints may be helpful:
>
> - Keep the atmosphere relaxed at mealtimes. Do not put pressure on your child to eat everything on his or her plate.
> - Serve small portions. You can always give second helpings.
> - Avoid too many snacks and excessive fluids between meals.
> - Be imaginative when preparing food. Cut sandwiches into decorative shapes and create "pictures" on the plate with fruit and vegetables.
> - Do not persist in offering rejected foods. Keep them off the menu for a week or two.
> - Avoid distractions, such as toys or television, at mealtimes.

WHAT MIGHT BE DONE?

If your child is reluctant to eat, there are practical ways in which you can help (*see* ENCOURAGING YOUR CHILD TO EAT, left). However, if the child fails to gain weight, loses weight, or has pica, you should consult the doctor. If the problem is caused by anxiety or emotional distress, the doctor may refer your child to a child psychologist or psychiatrist.

(WWW) ONLINE SITES: p.1028, p.1035

Encopresis

Inappropriate defecation after the age at which bowel control is usually attained

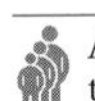
AGE Considered abnormal only after about the age of 4

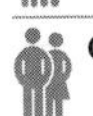
GENDER More common in boys

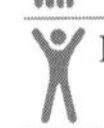
LIFESTYLE Stress is a risk factor

GENETICS Not a significant factor

Most children have achieved bowel control by the age of 3. If a child is still soiling by the age of 4, there may be a psychological or physical reason. Soiling problems, which are more common in boys, are known as encopresis. Sometimes, the behaviour is simply the result of inadequate toilet training. However, children occasionally begin soiling again after successful training. The most common cause of this recurrence is overflow of liquid faeces from above a hard, constipated stool (*see* CONSTIPATION IN CHILDREN, p.865). Some children pass normal faeces in unacceptable places, such as behind furniture. This soiling may be related to emotional stress.

WHAT MIGHT BE DONE?

A sympathetic approach to encopresis is vital, because scolding and criticizing a child often makes the problem worse. Usually, patient toilet training is all that is required. If you suspect that your child is constipated, you should change his or her diet to include more fibre.

If simple measures are not effective, you should consult your doctor. In the case of severe constipation, the doctor will probably advise on diet and may prescribe laxatives (p.924). Causes of emotional distress can often be identified after discussion with the child.

Encopresis usually disappears with unhurried toilet training once constipation has been treated or emotional problems have been addressed.

(WWW) ONLINE SITES: p.1028

Autism spectrum disorders

Severely impaired development of normal communication and social skills

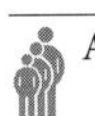
AGE Usually develop before the age of 3

GENDER More common in boys

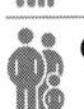
GENETICS Sometimes run in families

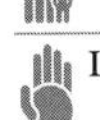
LIFESTYLE Not a significant factor

Autism was first identified in 1943 and is now known to affect between 2 and 4 of every 10,000 children in the UK. There are varying forms of autism known as autism spectrum disorders, and affected children have a wide range of symptoms. In general, there is a failure to develop language and communication skills, inability to form social relationships, and a marked need to follow routines. These disorders are more common in boys.

At least 2 in 3 autistic children have generalized learning disabilities (p.854). Rarely, affected children have normal or above-average intelligence, a form of autism known as Asperger's syndrome.

Autism spectrum disorders are possibly caused by abnormalities of the brain. The disorders sometimes run in families, which suggests that genetic factors may be involved. About 1 in 10 autistic children has a genetic abnormality, such as fragile X syndrome (p.822).

WHAT ARE THE SYMPTOMS?

Some autistic children show symptoms from birth, such as arching the back to avoid physical contact. In infancy, a child with autism may bang his or her head against the side of the cot. Other children may appear normal until they are about 12–18 months old, when the following symptoms become apparent:

- Failure to develop normal speech.
- Absence of normal facial expression and body language.
- Lack of eye contact.
- Tendency to spend time alone.
- Lack of imaginative play.
- Repetitive behaviour, such as rocking and hand flapping.
- Obsession with specific objects or particular routines.
- Severe learning difficulties.

Rarely, an autistic child has an exceptional skill, such as a particular aptitude for technical drawing, mathematics, or playing a musical instrument. About 1 in 3 affected children develops epilepsy (p.524). Children who have Asperger's syndrome may develop normal speech and language but have difficulty communicating with other people. These children are also rigid in their behaviour and cannot tolerate changes in routine.

ARE THERE COMPLICATIONS?

Autism spectrum disorders often have a devastating effect on family life. Bringing up an autistic child can be stressful, especially when the child is unable to show normal responsiveness and affection. Parents may find it difficult to take the child to public places because of his or her unusual or difficult behaviour. Other children in the family may feel neglected because an autistic sibling needs so much attention. A child with autism may also be at risk of self-harm.

WHAT MIGHT BE DONE?

Autism spectrum disorders are often first identified by parents who notice that their child's behaviour is different from that of other children in the same age group. The doctor will usually refer the child to a child psychiatrist. There are no specific tests to confirm the diagnosis. However, when a genetic disorder such as fragile X syndrome is suspected, blood tests may be performed to look for the genetic abnormality.

There is no cure for autism spectrum disorders. Treatment normally focuses on education designed to maximize a child's potential. Language and speech therapy (p.963) can improve communication skills. Behaviour therapy (p.969) can help to replace abnormal behaviours with more appropriate ones, and occupational therapy can improve physical skills. A highly structured daily routine is usually recommended.

WHAT IS THE PROGNOSIS?

Most children with autism spectrum disorders cannot lead independent lives and require long-term care, either from their parents or in a residential home. Some people with Asperger's syndrome achieve academic success, although they may always have poor social skills.

(WWW) ONLINE SITES: p.1027

Developmental delay

Delay of a child in achieving the abilities expected at a particular age

 AGE Usually apparent by the age of 5

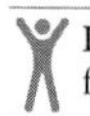 LIFESTYLE Lack of stimulation is a risk factor

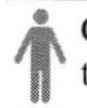 GENDER GENETICS Risk factors depend on the cause

There are significant stages in the first few years of life, known as developmental milestones, when a child is normally expected to have acquired certain basic physical, intellectual, and social skills. Children achieve these milestones at different ages but usually within an established typical age range. Failure to reach the milestones within this range is known as developmental delay.

WHAT ARE THE TYPES?

Delays may be of varying severity and can affect one or more area of development. Children are usually mobile by about 9 months, and most are walking by 15 months. A delay in walking frequently runs in families and often has no obvious cause; most children catch up eventually and continue to develop normally. However, children who have a severe underlying disability, such as cerebral palsy (p.846), will have long-term difficulties with mobility.

Some children are slow to develop movements that involve good hand–eye coordination or fine control, such as catching a ball or using a pencil. These children should be monitored carefully because they are at risk of experiencing specific learning disabilities (p.854) during their school years.

Delay in acquiring speech and language ranges from minor difficulties in increasing vocabulary (*see* SPEECH AND LANGUAGE DIFFICULTIES, p.854) to the severe communication problems often associated with autism spectrum disorders (opposite page). Sometimes, delay is due to a lack of stimulation in the child's environment. Hearing problems, which can be due to disorders such as chronic secretory otitis media (p.860), may also be a cause of delayed development in speech and language skills.

Certain basic accomplishments, such as learning to use the toilet unaided, are acquired only slowly in some children. Usually, these skills improve with time, but occasionally there may be underlying problems (*see* BEDWETTING, p.872, and ENCOPRESIS, opposite page).

Developmental delays that affect all areas of learning and general ability are usually caused by underlying disorders, such as Down's syndrome (p.821) or inborn errors of metabolism (p.867), but often the underlying cause cannot be identified. Such delays in development can lead later to a diagnosis of generalized learning disabilities (p.854).

WHAT MIGHT BE DONE?

Developmental delays are usually first noticed by parents who are concerned when a child does not reach the normal milestones for his or her age group. A delay may also be detected at routine developmental checkups during the first 5 years of life. If a problem is suspected, your doctor may arrange for a full developmental assessment, which normally includes hearing tests (*see* HEARING TESTS IN CHILDREN, p.859) and vision tests (*see* VISION TESTS IN CHILDREN, p.857). Tests may be performed on a sample of the child's blood to check for a genetic abnormality.

A child with delay in one area of development may only need encouragement to begin to catch up. Many children with mild delays develop normally over a period of time, especially if the cause is understimulation and the problem is given appropriate treatment. Other children benefit from help, such as speech therapy (p.963), in particular areas of development. A child with more severe delays will need specialized treatment.

(WWW) ONLINE SITES: p.1028

Generalized learning disabilities

Difficulties with all areas of learning experienced by children with significantly lower than average intelligence

AGE Usually becomes apparent in early childhood

GENETICS Risk factors depend on the cause

GENDER LIFESTYLE Not significant factors

A child with generalized learning disabilities has poor intellectual skills, leading to developmental delay (p.853). Generalized learning disabilities can affect speech, language, reading, and writing. Physical development may be affected, causing general clumsiness and poor hand–eye coordination. Behavioural problems may also develop.

There is often no obvious cause for mild generalized learning disabilities, which may not be noticeable until an affected child reaches school age. Severe learning disabilities usually have an obvious cause, such as the genetic disorders Down's syndrome (p.821) or fragile X syndrome (p.822).

WHAT MIGHT BE DONE?

Mild general learning disabilities are usually first suspected by parents or teachers when a child fails to develop skills at the same rate as his or her peers or is experiencing difficulties at school. In more severe cases, delays in development are usually detected at an early stage in childhood, often during routine developmental checkups.

If a child is thought to have generalized learning disabilities, the doctor will probably arrange for a full developmental assessment, including hearing tests (*see* HEARING TESTS IN CHILDREN, p.859) and vision tests (*see* VISION TESTS IN CHILDREN, p.857). Blood tests to check for evidence of genetic abnormalities may also be performed.

Most affected children have special educational needs and will benefit from attending classes or schools where they can have individual attention. Parents will be supported by a team of specialists, who may provide physiotherapy (p.961) and speech therapy (p.963).

Many children with mild generalized learning disabilities can do well if they receive appropriate education and support. Those who are severely affected usually need lifelong supervision.

(WWW) ONLINE SITES: p.1034

Specific learning disabilities

Difficulties in one or several areas of learning in a child of average or above average intelligence

AGE Usually become apparent between the ages of 3 and 7

GENDER More common in boys

GENETICS Sometimes run in families

LIFESTYLE Not a significant factor

A child whose development is delayed in one or several areas of learning but who has normal intelligence probably has a specific learning disability. Such disabilities are thought to affect up to 15 in 100 otherwise normally developed children and are a common cause of poor achievement at school. Specific learning disabilities are more common in boys.

Dyslexia is a common example of a specific learning disability and affects a child's ability to read or write. In dyscalculia, a child has specific problems with mathematics. Dyspraxia is a learning disability that affects coordination, particularly finely controlled movement, often leading to clumsiness.

In most cases, the cause of a particular learning disability is not known. However, such conditions sometimes run in families, suggesting that genetic factors may be involved. In some cases, specific learning disabilities are due to problems with vision or hearing.

WHAT ARE THE SYMPTOMS?

The symptoms of specific learning disabilities are usually first recognized in early school years and may include:

- Difficulty coping with reading, writing, and/or mathematics.
- Problems telling left from right.
- Poor coordination and difficulty with sports and other physical activities.

A child may also become frustrated and develop behavioural problems, such as extreme shyness or aggression.

WHAT MIGHT BE DONE?

If a specific learning disability is suspected, a full assessment of a child's academic and developmental skills will be made. Hearing tests (*see* HEARING TESTS IN CHILDREN, p.859) and vision tests (*see* VISION TESTS IN CHILDREN, p.857) may also be performed to rule out the presence of physical conditions that may cause delays in learning.

Parents and teachers should work together to encourage an affected child. In many cases, specialized teaching is necessary. Disorders causing impaired hearing or vision can often be treated successfully. Many children do well if the appropriate remedial treatment is given, but some continue to experience difficulties throughout life.

(WWW) ONLINE SITES: p.1034

Speech and language difficulties

The slow or abnormal development of understanding and expression of language

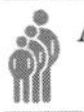
AGE Usually develop in early childhood

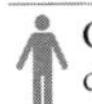
GENDER GENETICS LIFESTYLE Risk factors depend on the type

There is wide variation in the age at which speech and language skills are acquired, but most children are able to communicate verbally well before the age of 3. Many children have some type of speech and language difficulty in their early years, commonly only a minor impediment, such as a lisp, that rapidly improves with increasing maturity.

A common cause of delay in speech and language development is hearing impairment (*see* CHRONIC SECRETORY OTITIS MEDIA, p.860, and CONGENITAL DEAFNESS, p.859). Children who have cerebral palsy (p.846) and those with a cleft lip and palate (p.862) may have difficulty coordinating the movements of their mouth and tongue. Slowness in acquiring speech and language skills may be due to lack of intellectual stimulation or developmental delay (p.853). Severe generalized learning disabilities (opposite page) may cause speech and language difficulties.

Difficulties with fluency of speech, for example stuttering, affect about 1 in 100 children, especially boys, and sometimes run in families.

WHAT MIGHT BE DONE?

A speech or language difficulty may first be noticed by parents or teachers or at a routine developmental checkup. A full assessment of the child's development and hearing will then be made.

A child with a speech or language difficulty usually catches up with his or her peers when given appropriate guidance. Impaired hearing will be treated when possible. Stuttering can often be improved with speech therapy (p.963).

Once the underlying cause is treated, most speech and language difficulties improve. However, if there is a physical cause, such as cerebral palsy, the speech or language difficulty may persist.

(WWW) ONLINE SITES: p.1037

Attention deficit disorder

A behavioural disorder in which a child consistently has a high level of activity and/or difficulty attending to tasks

 AGE Usually develops in early childhood

 GENDER More common in boys

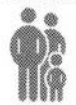 GENETICS Often runs in families

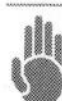 LIFESTYLE Not a significant factor

Attention deficit disorder (ADD), also known as attention deficit hyperactivity, or hyperkinetic, disorder, is a condition that affects up to 1 in 20 children in the UK. The disorder, which is more common in boys, should not be confused with the normal boisterous conduct of a healthy child. Children with ADD consistently show abnormal patterns of behaviour over a period of time. An affected child is likely to be restless, unable to sit still for more than a few moments, inattentive, and impulsive.

The causes of ADD are not fully understood. However, the disorder often runs in families, which suggests that genetic factors may be involved. ADD is not, as popularly believed, a result of poor parenting or abuse.

WHAT ARE THE SYMPTOMS?

The symptoms of ADD develop in early childhood, usually between the ages of 3 and 7, and may include:

- Inability to finish tasks.
- Short attention span and inability to concentrate in class.
- Difficulty following instructions.
- Tendency to talk excessively and frequently interrupt others.
- Difficulty waiting or taking turns.
- Inability to play quietly alone.
- Physical impulsiveness.

Children with ADD may have difficulty forming friendships. Self-esteem is often low because an affected child is frequently scolded and criticized.

WHAT MIGHT BE DONE?

The doctor will probably refer a child with suspected ADD to a child psychiatry team. The diagnosis is normally made following discussion with parents and observation of the child. However, ADD is often difficult to diagnose in preschool children. Parents have a key role in their child's treatment and are usually given training in techniques that help to improve the child's behaviour. These techniques are based on giving praise for good behaviour rather than criticism for inappropriate conduct. An affected child may also benefit from structured teaching in small groups.

For some children, the doctor may prescribe drugs that help to improve concentration and reduce disruptive behaviour (*see* CENTRAL NERVOUS SYSTEM STIMULANT DRUGS, p.918).

In most affected children, the disorder continues throughout adolescence, although the behavioural problems may become less severe in older children. A small proportion of those with ADD later develop conduct disorder (right), in which a child consistently displays antisocial and unruly behaviour.

(WWW) ONLINE SITES: p.1028

Conduct disorder

A behavioural disorder in which a child persistently behaves in an antisocial or disruptive manner

 AGE More common in late childhood and adolescence

 GENDER More common in boys

 GENETICS Sometimes runs in families

 LIFESTYLE An emotionally unstable home environment is a risk factor

Most children are mischievous from time to time, and some may become rebellious, especially as they reach adolescence. Conduct disorder is suspected only if a child or adolescent persists in antisocial or disruptive behaviour.

Many children with conduct disorder have failed to acquire a sense of right and wrong. They may have grown up in an unstable home environment in which there is family discord or violence and lack of parental supervision. Children with attention deficit disorder (left) are at increased risk of developing conduct disorder in later childhood.

Conduct disorder is more common in boys. The antisocial behaviour usually becomes more obvious towards adolescence, when an affected child may start to become aggressive and play truant from school. In some cases, a child will indulge in substance or alcohol abuse or become involved in criminal activities, such as theft, vandalism, assault, and arson. Children with conduct disorder often have low self-esteem and find it difficult to form relationships.

WHAT MIGHT BE DONE?

A diagnosis of conduct disorder is usually based on a psychiatric assessment of the child's behavioural patterns.

The treatment for conduct disorder is always aimed at the whole family. Therapy will be directed at overcoming conflicts or tensions within the family. Parents will be encouraged to reinforce good behaviour, and an aggressive child will be taught how to control his or her anger and to be considerate to others. However, only 1 in 3 children who has conduct disorder improves his or her behaviour. In most cases, antisocial behaviour persists throughout adult life.

(WWW) ONLINE SITES: p.1028

EYE AND EAR DISORDERS

Vision and hearing are important to a child's development because the eyes and ears collect information about the environment and play a key role in the acquisition of speech and language. Most eye and ear disorders are diagnosed during routine examinations in childhood.

KEY ANATOMY

Cornea
Retina
Pupil
Optic nerve
Lens
EYE

Inner ear
Middle ear
Outer ear
Eustachian tube
Eardrum
EAR

For more information on the structure and function of the eyes and ears, *see* pp.566–569 and pp.592–595.

The first article in this section covers congenital blindness, in which a child is born with impaired vision. The following articles discuss conditions such as strabismus, in which vision is affected due to misalignment of the gaze of the eyes, and amblyopia, in which a child's vision fails to develop normally. Both conditions can be treated successfully if they are diagnosed early. The remaining articles cover ear disorders. The most common cause of earache in children is acute otitis media. Repeated episodes of this middle-ear condition may lead to chronic secretory otitis media, which is discussed next. Eye and ear disorders that can affect people of any age are covered in other sections of the book (*see* EYES AND VISION, pp.566–591, and EARS, HEARING, AND BALANCE, pp.592–605).

Congenital blindness

Severely impaired vision that is present from birth

 AGE Present at birth

 GENETICS Sometimes runs in families

 GENDER LIFESTYLE Not significant factors

Vision plays a very important part in a child's early development. Impaired vision at birth can cause serious delay in development and may lead to learning disabilities, particularly when it is associated with other difficulties, such as congenital deafness (p.859).

About 9 in 10 children considered blind from birth do have some vision, even though it may be as little as recognition of light and dark or shapes.

WHAT ARE THE CAUSES?

In the developed world, half of all cases of congenital blindness run in families and may be due to a genetic disorder. Other important causes are congenital infections (p.817) such as the protozoal infection toxoplasmosis (p.307) and the viral infection rubella (p.294). These infections are transmitted from the mother to the developing fetus during pregnancy and may lead to impaired vision in a newborn baby. However, congenital rubella is now rare in the developed world due to routine immunization. A baby's eyes may also be affected by cataracts (p.573), in which the eye lenses are opaque, or glaucoma (p.575), in which the optic nerve is damaged due to increased pressure within the eyes. Congenital blindness may also be caused by damage to the brain as a result of lack of oxygen during birth.

WHAT ARE THE SYMPTOMS?

Parents usually become aware that their baby has a vision problem within a few weeks of birth. He or she may be less responsive than other babies, lying quietly to make the most of his or her hearing. Parents may also notice that their baby:

- Is unable to fix his or her eyes on a close object.
- Has random, jerky eye movements.
- Does not smile by the age of 6 weeks.
- Has abnormally large, cloudy eyes if glaucoma is present.

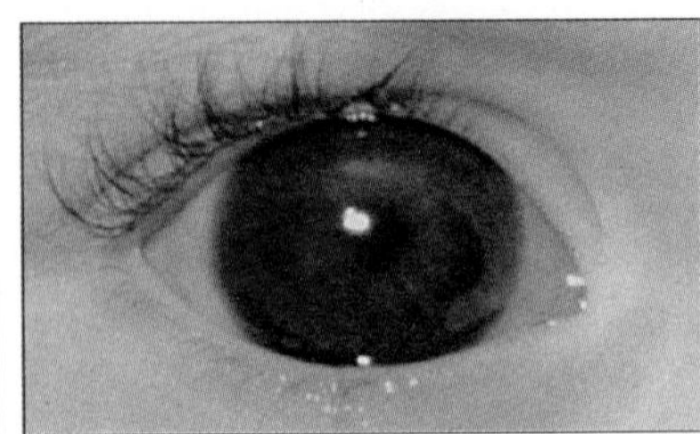

Congenital glaucoma
This child's eye appears enlarged and cloudy due to increased pressure within the eye caused by congenital glaucoma.

Parents may find it difficult to bond with a quiet baby who does not smile.

HOW IS IT DIAGNOSED?

If congenital blindness is not suspected by the baby's parents, it will probably be picked up during a routine examination in infancy. A child suspected of having impaired vision will be referred to a specialist for an examination and tests (*see* VISION TESTS IN CHILDREN, opposite page). His or her hearing will also be tested (*see* HEARING TESTS IN CHILDREN, p.859) because, if the child is severely visually impaired, he or she will need to rely on hearing.

WHAT IS THE TREATMENT?

It is possible to improve vision in only a small number of babies, such as those with cataracts or glaucoma. Early treatment of these conditions is important. Cataracts are usually removed surgically within the first month of life (*see* CATARACT SURGERY, p.573). Glaucoma may also be treated by surgery to allow fluid to drain from the eye.

If vision cannot be improved, much can be done to help a child to make maximum use of other senses or what little vision he or she has. If your child is diagnosed as blind, a team of specialists, including a teacher for the blind, will be available to give you and your child support and care. You will also be given advice on how to stimulate your child using speech, sounds, and touch and how to adapt your home so that your child is able to explore it safely and develop self-confidence. Some children require special schooling to learn braille, a system of raised dots that allows blind people to read and write.

Genetic counselling (p.272) is available for parents of an affected child who wish to have more children or for prospective parents who are blind.

WHAT IS THE PROGNOSIS?

Children treated for cataracts or glaucoma will probably still have impaired vision but often have enough sight to perform most activities unaided. Many blind or visually impaired children with no other disabilities go on to have successful personal and professional lives.

(WWW) ONLINE SITES: p.1031

Strabismus

Abnormal alignment of the gaze of one of the eyes, also known as crossed eyes or squint

 AGE Often occurs in early childhood

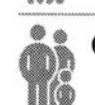 GENETICS Sometimes runs in families

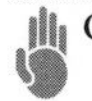 GENDER LIFESTYLE Not significant factors

Strabismus is a common condition in which only one eye points directly at the object being viewed. This abnormal alignment of the eyes causes the brain to receive conflicting images, which may result in double vision or, in children under the age of 8, suppression of the image from the misaligned eye.

Strabismus can be caused by any disorder of vision, such as longsightedness (*see* HYPERMETROPIA, p.586) or shortsightedness (*see* MYOPIA, p.586), and can run in families, suggesting a genetic factor. The condition may be caused by a structural difference between the muscles that control movement of the eyes. Very rarely, strabismus develops as a result of cancer of the eye (*see* RETINOBLASTOMA, p.858) or paralysis of the muscles in one eye caused by a serious underlying condition such as a tumour in the brain (*see* BRAIN AND SPINAL CORD TUMOURS IN CHILDREN, p.850).

Small babies often appear cross-eyed because of the arrangement of soft tissues around the eyes. This is normal and should not be confused with strabismus.

WHAT ARE THE SYMPTOMS?

If the condition is mild, the symptoms occur only when a child is tired, but in severe cases, they are present all the time. The symptoms of strabismus include:

- Misalignment of the gaze of one of the eyes.
- Poor vision in one of the eyes due to lack of use.

A child may cover or close the affected eye to see clearly and hold his or her head at an angle. Left untreated, strabismus may cause amblyopia (p.858), in which the vision in the affected eye does not develop normally.

(TEST) VISION TESTS IN CHILDREN

Vision tests in children are specifically tailored to age and ability and are routinely performed to look for defects that may delay normal development and learning. The need for glasses can be assessed in infants using tests such as retinoscopy, while older children may be asked to match shapes or letters. Once a child can read, a Snellen chart may be used to look for vision defects (*see* VISION TESTS, p.587).

RETINOSCOPY

This test can be performed on infants. Eyedrops are given about 30 minutes beforehand to dilate the pupils and prevent focusing. A beam of light is shone from an instrument called a retinoscope into each eye in turn. The effect of different lenses on the beam of light determines whether glasses are needed.

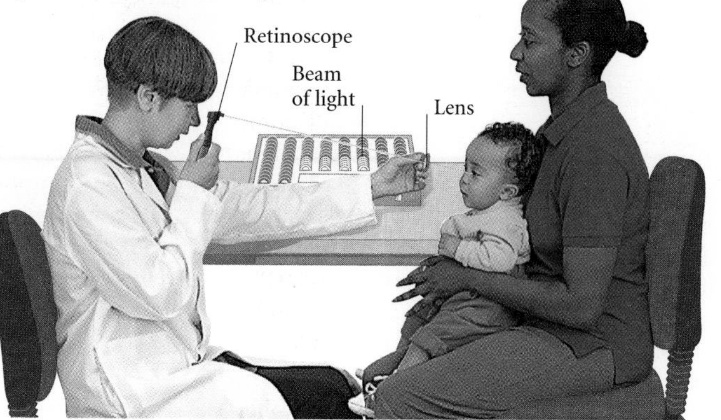

During the test
The test is performed in a darkened room. Each eye is tested individually.

LETTER MATCHING TEST

This test is designed for children of about 3 years of age. A child is given a card with letters printed on it. The doctor then holds up letters of decreasing size at a distance of 3 m (10 ft) and asks the child to identify the same letters on the card. By using an eye patch, each of the eyes can be tested separately.

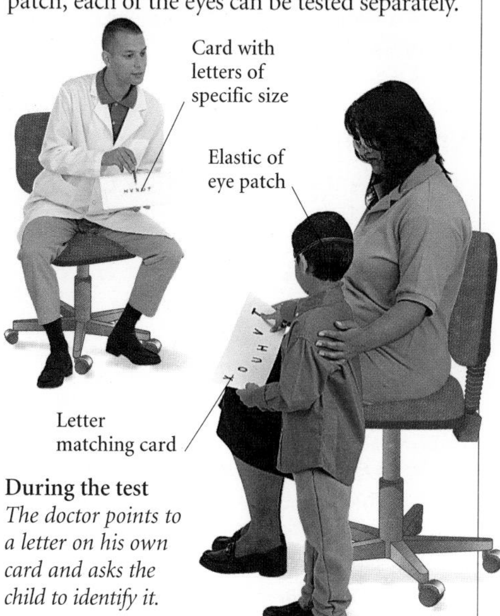

During the test
The doctor points to a letter on his own card and asks the child to identify it.

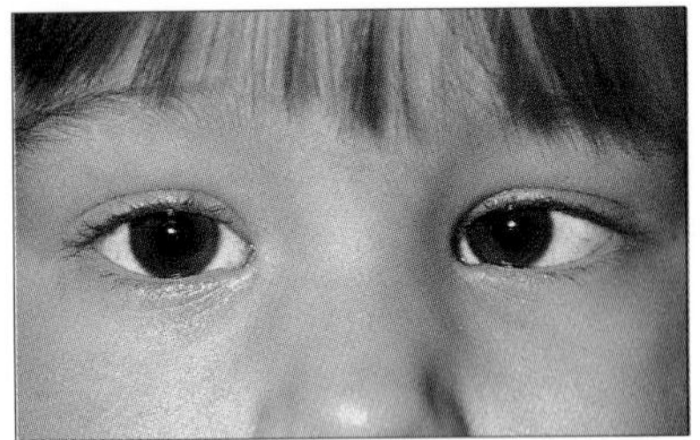

Strabismus
The gaze of this child's eyes is misaligned, a disorder known as strabismus, causing conflicting images to be sent to the brain.

WHAT MIGHT BE DONE?

The doctor will arrange for your child to have vision tests (*see* VISION TESTS IN CHILDREN, p.857). If the strabismus has developed suddenly, an imaging test, such as CT scanning (p.247), may be performed to look for a tumour.

The aim of treatment is to correct the strabismus. If your child has a vision disorder such as myopia, he or she may have to wear glasses, which should also correct strabismus. To treat amblyopia, your child may also be given a patch to wear over the unaffected eye for a period of time each day. Wearing the eye patch forces the child to use the weaker eye, which is essential for the normal development of vision. Your child will have regular checkups every 3 or 6 months until the strabismus is corrected. The treatment is usually successful, although the condition can recur. In some cases, surgery on the eye muscles may be necessary. In the rare cases in which the cause is a tumour, this will be removed.

(WWW) ONLINE SITES: p.1031

Amblyopia

Reduced vision that cannot be corrected by glasses

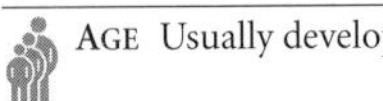
AGE Usually develops before the age of 5

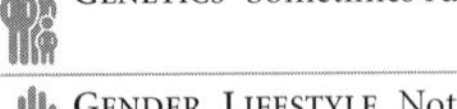
GENETICS Sometimes runs in families

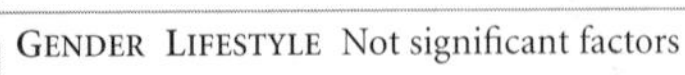
GENDER LIFESTYLE Not significant factors

Amblyopia develops in young children if each of the two eyes send a different image to the brain. The development of vision occurs until a child is about 5 years old and depends on the brain learning to combine the images from both eyes. If each eye produces a different image during this period, the brain responds by suppressing images it receives from the more unfocused eye, and vision does not develop normally. If the underlying cause is not treated by the age of 10, later attempts to correct vision will fail.

WHAT ARE THE CAUSES?

Any condition that causes each eye to send a different image to the brain may lead to amblyopia. Misalignment of the gaze of the eyes (*see* STRABISMUS, p.857) is the most common cause of amblyopia. Other causes include vision disorders in one eye, such as astigmatism (p.588), shortsightedness (*see* MYOPIA, p.586), and longsightedness (*see* HYPERMETROPIA, p.586). The condition sometimes runs in families, suggesting that genetic factors are involved.

WHAT MIGHT BE DONE?

If you suspect that your child cannot see clearly, you should consult the doctor without delay to minimize the risk of permanent visual impairment. Your child will probably be referred to an ophthalmologist, who will examine your child's eyes and assess vision (*see* VISION TESTS IN CHILDREN, p.857).

Treatment depends on the underlying cause of amblyopia. If your child has a vision disorder such as shortsightedness, this may be corrected by wearing glasses. If vision in one eye is reduced, wearing a patch over the good eye for at least 5 hours each day for several months forces the brain to process visual information from the weaker eye, whatever the underlying cause. If your child has to wear an eye patch to correct amblyopia, he or she will need support and encouragement, especially if vision in the affected eye is poor.

Left untreated, strabismus may lead to amblyopia. In some cases, an operation to correct strabismus is necessary to prevent amblyopia from developing.

WHAT IS THE PROGNOSIS?

The outlook for children with amblyopia depends on when the condition is detected and treatment to correct it begins. Amblyopia is usually at least partially reversible in children under the age of 10. Older children with the condition will probably already have some degree of permanent visual impairment.

(WWW) ONLINE SITES: p.1031

Retinoblastoma

A rare cancer of the retina, the light-sensitive membrane at the back of the eye

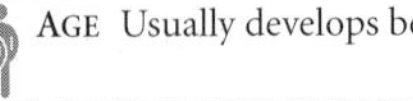
AGE Usually develops before the age of 2

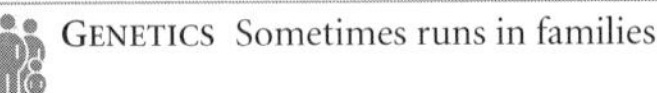
GENETICS Sometimes runs in families

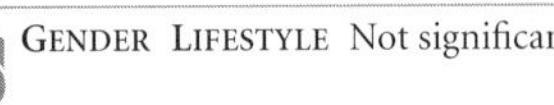
GENDER LIFESTYLE Not significant factors

In the UK, about 1 in 20,000 babies is affected with retinoblastoma, a rare cancer of the retina (the light-sensitive membrane at the back of the eye). The condition can develop in one or both of the eyes, usually before a child reaches 2 years of age. Of those affected, about 1 child in 5 has retinoblastoma in both eyes. About half of all cases are caused by an abnormal gene, which is located on chromosome 13 and is inherited in an autosomal dominant manner (*see* GENE DISORDERS, p.271). In the remaining cases, the cause is unknown.

The most common symptom is the development of a whitened area behind the pupil. Impaired vision caused by retinoblastoma may lead to strabismus (p.857). Left untreated, the cancer can spread to other parts of the body.

WHAT MIGHT BE DONE?

If the doctor suspects that a child has retinoblastoma, he or she will refer the child to a specialist, who will examine the eyes, possibly under general anaesthesia. The child may also have blood tests to look for the abnormal gene. If retinoblastoma is confirmed, CT scanning (p.247) or MRI (p.248) may be done to see if the cancer has spread.

The aim of treatment is to cure the cancer and, if possible, to retain vision

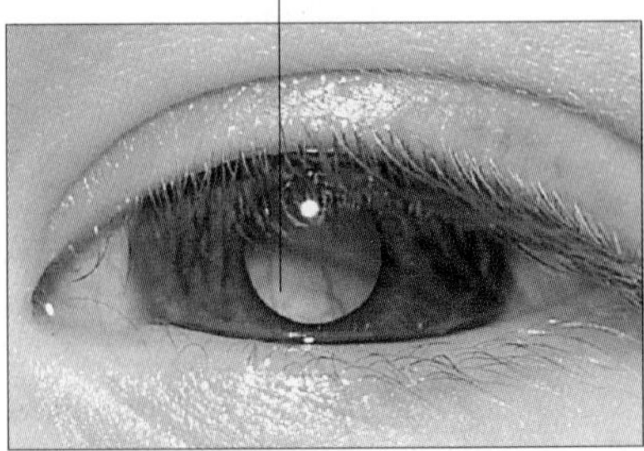

Retinoblastoma
The pale area seen through the pupil of this eye is a retinoblastoma, a rare cancer of the membrane at the back of the eye.

in the affected eyes. It is usually possible to destroy small cancerous tumours in the retina by freezing the tissue. However, surgical removal of the entire eye will probably be necessary to treat large tumours. Treatment with chemotherapy (p.280) and radiotherapy (p.281) may also be required if the cancer has spread.

What is the prognosis?

In most cases, the cancer can be cured, but the child's vision may be severely impaired. Genetic counselling (p.272) is available to relatives of an affected child and to adults treated for retinoblastoma in childhood. The siblings of an affected child should have regular eye tests.

(WWW) ONLINE SITES: p.1028, p.1032

Congenital deafness

Partial or total hearing loss that is present from birth

AGE Present at birth

GENETICS Risk factors depend on the cause

GENDER LIFESTYLE Not significant factors

Normally, a baby reacts to noise from birth, and even a fetus in the uterus is sensitive to sound. Hearing is particularly important for emotional contact between a baby and his or her family and for the development of speech and language skills. Congenital deafness is the rarest form of deafness; only about 2 in 1,000 babies are born with a hearing impairment that affects both ears. The condition varies from partial hearing loss to profound deafness.

What are the causes?

Congenital deafness is caused by the abnormal development of the inner ear or of the vestibulocochlear nerve, which transmits electrical impulses from the inner ear to the brain. In about half of all cases, the condition runs in families, suggesting that a genetic factor may be involved. Congenital deafness is also associated with the chromosome disorder Down's syndrome (p.821).

Certain infections, such as rubella or cytomegalovirus (CMV), can also cause congenital deafness if they are transmitted from the mother to the fetus during the early stages of development

(TEST) Hearing tests in children

Tests to detect impaired hearing are now routinely performed in childhood. These tests are tailored to the age of the child. Increasingly, screening of newborn babies is being carried out using tests such as oto-acoustic emission. Once a child has learned simple language, speech discrimination tests may be performed. By the age of 4, most children can manage a simple form of audiometry similar to that used to diagnose hearing impairment in adults (*see* HEARING TESTS, p.600).

Oto-acoustic emission test

This test detects the echo that is normally emitted by the inner ear in response to sound. An earpiece is placed in the ear canal, and a sound is played through it. The resulting echo is recorded. The test is painless.

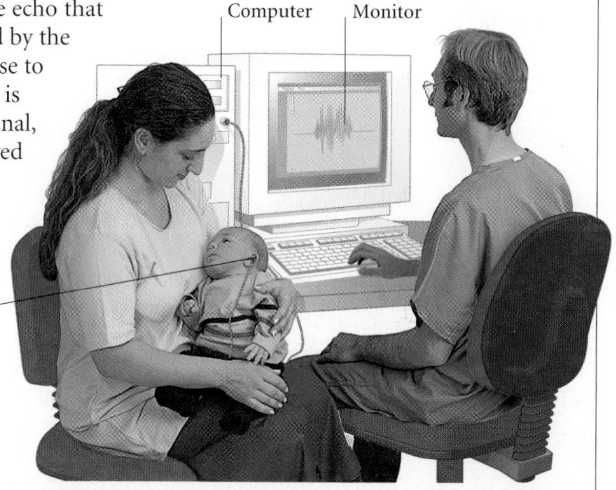

During the test
While the baby is quiet, a sound is played through the earpiece and the response is recorded.

(RESULTS)

Oto-acoustic emission
This normal tracing shows the echo emitted by the inner ear as sound is played through an earpiece. An echo is produced only if the inner ear is healthy and functioning normally.

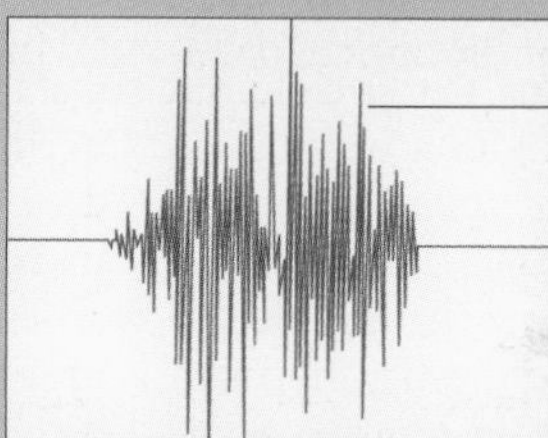

Speech discrimination tests

Speech discrimination tests can be used to detect hearing loss in young children who have a simple vocabulary. For example, the McCormick toy discrimination test is used in children of about 3 years old. The child is shown various toys and is then asked to identify pairs of toys that have similar-sounding names, such as tree and key.

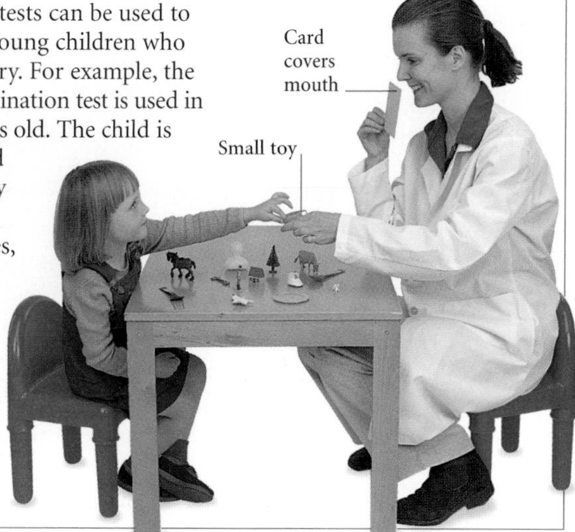

McCormick test
The doctor prevents the child from lip-reading by covering his or her mouth with a card and then asks the child to identify various toys.

(*see* CONGENITAL INFECTIONS, p.817). The development of hearing may also be affected if the mother takes certain drugs during pregnancy, particularly some types of antibiotic (p.885).

WHAT ARE THE SYMPTOMS?

The symptoms of congenital deafness may be noticed in the first few weeks or months after birth and include:

- Lack of response to loud noise.
- Failure to make normal baby sounds such as cooing by about 6 weeks of age or babbling by about 3 months.

You should take your baby to the doctor without delay if you suspect that he or she has impaired hearing.

WHAT MIGHT BE DONE?

In some hospitals, all newborn babies are routinely tested for congenital deafness by using oto-acoustic emission (*see* HEARING TESTS IN CHILDREN, p.859). Otherwise, a hearing test is performed only if a problem is suspected or if the baby is considered to be at particular risk, for example by having a family history of congenital deafness. An older baby may be tested by recording his or her response to loud sounds.

There is no cure for congenital deafness, but any hearing that a child has can be maximized with a hearing aid (p.601) or, in some children, using a cochlear implant (p.603). In all cases, it is important to ensure that a child can communicate. He or she may be taught sign language and lip-reading. Some children are able to learn to speak.

About half of all children with congenital deafness attend a normal school. Others, such as those with Down's syndrome, need to receive special schooling. Children who have congenital deafness and their families may find it helpful to contact a support group for advice.

CAN IT BE PREVENTED?

Immunization against rubella before starting a pregnancy reduces the risk to the developing fetus. You should not take drugs during pregnancy unless they are known to be safe for the fetus.

If the condition runs in your family, you may wish to consider genetic counselling (p.272), in which you will be advised about the risks of passing the condition on to your children.

(WWW) ONLINE SITES: p.1032

Acute otitis media in children

Infection of the middle ear, which often causes earache

 AGE More common under the age of 8

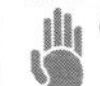 LIFESTYLE Passive smoking is a probable risk factor; more common in children who attend daycare centres

GENDER GENETICS Not significant factors

The most common cause of earache in children is acute otitis media, which is caused by infection in the middle ear. Children are at risk because the eustachian tubes, which connect the middle ear to the throat, are small and become obstructed easily. Acute otitis media is often part of infection of the respiratory system with a virus such as the common cold (p.288). Infection causes inflammation that may block one of the eustachian tubes, causing a build-up of fluid in the middle ear that may then become infected with bacteria.

About 1 in 5 children under the age of 4 has an episode of acute otitis media each year. There is some evidence to suggest that the condition is more common in children whose parents smoke. Children who attend daycare centres are also more susceptible, particularly if these are crowded. The condition is less common in children over the age of 8.

WHAT ARE THE SYMPTOMS?

The symptoms usually develop rapidly over several hours. A very young child may have difficulty locating the pain, and the only symptoms may be fever

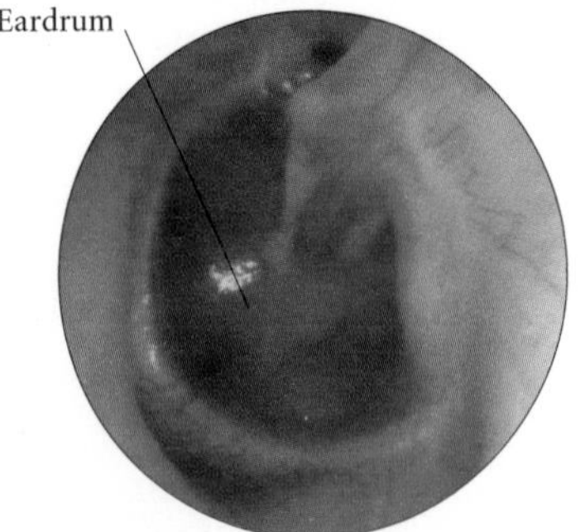

Acute otitis media

The eardrum shown above is bulging and inflamed as a result of the middle-ear infection acute otitis media.

and vomiting. In older children, symptoms may be more specific and include:

- Earache.
- Tugging or rubbing the painful ear.
- Temporary impaired hearing in the affected ear.

Left untreated, the eardrum may rupture, relieving the pain but causing a discharge of blood and pus. Recurrent infections in the middle ear may cause chronic secretory otitis media (below).

WHAT MIGHT BE DONE?

You should consult your child's doctor if liquid is discharged from the ear or if the earache lasts more than a few hours. He or she will examine your child's ears and may blow air into the affected ear using a special instrument to check that the eardrum is moving normally. Acute otitis media can clear up without treatment; however, the doctor will probably prescribe antibiotics (p.885) if he or she suspects that a bacterial infection is present. Paracetamol (*see* PAINKILLERS, p.912) may be given to relieve discomfort. The doctor will re-examine your child after a few days.

The symptoms usually clear up in a few days with appropriate treatment. A ruptured eardrum should heal within a few weeks. In some children, hearing is affected for more than 3 months until the fluid in the ear disappears.

(WWW) ONLINE SITES: p.1028, p.1031

Chronic secretory otitis media

A persistent collection of fluid in the middle ear

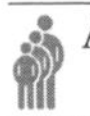 AGE More common under the age of 8

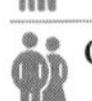 GENDER More common in boys

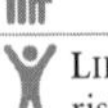 LIFESTYLE Passive smoking is a probable risk factor

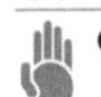 GENETICS Not a significant factor

In chronic secretory otitis media, the middle ear becomes filled with a thick, sticky, glue-like fluid. The condition is more common in boys and is the most common cause of impaired hearing in children under the age of 8. Since the disorder is persistent and usually occurs at a stage of a child's development when

TREATMENT GROMMET INSERTION

The ear disorder chronic secretory otitis media (opposite page) may be treated surgically by inserting a small plastic tube, called a grommet, into the eardrum. This tube ventilates the middle ear and allows fluid to drain away. After insertion of the grommet, hearing in the affected ear usually returns to normal, often within a few days. In most cases, the operation is performed on both ears under general anaesthesia as day surgery.

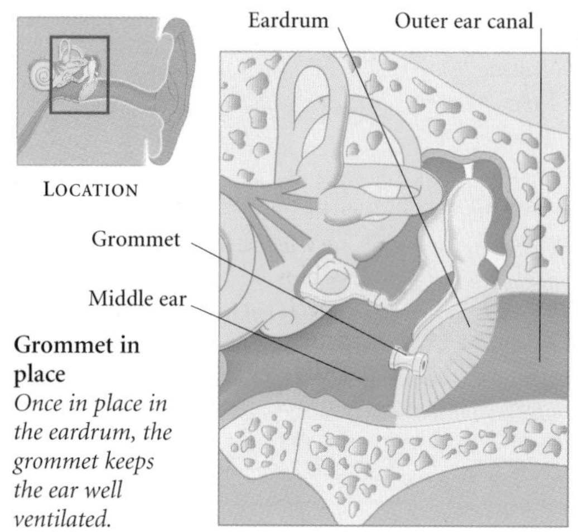

Grommet in place
Once in place in the eardrum, the grommet keeps the ear well ventilated.

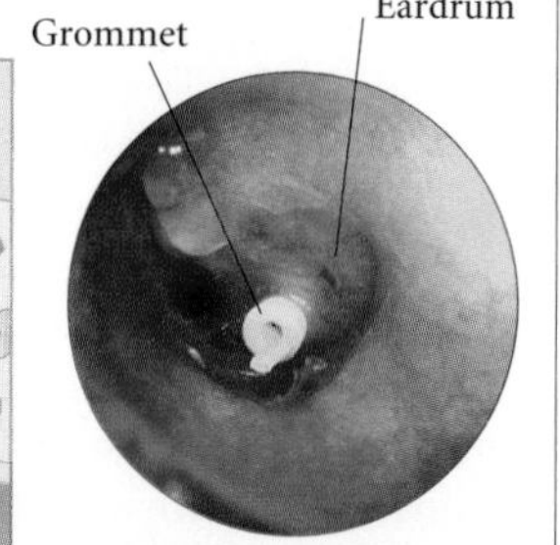

View of the eardrum
A grommet has been inserted into the eardrum above. Grommets usually fall out 6–12 months after insertion, and the hole in the eardrum closes.

good hearing is essential for learning to speak, it may cause a delay in speech development and in the normal acquisition of language skills.

WHAT ARE THE CAUSES?

The middle ear is normally ventilated by the eustachian tube (the narrow tube that connects the middle ear to the back of the throat). However, if this tube becomes blocked, possibly as a result of infection (*see* ACUTE OTITIS MEDIA IN CHILDREN, opposite page), the middle ear may fill with fluid. Often the blockage persists, causing chronic secretory otitis media. In some cases, the cause of the blockage is unknown. However, the disorder is thought to be more common in children whose parents smoke. Children who have asthma (p.839) or allergic rhinitis (p.466) are also more susceptible to chronic secretory otitis media. Children born with Down's syndrome (p.821) or a cleft lip and palate (p.862) are known to be at an increased risk of developing the disorder.

WHAT ARE THE SYMPTOMS?

In most cases, the symptoms of chronic secretory otitis media develop gradually and may initially go unnoticed. The symptoms often fluctuate and tend to be worse in the winter months. They may include:

- Partial deafness.
- Immature speech for the child's age.
- Behavioural problems due to frustration at being unable to hear well.

You may notice that your child is sitting close to the television or turning up the volume. His or her school performance may suffer because of difficulty hearing. If you suspect a hearing problem, you should consult the doctor without delay.

HOW IS IT DIAGNOSED?

The doctor will examine your child's ears and may then refer him or her to a specialist. Depending on the age of your child, various hearing tests may be performed to find out whether his or her hearing is impaired (*see* HEARING TESTS IN CHILDREN, p.859). The specialist may also perform a test in which air is blown into the affected ear using a special instrument. This test is carried out to measure the amount of movement of the eardrum, which is reduced in chronic secretory otitis media. Since the condition can fluctuate, the specialist will probably wish to examine your child again after about 3 months, when the tests will be repeated. An allergy test may also be recommended.

WHAT IS THE TREATMENT?

In most cases, chronic secretory otitis media clears up without treatment. If symptoms persist for several months, an operation may be advised. During the procedure, which is carried out under general anaesthesia, a small plastic tube called a grommet is inserted in the eardrum (*see* GROMMET INSERTION, left). The tube allows air to enter and circulate around the middle ear, drying it out. Some children with chronic secretory otitis media also have enlarged adenoids (p.842), which may be removed in the same operation (*see* TONSILLECTOMY AND ADENOIDECTOMY, p.843).

WHAT IS THE PROGNOSIS?

As a child grows, the eustachian tubes widen, allowing fluid to drain away from the middle ear more efficiently. As a result, the eustachian tubes are much less likely to become blocked. Chronic secretory otitis media is therefore rare in children over the age of 8.

WWW ONLINE SITES: p.1028, p.1031

Protruding ears

Prominent ears, which have no harmful effect on hearing

AGE Present at birth

GENETICS Sometimes runs in families

GENDER LIFESTYLE Not significant factors

Some children are born with ears that protrude instead of lying almost flat against the head. If the condition is particularly noticeable, a child may be self-conscious and experience psychological distress, usually from the teasing of other children. The condition sometimes runs in families, suggesting that a genetic factor is involved.

WHAT MIGHT BE DONE?

Protruding ears can be hidden by a suitable hairstyle. However, in extreme cases, cosmetic surgery may be recommended by your child's doctor. During the operation, a thin strip of skin from behind the ear is removed and then the the ear is drawn into the desired position. Scarring is hidden behind the ear. This surgery is not usually performed until a child is at least 5 years of age.

Disorders of the Digestive System

Throughout early childhood, attacks of diarrhoea and vomiting are common, and many children have episodes of constipation. Such disorders can often be treated successfully at home with self-help measures. Other rarer disorders may be due to a physical defect present at birth, and these disorders may require surgery.

The first two articles in this section cover problems with the mouth that affect babies: the physical defects of cleft lip and palate, which require surgery, and oral thrush, which is a common fungal infection. Two other digestive disorders that may affect babies, gastro-oesophageal reflux and pyloric stenosis, are covered next. Both can be treated successfully, but pyloric stenosis requires surgery.

A general article follows on vomiting and diarrhoea, including self-help measures for avoiding dehydration. There is also an article on cows' milk protein allergy. The section ends with articles on intussusception, a rare obstruction of the intestines, and constipation. Digestive disorders that affect adults only or affect adults and children are covered in the section on the digestive system (pp.620–669).

KEY ANATOMY

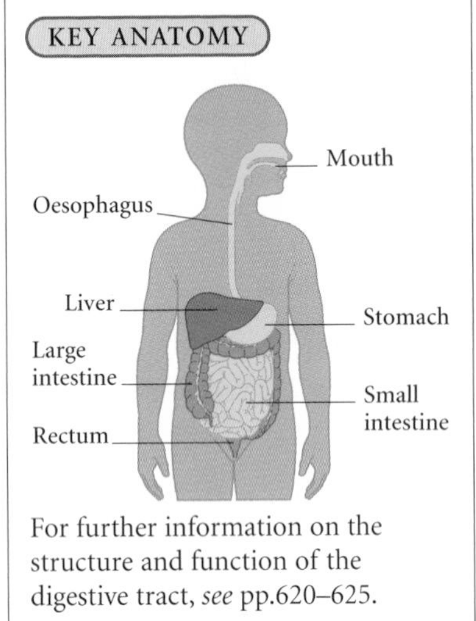

For further information on the structure and function of the digestive tract, *see* pp.620–625.

Cleft lip and palate

Splits in the upper lip and the roof of the mouth that are present at birth

 AGE Present at birth

 GENETICS Sometimes run in families

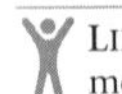 LIFESTYLE Heavy drinking and using some medical drugs in pregnancy are risk factors

 GENDER Not a significant factor

A cleft upper lip and palate are among the most common defects in babies and affect about 1 in 700 babies in the UK. These conditions may occur singly or together and are present at birth. These conditions can be upsetting for parents, but plastic surgery (p.952) produces excellent results in most cases.

The defects occur when the upper lip or roof of the mouth does not fuse completely in the fetus. In many cases, the cause is unknown, but the risk is higher if certain anticonvulsant drugs (p.914), such as phenytoin, are taken during pregnancy or if the mother is a heavy drinker. Cleft lip and/or palate sometimes run in families.

If a baby is severely affected, he or she may find it difficult to feed at first, and, if the condition is not treated early, speech may be delayed. Children with a cleft lip and/or palate are also susceptible to persistent build-up of fluid in the middle ear (*see* CHRONIC SECRETORY OTITIS MEDIA, p.860) that impairs hearing and may delay speech.

What might be done?

A cleft lip is usually repaired surgically by the age of 3 months, and a cleft palate is repaired at 6–15 months of age. While waiting for surgery, a plate may be fitted into the roof of the mouth if a baby has feeding problems. Following surgery, a child may have a hearing test (*see* HEARING TESTS IN CHILDREN, p.859) to check for hearing impairment caused by fluid build-up in the ear. A child may also need speech therapy (p.963) when he or she begins to talk. Plastic surgery often produces good results and allows speech to develop normally.

(WWW) ONLINE SITES: p.1027, p.1037

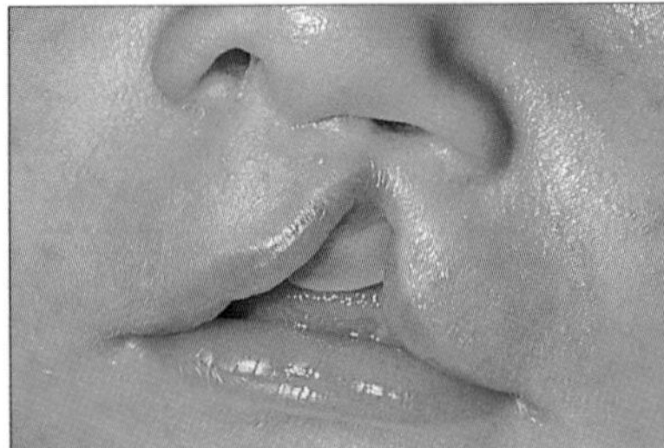

Cleft lip
This child has a split in the upper lip, known as a cleft lip. This can usually be repaired successfully with plastic surgery.

Oral thrush

A fungal mouth infection caused by an overgrowth of a yeast

 AGE Most common under 1 year of age

 GENDER GENETICS LIFESTYLE Not significant factors

Oral thrush is a common fungal infection in the first year of life. It produces white spots inside the mouth and may make a baby reluctant to feed. The infection is caused by an overgrowth of *Candida albicans*, a yeast naturally present in the mouth. The reason for the overgrowth is often unknown.

What are the symptoms?

In most cases, the symptoms of oral thrush include the following:

- Creamy yellow or white spots in the mouth that are difficult to rub off.
- Sore mouth that may make a baby reluctant to feed.

Oral thrush may be associated with a candida infection in the nappy area (*see* NAPPY RASH, p.829).

What might be done?

If you think your baby has oral thrush, you should arrange for him or her to see a doctor within 48 hours. The doctor will examine your baby's mouth and may take a mouth swab to check

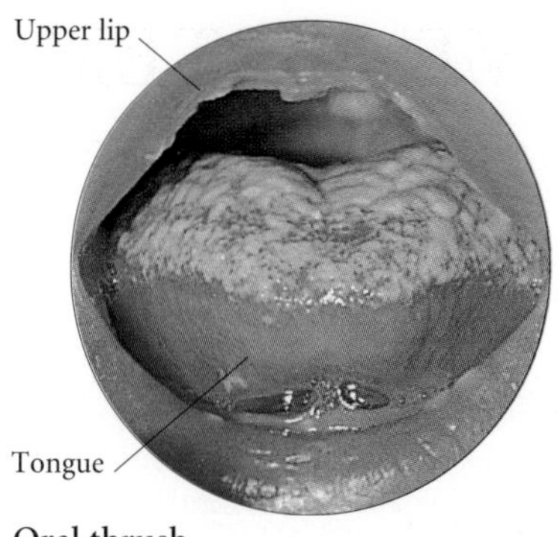

Oral thrush
The white patches on the tongue and the lining of this baby's mouth are caused by a common yeast infection, oral thrush.

for *Candida albicans.* He or she may prescribe antifungal drops and, to prevent reinfection if you breast-feed, an antifungal cream for your nipples (*see* PREPARATIONS FOR SKIN INFECTIONS AND INFESTATIONS, p.892). If you bottle-feed your baby, all the equipment should be thoroughly sterilized by boiling. Oral thrush often improves within days of starting treatment and clears up within a week, but the infection may recur.

(WWW) ONLINE SITES: p.1028, p.1033

Gastro-oesophageal reflux in infants

Regurgitation of the stomach contents caused by immaturity and weakness of the muscles around the stomach's entrance

 AGE Most common under 1 year of age

 GENDER GENETICS LIFESTYLE Not significant factors

Most babies bring up small amounts of milk after a feed. This regurgitation is normal and does not usually cause distress. However, if an infant regurgitates larger amounts of milk or food regularly, gastro-oesophageal reflux may be the cause. This condition occurs because the muscles at the entrance of a baby's stomach are not fully developed. As a result, the contents of the stomach, including acidic digestive juices, are able to pass back up the oesophagus (the tube between the throat and the stomach). Gastro-oesophageal reflux is more common in premature babies and those with cerebral palsy (p.846), who have poor overall muscle tone.

WHAT ARE THE SYMPTOMS?

The symptoms of gastro-oesophageal reflux are most noticeable after a feed and may include the following:

- Regurgitation of milk, usually more pronounced when the baby is lying flat or is crying.
- Coughing or wheezing if regurgitated milk is inhaled into the lungs.

If gastro-oesophageal reflux is severe, it may prevent the baby gaining weight. Severe reflux may also cause inflammation and bleeding of the lining of the oesophagus, which may make the vomit bloodstained. Sometimes, if milk is inhaled into the lungs, a chest infection, such as pneumonia (p.490), may develop. Rarely, a baby can stop breathing temporarily after inhaling milk.

If your baby regularly regurgitates more than a dribble of milk after feeding or if the vomit is bloodstained, contact a doctor as soon as possible.

HOW IS IT DIAGNOSED?

The doctor may be able to diagnose the condition from your baby's symptoms. However, if he or she is unsure of the diagnosis, a test may be carried out to monitor the amount of acid passing up the oesophagus from the stomach over 24 hours. This test involves passing a narrow tube into the baby's nose and down the oesophagus. The doctor may arrange for further tests, including a specialized X-ray (*see* BARIUM SWALLOW, p.637), to check for a structural abnormality in the oesophagus. If a baby has severe reflux with bloodstained vomit, endoscopy (*see* UPPER DIGESTIVE TRACT ENDOSCOPY, p.641) may be carried out to look for inflammation of the lining of the oesophagus.

WHAT IS THE TREATMENT?

In most cases, small, frequent feeds help to prevent gastro-oesophageal reflux, as does raising the head end of the cot after giving feeds. The doctor may prescribe a thickener or antacids (p.923) that should be to be added to your baby's milk. In more severe cases, drugs may be given to lower the production of acid in the stomach (*see* ULCER-HEALING DRUGS, p.923). With appropriate treatment, symptoms usually improve. Most babies outgrow gastro-oesophageal reflux by the age of 1 year to 18 months.

(WWW) ONLINE SITES: p.1028

Pyloric stenosis in infants

Narrowing of the outlet of the stomach in infancy, causing severe vomiting

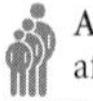 AGE Symptoms usually develop 3–8 weeks after birth

 GENDER Five times more common in boys

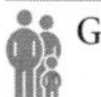 GENETICS Sometimes runs in families

 LIFESTYLE Not a significant factor

In pyloric stenosis, the ring of muscle that forms the outlet from the stomach to the duodenum (the first part of the small intestine) becomes thickened and narrowed due to excess growth of the muscle tissue. As a result, only a small amount of milk can pass into the duodenum, and the remainder builds up in the stomach until the baby vomits. The condition is five times more common in boys. The cause of pyloric stenosis is unknown, but it may run in families.

WHAT ARE THE SYMPTOMS?

The symptoms of pyloric stenosis develop gradually, usually between 3 and 8 weeks after birth, and may include:

- Persistent vomiting, which is sometimes projectile (ejected forcefully).
- Immediate hunger after vomiting.
- Infrequent bowel movements.

If vomiting is persistent or projectile, consult your doctor immediately.

WHAT MIGHT BE DONE?

The doctor will examine your baby's abdomen, usually during a feed, to feel for a swelling around the stomach outlet. If pyloric stenosis is suspected, your child will probably be admitted to hospital because affected babies frequently become dehydrated and may need to be given intravenous fluids. To confirm the diagnosis, ultrasound scanning (p.250) and/or specialized X-rays (*see* CONTRAST X-RAYS, p.245) of the abdomen may be carried out. The treatment for pyloric stenosis is a minor operation to widen the stomach outlet. Feeds can then be increased gradually until the baby's intake is normal. After surgery, most babies make a full recovery, and the condition does not usually recur.

(WWW) ONLINE SITES: p.1028

Vomiting and diarrhoea

Vomiting and the passage of loose stools caused by allergy, infection of the digestive tract, or an infection elsewhere in the body

 AGE Most common under the age of 5

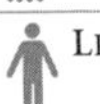 LIFESTYLE Risk factors depend on the cause

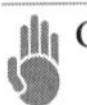 GENDER GENETICS Not significant factors

Attacks of vomiting and diarrhoea occur throughout childhood but are more common under the age of 5. There are many causes, some more serious than others, and it may be useful to assess your child (*see* SYMPTOM CHART: VOMITING IN CHILDREN, p.198, and SYMPTOM CHART: DIARRHOEA IN CHILDREN, p.200). Most cases improve within 24 hours, but prompt treatment with fluids is important because babies and young children become dehydrated easily.

WHAT ARE THE CAUSES?

Most episodes of vomiting and diarrhoea develop as a result of a viral or bacterial infection of the digestive tract (*see* GASTROENTERITIS, p.628). Vomiting and diarrhoea in young children may also be caused by an infection elsewhere in the body, such as the ear (*see* ACUTE OTITIS MEDIA IN CHILDREN, p.860).

Persistent diarrhoea in children aged between 1 and 3 years is often associated with inability to digest vegetables such as peas and carrots, which may be visible in the stools. This so-called "toddler's diarrhoea" is no cause for concern if your child is otherwise well. However, persistent diarrhoea that is accompanied by failure to gain weight should always be investigated by a doctor.

Persistent vomiting with diarrhoea is usually due to conditions such as cows' milk protein allergy (right) and sensitivity to the gluten in certain foods (*see* COELIAC DISEASE, p.658).

ARE THERE COMPLICATIONS?

If your child has vomiting and diarrhoea that lasts for several hours, he or she may become dehydrated. The symptoms may then also include:

- Abnormal drowsiness or irritability.
- Passing of small amounts of concentrated urine.
- Sunken eyes.
- In a baby, a sunken fontanelle (the soft spot on the top of a baby's head).

If a child with vomiting and diarrhoea develops symptoms of dehydration, you should seek medical help immediately.

WHAT MIGHT BE DONE?

Most cases of vomiting and diarrhoea clear up without treatment. Make sure your child drinks plenty of fluids, but avoid milk (except breast milk). Over-the-counter oral rehydration solutions (p.926) that contain the ideal balance of salts and minerals can help to prevent dehydration. If the symptoms persist for over 24 hours or become worse, consult a doctor. He or she will assess the level of hydration and check for infection. If your child is dehydrated, admission to hospital and treatment with intravenous fluids may be necessary, and antibiotics (p.885) may be prescribed if the child has a bacterial infection. If the disorder is found to be caused by food sensitivity, a modified diet will be recommended. Treatment is usually successful.

(WWW) ONLINE SITES: p.1028

Cows' milk protein allergy

An allergic reaction to the proteins present in cows' milk and cows' milk products

 AGE Usually develops during the first 6 months of life

 GENETICS Sometimes runs in families

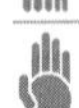 GENDER LIFESTYLE Not significant factors

An allergy to the proteins in cows' milk occurs in about 1 in 25 babies, usually during the first 6 months of life. Most babies are exposed to these proteins because they are present in formula and, if the mother consumes cows' milk products, in breast milk. If a baby has the allergy, his or her immune system reacts to cows' milk proteins, causing inflammation of the digestive tract. The cause is unknown, but the disorder may run in families, suggesting a genetic factor.

WHAT ARE THE SYMPTOMS?

The symptoms of cows' milk protein allergy vary and may include:

- Diarrhoea, with loose stools containing blood and/or mucus.
- Abdominal discomfort, causing the baby to cry and become irritable.
- Vomiting.
- Wheezing and coughing.
- Eczema (p.829) or an itchy, red rash (*see* URTICARIA, p.468).
- Failure to gain weight.

If you think that your baby is allergic to proteins in cows' milk, consult a doctor. Rarely, cows' milk protein allergy leads to anaphylaxis (p.469), a potentially life-threatening allergic reaction.

WHAT MIGHT BE DONE?

If the doctor suspects cows' milk protein allergy, you may be advised to exclude cows' milk temporarily from your child's diet under a dietitian's supervision. If you are breast-feeding, you will be told to exclude all milk products from your own diet. If symptoms disappear while your child is on the special diet and reappear when cows' milk is reintroduced, the diagnosis is confirmed and the special diet is continued. Treatment for cows' milk protein allergy is usually successful, and children rapidly put on weight on the modified diet. Your child will be tested every year to check whether the allergy is still present and a special diet is still required. The problem usually disappears by about the age of 3, but in a minority of affected children it continues in some form into adult life.

(WWW) ONLINE SITES: p.1027

Intussusception

A rare condition in which a segment of intestine slides inside the neighbouring part, causing an intestinal obstruction

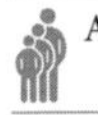 AGE Usually develops in early childhood

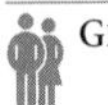 GENDER More common in boys

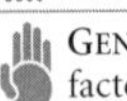 GENETICS LIFESTYLE Not significant factors

Intussusception is a rare condition, but it is the most common cause of intestinal obstruction in children under the age of 2. In intussusception, a section of the intestine "telescopes" into a neighbouring part, forming a tube within a tube. The condition usually affects the last part of the small intestine. If left untreated, the blood supply to the affected "telescoped" part may be cut off and cause tissue death in that section of intestine. The cause of intussusception is usually unknown. However, it may be associated with enlargement of the lymph nodes in the lining of the intestine, possibly due to a viral infection.

WHAT ARE THE SYMPTOMS?

The symptoms of intussusception are usually intermittent. Each episode develops suddenly and usually lasts for a few minutes. Symptoms may include:

- Severe abdominal pain, which may cause the child to cry and draw up his or her legs.
- Pale skin.
- Vomiting.
- After a few hours, passage from the rectum of bloodstained mucus that may resemble redcurrant jam.

Between the intermittent episodes of pain and vomiting, your child may feel ill and lethargic. If you suspect intussusception, seek medical attention at once. The disorder progresses rapidly, and prompt treatment is essential.

WHAT MIGHT BE DONE?

If your child's doctor suspects intussusception from the symptoms, he or she will arrange for your child to be admitted to hospital immediately.

In hospital, your child will probably be given intravenous fluids. A tube is passed through the nose and into the stomach to keep the stomach empty and to prevent vomiting. In order to confirm the diagnosis, your child may be given a contrast X-ray (p.245) of the intestines, known as a barium enema. In at least 7 in 10 cases, the gentle pressure of the barium solution relieves the intestinal

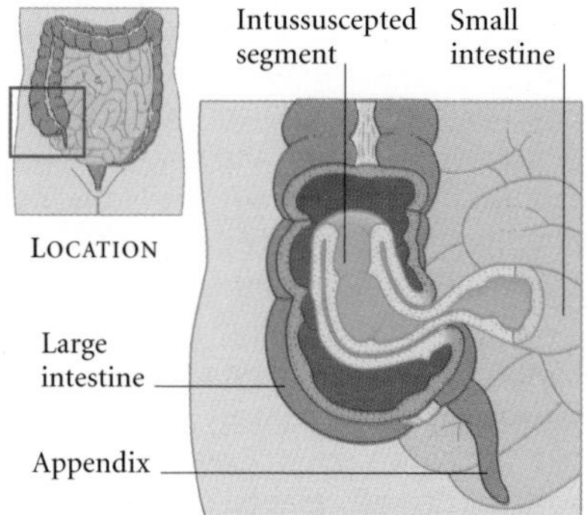

Intussusception
In this example of intussusception, the last part of the small intestine has passed into the adjacent section of large intestine and caused an obstruction.

obstruction. In some medical centres, air may be used instead of barium. In other cases, emergency surgery may be performed to relieve the obstruction and to remove the damaged intestine. Most affected children recover fully following treatment, and the condition recurs in fewer than 1 in 20 of all cases.

WWW ONLINE SITES: p.1028

Constipation in children

Difficult, infrequent, and sometimes painful passage of hard faeces

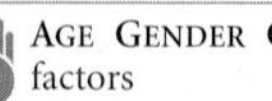

LIFESTYLE A low-fibre diet is a risk factor

AGE GENDER GENETICS Not significant factors

All children differ in their bowel habits. Some children pass faeces several times a day, and others may do so only once every few days. Both these situations are normal provided that the faeces are not too runny or so hard that they cause discomfort. The presence of hard faeces that are difficult or painful to pass indicates that your child has constipation, a common condition that affects people of all ages. Constipation in children is usually only a temporary problem, and very rarely indicates a more serious underlying disorder.

WHAT ARE THE CAUSES?

A common cause of temporary constipation is a change in diet, particularly if there is insufficient fibre or fluid in the diet. Constipation is rare in babies, but the condition may occur during the change from formula or breast milk to cows' milk. Sometimes, temporary constipation occurs during toilet training, when it is common for a toddler to try to avoid defaecation. This phase may be associated with a toddler passing faeces in inappropriate places (*see* ENCOPRESIS, p.852). Illnesses that cause high fever and vomiting can also cause temporary constipation due to dehydration.

Underlying disorders that may cause persistent constipation include cerebral palsy (p.846), in which there is brain damage that impairs muscular control. An abnormally tight anal sphincter may also cause constipation by preventing the release of faeces from the body.

WHAT ARE THE SYMPTOMS?

If your child has constipation, you may notice the following symptoms:

- Difficult passage of small or bulky hard, dry faeces.
- Infrequent defaecation.
- Soiling of clothes due to leakage of faeces associated with constipation.
- Sometimes, loss of appetite.

Your child may be afraid to pass faeces if he or she experiences severe discomfort during bowel movements, especially if a painful tear develops in the anal tissue (*see* ANAL FISSURE, p.669) caused by straining to pass stools. In these cases, constipation may become a severe and long-term problem.

WHAT CAN I DO?

In most cases, constipation in children does not require medical treatment. You should encourage your child to drink plenty of fluids. Adding a little sugar to drinks for a few days may help. If the child is over the age of 6 months, make sure that there is plenty of fibre in the diet from fresh fruit and vegetables. If constipation is linked to problems with toilet training, patience and time will usually solve the problem. Seek medical advice if constipation persists for a week despite self-help measures.

WHAT MIGHT THE DOCTOR DO?

The doctor will probably examine your child's abdomen and may perform a rectal examination, in which a gloved finger is gently inserted into the rectum. He or she may prescribe a short course of drugs to soften the faeces (*see* LAXATIVES, p.924) and reduce the discomfort of defaecation. Softened faeces will also allow an anal tear to heal. Once the pain of defaecation is relieved, your child should feel confident to pass faeces normally again. Rarely, surgery may be required to treat an anal sphincter that is abnormally tight.

If constipation persists, your child may need an abdominal X-ray (p.244) or a specialized contrast X-ray (p.245) of the bowel to exclude an underlying disorder. Severe constipation caused by a condition such as cerebral palsy may require lifelong treatment with laxatives. However, constipation usually clears up within 1–2 weeks of changing the child's diet or of laxative treatment.

WWW ONLINE SITES: p.1028, p.1035

ENDOCRINE AND METABOLIC DISORDERS

Some endocrine and most metabolic disorders in children are present from birth and are caused by an abnormal gene that is inherited from one or both parents. Most of these disorders are rare, but, when they do occur, they can adversely affect normal growth and development unless diagnosed and treated early.

Most of the disorders discussed in this section are caused by abnormalities in the production of enzymes that are vital for the metabolic (chemical) processes of the body. The first disorder covered is congenital adrenal hyperplasia, in which deficiency of an enzyme affects production of one or more hormones by the adrenal glands. As a result, important metabolic processes are disrupted and excessive production of male sex hormones may affect the formation of a female baby's genitals. The second article introduces a group of rare inherited metabolic disorders, known as inborn errors of metabolism. The articles that follow cover four of these disorders: phenylketonuria, galactosaemia, Tay–Sachs disease, and albinism. The section concludes with a general article on growth disorders. Endocrine and metabolic conditions such as diabetes mellitus that affect adults only or adults in addition to children are discussed in hormones and metabolism (pp.670–693) or in the section that covers the particular body system affected.

KEY ANATOMY

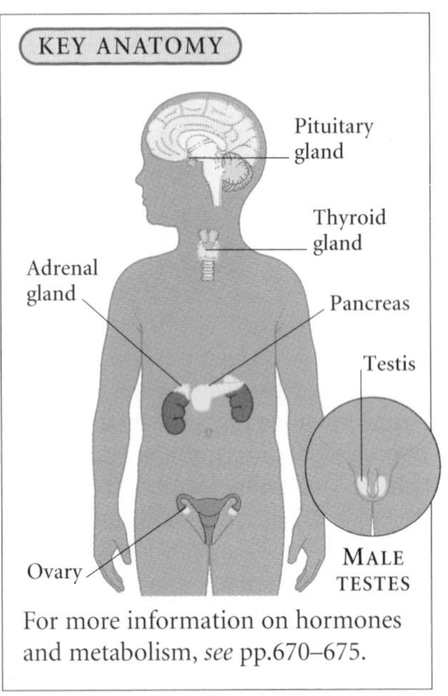

For more information on hormones and metabolism, *see* pp.670–675.

Congenital adrenal hyperplasia

In either sex, abnormally high production of male sex hormones by the adrenal glands

 AGE Present from birth

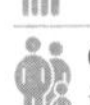 GENETICS Due to an abnormal gene inherited from both parents

 GENDER LIFESTYLE Not significant factors

Congenital adrenal hyperplasia is a rare inherited condition that affects around 1 in 5,000 babies in the UK. In congenital adrenal hyperplasia, the production of one or more hormones in the adrenal glands is abnormal.

In the most common form of congenital adrenal hyperplasia, there is a deficiency of an enzyme that is essential for the production of the adrenal hormones aldosterone, which maintains the salt and water balance in the body, and cortisol, which maintains glucose levels in the blood. As a result, these hormones may be absent or deficient. The condition also leads to excessive production of male sex hormones (androgens).

Congenital adrenal hyperplasia is caused by an abnormal gene that is inherited in an autosomal recessive manner (*see* GENE DISORDERS, p.271).

WHAT ARE THE SYMPTOMS?

The symptoms of congenital adrenal hyperplasia may be present at birth or may develop later in childhood or adolescence. Raised levels of androgens may lead to the following symptoms:

- In girls, an enlarged clitoris and external genitals that are fused, giving a masculinized appearance.
- In boys, a slight increase in pigmentation of the scrotum, which often goes unnoticed.
- Early puberty in boys.

Lack of aldosterone may cause a "salt-losing crisis" in which there is a sudden loss of salt and fluid. The symptoms of such a crisis may include:

- Lethargy.
- Vomiting.
- Loss of weight.

If it is not treated, the salt-losing crisis may lead to shock (p.414), which may be life-threatening. A lack of cortisol may cause low levels of glucose in the blood (*see* HYPOGLYCAEMIA, p.691).

WHAT MIGHT BE DONE?

Congenital adrenal hyperplasia is usually diagnosed in girls at birth from the appearance of the genitals. The disorder may become apparent in boys due to a salt-losing crisis in the first 2 years of life.

An affected child will have blood tests to measure the levels of hormones, salt, and glucose. If a baby has a salt-losing crisis, he or she will require emergency treatment in hospital with intravenous salt and glucose solutions. Cortisol and a drug that mimics the actions of aldosterone will also be given. A child who has congenital adrenal hyperplasia will require lifelong treatment to replace the deficient hormones and to normalize the production of androgens. Affected girls may need to have surgery to correct genital abnormalities.

With treatment, most children with congenital adrenal hyperplasia can lead normal lives. A pregnant woman who has previously given birth to a child with the disorder may be offered screening tests (*see* ANTENATAL GENETIC TESTS, p.787), and, if necessary, drug treatment may be prescribed to minimize the effects of the condition on a female fetus.

(WWW) ONLINE SITES: p.1033

Inborn errors of metabolism

Genetic disorders in which chemical processes in the body are disrupted or faulty

 AGE Present from birth

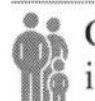 GENETICS Due to an abnormal gene usually inherited from both parents

 GENDER LIFESTYLE Not significant factors

Inborn errors of metabolism is a general term used to describe a group of genetic disorders in which the body chemistry (metabolism) is affected by an abnormal gene. In each disorder, this abnormal gene affects the production of a particular enzyme that is essential for specific metabolic processes. The disruption of these processes results in damage to one or more organs of the body, and the severity of a particular disorder depends on the chemical processes affected. Over 200 inborn errors of metabolism have been identified, but each disorder is extremely rare. Most of the abnormal genes that cause these inborn metabolic disorders are inherited in an autosomal recessive manner (*see* GENE DISORDERS, p.271).

WHAT ARE THE TYPES?

Many inborn errors of metabolism lead to a build-up of harmful chemicals that cause damage to one or more organs in the body. In phenylketonuria (right), the accumulation of phenylalanine causes brain damage. In galactosaemia (p.868), the sugar galactose builds up to a dangerously high level and causes damage to the liver and brain. In Tay–Sachs disease (p.868), chemical build-up in the brain results in fatal brain damage. In the milder condition albinism (p.868), a deficient enzyme affects the production of the pigment melanin, which gives colour to the skin, eyes, and hair, but there is no harmful chemical build-up.

The symptoms of inborn errors of metabolism are usually present at or soon after birth, although in some cases symptoms may not appear until later in childhood. The symptoms may include unexplained illness and failure to thrive in a newborn, and drowsiness, floppiness, seizures, and developmental delay (p.853) in older babies and children.

WHAT MIGHT BE DONE?

Couples planning to have children may be offered screening for the presence of an abnormal gene before beginning a pregnancy if there is a family history of an inborn error of metabolism or if a particular metabolic disorder is common in their ethnic group (*see* TESTS FOR ABNORMAL GENES, p.239). A pregnant woman can also be screened for the condition before the baby is born (*see* ANTENATAL GENETIC TESTS, p.787). In the UK, all newborn infants are routinely screened for phenylketonuria and the hormone disorder hypothyroidism (p.680) shortly after birth (*see* SCREENING FOR METABOLIC DISORDERS, below).

Some inborn errors of metabolism can be treated easily. For example, the diet of an affected child can be adapted to restrict the intake of substances, such as phenylalanine or galactose, that his or her body cannot process. If the missing enzyme is produced by white blood cells, the condition may sometimes be cured by a bone marrow transplant (p.454).

(TEST) SCREENING FOR METABOLIC DISORDERS

All newborn babies in the UK are screened shortly after birth for the condition phenylketonuria (right), an inborn error of metabolism, and also for the hormone disorder hypothyroidism (p.680). The baby's heel is pricked with a small needle to obtain a few drops of blood for testing, which are collected using a special card. The card is sent to a laboratory for analysis and the test results are available in a few days.

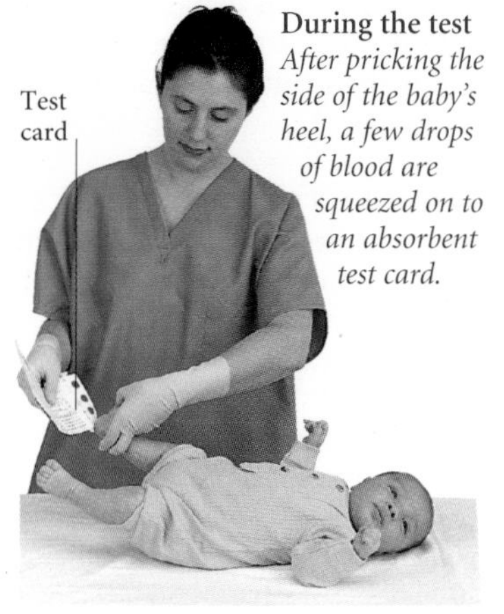

During the test *After pricking the side of the baby's heel, a few drops of blood are squeezed on to an absorbent test card.*

WHAT IS THE PROGNOSIS?

The outlook for inborn errors of metabolism depends on the disorder and how early it is diagnosed. Some disorders, such as albinism, rarely cause serious problems; others, such as galactosaemia, can be treated successfully if diagnosed soon after birth. However, there is no treatment for Tay–Sachs disease, which is usually fatal in early childhood.

(WWW) ONLINE SITES: p.1032, p.1033

Phenylketonuria

An inherited chemical defect that can cause brain damage

 AGE Present from birth

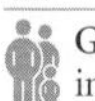 GENETICS Due to an abnormal gene inherited from both parents

 GENDER LIFESTYLE Not significant factors

Children with phenylketonuria lack the enzyme that is responsible for breaking down phenylalanine, which occurs naturally in most food containing protein. As a result, phenylalanine is converted into harmful substances that build up in the blood and may damage the developing brain. Although phenylketonuria is rare in the UK, affecting about 1 in 10,000 infants, all newborn babies are screened for the disorder because of the risk of serious brain damage. Like most inborn errors of metabolism, phenylketonuria is due to an abnormal gene that is inherited in an autosomal recessive manner (*see* GENE DISORDERS, p.271). If both parents carry the abnormal gene, there is a 1 in 4 chance that their baby will be affected.

WHAT ARE THE SYMPTOMS?

At birth, some babies with phenylketonuria have a red, itchy rash similar to eczema, but most affected infants appear healthy. The symptoms of the disorder usually develop gradually over 6–12 months and may include:

- Vomiting.
- Restlessness and sometimes seizures.
- Stale, unpleasant skin odour.
- Delay in development (*see* DEVELOPMENTAL DELAY, p.853).

If it is not treated, phenylketonuria may lead to serious brain damage, resulting in severe learning problems (*see* GENERALIZED LEARNING DISABILITIES, p.854).

What might be done?

In the UK, a blood test for phenylketonuria is given to all newborn babies (*see* SCREENING FOR METABOLIC DISORDERS, p.867). Early screening is important because prompt diagnosis and treatment are vital. If your baby is diagnosed as having phenylketonuria, he or she will probably be prescribed a special formula or milk substitute that is rich in protein but contains little phenylalanine. Your child should continue with a diet low in phenylalanine, at least throughout his or her childhood until the brain has stopped growing. Most doctors recommend that an affected person should follow a low-phenylalanine diet for life. Women with the condition who are planning a pregnancy are advised to follow a low-phenylalanine diet before conception and throughout pregnancy.

With early diagnosis and treatment, children with phenylketonuria develop normally, attend mainstream schools, and do not have reduced life expectancy.

(WWW) ONLINE SITES: p.1032, p.1033

Galactosaemia

An abnormal build-up of the sugar galactose, due to a deficient enzyme

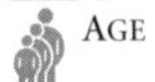 AGE Present from birth

 GENETICS Due to an abnormal gene inherited from both parents

 GENDER LIFESTYLE Not significant factors

Galactosaemia is a rare condition in which harmful amounts of galactose, a sugar that is present in milk, build up in a baby's body tissues. Normally, an enzyme in the liver converts galactose into glucose, but in galactosaemia this enzyme is missing. If the disorder is not treated, high levels of galactose accumulate, leading to serious damage to the liver, brain, and eyes. In the UK, the disorder affects about 1 in 62,000 infants. Galactosaemia is caused by an abnormal gene inherited in an autosomal recessive manner (*see* GENE DISORDERS, p.271).

What are the symptoms?

Symptoms of galactosaemia appear in the first few days of life, often after the baby's first milk feeds, and include:

- Vomiting and diarrhoea.
- Failure to gain weight.
- Yellow coloration of the skin and the whites of the eyes (*see* NEONATAL JAUNDICE, p.817).

If not treated, cataracts (p.573), chronic liver failure (p.650), and generalized learning disabilities (p.854) may develop.

What might be done?

If a newborn infant develops the above symptoms, the doctor may suspect galactosaemia and arrange for the baby's urine to be tested for the presence of galactose. If galactosaemia is confirmed, you will be advised to exclude galactose from your baby's diet and to use milk substitutes in feeds. Usually, a galactose-free diet is recommended throughout childhood and, in some cases, for life. With early treatment, most affected children develop normally, but some have mild learning difficulties.

(WWW) ONLINE SITES: p.1032, p.1033

Tay–Sachs disease

An inherited condition in which harmful chemicals accumulate in the brain

 AGE Present from birth

 GENETICS Due to an abnormal gene inherited from both parents

 GENDER LIFESTYLE Not significant factors

Tay–Sachs disease is a fatal childhood disorder that is most common in the Ashkenazi Jewish population, affecting about 1 in 2,500 people in this group. The condition is caused by the lack of a vital enzyme in the brain. Without the enzyme, abnormal chemicals build up, leading to progressive and fatal brain damage. Tay–Sachs disease is caused by an abnormal gene that is inherited in an autosomal recessive manner (*see* GENE DISORDERS, p.271).

What are the symptoms?

A baby who has Tay–Sachs disease often appears healthy at birth. The symptoms, which usually start to appear at 3–6 months of age, may include:

- Exaggerated startle response to noise.
- Muscle weakness and floppy limbs.
- Lack of awareness of surroundings.
- Deteriorating vision.

An affected baby may have seizures and gradually become paralysed during the first 6 months of life.

What might be done?

If the doctor suspects that your baby has Tay–Sachs disease, he or she may arrange for a blood test or a test on a sample of skin tissue to confirm that the enzyme is missing. The doctor will also examine the baby's eyes to look for the presence of an abnormal "cherry-red spot" on the retina (the layer of light-sensitive cells at the back of the eye). There is no cure for Tay–Sachs disease, but an affected child will be made as comfortable as possible by treating symptoms as they arise.

People who are at risk of having a child with Tay–Sachs disease, especially Ashkenazi Jews, can be screened for the abnormal gene (*see* TESTS FOR ABNORMAL GENES, p.239) before marriage or pregnancy. If both partners in a couple are found to be carriers of the Tay–Sachs gene, there is a 1 in 4 chance of their child being affected. The couple will be offered genetic counselling (p.272) to explain these risks and to discuss the options they may wish to consider. Affected couples may decide not to have children or to conceive a child using IVF treatment (*see* ASSISTED CONCEPTION, p.776), so that the embryo can be tested for the presence of the disease before implantation in the uterus.

Tay–Sachs disease is a fatal disorder, and children with the disease do not usually survive beyond the age of 5.

(WWW) ONLINE SITES: p.1032, p.1033

Albinism

An inherited condition in which there is inadequate production of the pigment that gives colour to skin, eyes, and hair

 AGE Present from birth

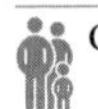 GENETICS Due to an abnormal gene

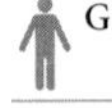 GENDER Risk factors depend on the type

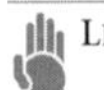 LIFESTYLE Not a significant factor

Albinism is a rare inherited disorder in which a baby is born with little or no colour in the skin, hair, and eyes or, more rarely, in the eyes only. Like other inborn errors of metabolism (p.867), the condition is caused by a fault in an enzyme that is essential for the production of the pigment melanin. In most cases, albinism is due to an abnormal gene that

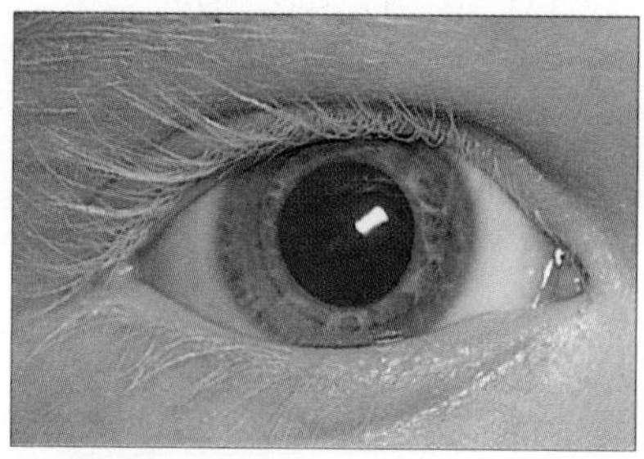

Albinism
The iris of this eye is pink and the eyebrows and eyelashes are white, due to absence of the brown pigment melanin.

is inherited in an autosomal recessive manner (*see* GENE DISORDERS, p.271) and affects the skin, hair, and eyes. A less common type, in which the abnormal gene is inherited in an X-linked recessive manner from the mother, affects only males. In this type of albinism, only the eyes are affected by lack of melanin. Albinism affects about 1 in 20,000 babies.

WHAT ARE THE SYMPTOMS?

The symptoms depend on the amount of melanin that is produced and vary from mild to severe. They may include:

- Unusual eye colour, ranging from pink to pale, watery blue.
- Dislike of bright light.
- Involuntary, jerky eye movements.
- Severe visual impairment.
- White hair and fair skin that does not tan normally.

Children with albinism are at increased risk of developing skin cancer (p.344) in later life from exposure to sunlight.

WHAT MIGHT BE DONE?

Albinism is usually diagnosed from the baby's appearance at birth. If albinism is suspected, a blood test is performed to confirm that the enzyme is missing. There is no medical treatment for the condition. However, tinted lenses can be worn to help with the aversion to bright light, and visual impairment can be corrected with glasses or, when the child is older, with contact lenses. The doctor will also recommend the use of sunscreens and sunblocks (p.893) and a hat to protect your child's skin in bright sunlight. People with albinism have a normal life expectancy. Parents of children with albinism may find it useful to contact support groups for advice.

WWW ONLINE SITES: p.1032

Growth disorders

Abnormally short or tall stature in babies and children due to a number of causes

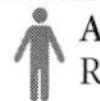

AGE GENDER GENETICS LIFESTYLE
Risk factors depend on the type

Children of the same age vary greatly in height due to factors such as diet, genetics, and ethnic background. In most cases, tall or short stature is not abnormal and is due to a family tendency to be taller or shorter than average or to reach final height later than usual. Tall or short stature is a cause for concern only if the child's height is well outside the average range for his or her age (*see* GROWTH CHARTS FOR CHILDREN, p.42). Abnormally short or tall stature may be caused by a number of disorders.

WHAT ARE THE TYPES?

Normal growth depends on a nutritionally adequate diet and good general health and is controlled by specific hormones. Disruption of any of these three important factors may lead to a growth disorder that results in a child having abnormally short or tall stature.

SHORT STATURE A child may be shorter than normal if his or her diet is inadequate. A long-term illness, such as cystic fibrosis (p.824) or severe asthma (*see* ASTHMA IN CHILDREN, p.839), may also result in poor growth. Crohn's disease (p.658), an inflammatory bowel condition, is another example of a long-term illness that may lead to short stature. Some babies who have severe intrauterine growth retardation (p.796) may be slightly below average height in later life.

Sometimes, short stature is caused by insufficient production of the hormones that are necessary for normal growth. In some children, the pituitary gland does not produce enough growth hormone (*see* HYPOPITUITARISM, p.678). Insufficient production of thyroid hormones is another cause of poor growth (*see* HYPOTHYROIDISM, p.680).

Short stature is also a characteristic feature of Turner's syndrome (p.823), a genetic disorder that only affects girls. In addition, short stature may occur as a result of a skeletal abnormality such as achondroplasia (p.833), an inherited disorder in which the bones of the legs and arms are shorter than normal.

TALL STATURE Children may be temporarily taller than others of the same age and sex if puberty occurs early (*see* ABNORMAL PUBERTY IN MALES, p.728, and ABNORMAL PUBERTY IN FEMALES, p.739). However, in these children, final height is usually normal. In rare cases, exaggerated growth caused by the overproduction of growth hormone results in excessive height, called gigantism. The overproduction may be due to a tumour in the pituitary gland (*see* PITUITARY TUMOURS, p.676). Boys with the chromosome disorder Klinefelter's syndrome (p.822) may also grow taller than normal due to a deficiency of sex hormones.

HOW IS IT DIAGNOSED?

Your child's height will be measured during routine checkups. If his or her height is consistently either lower or higher than the normal range, he or she will be measured more frequently. If growth rates continue to be abnormal, tests may be performed to check hormone levels and to look for underlying disorders, such as a genetic abnormality. In some cases, maturity of a child's bones may be assessed by taking X-rays (p.244) of the hand and wrist.

WHAT IS THE TREATMENT?

Treatment for growth disorders is most successful if started well before puberty when bones still have the potential for normal growth. Slow growth due to an inadequate diet in infancy usually improves if the diet is modified. Later in childhood, a growth disorder is likely to be the result of long-term illness, and careful control of the illness sometimes results in normal growth. Growth hormone deficiency is usually treated by hormone replacement. Hypothyroidism is treated by replacing thyroid hormone.

Abnormal early puberty is sometimes treated using drugs to halt the advancement of puberty. Gigantism caused by a pituitary gland tumour may be treated by surgical removal of the tumour.

If treated early, most children with a growth disorder reach a relatively normal height, but, if treatment is delayed until puberty, normal height is more difficult to achieve. Abnormal stature may cause a child to be self-conscious and unhappy, and he or she may need support such as counselling (p.971).

WWW ONLINE SITES: p.1028, p.1033

Disorders of the Reproductive and Urinary Systems

The two main causes of reproductive and urinary disorders in children are abnormal development of the affected systems in the fetus and infection. Prompt treatment of urinary tract infections is important because of the risk of kidney damage.

The first articles in this section cover two disorders of the male reproductive and urinary systems, hypospadias and undescended testis, which are present at birth. In hypospadias, the opening of the urethra (the passage that carries urine from the bladder to the outside of the body) is on the underside of the penis rather than the tip. Undescended testis is a condition in which one testis (or rarely both) fails to descend into the scrotum before birth. Urinary tract infections, which are more common in girls, are discussed next. All children who have these infections need prompt medical treatment because the kidneys can be damaged if the infection persists. An article follows on bedwetting, a common urinary problem in infancy. The section ends with an article on Wilms' tumour, a rare cancer of the kidney that can often be treated successfully. Circumcision (p.722) is discussed elsewhere.

KEY ANATOMY

Kidney
Ureter
Ovary
Uterus
Bladder
Urethra
Vagina
FEMALE

Kidney
Ureter
Bladder
Prostate
Urethra
Penis
Testis
MALE

For more on the urinary and male and female reproductive systems, *see* pp.694–697, pp.716–717, and pp. 730–733.

Hypospadias

An abnormality in which the opening of the urethra is on the underside of the penis rather than at the tip

AGE Present at birth

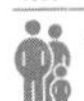
GENETICS Sometimes runs in families

LIFESTYLE Not a significant factor

Hypospadias is a common birth defect in which the opening of the urethra (the passage that carries urine from the bladder to outside the body) develops on the underside of the shaft of the penis instead of at the tip. Most commonly, the opening develops near the end of the penis, but in severe cases it can occur far back towards the scrotum. Sometimes, part of the foreskin may be missing and the penis curves downwards, a condition known as chordee. Hypospadias occurs in about 1 in 300 boys and can run in families, which suggests that a genetic factor is involved. If the condition is not treated early, an affected child may need to sit on the toilet to pass urine, unlike other boys, which may make him self-conscious.

What might be done?

Hypospadias is usually detected at birth and treated with surgery before the age of 2. During the operation, the foreskin is used to form an extension to the existing urethra so that it reaches the tip of the penis. It is therefore important that your son is not circumcised. If chordee is also present, this can be corrected during the same operation. Surgery usually allows the child to pass urine normally. Sexual activity and fertility in later life are unlikely to be affected.

(WWW) ONLINE SITES: p.1027

Undescended testis

A testis that fails to descend into the scrotum before birth

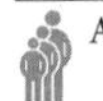
AGE Present at birth

GENETICS LIFESTYLE Not significant factors

Normally, the testes descend from the abdomen into the scrotum before birth. In about 3 in 100 boys, one testis (or rarely both) fails to move down. In 2 in 3 affected boys, an undescended testis moves to the scrotum within a year, but the rest may need surgery to correct the condition. If treatment is delayed, the future risk of cancer of the testis (p.719) is slightly increased. If both testes are undescended, treatment should be carried out promptly since there is a risk of impaired fertility in later life (*see* MALE INFERTILITY, p.777).

It can be difficult to determine if your son has an undescended testis because the testes of most young boys retract up into the abdomen in response to cold or touch. However, you should consult the doctor if you are concerned.

What might be done?

Examination of the testes is part of the routine check of a newborn boy. If a testis has not descended, regular checks will be carried out until 1 year of age. After this age, the testis is unlikely to descend spontaneously, and treatment is needed.

A drug may be given in a nasal spray to trigger the release of sex hormones to bring the testis into the scrotum, or a hormone that may cause the testis to descend can be injected. If drug treatment is unsuccessful, surgery is carried out between the ages of 2 and 3. After treatment, most boys develop normally, and sexual function is unaffected.

(WWW) ONLINE SITES: p.1028

Urinary tract infections in children

Infection of the urinary tract, which may lead to kidney damage

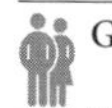 GENDER Overall more common in girls

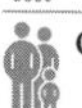 GENETICS Sometimes run in families

 AGE LIFESTYLE Not significant factors

Urinary tract infections develop when bacteria, normally present around the anus, pass up the urethra (the passage from the bladder to outside the body) and infect the bladder (*see* CYSTITIS, p.709) or kidneys (*see* PYELONEPHRITIS, p.698). Less commonly, a bacterial infection may be carried to the urinary tract in the bloodstream. Most urinary infections are easily treated, but they may scar the kidneys, increasing the risk of further infection, so treatment must be prompt. Urinary infections tend to be more common in girls, although newborn boys are more susceptible than newborn girls.

The kidney infection pyelonephritis is more common in children who have urinary reflux. In this condition, there is an abnormality of the ureters (the passages from the kidneys to the bladder) where they open into the bladder. This abnormality results in a small amount of urine flowing back up the ureters towards the kidneys when the bladder is emptied. Urinary reflux sometimes runs in families, suggesting a genetic factor.

WHAT ARE THE SYMPTOMS?

If your child is under the age of 2, he or she may be unable to describe any specific symptoms, but you may notice:

- Fever.
- Vomiting and/or diarrhoea.
- Irritability or drowsiness.

Older children often have more specific symptoms and can explain how they feel. In addition to the symptoms of young children, an older child may have:

- Frequent, urgent need to pass urine.
- Burning sensation on passing urine.
- Pain in the lower abdomen or side.
- Bedwetting (p.872) or daytime wetting after a period of dryness.

If you suspect that your child has developed an infection of the urinary tract, you should consult the doctor at once.

TEST DMSA SCANNING

To look for scarring in the kidneys, a type of radionuclide scanning (p.251) called dimercaptosuccinic acid (DMSA) scanning is used. In this procedure, which takes place in hospital, a small amount of radioactive DMSA is injected into a vein in the arm. After 2 hours, the DMSA collects in the kidneys and images of the organs are taken with a gamma camera. The scan takes about 30 minutes and is painless.

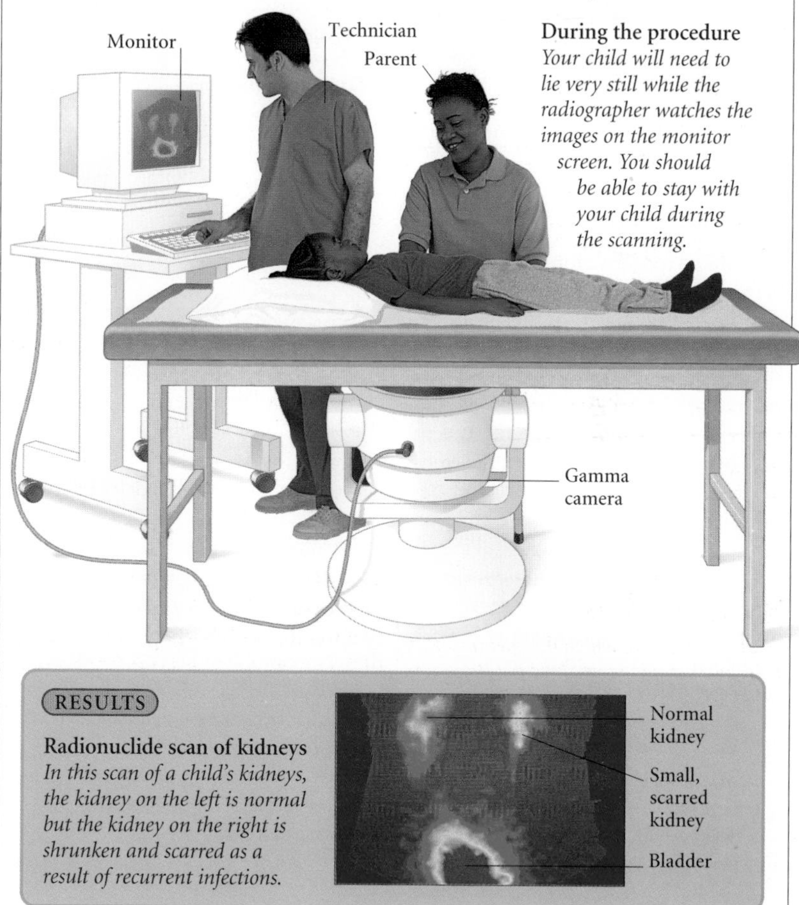

During the procedure
Your child will need to lie very still while the radiographer watches the images on the monitor screen. You should be able to stay with your child during the scanning.

Radionuclide scan of kidneys
In this scan of a child's kidneys, the kidney on the left is normal but the kidney on the right is shrunken and scarred as a result of recurrent infections.

WHAT MIGHT BE DONE?

The doctor will test a urine sample for evidence of infection. If the test indicates a possible infection, your child will be treated at once with antibiotics (p.885). The sample will be sent for laboratory testing to identify the bacteria responsible. The antibiotics may be changed when the results are known. If the symptoms suggest pyelonephritis, your child will probably be treated in hospital with intravenous antibiotics and fluids.

Your child may need to have radionuclide scanning (*see* DMSA SCANNING, above) or ultrasound scanning (p.250) to look for scarring in the kidneys or other abnormalities of the urinary tract. A specialized X-ray to check for urinary reflux may also be carried out. In this procedure, a dye is introduced into the bladder through a narrow tube. X-rays are then taken as the child passes urine. A child with urinary reflux will be given low-dose antibiotics until the age of 7, when the kidneys are no longer at risk. In severe cases, surgery may be needed.

With treatment, most children with a urinary tract infection make a full recovery. However, infections may recur, and your child should drink plenty of fluids. A few children who have recurrent infections due to reflux develop kidney failure (p.705) in later life.

WWW ONLINE SITES: p.1028, p.1033

Bedwetting

Involuntary emptying of the bladder during sleep, also known as enuresis

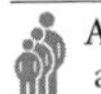
AGE Considered abnormal only over the age of 6 years

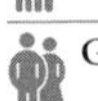
GENDER Slightly more common in boys

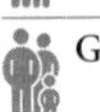
GENETICS Sometimes runs in families

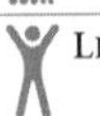
LIFESTYLE Emotional stress is a risk factor

Children normally stop wetting the bed between the ages of 3 and 6 years. Bedwetting is considered a problem only if it persists after the age of 6 or if it starts again after 6 months or more of dryness. At the age of 5, about 1 in 10 children wets the bed regularly. At the age of 10, the number is about 1 in 20. The problem is slightly more common in boys. Some children are late staying dry at night because the section of the nervous system that controls bladder function develops slowly. This developmental delay sometimes runs in families. Other children start to bedwet following stressful events such as divorce. Rarely, the condition develops because of an underlying disorder, such as diabetes mellitus (p.687) or a urinary tract infection (*see* URINARY TRACT INFECTIONS IN CHILDREN, p.871).

WHAT CAN I DO?

The most important factors in helping your child to stop bedwetting are praise, patience, and encouragement. Talking to your child may reveal worries that could be contributing to the problem. Routine visits to the toilet before bedtime are important, and it may be helpful to wake your child at your own bedtime so he or she can pass urine. A chart, on which a star is awarded after each dry night, is a visible reminder of progress. If your child is still wetting the bed after the age of 6 or begins to wet after 6 months or more of being dry at night, consult your doctor. If your child also has "accidents" during the day, the cause could be a bladder problem, which can be treated with antispasmodic drugs (p.926).

WHAT MIGHT THE DOCTOR DO?

Your doctor may test a urine sample to exclude diabetes mellitus or a urinary tract infection that may require treatment with antibiotics (p.885).

SELF-HELP OVERCOMING BEDWETTING

A child may be helped to overcome persistent bedwetting by using a pad and buzzer system. The pad, which can detect moisture, is placed in the bed and attached to a buzzer. When a child starts to pass urine, the buzzer is activated. The noise wakes the child, who can then get up and go to the bathroom before going back to sleep. After a few weeks, the child will wake automatically without the buzzer if he or she needs to pass urine.

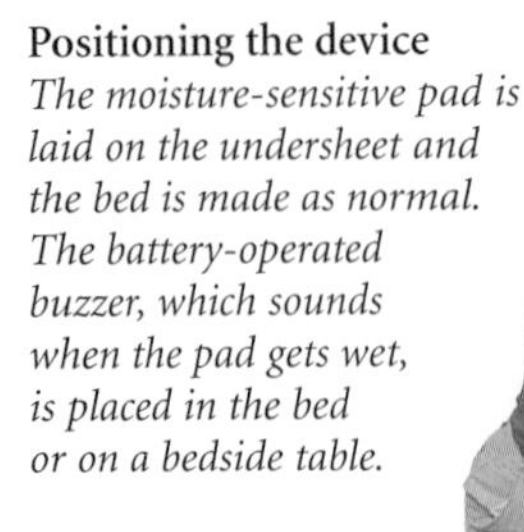
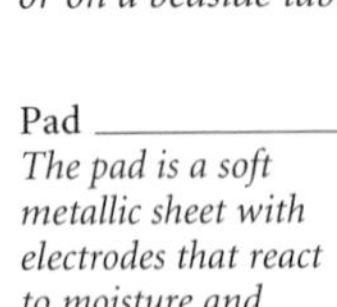
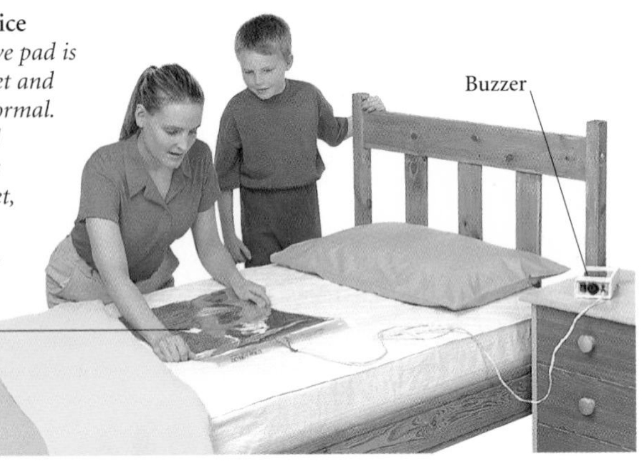

Positioning the device
The moisture-sensitive pad is laid on the undersheet and the bed is made as normal. The battery-operated buzzer, which sounds when the pad gets wet, is placed in the bed or on a bedside table.

Pad
The pad is a soft metallic sheet with electrodes that react to moisture and trigger the buzzer

Children may be helped to overcome persistent bedwetting with a special pad that triggers a buzzer when they start to pass urine (*see* OVERCOMING BEDWETTING, above). If your child goes away overnight, a nasal spray that contains desmopressin (*see* DRUGS THAT AFFECT BLADDER CONTROL, p.939) may be prescribed. If bedwetting persists, your child may be referred to a special clinic for advice. With patience and support, most children eventually stop bedwetting.

WWW ONLINE SITES: p.1028

Wilms' tumour

A rare cancer of the kidney, also known as a nephroblastoma

AGE Usually develops between birth and the age of 5

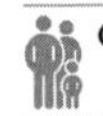
GENETICS Sometimes runs in families

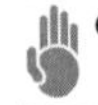
GENDER LIFESTYLE Not significant factors

Wilms' tumour is a rare type of kidney cancer, affecting fewer than 8 in 100,000 children. The tumour commonly develops before the age of 5, and it may be present at birth. Usually, one kidney is affected, but in about 1 in 10 children with the disease tumours occur in both kidneys. Wilms' tumour sometimes runs in families, but the cause is unknown.

WHAT ARE THE SYMPTOMS?

A tumour may be large before symptoms appear. Symptoms may include:

- Obvious swelling in the abdomen.
- Abdominal pain or discomfort.
- Occasionally, blood in the urine.

A child with these symptoms should be seen by a doctor immediately.

WHAT MIGHT BE DONE?

The doctor will examine your child and test a urine sample for the presence of blood. If the doctor suspects that there is a tumour in the kidney, further tests will be necessary. Ultrasound scanning (p.250) or CT scanning (p.247) of the kidneys may be performed. Other tests, such as a chest X-ray (p.490), may also be carried out to check if the cancer has spread elsewhere in the body.

Surgical removal of the affected kidney is the usual treatment for Wilms' tumour. The remaining healthy kidney can easily perform the work of both. To destroy any remaining cancerous cells, an affected child may have radiotherapy (p.281) and/or chemotherapy (p.280). In rare cases in which both the kidneys need to be removed, dialysis (p.707) or a kidney transplant (p.708) is necessary. Treatment has a high success rate, and about 8 in 10 affected children are free of the cancer after 5 years.

WWW ONLINE SITES: p.1028, p.1037

Treating Disease

This section provides an overview of a wide range of medical treatments, such as types of drug and surgery. It also covers rehabilitation, psychological, and complementary therapies. The section provides advice on home nursing and caring for the critically ill and dying. The final part illustrates the general principles of first aid for a range of injuries and disorders. Many of the articles direct you to online sites where further information can be found.

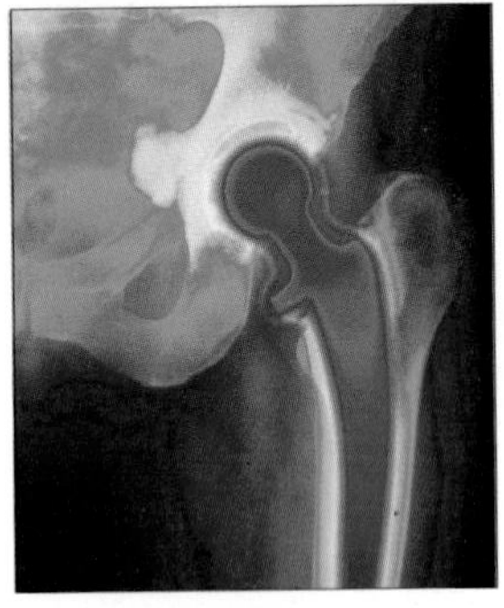

Artificial hip joint
Joints that have been damaged by disease can be replaced by artificial joints to relieve pain and to restore mobility.

INTRODUCTION

MEDICAL AND PHARMACEUTICAL RESEARCH has provided doctors with a broad range of effective treatments, including powerful drugs and precise new forms of surgery. Although there are many treatments that cure a disease or disorder, the majority are designed to relieve symptoms. Some treatments, such as immunizations, are given to prevent diseases developing. Treatments for sick, disabled, and elderly people are provided in hospital and at home by carers ranging from nurses and other professionals to relatives and friends.

When you are ill or injured, the first decision to be made is whether professional medical help is required. This may be obvious in an emergency but less so if the disorder is troublesome but not serious. Many minor problems disappear without treatment, and many others can be dealt with using home or over-the-counter remedies. Routine first-aid treatments can be used for trivial injuries, or while a person is waiting for medical assistance for serious injuries. However, if you are in doubt, or if a condition does not start to improve with self-help measures, you should seek medical advice.

In the past, people generally accepted the treatment suggested by their doctor without question. Today, with better education and access to medical information, people expect to be involved in decisions about their treatment. Most treatments fall into one of three broad categories: drugs, surgery, or some form of supportive therapy or care. In practice, many disorders require a combination of treatments used simultaneously or in sequence and often supported by nursing care.

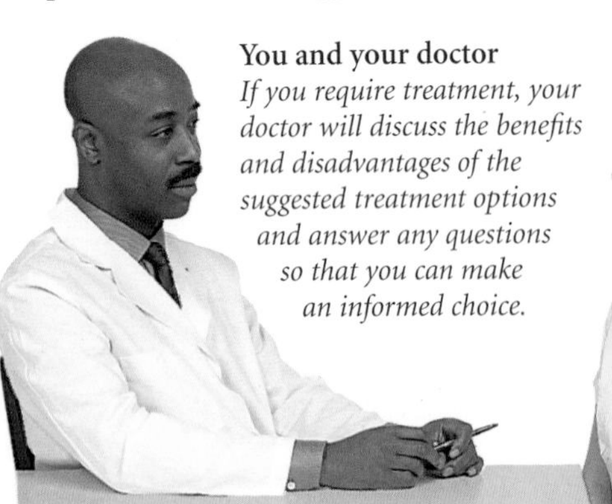

You and your doctor
If you require treatment, your doctor will discuss the benefits and disadvantages of the suggested treatment options and answer any questions so that you can make an informed choice.

Bacteria
Sample of ineffective antibiotic
Bacteria-free zone
Sample of effective antibiotic

Testing drugs
Drug prescriptions are tailored for each patient's needs. The sensitivity of an infectious organism to various antibiotics can be tested before prescribing.

AIMS OF TREATMENT

The purpose of treatment may be to cure a disorder, slow down its progress, relieve symptoms, or prevent an illness developing. Supportive treatments, such as physiotherapy and counselling, focus on speeding up recovery or helping people to come to terms with their illness and live as independently as possible. The optimal result of treatment is to cure an illness completely with minimum risk and side effects. Many drugs and surgical treatments are complete cures. For example, antibiotics cure by eliminating infection, and surgery can cure completely when used to repair an injury or replace a diseased organ with a transplant.

When no cure is available, the next option is relief of symptoms. Some drugs relieve symptoms common to several conditions. For example, painkillers relieve headache and muscle and joint pain regardless of whether the cause is a minor injury, a common cold, or a long-term condition such as arthritis.

Other drugs relieve symptoms that are specific to particular conditions. Bronchodilators are drugs that ease the wheezing that occurs in lung disorders such as asthma. Drugs may also be used to increase

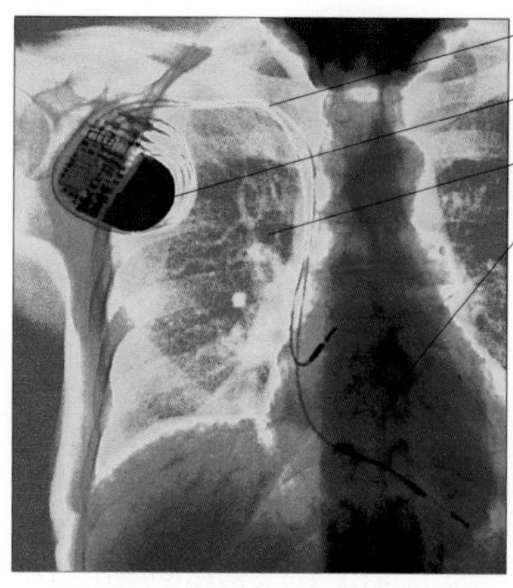

Regulating the heart
Some treatments, such as the fitting of an artificial pacemaker, help to control the effects of a disorder rather than treating the underlying cause.

the levels of substances in the body, such as hormones and neurotransmitters. For example, drugs that restore normal levels of dopamine, a neurotransmitter that acts on the part of the brain controlling movement, reduce symptoms of Parkinson's disease.

If a disease is incurable, treatment may be able to slow its progression. For example, immunosuppressant drugs may slow the progress of joint damage due to rheumatoid arthritis. Increasingly, doctors use drug treatments to prevent disease. For example, drugs that lower blood pressure reduce the risk of stroke.

Planning treatment

Before starting treatment, your doctor will discuss the available options with you. For minor illnesses or when there is only one suitable treatment, little discussion may be required. However, for a long-term disorder or one that is serious, there may be a choice between treatment with surgery or with drugs, or between different forms of surgery or different drugs. Your doctor will also discuss the risks or possible side effects of your treatment. Your consent will be needed before treatment can begin.

For most disorders, early diagnosis and treatment offer the best chance of a cure. Treatment that is started late may involve more risks and a longer recovery time. However, in the absence of a clear diagnosis, your doctor may wait for confirmation of the disorder rather than begin treatment that may turn out to be inappropriate. Before treating you, he or she will take into account your age and existing medical conditions and may ask you to make lifestyle changes, such as losing weight or giving up smoking.

In circumstances in which there is no prospect of a cure, there may be little benefit in radical treatment. For example, when a person has advanced cancer, chemotherapy and radiotherapy treatments may do little to prolong life and can cause debilitating side effects. The better option may be relief of symptoms and care given by professionals in a hospital or hospice or by carers and family at home.

Advances and improvements

Advances in medicine have led to new treatments that play a major part in improving life expectancy and reducing long-term illness. New technologies have brought about improvements in surgical techniques that minimize post-operative pain, reduce risks and

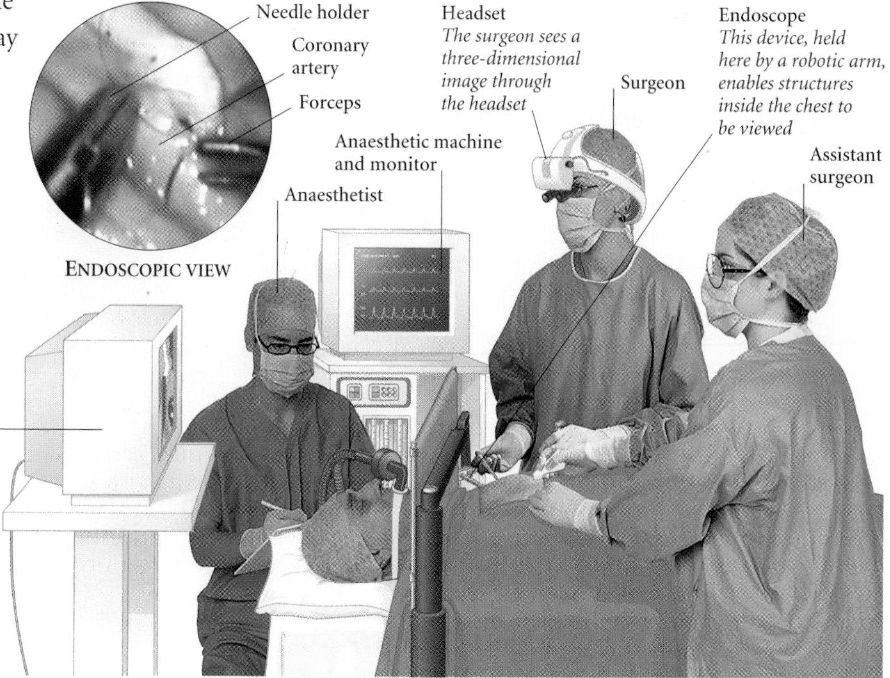

New surgical techniques
Advances in computer-guided surgery and three-dimensional viewing have made endoscopic surgery on the beating heart possible. These new techiques result in fewer complications than in standard open surgery.

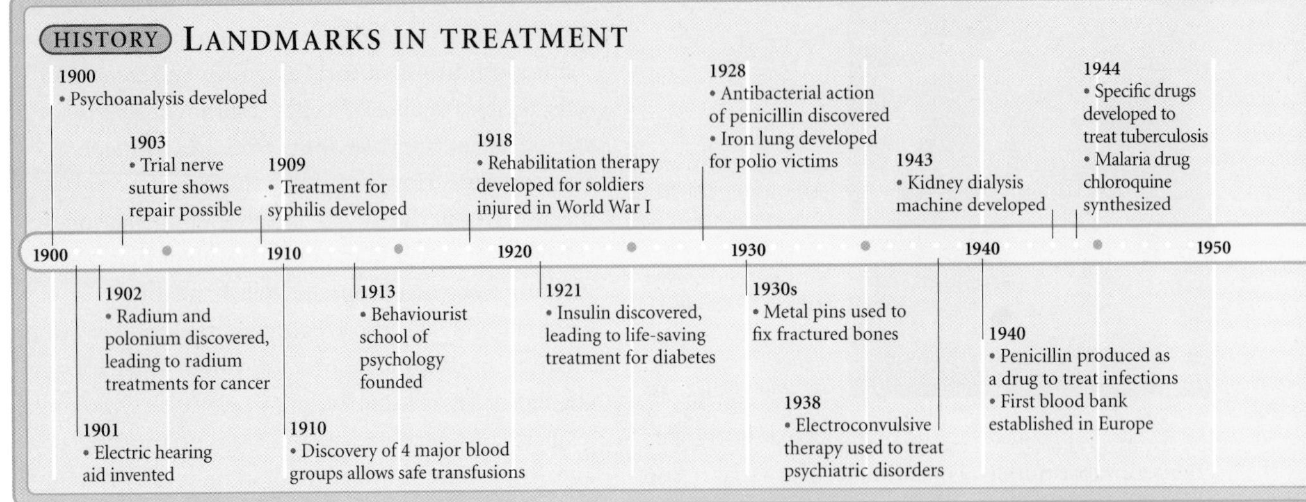

New technologies and discoveries
In the space of 100 years, new technologies and drug discoveries have provided treatments that have reduced the impact of many diseases. In particular, new types of surgery have made operations safer and shortened recovery times.

complications, and allow quicker recovery. However, before a new drug or technique is approved, it must be rigorously tested, and its effectiveness and safety and demonstrated in controlled trials.

Development of drugs

At one time, the only drugs available were substances extracted from plants and natural minerals such as salts. Over the past 100 years, medical research has produced safer and more reliably effective synthetic modifications of naturally occurring substances and some completely new drugs. Antibiotics and vaccines have revolutionized the treatment of infections.

Genetic engineering is now used to produce human insulin and other hormonal treatments. In addition, research into the underlying mechanisms of disease has produced tailor-made drugs that target a particular part of a disease process. For example, some treatments for high blood pressure block the action of particular hormones on the heart and blood vessels. The development of immunosuppressant drugs that reduce the body's rejection of new tissue has enabled transplant surgery to be carried out successfully.

Advances in surgery

About 30 years ago, major surgery inevitably required a large incision to open up the body. Conventional open surgery is still needed to treat many conditions, but there are now many less invasive techniques that result in fewer complications, less post-operative pain, and shorter recovery times. Surgery can be performed through a natural body opening or through a small incision using a viewing tube called an endoscope.

Surgical precision has been improved by advances in imaging and viewing techniques. In microsurgery, surgeons use a specialized microscope and tiny instruments to perform operations on minute structures, such as nerves and small blood vessels. For operations on delicate areas such as the brain, surgeons can wear a headset that displays three-dimensional images of the site of the operation. Technological advances also include the use of lasers and electrocautery equipment, which seal blood vessels as tissue is cut, reducing bleeding during surgery.

Home therapy
Although some treatments must be started in hospital, they can be continued at home by a visiting professional, such as a physiotherapist. The trend is for recovery and rehabilitation to take place at home.

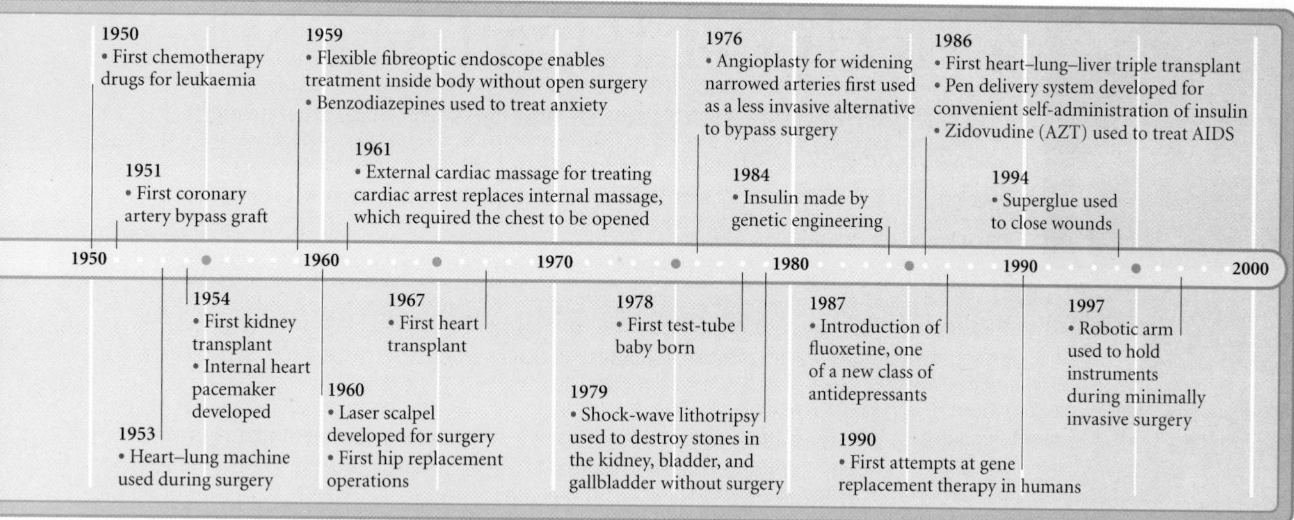

Changing attitudes to care

Treatment must be provided in a setting of effective care but, even in the case of serious illness, care no longer necessarily takes place in hospital. Complex treatments, such as kidney dialysis, can now be carried out at home by carers, and a number of surgical procedures take place in outpatient departments and doctors' surgeries, allowing the patient to return home for convalescence immediately after treatment.

Interest in complementary medicine is growing, and some people may not regard conventional medicine as the first choice of treatment for certain problems. For example, chiropractic may be used for back problems, and acupuncture for pain relief. Most complementary therapies have not been subjected to the same research and trials as conventional treatments, but there is good evidence for the effectiveness of some therapies, particularly acupuncture and biofeedback.

(ORGANIZATION) How this part of the book is organized

This part of the book describes drug treatments, surgery, supportive care and therapeutic treatments, and first aid. The drug treatment section covers the major drug groups, arranged primarily under the body systems that they are used to treat. Common brand-name and generic drugs are listed in the drug glossary at the end of the book.

Drug treatment p.878
Explains what drugs are and how they work; how drugs affect individual body cells; different routes of administration; how drugs are broken down in the body.

Understanding drugs p.880
The effects of drugs, including side effects, drug tolerance and dependence; advice on using medication safely and effectively.

Drug groups p.883
Covers the major drug groups; describes how drugs in each group work, how they are taken, and their main side effects; includes lists of common drugs.

Surgery p.940
Advances in surgical technology and methods; illustrates a typical operating room and common surgical instruments.

Having an operation p.942
What is involved when you have surgery; includes pre-operative preparation, types of anaesthesia, and post-operative care.

Types of surgery p.947
The major types of surgery and surgical techniques, including open and endoscopic surgery, microsurgery, laser treatment, plastic surgery, and transplant surgery.

Care and therapies p.954
Introduces the range of care and therapies used at home and in hospital, from emergency care to rehabilitation, and describes changing trends in caregiving.

Care of the sick p.956
The different settings in which care is given, including outpatient departments and day care in hospital and home care.

Rehabilitation therapies p.961
Physiotherapy and occupational and speech therapy used in rehabilitation.

Death and dying p.964
Preparations for death, including making a living will; caring for a terminally ill person; practical issues following a death.

Psychological therapies p.968
Psychoanalytic psychotherapy; behaviour, cognitive, person-centred, and group therapies; and counselling.

Complementary therapies p.972
The place of complementary therapies in treatment; different types of therapy.

First aid p.976
Key techniques to help you deal with a range of common emergencies.

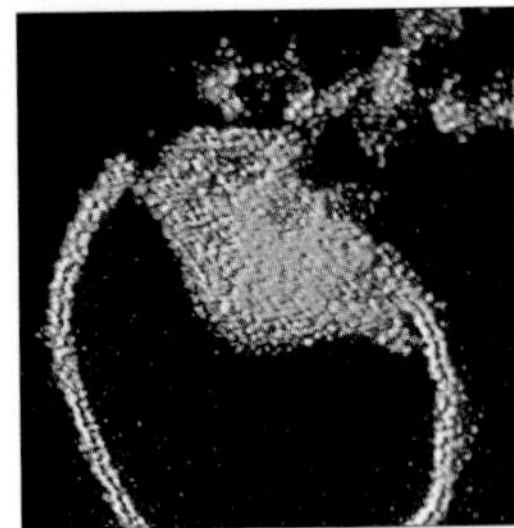

Drug killing a bacterium
A Staphylococcus aureus *bacterium is destroyed by an antibiotic drug.*

DRUG TREATMENT

MEDICINAL DRUGS ARE SUBSTANCES that can cure, arrest, or prevent disease, relieve symptoms, or help in the diagnosis of certain disorders. Over the past 50 years, the number of drugs available has increased enormously, and new drugs have been developed that are more effective in restoring health and saving lives than ever before. Researchers continue to improve the effectiveness of existing drugs and to develop treatments for as yet unconquered areas of medicine, such as cancer and HIV infection.

Modern drug therapy began when scientists discovered how to isolate the active ingredients in plant sources and how to create synthetic versions of those substances. This new technology, together with a better understanding of how the body functions both in health and in disease, has enabled the development of drugs that can target specific processes in the body.

Before any new drug is marketed, it is thoroughly tested. The effects that the drug has on people are measured either against the existing standard treatment or against a placebo (an inactive substance that looks and tastes exactly like the drug).

In the UK, drugs are approved and licensed by the Committee on Safety of Medicines (CSM). A new drug is approved only if it is shown to be safe and effective. The CSM can withdraw a drug from the market if it later proves to cause unacceptable side effects.

HOW DRUGS WORK

Drugs act in a variety of ways. Some kill or halt the spread of invading organisms, such as bacteria, fungi, and viruses. These drugs include antivirals, antifungals, and antibiotics. Other drugs, known as cytotoxic drugs, kill cells as they divide or prevent their replication. Cytotoxic drugs are mainly used in the treatment of cancer.

Some drugs simply supplement missing or low levels of natural body chemicals such as certain hormones or vitamins. Another group of drugs alters the effectiveness of certain body chemicals. These drugs work either by mimicking the action of natural chemicals to increase their effect or by blocking their action to decrease their effect (*see* HOW DRUGS ACT ON RECEPTORS, below). For example, beta-blockers slow the rate at which the heart beats by blocking the effects of chemicals that increase the heart rate.

Drugs may also affect the part of the nervous system that controls a particular process. For example, most drugs taken to relieve vomiting act on the vomiting centre in the brain.

HOW DRUGS ARE USED

There are various different ways in which drugs may be delivered to their intended site of action. Some, such as eyedrops or topical skin preparations, can be applied directly to the target area. These preparations tend to have a very localized effect and do not usually enter the bloodstream in significant quantities. Other preparations are introduced into the bloodstream, which circulates them to their target area in the body. These drugs may be delivered by different routes, depending on which is the most effective way to reach the target area and on how the drugs are metabolized (*see* DRUG METABOLISM, opposite page).

DRUG ACTION

HOW DRUGS ACT ON RECEPTORS

Many cells have specialized areas, known as receptors, on their outer walls. Natural chemical messengers, such as hormones, bind with these receptors to produce changes in cells and thereby affect body processes. In order to treat some disorders, it may be necessary to increase or decrease the effect of a particular natural chemical. Drugs called agonists bind with specific receptors to produce an effect similar to that of the natural chemical. Antagonist drugs inhibit the effect of the chemical by blocking the receptors.

Natural chemical
Agonist drug
Receptor
Change in the cell
Body cell
BEFORE DRUG
AFTER DRUG

Agonist drugs
An agonist drug mimics the action of body chemicals. It occupies an empty receptor and enhances the natural chemical's effect.

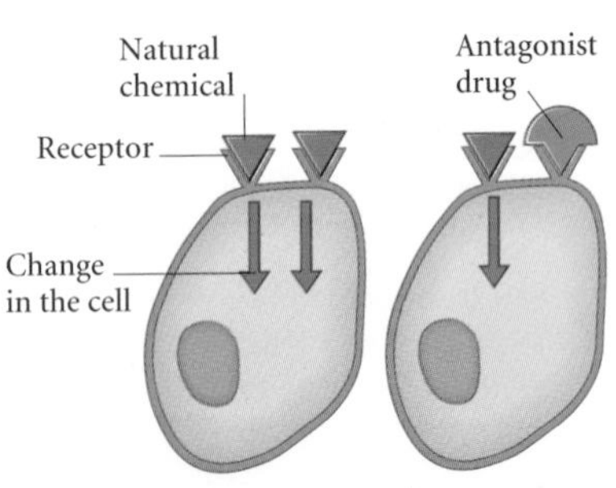

BEFORE DRUG
AFTER DRUG

Antagonist drugs
An antagonist drug occupies cell receptors, preventing the body chemicals from binding to them, thereby inhibiting their action.

(PROCESS) DRUGS IN YOUR BODY

Drugs can be introduced into the bloodstream by a number of different routes. Most commonly, they are taken orally in the form of pills, capsules, or liquids. However, if oral treatment is inappropriate, drugs may be given in other ways. For example, a suppository containing a drug can be inserted into the rectum. If an immediate effect is needed, intravenous injection or infusion ensures the rapid delivery of the drug. A long-lasting effect is achieved by administering a drug in a skin patch or as an implant just below the skin.

Nasal/sublingual/ buccal route
Drugs in a nasal spray, in a sublingual tablet (placed under the tongue), or in a buccal tablet (placed inside the cheek) are absorbed through the thin mucous membrane directly into the bloodstream.

Drug
Blood vessel
Mucus layer
Mucous membrane

Oral route
Drugs in pill, capsule, or liquid form are swallowed and pass into the digestive system. The drugs are then broken down in either the stomach or the intestines and are absorbed in the same way as food.

Intestinal lining
Drug
Blood vessel

Intravenous route
An injection into a blood vessel allows a drug to take effect very quickly. The drug enters the bloodstream directly and is rapidly circulated to the organ or tissues where it is needed.

Needle
Skin surface
Drug
Blood vessel

Intramuscular route
Drugs are injected into a muscle in the upper arm, thigh, or buttock and then disperse into the bloodstream.

Needle
Muscle
Drug in bloodstream

Subcutaneous route
Drugs implanted or injected into fatty tissue just below the skin disperse slowly into the bloodstream.

Implant
Drug
Fatty tissue

Transdermal route
Drugs are released continuously from an adhesive patch or a gel on the skin surface and pass through the skin into blood vessels.

Drug
Patch
Skin surface
Blood vessel

Rectal route
Drugs inserted into the rectum in suppositories, enemas, or foam are quickly absorbed by blood vessels in the rectal wall.

Drug
Rectal wall
Suppository

DRUG METABOLISM

Drugs that are taken orally are absorbed in the intestines and pass through the liver before entering the general circulation. Drugs that are administered by other routes enter the bloodstream before they pass through the liver. Once a drug has entered the bloodstream, it circulates to the site where its action is needed. Most drugs are metabolized (broken down or transformed) each time they pass through the liver. They are eventually excreted by the kidneys in urine and/or by the liver in bile, which is excreted in faeces.

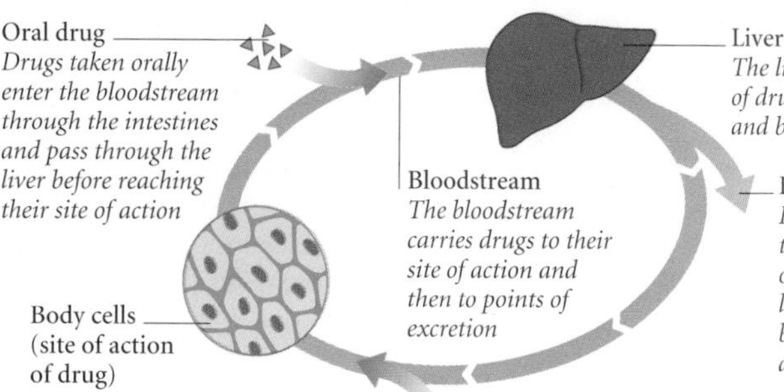

How drugs circulate
Oral drugs pass through the liver, where some may be inactivated before reaching their site of action. Drugs given by other routes bypass the liver initially.

UNDERSTANDING DRUGS

All drugs, even the familiar ones such as aspirin, may have potentially harmful as well as beneficial effects. Whether you are prescribed drug treatment or you choose remedies for yourself, you will gain most benefit from drugs if you understand how they are likely to act and how to use them safely and effectively.

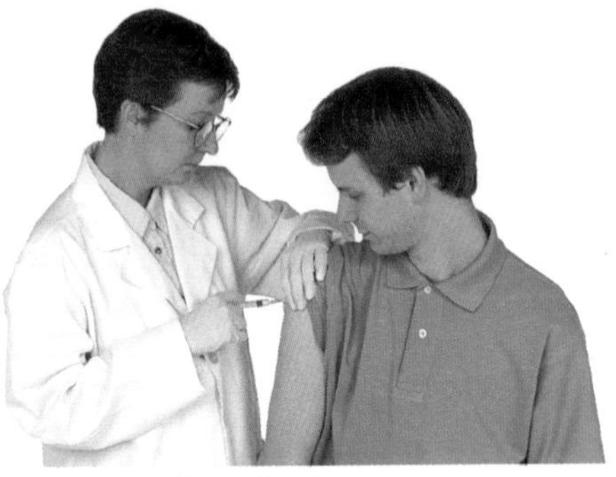

Courses of vaccination
Most drugs are used in the treatment of disease. However, vaccines may be given to prevent certain diseases, such as diphtheria or tetanus, from developing.

During the last century, advances in drug treatment have enabled doctors to cure many conditions, including a wide range of infectious diseases. Drug treatment can also be used to control symptoms in disorders such as epilepsy and to relieve common symptoms such as wheezing or itching. Today, there is a vast range of drugs available for many purposes. Some drugs can be bought over the counter at pharmacies or other retail outlets. Other types of drug require a doctor's prescription, and a few drugs are available only in hospitals. In order to make the best use of drug treatments and avoid any possible adverse effects, you must follow the instructions given by your doctor or pharmacist or those supplied by the manufacturer carefully. You may find it useful to discuss your treatment with your doctor or pharmacist so that you know when you can expect to feel an improvement and whether there could be any adverse effects.

The first article in this section covers the types of effect that various drugs may have on the body. The second article gives practical advice on how to use various types of medication safely and effectively along with a discussion on how to store drugs safely.

How drugs affect you

How drugs act on your body and their possible effects

A drug may have several types of effect on your body as well as the intended action. These include side effects, tolerance, and dependence. Interaction may also occur, in which drugs that are taken together enhance or reduce each other's actions. Many drugs can have a powerful psychological benefit called the placebo effect. A number of drugs have unwanted effects, which can be unpleasant or harmful, and your doctor will plan drug treatment to avoid or minimize these effects.

A drug's effects can vary from one individual to another. Drugs tend to have particularly strong effects on certain people, such as children and the elderly.

SIDE EFFECTS OF DRUGS

Almost all systemic drugs (drugs that affect the whole body) can cause side effects – undesired reactions resulting from a normal dose. Side effects occur because drugs act on cells throughout the body, not just in the area to be treated. For example, beta-blocker drugs (p.898) may be used in the treatment of hypertension (p.403). However, they may disrupt sleeping patterns as a side effect of their intended action.

Some side effects, such as the dry mouth caused by some antihistamines (p.906), are predictable because they result from the known chemical effects of a drug. However, drugs may also produce unpredictable reactions such as drug allergy (p.467). Any type of drug, including penicillins (*see* ANTIBIOTICS, p.885), can cause allergic reactions that can range in severity from a mild rash to severe breathing problems. Other unexpected reactions occur in people whose genetic make-up influences their body's ability to break down particular drugs. For example, some people of Mediterranean, African, or Southeast Asian origin inherit a condition called G6PD deficiency, which affects the chemistry of red blood cells. If these people take certain types of drug, such as sulphonamides, they may develop haemolytic anaemia (p.450), a condition in which red blood cells are destroyed prematurely. As a result, the blood does not carry enough oxygen to body tissues.

Most side effects are not serious, and they often disappear gradually as your body becomes used to a drug. However, for some drugs used to treat serious disorders, the side effects are severe and potentially fatal. For instance, certain cytotoxic drugs used to treat cancer (*see* ANTICANCER DRUGS, p.907) are toxic to the heart and can cause it to fail. A medical decision to use a drug depends on whether the overall benefit outweighs the risk of harmful effects.

DRUG TOLERANCE AND DEPENDENCE

If you take certain drugs for a long time, your body adapts to them in a process known as tolerance. With some drugs, tolerance may be useful, allowing the body to overcome side effects while still responding to the beneficial effects of the drug. For example, many people taking antidepressants (p.916) find that side effects such as a dry mouth disappear while the benefits remain. However, tolerance may make some drugs less effective so that a higher dose is needed to obtain the same result. The higher dose may increase side effects.

Dependence is a need for a drug. The need can be psychological, leading you to think that you cannot function normally without a certain drug. It can also be physical. For example, long-term use of laxatives (p.924) can make your body depend on them for bowel movements.

If you become dependent on certain drugs, such as benzodiazepines (*see* ANTIANXIETY DRUGS, p.916), your body may develop tolerance to them. If you then stop taking them, you may suffer unpleasant effects known as withdrawal symptoms, which are sometimes dangerous. It is also possible to become dependent on drugs that are not medicines, such as alcohol (*see* ALCOHOL DEPENDENCE, p.564) or nicotine.

PEOPLE AT SPECIAL RISK

The effects of a drug may differ from one person to another. This variation occurs because people's bodies absorb and excrete drugs at different rates. In addition, the same dose of a drug may reach different concentrations in the blood depending on factors such as body size and kidney function. Groups at higher risk of adverse effects include fetuses, babies (particularly breast-fed babies whose mothers are taking drugs), children, people who have liver or kidney disease, and elderly people.

FETUSES Most drugs that are taken during pregnancy pass across the placenta to the fetus. Many can harm the fetus, especially if taken during the first 12 weeks of pregnancy when the fetus's organs are developing. If you know or believe that you are pregnant, check with your doctor or pharmacist before taking any drug. If you take regular medication for a long-term condition such as diabetes mellitus (p.687) or epilepsy (p.524), discuss your treatment with your doctor if you are planning to have a baby. Often, the risk to mother and fetus from not treating a condition such as epilepsy is greater than the risk posed by the drug itself.

BREAST-FED BABIES If a woman takes drugs while breast-feeding, they may pass into her breast milk. Some drugs cause unwanted effects in the baby. For example, antianxiety drugs may make the baby drowsy and cause feeding difficulties. If you are breast-feeding, you should check with your doctor or pharmacist before taking any drug.

BABIES AND CHILDREN Drugs must be used with care in babies and children. Children's doses are usually smaller than doses for adults and are often calculated on the basis of a child's weight or age. It is very important to give children the correct dose. Never give a child a drug prescribed for an adult.

PEOPLE WITH LIVER OR KIDNEY DISEASE Most drugs are broken down by enzymes in the liver. The drugs are then eliminated by the liver itself or by the kidneys and excreted in the urine (*see* DRUGS IN YOUR BODY, p.879). However, if your liver or kidneys are not functioning well, toxic substances may build up in your blood, thereby increasing the risk of side effects. You may therefore need lower doses than normal. Alcohol also affects liver function, and thus the effect of some drugs may be altered if you drink heavily or regularly.

OLDER PEOPLE Older people are at increased risk of side effects. This risk may be due to the decline in the function of organs such as the liver and kidneys as the body ages, which causes toxins to accumulate faster in the body. Older people may need to take several drugs together to treat a number of disorders, and therefore may also be at increased risk of drug interactions.

(WWW) ONLINE SITES: p.1030

Managing your medication

Using prescription and over-the-counter medications safely and effectively

Drugs must always be used with care, and you should be especially careful if you give them to children. It is important that you understand what drugs you are taking and how they are likely to affect you. Drugs must be stored safely and should be disposed of when they have expired or are no longer useful.

HOW ARE DRUGS OBTAINED?

Some drugs may be bought over the counter, but others require a doctor's prescription. Certain over-the-counter (OTC) treatments, which include some herbal and homeopathic remedies, are intended simply to relieve symptoms such as pain, nasal congestion, coughing, or indigestion. It is always wise to consult a pharmacist to make sure you are buying the most effective remedy.

(COMPARISON) DRUG PREPARATIONS

Many drugs are available in different forms. Each form has advantages. For example, tablets and liquids are easy to self-administer. Creams, ointments, gels, and sprays act directly at the site of application. Nonoral forms, such as inhaled and injected drugs, bypass the digestive system, which may break them down, and therefore reach the site of action at full strength.

Ingredients of medications
Medications are designed to be absorbed easily and to act over a set period of time. The drugs are mixed with inactive ingredients that control these factors.

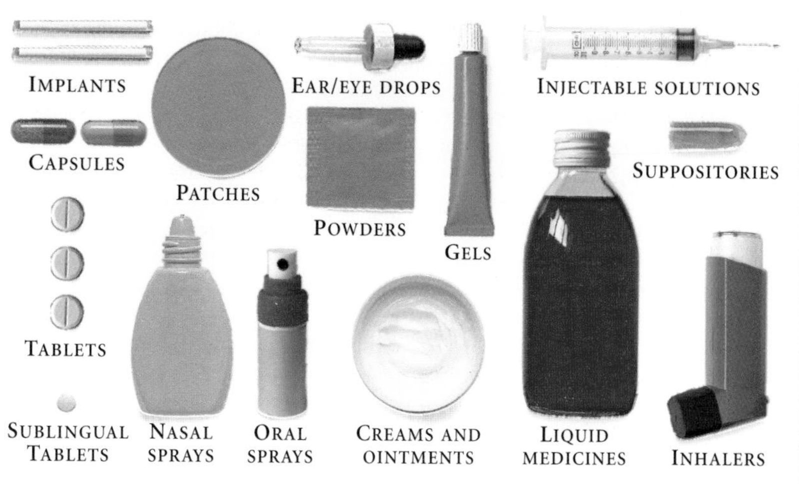

USING DRUGS SAFELY

Before taking any medication, make sure that you understand when and how to take it. Read the instructions carefully and discuss anything that you do not understand with your doctor or pharmacist. Find out whether the drug is likely to affect everyday tasks such as driving, whether you should take the drug with food or on an empty stomach, and what you should do if you miss or exceed a dose.

When you discuss your treatment with a doctor or pharmacist, let him or her know if you have recently taken any other medications, including complementary remedies, because these could affect your new treatment. In addition, you should say if you have previously taken any OTC or prescribed medication that has affected you adversely. If you are planning to have a baby or suspect that you may already be pregnant, consult your doctor before starting any treatment because some types of drug, such as retinoid drugs (p.890), can have harmful effects on a fetus.

TAKING DRUGS CORRECTLY When taking tablets or capsules, swallow them with plenty of water so that they do not become stuck in your oesophagus. If you are taking liquid medicine, shake the bottle before use to mix the ingredients thoroughly, and measure the doses carefully. Devise a routine for taking the correct doses at the correct time, especially if you take several drugs.

Make sure that you complete the full course of any treatment, even if your symptoms seem to have disappeared. Never take a drug prescribed for someone else or give your prescribed drug to anyone else. If you are using an OTC remedy, do not take the drug for more than a few days unless you are sure that the cause of your symptoms is a minor, short-lived illness, such as a cold.

DEALING WITH SIDE EFFECTS Seek medical help if you develop any unexpected side effects or symptoms that seem unrelated to your illness while taking either prescription or OTC drugs. If you have a severe reaction to a drug, such as difficulty in breathing, call for urgent medical attention. If you have a mild reaction from a prescription drug, see your doctor as soon as possible and ask whether you should stop the treatment. If you have a mild reaction from an OTC drug, stop taking it and consult your doctor before continuing.

SELF-ADMINISTRATION GIVING A CHILD MEDICINE

When giving liquid medicines to a baby or a young child, use a syringe or dropper to avoid spillage and ensure that you give the correct dose. If you are unsure how to use the syringe or dropper, ask your doctor to show you how to measure and give a dose of medicine. When treating the child, hold him or her securely to give reassurance and keep the child from struggling.

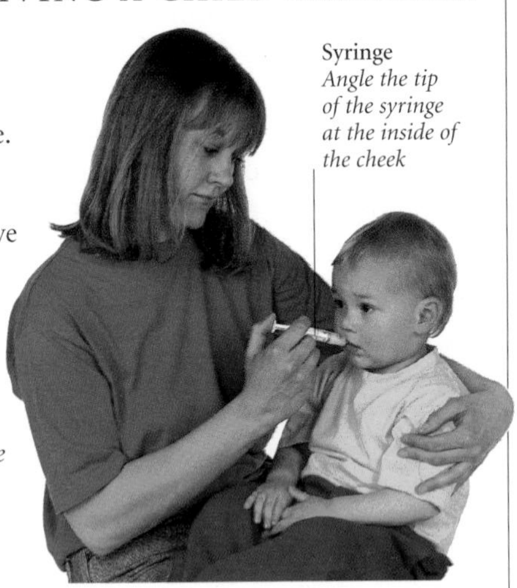

Giving medicine with a syringe
Place the tip of the syringe well inside the child's mouth and angle it towards the cheek. Slowly press the plunger, allowing the child time to swallow. Do not aim directly down the child's throat.

TAKING LONG-TERM MEDICATION If you need drug treatment that continues for a long time, such as medication to treat high blood pressure (*see* HYPERTENSION, p.403) or diabetes mellitus (p.687), you may be given a prescription that can be renewed so that you do not have to see your doctor each time. However, you will still need to see the doctor regularly so that he or she can monitor your condition and your response to treatment. Never stop taking your medication suddenly without consulting your doctor first. For some drugs, it is necessary to reduce the dose gradually so that your condition does not suddenly become worse. Gradual reduction of the dose of a drug also helps to prevent you from developing withdrawal symptoms.

If you are taking long-term medication, always talk to your pharmacist before using any additional drugs. If you need hospital treatment, tell the hospital staff which drugs you are taking, including OTC drugs or complementary remedies. Do not take your own medications while you are in hospital unless the staff specifically say that it is all right for you to do so. Some drugs, such as anticoagulants (*see* DRUGS THAT PREVENT BLOOD CLOTTING, p.904), can cause severe problems during surgery or emergency treatment or if they are taken with other drugs. If you are on long-term medication with particular drugs, such as corticosteroids (p.930), you should obtain a card, bracelet, or pendant that gives details of your medication. You should always carry this information with you so that it will be available to any medical staff who may need to treat you in an emergency.

GIVING DRUGS TO CHILDREN

Medicine for babies and toddlers usually comes in liquid form, which is easier for them to swallow. It is normally simpler to administer liquid medicine by syringe or dropper (*see* GIVING A CHILD MEDICINE, above). Older children may be given tablets, but if you need to crush them first, check with the pharmacist that this will not affect the absorption of the drug. A child who strongly dislikes medicine can hold his or her nose while taking it. Have a pleasant drink ready to wash away the taste afterwards.

HOW SHOULD DRUGS BE KEPT?

Follow storage directions to prevent drugs from deteriorating. Some drugs need to be stored in a cool, dry place and others in the refrigerator or away from light. Always keep medicines out of reach of children, preferably keeping unrefrigerated ones in a locked cabinet.

Do not keep medicines beyond their expiry dates because they may become ineffective or even harmful. Always dispose of drugs carefully.

(WWW) ONLINE SITES: p.1030

DRUGS FOR INFECTIONS AND INFESTATIONS

As recently as 50 years ago, infectious diseases were the leading cause of death in children and young adults. That picture has changed with the introduction of immunization against the major childhood diseases, antibiotics to kill bacteria, and a wide range of other anti-infective drugs.

This section describes the drugs that are used to protect the body against infectious disease as well as to control or cure infections and infestations once they have developed.

The first article discusses vaccines and immunoglobulins, which are given to provide immunity against certain infections and to prevent the spread of diseases. The next article describes antibiotics, a large group of drugs used widely to treat bacterial infections. In the UK, millions of prescriptions are written for these drugs each year.

The following articles in this section explain how drugs are used to treat infections caused by viruses, protozoa, and fungi. The information includes discussion of the prevention and cure of malaria and of recent advances made in the treatment of HIV infection and AIDS. The final article deals with drugs to eradicate parasitic worm infestations.

KEY ELEMENTS

FUNGI

BACTERIA

1mm

WORMS

PROTOZOA

VIRUSES

For more information on the structure and function of infectious organisms, *see* pp.284–287.

Vaccines and immunoglobulins

Preparations that immunize the body against certain infectious diseases

COMMON PREPARATIONS

VACCINES
- BCG • Diphtheria • Haemophilus b
- Hepatitis A • Hepatitis B • Influenza • Measles/Mumps/Rubella (MMR) • Meningococcus C
- Pertussis • Pneumococcus • Polio • Rabies
- Tetanus • Typhoid • Yellow fever

IMMUNOGLOBULINS
- Anti-D • Cytomegalovirus • Hepatitis B
- Normal immunoglobulin • Rabies
- Tetanus • Varicella–zoster

A variety of vaccines and immunoglobulins is available to provide protection against particular infectious diseases. The use of these preparations is known as immunization (p.45). Vaccines contain infectious organisms that have been modified or killed. Immunoglobulins contain antibodies (proteins made by white blood cells that neutralize or destroy infectious organisms) extracted from the blood of a person or an animal who has already had a specific disease. The body's own defence mechanism, the immune system, is able to combat many infections, but it cannot protect people against all infectious diseases. Immunization with vaccines or immunoglobulins is therefore used to give added protection. The incidence of a number of highly infectious diseases has declined dramatically worldwide since the introduction of immunization programmes. One disease, smallpox, has been eradicated worldwide.

HOW DO THEY WORK?

There are two forms of immunization, which are known as active immunization and passive immunization (*see* HOW IMMUNIZATION WORKS, p.884). In active immunization, vaccines are given to stimulate the immune system to produce its own antibodies. A different vaccine must be given for each disease because each type of infectious organism triggers the production of a specific type of antibody. Some vaccines contain live organisms that have been altered and made harmless. Others contain killed organisms, part of an organism, or a toxin (poison) made by bacteria. All forms of vaccine have the same effect of priming the body's immune system to produce appropriate antibodies so that the body is ready to fight off particular invading organisms. Passive immunization uses immunoglobulins and works by introducing donated antibodies into the blood. These antibodies destroy infectious organisms that are present or that enter the body shortly afterwards.

WHY ARE THEY USED?

Some highly infectious diseases cannot be treated effectively or can be so serious that prevention, in the form of active or passive immunization, is recommended. Active immunization with vaccines is used mainly to prevent diseases from spreading within a community. If most people are vaccinated, some diseases may eventually disappear. In developed countries, children are routinely given active immunization against a range of diseases, including measles (p.293), tetanus (p.302), and pertussis (whooping cough) (p.492), from the age of 2 months to 15 years (*see* ROUTINE IMMUNIZATIONS, p.45).

Other vaccines are used for specific groups of people. For example, immunization against influenza (p.289) is recommended for people who are at risk of becoming seriously ill if they develop the disease. Those at high risk

(DRUG ACTION) HOW IMMUNIZATION WORKS

The most commonly used method of immunization is known as active immunization or vaccination. This involves the introduction into the body of a harmless form of an infectious organism that stimulates the body to produce antibodies against that organism. To provide immediate protection, a method called passive immunization is used. This introduces into the body "ready-made" antibodies extracted from people or animals who already have immunity to the infection.

ACTIVE IMMUNIZATION

Many vaccines are made from weakened forms of a disease-causing organism; these are known as live vaccines. Others use an inactive form or just a part of the organism, such as a protein. Protection may be lifelong, or booster shots may be needed.

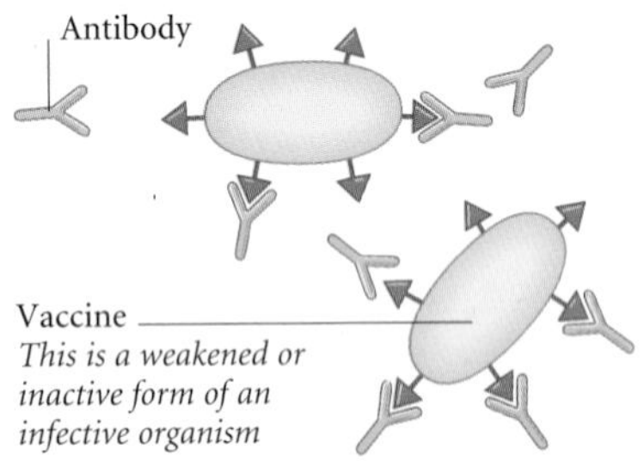

1 *Antibodies are formed in response to the organisms in the vaccine. A "memory" of these antibodies is retained by the immune system.*

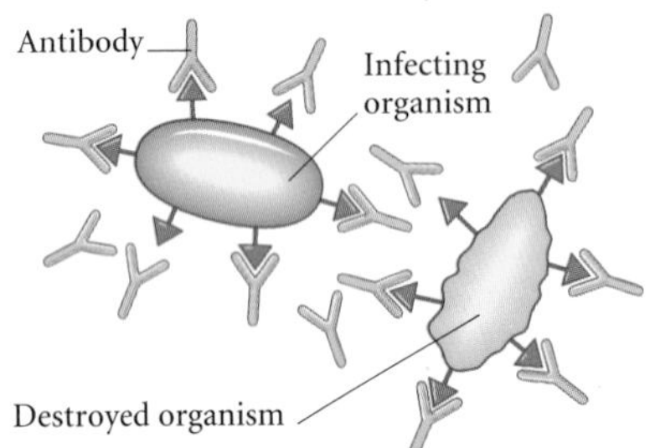

2 *If the same organism invades the body at a later date, the immune system will recognize it and will rapidly produce antibodies to destroy it.*

PASSIVE IMMUNIZATION

Immunity to an infectious organism can be achieved by the introduction of donated antibodies. This is needed if no active immunization is available or if rapid protection against an organism is vital, especially for people with weakened immune systems.

Donated antibody

1 *Antibodies taken from humans or animals with immunity to the infection are introduced into the body.*

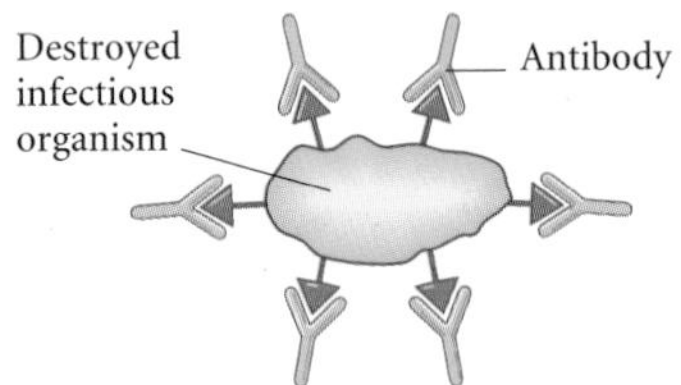

2 *When exposed to the infectious organism, the antibodies immediately destroy it. They also provide short-term protection against future infection.*

include elderly people, those who have reduced immunity because of diseases such as diabetes mellitus (p.687), and people with long-term heart or lung disease. There are many different types (strains) of influenza, and a specific vaccine is required for each one. New influenza vaccines are usually created each year to match the viral strains predicted to be most widespread.

Vaccines are also used for people who are at increased risk from certain infections. For example, people travelling to a developing country are advised to receive immunization against diseases that are common in that region (*see* TRAVEL IMMUNIZATIONS, p.86).

The main use of passive immunization with immunoglobulins is in cases where rapid protection against disease is necessary, for example after exposure to infection. This process is also used to provide antibodies against particular infections in people whose immune systems are suppressed due to disorders such as HIV infection and AIDS (p.297) or as a result of certain drug treatments (*see* IMMUNOSUPPRESSANTS, p.906).

HOW ARE THEY USED?

In most cases, vaccines are given by injection, although the polio vaccine may be given orally. Many vaccines provide lifelong immunity with one dose or a course of several doses, but some may not give full protection or may be effective for only a few months or years. The degree of protection given depends largely on the strength of the immune reaction a vaccine provokes. Additional doses, known as booster doses, may be needed at regular intervals to reinforce the effect of the original course of a vaccine and to maintain immunity.

Often, vaccines against more than one infection are given in a combined preparation, limiting the number of injections that are needed. For example, vaccines against diphtheria, pertussis, and tetanus (DPT) are given together.

Immunoglobulins are given by injection into a muscle or intravenously. They are effective for a short period only, and protection diminishes over several weeks, partly depending on the dose. If continued protection is needed, the treatment must be repeated.

WHAT ARE THE SIDE EFFECTS?

Some vaccines, such as the polio vaccine, cause few side effects. Others, such as the measles, mumps, and rubella vaccine, may produce mild forms of the diseases. Many vaccines may cause a red, slightly raised, tender area at the injection site and a mild fever or flu-like illness that lasts for a few days. Severe side effects, including the allergic reaction known as anaphylaxis (p.469), are rare. For most people, the risk of a reaction is far outweighed by the value of the protection given.

In some instances, vaccines should not be given. If you or your child has a fever, vaccination should be postponed until the fever has subsided. Vaccines containing live organisms should not be given during pregnancy or to people who have cancer or whose immune systems are suppressed.

Side effects of immunoglobulins are uncommon but may include tenderness at the injection site and fever. Repeated treatment with immunoglobulins can sometimes result in an allergic reaction, such as a rash.

Antibiotics

A group of drugs used primarily to treat infections caused by bacteria

Common drugs

Penicillins
• Amoxicillin • Ampicillin • Co-amoxiclav
• Flucloxacillin • Phenoxymethylpenicillin

Cephalosporins
• Cefaclor • Cefalexin • Cefazolin • Cefixime
• Cefoxitin • Ceftazidime • Cefuroxime

Macrolides
• Azithromycin • Clarithromycin • Erythromycin

Tetracyclines
• Doxycycline • Minocycline • Oxytetracycline
• Tetracycline

Aminoglycosides
• Amikacin • Gentamicin • Neomycin
• Streptomycin • Tobramycin

Sulphonamides
• Co-trimoxazole • Sulfadiazine

Quinolones
• Ciprofloxacin • Levofloxacin • Norfloxacin

Other antibiotics
• Chloramphenicol • Clindamycin • Fusidic acid
• Metronidazole • Trimethoprim • Vancomycin

DRUG ACTION How penicillins work

Penicillin antibiotics are used to treat many bacterial infections. Penicillins are bactericidal, which means that they actually destroy the bacteria causing infection. Most other types of antibiotic work by altering chemical activity in the bacteria, thereby preventing them from reproducing. The immune system is then able to overcome the remaining infection.

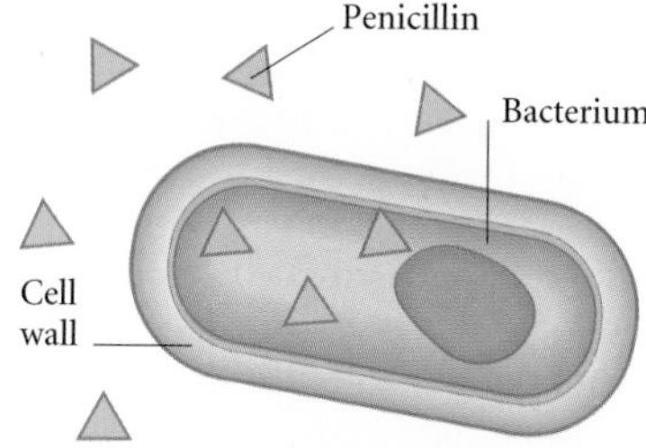

1 *Bacteria are single-celled organisms that have protective cell walls. The penicillin enters the bacterium, beginning a process that will destroy it.*

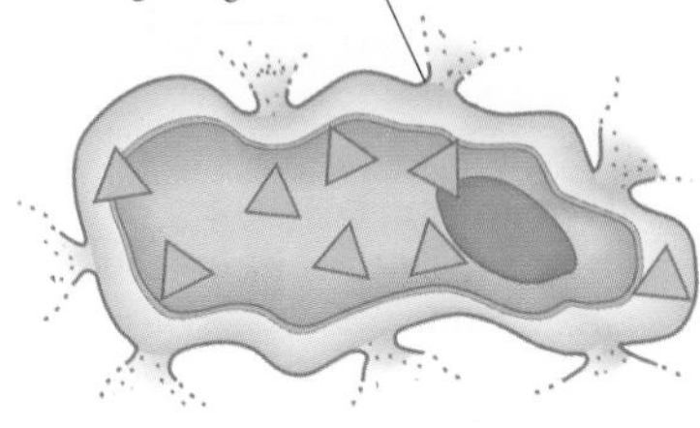

2 *The drug interferes with chemicals needed by the bacterium to form its cell walls. This causes the cell walls to disintegrate, and the bacterium dies.*

Antibiotics are among the most commonly prescribed drugs in the world. They are used to treat and prevent bacterial infections. The drugs work either by killing bacteria directly or by halting their multiplication so that the body's immune system is able to overcome the remaining infection.

Antibiotics are classified in groups, such as penicillins, cephalosporins, and tetracyclines, according to their chemical composition and the way in which they work. One of the most commonly used groups of antibiotics is penicillins (*see* How penicillins work, above). Some antibiotics work against a wide range of bacteria and are called broad-spectrum antibiotics. Other antibiotics work against only one or two types of bacteria and are known as narrow-spectrum antibiotics. Some also work against other types of infection, such as those caused by certain protozoa (*see* Antiprotozal drugs, p.888).

Why are they used?

Antibiotics are most commonly used for the short-term treatment of minor infections, such as infections of the ear, throat, or urinary tract. The drugs may also be used in the treatment of serious infections such as septicaemia (p.299) and bacterial meningitis (p.527).

On occasion, long-term treatment with low-dose antibiotics may be given to prevent infection in people whose immunity is reduced, such as those with HIV infection or AIDS (p.297) and people who are taking immunosuppressants (p.906). Long-term use of antibiotics may also be prescribed for other conditions, such as acne (p.340).

How are they used?

Most bacterial infections are treated with oral antibiotics. Eye and ear infections are often treated using antibiotic drops (*see* Drugs for eye and ear disorders, pp.919–921). To treat severe infections, when high doses of antibiotics are needed immediately, the drugs may be given by intramuscular injection or by intravenous injection or infusion.

If you have a bacterial infection, your doctor will probably prescribe a specific antibiotic that is effective against the bacterium most likely to be causing that infection. For certain conditions, such as pneumonia (p.490) or a wound infection, your doctor may carry out tests (*see* Tests for microorganisms, pp.234–235) to identify the infecting organism before prescribing a narrow-spectrum antibiotic. In the meantime, you will probably be treated with a broad-spectrum antibiotic. More than one antibiotic may be prescribed to reduce the risk of antibiotic resistance.

When you are taking antibiotics, you should continue treatment even after your symptoms start to improve. Finish the entire course as prescribed by your doctor in order to eradicate the infection. Bacterial resistance to antibiotics is increasing, due in part to overprescription and incorrect use.

Antibiotics are available by prescription only. The choice of antibiotic may be restricted if you are pregnant, have a history of drug allergy, have impaired kidney or liver function, or if you are taking other drugs that might interact with a particular antibiotic.

What are the side effects?

Antibiotics do not usually cause serious side effects. The most common is diarrhoea, although it is not usually severe. Antibiotics can alter the balance between normal bacteria and the yeast *Candida albicans* that occurs naturally in or on the body; this imbalance may lead to an overgrowth of the yeast (*see* Candidiasis, p.309). In some cases, antibiotics destroy harmless bacteria in the bowel that prevent the growth of disease-causing organisms. Rarely, this results in the potentially serious condition pseudomembranous colitis, which can cause diarrhoea and severe dehydration.

Penicillins may cause rashes and in some people a rare, life-threatening allergic reaction known as anaphylaxis (p.469). This is more common when the drugs are given by injection and occurs mainly in people who have previously had a mild allergic reaction to a penicillin. If you are allergic to one type of penicillin, you may be allergic to others in the same group. About 1 in 10 people who is allergic to penicillin is also allergic to cephalosporins. If you have an adverse reaction, such as a rash, stop taking the drug and see your doctor promptly. If you have previously had a reaction, tell your doctor.

Tetracyclines can cause changes to growing bones and teeth and are therefore not prescribed for young children or pregnant women. In some rare cases, aminoglycosides can damage the kidneys, cause severe skin rashes, and affect the sense of hearing and balance.

Quinolones occasionally cause convulsions and should not be taken by people with epilepsy. They are not suitable for children because they may damage growing tendons and joints.

Sulphonamides, one of the earliest classes of antibiotics to be developed, sometimes cause serious side effects, such as rashes and kidney damage.

Antituberculous drugs

Drugs used in the treatment of the bacterial infection tuberculosis

COMMON DRUGS

- Capreomycin • Cycloserine • Ethambutol
- Isoniazid • Pyrazinamide • Rifabutin
- Rifampicin • Streptomycin

Antituberculous drugs are antibiotics (p.885) used mainly or exclusively to treat tuberculosis, also known as TB (p.491). The initial infection usually develops in the lungs, but tuberculosis may spread to other parts of the body, such as the kidneys, lymph nodes, and sometimes the membranes covering the brain and spinal cord (*see* MENINGITIS, p.527). Usually, several antituberculous drugs are given together to prevent the development of drug resistance.

HOW ARE THEY USED?

If you are diagnosed with TB, the strain of bacteria causing the infection will be tested to determine its sensitivity to specific antituberculous drugs. While you are waiting for the results, which can take up to 2 months, your doctor will prescribe an initial combination of three or four drugs to be taken orally. The main drugs used are isoniazid, pyrazinamide, ethambutol, and rifampicin. The test results will identify the most effective drugs. Treatment with these drugs is usually continued for 6–9 months to ensure that your infection is eradicated. In some cases, this treatment may need to be continued for a longer period, depending on the organs that are affected. For example, treatment may need to continue for 12 months if the infection has led to meningitis.

It is important that you complete the course of drugs as instructed by your doctor. If you fail to do so, the bacteria may not be eradicated, and drug-resistant strains may develop, which can then be transmitted to other people.

WHAT ARE THE SIDE EFFECTS?

Antituberculous drugs may produce various side effects, including nausea, vomiting, rashes, and abdominal pain. Isoniazid, pyrazinamide, and rifampicin may damage the liver or kidneys; your doctor will regularly check your liver and kidney function. Rifampicin may turn urine and other body secretions red, but this effect is harmless. Isoniazid may affect the nerves, causing numbness or tingling in the hands or feet. Ethambutol may rarely damage the nerves in the eyes, causing vision problems. People taking the drug are usually advised to have regular vision tests. If you are taking ethambutol and develop blurred vision or are unable to distinguish colours, see your doctor promptly.

Antiviral drugs

Drugs that are used to treat certain infections caused by viruses

COMMON DRUGS

- Aciclovir • Amantadine • Famciclovir
- Foscarnet • Ganciclovir • Idoxuridine
- Interferon alfa • Ribavirin • Valaciclovir
- Zanamivir

Various drugs are available to treat viral infections. Although these drugs may not eliminate an infection, they are often effective in reducing its severity. Many viral illnesses are mild and clear up without treatment because healthy people can usually fight off infection quickly. Sometimes, antiviral drugs help to relieve symptoms and hasten recovery. However, because viruses invade body cells in order to multiply, antiviral drugs can damage body cells as well as the targeted viruses. Their use is therefore usually limited to treating severe or recurrent infections. Some antiviral drugs are more effective against certain viruses than others. A particular range of antivirals is used to treat HIV infection (*see* DRUGS FOR HIV INFECTION AND AIDS, opposite page).

WHY ARE THEY USED?

The main use for antivirals is in the treatment of infections that recur over a prolonged period. The drugs are also effective in treating or preventing infections in people with impaired immune systems who are at increased risk of severe illness and complications. In such cases, antiviral drugs may be life-saving.

Antiviral drugs such as aciclovir are most commonly used to treat herpes infections, particularly the herpes simplex infections (p.291), which typically cause recurrent attacks of cold sores and genital herpes. People who have frequent and severe recurrences of such infections may be given long-term antiviral drug treatment. Aciclovir is also effective against the varicella–zoster virus, which causes chickenpox (p.290) as well as shingles (*see* HERPES ZOSTER, p.290).

Some antivirals are used for specific infections, especially in people who are particularly vulnerable because their immunity is impaired by disease or by drug treatment such as chemotherapy (p.280). Amantadine may be prescribed to treat influenza (p.289) in unimmunized people who are at high risk of complications. A new drug, zanamivir, which is taken by inhaler, may shorten the duration of influenza but does not give protection against serious complications. Ganciclovir is used for severe cytomegalovirus infection (p.292), especially in people with reduced immunity.

Ribavirin can be used to treat babies with bronchiolitis (p.841), a serious lung infection. This drug can also be used to treat Lassa fever (*see* VIRAL HAEMORRHAGIC FEVERS, p.295). Interferon alfa (*see* INTERFERON DRUGS, p.907), a synthesized version of antiviral substances produced naturally in the body, can be used to treat chronic hepatitis (p.645) caused by hepatitis B and C viruses.

How do they work?

Viruses invade body cells, where they use human genetic material (DNA) to reproduce. Antiviral drugs act in various ways to block this process, either by causing changes within body cells to prevent the virus from replicating or by preventing the virus from entering cells. If treatment is started early, the drugs usually work rapidly and relieve symptoms within a few days. However, some viruses develop resistance to the effects of drugs, which can make particular infections difficult to treat.

How are they used?

The drugs used to treat herpes infections, such as aciclovir, can be applied as a topical preparation or taken orally, depending on the site and severity of the infection, or given by injection for urgent treatment of a serious infection. For mild infections, topical antivirals can be bought over the counter.

Amantadine is taken orally and can be given for up to 6 weeks as a preventive drug against influenza. Ganciclovir and interferon are given by injection in hospital. Ribavirin can be given by inhaler to babies with bronchiolitis and is given as an injection for Lassa fever.

What are the side effects?

Aciclovir does not usually produce side effects, although when taken orally it may cause nausea. Rarely, when given by injection, the drug can cause kidney damage and may produce symptoms such as confusion and seizures.

In some people, amantadine causes reactions such as dizziness, confusion, and insomnia. Ganciclovir may cause skin rashes and nausea. This drug can reduce red blood cell production, causing anaemia (p.446), and white blood cell production, increasing susceptibility to further infections. Ganciclovir may also lead to impairment of kidney function. Ribavirin can cause anaemia.

Interferon alfa commonly produces side effects, including nausea and flu-like symptoms such as tiredness, fever, and aching muscles. These effects are usually mild and may diminish with continued treatment. However, prolonged treatment can lead to decreased production of red and white blood cells. In rare cases, people taking interferon alfa may develop tremor.

Drugs for HIV infection and AIDS

A range of drugs that are used to treat HIV infection and its complications

Common drugs

Reverse transcriptase inhibitors
- Didanosine (ddI) • Efavirenz • Lamivudine
- Nevirapine • Stavudine • Zalcitabine (ddC)
- Zidovudine (AZT)

Protease inhibitors
- Indinavir • Nelfinavir • Ritonavir • Saquinavir

Other drugs for HIV
- Interferons

Recent advances in drug treatments for people with HIV infection and AIDS (p.297) have offered new hope by slowing or halting the progression of the disease and improving quality of life.

The human immunodeficiency virus (HIV) infects and gradually destroys white blood cells of the body's immune system, known as CD4 lymphocytes, which normally help to fight infections. People with HIV infection may remain symptom-free for many years, or they may experience frequent or prolonged mild infections. If a specific infection or tumour occurs, a person is said to have developed AIDS (acquired immunodeficiency syndrome). These conditions, called AIDS-defining illnesses, include a number of severe infections, such as pneumocystis infection (p.308), toxoplasmosis (p.307), and certain cancers, such as Kaposi's sarcoma (p.346) and non-Hodgkin's lymphoma (p.459).

Why are they used?

The drugs currently in use to treat HIV infection have made it possible to suppress the level of the virus in the blood, with the aim of reducing it so that the virus becomes undetectable. If this aim is achieved, the immune system can recover sufficiently to overcome or prevent infections. Experts believe that, in some people, the drugs may be able to prevent the progression of HIV infection to AIDS. Evidence to support this is very encouraging, and many people who use the newer drugs have shown a dramatic improvement in their condition.

Treatment of HIV infection involves two distinct groups of drugs: antiretroviral drugs, which act against the virus itself, and anti-infective drugs such as antibiotics (p.885), which are used to treat the diseases that develop as a result of reduced immunity.

Treatment with antiretroviral drugs is believed to be beneficial for anybody with HIV infection or AIDS, but expert opinion is still divided about the best time to begin this treatment. Current research suggests that drug treatment is likely to be effective for people who have recently been exposed to the virus and are showing initial symptoms of infection. Drug treatment is also recommended at a later stage in the disease for people with falling numbers of CD4 lymphocytes or rising virus levels and people with an AIDS-defining illness. It is generally believed that the earlier treatment begins, the greater the possibility of altering the course of the disease. However, the drugs have severe side effects that are difficult to tolerate over years of treatment.

People who have been in contact with blood or other body fluids from a person with HIV are given immediate treatment with antiretroviral drugs for 1 month. Antiretrovirals are also recommended for HIV-positive mothers during pregnancy to reduce the risk of the baby being born with the virus.

How do they work?

There are two main groups of antiretroviral drugs used in the treatment of HIV infection and AIDS: reverse transcriptase inhibitors and protease inhibitors. The drugs work by blocking the processes necessary for viral replication without significantly damaging the body cells that the virus has invaded. Reverse transcriptase inhibitors, such as zidovudine (AZT), alter the genetic material of the infected cell, which is needed by the virus to replicate, or the genetic material of the virus itself. Protease inhibitors, such as ritonavir, prevent the production of viral proteins necessary for replication.

How are they used?

Treatment of HIV infection and AIDS is subject to rapid change as knowledge about the virus increases. Currently, antiretroviral drugs are generally used in combination to destroy the virus more effectively and help to prevent the development of drug-resistant strains of HIV. The drugs are taken orally, and often many tablets must be taken daily. It is important to take the drugs on time each day to help to prevent the emergence of drug resistance in HIV.

WHAT ARE THE SIDE EFFECTS?

If you have HIV infection, your doctor will discuss your treatment options with you at length because the drugs have side effects that should be weighed against the benefits of treatment.

Antiretroviral drugs can cause nausea, vomiting, and diarrhoea, which may be very severe. Other serious side effects include inflammation of the pancreas (*see* ACUTE PANCREATITIS, p.652) and damage to the nerves, eyes, liver, or kidneys. Anaemia (p.446) may also develop. You need regular checkups and blood tests to look for warning signs of side effects. Pregnant women need expert advice on having treatment with antiretrovirals; these drugs can prevent transmission of HIV to the fetus but are potentially harmful to its development.

Antiprotozoal drugs

A group of drugs that is used to treat infections caused by protozoa

COMMON DRUGS

- Atovaquone • Co-trimoxazole • Diloxanide furoate • Mepracrine hydrochloride
- Metronidazole • Pentamidine • Pyrimethamine with sulfadiazine • Sodium stibogluconate
- Tinidazole

A range of drugs is used to treat infections caused by single-celled organisms called protozoa. Some antiprotozoals, such as metronidazole, are also used for bacterial infections. A specific group of these drugs is used to treat malaria, a serious disease caused by protozoa that affects millions of people worldwide (*see* ANTIMALARIAL DRUGS, right).

Antiprotozoals act in various ways, but most of the drugs work by preventing protozoa from multiplying.

WHY ARE THEY USED?

Antiprotozoal drugs are commonly used to treat infections such as trichomoniasis (p.767), which affects the vagina, and giardiasis (p.307), which affects the intestine. Metronidazole or tinidazole is often taken for these disorders. Another common use for antiprotozoals, particularly pyrimethamine with sulfadiazine, is to treat toxoplasmosis (p.307), an infection that can cause severe illness in fetuses and people with reduced immunity. Co-trimoxazole and pentamidine may be used for pneumocystis infection (p.308), a form of pneumonia that is potentially fatal in people whose immunity is reduced.

HOW ARE THEY USED?

For minor infections, antiprotozoals are usually taken for about a week. Severe infections may need treatment for several months, especially in people with reduced immunity, such as those who have HIV infection or AIDS (p.297).

Most antiprotozoals are taken orally, but some may be injected to treat severe infections. Pentamidine is administered by injection or taken through an inhaler. This drug is given only under the supervision of a doctor.

WHAT ARE THE SIDE EFFECTS?

Antiprotozoal drugs often cause side effects, including nausea, diarrhoea, and abdominal cramps. If you are taking metronidazole, you should avoid alcohol because it can cause vomiting. Another side effect of the drug is darkening of the urine. Pentamidine may cause a severe drop in blood pressure, either when it is administered or directly afterwards. In rare cases, pyrimethamine reduces red blood cell production, causing anaemia (p.446). If you have unusual bruising or bleeding while taking this drug, notify your doctor because these may be signs of a blood disorder.

Antimalarial drugs

A group of drugs that is used for the prevention and treatment of malaria

COMMON DRUGS

- Chloroquine • Doxycycline • Mefloquine
- Primaquine • Proguanil • Pyrimethamine with dapsone • Pyrimethamine with sulfadoxine
- Quinine • Proguanil with atovaquone

Antimalarial drugs are prescribed as a preventive measure against infection with malaria (p.305) and also as treatment if the disease develops. There are various types of antimalarial drug. Some are suitable only for treatment of the infection, while others are used for both prevention and treatment. Malaria is a serious infectious disease caused by protozoa that are transmitted to humans by the bites of infected mosquitoes. The protozoa travel through the blood to the liver, where they multiply before re-entering the blood and circulating throughout the body. At this stage, the symptoms of malaria appear.

No antimalarial provides complete protection against the disease because malarial protozoa continually develop drug resistance. For this reason, you should protect yourself from mosquito bites if you visit an area where malaria occurs. It is important to keep your body well covered and to use insect repellents and netting (*see* TRAVEL HEALTH, p.85).

HOW DO THEY WORK?

Antimalarial drugs are effective at different stages in the life cycle of the malarial protozoa. When taken to prevent malaria, the drugs act by killing the protozoa when they enter the liver. To treat malaria once symptoms have appeared, higher doses of drugs are given to destroy the protozoa when they are released from the liver into the blood. In some cases, the protozoa lie dormant in the liver and reactivate to cause recurrent episodes of malaria. These protozoa are difficult to eradicate and are treated with stronger drugs.

HOW ARE THEY USED?

The choice of antimalarial drug usually depends on which part of the world you are planning to visit or where you contracted the disease.

If you plan to visit a malarial area, you need to start preventive treatment up to 3 weeks before departure, continuing for 1–4 weeks after your return (the extact timings depend on the drugs taken). Antimalarials are usually taken orally, either once a day or once a week. To increase protection against the most widespread strains, combinations of drugs may be given. For example, pyrimethamine with dapsone may be taken together with chloroquine.

If you develop malaria, the drugs used for treatment may be taken orally or given by injection up to several times a day for several days. If you have recurrent bouts of malaria, your doctor will prescribe an oral antimalarial such as primaquine for 2–3 weeks or more to eradicate the protozoa.

WHAT ARE THE SIDE EFFECTS?

Antimalarial drugs can cause a number of side effects, including nausea, diarrhoea, headaches, rashes, and blood disorders. Quinine can cause ringing in the ears (*see* TINNITUS, p.602), blurred vision, and hot flushes. Mefloquine can cause some people to experience panic attacks, dizziness, hallucinations, and depression.

Several of the antimalarial drugs should not be taken in early pregnancy or while you are breast-feeding. Mefloquine and chloroquine should not be taken by people with epilepsy.

Antifungal drugs

A group of drugs that is used to treat infections caused by fungi

COMMON DRUGS

- Amphotericin • Clotrimazole • Econazole
- Fluconazole • Flucytosine • Griseofulvin
- Itraconazole • Ketoconazole • Miconazole
- Nystatin • Sulconazole • Terbinafine

Various drugs are available to treat fungal infections. These antifungal drugs have a wide range of uses because disorders resulting from fungal infections can occur on or in many different parts of the body. For example, treatment may be needed for infections of superficial areas such as the skin, nails, or genitals; rarely, internal organs, such as the heart or lungs, may also be infected.

Most antifungals work by damaging the walls of fungal cells. This causes vital substances within the cell to leak out, destroying the fungus.

WHY ARE THEY USED?

Antifungal preparations are frequently used to treat minor fungal infections of the skin, such as athlete's foot (p.353) and ringworm (p.352), or of the nails (*see* NAIL ABNORMALITIES, p.360). These types of drug are also effective against candidiasis (p.309), a common fungal infection that can affect moist areas of the body, in particular the mucous membranes that line the mouth (*see* ORAL THRUSH, p.862) and the vagina (*see* VAGINAL THRUSH, p.752).

Antifungal drugs may also be used for the long-term treatment of potentially serious fungal infections such as aspergillosis (p.309), which may affect the lungs and spread to other organs. People with reduced immunity, such as those who have HIV infection or AIDS (p.297), are at high risk from severe fungal infections, and in such cases antifungal drugs may be life-saving.

HOW ARE THEY USED?

If you have a fungal infection of the skin or scalp, your doctor may prescribe a cream or shampoo containing an antifungal such as ketoconazole. Symptoms normally start to improve within about a week. However, you should continue the treatment for at least 2 weeks after symptoms have disappeared to ensure that the infection has been eradicated. Nail infections are treated with a drug such as terbinafine, taken orally for several months. It may take much longer than this for the infected part of the nail to grow out.

Drugs used to treat vaginal thrush are available over the counter. The most commonly used drug is clotrimazole, which is inserted in the vagina either as a cream using a special applicator or in the form of a pessary. These preparations vary in strength and, while some may be effective after a single dose, others need to be used for 3 days. For recurrent vaginal thrush, your doctor may prescribe a drug to be taken orally, such as fluconazole. Oral thrush is treated by antifungal drugs given as lozenges, which are dissolved slowly in the mouth, or as gels or solutions applied directly to the affected area.

Serious infections of internal organs need to be treated with potent antifungal drugs, such as amphotericin, which are initially given intravenously. Further treatment with oral drugs may then be continued for months.

WHAT ARE THE SIDE EFFECTS?

Antifungal drugs used topically on the skin, scalp, or mucous membranes do not often cause side effects, although you may experience some local irritation. Nystatin used as a cream may stain clothing yellow.

If you are prescribed potent oral antifungal drugs to treat infections of internal organs, you may experience nausea and vomiting. Less frequently, serious side effects may occur, including kidney damage and blood disorders. Treatment with the drug ketoconazole may cause liver damage.

Anthelmintic drugs

A group of drugs that is used to eradicate parasitic worm infestations

COMMON DRUGS

- Albendazole • Diethylcarbamazine • Ivermectin
- Mebendazole • Praziquantel • Tiabendazole

Anthelmintic drugs are used to eradicate worm (helminth) infestations of the intestine or of the tissues of other organs, such as the lungs. The most common intestinal worm infestation occurring in the UK is threadworm (*see* THREADWORM INFESTATION, p.310).

Infestations affecting the intestines are treated with anthelmintics that kill or paralyse the worms, which then pass out of the body in the faeces. Worm infestations of other body tissues are treated with anthelmintic drugs that circulate in the bloodstream and are absorbed by the tissues, where they kill the worms by preventing them from obtaining essential nutrients.

HOW ARE THEY USED?

Many anthelmintic drugs are appropriate only for certain types of infestation. Your doctor will therefore need to identify the worm before prescribing the drug to be taken. In most cases, infestations are treated easily with a short course of oral drugs.

The most commonly used drug for intestinal infestations is mebendazole. Threadworms can often be eradicated with a single dose of mebendazole, provided that treatment is combined with good hygiene measures, such as careful handwashing, to prevent reinfestation. Your doctor may suggest that the whole family be treated with the drug at the same time, because threadworms can spread very rapidly to other people.

Worm infestations of the tissues, such as hydatid disease (p.313), which can affect the lungs, liver, or bones, may be treated with albendazole. Tissue infestations are difficult to eradicate, and it may be necessary to continue taking the drug for several weeks.

Anthelmintics usually do not cause side effects. However, sometimes the drugs produce diarrhoea, headaches, and dizziness. Albendazole may impair liver function; this may necessitate regular monitoring during treatment.

DRUGS ACTING ON THE SKIN

Drugs acting on the skin are commonly used to relieve dryness and itching, to reduce inflammation, or to treat skin infections and infestations. Most treatments are applied directly to the skin as ointments, creams, or gels. Treatment with oral drugs may be necessary if a skin condition is severe or widespread.

The first article in this section covers emollients and barrier preparations, which are widely used to moisturize the skin and to protect it against the effects of irritant substances. Retinoid drugs, discussed next, are used to treat specific disorders, such as severe acne.

The following two articles in this section cover antipruritic drugs, which are used to relieve itching, and topical corticosteroids, which may be given to reduce inflammation of the skin.

Preparations that are applied to the skin to treat infections and infestations are discussed next. Oral anti-infective drugs to treat the skin are described elsewhere (*see* DRUGS FOR INFECTIONS AND INFESTATIONS, pp.883–889).

The final article covers sunscreens and sunblocks, which protect the skin against the damaging effects of the sun. Drug treatments for other specific disorders are discussed elsewhere (*see* SKIN, HAIR, AND NAILS, pp.328–361).

KEY ANATOMY

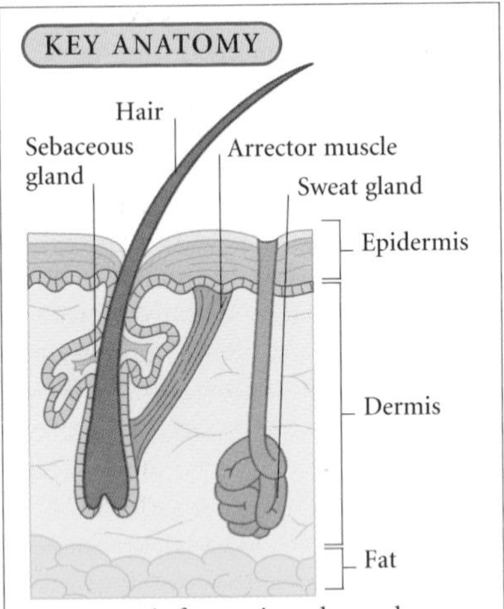

For more information about the structure and function of the skin, *see* pp.328–331.

Emollients and barrier preparations

Preparations that moisturize and protect the skin against water and other irritants

COMMON DRUGS

EMOLLIENTS
- Aqueous creams
- Petroleum jelly

BARRIER PREPARATIONS
- Dimeticone
- Zinc ointment

Emollients are commonly used to treat dry, scaly, or itchy skin that results from skin disorders such as eczema (p.333), contact dermatitis (p.335), seborrhoeic dermatitis (p.335), and psoriasis (p.332). Emollients increase the moisture content of the skin by forming an oily film that stops water from evaporating from the skin's surface, thereby soothing and softening the skin. Emollient preparations are available over the counter in the form of creams, ointments, lotions, bath additives, and washes.

Barrier preparations often contain water-repellent substances and are used to protect the skin from water and irritants. They are useful for protecting the skin around pressure sores (p.350) and leg ulcers (p.350). They can also be applied to the nappy area in babies to help to prevent nappy rash (p.829).

HOW ARE THEY USED?

Emollients and barrier preparations are available without a prescription. They should be rubbed gently on to clean, dry skin. However, the effects of the preparations are short-lived, and they may need to be applied frequently, especially after washing. Emollient bath additives and washes are used in place of normal soap. Occasionally, ingredients that are commonly added to emollient preparations, such as lanolin, irritate the skin. If sensitivity occurs, you should discontinue using the product. In some cases, emollients may need to be used for an extended period of time, such as in the treatment of severe psoriasis.

Retinoid drugs

A group of drugs used for skin conditions such as acne, psoriasis, and sun damage

COMMON DRUGS

- Acitretin
- Isotretinoin
- Tretinoin

Retinoid drugs are used to treat a number of skin conditions, including acne, psoriasis, and sun damage. These drugs are related chemically to vitamin A, which is needed to maintain healthy skin. Tretinoin and isotretinoin are used mainly in the treatment of severe acne (p.340). In addition, tretinoin may be used to treat mottling, fine wrinkles, and roughness in sun-damaged skin. However, the effects are only temporary, and the drug is not effective on deep wrinkles or for people over the age of 50. Acitretin is used mainly to treat some types of severe psoriasis (p.332), a condition in which the skin becomes red, thickened, and scaly.

HOW DO THEY WORK?

Retinoid drugs act on cells in the outer layers of the skin. The precise way in which tretinoin and isotretinoin work is unknown, but both drugs increase the rate at which the outer layers of skin are shed. This action helps to prevent acne by unblocking hair follicles clogged by sebum (oil) that might develop into blackheads or whiteheads. Isotretinoin also reduces the production of sebum by sebaceous glands in the skin.

Acitretin reduces the rate of production of keratin, a protein found in the outer layer of the skin. Keratin is produced in excessive amounts in the skin

WARNING

Retinoid drugs can damage a developing fetus. You should discuss your contraception needs with your doctor before starting treatment.

of people with psoriasis. Acitretin also has anti-inflammatory properties and may help to relieve the inflammation of the joints that is sometimes experienced by people who have severe psoriasis.

HOW ARE THEY USED?

Topical tretinoin preparations should be applied as a liquid, gel, or cream once or twice daily in a thin layer over the affected area. Skin affected by acne will probably improve after 2–3 weeks, although the maximum effect may not be apparent for 8–12 weeks. Skin that has been damaged by sun exposure is treated with a cream preparation. You will probably notice an improvement in your skin's condition after 2–4 weeks, but treatment may last up to 6 months.

Isotretinoin is available in capsule form and is prescribed only when acne is very severe. It should be taken daily with food. After 4 weeks, your doctor may adjust the dose, depending on how your skin has responded to the treatment. A 12–16 week course of the drug often clears up acne entirely. A repeat course is not usually recommended.

Acitretin, which is used to treat psoriasis, is only taken orally. If your doctor prescribes acitretin, it will have to be taken daily, and you will usually see an improvement in your skin after about 2–4 weeks. The full benefit is usually seen after 4–6 weeks. Your doctor will prescribe acitretin for no longer than 6–9 months, but treatment may resume after a 3–4 month break.

WHAT ARE THE SIDE EFFECTS?

Using topical preparations that contain tretinoin may cause your skin to peel and become red and inflamed.

If you are taking isotretinoin or acitretin, your skin may become dry, flaky, and itchy, and you may experience sore lips and eyes, nosebleeds, and hair loss. Acitretin and isotretinoin can also affect the liver, and your blood will be tested regularly during treatment to monitor liver function. Women who are taking these drugs may find that their periods become irregular.

All retinoid drugs can cause severe birth defects. Women should therefore avoid becoming pregnant while taking any of the drugs. Pregnancy should also be avoided for at least 1 month after completing treatment with tretinoin and isotretinoin and for at least 2 years after stopping treatment with acitretin. Long-term treatment with these drugs may lead to pain in the joints and bones. In very rare cases, the treatment may also result in thinning or thickening of the bones in the spine, knees, and ankles.

(SELF-ADMINISTRATION) APPLYING OINTMENTS, CREAMS, AND GELS

When applying medication in the form of ointments, creams, or gels, it is important to use the correct amount. Too much may increase the chance of side effects, whereas too little may not achieve the desired effect. The fingertip unit is a simple measure that can help you to work out how much medication you need to apply over an area of skin.

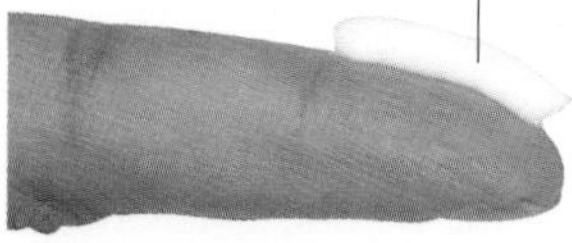

One fingertip unit of cream

A fingertip unit
One unit is the amount of the preparation that can be squeezed in a line onto the tip of the index finger as far as the first joint.

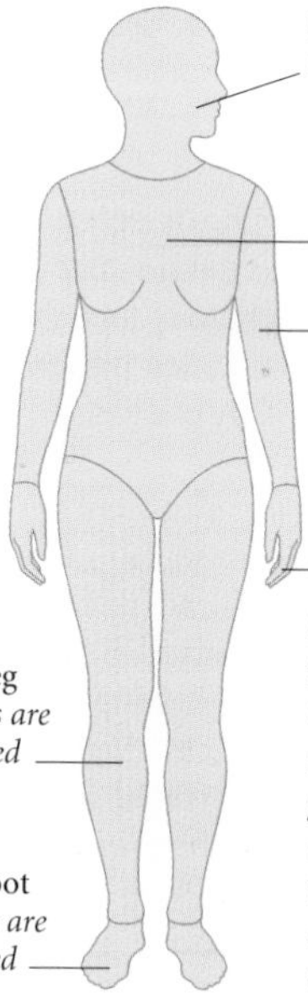

Face and neck
2.5 units are required

Trunk
7 units are required for front or back

One arm
3 units are required

One hand (both sides)
1 unit is required

One leg
6 units are required

One foot
2 units are required

Measuring with fingertip units
Using the measures shown here as a guide, apply an amount of cream that is proportional to the area of skin that you need to cover.

Antipruritic drugs

Drugs used to control itching, a condition also known as pruritus

COMMON DRUGS

TOPICAL CORTICOSTEROIDS
• Hydrocortisone

ANTIHISTAMINES
• Antazoline • Diphenhydramine • Mepyramine

LOCAL ANAESTHETICS
• Benzocaine • Lidocaine • Tetracaine

SOOTHING PREPARATIONS
• Calamine lotion • Emollients

Antipruritic drugs are used to relieve itching, a symptom with a variety of possible causes, including inflammation or dryness of the skin, allergy, hormone deficiency in older women, exposure to irritant substances, and skin infections and infestations. Scratching the skin may cause further inflammation and itching, which may continue after the initial cause of the itching has disappeared. This cycle may be broken by the use of antipruritics, which can be applied to the skin or taken orally. Most antipruritic drugs are available over the counter. However, itching should be investigated by your doctor in case there is an underlying cause that needs specific treatment. If you have an infection or infestation, you may be prescribed an alternative treatment (*see* PREPARATIONS FOR SKIN INFECTIONS AND INFESTATIONS, p.892).

WHAT ARE THE TYPES?

The main types of antipruritic drug include topical corticosteroids (p.892), antihistamines (p.906), local anaesthetics, and soothing preparations, such as emollients (*see* EMOLLIENTS AND BARRIER PREPARATIONS, opposite page). A topical corticosteroid can help to relieve itching caused by skin inflammation; antihistamines may be used to relieve itching caused by an allergic reaction; local anaesthetics numb small areas of skin, reducing itchiness caused by insect bites or stings; and soothing preparations ease itching caused by a variety of disorders, including eczema (p.333).

TOPICAL CORTICOSTEROIDS A corticosteroid preparation may be applied to the skin to reduce inflammation and thereby relieve itching caused by skin

> WARNING
>
> Do not apply an antipruritic drug to broken or infected skin except on the advice of a doctor.

conditions such as psoriasis (p.332), contact dermatitis (p.335), or eczema. Their exact mechanism is unknown, but corticosteroids are thought to reduce the production of substances called prostaglandins that trigger inflammation.

ANTIHISTAMINES Topical ointments or creams that contain antihistamine are commonly used for localized itching, such as that caused by an insect bite or sting (p.995). Widespread itching that is caused by a disorder such as chickenpox (p.290) can often be treated more effectively with an oral antihistamine.

Antihistamines relieve itching by inhibiting the action of histamine, which is produced by body tissues in response to tissue damage or the presence of an allergen (a substance that triggers an allergic reaction, such as wasp venom). Histamine causes itching, swelling, and other symptoms of allergic reaction.

Topical antihistamines may themselves cause an allergic skin reaction, and you should stop using the product if additional irritation occurs. Certain oral antihistamines may make you feel drowsy, which can be useful if itching has prevented you from sleeping.

LOCAL ANAESTHETICS Small regions of skin irritation, such as those caused by insect stings or bites, may be soothed using a local anaesthetic cream or spray. These products stop itching by blocking the transmission of impulses along the nerves in the affected area. Local anaesthetics are inappropriate for widespread itching and can worsen symptoms by causing an allergic reaction in the skin.

SOOTHING PREPARATIONS Itching, such as that caused by insect bites and stings, sunburn (p.357), or an allergic rash such as urticaria (p.468), can often be soothed using calamine lotion or cream or an emollient. Emollient preparations reduce moisture loss from the skin, preventing dryness and easing itching, and can be used to relieve the symptoms of eczema, psoriasis, and other dry skin conditions.

Topical corticosteroids

Drugs related to natural hormones that are applied directly to the skin to reduce inflammation

COMMON DRUGS

VERY POTENT CORTICOSTEROIDS
- Clobetasol • Fluocinonide • Halcinonide

POTENT CORTICOSTEROIDS
- Beclometasone • Betamethasone
- Desoximetasone • Fluocinolone • Fluticasone
- Mometasone • Triamcinolone

MODERATELY POTENT CORTICOSTEROIDS
- Alclometasone

MILD CORTICOSTEROIDS
- Hydrocortisone

Corticosteroids (p.930) are chemically similar to the natural hormones produced by the adrenal glands. They are used topically as cream or ointment preparations to relieve skin inflammation and itching caused by conditions such as eczema (p.333), contact dermatitis (p.335), seborrhoeic dermatitis (p.335), and, less commonly, for psoriasis (p.332). If inflammation is caused by a bacterial or fungal infection of the skin, topical corticosteroids may be used in conjunction with an anti-infective preparation (*see* PREPARATIONS FOR SKIN INFECTIONS AND INFESTATIONS, right).

When applied directly to the skin, corticosteroids are absorbed into the underlying layers of tissue, where they reduce inflammation and relieve itching. The exact mechanism of corticosteroid action is unknown, but these drugs are thought to act by inhibiting the release of prostaglandins, which are substances that trigger inflammation.

HOW ARE THEY USED?

Your doctor will prescribe a corticosteroid cream or ointment that is potent enough to relieve your symptoms while minimizing the risk of side effects. You should follow your doctor's instructions on how often to apply the cream or ointment (usually once or twice a day) and make sure that you use the correct amount (*see* APPLYING OINTMENTS, CREAMS, AND GELS, p.891). Some mild topical corticosteroid preparations are available over the counter.

> WARNING
>
> Do not use a topical corticosteroid on your face or on a baby's skin except on the advice of a doctor.

WHAT ARE THE SIDE EFFECTS?

Mild topical corticosteroid preparations used sparingly and for a short time do not usually cause side effects. However, prolonged use of these preparations can cause permanent changes to the skin. Most commonly, the treated skin becomes thin and easily damaged. If corticosteroids are applied to infected skin, the condition may worsen.

More potent topical corticosteroids used long-term may rarely cause more severe side effects, such as increased blood pressure and a susceptibility to bruising. If you are using potent topical corticosteroids, your doctor will review your condition regularly. Do not stop using corticosteroids without first consulting your doctor.

Preparations for skin infections and infestations

Preparations applied directly to the skin to treat skin infections and infestations

COMMON DRUGS

ANTISEPTIC PREPARATIONS
- Chlorhexidine • Triclosan

ANTIBIOTICS
- Fusidic acid • Mupirocin • Neomycin

ANTIVIRAL DRUGS
- Aciclovir • Penciclovir

ANTIFUNGAL DRUGS
- Clotrimazole • Econazole • Ketoconazole
- Miconazole • Nystatin • Terbinafine
- Tioconazole

ANTIPARASITIC DRUGS
- Benzyl benzoate • Lindane • Malathion
- Permethrin

Topical anti-infective or antiparasitic skin preparations are used to prevent or treat a number of skin infections and infestations. These preparations contain an active ingredient, which is mixed with a cream, ointment, lotion, or detergent base. The preparations are easy to apply and are formulated so that the drug remains on the surface of the skin, where its effect is needed. Some preparations that are used to treat skin infections and infestations may themselves irritate or inflame the skin or result in an allergic reaction, and, if this occurs, treatment should be discontinued.

WHAT ARE THE TYPES?

Topical treatments for skin infections include antiseptic preparations, which are effective against a wide range of microorganisms; antibiotics (p.885), used to prevent or treat infection with bacteria; and antiviral drugs (p.886) and antifungal drugs (p.889), used to treat viral and fungal infections respectively. Antiparasitic drugs are commonly used to treat skin infestations.

ANTISEPTIC PREPARATIONS These preparations contain chemicals that kill or prevent the growth of microorganisms that can cause infection in damaged skin. Antiseptic solutions and creams can be bought over the counter. Antiseptic solutions are added to water and used to clean broken skin; creams should be applied to wounds after they have been thoroughly cleansed. Antiseptics are also included in some shampoos and soaps to prevent minor scalp and skin problems, but they are of doubtful benefit.

ANTIBIOTICS These drugs are used in topical preparations to treat bacterial infections of the skin, such as infected eczema (p.333) or impetigo (p.351). Severe burns may also be treated with a topical antibiotic in order to prevent infection. In some cases, a preparation containing two or more antibiotics is used to make sure that all bacteria are eradicated. You should always follow your doctor's instructions on how long to continue using a topical antibiotic preparation. Stopping early may allow a skin infection to recur.

ANTIVIRAL DRUGS Some topical antivirals used to treat conditions such as cold sores (p.354), which are caused by herpes viruses, can be bought over the counter. These drugs are most effective used early in an attack. Most common viral infections that cause a rash, such as rubella (p.294), do not need treatment, and many in fections in the skin, such as warts (p.354), do not respond to topical antiviral drugs. However, herpes zoster (p.290) and genital herpes (p.767) are treated effectively with oral antivirals.

ANTIFUNGAL DRUGS These drugs are used to treat fungal infections, including athlete's foot (p.353), ringworm (p.352), thrush (*see* VAGINAL THRUSH, p.752, and ORAL THRUSH, p.862), and fungal nail infections (*see* NAIL ABNORMALITIES, p.360). Treatment of nail infections may need to be continued for several months to allow healthy nail to grow. Some topical antifungals can be bought over the counter. However, some fungal infections do not respond to topical preparations and require treatment with oral drugs.

ANTIPARASITIC DRUGS Topical antiparasitic drugs are used to destroy adult parasites and their eggs and to treat infestations, including head lice (p.831), pubic lice (p.768), and scabies (p.355).

Infestations of head lice are treated with an antiparasitic lotion or cream rinse that is washed off later. For pubic lice, your doctor will prescribe a lotion or cream to apply to the pubic area. Scabies is treated with a lotion or cream applied all over the body and washed off after 8–24 hours. All members of a household affected by head lice or scabies should be treated at the same time to avoid reinfestation. In the case of infestation with pubic lice, sexual partners should be checked for lice and treated simultaneously if necessary.

Sunscreens and sunblocks

Preparations containing chemicals that help to protect the skin from the damaging effects of the sun's ultraviolet radiation

COMMON DRUGS

- Aminobenzoic acid • Dioxybenzone
- Oxybenzone • Padimate O
- Para-aminobenzoic acid • Titanium dioxide
- Zinc oxide

Sunscreens and sunblocks contain a variety of chemicals that help to protect the skin from the damaging effects of ultraviolet (UV) radiation present in sunlight. UV radiation is composed of UVA and UVB rays, both of which age the skin. In addition, UVA rays cause tanning, and UVB rays cause burning (*see* SUNBURN, p.357). Excessive exposure to sunlight also increases the risk of skin cancer (p.344). The sun's rays can cause cancerous changes to occur in the skin because they progressively damage the genes that control important functions in the skin, such as cell division.

Using sunscreens or sunblocks protects against these harmful effects and is advisable for anyone spending time in the sun. The use of these preparations is particularly important for people with fair skin and young children, whose skin is more vulnerable to sun damage (*see* SAFETY IN THE SUN, p.80).

If your skin becomes sensitive to the sun (*see* PHOTOSENSITIVITY, p.338), you may need to use sunscreen or sunblock even when you are not exposed to strong sunlight. UV sensitivity may develop in people who are taking certain types of drug, such as some oral contraceptives (*see* CONTRACEPTION, p.69), antibiotics (p.885), and thiazide diuretics (*see* DIURETIC DRUGS, p.902).

HOW DO THEY WORK?

Sunscreens protect the skin by absorbing UVB rays, thereby reducing the amount that enters the skin; sunblocks provide a physical barrier that reflects or scatters UVA and UVB rays. Substances in sunscreens that absorb UVB rays include para-aminobenzoic acid (PABA) and padimate O. Sunblocks contain chemicals such as zinc oxide and titanium dioxide, which are opaque and therefore reflect and scatter both UVB and UVA rays. Sunscreens are graded using a sun protection factor (SPF), which is a measure of the level of protection they provide against UVB rays. The higher the rating, the greater the protection against this type of radiation. However, even sunscreens with a high SPF do not provide complete UVB protection.

HOW ARE THEY USED?

Sunscreens and sunblocks are available as creams, lotions, gels, and sprays. All products need to be applied frequently and generously to maintain protection, especially after swimming. You may experience irritation or an allergic rash when using certain sun protection products, particularly those containing PABA.

CAUTION

Reapply sunscreens regularly, particularly after swimming or if you are sweating.

DRUGS FOR MUSCULOSKELETAL DISORDERS

Pain in the bones, muscles, or joints is a common problem. In many cases, it is due to a minor muscular injury, and drugs are used to relieve the pain while the problem gets better. More serious disorders may cause persistent pain or disability, and long-term medication is needed to control the symptoms.

The first two articles in this section cover nonsteroidal anti-inflammatory drugs and locally acting corticosteroids. These drugs can relieve symptoms of musculoskeletal disorders, such as inflammation and pain, but have no effect on the underlying causes.

Drugs used to treat specific joint and bone disorders are discussed in the next two articles. Antirheumatic drugs are commonly used to treat rheumatoid arthritis. They can slow or halt joint damage, thereby preventing the disability that may be the long-term result of this disorder. The next article covers drugs for bone disorders. These drugs prevent or halt the abnormal growth or breakdown of bone that occurs in bone disorders such as Paget's disease and osteoporosis.

The final article in this section covers muscle relaxants, drugs that are used to relieve muscle spasms resulting from a variety of disorders.

KEY ANATOMY

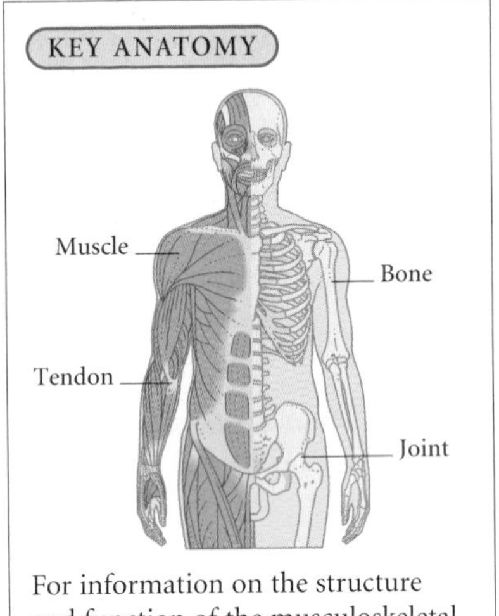

For information on the structure and function of the musculoskeletal system, *see* pp.362–367.

Nonsteroidal anti-inflammatory drugs

A group of drugs that are used to relieve pain and inflammation, particularly in muscles, ligaments, and joints

COMMON DRUGS

• Aspirin • Diclofenac • Diflunisal • Etodolac • Fenoprofen • Flurbiprofen • Ibuprofen • Indometacin • Ketoprofen • Ketorolac • Mefenamic acid • Nabumetone • Naproxen • Piroxicam • Rofecoxib • Sulindac

Nonsteroidal anti-inflammatory drugs (NSAIDs) are non-opioid painkillers (p.912) that are used to relieve the discomfort and inflammation caused by a variety of musculoskeletal disorders. These drugs are also commonly used to treat other types of pain and inflammation, such as headache (p.518).

Although it is technically an NSAID, aspirin is not usually classed with other types of NSAID because it has only a limited anti-inflammatory effect at normal doses. For this reason, NSAIDs with a more powerful anti-inflammatory action are normally prescribed to treat inflammatory conditions.

NSAIDs may be used for conditions that develop suddenly, such as ligament damage and muscle strains and tears (p.395). They usually reduce symptoms within a few hours. NSAIDs are also used to relieve pain and inflammation caused by long-term musculoskeletal disorders, such as osteoarthritis (p.374) and rheumatoid arthritis (p.377). When used to treat these conditions, NSAIDs can rapidly relieve pain, but they may take about 2 weeks to reduce inflammation. Although NSAIDs are effective in alleviating symptoms, they do not cure the underlying condition.

NSAIDs work by limiting the release of prostaglandins, chemicals occurring naturally in the body that cause pain and trigger the inflammatory response (*see* HOW NSAIDS WORK, opposite page). However, prostaglandins also have a protective action in the stomach lining, and blocking their production with NSAIDs may lead to stomach irritation.

HOW ARE THEY USED?

NSAIDs are most commonly taken orally, although occasionally they may be applied as a gel or given by injection. Certain NSAIDs are available in a slow-release form, which may be effective for up to 24 hours. This reduces the need to take pills frequently when long-term conditions are being treated. Slow-release NSAIDs also provide a more constant level of pain relief. For many conditions, these drugs are used with other treatments, such as physiotherapy (p.961). Some NSAIDs, such as ibuprofen, can be bought over the counter.

WHAT ARE THE SIDE EFFECTS?

NSAIDs have varying potential to irritate the stomach lining. If you are given certain NSAIDs, such as ibuprofen, for long-term use, you may also be given an antiulcer drug (*see* ULCER-HEALING DRUGS, p.923) to protect your stomach lining. A recently developed group of NSAIDs, cyclo-oxygenase 2 inhibitors (COX-2 inhibitors) such as rofecoxib, are thought to have a less damaging effect on the stomach lining than some other types of NSAID.

NSAIDs may cause allergic reactions (*see* DRUG ALLERGY, p.467), including rashes and a condition known as angio-oedema (p.469), in which temporary, painless swellings develop in the skin and mucous membranes. Some people may develop photosensitivity (p.338), in which the skin becomes abnormally sensitive to sunlight. People who have asthma (p.483) or a kidney disorder are advised not to take NSAIDs because the drugs can make these conditions worse.

DRUG ACTION How NSAIDs work

Nonsteroidal anti-inflammatory drugs (NSAIDs) are used to treat a variety of conditions, including inflammatory disorders such as rheumatoid arthritis (p.377). The inflammatory response is triggered by substances called prostaglandins, which are released when tissue is damaged. NSAIDs reduce inflammation by blocking the production of prostaglandins.

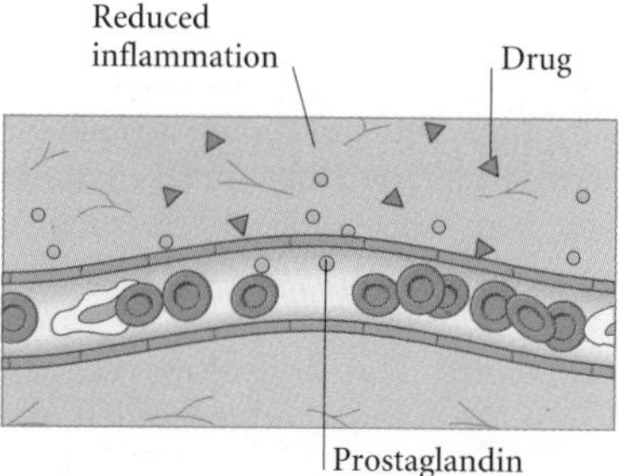

Before drug
Prostaglandins are released in damaged tissue, causing the blood vessels to widen and leak fluid. White cells move into the tissue. The area becomes red and swollen.

After drug
NSAIDs limit the release of prostaglandins, thereby reducing the inflammation. The leaky blood vessels return to normal, and swelling and redness subside.

Locally acting corticosteroids

Drugs that are injected directly into body tissues to reduce inflammation

Common drugs

- Betamethasone • Dexamethasone
- Hydrocortisone • Methylprednisolone
- Prednisolone • Triamcinolone

Locally acting corticosteroids are anti-inflammatory drugs that are injected into a specific area of the body to reduce inflammation in that area. The drugs block the immune response that triggers production of natural chemicals that cause inflammation and pain. Corticosteroids can be injected into joints to relieve inflammation due to conditions such as rheumatoid arthritis (p.377). Injections can also be given around ligaments and tendons to relieve conditions such as tennis elbow (p.389). A local anaesthetic may be injected with a corticosteroid to relieve pain quickly.

Side effects do not often occur with injected corticosteriods; if they do, they are usually limited to the site of injection. These local side effects can include thinning of the skin or fat at the injection site, which may produce a dimple. There may be a temporary increase in pain; rarely, the area becomes infected.

Antirheumatic drugs

Drugs that are used to slow or stop the joint damage that often results from long-term inflammation

Common drugs

Immunosuppressants
- Azathioprine • Cyclophosphamide
- Ciclosporin • Methotrexate

Gold-based drugs
- Auranofin • Sodium aurothiomalate

Other antirheumatic drugs
- Hydroxychloroquine • Penicillamine
- Sulfasalazine

Antirheumatic drugs slow or halt the progress of long-term inflammatory disorders of the joints and connective tissues. They are most commonly used to treat rheumatoid arthritis (p.377). In this disorder, the immune system attacks the body's own tissues, primarily the joints, causing them to become swollen, stiff, and painful. These drugs are often used together with a nonsteroidal anti-inflammatory drug (opposite page).

What are the types?

Antirheumatic drugs include immunosuppressants (p.906) and gold-based drugs, as well as a number of others. The way many of these drugs work is unclear. Immunosuppressants suppress the body's inflammatory responses; the use of other types of drug leads to a decline in the inflammation around the joints. Most antirheumatic drugs need to be taken for at least 6 weeks before there is an improvement in symptoms.

Immunosuppressants Drugs in this group may be used to treat severe rheumatoid arthritis. They are usually taken orally but may be injected. The drugs work by suppressing the body's immune response. If you are taking these drugs, you will have regular blood tests to ensure that the level of white blood cells does not fall too low, which can lead to increased susceptibility to infection.

Gold-based drugs These drugs are usually given by injection into a muscle. In some people, gold-based drugs cause side effects, such as a rash and diarrhoea. Rarely, the drugs affect the kidneys, and regular urine tests are performed during treatment to detect complications. Gold-based drugs also occasionally suppress blood cell production in the bone marrow, which may cause serious problems such as abnormal bleeding. For this reason, regular blood tests are needed.

Other antirheumatic drugs Other commonly used drugs that are thought to have an immunosuppressant effect are sulfasalazine, hydroxychloroquine, and penicillamine. Recently developed drugs include agents that suppress a natural chemical in the blood known as tumour necrosis factor. This factor is present at excessive levels in people who have rheumatoid arthritis.

Sulfasalazine is a combination of an antibiotic and a form of aspirin and is taken orally. Side effects may include rashes, nausea and vomiting, and blood disorders such as anaemia (p.446).

Hydroxychloroquine is an antimalarial drug (p.888) that may also be used to treat systemic lupus erythematosus (p.461), a disorder that causes inflammation in many body tissues, including

> **WARNING**
>
> If you are taking an antirheumatic drug, you should report any sign of infection, such as a sore throat, or any unusual bleeding to your doctor immediately.

joints and muscles. Hydroxychloroquine is taken orally. Possible side effects include headaches and stomach upsets. Very rarely, eye damage may occur after prolonged treatment and eye examinations are needed periodically.

Penicillamine may be used to treat rheumatoid arthritis when inflammation affects other areas of the body in addition to the joints. It has similar side effects to gold-based drugs.

Drugs for bone disorders

Drugs used to treat disorders affecting bone formation, replacement, and repair

COMMON DRUGS

OESTROGEN AND COMPOUNDS WITH OESTROGEN-LIKE EFFECTS
• Conjugated oestrogens • Raloxifene
• Tibolone

BISPHOSPHONATES
• Alendronate • Etidronate

CALCITONIN

CALCIUM AND VITAMIN D
• Calciferol • Calcitriol • Calcium carbonate
• Ergocalciferol • Vitamin D

The body constantly breaks down and rebuilds bone. Disorders can develop if the balance between breakdown and renewal is upset. Drugs that affect bone growth are used to treat disorders in which either too much bone is broken down or bone grows abnormally. For example, in osteoporosis (p.368), bone is broken down faster than it is replaced; in Paget's disease of the bone (p.370), there is abnormal bone formation.

WHAT ARE THE TYPES?

Drugs used to treat bone disorders include oestrogen and compounds with oestrogen-like effects, bisphosphonate drugs, and the hormone calcitonin. Calcium and vitamin D are also used.

OESTROGEN The sex hormone oestrogen and compounds with oestrogen-like effects slow the breakdown of bone and may be used to prevent osteoporosis or to slow its progress. Oestrogen is commonly prescribed to postmenopausal women as hormone replacement therapy (p.937). It is either taken on its own or with the hormone progestogen. A newly developed drug, tibolone, combines the effects of both oestrogen and progestogen. Oestrogens can be applied to the skin as a patch or gel, or taken orally. Side effects include weight gain, headache, and depression.

BISPHOSPHONATES These drugs may be used to treat osteoporosis and Paget's disease. They work by reducing abnormally high rates of bone breakdown and renewal. The drugs are taken orally. They may cause side effects such as nausea, diarrhoea, and indigestion.

CALCITONIN This drug slows the rate of bone breakdown and renewal. It may be used to treat Paget's disease and to reduce the risk of osteoporotic fractures in postmenopausal women. Calcitonin may be given as a nasal spray or by self-injection several times a week. Side effects may include irritation at the injection site, nausea, and hot flushes.

CALCIUM AND VITAMIN D These substances are essential for maintaining healthy bone. Supplements may be used to treat bone disorders. Postmenopausal women require a daily calcium intake of 1,200 mg–1,500 mg, much of which can be obtained in the diet. Calcium supplements may cause constipation.

Vitamin D helps the body to absorb calcium from food. Deficiency is rare but can cause rickets in children and osteomalacia in adults (*see* OSTEOMALACIA AND RICKETS, p.370). Taken at the recommended dose, vitamin D supplements usually cause no side effects.

Muscle relaxants

A group of drugs that are used to treat muscular stiffness and cramps

COMMON DRUGS

• Baclofen • Botulinum toxin • Dantrolene
• Diazepam • Quinine • Tizanidine

Muscle relaxants are used for the relief of muscle spasm, a painful, involuntary contraction of one or more muscles. These drugs are also used to ease the movement of limbs that are stiff because of nervous system disorders such as multiple sclerosis (p.541) and cerebral palsy (p.846). Muscle relaxants are sometimes prescribed for the treatment of conditions such as night-time muscle cramps (p.388) and torticollis (p.388), in which muscles in the neck contract, pulling the head over to one side. Certain muscle relaxants are used to paralyse muscles during surgery carried out under general anaesthesia (*see* HAVING MAJOR SURGERY, p.943).

HOW DO THEY WORK?

Muscle relaxant drugs work in a variety of ways. Some muscle relaxants, such as tizanidine, baclofen, and the antianxiety drug diazepam, work by reducing transmission of nerve signals from the brain and spinal cord to the muscles, causing the muscles to relax.

Dantrolene relieves spasm by acting directly on muscles and making them less sensitive to nerve signals from the brain and spinal cord. Botulinum toxin relaxes muscles by blocking the transmission of signals from nerve endings to muscle cells. The way in which quinine works is not fully understood.

HOW ARE THEY USED?

Doses of muscle relaxants need careful adjustment. Too little has no effect, and too much may lead to muscle weakness. For long-standing conditions such as multiple sclerosis, doses begin at a low level and are increased gradually to reach a balance between symptom control and muscle strength.

Involuntary contractions of the neck and facial muscles can be relieved by injecting tiny amounts of botulinum toxin directly into the affected area. A single injection is usually effective for about 3 months. Quinine taken at bedtime, also in tiny amounts, helps to prevent cramp developing in the night.

WHAT ARE THE SIDE EFFECTS?

A common side effect of many muscle relaxants is drowsiness, which usually decreases as treatment progresses. With long-term use, the body may become dependent on a muscle relaxant; if the drug is withdrawn suddenly, muscle spasms may become worse than they were before treatment began.

Dantrolene can cause diarrhoea. This drug may also cause severe liver problems, as may tizanidine. If you are taking either of these drugs, your doctor will carry out regular blood tests to check that your liver function is normal.

DRUGS FOR CARDIOVASCULAR DISORDERS

Disorders of the cardiovascular system are a major cause of poor health and early death in the developed world. In some cases, cardiovascular disorders can be improved by changes in lifestyle, such as improving diet or giving up smoking. In other cases, cardiovascular disorders require treatment with drugs that act on the blood vessels, the heart, or the kidneys.

The opening article in this section discusses drugs that are used to treat high blood pressure, a disorder that affects 1 in 5 people in developed countries. A number of these drugs are effective not only in lowering blood pressure but also in the treatment of heart failure, angina, and coronary artery disease.

The next article gives an overview of the types of drug that may be used in the treatment of arrhythmias, a group of disorders in which the heart beats extremely rapidly or with an abnormal rhythm.

Specific classes of drugs are discussed in separate articles. Beta-blockers and calcium channel blockers are used to treat certain arrhythmias; these drugs and nitrates also treat coronary artery disease; diuretics, ACE inhibitors, and beta-blockers are helpful in treating congestive heart failure; and all are useful in lowering high blood pressure.

Lipid-lowering drugs, which are used to reduce the risk of heart attack by lowering levels of fats in the blood, are discussed elsewhere (*see* DRUGS ACTING ON THE ENDOCRINE SYSTEM AND METABOLISM, pp.930–935).

KEY ANATOMY

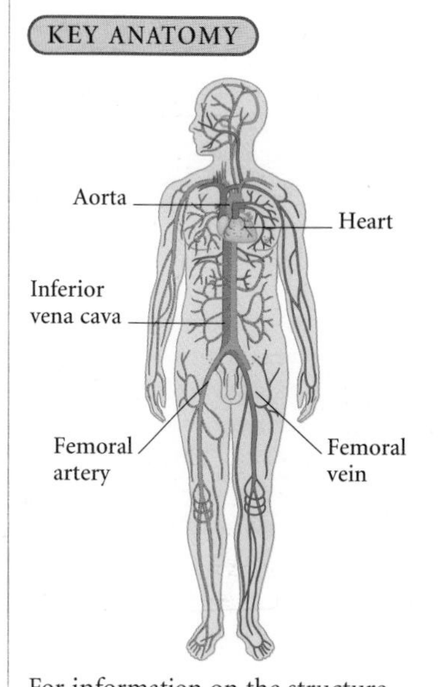

For information on the structure and function of the cardiovascular system, *see* pp.396–401.

Antihypertensive drugs

Drugs used to treat high blood pressure, a condition also known as hypertension

COMMON DRUGS

ACE INHIBITOR DRUGS (p.900)

ALPHA-BLOCKER DRUGS
• Doxazosin • Prazosin • Terazosin

ANGIOTENSIN II BLOCKER DRUGS
• Candesartan • Irbesartan • Losartan • Valsartan

BETA-BLOCKER DRUGS (p.898)

CALCIUM CHANNEL BLOCKER DRUGS (p.900)

CENTRALLY ACTING DRUGS
• Clonidine • Methyldopa • Moxonidine

DIURETIC DRUGS (p.902)

OTHER ANTIHYPERTENSIVE DRUGS
• Hydralazine • Minoxidil • Nitroprusside

High blood pressure (*see* HYPERTENSION, p.403) requires treatment mainly because it increases the risk of both coronary artery disease (p.405) and stroke (p.532). Antihypertensive drugs are most often used when changes in your lifestyle, such as improving your diet, doing more exercise, and giving up smoking, fail to produce an adequate fall in blood pressure over a short period of time. Antihypertensives are also used to treat hypertension in pregnancy (*see* PRE-ECLAMPSIA AND ECLAMPSIA, p.794).

WHAT ARE THE TYPES?

There are many different types of antihypertensive drug. The types that are most commonly used are beta-blockers (p.898), ACE inhibitor drugs (p.900), calcium channel blocker drugs (p.900), and diuretic drugs (p.902). Less commonly, alpha-blocker drugs, angiotensin II blocker drugs, centrally acting drugs, and other drugs, including diazoxide, hydralazine, and minoxidil, are used.

Most types of antihypertensive drug reduce high blood pressure by increasing the diameter of the blood vessels (a process known as vasodilation) or by reducing the force with which the heart pumps the blood. ACE inhibitors, alpha-blockers, angiotensin II blockers, calcium channel blockers, and centrally acting drugs act in a variety of ways to cause vasodilation. Beta-blockers lower blood pressure by reducing the force with which the heart pumps. This effect is achieved by blocking the action of substances produced naturally by the body that increase heart rate and blood pressure. Diuretics cause the kidneys to excrete more water and salts than usual, which reduces the volume of blood that is present in the circulation and thereby lowers blood pressure.

HOW ARE THEY USED?

Antihypertensives are normally taken orally over long periods of time and often for life. However, in some cases it is possible to reduce the dose gradually and eventually stop the drugs if blood pressure returns to normal following long-term changes in weight or lifestyle. The choice of drug depends on several factors, including age and other medical conditions that might be present. Certain drugs are especially likely to cause side effects in elderly people.

If you have mild or moderate hypertension, you will usually be prescribed a single drug, such as a diuretic or a beta-blocker. These drugs are not suitable for everyone. For example, they may make the control of diabetes mellitus (p.687) more difficult. In such circumstances, an ACE inhibitor or a calcium channel blocker may be used instead. If your blood pressure is not controlled adequately by a single drug, you may be given a diuretic in combination with either one or two other types of antihypertensive drugs in order to reduce blood pressure to a safe level.

You may be given alpha-blockers, angiotensin II blockers, or centrally acting drugs if other drugs or combinations of drugs have not reduced your blood pressure sufficiently or if other antihypertensives are unsuitable.

Unless you have severe hypertension, your doctor will usually start you on a low dose of a drug. The dose is then gradually increased until your blood pressure is normal or until you experience side effects. Your blood pressure will be monitored frequently until it is stable at a safe level.

WHAT ARE THE SIDE EFFECTS?

All antihypertensive drugs, in particular ACE inhibitors and alpha-blockers, can cause a sudden drop in blood pressure (*see* HYPOTENSION, p.414) when you first take them. This drop in blood pressure can cause light-headedness. The drugs may also cause drowsiness. If you experience these side effects, your doctor may reduce the dose or may give you a different drug. You should not stop taking an antihypertensive without first consulting your doctor.

Other side effects are associated with specific types of antihypertensive. Several types, especially beta-blockers and some diuretics, may cause impotence; ACE inhibitors sometimes cause a dry cough; calcium channel blockers may cause swollen ankles, flushing, and headaches. Long-term use of diuretics may increase the risk of gout (p.380). Minoxidil may result in excessive hair (p.359) and hydralazine may cause palpitations.

> **WARNING**
>
> Do not suddenly stop taking an antihypertensive drug without first consulting your doctor. Abrupt withdrawal of the drug could cause a rapid increase in blood pressure.

Antiarrhythmic drugs

Drugs used to treat abnormal heart rates and rhythms (arrhythmias)

COMMON DRUGS

BETA-BLOCKER DRUGS (p.898)

CALCIUM CHANNEL BLOCKER DRUGS (p.900)
- Verapamil

DIGITALIS DRUGS (p.901)
- Digoxin

OTHER ANTIARRHYTHMIC DRUGS
- Adenosine • Amiodarone • Bretylium
- Disopyramide • Flecainide • Lidocaine
- Mexiletine • Moracizine • Procainamide
- Propafenone • Quinidine

Abnormalities in heart rhythm and rate, known as arrhythmias (p.415), are caused by a disturbance in the electrical signals that control heart action. Often, minor disturbances do not need treatment. However, some arrhythmias do require treatment to restore normal heart rhythm, thereby reducing symptoms such as palpitations, shortness of breath, light-headedness, and chest pain.

Antiarrhythmics are commonly prescribed to treat the arrhythmias atrial fibrillation (p.417) and supraventricular tachycardia (p.416), both of which cause the heart to beat very rapidly. They are also used to treat ventricular arrhythmia, which may develop after a heart attack (*see* MYOCARDIAL INFARCTION, p.410) and, if left untreated, may lead to cardiac arrest (p.419).

Commonly used antiarrhythmics include beta-blockers (right), the calcium channel blocker drug verapamil, and the digitalis drug digoxin. There are various other types of antiarrhythmics, some of which are mostly used to treat ventricular arrhythmias.

HOW ARE THEY USED?

Once an antiarrhythmic is required, you may have to take the drug indefinitely. For long-term treatment, the drugs are given orally, and initially you may need to take several doses a day. When your heartbeat has been stabilized, your doctor will probably test the drug levels in your blood in order to correct the dose.

The type of drug your doctor selects depends on which form of arrhythmia you have. For example, a beta-blocker, calcium channel blocker, or the digitalis drug digoxin may be useful in reducing a rapid heart rate in atrial fibrillation; another drug such as quinidine or procainamide may be necessary to restore regular heart rhythm.

If you have developed arrhythmia suddenly and the condition is severe, you may be given a drug such as adenosine intravenously as an emergency measure to restore normal heart activity. When the initial symptoms have been brought under control, your doctor may prescribe drugs for long-term treatment to prevent future attacks.

WHAT ARE THE SIDE EFFECTS?

Many types of antiarrhythmic drug reduce blood pressure, and this may cause light-headedness when you stand up. You may also experience nausea and blurred vision.

Other side effects are specific to certain drugs. For example, amiodarone may cause skin sensitivity to sunlight and may also affect the function of the thyroid gland and lungs. If you are taking the digitalis drug digoxin, contact your doctor immediately if you experience nausea, diarrhoea, vomiting, or any visual disturbances. These symptoms indicate that the dose is too high.

You should tell your doctor if you are taking other drugs because of the risk of an adverse interaction with an antiarrhythmic. You should not stop taking an antiarrhythmic without consulting your doctor because abrupt withdrawal of the drug may make your condition worse.

Beta-blocker drugs

Drugs that block the transmission of certain nerve impulses and are used to treat disorders of the heart and circulation

COMMON DRUGS

- Acebutolol • Atenolol • Bisoprolol • Carvedilol
- Esmolol • Labetalol • Metoprolol • Nadolol
- Oxprenolol • Pindolol • Propranolol • Sotalol
- Timolol

Beta-blocker drugs, or beta-adrenergic blocking agents, are widely prescribed to treat disorders of the heart and circulation and also to treat other conditions. Cardioselective beta-blockers act mainly on the heart. Other beta-blockers act on blood vessels throughout the body and on other target tissues such as the cells that secrete fluid in the eye.

WHY ARE THEY USED?

Beta-blockers are most commonly used in the treatment of high blood pressure (*see* HYPERTENSION, p.403). They are also used to treat disorders of the heart, including angina (p.407), which is a disabling chest pain caused by too little oxygen reaching the heart muscle; to prevent the recurrence of a heart attack (*see* MYOCARDIAL INFARCTION, p.410); to correct some irregularities of the heartbeat (*see* ARRHYTHMIAS, p.415); and in the treatment of certain forms of heart failure (*see* CHRONIC HEART FAILURE, p.413).

Beta-blockers are used to treat or prevent other conditions, such as recurrent migraine (p.518), which is thought to be caused by constriction and rebound widening of blood vessels in the head. They are also used for glaucoma (p.575), in which pressure in the eye is increased by a build-up of excess fluid. Some beta-blockers are used to control physical symptoms of anxiety, such as tremor. The drugs also help in the treatment of hyperthyroidism (p.679) by reducing the symptoms caused by the excess production of thyroid hormone, such as sweating, tremor, and rapid heart rate.

HOW DO THEY WORK?

Beta-blockers work by blocking the action of epinephrine (adrenaline) and norepinephrine (noradrenaline), two chemicals produced by the body that increase heart rate and raise the blood pressure. Cardioselective beta-blockers are especially effective at slowing heart rate and reducing the force of the heartbeat, thereby reducing the workload of the heart. These actions make beta-blockers effective in the treatment of angina, hypertension, and some types of arrhythmia. Other beta-blockers have a more widespread action and block many of the effects that norepinephrine has throughout the body, such as narrowing blood vessels and causing tremor and sweating. As a result, they may be effective in treating some physical symptoms caused by this chemical, such as tremor. Beta-blockers do not treat the underlying causes of these conditions.

Beta-blockers are used for migraine because they block the effects of norepinephrine on blood vessels in the head. They also reduce fluid formation, and thus pressure, in the eyeball, and so are used to treat glaucoma.

HOW ARE THEY USED?

If you have angina, high blood pressure, or recurrent migraine, you may be given long-term treatment with oral beta-blockers. Your doctor may initially prescribe a low dose and increase it until the desired effect is reached. If you have glaucoma, you may be prescribed eyedrops that contain the beta-blocker timolol. A beta-blocker may be given intravenously in hospital if you experience sudden severe angina or if you have a heart attack.

Beta-blockers are also used along with other types of drug, especially in the treatment of angina, high blood pressure, and some types of heart failure.

WHAT ARE THE SIDE EFFECTS?

Beta-blockers can exacerbate some respiratory disorders and are not normally given to people who have a history of chronic obstructive pulmonary disease or asthma. However, if treatment with these drugs is necessary, cardioselective beta-blockers can sometimes be used. Since beta-blockers can mask some of the symptoms of hypoglycaemia (low blood glucose), which is a serious condition that must be recognized and treated immediately, they may not be suitable for people who need to take insulin for diabetes mellitus (p.687).

If you are taking a beta-blocker, your sleeping pattern may be disrupted, and your hands and feet may feel cold because the blood circulation in the extremities is reduced. Men sometimes experience impotence, but normal sexual function usually returns when the drug is stopped. Rarely, beta-blockers cause rashes and dry eyes. All these side effects tend to be more common and more severe in elderly people.

If you need to stop taking a beta-blocker, your doctor will advise you on how to reduce the dose gradually to avoid rebound high blood pressure, a recurrence of angina, or a heart attack.

WARNING

Do not suddenly stop taking a beta-blocker drug without consulting your doctor. Abrupt withdrawal of the drug could cause a rise in blood pressure, worsening of angina, or an increased risk of a heart attack.

Nitrate drugs

A group of drugs used to prevent and treat angina (chest pain) caused by coronary artery disease

COMMON DRUGS

- Glyceryl trinitrate • Isosorbide dinitrate
- Isosorbide mononitrate

Nitrate drugs are often used in conjunction with various other drugs in the treatment of angina (p.407), a disabling chest pain that occurs when too little oxygen reaches the heart muscle.

Nitrates may be prescribed to prevent angina attacks or to relieve the symptoms of an attack when it happens. However, nitrates do not treat the underlying cause of angina, which is usually narrowing of the coronary arteries due to build-up of fatty deposits (*see* CORONARY ARTERY DISEASE, p.405).

HOW DO THEY WORK?

Nitrates cause blood vessels in the body to dilate (widen), making it easier for the heart to pump blood around the body. This reduces the oxygen requirement of the heart muscle. Nitrates also make the coronary arteries dilate, which improves the blood supply to the heart muscle.

HOW ARE THEY USED?

Nitrates may be used either to provide rapid relief from an angina attack or to prevent an attack occurring. "Reliever" nitrates provide fast relief from chest pain in the event of an angina attack, but are effective for only 20–30 minutes. These drugs are available as tablets that you place under your tongue or between your upper lip and gum, and as an aerosol spray that is sprayed under the tongue (*see* USING SUBLINGUAL SPRAYS, p.900). Your doctor may advise you to use a fast-acting nitrate just before exerting yourself.

A long-acting nitrate takes more time to become effective than a fast-acting nitrate but it may continue to have an effect for several hours. Long-acting nitrates may be prescribed as skin patches, ointment, or tablets, usually taken twice a day. Skin patches, which may be applied to the chest, back, abdomen, or thigh, are useful if you have angina at night. Skin patches should be applied to a different part of

SELF-ADMINISTRATION USING SUBLINGUAL SPRAYS

Sublingual sprays are used when immediate drug action is needed. For example, they are used to relieve the symptoms of an angina attack. The drugs are absorbed into the blood through the tongue's rich supply of blood vessels. This is a much faster route than absorption from the digestive tract, which occurs when drugs are taken orally.

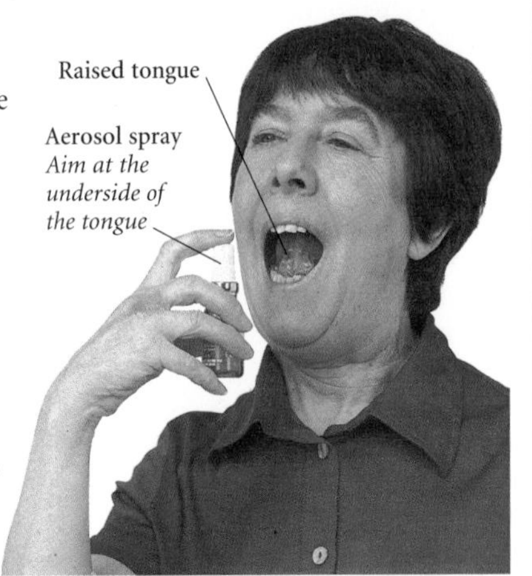

Using the spray
With an open mouth, touch the roof of your mouth with your tongue and spray on to the underside of your tongue. Avoid inhaling through your mouth at the same time as you spray the drug.

the skin each day. Nitrate drugs may also be administered intravenously in hospital as an emergency treatment to relieve an angina attack.

What are the side effects?

Nitrates commonly cause a throbbing headache and flushing. They can also cause a fall in blood pressure, resulting in light-headedness when you stand up.

If you are using a long-acting nitrate, you may develop tolerance, resulting in a reduction of the drug's effectiveness. Tolerance can be avoided by interrupting use of a skin patch or an ointment for 4–8 hours each day. Usually, long-acting nitrate pills allow levels of the drug in the blood to fall overnight.

Calcium channel blocker drugs

A group of drugs used to treat several disorders of the heart and circulation

Common drugs

- Amlodipine • Diltiazem • Felodipine
- Isradipine • Nicardipine • Nifedipine
- Verapamil

Calcium channel blocker drugs may be prescribed to treat angina (p.407), a disabling chest pain that occurs when too little oxygen reaches the heart muscle. These drugs may also be used in the treatment of high blood pressure (*see* HYPERTENSION, p.403). The calcium channel blocker, verapamil, is used to treat some abnormal heart rhythms (*see* ARRHYTHMIAS, p.415). Nifedipine may be used to treat Raynaud's phenomenon (p.436), a disorder in which spasm of arteries in the hands or feet restricts the blood supply to the fingers or toes, causing them to become painful, tingle, and become pale. Certain other calcium channel blockers may be taken regularly to reduce the frequency of attacks of migraine (p.518), in which blood vessels in the head constrict and then widen, causing severe headache.

How do they work?

Muscle cells need calcium to contract. Calcium channel blockers reduce the amount of calcium entering the muscle cells in blood vessel walls. This action causes the muscle cells to relax and the blood vessels to widen, thereby reducing blood pressure. This widening of blood vessels is thought to be the reason why calcium channel blockers work in the treatment of Raynaud's phenomenon and in the prevention of migraine attacks. Since the drugs reduce the amount of calcium that enters heart muscle cells, they reduce both the force and the rate of the heartbeat and therefore help to relieve angina.

WARNING

Do not suddenly stop taking a calcium channel blocker drug without first consulting your doctor. Abrupt withdrawal could cause worsening of your angina.

Verapamil also slows down the flow of electrical impulses through the heart and thus slows the heartbeat. It may be used in treating some arrhythmias in which the heart beats excessively fast.

How are they used?

Calcium channel blockers may be used alone or in combination with other drugs that are used in the treatment of angina, hypertension, or certain types of arrhythmia. Usually, the drugs are initially prescribed at a low dose, and the dose is gradually increased to an effective level. The ideal dose for you will be one that is high enough to allow the drug to be effective without causing troublesome side effects.

What are the side effects?

The most common side effects of calcium channel blockers are headache, light-headedness, flushing, and swollen ankles. Constipation can sometimes be a problem, particularly if you are taking verapamil. If you are constipated, you may find it helpful to eat more dietary fibre and drink plenty of fluids. Grapefruit may increase the effects of some of these drugs and should be avoided. Occasionally, taking calcium channel blockers can cause nausea, palpitations, excessive tiredness, and rashes. Calcium channel blockers are generally avoided for people with heart failure because the drugs can make symptoms worse.

ACE inhibitor drugs

A group of drugs used to treat heart failure and high blood pressure

Common drugs

- Captopril • Enalapril • Fosinopril • Lisinopril
- Moexipril • Perindopril • Quinapril • Ramipril
- Trandolapril

Angiotensin converting enzyme (ACE) inhibitor drugs are commonly used in the treatment of chronic heart failure (p.413), in which the efficiency of the heart in pumping blood around the body is reduced. ACE inhibitors are also used to treat high blood pressure (*see* HYPERTENSION, p.403), especially when it occurs in people who have diabetes mellitus (p.687), or when other antihypertensive drugs (p.897) prove to be ineffective or cause unacceptable side effects. ACE inhibitors may also be used to treat diabetic kidney disease (p.705). In this disorder, the small blood vessels in the filtering units of the kidneys are damaged and, as a result of this, protein leaks into the urine.

How do they work?

ACE inhibitors prevent the normal formation in the body of angiotensin II, a hormone that causes constriction (narrowing) of blood vessels (*see* How ACE inhibitor drugs work, below). By reducing the amount of angiotensin II present in the blood, ACE inhibitors allow blood vessels to dilate (widen). This widening of the blood vessels reduces blood pressure, which makes it easier for the heart to pump blood and therefore alleviates heart failure.

The mechanism by which ACE inhibitor drugs are effective in relieving diabetic kidney disease is not entirely understood. ACE inhibitors are not given to people with certain other types of kidney damage because they may make the condition worse.

How are they used?

ACE inhibitors are sometimes prescribed in combination with diuretic drugs (p.902) or beta-blockers (p.898) to reduce blood pressure when a single drug is not sufficiently effective.

You will probably need to take these drugs for several months at least, and sometimes years. Before you are given an ACE inhibitor to treat heart failure or high blood pressure, you may have a blood test to check that your kidney function is normal. Your doctor is likely to prescribe a low oral dose of the drug initially. The dose is gradually increased over several weeks until an effective level is reached. You may be advised to take the first dose at bedtime because it may cause your blood pressure to fall rapidly, making you feel light-headed. If you are elderly or taking another drug for high blood pressure, such as a diuretic, your doctor may suggest that you try a small dose while still in the doctor's surgery so that you can be monitored in case you have a sudden drop in blood pressure.

> **WARNING**
>
> If you are taking an ACE inhibitor drug, do not take a nonsteroidal anti-inflammatory drug (p.894) without first consulting your doctor because the combination may increase the risk of kidney damage.

What are the side effects?

Light-headedness can occur if there is a temporary fall in blood pressure and not enough blood reaches the brain. If light-headedness persists, you should consult your doctor. He or she may wish to adjust your dose. You should not drive or undertake hazardous tasks until you know how you are affected by the drug.

Other common side effects include a persistent dry cough, muscle cramps, diarrhoea, and occasionally the skin condition urticaria (p.468). A rare but serious side effect is kidney damage.

Digitalis drugs

A group of plant-derived drugs used to treat certain heart disorders

Common drugs

• Digitoxin • Digoxin

Digitalis drugs are members of a group of plant-derived drugs called cardiac glycosides. Today, the most commonly used drug belonging to this group is digoxin. Digitalis drugs may be used to treat chronic heart failure (p.413), in which the heart fails to pump blood around the body effectively. These drugs act by increasing the strength of the heart's contraction. They also slow down an abnormally rapid heart rate and allow the heart to pump more blood with each beat. This action results in an improved flow of blood to organs throughout the body.

Digitalis drugs may also be used to treat a very rapid, irregular heartbeat, such as atrial fibrillation (p.417). However, in this condition, digitalis drugs may slow the heart rate without correcting the irregularity.

How are they used?

You will normally be prescribed oral digitalis drugs. You may be given a large initial dose so that the drug becomes effective quickly. If your heart failure is life-threatening, very rapid treatment will be needed, and the drug may be administered by infusion into a vein.

While you are taking a digitalis drug, your doctor will monitor your heart

DRUG ACTION How ACE inhibitor drugs work

Angiotensin converting enzyme (ACE) inhibitors are used to reduce high blood pressure and relieve heart failure. They work by blocking the action of an enzyme in the blood that is responsible for converting a chemical known as angiotensin I into angiotensin II. Angiotensin II stimulates blood vessels to constrict (narrow), and its absence permits them to dilate (widen). This effect on blood vessels throughout the body causes a fall in blood pressure and relieves heart failure by allowing the heart to pump blood more easily.

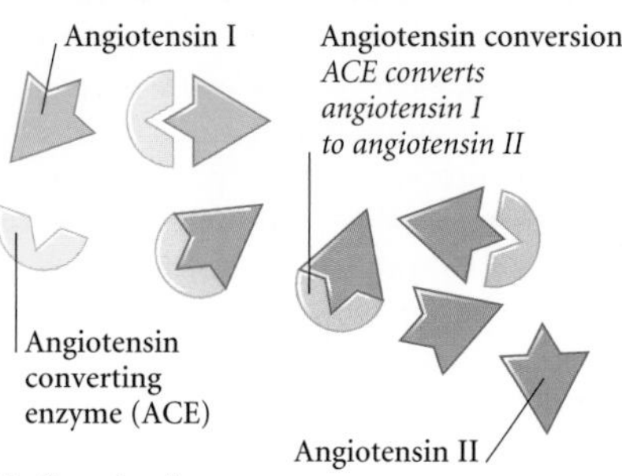

Before the drug
Angiotensin I is converted to angiotensin II by an enzyme known as ACE. The presence of angiotensin II in the bloodstream causes blood vessels to constrict.

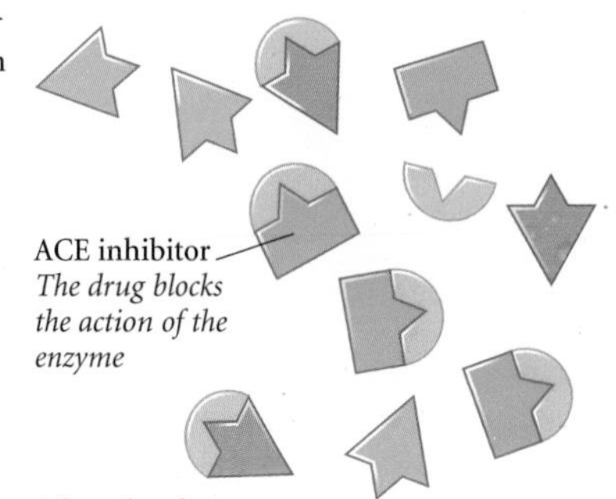

After the drug
ACE inhibitor drugs block enzyme activity, thereby reducing the rate of formation of angiotensin II. This action allows the blood vessels to dilate.

> **WARNING**
>
> Contact your doctor immediately if you experience nausea, vomiting, diarrhoea, or visual disturbances while you are taking the digitalis drug digoxin.

rate regularly and may also arrange for blood tests to check levels of the drug in your blood. You may need to take the drug for a prolonged period.

WHAT ARE THE SIDE EFFECTS?

You are most likely to experience side effects if the dose you are taking is too high. These side effects often develop slowly and may include nausea, vomiting, diarrhoea, abdominal pain, and headache. You may also experience loss of appetite, fatigue, and visual disturbances, such as seeing coloured haloes around lights. In rare cases, drowsiness, confusion, hallucinations, and delirium may occur. You should report any of these side effects to your doctor.

Diuretic drugs

Drugs that increase the volume of urine and that are used to remove excess fluid from the body

COMMON DRUGS

THIAZIDE DRUGS
- Bendroflumethazide (bendrofluazide)
- Chlorothiazide • Chlortalidone
- Hydrochlorothiazide
- Indapamide • Metolazone

LOOP DIURETIC DRUGS
- Bumetanide • Furosemide (frusemide)
- Torasemide

POTASSIUM-SPARING DIURETIC DRUGS
- Amiloride • Spironolactone • Triamterene

OTHER DIURETIC DRUGS
- Acetazolamide • Mannitol

Diuretic drugs are commonly used in the treatment of high blood pressure (*see* HYPERTENSION, p.403) and chronic heart failure (p.413). Diuretics are also used to treat other conditions in which excess fluid accumulates in the body, such as liver or kidney disorders and glaucoma (p.575). Some diuretics may be used to prevent altitude sickness (p.324) and to treat the inner ear condition Ménière's disease (p.604).

HOW DO THEY WORK?

Diuretics act on the kidneys to increase the volume of water that is excreted from the body as urine. Water, salts (such as sodium and potassium), and waste products are removed from the blood as it passes through small tubules in the kidneys. Most of the water and salts are reabsorbed into the bloodstream. What is not reabsorbed is then excreted, along with waste products, as urine. Diuretics reduce the reabsorption of water and salts into the blood, thereby increasing the volume of urine that is produced. This action of diuretics relieves the accumulation of fluid that occurs in the body due to heart failure, and the reduced blood volume helps to reduce blood pressure. Some diuretics also dilate (widen) blood vessels in the body, which also has the effect of lowering blood pressure.

WHAT ARE THE TYPES?

The diuretic drugs that are most frequently prescribed are thiazide drugs, loop diuretic drugs, and potassium-sparing diuretic drugs, which vary in their potency. Different types of diuretic affect reabsorption at different sites along the kidney tubules. The type of diuretic that your doctor prescribes is likely to depend on the condition being treated, your age, and any other existing medical conditions that you may have.

THIAZIDES These are the most commonly used diuretics for the treatment of high blood pressure. Thiazides lower blood pressure by reducing blood volume as well as by dilating (widening) blood vessels. These types of diuretic are usually taken orally once a day and have an effect at low doses.

Thiazides generally cause few side effects. However, the increased frequency with which you need to pass urine may be inconvenient. This effect is most noticeable at the start of treatment. You may find it convenient to take the diuretic early in the morning so that your sleep is not interrupted at night by a frequent need to go to the toilet.

Occasionally, thiazide diuretics cause light-headedness due to a drop in blood pressure. Thiazides can cause excessive loss of potassium from the body, which can result in confusion, weakness, and, in rare cases, an abnormal heart rhythm. Blood tests are used to monitor the levels of potassium in the body. To correct low levels, you may be given a potassium supplement or a potassium-sparing diuretic either in place of or in combination with a thiazide.

Thiazides may also cause increased levels of uric acid in the blood. When the level of uric acid becomes too high, crystals may be deposited in the joints, which may cause the painful condition gout (p.380). Thiazides are sometimes avoided in people with diabetes mellitus (p.687) because they may make control of the condition more difficult. In addition, these drugs can cause the skin to become sensitized to sunlight (*see* PHOTOSENSITIVITY, p.338).

LOOP DIURETICS These diuretics have a more powerful effect than thiazides and are used to treat the accumulation of fluid due to heart failure, some kidney disorders, and some liver disorders. They may also be given as an injection for the emergency treatment of acute heart failure in hospital.

Loop diuretics cause the production of urine to increase dramatically. In men with an enlarged prostate gland (p.725), this problem may lead to urinary retention (p.713). The drugs may also cause nausea. In addition, loop diuretics can deplete the body's supply of potassium. If you are affected by potassium loss, your doctor may prescribe a potassium supplement or a potassium-sparing diuretic to be taken in combination with a loop diuretic.

POTASSIUM-SPARING DIURETICS Most of these drugs are mild diuretics and are used either alone or in combination with a thiazide or loop diuretic if potassium depletion has occurred. The side effects of potassium-sparing diuretics may include digestive disturbances, such as flatulence and nausea, a dry mouth, and rashes. One drug, spironolactone, may cause breast enlargement in men (*see* GYNAECOMASTIA, p.729).

OTHER DIURETIC DRUGS Mild diuretics, such as acetazolamide, are occasionally used to prevent altitude sickness and attacks of dizziness associated with the inner ear condition Ménière's disease and to relieve the excessive pressure in the eye that occurs in glaucoma.

DRUGS FOR BLOOD AND IMMUNE SYSTEM DISORDERS AND CANCER

Improved understanding of blood and immune system disorders has led to advances in certain drug treatments. For example, there are now drugs that reduce the risk of heart attacks caused by blood clots. Recently developed drugs that act on the immune system also allow some forms of cancer to be controlled.

There are a number of potentially serious disorders that alter the clotting mechanism of the blood, resulting in either abnormal bleeding or the formation of unwanted clots. The first articles in this section describe the drugs that help to keep the clotting factors of the blood at normal levels.

The body's immune system combats disease by activating white blood cells and proteins in the blood against infections and cancers. Sometimes, this system malfunctions and needs to be treated with drugs. Types of drug used to treat immune system malfunction include antiallergy drugs, which counter overreaction of the immune system; immunosuppressants, which prevent the immune system attacking the body's own tissues; and interferon drugs, which boost immunity. Drugs for the immune deficiency disease AIDS are discussed elsewhere (*see* DRUGS FOR HIV INFECTION AND AIDS, p.887). The final article in this section describes anticancer drugs, which can destroy cancerous cells or prevent them from spreading elsewhere in the body. The use of anticancer drugs is known as chemotherapy (p.280).

KEY ELEMENTS

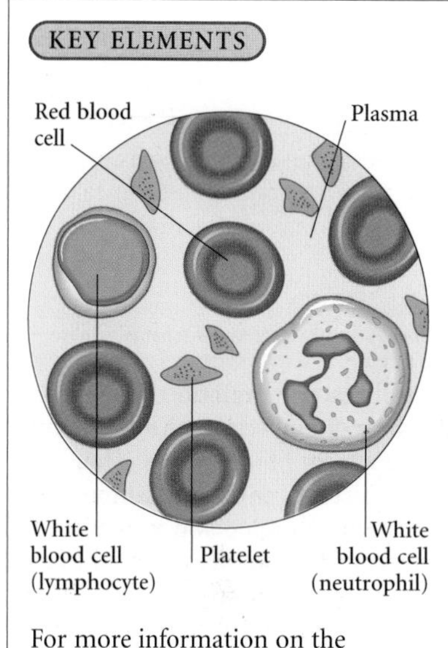

For more information on the structure and function of blood, *see* pp.440–442.

Drugs that promote blood clotting

Drugs used to treat disorders in which blood fails to clot normally

COMMON DRUGS

BLOOD PRODUCTS
• Factor VIII • Factor IX • Fresh frozen plasma

VITAMIN K
• Phytomenadione

ANTIFIBRINOLYTIC DRUGS
• Aprotinin • Etamsylate • Tranexamic acid

Several types of disorder cause spontaneous internal bleeding or excessive bleeding after even minor injuries (*see* BLEEDING DISORDERS, p.451). These disorders are usually treated with drugs that promote blood clotting or slow the breakdown of existing clots.

WHAT ARE THE TYPES?

The three main types of drug that are used to promote the formation of blood clots and to prevent or reduce abnormal bleeding are blood products, vitamin K, and antifibrinolytic drugs.

BLOOD PRODUCTS Normal blood clotting depends on the presence in the blood of certain proteins called clotting factors. People who lack one of these clotting factors (often due to an inherited disorder) may be given specific blood products, which are concentrated supplements of the missing protein. For example, a blood product called Factor VIII is needed for the treatment of the inherited bleeding disorder haemophilia (*see* HAEMOPHILIA AND CHRISTMAS DISEASE, p.452), in which a defective gene causes a deficiency of natural Factor VIII in the blood. Another blood product, fresh frozen plasma, is given to counteract abnormally prolonged or severe bleeding due to causes such as an excessive dose of anticoagulants (*see* DRUGS THAT PREVENT BLOOD CLOTTING, p.904).

All blood products are administered intravenously, either in hospital or at home, and may be used regularly as a preventive treatment or given when abnormal bleeding occurs.

Some people experience side effects, including chills and fever, when being given blood products. These side effects may result from an allergic reaction.

VITAMIN K This vitamin is essential for the production of several vital blood-clotting factors. Newborn babies (who are born with no stores of vitamin K) and people who are deficient in vitamin K may need a supplement, which is either given by injection or taken orally. Vitamin K is also used to reverse the effect of an excessive dose of oral anticoagulants. No side effects are known to be associated with its use.

ANTIFIBRINOLYTIC DRUGS These drugs may be used when bleeding is difficult to control, as may occur after surgery, or to reduce menstrual bleeding that is excessively heavy (*see* MENORRHAGIA, p.735). Antifibrinolytic drugs affect the clotting process of blood by slowing the breakdown of existing clots. The drugs may be injected or given by infusion into a vein if bleeding must be stopped urgently or may be taken orally for the treatment of menorrhagia. Side effects such as headaches, diarrhoea, nausea, and vomiting are sometimes experienced by people who are taking these drugs. Occasionally, the drug aprotinin causes an allergic reaction.

Drugs that prevent blood clotting

Drugs used to prevent unwanted blood clots developing or to stabilize existing blood clots

COMMON DRUGS

ANTIPLATELET DRUGS
• Aspirin • Dipyridamole • Ticlopidine

ORAL ANTICOAGULANTS
• Warfarin

INJECTED ANTICOAGULANTS
• Certoparin • Dalteparin • Danaparoid
• Enoxaparin • Heparin • Tinzaparin

Drugs may be prescribed to prevent unwanted blood clots (thrombi) from developing in blood vessels. They may also be used to prevent existing blood clots from enlarging and to reduce the risk of an embolism, in which a piece of an existing clot in a vein breaks off and travels to a vital organ. Thrombolytic drugs (right) are used when a blood clot needs to be dissolved rapidly.

WHAT ARE THE TYPES?

Antiplatelet drugs and anticoagulants are used to prevent blood clots from forming. In general, antiplatelet drugs are used to prevent clots from forming in arteries and anticoagulants are prescribed to prevent clots from forming or enlarging in veins or within the heart.

ANTIPLATELET DRUGS These drugs are used to help prevent blood clots from forming in the arteries. The drugs work by reducing the tendency of platelets, a type of blood cell that plays a vital role in the clotting process, to stick together. If you have symptoms of coronary artery disease, such as angina (p.407), or have had a heart attack (*see* MYOCARDIAL INFARCTION, p.410), a stroke (p.532), or a transient ischaemic attack (p.531), you may need to take an antiplatelet drug for the rest of your life.

Aspirin is the most commonly prescribed antiplatelet drug. However, you should not take aspirin if you are pregnant or breast-feeding.

ORAL ANTICOAGULANTS These drugs are given as a long-term treatment to prevent deep vein thrombosis (p.437), in which a blood clot forms in a vein, and pulmonary embolism (p.495), in which a piece of a clot breaks off and travels to the lungs, where it lodges. Oral anticoagulants may also be given to people with the heart rhythm disorder atrial fibrillation (p.417), in which a blood clot may form in the heart. If the clot fragments, a piece may reach the brain and cause a stroke. Warfarin is the most frequently used oral anticoagulant.

> **WARNING**
>
> Contact your doctor immediately if you are taking an oral anticoagulant and you have nosebleeds or you notice blood in your urine.

Oral anticoagulants act by preventing the formation of clotting factors, the proteins that are essential for normal blood clotting. The drugs usually take 48–72 hours to become effective.

While you are taking oral anticoagulants, you will need frequent blood tests for the first few days and then regular tests throughout your treatment so that the dose can be adjusted to your particular needs. If the dose is too high, these drugs can sometimes cause abnormal bleeding. For this reason, you should consult your doctor immediately if you develop symptoms such as nosebleeds or blood in your urine. To treat abnormal bleeding, your doctor may prescribe drugs that reverse the effect of the anticoagulants (*see* DRUGS THAT PROMOTE BLOOD CLOTTING, p.903).

Oral anticoagulants may cause other side effects, including rashes, diarrhoea, easy bruising, hair loss, and impaired liver function. You should avoid drinking alcohol and making any sudden changes to your diet, both of which may affect the action of anticoagulants. Since many drugs interact with anticoagulants, you should not take other medications, particularly aspirin, without first consulting your doctor. It is very important that you inform your doctor if you plan to become pregnant because certain anticoagulants can cause abnormalities in a developing fetus. You should not discontinue anticoagulant drug treatment suddenly. You will be given an anticoagulant treatment card or a medical alert bracelet or pendant, which you should always carry with you to inform health professionals in case of an emergency.

INJECTED ANTICOAGULANTS If blood clotting must be controlled quickly, an anticoagulant, such as heparin, may be given by injection or infusion so that it can take effect immediately. These fast-acting injected anticoagulants are used to treat disorders such as pulmonary embolism before oral anticoagulants take effect. Injected anticoagulants are given as a preventive measure before orthopaedic surgery, and they may also be given before surgery to people who are at particular risk of blood clotting because of problems such as excessive weight. The drugs are often prescribed for people who are immobilized during treatment in hospital.

Some newly developed, longer-acting drugs, such as tinzaparin, which need be given only once a day, can be self-administered at home for the treatment of deep vein thrombosis. Injected anticoagulants may cause side effects, such as skin rashes, in some people.

Thrombolytic drugs

A group of drugs, also known as fibrinolytics, used to dissolve blood clots

COMMON DRUGS

• Alteplase • Anistreplase • Reteplase
• Streptokinase • Urokinase

Thrombolytic drugs act rapidly to dissolve unwanted blood clots (thrombi) that have formed in blood vessels in the body. These drugs are most commonly given as an emergency treatment for heart attacks (*see* MYOCARDIAL INFARCTION, p.410) or for certain types of stroke (p.532) and can significantly increase a person's chance of survival.

A heart attack is usually caused by a blood clot blocking one of the coronary arteries, which supply blood to the heart muscle. Left untreated, such a clot can cause irreversible damage to the heart, which can be fatal. Strokes are usually caused by a blood clot blocking the supply of blood to an area of the brain.

Thrombolytics may be used to dissolve a blood clot in a vein deep within the body, often in the legs (*see* DEEP VEIN THROMBOSIS, p.437). These fast-acting drugs may also be used to treat pulmonary embolism (p.495), in which a blood clot breaks off from a distant vein and lodges in the lungs.

Thrombolytic drugs work by dissolving the mesh of fibrin, a stringy protein that binds a blood clot together (*see* HOW THROMBOLYTIC DRUGS WORK, below). When the blood clot has been dissolved by the drugs, normal blood flow to the affected area is restored.

HOW ARE THEY USED?

Thrombolytics are given by injection or by infusion. In the treatment of a heart attack, the drugs must be given within 6 hours of the start of the attack to be effective. In the case of a stroke, the drugs must be given within 3 hours of the onset of symptoms.

DRUG ACTION

HOW THROMBOLYTIC DRUGS WORK

Thrombolytic drugs are used to dissolve unwanted blood clots, known as thrombi. A blood clot consists of blood cells and platelets that are held together by a mesh of fibrin strands. Thrombolytics dissolve the fibrin strands, thereby breaking up the blood clot.

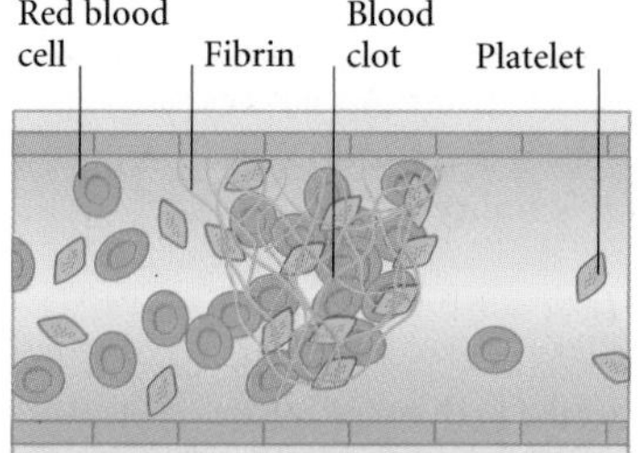

Before drug
A clot, made up of red and white blood cells and platelets bound together by strands of fibrin, has formed in a blood vessel, restricting blood flow.

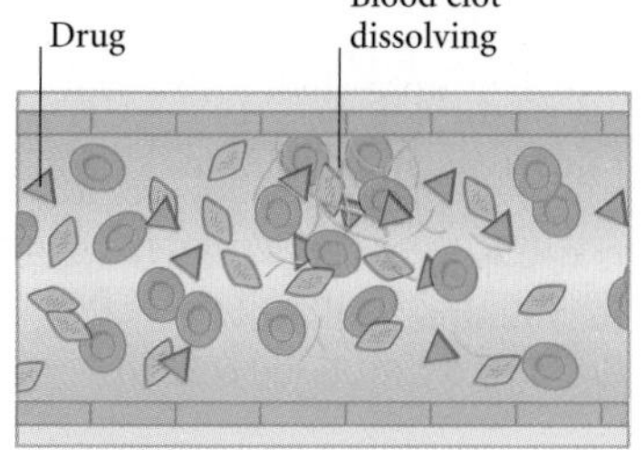

After drug
The thrombolytic drug dissolves the fibrin strands that bind the blood clot together. The clot is broken down and normal blood flow resumes.

Thrombolytics may cause side effects such as nausea and vomiting, as well as increased susceptibility to bruising and bleeding. Anistreplase and streptokinase, two of the most frequently used thrombolytics, can cause allergic reactions, often in the form of a rash. Occasionally, a life-threatening allergic reaction called anaphylaxis (p.469) occurs.

Antiallergy drugs

Drugs used to prevent and treat allergic conditions and allergic reactions

COMMON DRUGS

ANTIHISTAMINES (p.906)

MAST CELL STABILIZERS
• Nedocromil sodium • Sodium cromoglicate

CORTICOSTEROIDS (p.930)

LEUKOTRIENE ANTAGONISTS
• Montelukast • Zafirlukast

ALLERGEN EXTRACTS

OTHER ANTIALLERGY DRUGS
• Epinephrine (adrenaline)

Antiallergy drugs are used in the treatment of a variety of allergic disorders, such as allergic conjunctivitis (p.570), hay fever (*see* ALLERGIC RHINITIS, p.466), and atopic eczema (p.334). Antiallergy drugs can be used to prevent an allergic response from occurring or to relieve the symptoms of allergy, such as sneezing.

WHAT ARE THE TYPES?

Several groups of drugs are used to treat allergic reactions. The most commonly used are antihistamines (p.906), mast cell stabilizers, corticosteroids (p.930), leukotriene antagonists, allergen extracts, and the drug epinephrine (adrenaline).

ANTIHISTAMINES These drugs are most commonly used to relieve the symptoms of hay fever. Antihistamines are also used to treat allergic rashes such as urticaria (p.468) and are effective in relieving itching due to insect bites. The drugs work by blocking the action of histamine, a chemical that is released by the body in an allergic reaction.

MAST CELL STABILIZERS These may be prescribed to prevent allergic reactions. The drugs block the release of histamine, a chemical that is stored in mast cells (a type of white blood cell), which are present in blood and most body tissues. Histamine is released from these cells in allergic reactions. The most commonly used mast cell stabilizer is sodium cromoglicate, which is given for allergic conjunctivitis, hay fever, asthma in children (p.839), and exercise-induced asthma (p.483) in adults. Since these drugs cannot be absorbed when taken orally, they are used topically in the form of eyedrops, nasal sprays, or inhalers. Mast cell stabilizers are taken regularly as preventive treatment; they do not relieve symptoms.

CORTICOSTEROIDS These drugs reduce inflammation caused by allergic reactions. They may be included in skin creams used to treat atopic eczema (*see* TOPICAL CORTICOSTEROIDS, p.892) and in nasal sprays to relieve the symptoms of hay fever (*see* CORTICOSTEROIDS FOR RESPIRATORY DISEASE, p.911). For severe or persistent allergies, corticosteroids may be given orally or intravenously.

LEUKOTRIENE ANTAGONISTS When used with corticosteroids, these drugs help to prevent asthma attacks. They block the action of leukotrienes, chemicals that cause airway inflammation in asthma.

ALLERGEN EXTRACTS Substances that can cause allergic reactions, such as bee venom or grass pollen, are called allergens. Tiny amounts of an allergen may be used to desensitize a person who has a severe allergy to that substance. The treatment is usually given as a series of weekly injections containing gradually increasing doses. Treatment may last for several months. Allergen extracts can themselves cause life-threatening allergic reactions and are given only where emergency treatment is available.

EPINEPHRINE (ADRENALINE) This drug is used to treat anaphylaxis (p.469), a life-threatening allergic reaction. The drug reverses the swelling of the throat, narrowing of the airways, and drop in blood pressure that occurs in anaphylaxis. Epinephrine is injected in repeated doses until the condition improves. If you are at risk of anaphylaxis because of a severe allergy, you should carry a syringe prefilled with epinephrine for emergency treatment (*see* EMERGENCY AID FOR ANAPHYLAXIS, p.469).

DRUG ACTION HOW ANTIHISTAMINES WORK

Antihistamine drugs are used to prevent or relieve the symptoms of allergic reactions, such as a rash. Allergens, such as grass pollen, can trigger the release of the chemical histamine from body cells. This chemical acts on small blood vessels, glands, and other tissues, causing the symptoms of allergy. The drugs work by blocking the action of histamine.

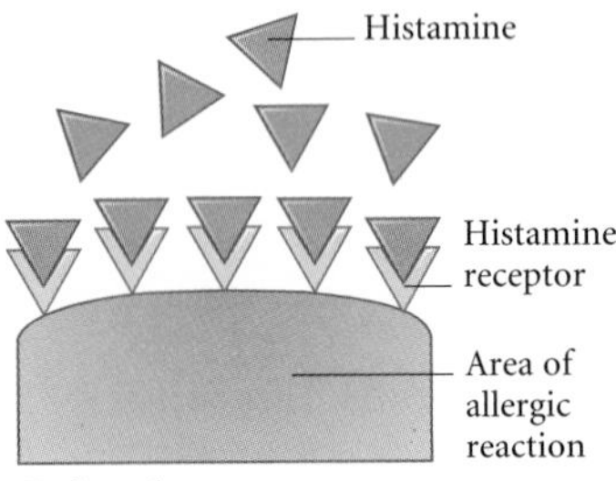

Before drug
Histamine is released in response to an allergen and attaches to sites on tissue cells known as histamine receptors. This causes an allergic reaction in the tissue.

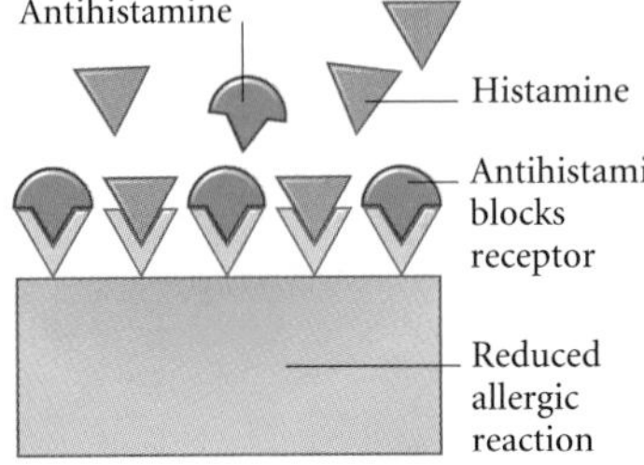

After drug
The antihistamine drug occupies some of the histamine receptors, thereby preventing histamine from attaching to them. This reduces the severity of allergic symptoms.

Antihistamines

Drugs that block the effects of histamine, a chemical released during allergic reactions

COMMON DRUGS

SEDATING ANTIHISTAMINES
- Alimemazine (trimeprazine)
- Azatadine • Brompheniramine
- Chlorphenamine (chlorpheniramine)
- Clemastine • Cyproheptadine
- Diphenhydramine • Promethazine

NONSEDATING ANTIHISTAMINES
- Acrivastine • Cetirizine • Loratadine
- Terfenadine

Antihistamines are used mainly to prevent or relieve symptoms of allergies, such as hay fever (*see* ALLERGIC RHINITIS, p.466), and to treat allergic rashes, such as urticaria (p.468). These drugs are also effective in relieving itching and irritation due to insect bites or stings. Antihistamines are sometimes included in cold and flu remedies (p.910) because they dry up mucus. Since some types of antihistamine also depress the vomiting reflex in the brain, these drugs may also be taken to relieve nausea, vomiting, vertigo, and motion sickness (*see* ANTIEMETIC DRUGS, p.922). Certain antihistamines have a sedative effect and are recommended if you have regular night-time itching.

Antihistamines are normally taken orally, but some types are available for topical use as nasal sprays, eyedrops, or skin lotions. Antihistamines may also be given by injection as emergency treatment for the life-threatening allergic reaction anaphylaxis (p.469).

HOW DO THEY WORK?

Antihistamines prevent or relieve the symptoms of an allergic reaction by blocking the action of histamine, a chemical that is released from certain cells in the blood and body tissues when they are exposed to an allergen (*see* HOW ANTIHISTAMINES WORK, above). The effects of histamine include widening of the small blood vessels in the affected area, often the skin, nose, and eyes, leading to redness and swelling and increased production of mucus. By blocking the action of histamine, antihistamine drugs can reduce some of the symptoms of allergies, such as swelling, rash, itching, runny nose, and sneezing.

WHAT ARE THE SIDE EFFECTS?

Many antihistamines make you drowsy and cause problems with coordination. If you are affected, you should not drive or operate machinery. However, in some children, the drugs cause hyperactive behaviour. All types of antihistamine can cause difficulty in passing urine, and the drugs should not be taken by men who have prostate problems. You should not drink alcohol while you are taking antihistamines because this will increase the sedative effect of the drugs.

Immunosuppressants

Drugs used to reduce the activity of the body's immune system

COMMON DRUGS

CORTICOSTEROIDS
- Prednisolone

CYTOTOXIC IMMUNOSUPPRESSANTS
- Azathioprine • Cyclophosphamide
- Methotrexate

OTHER IMMUNOSUPPRESSANTS
- Ciclosporin • Tacrolimus

Immunosuppressants reduce the level of activity of the body's immune system. The immune system works to protect the body against infection and helps to destroy diseased cells. However, in certain conditions, known as autoimmune disorders (p.461), the immune system acts against the body's healthy tissues, and immunosuppressant drugs may be required to protect them from permanent damage. Immunosuppressants are also given just before transplant surgery (p.952) and afterwards for life to prevent the immune system from attacking and rejecting the new organ. The drugs are also used to treat some cancers.

People who are taking immunosuppressant drugs are at increased risk of infection because the drugs reduce the body's ability to fight disease.

WHAT ARE THE TYPES?

The main types of drug used to suppress the activity of the immune system are corticosteroids (p.930) and cytotoxic immunosuppressants. Other immunosuppressants that are commonly used include ciclosporin and tacrolimus.

CORTICOSTEROIDS You may be given oral corticosteroid drugs if you have an autoimmune disorder such as systemic lupus erythematosus (p.461). Corticosteroids weaken the immune system by affecting the activity of white blood cells, which are an essential component of the immune response.

Prolonged use of oral corticosteroids may cause acne, the development of a moon-shaped face, and weight gain. The drugs also increase the risk of developing osteoporosis (p.368), high blood pressure (*see* HYPERTENSION, p.403), and diabetes mellitus (p.687), and may make some otherwise minor infections, such

WARNING

When taking immunosuppressant drugs, it is important that you report any signs of infection, such as a sore throat or fever, or any unusual bruising or bleeding to your doctor immediately.

as chickenpox (p.290), life-threatening. You should not stop taking corticosteroids suddenly. Your pharmacist or doctor will issue a card giving details of your treatment, which you should carry at all times to inform health professionals in case of a medical emergency.

CYTOTOXIC IMMUNOSUPPRESSANTS If corticosteroids are ineffective, autoimmune disorders, such as rheumatoid arthritis, may be treated with cytotoxic immunosuppressants. This type of drug may also be used with corticosteroids so that the corticosteroid dose can be reduced. Some cytotoxic immunosuppressants are used to treat cancers, such as leukaemia (p.453), and to prevent the rejection of tissue grafts or organ transplants. The drugs suppress the immune system by stopping the growth of new white blood cells in the bone marrow.

Cytotoxic immunosuppressant drugs can cause side effects including nausea, vomiting, diarrhoea, hair loss, and sterility. They may also cause easy bruising and abnormal bleeding, such as nosebleeds. You will need regular blood tests to monitor the drug's effects.

OTHER IMMUNOSUPPRESSANTS Ciclosporin and tacrolimus are drugs that may be given to prevent the rejection of a transplanted organ. Ciclosporin may also be used to treat autoimmune disorders, such as rheumatoid arthritis, when other drugs are ineffective. The drugs work in similar ways by blocking the action of white blood cells that are involved in the immune response.

Ciclosporin and tacrolimus are often given as intravenous infusions before a transplant operation and are taken orally afterwards. These drugs may cause side effects such as tiredness, gastrointestinal upsets, and excessive hair growth. They can also cause high blood pressure and kidney damage, and regular blood tests are needed to check kidney function.

Interferon drugs

A group of drugs that limit viral infection or destroy cancerous cells

COMMON DRUGS

• Interferon alfa • Interferon beta

Interferons are a group of proteins produced naturally in the body in response to viral infections. Synthetic versions that mimic the action of these natural interferons are used as drugs to treat a number of disorders. There are two types of synthetic interferon: interferon alfa and interferon beta. They each have a slightly different chemical structure and different medical uses.

Interferon alfa is used to treat people who have the persistent viral infections hepatitis B or C (*see* ANTIVIRAL DRUGS, p.886). It is also used in the treatment of certain types of cancer (*see* ANTICANCER DRUGS, right). Interferon beta reduces the frequency and severity of relapses in some people with multiple sclerosis (p.541), although it has not been shown to affect the eventual degree of disability caused by the disorder.

How do they work?

Interferons bind to body cells, thereby activating the immune response. Their main effect is to increase the activity of white blood cells, which are important components of the body's immune system. Interferons are also able to slow down the multiplication of cancerous cells and to reduce or prevent the replication of certain viruses, such as the hepatitis virus, inside infected cells.

Interferons are given only by injection, and in most cases the drugs can be self-administered. Your doctor or nurse will teach you how to inject yourself.

What are the side effects?

The most common side effect of interferon drugs is a flu-like syndrome, in which you may have a fever, muscular aches, and a headache. Other possible side effects are nausea, tiredness, and depression. Redness and swelling at the site of injection is common. Interferons may also cause liver and kidney problems. If you are taking an interferon drug, your doctor will arrange for regular blood and urine tests to monitor changes in body functions.

Anticancer drugs

A group of drugs used to destroy or slow the growth of cancerous cells

COMMON DRUGS

CYTOTOXIC DRUGS
• Bleomycin • Busulfan • Carboplatin
• Chlorambucil • Cisplatin • Cyclophosphamide
• Cytarabine • Dacarbazine • Doxorubicin
• Etoposide • Fluorouracil
• Hydroxycarbamide (hydroxyurea)
• Irinotecan • Melphalan • Mercaptopurine
• Methotrexate • Paclitaxel • Procarbazine
• Temozolomide • Tioguanine • Vincristine

HORMONES AND HORMONE ANTAGONISTS
• Aminoglutethimide • Diethylstilbestrol
• Flutamide • Goserelin • Leuprorelin
• Medroxyprogesterone • Megestrol • Octreotide
• Tamoxifen

OTHER DRUGS
• Aldesleukin • Interferon alfa • Rituximab

Cancers are a broad group of diseases in which abnormal body cells form and multiply, interfering with the function of surrounding tissues. Cancerous cells may affect vital organs and can spread to other parts of the body through the bloodstream. Anticancer drugs either destroy the cancer cells or prevent them from spreading. Treatment with these drugs, which is known as chemotherapy (p.280), is normally managed by an oncologist, a doctor who is a specialist in the medical treatment of cancer.

Anticancer drugs may be given with the aim of curing the cancer, prolonging life, or relieving symptoms. In some cases, chemotherapy is used in combination with surgery and/or radiotherapy (p.281). Anticancer drugs may be used to shrink the tumour before the other treatments, or they may be used after surgery or radiotherapy to prevent the growth of cancer cells that may have spread around the body.

What are the types?

The group of drugs most commonly used to treat cancer are cytotoxic drugs, which damage or destroy both cancerous and healthy body cells. Some hormonal drugs, such as the synthetic female sex hormones medroxyprogesterone and megestrol, are also used to treat certain forms of cancer, as are hormone antagonist drugs, which work by blocking the effects of hormones that stimulate cancer growth. Drugs that mimic parts of the immune system are also used.

How chemotherapy treatment works
Anticancer drugs (chemotherapy) may be given in a series of treatments. The drugs kill cancer cells, but they also destroy some normal cells. For this reason, there are recovery periods between treatments during which the number of normal cells is allowed to rise again. Treatment is stopped when no cancer cells are detectable.

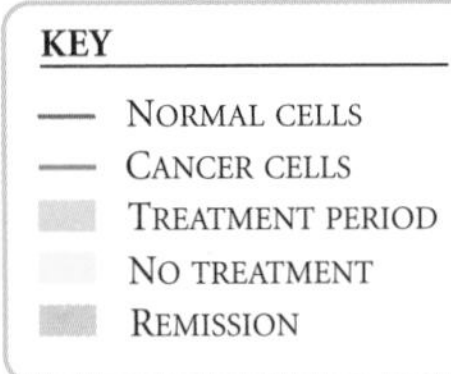

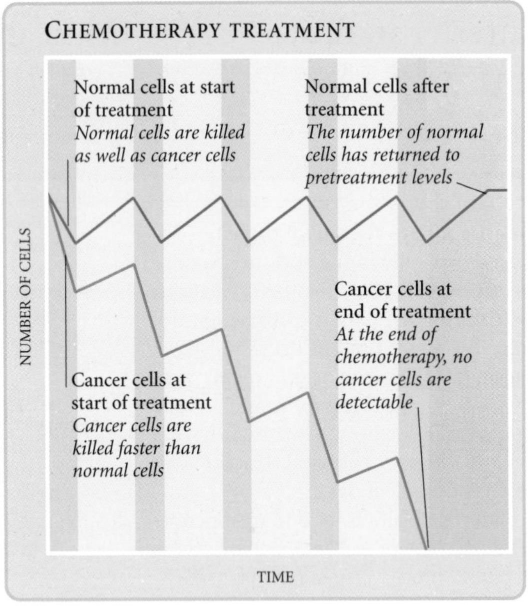

CYTOTOXIC DRUGS There are several types of cytotoxic drug, which kill cells or prevent cancer cells from increasing in number. The drugs either act directly on the cells' genetic material, DNA, or prevent the cells from using the nutrients they need to divide normally. The effect of the drugs is concentrated on areas of tissue where cells are rapidly dividing, and they are therefore effective in treating rapidly growing cancers, such as those of the lymphatic system (*see* LYMPHOMA, p.459), various forms of leukaemia (p.453), many childhood cancers, and some types of cancer of the testis (p.719). The drug methotrexate may also be used to treat severe psoriasis (p.332). Cytotoxic drugs are usually administered in hospital. Several short courses of the drugs are given over a number of weeks, with drug-free periods in between to allow time for the normal body cells to recover.

Cytotoxic drugs tend to cause severe side effects because they affect any area of the body where there is rapid cell division, including the bone marrow, the hair follicles, and the lining of the mouth and the intestines. Damage to the bone marrow may reduce the numbers of red and white blood cells and platelets in the blood. Some anticancer drugs may also cause folic acid deficiency. These problems can lead to anaemia (p.446), an increased susceptibility to infection, and reduced ability of the blood to clot. Nausea and vomiting are particularly common side effects of cytotoxic drugs and may be severe. Certain drugs may cause mouth ulcers and hair loss.

The severity of many side effects can be reduced by additional treatment with other drugs. For example, antiemetic drugs (p.922) may be given for nausea and vomiting. Most side effects are temporary and do not result in long-term damage. However, some types of cytotoxic drug can cause irreversible damage to the ovaries, which leads to premature menopause, or to the testes, resulting in abnormal or reduced sperm production. Men who wish to have children in the future can arrange to have their sperm frozen and stored before treatment. For women, the harvesting of ovarian tissue or eggs for future use is a possibility.

If you are taking cytotoxic drugs, you will have regular blood tests, including a blood count, before each course of treatment to measure the levels of different types of blood cell. You should see your doctor immediately if you develop new symptoms, such as a sore throat, because these symptoms may be a sign of a very low number of white blood cells.

WARNING

Many anticancer drugs are potentially harmful to a developing fetus. You should consult your doctor about your contraception needs before starting treatment.

HORMONES AND HORMONE ANTAGONISTS Treatment with hormones may be suitable for certain types of cancer whose growth is influenced by hormones. This type of treatment may be used following surgery or radiotherapy to prevent any remaining cancer cells from growing and spreading. The treatment may involve the use a hormone that halts the progression of the cancer. For example, megestrol is used to slow the progression of cancer of the uterus (p.748).

Alternatively, a hormone antagonist drug may be used. Drugs of this type oppose the effects of the hormone that stimulates the growth of the cancer. For example, hormone antagonists such as tamoxifen are often effective in halting the progression of certain types of breast cancer (p.759) that are stimulated by the female sex hormone oestrogen. The drug blocks the action of oestrogen on breast cells. The growth of cancerous cells that have spread from a cancer in the prostate gland may be slowed by using the drug goserelin, which blocks the secretion of the male sex hormone testosterone.

Hormonal drugs are usually taken orally, and sometimes treatment is continued for several years. Most of these drugs have milder side effects than cytotoxic drugs. However, treatment with tamoxifen slightly increases the risk of developing cancer of the uterus; you should report abnormal vaginal bleeding to your doctor immediately.

OTHER ANTICANCER DRUGS This group of anticancer drugs includes interferon alfa (*see* INTERFERON DRUGS, p.907) and aldesleukin, which is commonly used to treat the AIDS-related skin cancer Kaposi's sarcoma (p.346). Aldesleukin is also used in the treatment of some types of lymphoma and leukaemia, and for advanced kidney cancer (p.704). The drug may kill the cancer cells or stimulate an immune response against them. Rituximab is a monoclonal antibody that can be used as an anticancer drug or as an immunosuppressant (p.906).

Common side effects of interferon drugs include nausea and flu-like symptoms. Aldesleukin may cause shortness of breath and dizziness and can sometimes affect the function of organs such as the liver and kidneys. Rituximab can produce chills and fever, vomiting, and allergic reactions such as rashes.

DRUGS FOR RESPIRATORY DISORDERS

Conditions affecting the airways and lungs range from minor illnesses, such as the common cold, to serious long-term disorders, such as asthma. The discomfort of coughs and colds may be eased with over-the-counter remedies. However, the symptoms of long-term disorders, such as shortness of breath, can be severe and require specific medical treatment.

This section describes some of the drugs used to treat both common illnesses, such as coughs and colds, and more serious conditions that affect the airways and lungs.

The first three articles in this section discuss drugs used to treat common symptoms of upper respiratory tract infections, such as nasal congestion, cough, and fever. The next article discusses bronchodilator drugs, which widen the airways of the lungs and are used to treat respiratory conditions in which breathing becomes difficult, such as asthma (p.483) and chronic obstructive pulmonary disease (p.487). The final article in this section covers the use of corticosteroids in the treatment of respiratory conditions, including their use in preventing attacks of asthma. Drugs used for hay fever and other allergic disorders that affect the respiratory system are described elsewhere (*see* ANTIALLERGY DRUGS, p.905), as are antibiotics used in the treatment of respiratory infections (*see* DRUGS FOR INFECTIONS AND INFESTATIONS, pp.883–889).

KEY ANATOMY

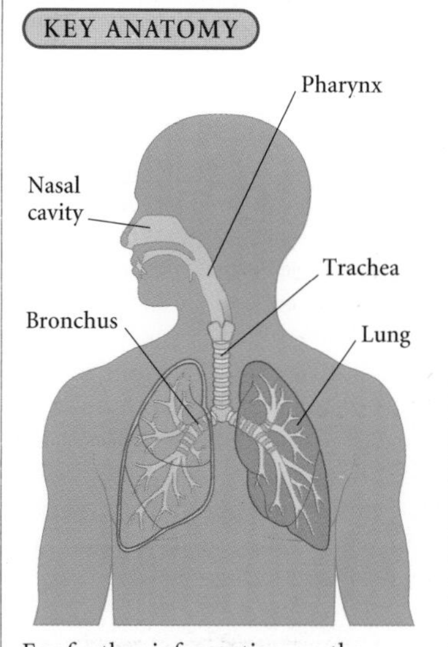

For further information on the structure and function of the respiratory system, *see* pp.470–473.

Decongestants

Drugs that are used to reduce swelling of the membranes lining the nose and sinuses

COMMON DRUGS

- Ephedrine • Oxymetazoline • Phenylephrine
- Phenylpropanolamine • Pseudoephedrine
- Xylometazoline

Decongestants act to relieve congestion in the nose and sinuses. A blocked nose or sinuses (*see* SINUSITIS, p.475) may be caused by a viral infection, such as the common cold (p.288), or by an allergic condition, such as hay fever (*see* ALLERGIC RHINITIS, p.466).

Infections and allergic reactions can cause inflammation of the delicate lining of the nose or sinuses. The blood vessels in the lining enlarge, and increased volumes of fluid pass into the mucous membranes, which swell and produce excessive amounts of mucus. Decongestants act directly on the blood vessels to constrict them and reduce the swelling and mucus secretion.

Decongestants are available as sprays or drops that are used in the nose or as oral pills or capsules. Some cold and flu remedies (p.910) that are available over the counter also contain a small amount of decongestant. You can spray or insert decongestant drops directly into your nose to provide rapid relief. When taken orally, decongestants work more slowly, but the effects last longer.

Decongestant sprays or drops should be used in moderation and for no longer than a week. After that time, they lose their capacity to constrict blood vessels. When the last effective dose wears off, the blood vessels widen again, and congestion may become worse.

Used sparingly, decongestant sprays or drops have few side effects. If you have heart disease, high blood pressure, or take antidepressant drugs (p.916), you should check with your doctor or pharmacist before taking oral decongestants because they sometimes cause a rapid, irregular heartbeat and raise blood pressure. Decongestants may also cause slight tremor in the hands.

CAUTION

Avoid using decongestants for longer than a week because the drugs may become ineffective or worsen your condition.

Cough remedies

Preparations containing various drugs used to treat coughing

COMMON DRUGS

- Codeine • Dextromethorphan • Guaifenesin
- Pholcodine

Coughing is a natural reflex action that helps to clear the lungs of sputum produced by infections. The effectiveness of cough medicines is doubtful, which is why doctors rarely prescribe them for minor respiratory disorders. However, there are many cough remedies that are available over the counter. Almost all of these remedies are syrups to which a variety of drugs and flavourings have been added. Most of these preparations are of little medicinal value, although some may have soothing properties.

The main groups of drugs used to treat coughs are expectorants, mucolytics, and suppressants. Expectorants are supposed to encourage productive coughs (which produce sputum), but their benefit is not proven.

Mucolytic preparations make sputum less sticky and easier to cough up, but they are of little benefit to most people.

However, mucolytic drugs are used in the treatment of cystic fibrosis (p.824), an inherited condition in which large amounts of abnormally thick, sticky sputum are produced.

Cough suppressant remedies, which often contain drugs such as codeine or pholcodine, are usually effective in relieving a troublesome cough. These drugs can cause drowsiness, which may be helpful if a cough interrupts sleep at night. However, if you feel drowsy after taking the drugs, you should not drive or operate machinery. Cough suppressants should be taken according to your doctor's or the manufacturer's instructions. The use of suppressants is not advised for a cough that is producing large amounts of sputum because preventing the expulsion of sputum can delay recovery from an infection.

Cold and flu remedies

Preparations containing drugs that ease the symptoms of colds and flu

COMMON DRUGS

PAINKILLERS
• Aspirin • Ibuprofen • Paracetamol

DECONGESTANTS
• Ephedrine • Oxymetazoline • Phenylephrine
• Phenylpropanolamine • Pseudoephedrine
• Xylometazoline

There are no cures for the common cold (p.288) or influenza (p.289), but there are various remedies that may suppress the symptoms and ease discomfort. Most of these remedies are combinations of drugs, which may include a painkiller (p.912), such as paracetamol or ibuprofen, to lower fever and relieve muscle aches, sore throat, and headache; decongestants (p.909) to relieve congestion; caffeine, which acts as a mild stimulant; and vitamin C. Generally, doctors advise taking single drugs to treat individual symptoms rather than medicines that contain several different types of drug, some of which are not necessary. Antiviral drugs (p.886) may occasionally be used to treat influenza.

HOW ARE THEY USED?

Dosages for cold and flu remedies tend to vary. It is important to follow the instructions given with the product and not to exceed the recommended daily dose of paracetamol because high doses can cause liver damage. Children under the age of 12 should not be given aspirin because this drug is linked with Reye's syndrome (p.849). You should avoid taking cold and flu remedies containing aspirin or ibuprofen if you have asthma (p.483), a peptic ulcer (p.640), indigestion (p.626), or gout (p.380).

> WARNING
>
> Do not give aspirin to children under 12 years because it increases the risk of Reye's syndrome, a rare brain and liver disorder.

Bronchodilator drugs

Drugs that widen the airways of the lungs to ease breathing difficulties

COMMON DRUGS

SYMPATHOMIMETICS
• Bambuterol • Formoterol • Salbutamol
• Salmeterol • Terbutaline

ANTICHOLINERGICS
• Atropine • Ipratropium bromide

XANTHINES
• Aminophylline • Theophylline

Bronchodilator drugs are used to dilate (widen) the bronchi (airways) inside the lungs (*see* HOW BRONCHODILATOR DRUGS WORK, right). Widening the airways prevents or relieves the wheezing, tightness of the chest, and shortness of breath that can result from conditions such as asthma (p.483) and chronic obstructive pulmonary disease (p.487), a progressive disease of the lungs most often caused by smoking.

Many bronchodilator drugs are inhaled through a metered-dose inhaler, a small aerosol pump that delivers a controlled amount of the drug to be inhaled into the lungs. Spacers, which are plastic chambers into which a dose of the drug is released before it is inhaled, and breath-activated inhalers are also available. You may prefer to use a spacer if you have difficulty using an inhaler on its own (*see* TAKING INHALED ASTHMA DRUGS, p.485). If you have severe shortness of breath, you may need to take bronchodilator drugs by means of a nebulizer, a device that delivers the drug in aerosol form through a mask or a mouthpiece. Certain bronchodilators are taken orally on a regular basis to prevent asthma attacks occurring.

During any discussion about your bronchodilator treatment, you should let your doctor know if you are pregnant or breast-feeding.

WHAT ARE THE TYPES?

Bronchodilator drugs are divided into three main groups: sympathomimetics, anticholinergics, and xanthines. When inhaled, some sympathomimetics take effect within 10 minutes and are often

DRUG ACTION

HOW BRONCHODILATOR DRUGS WORK

Bronchodilator drugs are often used to prevent or relieve wheezing and shortness of breath caused by disorders such as asthma. In these conditions, the bronchi (airways in the lungs) become abnormally narrowed because muscles in their walls contract. Bronchodilators work by widening the airways and thereby increasing the air flow.

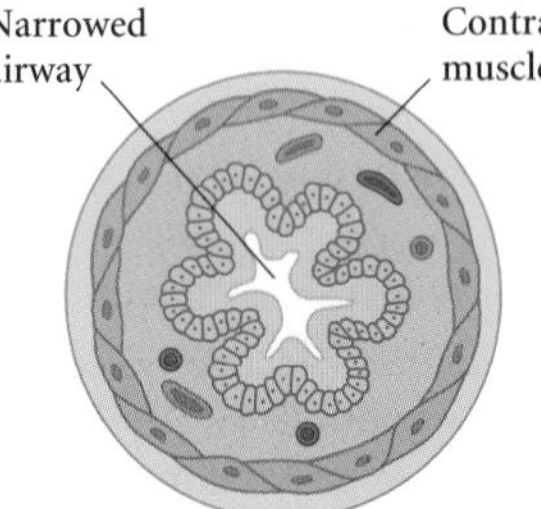

Before drug
The airway narrows as the muscle layer in its walls contracts. The flow of air to the lungs becomes reduced.

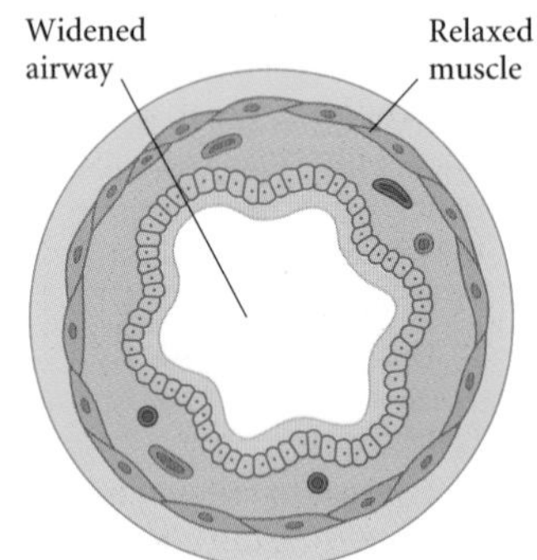

After drug
The drugs act on the muscle cells of the airway. The muscles relax, and the airway widens, increasing air flow.

used for rapid relief from shortness of breath; anticholinergics and xanthines are slower acting. Two or more types of drug may be used simultaneously.

SYMPATHOMIMETICS The drugs in this group are the most commonly used bronchodilators. They work by acting on nerve endings in the muscles in the walls of the airways, causing the muscles to relax and the airways to widen.

Sympathomimetics are usually inhaled and are of two types: short-acting and longer-acting. Short-acting sympathomimetics, such as salbutamol, act within minutes and remain effective for 4–6 hours. Other types, such as salmeterol and formoterol, are slower acting and longer lasting, taking up to 4 hours to act and lasting for about 12 hours.

Usually, inhaled sympathomimetics are used at the first sign of symptoms or to prevent symptoms developing, for instance before physical activity. If you take these drugs, you may experience slight tremor, agitation, insomnia, and, rarely, a rapid heartbeat.

ANTICHOLINERGICS The drugs in this group are often used in combination with sympathomimetics to treat chronic obstructive pulmonary disease. Anticholinergics work in a similar way to sympathomimetics: they stop the constriction of airways. These drugs may cause some side effects, including a dry mouth, difficulty in passing urine, and blurred vision. In rare cases, anticholinergics may trigger an attack of acute glaucoma (p.575), a disorder of the eye that can cause permanent damage to vision and needs immediate treatment.

XANTHINES These bronchodilator drugs have a prolonged action, which makes them useful in preventing night-time asthma attacks. Xanthines act on the muscle cells of the airway walls, causing the airways to widen.

Oral xanthines may be taken daily as a preventive measure. If you have a severe attack of shortness of breath, you may be given aminophylline intravenously through a drip. These drugs sometimes cause nausea and headache and, taken in high doses, occasionally produce a rapid and irregular heartbeat. For this reason, xanthines are used less commonly than other bronchodilators.

Corticosteroids for respiratory disease

A group of anti-inflammatory drugs used to treat several respiratory disorders

COMMON DRUGS

- Beclometasone • Budesonide • Fluticasone
- Hydrocortisone • Prednisolone

Corticosteroids (p.930) are drugs that are related to natural hormones. When used to treat respiratory disorders, these drugs reduce or prevent inflammation of the airways. Corticosteroids are frequently prescribed to prevent attacks of asthma (p.483). They are also occasionally prescribed for people with chronic obstructive pulmonary disease (p.487). In addition, corticosteroids are sometimes helpful in preventing or treating inflammation of the nasal passages in allergic conditions such as hay fever (*see* ALLERGIC RHINITIS, p.466).

Less commonly, corticosteroids are used to treat people with sarcoidosis (p.498) and fibrosing alveolitis (p.497), disorders in which the tissues of the lungs become inflamed.

HOW DO THEY WORK?

The lining of the airways in the lungs becomes inflamed in asthma. This reaction causes the airways to narrow and restricts air flow. Corticosteroids reduce inflammation by blocking the action of certain natural chemicals in the body, called prostaglandins, that are normally responsible for triggering the inflammatory response. Reducing inflammation widens the airways and thereby relieves or prevents asthma attacks. When they are used in treating hay fever, corticosteroid drugs act on the lining of the nose to reduce inflammation. In people with sarcoidosis or fibrosing alveolitis, the reduction in inflammation produced by corticosteroid treatment slows down and minimizes damage to lung tissues.

HOW ARE THEY USED?

Your doctor may prescribe an inhaled corticosteroid if you are experiencing attacks of asthma or if you find that you need to use bronchodilator drugs (opposite page) more than a few times a week. Regular use of inhaled corticosteroid drugs can prevent asthma attacks occurring, and, over time, it may be possible to reduce the dose. If you have a severe asthma attack, you may need to take an oral corticosteroid drug for a few days. Long-term use of low-dose oral corticosteroids is usually necessary only if you have severe asthma that cannot be controlled by inhaled drugs. If you are admitted to hospital with a severe attack, you may be given an intravenous corticosteroid. To treat hay fever, corticosteroids are taken as a nasal spray. People who have fibrosing alveolitis or sarcoidosis will probably be prescribed long-term treatment with oral corticosteroids.

If you have been taking oral corticosteroid drugs for more than a few weeks, it is important not to stop taking them suddenly. If these drugs are taken for a prolonged period of time, they can suppress the body's own production of corticosteroids, which are needed to fight infection. The dose should therefore be reduced gradually in order to allow the body to restore normal levels of corticosteroid production.

If you are prescribed an oral corticosteroid for longer than a few weeks, your doctor or pharmacist will give you a treatment card to carry with you at all times in case of an emergency.

WHAT ARE THE SIDE EFFECTS?

The side effects from inhaled corticosteroids are usually minimal because the drugs act directly on the airways with little effect elsewhere in the body. The most common side effect is oral thrush (*see* CANDIDIASIS, p.309), a fungal infection more commonly associated with other areas of the body. To avoid this infection, rinse your mouth with cold water after using your inhaler.

Your doctor will prescribe the lowest dose for your condition to reduce the risk of side effects. However, if oral corticosteroids are taken on a long-term basis, there is a risk of side effects, including an increased susceptibility to infections, osteoporosis (p.368), cataracts (p.573), bruising, acute glaucoma (p.575), and slowed growth in children.

WARNING

Do not suddenly stop taking oral corticosteroids without first consulting your doctor.

DRUGS ACTING ON THE BRAIN AND NERVOUS SYSTEM

Many of the drugs that act on the brain and nervous system relieve symptoms such as pain, insomnia, and anxiety. Others treat the underlying disorders that are causing the symptoms. As understanding of the chemical changes that cause disorders such as depression improves, treatment is becoming more effective.

The opening article in this section describes groups of drugs known as painkillers. Most of these drugs work by preventing pain signals from being produced or altering the way in which the brain perceives pain. Drugs for migraine are covered next, followed by general anaesthetic drugs, which induce unconsciousness so that no pain can be felt during surgery. Local anaesthetic drugs, which block the transmission of pain signals in a specific body part, are then discussed.

The next articles in this section cover anticonvulsant drugs, sleeping drugs, and antianxiety drugs. Most work by reducing electrical activity in the brain to relieve symptoms but do not treat the underlying disorder.

Antidepressant drugs, which are described next, work by increasing levels of chemicals in the brain that regulate mood. Reduced levels of these chemicals can usually be found in people who are depressed.

In the final articles, antipsychotic drugs, mood-stabilizing drugs, and central nervous system stimulants are described. All of these drugs work by altering chemical activity in the brain.

KEY ANATOMY

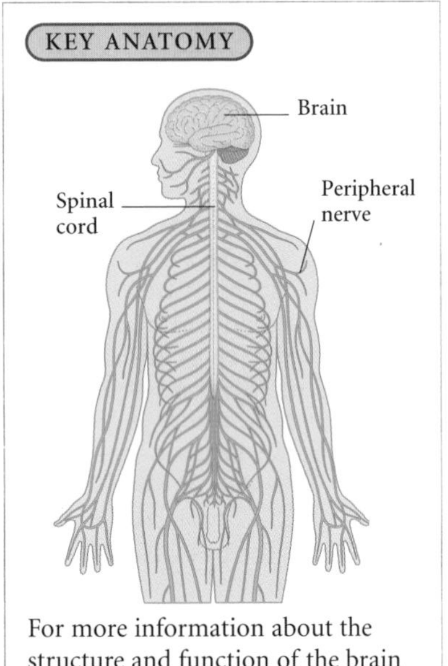

For more information about the structure and function of the brain and nervous system, *see* pp.508–515.

Painkillers

Drugs of varying potency that are used to relieve pain

COMMON DRUGS

OPIOID PAINKILLERS
- Codeine • Fentanyl • Meperidine • Methadone
- Morphine • Pentazocine • Tramadol

NONOPIOID PAINKILLERS
- Aspirin • Diclofenac • Etodolac • Fenoprofen
- Ibuprofen • Indometacin • Ketoprofen
- Ketorolac • Mefenamic acid • Naproxen
- Paracetamol • Piroxicam

COMBINATION PAINKILLERS
- Aspirin with codeine • Dextropropoxyphene with paracetamol • Dihydrocodeine with paracetamol • Paracetamol with codeine

Painkillers work in two different ways, depending on the type of preparation. Some drugs block the nerve pathways that transmit pain signals from a part of the body to the brain. Other painkillers reduce the perception of pain by preventing further transmission of pain signals once they reach the brain. However, pain relief for most long-term disorders depends on treatment of the underlying cause.

WHAT ARE THE TYPES?

The two main types of painkiller are opioid (narcotic) and nonopioid (non-narcotic). A number of commonly used painkillers are combinations of more than one drug. Opioid painkillers are mainly used to relieve severe pain. Nonopioid painkillers, most of which are nonsteroidal anti-inflammatory drugs (p.894), may be used to ease mild to moderate pain. Combinations of two or more painkillers and, in some cases, another drug may provide greater pain relief than a single drug.

OPIOID PAINKILLERS These drugs are the strongest painkillers available. They may be given for pain during a heart attack (*see* MYOCARDIAL INFARCTION, p.410) or following surgery or serious injury. They are also widely used in pain relief for cancer (p.283). Opioids act on the brain, altering the perception of pain. These drugs work in a similar way to natural substances called endorphins, which are released in the brain in response to pain. Opioids bind to the same receptors in the brain as endorphins and stop the transmission of pain signals from cell to cell (*see* HOW OPIOID PAINKILLERS WORK, opposite page).

Prolonged use of opioids may lead to dependence. However, you are very unlikely to become dependent if you take the drugs for a few days to relieve severe pain. Dependence is also not usually a cause for concern in the treatment of pain in a terminally ill person. However, prolonged use leads to tolerance, which means that progressively higher doses are needed to achieve the same level of pain relief.

Opioids may be taken orally or, if the pain is extremely severe or accompanied by vomiting, may be given by injection. Side effects include constipation, nausea, vomiting, and drowsiness. Larger doses can depress breathing and may also cause confusion and impaired consciousness. Overdose may be fatal.

NONOPIOID PAINKILLERS These types of drug are less potent than opioids, and a number are available over the counter. They include paracetamol and nonsteroidal anti-inflammatory drugs (NSAIDs) such as aspirin and ibuprofen. Nonopioids are used mainly for pain

> **WARNING**
>
> Do not give aspirin to children under 12 years because it increases the risk of Reye's syndrome, a rare brain and liver disorder.

such as headache or menstrual pain and also lower fever and reduce inflammation in conditions such as arthritis.

Side effects are rarely a problem if you take nonopioid painkillers occasionally and at the doses recommended for pain relief. However, when used repeatedly, aspirin and other NSAIDs may damage the lining of the stomach and intestines, resulting in peptic ulcers (p.640), and may lead to bleeding in the digestive tract. Taking NSAIDs with food may reduce these side effects, which are less likely to occur with the new group of NSAIDs known as COX2 inhibitors. Some people who have asthma are sensitive to particular NSAIDs, which may make their asthma worse.

Paracetamol relieves pain and lowers fever, but, unlike NSAIDs, it does not reduce inflammation. The drug works by blocking pain impulses in the brain. Paracetamol is dangerous if taken in doses above the recommended maximum daily intake. Overdose can cause severe liver and, rarely, kidney damage.

COMBINATION PAINKILLERS Combination painkillers, which may contain other types of drug, are available as over-the-counter remedies for headaches, backache, menstrual pain, and other minor disorders. However, caffeine, an ingredient included in some remedies, may itself cause headaches.

> **DRUG ACTION**
>
> ### How opioid painkillers work
>
> Opioid drugs are often used to relieve severe pain. Pain signals are transmitted along nerves from the source of pain to the brain. Opioids block the transmission of pain signals in the brain, and thus reduce the sensation of pain.

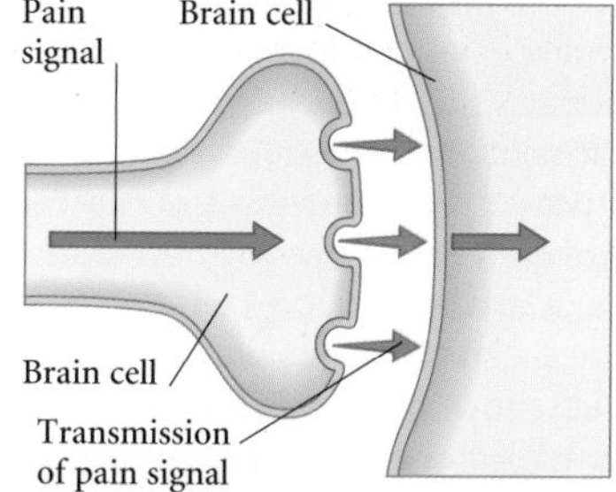

Before the drug
On reaching the brain, the pain signal is transmitted from one brain cell to the next until it reaches the part of the brain that interprets the signal as pain.

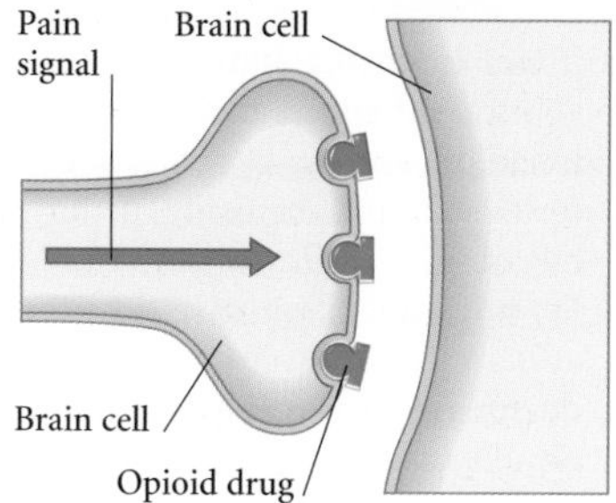

After the drug
Opioid painkillers block transmission of the pain signal in the brain, thereby reducing the sensation of pain.

Antimigraine drugs

Drugs that are used in the prevention and treatment of migraine

Common drugs

Drugs to prevent migraine
• Amitriptyline • Clonidine • Cyproheptadine
• Methysergide • Nifedipine • Propranolol
• Sodium valproate • Verapamil

Drugs to relieve migraine
• Ergotamine • Naratriptan • Rizatriptan
• Sumatriptan • Zolmitriptan

Painkillers (opposite page)
• Aspirin • Codeine • Paracetamol

Migraine attacks (*see* MIGRAINE, p.518) produce severe headaches and are often accompanied by nausea and vomiting. These symptoms may be preceded by visual disturbances. Some drugs used to treat migraine are taken regularly to prevent attacks, while others are taken during an attack to alleviate the symptoms. Painkillers (opposite page) may help to relieve headaches.

How do they work?

During a migraine attack, blood flow inside the brain changes. Initially, the blood vessels narrow, reducing blood flow. After this initial phase, the vessels rapidly widen, and a severe headache develops. Drugs that are used to prevent migraine, such as propranolol (*see* BETA-BLOCKER DRUGS, p.898), prevent these changes in blood vessel size. However, the exact mechanism by which they work is not understood.

Triptan drugs, such as sumatriptan and naratriptan, and ergotamine relieve the symptoms of a migraine attack by returning widened blood vessels to their normal size. Painkillers can provide some relief but do not shorten the duration of a migraine attack.

How are they used?

Most people who experience migraines have attacks infrequently and can control the pain by taking drugs such as paracetamol, aspirin, or codeine. If you experience frequent, severe migraine attacks, your doctor may recommend that you use a preventive drug, such as the beta-blocker propranolol, to be taken daily for a few months.

Severe migraine that is not relieved by painkillers may respond to triptans or ergotamine. You should take these antimigraine drugs as soon as you notice migraine symptoms developing. Triptans and ergotamine can be taken orally, but if you regularly experience episodes of very severe migraine, especially if they are accompanied by nausea and vomiting, your doctor may prescribe triptans in a form that can be given by injection. Ergotamine is also available as an aerosol spray or in the form of a suppository.

There are various over-the-counter preparations for migraine. These may contain one or more painkillers and an antiemetic drug (p.922) to help to relieve nausea and vomiting.

What are the side effects?

You may experience side effects when taking drugs to treat migraine. Taking propranolol may cause cold hands and feet and tiredness. Triptans can make you feel drowsy and can sometimes cause flushing, dizziness, tingling sensations, and chest pain. Ergotamine may cause nausea, vomiting, abdominal pain, diarrhoea, and muscle cramps. Excessive use of triptans or ergotamine may reduce their effectiveness. You should not exceed the recommended dose of any antimigraine drug.

General anaesthetics

Drugs that act on the brain to induce unconsciousness for surgery

COMMON DRUGS

INJECTED ANAESTHETICS
• Etomidate • Ketamine • Propofol • Thiopental

INHALED ANAESTHETICS
• Enflurane • Halothane • Isoflurane
• Nitrous oxide

General anaesthetics induce and maintain unconsciousness and thus are used to prevent all sensations in individuals undergoing surgery (*see* HAVING A GENERAL ANAESTHETIC, p.944). The drugs are rapidly absorbed by the brain and produce unconsciousness by reducing the flow of nerve impulses in the brain.

HOW ARE THEY USED?

General anaesthetics are administered either by injection into a vein in the arm or back of the hand or by inhalation. They are usually given together with an injected muscle relaxant that relaxes all muscles in the body, including those of the throat and respiratory system. Consequently, breathing has to be assisted artificially and vital body functions, such as heart rate and blood pressure, are carefully monitored during a general anaesthetic.

An injected drug, such as etomidate or propofol, is initially used to induce anaesthesia, but the drug's effect wears off within a few minutes. For this reason, inhaled anaesthetics are usually given continuously to maintain unconsciousness throughout surgery. Various anaesthetics are often combined so that only a minimum dose of each drug is needed to maintain unconsciousness. This technique reduces the potential for side effects from any of the drugs.

For minor surgical procedures, an injected general anaesthetic is sometimes used without inhaled anaesthetics.

WHAT ARE THE SIDE EFFECTS?

The most common side effects that you may experience on regaining consciousness after a general anaesthetic are nausea and tiredness. Rarely, some inhaled anaesthetic drugs may cause liver damage if given repeatedly. Your doctor or anaesthetist will ask if you have had a general anaesthetic within the last 3 months and whether you have had adverse reactions to an anaesthetic.

Certain other drugs, such as those used to treat high blood pressure, may interact with anaesthetics. Inform your anaesthetist about any drugs that you have been taking, whether prescription, over-the-counter, or recreational.

Local anaesthetics

Drugs that block pain sensations in a limited region of the body

COMMON DRUGS

• Benzocaine • Bupivacaine • Lidocaine
• Tetracaine

Local anaesthetics are used to block sensation in a specific area of the body. They have a wide range of uses, including the prevention of pain during minor surgical procedures or diagnostic tests. The drugs are also used to produce regional anaesthesia, sometimes called a nerve block, in which a large area of the body is anaesthetized. Local anaesthetics vary in potency and in the duration of their effect. They work by temporarily preventing the conduction of pain signals along nerve fibres.

HOW ARE THEY USED?

A local anaesthetic may be injected directly into the site at which sensation needs to be blocked (*see* HAVING A LOCAL ANAESTHETIC, p.942). For example, local anaesthesia may be used to numb a small area of skin before the removal of a mole. Local anaesthetics may also be applied to the skin or the mucous membranes as a cream, gel, or spray. Some products that contain a local anaesthetic are available over the counter; these include throat lozenges and suppositories or ointments used to relieve painful haemorrhoids (p.668).

Regional anaesthesia is used to anaesthetize a large area of the body. The drug is usually injected at a site close to a nerve or bundle of nerves that supplies a specific area of the body (*see* HAVING A REGIONAL ANAESTHETIC, p.945). The anaesthetic then numbs the entire area supplied by that nerve or nerve bundle. One example of this type of anaesthesia is epidural anaesthesia, in which a local anaesthetic is injected into the space around the spinal cord. This procedure anaesthetizes the whole of the lower body and is sometimes used as a form of pain relief during labour (*see* EPIDURAL ANAESTHESIA IN LABOUR, p.801).

WHAT ARE THE SIDE EFFECTS?

Some local anaesthetics applied to the skin can cause an allergic reaction if they are used repeatedly. If a large dose of local anaesthetic becomes absorbed into the bloodstream, it may lead to symptoms such as dizziness.

Following an epidural anaesthetic, you may have a headache or backache that can last for several days.

Anticonvulsant drugs

Drugs used to prevent and treat epileptic seizures and other types of seizures

COMMON DRUGS

BENZODIAZEPINES
• Diazepam • Clonazepam • Lorazepam

OTHER ANTICONVULSANT DRUGS
• Carbamazepine • Ethosuximide • Gabapentin
• Lamotrigine • Phenobarbital • Phenytoin
• Primidone • Sodium valproate • Topiramate

Anticonvulsant drugs are mainly used to prevent recurrent seizures caused by epilepsy (p.524) and as an emergency treatment for prolonged seizures. Left untreated, prolonged seizures may cause brain damage. Rarely, an anticonvulsant drug is used for seizures not due to epilepsy, such as febrile convulsions (p.849), which can occur in children. Some anticonvulsant drugs are used to treat pain due to nerve damage, such as trigeminal neuralgia (p.546), which causes severe pain on one side of the face.

WARNING

- If you are taking anticonvulsants, you should report any sign of infection, such as a sore throat or fever, a rash, bruising, or bleeding, to your doctor.
- Do not stop taking an anticonvulsant without consulting your doctor. Abrupt withdrawal could rapidly worsen seizures.
- Anticonvulsants can harm a developing fetus. If you are planning a pregnancy, you should discuss this with your doctor.

How do they work?

Anticonvulsants have a direct effect on electrical activity in the brain. A seizure occurs when excessive electrical activity spreads from one part of the brain to other areas, causing uncontrolled stimulation of nerves supplying many parts of the body. Anticonvulsants reduce these abnormally high levels of electrical activity and thereby prevent or reduce the muscle spasms that are characteristic of a seizure. The mechanism by which anticonvulsants relieve nerve pain in disorders such as trigeminal neuralgia is not clearly understood.

How are they used?

If you have recurrent seizures, you are likely to need anticonvulsants for a prolonged period to reduce the frequency and severity of your seizures or, if possible, to prevent them altogether. Your doctor will initially prescribe a single drug that is appropriate for the type of seizure that you have. For example, if you experience absence (petit mal) epileptic seizures, in which brief periods of detachment from reality occur, your doctor will usually give you either ethosuximide or sodium valproate. If seizures are tonic-clonic (characterized by uncontrolled movement of the limbs and trunk) or partial (involving minor twitching movements), your treatment may be with sodium valproate, phenytoin, lamotrigine, or carbamazepine. Drugs such as gabapentin may be used if other anticonvulsants do not control seizures or cause severe side effects.

If a seizure is prolonged, diazepam may be given by intravenous injection, or as a liquid that is administered into the rectum. Once the seizure has been brought under control, intravenous infusions of phenytoin or another drug may be given for a few hours afterwards to prevent seizures from recurring.

The dose of an anticonvulsant is adjusted so that the drug is effective without causing unwanted side effects. You may find that you have occasional seizures while taking anticonvulsants. If this is the case, your doctor may try another drug, either as an alternative or as an additional treatment.

Some people with epilepsy will eventually stop having seizures naturally, usually about 10 years after onset. Your doctor will usually stop treatment only if you have not had a seizure for at least 2 years. The drug will then gradually be withdrawn over a few months to reduce the risk of seizures beginning again.

If you have epilepsy you will probably be given a card, bracelet, or pendant giving the details of your condition and treatment. It is advisable to carry this identification with you at all times for others to refer to if you have a seizure.

Diazepam in liquid form may also be given into the rectum during an isolated seizure that is not due to epilepsy, such as a febrile convulsion. Trigeminal neuralgia may need long-term treatment with an oral anticonvulsant.

What are the side effects?

Anticonvulsants can affect memory and coordination and may induce lethargy and impair concentration. You should consult your doctor if you develop an infection, because some anticonvulsants reduce the effectiveness of the immune system. If you are planning to become pregnant, you should also arrange to see your doctor to discuss your treatment needs during pregnancy.

Sleeping drugs

Drugs that reduce nerve cell activity in the brain and are used to treat insomnia

Common drugs

Benzodiazepines
- Flurazepam • Nitrazepam • Temazepam

Antihistamines (p.906)

Other sleeping drugs
- Amobarbital sodium • Chloral hydrate
- Zolpidem • Zopiclone

Sleeping drugs may be prescribed to reestablish sleep patterns after a period of insomnia (p.554) or when insomnia is the result of a stressful event, such as a death in the family. They may also be used if you need to adjust your sleep patterns to suit your work. However, sleeping drugs do not treat the cause of insomnia, which may be depression (p.554) or anxiety (*see* Anxiety disorders, p.551). You should not drink alcohol when taking sleeping drugs because the sedative effect is enhanced.

Many sleeping drugs cause dependence, and they are usually prescribed only for a week or two when other measures to treat insomnia have failed.

> **WARNING**
>
> Sleeping drugs can affect your ability to drive or to operate machinery; these effects may persist the following day.

What are the types?

Many sleeping drugs belong to a group of drugs called benzodiazepines, which are also used to treat anxiety disorders. Over-the-counter remedies containing an antihistamine (p.906) are also available to treat insomnia. If insomnia is caused by depression, your doctor may prescribe antidepressant drugs (p.916) to relieve the symptoms of depression, including insomnia. In the past, barbiturates were commonly used to treat insomnia. However, these drugs may cause serious side effects and dependence and are no longer recommended for treating sleeping problems.

Benzodiazepines These drugs reduce the level of activity in the brain, causing drowsiness. If your doctor prescribes a benzodiazepine, you will usually have only a limited supply and be advised not to take the drug every night. This is because prolonged use may result in dependence and tolerance, in which progressively larger doses of the drug are needed to produce the same effect. When you take benzodiazepines, side effects such as confusion, dizziness, and poor coordination may develop even between doses. If you are elderly, you should take particular care because these drugs can increase the risk of falling. You may also experience withdrawal symptoms when you stop taking benzodiazepines, including a recurrence of insomnia and increased dreaming, restlessness, and anxiety. It is possible to minimize withdrawal symptoms by reducing the dose gradually.

Antihistamines Some sleep preparations containing an antihistamine may be purchased over the counter. These preparations do not cause dependence and have only a few minor side effects. However, you should not take any of these preparations for longer than a few days without first consulting your doctor. Antihistamines sometimes cause a dry mouth and blurred vision.

OTHER SLEEPING DRUGS Zolpidem and zopiclone reduce electrical activity in the brain, so that falling asleep is easier. Their effects are brief and they are less likely to cause dependence, but they are not recommended for long-term use.

The sleeping drugs chloral hydrate and amobarbital sodium are nowadays used only if other drugs prove unsuccessful. Chloral hydrate may irritate the stomach and cause nausea.

Antianxiety drugs

Drugs that are used to reduce and control the symptoms of stress and anxiety

COMMON DRUGS

BENZODIAZEPINES
• Chlordiazepoxide • Diazepam • Lorazepam
• Oxazepam

BETA-BLOCKER DRUGS
• Atenolol • Propranolol

OTHER ANTIANXIETY DRUGS
• Buspirone

Antianxiety drugs, sometimes known as anxiolytics or minor tranquillizers, are used to treat anxiety disorders (p.551), in which feelings of foreboding and fear may be accompanied by physical symptoms such as palpitations and tremor. The underlying cause of the anxiety may also need to be treated at the same time, possibly using one or more psychological therapies (pp.968–971). Some drugs are used specifically to relieve the physical symptoms of anxiety. For example, they may be prescribed for people who are nervous about giving a public performance or to calm a person who is anxious before an operation.

WHAT ARE THE TYPES?

Several types of drug are used in the treatment of anxiety. Benzodiazepines are the drugs most commonly prescribed for the short-term treatment of psychological symptoms of anxiety.

Where physical symptoms, such as muscle tremor, are the main problem, beta-blocker drugs (p.898) may be used instead. Buspirone is sometimes prescribed to treat anxiety because it is less sedating than benzodiazepines.

BENZODIAZEPINES These drugs may be used for the treatment of severe anxiety. They reduce agitation and make you feel relaxed. However, doctors only prescribe short courses of benzodiazepines to avoid causing dependence.

Benzodiazepines slow mental activity by reducing the signals between brain cells. They often cause drowsiness, and for this reason are also used as sleeping drugs (p.915). You should not drink alcohol while taking benzodiazepines because it increases the sedative effect. These drugs can also cause confusion, dizziness, lethargy and poor coordination. Benzodiazepines should not be taken for more than 1–2 weeks. If they are taken for longer, stopping the treatment may cause withdrawal symptoms such as excessive anxiety and insomnia.

BETA-BLOCKER DRUGS Physical symptoms that can occur with anxiety may be reduced with beta-blockers. These drugs should only be used occasionally and are not suitable for long-term treatment.

The drugs block the actions of two hormones, epinephrine (adrenaline) and norepinephrine (noradrenaline), that produce the physical symptoms of anxiety. Beta-blockers reduce heart rate and may prevent palpitations. They can also be used to reduce muscle tremor. If you take a beta-blocker, you may find that your sleep is disturbed and that your hands and feet feel cold. People who have respiratory disorders such as asthma should not take beta-blockers because the drugs may exacerbate their breathing difficulties.

OTHER ANTIANXIETY DRUGS The most common of the other drugs used to reduce anxiety is buspirone, which is less addictive than the benzodiazepines and has a less sedative effect. Buspirone can take up to 2 weeks to become fully effective and is therefore not used when immediate relief from stress or anxiety is needed. You may experience side effects, such as nervousness, headache, and dizziness, when taking buspirone. The drug may also affect your ability to drive or operate machinery.

WARNING

Benzodiazepine drugs often cause drowsiness and may affect your ability to drive vehicles or operate machinery.

Antidepressant drugs

Drugs that are used to treat the symptoms of depression

COMMON DRUGS

SELECTIVE SEROTONIN REUPTAKE INHIBITORS
• Citalopram • Fluoxetine • Fluvoxamine
• Paroxetine • Sertraline

TRICYCLICS
• Amitriptyline • Clomipramine • Imipramine

MONOAMINE OXIDASE INHIBITORS
• Phenelzine • Tranylcypromine

OTHER ANTIDEPRESSANT DRUGS
• Maprotiline • Nefazodone • Trazodone
• Venlafaxine

Antidepressant drugs help to relieve many of the symptoms of depression (p.554), such as despair, lethargy, poor appetite, insomnia, and thoughts of suicide. Antidepressants are effective in about 2 in 3 people who take them.

People who are depressed have been shown to have reduced levels of certain chemicals called neurotransmitters in the brain. Serotonin and norepinephrine (noradrenaline) are two neurotransmitters that are thought to increase brain activity and improve mood. They are usually reabsorbed by brain cells and inactivated by an enzyme called monoamine oxidase. In a depressed person, levels of serotonin or norepinephrine are frequently lower than normal. Antidepressants work by helping to restore these chemicals to normal levels.

Antidepressants are taken orally and usually take 1–3 weeks to have an effect on depression. Side effects may develop immediately but gradually lessen. Your doctor will usually advise you to take an antidepressant for at least 6 months after your depression has lifted to prevent symptoms recurring and then to reduce the dose gradually. You should avoid alcohol while you are taking these drugs because it enhances the sedative effect.

Lithium, a mood-stabilizing drug (p.918), may be used on its own or with an antidepressant in severe depression.

WARNING

Antidepressant drugs can cause drowsiness and may affect your ability to drive vehicles or operate machinery.

WHAT ARE THE TYPES?

Most of the drugs used to treat depression belong to one of three main groups: selective serotonin reuptake inhibitors (SSRIs), tricyclics, and monoamine oxidase inhibitors (MAOIs). There are also several other types of antidepressant. All of these drugs treat depression by increasing levels of the neurotransmitters in the brain that lift mood.

SSRIs These drugs are the most commonly used type of antidepressant. They may also be used to treat phobias (p.552) and panic attacks (*see* ANXIETY DISORDERS, p.551). SSRIs cause fewer side effects than other types of antidepressant and are less toxic if more than the prescribed amount is taken. The drugs work by blocking the reabsorption of the neurotransmitter serotonin, leaving more of the chemical to stimulate brain cells (*see* HOW SSRIS WORK, right). SSRIs may cause side effects, including diarrhoea, nausea and vomiting, reduced sex drive, and headache. They may also cause restlessness and anxiety.

TRICYCLICS Tricyclics are often used to treat depression and are sometimes used as a treatment for pain from damaged nerves in conditions such as trigeminal neuralgia (p.546). The drugs interfere with the reabsorption of both serotonin and norepinephrine in the brain. As a result, levels of these mood-lifting chemicals increase. It is not well understood how tricyclics relieve pain in trigeminal neuralgia.

Tricyclics cause a number of side effects, including a dry mouth, blurred vision, constipation, and difficulty in passing urine. The side effects are usually worse when the drug is first started and become less of a problem as you get used to the drug. Tricyclics are dangerous if you exceed the usual dose. They may cause seizures and heart rhythm irregularities, which can be fatal.

MAOIs These drugs are usually only used when other types of antidepressant drug are ineffective. They work by blocking the activity of monoamine oxidase (the enzyme that makes serotonin and norepinephrine inactive) in brain cells. The side effects of MAOIs may include light-headedness, drowsiness, insomnia, headache, a dry mouth, constipation, and other digestive disturbances. These drugs interact with other drugs and some foods, including cheese and meat extracts. It is therefore important that you follow your doctor's instructions. If you plan to stop taking an MAOI, the dose should be reduced gradually to reduce the chance of dangerous changes in blood pressure.

OTHER ANTIDEPRESSANT DRUGS There are two other drugs, maprotiline and trazodone, that are related to tricyclic antidepressants. Maprotiline is used to treat both depression and anxiety when sedation is required. Trazodone is also used to treat depression when sedation is required. It is less likely to cause heart rhythm problems than other tricyclics.

Venlafaxine blocks the reuptake of serotonin and norepinephrine. It has fewer side effects than most antidepressants, but you should see your doctor if you develop a rash while taking the drug. Nefazodone works in a similar way to SSRIs but also works by blocking serotonin receptors.

DRUG ACTION HOW SSRIS WORK

SSRI drugs are often used to treat depression. Depression is associated with low levels of serotonin, a chemical that acts on certain brain cells involved in thoughts and mood.

Nerve cells in the brain constantly release and reabsorb the chemical serotonin. SSRIs reduce the rate of reabsorption, resulting in higher levels of serotonin in the brain.

Before the drug
Nerve impulses stimulate the release of serotonin from nerve endings in brain cells. The serotonin stimulates other brain cells. It is then reabsorbed and stored in the nerve endings, ready to be released again.

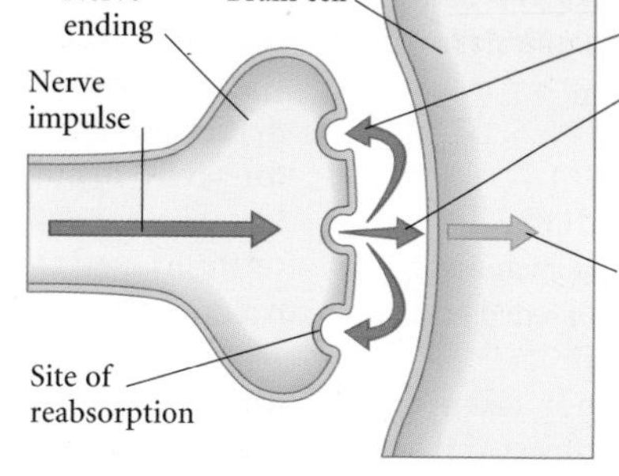

After the drug
The drug blocks some of the reabsorption sites on the nerve endings, reducing the amount of serotonin that is absorbed. This leaves higher levels of serotonin available in the brain, which increases brain cell stimulation.

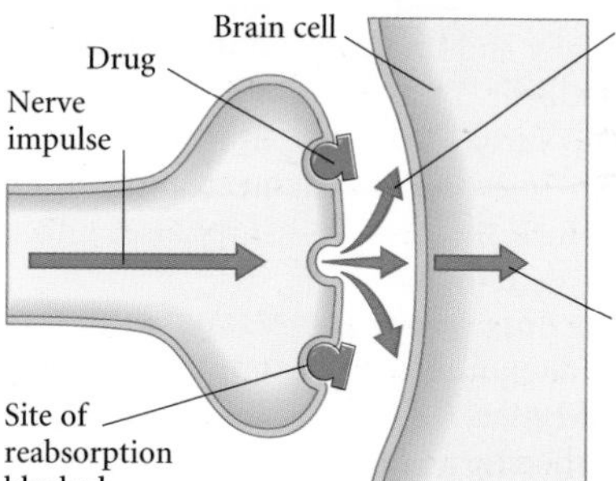

Antipsychotic drugs

Drugs used to treat schizophrenia and other severe psychiatric disorders

COMMON DRUGS

• Chlorpromazine • Clozapine • Droperidol
• Fluphenazine • Haloperidol • Loxapine
• Olanzapine • Pimozide • Promazine
• Risperidone • Sertindole • Thioridazine
• Trifluoperazine

Antipsychotic drugs are used to control symptoms such as hallucinations and disturbed patterns of thought in schizophrenia (p.560) and other psychotic disorders. Some of these drugs are also used to stabilize mood in people with bipolar affective disorder (p.557), also known as manic-depressive disorder, although people with this condition are also likely to be treated with a mood-stabilizing drug (p.918) such as lithium. Occasionally, an antipsychotic drug is used to control vomiting or uncontrollable hiccups where other treatments have failed. Antipsychotic drugs may also be prescribed to treat severe anxiety.

How do they work?

Many antipsychotic drugs block the action of the neurotransmitter (brain chemical) dopamine. This chemical is released in the brain at higher than normal levels in people with psychotic disorders and is believed to play a part in producing symptoms. Some antipsychotic drugs also block the action of serotonin and other chemicals involved in regulating mood.

How are they used?

The type of antipsychotic drug prescribed will depend on factors such as how much sedation is needed and your susceptibility to side effects.

The drugs are usually taken orally, although they may be injected if a person is very agitated. A low dose of the drug is prescribed initially, and the dose is then increased gradually until the symptoms are under control. A depot injection, which is an injection deep into a muscle from which the drug is slowly released, may be used so that you do not have to take the drug every day. Depot injections provide enough of the drug to last up to 4 weeks.

If you have bipolar affective disorder, your doctor may prescribe lithium or another mood-stabilizing drug. These drugs take time before they become fully effective. For this reason, you may initially be given a short course of an antipsychotic drug that acts rapidly to make you feel calmer until the mood-stabilizing drug reaches its full effect.

What are the side effects?

Antipsychotics may cause a dry mouth, blurred vision, and dizziness due to lowering of blood pressure, and some may make you feel drowsy. They may also cause restlessness and, rarely, movement disorders such as parkinsonism (see Parkinson's disease and parkinsonism, p.539). These side effects tend to disappear when you stop taking the drug, but certain antipsychotic drugs may occasionally cause permanent side effects after more than a year of use, such as repeated jerking movements of the mouth, face, and tongue.

You should never suddenly stop taking any antipsychotic drug without first consulting your doctor. If you need to stop taking the drug, the dose will be reduced gradually by your doctor.

Mood-stabilizing drugs

Drugs used to treat severe psychiatric disorders involving excessive mood swings

Common drugs

- Carbamazepine • Lithium • Sodium valproate

Mood-stabilizing drugs are used for the treatment of bipolar affective disorder (p.557), which is also known as manic-depressive disorder, and less commonly for severe depression (p.554). In bipolar affective disorder, cycles of mania (elation) and severe depression may occur. Lithium is the drug most commonly used to treat this disorder and can control or reduce the intensity of mania. It may also prevent or reduce the frequency of attacks and lift depression. Two other drugs, carbamazepine and sodium valproate, may be used as mood stabilizers if lithium is ineffective in treating bipolar affective disorder or if it causes unacceptable side effects.

How are they used?

Lithium is taken orally. It takes a few days before the drug's effects are noticeable and up to 3 weeks for it to take full effect. For this reason, a rapidly acting antipsychotic drug (p.917) is often prescribed at the same time for initial control of mania. Lithium will then be continued to prevent further episodes.

Treatment with lithium can cause nausea, diarrhoea, tremor, and excessive thirst. These side effects usually reduce in severity if treatment is continued. If the dose is too high, lithium can cause blurred vision, confusion, and seizures. Carbamazepine and sodium valproate may be given if lithium is unsuitable. These drugs may cause memory and coordination problems. For this reason, your doctor will carry out blood tests to measure drug levels during treatment with mood-stabilizing drugs.

If you are taking lithium, you will be given a treatment card, bracelet, or pendant, which you should carry with you at all times. You should be careful not make changes in your diet that might alter the amount of salt you take in because this may affect lithium levels in your body. It is also important to avoid dehydration, which may occur if you develop diarrhoea or vomiting or travel to a region with a hot climate.

Central nervous system stimulant drugs

Drugs that are used to increase mental alertness and wakefulness

Common drugs

- Caffeine • Dexamfetamine
- Methylphenidate

Central nervous system (CNS) stimulant drugs act by increasing activity in the brain, which increases wakefulness and mental alertness. Their main use is in the treatment of narcolepsy (p.526), a disorder in which a person experiences recurrent episodes of involuntary sleep during the day. Some CNS stimulants, including methylphenidate, are used to improve the attention span of children who have a behavioural problem known as attention deficit disorder (p.855).

How do they work?

CNS stimulants improve concentration and increase wakefulness by acting on a part of the brain that regulates mental alertness. These stimulants promote the release of certain chemicals in the brain (neurotransmitters) that increase nerve activity in this part of the brain.

How are they used?

CNS stimulants are given orally long-term for the treatment of narcolepsy. Doctors avoid prescribing CNS stimulants over a prolonged period for a child because they may slow growth. Children taking methylphenidate may need to have blood tests at regular intervals, because this drug can reduce the effectiveness of the immune system, thereby increasing the risk of infection.

What are the side effects?

While you are taking CNS stimulants, you may experience reduced appetite, tremor, and palpitations. These drugs can also cause restlessness, sleeplessness, anxiety, shaking, and sweating. Some CNS stimulants produce symptoms similar to those of schizophrenia (p.560), such as hallucinations. Other side effects include rashes and allergies. If you take a CNS stimulant long-term, stopping treatment may cause withdrawal symptoms, including lethargy, depression, and increased appetite.

DRUGS FOR EYE AND EAR DISORDERS

Eye and ear problems need prompt attention because they affect our most important senses. Many infections and chronic (long-term) conditions can be treated effectively with drugs. Medication for eye and ear disorders can often be administered easily as drops or ointments.

KEY ANATOMY

Pupil Lens Retina Optic nerve Cornea

EYE

Inner ear Middle ear Outer ear Eardrum

EAR

For more information on the structure and function of the eyes and ears, *see* pp.566–569 and pp.592–595.

Most eye and ear disorders are minor and clear up rapidly with appropriate treatment. More serious and persistent problems may need medical attention and long-term use of drugs.

The first article in this section discusses drugs used to treat infections and inflammation of the eye. It also covers artificial tears, which relieve dry eyes, and mydriatics, a group of drugs that are used in the treatment of the inflammatory disorder uveitis.

Drugs that are used for glaucoma, a potentially serious condition if left untreated, are described in the next article. These drugs work in a variety of ways to relieve excess accumulation of fluid in the eye. As a result, the pressure that can damage the optic nerve is relieved, thereby diminishing the likelihood of partial or complete loss of vision.

The final article in this section discusses drugs used to treat disorders of the ear. These drugs range from treatments for bacterial infections and excess earwax to treatments for nausea and vomiting, symptoms that are commonly seen in inner ear disorders and can affect the balance mechanism. Drugs that relieve nausea and vomiting are discussed further elsewhere (*see* ANTIEMETIC DRUGS, p.922).

Drugs acting on the eye

Drugs that are used to treat a variety of disorders affecting the eye

COMMON DRUGS

ANTI-INFECTIVE DRUGS
• Aciclovir • Chloramphenicol • Ciprofloxacin • Gentamicin • Neomycin • Polymyxin B

ANTI-INFLAMMATORY DRUGS
• Betamethasone • Dexamethasone • Nedocromil sodium • Prednisolone • Sodium cromoglicate

ARTIFICIAL TEARS
• Hydroxyethylcellulose • Hypromellose • Polyvinyl alcohol

MYDRIATICS
• Atropine • Cyclopentolate • Phenylephrine

Many eye disorders can be treated by applying drugs directly to the eye in the form of eyedrops (*see* USING EYEDROPS, right) or ointments (*see* USING EYE OINTMENT, p.920). Minor eye problems, such as dryness or irritation due to allergy, can often be relieved with over-the-counter remedies. Drugs for eye infections and for other serious conditions, such as uveitis (p.574) or scleritis (p.574), in which the eye is inflamed, are available only on prescription.

WHAT ARE THE TYPES?

The main types of drug used to treat eye disorders are anti-infective drugs and anti-inflammatory drugs. Anti-infective drugs are commonly used to treat bacterial, viral, and, less commonly, fungal infections of the eye. Anti-inflammatory drugs are used to relieve the redness and swelling that may develop as a result of infection, allergic reactions, or autoimmune disorders (in which the immune system attacks the body's own tissues). Artificial tears are used to relieve dryness of the eyes (*see* KERATOCONJUNCTIVITIS SICCA, p.585). Mydriatrics dilate (widen) the pupil and are most commonly used to treat uveitis.

ANTI-INFECTIVE DRUGS There are two main groups of drugs used to treat eye infections. Antibiotics (p.885), such as chloramphenicol, may be used to treat bacterial infections such as conjunctivitis (p.570) and blepharitis (p.583).

SELF-ADMINISTRATION USING EYEDROPS

Eyedrops deliver a drug directly to the area where its effect is needed. Always wash your hands before using the drops and do not touch the eye or the skin around it with the dropper. If you wear contact lenses, check with your doctor or pharmacist before using eyedrops because some preparations may be unsuitable.

Instilling the drops
Tilt your head backwards and draw the lower lid away from the affected eye. Drop the eyedrops on to the inside of your lower lid. Try to avoid blinking immediately.

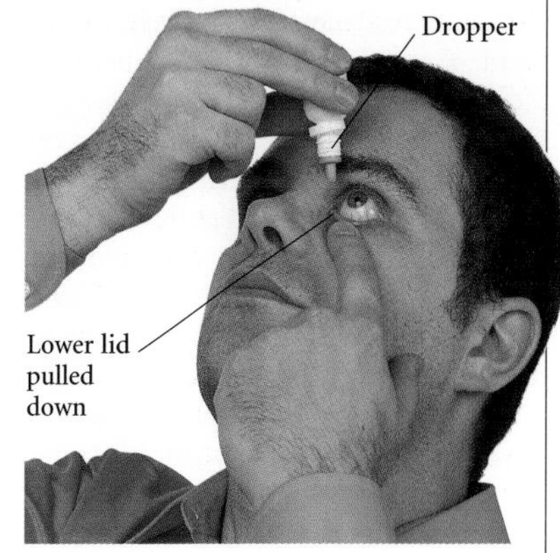

SELF-ADMINISTRATION USING EYE OINTMENT

Medication in the form of eye ointment may have a longer-lasting effect than if applied as eyedrops. To reduce the risk of contaminating the eye, always wash your hands before applying the ointment and do not touch the affected eye with your fingers or the tube.

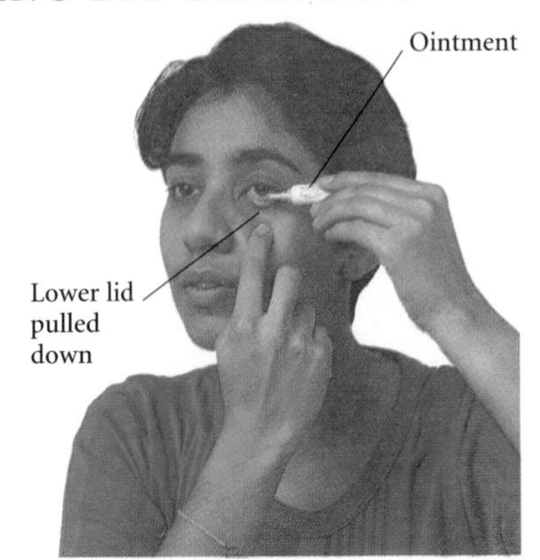

Correct application of ointment
Squeeze a thin line of ointment along the inside of the lower eyelid. Close your eye briefly after application. You may find that the ointment makes your vision blurred for a few minutes.

Antiviral drugs (p.886), such as aciclovir, are used to treat corneal ulcers (p.571) that occur as a result of infection with herpes viruses.

Antibiotics are usually applied as eyedrops or ointment directly on to the site of infection in the eye. However, if a bacterial infection is severe, it may be necessary to take oral antibiotics as well as using eyedrops. Viral infections of the eye may be treated with both antiviral eyedrops and oral antiviral drugs.

When using antibiotic eyedrops or ointment, you may experience temporary stinging or itching. You may also notice a bitter taste as the eyedrops run down inside the tear ducts and into your nose and mouth.

ANTI-INFLAMMATORY DRUGS The drugs most commonly prescribed to treat the inflammation that accompanies many eye disorders are corticosteroids (*see* TOPICAL CORTICOSTEROIDS, p.892) and antiallergy drugs (p.905).

Corticosteroids are applied as eyedrops or as ointment squeezed just inside the eyelids. If you are predisposed to develop chronic glaucoma (p.576), in which the pressure of fluid in the eye becomes abnormally high, the use of corticosteroids may slightly increase your risk of developing drug-induced glaucoma (p.575). Corticosteroids are available on prescription and must be used under the supervision of a doctor.

Short-term inflammation caused by allergy is often treated with antihistamine or sodium cromoglicate eyedrops. Some antiallergy eyedrops, such as those used to treat eye irritation associated with hay fever (*see* ALLERGIC RHINITIS, p.466), are available over the counter. Antiallergy drugs may cause side effects such as blurred vision and headache.

ARTIFICIAL TEARS Eyedrops containing chemicals to relieve dryness are available for people whose eyes do not produce enough natural tear fluid. Artificial tears form a moist film on the cornea (the transparent front part of the eye), soothing and rehydrating the surface of the eyes. You can buy artificial tear preparations over the counter. They may be applied as often as necessary.

MYDRIATICS These drugs are used to treat uveitis, an inflammatory condition affecting the iris (the coloured part of the eye) and the muscles that control focusing. If the iris becomes inflamed, there is a danger that it may stick to the lens of the eye. Most mydriatics, such as atropine and cyclopentolate, relax the ring of muscles in the iris, causing dilation of the pupil. Mydriatics may also be used to dilate the pupil during eye examinations and eye surgery.

Mydriatics are usually prescribed as eyedrops or eye ointment. While using a mydriatic drug, you may find that bright lights cause discomfort, and you may also have difficulty in focusing. These drugs can cause contact dermatitis (p.335) and various other side effects, including dry mouth, constipation, and difficulty in passing urine. Certain mydriatics, such as phenylephrine, can raise blood pressure and are therefore unsuitable for people who have high blood pressure (*see* HYPERTENSION, p.403).

Drugs for glaucoma

Drugs that are used to reduce abnormally high pressure inside the eye

COMMON DRUGS

MIOTICS
• Carbachol • Pilocarpine

CARBONIC ANHYDRASE INHIBITORS
• Acetazolamide • Dorzolamide

BETA-BLOCKER DRUGS
• Betaxolol • Carteolol • Levobunolol
• Metipranolol • Timolol

OTHER DRUGS
• Apraclonidine • Brimonidine • Dipivefrine
• Latanoprost • Mannitol

Fluid is produced in the front part of the eye to maintain its shape and to nourish the tissues. To achieve a steady pressure, the fluid drains from the eye at the same rate at which it is produced. In glaucoma, abnormally high pressure develops in the eye because of an excessive build-up of fluid. This build-up is due to a defect in the internal drainage system between the iris (the coloured part of the eye) and the cornea (the transparent outer part of the front of the eye). High pressure can be relieved by surgery or by using drugs that either increase fluid drainage from the eye or reduce the production of fluid.

Prompt treatment is necessary when glaucoma occurs suddenly (*see* ACUTE GLAUCOMA, p.575) to avoid permanent damage to the eye. If the condition develops gradually (*see* CHRONIC GLAUCOMA, p.576), it may be treated by long-term use of drugs to reduce and maintain normal pressure in the eye.

WHAT ARE THE TYPES?

The types of drug most commonly used in the treatment of glaucoma are miotics, carbonic anhydrase inhibitors, and beta-blocker drugs. These act in various ways to lower pressure in the eye.

MIOTICS Both acute and chronic glaucoma can be treated using a miotic, such as pilocarpine. Miotic drugs cause the pupil (the circular opening in the centre of the eye) to constrict, thereby moving the iris away from the cornea. This increases the size of the opening (the drainage angle) through which fluid flows out of the eye. Miotics are usually administered as eyedrops.

While taking miotics, you may find it harder to see in dim light because the drugs constrict the pupil, thereby reducing the amount of light that enters the eye. You may also experience irritation of the eye, blurred vision, and headache.

CARBONIC ANHYDRASE INHIBITORS This type of drug is often used in cases of acute glaucoma. The drugs may also be used to treat chronic glaucoma if other drugs are not effective. Carbonic anhydrase inhibitors rapidly reduce fluid pressure inside the eye by blocking the effect of an enzyme necessary for fluid production. Some carbonic anhydrase inhibitors may be given as eyedrops, while others, such as acetazolamide, are given by intravenous or by intramuscular injection or are taken orally.

Carbonic anhydrase inhibitors used as eyedrops may cause stinging, itching, and inflammation of the eye. If you are having this type of drug by injection or taking it orally, you may experience loss of appetite, drowsiness, painful tingling in the hands and feet, and mood changes. Rarely, carbonic anhydrase inhibitors can cause the formation of kidney stones (p.701).

BETA-BLOCKER DRUGS In chronic glaucoma, a beta-blocker such as timolol may be used to decrease the amount of fluid produced inside the eye. The drug works by blocking the transmission of nerve signals that stimulate the production of fluid by certain cells in the eye.

Rarely, beta-blockers may slow your heart rate and lower blood pressure. Beta-blocker eyedrops are not usually prescribed for people who have asthma or certain heart conditions.

OTHER DRUGS Various other drugs are used to treat glaucoma. For example, latanoprost increases the drainage of fluid from the eye and may be given as eyedrops for chronic glaucoma.

Brimonidine works by both increasing the flow of fluid from the eye and by decreasing the production of fluid.

Mannitol encourages excess fluid to be absorbed from the eye into surrounding blood vessels. The drug may be given by intravenous infusion as emergency treatment for acute glaucoma or to relieve pressure within the eye just prior to surgery.

Drugs acting on the ear

Drugs that are used to treat disorders of the outer, middle, or inner ear

COMMON DRUGS

ANTIBIOTICS AND ANTIFUNGALS
- Chloramphenicol • Clioquinol • Clotrimazole
- Gentamicin • Neomycin

ANTI-INFLAMMATORY DRUGS
- Aluminium acetate • Betamethasone
- Dexamethasone • Hydrocortisone
- Prednisolone • Triamcinolone

EARWAX SOFTENERS
- Docusate • Olive oil • Sodium bicarbonate
- Urea • Hxydrogen peroxide

OTHER DRUGS
- Betahistine • Hyoscine • Prochlorperazine

Drugs can be used to treat conditions affecting the outer, middle, or inner ear. They may also be used to relieve the symptoms that accompany these conditions, such as pain, inflammation, and nausea. The drugs can be applied topically in the form of drops (*see* USING EARDROPS, right) or sprays or they can be taken orally.

SELF-ADMINISTRATION

USING EARDROPS

It is usually easier to have someone else apply eardrops for you than to do it yourself. If the eardrops are being kept in the fridge, allow them to warm to room temperature before they are applied.

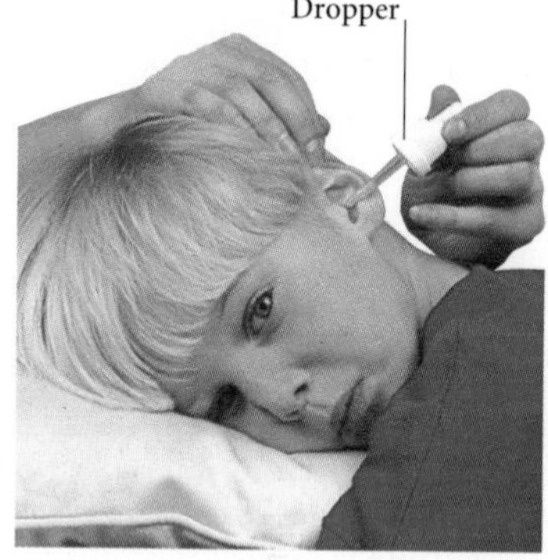

Instilling eardrops
Tilt the head and squeeze the eardrops into the ear canal. Keep the head tilted for a minute to let the eardrops settle.

WHAT ARE THE TYPES?

Several types of drug are used to treat ear disorders, including antibiotics (p.885), antifungals (p.889), anti-inflammatory drugs, and earwax softeners. Antibiotics are prescribed for bacterial infections, sometimes in combination with anti-inflammatory drugs, such as aluminium acetate, or mild corticosteroid drugs (*see* TOPICAL CORTICOSTEROIDS, p.892). Earwax softeners loosen excess earwax so that it can be removed easily. Various other drugs are used to treat symptoms that accompany disorders of the balance mechanism in the inner ear.

ANTIBIOTICS AND ANTIFUNGALS If you have a bacterial or fungal infection of your outer ear, such as otitis externa (p.596), your doctor will probably prescribe antibiotic or antifungal eardrops, which act directly on the infected area of the ear. Infections of the middle ear, such as otitis media (p.597), may be treated with oral antibiotics.

ANTI-INFLAMMATORY DRUGS The anti-inflammatory drugs most commonly prescribed are corticosteroid eardrops. Eardrops containing aluminium acetate are sometimes used to treat mild inflammation of the outer ear. You may notice a slight stinging sensation as the eardrops are applied.

EARWAX SOFTENERS If excess wax builds up in your ear canal (*see* WAX BLOCKAGE, p.597), your doctor will probably recommend an over-the-counter product or olive oil to soften the wax. This will make it easier to syringe the ear. However, some commercially prepared earwax softeners and removers can cause mild irritation of the skin inside the ear.

OTHER DRUGS Nausea, vomiting, and vertigo are common symptoms of inner-ear disorders such as Ménière's disease (p.604) and labyrinthitis (p.604). Mild symptoms may be relieved by treatment with antihistamines (p.906). However, if these drugs are ineffective, you may be prescribed the antiemetic drug prochlorperazine. Betahistine is used specifically to treat the nausea, dizziness, and ringing in the ears (*see* TINNITUS, p.602) that occur in Ménière's disease. Antiemetic drugs are usually taken orally, but if you are vomiting repeatedly, the drugs may be administered as an injection or by suppository or skin patch.

Drugs for digestive disorders

Minor digestive problems, such as indigestion, constipation, or bouts of vomiting or diarrhoea, are common and short-lived, and most do not require treatment. However, drugs may sometimes be used to relieve digestive symptoms and treat specific disorders. Many of these drugs are available over the counter.

The first articles in this section discuss drugs that act on the upper digestive tract. These include antiemetics, which relieve nausea and vomiting; antacids, which relieve indigestion; and ulcer-healing drugs, which are used to treat peptic ulcers. Drugs that act on the lower digestive tract are described next. These include aminosalicylate drugs, which are used to treat long-term inflammation of the intestines; antidiarrhoeal drugs, which relieve diarrhoea; and laxatives, which are used to relieve constipation or to clear the intestine before a medical procedure. Antispasmodic drugs and motility stimulants, used to treat disorders caused by abnormal muscle action in the digestive tract, are discussed in the following article. The final article covers oral rehydration solutions, which replace water and other essential substances that are lost in vomiting and diarrhoea.

KEY ANATOMY

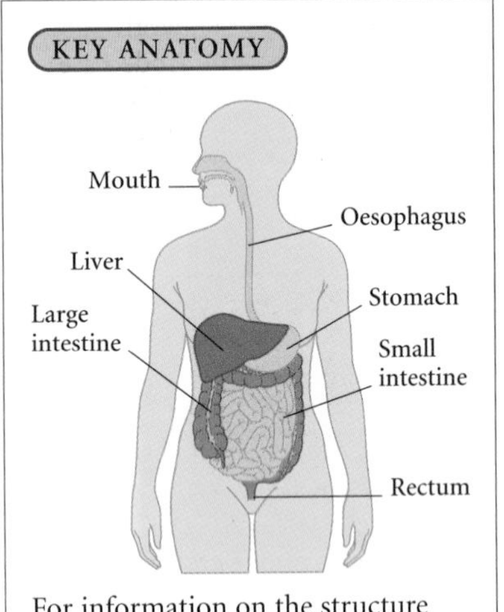

For information on the structure and function of the digestive system, *see* pp.620–625.

Antiemetic drugs

A group of drugs used to prevent or relieve nausea and vomiting

COMMON DRUGS

ANTIHISTAMINES
- Cyclizine • Dimenhydrinate
- Meclozine • Promethazine

PHENOTHIAZINES
- Perphenazine • Prochlorperazine
- Trifluoperazine

SEROTONIN ANTAGONISTS
- Granisetron • Ondansetron

OTHER DRUGS
- Droperidol • Hydroxyzine
- Hyoscine hydrobromide • Metoclopramide

Antiemetic drugs are used to treat nausea and vomiting, which are caused by stimulation of the vomiting centre in the brain. The drugs suppress signals passing to and from the vomiting centre. They are used to prevent or relieve nausea and vomiting due to motion sickness (p.604), migraine (p.518), and the inner ear disorders Ménière's disease (p.604) and labyrinthitis (p.604). Antiemetics can also relieve the nausea and vomiting that often occur during treatment with anticancer drugs (p.907) or after a general anaesthetic (p.944). They may be given for severe vomiting in pregnancy (*see* HYPEREMESIS, p.789).

If you need an antiemetic for any reason other than to prevent or relieve motion sickness, consult your doctor so that he or she can determine the cause of the vomiting and the correct treatment. Do not take antiemetics during pregnancy except on medical advice.

What are the types?

Antiemetic drugs can be classified into three main types: antihistamines, phenothiazines, and serotonin antagonists. Other common drugs include metoclopramide and hyoscine hydrobromide. Antiemetics are normally taken orally, but they may be given by injection or as a suppository if vomiting is severe.

ANTIHISTAMINES These drugs may be taken to ease nausea caused by Ménière's disease and labyrinthitis and to prevent motion sickness. Some antihistamines for motion sickness can be bought over the counter. Side effects include drowsiness, blurred vision, dry mouth, and difficulty passing urine. The drugs may affect your driving ability.

PHENOTHIAZINES These drugs may be used to treat severe vomiting in pregnancy or vomiting that is caused by anaesthetics. Phenothiazines may cause side effects such as dizziness, restlessness, muscle spasms, and tremor.

SEROTONIN ANTAGONISTS This group of drugs is used mainly to relieve severe vomiting caused by chemotherapy for certain types of cancer. Serotonin antagonists, which include granisetron and ondansetron, are extremely effective, and have made chemotherapy more tolerable than it was in the past. The serotonin antagonist is started a few hours before chemotherapy begins and is continued for about an hour after the final dose of chemotherapy drugs is given. Serotonin antagonists may also be used to prevent vomiting that follows surgery carried out under general anaesthesia; the drugs are administered by injection immediately after the operation. Serotonin antagonists cause very few side effects.

OTHER DRUGS Metoclopramide is used to relieve nausea and vomiting, such as that caused by chemotherapy or associated with migraine. Side effects include muscle spasms, especially of the face.

Hyoscine hydrobromide may be prescribed to treat nausea associated with Ménière's disease and labyrinthitis. The drug may also be used to relieve motion sickness. It is available over the counter. Side effects may include a dry mouth, difficulty passing urine, drowsiness, and dizziness. You should not take hyoscine hydrobromide if you need to drive.

DRUG ACTION HOW ANTACIDS WORK

Antacids are used to treat symptoms caused by acid in the digestive juices. This acid may inflame eroded areas in the layer of mucus that lines the stomach, irritating the stomach walls.

Antacids are mild alkaline substances that are taken orally. They work by neutralizing acidity in the digestive juices, thereby allowing eroded areas in the mucus layer to recover.

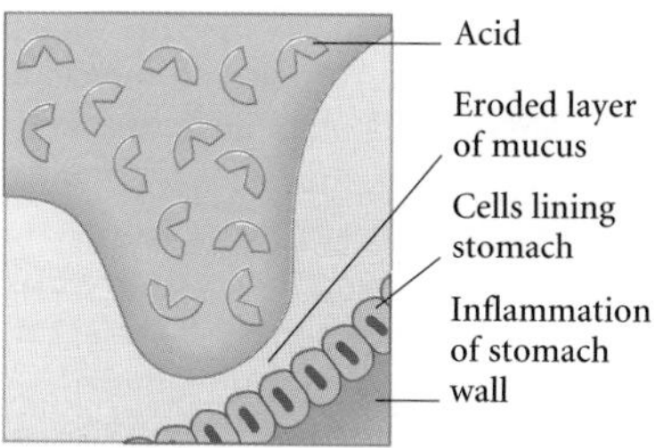

Before drug
The digestive juices contain acid, which may inflame eroded areas in the mucus layer and irritate the stomach lining.

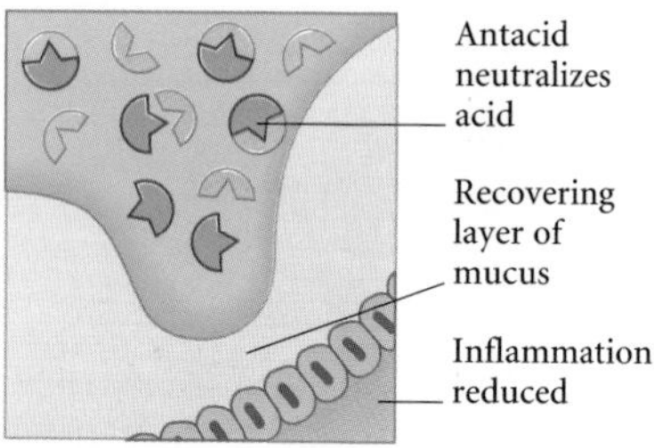

After drug
The antacid combines with some of the stomach acid and neutralizes it, reducing irritation of the stomach lining.

Antacids

Drugs that neutralize excess acid to relieve indigestion or help peptic ulcers to heal

COMMON DRUGS

• Activated dimeticone • Alginates • Aluminium hydroxide • Calcium carbonate • Magaldrate • Magnesium hydroxide • Sodium bicarbonate

Antacids are used to relieve upper abdominal discomfort caused by irritation of the stomach or duodenum (*see* INDIGESTION, p.626). Antacids can also relieve the discomfort caused by gastro-oesophageal reflux (p.636), in which stomach acid is regurgitated into the oesophagus. They may also help to ease symptoms due to peptic ulcers (p.640).

Antacid preparations may contain either aluminium or magnesium salts, both of which neutralize stomach acid (*see* HOW ANTACIDS WORK, above). Some contain additional ingredients such as activated dimeticone, which disperses bubbles of gas to reduce bloating, or alginates, which provide a protective coating for the oesophagus if regurgitation of the stomach contents occurs. If indigestion persists for more than a week, see your doctor.

WHAT ARE THE SIDE EFFECTS?

Most antacid preparations have very few side effects. However, antacids containing aluminium can occasionally cause constipation, while those that contain magnesium may cause diarrhoea. The antacid sodium bicarbonate may produce excess gas in the stomach, which can cause abdominal bloating. Sodium bicarbonate may cause fluid retention in people who have kidney disease or chronic heart failure (p.413) and should therefore be avoided by anyone with these conditions.

Consult your doctor before using antacids if you are already taking other medication; antacids can interfere with the body's absorption of certain drugs.

Ulcer-healing drugs

Drugs that reduce the secretion of acid by the stomach, helping peptic ulcers to heal

COMMON DRUGS

PROTON PUMP INHIBITORS
• Lansoprazole • Omeprazole

H_2 BLOCKERS
• Cimetidine • Famotidine • Nizatidine • Ranitidine

OTHER DRUGS
• Bismuth • Misoprostol • Sucralfate

Ulcer-healing drugs are used to treat peptic ulcers (p.640), which are eroded areas in the lining of the stomach or duodenum. One group of these drugs, called proton pump inhibitors, is used in combination with two antibiotics (p.885) to heal ulcers that are caused by the bacterium *Helicobacter pylori* (*see* HELICOBACTER PYLORI INFECTION, p.639). Ulcer-healing drugs may also be given without antibiotics to treat peptic ulcers and other digestive disorders that are not due to *H. pylori*, such as nonulcer dyspepsia (p.626).

WHAT ARE THE TYPES?

The two main groups of ulcer-healing drugs are proton pump inhibitors and H_2 blockers. Both of these types of drug work by reducing the production of acid in the stomach. Other drugs used to treat ulcers include misoprostol, sucralfate, and bismuth, which work by protecting the stomach lining from stomach acids. Ulcer-healing drugs are usually taken orally.

PROTON PUMP INHIBITORS Drugs in this group are given initially as a 4–6 week course, usually to reduce stomach acid and as part of the treatment regimen for ulcers caused by *H. pylori*. Antibiotics are included in this regimen for the first week or two. You may need to continue taking a lower dose of a proton pump inhibitor indefinitely to prevent ulcers from recurring. Proton pump inhibitors do not usually cause serious side effects, but you may have headaches, constipation, or diarrhoea. Other side effects may include dizziness, blurred vision, rashes, and muscle aches.

H_2 BLOCKERS These drugs are usually given as an initial course of 4–6 weeks to reduce stomach acid. You may then have to continue taking a lower dose to prevent ulcers from recurring. Some H_2 blockers can be bought over the counter for short-term treatment. Side effects are rare, but you may experience dizziness, tiredness, and rashes. In elderly people, the drugs can cause confusion.

OTHER DRUGS Your doctor may prescribe misoprostol if you need to take nonsteroidal anti-inflammatory drugs (p.894), such as ibuprofen, long term. These drugs may cause peptic ulcers if taken for a long time, and misoprostol prevents ulceration by protecting the lining of the stomach. Misoprostol can cause diarrhoea, which is sometimes severe. Less common side effects may include abdominal pain, nausea and vomiting, and flatulence. Do not take misoprostol if you are or may be pregnant; it can cause fetal abnormalities.

Sucralfate coats the ulcer, providing a barrier against stomach acid. This drug can cause constipation and indigestion. Less common side effects include diarrhoea, nausea, dizziness, and insomnia.

Bismuth seems to combat bacteria and protect ulcers from stomach acids. Side effects include a darkened tongue, black faeces, nausea, and vomiting.

Aminosalicylate drugs

A group of drugs used to reduce persistent inflammation of the intestines

COMMON DRUGS

- Balsalazide • Mesalazine • Olsalazine
- Sulfasalazine

Aminosalicylates are a group of anti-inflammatory drugs, chemically related to aspirin, that are used to treat persistent inflammation of the digestive tract. They work by suppressing the body's production of prostaglandins, which are naturally occurring chemicals that cause tissue inflammation. Aminosalicylates are often used to treat Crohn's disease (p.658), in which there is inflammation of parts of the digestive tract. They are also given to treat ulcerative colitis (p.659), in which only the large intestine is inflamed. The drugs can also be used to help to prevent attacks of these conditions.

Aminosalicylates are usually taken orally but may be given as enemas or suppositories if inflammation mainly affects the lower part of the large intestine. Treatment is started with a high dose. Dosage is then reduced to a lower level for long-term use.

WHAT ARE THE SIDE EFFECTS?

Aminosalicylates can cause side effects such as nausea, vomiting, abdominal pain, headache, rashes, and diarrhoea. Taking these drugs can also sometimes cause increased susceptibility to infections or abnormal bleeding.

CAUTION

If you are taking aminosalicylates, you should report any sign of infection, such as a sore throat, or any unusual bleeding or bruising to your doctor immediately.

Antidiarrhoeal drugs

Drugs that stop diarrhoea by slowing the passage of the intestinal contents or regulating the action of the intestine

COMMON DRUGS

OPIOIDS
- Codeine phosphate • Diphenoxylate
- Loperamide

BULK-FORMING AGENTS
- Bran • Ispaghula • Methylcellulose

ADSORBENTS
- Kaolin

Antidiarrhoeal drugs are used to relieve diarrhoea (p.627), which is the frequent passing of loose, watery faeces. They may be used as a short-term measure to control a sudden attack of diarrhoea or long term for diarrhoea that persists due to disorders such as diverticular disease (p.663) or irritable bowel syndrome (p.655). Some drugs also relieve abdominal pain associated with diarrhoea.

In most cases, an attack of diarrhoea clears up in about 48 hours and drug treatment is not normally required. Drinking plenty of fluids, but not milk, to compensate for the water that the body loses in diarrhoea is usually all that is needed. However, infants and young children are at higher risk of dehydration and may need to be given oral rehydration solutions (p.926). If an attack of diarrhoea lasts longer than 48 hours, consult your doctor. Do not give antidiarrhoeal drugs to children.

WHAT ARE THE TYPES?

The main types of antidiarrhoeal drug are opioids, bulk-forming agents, and adsorbents. All types of antidiarrhoeal drug should be taken with plenty of water to prevent constipation.

OPIOIDS These drugs reduce the muscle contractions of the intestine. As a result, the intestine moves faeces more slowly and therefore has more time to absorb water from food residue. Opioid drugs may also help to relieve pain in the lower abdomen associated with frequent contractions of the intestinal muscle.

Most opioid drugs can be obtained only on prescription. However, some opioids, such as loperamide, can be bought over the counter for the short-term treatment of diarrhoea.

BULK-FORMING AGENTS These preparations absorb water, resulting in larger and firmer stools produced at less frequent intervals. Bulk-forming agents are often given to regulate intestinal action over a long period if you have had an operation on your intestine, such as a colectomy (p.665), or if you have persistent diarrhoea due to a disorder such as diverticular disease. Since they help to regulate intestinal action, bulk-forming agents are sometimes also used as laxatives (below). Some types are available over the counter, others only on prescription. All types are usually supplied as granules, powder, or capsules. Do not take a bulk-forming agent when taking opioids; the combination could cause faeces to obstruct the intestine. Drink plenty of water when taking a bulk-forming agent.

ADSORBENTS These are substances that attract and bind to irritants in the intestine, such as harmful microorganisms. As the adsorbents are moved through the intestine and excreted, the irritants are carried with them. Like bulk-forming agents, adsorbents are used to control the consistency of the faeces and to regulate intestinal action. They are usually used to treat mild diarrhoea. The adsorbent kaolin can be purchased over the counter.

Laxatives

Drugs used to relieve constipation or clear the intestine before a medical procedure

COMMON DRUGS

BULK-FORMING AGENTS
- Bran • Ispaghula • Methylcellulose

OSMOTIC LAXATIVES
- Lactulose • Magnesium salts • Phosphates
- Sodium citrate

FAECAL SOFTENERS/LUBRICANTS
- Liquid paraffin

STIMULANT LAXATIVES
- Bisacodyl • Dantron • Docusate • Glycerol
- Senna • Sodium picosulfate

Laxatives make faeces pass more easily through the intestines. They are most commonly used to treat constipation (p.628), the difficult, infrequent passing of stools that are hard and dry. However, laxatives may be prescribed for other reasons. For example, they may be given to clear the intestine before a colonoscopy (p.661), in which an instrument for viewing the colon is passed through the anus. Laxatives may also be prescribed to counteract the constipating effect of other drugs such as morphine or codeine.

Laxatives can be purchased over the counter. If you are taking laxatives for constipation, use them only until your bowel movements have returned to normal. If the constipation continues for more than a few days, you should see your doctor. Do not take more than the recommended dose because some laxatives can cause severe abdominal pain. Never give laxatives to children without first consulting your doctor.

What are the types?

Laxatives can be classified into different types, depending on how they work. Bulk-forming agents, osmotic laxatives, and faecal softeners all make stools softer and easier to pass. Stimulant laxatives make the intestinal muscles move faeces more rapidly. Most laxatives are taken orally, but some osmotic and stimulant laxatives may be administered as enemas or suppositories.

BULK-FORMING AGENTS These preparations cause the faeces to retain water, keeping them soft and increasing their volume, and thereby stimulating intestinal muscle action. They are mainly available as granules or powders that are taken orally. It may take several days for these agents to have their full effect.

Bulk-forming agents are mostly prescribed to treat long-term constipation. For example, they may be used in the treatment of irritable bowel syndrome (p.655) or diverticular disease (p.663). You may also be given bulk-forming agents to make passing stools easier after childbirth or abdominal surgery.

Bulk-forming laxatives are the safest type of preparation for the long-term treatment of constipation because their action is similar to the natural action of fibre in food (*see* DIET AND HEALTH, pp.48–54). You should be sure to drink plenty of water when taking these laxatives because the bulky stools may otherwise eventually block the intestine. Side effects of bulk-forming laxatives may include excess intestinal gas and abdominal pain and bloating.

DRUG ACTION

How bulk-forming laxatives work

Bulk-forming agents are often used as laxatives and are used mainly to treat constipation, when faeces are hard and painful to pass. Bulk-forming agents act on the large intestine, causing faecal matter to retain water as it moves through the intestine. This makes faeces softer and easier to pass.

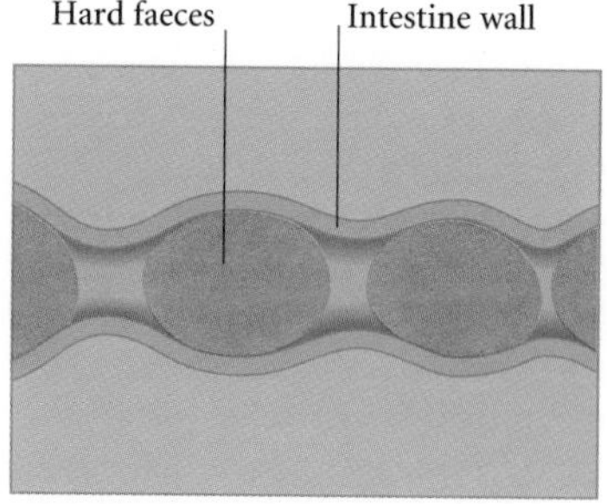

Before drug
Faecal matter does not retain much water as it passes slowly through the intestine, resulting in dry, hard faeces that are difficult to pass.

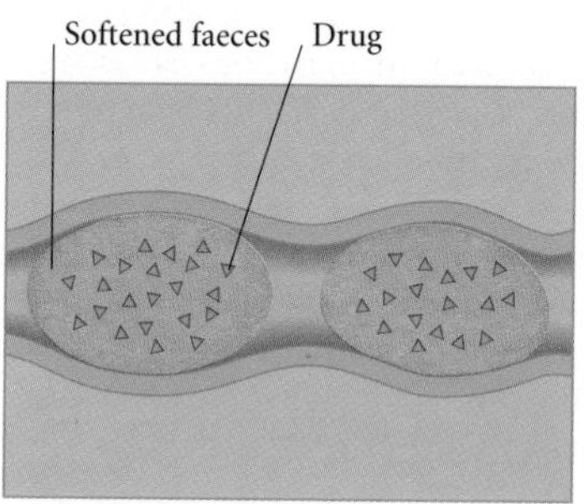

After drug
The bulk-forming agent mixes with faecal matter, causing it to retain water as it passes through the intestine. This produces faeces that are soft and bulky.

OSMOTIC LAXATIVES These drugs work by preventing the body from removing water from faeces. As a result, the faeces stay soft, but they do not increase in bulk as happens with bulk-forming laxatives. Osmotic laxatives are available only on prescription. The most commonly prescribed osmotic laxative is lactulose, which is a synthetic form of sugar that the body does not absorb. Lactulose can cause side effects such as intestinal gas and abdominal cramps, which may gradually lessen with continued use. In elderly people, long-term use of lactulose can eventually cause dehydration and lead to a chemical imbalance in the blood.

Other drugs that keep water in the intestines, including magnesium salts, phosphates, and sodium citrate, may be used to achieve rapid bowel evacuation, particularly before procedures such as colonoscopy, radiological investigation, or surgery on the lower digestive tract. Some of these laxatives are taken orally, others are given by enema. They work by drawing water into the gut from the body and therefore may cause dehydration. You should be sure to drink plenty of water when taking these laxatives. Side effects may include intestinal gas and abdominal bloating.

FAECAL SOFTENERS These laxatives act by softening faeces. They also lubricate faecal matter, enabling it to pass more easily through the intestine. Docusate can be taken orally as liquid or capsules, or used as an enema. Liquid paraffin (mineral oil) is a commonly used faecal softener that is taken orally. It is available over the counter, but you should not take this laxative over a long period because it can cause anal irritation. Liquid paraffin can also prevent your body from absorbing certain vitamins, which may lead to nutritional deficiencies (p.630) in the long term.

STIMULANT LAXATIVES These laxatives stimulate the intestinal muscles to contract more strongly, resulting in more frequent bowel movements. Stimulant laxatives are sometimes used to clear the intestines quickly if other drugs have failed to work. Some of these drugs can be bought over the counter. You should not take stimulant laxatives regularly because your body may come to depend on them to stimulate bowel movements. Side effects commonly include abdominal cramps and diarrhoea. Dantron may colour the urine red.

CAUTION

When taking a bulk-forming laxative such as bran, be sure to drink plenty of water; otherwise, the bulky faeces that are produced may cause an intestinal blockage.

Antispasmodic drugs and motility stimulants

Drugs used to relieve muscle spasms in the intestine or to stimulate the passage of food through the digestive tract

COMMON DRUGS

DIRECT SMOOTH-MUSCLE RELAXANTS
• Alverine • Mebeverine • Peppermint oil

ANTICHOLINERGIC DRUGS
• Atropine • Dicycloverine (Dicyclomine)
• Hyoscine • Propantheline

MOTILITY STIMULANT DRUGS
• Domperidone • Metoclopramide

Antispasmodics and motility stimulants regulate the waves of muscular contraction that propel food through the digestive tract. Both these types of drug are used to treat conditions caused by abnormal muscle action in the digestive tract, including irritable bowel syndrome (p.655) and diverticular disease (p.663). In some cases, these drugs may be used to relieve the symptoms of nonulcer dyspepsia (p.626). Motility stimulants are also used to treat gastro-oesophageal reflux (p.636), a condition in which acidic stomach contents are regurgitated into the oesophagus.

Changes in diet, such as altering the amount of fibre eaten, may help to regulate intestinal contractions in people with conditions such as irritable bowel syndrome. Other changes in lifestyle, such as decreasing your alcohol intake and learning how to reduce stress, may also help. Your doctor may initially suggest that you make such changes to see whether they bring about an improvement. However, if self-help measures are not effective, your doctor may recommend that you take antispasmodic drugs or motility stimulants.

WHAT ARE THE TYPES?

Antispasmodic drugs can be classified into two groups: direct smooth-muscle relaxants and anticholinergic drugs. Both types of drug may be used to relieve the abdominal pain that occurs in gastrointestinal conditions such as irritable bowel syndrome and diverticular disease. Motility stimulants are usually given to relieve some of the symptoms caused by nonulcer dyspepsia and gastro-oesophageal reflux.

DIRECT SMOOTH-MUSCLE RELAXANTS These drugs have a direct action on the intestinal wall, which contains smooth muscle. Direct smooth-muscle relaxants work by causing the muscle to relax, thereby relieving painful intestinal cramps. The drugs are taken orally. Some preparations containing low doses of direct smooth-muscle relaxants are available over the counter.

It is important to drink plenty of water if you are taking direct smooth-muscle relaxants because otherwise an intestinal blockage may occur. These drugs occasionally cause headache or nausea. Peppermint oil capsules can irritate the mouth or oesophagus; for this reason, they should always be swallowed whole with plenty of water.

ANTICHOLINERGIC DRUGS These drugs help to reduce muscle spasm by lessening the transmission of nerve signals to the intestinal wall. Anticholinergics are usually taken orally and are available by prescription only.

Side effects of anticholinergic drugs may include headache, constipation, a dry mouth, flushed skin, and blurred vision. These drugs may also cause difficulty in passing urine. Children and elderly people in particular are at risk of developing side effects.

MOTILITY STIMULANT DRUGS Motility stimulants work primarily by causing the contents of the stomach to empty into the small intestine more rapidly than would otherwise happen. In this way, they help to prevent the occurrence of gastro-oesophageal reflux and relieve attacks of nonulcer dyspepsia. Motility stimulant drugs also cause the muscular valve between the stomach and the oesophagus to close with more force. This also helps to prevent gastro-oesophageal reflux from occurring.

Motility stimulant drugs are usually taken orally. They are available by prescription only. These drugs may cause a number of different side effects, including abdominal cramps and diarrhoea, headaches, and dizziness. Metoclopramide and domperidone may occasionally cause uncontrollable muscle spasms, particularly of the face, tongue, mouth, and neck. These muscle spasms are more likely to occur in children and young adults, particularly women. Both drugs are also used to relieve nausea and vomiting (*see* ANTIEMETIC DRUGS, p.922)

> **CAUTION**
>
> When taking a direct smooth-muscle relaxant such as alverine, drink plenty of water to prevent intestinal blockage. Do not take these drugs before going to bed.

Oral rehydration solutions

Preparations used to treat dehydration resulting from diarrhoea and vomiting

Oral rehydration solutions are made up of water and essential minerals, such as sodium and potassium, that are lost during severe attacks of diarrhoea (p.627) or vomiting. Usually, drinking plenty of fluids to replace the water that the body loses in diarrhoea or vomiting is the only treatment needed for adults. However, it may be necessary to give oral rehydration solutions to treat fluid loss that occurs in infants and young children. These groups are at a higher risk of dehydration because any water lost accounts for a higher proportion of the total water content in their bodies.

Rehydration solutions contain the minerals sodium, which is necessary for the body to retain water, and potassium, which is vital for the functioning of nerves and muscle. Both these minerals may be lost very quickly and in large amounts as a result of diarrhoea and vomiting. Oral rehydration solutions also contain glucose, a sugar that improves the absorption of sodium and water through the wall of the intestine and into the bloodstream.

Rehydration solutions can be purchased over the counter as soluble tablets or as powder for reconstitution with water. Some are flavoured to make them more palatable.

You should make sure that you store any unused rehydration solution in a refrigerator. However, if this is kept for longer than 24 hours it should then be discarded. When used according to instructions, oral rehydration solutions do not cause side effects.

VITAMIN AND MINERAL SUPPLEMENTS

A well-balanced diet should contain adequate amounts of all vitamins and minerals required for health. For most people, supplements are unnecessary, and high doses may even be harmful. However, certain groups of people are vulnerable to vitamin or mineral deficiencies. Doctors may prescribe vitamin or mineral supplements for people in these groups to prevent a deficiency or to treat a deficiency that has already developed.

Groups who are particularly prone to developing vitamin and mineral deficiencies include young children, pregnant women, and elderly people, especially those who live alone. Those who are seriously ill due to injury or long-term illness, or those who have disorders that impair their ability to absorb nutrients from the digestive tract (*see* MALABSORPTION, p.656), are also at increased risk of deficiencies, not only of vitamins and minerals but also of other nutrients (*see* NUTRITIONAL DEFICIENCIES, p.630). These people may require dietary supplementation with extra proteins, carbohydrates, and fats as well as vitamins and minerals. In the case of individuals who are unable to eat and drink normally because of illness, such as a stroke or other neurological disorder, which prevents them from swallowing, nutrients sometimes have to be given in a liquid form by tube, either through the nose down to the stomach or directly into the stomach. More rarely, in people who have very severe intestinal disorders, nutrients may be administered directly into the bloodstream through a vein.

The body needs some nutrients, such as carbohydrates, proteins, and fats, in relatively large quantities but requires vitamins and minerals in only small amounts. The articles in this section describe the vitamins and minerals that doctors most commonly prescribe as dietary supplements. The first article deals with vitamins and the second with minerals.

Vitamins

Chemical compounds that enable the body to carry out essential functions

Vitamins are complex chemicals that are essential for the normal growth, development, and functioning of the body. The principal source of most vitamins, except vitamin D and vitamin K, is a balanced diet (*see* GOOD SOURCES OF VITAMINS AND MINERALS, p.51).

Most people do not need vitamin supplements. However, these treatments may be prescribed for people who have conditions such as alcohol dependence (p.564) that deplete the body's supply of certain vitamins. Supplements may also be prescribed for people who need larger than normal quantities of certain vitamins because they are recovering from serious injuries or they are taking medications that affect the action or absorption of particular vitamins.

WHAT ARE THE TYPES?

Many types of vitamin are necessary for the maintenance of good health. They are broadly categorized into two main groups: fat-soluble and water-soluble. Fat-soluble vitamins, such as A, D, E, and K, are not readily excreted in urine. They are stored in fatty body tissues, such as the liver, for long periods and do not normally need to be supplemented by a daily intake. Water-soluble vitamins, which include B, C, and folic acid, are rapidly excreted in urine. The body cannot hold long-term reserves of these vitamins, and they must be replaced on a daily basis through food sources to prevent deficiencies.

VITAMIN A This vitamin is required for growth, healthy skin and surface tissues, and good eyesight and night vision. Vitamin A is also necessary for fertility in both sexes. Supplements may be prescribed for people with conditions that can cause deficiency of this vitamin, such as certain intestinal disorders. Diets that are too low in fat may also lead to vitamin A deficiency.

Taking excessive doses of vitamin A can cause dry skin, nosebleeds, and hair loss. You should not take vitamin A supplements if you are either pregnant or planning to become pregnant because taking too much of this vitamin may cause fetal abnormalities.

> WARNING
>
> Vitamin A may harm a developing fetus. Do not take supplements if you are pregnant or planning to conceive, except on medical advice.

VITAMIN B_1 (THIAMINE) This vitamin is necessary for the normal functioning of the brain and peripheral nerves, the heart, and the muscles. Thiamine is present in unprocessed food, and most people should be able to obtain enough by eating a balanced diet. A severe lack of thiamine can cause certain deficiency diseases, such as beriberi, which affects the nervous system. Your doctor may prescribe supplements for conditions in which severe thiamine deficiency can occur, such as alcohol dependence (p.564) or alcohol-related liver disease (p.646).

The risk of developing side effects from thiamine supplements is very low. However, in some cases this vitamin may cause serious allergic reactions.

VITAMIN B_3 (NIACIN) This vitamin, also known as nicotinic acid, plays a vital role in the activities of many enzymes involved in digestion. Niacin is also essential for the production of the sex hormones oestrogen, progesterone, and testosterone. Severe niacin deficiency can result in the skin disorder pellagra. You may be prescribed niacin supplements if you have alcohol-related liver disease or a bowel disorder that results in poor absorption of food, a condition known as malabsorption (p.656).

Large doses of niacin inhibit the body's synthesis of some fats and are used to treat high levels of cholesterol and triglycerides (*see* LIPID-LOWERING DRUGS, p.935). Niacin may cause some side effects, including itching, flushing, and headaches. If excessive amounts of niacin are taken, liver damage and gout (p.380) can occur as a result.

VITAMIN B_6 (PYRIDOXINE) Vitamin B_6 helps the body to process proteins, fats, and carbohydrates in food and is needed to help the central nervous system to function correctly. Supplements may be given to relieve the symptoms of premenstrual syndrome (p.736), but there is little evidence that this treatment is effective. Supplements may also be given to relieve morning sickness during pregnancy (*see* COMMON COMPLAINTS OF NORMAL PREGNANCY, p.784). Excessive doses may lead to nerve damage, which can result in numbness and impaired physical coordination.

VITAMIN B_{12} (COBALAMIN) This vitamin is essential for the formation of red blood cells. The most common cause of vitamin B_{12} deficiency is pernicious anaemia (*see* MEGALOBLASTIC ANAEMIA, p.448), in which a substance necessary for the absorption of vitamin B_{12} is not produced by the body. Vegan diets may also result in deficiency because the best dietary sources of vitamin B_{12} are animal products such as eggs and milk.

Treatment for pernicious anaemia involves regular injections of hydroxycobalamin (a synthesized form of the vitamin). Side effects are very uncommon but can include itching, flushing, and nausea. If deficiency results from a vegan diet, oral supplements of cobalamin may be required.

FOLIC ACID This vitamin is needed for nervous system function and for the formation of red blood cells. Dietary sources include green leafy vegetables, liver, and nuts. Supplements may be advised if you are taking certain drugs, including some antimalarials (p.888) or anticonvulsant drugs (p.914), which deplete folic acid. Folic acid also lowers levels of the amino acid homocysteine, high levels of which may increase the risk of coronary artery disease (p.405).

Women are advised to take folic acid supplements if they are planning to become pregnant and for at least the first 12 weeks of pregnancy to reduce the risk of neural tube defects (p.844) in the fetus, such as spina bifida. The vitamin has no harmful side effects.

> **WARNING**
>
> Do not exceed the prescribed dose of vitamin D. Excessive intake can cause a dangerous rise in the level of calcium in the blood.

VITAMIN C This vitamin is needed for the formation of bones, teeth, ligaments, and blood vessels. It is found in fresh fruit and vegetables, and therefore severe deficiency is uncommon. If it does occur, a severe deficiency causes a disorder called scurvy, which is rare in developed countries. However, mild deficiency is common among people who eat a poor diet, and particularly among elderly people living alone.

Supplements of vitamin C may be prescribed after serious injury or burns because the vitamin is used up more quickly than normal during the healing process. In some cases, iron supplements are combined with vitamin C because the vitamin improves the efficiency of iron absorption by the body.

VITAMIN D This vitamin helps to regulate the amount of calcium in the body. The body's requirements for the vitamin are usually met by normal diet and exposure to sunlight, which the body needs to make vitamin D. A vitamin D deficiency can cause a disorder in which the bones become weak and soft (*see* OSTEOMALACIA AND RICKETS, p.370).

Vitamin D supplements may be given to increase calcium levels in people with hypoparathyroidism (p.683); in this disorder the body produces too little of a hormone called parathyroid hormone, which controls levels of calcium in the blood. Supplements are sometimes given to elderly people and to premature infants, who may not obtain enough dietary vitamin D. They may also be given in combination with calcium to prevent or treat osteoporosis (p.368).

Taking high doses of vitamin D may increase levels of calcium in the body, which may lead to calcium deposits in soft tissues, impaired kidney function, or impaired growth in children.

VITAMIN E This vitamin is an important antioxidant, meaning that it protects cell membranes from the damaging effects of particles known as free radicals, which are thought to cause tissue damage. Premature babies are deficient in vitamin E and may develop a form of anaemia if they do not receive supplements. Deficiency also occurs in people who cannot absorb fat, especially those with cystic fibrosis (p.824). Supplements may be prescribed to treat malabsorption in children, heart disease, and, in women, fibrocystic breast disease (*see* BREAST LUMPS, p.754), although its effectiveness has not been proved. Vitamin E is also used in skin creams. Overly high doses of vitamin E can cause diarrhoea and abdominal pain.

VITAMIN K This vitamin is essential for the formation of blood clotting factors, substances that are necessary for blood to clot and seal off damaged blood vessels. Most of the required amount is produced by bacteria in the intestines, but the body also obtains some vitamin K from dietary sources, such as green leafy vegetables, eggs, and liver.

Newborn babies lack the intestinal bacteria that produce vitamin K and, as a result, are at risk of developing a condition called haemorrhagic disease of the newborn, which results in easy bruising and internal bleeding. For this reason, newborn babies are given vitamin K routinely. Supplements may be given to older children and adults taking antibiotics for long periods because these drugs destroy the intestinal bacteria that produce vitamin K. In addition, people who are unable to absorb nutrients, or those who experience abnormal bleeding as a side effect of oral anticoagulant drugs (*see* DRUGS THAT PREVENT BLOOD CLOTTING, p.904), may be given supplements of this vitamin.

MULTIVITAMINS Preparations containing a combination of vitamins are used to treat people who have nutritional deficiencies, alcoholism, and other conditions in which dietary vitamin intake is insufficient. Some of these multivitamin preparations contain iron and other minerals. Multivitamins can be purchased over the counter, usually in the form of oral liquid, tablets, or capsules to be taken once daily.

Minerals

Chemical elements that enable the body to perform essential functions

Minerals are chemical elements that are necessary to maintain health. The body does not manufacture minerals and therefore it must obtain them from dietary sources (*see* GOOD SOURCES OF VITAMINS AND MINERALS, p.51).

Your doctor may prescribe mineral supplements if you have a medical condition that interferes with the ability of your body to absorb minerals (*see* MALABSORPTION, p.656) or if you need extra amounts of certain minerals, as may happen in pregnancy. Most people should not need mineral supplements because a balanced diet usually provides sufficient amounts. You should not take mineral supplements unless you need them because excessive doses of some minerals can be toxic.

WHAT ARE THE TYPES?

Many minerals are necessary to maintain good health. The most important minerals prescribed to treat deficiencies include iron, calcium, magnesium, zinc, fluoride, iodine, and phosphorus.

IRON This mineral is a vital component of haemoglobin, the oxygen-carrying pigment in blood. A correctly balanced diet usually provides sufficient supplies of iron but deficiency sometimes occurs in women with heavy menstrual periods (*see* MENORRHAGIA, p.735), pregnant women, and women who have recently given birth. Vegans, and people who have persistent blood loss due to conditions such as a peptic ulcer (p.640), may also be deficient in iron.

Iron is usually taken orally as a liquid or tablets and can be purchased over the counter. Side effects of taking iron supplements may include darker stools, constipation or diarrhoea, nausea, and abdominal pain. In certain cases when the body cannot absorb sufficient iron from the digestive tract, for example following extensive bowel surgery, injections of iron may be needed. Although these injections are given deep into muscle, staining of the skin at the injection site may result.

> **WARNING**
>
> Iron swallowed in relatively small amounts can cause potentially fatal poisoning in children. Keep your medicines in a safe place and seek urgent medical help if you suspect that a child has taken any tablets.

CALCIUM This mineral is essential for the formation and maintenance of the bones and teeth, as well as for muscle contraction and the transmission of nerve impulses. Dairy products in the diet usually provide sufficient calcium.

Oral supplements are sometimes prescribed for women who are pregnant or breast-feeding because both fetal bone formation and maternal milk production require large amounts of calcium. Elderly people may need supplements because the body absorbs calcium less efficiently with age. Calcium supplements may also be prescribed to prevent bone disorders such as osteoporosis (p.368) and to increase blood levels of calcium in people who have hypoparathyroidism (p.683) or kidney failure (p.705). In addition, calcium may be given by intravenous injection to treat cardiac arrest (p.419). Severe calcium deficiency leads to cramps and muscle spasms and may be treated with calcium injections. Side effects of calcium include constipation and nausea.

MAGNESIUM This mineral is needed for healthy teeth and bones, muscle action, and transmission of nerve impulses. Magnesium supplements may be prescribed for certain conditions that can interfere with the absorption of magnesium from food, including alcohol dependence (p.564), repeated vomiting, or long-term diarrhoea. Excessive doses of magnesium may cause nausea, vomiting, diarrhoea, and dizziness.

ZINC This mineral is used for growth and to help wounds to heal efficiently. Zinc deficiency is rarely seen in developed countries; it usually occurs only in malnourished elderly people, and may also occur in people with severe burns or other traumatic injury because zinc is used up rapidly in the healing process. In these cases, zinc supplements are sometimes prescribed. Zinc is usually taken orally but may also be given as a topical treatment for skin disorders, such as nappy rash. Taking overly large doses of oral zinc may cause side effects such as fever, nausea, vomiting, headaches, and abdominal pain.

FLUORIDE The mineral fluoride helps to prevent tooth decay and makes bones stronger. Water is very often the main dietary source because fluoride occurs naturally in some water supplies or is added to the drinking water in many areas. Fluoride is also an ingredient in most toothpastes. Your dentist may recommend fluoride supplements in the form of drops or tablets if the water in your area is not fluoridated or if you are susceptible to dental caries (p.609). If you take excessive amounts of fluoride, you may develop a condition known as fluorosis, in which the tooth enamel becomes brown or mottled (*see* DISCOLOURED TEETH, p.612).

IODINE This mineral is essential for the formation of thyroid hormones, which control the rate at which the body uses energy and which are vital for normal growth in childhood. Supplements are rarely needed because sufficient iodine is usually present in the diet. Important sources of iodine include seafood, bread, and dairy products. Radioactive iodine may be given to people with a goitre (p.680) or hyperthyroidism (p.679) in order to shrink the thyroid gland. Excessive amounts of iodine can suppress the activity of the thyroid gland, leading to hypothyroidism (p.680).

PHOSPHORUS The mineral phosphorus is an essential part of the diet. It is present in many foods, including cereals, dairy products, eggs, and meat. Much of the phosphorus contained in the body is combined with calcium to form the structure of the bones and teeth. Hypophosphataemia, in which the body contains an abnormally low level of phosphorus, may occur in some forms of kidney disease, hyperparathyroidism (p.682), and malabsorption.

Deficiencies of this mineral can be treated with phosphate supplements. In addition, hypercalcaemia, in which blood levels of calcium are abnormally high, may be treated using phosphates. Diarrhoea is a potential side effect of taking phosphate supplements.

DRUGS ACTING ON THE ENDOCRINE SYSTEM AND METABOLISM

Disorders of the endocrine system and metabolism, such as diabetes mellitus and hypothyroidism, may have wide-ranging, serious effects, and in some cases may be fatal if left untreated. Drug treatments can control the symptoms of these disorders and in many cases restore normal health to affected people.

The first article in this section covers corticosteroids, which are synthetic hormones that are chiefly used to treat inflammation in a variety of disorders and may also be used as hormone replacement therapy. The next four articles discuss drugs that control levels of insulin, thyroid hormones, and sex hormones in the body. Drugs that replace, inhibit, or stimulate some of the many hormones produced by the pituitary gland, which is the major hormone-secreting gland in the body, are covered next. The final article looks at lipid-lowering drugs, which control disorders in which the blood contains excessive levels of lipids (fats and related substances).

Topical corticosteroids (p.892), which are used to treat certain skin disorders, are covered elsewhere, as are locally acting corticosteroids (p.895), which are used in the treatment of inflamed joints or muscles.

KEY ANATOMY

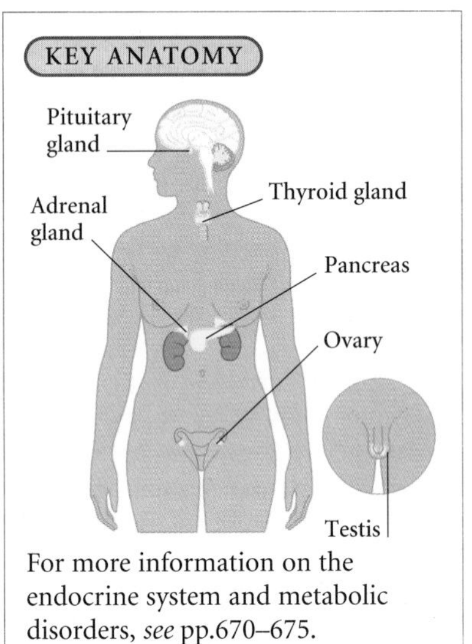

For more information on the endocrine system and metabolic disorders, *see* pp.670–675.

Corticosteroids

Drugs similar to the natural corticosteroid hormones produced by the adrenal gland

COMMON DRUGS

- Beclometasone • Betamethasone • Cortisone
- Dexamethasone • Fludrocortisone
- Fluocinolone • Fluticasone • Hydrocortisone
- Methylprednisolone • Prednisolone
- Triamcinolone

Corticosteroids are related to corticosteroid hormones produced by the body. The production of corticosteroid hormones by the adrenal glands is regulated by corticotropin, a pituitary hormone.

The main use for corticosteroid drugs is in the treatment of inflammatory conditions that may affect the joints, skin, digestive tract, respiratory system, eyes, and ears. These drugs are also prescribed as replacement therapy if the body is unable to produce sufficient natural corticosteroid hormones on its own (*see* ADDISON'S DISEASE, p.686, and HYPOPITUITARISM, p.678).

In addition, corticosteroids may be given as long-term treatment following transplant surgery because their action suppresses the body's immune system. This action helps to prevent rejection of the transplanted organs or tissue.

HOW DO THEY WORK?

Corticosteroids reduce inflammation by blocking the production of natural substances that trigger inflammation, such as prostaglandins. The drugs suppress the immune system by reducing the production and effectiveness of certain white blood cells that are an important part of the body's immune response.

HOW ARE THEY USED?

Corticosteroids can be given in a variety of ways. The drugs may be injected directly into body tissues near inflamed areas such as tendons (*see* LOCALLY ACTING CORTICOSTEROIDS, p.895). Used in this way, they may improve symptoms in joint disorders such as osteoarthritis (p.374). Frequent injections are avoided because of the risk of side effects.

Topical corticosteroids (p.892) in the form of creams or ointments are used to reduce inflammation and itching in some skin conditions. Oral corticosteroids are used for severe rheumatoid arthritis (p.377) and respiratory disorders such as asthma (p.483), sarcoidosis (p.498), and fibrosing alveolitis (p.497). Oral corticosteroids are also used after transplant surgery (*see* IMMUNOSUPPRESSANTS, p.906) and to treat Addison's disease and hypopituitarism. The drugs may also be injected into the bloodstream to treat severe Addison's disease or the dangerous allergic reaction anaphylaxis (p.469). In addition, the drugs can be given by inhaler to prevent asthma attacks (*see* CORTICOSTEROIDS FOR RESPIRATORY DISEASE, p.911).

WHAT ARE THE SIDE EFFECTS?

Short-term use of corticosteroids rarely produces side effects. Such effects are also rare in long-term corticosteroid replacement therapy for Addison's disease and hypopituitarism because the drugs replace the natural hormones that the body lacks. Doctors use corticosteroids as sparingly as possible for other conditions because of side effects.

Prolonged use of strong topical corticosteroid drugs can damage the skin in the affected areas, causing thinning, wrinkling, and loss of pigmentation. Particular care is needed when using these drugs on the face or on a baby's skin. Locally injected or inhaled corticosteroids are unlikely to cause serious side effects, but both may cause local problems. For example, inhaled drugs may cause minor throat infections.

Long-term treatment with oral corticosteroids may cause easy bruising, acne, a moon-shaped face, and weight gain (*see* CUSHING'S SYNDROME, p.684). Prolonged use of these drugs can also cause raised blood pressure and osteoporosis (p.368). Children who are taking corticosteroids will have their height carefully monitored during treatment, as the drugs can slow growth. The risk of infections, particularly of viral infections such as chickenpox, is increased by corticosteroids because the drugs suppress the immune system.

Corticosteroids suppress the body's own production of corticosteroid hormones. As a result, the body may not be able to produce sufficient corticosteroid hormones if treatment is stopped suddenly. An abrupt withdrawal from long-term, high-dose corticosteroids can lead to a rapid fall in blood pressure and, in some cases, shock (p.414), which can be fatal. If your doctor prescribes corticosteroid drugs for you for more than 3 weeks, you will be given a medical alert card that gives details of your medication to inform any health professional who treats you. You will also be warned to avoid coming into contact with anyone with chickenpox or shingles because of the risk of a severe infection. If you develop an infection or if you sustain injuries, a higher dose of corticosteroids may be needed.

Drugs for diabetes mellitus

Drugs used to treat diabetes mellitus that control blood glucose (sugar) levels

COMMON DRUGS

INSULIN

SULPHONYLUREA DRUGS
• Chlorpropamide • Glibenclamide
• Glimepiride • Glipizide • Tolbutamide

OTHER DRUGS FOR DIABETES
• Acarbose • Glucagon • Metformin
• Repaglinide • Rosiglitazone

In diabetes mellitus (p.687), levels of blood glucose are too high because the body produces too little or is resistant to the action of the hormone insulin, which is secreted by the pancreas and regulates blood glucose. Drugs for diabetes mellitus keep blood glucose at normal levels.

There are two types of diabetes mellitus. In type 1 diabetes, the body does not produce sufficient insulin, and synthetic insulin is needed. In type 2 diabetes, the body tissues have reduced sensitivity to the action of insulin. Mild forms of type 2 diabetes may be controlled by making changes to the diet and without having to use drugs.

WHAT ARE THE TYPES?

The main drugs for diabetes mellitus are insulin, which is always given for type 1 diabetes, and antidiabetic drugs, which are used to treat type 2 diabetes. The most common antidiabetic drugs are sulphonylurea drugs and metformin, but the drugs acarbose or repaglinide may also be prescribed. If antidiabetic drugs are ineffective, insulin may be used to treat cases of type 2 diabetes.

INSULIN Injections of insulin are given to replace missing natural insulin. This insulin replacement mimics the body's normal patterns of insulin production, maintaining low background levels of insulin with peaks at meal times when glucose enters the blood. All insulin was once extracted from pork or beef pancreas and modified for human use, but most insulin is now genetically engineered to be identical to human insulin.

There are several types of insulin preparation whose durations of action differ. Short-acting insulins are taken 15–30 minutes before meal times, giving high levels of insulin in the blood to coincide with high levels of glucose. Longer-acting insulins are taken once or twice a day. Many people take a combination of both types. The dose will be tailored to your individual needs.

Since insulin is destroyed by stomach acids it cannot be taken orally and is always injected. Your doctor or nurse will teach you how to inject insulin (*see* INJECTING INSULIN, p.688), and you will be shown how to measure your blood glucose levels (*see* MONITORING YOUR BLOOD GLUCOSE, p.689). You should measure your glucose levels at regular intervals during the day to see whether your insulin dose is at the correct level. For type 1 diabetes that is hard to control, continuous and timed doses of insulin can be given by a pump.

Taking excess insulin or too little food may cause hypoglycaemia (p.691), in which blood glucose levels are abnormally low. You will be taught how to recognize symptoms of this condition,

DRUG ACTION

HOW SULPHONYLUREA DRUGS WORK

Sulphonylurea drugs are used to treat type 2 diabetes. In this type of diabetes, body tissues have reduced sensitivity to insulin. Sulphonylurea drugs stimulate cells in the pancreas to secrete more insulin to compensate for the reduced sensitivity.

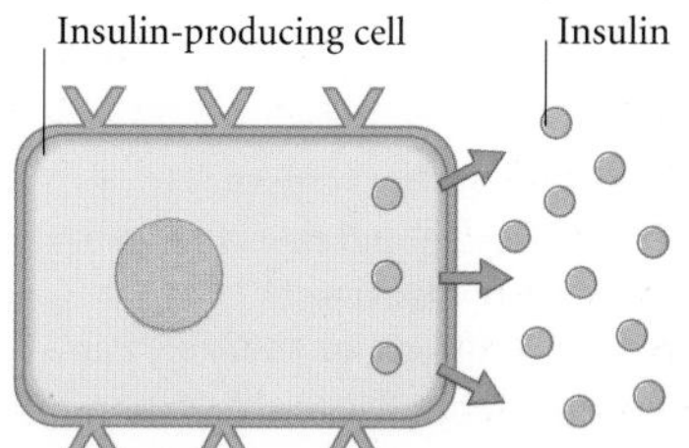

Before drug
The amount of insulin made by the insulin-secreting cells in the pancreas is not sufficient for the body's needs.

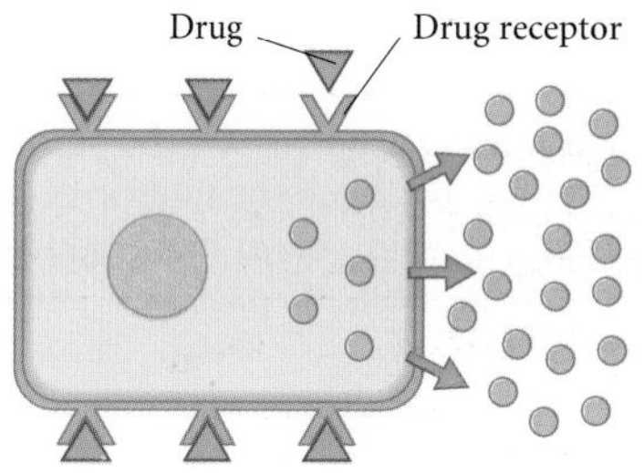

After drug
The sulphonylurea drug acts on the insulin-producing cells, stimulating them to increase production of insulin.

which include sweating, hunger, faintness, and anxiety. If you have an attack of hypoglycaemia, you should eat or drink something sweet immediately. An injection of glucagon, which increases blood glucose levels, may be given for severe hypoglycaemia.

Common injection sites for insulin include the abdomen and thighs. Some preparations contain an additive that can cause soreness and inflammation at the injection site when you start using insulin, but this is usually temporary.

SULPHONYLUREA DRUGS If changes in diet fail to control type 2 diabetes, you may be prescribed sulphonylurea drugs, which stimulate the insulin-producing cells in the pancreas to increase insulin production (*see* HOW SULPHONYLUREA DRUGS WORK, p.931). This helps to compensate for the low sensitivity of body tissues to insulin that occurs in type 2 diabetes. Sulphonylurea drugs are usually taken orally once or twice a day, and treatment is combined with dietary restrictions. However, in some people, weight gain is a side effect of these drugs.

OTHER DRUGS FOR DIABETES The drug metformin is often given to overweight people if dietary changes have not controlled their diabetes. Metformin can be used together with sulphonylurea drugs or rosiglitazone to increase the sensitivity of body tissue to insulin. Metformin also increases the utilization of glucose by the tissues.

Metformin is less likely to cause an attack of hypoglycaemia than sulphonylurea drugs, but it may initially cause nausea, diarrhoea, abdominal bloating, low appetite, and facial flushing. These side effects often stop after a few weeks.

Your doctor may prescribe either of the drugs acarbose and repaglinide for mild type 2 diabetes together with other treatments. Acarbose slows the absorption of glucose from the intestines and prevents a rapid rise in blood glucose levels after meals. Repaglinide stimulates the release of insulin from the pancreas. These drugs cause side effects in some people, including flatulence, abdominal discomfort, and diarrhoea.

Drugs for hypothyroidism

Synthetic thyroid hormones used to treat underactivity of the thyroid gland

COMMON DRUGS

• Levothyroxine (thyroxine) • Liothyronine

In hypothyroidism (p.680), the thyroid gland produces insufficient amounts of thyroid hormones, particularly thyroxine, causing symptoms such as tiredness and weight gain. This disorder can be caused by inflammation of the thyroid gland, known as thyroiditis (p.681), which may be either a short-term or long-term condition. Hypothyroidism may also be the result of previous radioiodine treatment for overactivity of the thyroid gland (*see* DRUGS FOR HYPERTHYROIDISM, right), or it may be present from birth (*see* INBORN ERRORS OF METABOLISM, p.867). Hypothyroidism usually needs lifelong treatment with synthetic thyroid hormones.

HOW ARE THEY USED?

Newborn babies who have hypothyroidism may initially need injections of the hormones. In adults, synthetic thyroid hormones are taken orally every day. Drugs are started at a low dose and the dose is increased gradually until an effective level is reached without causing side effects. The drugs take a few weeks to become effective, and it may take up to 6 months for symptoms to disappear completely.

WHAT ARE THE SIDE EFFECTS?

Given at the correct dose, synthetic thyroid hormones cause no side effects. To ensure that the correct dose is maintained, you will have regular blood tests. If the dose that you are given initially is too high, you may develop symptoms of hyperthyroidism (p.679), which may include tremor, weight loss, and rapid, sometimes irregular heartbeat. These symptoms will disappear once the correct dose for you has been established.

Drugs for hyperthyroidism

Drugs that are used to treat overactivity of the thyroid gland

COMMON DRUGS

ANTITHYROID DRUGS
• Carbimazole • Propylthiouracil

RADIOIODINE

Hyperthyroidism (p.679) is a disorder in which an overactive thyroid gland secretes excessive amounts of thyroid hormones. The symptoms of hyperthyroidism include weight loss, persistent tremor, and rapid, sometimes irregular heartbeat. Drugs for hyperthyroidism reduce the activity of the thyroid gland.

WHAT ARE THE TYPES?

An overactive thyroid gland may be treated using either antithyroid drugs or radioiodine. The drugs take several weeks to become effective, and a beta-blocker drug (p.898) may be prescribed in the interim. Beta-blockers are used to control symptoms of hyperthyroidism such as rapid heartbeat and tremor.

ANTITHYROID DRUGS These drugs are used for long-term treatment of hyperthyroidism. Rarely, they may be used in preparation for surgery to remove all or part of an overactive thyroid gland. The drugs decrease the production of thyroid hormones (*see* HOW ANTITHYROID DRUGS WORK, opposite page).

Carbimazole is the antithyroid drug that is most commonly used. Antithyroid drugs are taken on a daily basis. Symptoms of hyperthyroidism should begin to improve after about 10–20 days, and levels of thyroid hormones are usually reduced to normal over a period of 2–3 months. Drug treatment usually continues for 12–18 months, in which time the underlying disorder that is responsible for the hyperthyroidism may have cleared up.

During the treatment of hyperthyroidism, blood tests are performed on a regular basis to monitor levels of thyroid hormones in the blood so that the dose of antithyroid drugs can be adjusted if necessary. These tests are necessary to ensure that thyroxine levels do not become too high or too low.

The side effects of antithyroid drugs are usually minor and include nausea, headache, rashes, itching, and joint pains. Reduced production of white blood cells is a rare but potentially serious side effect that can occur during treatment with carbimazole. Decreased levels of these cells reduce the body's ability to fight infection. If you develop symptoms of an infection or a severe sore throat while taking carbimazole, inform your doctor immediately.

RADIOIODINE A radioactive form of iodine, called radioiodine, may be used to treat an overactive thyroid gland. Normally, the thyroid gland uses iodine

WARNING

If you are taking carbimazole and have symptoms of an infection, or a severe sore throat, you should contact your doctor at once. Do not take any more tablets until your doctor tells you it is safe to do so.

DRUG ACTION

How antithyroid drugs work

Antithyroid drugs are used to treat hyperthyroidism, in which the thyroid gland produces excessive quantities of hormones. Active hormones are formed when iodine combines with precursor (inactive) hormone. Antithyroid drugs block this combination, reducing the formation of thyroid hormones.

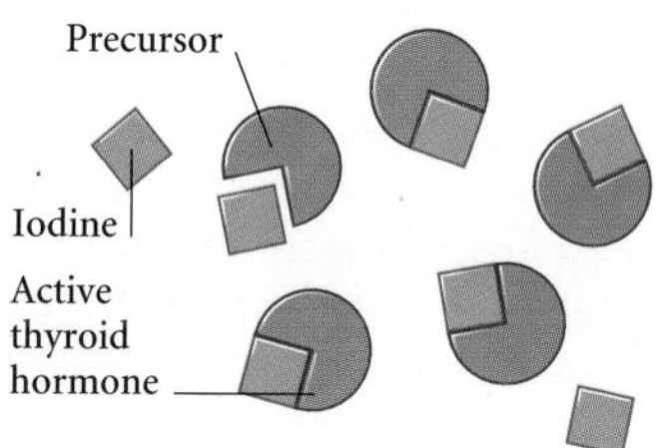

Before drug
Active thyroid hormone is formed when iodine binds to precursor (inactive) hormones in the thyroid gland.

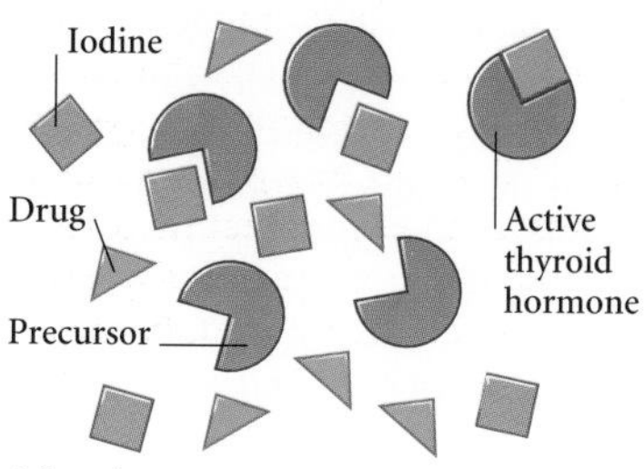

After drug
The drug prevents iodine binding to precursors, reducing the amount of active thyroid hormone produced.

from the diet to produce thyroid hormones. If radioiodine is given, it is taken up by the thyroid gland instead of normal iodine. The radioiodine then destroys part of the thyroid tissue, thereby reducing hormone production.

After treatment, levels of thyroid hormone should return to normal within 2–3 months. If the levels are still high after 4 months, you will probably be given a second dose of radioiodine.

Following this treatment, you may eventually develop the symptoms of hypothyroidism (p.680), such as dry, thickened skin, hair thinning, weight gain, and tiredness, because your thyroid gland has become underactive. Your doctor will regularly monitor the levels of thyroid hormones in your blood. If hormone levels become too low, you will need to take synthetic thyroid hormones to compensate (*see* DRUGS FOR HYPOTHYROIDISM, opposite page); it will be necessary to continue this treatment for the rest of your life. When given in correct doses, drugs for hypothyroidism cause no side effects.

Radioiodine treatment is not given during pregnancy because there is a risk of damage to the developing fetus.

Radioactive iodine may also be used following surgery to treat thyroid cancer (p.681) but at a much higher dose since the intention is to destroy any remaining thyroid tissue that may be cancerous. After undergoing this treatment, you will need to take synthetic thyroid hormones for life.

Sex hormones and related drugs

Drugs that are used to increase levels of female and male sex hormones or block their release or action

Common drugs

Female sex hormones
• Estradiol • Ethinylestradiol • Levonorgestrel • Medroxyprogesterone • Mestranol • Norgestrel • Tibolone

Anti-oestrogens
• Clomifene • Tamoxifen

Danazol

Male sex hormones
• Mesterolone • Testosterone

Antiandrogens
• Bicalutamide • Cyproterone acetate • Finasteride • Flutamide

Gonadorelin and gonadorelin analogues
• Buserelin • Gonadorelin • Goserelin • Leuprorelin • Nafarelin • Triptorelin

Various forms of sex hormones and sex hormone antagonists (chemicals that block the release or action of hormones) are used to treat disorders in which there are abnormally high or low levels of sex hormones in the body.

A brain area called the hypothalamus produces gonadotrophin-releasing hormone. This hormone then stimulates the further production of follicle-stimulating hormone (FSH) and luteinizing hormone (LH) by the pituitary gland, which is located at the base of the brain. FSH and LH, in turn, regulate sexual development by stimulating the release of the sex hormones: testosterone by the testes in males, and oestrogen and progesterone by the ovaries in females.

What are the types?

The hormones and drugs used to treat hormonal disorders in women include forms of the female hormones oestrogen and progesterone. Anti-oestrogens are sex hormone antagonists and may be used to block the action of oestrogen. The male hormone testosterone is used to treat certain hormonal disorders in boys and men; male sex hormone antagonists called antiandrogens may also be necessary to block the action of testosterone. Gonadorelin, a synthetic form of gonadotrophin-releasing hormone, and gonadorelin analogues, which block the release of gonadotrophin, are also used to treat hormonal disorders.

FEMALE SEX HORMONES Synthetic forms of the hormones oestrogen and progesterone have several uses. By far the most widespread use is as oral contraceptives (*see* CONTRACEPTION, p.69), in which the two hormones are taken together, or progesterone is taken alone, to prevent pregnancy. Oestrogen and progesterone are used in lower doses in hormone replacement therapy (p.937) to relieve the symptoms of the menopause and prevent long-term problems, such as osteoporosis (p.368). At higher doses, synthetic oestrogen and progesterone are prescribed to treat menstrual disorders such as heavy periods (*see* MENORRHAGIA, p.735).

The drugs may be administered by injection, taken orally, or used as skin patches, depending on the type of drug and the reason for its use. Side effects are most likely to occur at the higher doses and may include fluid retention, headache, nausea, weight gain, and depression. In addition, premenopausal women may experience some bleeding between periods while taking synthetic sex hormone drugs.

ANTI-OESTROGENS Clomifene is often used to treat infertility in women (*see* FEMALE INFERTILITY, p.775). Tamoxifen is used to treat and possibly prevent breast cancer (p.759). Prolonged use of anti-oestrogen drugs can cause various side effects. For example, some women experience vaginal bleeding, irregular periods or the suppression of menstruation, and hot flushes. Other possible side effects of anti-oestrogens include weight gain, nausea, vomiting, breast tenderness, and dizziness. More rarely, you may have visual disturbances while taking these drugs.

MALE SEX HORMONES Synthetic forms of male sex hormones are used to treat certain conditions caused by low levels of testosterone, including delayed puberty in boys (*see* ABNORMAL PUBERTY IN MALES, p.728) and decreased libido in men (*see* DECREASED SEX DRIVE, p.769). Given in low doses, synthetic testosterone mimics the action of the natural hormone, and side effects are rare.

ANTIANDROGENS Some antiandrogens, such as finasteride, are used to treat an enlarged prostate gland (p.725); others, such as flutamide, are used in the treatment of prostate cancer (p.726). In addition, virilization (p.740), in which women develop a number of masculine characteristics such as excessive facial and body hair, may also be treated using one of these drugs, usually cyproterone acetate. Antiandrogens act by blocking the action of the natural male sex hormones. A common side effect of treatment with antiandrogens is tiredness. The drugs can also affect liver function and are not normally given to anyone with a history of liver problems.

DANAZOL This drug inhibits pituitary gonadotrophins and so prevents ovulation. It is used to treat endometriosis (p.742) and menorrhagia. Side effects of danazol include hirsutism (excessive hair growth), acne, and voice changes, as well as changes in libido and disturbances to the menstrual cycle.

GONADORELIN AND GONADORELIN ANALOGUES Gonadorelin is a synthesized version of a natural hormone called gonadotrophin-releasing hormone. This drug is used to treat infertility and endometriosis in women. In infertility treatment, it is injected in short courses to stimulate LH and FSH secretion. Given in this way, the drug has few side effects. However, if given for longer periods, gonadorelin can reduce libido and cause rashes and hot flushes. Gonadorelin analogues are prescribed for certain female reproductive disorders, such as endometriosis; menstrual disorders, including heavy periods; and breast pain (p.756) associated with menstruation. These drugs may also be used to treat prostate cancer and, rarely, the excessive growth of breast tissue in men (*see* GYNAECOMASTIA, p.729). In a similar way to gonadorelin, their initial effect is to stimulate the release of LH and FSH from the pituitary gland. When given over a long period of time, gonadorelin analogues reduce production of these hormones. This, in turn, inhibits the release of oestrogen, progesterone, and testosterone. Gonadorelin analogues are given by injection or as a nasal spray. Side effects may include acne, nausea and vomiting, and headache. In premenopausal women these drugs may cause bleeding between periods, hot flushes, and increased sweating.

Pituitary drugs

Drugs that replace, stimulate, or inhibit some of the hormones produced by the pituitary gland

COMMON DRUGS

GROWTH HORMONE
- Somatropin

GROWTH HORMONE ANTAGONISTS
- Bromocriptine • Lanreotide • Octreotide

PROLACTIN INHIBITORS
- Bromocriptine • Cabergoline

DRUGS FOR DIABETES INSIPIDUS
- Desmopressin • Vasopressin

The pituitary gland, located at the base of the brain, produces a number of hormones. These hormones include growth hormone, prolactin, which controls the production of breast milk in women, and vasopressin, which regulates the function of the kidneys.

Drugs for pituitary disorders work in various ways. Some drugs are synthetic hormones that replace missing natural hormones, and others, known as antagonists, reduce the production or action of pituitary hormones.

Drugs that act on the hormones produced directly by the pituitary gland are discussed below. Other drugs whose action on the pituitary gland affects the production of hormones in other parts of the body are discussed elsewhere. These drugs include sex hormones and related drugs (p.933), drugs for infertility (p.936), corticosteroids (p.930), and drugs for labour (p.938).

WHAT ARE THE TYPES?

A number of drugs are used to treat pituitary disorders. Growth hormone and growth hormone antagonists are given to adjust levels of growth hormone that are either too low or too high. Prolactin inhibitors reduce levels of prolactin. The pituitary disorder diabetes insipidus (p.678), which results from insufficient vasopressin, is treated by replacement of the hormone with a synthetic equivalent.

GROWTH HORMONE If the pituitary gland does not secrete sufficient growth hormone during childhood, a synthetic form of the hormone can be prescribed to replace it. Low levels of growth hormone in childhood can cause impaired growth (*see* GROWTH DISORDERS, p.869). If a child begins the treatment at an early age, normal growth usually takes place. The drug is usually administered by injection 3–7 times a week, depending on the body's response. Treatment normally continues for several years until the child reaches adult height. Side effects may include aching muscles and joints and headaches.

GROWTH HORMONE ANTAGONISTS If too much growth hormone is produced by the pituitary gland, adults may be given growth hormone antagonists such as octreotide. Excess growth hormone can cause abnormal enlargement of certain parts of the body, particularly facial features, hands, and feet, a condition known as acromegaly (p.677). In adults, overproduction of growth hormone is most commonly caused by a pituitary tumour (p.676). Drugs that block the production of growth hormone may be prescribed as a temporary measure prior to surgery or radiotherapy; where surgery is not possible, they may be given long term.

The drugs octreotide and lanreotide are given by injection. Bromocriptine is taken orally. Possible side effects of octreotide and lanreotide include diarrhoea and cramping abdominal pain. Bromocriptine can cause nausea, vomiting, dizziness, and confusion.

PROLACTIN INHIBITORS These drugs are used to treat disorders in which excessive amounts of prolactin are produced by the pituitary gland. Excess prolactin may cause the production of breast milk in women who are not breast-feeding, and also in men. Overproduction of prolactin is often caused by a pituitary tumour called a prolactinoma (p.677). Drugs for a prolactinoma can be very effective, and surgery to remove the tumour may not be needed. The drugs bromocriptine and cabergoline may be used to suppress milk production in women who have given birth but for whom breast-feeding is inappropriate.

Prolactin inhibitors are most commonly taken orally. Side effects such as nausea and vomiting sometimes occur.

DRUGS FOR DIABETES INSIPIDUS You may be given vasopressin or a synthetic form of this hormone (desmopressin) if you have cranial diabetes insipidus (p.678). In this disorder, the pituitary gland produces insufficient vasopressin to regulate kidney function, which controls the amount of water retained in the body. It may also be given orally or as a nasal spray, usually twice a day.

Vasopressin or desmopressin may cause some side effects, including nausea, belching, and abdominal cramps.

Lipid-lowering drugs

Drugs used to reduce the level of lipids (fats and related substances) in the blood

COMMON DRUGS

STATINS
- Atorvastatin • Fluvastatin
- Pravastatin • Simvastatin

ANION-EXCHANGE RESINS
- Colestyramine • Colestipol

FIBRATES
- Bezafibrate • Fenofibrate • Gemfibrozil

NICOTINIC ACID

OTHER LIPID-LOWERING PRODUCTS
- Fish oil • Ispaghula

Lipid-lowering drugs reduce excessive levels of lipids, particularly cholesterol and triglycerides, in the bloodstream. Blood contains several types of lipids that are needed for normal body function. However, if lipids are present in excess, they can build up in the arteries (*see* ATHEROSCLEROSIS, p.402), and can cause serious disorders such as coronary artery disease (p.405), heart attack (*see* MYOCARDIAL INFARCTION, p.410), and stroke (p.532). In addition, high levels of triglycerides can sometimes result in inflammation of the pancreas (*see* ACUTE PANCREATITIS, p.652).

Elevated blood lipid levels can be reduced to some extent by weight loss, which will mean making changes to the diet (*see* DIET AND HEALTH, pp.48–54) and exercising. However, for some people, especially those with a family history of high blood lipid levels (*see* INHERITED HYPERLIPIDAEMIAS, p.692), drug treatment is also needed to lower the lipid levels. Drugs to reduce lipid levels may also be given to people with angina (p.407) to reduce the risk of having a heart attack, and after a heart attack to minimize the risk of further attacks.

WHAT ARE THE TYPES?

The main types of lipid-lowering drug include statins, anion-exchange resins, fibrates, and nicotinic acid and its derivatives. These drugs work in different ways to lower the levels of lipids in the blood. In addition, the natural dietary products ispaghula, which is a soluble fibre, or fish oil may be recommended.

Your doctor's choice of drug treatment will depend on which type of lipid is causing your condition. In some instances, your doctor may prescribe a combination of drugs. Lipid-lowering drugs are taken orally on a daily basis, and most need to be taken long term.

STATINS These drugs reduce the formation of cholesterol and triglycerides in the body. The side effects that may occur while taking statins include nausea, headaches, abdominal pain, and either diarrhoea or constipation. The drugs may also cause inflammation of the muscles. You should inform your doctor if you develop any unexplained muscle pain, tenderness, or weakness. You should also tell your doctor if you are planning a pregnancy, are pregnant, or are breast-feeding because statins can harm a fetus or baby.

ANION-EXCHANGE RESINS These drugs lower blood cholesterol levels by reducing fat absorption from the intestines. Anion-exchange resins may be used in combination with other lipid-lowering drugs, such as fibrates and statins. If you are being treated with other lipid-lowering drugs, you should take them at least 1 hour before or 3–4 hours after taking an anion-exchange resin because the resin can interfere with the absorption of other drugs.

Anion-exchange resins have few side effects, although they sometimes cause nausea, abdominal discomfort, and constipation. Supplements of vitamins A, D, and K may be necessary in long-term treatment with anion-exchange resins because the drugs reduce the body's absorption of these vitamins.

FIBRATES These drugs are effective in lowering levels of both cholesterol and triglycerides in the blood. Fibrates are unsuitable if you have a disorder of the kidneys, liver, or gallbladder. The drugs occasionally cause side effects, including muscle pain, nausea, headache, and impotence. Muscle pain may be more common if you have a disorder of the kidneys or are also receiving a statin. Fibrates can harm a fetus or baby, and it is important to tell your doctor if you are planning a pregnancy, are pregnant, or are breast-feeding.

NICOTINIC ACID Excessively high levels of cholesterol or triglycerides in the blood may be reduced by treatment with nicotinic acid. However, nicotinic acid often causes side effects and is generally used only when other drugs have proved ineffective. The side effects may include facial flushing, unsteadiness, headache, nausea and vomiting, and itching. Muscle pain may develop if this drug is used together with a statin. Women who are planning a pregnancy or who are pregnant or breast-feeding should avoid nicotinic acid because it may harm a fetus or baby.

OTHER LIPID-LOWERING PRODUCTS The natural products ispaghula and fish oil can reduce blood lipid levels when they are incorporated into the daily diet. Ispaghula is a non-absorbable fibre that helps to reduce high blood cholesterol levels, although its effectiveness is small compared with that of other drugs. Fish oil helps to reduce the triglyceride levels in the blood. It occurs naturally in oily fish, such as mackerel, and is available as a dietary supplement.

DRUGS ACTING ON THE REPRODUCTIVE AND URINARY SYSTEMS

Recent advances in our understanding of how the reproductive and urinary systems function, in particular the role of hormones, have led to improved drug treatments for conditions such as infertility and prostate disorders. Drugs can also prevent problems of the menopause or labour.

KEY ANATOMY

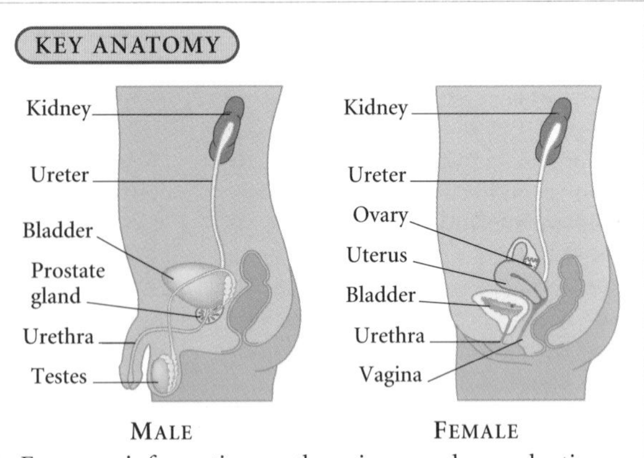

For more information on the urinary and reproductive systems, *see* pp.694–697, pp.716–717, and pp. 730–733.

Drugs are used to increase the likelihood of conception if infertility is due to hormonal imbalances. These drugs are discussed in the first article of this section. The second article covers hormone replacement therapy, which helps to reduce the symptoms of the menopause, which occurs when levels of sex hormones decline.

The next article covers drugs for labour, which are most often used to prevent premature labour or to induce or hasten labour. They may also be used to prevent bleeding after delivery.

In the following article, the various drug treatments for prostate disorders, including prostate cancer, are covered.

The final article in this section deals with drugs that affect bladder control. These drugs are used to treat urinary incontinence and urinary retention.

Further information on drugs for the male and female reproductive and urinary systems, including articles on contraception (p.69) and on the use of sex hormones and related drugs (p.933), can be found elsewhere. In addition, antibiotics (p.885) are widely used in the treatment of infections of the reproductive and urinary systems.

Drugs for infertility

Drugs that are used to treat couples who are unable to conceive

COMMON DRUGS

ANTI-OESTROGENS
• Clomifene

GONADORELIN

GONADOTROPHINS
• Follitropin • Human chorionic gonadotrophin
• Menotrophin • Urofollitropin

GONADORELIN ANALOGUES
• Buserelin • Goserelin • Leuprorelin • Nafarelin

Drugs can be used to help a woman to become pregnant when a couple's inability to conceive is caused by a hormonal imbalance in either the male or the female (*see* INFERTILITY, pp.774–777).

Fertility is influenced by hormones produced in the brain by the hypothalamus and the pituitary gland. The hypothalamus secretes gonadotrophin-releasing hormone, which regulates the release of gonadotrophin hormones from the pituitary gland. The main gonadotrophin hormones are known as follicle-stimulating hormone (FSH) and luteinizing hormone (LH). These hormones control fertility. In females, FSH stimulates the ripening of eggs, and LH triggers ovulation (release of the egg). In males, FSH and LH regulate sperm production. An imbalance or deficiency of these hormones may lead to infertility. In such cases, drugs may be used to stimulate the ovaries to produce eggs or, less commonly, to stimulate a man to produce more sperm.

In women, drugs may also be used to stimulate the ovaries to produce more eggs than normal as part of techniques called assisted conception (p.776), such as in vitro fertilization (IVF).

Women who are having treatment with fertility drugs are monitored using blood tests and ultrasound scanning (p.250) because there is a small risk that the ovaries may become overstimulated, which can be a life-threatening condition. Symptoms of overstimulation can include nausea, vomiting, and abdominal pain and swelling. Infertility treatment also increases the likelihood of multiple pregnancy.

Treatments for infertility may not be effective immediately and often need to be continued for several months to increase the likelihood of conception.

WHAT ARE THE TYPES?

In females, low levels of FSH and LH can be boosted using an anti-oestrogen (also known as an oestrogen antagonist), such as clomiphene. Alternatively, a synthetic version of gonadotrophin-releasing hormone, called gonadorelin, may be prescribed to achieve a similar result. Synthetic gonadotrophin hormones may also be given to influence fertility directly in both males and females. A gonadorelin analogue may sometimes be given in conjunction with gonadotrophin drugs in the treatment of female infertility.

ANTI-OESTROGENS The naturally occurring hormone oestrogen suppresses the production of FSH and LH. Treatment with an oral anti-oestrogen, such as clomifene, blocks this effect and stimulates the pituitary gland to produce more FSH and LH, encouraging ovulation.

If you are taking clomifene, you may notice side effects such as visual disturbances, headache, nausea, hot flushes, and abdominal pain. If you take the drug for longer than 6 months, there may be an increased risk of cancer of the ovary (p.744) developing later on.

GONADORELIN This drug is a synthetic version of the gonadotrophin-releasing hormone that is produced by the hypothalamus and that stimulates the release of the gonadotrophin hormones FSH and LH. Gonadorelin may be used to stimulate FSH and LH secretion and is used particularly for treating infertility in women. Gonadorelin is administered by injection. Side effects may include hot flushes, sweating, and vaginal dryness.

GONADOTROPHINS Men and women who produce very low levels of FSH or LH may be given injections of synthetic FSH, such as follitropin, or human chorionic gonadotrophin (HCG), a hormone that mimics the action of LH. Gonadotrophins can also be used with the anti-oestrogen clomifene or used alone if treatment with clomifene is unsuccessful. These synthetic hormones can be used to stimulate the production of several eggs in women who are having assisted conception. In men, synthetic gonadotrophins can be used to increase production of sperm. Several monthly courses of the drugs may be needed. Possible side effects include headaches, tiredness, and mood changes. In men, the breasts may enlarge.

GONADORELIN ANALOGUES These drugs are sometimes given to women undergoing assisted conception who are also being given synthetic gonadotrophins. When given intermittently, gonadorelin analogues have a similar effect to gonadorelin and stimulate the release of FSH and LH. However, when these drugs are taken continuously, they block the effects of natural gonadotrophin-releasing hormone, which reduces the production of FSH and LH. Blocking the production of natural gonadotrophins makes it easier for doctors to control the action of synthetic gonadotrophins. Gonadorelin analogues are given by injection or as a nasal spray. Side effects include hot flushes, itching, loss of libido, nausea, and vomiting.

Hormone replacement therapy

Drugs that act in a similar way to female sex hormones and that are used to reduce symptoms associated with the menopause

COMMON DRUGS

OESTROGENS
- Conjugated oestrogens • Dienestrol • Estradiol • Estrone • Estropipate • Ethinylestradiol • Mestranol • Tibolone

PROGESTOGENS
- Levonorgestrel • Medroxyprogesterone • Norethisterone • Norgestrel

At the menopause, there is a decline in the levels of the sex hormone oestrogen (*see* HEALTH AT THE MENOPAUSE, p.36). Hormone replacement therapy (HRT) can be used to restore oestrogen to premenopausal levels. Reduced oestrogen levels may lead to symptoms such as hot flushes and vaginal dryness. In the long term, low levels of oestrogen may increase the risk of osteoporosis (p.368) and heart disease. Menopausal symptoms may be particularly severe after surgical removal of the ovaries or following radiotherapy of the pelvic area in the treatment of cancer. Whether they occur naturally or after surgery or radiotherapy, the symptoms of the menopause are usually relieved by HRT.

HRT usually consists of a combination of oestrogen and a progestogen (a synthetic form of the hormone progesterone). Oestrogen that is taken alone is associated with a higher than normal risk of cancer of the uterus (p.748). For this reason, most women are also prescribed a progestogen, which gives protection against uterine cancer. In the case of women who have had a hysterectomy (p.747), usually oestrogen alone is prescribed. A newly developed drug, tibolone, combines the action of both oestrogen and progestogen in a single preparation.

HOW IS IT USED?

HRT is usually given in the form of tablets, skin patches, or as a combination of the two. Tablets are taken daily; patches are usually changed twice a week and should be placed on a different area of skin each time. Other forms of HRT include a gel that is rubbed into the skin daily. Oestrogen creams, applied to the vagina for several weeks to treat vaginal dryness, may also be used. Courses of treatment with creams can be repeated if necessary, but if creams are used in the long term, you will need to take an oral progestogen as protection against cancer of the uterus.

If you are still having periods or if it is less than one year since your last period, HRT will be given in a dose that mimics the monthly cycle of natural hormones. As a result, you should have regular monthly bleeding, although it may be irregular initially. After taking HRT for a year, you may be given oestrogen and a progestogen continuously, which should stop further periods.

Women who are taking HRT during the menopause may need to continue using contraception (p.69) if they wish to avoid becoming pregnant.

Women who take HRT are often recommended to continue treatment for at least 5–10 years after the menopause. Treatment for longer may be associated with a slightly increased risk of breast cancer (p.759). The level of risk returns to normal within about 5 years of stopping HRT. Some women are at a higher than normal risk of developing deep vein thrombosis (p.437), particularly if they have severe varicose veins or are

SELF-ADMINISTRATION

USING SKIN PATCHES

Adhesive skin patches are a simple and effective way to deliver drugs, such as HRT, gradually into the body. Drugs that are administered in this way are released slowly and steadily and are absorbed directly into the bloodstream.

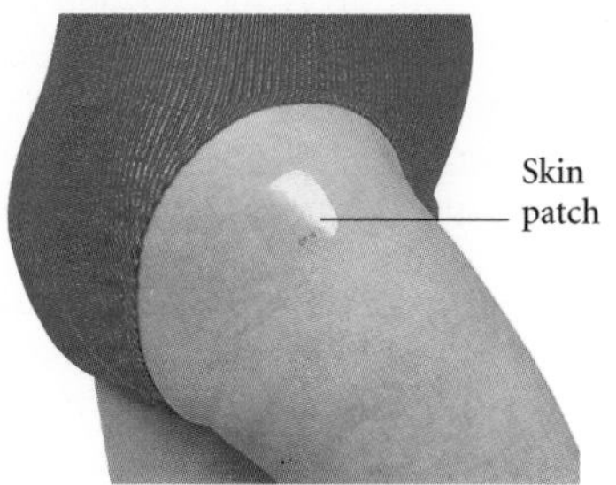

Using skin patches
Patches should always be placed on an area of dry, unbroken skin. Patches given for HRT are usually placed on the lower abdomen or upper thigh.

very overweight. Your doctor will discuss the particular risks and benefits of HRT that may apply to you. After counselling, many women choose to take HRT for more than 5–10 years.

What are the side effects?

If you are taking oestrogen, you may experience side effects including nausea, headaches, and mood swings. Oestrogen may also cause breast tenderness, fluid retention, fluctuating weight, and eye irritation when wearing contact lenses. Progestogens can produce similar side effects to oestrogen, and occasionally cause acne and skin rashes. Such side effects are usually temporary and disappear after 1–2 months of treatment.

Drugs for labour

Drugs that are used to prevent or start labour or for associated problems

COMMON DRUGS

UTERINE STIMULANT DRUGS
• Carboprost • Dinoprostone • Ergometrine
• Oxytocin

UTERINE MUSCLE RELAXANT DRUGS
• Salbutamol • Ritodrine • Terbutaline

MAGNESIUM

Drugs may be used during labour, either as a routine part of medical care or to treat specific problems. Among the most commonly used drugs during childbirth are epidural anaesthetics (*see* EPIDURAL ANAESTHESIA IN LABOUR, p.801).

It may be necessary to use drugs to induce labour (start labour artificially) if the health of the mother or the fetus is at risk. The most common reasons for the induction of labour (p.797) include continuation of pregnancy beyond the due delivery date or complications, such as poor growth of the baby. Drugs may also be given to speed up labour if it does not progress as quickly as it should or to prevent bleeding after delivery.

If labour starts early (before the 34th week of pregnancy), drugs are often used to stop or delay delivery.

What are the types?

Drugs are used during labour either to stimulate contractions of the uterus or to relax the uterus. The most commonly used drugs are known as uterine stimulants. These drugs induce labour by starting contractions or speed up labour by strengthening contractions. Uterine stimulants may also be used for the termination of pregnancy (p.789). Drugs that relax the uterus to delay premature labour are called uterine muscle relaxants. Magnesium may be used to prevent seizures during labour in women with the condition pre-eclampsia (*see* PRE-ECLAMPSIA AND ECLAMPSIA, p.794).

UTERINE STIMULANT DRUGS If labour is going to be induced or if it is necessary to terminate pregnancy, a pessary that contains a prostaglandin uterine stimulant, such as carboprost, may be inserted into the vagina. Prostaglandins not only stimulate contractions but also soften and widen the cervix. Prostaglandins may also be administered in the form of gel. During treatment with a prostaglandin, you may experience some side effects, such as nausea, vomiting, diarrhoea, and hot flushes.

Oxytocin, another uterine stimulant, is given by infusion into a vein to induce labour or to speed up prolonged labour by increasing the strength, duration, and frequency of contractions. The dose will be adjusted carefully, as excess oxytocin may result in painful, continuous contractions, nausea, and vomiting.

A combination of oxytocin and ergometrine, another uterine stimulant drug, is given by intramuscular injection to most women just as the baby is delivered. The drugs cause strong uterine contractions that hasten delivery of the placenta and also constrict the blood vessels in the uterus to reduce bleeding after delivery. A common side effect of ergometrine is nausea. In rare cases, headache, light-headedness, and ringing in the ears may occur.

UTERINE MUSCLE RELAXANT DRUGS If labour begins prematurely, the doctor may give you drugs, such as ritodrine or terbutaline, to relax the muscles of your uterus, thereby preventing further contractions. Uterine muscle relaxants are given continuously by infusion into a vein. However, even with this method of administration, the drugs often become less effective after about 48 hours. Uterine muscle relaxants may have side effects such as nausea, hot flushes, and rapid heartbeat; your blood pressure may drop, causing light-headedness.

MAGNESIUM This mineral may be used to prevent seizures that can occur during labour in women with pre-eclampsia. It may also be used to stop premature labour, especially in multiple pregnancy (p.792). Side effects may include flushing, sweating, and low blood pressure.

Drugs for prostate disorders

Drugs that are used to treat disorders affecting the prostate gland

COMMON DRUGS

ALPHA-BLOCKER DRUGS
• Alfuzosin • Doxazosin • Tamsulosin • Terazosin

ANTIANDROGEN DRUGS
• Bicalutamide • Cyproterone • Finasteride
• Flutamide

GONADORELIN ANALOGUES
• Goserelin • Leuprorelin

OESTROGENS
• Diethylstilbestrol

The main disorders that affect the prostate are noncancerous enlargement of the prostate (*see* ENLARGED PROSTATE GLAND, p.725), prostate cancer (p.726), and infection (*see* PROSTATITIS, p.724). Drugs may be used to treat all of these conditions, sometimes in conjunction with surgery or other treatments.

An enlarged prostate gland constricts the urethra, the tube along which urine flows from the bladder. There may also be obstruction if the muscle at the outlet of the bladder fails to relax. This can cause problems, such as a frequent urge to pass urine but difficulty in doing so. Prostate cancer can cause similar difficulties in passing urine. In some cases, prostate cancer may spread and affect other parts of the body.

Infection of the prostate may cause symptoms including fever and pain in the lower back, around the anus, or around the base of the penis. You may also have other symptoms, including frequent, painful passing of urine and discoloured semen that contains blood.

What are the types?

The main types of drug used to treat prostate disorders are alpha-blockers and antiandrogens. Alpha-blockers are used to improve the flow of urine from the bladder. Antiandrogens are used to treat both noncancerous and cancerous enlargement of the prostate. Gonadorelin analogues and oestrogens may also be used to treat prostate cancer.

Prostate infections are usually treated with a course of antibiotics (p.885). The course of treatment may need to be continued for several weeks before the infection clears up completely.

ALPHA-BLOCKER DRUGS Drugs of this type, such as doxazosin and alfuzosin, relax the ring of muscle at the outlet of the bladder, thereby improving urine flow. Alpha-blockers are taken orally and may need to be used indefinitely because symptoms often recur when the drugs are stopped. Alpha-blockers may lower blood pressure, leading to light-headedness. The drugs may also cause drowsiness, tiredness, mood changes, a dry mouth, headache, and nausea.

ANTIANDROGEN DRUGS Androgens are male sex hormones that play an important but incompletely understood role in the development of noncancerous enlargement of the prostate gland and of prostate cancer. Antiandrogens work by counteracting the effects of androgens.

The main antiandrogen used for noncancerous enlargement of the prostate is finasteride, a drug which shrinks the enlarged gland by blocking the production of testosterone, needed for the growth of tumours. This drug can be used as an alternative to alpha-blockers but may take several months to have beneficial effects. Other antiandrogens, such as bicalutamide, are used in the treatment of prostate cancer.

Antiandrogens are taken orally. They are usually used on a long-term basis for prostate enlargement but may be given either short or long term for cancer. The side effects of antiandrogens may include reduced libido, impotence, and breast tenderness.

GONADORELIN ANALOGUES These drugs are commonly used to treat prostate cancer that has spread beyond the prostate gland. They affect the release of gonadotrophin hormones from the pituitary gland in the brain, thereby reducing the production of testosterone, which promotes the growth of prostate tumours. Gonadorelin analogues are given either by injection or as an implant under the skin. They may initially make symptoms worse. This effect may be treated with an antiandrogen, such as flutamide. Gonadorelin analogues may cause hot flushes, itching, loss of libido, nausea, and vomiting.

OESTROGENS These are female sex hormones that were once used widely in the treatment of prostate cancer. They act by suppressing the production of the natural hormone testosterone, which is needed for tumour growth. Oestrogens are rarely used now because their side effects may include breast enlargement, impotence, nausea, and fluid retention. Oestrogens also slightly increase the risk of deep vein thrombosis (p.437).

Drugs that affect bladder control

Drugs for disorders that affect the ability of the bladder to store or expel urine

COMMON DRUGS

ANTICHOLINERGIC DRUGS
• Flavoxate • Imipramine • Oxybutynin
• Propantheline • Tolterodine

DESMOPRESSIN

ALPHA-BLOCKER DRUGS
• Alfuzosin • Doxazosin • Tamsulosin • Terazosin

OTHER DRUGS FOR BLADDER DISORDERS
• Finasteride • Imipramine

Drugs may be used to treat disorders that affect the normal functioning of the bladder. These disorders fall into two main groups: urinary incontinence (p.710), in which there is involuntary leakage of urine; and urinary retention (p.713), in which there is difficulty emptying the bladder.

Urinary incontinence may occur for many reasons, including involuntary contractions of the muscle of the bladder wall, loss of nerve control due to a disorder such as stroke (p.532), or poor muscle tone at the bladder outlet, which is common in postmenopausal women. Bedwetting (p.872) is a common form of incontinence in young children. Normally, bedwetting stops by the age of 6, but some children do not gain full bladder control until they are older.

Urinary retention can also occur for a variety of reasons, including damage to nerves supplying the muscle of the bladder wall or an obstruction that prevents the outflow of urine from the bladder, which is commonly caused by an enlarged prostate gland (p.725).

WHAT ARE THE TYPES?

Anticholinergic drugs are used to treat incontinence. Desmopressin may occasionally be used to treat bedwetting in children. Urinary retention may be treated with alpha-blocker drugs.

DRUGS FOR INCONTINENCE You may be prescribed an anticholinergic drug such as oxybutynin if you have frequent, sudden urges to pass urine and cannot control your bladder. Anticholinergic drugs work by relaxing the muscle in the bladder wall. This increases the bladder's capacity and reduces the urge to pass urine. If you are taking anticholinergic drugs, you may have side effects such as a dry mouth, blurred vision, constipation, and nausea.

Bedwetting in children is sometimes treated with desmopressin, which is a synthetic version of a natural hormone produced by the pituitary gland that reduces urine production. Desmopressin may be given either orally or as a nasal spray. Side effects of the drug may include fluid retention, salt imbalance, nausea, and headache. Rarely, desmopressin can cause seizures.

Other drugs that may be helpful for overcoming bedwetting in children are tricyclic antidepressants (p.916) such as imipramine. This type of drug is given in small doses and is rarely used for longer than 3 months.

DRUGS FOR URINARY RETENTION Alpha-blockers, such as doxazosin, may be used to treat urinary retention that develops gradually due to noncancerous enlargement of the prostate gland. The drugs work by relaxing the muscles at the bladder outlet, allowing urine to flow out more easily. Alpha-blockers sometimes cause drowsiness, headache, dry mouth, nausea, and mood changes. They may also lower blood pressure, resulting in light-headedness.

In some cases, the antiandrogen drug finasteride (*see* DRUGS FOR PROSTATE DISORDERS, left) may be used to shrink the prostate gland and allow urine to flow more easily. However, the benefits of this drug are often slow to develop.

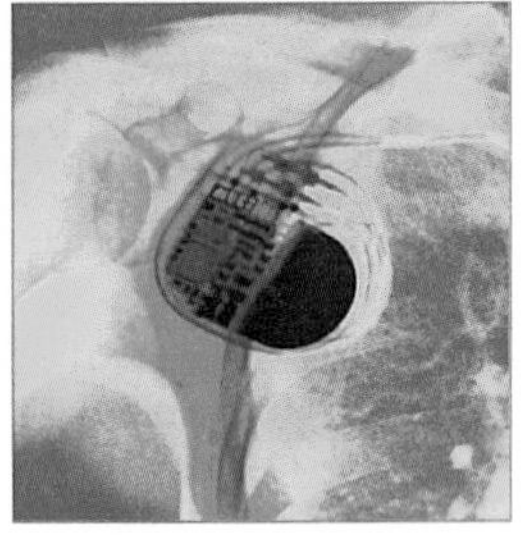

Heart pacemaker
Surgery sometimes involves implanting semipermanent artificial devices.

SURGERY

ADVANCES IN TECHNOLOGY have changed surgery from a risky procedure, often used only as a last resort, to a safe and effective treatment with many applications. New surgical techniques and improved anaesthetic drugs have reduced risks, increased success rates, and shortened recovery times. Many new types of surgery are far less invasive than techniques used previously, and a stay in hospital is now often unnecessary. These improvements have done much to reduce most people's anxiety about having an operation.

Surgery now has such a wide range of applications that it has become the first choice treatment for many disorders, often bringing about immediate relief or even a complete cure.

Surgical procedures can be used to remove, repair, or replace damaged tissue anywhere in the body. A surgeon can take out a diseased body part, such as an inflamed appendix, or remove a tumour. Broken bones and torn tendons can be repaired following an accident. Diseased body organs, such as kidneys, can now be replaced with healthy donor organs, and artificial body parts, such as heart valves, can be implanted. Artificial hip replacement is now a routine operation.

Surgery can also be used to improve the efficiency of body functions. For example, blood flow to the heart muscle can be substantially improved by an operation to bypass blocked blood vessels using grafted lengths of veins taken from another part of the body.

SURGICAL ADVANCES

In recent years, advances in surgical techniques have changed the way in which operations are performed. The most dramatic change has been the development of endoscopic surgery, in which a tube-like viewing instrument called an endoscope is used. The endoscope is inserted through a small incision made in the body or through a natural body opening. Recovery time from endoscopic surgery is much shorter than after open surgery, in which larger incisions are made in the skin. Endoscopes can be used to take samples of diseased tissue, which are sent for laboratory examination, to remove diseased body tissues, such as the gallbladder, and to repair tissue damage, such as a hernia.

Surgeons now use microscopes and tiny instruments to carry out detailed work on minute structures, such as blood vessels. Lasers are increasingly being used for delicate operations on the eye, to remove skin blemishes, and to destroy tumours without damaging surrounding tissue.

Today, a wide range of body organs can be transplanted, largely due to the development of immunosuppressant drugs, which help the body to accept new organs by reducing the likelihood of rejection after transplant surgery.

There have been improvements in care and monitoring before, during, and after an operation, as well as new anaesthetic drugs that have fewer side effects. Thanks to these developments, many people who might once have been considered too ill for surgery can be operated on successfully.

CHOICES IN SURGERY

Advances in surgery mean that any operation now involves decisions that the patient and doctor need to make together. Many minor procedures can now be done in the doctor's surgery rather than in hospital, and operations such as cataract removal, which used to require general anaesthesia, are now offered under local anaesthesia. Where the operation takes place and the type of anaesthesia used largely depend on age, general state of health, personal preference, and whether care can be provided at home following surgery.

PROCEDURE UNDERGOING SURGERY

All types of surgery follow set procedures before, during, and after the operation. Before anaesthesia and surgery, you are given a preoperative assessment. Afterwards, your condition is assessed by your doctor before you are allowed to go home. Major surgery is always carried out in hospital, but minor operations may be performed in the doctor's surgery or in an outpatient clinic.

A surgical procedure
Before surgery, a physical assessment will check your fitness for anaesthesia and surgery. Your recovery time depends on your general state of health and the type of surgery you have.

SURGERY IS REQUIRED → Preoperative assessment of your physical health → You are given a local, regional, or general anaesthetic → Surgery is performed → Assessment of your condition after surgery → You return home the same day or after a period of recovery in hospital

SETTING THE OPERATING THEATRE

An operating theatre is specially designed to provide a clean environment in which the operating team can perform surgery efficiently. To help to reduce the risk of wound infection, the walls and floors are easily washable, and a special ventilation system provides a constant supply of filtered air. All instruments that come into contact with the operation site are sterile. The lamps over the operating table can be adjusted to focus directly on the operation site, and all equipment is positioned for ease of access. An independent electricity supply keeps lights and machinery running in the event of a power failure.

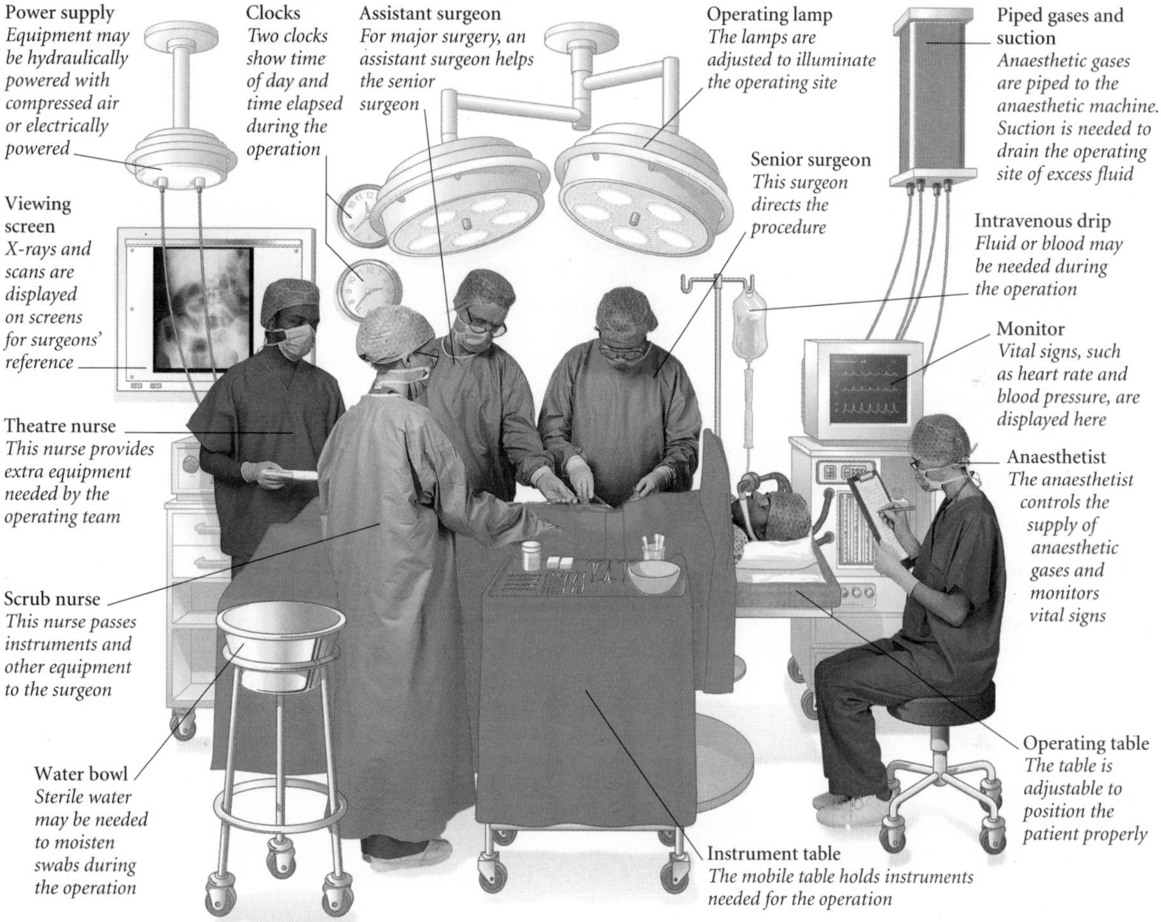

Power supply
Equipment may be hydraulically powered with compressed air or electrically powered
Clocks
Two clocks show time of day and time elapsed during the operation
Assistant surgeon
For major surgery, an assistant surgeon helps the senior surgeon
Operating lamp
The lamps are adjusted to illuminate the operating site
Piped gases and suction
Anaesthetic gases are piped to the anaesthetic machine. Suction is needed to drain the operating site of excess fluid
Viewing screen
X-rays and scans are displayed on screens for surgeons' reference
Senior surgeon
This surgeon directs the procedure
Intravenous drip
Fluid or blood may be needed during the operation
Monitor
Vital signs, such as heart rate and blood pressure, are displayed here
Theatre nurse
This nurse provides extra equipment needed by the operating team
Anaesthetist
The anaesthetist controls the supply of anaesthetic gases and monitors vital signs
Scrub nurse
This nurse passes instruments and other equipment to the surgeon
Operating table
The table is adjustable to position the patient properly
Water bowl
Sterile water may be needed to moisten swabs during the operation
Instrument table
The mobile table holds instruments needed for the operation

SURGICAL INSTRUMENTS

All surgical instruments used for an operation are sterilized to prevent infection. Reusable items are sterilized by exposure to high-pressure steam. Disposable items, such as scalpel blades and needle and thread, are supplied in sealed, sterile packs.

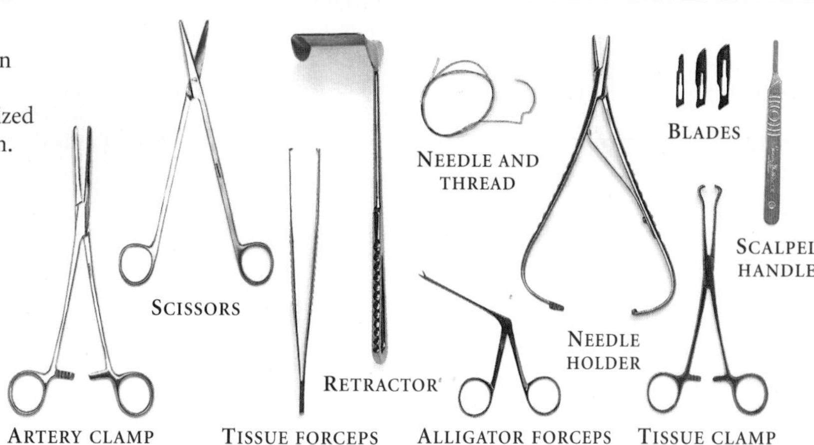

Essential surgical equipment
Surgical instruments are used to cut or manipulate body tissue. Scalpels and scissors cut tissue, retractors hold incisions open, and forceps and clamps hold tissue still and prevent leakage from arteries or veins.

NEEDLE AND THREAD
BLADES
SCALPEL HANDLE
SCISSORS
NEEDLE HOLDER
RETRACTOR
ARTERY CLAMP
TISSUE FORCEPS
ALLIGATOR FORCEPS
TISSUE CLAMP

HAVING AN OPERATION

Many people face having an operation at some point in their lives. While some operations require a stay in hospital as an inpatient, an increasing number of procedures can be performed as day surgery. Advances in surgical procedures and anaesthesia have made having an operation safer than ever, with shorter recovery times and fewer side effects.

The first article covers minor surgical procedures that may be carried out in your doctor's surgery or in hospital on an outpatient basis. The second article outlines what you can expect to take place when you have major surgery, including your recovery afterwards. Major surgery is always performed in hospital. All hospitals and surgical procedures vary, but there are certain routines that are common to all, such as a thorough physical assessment before an operation to check your overall fitness for anaesthesia and surgery. This assessment may take place weeks or days before you are admitted to hospital. The final article discusses convalescence once you have returned home after major surgery. Different types of surgery are described in a separate section (*see* TYPES OF SURGERY, pp.947–953).

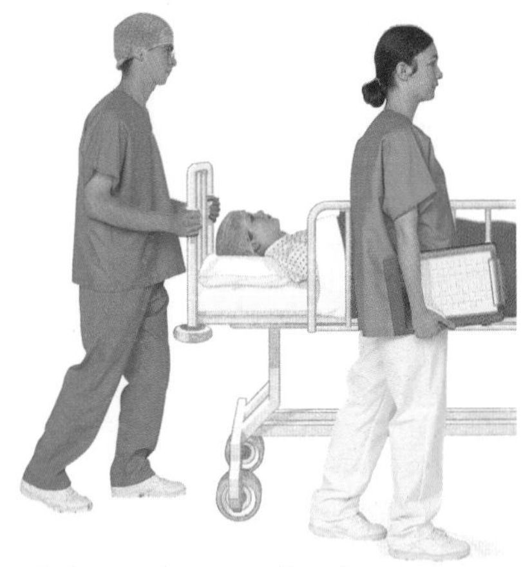

Going to the operating theatre
After you have been given premedication drugs to make you feel calm and to dry mucous secretions, you will be taken to the operating theatre accompanied by a nurse.

Having minor surgery

Minor surgical procedures that take a short time to perform and usually require only local anaesthesia

Minor surgical procedures are those that can be done quickly, usually with only a local anaesthetic (*see* HAVING A LOCAL ANAESTHETIC, right). Examples of these procedures include removal of moles, drainage of cysts or abscesses, and vasectomy (p.721). Most minor surgical procedures involve instruments. However, in some situations no instruments are needed, such as in the manipulation of a simple fracture (p.392).

Minor surgery is usually carried out in hospital as a day case or on an outpatient basis, or your doctor may carry out the procedure in his or her surgery.

WHAT DOES IT INVOLVE?

A minor operation that involves little blood loss requires only minimal preparation when performed on a healthy individual. The doctor will usually discuss the procedure with you, carry out a brief physical examination, and ask you to sign a consent form.

You may be given a local anaesthetic, usually by injection. Anaesthetic creams and sprays can also be used, but these are much less effective than injected anaesthetics. However, they may be used to numb the skin before giving a local anaesthetic injection to a child.

The doctor then scrubs up, puts on a sterile gown and mask, and uses an antiseptic liquid to clean the part of your body that requires surgery. The affected area will then be covered with a sterile drape to prevent bacteria on the surrounding skin from entering the wound.

Once the skin around the affected area is clean and anaesthetized, the doctor carries out the procedure. Some procedures involve cutting through the skin and leave a wound, which is closed after surgery using stitches (sutures), tape, staples, or glue (*see* REJOINING TISSUE, p.948). Other procedures do not leave a wound, and the area may simply be covered with a light gauze or bandage.

PROCEDURE HAVING A LOCAL ANAESTHETIC

A local anaesthetic is used to prevent pain during minor procedures such as removing moles or stitching cuts. The anaesthetic drug numbs the nerve endings around the site where it is administered. A local anaesthetic is usually given by injection, although it may also be applied in a cream or as a spray.

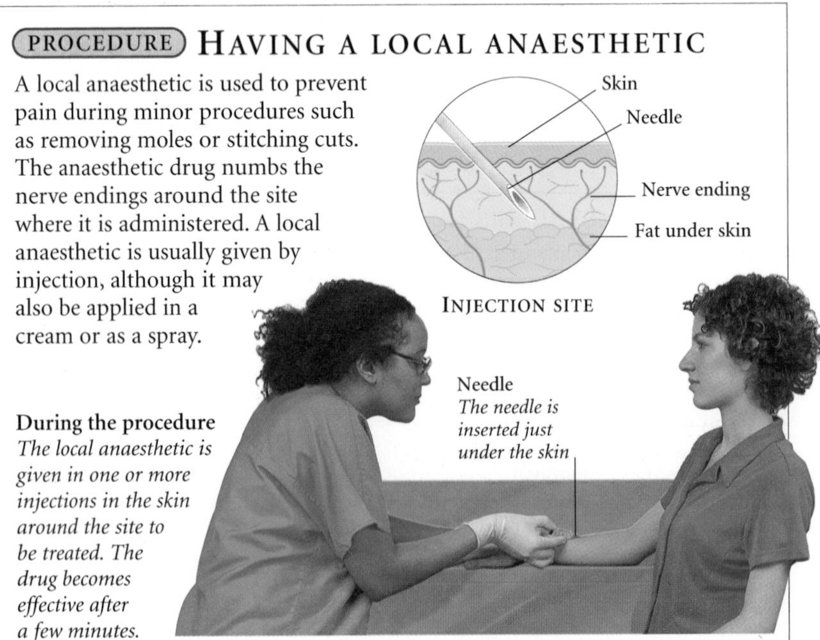

Needle
The needle is inserted just under the skin

During the procedure
The local anaesthetic is given in one or more injections in the skin around the site to be treated. The drug becomes effective after a few minutes.

What happens after surgery? If there is a wound, your doctor or a nurse will give you instructions on how to look after it in order to keep it clean and free of infection until it has healed.

When the local anaesthetic wears off, you may need to take painkillers (p.912) to relieve any discomfort and a course of antibiotics (p.885) to prevent infection. Your doctor will prescribe these drugs for you if necessary.

After some minor procedures, you may feel uncomfortable or a little faint, and you may need someone to take you home. You are usually given a follow-up appointment so that the doctor can check that the procedure has been successful and that the wound is healing. If you have stitches, they may need to be removed, but some types of stitch dissolve on their own after several days.

(WWW) ONLINE SITES: p.1037

Having major surgery

Major surgical procedures carried out under general or regional anaesthesia

Major surgery always takes place in hospital and usually involves a procedure performed on tissue deep inside the body. For example, surgery to remove a section of intestine, implant an artificial hip, or bypass a coronary artery would be considered major surgery (*see* TYPES OF SURGERY, pp.947–953).

Before you undergo a major surgical procedure, your doctor will discuss with you why surgery is necessary, exactly what the procedure involves, where the operation will take place, and how long it will take. You will be fully informed about possible risks associated with the operation, and you will be asked to sign a consent form to say that you understand the risks and agree to surgery.

Before the procedure is performed, your general health and fitness for surgery will be assessed. On the day of the operation, you will be prepared for surgery and given an anaesthetic. Usually, major surgery is performed under general anaesthesia (*see* HAVING A GENERAL ANAESTHETIC, p.944). However, an increasing number of procedures are now carried out under regional anaesthesia (*see* HAVING A REGIONAL ANAESTHETIC, p.945), in which you remain fully conscious but free of pain. A sedative may be given along with regional anaesthesia to help to keep you calm and reduce anxiety. The type of anaesthesia you have depends largely on the nature of the procedure, but your general health and age may also play a part.

After the operation has been completed, there is a recovery period. For most major surgical procedures, a stay in hospital of several days is required. However, some relatively uncomplicated procedures, such as female sterilization (p.743), are sometimes carried out as day surgery. This is particularly likely if the procedures are performed using modern minimally invasive techniques (*see* ENDOSCOPIC SURGERY, p.948).

Your doctor will be able to advise you on how long it will take for you to recover from your operation. There may be particular practical issues that you wish to clarify with the doctor. For example, you may want to check whether further treatment will be needed after the operation and how long it is likely to be before you are able to carry out your normal day-to-day activities.

Preoperative assessment

Before you undergo a major surgical procedure, you will be given a preoperative assessment. The main purpose of this assessment is to find out whether you have an underlying medical condition, such as heart disease, that may require special precautions during the operation in order to minimize the risk of complications developing.

During the preoperative assessment, a doctor reviews your medical history and performs a physical examination. Routine tests, such as blood tests, will also be carried out, together with any other investigations that may be needed because of your age, general health, or underlying condition.

You will also be seen by an anaesthetist, who checks your suitability for anaesthesia, discusses how the anaesthetic will be administered, and answers any questions you may have.

Medical history and examination

You will be asked about your current condition and about other serious illnesses or allergies you have experienced in the past (*see* MEDICAL HISTORY, p.218). You will also be asked about any medications you are taking because these may affect the safety of the surgery. You will then be given a full medical examination, during which the doctor will listen to your chest and back with a stethoscope (*see* PHYSICAL EXAMINATION, p.219), to help to identify any underlying medical conditions that may increase the risk of complications occurring during or following the operation.

Routine tests You may have a number of routine tests, many of which require a sample of blood or occasionally urine to be taken. Blood tests usually require no more than two or three small tubes of blood to be withdrawn through a single needle (*see* BLOOD SAMPLES, p.221). The most common blood test measures the level of haemoglobin in your blood (*see* BLOOD CELL TESTS, p.226). Haemoglobin is an oxygen-carrying pigment found in red blood cells. If you lose a small amount of blood during surgery, it is important that your body still has adequate reserves of haemoglobin to compensate. Your blood group will also be checked (*see* BLOOD TYPING, p.227). A sample of blood may be saved for cross-matching against blood from the blood bank if you need to have a blood transfusion (p.447) during surgery. The levels of certain chemicals, such as urea and salts, in your blood may be measured because they reflect the function of internal organs such as the kidneys (*see* ROUTINE BLOOD CHEMISTRY, p.229).

Other presurgical investigations

Depending on the outcome of your initial physical examination, your doctor may decide that other investigations are needed before you undergo surgery. For example, if your medical history suggests that you may have heart disease, your doctor may arrange for an ECG (p.406) to assess the condition of your heart and make a diagnosis. If there is a possibility that you have a heart or lung disorder, a chest X-ray (p.490) may also be performed. The results of these tests may influence how the surgery is carried out and the level of monitoring that is required during the operation. In some cases, these initial test results indicate the need for further investigations, such as exercise testing (p.407), which evaluates the flow of blood to the heart while at a person is rest and during the physical stress of exercise.

Preparations for surgery

On the day of your surgery, you will be prepared for the operation and given premedication drugs. You will then be given the anaesthetic.

You should not eat or drink for at least 6 hours before an operation under general anaesthesia. If you have food in your stomach, there is an increased risk of vomiting while you are unconscious. If the acidic contents of the stomach are inhaled, serious damage to your lungs may result. You may also need to fast if you are having a regional anaesthetic in case it becomes necessary to give you a general anaesthetic during surgery.

GENERAL PREPARATIONS If there is a particular risk of infection occurring during the operation, such as bacteria spreading from the intestine during intestinal surgery, a course of antibiotics (p.885) may be prescribed. These may be given initially by injection. An hour or two before your operation, you will be asked to remove all jewellery and to change into a surgical gown. You will be asked to remove dentures, if you have them, or to point out loose teeth or crowns, which could be damaged when the breathing tube for anaesthetic gases is inserted. If a surgical incision is to be made in an area of skin that is covered with hair, the area may be shaved to make the skin easier to clean. The surgeon may mark the skin over the site of the operation to indicate where the incision should be made.

PREMEDICATION An hour or so before your anaesthetic, you will be given premedication drugs to help you to feel calm and to dry mucous secretions. These drugs may be administered by injection or by mouth. A nurse will then take you to the operating theatre.

ANAESTHESIA When you arrive in the operating theatre, you will be given an anaesthetic. For longer operations carried out under general anaesthesia, the anaesthetic is given in two parts. First, an anaesthetic is injected into a vein on the back of your hand. Although this injection induces anaesthesia rapidly, it is not long-lasting. Second, inhaled gases are given to maintain unconsciousness. For shorter operations, a single injected or inhaled anaesthetic may be used. The initial anaesthetic drug is injected into a thin plastic tube called a catheter. This tube is inserted into a vein either in the back of your hand or in your arm, and the anaesthetic drug causes almost immediate loss of consciousness.

The anaesthetist then inserts a breathing tube, called an endotracheal tube, through your mouth and down into your trachea (windpipe). The tube is connected to a ventilator, which regulates the speed and depth of breathing throughout surgery. You will be given a mixture of gases to breathe, including oxygen and an inhaled anaesthetic. You will also be given a drug through the catheter that relaxes your muscles and therefore makes it possible for the surgeon to cut and move muscles easily. By doing this, the surgeon can obtain a clear view of the operating area.

If you are having a regional anaesthetic, the anaesthetic drug is given by injection. The site of the injection varies according to the procedure that is to be performed, and for some types of regional anaesthesia, such as epidural or spinal anaesthesia, the skin around the injection site will be numbed first with a local anaesthetic.

PROCEDURE Having a general anaesthetic

General anaesthesia is used in surgery to induce unconsciousness and thereby to prevent pain. First, a rapidly acting drug is injected through a catheter into a vein in the back of your hand or in your arm. A drug given at the same time relaxes the muscles. Once unconscious, you are given a mixture of gases, including oxygen, through a tube inserted into your trachea (windpipe).

Syringe
Drugs or fluids are delivered from the syringe

Intravenous catheter
The catheter tip is within the vein

Skin

Fatty tissue

Vein

DETAIL OF CATHETER

Catheter

1 *A fast-acting general anaesthetic is injected through a catheter into a vein in the back of your hand. You become unconscious within seconds.*

Anaesthetic machine
The flow, concentration, and mixture of gases are regulated by the machine

Monitor
The monitor displays your heart rate, blood pressure, and the amount of oxygen in your blood

Endotracheal tube

ECG leads
Leads on your chest connect to the monitor

Record
The anaesthetist records vital signs and drugs used

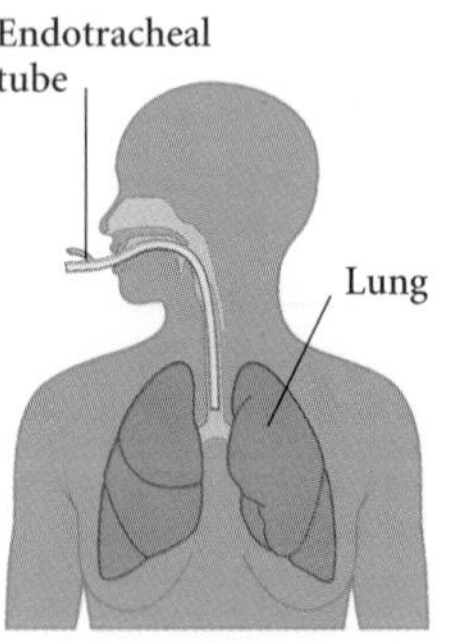

SITE OF TUBE

2 *A mixture of oxygen and anaesthetic gases is given to keep you unconscious. These gases are delivered directly into the lungs through an endotracheal tube, which is inserted down the throat into the trachea.*

IN THE OPERATING THEATRE

As soon as you are anaesthetized, the surgeon or assistant surgeon uses an antiseptic solution to clean the appropriate area of your skin. The solution used may leave pink or brown stains on the skin for a short time after the operation. The remaining nonsterile parts of your skin are covered with sterile drapes, and the procedure is then carried out.

When the procedure is completed, the wound is closed up (*see* REJOINING TISSUE, p.948) by the surgeon. For some types of wound, you may have internal stitches as well as those that are visible on your skin. If you have been given a general anaesthetic, the proportion of anaesthetic gases you are breathing will be reduced and the proportion of oxygen you are given will be increased to allow you to wake up.

IN THE RECOVERY ROOM

As soon as you show signs of breathing on your own, the anaesthetist will remove the endotracheal tube. You may hear someone telling you the operation is over, but you will probably wake up only briefly. You will then be moved to the recovery room. If you have had a general anaesthetic, the recovery room is probably the first place that you will remember after the operation. For the first hours after a major operation, your temperature, blood pressure, and pulse are checked frequently. When you are taken back to the ward, usually when you are fully awake, these checks are repeated, but less frequently.

Some major surgery requires intensive nursing care afterwards, and you may be transferred to an intensive care unit (p.958) rather than taken directly back to the ward. You will be transferred to the ward when you are no longer dependent on specialized equipment and medical personnel.

BACK TO THE WARD

After major surgery, you will be transferred to the ward so that you can be monitored and given any further treatment that you may need. Postoperative monitoring is carried out in order to identify any complications as early as possible. If necessary, you will be given pain relief. Generally, the more extensive the operation, the longer it will take for you to recover. Usually, your recovery is faster and complications are less likely to occur if you start moving around as soon as possible after the effects of the anaesthetic have worn off.

If you have had a general anaesthetic, you are likely to remain drowsy for a number of hours. After regional anaesthesia, you will not experience the drowsiness that normally follows general anaesthesia. However, the numbing effects of a regional anaesthetic usually take several hours to wear off.

TREATMENT AND MONITORING You may be attached to tubes and equipment that monitor your condition or help you to perform particular bodily processes. For example, you may be attached to an ECG machine that monitors your heart function. You may have a urinary catheter if surgery has involved the bladder or nearby organs, such as the prostate gland. The catheter enables medical staff to monitor the amount of urine that you produce. An intravenous drip may be placed in your arm or the back of your hand to deliver fluids and medication if necessary. Fluids help to prevent you becoming dehydrated until you are able to eat and drink normally. After certain procedures, there may be a tube called a drain coming from a small hole in the skin near the surgical wound. This tube is often attached to a vacuum bottle and allows excess tissue fluid or blood to drain away from the operation site. It is usually removed after a few days. You may also have a tube called a central line coming from the side of your neck or just below your collarbone. This tube is held in place by stitches and is used to monitor your fluid balance and blood pressure and to give you extra fluids or drugs if these are needed. This tube will be removed as soon as continuous monitoring and fluids are no longer necessary.

PAIN RELIEF You may not feel much pain when you wake up because of the effects of the drugs you have received during anaesthesia, and because the surgeon may inject a local anaesthetic into the edges of the surgical wound. After a few hours, you may become more uncomfortable and require painkillers (p.912). These drugs may be administered orally or by injection, depending

PROCEDURE HAVING A REGIONAL ANAESTHETIC

A regional anaesthetic blocks the transmission of pain along a nerve or group of nerves. The anaesthetic is injected around targeted nerves, and you remain awake throughout the procedure. Regional anaesthesia can be used in many parts of the body. A spinal nerve block, shown here, anaesthetizes the whole of the lower body below the site of injection.

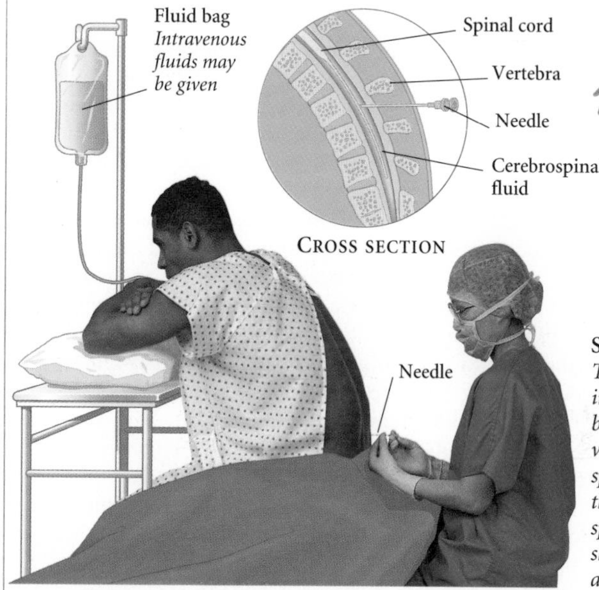

Spinal anaesthesia
The anaesthetist inserts a needle between two of the vertebrae in the lower spine until it reaches the fluid bathing the spinal nerves. He or she then injects the anaesthetic.

on the drug, the severity of your pain, and your ability to absorb the medication. You may be able to administer your own painkillers in small, safe doses as often as you need to using a patient-controlled analgesic pump attached to a tube that is inserted into a blood vessel in your arm. This type of pump has a built-in device to prevent you receiving too much medication.

OTHER TREATMENTS Some major surgery may necessitate other treatments to prevent complications. For example, blood clots may develop in the legs (*see* DEEP VEIN THROMBOSIS, p.437) if you are immobile for long periods of time. These clots may break off and travel to the heart or lungs, which may be life-threatening. If clots are likely to form, your doctor will prescribe injections of a drug that reduces blood clotting (*see* DRUGS THAT PREVENT BLOOD CLOTTING, p.904), which are usually given into the skin of the abdomen. You may also need to wear support stockings for a few days until you are fully mobile.

If you have had an operation on an infected area such as an abscess, you may be given antibiotics. Depending on the type of operation you have had, you may be offered physiotherapy (p.961) or other treatment while in hospital to help you to return to full mobility.

LEAVING THE HOSPITAL

You will be discharged from hospital when you no longer need close monitoring or special treatment. You usually need to be eating and drinking normally without the aid of tubes and to be able to pass urine without a catheter. The medical staff need to be satisfied that you have someone to accompany you home and that you will be adequately looked after if you are unable take care of yourself. Home nursing (*see* HOME CARE, p.960) may need to be organized in advance. If you require special aids, such as a bath lift, you may be assessed by an occupational therapist (*see* OCCUPATIONAL THERAPY, p.962) before you are discharged from hospital.

Before you leave hospital, you will be provided with any medication that you need, and a follow-up appointment will be made to check on your progress and, if necessary, to remove stitches.

(WWW) ONLINE SITES: p.1037

Convalescence after major surgery

The period of adjustment and recovery following a major operation

After surgery, there may be a period of time before you are able to return to work and resume your normal activities. This period of convalescence often involves some bed rest, and you may need help with day-to-day tasks. In addition to physical recovery, convalescence following major surgery may also involve a period of psychological adjustment. It is not unusual to feel emotional or depressed after surgery, and many people find counselling (p.971) helpful.

Recent developments in surgical technique, for example endoscopic surgery (p.948), and improvements in the control and relief of pain have shortened the time needed for convalescence. In most cases, the older you are, the more extensive the surgery, and the poorer your general health, the more time you will need to convalesce.

You are likely to need a period of rest after surgery and may be in enough discomfort to restrict movement. However, this must be balanced with the need for you to gradually increase your level of activity in order to regain your strength and reduce the risk of deep vein thrombosis (p.437). If your muscles are weak from lack of use, such as after surgery on bones or joints, you may be offered regular physiotherapy (p.961) to regain mobility and muscle strength. You may also need help from a specialist nurse to make temporary or permanent lifestyle changes, such as learning how to manage a colostomy (p.666).

RESUMING ACTIVITY

To help you recover as quickly as possible after surgery, it is important to try to be as physically active as you can. Make sure that you have appropriate medication to allow you to move around without excessive pain. After some types of surgery, particularly operations on the abdomen, it may hurt to cough, and secretions may remain in the lungs. In this case, you will be shown breathing exercises and how to reduce discomfort when you cough before you leave hospital, and you should continue to use these techniques during convalescence. As you recover from surgery, you should gradually be able to resume many of your day-to-day activities. With time, you will be able to return to your normal lifestyle, resume sexual activity, and drive again.

WORK You should follow your doctor's advice on when to return to work, taking into account the progress of your recovery and the nature of your occupation. Manual work naturally requires a higher level of physical fitness than office work. You may be able to arrange to resume your work duties gradually. For many people, travelling to and from work may be the most demanding part of the day.

SEX Few surgical operations require you to abstain from sexual activity afterwards for physical reasons, but your surgeon will tell you if there is a particular risk. However, sometimes you may wish to avoid sex for reasons of comfort as well as from medical necessity, such as after surgery on a hernia (p.661) in the groin. You may also need time for your sexual feelings to return to normal, since it is very common for sex drive to disappear during a period of illness. If you have sexual problems that continue for some time after surgery, consult your doctor.

DRIVING You may be advised not to drive if your operation or medical condition could affect your concentration or your ability to drive safely, for example if you are unable to wear a seat belt or stop quickly in an emergency. It may be unsafe for you to drive while you are taking certain painkillers or other drugs. Your doctor will advise you when you can start driving again.

IDENTIFYING COMPLICATIONS

Something may be seriously wrong if you suddenly feel ill or if a symptom that was improving begins to get worse. Symptoms such as fever, shortness of breath, coughing, bleeding or a new discharge from the surgical wound, or pain in the legs, chest, or operation site that becomes worse may indicate a problem. If you develop any of these symptoms, you should seek advice promptly from your doctor or a contact at the hospital, who can distinguish between normal postoperative symptoms and serious complications.

(WWW) ONLINE SITES: p.1037

TYPES OF SURGERY

Surgery at its most basic level consists of cutting through body tissues, treating a problem, and sewing up the wound. However, the development of surgical techniques using new technology, such as microsurgery and laser treatment, has enabled more complex operations to be performed with increasing precision.

Open surgery, in which internal body structures are accessed through large incisions, is the most common type of surgery and is discussed in the opening article. However, an increasing number of operations are now performed using endoscopic surgery, which is discussed next. Endoscopic surgery requires only a small incision or none at all. Further articles cover other specialized surgical techniques, including microsurgery and laser treatment, both of which are used in plastic surgery to reconstruct or repair tissues. Microsurgery can be performed on tiny structures, such as the nerves. Laser treatment has many uses, such as removing birthmarks and repairing delicate parts of the eye. The final article discusses transplant surgery, which enables diseased and failing body parts to be replaced with healthy ones.

What happens before, during, and after surgery is covered elsewhere (*see* HAVING AN OPERATION, pp.942–946).

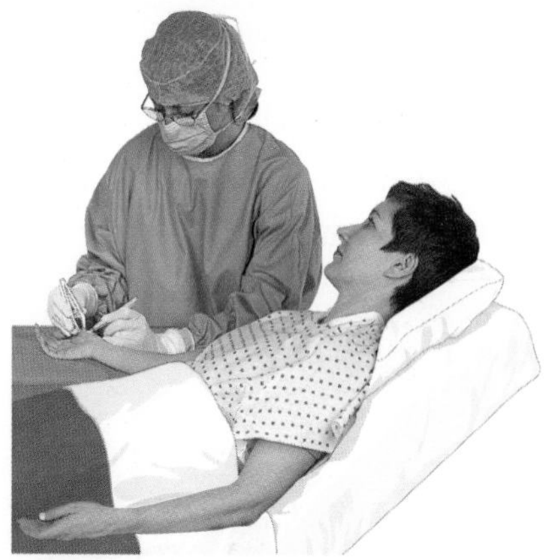

A surgical procedure
Almost all surgical procedures involve cutting through tissues and then securing the tissue edges together to promote healing, reduce bleeding, and prevent infection.

Open surgery

Surgical procedures in which internal body structures are accessed by large incisions made in the skin

Most operations are carried out using open surgery. In this type of surgery, an incision is made in the skin large enough to allow the surgeon to see clearly the internal body parts that require treatment and the surrounding tissues. A large incision provides easy access, but it may leave an obvious scar.

Open surgery is used for all internal organ transplant operations and for caesarean sections (p.802). Open surgery may also be necessary for the removal of certain types of tumour or in cases in which the extent of the problem is not known. Sometimes, open surgery may need to be performed urgently in order to deal promptly with an emergency such as internal bleeding.

WHAT HAPPENS DURING THE OPERATION?

There are a number of open surgery procedures, such as a caesarean section, that may be performed under regional anaesthesia (*see* HAVING A REGIONAL ANAESTHETIC, p.945). However, most open surgery is carried out under general anaesthesia (*see* HAVING A GENERAL ANAESTHETIC, p.944). Once you are fully anaesthetized, the surgeon makes an incision through the skin and the layers of fat and muscle below it. The skin and muscles may be held back by clamps, and organs and tissues that are not being operated on are pulled out of the way by retractors. When the area to be treated is clearly visible, the surgeon is able to carry out the procedure.

Blood vessels that have to be severed during surgery are sealed in order to prevent serious loss of blood. This is done using electrocautery, a process in which blood vessels are sealed by an electric current applied through a pen-like instrument, or by tying off the severed ends of the vessels with synthetic thread. Lasers are also sometimes used during open surgery to seal blood vessels (*see* LASER TREATMENT, p.951).

The operation site is kept free of blood and other fluids to ensure that the surgeon can see clearly what he or she is doing. Sponges and suction tubes are positioned around the area to remove fluids. The number of sponges used is counted carefully and is checked after the operation to make sure that they have all been removed. The surgeon checks that there is no internal bleeding before he or she sews up the wound (*see* REJOINING TISSUE, p.948). The wound may be covered with a sterile dressing.

WHAT ARE THE RISKS?

All surgical procedures, whether major or minor, involve some risk. For example, there may be an adverse reaction to the anaesthetic, excessive bleeding, formation of blood clots, or infection.

A general anaesthetic can provoke changes in heart rhythm during or after surgery. The risk of this is higher if you are elderly, have a heart problem, or are overweight. In rare cases, an allergic reaction to the anaesthetic may occur.

Rarely, if blood vessels are not fully sealed, excessive bleeding may occur during the operation, or there may be persistent bleeding afterwards. In either case, a blood transfusion (p.447) may be required. A supply of cross-matched (compatible) blood is made available for each person having major surgery.

After surgery, blood has an increased tendency to clot, which may lead to the formation of blood clots in the deep veins of the legs (*see* DEEP VEIN THROMBOSIS, p.437). These blood clots may cause pain and swelling in the leg, and they can sometimes travel to the lungs. If a blood clot becomes lodged in an artery that supplies a lung, it can cause chest pain and shortness of breath and may be life-threatening (*see* PULMONARY EMBOLISM, p.495). To reduce the risk of blood clots developing, you will be encouraged to move around as soon as

(TECHNIQUE) REJOINING TISSUE

Tissues are rejoined after surgery to promote healing, stop bleeding, and prevent infection. There are various rejoining techniques and materials that can be used depending on the site and the type of tissue. Some materials are designed to dissolve as the tissues heal, and these are particularly useful for internal use. Materials that do not dissolve are used if healing is likely to take a long time or needs assessment before the stitches are removed.

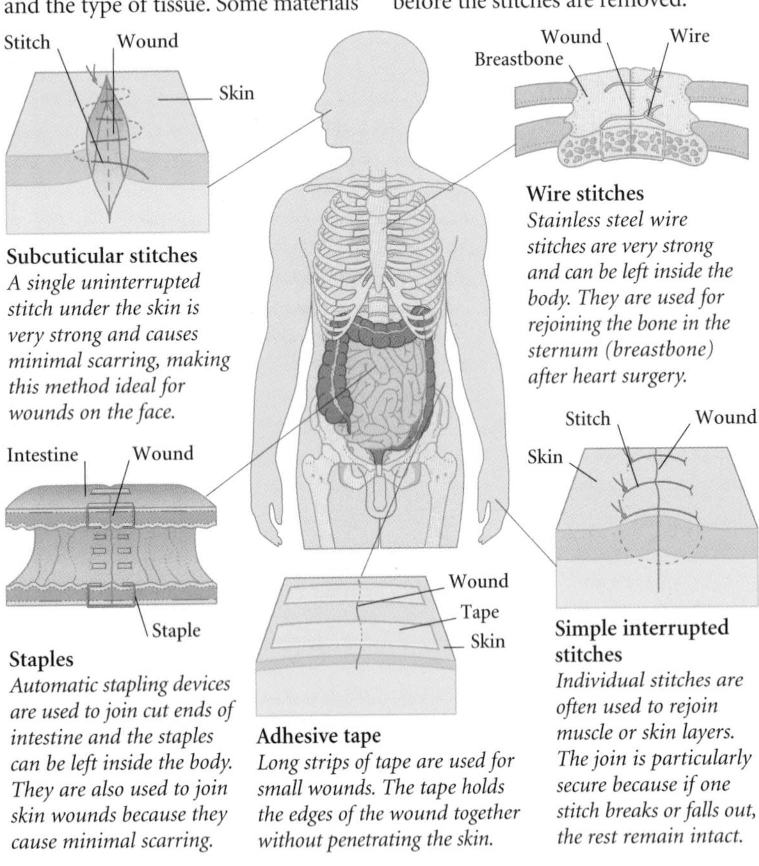

Subcuticular stitches
A single uninterrupted stitch under the skin is very strong and causes minimal scarring, making this method ideal for wounds on the face.

Wire stitches
Stainless steel wire stitches are very strong and can be left inside the body. They are used for rejoining the bone in the sternum (breastbone) after heart surgery.

Staples
Automatic stapling devices are used to join cut ends of intestine and the staples can be left inside the body. They are also used to join skin wounds because they cause minimal scarring.

Adhesive tape
Long strips of tape are used for small wounds. The tape holds the edges of the wound together without penetrating the skin.

Simple interrupted stitches
Individual stitches are often used to rejoin muscle or skin layers. The join is particularly secure because if one stitch breaks or falls out, the rest remain intact.

you can after the operation. Treatment with drugs such as heparin (see DRUGS THAT PREVENT BLOOD CLOTTING, p.904) may be given during and after surgery to thin the blood. Painkillers (p.912) may also help to prevent the formation of blood clots by allowing you to move around more easily without pain.

Infection may occur if bacteria or other microorganisms enter a wound during or after surgery, preventing or delaying the healing process and causing tissue damage and fever. The risk of infection is minimized by performing the operation in a highly sterile environment with instruments that have been carefully sterilized. Antibiotics (p.885) are often given before, during, or after surgery to help to prevent infection.

(WWW) ONLINE SITES: p.1037

Endoscopic surgery

Surgical procedures that use a viewing instrument inserted through a natural body opening or through skin incisions

Endoscopic surgery is a technique that enables various procedures to be performed without making large incisions in the skin. An endoscope is a tube-like viewing instrument with a light source. Some endoscopes have a built-in miniature camera. Endoscopes are inserted either through a natural body opening, such as the anus, or through a small incision, depending on the site to be accessed. Endoscopic surgery performed through skin incisions is often referred to as minimally invasive surgery (see HAVING MINIMALLY INVASIVE SURGERY, opposite page). Endoscopes may be flexible or rigid (see FLEXIBLE ENDOSCOPY, p.255, and RIGID ENDOSCOPY, p.256) and are used to provide a view of the inside of body cavities, either directly through the endoscope or on a screen.

Endoscopes may be used to carry out treatment, to examine a particular area, or to take tissue samples. Tiny instruments, such as forceps and scissors, are passed through small incisions in the skin or through side channels in the endoscope to reach the operating site. These instruments are operated by the surgeon, who is guided by the view through the endoscope or on the screen.

Since endoscopic surgery may not involve any incisions or only require small ones, the length of stay in hospital and recovery time are shorter than for open surgery. Bleeding from any small incisions that have been made is minimal. Therefore, the wounds heal more quickly and are less likely to become infected than the large incisions that are needed in open surgery.

WHEN IS IT USED?

Endoscopic surgery may be used to operate inside any part of the body that is large enough for the instruments to be inserted into and moved around. Suitable sites include the chest, abdominal cavity, pelvic cavity, digestive tract, large joints, such as the knee and hip, and the nasal sinuses. Endoscopes have different names according to the part of the body in which they are used. For example, laparoscopes are used in the abdominal cavity, bronchoscopes are used to look in the lungs, and colonoscopes are used inside the colon.

If you have symptoms that suggest a disorder of the reproductive system, digestive tract, lungs, sinuses, or bladder, an endoscope may be inserted through the vagina, anus, mouth, nose, or urethra in order to investigate the affected area. Endoscopy through natural openings may be repeated safely many times and can be used to monitor a condition such as a peptic ulcer (p.640).

When the area under investigation cannot be accessed through a natural body opening, small incisions need to be made for the endoscope and other instruments. For example, if you have a disorder of the gallbladder, appendix, or some parts of the female reproductive

(PROCEDURE) HAVING MINIMALLY INVASIVE SURGERY

Minimally invasive surgery allows the surgeon to examine and treat disorders in body cavities, such as the abdomen, through small incisions. An endoscope (a tube-like viewing instrument with a light source and a camera) is inserted through one incision to provide a view of the cavity.

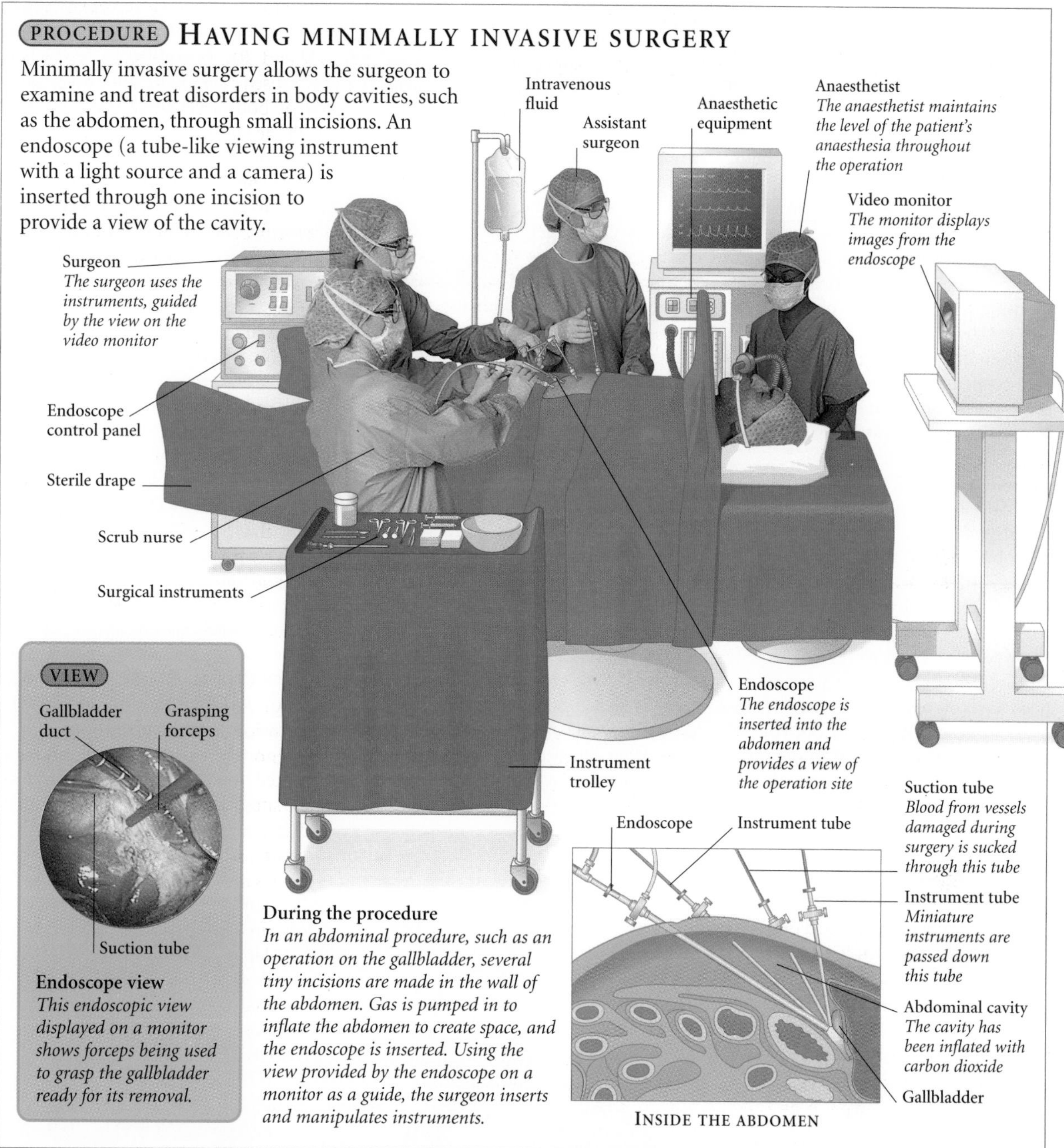

Endoscope view
This endoscopic view displayed on a monitor shows forceps being used to grasp the gallbladder ready for its removal.

During the procedure
In an abdominal procedure, such as an operation on the gallbladder, several tiny incisions are made in the wall of the abdomen. Gas is pumped in to inflate the abdomen to create space, and the endoscope is inserted. Using the view provided by the endoscope on a monitor as a guide, the surgeon inserts and manipulates instruments.

system, such as the fallopian tubes, a laparoscope may be inserted through an incision in the abdomen to carry out investigations or treatment (*see* LAPAROSCOPY, p.742). Laparascopes are also used in female sterilization (p.743). If you have a disorder of the joints, such as arthritis, or a damaged cartilage or ligament, an arthroscope inserted through a small incision may be used to view and possibly to operate on the affected joint (*see* ARTHROSCOPY, p.386).

WHAT HAPPENS DURING THE OPERATION?

Endoscopic surgery through natural openings in the body, such as the throat or anus, may not need an anaesthetic or may take place under sedation or local anaesthesia. This means that you remain conscious, but the area being operated on is numb (*see* HAVING A LOCAL ANAESTHETIC, p.942, and HAVING A REGIONAL ANAESTHETIC, p.945). In some cases, you may be given a drug to help you to relax before the procedure takes place. After the endoscope has been inserted into the body opening, surgical instruments may be introduced through specific channels in the endoscope.

The majority of endoscopic surgical procedures through incisions are performed under general anaesthesia (*see* HAVING A GENERAL ANAESTHETIC, p.944). An incision about 13 mm (½ in) long is made for the endoscope, and then further tiny incisions are made so that instruments, such as lasers (*see* LASER TREATMENT, opposite page) and scissors, can be inserted if needed. In a laparoscopic operation on the abdomen, a tube is inserted through an incision, and gas is pumped through it to inflate the abdominal cavity, giving the surgeon a better view and more operating space.

The surgeon looks at the procedure through an eyepiece on the endoscope and also observes a magnified image of the operating site transmitted to a video monitor. The surgeon's colleagues can also watch the procedure on the screen.

When the operation is complete, the endoscope and all the instruments are removed. The incisions are then closed, often with a single stitch.

WHAT ARE THE RISKS?

The risk of damage to a body organ or blood vessel is slightly greater with endoscopic surgery than it is with open surgery (p.947) because the surgeon has to work in a more restricted area. As with all types of surgery, there is a risk of an adverse reaction to the anaesthetic. During the operation, the surgeon may need to access a larger area and perform open surgery. For this reason, you will be asked for your consent to open surgery before an endoscopic operation.

(WWW) ONLINE SITES: p.1037

Microsurgery

Surgical procedures that use magnifying equipment and tiny surgical instruments to operate on small or delicate structures

Microsurgery makes it possible to perform operations on extremely small or delicate tissues in the body. In this form of surgery, a surgeon uses a binocular microscope to view the operating site and specially adapted small operating instruments. Using microsurgery, delicate surgical procedures can be carried out that would be difficult or impossible with other surgical techniques.

WHEN IS IT USED?

Microsurgery is most commonly used to operate on tissues such as nerves and blood vessels and on small structures in the eye, middle ear, and reproductive system. For example, microsurgery can be used to repair a detached retina (*see* RETINAL DETACHMENT, p.578). It can also be used to remove the diseased eye lens of someone with a cataract and replace it with an artificially made lens (*see* CATARACT SURGERY, p.573). In the disorder otosclerosis (p.598), deafness may occur when a bone in the middle ear becomes diseased and is unable to transmit sound. Hearing can be restored using microsurgery to replace the diseased bone with an artificial substitute.

During an operation to reattach a severed limb or digit, microsurgery is used to reconnect severed nerves and blood vessels. Microsurgery is also used to try to reverse two sterilization procedures: tubal ligation in women (*see* FEMALE STERILIZATION, p.743) and vasectomy (p.721) in men. Sterilization in women involves cutting or sealing the fallopian tubes. In a vasectomy, the narrow tubes that carry sperm from the testes to the penis are severed, preventing the release of sperm. In both cases, microsurgery procedures can be used to rejoin the sealed or severed tubes accurately, and, in many cases, a person's reproductive function can be restored.

WHAT HAPPENS DURING THE OPERATION?

Microsurgery is normally carried out under general anaesthesia (*see* HAVING A GENERAL ANAESTHETIC, p.944). However, regional or local anaesthesia (*see* HAVING A REGIONAL ANAESTHETIC, p.945, and HAVING A LOCAL ANAESTHETIC, p.942) may be used for some minor procedures, such as cataract operations.

During the operation, the surgeon views the operating site through a binocular microscope, which is operated

PROCEDURE HAVING MICROSURGERY

Microsurgery is a technique that allows delicate operations to be performed on very small structures in the body. The technique is used for a number of procedures, such as repairing damaged blood vessels and nerves. Microsurgery is also frequently used to remove the eye lens of someone with a cataract and to operate on the tiny bones in the middle ear.

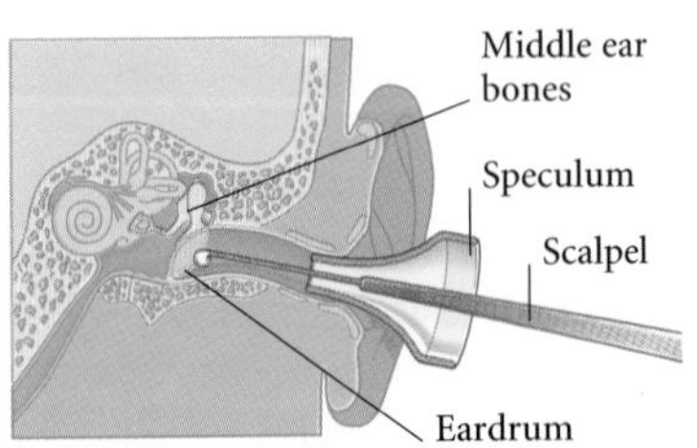

During the procedure
The surgeon views the operating site through a powerful microscope and uses extremely small instruments. Here an operation is being carried out on delicate structures inside the ear.

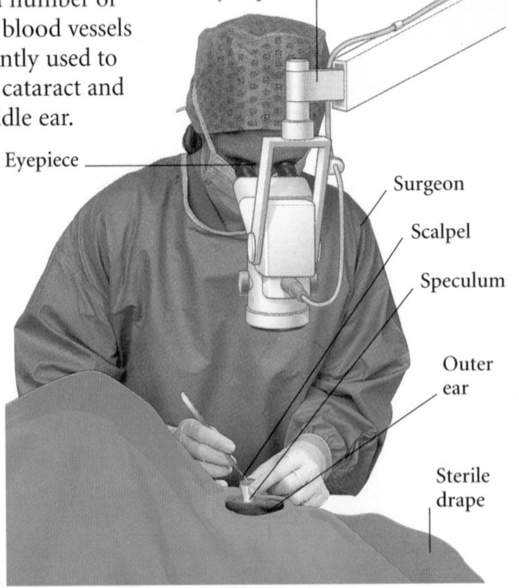

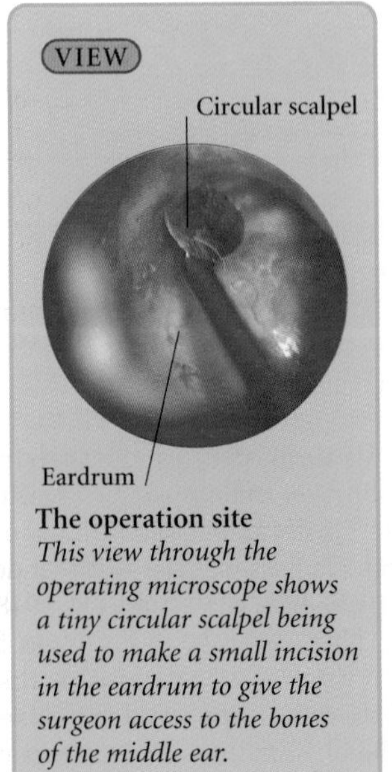

The operation site
This view through the operating microscope shows a tiny circular scalpel being used to make a small incision in the eardrum to give the surgeon access to the bones of the middle ear.

using foot pedals. This leaves his or her hands free to use small precision instruments, including scissors, forceps, and clamps (*see* HAVING MICROSURGERY, opposite page). To repair nerves and blood vessels, small needles and fine thread are used to make tiny stitches.

WHAT ARE THE RISKS?

Any type of surgery involves some risk, whether from a reaction to the anaesthetic, excessive bleeding, formation of blood clots, or infection. Some microsurgical operations take longer to carry out than other similar surgical procedures, which means that the time under anaesthesia is longer. This increases the risk of adverse reaction to the anaesthetic and may extend the recovery time from anaesthesia. The risk of infection may be greater with microsurgery since the operating site is exposed for a relatively long time compared with other procedures.

There is a high success rate for many of the most routine microsurgical procedures, such as cataract removal and repair of retinal detachment. However, some procedures, such as reattachment of severed limbs or reversal of female sterilization, have lower success rates, which are partly determined by the extent of the tissue damage. Nevertheless, without microsurgery, operations such as these could not be attempted.

(WWW) ONLINE SITES: p.1037

Laser treatment

Procedures using intense beams of light to cut, join, or destroy tissue

Light from a laser can cut or destroy tissue or repair damaged tissue by fusing together torn edges. This ability allows lasers to be used in a number of surgical procedures in place of scalpels, scissors, and stitches.

A wide range of lasers is used for various purposes, including treatment of skin problems, operations on the eye, and internal operations that are carried out in conjunction with endoscopes (*see* ENDOSCOPIC SURGERY, p.948).

Since laser beams can be focused precisely, small sections of tissue can be treated without causing damage to the surrounding tissues. Lasers produce differing wavelengths of light that are absorbed by different types of tissue. For example, a wavelength of light that is absorbed by melanin (the dark pigment that gives skin its colour) may be effective in removing a mole caused by the overproduction of melanin. A wavelength that is absorbed by blood causes clotting to occur and prevents bleeding from tissues cut during treatment.

Lasers generate intense heat, and laser treatment is therefore given in short bursts to avoid burning.

WHEN IS IT USED?

Laser treatment is commonly used in gynaecological procedures. A laser beam can be directed into the body through an endoscope to remove scar tissue inside the fallopian tubes, which may be a cause of infertility. Lasers are also used to remove cysts that form in the pelvic area due to endometriosis (p.742) and to destroy abnormal cells on the cervix that, if left untreated, may develop into cancer (*see* CERVICAL DYSPLASIA, p.749).

Small tumours or precancerous cells in other internal body areas, such as the larynx or inside the digestive tract, can be destroyed by laser beams directed through an endoscope. The technique can also be used to open arteries that have been narrowed by fatty deposits (*see* ATHEROSCLEROSIS, p.402). In ophthalmic surgery, laser beams can be used to seal small tears in the retina, the light-sensitive cells at the back of the eye (*see* RETINAL DETACHMENT, p.578).

Laser treatment is often used on the skin, especially on the face, for reducing scar tissue and birthmarks (p.828), noncancerous moles (p.343), wrinkles, or

(PROCEDURE) LASER TREATMENT ON THE SKIN

Lasers can be used to remove tattoos and birthmarks from the skin by destroying cells with a particular colour, such as cells in red birthmarks. A laser beam can also be used to reduce the severity of scars and the effects of aging, such as wrinkles, by removing the top layer of cells to smooth the skin. The beam of high-intensity light is precise and does not cause damage to surrounding cells.

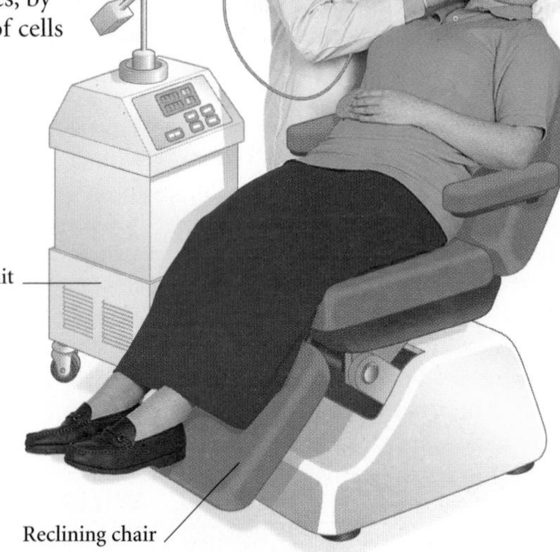

Treating a birthmark
To treat a birthmark on the face, a hand-held laser is used to give several short bursts of laser light. Local anaesthesia is normally used, and each treatment lasts about 20 minutes.

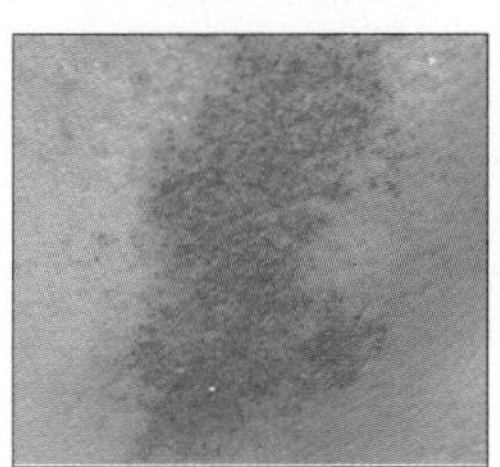
BEFORE TREATMENT

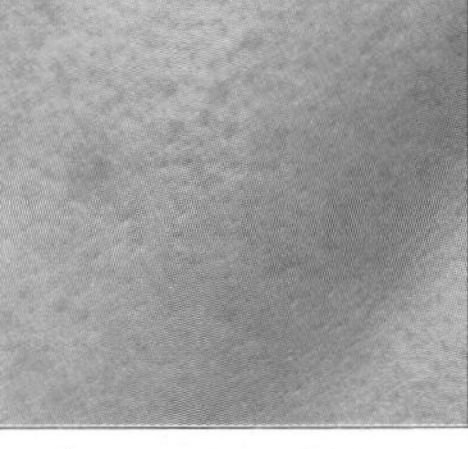
AFTER TREATMENT

Effect of treatment
Laser treatment destroys the cluster of blood vessels under the skin that make up the birthmark. In some cases, a course of several treatments is needed before noticeable improvement is seen and the birthmark disappears completely.

tattoos (*see* LASER TREATMENT ON THE SKIN, p.951). The results depend on the extent of the problem but in most cases scarring is minimal, and the appearance of the skin is much improved.

External laser treatment can also be used to treat conditions such as spider veins and to remove warts (p.354) on the skin and genital warts (p.768).

WHAT HAPPENS DURING THE TREATMENT?

Most forms of laser treatment are performed under either local or general anaesthesia, depending on the type of surgery and the area to be treated. However, for minor skin conditions, laser treatment causes little discomfort and may be performed without anaesthesia. There may be some swelling, redness, and blistering, which usually disappear within a week. Large areas of skin may need to be treated over several sessions.

WHAT ARE THE RISKS?

Occasionally, laser treatment may cause scarring, or there may be incomplete removal of damaged tissue. Skin treated by laser may also be vulnerable to infection until it has healed completely. The intense heat of the laser can sometimes lead to coarsening of the skin.

(WWW) ONLINE SITES: p.1037

Plastic surgery

Procedures used to repair and reconstruct skin and underlying tissue or alter its appearance

Skin or tissue that has been damaged or destroyed as a result of disease or injury or that has been malformed since birth can often be repaired or reconstructed using plastic surgery. The aim of plastic surgery is to restore the appearance and function of the affected area as much as possible with minimal visible scarring. A form of plastic surgery known as cosmetic surgery may be used in healthy people to disguise the signs of aging or to change the shape of part of the body. Cosmetic surgery may also be used following disease or injury. For example, skin grafting (p.318) can improve the appearance of burned skin, and breast reconstruction is often carried out after a mastectomy has been performed (*see* SURGERY FOR BREAST CANCER, p.761). Some congenital conditions, such as a cleft lip and palate (p.862), can be corrected by plastic surgery. Finally, plastic surgery can also be used in sex change operations to create or remove breasts and male and female genitals.

Before you have plastic surgery, it is important to obtain as much information as possible about the risks of the procedure and the likelihood of a good outcome. You should also check that the surgeon is well qualified and experienced in the techniques to be used.

WHAT HAPPENS DURING THE OPERATION?

In most plastic surgery, general anaesthesia is needed (*see* HAVING A GENERAL ANAESTHETIC, p.944). However, minor procedures, such as removing a mole, may be performed under local anaesthesia (*see* HAVING A LOCAL ANAESTHETIC, p.942). Various surgical techniques may be used, depending on the nature of the operation. A technique that is commonly used in plastic surgery is skin grafting, in which a piece of healthy skin is detached from one part of the body and is placed over a damaged area in another part. Another commonly used technique is the skin and muscle flap, in which a section of skin and underlying muscle is moved from one area of the body to replace damaged tissue in another area. This technique may be used together with an implant to reconstruct a breast following a mastectomy.

Cosmetic surgery uses a range of techniques that are either the same or similar to those used in plastic surgery to alter a person's appearance. For example, in cosmetic surgery the techniques used to alter breast size are similar to those used to reconstruct a breast following a mastectomy.

WHAT ARE THE RISKS?

Plastic surgery carries the risks of infection and bleeding that all other types of surgery share. Swelling and bruising after the operation are also common. When skin is grafted, the graft sometimes fails to attach properly to the new area, and the procedure needs to be repeated.

There is also the risk that plastic surgery may not produce as satisfactory an effect as initially expected, and sometimes scars remain afterwards.

(WWW) ONLINE SITES: p.1037

Transplant surgery

Operations carried out to replace failing body organs or tissues with healthy ones

Diseases can occasionally cause major organs, such as the heart, kidneys, or liver, to fail irreversibly. Dialysis (p.707) can take over the functions of the kidneys but may lead to a deterioration in health. Dialysis also has to be carried out frequently and is time-consuming. Replacing the diseased organ with a transplanted one is usually the best long-term treatment. In the case of a failing heart or liver, a transplant may be the only chance of survival if the organ has deteriorated significantly.

Many body organs and tissues can be transplanted. Kidney transplants are now common, and liver, heart, lung, cornea, and bone marrow transplants are performed routinely. Transplants of the intestines and pancreas are carried out less often. More than one organ may be transplanted at the same time, as in the case of heart and lung transplants.

Transplants are carried out not only to treat life-threatening conditions but also to improve quality of life when a condition is not potentially fatal. For example, a damaged cornea that causes loss of vision can be repaired by a corneal graft to restore sight.

Organ and tissue transplants can be carried out only if a suitable donor organ can be found at the right time and if the person receiving the transplant has no other medical problems that could hinder his or her recovery.

WHO ARE THE DONORS?

Transplants are usually performed only when the tissue type and blood group of the donor and recipient are similar. This is necessary because the recipient's immune system will attack any organ it identifies as "foreign", a process known as rejection. Most transplant organs are removed from donors who have very recently been declared dead and who are unrelated to the recipient. However, bone marrow and single kidneys can be taken from living donors without damaging their health. Bone marrow is always taken from a living donor. When bone marrow or kidneys are donated by a close, living, genetic relative, often a brother or sister, the transplants are

TECHNIQUE SURGERY USING A HEART–LUNG MACHINE

A heart–lung machine takes over the function of the heart and the lungs. This allows the surgeon to operate on the heart during certain major chest operations, such as coronary artery bypass grafts, a heart transplant, or heart valve replacements. The heart is cooled and paralysed to stop it beating during surgery, and blood is diverted to the heart–lung machine, which oxygenates the blood, removes carbon dioxide, and then returns the blood to the body. Afterwards, the heart is restarted with an electric shock and the circulation is restored.

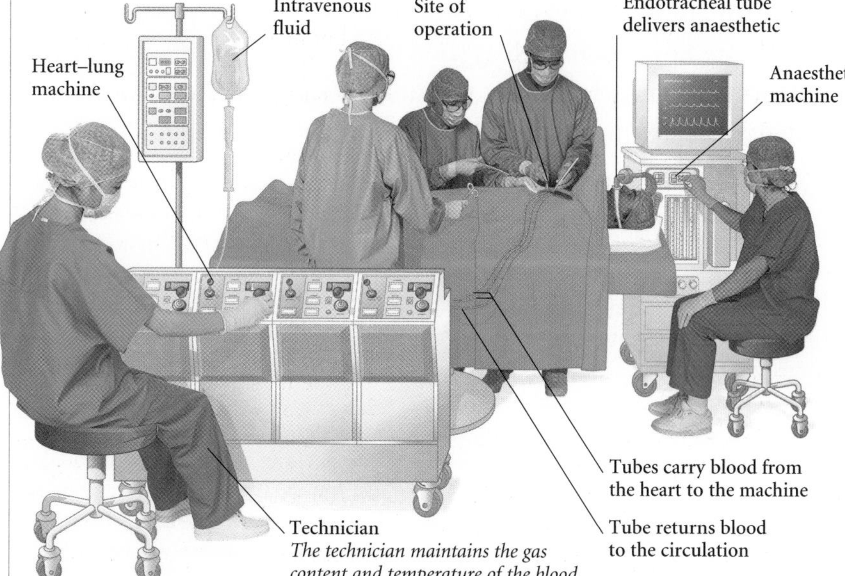

Technician
The technician maintains the gas content and temperature of the blood

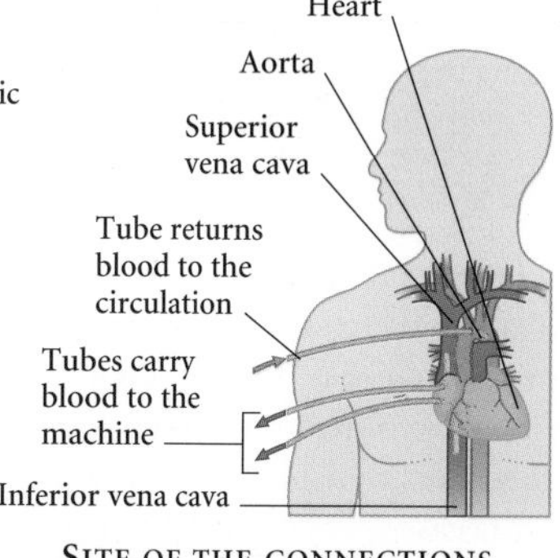

SITE OF THE CONNECTIONS

During the operation
Tubes from the heart–lung machine are inserted into the blood vessels entering and leaving the heart to divert blood through the machine. The heart is then stopped and the operation performed. Afterwards, the heart is restarted and disconnected from the machine.

far less likely to be rejected by the recipient because the tissue types are likely to match more closely.

In the case of organ transplants from a donor who has recently died, most come from people in whom brain function has ceased irreversibly but whose other organs have been kept functioning by a life-support machine.

WHAT HAPPENS DURING THE OPERATION?

Most transplant surgery requires general anaesthesia (*see* HAVING A GENERAL ANAESTHETIC, p.944).

In an organ transplant, the organ to be transplanted is removed from the donor and chilled in a salt-containing solution until it reaches the operating room. This prolongs the time the organ can safely be deprived of its normal blood supply by a few hours. In most cases, the diseased organ is replaced by the donor organ. However, in kidney transplants (p.708) the defective organ may be left in place and the new kidney placed in the pelvis, where it is connected to the appropriate blood vessels. During a heart transplant (p.427), the major blood vessels are connected to a heart–lung machine to oxygenate the blood and remove the carbon dioxide from it while the heart transplant is being carried out (*see* SURGERY USING A HEART–LUNG MACHINE, above).

To perform a bone marrow transplant (p.454), cells from the centre of certain bones are collected from the living donor. These bone marrow cells are then transfused directly into one of the recipient's veins after his or her abnormal bone marrow has been destroyed. Alternatively, cells may be collected from the recipient's own bone marrow during a period when his or her underlying disease is in remission and frozen for later use. The stored bone marrow cells may then be thawed and used to replace abnormal bone marrow in the recipient's body if the disease recurs.

After a transplant, you will probably spend several days in a critical care unit (p.958). With all transplants except the cornea, you will need to take immunosuppressant drugs (p.906) indefinitely to prevent your immune system from rejecting the new organ or tissue. You should be able to leave hospital after a few weeks if the transplant has been successful. Recovery time for a corneal graft is shorter, and it is usually possible to go home after a few days.

WHAT ARE THE RISKS?

Transplant surgery, like other forms of major surgery, involves a risk of excessive bleeding and an adverse reaction to the anaesthetic. Transplant surgery carries a higher risk of infection than other types of surgery because immunosuppressant drugs interfere with the body's natural defences. However, the greatest risk of this type of surgery is that the transplanted organ will be rejected by the immune system and that this will cause the organ to fail.

Following a major transplant operation, the chances of long-term survival improve significantly once the first year after the operation has passed. However, survival depends on the transplanted organ not being rejected and on the recipient remaining free of a serious infection. The best outcomes are usually in people who were otherwise healthy when the original organ failed.

(WWW) ONLINE SITES: p.1037

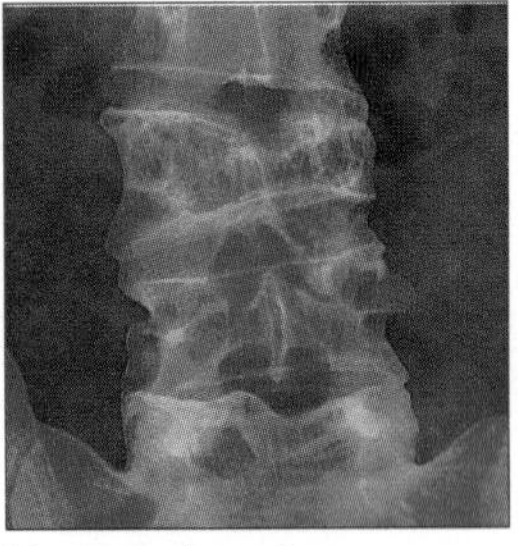

Treating the spine
Either conventional or complementary therapies may be used to relieve back pain.

Care and Therapies

In spite of advances in the prevention and early detection of disease, most of us need treatment from time to time to relieve symptoms or cure an illness. Patterns of medical care have changed recently: although major surgery and treatment for serious short-term illness still take place in hospital, people are now discharged as soon as possible. In addition, many long-term treatments and procedures now take place in the home or in an outpatient department without the need for admission to hospital.

The range of care and therapies that is available today to treat illness and injury is extensive. The first choice for most people is treatment recommended by their doctor, usually with drugs or, in some cases, with therapies such as physiotherapy or occupational therapy. However, complementary therapies, such as homeopathy, acupuncture, and hypnotherapy, are increasingly popular and are often used in conjunction with conventional treatments. Your doctor may suggest one of these therapies if he or she feels that it may be useful.

Location of care

The current emphasis is on providing care and therapies either in the home or in outpatient departments rather than in hospital. There are two reasons for this trend. The first is that the cost of hospital care is far greater than the cost of care as an outpatient. Secondly, visiting an outpatient department or receiving care in familiar surroundings is, for most people, preferable to being in hospital. However, there are times when hospital facilities and a skilled medical team are essential, as in the case of severe illness or injury or when a person who has a long-term illness cannot be cared for at home.

Choice of therapies

The type of care or therapy that is most appropriate for an individual depends on the severity of the illness or injury. Choice is an important element, and health-care professionals always try to consider the wishes of the individual. At one extreme, a person with an acute illness or a serious injury may require emergency admission to hospital and treatment in an intensive care unit. At the other extreme, a person who has strained a muscle may only need to have a short course of physiotherapy in a local outpatient department.

Therapies such as physiotherapy and occupational therapy are used to rehabilitate a person, usually following an acute illness or injury. They also help a person to remain independent during a long-term illness. Of equal importance are psychological therapies that are used to treat mental health problems, such as depression.

Complementary therapies have been used for centuries, but many have seen a surge in popularity in recent years. Although there is scepticism about the effectiveness of some therapies, doctors are becoming aware of the benefits of others. However, doctors tend to restrict their use of complementary therapies to the ones that, like all conventional medical treatments, are backed by sound evidence from controlled trials.

(PROCEDURE) Care at home

If you have an illness or disability that does not require admission to hospital, you will probably be cared for at home by a partner, close friend, or relative. Helping you with daily tasks, such as washing and dressing, does not necessarily require particular nursing skills. However, if you are very disabled, these tasks may require extra time and patience.

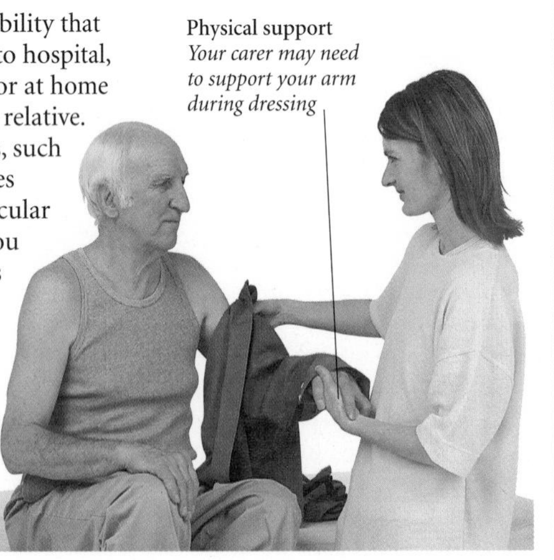

Physical support
Your carer may need to support your arm during dressing

Dressing and undressing
If you have a disability, such as a weak limb following a stroke, you may require help from your carer to dress and undress.

Care of the dying

Over the last few decades, there has been an increasing awareness that a person who is dying has unique needs. As a result, caring for people with a terminal illness has become a medical speciality. The medical and nursing care that addresses the needs of people who are dying is known as palliative care, and its main focus is on relieving distressing symptoms, such as pain and shortness of breath, with drugs and other techniques. The overall aim of palliative care is to provide a comfortable and dignified death while giving support to the partner and/or family of the dying person.

TREATMENT PROFESSIONAL CARE AND THERAPY

A variety of care and therapies are used to treat illness and disability. These range from high-technology medicine, such as that provided in an intensive care unit in hospital, to treatments that aid rehabilitation. In addition, complementary therapies, such as chiropractic (a manipulative therapy) and acupuncture, are now being used more widely.

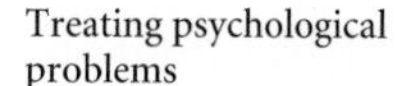

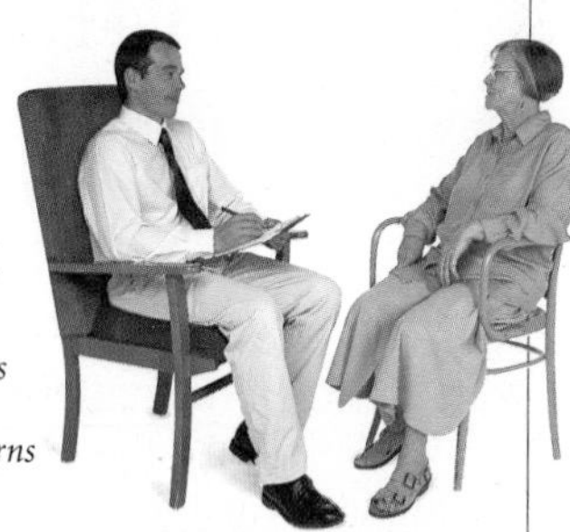

Treating psychological problems
Mental health problems may be treated with psychological therapies, such as helping people to identify and address their difficulties by changing thought and behaviour patterns

PSYCHOLOGICAL THERAPY

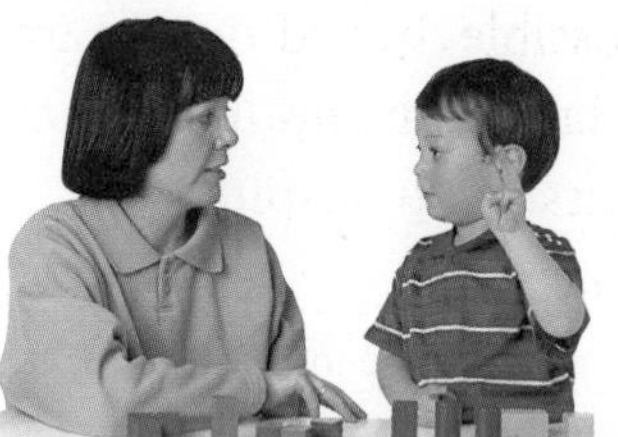

SPEECH THERAPY

Helping speech problems
People with speech and communication difficulties can be helped by speech therapy. Children may be given play therapy to help to develop their speech

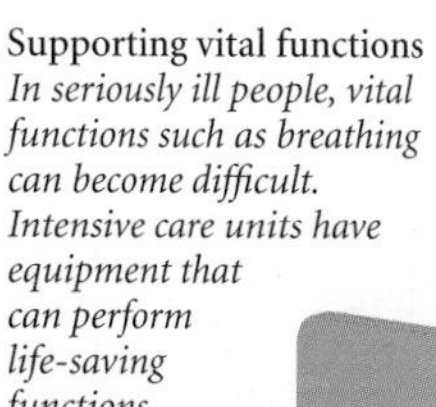

Supporting vital functions
In seriously ill people, vital functions such as breathing can become difficult. Intensive care units have equipment that can perform life-saving functions

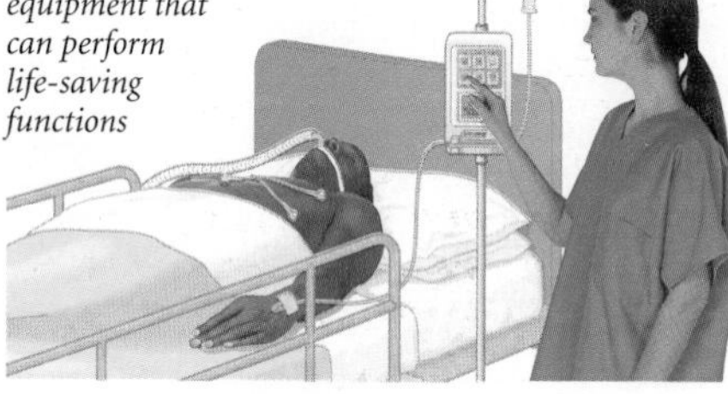

INTENSIVE CARE

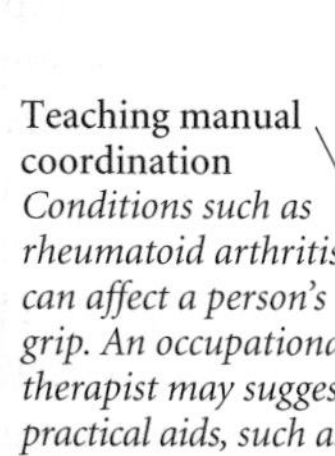

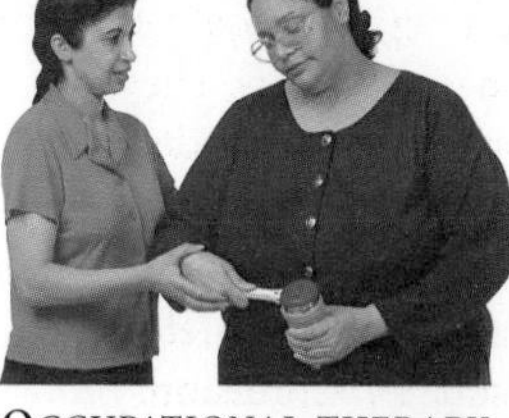

OCCUPATIONAL THERAPY

Teaching manual coordination
Conditions such as rheumatoid arthritis can affect a person's grip. An occupational therapist may suggest practical aids, such as a jar opener

Treating medical emergencies
An emergency, such as a cardiac arrest, may be treated at the scene by paramedics using life-saving equipment and resuscitation techniques

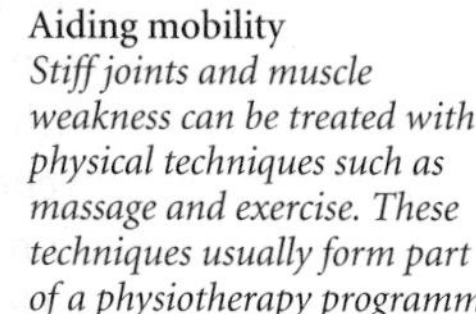

Aiding mobility
Stiff joints and muscle weakness can be treated with physical techniques such as massage and exercise. These techniques usually form part of a physiotherapy programme

PHYSIOTHERAPY

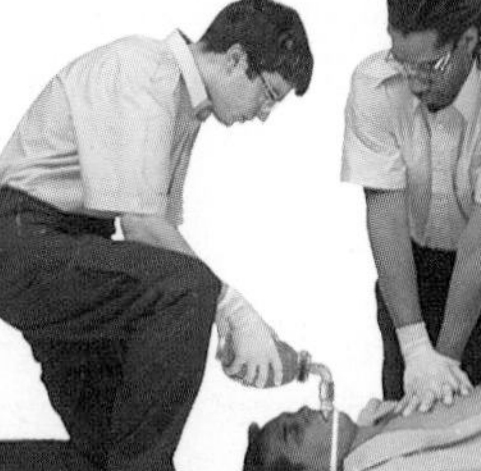

EMERGENCY CARE

COMPLEMENTARY THERAPIES

Although doctors do not always fully understand exactly how complementary therapies work, many therapies are used in addition to conventional medicines and surgery. Some therapies may be especially helpful for conditions such as migraine and eczema, which are often difficult to treat conventionally.

Effective complementary therapies
Manipulative therapies, which are used mainly to relieve disorders of the spine such as back and neck pain, and acupuncture, which has been shown to be useful in all types of pain relief, are two therapies that are often effective.

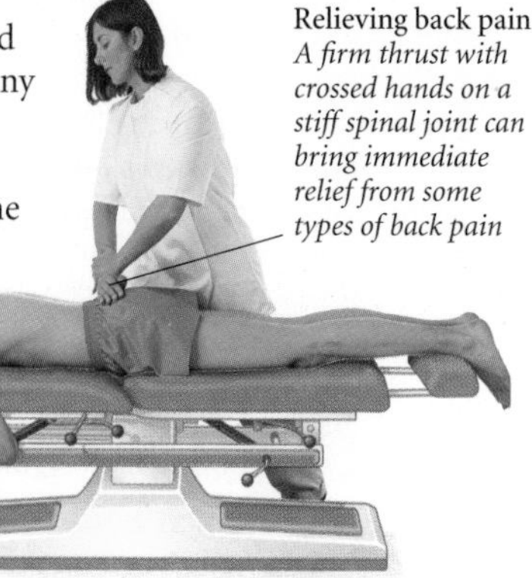

Relieving back pain
A firm thrust with crossed hands on a stiff spinal joint can bring immediate relief from some types of back pain

MANIPULATIVE THERAPY

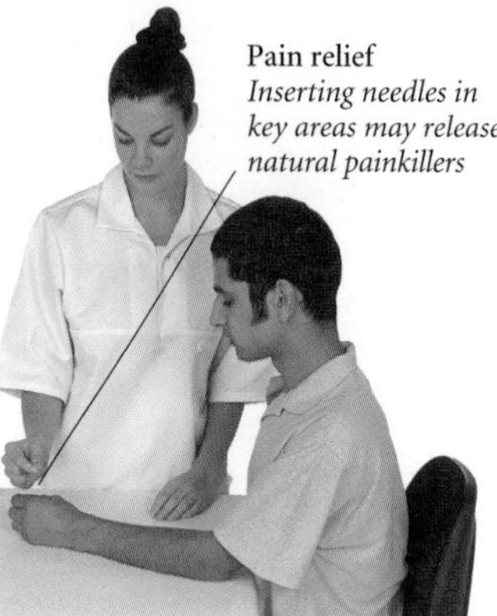

Pain relief
Inserting needles in key areas may release natural painkillers

ACUPUNCTURE

CARE OF THE SICK

Many people are referred for treatment or need nursing care at some time in their lives, but increasingly this takes place without a stay in hospital. The high cost of care in hospital and advances in medical techniques have created a trend for treatment on day wards and in outpatient clinics and for nursing care at home.

The first article in this section looks at ways of accessing hospital care, either through accident and emergency services or, more usually, when you are referred to a specialist for treatment.

Outpatient treatment, also known as ambulatory care, is provided in a number of settings. The development of less invasive surgical techniques has enabled many treatments that would once have required a hospital stay to be carried out on an outpatient basis.

The article on hospital care looks at the various reasons why you might be admitted to hospital and provides an overview of ward routines and staffing. The different levels of care, from routine care on a general ward to intensive care for people who are critically ill, are also described here.

Finally, the advantages of nursing care in the home are discussed, with particular emphasis on the need for support for long-term carers.

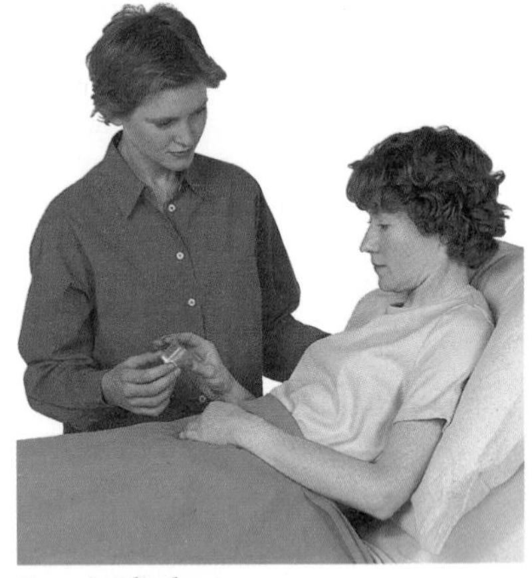

Care in the home
Drugs and other treatments that do not require specialized equipment or medical expertise can often be delivered just as effectively at home as in hospital.

Accessing hospital care

Being referred to hospital for secondary or tertiary care by your GP or going straight to hospital in an emergency

Most health problems can be diagnosed and treated at primary health care level by general practitioners (GPs). However, if you have an injury or an illness that requires special tests and/or expertise you may need treatment that can only be provided by a specialist in hospital.

The usual way of accessing hospital care is by referral from a GP, but people also have direct access to hospital treatment when they go to an accident and emergency department. Hospital clinics for the treatment of sexually transmitted infections, called STI clinics or genitourinary medicine clinics, are also run on the basis of self-referral.

REFERRAL BY YOUR GP

If your doctor thinks that your condition may be serious and requires urgent treatment, you should have only a short wait to see a consultant, and treatment should be arranged promptly. For less urgent problems you will probably have to wait longer for treatment. Waiting times vary from one region to the next and for different types of treatment, but you should not have to wait for more than 6 months for a first appointment with a consultant and for longer than 18 months for subsequent treatment.

If you are faced with a long wait for the treatment you need in your area, you can ask your GP to consider referring you to another hospital where the waiting time is shorter. You can also get information about which hospitals have the shortest waiting times for particular treatments from the Health Information Service helpline, which gives details of waiting times in all parts of the country.

GOING STRAIGHT TO HOSPITAL

People with urgent medical problems may be treated in the accident and emergency department of a hospital, and are sometimes admitted to hospital for further care if it is needed.

You may be taken to hospital by ambulance after an accident or because your condition causes concern, or your doctor may arrange emergency admission. For example, if you have severe chest pain that suggests a heart attack, you may be taken straight to hospital by ambulance. If your condition is serious, paramedics may stabilize your condition or begin treatment on the way (*see* INSIDE AN AMBULANCE, right).

Many people go to the accident and emergency department themselves after an accident or because they have severe symptoms, such as bleeding. However, every year thousands of people arrive at hospital with minor health problems that could be easily have been dealt with by their GP. If your injuries or symptoms are not severe, you should consider waiting to see your GP or calling the NHS helpline, NHS Direct, for advice.

(WWW) ONLINE SITES: p.1026

Outpatient and day care treatment

Hospital treatment that does not require an overnight stay

Many hospital treatments are now carried out without the need for hospital admission. For example, you may be treated in a hospital outpatient clinic or admitted to a day ward and discharged on the same day as your treatment. This form of treatment is sometimes called ambulatory care and can take place in a variety of settings, including local, community, and cottage hospitals, and GP hospitals, where GPs treat their own patients. Most first consultations with a specialist take place in an outpatient department. You may also need to go to an outpatient clinic or spend time on a day ward for more complex tests such as coronary angiography (p.408).

WHAT TREATMENT CAN BE PROVIDED?

Many elements of hospital care, including giving specialist advice, prescribing drugs, and monitoring a person's condition, can be provided on a day care basis. In addition, a wide range of complex tests and treatments, including some surgical procedures and operations, can be carried out successfully in outpatient clinics or in day care units.

Many minor surgical procedures that do not need a general anaesthetic, such as the removal of skin lesions and cysts or cataract surgery (p.573) on the eye, can be performed as day cases.

In addition, an increasing number of operations can now be carried out as day cases using techniques that require only tiny incisions in the body or no incisions at all. For example, female sterilization (p.743) and hernia repairs (p.662) can be performed by endoscopic surgery (p.948), in which a viewing tube is inserted through a natural body opening or a tiny incision in the skin. Even if you have a general anaesthetic, you may not need to stay in hospital overnight.

Hospital care

Medical and nursing care that require a stay in hospital

Outpatient or day care treatment (left) is the preferred option for many procedures, but complicated treatments and severe illness may still require hospital admission. Hospitals provide specialized medical and nursing care as well as expertise, treatments, and technology not available elsewhere. A stay in hospital is always necessary for major surgery. You

SETTING INSIDE AN AMBULANCE

Most emergency ambulances are fully equipped with first aid and resuscitation equipment. The ambulance is staffed by paramedics who are trained in first aid procedures and resuscitation techniques. Paramedics are able to carry out life-saving treatment at the scene of an accident, in a person's home, and during the trip to hospital. The forms of emergency treatment that they can provide include setting up intravenous infusions, administering oxygen or drugs such as painkillers, and beginning artificial respiration. Defibrillation, in which electric shocks are used to treat abnormal heart rhythms, can also be performed.

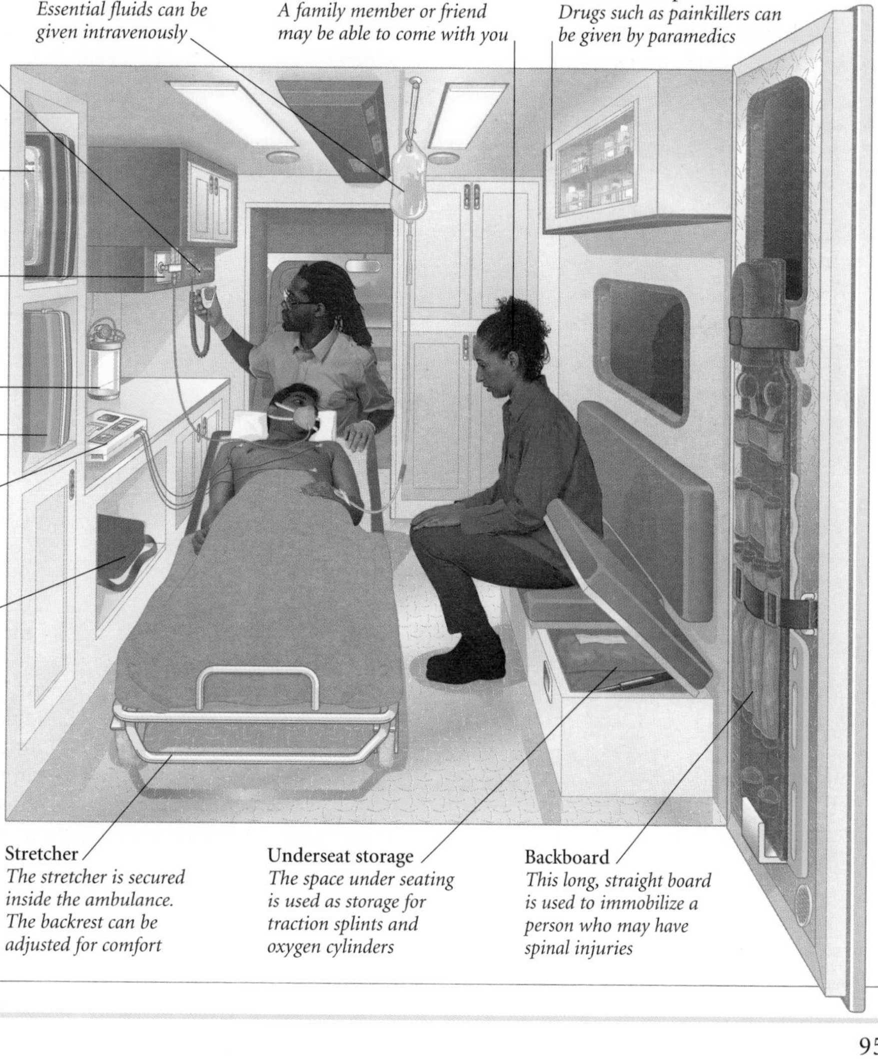

Radio/telephone
Communication between the paramedics, the hospital, and other emergency services is vital

Intravenous fluids
Essential fluids can be given intravenously

Relative
A family member or friend may be able to come with you

Medication cupboard
Drugs such as painkillers can be given by paramedics

Obstetric kit
A special emergency kit for delivering a baby is always kept on board the ambulance

Oxygen supply
Both piped and portable oxygen are available to treat a person with breathing difficulties

Suction equipment
This equipment is used to remove secretions from the mouth and airways

First aid supplies
All ambulances carry supplies such as bandages, dressings, and sterile gloves

ECG monitor
The monitor shows a tracing of electrical activity of the heart and can detect abnormalities

Defibrillator
This equipment delivers brief electric shocks to the heart to re-establish a normal heartbeat

Stretcher
The stretcher is secured inside the ambulance. The backrest can be adjusted for comfort

Underseat storage
The space under seating is used as storage for traction splints and oxygen cylinders

Backboard
This long, straight board is used to immobilize a person who may have spinal injuries

Inside the ambulance
Specialized equipment and supplies are stored securely on either side of the ambulance to allow room for the patient, paramedic, and stretcher.

may also need to be kept in hospital after minor surgery if you have a long-term disorder, such as a heart or lung disease, that increases the risk of complications.

You may need to be treated in hospital if you develop a serious illness or sustain a severe injury, or if you have a flare-up of an existing disorder, such as asthma (p.483). An elderly person may need time in hospital if his or her general health is poor. Children may be admitted to hospital for all of the above reasons or in particular circumstances, for example if a non-accidental injury is suspected. If a doctor is unsure about the cause of a child's symptoms, such as a high temperature or abdominal pain, the child may be need to be admitted to hospital for investigations.

You may need to be cared for in hospital if you are living alone and become too ill to look after yourself adequately. A hospital stay can be anything from one night to weeks or, rarely, months but the trend is towards early discharge. People with a long-term or terminal illness are more commonly cared for in a hospice or a nursing home.

WHAT ARE THE TYPES OF CARE?

Most routine operations and procedures can be arranged in a hospital near your home, but some conditions may need treatment in a specialist centre. For example, end-stage kidney failure (p.708), some types of cancer, and rare metabolic disorders are sometimes treated in hospitals that have particular expertise in these disorders. In addition, there are specialist hospitals for people who have long-standing mental health problems, although, whenever possible, care is arranged in the community using NHS and Social Services support services.

Routine admissions are to a general medical ward, but, if you are severely ill, you may need to be treated in an intensive care unit (below). Usually, children are cared for on children's wards in general hospitals, although there are some hospitals specifically for children.

GENERAL MEDICAL WARDS Most people are admitted to a general medical ward, which provides a wide range of routine care, or to a general surgical ward if they are to have surgery. There are also

SETTING INTENSIVE CARE UNIT

Most hospitals have an intensive care unit, sometimes called an intensive treatment unit, that is devoted to caring for people in a critical or unstable condition who need continuous monitoring. Frequently, patients in these units require mechanical ventilation, in which a machine takes over or assists with breathing. Blood pressure is checked continuously and heart rate and rhythm are monitored by an ECG machine. Fluids are given intravenously. If nutrients are required, they are supplied to the stomach through a tube.

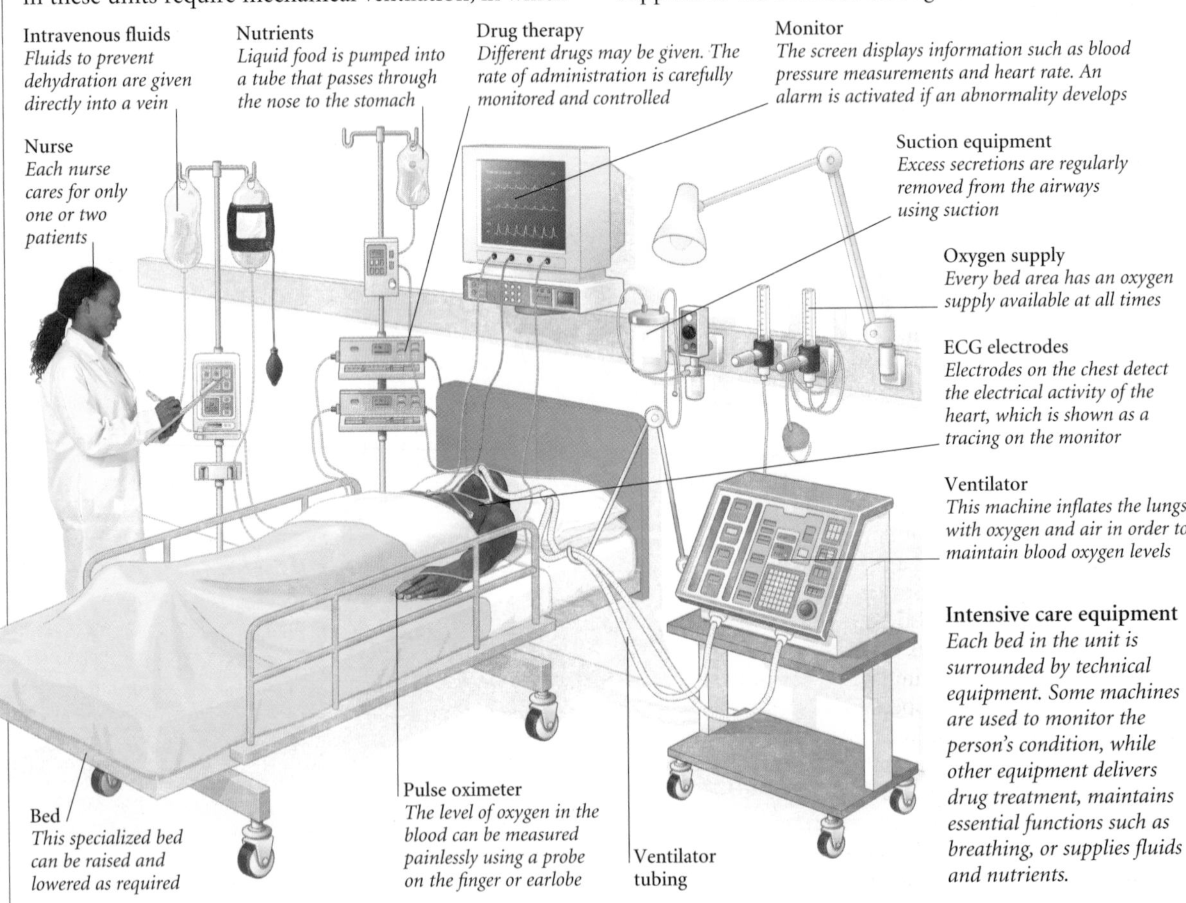

Intensive care equipment
Each bed in the unit is surrounded by technical equipment. Some machines are used to monitor the person's condition, while other equipment delivers drug treatment, maintains essential functions such as breathing, or supplies fluids and nutrients.

wards that are designated for a particular branch of medicine or type of disease, such as oncology wards for cancer and coronary wards for heart disease. The head of nursing on a ward is a sister, or a charge nurse if a man; either person may be called a ward manager.

You are usually allocated to a team of nurses who will be responsible for your care. Any medication that is needed will be given on a regular schedule, although drugs such as painkillers (p.912) will be given as and when they are needed. Your temperature, pulse, and blood pressure will be measured at regular intervals and recorded on charts so that your doctor can monitor your progress.

A particular consultant, with a team of doctors, is in charge of your treatment in hospital. Decisions about your care are made on medical rounds, when this team of professionals will examine you and discuss your condition. This is usually the best opportunity for you to ask questions about the results of tests, your treatments, and progress.

Most wards allow visiting for most of the day, but visitors may be advised to avoid early morning visits when staff are busiest. Visiting may be restricted until you have fully recovered from a general anaesthetic (*see* HAVING A GENERAL ANAESTHETIC, p.944).

INTENSIVE CARE UNITS People who are critically ill are usually admitted to an intensive care unit. These units differ from general wards in that they have a higher ratio of nurses to patients. They are also fully equipped with specialized equipment for treating and monitoring people who are seriously ill.

Admission to an intensive care unit is often necessary for monitoring after major surgery, such as transplant surgery (p.952) or heart surgery, or during a serious acute illness, such as a severe attack of asthma (p.483) or septicaemia (p.299). Intensive care may also be required after a person sustains a head injury (p.521) or other major injury.

Some intensive care units specialize in treating particular conditions. For example, if you have had a heart attack (*see* MYOCARDIAL INFARCTION, p.410), you will be treated in a coronary care unit where your treatment can be monitored continuously. Some hospitals have separate intensive care units for people with serious kidney, liver, or nervous system disorders. Newborn babies who are premature or ill are usually monitored and treated in a special care baby unit, also called a neonatal unit (*see* SPECIAL CARE BABY UNIT, above).

SETTING SPECIAL CARE BABY UNIT

Premature or seriously ill babies need intensive treatment and monitoring in a special care baby unit. The normal mechanisms that regulate breathing and body temperature may not be fully developed in a premature baby. A heater keeps the baby's body at a constant temperature, and the baby may be attached to a ventilator if he or she needs assistance to breathe.

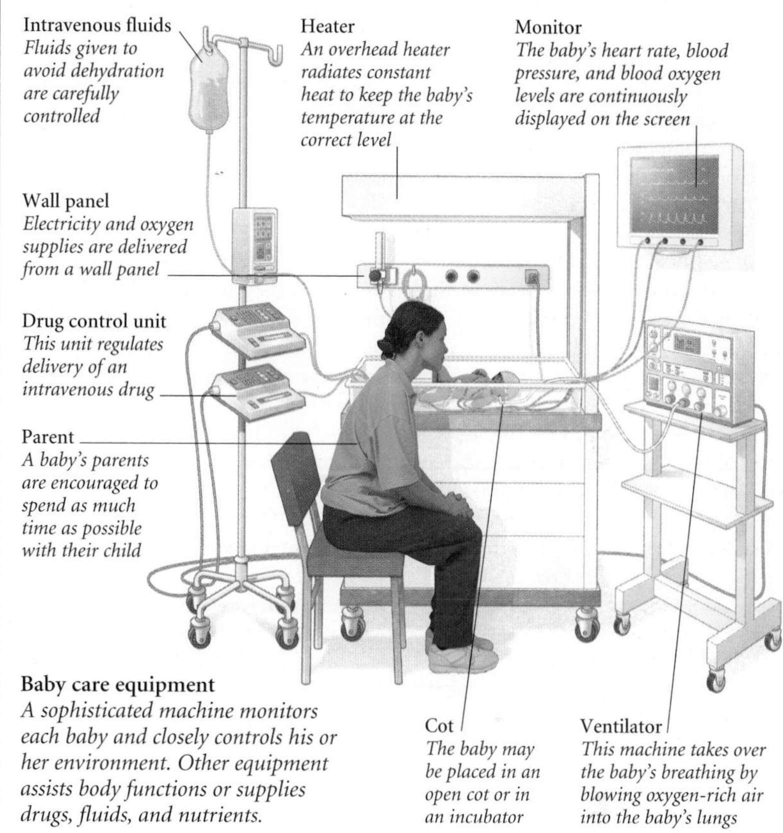

CHILDREN'S WARDS Children are almost always admitted to children's wards, staffed by doctors and nurses who specialize in the treatment of children. There is often a playroom attached to the unit to allow sick children the stimulation and company of other children. Play therapists and teachers may visit to provide educational support. Usually, a child's main concern is being separated from the family, and parents are encouraged to spend as much time as possible with their child. There are usually facilities for parents to stay overnight.

LEAVING HOSPITAL

The decision to discharge you from hospital will be made by your consultant after discussion with other members of the medical team and with you and your family. Ideally, your discharge will be planned in advance to allow time for any drugs that are needed to be prescribed and issued and any necessary follow-up care to be arranged.

After discharge from hospital, most people need no further care apart from follow-up appointments at an outpatient clinic or in a GP's surgery to check on their recovery. However, if you have a long-term disease or a disability as a result of illness, you may need rehabilitation, such as physiotherapy (p.961) or occupational therapy (p.962), at an outpatient clinic or in your own home.

(WWW) ONLINE SITES: p.1026

Home care

Nursing care and medical treatment delivered in a person's own home

As part of the trend away from hospital admission, many people are now treated at home. Even when hospital treatment is unavoidable, time spent in hospital is kept to the minimum, and care is often transferred to the home. Depending on your circumstances, you may be cared for by visiting health-care professionals working with family carers or friends.

Apart from the comfort and convenience of familiar surroundings, one of the main advantages of home care is that it reduces the risk of infections that are sometimes acquired in hospital.

Home care may be required for only a short period of time, such as after minor surgery, or may need to be established on a long-term basis for a person who has a long-standing illness, such as multiple sclerosis (p.541) or Alzheimer's disease (p.536). Some people with a terminal illness choose to be at home for the final weeks of their lives (*see* CARING FOR A TERMINALLY ILL PERSON, p.965).

PREPARING THE HOME

Depending on the severity of your illness and the extent of your disability, you may be advised to make practical adaptations to your home. Usually, an occupational therapist (*see* OCCUPATIONAL THERAPY, p.962) suggests which changes need to be made.

If you are only temporarily immobilized following an injury such as a leg fracture, you may need to have wheelchair ramps placed over steps. If you are likely to be permanently immobile, doorways can be widened and equipment, such as a lift to manoeuvre you from a chair to the bed or into the bath, can be installed to minimize the physical strain on your carer.

WHAT CARE CAN BE PROVIDED?

A growing number of treatments can now be carried out at home, including drug treatments, basic and specialist nursing care, and rehabilitation. You or your carer can be shown how to manage many simple and some more complex procedures yourselves on a day-to-day basis, while remaining under the overall supervision of visiting professionals.

DRUG TREATMENT Drugs are usually given orally, but some are given as injections or using a nebulizer that delivers drugs in aerosol form through a mask. Some painkillers, anticancer drugs, and antinausea drugs may be given by continuous infusion using a syringe pump. Injected, nebulized, and infusion drugs are usually first given by a nurse, but you or your carer may be shown how to administer them. If you have a heart or lung disorder, you may have oxygen at home to help to relieve breathlessness (*see* HOME OXYGEN THERAPY, p.507).

NURSING CARE Nursing help at home may include help with washing and getting dressed, changing wound dressings, monitoring healing, and helping to prevent pressure sores (p.350) in a person who is confined to bed. Specialized support may be needed. For example, a person with a stoma, an opening from the bowel that has been surgically created in the wall of the abdomen (*see* COLOSTOMY, p.666), will be shown how to manage it by a visiting stoma nurse.

REHABILITATION After major surgery or a disabling illness such as a stroke, you may need intensive rehabilitation to restore as much function as possible. A physiotherapist will arrange a programme of massage and exercise (*see* PHYSIOTHERAPY, p.961). You may also have occupational therapy (p.962) or speech therapy (p.963), depending on which skills you have lost.

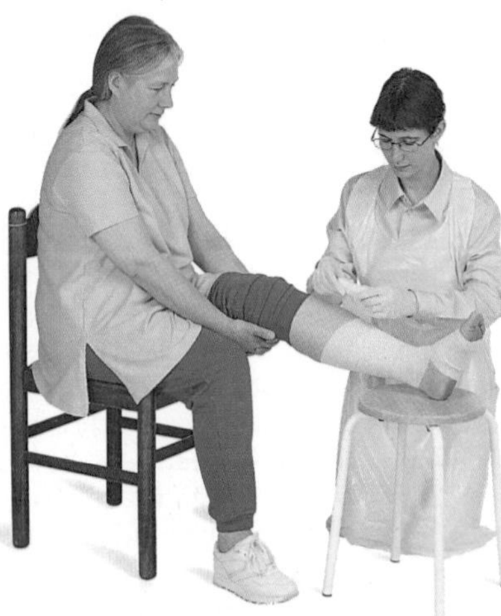

Changing a dressing
If necessary, a nurse can visit you regularly in your own home to change dressings and monitor the healing of a wound.

TECHNICAL TREATMENTS Advances in technology have made some kinds of medical equipment much easier to use. As a result, treatments such as kidney dialysis (p.707) can sometimes be carried out at home. If you are unable to eat, nasogastric feeding, in which liquid nutrients are pumped through a nasal tube to the stomach, may also be performed in your own home.

YOU AS CARER

As the partner, relative, or friend of a person who is ill, you may have made a conscious decision to become a carer. However, sometimes the role is taken on gradually as an ill, disabled, or elderly person becomes less able to cope. The role of carer can be physically and emotionally demanding, and you may find yourself neglecting your own health because of your other responsibilities. You may also feel resentful because the demands of caring inevitably lead to a loss of freedom. It is important that you do not ignore your own need for support. Joining a local support group to share experiences with people in a similar situation can make a difference. Making time for yourself is important. It may be possible to organise a short period of respite care for the person you care for in a residential home, nursing home, or local hospital.

Eventually, some carers find that they have to re-evaluate their role. There is no shame in admitting that you are having difficulty in coping, and it may be helpful to discuss the problem with your doctor or social worker.

MOVING INTO LONG-TERM CARE

The preferred option is to support care at home and in the community for as long as possible, but sometimes this is no longer viable. Eventually, long-term care may be needed for people with severe mental health problems, physical and/or learning difficulties, a degenerative disease such as multiple sclerosis, or a terminal illness. Elderly people who are physically frail or mentally impaired may also need to move into long-term care. The choice is usually between a specialist hospital, a hospice, a residential home for people with a fair degree of independence, or a nursing home for those who need full nursing care.

(WWW) ONLINE SITES: p.1033

REHABILITATION THERAPIES

Rehabilitation therapies aim to allow people to live independent lives, either after an illness or injury or because of a problem present since birth. Some therapies are used to treat children with developmental problems. Although some of these therapies may be started in hospital, treatment frequently continues at home.

This section describes three major types of therapy used in rehabilitation: physiotherapy, occupational therapy, and speech and language therapy. Rehabilitation may involve more than one type of therapy, and usually a programme is developed to meet an individual's needs and circumstances. The goal of physiotherapy is to improve mobility and maintain the normal function of the body using physical techniques, such as exercise, massage, hydrotherapy, heat and cold treatments, and ultrasound therapy.

Occupational therapy helps people who have physical or mental illnesses to cope with everyday living and allows those affected to remain as independent as possible. Speech therapy may be used to help people with communication problems or who have swallowing difficulties after a stroke.

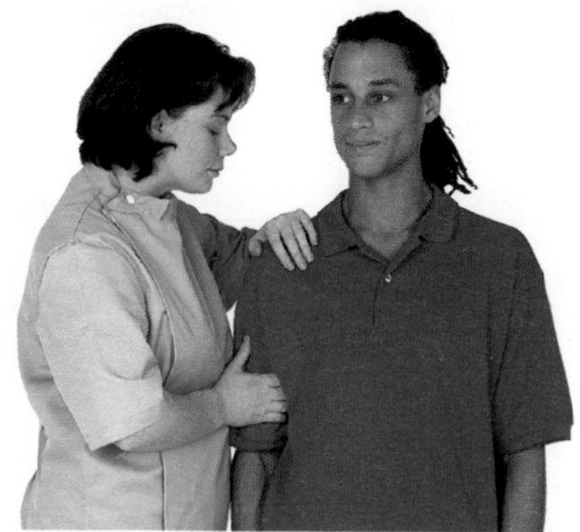

Assisting recovery
A variety of rehabilitation therapies can be used to relieve pain, speed the process of recovery, and help an individual to regain independence after an injury or illness.

Physiotherapy

The use of physical techniques, such as exercise and massage, to restore or maintain mobility and function

Physiotherapy is used to restore muscle strength and flexibility and to improve physical mobility after surgery, injury, or illness. It may also be used to help a person with a long-term disorder, such as arthritis (p.374), to maintain normal use of the body. In addition, physiotherapy can help to relieve pain and prevent complications from developing following an operation or an illness.

Physiotherapy is often combined with other types of treatment, such as drugs and occupational therapy (p.962).

WHAT DOES IT INVOLVE?

The physiotherapist starts by taking a detailed medical history and evaluating your condition. Assessment may involve determining the strength and flexibility of your muscles, how well you are able to get in and out of bed, and whether you are able to walk unaided or need to use a walking stick, walking frame, or wheelchair. The physiotherapist draws up a treatment plan using one or more physiotherapy techniques. These may include exercise, heat and cold treatments, massage, hydrotherapy, electrical stimulation, ultrasound, and gait training. A form of therapy called chest physiotherapy (p.962) may be used to prevent chest infections in people who are vulnerable because of illness or surgery.

EXERCISE Usually, the aim of exercise therapy is to strengthen weak muscles and increase flexibility. Exercise therapy is useful for anyone who has reduced movement in a limb. For example, this may occur after a person is confined to bed following knee surgery, after the limb has been immobilized to treat a fracture, or after a stroke. Anyone who has been confined to bed with a serious or long-term illness is likely to have lost muscle bulk and will also benefit from exercise. Your physiotherapist may show you exercises that you can do on your own, or, if you are unable to move a joint or limb, the physiotherapist may manipulate it to extend your range of movement. Equipment such as weights, treadmills, and exercise bicycles may be used in an exercise programme.

HEAT AND COLD TREATMENTS A physiotherapist often uses heat to treat muscle injuries and joint stiffness caused by excessive exercise or arthritis. The application of hot packs to the affected area stimulates blood flow, relaxes tense muscles, and relieves pain. Cold treatments using ice or cold packs may be used to reduce pain and swelling.

MASSAGE A physiotherapist uses his or her hands or specialized massage tools to knead muscles and stroke the body using circular or long, sweeping movements. Massage stimulates blood flow, which helps to reduce inflammation and relieve fluid retention and may also improve the suppleness of the skin. Massage techniques are also used by physiotherapists to promote relaxation, which in turn helps to relieve localized pain and muscle spasm.

HYDROTHERAPY This form of therapy usually takes place in a heated pool and uses water to support the body, making movements easier or providing resistance to motion during exercise. Gentle exercise can help to improve muscle strength, flexibility, and general fitness. Hydrotherapy is helpful if you are unable to bear weight on a limb because of injury or a disorder such as arthritis.

ELECTRICAL STIMULATION In this type of therapy, a mild electric current is passed through pads applied to the surface of the skin to generate heat, which relieves stiffness and improves mobility in joints affected by injury or illness.

ULTRASOUND This form of therapy uses high-energy sound waves to create heat in the tissues, which helps to relieve pain and inflammation. This technique

TECHNIQUE CHEST PHYSIOTHERAPY

Several techniques, including chest clapping and breathing exercises, are used in chest physiotherapy to prevent the accumulation of mucus in the lungs, which may otherwise lead to a chest infection. Chest physiotherapy is commonly used in elderly people who have had major surgery and in children with the inherited disorder cystic fibrosis.

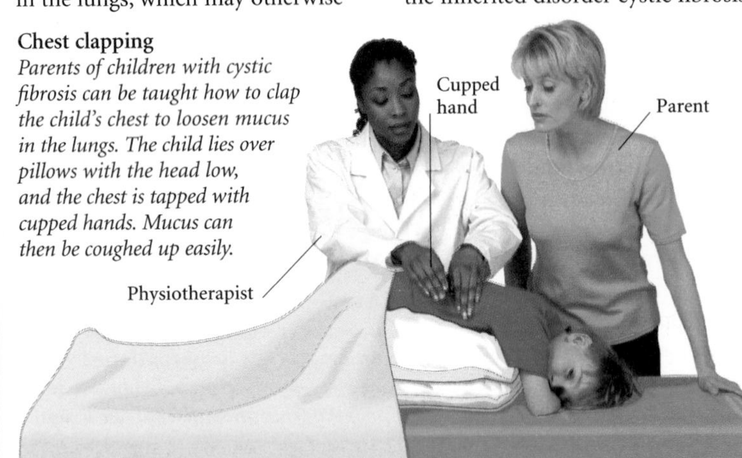

Chest clapping
Parents of children with cystic fibrosis can be taught how to clap the child's chest to loosen mucus in the lungs. The child lies over pillows with the head low, and the chest is tapped with cupped hands. Mucus can then be coughed up easily.

is often used to treat soft tissue injuries involving a ligament, tendon, or muscle and may be given in several sessions. A gel is applied to the skin, and an ultrasound probe is then placed on the skin and moved over the area being treated. After each session of ultrasound therapy, you may experience a slight tingling sensation in the affected area.

GAIT TRAINING This training is used to help a person to walk again after an injury or an illness such as a stroke (p.532) or if the person has a long-term disability. The type of equipment used supports the upper body while a person builds up strength in his or her legs.

CHEST PHYSIOTHERAPY This form of physiotherapy is used to help prevent chest infections in people who have had major surgery or who have an illness that prevents them from clearing their lungs. In particular, elderly people who have had a major operation and children with the inherited disorder cystic fibrosis (p.824) may accumulate mucus in their lungs, which may cause infections. You may be shown breathing and coughing exercises that help to expand the chest and fill the lungs with air. Some techniques involve lying in a position that allows mucus to drain from the lungs while the chest is tapped with cupped hands (*see* CHEST PHYSIOTHERAPY, above). If your child needs regular chest physiotherapy, you may be taught to use these techniques at home.

WHAT CAN I EXPECT?

You may need only a brief course of physiotherapy after a minor injury, but long-term therapy may be required after a major injury or illness. Physiotherapy helps to slow the progression of long-term disorders, such as cystic fibrosis, and reduce complications.

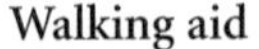
(WWW) ONLINE SITES: p.1036

Occupational therapy

Treatment to encourage independence following a physical illness or injury or in people with a mental health disorder

The purpose of occupational therapy is to help a person with a physical or mental health problem to be as independent as possible. The therapy is tailored to each individual's needs and may include help with daily tasks, such as dressing, bathing, driving, food preparation, and going to the toilet. It can also help a person who is returning to work after a long illness or severe injury and help children with a disability to develop their full potential. Usually, referral for occupational therapy comes from your own doctor or a hospital doctor. Occupational therapy is incorporated in a comprehensive treatment plan, which may also include drugs and physiotherapy (p.961).

WHEN IS IT USED?

Occupational therapy is used to help people cope with everyday living if simple tasks have become difficult because of a long-term disorder, such as multiple sclerosis (p.541) or arthritis (p.374). It is also used to aid recovery following hand or upper arm injuries or after a major illness, such as a stroke (p.532). An occupational therapist teaches a person how to conserve energy by using specialized techniques for daily tasks. A person may be shown how to use different muscles to carry out actions or to work with a variety of specialized aids.

Children who have learning difficulties or problems with coordination can benefit from occupational therapy. This therapy also helps elderly people to remain independent and active and may make enough difference to allow a person to stay in his or her own home.

In addition, occupational therapy is useful for people with a mental health problem such as schizophrenia (p.560). Once the main symptoms of the illness are under control, occupational therapy can help a person to adjust to living in the community by gradually increasing his or her independence, providing support, and preventing a relapse.

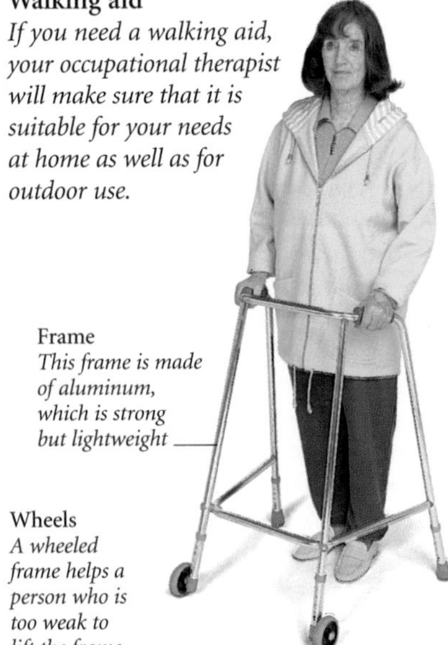

Walking aid
If you need a walking aid, your occupational therapist will make sure that it is suitable for your needs at home as well as for outdoor use.

Frame
This frame is made of aluminum, which is strong but lightweight

Wheels
A wheeled frame helps a person who is too weak to lift the frame

WHAT DOES IT INVOLVE?

At your first consultation, the occupational therapist starts by assessing your current health problems and past medical history. The therapist may arrange to visit you at home to observe how you manage with routine activities, such as dressing and bathing. The therapist may also ask you to perform specific tasks, such as making a hot drink. If your child needs to have occupational therapy, he or she is likely to be assessed by an occupational therapist who specializes in treating children.

Your occupational therapist will plan a therapy programme based on his or her initial assessment. The programme may include therapeutic activities and practical exercises to improve your performance of daily tasks. Your therapist may suggest or provide you with specialized equipment to make tasks easier.

PRACTICAL WORK If you need to build muscle strength, stamina, and concentration, your occupational therapist may recommend an activity such as a handicraft or cooking. For example, you may initially find it difficult to write following a stroke. Practical activities such as woodwork can help to improve your strength and fine muscle control, which may help you to regain near-normal dexterity and coordination.

HELP WITH AIDS AND EQUIPMENT Your occupational therapist can provide a wide range of equipment to help you to increase your independence. For example, items such as slings or splints can help provide support for a weakened part of the upper body. If you have a long-term disorder that restricts mobility, you may need to use a walking aid. Some adaptations to your home, such as raised chairs, handrails, or a stairlift, may be necessary. You may be offered specially adapted devices that can help to make everyday tasks, such as opening jars, dressing, and eating, easier.

WHAT CAN I EXPECT?

Your occupational therapist may see you several times to check your progress and to ensure that your treatment is effective. Depending on the extent of your disability, you will be helped to regain as much of your independence as possible.

(WWW) ONLINE SITES: p.1036

Speech therapy

Treatment to help people develop, improve, or recover their ability to speak

Speech therapy is used to help children and adults who have verbal communication problems. Speech therapy can benefit children whose speech is delayed by impaired hearing or learning difficulties or by physical problems, such as a cleft lip and palate (p.862).

People with a fluency problem, such as stuttering, may be given speech therapy, as may people who forget words or who have problems with comprehension or swallowing after a stroke (p.532). A speech problem with a physical cause, such as cancer of the larynx (p.481), may be helped by exercises or artificial aids.

WHAT DOES IT INVOLVE?

At your first appointment, your speech therapist will assess the extent of your speech problem and evaluate the effect that it has on your daily life. For children, the assessment is usually through observation of play. Adults are assessed on their ability to carry on a conversation and to perform tasks such as describing a picture. Part of the assessment conversation may be recorded on a computer and analysed later. This recording is used to determine whether your speech patterns, vocabulary, and the pitch, range, and volume of your voice are within normal ranges. If you find swallowing difficult as a result of a stroke, your speech therapist will advise you on eating and drinking safely.

The approach used in speech therapy depends on the problem, its cause, and the age of the person affected. Play therapy is often used to help children to improve their speech and is likely to be combined with other approaches, such as voice exercises. Parents or carers are taught useful games and exercises so that the child's speech improvement can continue at home.

Adults may be taught voice exercises or how to use artificial devices to aid communication. Speech difficulties that have been caused by a neurological problem such as a stroke may be helped by learning other ways of communicating. For example, you may be given a chart to indicate your basic needs until you are able to speak again.

PLAY THERAPY Children are frequently treated for speech problems using play therapy and games and by encouraging them to use both verbal and nonverbal communication. The speech therapist may also teach parents or carers how to encourage speech development at home by playing games that incorporate verbal description or naming.

EXERCISES If you have a condition that affects your mouth, tongue, or larynx (voice box), you may be given exercises that help to improve your articulation. For disorders that affect your fluency, you may be shown exercises to help you to control your speech and make you feel less anxious. If you have speech difficulties as a result of brain damage, such as a stroke, you may need to do exercises, such as describing pictures, to improve your word-retrieval abilities. In cases in which the larynx has been damaged or removed to treat cancer, a person can be taught to produce speech sounds by trapping air in the oesophagus and gradually releasing it.

USE OF ARTIFICIAL DEVICES There are a number of different electronic voice-synthesizers and artificial voice aids that may be used if speech difficulties are the result of a major physical problem. For example, if the larynx has been removed as part of treatment for cancer, a person may be taught to speak using a hand-held electromechanical device that generates sounds when it is held against the neck. Alternatively, a device called a tracheoesophageal implant may be fitted. The device is inserted between the windpipe and the oesophagus and uses inhaled air to produce sound. The sounds produced by the device can be converted into normal speech sounds using the lips, tongue, and teeth.

WHAT CAN I EXPECT?

Some problems, such as mild articulation problems, may improve with only a few weekly sessions of speech therapy. For other, more serious problems, regular speech therapy sessions over several months or years may be needed. Early treatment for children is particularly important because delayed speech affects the ability to relate to other people and may cause learning difficulties.

(WWW) ONLINE SITES: p.1036, p.1037

Death and dying

For many people, coming to terms with death is the most difficult challenge of their lives. Death may come peacefully at the end of a long life, be unexpected, or result from an incurable, progressive illness. In some cases of disease or injury, a point is reached when a cure becomes impossible and the goal of medical care changes.

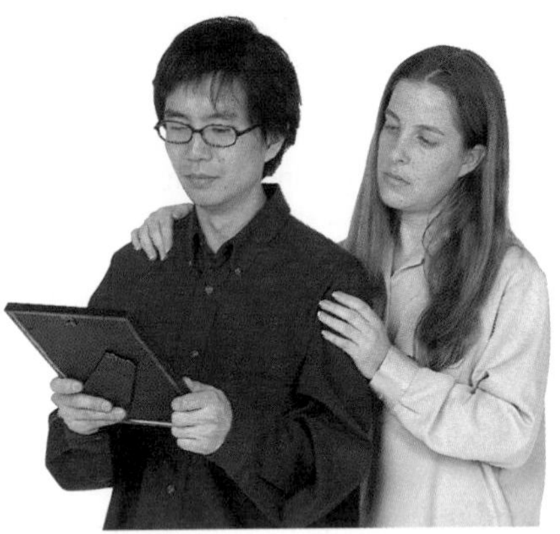

After a death
Coming to terms with a death may be a slow and difficult process. It is important to address your feelings and accept practical and emotional support from other people.

During the last weeks of life, active treatment of a disease itself is usually stopped, and treatment is directed at the relief of symptoms and making the most of the life that remains. This section initially addresses preparations for death, taking into account personal choices and values. Caring for a person who has a terminal illness is covered next. With the support of professionals who are skilled in terminal care, it is usually possible for family and friends to improve the quality of life of a dying person during the final stages of illness.

Finally, the period following death is discussed. This is a time when there are many practical issues to consider, such as arranging the funeral and registering the death, at the same time as dealing with grief. Bereavement is covered in more detail elsewhere (*see* LOSS AND BEREAVEMENT, p.76).

Practical preparations for death

Personal and practical decisions affecting a dying person that can be made before death occurs

A person who has come to terms with a terminal illness may wish to become involved in planning the final stages of his or her life and deciding what should happen after death. These preparations may include thinking about where to die, specific personal wishes concerning final medical care, planning burial arrangements, and arranging finances and updating a will. There will probably be many questions that a terminally ill person would like answered, such as when death might occur, how it will happen, and what it will feel like. A person who is facing death should be given every opportunity to ask health-care professionals about these concerns, and should be encouraged to discuss these issues with family and friends.

Children close to the dying person need special support and consideration. Very young children may not realize that death is permanent, but more than half will have come to understand this fact by about the age of 5. Try to keep children involved and informed because what they imagine is often worse than reality.

Making choices

Many people who are terminally ill have strong views about whether they would prefer to die in hospital, in a hospice, or in their own home. Ideally, the individual's personal attitudes and preferences should be established at an early stage so that terminal care can be planned with his or her involvement and cooperation. If a dying person decides to be nursed at home, care can often be carried out by family members or close friends with the ongoing support and advice of health-care professionals.

Living wills

Every adult, whether dying in hospital or at home, has the right to certain choices about his or her medical care. For example, an individual may wish to state how far he or she wants the hospital medical team to proceed with resuscitation if heartbeat or breathing suddenly stops. A living will, also known as an advance directive, is a document in which these preferences are expressed. Doctors caring for a person who has written a living will should be made aware of its existence, and the document should be consulted when the person is no longer able to make decisions. A living will is only legally binding for refusal of medical treatment, and it must have been voluntarily completed by a person who was mentally sound and fully understood the consequences of his or her decisions. To strengthen the validity of a living will, the document should be prepared with the help of a solicitor, a doctor, and family members.

(WWW) ONLINE SITES: p.1029

(SELF-HELP) Writing a living will

A living will, also known as an advance directive, is a written document that expresses your personal values, beliefs, and wishes related to medical treatment and dying. You could include any or all of the following issues in your living will:

- The name of a nominated person who knows your wishes and intentions, and who will assist in making critical medical decisions if you cannot do so.
- If desired, refusal of a particular treatment or procedure, such as tube feeding, intravenous infusions, blood transfusions, or antibiotic therapy.
- Specified circumstances in which no life-sustaining treatment, such as resuscitation or mechanical ventilation, should be given.
- Your wishes regarding organ donation after your death.

Caring for a terminally ill person

Relieving distress and discomfort during the final stages of life

For all people with a terminal illness, there comes a time when treatment for the disease itself no longer has a realistic chance of producing a cure and may cause harmful or unpleasant side effects. From this point, active treatment may be gradually withdrawn, and care is focused on achieving a dignified death for the person, avoiding distressing symptoms, and providing a reassuring and comfortable environment in which to spend the last days or weeks of life. Such measures are known as palliative care.

Once it is established that an illness is in its final stages, issues such as where death will take place, how pain will be controlled, and fear of death itself will undoubtedly cause anxiety for both the affected person and his or her family. To address these issues, health care professionals trained to relieve the distress caused by terminal illness usually work in partnership with the family.

Caring for a child with a terminal illness

Caring for a dying child is an intensely emotional and harrowing experience for everyone involved. Many children are looked after at home during the final stages of an illness because parents wish to carry out the care themselves. Effective communication is vital, and it is particularly important that parents are able to discuss the illness openly and honestly with the child.

There is a network of children's hospices and specialist nurses trained to help parents come to terms with the experience of caring for a dying child. These specialists are also able to address particular problems, such as difficulty in assessing pain and distress in children who are too young or too ill to communicate effectively. Parents can be taught to recognize nonverbal cues, such as facial expressions and body language, that may indicate that a child is in pain.

The parents of a dying child may find it helpful to contact specialist support groups and to meet other parents who are in a similar situation.

Accepting death

One of the most difficult aspects of terminal illness for both the dying person and his or her family and friends is the acceptance of imminent death. When a terminal illness is first diagnosed, many affected people express disbelief and anger. Normally, these feelings of denial are gradually replaced by acceptance.

For the terminally ill person, fear of being in pain and overwhelming anxiety about the moment of death may contribute to depression (*see* MENTAL PROBLEMS DUE TO PHYSICAL ILLNESS, p.558). Anxiety and depression can often be relieved by open and honest discussion, but in some cases, the doctor may prescribe antianxiety drugs (p.916) or antidepressant drugs (p.916). Family members and friends may also benefit from emotional support.

Relieving symptoms

Many people who have a terminal illness experience some degree of pain. Depending on the nature of the illness, a dying person may also have other symptoms, such as shortness of breath and nausea. In most people, distressing symptoms can be relieved using drug therapy or, in some cases, simple practical measures (*see* RELIEVING SYMPTOMS IN A TERMINALLY ILL PERSON, p.966).

CONTROLLING PAIN Most pain can be relieved with painkillers (p.912). Treatment is aimed at achieving maximum pain control with minimum side effects (*see* PAIN, p.516). In some cases, even if pain is well controlled, there can still be sudden episodes of severe "breakthrough" pain that may often be related to movement. However, with careful planning, this occasional pain can often be anticipated and avoided.

RELIEVING SHORTNESS OF BREATH A terminally ill person may experience difficulty breathing. This problem may be due to a lung disorder, such as pneumonia (p.490) or pulmonary embolism (p.495), or to a build-up of fluid in or around the lungs. Shortness of breath may also result from anaemia (p.446), in which the oxygen-carrying pigment of the blood is reduced. If there is an underlying infection, antibiotics (p.885) may help to relieve the symptoms. In many cases, shortness of breath can be alleviated by small doses of an opiate painkiller, such as morphine. Opiate drugs may also help to relieve anxiety, which often aggravates shortness of breath. The possibility of addiction to prescribed opiate drugs is not a cause for concern in the treatment of a person with a terminal illness.

CONTROLLING NAUSEA AND VOMITING Nausea and vomiting may be a symptom of the disease itself or may be a side effect of certain drugs, such as strong painkillers or anticancer drugs (p.907). However, antiemetic drugs (p.922) usually relieve nausea and vomiting if given regularly. Antiemetics are usually taken orally, but, if vomiting is severe, they can be given as an injection or as a suppository. If severe vomiting is causing distress, the stomach contents can be removed at regular intervals through a tube that is passed down the nose to the stomach and left in place.

Sometimes, acupressure bands, which are available over the counter, and acupuncture (p.973) may be helpful. Acupressure bands are placed on the wrists so that pressure is applied to a specific area. Acupuncture involves the insertion of fine needles into the skin at particular points around the body.

PREVENTING THIRST Regular intake of fluid, even if this is only sips of iced water, should be encouraged to help to prevent the discomfort of thirst and dehydration. However, if swallowing is difficult, an intravenous infusion of fluids may occasionally be required in order to avoid dehydration.

CARING FOR THE SKIN The skin should be kept clean and dry for hygiene and comfort. A regular change of position prevents sore skin (*see* PRESSURE SORES, p.350). However, if movement is severely restricted, specially designed beds and mattresses that aid nursing and provide extra comfort may be available.

PREVENTING DIGESTIVE PROBLEMS Constipation (p.628) is common in a terminally ill person and may lead to bloating and abdominal discomfort. Constipation is usually due to the person's reduced mobility but may also be a side effect of certain drugs. The doctor may prescribe laxatives (p.924),

TREATMENT RELIEVING SYMPTOMS IN A TERMINALLY ILL PERSON

Certain symptoms are often experienced during the final stages of a terminal illness. The most common are pain, a dry mouth, shortness of breath, nausea, and anxiety. These symptoms can usually be relieved using drugs or complementary therapies, which often require the support of professionals. However, there are also practical measures that can be performed by carers to make a person as comfortable as possible.

ALLEVIATING PAIN

In the majority of people, pain can be effectively controlled, both at home and in a hospital or hospice, by using oral or injectable painkillers (p.912), such as morphine. Alternatively, painkillers can be administered as a continuous infusion using a portable syringe pump.

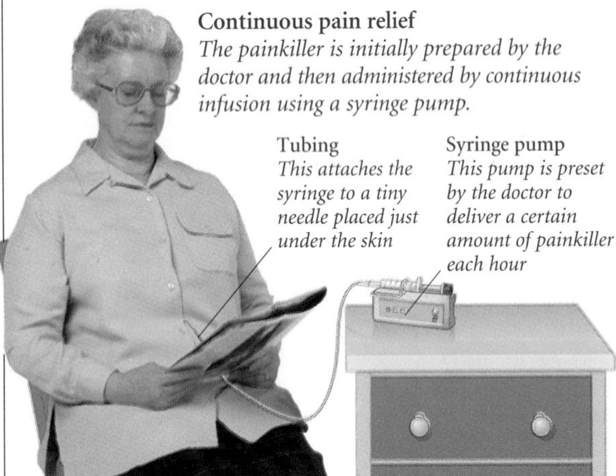

Continuous pain relief
The painkiller is initially prepared by the doctor and then administered by continuous infusion using a syringe pump.

RELIEVING A DRY MOUTH

Dryness of the lips and tongue often develops if a person is not drinking much fluid. You can help to keep the person's mouth moist by administering mouthwashes and regularly brushing his or her teeth. Fresh or canned pineapple is very effective for treating a furred tongue.

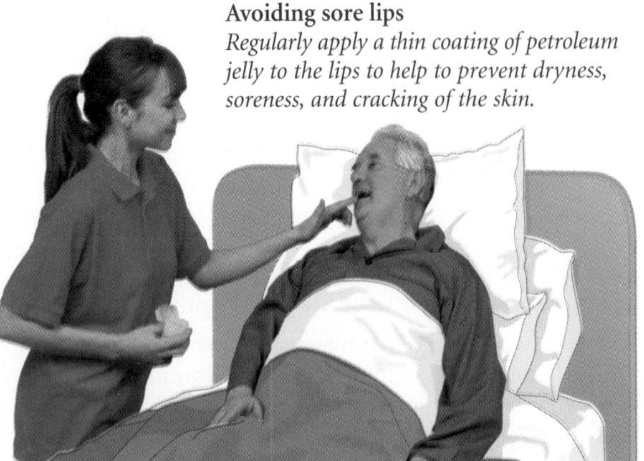

Avoiding sore lips
Regularly apply a thin coating of petroleum jelly to the lips to help to prevent dryness, soreness, and cracking of the skin.

AVOIDING NAUSEA

About half of all people who have a terminal illness feel nauseated, which may in turn lead to vomiting and loss of appetite. In some cases, antiemetic drugs (p.922) are prescribed by the doctor to relieve nausea and vomiting. Large, heavy meals are inappropriate for a person who is very ill, and food smells should be kept to a minimum.

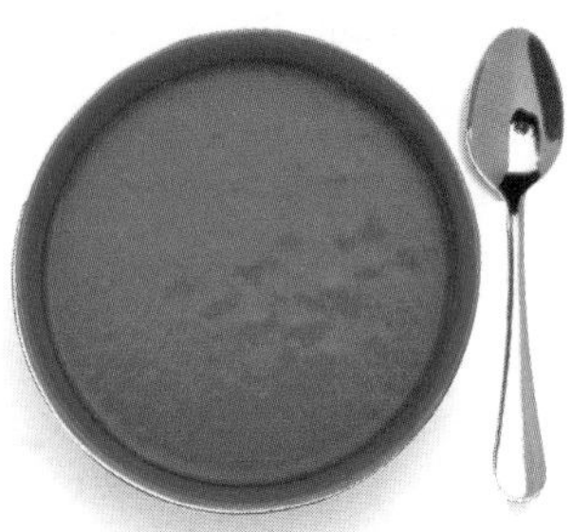

Palatable foods
A person who feels nauseated should not be pressed to eat regular meals. He or she may find snacks or nourishing fluids, such as soups, more palatable.

MINIMIZING ANXIETY

Complementary therapies, such as aromatherapy and massage, are effective methods of relieving anxiety and discomfort. Gentle massage can trigger the release of endorphins, the body's natural painkillers. Touch also encourages feelings of well-being and comfort.

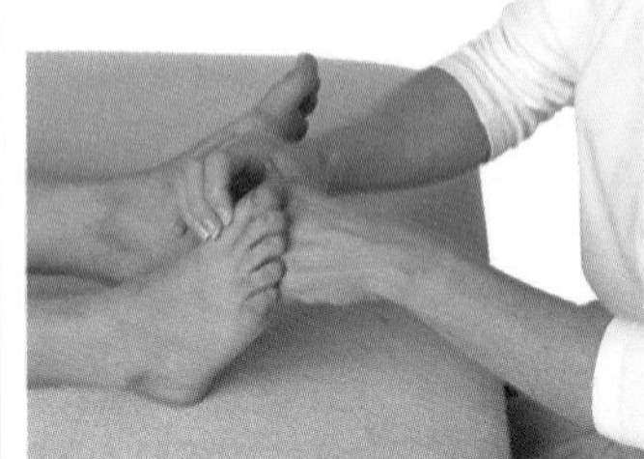

Foot massage
Massaging the feet can aid relaxation, relieve stress, and promote sleep. Using a massage oil or body lotion, apply gentle pressure to the sole of each foot in turn using your thumbs or knuckles.

EASING SHORTNESS OF BREATH

Severe shortness of breath can be alarming for both the person who is ill and for his or her family. Positioning the person comfortably and administering continuous or intermittent oxygen through a face mask usually helps to relieve shortness of breath. Use a portable electric fan to keep the air circulating around the room.

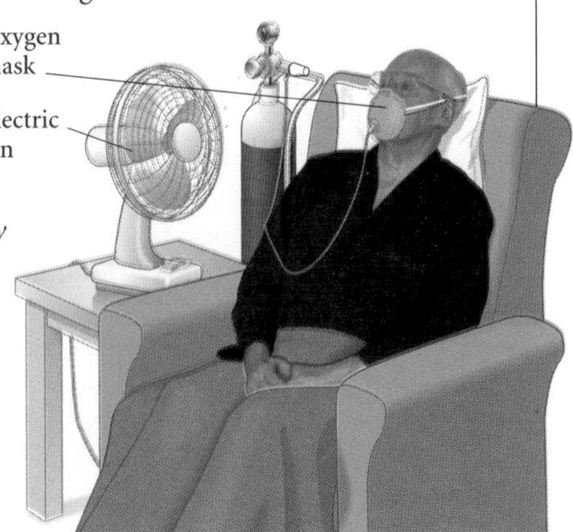

Helping with breathing
Careful positioning is important to allow the person's chest to expand freely for breathing. Many people are more comfortable sitting upright, either in a chair or in a bed, well supported by firm pillows.

either as pills or as suppositories, to help to prevent it. Diarrhoea (p.627) is rare unless there is an underlying bowel disorder, although "overflow" diarrhoea can be a complication of constipation.

THE LAST STAGE OF TERMINAL ILLNESS

The final stage of a terminal illness can be emotionally and physically exhausting for the family and other carers. If a dying person is conscious and alert, he or she may be able to participate in care and help with basic tasks, such as washing, ensuring an adequate fluid intake, and assessing how much pain relief is required. Familiar faces and reassuring surroundings are a great comfort to a dying person. Many people choose to die at home, and visiting hospice services and nurses may be arranged to care for and support the family.

As death approaches, a dying person may spend increasing amounts of time asleep. He or she may become confused and may slip into unconsciousness and then need full nursing care. If care is taking place at home, the community nurses will increase their practical and emotional support for the family. In particular, they may provide help at night, if possible, so that carers are able to have a break. If the family feels unable to cope at home, a dying person can be admitted to a hospice or hospital during the final days of his or her illness.

During the final stage of terminal illness, drug treatment is reviewed and medication that is no longer needed may be stopped. Painkillers will probably be continued, even if the person appears to be unresponsive, because he or she may still feel some discomfort. Drugs that were being given orally may be given by injection at this stage.

As the moment of death approaches, the pattern of breathing may change and may become noisier. Often, the person is deeply unconscious at this point, although some people remain conscious until the moment when their breathing ceases and death occurs.

For everyone concerned, the period leading up to a person's death is a traumatic experience. However, helping to provide a peaceful death can make the grieving process easier for the people who have been bereaved.

(WWW) ONLINE SITES: p.1029

What happens after a death

Practical procedures and emotional experiences that follow a death

Although the time following a death is emotionally distressing for the bereaved family, there are certain practical procedures that must be followed. If family members feel unable to cope with these matters, professional help is available. In many cases, the procedures have already been discussed within the family, and the deceased may have been involved in some of the planning before his or her death (*see* PRACTICAL PREPARATIONS FOR DEATH, p.964). This helps to relieve the strain of decision-making for relatives.

Organ donation may or may not have been talked about before a death. The family may be approached by a member of the nursing or medical staff to discuss their own views and those of their deceased relative, if known. Although it may be distressing to have to consider such issues so soon after a death, organ donation is often a comforting experience for the family in the long term.

REGISTERING THE DEATH

The doctor who has been caring for the deceased usually issues a death certificate, which states the cause of death. Staff at the hospital, your doctor, or the doctor employed by the funeral directors will give advice on how and where to register the death. In certain circumstances, such as when there is no next of kin, the doctor refers the death to the coroner, who then deals with the death certificate. In some circumstances, the coroner may decide that a postmortem examination is needed to confirm the cause of death; this is likely if the death was associated with certain work-related disorders, such as asbestos-related diseases (p.501), or occurred soon after an operation or medical procedure. In rare cases, in which a death was unexpected or appears not to have been due to natural causes, an inquest may be needed.

ARRANGING THE FUNERAL

Most families ask a funeral director to take care of the practical arrangements. Funeral directors are able to offer advice and suggestions for the funeral and give information about the formal procedures involved. Sometimes, the funeral arrangements can be made in advance with the participation of the dying person and his or her family. Funeral directors can also make preparations that enable family members to see the deceased for a last time, especially if they did not have the opportunity to say goodbye at the time of death.

Funerals can be arranged to suit personal preferences, religions, and cultural practices, but such requirements should be discussed and clarified at an early stage. Some people wish to be cremated, while others prefer a burial. The funeral service functions as both a memorial to the deceased person and the beginning of the acceptance of the death on the part of the bereaved.

THE EXPERIENCE OF GRIEVING

Although nearly everyone experiences bereavement at some time in life, the grief that follows a death can be a lonely and isolating experience (*see* LOSS AND BEREAVEMENT, p.76). After the initial shock and disbelief, overwhelming feelings of sadness and anger are common. A bereaved person may experience an irrational need to search for the person who has died. It can be difficult to accept the loss, especially for someone who has not seen the body after death.

During the first few months after the death, when these experiences are often at their most intense, it may seem that the world outside expects you to be getting over the loss. Although it can help to continue to work and maintain daily routines, the understanding and support of friends and family is especially important at this time. You may also find it helpful to contact an organisation that helps people to come to terms with their bereavement.

Eventually, perhaps over a number of years, nearly all bereaved people adjust to their loss. Keeping alive the memory of the person who has died is an important part of this adjustment process. Painful memories and feelings relating to the death may come back at times, especially on occasions such as anniversaries and family events. However, there usually comes a time when positive feelings about the person's life eclipse the memory of his or her death.

(WWW) ONLINE SITES: p.1029

PSYCHOLOGICAL THERAPIES

Many mental health problems, including depression, personality disorders, addictions, and eating disorders, may be helped by psychological therapies. There is a variety of therapies available, some of which explore a person's past while others focus on current behaviour or thought processes. The person in therapy is often encouraged to take an active role in the treatment.

The treatment of mental health problems with psychological therapy, or psychotherapy, was developed by Sigmund Freud at the end of the 19th century. Since that time, a number of different forms of psychological therapy have evolved. Some of the major types of therapy are described in this section, beginning with forms of psychoanalytic-based psychotherapy, in which the therapist tries to give a person insight into the effect of past experiences. The next two articles look at behaviour and cognitive therapies, which are based on changing the way people act or think. Both person-centred therapy and group therapy emphasize supporting the individual and helping people to achieve self-awareness and understanding. In the last article in this section, counselling is discussed. Counselling can help people who need to learn how to cope with personal problems and crises.

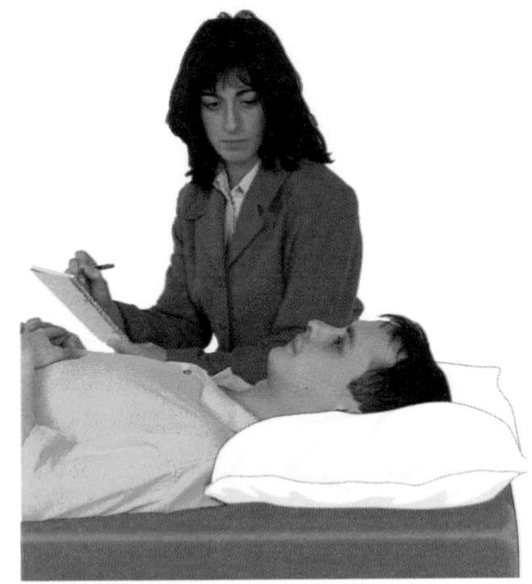

Psychoanalysis
In psychoanalytic-based psychotherapy, your therapist encourages you to talk freely about your past experiences. You work together to resolve your problems.

Psychoanalytic-based psychotherapy

Treatment that may help a person to overcome psychological problems by uncovering suppressed feelings

Psychoanalytic-based therapy tries to help people to identify, confront, and eventually work through their psychological problems. The therapy, which is also called psychoanalysis, is based on the theory that some painful feelings and memories are suppressed and confined to an unconscious part of the mind, and that these feelings may resurface as psychological problems.

In psychoanalytic-based psychotherapy, you are encouraged to talk freely about your past experiences and express openly the emotions that these recollections cause. Your therapist interprets the information you give to help you to gain insight into your psychological history and problems.

Classical psychoanalysis, as developed by Sigmund Freud, is the most intensive form and involves seeing a therapist several times a week for years. Today, other forms of psychoanalysis that are less time-consuming than classical psychoanalysis are available.

WHEN IS IT USED?

The various forms of psychoanalytic-based psychotherapy may be helpful for people in whom the cause of their psychological problems is not immediately apparent. The aim of the therapy is to increase a person's awareness of the way in which past experiences may have shaped his or her present moods and behaviour. For this reason, psychoanalytic-based therapy is most commonly used to help people who have a long history of depression (p.554).

WHAT DOES IT INVOLVE?

During classical psychoanalysis, you will probably lie on a couch while your therapist, who sits just out of your view, waits for you to reveal information. The therapist will encourage you to talk freely about whatever comes to mind. This technique, known as free association, helps your therapist to uncover painful feelings or memories that you may have repressed. You may have 3–6 sessions per week, each session lasting for up to 1 hour, for 3–5 years.

In the newer forms of treatment, you usually sit facing your therapist. These sessions last for 30 minutes to 1 hour and take place once or twice a week. Therapy usually continues for a period of 6 months to 2 years.

All forms of psychoanalytic-based psychotherapy use similar basic techniques and methods. The therapist interprets your memories and dreams, and the feelings you express, and uses the interpretation as a basis for discussion. The difference between the classical and the newer forms lies in the role of the therapist. In the newer forms, the therapist is more active in helping you to reveal information about your past.

A good relationship between you and your therapist is vital to successful treatment because you work together to resolve your problems over a relatively long period of time.

WHAT CAN I EXPECT?

Classical psychoanalysis is a time-consuming process, which you may find emotionally distressing at times. During the course of treatment, you may experience periods of vulnerability and despair when unwelcome feelings resurface before you feel able to deal with them. Supporters of psychoanalysis feel that the self-understanding that results from such distress leads to a resolution of psychological problems that outweighs the level of distress itself.

You might find the newer, briefer forms of therapy more acceptable than classical psychoanalysis because therapy with a time limit may motivate you to tackle specific issues by identifying and working through the underlying cause. You may find that your psychological problems are more likely to recur with shorter-term therapy, but you may be able to avoid this problem by obtaining support from group therapy (p.970) when your psychoanalytic-based therapy has come to an end.

(WWW) ONLINE SITES: p.1029

Behaviour therapy

Techniques for changing inappropriate behaviour by substituting new behaviour

The aim of behaviour therapy is to alter abnormal or maladjusted behaviour associated with certain psychological conditions. The therapist works to modify a person's current behaviour but does not explore the underlying reasons, as would occur in psychoanalytic-based therapy (opposite page).

Treatment is based on two ideas: desirable behaviour can be encouraged by using a system of rewards, and exposure to a feared experience or object under conditions where you feel safe will make it less threatening. Behaviour therapy is often used in combination with cognitive therapy (p.970), which explores and changes the thought processes that lead to abnormal behaviour.

TECHNIQUE DESENSITIZATION THERAPY

Desensitization therapy may help you to overcome a phobia. With the help of relaxation exercises in weekly sessions for several months, you will face the object or circumstance that you fear. You learn to overcome your phobia by facing the focus of it in its least distressing form and gradually working towards more direct contact.

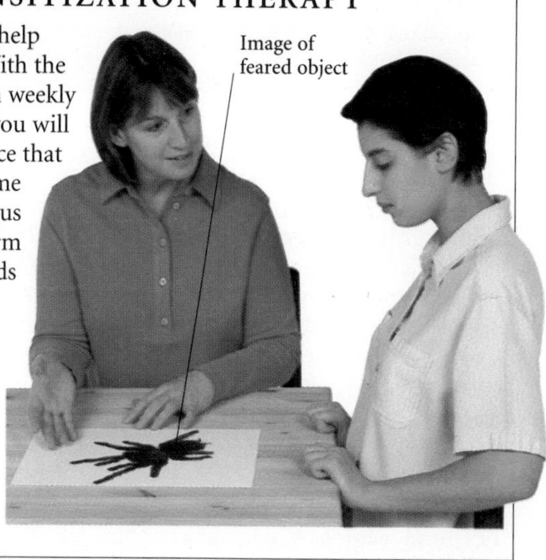
Image of feared object

During a session
The therapist helps you to face your phobia. In this case, a picture of a spider is used as the least distressing form of exposure for someone with an intense fear of spiders.

When is it used?

Behaviour therapy is useful in the treatment of a person with a phobia (p.552), which is an irrational fear that occurs in response to a particular object, creature, or circumstance. For example, a person may have an overwhelming fear of insects or air travel. Some people have a complex phobia, such as agoraphobia, which typically involves multiple fears about being trapped in crowds or being alone in open spaces.

People who have habitual behaviour, such as frequent, repeated hand-washing (*see* OBSESSIVE-COMPULSIVE DISORDER, p.553), or who lack assertiveness can also benefit from this therapy.

Behaviour therapy can also be used to treat certain eating disorders, such as anorexia nervosa (p.562) and bulimia (p.563), and it may help people with an anxiety-related problem such as panic attacks (*see* ANXIETY DISORDERS, p.551).

What does it involve?

Behaviour therapy begins with the therapist making a detailed analysis of your behaviour by interviewing you at length. You may be asked to rate the severity of your symptoms on a scale of 1 (mild) to 10 (extremely severe). Improvement may also be measured in this way. The therapist will discuss with you the best approach to overcoming your problem. The techniques that might be used include desensitization, and flooding, assertiveness training, and response prevention. Since changing ingrained behaviour often causes anxiety, you will probably also be taught to use relaxation techniques, such as breathing exercises, to help you cope.

DESENSITIZATION AND FLOODING Both desensitization and flooding are used to treat phobias. Desensitization involves gradually increasing exposure to the object or circumstance of the phobia (*see* DESENSITIZATION THERAPY, above) and uses relaxation techniques to help you deal with the anxiety. For example, if you have agoraphobia, in early sessions you might walk just outside your house with the therapist. As sessions continue, you may try walking from the house to the end of the street with your therapist until, over time, you can travel alone without anxiety.

Flooding forces you to confront the focus of your fear directly for prolonged periods. You will be supported throughout by your therapist. After you have confronted the object or circumstance of your phobia, either gradually or in one step, the distress associated with it is reduced and may eventually disappear completely.

ASSERTIVENESS TRAINING This therapy uses role-play to demonstrate the appropriate responses to different situations, for example someone acting aggressively towards you. Your therapist shows you an appropriate response and, by copying it, you become more confident in your ability to react to real situations.

RESPONSE PREVENTION This technique is used in the treatment of compulsive rituals, such as repeated hand-washing. You are encouraged to resist the urge to carry out the action, even though resistance results in intense anxiety. The therapist gives you support and suggests relaxation techniques. If you continue to successfully resist the compulsion, eventually the anxiety will lessen.

What can I expect?

You may find that improvement is slow at first and that it is difficult to avoid returning to your unwanted behaviour when your therapist is not there to support you. Group therapy (p.970) may be recommended to provide extra support when individual therapy ends.

Improvements in your behaviour can be maintained after your therapy has finished by carrying on with the techniques that you have learned.

Cognitive therapy

An approach to overcoming psychological problems that aims to change inappropriate attitudes and thoughts

Cognitive therapy is based on the idea that some psychological problems are maintained by inappropriate ways of thinking. It helps people to recognize and understand their current thought patterns and shows them ways to consciously change the way they think. Cognitive therapy does not look into past events and is often used in conjunction with behaviour therapy (p.969).

WHEN IS IT USED?

People who suffer depression (p.554) or those who lack confidence often benefit from cognitive therapy because it helps them to identify and change the thoughts that contribute to their low mood or self-esteem. Such thoughts may include "I am a failure", and "no one likes me because I'm ugly".

By pointing out inconsistencies in thinking, cognitive therapists can help people who have extreme concerns about their body shape, such as those with anorexia nervosa (p.562). Similarly, when it is used with behaviour therapy, cognitive therapy helps people to break habitual patterns of thought and/or behaviour (*see* OBSESSIVE–COMPULSIVE DISORDER, p.553).

In conjunction with drug treatment, cognitive therapy has been found to help some people with schizophrenia (p.560) to cope better with some of their symptoms, such as hearing voices.

WHAT DOES IT INVOLVE?

At the initial session, your therapist assesses your problem, and together you decide on an approach to solve it.

People undergoing cognitive therapy are often asked to keep a diary of their thoughts. For example, someone suffering from anxiety might be asked to record the thoughts that precede and accompany an anxiety attack.

During a therapy session, the therapist helps you to analyse the thoughts you have recorded and asks if you now feel they were appropriate to the circumstances. Once you identify those thoughts that are inappropriate, it then becomes possible to change them.

In some people, attempts to change ingrained ways of thinking may produce anxiety. To help people cope with anxiety, the cognitive therapist may teach relaxation techniques, such as breathing exercises.

You will probably see your therapist weekly for sessions lasting about 45 minutes to 1 hour. If you have a specific problem, such as stopping an unwanted habit, your therapy may only last for a matter of weeks. For more complex problems, such as low self-esteem, you may see your therapist for months.

WHAT CAN I EXPECT?

Once therapy is finished, you will probably need to make a conscious effort to analyse and challenge your thoughts for a while. However, many people find that their new thought patterns eventually become incorporated unconsciously.

(WWW) ONLINE SITES: p.1029

Person-centred therapy

A process that aims to increase a person's self-esteem and encourages self-reliance

Person-centred therapy is based on the concept that an individual's behaviour arises from their inner feelings and self-image rather than from their responses to people or past experiences. Person-centred therapists avoid interpreting or explaining the information a person gives them, in contrast to therapists in psychoanalytic-based therapies (p.968). Instead, the therapist gives a person support as he or she develops greater self-esteem and self-reliance.

The person-centred therapist is non-directive and helps to clarify a person's feelings and thoughts rather than telling him or her what to do or think. Most forms of person-centred therapy follow this approach, apart from Gestalt therapy, in which the therapist helps an person to reach increased self-awareness by directing them through a series of exercises or experiences.

WHEN IS IT USED?

Person-centred therapy may be used to treat long-term depression (p.554) and low self-esteem. This therapy is also used in crisis intervention to help people who are becoming increasingly overwhelmed by multiple stressful events. These events may be a combination of stresses such as problems at work, the failure of a marriage, or a physical or sexual assault. Person-centred therapy can be helpful in providing support, especially to individuals who need to work through their difficulties in an environment that feels safe.

Person-centred therapy is not often recommended for people with severe disorders, such as schizophrenia (p.560), in which the individual has no insight into his or her behaviour. Nor is this therapy considered appropriate for a person with severe mood swings (*see* BIPOLAR AFFECTIVE DISORDER, p.557) or obsessive–compulsive disorder (p.553).

WHAT DOES IT INVOLVE?

You and your therapist sit face to face while you speak about yourself, your relationships, and your environment. From time to time, your therapist summarizes what you have said but does not judge or interpret it.

In Gestalt therapy, the therapist plays a more active role. For example, if you are very introverted, he or she may ask you to act the role of an extrovert to help you to accept that you are capable of this type of expression.

You will probably see your therapist for a weekly session of about 1 hour. The duration of the treatment depends on the time it takes you to feel more confident and in control of your life. It may take months if you are trying to overcome a specific crisis, such as the loss of a loved one. However, if you have a less specific problem, such as long-term depression, it may take more than a year.

(WWW) ONLINE SITES: p.1029

Group therapy

Interaction with a small group of people to share experiences and feelings and gain insight or support

Group therapy is thought to be helpful in improving a person's ability to cope with and solve problems by discussing his or her experiences and emotions with a small group of people.

Each group session has one or more therapists who primarily help to guide the interaction that takes place. You may join a group directly or be referred to one in the course of individual therapy.

TECHNIQUE HAVING GROUP THERAPY

Group therapy encourages people to share problems and feelings with others, and some people find that it provides better motivation for change than individual therapy. Supportive group therapy may help you to overcome lack of self-esteem or confidence or an addiction. Therapy in groups of people with diverse problems may be useful because the relationships within the group raise issues and help to solve problems.

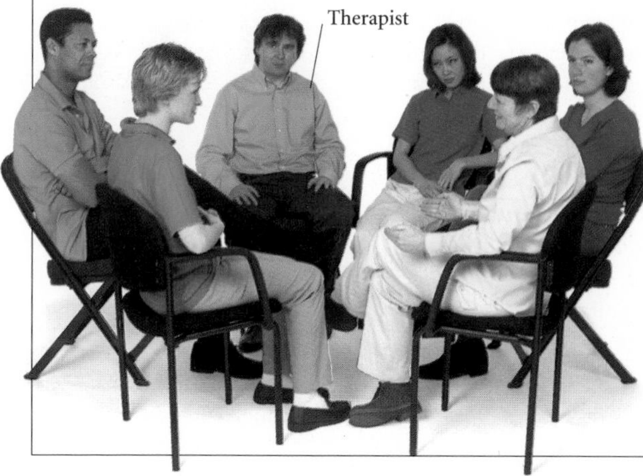

During a session
A therapist and up to 12 group members sit informally in a circle. The therapist directs group discussions and encourages one member at a time to talk in front of the group about their problems or feelings. The group may also be coached through role-play sessions.

Group therapy may use techniques from other forms of psychotherapy, such as psychoanalytic-based therapy (p.968), behaviour therapy (p.969), cognitive therapy (opposite page), and person-centred therapy (opposite page).

WHEN IS IT USED?

Group therapy is used to treat a wide range of problems. For instance, it is helpful for people with irrational fears, those who have suffered serious physical or sexual assault, and those with addictions or habits that they are trying to break. It is also used to support and continue the therapy of people who have finished individual therapy.

Group therapy is not suitable for people who particularly need personal attention and privacy in which to examine their own experiences and feelings. It is also unsuitable for people who are shy or extremely introverted, or for those with severe disorders, such as schizophrenia (p.560) or bipolar affective disorder (p.557).

WHAT DOES IT INVOLVE?

There are two main types of group therapy. One is supportive therapy, in which people with similar problems share their experiences and learn how to cope from each other. In the other type of group therapy, people with diverse problems are brought together. The therapist conducts the sessions so that the interactions among the group members can be explored, with the aim of enabling individual members to develop increased self-understanding. The group setting also allows an individual to test out opinions or newly learned ways of thinking in the group before applying them to everyday life.

Supportive groups are usually run as open groups. The number of meetings is unlimited and members may join and leave when they choose. By contrast, mixed groups are usually run as closed groups. The therapist selects the members, who meet for a limited number of sessions, sometimes as few as six.

Groups usually meet weekly for sessions of 1–2 hours (*see* HAVING GROUP THERAPY, above).

WHAT CAN I EXPECT?

It may take several sessions before you feel completely at ease in the group. You may also find that it will take some time before what you have learned in the group becomes part of your usual behaviour and thoughts. Some people find group therapy more useful than individual therapy, particularly if their problems relate to difficulties in interacting with other people or if they appreciate uncritical group support.

Counselling

Support in identifying and addressing personal problems

People who are having trouble coping with their problems may use counselling to provide support and relieve distress. Counsellors act as a sounding board and encourage people to express their feelings, allowing them to take the lead in dealing with their problems.

Counselling can help support people who are sad, worried, or facing a crisis. You may find it helpful if you are having difficulty dealing with bereavement or if you are facing a terminal illness. However, if you have more deep-seated psychological problems, you may need a form of therapy in which the therapist plays a stronger and more active role, such as behaviour therapy (p.969) or cognitive therapy (opposite page).

For some problems, you may need a specific form of support. For example, you may require relationship counselling if you are in a troubled relationship or debt counselling if you are continually in financial difficulty.

WHAT DOES IT INVOLVE?

At the first session, which may take one hour or longer, the counsellor asks you about yourself and your background to build up a clear picture of you and your problem. You may also discuss what you want counselling to achieve.

At counselling sessions, which are usually held once a week, you decide, with the counsellor's guidance, what you discuss and the pace at which you discuss it. Your counsellor may suggest problem-solving exercises to help you deal with your problems one by one.

Counselling may be short-term if you are dealing with a situation such as a bereavement, or long-term to help with a more complex problem.

WHAT CAN I EXPECT?

You may find that talking about your problems is enough to help you to find a solution. With your counsellor's support, you should be able to develop ways to solve your problems. In counselling, it is often easier than in some other therapies to see whether specific goals have been achieved.

(WWW) ONLINE SITES: p.1029

COMPLEMENTARY THERAPIES

A growing number of people now use complementary therapies for the treatment of a wide range of physical and psychological problems. In the past, these therapies were often described as "alternative" treatments, but now they are increasingly accepted and used to complement conventional medicine.

As their popularity increases, a number of complementary treatments are now being subjected to the rigorous testing and clinical trials that all conventional medical treatments have to undergo before acceptance. Trials have shown that the manipulative therapies chiropractic and osteopathy can be effective treatment for back and neck pain. Sometimes, therapies are found to relieve symptoms, but the reasons why they work remain controversial.

This section begins with an overview of the many types of complementary therapy that are available and gives advice about how to choose a therapist. Separate articles provide information about some of the most common forms of therapy. Each article discusses what the treatment is used for and which conditions are the most suitable for treatment before going on to describe how the treatment is carried out and the results that can be expected.

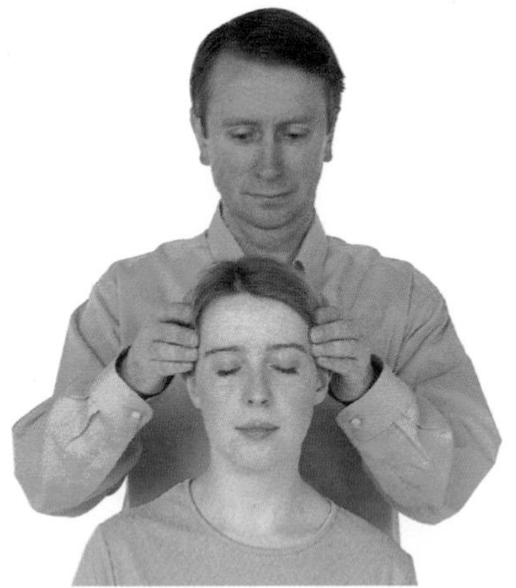

Massage
A complementary therapist may use gentle massage to relieve certain stress-related symptoms, such as tension headaches.

Complementary therapy choices

The place of complementary therapies in the treatment of disorders

Anyone who is interested in using complementary medicine to overcome an illness or maintain health is faced with a wide and often bewildering range of choices. There are many different complementary therapies available, but not all of them are supported by scientific evidence. For example, a form of therapy known as biofeedback (p.975) has been shown to reduce stress levels and blood pressure. By contrast, the effectiveness of reflexology, in which points on the feet are stimulated to treat a variety of disorders, is not supported by scientific research. For this reason, complementary therapies have varying degrees of medical acceptance.

Most complementary therapies aim to treat the whole person rather than just the symptoms of an illness and take account of a person's lifestyle and personality as well as his or her symptoms and medical history. Complementary therapists are often able to offer people more time than conventional doctors, and this extra attention may explain the popularity of these therapies.

WHAT ARE THE TYPES OF THERAPY?

The treatments used in complementary medicine fall into three broad categories: treatments based on movement and touch, such as massage, manipulative therapies (opposite page), acupuncture (opposite page), reflexology, and shiatsu; treatments using a medicinal approach, such as homeopathy (p.974), Chinese herbalism, and naturopathy; and those with a psychological basis, for example biofeedback, hypnotherapy (p.974), and meditation.

People tend to think of complementary therapies as being harmless, but certain herbs and preparations used in some therapies contain active ingredients that can be dangerous if used without sufficient care or in combination with prescription drugs.

WHEN SHOULD I SEE A THERAPIST?

It is very important to consult a medical doctor before you begin any type of complementary therapy. When you see a therapist, tell him or her about any medical treatment that you are already receiving (and vice versa).

Complementary therapies are often useful for treating persistent conditions, such as eczema (p.333); for easing lower back pain (p.381); and for alleviating stress (p.74) and anxiety (*see* ANXIETY DISORDERS, p.551). However, complementary therapies are not suitable for treating suddenly occurring conditions, such as an infection, or for use in emergencies, such as an asthma attack.

HOW DO I CHOOSE A THERAPIST?

Your choice of therapist will probably be determined in the first instance by your reason for seeking treatment. For example, if you want to stop smoking, you may feel that hypnotherapy can help, and, if you have back pain, you may choose a manipulative therapy.

You should find out if the therapist belongs to a professional organization and if there is a code of practice for the particular therapy. The therapies that are generally accepted by conventional medicine are those provided by practitioners who have passed examinations that allow them to be licensed and join a professional organization. You should avoid therapists who do not belong to a recognized organization or who make excessive claims for the treatment.

In the case of therapies that are more readily accepted medically, for example manipulation and acupuncture, your doctor may know of an accredited practitioner and refer you for treatment.

(WWW) ONLINE SITES: p.1029

Acupuncture

Stimulating points on the body, mainly by using needles, to relieve pain and help the body to heal itself

Acupuncture originated thousands of years ago as part of the system of traditional Chinese medicine. The technique treats disorders by stimulating various points on the body that are known as acupoints. Most commonly, acupuncture is performed with fine needles that are inserted into the skin. Acupuncture is gaining acceptance in mainstream medicine, particularly for pain relief, and some medical doctors now practise acupuncture themselves. Doctors who use acupuncture tend to use tender points on the body to guide their treatment instead of traditional acupoints.

A reputable, qualified acupuncturist always uses disposable needles or reusable needles that have been sterilized. This is important because of the risk of contracting acute hepatitis (p.644), HIV infection (*see* HIV INFECTION AND AIDS, p.297), or other blood-borne infections from contaminated needles.

HOW DOES IT WORK?

Research has shown that acupuncture can trigger the release of pain-killing chemicals called endorphins from nerve terminals in the brain. The procedure may also prevent pain messages from travelling to the brain by stimulating nerves around the site of the pain. The use of acupuncture in Chinese medicine is founded on the belief that an imbalance in the body's flow of energy gives rise to illness. Needles are inserted to relieve blockages and restore energy flow along one or more of the body's 14 meridians (energy channels).

WHAT IS IT USED FOR?

The most common use of acupuncture in conventional medicine is for pain relief, and the therapy is frequently used in pain clinics. In addition, acupuncture has been used successfully as an anaesthetic for dental and surgical procedures and during labour. Addictions have also been treated successfully by acupuncture. Other conditions that may respond to this therapy include hay fever (*see* ALLERGIC RHINITIS, p.466), migraine (p.518), and lower back pain (p.381).

WHAT HAPPENS IN A SESSION?

On your first visit to a traditional acupuncturist, he or she asks about your medical history and lifestyle. The acupuncturist assesses your condition by looking at your tongue and feeling 12 pulses, six in each wrist. Each pulse is believed to give information about the health of a particular body area. If the acupuncturist is a doctor, he or she will probably assess you by performing a physical examination and looking at your medical records.

The acupuncturist will ask you to remove clothing that is covering acupoints and to lie on an examining table. Between six and 12 acupoints may be used at any one time, depending on the condition being treated. A slight pricking sensation may be felt as the needles are inserted, but a competent acupuncturist should not cause any pain. The acupuncturist may rotate the needles for a few seconds to stimulate the acupoints. You may experience numbness and a slight ache while the needles are in place. Medical doctors who practice acupuncture may apply electrical stimulation to needles placed at selected acupoints.

The needles may be left in place for as little as a few seconds or as long as an hour, but 20–30 minutes is usual in most cases. The needles are then withdrawn quickly and gently.

WHAT CAN I EXPECT?

You may feel temporarily light-headed and drowsy just after treatment with acupuncture. The number of sessions you need varies according to the condition for which you are being treated. Some change in your condition is usually noticeable after about five sessions.

(WWW) ONLINE SITES: p.1029

Manipulative therapies

Manipulation of bones and muscles to treat disorders of the spine and joints

Manipulation as a treatment dates back to the second half of the 19th century, when two new techniques were developed based on the belief that many illnesses were due to misalignment of the spine. Such treatment was used for a broad spectrum of disease. Today, these two manipulative therapies, osteopathy and chiropractic, are used mainly to treat disorders of the musculoskeletal system, particularly of the joints and spine. Although regarded as separate practices, osteopathy and chiropractic share many similar techniques.

In the UK, osteopathy and chiropractic are regulated by their own councils, which were set up in the 1990s. These councils supervise education and professional standards of practitioners.

(TECHNIQUE) HAVING CHIROPRACTIC

Chiropractic is a manipulative therapy, used mainly on the spine, that is effective in the treatment of disorders such as lower back pain. The therapist manipulates the vertebrae (bones of the spine) by adjusting the position of the bones in relation to each other.

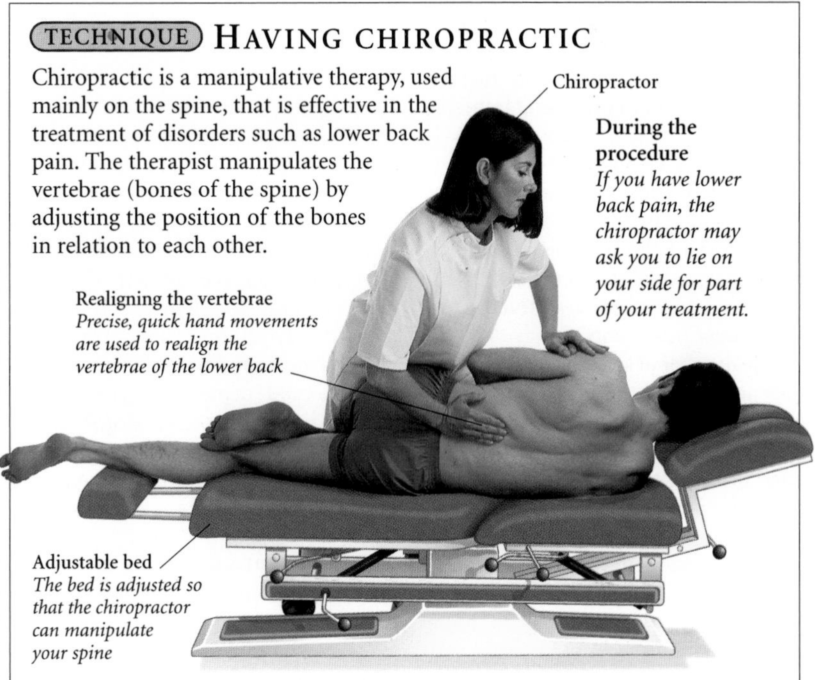

What is it used for?

In the UK, many people consult practitioners of osteopathy and chiropractic because of lower back pain (p.381) or neck pain. There is now good scientific evidence that these conditions can be treated successfully with either of these manipulative therapies.

What happens in a session?

A manipulative therapist will ask about your medical history in a similar way to a doctor. He or she will then give you a physical examination, looking for changes in muscle tension and skin tone, and for any restriction of the normal range of movement of the spine and other joints. The examination may include taking your blood pressure and testing your spinal reflexes. Chiropractors often include X-rays in their preliminary assessment, but osteopaths are less likely to do so.

The first consultation may last for 30–60 minutes, after which a treatment plan will be suggested. Treatment may involve a number of manipulative techniques, the best known of which is a sharp pushing movement called the "high velocity thrust". Chiropractors usually work directly on the spine (*see* HAVING CHIROPRACTIC, p.973), while osteopaths also manoeuvre the limbs. Both types of therapist may use prolonged pulling on a limb to relieve pain around a joint or increase its range of movement. A full course of treatment may take several weeks and include exercises for you to practise at home.

What can I expect?

Immediately after your first treatment session, you may experience temporary discomfort in the manipulated joints, headache, and fatigue, but these reactions tend to become less severe after subsequent treatments.

The number of sessions that you need depends on the condition being treated and how well you respond to treatment. Some short-term conditions improve after the first two or three treatment sessions. For example, if you have injured your back slightly while playing sport, you may find that you need only a few sessions. For long-standing conditions, the improvement may be more gradual, taking place over several sessions. Misalignment of the spine due to years of bad posture may take months of treatment to correct. In these cases, most therapists recommend regular maintenance visits once the condition has been treated successfully to prevent the problem from recurring.

(WWW) ONLINE SITES: p.1029

Homeopathy

The use of very dilute forms of natural substances to stimulate the body's defences against a disease

The basic principle of homeopathy is that the body's immune system can be stimulated to overcome an illness by administering a substance in a very dilute form that at full strength would produce the same symptoms as those of the illness to be treated.

Homeopathic remedies are prepared by a process of repeated dilution known as potentiation. The remedy is shaken after each stage of dilution. Eventually, the remedy becomes so dilute that only a few molecules, if any, of the original substance remain. The belief is that the more dilute a remedy is, the more potent it becomes, although how this can be the case is not fully understood.

There are more than 2,000 homeopathic remedies, most of which can be bought from a chemist without a prescription. Some remedies may contain several homeopathic preparations.

What is it used for?

Homeopathy is used to treat a range of physical and some psychological conditions. Physical conditions may include infections, such as the common cold (p.288); allergic conditions, such as hay fever (*see* ALLERGIC RHINITIS, p.466); skin conditions, such as eczema (p.333); and gynaecological problems, such as premenstrual syndrome (p.736). Common psychological conditions that are treated include mild depression (p.554) and anxiety disorders (p.551). Homeopathy is not suitable for sudden-onset conditions that may be life-threatening, such as asthma attacks and appendicitis.

What happens in a session?

Your first appointment with the homeopath usually lasts 1–2 hours. He or she will want to build a complete picture of you and your lifestyle and will ask you about your symptoms and medical history, family circumstances, emotional state, diet, and medications that you are taking. All of these factors influence the homeopath's choice of remedy.

The homeopath may give you a remedy during the consultation or write a prescription for you to take to a homeopathic chemist. He or she may also advise you on your lifestyle and diet. You may be asked to avoid caffeine, tobacco, and substances found in very sweet or spicy foods that are thought to counteract the action of some remedies.

The number and frequency of your follow-up visits depends on your symptoms. For most conditions the first follow-up visit is usually 4–8 weeks after starting treatment.

What can I expect?

Homeopathic remedies are so dilute that they should not result in side effects. However, you may find that your symptoms become worse temporarily about 10–14 days after you begin taking the remedy. This effect is thought to be due to the initial stimulation of your body's defence system and may last anything from a few hours to a few days.

The remedies for some conditions may take effect after only a few days of treatment. Long-term conditions, such as eczema, may take weeks or months before showing signs of improvement. If there is no improvement, it is important that you see your doctor.

(WWW) ONLINE SITES: p.1029

Hypnotherapy

Production of a trance-like state in which suggestions are made to help to reduce anxiety or change behaviour patterns

Hypnosis induces a deep state of relaxation. It is accepted by many doctors as an effective way to help people overcome stress-related disorders or to change behaviour patterns. Some hypnotherapists are medically qualified.

The hypnotherapist induces a state of trance in which breathing and heartbeat slow and brain activity is similar to that during meditation. While in this state, a person is relaxed and more open to suggestion. The hypnotherapist can take advantage of this to introduce positive ideas that may affect behaviour.

WHAT IS IT USED FOR?

Hypnotherapy has been shown to be useful for relaxation and is mainly used to treat people who suffer from anxiety and panic attacks (*see* ANXIETY DISORDERS, p.551). This form of therapy may also be used to help to overcome an irrational fear that is affecting your life (*see* PHOBIAS, p.552). Treatment with hypnotherapy may be helpful if you have a condition related to stress, such as irritable bowel syndrome (p.656) or migraine (p.518). You may also want to consider hypnosis to help you to change undesirable patterns of behaviour. For example, some people use hypnotherapy to help them to give up smoking.

WHAT HAPPENS IN A SESSION?

The hypnotherapist begins by asking about your physical and mental health and your motivation to change the unwanted behaviour. Different methods can be used to induce a trance, but you will probably be encouraged to lie back on a couch or in a chair. You may be asked to visualize something pleasant or to look at a certain object while the hypnotherapist slowly repeats a series of monotonous statements. When you are in a trance, the therapist makes suggestions aimed at changing your current behaviour, if this is the goal of the treatment. For example, if you are trying to stop smoking, the therapist may tell you that you no longer desire cigarettes. After a while you are brought slowly out of the trance, possibly by being asked to count backwards from 10 to 1.

The first session lasts about 1 hour; follow-up sessions may be shorter. The number of sessions needed depends on whether you respond well to hypnosis and how quickly improvement is seen. On average, 6–12 sessions are required to bring about a positive result.

WHAT CAN I EXPECT?

You may find that you experience an improvement in the problem you are trying to overcome after the first session. For example, if you are trying to stop smoking, you may find that your craving for tobacco is less strong. The time it takes to see an improvement depends on your motivation, how susceptible you are to hypnosis, and how deeply rooted your problems are.

(WWW) ONLINE SITES: p.1029

Biofeedback

Consciously altering biological functions to gain control over physical conditions, such as high blood pressure or anxiety

In biofeedback, body functions that are not normally under conscious control, such as heart rate and skin temperature, are monitored and translated into visual or auditory signals using special equipment. A person is taught relaxation techniques, such as deep breathing, to alter these functions. After several sessions, the person is able to produce a relaxed state at will without using the biofeedback equipment.

Although it is not yet known how the mind is able to influence the body's involuntary workings, biofeedback has been studied extensively, and results show that it can be effective for some situations. Biofeedback is generally well accepted by conventional medicine.

WHAT IS IT USED FOR?

Biofeedback is used most frequently for stress-related conditions, such as panic attacks (*see* ANXIETY DISORDERS, p.551), high blood pressure (*see* HYPERTENSION, p.403), tension headaches (p.518), irritable bowel syndrome (p.656), insomnia (p.554), and migraine (p.518). This type of therapy may also help muscle and joint pain and disorders caused by poor control over muscles, such as urinary incontinence (p.710).

WHAT HAPPENS IN A SESSION?

During your first session, the biofeedback practitioner may ask you about your general health, the history of your condition, and any medication that you are taking. He or she will show you how the biofeedback equipment works and attach electrodes to your skin, often on your scalp, arm, or fingers (*see* HAVING BIOFEEDBACK TRAINING, below). Your responses are relayed along wires to the biofeedback equipment and displayed on a dial or a monitor, sometimes as computer-generated images or sound waves. You are shown relaxation techniques, such as meditation, and taught to recognize biofeedback signals that indicate that you are relaxed. You can then practise producing these signals by using relaxation techniques.

Six to seven half-hour sessions are usually needed to produce a relaxed state at will. For long-term conditions, such as phobias (p.552), improvement may take weeks or months to achieve.

(WWW) ONLINE SITES: p.1029

(TECHNIQUE) HAVING BIOFEEDBACK TRAINING

Biofeedback training teaches you how to enter a relaxed state at will. Biofeedback equipment gives you information about your physical state, such as your heart rate, stress levels, and muscle tension. This changing information is constantly fed back to you as you try to practise various relaxation techniques. Over time, you learn consciously to control your body responses so that you can remain calm in stressful situations.

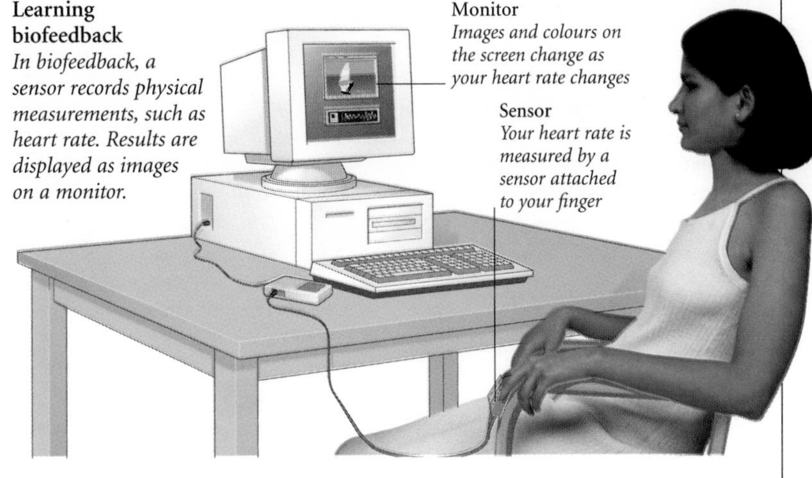

Learning biofeedback
In biofeedback, a sensor records physical measurements, such as heart rate. Results are displayed as images on a monitor.

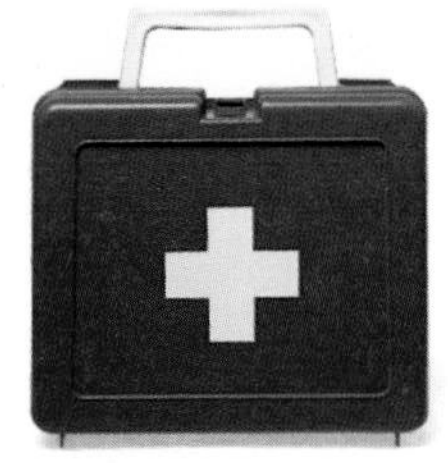

First-aid box
A first-aid box should be clearly marked with a cross so that it is easily recognized.

First Aid

FIRST AID IS THE IMMEDIATE CARE given to a person following an injury or sudden illness before medical help arrives. It can make the difference between life and death. The aim of first aid is to preserve life, to prevent the condition from worsening, and to promote as fast a recovery as possible. However, remember that you will not be able to help the person if you become a victim yourself. Always put your own safety first.

To be able to give effective first aid, you must follow a systematic plan and establish immediate priorities. This section aims to provide you with clear instructions to help you to handle common emergency situations. However, there is no substitute for professional training. The best way to prepare for a real-life emergency is to take a practical course in first aid.

FIRST AID PRIORITIES

Your top priority in an emergency is to get medical assistance by calling 999. If possible, ask a bystander to make the call for you. The caller should give the control officer as much information as possible about the situation and the condition of the victim. Let the control officer be the first to hang up the phone to ensure that all necessary information has been communicated.

As a first-aid provider, you must also check the scene for possible dangers to you, the victim, or bystanders, such as fire, dangerous fumes, or electrical power lines. Eliminate the danger if you can or remove the victim from the situation. If you cannot do so safely, phone for help immediately.

If you can approach the victim safely, you should aim to assess his or her condition and give appropriate first aid. If you do not feel qualified to give first aid, wait for professional help to arrive. Meanwhile, remain calm and reassure the victim.

TAKING A FIRST-AID COURSE

You can take a first-aid course at any local branch of the British Red Cross, St John Ambulance, or St Andrew's Ambulance Association. On successful completion of a course, you will receive a certificate that is effective for 3 years, after which time you will need to refresh your skills and take the test once again. First-aid training in some skills, such as artificial respiration, is valid for only 1 year.

(WWW) ONLINE SITES: p.1032

(EQUIPMENT) HOME FIRST-AID KIT

Having the correct supplies can make a big difference in an emergency, and you should always keep a supply of essential first-aid materials at home and in the car. Store the items in a first-aid kit or in a similar type of airtight container in a dry place. The kit should be easily accessible in an emergency but kept away from other medicines and out of the reach of children. Ideally, the kit should be small enough for you to carry easily. Check and replenish the first-aid kit regularly so that the contents are always kept up to date.

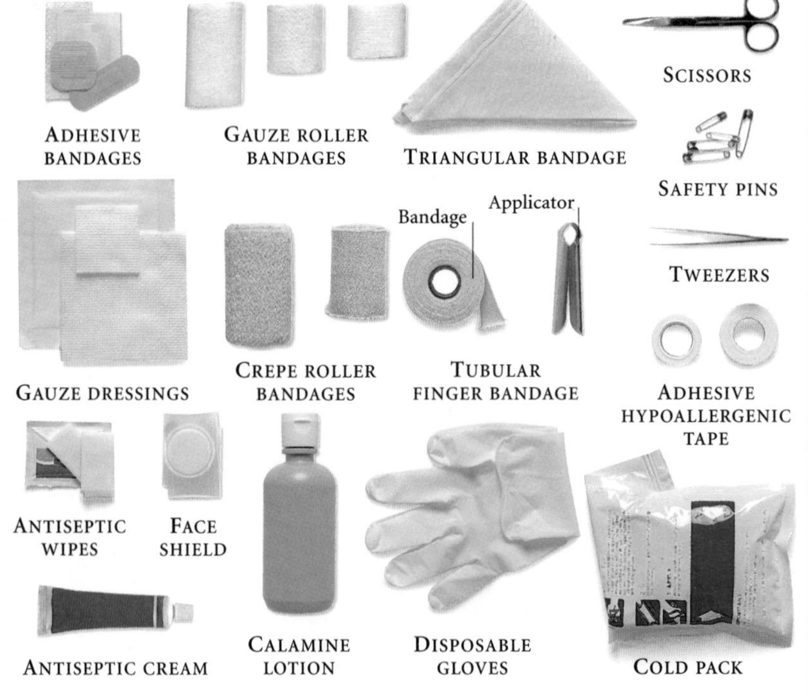

Contents of the first-aid kit
Most of the items shown here are essential items to include in your first-aid kit. The face shield, which enables you to give artificial respiration hygienically, is an optional item that you may wish to include if you are trained in first aid.

PROCEDURE ACTION IN AN EMERGENCY

When faced with an emergency, there are several important guidelines to bear in mind. If possible, you should send someone for an ambulance while you deal with the situation. Before trying to help someone, you must be certain that you are not putting yourself in any possible danger. After you have made sure that the scene is safe, the next step is to check the victim's condition and carry out the appropriate first-aid treatment.

START HERE

EMERGENCY ACTION!
If you have a helper, send him or her to call an ambulance.

Is the scene safe to enter or can you make it safe, either by removing the danger from the victim or by removing the victim from the danger?

YES

NO

EMERGENCY ACTION!
Call an ambulance if someone has not already done so.

Is the victim visibly conscious, or, if not, does he or she respond when you speak loudly or tap him or her gently?

YES

NO

Is the victim breathing? (*see* ABC OF RESUSCITATION, p.978)

YES

NO

EMERGENCY ACTION!
- Check the victim for serious injuries and treat as appropriate.
- Call an ambulance if someone has not already done so.

Is the victim a child or infant?

YES

NO

EMERGENCY ACTION!
Call an ambulance if someone has not already done so.

EMERGENCY ACTION!
Give artificial respiration (p.982). Continue until the victim shows signs of recovery or help arrives.

Is there a pulse? (*see* ABC OF RESUSCITATION, p.978)

YES

NO

EMERGENCY ACTION!
- Give cardiopulmonary resuscitation (p.985) for 1 minute.
- Call an ambulance if someone has not already done so.
- Continue with treatment until child shows signs of recovery or help arrives.

EMERGENCY ACTION!
- Give artificial respiration (pp.982–983) for 1 minute.
- Call an ambulance if someone has not already done so.
- Continue with treatment until child shows signs of recovery or help arrives.

Is there a pulse? (*see* ABC OF RESUSCITATION, p.978)

YES

NO

EMERGENCY ACTION!
Start cardiopulmonary resuscitation (p.984). Continue until the victim shows signs of recovery or help arrives.

FIRST-AID PROCEDURES

Knowing how to deal with a major emergency could make the difference between life and death. However, even when someone's life is not at risk, knowing the correct first-aid procedure can prevent permanent physical damage, avoid complications, or help someone to make the fastest possible recovery.

The first rule of first aid is "Do no further harm", and to be able to do this you need to be familiar with the correct techniques. There is no real substitute for professional first-aid training, but the information given in this section should help you to make appropriate decisions in an emergency. You should never attempt treatment if you do not feel confident; get help instead. Also remember that you will be most effective if you stay calm.

The first articles describe the most important principles of dealing with emergencies in which a person's life may be at immediate risk. They cover checking for breathing and circulation and describe life-saving techniques that may be needed, such as artificial respiration if breathing has stopped and cardiopulmonary resuscitation if both breathing and heartbeat are absent. Although you may not get the breathing or heartbeat to start again, using these techniques will ensure that the body receives enough oxygen and that circulation continues to vital organs, such as the brain, to keep the person alive until medical help arrives.

The next group of articles describe how to deal with serious injuries or situations that could be life-threatening if not treated, such as severe bleeding and major burns. The final articles cover injuries that are unlikely to be life-threatening, such as sprains and strains and insect bites, but for which correct treatment is still important. Techniques for some specific injuries are covered elsewhere (*see* SERIOUS INJURIES AND ENVIRONMENTAL DISORDERS, pp.314–327).

ABC of resuscitation

The ABC of resuscitation is the most important principle of first aid. The "ABC" stands for Airway, Breathing, and Circulation. The ABC of resuscitation is a procedure that enables you to assess whether a victim who has collapsed needs artificial respiration or cardiopulmonary resuscitation (CPR), which are both life-saving techniques. The *airway* must be opened, the victim must be checked to establish if *breathing* is present, and the pulse must be checked to assess whether there is *circulation*. If breathing has stopped, you must give artificial respiration at once. If there is no pulse, you must begin cardiopulmonary resuscitation immediately. If the victim is unconscious, always follow the ABC sequence before giving any other treatment.

A: Airway

To open the airway, place one hand on the victim's forehead, and place two fingers of your other hand under the chin. Tilt the head back by pressing down on the forehead while you lift the chin. For an infant, use only one finger to lift the chin.

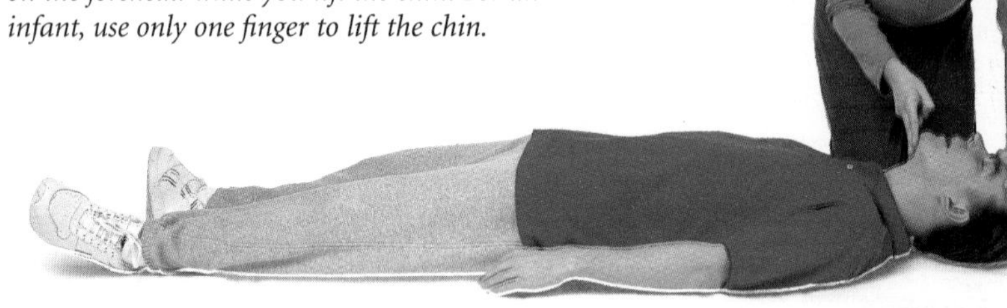

B: Breathing

To check for breathing, watch the chest for movement, listen for breath, and feel for breath on your cheek for up to 10 seconds. If breathing is absent, give 2 slow breaths of artificial respiration (pp.982–983).

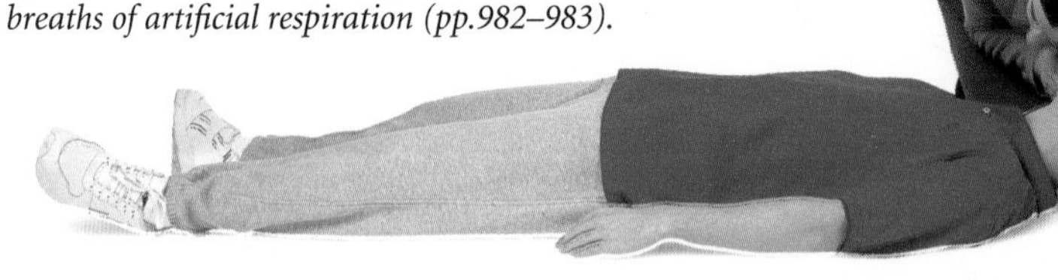

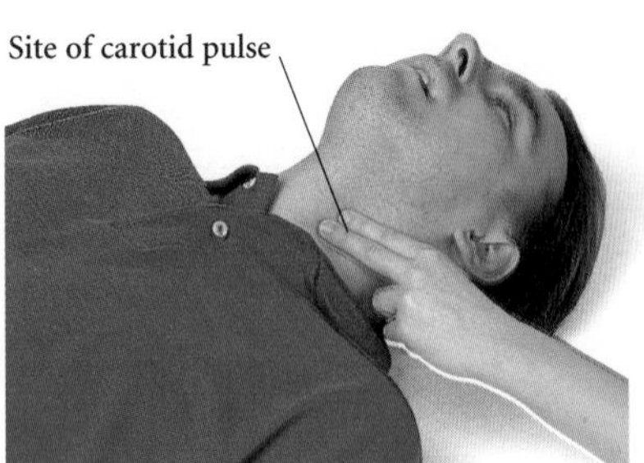

ADULT OR CHILD

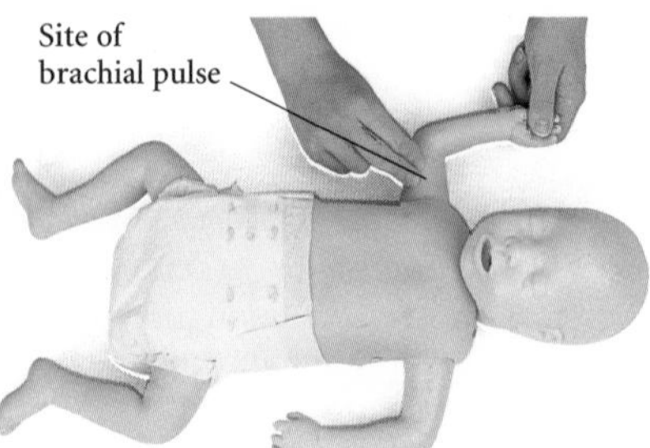

INFANT

C: Circulation

To assess circulation in an adult or a child, check the carotid pulse, in the neck, for up to 10 seconds by pressing the hollow between the trachea (windpipe) and the large neck muscle with two fingers. For an infant, use two fingers to check the brachial pulse, on the inside of the arm. If the pulse is absent and there are no signs of recovery, start cardiopulmonary resuscitation (pp.984–985).

Recovery position for adults and children

The recovery position is a secure position in which to place an unconscious adult or child while waiting for help to arrive. If an unconscious victim is lying on his or her back, the tongue may fall to the back of the throat and block the airway. This obstruction of the airway may cause breathing, and soon afterwards the heart, to stop. The recovery position keeps the head, neck, and back aligned, keeps the airway open, and allows fluid to drain out of the mouth if the victim vomits. You may not need to follow all of the steps if the person was found lying on his or her front or side.

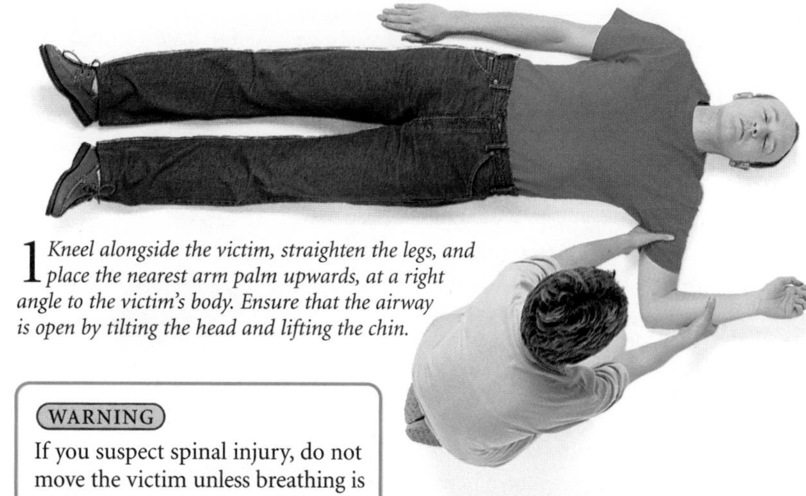

1 *Kneel alongside the victim, straighten the legs, and place the nearest arm palm upwards, at a right angle to the victim's body. Ensure that the airway is open by tilting the head and lifting the chin.*

WARNING

If you suspect spinal injury, do not move the victim unless breathing is impeded or he or she needs to be removed from danger.

2 *Bring the arm furthest from you across the victim's chest. Place the back of that hand under his or her near cheek. Pull the far leg into a bent position, with the foot on the floor at first, then pull the knee towards you.*

Hold victim's hand in place

3 *Continue to pull the upper leg towards you so that the victim rolls forwards on to his or her side. If necessary, support the victim with your knees. Tilt the head back to maintain an open airway.*

Head tilted back slightly

4 *It may be necessary to adjust the victim's hand under his or her head and bend the upper leg so that it supports the body and is positioned at a right angle to the hip, if possible.*

Leg bent

Keep victim's hand supporting the head

5 *Call an ambulance. Regularly monitor and record the victim's breathing and pulse (see* ABC OF RESUSCITATION, *opposite page).*

Recovery position for infants

The recovery position is the safest position in which to hold an unconscious infant until medical help arrives. This position prevents the tongue from falling towards the back of the throat and blocking the airway. The recovery position also allows fluid to drain from the mouth. You should keep the head, neck, and back aligned at all times.

WARNING

If you suspect spinal injury, do not move an infant unless the breathing is impeded or he or she needs to be removed from danger.

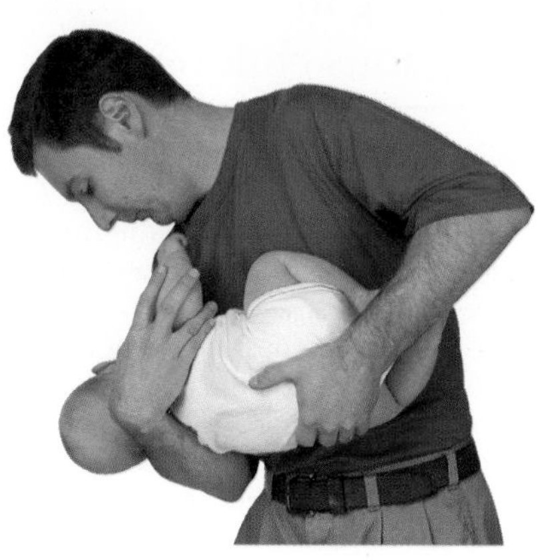

How to hold an infant correctly
Hold the unconscious infant securely in your arms so that the head is lower than the body. The infant's head should be tilted back to keep the airway open.

Choking in conscious adults

Choking is due to an obstruction of the airway, usually by food or a foreign body. A victim who is choking may cough and gasp at first, and the face may redden. He or she may point to or grasp at the throat. If the airway is totally blocked, the victim may produce high-pitched noises, be unable to cough, or have only a weak cough. If coughing does not clear the blockage, you need to give first aid to prevent suffocation. Usually, you can do this by using the techniques shown here.

1 *Encourage the victim to cough up the object. Bend the victim forwards and give his or her back 5 sharp slaps between the shoulder blades.*

2 *If the victim continues to cough without clearing the object, stand behind him or her, make a fist, and, with your thumb towards his or her abdomen, position your fist in the middle of the victim's abdomen, just below the breastbone. Place your other hand over your fist and pull sharply inwards and upwards to give an abdominal thrust. Give up to 5 of these thrusts. If these are unsuccessful, go through a repeat cycle of slaps and thrusts.*

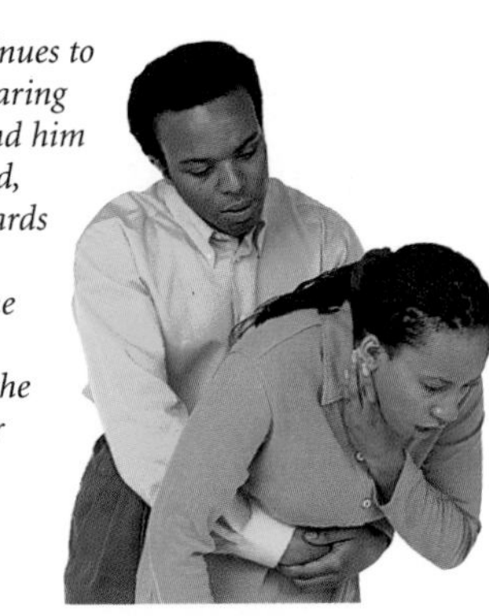

3 *Call an ambulance if the obstruction does not clear or if the victim loses consciousness (see* CHOKING IN UNCONSCIOUS ADULTS*, below).*

Choking in unconscious adults

If a person's airway has become completely blocked, he or she will be unable to breathe and will become unconscious. If an adult loses consciousness while you are giving first-aid treatment for choking, or if you find an unconscious person and you know that the person has choked, urgent treatment is essential.

1 *If you have a helper, send him or her to call an ambulance. If the victim has lost consciousness while undergoing treatment, or is found unconscious and is known to have choked, lay him or her on a firm surface and open the airway by pressing the forehead down with one hand and lifting the chin with two fingers of the other. If you can see the obstruction clearly, attempt to pick it out.*

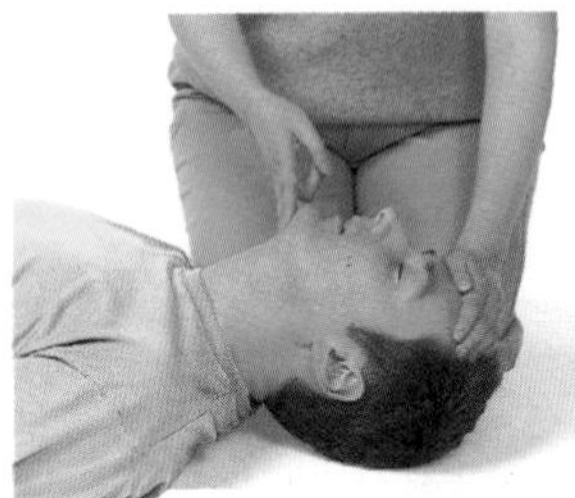

2 *Attempt up to 5 slow breaths of artificial respiration (p.982). If the breaths do not go in, proceed to Step 3. Call an ambulance if it has not already been called.*

3 *Turn the victim on to his or her side and give up to 5 sharp back slaps with the flat of your hand between the shoulder blades. Afterwards, you should recheck the mouth and remove any obvious obstruction.*

4 *Kneel astride the victim and place the heel of one hand just above the navel. Place your other hand on top and, with your fingers lifted off the chest, give up to 5 quick thrusts inwards and upwards. Check the mouth. If still unsuccessful, attempt 5 breaths of artificial respiration. If breaths do not go in, repeat Steps 3–4 until medical help arrives.*

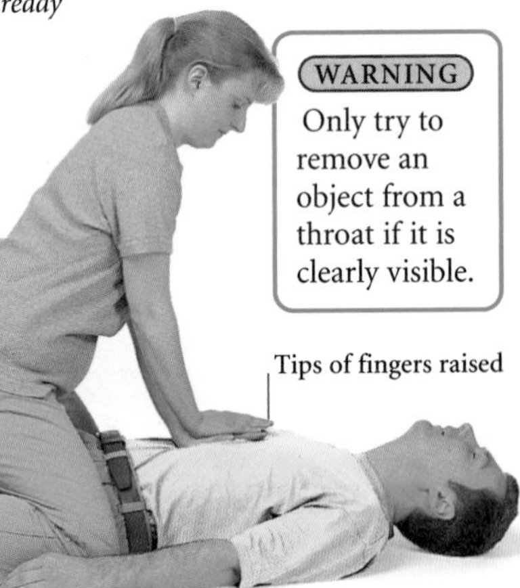

WARNING

Only try to remove an object from a throat if it is clearly visible.

5 *If breathing resumes, place the victim in the recovery position (p.979) and monitor the breathing and pulse regularly (see* ABC OF RESUSCITATION*, p.978) until help arrives.*

Choking in conscious children

Children often put small objects in their mouths, which may cause choking. A child who is choking will have difficulty in speaking and breathing. He or she will show signs of distress, and the face and neck will become flushed. Do not feel blindly in the child's throat to look for a blockage. If the child becomes unconscious during first aid for choking, you should follow the instructions on choking in unconscious children (opposite).

1 *If the child can still breathe, encourage coughing because this will help to dislodge the obstruction.*

2 *If the child stops coughing or breathing, bend him or her forwards and give up to 5 sharp back slaps between the shoulder blades. Check the mouth, and remove the obstruction if you can see it clearly.*

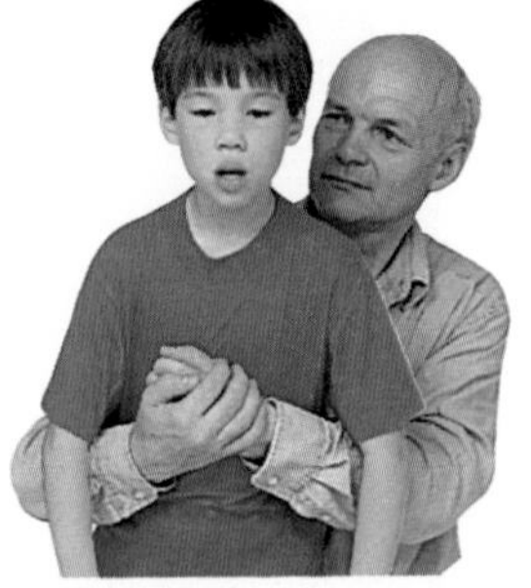

3 *If slaps fail, kneel behind the child and place a fist against the lower breastbone. Hold the fist in the other hand and press the chest with an inward thrust up to 5 times. Check the mouth.*

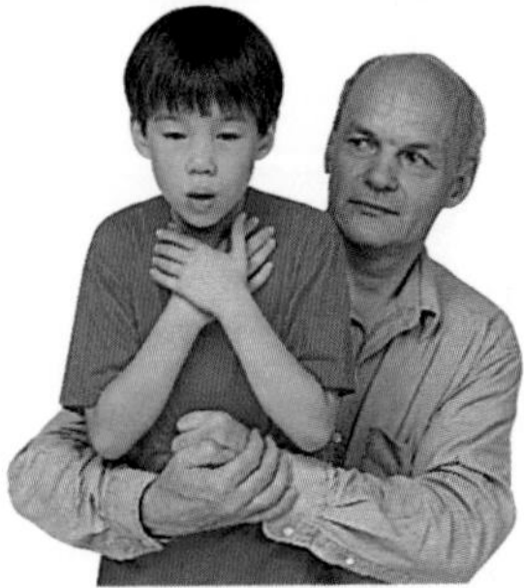

4 *If chest thrusts fail, give up to 5 abdominal thrusts by pressing the fist this time into the child's central upper abdomen. If this fails, call an ambulance and repeat Steps 2–4 until help arrives.*

Choking in unconscious children

If a child's airway has become totally blocked, he or she will be unable to breathe and will lose consciousness. If a child becomes unconscious while you are giving treatment for choking, or if you find an unconscious child who is known to have choked, urgent first-aid treatment is essential. It is important that you do not feel blindly in the child's throat for the obstruction.

1 *Open the child's airway and check if he or she is breathing. Ask a helper to call an ambulance. Remove any obvious obstruction in the child's mouth, but do not feel blindly in the throat.*

2 *If the breathing has stopped, try to give up to 5 slow breaths of artificial respiration (p.982). If the child is still not breathing, proceed to step 3.*

3 *Turn the child on to his or her side and give 5 back slaps between the shoulder blades. Check the mouth and remove any obvious obstruction. If unsuccessful, proceed to step 4.*

4 *Turn the child on to his or her back. Give up to 5 sharp inward chest thrusts with one hand on the child's lower breastbone. Check the mouth again for the obstruction.*

5 *If still unsuccessful, position your hand halfway between the child's navel and breastbone, and give up to 5 upward abdominal thrusts with one hand. Check the mouth again.*

6 *If the airway is still obstructed, give 5 breaths of artificial respiration. If unsuccessful, repeat steps 3–6 in cycles until an ambulance arrives. If the child begins to breathe again, position him or her in the recovery position (p.979).*

WARNING

Only attempt to remove an object from a throat if you can see the object clearly.

Choking in infants

Infants (0–12 months) can easily choke on small objects. A choking infant may squeak, the face may turn red then blue, and he or she may appear to cry without making a noise. If the airway is totally blocked, the baby will lose consciousness. You must relieve a blocked airway before giving any other treatment.

1 *If the infant has a strong cough, let him or her continue. If the child becomes too weak or tired to cough, go to Step 2. Ask a helper to call an ambulance.*

WARNING

- Never shake a choking infant.
- Only try to remove an object from an infant's throat if you can see the obstruction clearly.

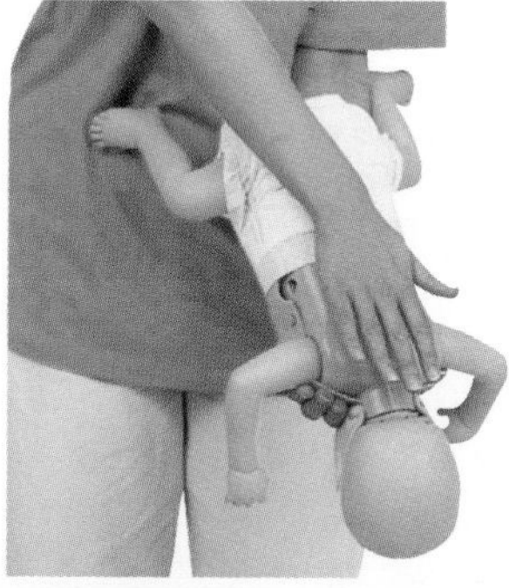

2 *Lay the infant face down on your forearm or lap with the head lower than the trunk, supporting the infant's chin and shoulders with your hand. Give up to 5 sharp back slaps between the infant's shoulders.*

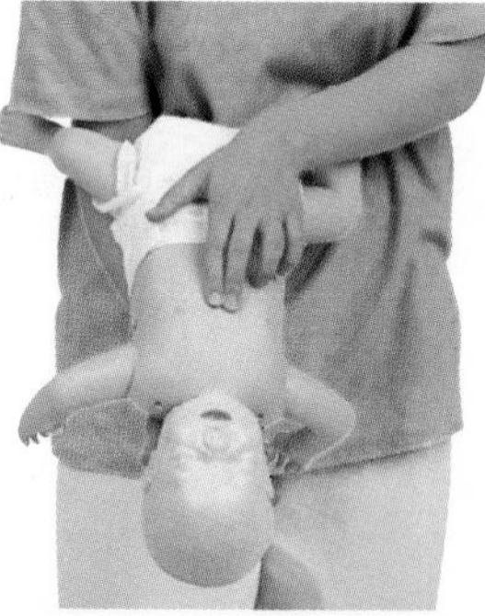

3 *If back slaps are not effective, lay the infant face up along your arm or knee. Place 2 fingers on the lower half of the breastbone. Give 5 sharp chest thrusts, one every 3 seconds.*

4 *Call an ambulance if a helper has not already done so. Continue alternating between back slaps and chest thrusts.*

5 *If the infant becomes unconscious, open his or her mouth, and, placing your finger on the tongue to allow you a clear view of the back of the mouth, remove any obvious obstruction.*

6 *Tilt the head back to open the airway and give 2 breaths of artificial respiration (p.983). If unsuccessful, retilt the infant's head and try again.*

7 *If the breaths still do not go in, repeat Steps 2–6 until medical help arrives or the infant starts breathing. If he or she starts breathing, place in the recovery position (p.979) and monitor the breathing and pulse (see ABC OF RESUSCITATION, p.978) until help arrives.*

Artificial respiration for adults and children

Artificial respiration is a way to force your exhaled air into the lungs of a victim who is not breathing. If breathing has stopped, the person will be unconscious, the chest will not rise or fall, and you will not be able to feel or hear breath. The face may be greyish blue. If a person is not breathing, you must give artificial respiration immediately. If the pulse is absent, indicating that the heart has stopped, you need to give artificial respiration and chest compressions (*see* CARDIOPULMONARY RESUSCITATION, pp.984–985). In most instances, artificial respiration can be given using the mouth-to-mouth technique shown on the right, but, if the victim has sustained a mouth or jaw injury, you may need to use mouth-to-nose respiration (*see* ARTIFICIAL RESPIRATION – MOUTH OR JAW INJURIES, below). Use a face shield or mask if one is available.

1 *If you have a helper, ask him or her to call an ambulance. If you are alone and the victim is an adult, call an ambulance before proceeding to Step 2. If the victim is a child, go to Step 2 immediately.*

2 *Lay the victim flat on his or her back. If you do not suspect spinal injury, open the airway by pressing down on the forehead with one hand and lifting the chin with two fingers of your other hand. In case of suspected spinal injury, use a modified method (see* OPENING THE AIRWAY – SPINAL INJURY*, below).*

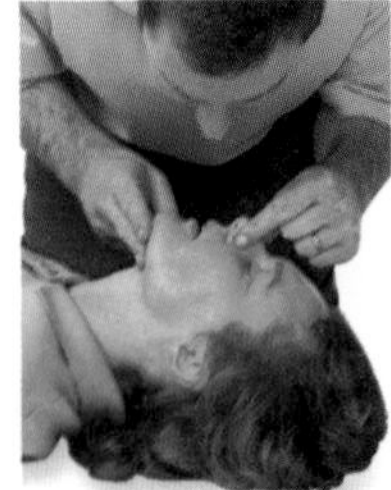

3 *Pinch the victim's nose closed with your thumb and index finger. Take a deep breath, then place your open mouth tightly around the victim's mouth to make a good seal.*

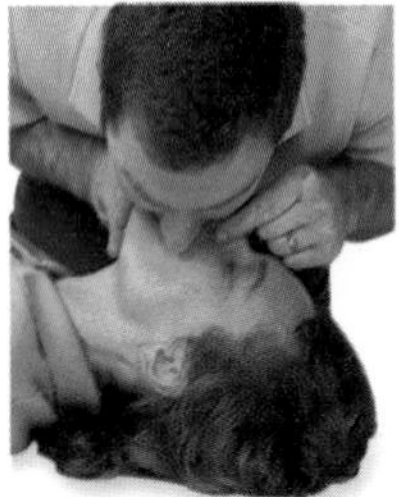

4 *Blow air into the victim's mouth for about 1½ seconds. Remove your lips, keeping your hands in the same position. Take a breath yourself, then give another 1½-second breath.*

5 *Look at the victim's chest. If there is no rise and fall, retilt the head and try again, checking that you make a good seal around the mouth. If you still cannot get air in, assume the airway is obstructed and treat as for choking (see* CHOKING IN UNCONSCIOUS ADULTS, *p.980, and* CHOKING IN UNCONSCIOUS CHILDREN, *p.981). If the chest does rise and fall, go to Step 6.*

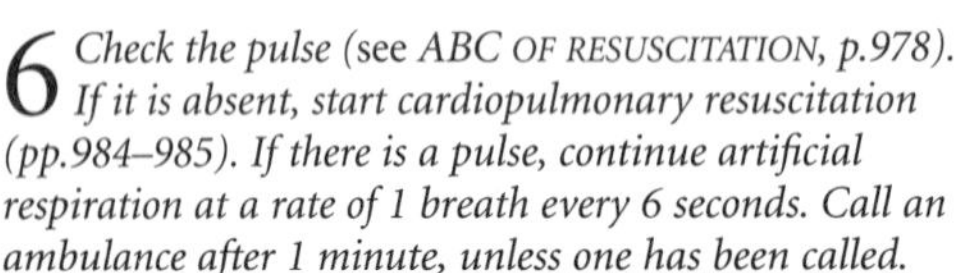

6 *Check the pulse (see* ABC OF RESUSCITATION, *p.978). If it is absent, start cardiopulmonary resuscitation (pp.984–985). If there is a pulse, continue artificial respiration at a rate of 1 breath every 6 seconds. Call an ambulance after 1 minute, unless one has been called.*

7 *Continue to give artificial respiration at a rate of 10 breaths per minute. Check the pulse and look for other signs of recovery after each cycle.*

(ALTERNATIVE) OPENING THE AIRWAY – SPINAL INJURY

If you need to administer artificial respiration to a victim who has a suspected spinal injury, try to open the airway without tilting the head back or tilting it only very slightly. This technique, which is known as the modified chin lift, minimizes movement to the head and neck.

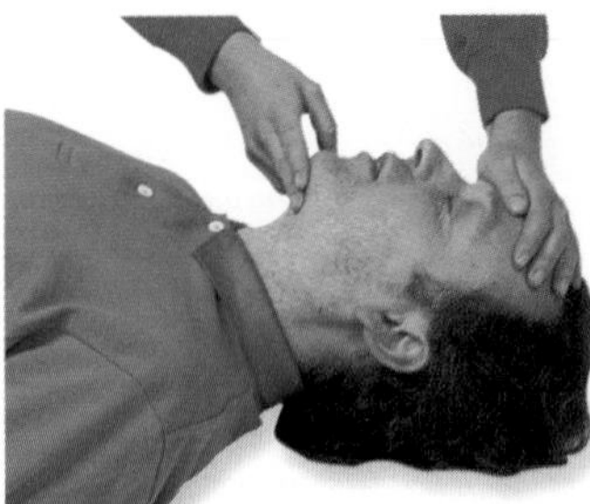

Opening the airway
Place one hand on the victim's forehead and gently lift the chin with the fingers of your other hand, then proceed with artificial respiration. If air does not go in you may need to tilt the head back very slightly by pressing on the forehead.

(SPECIAL CASE) ARTIFICIAL RESPIRATION – MOUTH OR JAW INJURIES

This technique should be used if there are injuries to the victim's mouth or jaw that make it difficult to use the mouth-to-mouth technique. In mouth-to-nose respiration, the victim's mouth is closed to stop air from escaping as you blow air into the lungs through the nose.

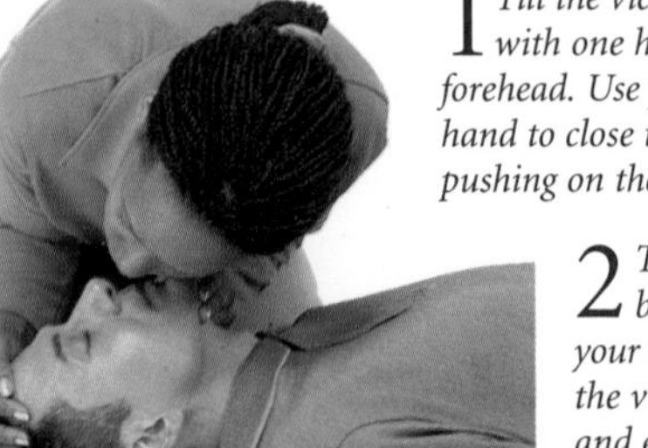

1 *Tilt the victim's head back with one hand on the forehead. Use your other hand to close the mouth by pushing on the chin.*

2 *Taking a deep breath, seal your mouth around the victim's nose and exhale. Open the victim's mouth between breaths to let air out.*

Artificial respiration for infants

An infant (aged 0–12 months) who is not breathing needs to be given artificial respiration, in which you blow your exhaled air into the infant's lungs. If the breathing has stopped, the infant will be unconscious, the chest will not rise or fall, and you will not be able to feel or hear breathing. The skin may become greyish blue. If you find an infant in this condition, you need to start artificial respiration immediately. An infant who also does not have a pulse needs to be given chest compressions with artificial respiration (*see* CARDIOPULMONARY RESUSCITATION FOR INFANTS, p.985). When you give artificial respiration to an infant, be careful not to blow too hard or the air will go into the stomach.

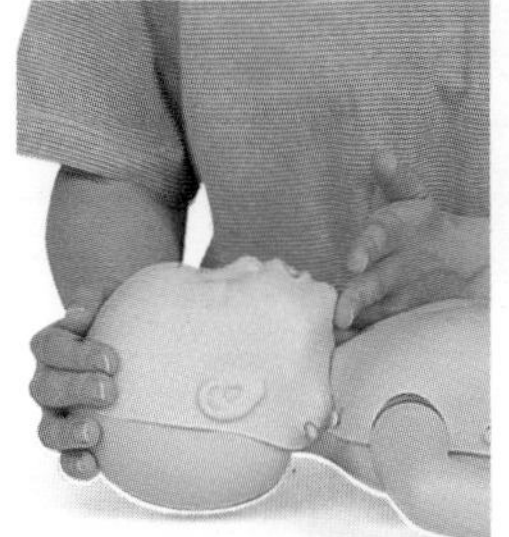

1 *Send a helper to call an ambulance. Place the infant on his or her back on a firm surface. Push down lightly on the baby's forehead to tilt the head back, and lift the baby's chin slightly with one finger of your other hand.*

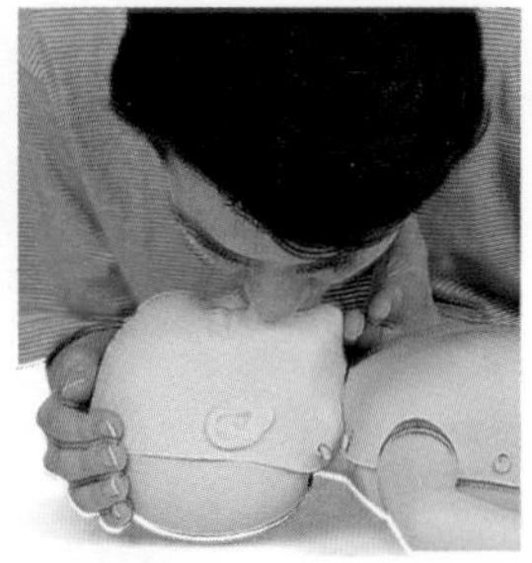

2 *Place your lips in a tight seal around the infant's mouth and nose. Give 2 slow, gentle breaths, each lasting about $1^1/_2$ seconds. Pause for a breath yourself after each breath. If the chest does not rise and fall, treat as for choking in infants (p.981); otherwise, go to Step 3.*

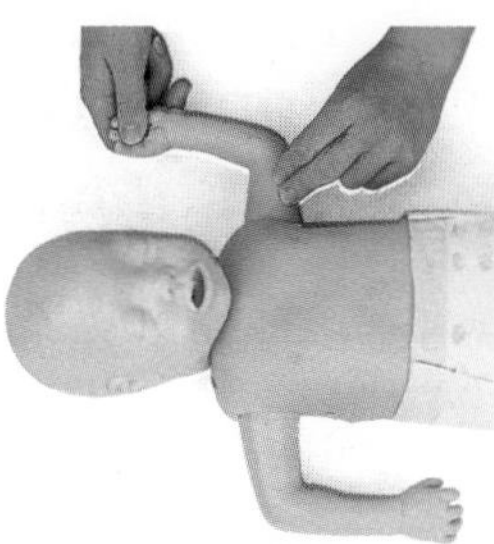

3 *Check for a pulse on the inner part of the arm (see* ABC OF RESUSCITATION, *p.978). You should also look for other signs of recovery in the infant, such as swallowing and the return of normal colour to the skin.*

4 *If you are unable to feel a pulse, start cardiopulmonary resuscitation (p.985). If a pulse is present but there are no signs of recovery, continue to give artificial respiration at a rate of 1 breath every 3 seconds. Check the pulse after 1 minute. If it is absent, proceed with cardiopulmonary resuscitation.*

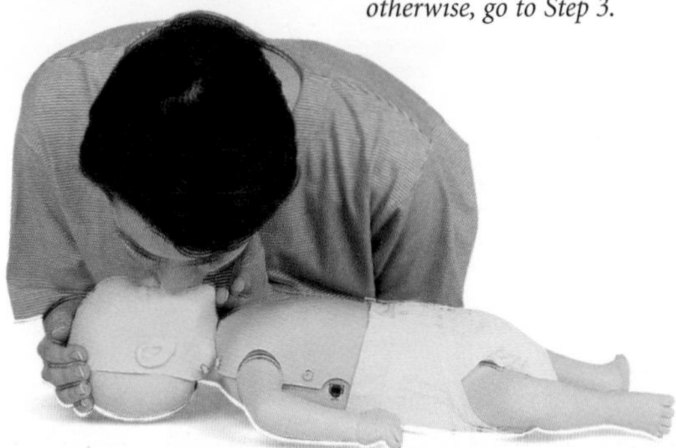

5 *Call an ambulance unless one has been called. Continue artificial respiration at the rate of 20 breaths per minute until help arrives. Check the pulse and look for signs of recovery after every cycle. If necessary, start cardiopulmonary resuscitation (p.985).*

Unconsciousness

Unconsciousness results from an interruption in the normal activity of the brain. It is a potentially life-threatening condition that needs immediate medical help. A victim is likely to be unconscious if he or she does not respond to loud noises or being tapped or shaken gently. The person's eyes will remain closed, and he or she will make no sound or movement. If an unconscious victim is lying on his or her back, the tongue may fall back and block the airway. First-aid priorities are to maintain an open airway and to check for and treat obvious injuries.

1 *If you have a helper, send him or her to call an ambulance. If you need to leave the victim alone to call for help, place the person in the recovery position (p.979). However, if you suspect spinal injury, do not move the person.*

2 *Check the victim's breathing and pulse and be prepared to resuscitate if necessary (*see *ABC OF RESUSCITATION, p.978).*

3 *Control any external bleeding (*see *SEVERE BLEEDING, p.986) and check for and support suspected fractures (p.992). Look for clues to the cause of the victim's condition, such as needle marks, warning bracelets, or cards. Ask bystanders for any information to give to the medical services.*

WARNING

- Do not move the victim unnecessarily in case there is spinal injury.
- Do not leave the victim alone except to call an ambulance.
- Do not try to give an unconscious victim anything to eat or drink.

4 *Stay with the victim until medical help arrives. Monitor the victim's breathing and pulse at regular intervals. In addition, you should periodically check whether the victim is regaining consciousness by asking simple, direct questions or tapping or shaking the person gently.*

Cardiopulmonary resuscitation for adults

An unconscious victim who is not breathing and has no pulse needs to be given cardiopulmonary resuscitation (CPR) because the heart has stopped beating. CPR is a life-saving technique in which artificial respiration is combined with chest compressions. Chest compressions force blood out of the heart and around the body, ensuring that the oxygen supplied by artificial respiration reaches the brain and other vital organs. Do not stop giving CPR until the victim's heart starts beating or medical help arrives. If you are too tired to continue, try to find another trained person to take over from you until medical help arrives.

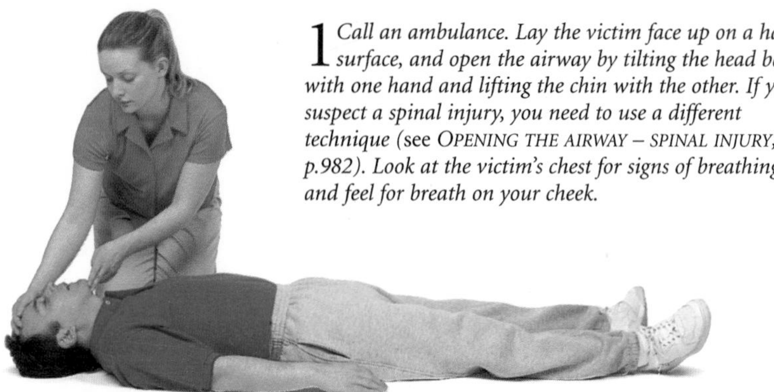

1 *Call an ambulance. Lay the victim face up on a hard surface, and open the airway by tilting the head back with one hand and lifting the chin with the other. If you suspect a spinal injury, you need to use a different technique (see* OPENING THE AIRWAY – SPINAL INJURY, *p.982). Look at the victim's chest for signs of breathing and feel for breath on your cheek.*

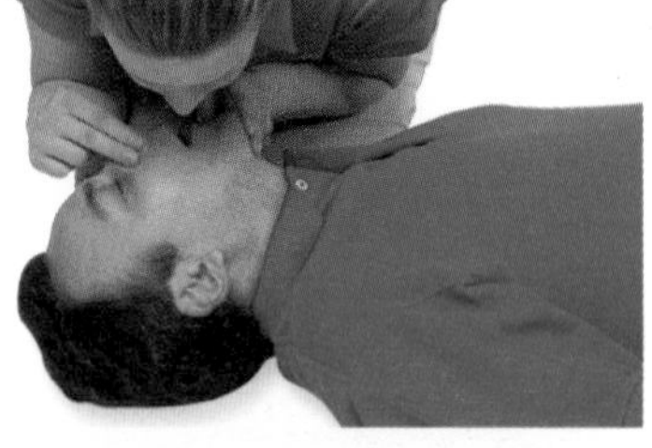

2 *If the victim is not breathing, pinch the nostrils shut with one hand, and keep the chin tilted with the other. Seal your mouth over the victim's mouth, and give 2 breaths of artificial respiration (p.982). Pause for a breath yourself between the breaths.*

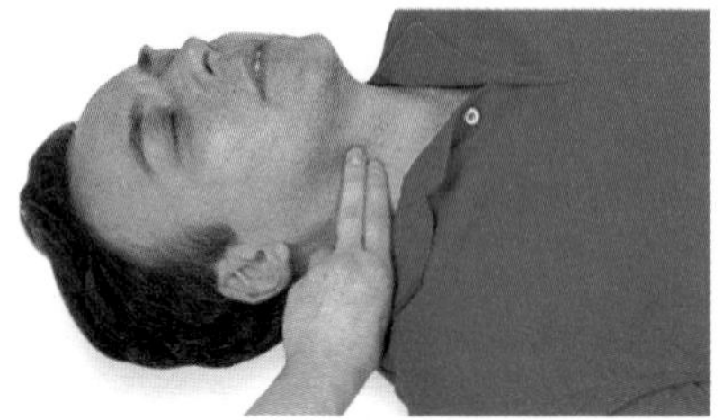

3 *Check the pulse at the neck for up to 10 seconds, and look for signs of recovery, such as return of skin colour or breathing. If a pulse is present, continue artificial respiration. If you cannot find a pulse and there are no signs of recovery, begin CPR (see Step 4).*

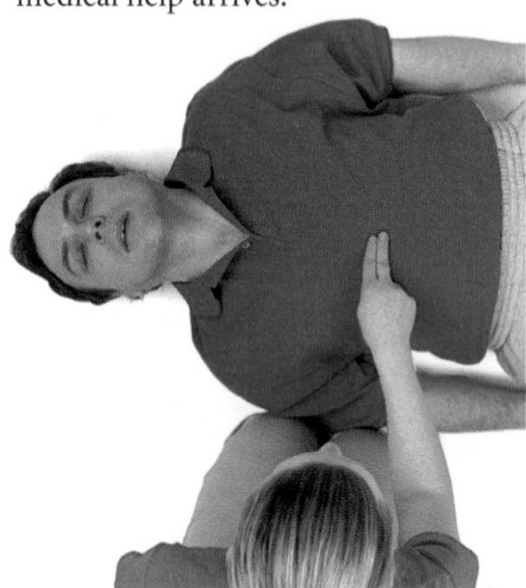

4 *Kneel to one side of the victim and with your lower hand locate the lowest rib on that side. Slide your fingers along the rib to where it meets the breastbone. Place your middle finger on this point and your index finger just above it.*

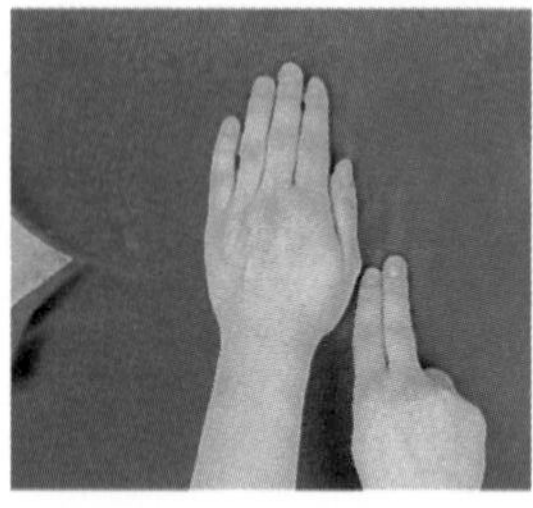

5 *Place the heel of your other hand just above your index finger on the breastbone. This is the area of the chest where you must apply pressure.*

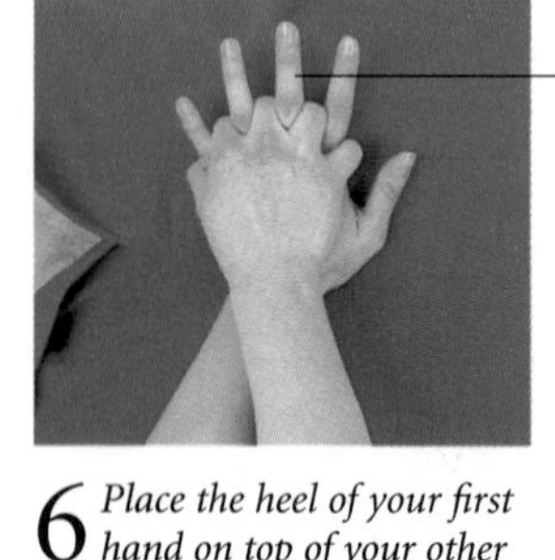

6 *Place the heel of your first hand on top of your other hand. Interlock the fingers, so that the fingers of the bottom hand are raised off the chest.*

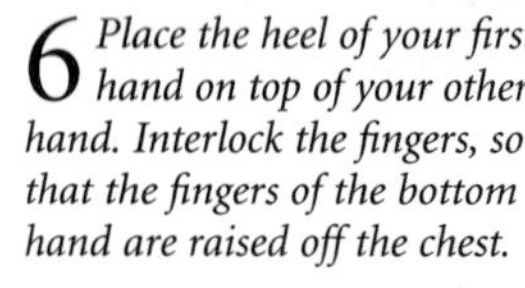

Shoulders above centre of victim's chest

Elbows locked

7 *With your shoulders directly above the victim and your elbows straight, apply pressure downwards, depressing the breastbone 4–5 cm (1½–2 in), then release the pressure without moving your hands. Compress the chest in this manner 15 times at a rate of about 15 compressions in 10 seconds, maintaining an even rhythm. Then give 2 breaths of artificial respiration.*

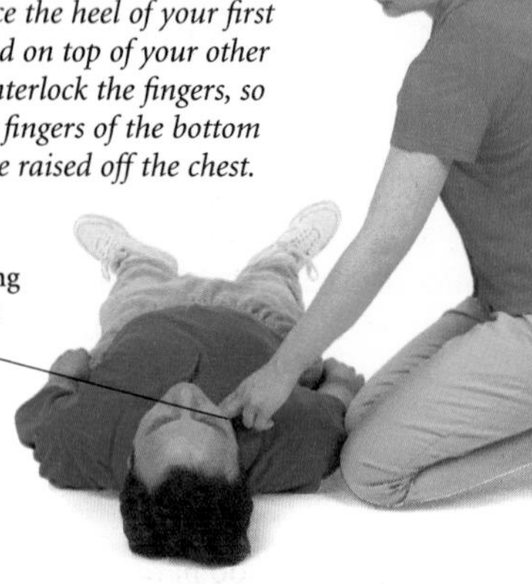

8 *Alternate 15 chest compressions with 2 breaths of artificial respiration. After 4 cycles of compressions and breaths, and every few minutes thereafter, check the pulse and breathing. If they are absent, continue CPR. If pulse and breathing return at any time, stop CPR but continue to monitor the pulse and breathing until help arrives.*

Cardiopulmonary resuscitation for children

If a child seems lifeless and you cannot find a pulse, he or she needs cardiopulmonary resuscitation (CPR) to force oxygenated blood from the heart and around the body. Like CPR for adults, CPR for children consists of alternating chest compressions and artificial respiration. However, the chest compressions are given with slightly less pressure than for adults, and the rate at which you do compressions and breaths is different.

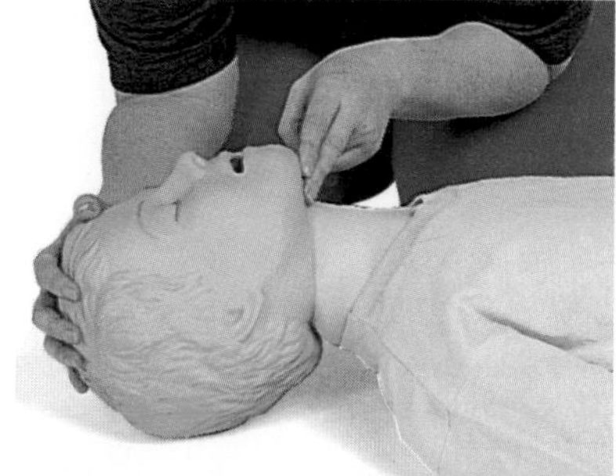

1 *Ask a helper to call an ambulance. Lay the child face up on a firm surface. Open the airway by tilting the head back slightly, or use a modified technique if you suspect that there is a spinal injury (see* OPENING THE AIRWAY – SPINAL INJURY, *p.982.)*

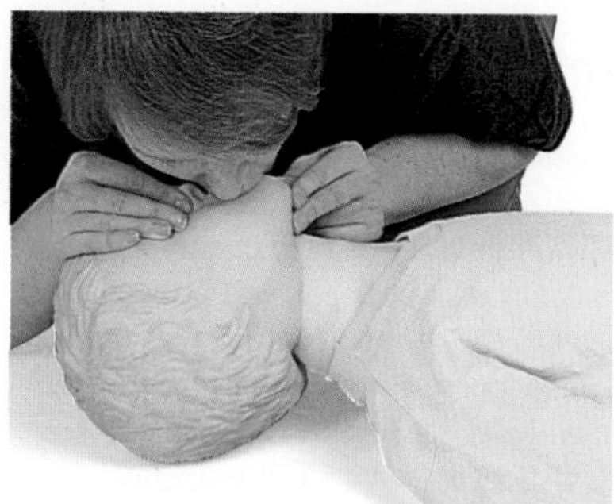

2 *If there are no signs of breathing, such as chest movement or the feel of breath on your cheek, pinch the child's nose shut and seal your lips over the mouth. Give 5 breaths of artificial respiration (p.982), pausing to take a breath yourself between each one.*

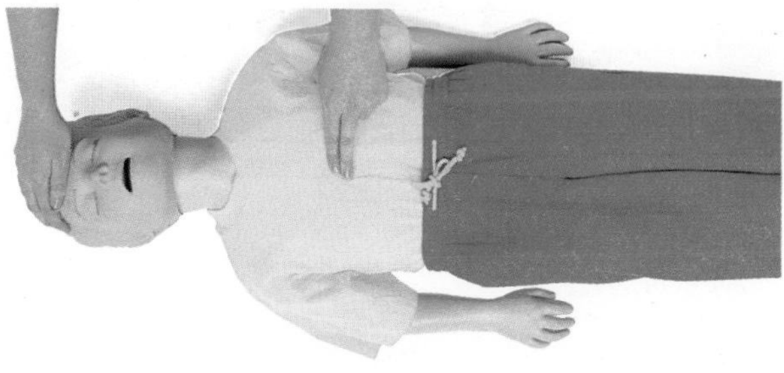

3 *Feel for a pulse in the child's neck for up to 10 seconds and look for signs of recovery, such as the return of skin colour or breathing. If there is a pulse, continue with artificial respiration. If there is no pulse, and the child shows no signs of recovery, commence CPR (see Step 4).*

4 *Place the middle finger of your lower hand on the end of the breastbone where the ribs meet and place your index finger just above it.*

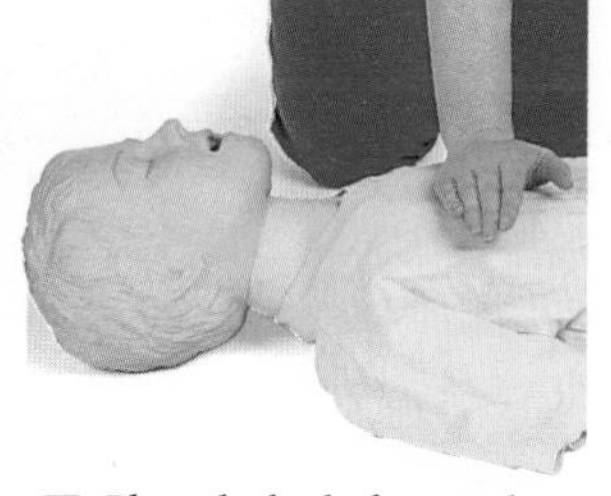

5 *Place the heel of your other hand on the breastbone next to your fingers. With the heel of your hand, press down sharply on the chest, to a depth of 2.5–4 cm (1–1½ in), 5 times in 3 seconds. Count from 1 to 5 to maintain an even rhythm.*

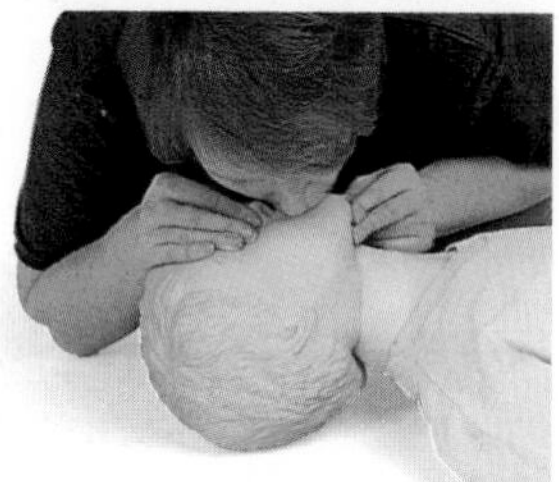

6 *Give 1 breath of artificial respiration. Repeat chest compressions and breaths for 1 minute. Call an ambulance if one has not been called. Repeat the cycle until the child recovers or help arrives. Recheck the pulse and breathing every few minutes.*

Cardiopulmonary resuscitation for infants

If a baby under 1 year old seems lifeless and has no pulse, he or she needs cardiopulmonary resuscitation (CPR) to distribute oxygen to the brain and other vital organs. CPR alternates chest compressions and artificial respiration. To avoid injury to the infant, chest compressions are given with 2 fingers only, taking care not to press too hard. When giving breaths of artificial respiration, you must not blow too hard.

1 *If you have a helper, send him or her to call an ambulance. Place the infant face up on a hard surface. Tilt the head back slightly with one hand and lift the chin with one finger of the other hand. Look, listen, and feel for evidence of breathing.*

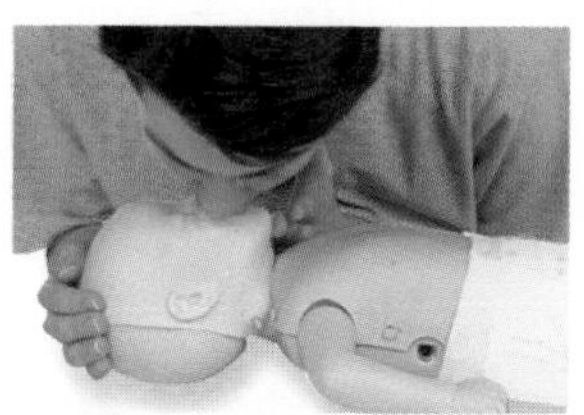

2 *If the baby is not breathing, seal your lips over the mouth and nose. Give 5 slow, gentle breaths of artificial respiration (p.983), pausing to breathe yourself between the breaths.*

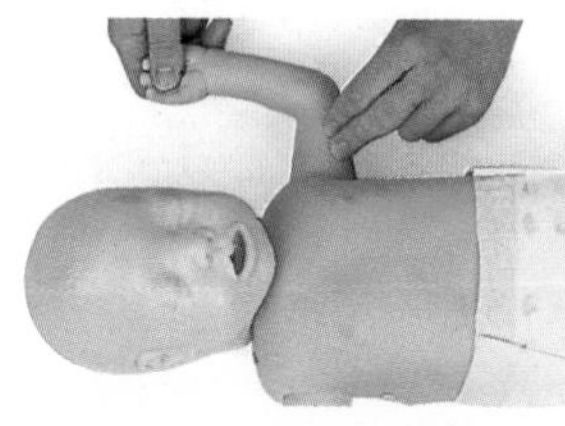

3 *Feel for a pulse on the inside of the upper arm for 5–10 seconds and look for signs of recovery, such as restored skin colour or breathing. If there is a pulse but no breathing, continue giving artificial respiration. If there is no breathing or pulse, start CPR (see Step 4).*

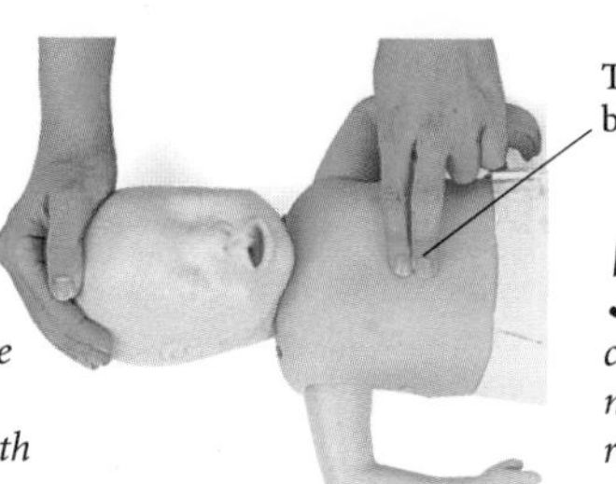

4 *With one hand on the baby's head, position 2 fingers of your other hand on the breastbone, a finger's width below the nipples. Press down sharply on the breastbone, to a depth of 1–2.5 cm (½–1 in), 5 times in 3 seconds.*

5 *Seal your lips over the infant's mouth and nose and give 1 breath. Check for breathing. Repeat chest compressions and breaths for 1 minute. If a helper has not already done so, call an ambulance. If the infant recovers at any time, stop CPR but monitor the breathing and pulse until medical help arrives.*

Severe bleeding

Severe bleeding is dramatic and distressing and can be life-threatening. Although you must try to stop bleeding as quickly as possible, you must also be alert to the general condition of the victim. A person who is bleeding heavily may lose consciousness (*see* UNCONSCIOUSNESS, p.983) and is also likely to develop shock (opposite page). Severe bleeding from an injury to the face or neck can cause choking (pp.980–981). Any of these conditions may require immediate treatment. Before and after treating bleeding, wash your hands well. Wear disposable gloves if they are available. Follow the procedure on the right to stop bleeding unless there is an object protruding from the wound (*see* SEVERE BLEEDING – EMBEDDED OBJECT, below).

1 *Place a sterile dressing (p.996), pad, or clean cloth over the wound and press firmly in place for at least 10 minutes or longer if necessary until the bleeding stops. If no clean dressing is available, ask the victim to apply pressure with the fingers or palm of his or her own hand.*

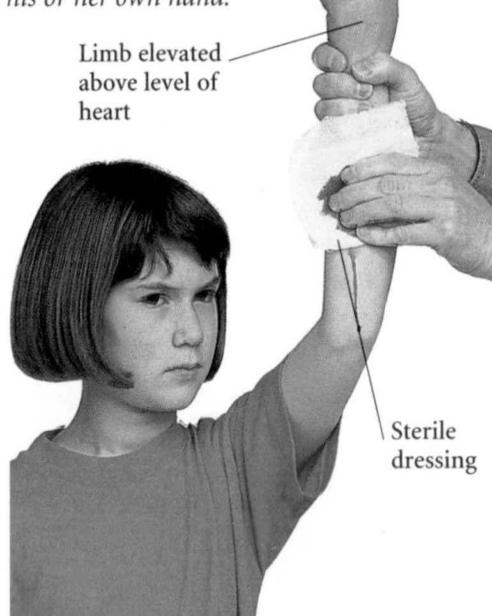

2 *If the bleeding does not stop, raise the injured part above the level of the heart, if possible, and continue to apply pressure. However, if you suspect a fracture (p.992), do not move the injured part.*

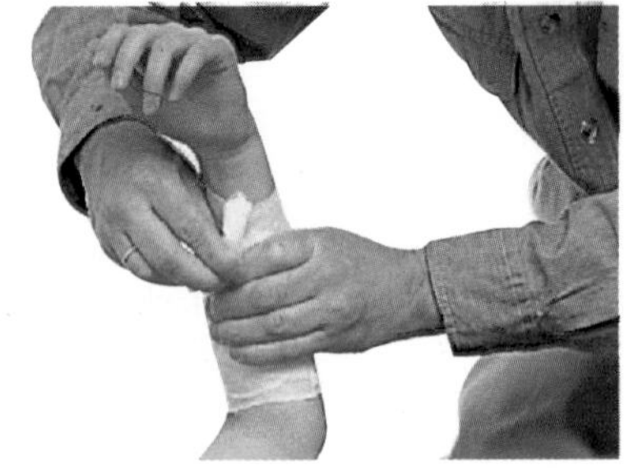

3 *Leaving any original pad in place, apply a pressure bandage (see* DRESSINGS AND BANDAGES, *pp.996–998). If blood seeps through the dressing, place another bandage on top. If the bleeding continues, use indirect pressure to stop bleeding (below).*

4 *Call an ambulance. Watch for signs of shock (opposite page), and treat if necessary. Continue to check the dressing for seepage of blood.*

WARNING

- Do not apply a tourniquet. This can make the bleeding worse and may result in tissue damage.
- Do not remove a foreign body embedded in a wound.

SPECIAL CASE SEVERE BLEEDING – EMBEDDED OBJECT

If a foreign body is embedded in a wound, do not attempt to remove it. You may be able to stop the bleeding by applying pressure on either side of the object or by using indirect pressure. The wound should be bandaged so that no pressure is placed on the object.

1 *If blood is gushing out of the wound, use indirect pressure to stop the bleeding (right). Otherwise, try to stop the bleeding by applying pressure on either side of the object.*

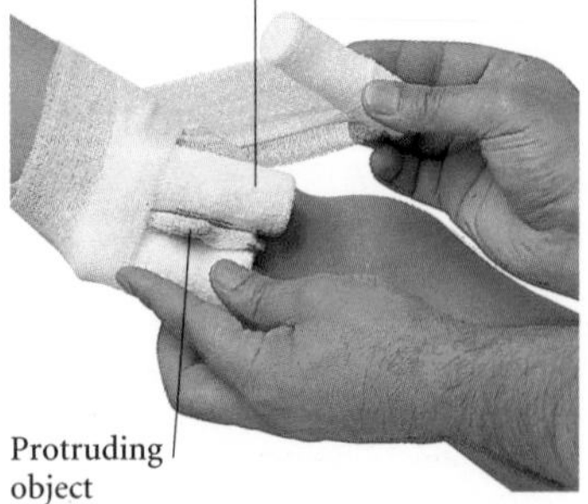

2 *When bleeding has slowed, place a piece of gauze over the wound to prevent infection. Build up padding to the same height as the protruding object. Bandage around the padding without pressing on the object.*

TECHNIQUE INDIRECT PRESSURE TO STOP BLEEDING

Indirect pressure can be used to stem bleeding from a limb when the flow of blood is too great to slow by direct pressure or if an object is protruding from the wound. To stop the bleeding in this situation, you can press on a main artery above the site of the bleeding, at places called pressure points. The pressure points that you will most probably need to use are on the brachial and femoral arteries, in the arms and legs, respectively.

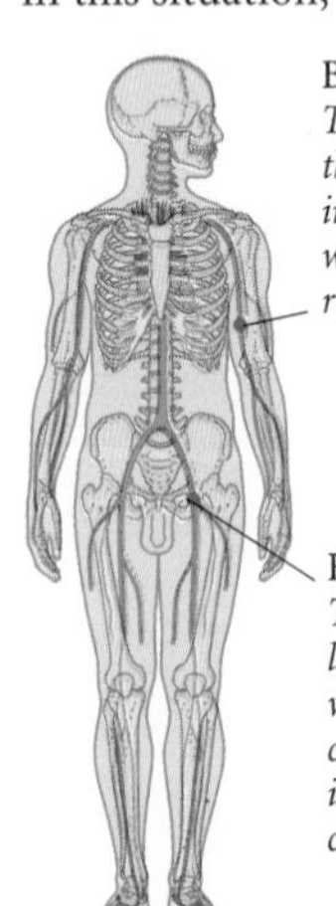

1 *Find the pressure point by feeling for a pulse with your fingertips. To feel for the femoral artery in the leg, first have the person lying down.*

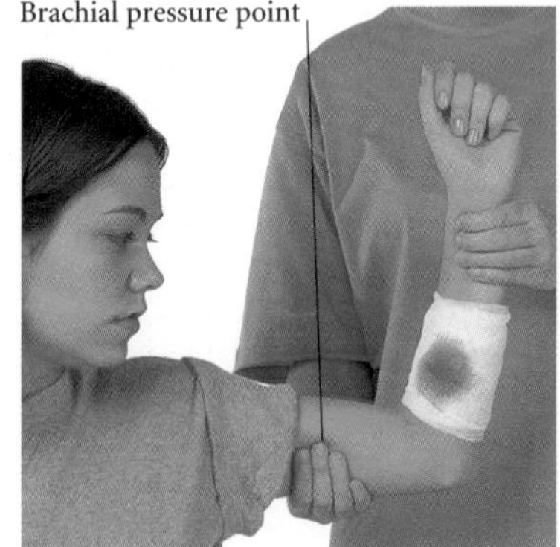

2 *Press against the artery for up to 10 minutes, until the blood supply to the lower part of the limb is greatly reduced. Use your fingertips to press against the brachial artery in the arm (as shown here). For the femoral artery, use your thumbs or the heel of your hand.*

Shock

Shock can occur as a result of any severe injury or illness that dramatically reduces the flow of blood around the body, such as a heart attack or severe bleeding. It can also be due to loss of body fluids from burns or severe diarrhoea and vomiting. If shock is not treated rapidly, vital organs such as the brain and heart may fail.

The first signs of shock may include a rapid pulse; greyish-blue skin, especially on the lips; and sweating with cold, clammy skin. Later symptoms include excessive thirst and nausea and vomiting. The victim may start to feel weak or dizzy and develop rapid, shallow breathing and a faint pulse. Eventually he or she may become restless, gasp for air, and lose consciousness. It is essential to call for medical help as soon as you notice early signs of shock, and to keep the victim warm and comfortable.

WARNING

- Do not leave the victim alone, except to call an ambulance.
- Do not let the victim eat or drink unless he or she has diabetes and is hypoglycaemic.

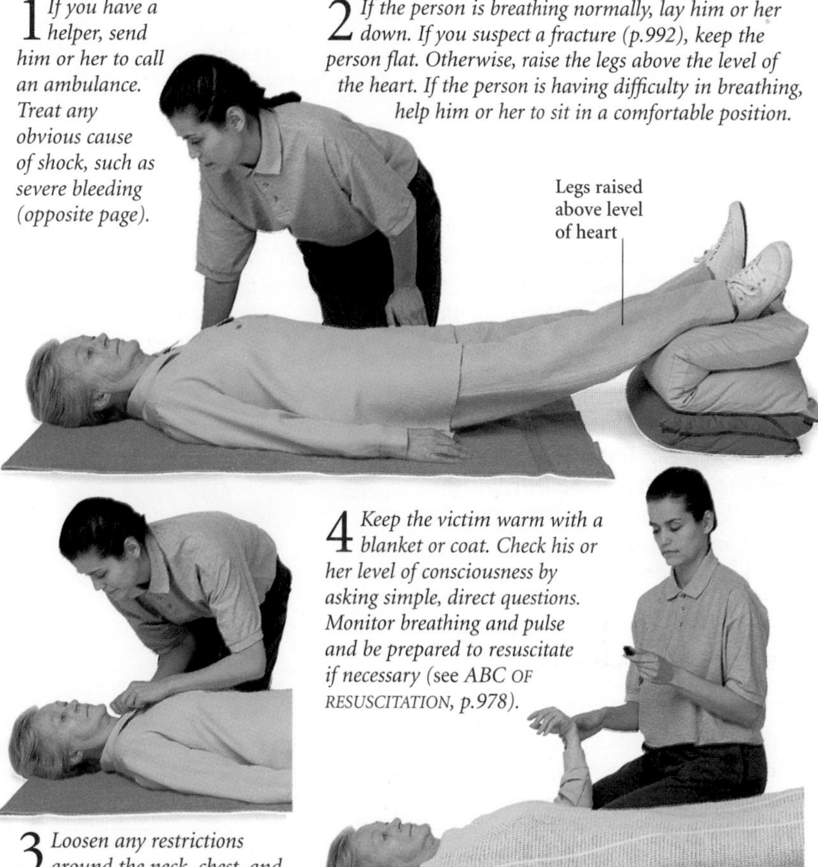

1 If you have a helper, send him or her to call an ambulance. Treat any obvious cause of shock, such as severe bleeding (opposite page).

2 If the person is breathing normally, lay him or her down. If you suspect a fracture (p.992), keep the person flat. Otherwise, raise the legs above the level of the heart. If the person is having difficulty in breathing, help him or her to sit in a comfortable position.

Legs raised above level of heart

3 Loosen any restrictions around the neck, chest, and waist, and remove the victim's shoes. Call an ambulance if a helper has not already done so.

4 Keep the victim warm with a blanket or coat. Check his or her level of consciousness by asking simple, direct questions. Monitor breathing and pulse and be prepared to resuscitate if necessary (see ABC OF RESUSCITATION, p.978).

Anaphylactic shock

Anaphylactic shock is a life-threatening allergic reaction to a specific food, drug, or insect sting. It can develop within seconds or a few minutes. The victim may be anxious and may have puffiness around the eyes, swelling of the face, lips, and tongue, and an itchy, red skin rash. He or she may develop wheezing and severe breathing difficulties and may lose consciousness. A victim with anaphylactic shock needs an injection of epinephrine (adrenaline) and must be given oxygen as quickly as possible. If a person is aware of having an allergy and carries a supply of epinephrine, you can help him or her to use this supply. Otherwise, first aid is limited to keeping the person comfortable and, if necessary, helping him or her to breathe until medical help arrives.

WARNING

Do not leave the victim alone, except to call an ambulance.

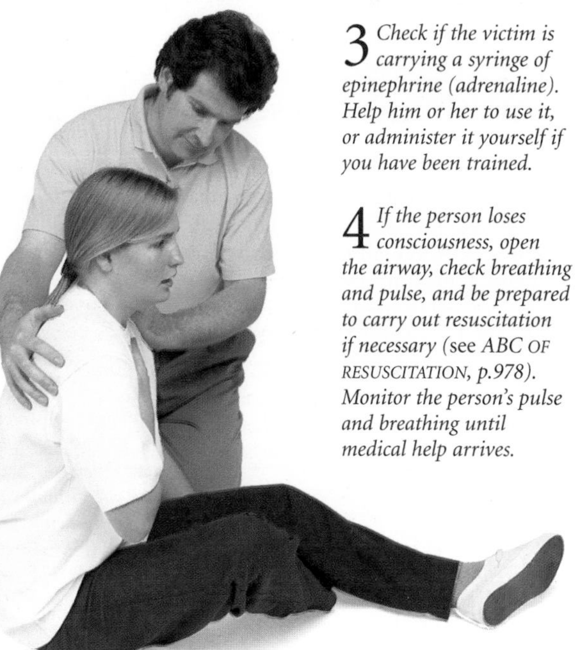

1 Call an ambulance or send a helper to do so immediately. If possible, provide the emergency services with details of the cause of the allergic reaction.

2 If the victim is conscious, help him or her to sit up in the position that makes breathing easiest.

3 Check if the victim is carrying a syringe of epinephrine (adrenaline). Help him or her to use it, or administer it yourself if you have been trained.

4 If the person loses consciousness, open the airway, check breathing and pulse, and be prepared to carry out resuscitation if necessary (see ABC OF RESUSCITATION, p.978). Monitor the person's pulse and breathing until medical help arrives.

Severe burns

A severe burn may involve all layers of the skin. If it is very severe, it may also destroy the tissues underlying the skin. The affected area may appear red and may have blisters that weep clear fluid. In some cases, the area may be brown or charred. If the burn extends to very deep tissues, the skin may be white. If the nerve endings have been damaged, there may be a loss of feeling in the injured area. The immediate response for a serious burn is to cool the area rapidly in order to minimize damage and prevent the loss of body fluids and the onset of shock (p.987). It is also essential to protect the wound from infection. The larger and deeper the burn, the greater the risk of shock or infection. A victim burned in a fire will probably have suffered damage to the airway. You should monitor his or her breathing regularly.

WARNING

- Do not touch the burn.
- Do not apply anything to the burn other than cool liquid, preferably cool water or otherwise a cold drink.
- Do not apply ice or iced water directly to the burned area.
- Do not burst blisters.

1 *If possible, remove the victim from the source of the burn and put out any flames on the person's clothing. If you have a helper, send him or her to call an ambulance.*

2 *Lay the victim down. Watch for signs of difficulty breathing. Be ready to resuscitate if necessary (see ABC OF RESUSCITATION, p.978).*

3 *If possible, raise the burned area above the level of the heart. Do not touch the burn or try to remove anything that is sticking to it. Call an ambulance if a helper has not already done so.*

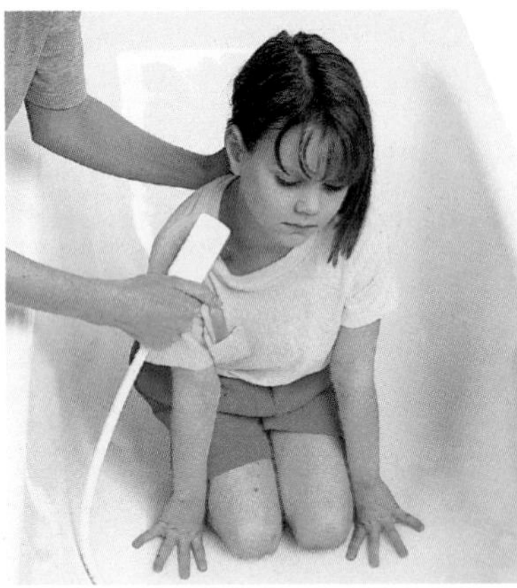

4 *Douse the burn with plenty of cool water, immerse it in water, or cover it with cold, wet towels for at least 10 minutes or until the burn has cooled down. If no tap water is available, use any other suitable source, including a garden hose, shower, or a cold, canned drink.*

5 *Once the burn has cooled, gently remove or cut away any clothing (unless sticking to the burn), shoes, belts, or jewellery before the area starts to swell or blister. Do not touch blisters. If pain persists, cool the area again.*

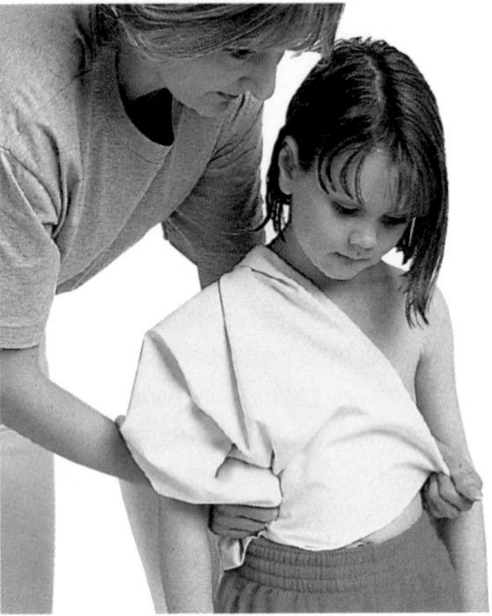

6 *Cover the burn with a prepacked sterile dressing (p.996) or improvise a dressing with clean, nonfluffy material, such as part of a pillowcase or a clean sheet. Loosely bandage in place but do not apply adhesive dressings or adhesive tape to the affected skin. Facial burns do not need to be covered.*

7 *Record details of the injuries and try to establish the cause. Reassure the victim while you wait for medical help, and monitor breathing and pulse (see ABC OF RESUSCITATION, p.978). If the burn is extensive, watch for signs of shock (p.987), such as rapid pulse and cool, moist skin, and be prepared to treat appropriately.*

Minor burns and scalds

A minor burn involves damage to only the top layers of skin. The injured area may be red and painful and may swell and blister. Although minor burns can be painful, most heal well within a few days if treated promptly with appropriate first-aid measures. Medical attention is usually not required. However, if you are unsure about the severity of a burn, you should always seek medical advice.

WARNING

- Do not apply anything other than cool liquid to the injury to stop the burning.
- Do not burst blisters.

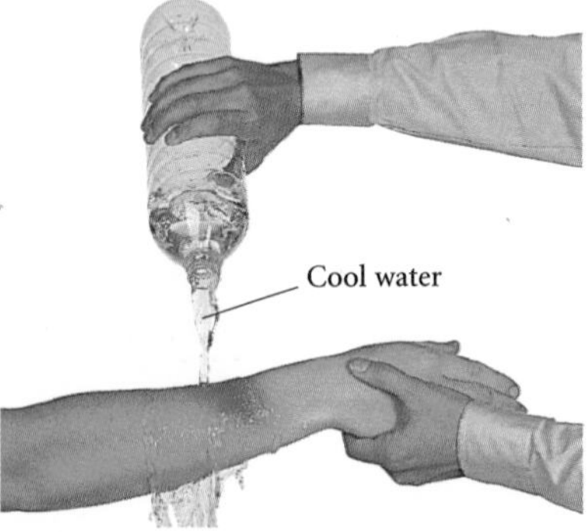

1 *Pour cool water over the injured area for at least 10 minutes to stop the burning and relieve the pain. If no water is available, use any suitable cold liquid, such as milk or a canned drink.*

2 *Once the burn has cooled, gently remove constricting clothing, shoes, belt, or jewellery from the affected area before it begins to swell.*

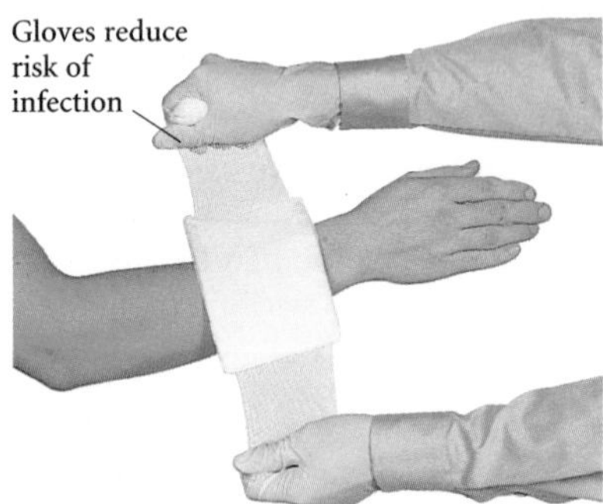

3 *Cover the burned area with a sterile dressing (p.996) or any clean, nonfluffy material. Bandage the dressing loosely in place. Do not apply creams, lotions, adhesive dressings, or tape to affected skin.*

4 *Check the wound daily for signs of infection, such as increasing pain, swelling, redness, or pus. If you suspect infection, contact your doctor at once.*

Major seizures

A major seizure (convulsion) is a result of an electrical disturbance in the brain and consists of muscular spasms and loss of body control. Seizures that are recurrent usually indicate the brain disorder epilepsy (p.524). During a major seizure, a person falls unconscious, often letting out a cry. The body becomes rigid, the back arches, the jaw is clenched, the eyes roll upwards, and the tongue may be bitten. The breathing becomes noisy and, in some cases, temporarily ceases. Convulsive shaking movements of the body may then follow, and may last for 1–3 minutes. The victim finally recovers consciousness within a few minutes but is left dazed and sleepy. Anyone who is giving first aid should protect the victim from injuring him- or herself during a major seizure and remain present until recovery is complete.

WARNING
- Do not use force to restrain the victim.
- Do not put anything in the victim's mouth.

1 *Attempt to support the victim if you see him or her falling. If bystanders are present, ask them to move away and remove any objects from around the victim.*

2 *Lay the victim down. Loosen clothing around his or her neck, and try to protect the head with something soft, such as a piece of folded clothing.*

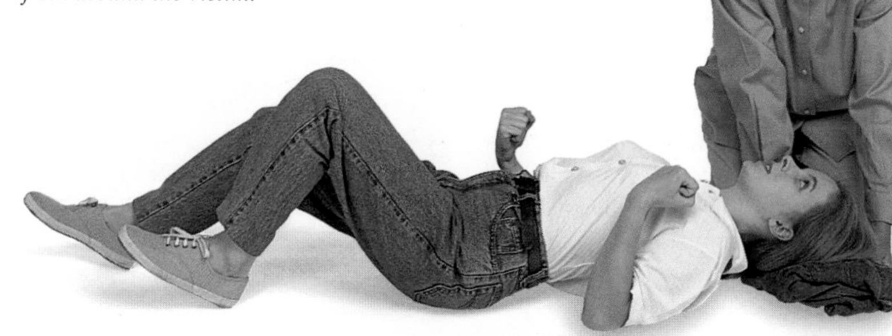

3 *When the seizures have finished, place the victim in the recovery position (p.979). Check his or her breathing and pulse (see* ABC OF RESUSCITATION, *p.978).*

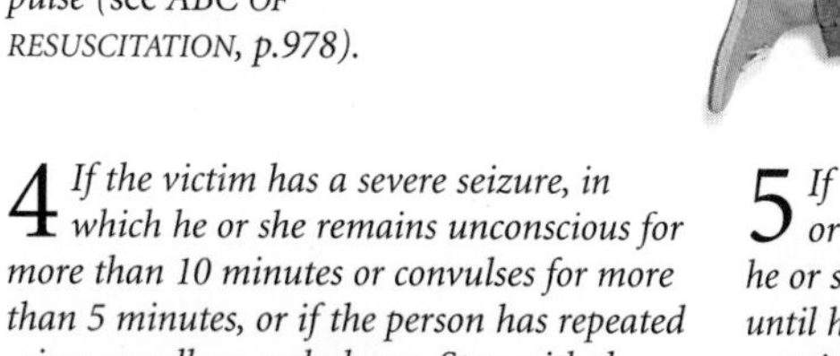

4 *If the victim has a severe seizure, in which he or she remains unconscious for more than 10 minutes or convulses for more than 5 minutes, or if the person has repeated seizures, call an ambulance. Stay with the victim and monitor breathing and pulse until the ambulance arrives.*

5 *If the victim has not had a severe seizure or repeated seizures and you know that he or she has epilepsy, stay with the person until he or she has recovered. If you are not certain that the person has epilepsy, call an ambulance and stay with the victim until the ambulance arrives.*

Febrile convulsions

Febrile convulsions are seizures that can occur in young children as a result of a very high temperature. They are most common in children under the age of 5. During a febrile convulsion, the eyes may roll back, the head and body may jerk, and the child may hold his or her breath. His or her back may arch, the legs and arms may become stiff, and the fists may clench. It is essential to lower the child's temperature and protect him or her from injury. Although alarming for parents, febrile convulsions are rarely dangerous.

WARNING
- Do not use force to restrain the victim.
- Do not put anything in the victim's mouth.

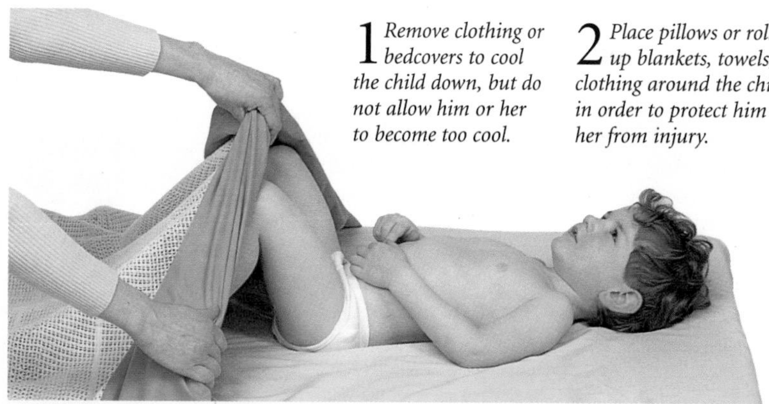

1 *Remove clothing or bedcovers to cool the child down, but do not allow him or her to become too cool.*

2 *Place pillows or rolled-up blankets, towels, or clothing around the child in order to protect him or her from injury.*

3 *Once the convulsions have stopped, sponge the child all over with tepid water, working from the head down. Do not dry the child; instead, allow the moisture to evaporate from his or her skin. Monitor the child's temperature at regular intervals, and stop cooling as soon as the temperature has reached normal (37°C/98.6°F).*

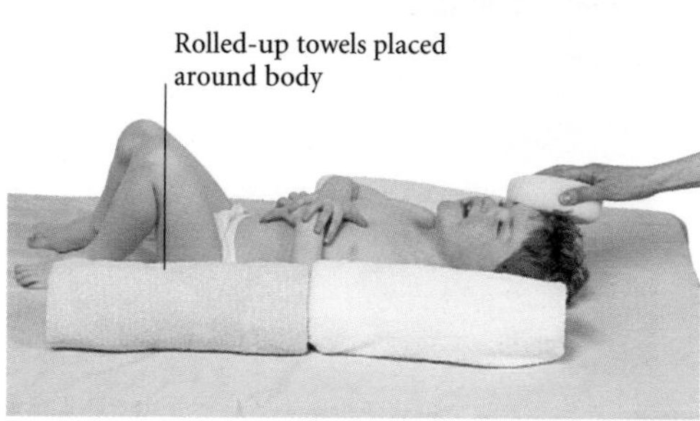

Spinal injury

The main risk when dealing with someone who has spinal injury is that any movement may damage the spinal cord. The most dangerous injuries are those to the neck, but any spinal injury is potentially serious, and you should seek emergency help immediately. When calling the emergency services, try to tell them how the injury to the spine occurred. If you suspect an injury to the spinal cord, it is vital to keep the victim still until a doctor arrives. Signs of possible damage to the spinal cord include a burning sensation or tingling in a limb or loss of feeling in a limb. The victim may also have breathing difficulties.

> **WARNING**
> Do not move the victim from the position in which he or she was found unless the person is in danger or loses consciousness and needs resuscitation. If you do have to move the victim, use the log-roll technique (below).

1 Call an ambulance. Reassure the victim and keep him or her as still as possible. If the victim was found face down, and you have to move him or her, get other people to help you to turn the victim over (see TURNING A VICTIM WITH SUSPECTED SPINAL INJURY, below*). If the victim was found on his or her back, proceed to Step 2.*

2 The safest position for a victim with a suspected spinal injury is with the head, neck, and spine aligned. To check alignment, make sure that the victim's nose is in line with his or her navel.

3 If you need to realign the victim, kneel by the victim's head, place your hands firmly over his or her ears, and move the head slowly into position. Stay in this position until the ambulance arrives.

4 If you have a helper, extra stability can be provided by getting him or her to place rolled-up clothes, towels, or blankets on either side of the victim's head and shoulders to minimize movement.

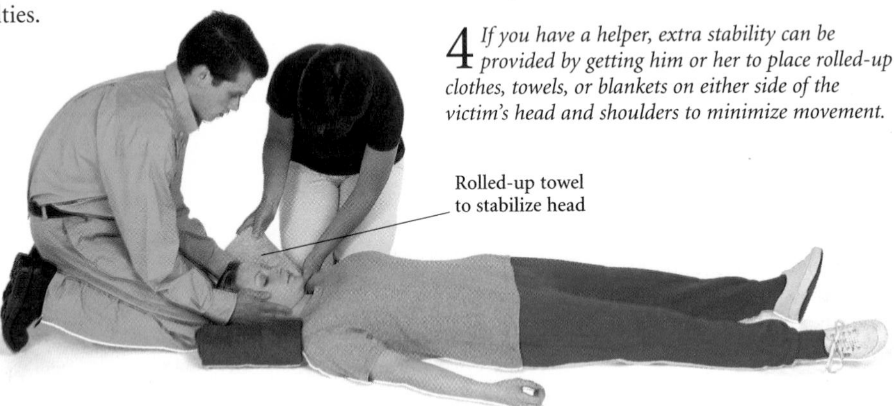

SPECIAL CASE: TURNING A VICTIM WITH SUSPECTED SPINAL INJURY

A technique called the log roll must be used if you suspect a spinal injury and need to turn the victim on to his or her back to open the airway (*see* OPENING THE AIRWAY – SPINAL INJURY, p.982) before giving artificial respiration or cardiopulmonary resuscitation. You will need to have several helpers, working as a team, to ensure that the entire body is rolled over at once.

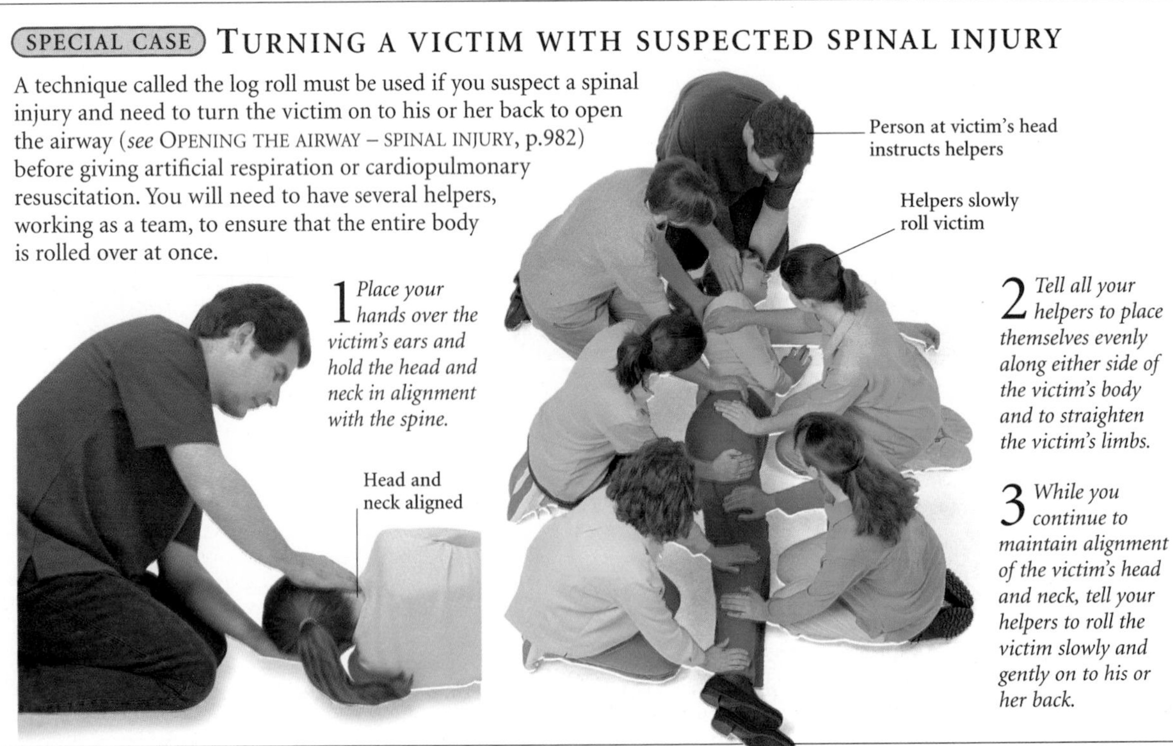

1 Place your hands over the victim's ears and hold the head and neck in alignment with the spine.

2 Tell all your helpers to place themselves evenly along either side of the victim's body and to straighten the victim's limbs.

3 While you continue to maintain alignment of the victim's head and neck, tell your helpers to roll the victim slowly and gently on to his or her back.

Head injury

It is usually difficult to determine the extent of damage in head injuries, and proper assessment by trained medical staff is required. You should suspect a serious head injury if there is bleeding or bruising at the site of the wound or a depression in the scalp. A person who has hit his or her head may have sustained a head injury even when there is no visible wound.

The victim of a head injury may feel dazed or nauseated and may have a headache or have some memory loss. Shock may cause pale and clammy skin. Leakage of blood or watery fluid from the nose or ears indicates a possible fracture of the skull. The victim may be unconscious or may gradually become less responsive over a period of time (*see* UNCONSCIOUSNESS, p.983).

> **WARNING**
>
> Call an ambulance immediately if the victim is unconscious or appears confused, or if blood or watery fluid is leaking from the ears or nose.

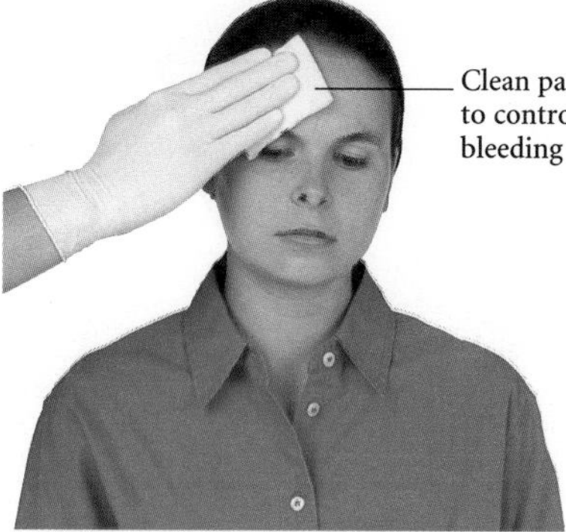

1 *Before treating bleeding from a wound, wash your hands thoroughly. Put on rubber gloves if possible. If there is a scalp wound, replace any skin flaps. Press a clean pad firmly and evenly over the wound to control the blood flow.*

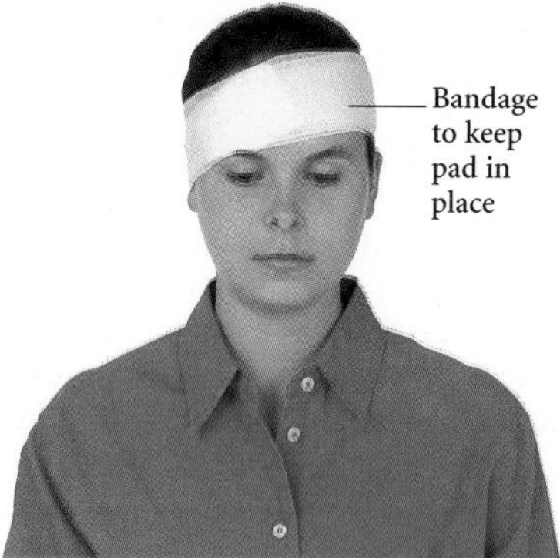

2 *When the bleeding has been controlled, secure a bandage around the victim's head in order to keep the pad in position over the wound. It is important to secure the bandage well away from the wound and also away from the eyes if possible.*

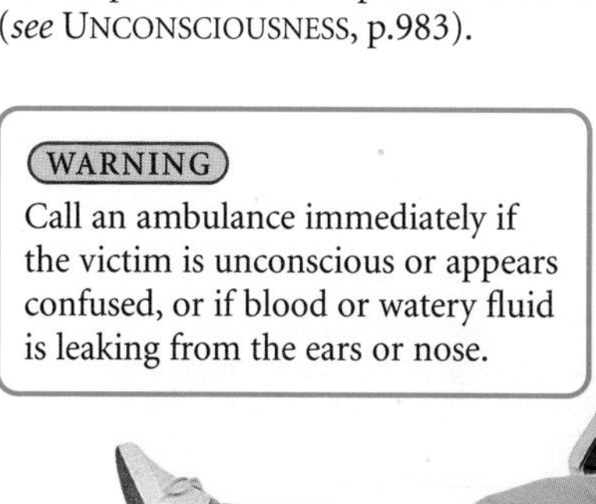

3 *Check that the victim is fully conscious by asking simple, direct questions. If the person is alert and responds normally to your questions, lay him or her down in a comfortable position with the head and shoulders supported. Arrange for transport to hospital for medical assessment. If the person does not respond or seems confused, proceed to Step 4.*

4 *Call an ambulance. If you need to leave the person to make the call yourself, place him or her in the recovery position (p.979). While waiting for medical help, monitor the victim's breathing and pulse (see* ABC OF RESUSCITATION, *p.978) and be ready to resuscitate if necessary.*

Sprains and strains

Sprains are injuries in which ligaments and other tissues that surround a joint are stretched or torn. In strains, muscles or tendons are overstretched and damaged. Both sprains and strains may lead to pain, swelling, deformity, and discoloration in the injured area. A severe sprain or strain can produce symptoms similar to those of a fracture. If you are in any doubt about the cause of the injury, treat as you would for a fracture (p.992). Otherwise, follow the "RICE" procedure: rest, ice, compression, and elevation. When you apply compression, you must make sure that you do not obstruct the blood supply to the tissues surrounding the injured area.

1 *Try to make the victim comfortable by steadying and supporting the injured part. Rest an injured limb on your knee or in your lap if it helps.*

2 *Apply a cold compress or an ice pack to the affected area for several minutes to reduce any swelling, bruising, and pain. Do not apply ice directly to the skin.*

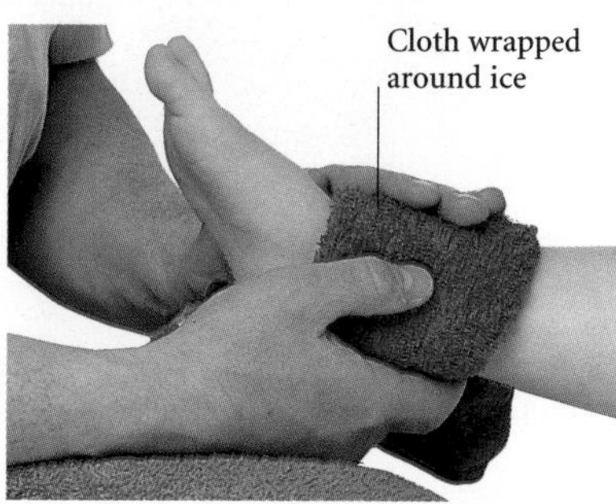

3 *Use a thick layer of padding, such as cotton, to apply gentle, even pressure to the injured area. Secure it in place with a bandage, making sure that it is not too tight (see* DRESSINGS AND BANDAGES, *pp.996–998).*

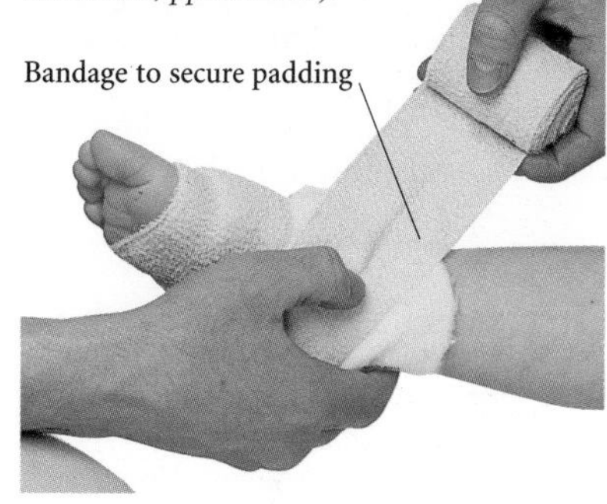

4 *Raise and support the limb to help to reduce bruising and swelling. Advise the victim to rest the limb and to see a doctor.*

Upper limb fractures

Upper limb fractures may involve any of the bones in the arm or the collarbone. You should suspect a fracture if the person cannot move the injured part or it is misshapen or very painful. There is likely to be swelling and bruising and possibly bleeding and a visible wound. A person with an upper limb fracture is usually able to walk and can be taken to hospital. The injured part must be kept as still as possible. This is to reduce pain but also to prevent further damage to nerves and blood vessels, especially in the region of the elbow.

WARNING

Do not give the victim anything to eat or drink, in case he or she needs a general anaesthetic.

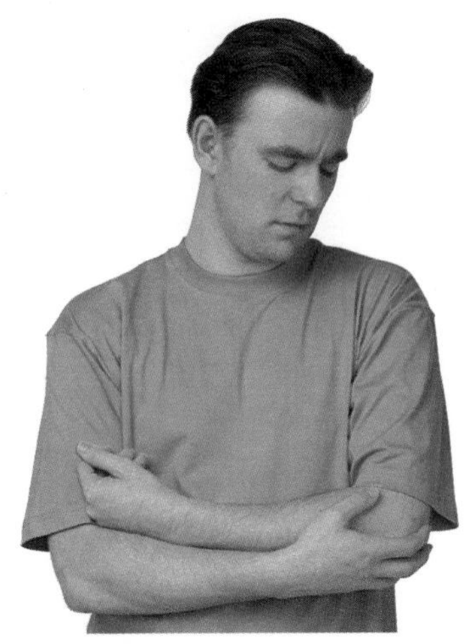

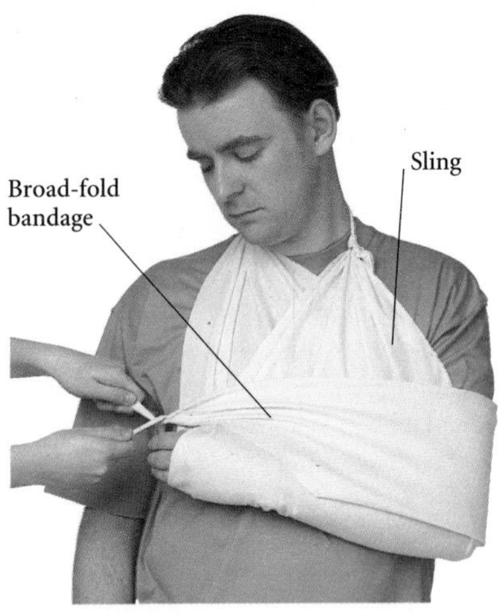

1 *Sit the victim down. If necessary, treat bleeding (see* SEVERE BLEEDING, *p.986).*

2 *Tell the victim to hold the injured arm across his or her chest in the position that is most comfortable. Ask the victim to support his or her arm or wrist, if possible. Alternatively, support it yourself.*

3 *Place the arm on the injured side in a sling (p.998) and insert soft padding between the arm and the chest. If the arm has to be kept still, tie a broad-fold bandage around the chest and over the sling.*

4 *Take or send the victim to hospital, keeping him or her seated if possible.*

Lower limb fractures

Fracture of a lower limb bone is a serious injury needing immediate treatment in hospital. It is important that the victim does not put any weight on the injured limb. A person who has a lower limb fracture is likely to be in severe pain and may not be able to move the affected part of the limb. The area around the fracture may be swollen and bruised, and there may be a visible wound with bleeding. If the femur (thigh bone) has been fractured, the affected leg may be turned outwards and may appear shorter than the uninjured leg. Fractures of the shaft of the femur usually involve severe internal bleeding. If there is serious bleeding, the victim may develop signs of shock (p.987), including a rapid pulse, pale or greyish-blue colouring, and sweaty, clammy, cold skin.

WARNING

- Do not move the victim unless he or she needs to be removed from a source of danger.
- Do not give the victim anything to eat or drink, in case he or she needs a general anaesthetic.

1 *Help the victim to lie down, and treat any bleeding (see* SEVERE BLEEDING, *p.986).*

2 *Put plenty of padding, such as rolled-up blankets or towels or folded newspaper, on both sides of the injured leg. If you have a helper, send him or her to call an ambulance.*

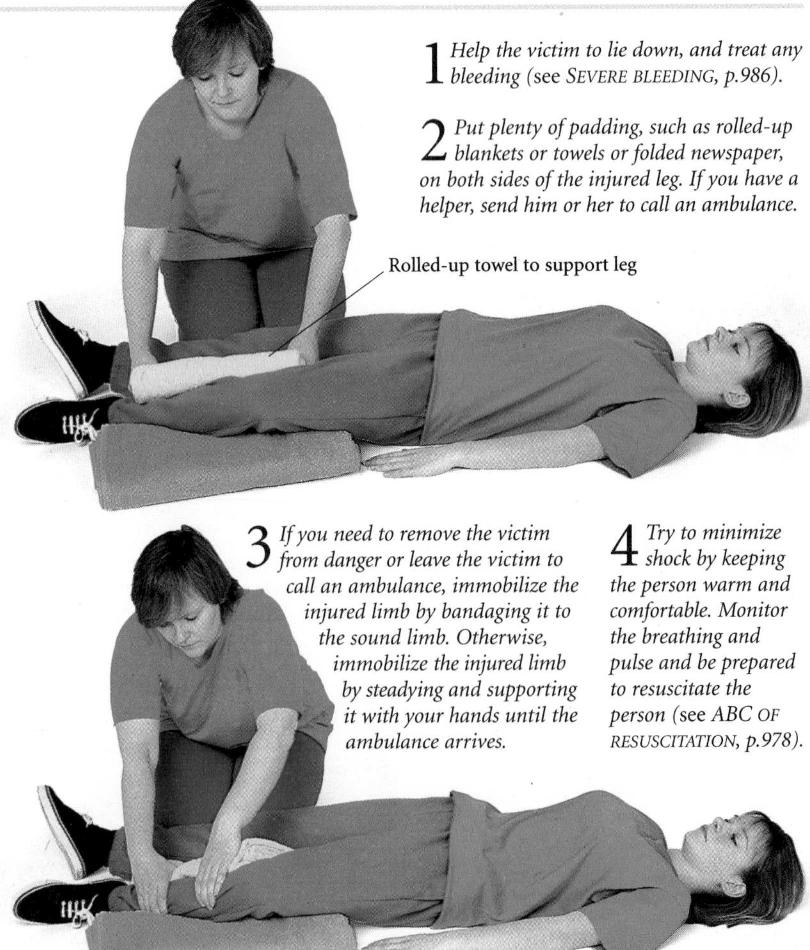

3 *If you need to remove the victim from danger or leave the victim to call an ambulance, immobilize the injured limb by bandaging it to the sound limb. Otherwise, immobilize the injured limb by steadying and supporting it with your hands until the ambulance arrives.*

4 *Try to minimize shock by keeping the person warm and comfortable. Monitor the breathing and pulse and be prepared to resuscitate the person (see* ABC OF RESUSCITATION, *p.978).*

Eye wound

All eye injuries are potentially serious and need prompt medical attention in order to minimize the risk of infection, scarring, or impaired vision. The victim may experience extreme pain, and the eyelids may go into spasm. There may be a visible wound to the eyeball, or the affected eye may be bloodshot and may bleed or leak clear fluid.

WARNING
- Do not touch the affected eye or allow the victim to touch it.
- Do not remove a foreign body embedded in the eye.

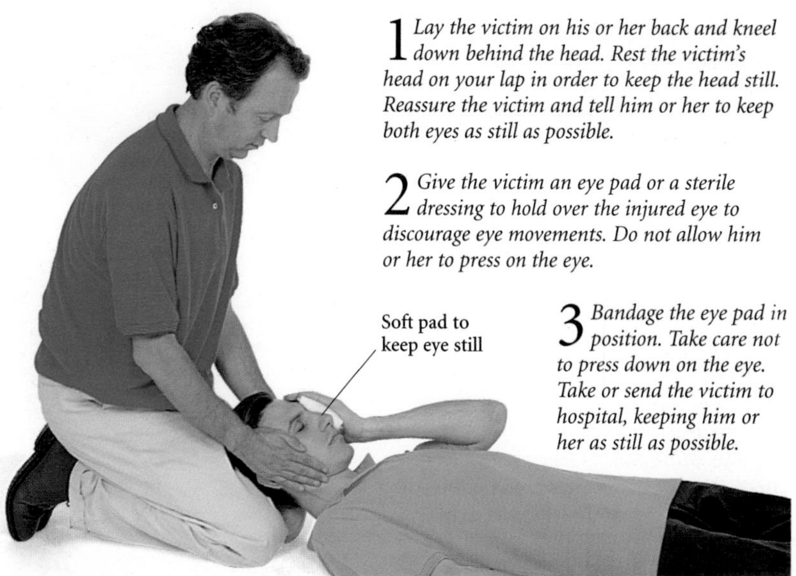

1 *Lay the victim on his or her back and kneel down behind the head. Rest the victim's head on your lap in order to keep the head still. Reassure the victim and tell him or her to keep both eyes as still as possible.*

2 *Give the victim an eye pad or a sterile dressing to hold over the injured eye to discourage eye movements. Do not allow him or her to press on the eye.*

Soft pad to keep eye still

3 *Bandage the eye pad in position. Take care not to press down on the eye. Take or send the victim to hospital, keeping him or her as still as possible.*

Foreign body in the eye

A foreign body in the eye may cause irritation, redness, watering, and blurred vision. An object floating on the white of the eye can usually be removed easily. However, anything that sticks to the eye, penetrates the eyeball, or rests on the coloured part of the eye should be treated as an eye wound (above).

WARNING
- Do not touch the affected eye or allow the victim to touch it.
- Do not remove a foreign body embedded in the eye.

1 *Sit the victim down so that he or she is facing the light. Using your finger and thumb, gently separate the upper and lower eyelids. Examine every part of the eye.*

2 *If you can see a foreign body floating on the white of the eye, try to flush it out with clean water. Tilt the head so that the damaged eye is lower than the uninjured one. Pour water into the corner of the injured eye, allowing it to drain away without it getting into the uninjured eye. Blinking under water may also make the foreign body float clear.*

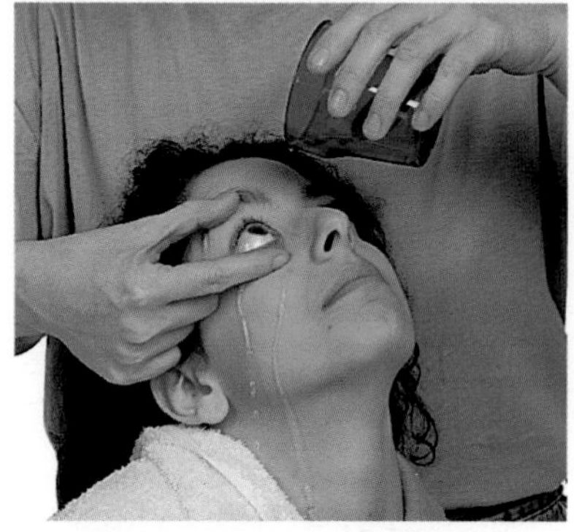

3 *If flushing out the eye with water is unsuccessful, try using the corner of a clean, dampened handkerchief or tissue to lift the foreign body off the white of the eye.*

4 *If the object is under the upper eyelid and you cannot remove it using a tissue, ask the victim to grasp the lashes and pull the upper lid over the lower one. This may help to brush the object out of the eye.*

5 *If you are not able to remove the foreign object from the eye, take the victim to hospital.*

Chemicals in the eye

Chemical injuries to the eye can cause serious damage, including blindness, if they are not treated quickly. Follow the steps shown here except if a person has been exposed to CS gas. To help to disperse CS gas, do not flush out the eye but turn the victim's head to the wind.

WARNING
Do not touch the affected eye or allow the victim to touch it.

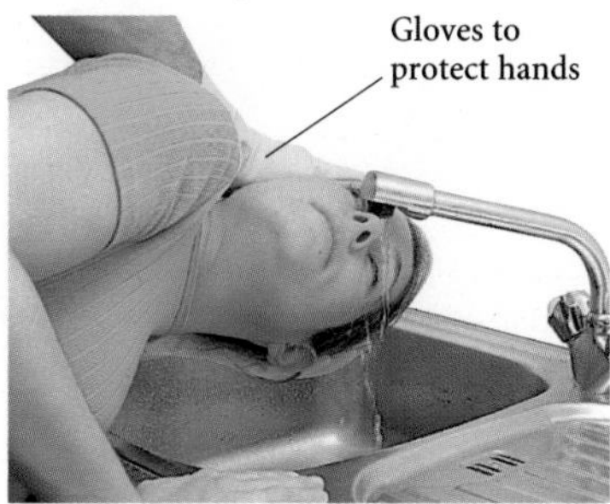

Gloves to protect hands

1 *Hold the victim's head under a running tap so that water runs over the eye for at least 10 minutes. Make sure that the contaminated rinsing water does not splash you or the victim. If it is easier, use a jug or glass to pour the water.*

2 *If the victim is unable to open the eye, gently pull his or her eyelids apart in order to clean all parts of the eye and eyelids.*

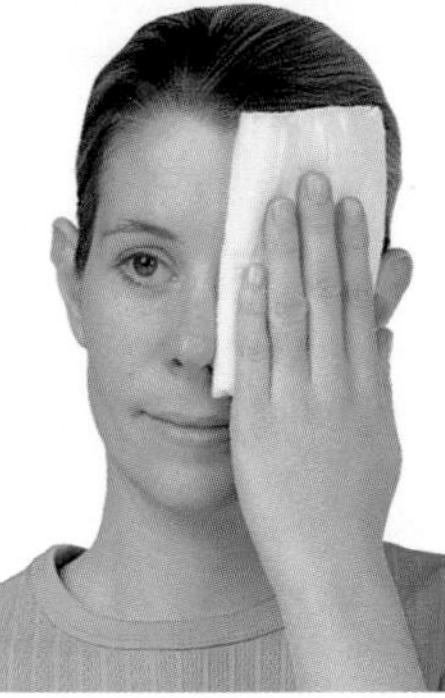

3 *Ask the victim to hold a sterile pad, or a pad made from clean, nonfluffy material, over the injured eye. If possible, identify the chemical. Take or send the victim to hospital.*

Swallowed poisons

Poisoning can be caused by swallowing toxic chemicals or poisonous plants or by overdosing on recreational or medicinal drugs. Common symptoms include pain in the abdomen or chest, nausea, vomiting, diarrhoea, breathing difficulties, and dizziness. There may be signs of burning around the mouth and lips. The victim may appear sluggish and confused, and he or she may lose consciousness. Rarely, certain poisons can cause anaphylactic shock (p.987), which is a life-threatening allergic reaction. The warning signs of anaphylactic shock include swelling of the face and neck and red, blotchy skin.

If you suspect poisoning, you must seek immediate medical assistance. Aim to provide the emergency services with as much information as you can about the poisoning, including the type of substance that was swallowed, the amount, and how long ago it was swallowed.

WARNING

Do not try to induce vomiting unless you are advised to do so by a medical professional.

1 If the victim is conscious, ask questions to obtain as much information as possible about the poisoning. If the victim is unconscious, go to Step 3.

2 Call your doctor or your local poison centre for further instructions. Give as much information as you can about the possible cause of the poisoning. Stay with the victim and monitor his or her condition. If he or she develops signs of shock or breathing difficulties, call an ambulance.

3 If the victim is unconscious or loses consciousness, check breathing and pulse and be prepared to resuscitate if necessary (see ABC OF RESUSCITATION, p.978).

4 Place the victim in the recovery position (p.979) unless you suspect that he or she has a spinal injury. Call an ambulance and then return to the victim. If alcohol poisoning is a possibility, keep the victim warm with a blanket.

Poisonous bites and stings

In various parts of the world, there are certain animals, such as snakes, spiders, and scorpions, that have a venomous bite or sting. One poisonous snake, the adder, is native to the UK. A venomous bite or sting can cause severe pain and burning at the site of the wound, with swelling and discoloration. Spider bites and scorpion stings may also cause vomiting, sweating, breathing problems, and an irregular heartbeat. With prompt hospital treatment, most victims of bites and stings recover rapidly. It is important to note the appearance of a snake responsible for a bite in order that the appropriate antivenom can be given.

WARNING

- Do not attempt to identify a venomous snake or spider by handling it.
- Do not apply a tourniquet to the affected limb or try to suck the venom from the bite.

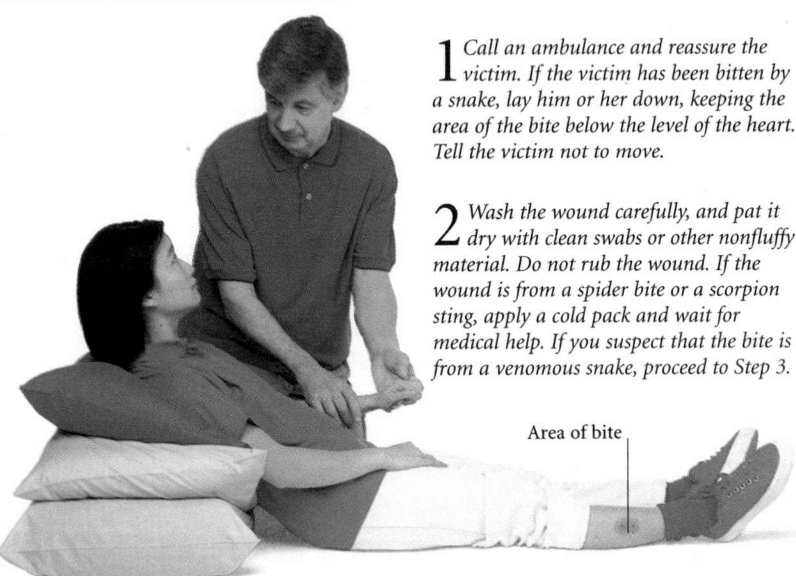

1 Call an ambulance and reassure the victim. If the victim has been bitten by a snake, lay him or her down, keeping the area of the bite below the level of the heart. Tell the victim not to move.

2 Wash the wound carefully, and pat it dry with clean swabs or other nonfluffy material. Do not rub the wound. If the wound is from a spider bite or a scorpion sting, apply a cold pack and wait for medical help. If you suspect that the bite is from a venomous snake, proceed to Step 3.

3 Minimize the victim's movement to stop the venom from spreading further around the body. Immobilize an injured arm with a sling (p.998), and immobilize an injured leg by binding it to the uninjured leg.

4 Keep the victim calm while waiting for the ambulance. Regularly monitor the victim's breathing and pulse and be ready to resuscitate if necessary (see ABC OF RESUSCITATION, p.978).

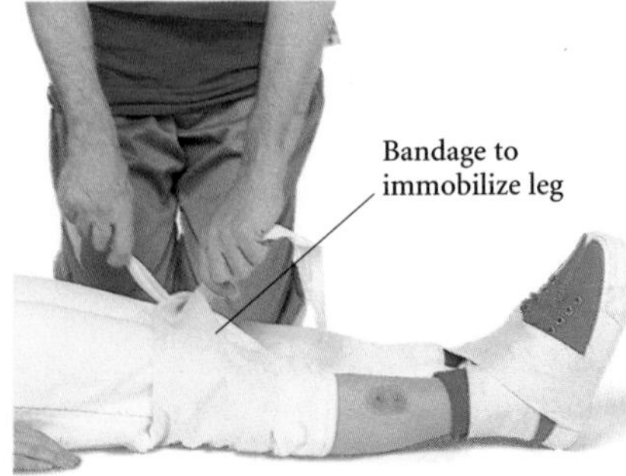

Human and animal bites

Bites from humans or animals carry a high risk of transmitting infection. Even a small bite should be assessed by a doctor as soon as possible in case treatment with antibiotics (p.885) or an injection against tetanus (p.302) is required. In many countries, although not in the UK, injections against rabies (p.296) may be needed. First aid consists of controlling bleeding and keeping the wound clean.

1 Remove the victim from danger if it is safe to do so. If bitten by an animal, do not try to capture it.

Sterile dressing

Rubber gloves for protection

2 If the wound is superficial, wash it with soap and water, pat dry, and apply a sterile dressing (p.996). If the wound is serious, treat as for severe bleeding (p.986) and take or send the victim to hospital for treatment.

WARNING

Severe infections can be transmitted by animal bites. Medical assessment is essential in all cases.

Tick bites

Ticks are tiny, spider-like creatures that live by attaching themselves to animals (including humans) and sucking their blood. They are found in woodlands and grasslands and are most active during the summer. An unfed tick is small and may not be noticed because the bite is usually painless. When a tick feeds, it becomes engorged with blood and is then usually easy to see. Some ticks can transmit diseases, including Lyme disease (p.303). People who visit the US may be at risk of contracting Rocky Mountain spotted fever (p.304) from tick bites. It is therefore important to remove a tick as soon as possible.

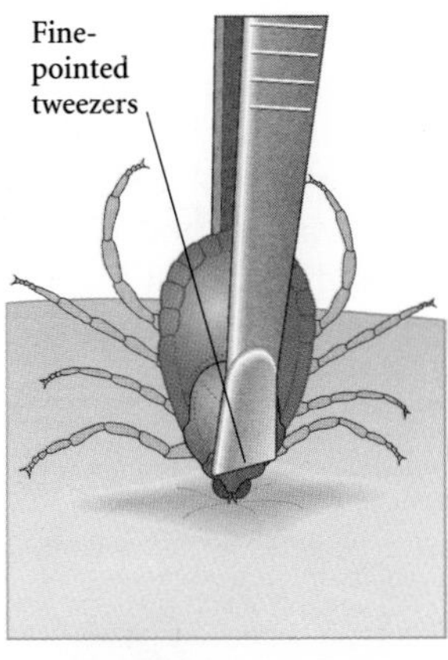

1 If you find a tick embedded in the skin, use a pair of fine-pointed tweezers to grasp the tick's head or mouthparts at the point where it is attached.

2 Lever the tick steadily and firmly out of the skin with a slight rocking motion. Do not twist or jerk as you pull. Once the tick has been removed, preserve it in a jar of alcohol and take it to show your doctor.

3 Wash your hands thoroughly, then apply an antiseptic to the wound. Place a light dressing or waterproof plaster on the wound.

4 If a rash appears at the site of the bite or if flu-like symptoms develop days or weeks after the bite, see a doctor in case you have been infected.

WARNING

Do not apply a hot match, alcohol, or any other substance to the tick in an attempt to remove it. The tick may become more firmly embedded and even more likely to transmit disease.

Insect stings

Stings from bees, wasps, and hornets are painful and uncomfortable but are not usually life-threatening. There may be a sharp pain followed by temporary swelling, soreness, and itching. A few people are allergic to insect stings, and, in severe cases, a single sting can lead to life-threatening anaphylactic shock (p.987). Signs of this condition include swelling of the face, lips, and tongue; wheezing and difficulty in breathing; and a rash that may appear anywhere on the body. The victim may lose consciousness.

1 If there are signs of anaphylactic shock or the bite is in the mouth or throat, call an ambulance. Give a victim stung in the mouth a piece of ice to suck or cold water to sip. If there is no indication of shock and the sting is still in the skin, proceed to Step 2.

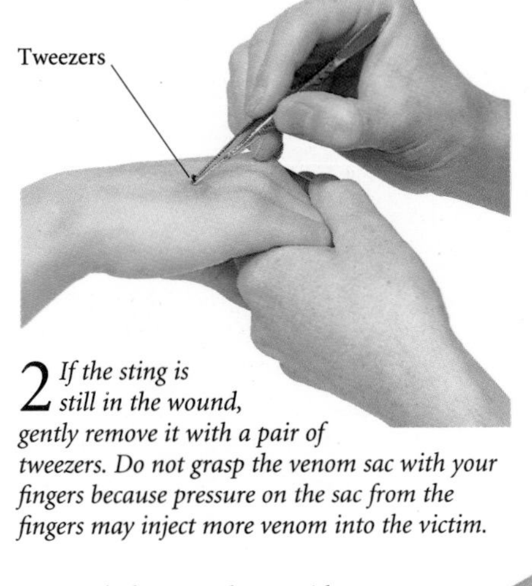

2 If the sting is still in the wound, gently remove it with a pair of tweezers. Do not grasp the venom sac with your fingers because pressure on the sac from the fingers may inject more venom into the victim.

3 Wash the injured area with soap and water, then pat dry. Cover the wound with a piece of clean cloth or gauze, and secure the material in place (see DRESSINGS AND BANDAGES, *pp.996–998).*

WARNING

Get help at once if the victim is allergic to stings.

4 Apply a cold compress on top of the cloth or gauze to reduce pain and swelling. Advise the victim to seek medical help if symptoms persist.

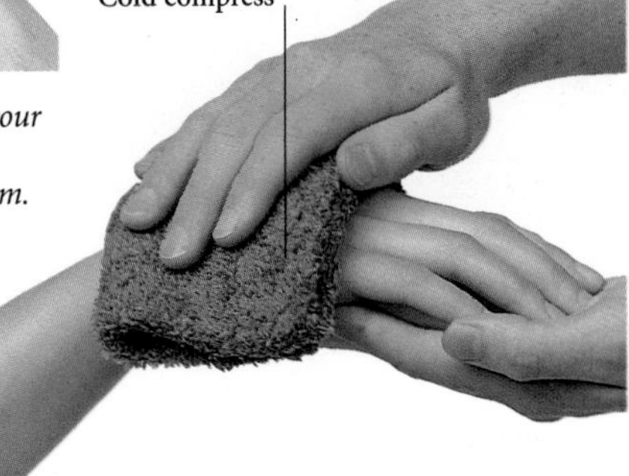

DRESSINGS AND BANDAGES

A dressing is a protective covering or pad placed directly on to a wound to absorb blood and other fluids and to prevent infection. A bandage is a piece of fabric used to wrap or cover any part of the body. Bandages may be used to keep dressings in place, to apply pressure, or to provide support for an injured body part.

If you need to apply a dressing to a wound, use a prepacked sterile dressing, if possible, in order to minimize the risk of infection. If no sterile dressing is available, you can use almost any clean, dry, absorbent fabric, such as a clean handkerchief or a pillow case or a sheet torn to an appropriate size.

Bandages come in several materials. Those made of open-weave material such as gauze are useful for holding light dressings in place; bandages made of elastic material are preferable for applying pressure to a wound to stop bleeding or to support a strain or sprain. Bandages also come in various shapes. Roller bandages are the most versatile and can be used for securing dressings on most parts of the body or for supporting an injured limb. Tubular bandages are used specifically for finger or toe injuries, and triangular bandages are used to make slings for supporting an injured arm or shoulder. You should include various sizes and types of dressing and bandage in your home first-aid kit (p.976).

The articles in this section show the first-aid techniques that should enable you to cope with most situations in which you need to apply a dressing or bandage. The first article shows how to apply a sterile dressing and how to secure the dressing with a roller bandage. The next two articles show the special methods needed to apply a roller bandage around an elbow or knee or to the wrist or ankle. The last two articles show how to bandage a finger or toe and how to put on a sling.

Sterile dressings

Choose a dressing that is large enough to cover an area 2.5 cm (1 in) beyond the edges of the wound. Before touching the dressing, wash your hands thoroughly. Ideally, wear disposable plastic gloves. Once you have placed the dressing over the wound, secure it using a roller bandage, taking care not to bandage so tightly that you impede the circulation. Leave the dressing in place unless the wound needs cleaning.

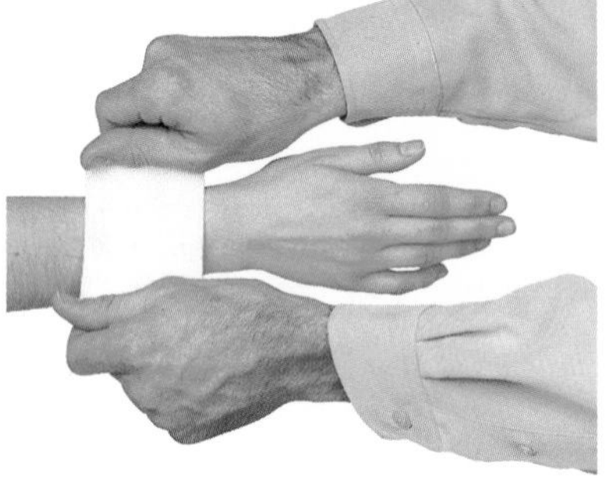

1 Grasping the edges of the dressing with the gauze face down, hold it directly over the wound, then lower it into place.

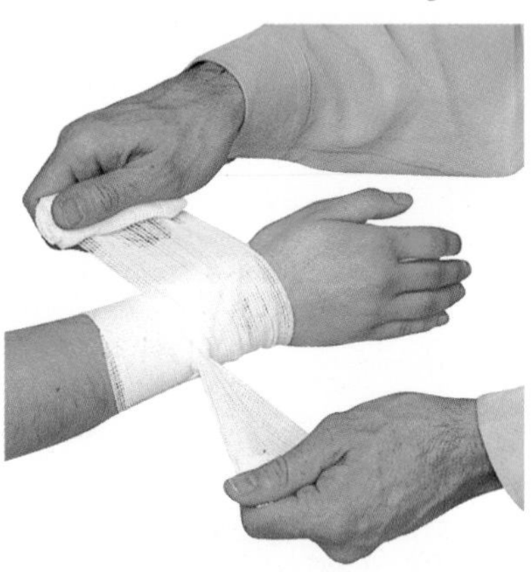

2 Hold the dressing in place by making several turns around it with a roller bandage. Keep hold of the free end. Continue to make turns, overlapping each preceding strip by about three-quarters of its width, until the dressing is completely covered.

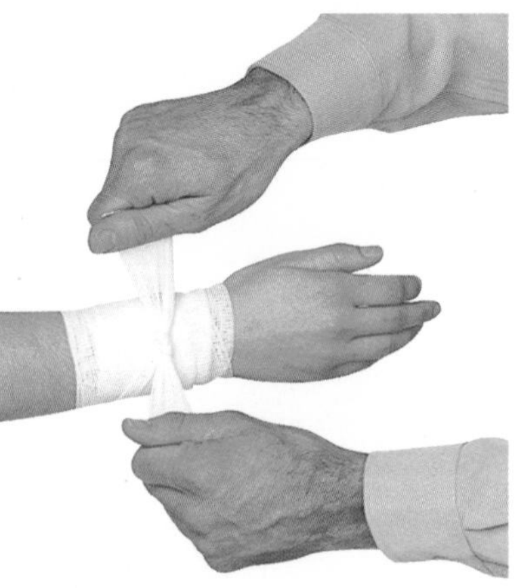

3 Cut the bandage and secure it by tying the ends or by using tape. If blood seeps through, apply another bandage over the top. Check the circulation and, if necessary, loosen the bandage (see CHECKING CIRCULATION AFTER BANDAGING, right).

(TECHNIQUE) CHECKING CIRCULATION AFTER BANDAGING

Immediately after bandaging a limb, check the circulation to make sure that the bandage is not too tight. Recheck the circulation every 10 minutes, because an injured limb may swell. Loosen a tight bandage at once, otherwise tissues may be permanently damaged.

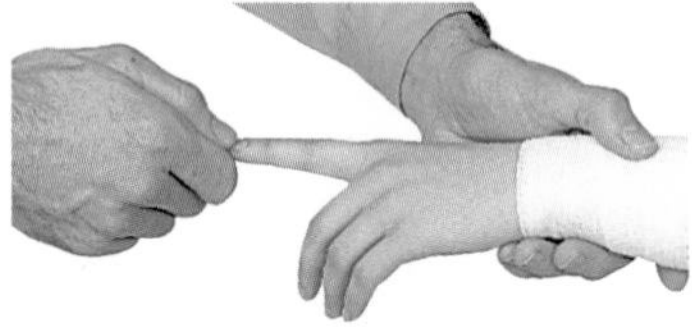

1 Press on a nail or on the skin of the hand or foot until the area turns pale. If the skin colour does not return immediately when the pressure is released, the bandage may be too tight.

2 To loosen a tight bandage, unwind it for a few turns. Wait for colour to return, then rewind the bandage more loosely. Check circulation as in Step 1.

3 Every 10 minutes, check fingers or toes for signs of impaired circulation, such as pale, cold skin, numbness, or inability to move the limb. If any of these signs are present, loosen the bandage immediately.

Elbow and knee bandages

A roller bandage applied in a figure of eight can be used to support a strain or sprain of the elbow or knee, or to hold a dressing in place at or near these joints. It is important to bandage adequately on either side of the elbow or knee as well as around the joint itself in order to provide even pressure over the entire injured area. The method shown here for bandaging the elbow can also be used for an injured knee.

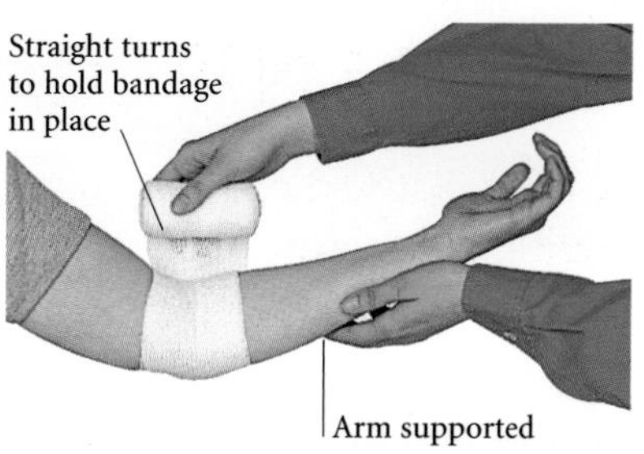

1 *Support the injured arm with one hand, keeping the elbow slightly flexed if possible. Starting at the crook of the elbow, unroll the bandage down towards the inner side of the arm and around the elbow joint. Wind the bandage around the joint several times to keep the end in place.*

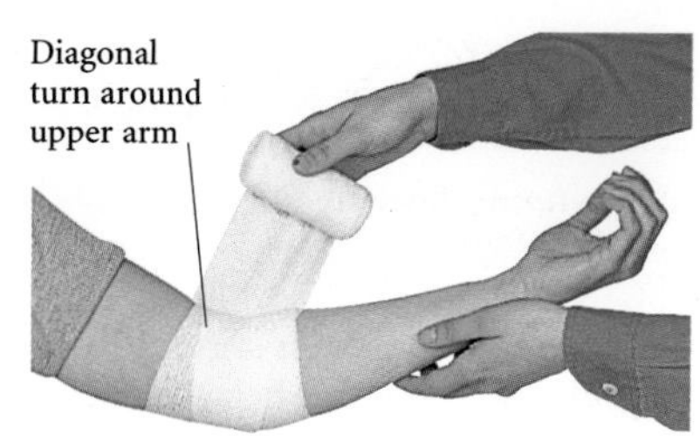

2 *Continue to unroll the bandage slowly, bringing it around the elbow joint at a slight angle so that you make a diagonal turn around the upper arm. This new turn should cover the top half of the previous layers from your initial turns. Continue to support the injured arm.*

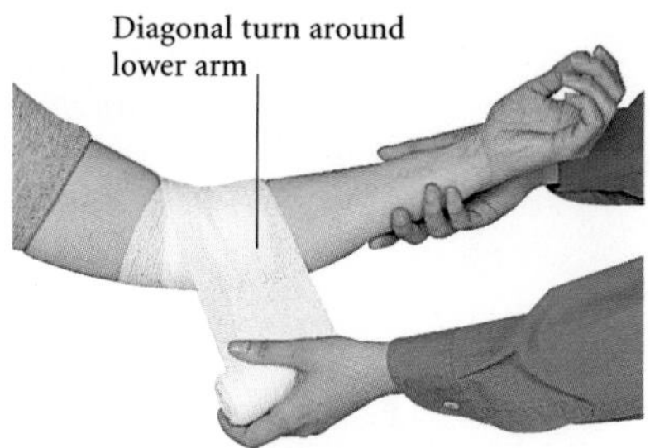

3 *Bring the bandage down around the outside of the elbow and up to make a diagonal turn around the forearm. The bandage should cover the lower half of the bandage from your first straight turns.*

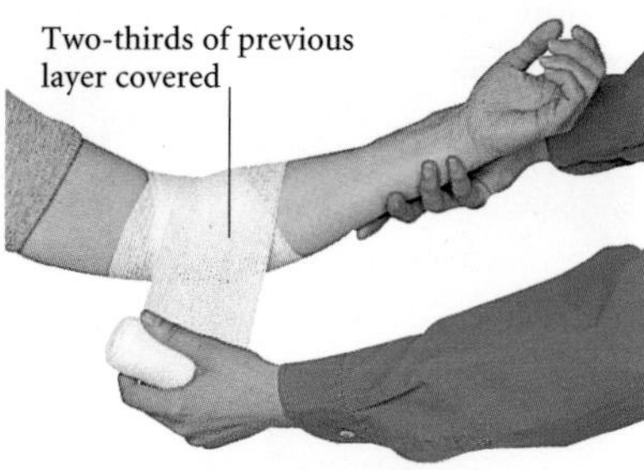

4 *Continue to wrap the bandage diagonally in a figure of eight above and below the joint. Each time you wrap the bandage around the joint, try to cover about two-thirds of the previous layer.*

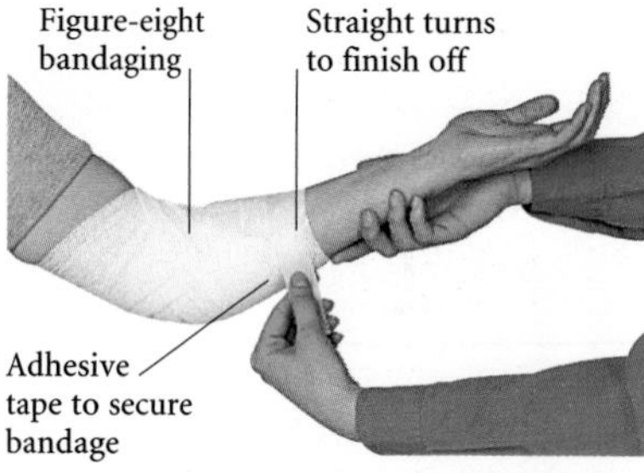

5 *To finish off, make two straight turns around the forearm and secure the end. Check the circulation and loosen the bandage if necessary (see CHECKING CIRCULATION AFTER BANDAGING, opposite page).*

Hand and foot bandages

You may need to apply a bandage to a hand or foot to provide support for a sprain or strain or to hold a dressing in place. The method shown here uses a roller bandage applied in diagonal fashion and can be used for either a hand or a foot. When bandaging a foot, substitute the big toe for the thumb and leave the heel unbandaged. The fingertips or toes should not be covered so that you can check the circulation.

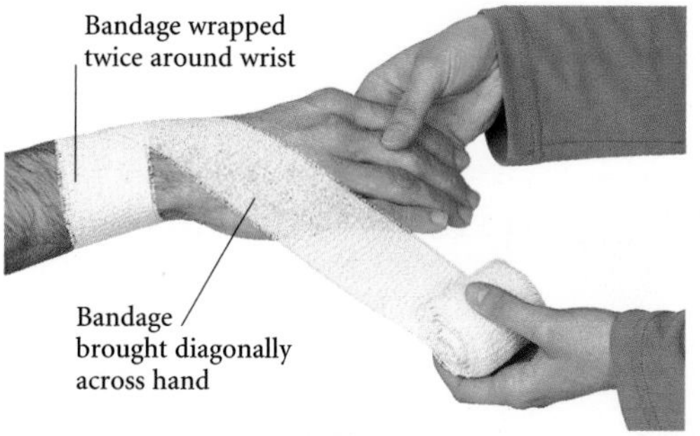

1 *Place the end of the bandage on the underside of the wrist at the base of the thumb and secure in place by wrapping the bandage around the wrist twice. Then bring the bandage diagonally across the back of the victim's hand in the direction of the little finger.*

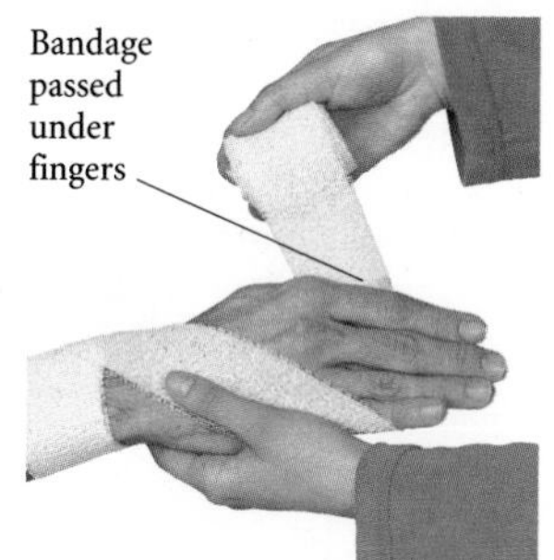

2 *Take the bandage under and across all the fingers so that the upper edge of the bandage touches the index finger about halfway up its length.*

3 *Take the bandage diagonally across the back of the hand, then around the wrist and back over the hand towards the little finger as in Step 1. Continue bandaging in this manner, trying to cover two-thirds of the previous layer with each new turn of the bandage. Leave the thumb and fingertips free.*

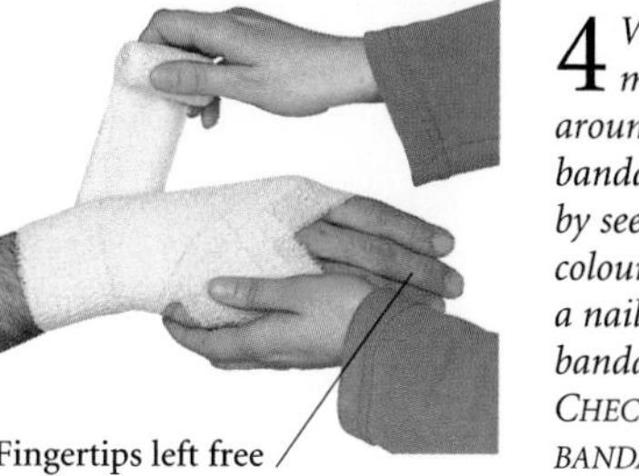

4 *When the hand is covered, make two straight turns around the wrist and secure the bandage. Check the circulation by seeing how long it takes for colour to return after pressing on a nail or the skin. Loosen the bandage if necessary (see* CHECKING CIRCULATION AFTER BANDAGING, *opposite page).*

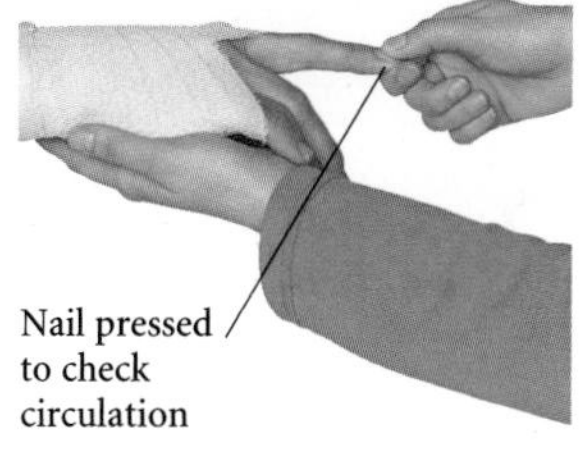

Finger or toe bandages

An injured finger or toe can be easily bandaged by using a piece of seamless, tube-shaped gauze. The tubular gauze is supplied on a roll and is cut to the appropriate size before being applied to the injured finger or toe. Each roll of gauze comes with a special applicator that enables you to slip the gauze into the correct position over the injured digit. Although tubular finger or toe dressings are suitable for most minor injuries, they cannot apply enough pressure to control heavy bleeding.

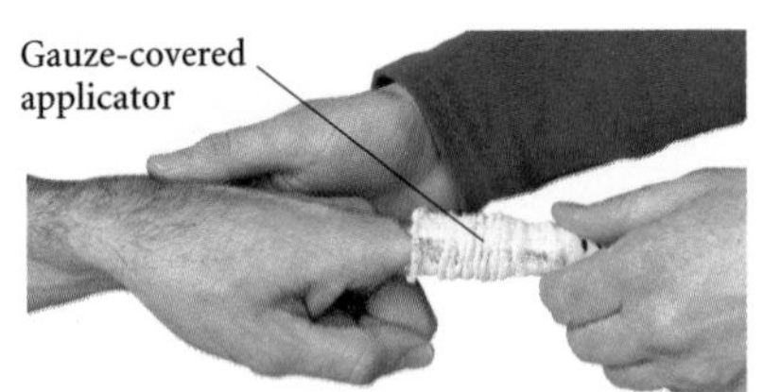

1 Cut a length of tubular gauze two-and-a-half times longer than the finger. Push the gauze on to the applicator, then gently place the applicator over the finger.

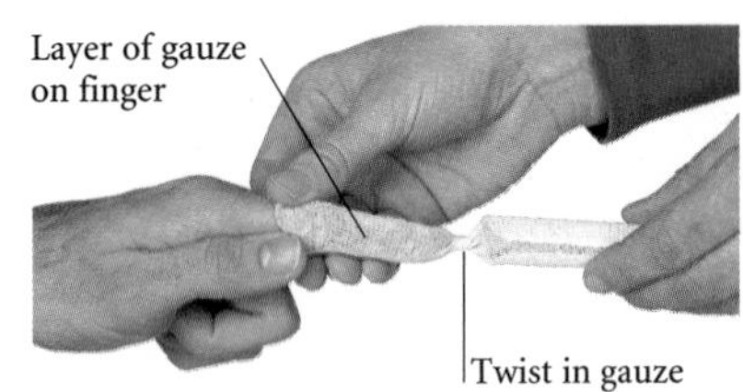

2 Hold the gauze in place at the base of the finger and pull the applicator off, leaving a layer of gauze behind. Hold the applicator just beyond the fingertip and twist it twice.

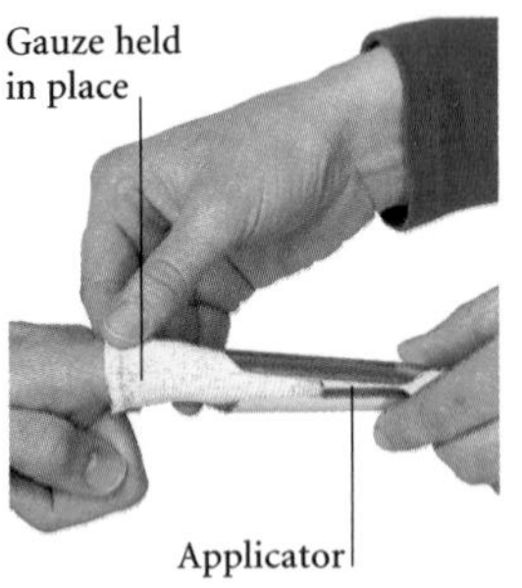

3 Continue to hold the gauze in place with one hand, and push the applicator back over the injured finger very gently, until the finger is covered with the rest of the tubular gauze. Remove the applicator from the finger.

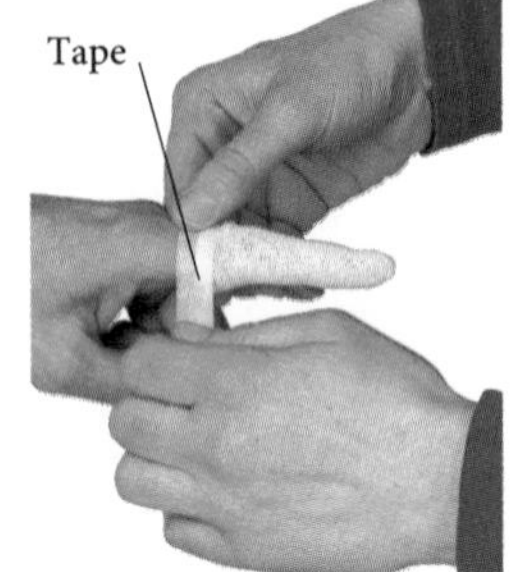

4 Secure the end of the gauze to the finger with a small piece of adhesive tape. Do not apply tape all the way around the finger. Regularly check the skin below the bandage for signs of impaired circulation such as pale or cool skin, and, if necessary, reapply the adhesive tape more loosely.

Slings

A sling is a triangular bandage, tied at the shoulder, that is used to support and immobilize an injured shoulder, arm, wrist, or hand. In an emergency, if no bandage is available, a sling can be made from a piece of cotton fabric measuring about 100 sq. cm (40 sq. in), which is then either cut in half or folded diagonally into a triangular shape.

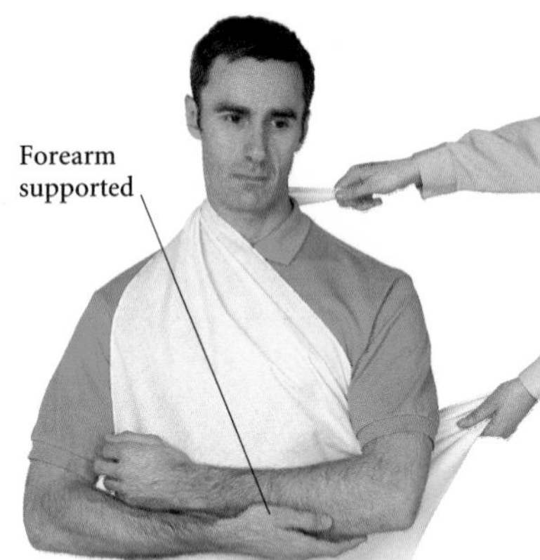

1 Support the arm on the injured side under the forearm or allow the victim to support it. Pass one end of the bandage under the elbow on the injured side and pull the bandage across to the opposite shoulder.

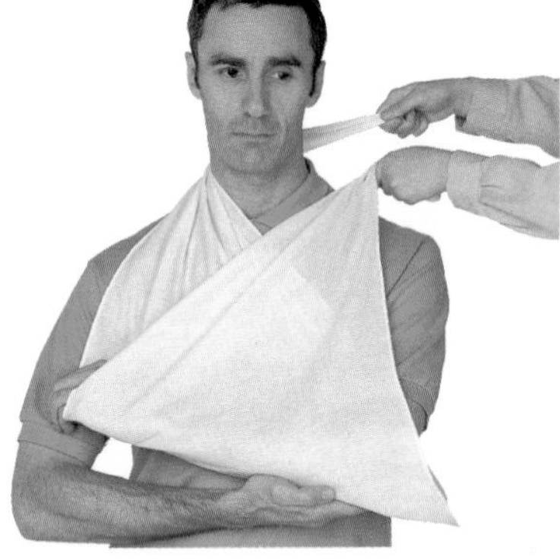

2 Spread the bandage out flat against the front of the victim's body, then bring the lower half of the bandage up over the forearm to meet the other end of the bandage at the shoulder.

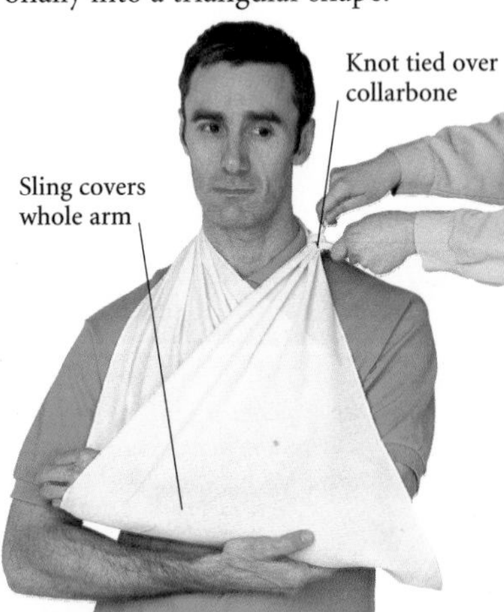

3 Tie a knot at the hollow over the victim's collarbone on the injured side of the body. Tuck both ends of the bandage under the knot to act as padding.

4 Fold the point forwards at the elbow. Tuck any loose bandage underneath it.

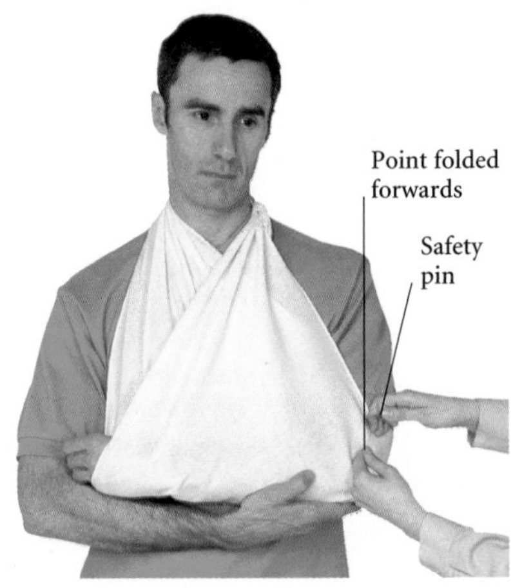

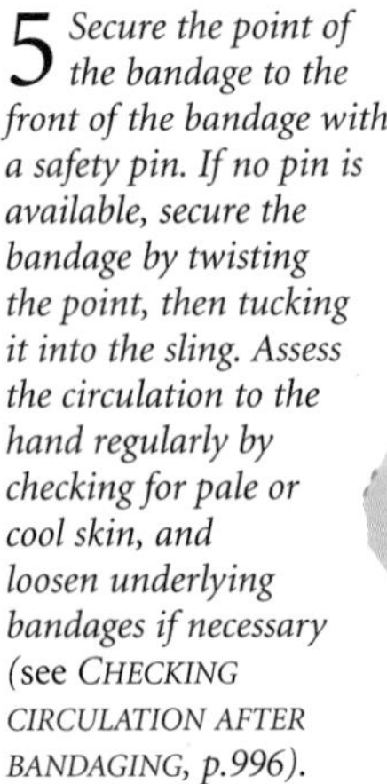

5 Secure the point of the bandage to the front of the bandage with a safety pin. If no pin is available, secure the bandage by twisting the point, then tucking it into the sling. Assess the circulation to the hand regularly by checking for pale or cool skin, and loosen underlying bandages if necessary (see *CHECKING CIRCULATION AFTER BANDAGING, p.996**).*

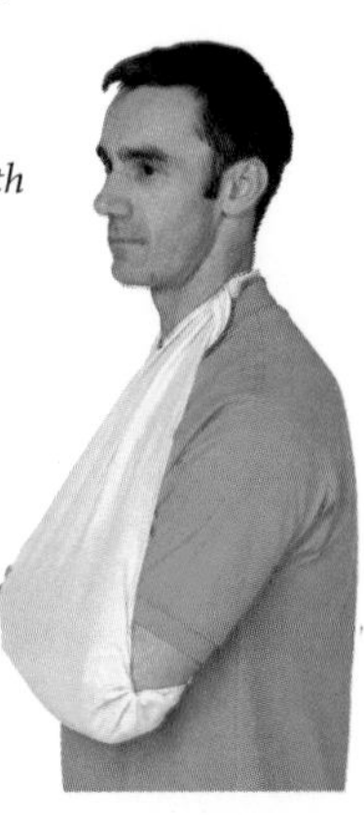

SECURING WITHOUT A PIN

Drug Glossary, Useful Online Sites and Addresses, and Index

This final reference section begins with a drug glossary, which lists by generic and brand name the most common prescription and over-the-counter drugs and gives a brief description of their uses. The glossary is followed by a list of support groups and organizations that can provide further information on medical problems and other health issues. The list includes online and e-mail addresses. The section ends with a comprehensive index.

DRUG GLOSSARY

Drugs are critically important in the treatment of almost every medical condition, whether it is an acquired or inherited disease or an injury. This glossary provides a quick reference to many of the brand-name and generic drugs that are commonly used today and briefly refers to the disorders that they treat.

Almost all of the drugs in use today were developed in a laboratory and are commercially manufactured using either chemical or genetic engineering processes. Many of these drugs are copies of naturally occurring chemicals, but a few are still obtained directly from natural sources, such as plants.

The drug glossary includes the names of over 2,500 generic and brand-name drugs currently used in the UK. Drugs frequently have more than one name. The generic name is used by doctors and pharmacists for the major active ingredient in a drug, but the same drug may also have a brand (proprietary) name chosen by the manufacturer. This brand name is often the name by which the drug is better known. If a generic drug is produced by several manufacturers, it will have a number of brand names.

In this glossary, brand-name drugs are indicated by an initial capital letter, and their generic name or generic components are included in their entry. Generic names of drugs are listed without an initial capital letter. These entries cross-refer to articles about drugs in the section Treating Disease or to descriptions of particular disorders in the section Your Body and Disease.

Some drugs can only be obtained with a doctor's prescription, while others can be purchased without a prescription and are known as over-the-counter drugs. A few drugs are only available for use in hospitals.

Also included in this glossary are some general terms, such as amino acid, which are often referred to in connection with drug treatments. These are listed in italic typeface.

A

ABACAVIR an antiviral drug used to treat HIV infection (*see* DRUGS FOR HIV INFECTION AND AIDS, p.887)

ABCIXIMAB an antiplatelet drug (*see* DRUGS THAT PREVENT BLOOD CLOTTING, p.904)

ABIDEC a brand-name multivitamin (*see* VITAMINS, p.927)

ACAMPROSATE an alcohol abuse deterrent (*see* ALCOHOL DEPENDENCE, p.564)

ACARBOSE an oral drug for diabetes mellitus (p.931)

ACCOLATE a brand name for zafirlukast

ACCUPRO a brand name for quinapril

ACCURETIC a brand-name antihypertensive drug (p.897) containing quinapril and hydrochlorothiazide

ACEBUTOLOL a beta-blocker drug (p.898)

ACECLOFENAC a nonsteroidal anti-inflammatory drug (p.894)

ACEMETACIN a nonsteroidal anti-inflammatory drug (p.894)

ACENOCOUMAROL (nicoumalone) an anticoagulant (*see* DRUGS THAT PREVENT BLOOD CLOTTING, p.904)

ACEPRIL a brand name for captopril

ACETAZOLAMIDE a diuretic drug (p.902), a carbonic anhydrase inhibitor for glaucoma (p.920), and an anticonvulsant (p.914)

ACETOMENAPHTHONE another name for vitamin K

ACETYLCHOLINE a mydriatic drug (*see* DRUGS ACTING ON THE EYE, p.919)

ACETYLCYSTEINE a substance used in artificial tears (*see* DRUGS ACTING ON THE EYE, p.919), and a drug used to treat paracetamol overdose (*see* DRUG OVERDOSE AND ACCIDENTAL INGESTION, p.321)

ACEZIDE a brand-name antihypertensive drug (p.897) containing captopril and hydrochlorothiazide

ACICLOVIR an antiviral drug (p.886)

ACI-JEL a brand-name drug used to restore vaginal acidity

ACIPIMOX a lipid-lowering drug (p.935)

ACITAK a brand name for cimetidine

ACITRETIN a retinoid drug (p.890) used to treat psoriasis (p.332)

ACLARUBICIN an anticancer drug (p.907)

ACNECIDE a brand name for benzoyl peroxide

ACNIDAZIL a brand-name drug used to treat acne (p.340) containing benzoyl peroxide and miconazole

ACNISAL a brand name for salicylic acid

ACRIVASTINE an antihistamine (p.906)

ACTAL a brand-name antacid (p.923) containing alexitol

ACTIFED COMPOUND a brand-name cough remedy (p.909) containing dextromethorphan, pseudoephedrine, and triprolidine

ACTIFED EXPECTORANT a brand-name cough remedy (p.909) containing guaifenesin, pseudoephedrine, and triprolidine

ACTINAC a brand-name drug used to treat acne (p.340) containing chloramphenicol, hydrocortisone, allantoin, butoxyethyl nicotinate, and sulphur

ACTINOMYCIN D *see* dactinomycin

ACTIVATED CHARCOAL a substance used to treat swallowed poisons (*see* DRUG OVERDOSE AND ACCIDENTAL INGESTION, p.321)

ACULAR a brand name for ketorolac

ACUPAN a brand name for nefopam

ADALAT a brand name for nifedipine

ADALAT RETARD a brand name for nifedipine

ADAPALENE a retinoid-like drug (p.890) used to treat acne (p.340)

ADCORTYL a brand name for triamcinolone

ADENOSINE an antiarrhythmic drug (p.898)

ADIZEM-XL a brand name for diltiazem

ADRENALINE *see* epinephrine

AEROBEC a brand name for beclometasone

AEROCROM a brand name for sodium cromoglicate and salbutamol

AEROLIN a brand name for salbutamol

AFRAZINE a brand name for oxymetazoline

AILAX a brand name for co-danthramer

AIROMIR a brand name for salbutamol

AKINETON a brand name for biperiden

AKNEMIN a brand name for minocycline

ALBENDAZOLE an anthelmintic drug (p.889)

ALCLOMETASONE a topical corticosteroid (p.892)

ALDACTIDE a brand-name diuretic drug (p.902) containing spironolactone and hydroflumethiazide

ALDACTONE a brand name for spironolactone

ALDARA a brand name for imiquimod

ALDESLEUKIN a cytokine anticancer drug (p.907)

ALDOMET a brand name for methyldopa

ALENDRONATE a drug for bone disorders (p.896)

ALEXITOL an antacid (p.923)

ALFACALCIDOL a form of vitamin D

ALFAD a brand name for alfacalcidol

ALFENTANIL an opioid painkiller used as a general anaesthetic (p.914)

ALFUZOSIN an alpha-blocker drug used to treat prostate disorders (p.938)

ALGESAL a brand name for diethylamine salicylate

ALGICON a brand-name antacid (p.923) containing aluminium hydroxide, magnesium carbonate, potassium bicarbonate, and magnesium alginate

ALIMEMAZINE (trimeprazine) an antihistamine (p.906)

ALKA-SELTZER a brand-name preparation for digestive upsets containing aspirin, sodium, sodium bicarbonate, and citric acid

ALKERAN a brand name for melphalan

ALLANTOIN a mild antibacterial substance

ALLEGRON a brand name for nortriptyline

ALLER-EZE a brand name for clemastine

ALLOPURINOL a drug used to prevent attacks of gout (p.380)

ALOMIDE a brand name for lodoxamide

ALPHADERM a brand-name topical corticosteroid (p.892) containing hydrocortisone and urea

ALPHAGAN a brand name for brimonidine

ALPHAPARIN a brand name for certoparin

ALPHA-TOCOPHERYL ACETATE a form of vitamin E

ALPHAVASE a brand name for prazosin

ALPHOSYL a brand-name drug used to treat psoriasis (p.332) and eczema (p.333) containing coal tar and allantoin

ALPRAZOLAM a benzodiazepine antianxiety drug (p.916)

ALPROSTADIL a drug used to treat congenital heart disease (p.836) in newborn babies and male impotence (p.770)

ALTACITE PLUS a brand-name antacid (p.923) containing hydrotalcite and dimeticone

ALTEPLASE a thrombolytic drug (p.904)

ALTRETAMINE a cytotoxic anticancer drug (p.907)

ALU-CAP a brand name for aluminium hydroxide

ALUDROX a brand name for aluminium hydroxide

ALUMINIUM ACETATE an astringent used to treat inflammation of the outer ear canal (*see* DRUGS ACTING ON THE EAR, p.921) and the skin

ALUMINIUM CHLORIDE an active ingredient in antiperspirants

ALUMINIUM HYDROXIDE an antacid (p.923)

ALVEDON a brand name for paracetamol

ALVERCOL a brand-name drug used to treat irritable bowel syndrome (p.655) containing sterculia and alverine

ALVERINE an antispasmodic drug (p.926)

AMANTADINE an antiviral drug (p.886) also used to treat Parkinson's disease and parkinsonism (p.539)

AMARYL a brand name for glimepiride

AMBISOME a brand name for amphotericin

AMETHOCAINE *see* tetracaine

AMETOP a brand name for tetracaine (amethocaine)

AMIAS a brand name for candesartan

AMIFOSTINE a drug used to reduce the risk of infection in patients taking anticancer drugs (p.907)

AMIKACIN an aminoglycoside antibiotic (p.885)

AMILORIDE a potassium-sparing diuretic drug (p.902)

AMILOSPARE a brand name for amiloride

AMINO ACID a compound from which proteins are synthesized; some amino acids are produced by the body, but others must be included in the diet.

AMINOBENZOIC ACID a drug used in sunscreens (*see* SUNSCREENS AND SUNBLOCKS, p.893)

AMINOGLUTETHIMIDE a hormonal anticancer drug (p.907) also used to treat Cushing's syndrome (p.684)

AMINOPHYLLINE a xanthine bronchodilator drug (p.910)

AMIODARONE an antiarrhythmic drug (p.898)

AMISULPRIDE an antipsychotic drug (p.917)

AMITRIPTYLINE a tricyclic antidepressant (p.916) and antimigraine drug (p.913)

AMIX a brand name for amoxicillin

AMLODIPINE a calcium channel blocker drug (p.900)

AMMONIUM CHLORIDE a drug that increases the body's acidity and is used as an expectorant in cough remedies (p.909)

AMOBARBITAL a barbiturate sleeping drug (p.915)

AMOROLFINE an antifungal drug (p.889)

AMOXAPINE a tricyclic antidepressant (p.916)

AMOXICILLIN a penicillin antibiotic (p.885)

AMOXIL a brand name for amoxicillin

AMPHOCIL a brand name for amphotericin

AMPHOTERICIN an antifungal drug (p.889)

AMPICILLIN a penicillin antibiotic (p.885)

AMSACRINE an anticancer drug (p.907)

AMSIDINE a brand name for amsacrine

AMYTAL a brand name for amobarbital

ANACAL a brand-name preparation for haemorrhoids (p.668) containing heparinoid

ANADIN 500 a brand-name painkiller (p.912) containing aspirin and caffeine

ANADIN EXTRA a brand-name painkiller (p.912) containing aspirin, paracetamol, and caffeine

ANADIN PARACETAMOL a brand name for paracetamol

ANAFLEX a brand name for polynoxylin

ANAFRANIL a brand name for clomipramine

ANAFRANIL SR a brand name for clomipramine

ANASTROZOLE a hormonal anticancer drug (p.907)

ANBESOL a brand-name topical liquid used to treat mouth ulcers (p.632) and discomfort during teething (p.819) containing lidocaine (lignocaine) and cetylpyridinium

ANDREWS ANTACID a brand-name antacid (p.923) containing calcium carbonate and magnesium carbonate

ANDROCUR a brand-name for cyproterone acetate

ANETHAINE a brand name for tetracaine (amethocaine)

ANGETTES-75 a brand name for aspirin

ANGILOL a brand name for propranolol

ANGIOPINE MR a brand name for nifedipine

ANGIOZEM a brand name for diltiazem

ANGITIL SR a brand name for diltiazem

ANHYDROL FORTE a brand name for aluminium chloride

ANISTREPLASE a thrombolytic drug (p.904)

ANODESYN a brand-name preparation for haemorrhoids (p.668) containing allantoin, lidocaine (lignocaine), and ephedrine

ANQUIL a brand name for benperidol

ANTABUSE a brand name for disulfiram

ANTAZOLINE an antihistamine (p.906)

ANTEPSIN a brand name for sucralfate

ANTHISAN a brand-name antihistamine cream (p.906)

ANTI-D IMMUNOGLOBULIN a drug used to prevent sensitization to Rhesus antigen

ANTIHAEMOPHILIC FACTOR another name for factor VIII (*see* DRUGS THAT PROMOTE BLOOD CLOTTING, p.903)

ANTIPRESSAN a brand name for atenolol

ANTURAN a brand name for sulfinpyrazone

ANTIZOL a brand name for fomepizole

ANUGESIC-HC a brand-name preparation for haemorrhoids (p.668) containing hydrocortisone, benzyl benzoate, bismuth, Peru balsam, pramocaine, and zinc oxide

ANUSOL-HC a brand-name preparation for haemorrhoids (p.668) containing benzyl benzoate, hydrocortisone, bismuth, Peru balsam, and zinc oxide

APOMORPHINE a drug used to treat Parkinson's disease (*see* PARKINSON'S DISEASE AND PARKINSONISM, p.539)

APP a brand-name antispasmodic drug (p.926) containing homatropine, bismuth, calcium, magnesium, and aluminium hydroxide

APRACLONIDINE a drug for glaucoma (p.920)

APRINOX a brand name for bendroflumethiazide (bendrofluazide)

APROTININ an antifibrinolytic drug (*see* DRUGS THAT PROMOTE BLOOD CLOTTING, p.903)

APROVEL a brand name for irbesartan

APSOLOL a brand name for propranolol

APSTIL a brand name for diethylstilbestrol

AQUABAN a brand-name diuretic drug (p.902) containing ammonium chloride and caffeine

AQUADRATE a brand name for urea

AREDIA a brand name for pamidronate

ARGIPRESSIN synthetic vasopressin

ARICEPT a brand name for donepezil

ARIDIL a brand-name diuretic drug (p.902) containing amiloride and furosemide (frusemide)

ARPIMYCIN a brand name for erythromycin

ARRET a brand name for loperamide

ARTHROFEN a brand name for ibuprofen

ARTHROSIN a brand name for naproxen

ARTHROTEC a brand-name antirheumatic drug (p.895) containing diclofenac with misoprostol

ARTHROXEN a brand name for naproxen

ARTICAINE a local anaesthetic (p.914)

ARYTHMOL a brand name for propafenone

ASACOL a brand name for mesalazine

ASCABIOL a brand name for topical benzyl benzoate

ASCORBIC ACID another name for vitamin C

ASENDIS a brand name for amoxapine

ASILONE a brand-name antacid (p.923) containing aluminium hydroxide, magnesium oxide, and dimeticone

ASMAVEN a brand name for salbutamol

ASPARAGINASE an anticancer drug (p.907)

ASPAV a brand-name painkiller (p.912) containing aspirin and papaveretum

ASPIRIN a nonopioid painkiller (p.912) and antiplatelet drug (*see* DRUGS THAT PREVENT BLOOD CLOTTING, p.904)

ASPRO CLEAR a brand name for soluble aspirin

ATENIX a brand name for atenolol

ATENOLOL a beta-blocker drug (p.898)

ATIVAN a brand name for lorazepam

ATORVASTATIN a lipid-lowering drug (p.935)

ATOVAQUONE an antiprotozoal (p.888) and antimalarial drug (p.888)

ATRACURIUM a muscle relaxant used in general anaesthesia (*see* HAVING MAJOR SURGERY, p.943)

ATROPINE an antispasmodic drug (p.926), anticholinergic bronchodilator (p.910), and mydriatic (*see* DRUGS ACTING ON THE EYE, p.919)

ATROVENT a brand name for ipratropium bromide

AUDICORT a brand-name drug acting on the ear (p.921) containing neomycin and triamcinolone

AURANOFIN an antirheumatic drug (p.895)

AUREOCORT a brand-name topical corticosteroid (p.892) containing chlortetracycline and triamcinolone

AUREOMYCIN a brand name for chlortetracycline

AUROTHIOMALATE an antirheumatic drug (p.895)

AVLOCLOR a brand name for chloroquine

AVOMINE a brand name for promethazine

AXID a brand name for nizatidine

AXSAIN a brand name for capsaicin

AZACTAM a brand name for aztreonam

AZAMUNE a brand name for azathioprine

AZAPROPAZONE a nonsteroidal anti-inflammatory drug (p.894)

AZATADINE an antihistamine (p.906)

AZATHIOPRINE an antirheumatic drug (p.895) and cytotoxic immunosuppressant drug (p.906)

AZELAIC ACID a drug used to treat acne (p.340)

AZELASTINE an antihistamine (p.906)

AZIDOTHYMIDINE (AZT, zidovudine) an antiviral drug used to treat HIV infection (*see* DRUGS FOR HIV INFECTION AND AIDS, p.887)

AZITHROMYCIN a macrolide antibiotic (p.885)

AZLOCILLIN a penicillin antibiotic (p.885)

AZT *see* azidothymidine

AZTREONAM an antibiotic (p.885)

B

BACITRACIN a topical antibiotic (*see* PREPARATIONS FOR SKIN INFECTIONS AND INFESTATIONS, p.892)

BACLOFEN a muscle relaxant (p.896)

BACLOSPAS a brand name for baclofen

BACTROBAN a brand name for mupirocin

BALSALAZIDE an aminosalicylate drug (p.924)

BAMBEC a brand name for bambuterol

BAMBUTEROL a sympathomimetic bronchodilator drug (p.910)

BARATOL a brand name for indoramin

BASILIXIMAB an immunosuppressant (p.906)

BAXAN a brand name for cefadroxil

BAYCARON a brand name for mefruside

BAZUKA a brand-name preparation used to treat verrucas (*see* WARTS, p.354) containing salicylic acid and lactic acid

BECLAZONE a brand name for beclometasone

BECLOFORTE a brand name for beclometasone

BECLOMETASONE a corticosteroid (p.930)

BECODISKS a brand name for beclometasone

BECONASE a brand name for beclometasone

BECOSYM a brand-name vitamin B complex preparation

BECOTIDE ROTACAPS a brand name for beclometasone

BEECHAMS POWDERS a brand-name cold and flu remedy (p.910) containing aspirin and caffeine

BEECHAMS POWDERS CAPSULES a brand-name cold and flu remedy (p.910) containing paracetamol, caffeine, and phenylephrine

BELLADONNA an antispasmodic drug (p.926)

BENDROFLUAZIDE *see* bendroflumethiazide

BENDROFLUMETHIAZIDE (bendrofluazide) a thiazide diuretic drug (p.902)

BENEMID a brand name for probenecid

BENORAL a brand name for benorilate

BENORILATE a nonsteroidal anti-inflammatory drug (p.894)

BENPERIDOL an antipsychotic drug (p.917)

BENSERAZIDE a drug used to enhance the effect of levodopa in the treatment of Parkinson's disease (p.539)

BENYLIN a brand-name cough remedy (p.909) containing diphenhydramine and menthol

BENZALKONIUM CHLORIDE a skin antiseptic (*see* PREPARATIONS FOR SKIN INFECTIONS AND INFESTATIONS, p.892)

BENZAMYCIN a brand-name drug containing erythromycin and benzoyl peroxide used to treat acne (p.340)

BENZHEXOL *see* trihexyphenidyl

BENZOCAINE a local anaesthetic (p.914)

BENZOYL PEROXIDE a drug used to treat acne (p.340) and ringworm (p.352)

BENZTHIAZIDE a thiazide diuretic drug (p.902)

BENZTROPINE an anticholinergic drug used to treat parkinsonism (*see* PARKINSON'S DISEASE AND PARKINSONISM, p.539)

BENZYDAMINE a painkiller (p.912)

BENZYL BENZOATE an antiparasitic drug (*see* PREPARATIONS FOR SKIN INFECTIONS AND INFESTATIONS, p.892)

BENZYLPENICILLIN a penicillin antibiotic (p.885)

BERACTANT a drug used to mature the lungs of premature babies with respiratory distress syndrome (*see* PROBLEMS OF THE PREMATURE BABY, p.816)

BERKOLOL a brand name for propranolol

BERKOZIDE a brand name for bendroflumethiazide (bendrofluazide)

BEROTEC a brand name for fenoterol

BETA-ADALAT a brand-name antihypertensive drug (p.897) containing nifedipine and atenolol

BETACAP a brand name for betamethasone

BETA-CARDONE a brand name for sotalol

BETACAROTENE a source of vitamin A

BETADINE a brand name for povidone iodine

BETAFERON a brand name for interferon beta

BETAGAN a brand name for levobunolol

BETAHISTINE a drug used to treat Ménière's disease (p.604)

BETALOC a brand name for metoprolol

BETAMETHASONE a corticosteroid (p.930)

BETA-PROGRANE a brand name for propranolol

BETAXOLOL a beta-blocker (p.898), antihypertensive drug (p.897), and drug for glaucoma (p.920)

BETHANECHOL a drug for urinary retention (*see* DRUGS THAT AFFECT BLADDER CONTROL, p.939) and a stimulant laxative (p.924)

BETNESOL a brand name for betamethasone

BETNOVATE a brand name for betamethasone

BETNOVATE-C a brand-name preparation for eczema (p.333) containing betamethasone and clioquinol

BETNOVATE-N a brand-name preparation for eczema (p.333) containing betamethasone and neomycin

BETNOVATE-RECTAL a brand-name preparation for haemorrhoids (p.668) containing betamethasone, lidocaine (lignocaine), and phenylephrine

BETOPTIC a brand-name drug for glaucoma (p.920) containing betaxolol

BETTAMOUSSE a brand name for betamethasone

BEZAFIBRATE a lipid-lowering drug (p.935)

BEZALIP-MONO a brand name for bezafibrate

BICALUTAMIDE an antiandrogen (*see* SEX HORMONES AND RELATED DRUGS, p.933, and DRUGS FOR PROSTATE DISORDERS, p.938) used as an anticancer drug (p.907)

BINOVUM a brand-name oral contraceptive (*see* CONTRACEPTION, p.69) containing ethinylestradiol and norethisterone

BIORAL a brand name for carbenoxolone

BIOTIN a member of the vitamin B complex

BIPERIDEN an anticholinergic drug used to treat parkinsonism (*see* PARKINSON'S DISEASE AND PARKINSONISM, p.539)

BISACODYL a stimulant laxative (p.924)

BISMAG a brand-name antacid (p.923) containing sodium bicarbonate and magnesium carbonate

BISMUTH a metal used as an ulcer-healing drug (p.923) and for haemorrhoids (p.668)

BISODOL a brand-name antacid (p.923) containing sodium bicarbonate, calcium carbonate, and magnesium carbonate

BISOPROLOL a beta-blocker drug (p.898)

BLEMIX a brand name for minocycline

BLEOMYCIN a cytotoxic anticancer drug (p.907)

BOCASAN a brand-name antimicrobial mouthwash containing sodium perborate

BONEFOS a brand name for sodium clodronate

BONJELA a brand name for choline salicylate

BONJELA PASTILLES brand-name pastilles for mouth ulcers (p.632) containing lidocaine (lignocaine) and aminacrine, an antiseptic

BOOTS NIROLEX LOZENGES a brand-name cough remedy (p.909) containing dextromethorphan and menthol

BOTULINUM TOXIN a muscle relaxant (p.896)

BRADOSOL a brand name for benzalkonium chloride

BRASIVOL a brand-name topical paste for acne (p.340)

BRETYLIUM an antiarrhythmic drug (p.898)

BREVINOR a brand-name oral contraceptive (*see* CONTRACEPTION, p.69) containing ethinylestradiol and norethisterone

BRICANYL a brand name for terbutaline

BRIMONIDINE a drug for glaucoma (p.920)

BRITAJECT a brand name for apomorphine

BRITLOFEX a brand name for lofexidine

BROFLEX a brand name for trihexyphenidyl (benzhexol)

BROLENE a brand name for propamidine isethionate

BROMAZEPAM a benzodiazepine antianxiety drug (p.916)

BROMOCRIPTINE a pituitary drug (p.934) and drug used to treat parkinsonism (*see* PARKINSON'S DISEASE AND PARKINSONISM, p.539)

BROMPHENIRAMINE an antihistamine (p.906)

BRONCHODIL a brand name for reproterol

BRUFEN a brand name for ibuprofen

BUCCASTEM a brand name for prochlorperazine

BUCLIZINE an antihistamine antiemetic drug (p.922)

BUDESONIDE a corticosteroid (p.930)

BUMETANIDE a loop diuretic drug (p.902)

BUPIVACAINE a long-lasting local anaesthetic (p.914)

BUPRENORPHINE an opioid painkiller (p.912)

BURINEX a brand name for bumetanide

BURINEX A a brand-name diuretic (p.902) containing bumetanide and amiloride

BURINEX K a brand-name diuretic (p.902) containing bumetanide and potassium

BURNEZE a brand name for benzocaine

BUSCOPAN a brand name for hyoscine

BUSERELIN a gonadorelin analogue (*see* SEX HORMONES AND RELATED DRUGS, p.933, and DRUGS FOR INFERTILITY, p.936)

BUSPIRONE a nonbenzodiazepine antianxiety drug (p.916)

BUSULFAN a cytotoxic anticancer drug (p.907)

BUTACOTE a brand name for phenylbutazone

BUTOBARBITAL a barbiturate sleeping drug (p.915)

C

CABERGOLINE a drug for infertility (p.936) and to stop milk production in women who do not want to breast-feed (*see* PITUITARY DRUGS, p.934)

CACIT a brand name for calcium carbonate

CAFERGOT a brand-name antimigraine drug (p.913) containing ergotamine and caffeine

CAFFEINE a stimulant in coffee, tea, and cola that is added to some painkillers (p.912)

CALABREN a brand name for glibenclamide

CALADRYL a brand-name topical antihistamine (p.906) containing calamine, diphenhydramine, and camphor

CALAMINE a substance containing zinc oxide and liquid paraffin that is used to soothe irritated skin and relieve itching

CALCICARD CR a brand name for diltiazem

CALCIFEROL a form of vitamin D

CALCIJEX a brand name for calcitriol

CALCIPARINE a brand name for heparin

CALCIPOTRIOL a drug for psoriasis (p.332)

CALCITONIN a drug for bone disorders (p.896)

CALCITONIN, SALMON (salcatonin) a drug for bone disorders (p.896)

CALCITRIOL a form of vitamin D

CALCIUM a mineral (p.929)

CALCIUM ACETATE a form of calcium

CALCIUM CARBONATE a form of calcium and an antacid (p.923)

CALCIUM CHLORIDE a form of calcium

CALCIUM FOLINATE a drug used to reduce the side effects of methotrexate

CALCIUM GLUCONATE a form of calcium

CALCIUM RESONIUM a brand name for polystyrene sulphonate

CALCORT a brand name for deflazacort

CALGEL a brand-name teething gel (*see* TEETHING, p.819) containing lidocaine (lignocaine) and cetylpyridinium

CALIMAL a brand name for chlorphenamine (chlorpheniramine)

CALMURID HC a brand-name preparation for eczema (p.333) containing hydrocortisone, lactic acid, and urea

CALPOL a brand name for paracetamol

CAM a brand name for ephedrine

CAMCOLIT a brand name for lithium

CAMPHOR a topical antipruritic drug (p.891)

CAMPRAL EC a brand name for acamprosate

CAMPTO a brand name for irinotecan

CANDESARTAN an angiotensin II blocker antihypertensive drug (p.897)

CANESTEN a brand name for clotrimazole

CANESTEN HC a brand-name antifungal drug (p.889) containing clotrimazole and hydrocortisone

CANRENOATE a potassium-sparing diuretic drug (p.902)

CAPASTAT a brand name for capreomycin

CAPOZIDE a brand-name antihypertensive drug (p.897) containing captopril and hydrochlorothiazide

CAPREOMYCIN an antituberculous drug (p.886)

CAPRIN a brand name for aspirin

CAPSAICIN a topical painkiller (p.912)

CAPTOPRIL an ACE inhibitor drug (p.900)

CARACE a brand name for lisinopril

CARBACHOL a drug for glaucoma (p.920) and urinary retention (*see* DRUGS THAT AFFECT BLADDER CONTROL, p.939)

CARBALAX a brand-name preparation for constipation (p.628) containing sodium acid phosphate and sodium bicarbonate

CARBAMAZEPINE an anticonvulsant (p.914), antipsychotic (p.917), and mood-stabilizing drug (p.918)

CARBARYL a treatment for head lice (p.831)

CARBELLON a brand-name drug used to treat indigestion (p.626) containing magnesium hydroxide, charcoal, and peppermint oil

CARBENOXOLONE an ulcer-healing drug (p.923)

CARBIDOPA a substance that enhances the effect of levodopa

CARBIMAZOLE an antithyroid drug (*see* DRUGS FOR HYPERTHYROIDISM, p.932)

CARBOCISTEINE a mucolytic drug (*see* COUGH REMEDIES, p.909)

CARBO-DOME a brand name for coal tar

CARBOPLATIN a cytotoxic anticancer drug (p.907)

CARBOPROST a uterine stimulant (*see* DRUGS FOR LABOUR, p.938)

CARDENE a brand name for nicardipine

CARDILATE MR a brand name for nifedipine

CARDINOL a brand name for propranolol

CARDURA a brand name for doxazosin

CARISOPRODOL a muscle relaxant (p.896)

CARMUSTINE a cytotoxic anticancer drug (p.907)

CARNITINE an amino acid used as a nutritional supplement

CARNITOR a brand name for carnitine

CARTEOLOL a beta-blocker drug (p.898)

CARVEDILOL a beta-blocker drug (p.898)

CARYLDERM a brand name for carbaryl

CASCARA a stimulant laxative (p.924)

CASTOR OIL a stimulant laxative (p.924)

CATAPRES a brand name for clonidine

CATARRH-EX a brand-name decongestant (p.909) containing pseudoephedrine and paracetamol

CAVERJECT a brand name for alprostadil

CEDOCARD a brand name for isosorbide dinitrate

CEFACLOR a cephalosporin antibiotic (p.885)

CEFADROXIL a cephalosporin antibiotic (p.885)

CEFALEXIN a cephalosporin antibiotic (p.885)

CEFAMANDOLE a cephalosporin antibiotic (p.885)

CEFAZOLIN a cephalosporin antibiotic (p.885)

CEFIXIME a cephalosporin antibiotic (p.885)

CEFODIZIME a cephalosporin antibiotic (p.885)

CEFOTAXIME a cephalosporin antibiotic (p.885)

CEFOXITIN a cephalosporin antibiotic (p.885)

CEFPIROME a cephalosporin antibiotic (p.885)

CEFPODOXIME a cephalosporin antibiotic (p.885)

CEFPROZIL a cephalosporin antibiotic (p.885)

CEFRADINE a cephalosporin antibiotic (p.885)

CEFROM a brand name for cefpirome

CEFTAZIDIME a cephalosporin antibiotic (p.885)

CEFTRIAXONE a cephalosporin antibiotic (p.885)

CEFUROXIME a cephalosporin antibiotic (p.885)

CELANCE a brand name for pergolide

CELECTOL a brand name for celiprolol

CELEVAC a brand name for methylcellulose

CELIPROLOL a beta-blocker drug (p.898)

CELLCEPT a brand name for mycophenolate mofetil

CEPOREX a brand name for cefalexin

CEREBROVASE a brand name for dipyridamole

CEREZYME a brand name for imiglucerase

CERTOPARIN an anticoagulant (*see* DRUGS THAT PREVENT BLOOD CLOTTING, p.904)

CERUMOL a brand-name preparation for ear wax removal (*see* DRUGS ACTING ON THE EAR, p.921)

CETIRIZINE an antihistamine (p.906)

CETRIMIDE a skin antiseptic (*see* PREPARATIONS FOR SKIN INFECTIONS AND INFESTATIONS, p.892)

CETRORELIX a drug for infertility (p.936)

CETROTIDE a brand name for cetrorelix

CETYLPYRIDINIUM a skin antiseptic (*see* PREPARATIONS FOR SKIN INFECTIONS AND INFESTATIONS, p.892)

CHIMAX a brand name for flutamide

CHLORACTIL a brand name for chlorpromazine

CHLORAL HYDRATE a sleeping drug (p.915)

CHLORAMBUCIL a cytotoxic anticancer drug (p.907)

CHLORAMPHENICOL an antibiotic (p.885)

CHLORDIAZEPOXIDE a benzodiazepine antianxiety drug (p.916)

CHLORHEXIDINE a skin antiseptic (*see* PREPARATIONS FOR SKIN INFECTIONS AND INFESTATIONS, p.892)

CHLORMETHINE (mustine) an anticancer drug (p.907)

CHLOROMYCETIN a brand name for chloramphenicol

CHLOROQUINE an antimalarial (p.888) and antirheumatic drug (p.895)

CHLOROTHIAZIDE a thiazide diuretic drug (p.902)

CHLOROXYLENOL a skin antiseptic (*see* PREPARATIONS FOR SKIN INFECTIONS AND INFESTATIONS, p.892)

CHLORPHENAMINE (chlorpheniramine) an antihistamine (p.906)

CHLORPHENIRAMINE *see* chlorphenamine

CHLORPROMAZINE a phenothiazine antipsychotic drug (p.917) and antiemetic drug (p.922)

CHLORPROPAMIDE an oral drug for diabetes mellitus (p.931)

CHLORTALIDONE a thiazide diuretic drug (p.902)

CHLORTETRACYCLINE a tetracycline antibiotic (p.885)

CHOLINE SALICYLATE a painkiller (p.912)

CHOLINE THEOPHYLLINATE a xanthine bronchodilator drug (p.910)

CHORIONIC GONADOTROPHIN, HUMAN a drug for infertility (p.936)

CHROMIUM a mineral

CICLOSPORIN an immunosuppressant drug (p.906)

CIDOFOVIR an antiviral drug (p.886)

CILASTATIN a drug used with imipenem to increase its effectiveness

CILAZAPRIL an ACE inhibitor drug (p.900)

CILEST a brand-name oral contraceptive (*see* CONTRACEPTION, p.69) containing ethinylestradiol and norgestimate

CIMETIDINE an ulcer-healing drug (p.923)

CINAZIERE a brand name for cinnarizine

CINCHOCAINE a local anaesthetic (p.914)

CINNARIZINE an antihistamine antiemetic drug (p.922)

CINOBAC a brand name for cinoxacin

CINOXACIN a quinolone antibiotic (p.885)

CIPRAMIL a brand name for citalopram

CIPROFIBRATE a lipid-lowering drug (p.935)

CIPROFLOXACIN a quinolone antibiotic (p.885)

CIPROXIN a brand name for ciprofloxacin

CISATRACURIUM a muscle relaxant used in general anaesthesia (*see* HAVING MAJOR SURGERY, p.943)

CISPLATIN a cytotoxic anticancer drug (p.907)

CITALOPRAM a selective serotonin reuptake inhibitor (SSRI) antidepressant drug (p.916)

CITRAMAG a brand name for magnesium citrate

CLADRIBINE a cytotoxic anticancer drug (p.907)

CLARITHROMYCIN an antibiotic (p.885)

CLARITYN a brand name for loratadine

CLAVULANIC ACID a substance given with amoxicillin or ticarcillin to make them more effective

CLEMASTINE an antihistamine (p.906)

CLEXANE a brand name for enoxaparin

CLIMAGEST a brand-name preparation containing estradiol and norethisterone, used in hormone replacement therapy (p.937)

CLIMAVAL a brand name for estradiol

CLIMESSE a brand-name preparation containing estradiol and norethisterone, used in hormone replacement therapy (p.937)

CLINDAMYCIN an antibiotic (p.885)

CLINITAR a brand name for coal tar

CLINORIL a brand name for sulindac

CLIOQUINOL an antibiotic (p.885) and antifungal drug (p.889)

CLOBAZAM a benzodiazepine antianxiety drug (p.916)

CLOBETASOL a topical corticosteroid (p.892)

CLOBETASONE a topical corticosteroid (p.892)

CLOBURATE a brand name for clobetasone

CLODRONATE an anticancer drug (p.907)

CLOFAZIMINE an antibiotic (p.885) used to treat Hansen's disease (p.302)

CLOMETHIAZOLE a sleeping drug (p.915)

CLOMID a brand name for clomifene

CLOMIFENE a drug for infertility (p.936)

CLOMIPRAMINE a tricyclic antidepressant (p.916)

CLONAZEPAM a benzodiazepine anticonvulsant drug (p.914)

CLONIDINE an antihypertensive drug (p.897) and antimigraine drug (p.913)

CLOPAMIDE a thiazide diuretic drug (p.902)

CLOPIDOGREL an antiplatelet drug (*see* DRUGS THAT PREVENT BLOOD CLOTTING, p.904)

CLOPIXOL a brand name for zuclopenthixol

CLORAL BETAINE a sleeping drug (p.915)

CLORAZEPATE a benzodiazepine antianxiety drug (p.916)

CLOTAM a brand name for tolfenamic acid

CLOTRIMAZOLE an antifungal drug (p.889)

CLOZAPINE an antipsychotic drug (p.917)

CLOZARIL a brand name for clozapine

COAL TAR a substance used to treat psoriasis (p.332) and eczema (p.333)

CO-AMILOFRUSE a diuretic drug (p.902) containing amiloride and furosemide (frusemide)

CO-AMILOZIDE a diuretic drug (p.902) containing amiloride and hydrochlorothiazide

CO-AMOXICLAV a penicillin antibiotic (p.885) containing amoxicillin and clavulanic acid

COBADEX a brand name for hydrocortisone

CO-BENELDOPA a drug used to treat Parkinson's disease (*see* PARKINSON'S DISEASE AND PARKINSONISM, p.539) containing levodopa and benserazide

CO-BETALOC a brand-name antihypertensive drug (p.897) containing hydrochlorothiazide and metoprolol

CO-CARELDOPA a drug used to treat Parkinson's disease (*see* PARKINSON'S DISEASE AND PARKINSONISM, p.539) containing carbidopa and levodopa

CO-CODAMOL a painkiller (p.912) containing codeine and paracetamol

CO-CODAPRIN a painkiller (p.912) containing aspirin and codeine

CODAFEN CONTINUS a brand-name nonsteroidal anti-inflammatory drug (p.894) containing codeine and ibuprofen

CODALAX a brand name for co-danthramer

CO-DANTHRAMER a stimulant laxative (p.924) containing dantron and poloxamer

CO-DANTHRUSATE a stimulant laxative (p.924) containing dantron and docusate

CODEINE an opioid painkiller (p.912), cough suppressant (*see* COUGH REMEDIES, p.909), and antidiarrhoeal drug (p.924)

CO-DERGOCRINE MESYLATE a vasodilator used to improve blood flow to the brain in senile dementia (p.535)

CODIS a brand-name painkiller (p.912) containing aspirin and codeine

CO-DYDRAMOL a painkiller (p.912) containing paracetamol and dihydrocodeine

CO-FLUAMPICIL a penicillin antibiotic (p.885) containing flucloxacillin and ampicillin

CO-FLUMACTONE a diuretic drug (p.902) containing hydroflumethiazide and spironolactone

COGENTIN a brand name for benztropine

COLAZIDE a brand name for balsalazide

COLCHICINE a drug used to treat gout (p.380)

COLD CREAM an antipruritic drug (p.891)

COLECALCIFEROL a form of vitamin D

COLESTIPOL a lipid-lowering drug (p.935)

COLESTYRAMINE a lipid-lowering drug (p.935)

COLFOSCERIL PALMITATE a drug used to mature the lungs of premature babies with respiratory distress syndrome (*see* PROBLEMS OF THE PREMATURE BABY, p.816)

COLIFOAM a brand name for hydrocortisone

COLISTIMETHATE an antibiotic (p.885)

COLISTIN an antibiotic (p.885)

COLLODION a substance that dries to form a sticky film, protecting broken skin

COLOFAC a brand name for mebeverine

COLOMYCIN a brand name for colistin

COLPERMIN a brand name for peppermint oil

CO-MAGALDROX an antacid (p.923) containing aluminium hydroxide and magnesium hydroxide

COMBIVENT a brand-name inhaler (*see* BRONCHODILATOR DRUGS, p.910) containing ipratropium bromide and salbutamol

COMBIVIR a brand-name preparation containing lamivudine and zidovudine used to treat HIV infection (*see* DRUGS FOR HIV INFECTION AND AIDS, p.887)

CO-METHIAMOL a nonopioid painkiller (p.912) containing paracetamol and methionine

COMPOUND W a brand-name treatment for warts (p.354) containing salicylic acid

COMTESS a brand name for entacapone

CONCAVIT a brand-name multivitamin (*see* VITAMINS, p.927)

CONCORDIN a brand name for protriptyline

CONDYLINE a brand name for podophyllotoxin

CONJUGATED OESTROGENS female hormones used to prevent osteoporosis in post-menopausal women (*see* DRUGS FOR BONE DISORDERS, p.896) and used in hormone replacement therapy (p.937)

CONOTRANE a brand-name skin cream (*see* EMOLLIENTS AND BARRIER PREPARATIONS, p.890) containing benzalkonium chloride and dimeticone

CONTAC 400 a brand-name cough remedy (p.909) containing phenylpropanolamine and chlorphenamine (chlorpheniramine)

CONTAC COUGH CAPS a brand-name cough remedy (p.909) containing dextromethorphan

CONTIMIN a brand name for oxybutynin

CONVULEX a brand name for sodium valproate

CO-PHENOTROPE an antidiarrhoeal drug (p.924) containing diphenoxylate and atropine

COPPER a mineral

CO-PRENOZIDE an antihypertensive drug (p.897) containing oxprenolol and cyclopenthiazide

CO-PROXAMOL an opioid painkiller (p.912)

CORACTEN a brand name for nifedipine

CORDARONE X a brand name for amiodarone

CORDILOX a brand name for verapamil

CORGARD a brand name for nadolol

CORGARETIC a brand-name antihypertensive drug (p.897) containing nadolol and bendroflumethiazide (bendrofluazide)

CORLAN a brand name for hydrocortisone

CORO-NITRO a brand name for glyceryl trinitrate

CORSODYL a brand name for oral preparations containing chlorhexidine

CORTICOTROPIN a hormone used to test adrenal-gland function

CORTISOL *see* hydrocortisone

CORTISONE a corticosteroid (p.930)

CORTISYL a brand name for cortisone

COSALGESIC a brand name for co-proxamol

CO-SIMALCITE an antacid (p.923) containing hydrotalcite and dimeticone

COSOPT a brand-name preparation containing dorzolamide and timolol, used to treat glaucoma (*see* DRUGS FOR GLAUCOMA, p.920)

CO-TENIDONE an antihypertensive drug (p.897) containing atenolol and chlortalidone

CO-TRIAMTERZIDE a diuretic drug (p.902) containing hydrochlorothiazide and triamterene

CO-TRIMOXAZOLE an antibiotic (p.885) and antiprotozoal drug (p.888)

COVERSYL a brand name for perindopril

COZAAR-COMP a brand-name antihypertensive drug (p.897) containing losartan and hydrochlorothiazide

CREAM OF MAGNESIA a brand name for magnesium hydroxide

CREMALGIN a brand-name topical nonsteroidal anti-inflammatory drug (p.894)

CREON a brand-name preparation containing pancreatin

CRISANTASPASE an anticancer drug (p.907)

CRIXIVAN a brand name for indinavir

CROMOGEN a brand name for sodium cromoglicate

CROMOGLICATE an antiallergy drug (p.905)

CROTAMITON an antipruritic drug (p.891)

CRYSTAPEN a brand name for benzylpenicillin

CUPANOL a brand name for paracetamol

CUPLEX a brand-name preparation for warts (p.354) containing copper acetate, lactic acid, and salicylic acid

CUPROFEN a brand name for ibuprofen

CURATODERM a brand name for tacalcitol

CUTIVATE a brand name for fluticasone

CYANOCOBALAMIN a form of vitamin B_{12}

CYCLIMORPH a brand-name opioid painkiller (p.912) containing morphine and cyclizine

CYCLIZINE an antihistamine (p.906) used as an antiemetic drug (p.922)

CYCLOGEST a brand name for progesterone

CYCLOPENTHIAZIDE a thiazide diuretic (p.902)

CYCLOPENTOLATE a mydriatic drug used in eye examinations (*see* DRUGS ACTING ON THE EYE, p.919)

CYCLOPHOSPHAMIDE a cytotoxic anticancer drug (p.907)

CYCLO-PROGYNOVA a brand-name preparation containing estradiol and levonorgestrel used in hormone replacement therapy (p.937)

CYCLOSERINE an antituberculous drug (p.886)

CYMALON a brand-name preparation for cystitis (p.709) containing sodium bicarbonate, citric acid, sodium citrate, and sodium carbonate

CYMEVENE a brand name for ganciclovir

CYPROHEPTADINE an antihistamine (p.906) and antimigraine drug (p.913)

CYPROSTAT a brand name for cyproterone acetate

CYPROTERONE ACETATE a synthetic sex hormone (*see* SEX HORMONES AND RELATED DRUGS, p.933) used to treat acne (p.340), prostate cancer (p.726), virilization (p.740) in women, and male sexual disorders

CYSTOLEVE a brand name for sodium citrate

CYSTOPURIN a brand name for potassium citrate

CYSTRIN a brand name for oxybutynin

CYTARABINE a cytotoxic anticancer drug (p.907)

CYTOTEC a brand name for misoprostol

D

DACARBAZINE a cytotoxic anticancer drug (p.907)

DACLIZUMAB an immunosuppressant drug (p.906)

DACTINOMYCIN a cytotoxic anticancer drug (p.907)

DAKTACORT a brand-name antifungal drug (p.889) containing miconazole and hydrocortisone

DAKTARIN a brand name for miconazole

DALACIN C a brand name for clindamycin

DALIVIT a brand-name multivitamin (*see* VITAMINS, p.927)

DALMANE a brand name for flurazepam

DALTEPARIN an injected anticoagulant (*see* DRUGS THAT PREVENT BLOOD CLOTTING, p.904)

DANAPAROID an injected anticoagulant (*see* DRUGS THAT PREVENT BLOOD CLOTTING, p.904)

DANAZOL a drug used to treat endometriosis (p.742) and menstrual disorders (*see* SEX HORMONES AND RELATED DRUGS, p.933)

DANERAL-SA a brand name for pheniramine

DANOL a brand name for danazol

DANTRIUM a brand name for dantrolene

DANTROLENE a muscle relaxant (p.896)

DANTRON a stimulant laxative (p.924)

DAPSONE an antibiotic (p.885)

DARAPRIM a brand name for pyrimethamine

DAUNORUBICIN a cytotoxic anticancer drug (p.907)

DAY NURSE a brand-name cold and flu remedy (p.910) containing dextromethorphan, paracetamol, and phenylpropanolamine

DDAVP a brand name for desmopressin

DEBRISOQUINE an antihypertensive drug (p.897)

DECADRON a brand name for dexamethasone

DE-CAPEPTYL SR a brand name for triptorelin

DEFLAZACORT a corticosteroid (p.930)

DELFEN a brand name for nonoxinol '9'

DELTACORTRIL ENTERIC a brand name for prednisolone

DELTASTAB a brand name for prednisolone

DEMECLOCYCLINE a tetracycline antibiotic (p.885)

DEMIX a brand name for doxycycline

DE-NOL a brand name for bismuth

DENTOMYCIN a brand name for minocycline

DEPIXOL a brand name for flupentixol

DEPO-MEDRONE a brand name for methylprednisolone

DEPONIT a brand name for glyceryl trinitrate

DEPO-PROVERA a brand name for medroxyprogesterone

DEPOSTAT a brand name for gestonerone

DEQUACAINE a brand-name throat antiseptic containing benzocaine and dequalinium

DEQUADIN a brand name for dequalinium

DEQUALINIUM an antibiotic (p.885)

DERBAC-M a brand name for malathion

DERMACORT a brand-name topical corticosteroid (p.892) containing hydrocortisone

DERMIDEX a brand-name topical local anaesthetic (p.914)

DERMOVATE a brand name for clobetasol

DERMOVATE-NN a brand-name topical corticosteroid (p.892) containing nystatin, clobetasol, and neomycin

DESFERRIOXAMINE an antidote for iron poisoning (*see* DRUG OVERDOSE AND ACCIDENTAL INGESTION, p.321)

DESFLURANE a general anaesthetic (p.914)

DESIRUDIN an anticoagulant (*see* DRUGS THAT PREVENT BLOOD CLOTTING, p.904)

DESMOPRESSIN a pituitary hormone (*see* PITUITARY DRUGS, p.934)

DESOGESTREL a progestogen (*see* SEX HORMONES AND RELATED DRUGS, p.933)

DESOXIMETASONE a topical corticosteroid (p.892)

DESTOLIT a brand name for ursodeoxycholic acid

DETECLO a brand-name tetracycline antibiotic (p.885) containing tetracycline, chlortetracycline, and demeclocycline

DETRUNORM a brand name for propiverine hydrochloride

DETRUSITOL a brand name for tolterodine

DETTOL a brand-name liquid skin antiseptic (*see* PREPARATIONS FOR SKIN INFECTIONS AND INFESTATIONS, p.892) containing chloroxylenol

DEXAMETHASONE a corticosteroid (p.930)

DEXAMFETAMINE an amfetamine (*see* CENTRAL NERVOUS SYSTEM STIMULANT DRUGS, p.918)

DEXA-RHINASPRAY DUO a brand-name nasal spray used to treat allergic rhinitis (p.466) containing dexamethasone, neomycin, and tramazoline

DEXEDRINE a brand name for dexamfetamine

DEXKETOPROFEN a nonsteroidal anti-inflammatory drug (p.894)

DEXTROMETHORPHAN a cough suppressant (*see* COUGH REMEDIES, p.909)

DEXTROMORAMIDE an opioid painkiller (p.912)

DEXTROPROPOXYPHENE an opioid painkiller (p.912)

DF 118 a brand name for dihydrocodeine

DHC CONTINUS a brand name for dihydrocodeine

DIABETAMIDE a brand name for glibenclamide

DIABINESE a brand name for chlorpropamide

DIALAR a brand name for diazepam

DIAMICRON a brand name for gliclazide

DIAMORPHINE an opioid painkiller (p.912)

DIAMOX a brand name for acetazolamide

DIANETTE a brand-name oral contraceptive (*see* CONTRACEPTION, p.69) containing cyproterone acetate and ethinylestradiol, also used to treat acne (p.340)

DIARPHEN a brand-name antidiarrhoeal drug (p.924) containing diphenoxylate and atropine

DIARREST a brand-name antidiarrhoeal drug (p.924) containing dicycloverine (dicyclomine) and codeine

DIASORB a brand name for loperamide

DIAZEMULS a brand name for diazepam

DIAZEPAM a benzodiazepine antianxiety drug (p.916), muscle relaxant (p.896), and anticonvulsant drug (p.914)

DIAZOXIDE an antihypertensive drug (p.897) and drug used to treat hypoglycaemia (p.691)

DICLOFENAC a nonsteroidal anti-inflammatory drug (p.894)

DICLOFLEX a brand name for diclofenac

DICLOMAX RETARD a brand name for diclofenac

DICOBALT EDETATE an antidote for cyanide poisoning (*see* DRUG OVERDOSE AND ACCIDENTAL INGESTION, p.321)

DICONAL a brand name for dipipanone

DICYCLOMINE *see* dicycloverine

DICYCLOVERINE (dicyclomine) an antispasmodic drug (p.926)

DICYNENE a brand name for etamsylate

DIDANOSINE (ddI) an antiviral drug used to treat HIV infection (*see* DRUGS FOR HIV INFECTION AND AIDS, p.887)

DIDRONEL PMO a brand-name drug for bone disorders (p.896) containing etidronate and calcium carbonate

DIENESTROL an oestrogen (*see* SEX HORMONES AND RELATED DRUGS, p.933, and HORMONE REPLACEMENT THERAPY, p.937)

DIETHYLAMINE SALICYLATE a counter-irritant applied to the skin

DIETHYLCARBAMAZINE an anthelmintic drug (p.889)

DIETHYLSTILBESTROL an oestrogen (*see* SEX HORMONES AND RELATED DRUGS, p.933), hormonal anticancer drug (p.907), and drug for prostate disorders (p.938)

DIETHYLTOLUAMIDE (DEET) a mosquito repellent (*see* TRAVEL HEALTH, p.85)

DIFFERIN a brand name for adapalene

DIFFLAM a brand name for benzydamine

DIFLUCAN a brand name for fluconazole

DIFLUCORTOLONE a topical corticosteroid (p.892)

DIFLUNISAL a nonsteroidal anti-inflammatory drug (p.894)

DIGIBIND a brand-name antidote for digoxin overdose (*see* DRUG OVERDOSE AND ACCIDENTAL INGESTION, p.321)

DIGITOXIN a digitalis drug (p.901)

DIGOXIN a digitalis drug (p.901)

DIHYDROCODEINE an opioid painkiller (p.912)

DIHYDROERGOTAMINE an antimigraine drug (p.913)

DIHYDROTACHYSTEROL a form of vitamin D

DIJEX a brand name for didanosine

DILOXANIDE FUROATE an antiprotozoal drug (p.888)

DILTIAZEM a calcium channel blocker drug (p.900)

DILZEM a brand name for diltiazem

DIMENHYDRINATE an antihistamine (p.906) used as an antiemetic drug (p.922)

DIMERCAPROL an antidote for heavy metal poisoning (*see* DRUG OVERDOSE AND ACCIDENTAL INGESTION, p.321)

DIMETICONE a silicone-based substance used in emollients and barrier preparations (p.890) and as an antifoaming agent with antacids (p.923)

DIMETRIOSE a brand name for gestrinone

DIMOTANE a brand name for brompheniramine

DIMOTAPP a brand-name cough remedy (p.909) containing phenylephrine, phenylpropanolamine, and brompheniramine

DINDEVAN a brand name for phenindione

DINOPROST a prostaglandin used to terminate pregnancy and induce labour (*see* DRUGS FOR LABOUR, p.938)

DINOPROSTONE a prostaglandin used to terminate pregnancy and induce labour (*see* DRUGS FOR LABOUR, p.938)

DIOCALM a brand-name antidiarrhoeal drug (p.924) containing morphine and attapulgite, an adsorbent

DIOCALM ULTRA a brand name for loperamide

DIOCTYL a brand name for docusate

DIODERM a brand name for hydrocortisone

DIORALYTE brand-name oral rehydration tablets (p.926) containing sodium bicarbonate, glucose, potassium chloride, and sodium chloride

DIOVOL a brand-name antacid (p.923) containing aluminium hydroxide, magnesium hydroxide, and dimeticone

DIPENTUM a brand name for olsalazine

DIPHENHYDRAMINE an antihistamine (p.906), antiemetic drug (p.922), and antipruritic drug (p.891)

DIPHENOXYLATE an opioid antidiarrhoeal drug (p.924)

DIPHENYLPYRALINE an antihistamine (p.906)

DIPIPANONE an opioid painkiller (p.912)

DIPIVEFRINE a drug for glaucoma (p.920)

DIPROBASE a brand-name emollient (*see* EMOLLIENTS AND BARRIER PREPARATIONS, p.890)

DIPROSALIC a brand-name topical corticosteroid (p.892) containing betamethasone and salicylic acid

DIPROSONE a brand name for betamethasone

DIPYRIDAMOLE an antiplatelet drug (*see* DRUGS THAT PREVENT BLOOD CLOTTING, p.904)

DIRYTHMIN SA a brand name for disopyramide

DISIPAL a brand name for orphenadrine

DISOPYRAMIDE an antiarrhythmic drug (p.898)

DISPRIN a brand name for soluble aspirin

DISPRIN EXTRA a brand-name soluble painkiller (p.912) containing aspirin and paracetamol

DISPROL a brand name for paracetamol

DISTACLOR MR a brand name for cefaclor

DISTALGESIC a brand name for co-proxamol

DISTAMINE a brand name for penicillamine

DISTIGMINE a parasympathomimetic drug used to treat urinary retention (*see* DRUGS THAT AFFECT BLADDER CONTROL, p.939) and myasthenia gravis (p.549)

DISULFIRAM an alcohol abuse deterrent (*see* ALCOHOL DEPENDENCE, p.564)

DITHRANOL a drug for psoriasis (p.332)

DITHROCREAM a brand name for dithranol

DITROPAN a brand name for oxybutynin

DIUMIDE-K CONTINUS a brand-name loop diuretic drug (p.902) and antihypertensive drug (p.897) containing furosemide (frusemide) and potassium

DIUREXAN a brand name for xipamide

DIXARIT a brand name for clonidine

DOBUTAMINE a drug used to treat acute heart failure (p.412) and shock (p.414)

DOCETAXEL an anticancer drug (p.907)

DOCUSATE a faecal softener, laxative (*see* LAXATIVES, p.924), and ear wax softener (*see* DRUGS ACTING ON THE EAR, p.921)

DOLMATIL a brand name for sulpiride

DOLOBID a brand name for diflunisal

DOLOXENE a brand name for dextropropoxyphene

DOMICAL a brand name for amitriptyline

DOMPERIDONE an antiemetic drug (p.922) and motility stimulant (p.926)

DONEPEZIL a drug used to treat Alzheimer's disease (p.536)

DOPAMINE a drug used to treat acute heart failure (p.412), kidney failure (p.705), and shock (p.414)

DOPEXAMINE a drug used to treat chronic heart failure (p.413)

DORALESE a brand name for indoramin

DORZOLAMIDE a carbonic anhydrase inhibitor drug for glaucoma (p.920)

DOSTINEX a brand name for cabergoline

DOSULEPIN (dothiepin) a tricyclic antidepressant (p.916)

DOTHAPAX a brand name for dosulepin (dothiepin)

DOTHIEPIN *see* dosulepin

DOVONEX a brand name for calcipotriol

DOXAPRAM a drug used to stimulate respiration in respiratory failure (p.507)

DOXAZOSIN an alpha-blocker antihypertensive drug (p.897), drug for prostate disorders (p.938), and drug that affects bladder control (p.939)

DOXEPIN a tricyclic antidepressant (p.916)

DOXORUBICIN a cytotoxic anticancer drug (p.907)

DOXYCYCLINE a tetracycline antibiotic drug (p.885) and antimalarial (p.888)

DOXYLAMINE an antihistamine (p.906)

DOZIC a brand name for haloperidol

DRAMAMINE a brand name for dimenhydrinate

DRAPOLENE a brand-name skin antiseptic (*see* PREPARATIONS FOR SKIN INFECTIONS AND INFESTATIONS, p.892) containing benzalkonium chloride and cetrimide

DRICLOR a brand name for aluminium chloride

DRISTAN NASAL SPRAY a brand-name nasal decongestant (p.909) containing oxymetazoline and chlorphenamine (chlorpheniramine)

DROGENIL a brand name for flutamide

DROLEPTAN a brand name for droperidol

DROPERIDOL a butyrophenone antipsychotic drug (p.917) and antiemetic drug (p.922)

DRYPTAL a brand name for furosemide (frusemide)

DULCO-LAX a brand name for bisacodyl

DUOFILM a brand-name preparation used to treat warts (p.354) containing lactic acid, salicylic acid, and collodion

DUOVENT a brand-name bronchodilator drug (p.910) containing fenoterol and ipratropium bromide

DUPHALAC a brand name for lactulose

DUPHASTON a brand name for dydrogesterone

DURAGEL a brand name for nonoxinol '9'

DUROGESIC a brand name for fentanyl

DUTONIN a brand name for nefazodone

DYAZIDE a brand-name diuretic drug (p.902) containing hydrochlorothiazide and triamterene

DYDROGESTERONE a female sex hormone (*see* SEX HORMONES AND RELATED DRUGS, p.933)

DYSMAN a brand name for mefenamic acid

DYSPAMET a brand name for cimetidine

DYTAC a brand name for triamterene

DYTIDE a brand-name diuretic drug (p.902) containing benzthiazide and triamterene

E

EAREX a brand-name preparation for ear wax removal (*see* DRUGS ACTING ON THE EAR, p.921)

EBUFAC a brand name for ibuprofen

ECONACORT a brand-name antifungal drug (p.889) containing econazole and hydrocortisone

ECONAZOLE an antifungal drug (p.889)

ECONOMYCIN a brand name for tetracycline

ECOSTATIN a brand name for econazole

ECOTHIOPATE a drug for glaucoma (p.920)

EDRONAX a brand name for reboxetine

EDROPHONIUM a drug used in the diagnosis of myasthenia gravis (p.549)

EFALITH a brand-name ointment for seborrhoeic dermatitis (p.335)

EFAMAST a brand name for gamolenic acid

EFAVIRENZ an antiviral drug used to treat HIV infection (*see* DRUGS FOR HIV INFECTION AND AIDS, p.887)

EFCORTELAN a brand name for hydrocortisone

EFCORTESOL a brand name for hydrocortisone

EFFERCITRATE a brand name for potassium

EFORMOTEROL *see* formoterol

ELANTAN a brand name for isosorbide mononitrate

ELAVIL a brand name for amitriptyline

ELECTROLADE brand-name oral rehydration powder (p.926) containing potassium, sodium chloride, sodium bicarbonate, and glucose

ELLESTE DUET a brand-name preparation for menopausal problems (p.737) containing estradiol and norethisterone

ELLESTE SOLO a brand name for estradiol

ELOCON a brand name for mometasone

ELTROXIN a brand name for levothyroxine (thyroxine)

ELUDRIL a brand name for chlorhexidine

ELYZOL a brand name for metronidazole

EMCOR a brand name for bisoprolol

EMESIDE a brand name for ethosuximide

EMFLEX a brand name for acemetacin

EMINASE a brand name for anistreplase

EMLA a brand-name local anaesthetic (p.914) containing lidocaine (lignocaine) and prilocaine

ENALAPRIL an ACE inhibitor drug (p.900)

EN-DE-KAY a brand name for fluoride

ENDOXANA a brand name for cyclophosphamide

ENFLURANE a general anaesthetic (p.914)

ENO'S a brand-name antacid (p.923)

ENOXAPARIN an injected anticoagulant (*see* DRUGS THAT PREVENT BLOOD CLOTTING, p.904)

ENOXIMONE a drug used to treat chronic heart failure (p.413)

ENTACAPONE a drug used to treat parkinsonism (*see* PARKINSON'S DISEASE AND PARKINSONISM, p.539)

ENTOCORT CR a brand name for budesonide

EPANUTIN a brand name for phenytoin

EPHEDRINE a decongestant (p.909)

EPILIM a brand name for sodium valproate

EPINEPHRINE (adrenaline) a drug used to treat cardiac arrest (p.419) and anaphylaxis (p.469)

EPIPEN a brand name for epinephrine (adrenaline)

EPIRUBICIN a cytotoxic anticancer drug (p.907)

EPIVIR a brand name for lamivudine

EPOETIN (erythropoietin) a kidney hormone used to treat anaemia due to kidney failure (p.705) or chemotherapy (p.280)

EPOGAM a brand name for gamolenic acid

EPOPROSTENOL a prostaglandin used to treat pulmonary hypertension (p.505)

EPPY a brand name for epinephrine (adrenaline)

EPREX a brand name for epoetin (erythropoietin)

EPTIFIBATIDE a drug for prevention of myocardial infarction (p.410)

EQUAGESIC a brand-name nonopioid painkiller (p.912) and antianxiety drug (p.916) containing meprobamate and aspirin

ERGOCALCIFEROL a form of vitamin D

ERGOMETRINE a uterine stimulant (*see* DRUGS FOR LABOUR, p.938)

ERGOTAMINE an antimigraine drug (p.913)

ERWINASE a brand name for crisantaspase

ERYCEN a brand name for erythromycin

ERYMAX a brand name for erythromycin

ERYTHROCIN a brand name for erythromycin

ERYTHROMYCIN a macrolide antibiotic (p.885)

ERYTHROPED a brand name for erythromycin

ERYTHROPOIETIN (*see* epoetin)

ESKAMEL a brand-name treatment for acne (p.340) containing resorcinol and sulphur

ESKORNADE a brand-name cough remedy (p.909) containing phenylpropanolamine and diphenylpyraline

ESMOLOL a beta-blocker drug (p.898)

ESTRACOMBI a brand-name preparation for menopausal problems (p.737) containing estradiol and norethisterone

ESTRADERM TTS a brand-name preparation for menopausal problems (p.737) containing estradiol

ESTRADIOL an oestrogen (*see* SEX HORMONES AND RELATED DRUGS, p.933, and HORMONE REPLACEMENT THERAPY, p.937)

ESTRAMUSTINE a cytotoxic anticancer drug (p.907)

ESTRAPAK a brand-name preparation for menopausal problems (p.737) containing estradiol and norethisterone

ESTRIOL an oestrogen (*see* SEX HORMONES AND RELATED DRUGS, p.933)

ESTRONE an oestrogen (*see* SEX HORMONES AND RELATED DRUGS, p.933, and HORMONE REPLACEMENT THERAPY, p.937)

ESTROPIPATE an oestrogen (*see* SEX HORMONES AND RELATED DRUGS, p.933, and HORMONE REPLACEMENT THERAPY, p.937)

ETACRYNIC ACID a loop diuretic drug (p.902)

ETAMSYLATE an antifibrinolytic (*see* DRUGS THAT PROMOTE BLOOD CLOTTING, p.903)

ETHAMBUTOL an antituberculous drug (p.886)

ETHINYLESTRADIOL an oestrogen (*see* SEX HORMONES AND RELATED DRUGS, p.933, and HORMONE REPLACEMENT THERAPY, p.937)

ETHOHEPTAZINE an opioid painkiller (p.912)

ETHOSUXIMIDE an anticonvulsant drug (p.914)

ETIDRONATE a drug for bone disorders (p.896)

ETODOLAC a nonsteroidal anti-inflammatory drug (p.894)

ETOMIDATE a general anaesthetic (p.914)

ETOPOSIDE a cytotoxic anticancer drug (p.907)

ETYNODIOL a progestogen (*see* SEX HORMONES AND RELATED DRUGS, p.933) and oral contraceptive drug (*see* CONTRACEPTION, p.69)

EUCARDIC a brand name for carvedilol

EUGLUCON a brand name for glibenclamide

EUGYNON-30 a brand-name oral contraceptive (*see* CONTRACEPTION, p.69) containing ethinylestradiol and levonorgestrel

EURAX a brand name for crotamiton

EURAX-HYDROCORTISONE a brand-name topical corticosteroid (p.892) containing hydrocortisone and crotamiton

EVISTA a brand name for raloxifene

EVOREL a brand name for estradiol

EXELDERM a brand name for sulconazole

EXELON a brand name for rivastigmine

EX-LAX a brand name for senna

EXOCIN a brand name for ofloxacin

EXPULIN a brand-name cough remedy (p.909) containing chlorphenamine (chlorpheniramine), menthol, pholcodine, and pseudoephedrine

EXPULIN DECONGESTANT a brand-name decongestant (p.909) containing chlorphenamine (chlorpheniramine), ephedrine, and menthol

EXTEROL a brand-name preparation for ear wax removal (*see* DRUGS ACTING ON THE EAR, p.921) containing urea

F

FACTOR VIIa a blood product used to promote blood clotting (*see* DRUGS THAT PROMOTE BLOOD CLOTTING, p.903)

FACTOR VIII a blood product used to promote blood clotting (*see* DRUGS THAT PROMOTE BLOOD CLOTTING, p.903)

FACTOR IX a blood product used to promote blood clotting (*see* DRUGS THAT PROMOTE BLOOD CLOTTING, p.903)

FAMCICLOVIR an antiviral drug (p.886)

FAMOTIDINE an ulcer-healing drug (p.923)

FAMVIR a brand name for famciclovir

FANSIDAR a brand-name antimalarial drug (p.888) containing pyrimethamine and sulfadoxine

FARLUTAL a brand name for medroxyprogesterone

FASIGYN a brand name for tinidazole

FAVERIN a brand name for fluvoxamine

FECTRIM a brand name for co-trimoxazole

FEFOL a brand name for folic acid with iron

FELBINAC a nonsteroidal anti-inflammatory drug (p.894)

FELDENE a brand name for piroxicam

FELODIPINE a calcium channel blocker drug (p.900)

FEMAPAK a brand-name preparation for menopausal problems (p.737) containing estradiol and dydrogesterone

FEMARA a brand name for letrozole

FEMATRIX a brand name for estradiol

FEMERON a brand name for miconazole

FEMIGRAINE a brand-name antimigraine drug (p.913) containing aspirin and cyclizine

FEMINAX a brand-name painkiller (p.912) containing paracetamol, codeine, hyoscine, and caffeine

FEMODENE a brand-name oral contraceptive (*see* CONTRACEPTION, p.69) containing ethinylestradiol and gestodene

FEMOSTON a brand-name preparation for menopausal problems (p.737) containing estradiol and dydrogesterone

FEMSEVEN a brand name for estradiol

FEMULEN a brand-name oral contraceptive (*see* CONTRACEPTION, p.69) containing etynodiol

FENBID a brand name for ibuprofen

FENBUFEN a nonsteroidal anti-inflammatory drug (p.894)

FENBUZIP a brand name for fenbufen

FENOFIBRATE a lipid-lowering drug (p.935)

FENOKET a brand name for ketoprofen

FENOPROFEN a nonsteroidal anti-inflammatory drug (p.894)

FENOPRON a brand name for fenoprofen

FENOTEROL a sympathomimetic bronchodilator drug (p.910)

FENTAMOX a brand name for tamoxifen

FENTANYL an opioid painkiller (p.912)

FENTAZIN a brand name for perphenazine

FENTICONAZOLE an antifungal drug (p.889)

FEOSPAN a brand name for iron

FERFOLIC SV a brand name for folic acid and ferrous gluconate

FERRIC AMMONIUM CITRATE a form of iron

FERROGRAD a brand name for iron

FERROGRAD C a brand name for iron and vitamin C

FERROGRAD FOLIC a brand name for folic acid and iron

FERROUS FUMARATE a form of iron

FERROUS GLUCONATE a form of iron

FERROUS GLYCINE SULPHATE a form of iron

FERROUS SULPHATE a form of iron

FERSADAY a brand name for iron

FERSAMAL a brand name for iron

FEXOFENADINE an antihistamine (p.906)

FIBRINOLYSIN an enzyme that breaks down blood clots; used to treat wounds

FIBRO-VEIN a brand name for sodium tetradecyl sulphate

FILAIR a brand name for beclometasone

FILGRASTIM a drug that stimulates the production of white blood cells

FINASTERIDE a drug used to treat benign prostatic hypertrophy (*see* DRUGS FOR PROSTATE DISORDERS, p.938)

FLAGYL a brand name for metronidazole

FLAMATROL a brand name for piroxicam

FLAMAZINE a brand name for silver sulfadiazine

FLAVOXATE an anticholinergic drug used to treat urinary incontinence (*see* DRUGS THAT AFFECT BLADDER CONTROL, p.939)

FLECAINIDE an antiarrhythmic drug (p.898)

FLEXIN CONTINUS a brand name for indometacin

FLIXONASE a brand name for fluticasone

FLOMAX MR a brand name for tamsulosin

FLORINEF a brand name for fludrocortisone

FLOXAPEN a brand name for flucloxacillin

FLUANXOL a brand name for flupentixol

FLUCLOXACILLIN a penicillin antibiotic (p.885)

FLUCONAZOLE an antifungal drug (p.889)

FLUCYTOSINE an antifungal drug (p.889)

FLUDARABINE a cytotoxic anticancer drug (p.907)

FLUDROCORTISONE a corticosteroid (p.930)

FLUDROXYCORTIDE (flurandrenolone) a topical corticosteroid (p.892)

FLUMAZENIL an antidote for benzodiazepine overdose (*see* DRUG OVERDOSE AND ACCIDENTAL INGESTION, p.321)

FLUMETASONE a corticosteroid (p.930)

FLUNISOLIDE a corticosteroid (p.930)

FLUNITRAZEPAM a benzodiazepine sleeping drug (p.915)

FLUOCINOLONE a topical corticosteroid (p.892)

FLUOCINONIDE a topical corticosteroid (p.892)

FLUOCORTOLONE a topical corticosteroid (p.892)

FLUOR-A-DAY a brand name for fluoride

FLUORESCEIN a substance used to stain the eye before examination

FLUORIDE a mineral (p.929) used to prevent dental caries (p.609)

FLUORIGARD a brand name for fluoride

FLUOROMETHOLONE a corticosteroid used to treat eye disorders (*see* DRUGS ACTING ON THE EYE, p.919)

FLUOROURACIL a cytotoxic anticancer drug (p.907)

FLUOXETINE a selective serotonin reuptake inhibitor (SSRI) antidepressant (p.916)

FLUPENTIXOL an antipsychotic drug (p.917)

FLUPHENAZINE an antipsychotic drug (p.917)

FLURANDRENOLONE *see* fludroxycortide

FLURAZEPAM a benzodiazepine sleeping drug (p.915)

FLURBIPROFEN a nonsteroidal anti-inflammatory drug (p.894)

FLUREX a brand-name cold and flu remedy (p.910) containing paracetamol, phenylephrine, and dextromethorphan

FLUTAMIDE an antiandrogen (*see* SEX HORMONES AND RELATED DRUGS, p.933, and DRUGS FOR PROSTATE DISORDERS, p.938) used as an anticancer drug (p.907)

FLUTICASONE a corticosteroid (p.930)

FLUVASTATIN a lipid-lowering drug (p.935)

FLUVOXAMINE a selective serotonin reuptake inhibitor (SSRI) antidepressant (p.916)

FOLATE SODIUM a form of folic acid

FOLIC ACID a vitamin (p.927)

FOLINIC ACID a form of folic acid used to decrease the toxicity of methotrexate

FOLLICLE-STIMULATING HORMONE (FSH) a natural hormone used as a drug for infertility (p.936)

FOLLITROPIN ALFA a drug for infertility (p.936)

FOLLITROPIN BETA a drug for infertility (p.936)

FOMEPIZOLE an antidote for ethylene glycol (antifreeze) poisoning (*see* DRUG OVERDOSE AND ACCIDENTAL INGESTION, p.321)

FORMESTANE an anticancer drug (p.907)

FORMOTEROL (eformoterol) a sympathomimetic bronchodilator (p.910)

FORTAGESIC a brand-name painkiller (p.912) containing pentazocine and paracetamol

FORTRAL a brand name for pentazocine

FORTUM a brand name for ceftazidime

FOSCARNET an antiviral drug (p.886) used to treat herpes simplex infections (p.291) and retinitis in people with HIV infection and AIDS (p.297)

FOSCAVIR a brand name for foscarnet

FOSFESTROL a female sex hormone (*see* SEX HORMONES AND RELATED DRUGS, p.933) and anticancer drug (p.907)

FOSINOPRIL an ACE inhibitor drug (p.900)

FRAGMIN a brand name for dalteparin

FRAMYCETIN an aminoglycoside antibiotic (p.885)

FRANGULA a mild stimulant laxative (p.924)

FRANOL a brand-name bronchodilator drug (p.910) containing ephedrine and theophylline

FRISIUM a brand name for clobazam

FROBEN a brand name for flurbiprofen

FROOP a brand name for furosemide (frusemide)

FRU-CO a brand-name diuretic drug (p.902) containing amiloride and furosemide (frusemide)

FRUMIL a brand-name diuretic drug (p.902) containing amiloride and furosemide (frusemide)

FRUSEMIDE *see* furosemide

FRUSENE a brand-name diuretic drug (p.902) containing furosemide (frusemide) and triamterene

FSH *see* follicle-stimulating hormone

FUCIBET a brand-name topical corticosteroid (p.892) containing betamethasone and fusidic acid

FUCIDIN a brand name for fusidic acid

FUCIDIN H a brand-name topical corticosteroid (p.892) containing fusidic acid and hydrocortisone

FUCITHALMIC a brand name for fusidic acid

FULL MARKS a brand name for phenothrin

FUNGILIN a brand name for amphotericin

FUNGIZONE a brand name for amphotericin

FURADANTIN a brand name for nitrofurantoin

FURAMIDE a brand name for diloxanide furoate

FUROSEMIDE (frusemide) a loop diuretic drug (p.902)

FUSIDIC ACID an antibiotic (p.885)

FYBOGEL a brand name for ispaghula

FYNNON CALCIUM ASPIRIN a brand-name painkiller (p.912)

G

GABAPENTIN an anticonvulsant drug (p.914)

GABITRIL a brand name for tiagabine

GALCODINE a brand name for codeine

GALENPHOL a brand name for pholcodine

GALFER a brand name for iron

GALFER FA a brand name for folic acid and iron

GALLAMINE a muscle relaxant (p.896) used in general anaesthesia (*see* HAVING MAJOR SURGERY, p.943)

GALPSEUD a brand name for pseudoephedrine

GAMANIL a brand name for lofepramine

GAMMA GLOBULIN an immunoglobulin (*see* VACCINES AND IMMUNOGLOBULINS, p.883)

GAMOLENIC ACID a drug used to treat breast pain (p.756) and eczema (p.333)

GANCICLOVIR an antiviral drug (p.886)

GANDA a brand-name drug for glaucoma (p.920) containing epinephrine (adrenaline) and guanethidine

GARAMYCIN a brand name for gentamicin

GARDENAL a brand name for phenobarbital

GASTROBID CONTINUS a brand name for metoclopramide

GASTROCOTE a brand-name antacid (p.923)

GASTROFLUX a brand name for metoclopramide

GASTROMAX a brand name for metoclopramide

GAVISCON a brand-name antacid (p.923)

GELCOSAL a brand-name preparation for psoriasis (p.332) and eczema (p.333)

GELCOTAR a brand name for coal tar

GEMCITABINE a cytotoxic anticancer drug (p.907)

GEMEPROST a drug used in labour (*see* DRUGS FOR LABOUR, p.938)

GEMFIBROZIL a lipid-lowering drug (p.935)

GENOTROPIN a brand name for somatropin

GENTAMICIN an aminoglycoside antibiotic (p.885)

GENTICIN a brand name for gentamicin

GENTISONE HC a brand-name aminoglycoside antibiotic (p.885) containing gentamicin and hydrocortisone

GESTODENE a progestogen and oral contraceptive (*see* CONTRACEPTION, p.69)

GESTONE a brand name for progesterone

GESTONORONE (gestronol) a progestogen used to treat an enlarged prostate gland (p.725)

GESTRINONE a drug used to treat endometriosis (p.742)

GLANDOSANE a brand-name artificial saliva

GLIBENCLAMIDE an oral drug for diabetes mellitus (p.931)

GLICLAZIDE an oral drug for diabetes mellitus (p.931)

GLIMEPIRIDE an oral drug for diabetes mellitus (p.931)

GLIPIZIDE an oral drug for diabetes mellitus (p.931)

GLIQUIDONE an oral drug for diabetes mellitus (p.931)

GLUCAGEN a brand name for glucagon

GLUCAGON a pancreatic hormone used to treat hypoglycaemia (*see* DRUGS FOR DIABETES MELLITUS, p.931)

GLUCOBAY a brand name for acarbose

GLUCOPHAGE a brand name for metformin

GLURENORM a brand name for gliquidone

GLUTARALDEHYDE a topical preparation for treating warts (p.354)

GLUTAROL a brand name for glutaraldehyde

GLYCEROL a diuretic drug (p.902), laxative (p.924), and drug for glaucoma (p.920), also used to soften earwax (*see* DRUGS ACTING ON THE EAR, p.921) and as an ingredient in topical preparations

GLYCERYL TRINITRATE a nitrate drug (p.899) used to treat angina (p.407)

GLYCOPYRRONIUM BROMIDE a drug used to dry secretions during general anaesthesia (*see* HAVING MAJOR SURGERY, p.943)

GLYTRIN a brand name for glyceryl trinitrate

GOLD a metal used as an antirheumatic drug (p.895)

GOLDEN EYE a brand name for propamidine isethionate

GONADORELIN a hypothalamic hormone that regulates sex hormones (*see* SEX HORMONES AND RELATED DRUGS, p.933) and a drug for infertility (p.936)

GONADOTROPHIN, HUMAN CHORIONIC a drug for infertility (p.936)

GOSERELIN a hormonal anticancer drug (p.907) and gonadorelin analogue (*see* SEX HORMONES AND RELATED DRUGS, p.933, DRUGS FOR INFERTILITY, p.936, and DRUGS FOR PROSTATE DISORDERS, p.938)

GRAMICIDIN an aminoglycoside antibiotic (p.885)

GRANEODIN a brand-name aminoglycoside antibiotic (p.885) containing gramicidin and neomycin

GRANISETRON an antiemetic drug (p.922)

GREGODERM a brand-name antibiotic (p.885) and antifungal drug (p.889) containing neomycin, polymyxin B, nystatin, and hydrocortisone

GRISEOFULVIN an antifungal drug (p.889)

GRISOVIN a brand name for griseofulvin

GROWTH HORMONE *see* somatropin

GTN 300 MCG a brand name for glyceryl trinitrate

GUAIFENESIN an expectorant (*see* COUGH REMEDIES, p.909)

GUANETHIDINE an antihypertensive drug (p.897), also used as a drug for glaucoma (p.920)

GUANOR EXPECTORANT a brand-name cough remedy (p.909) containing diphenhydramine, ammonium chloride, and menthol

GUAREM a brand name for guar gum

GUAR GUM a drug for diabetes mellitus (p.931)

GYNO-DAKTARIN a brand name for miconazole

GYNOL II a brand name for nonoxinol '9'

GYNO-PEVARYL a brand name for econazole

H

HAELAN a brand name for fludroxycortide (flurandrenolone)

HALCIDERM TOPICAL a brand name for halcinonide

HALCINONIDE a topical corticosteroid (p.892)

HALDOL a brand name for haloperidol

HALIBUT LIVER OIL a natural fish oil rich in vitamin A and vitamin D

HALOPERIDOL a butyrophenone antipsychotic drug (p.917)

HALOTHANE a gas used to induce general anaesthesia (*see* GENERAL ANAESTHETICS, p.914, AND HAVING MAJOR SURGERY, p.943)

HALYCITROL a brand name for vitamin A and vitamin D

HARMOGEN a brand name for estropipate

HAY-CROM a brand name for sodium cromoglicate

HAYMINE a brand-name cough remedy (p.909) containing chlorphenamine (chlorpheniramine) and ephedrine

HEDEX a brand name for paracetamol

HEDEX EXTRA a brand-name nonopioid painkiller (p.912) containing paracetamol and caffeine

HELICLEAR a brand-name ulcer-healing drug (p.923) containing lansoprazole, amoxicillin, and clarithromycin

HEMINEVRIN a brand name for clomethiazole

HEPARIN an injected anticoagulant (*see* DRUGS THAT PREVENT BLOOD CLOTTING, p.904)

HEPARINOID a topical nonsteroidal anti-inflammatory drug (p.894)

HEP-FLUSH a brand name for heparin

HEXACHLOROPHENE a skin antiseptic (*see* PREPARATIONS FOR SKIN INFECTIONS AND INFESTATIONS, p.892)

HEXALEN a brand name for altretamine

HEXAMINE *see* methenamine

HEXETIDINE an oral antiseptic

HEXOPAL a brand name for nicotinic acid

HIBITANE a brand name for chlorhexidine

HIOXYL a brand name for hydrogen peroxide

HIPREX a brand name for methenamine

HIRUDOID a brand name for heparinoid

HISTAFEN a brand name for terfenadine

HISTALIX a brand-name cough remedy (p.909) containing diphenhydramine, ammonium chloride, and menthol

HIVID a brand name for zalcitabine

HOMATROPINE a mydriatic drug (*see* DRUGS ACTING ON THE EYE, p.919)

HUMALOG a brand name for insulin lispro

HUMAN ACTRAPID a brand name for insulin

HUMAN CHORIONIC GONADOTROPHIN a gonadotrophin hormone (*see* SEX HORMONES AND RELATED DRUGS, p.933), and drug for infertility (p.936)

HUMAN INSULATARD a brand name for insulin

HUMAN MENOPAUSAL GONADOTROPHIN a drug for infertility (p.936)

HUMAN MIXTARD a brand name for insulin

HUMAN MONOTARD a brand name for insulin

HUMAN ULTRATARD a brand name for insulin

HUMAN VELOSULIN a brand name for insulin

HUMATROPE a brand name for somatropin

HUMULIN a brand name for insulin

HYALASE a brand name for hyaluronidase

HYALURONIDASE a drug used to increase the absorption of injected fluids

HYDRALAZINE an antihypertensive drug (p.897)

HYDROCHLOROTHIAZIDE a thiazide diuretic drug (p.902)

HYDROCORTISONE a corticosteroid (p.930)

HYDROCORTISTAB a brand name for hydrocortisone

HYDROCORTONE a brand name for hydrocortisone

HYDROFLUMETHIAZIDE a thiazide diuretic drug (p.902)

HYDROGEN PEROXIDE an antiseptic (*see* PREPARATIONS FOR SKIN INFECTIONS AND INFESTATIONS, p.892)

HYDROMORPHONE an opioid painkiller (p.912)

HYDROSALURIC a brand name for hydrochlorothiazide

HYDROTALCITE an antacid (p.923)

HYDROXOCOBALAMIN a form of vitamin B_{12}

HYDROXYAPATITE a drug for bone disorders (p.896)

HYDROXYCARBAMIDE (hydroxyurea) a cytotoxic anticancer drug (p.907)

HYDROXYCHLOROQUINE an antirheumatic drug (p.895)

HYDROXYPROGESTERONE a progestogen (*see* SEX HORMONES AND RELATED DRUGS, p.933) used to prevent miscarriage (p.791)

HYDROXYUREA *see* hydroxycarbamide

HYDROXYZINE a nonbenzodiazepine antianxiety drug (p.916), antipruritic drug (p.891), and antiemetic drug (p.922)

HYGROTON a brand name for chlortalidone

HYOSCINE an antispasmodic drug (p.926)

HYPOTEARS a brand name for polyvinyl alcohol

HYPOVASE a brand name for prazosin

HYPROMELLOSE a substance used in artificial tears (*see* DRUGS ACTING ON THE EYE, p.919)

HYPURIN a brand name for insulin

HYTRIN a brand name for terazosin

I

IBUGEL a brand name for ibuprofen

IBULEVE a brand-name for ibuprofen

IBUPROFEN a nonsteroidal anti-inflammatory drug (p.894) and nonopioid painkiller (p.912)

IBUSPRAY a brand name for ibuprofen

ICHTHAMMOL a drug included in skin preparations for eczema (p.333)

IDARUBICIN a cytotoxic antibiotic used as an anticancer drug (p.907)

IDOXURIDINE an antiviral drug (p.886)

IFOSFAMIDE a cytotoxic anticancer drug (p.907)

IKOREL a brand name for nicorandil

ILOSONE brand name for erythromycin

ILUBE a brand-name artificial tears preparation (*see* DRUGS ACTING ON THE EYE, p.919) containing acetylcysteine and hypromellose

IMBRILON a brand name for indometacin

IMDUR a brand name for isosorbide mononitrate

IMIDAPRIL an ACE inhibitor drug (p.900)

IMIGLUCERASE a drug used to treat Gaucher's disease, an inborn error of metabolism (p.867)

IMIGRAN a brand name for sumatriptan

IMIPENEM an antibiotic (p.885)

IMIPRAMINE a tricyclic antidepressant (p.916) and anticholinergic drug used to treat urinary incontinence (*see* DRUGS THAT AFFECT BLADDER CONTROL, p.939)

IMIQUIMOD a drug to treat genital warts (p.768)

IMMUKIN a brand name for interferon gamma

IMMUNOGLOBULIN a preparation injected to prevent infectious diseases (*see* VACCINES AND IMMUNOGLOBULINS, p.883)

IMMUNOPRIN a brand name for azathioprine

IMODIUM a brand name for loperamide

IMURAN a brand name for azathioprine

INDAPAMIDE a thiazide-like diuretic (p.902)

INDERAL a brand name for propranolol

INDERAL-LA a brand name for propranolol

INDERETIC a brand-name antihypertensive drug (p.897) containing propranolol and bendroflumethiazide (bendrofluazide)

INDEREX a brand-name antihypertensive drug (p.897) containing propranolol and bendroflumethiazide (bendrofluazide)

INDINAVIR an antiviral drug used to treat HIV infection (*see* HIV INFECTION AND AIDS, p.887)

INDOCID a brand name for indometacin

INDOLAR a brand name for indometacin

INDOMETACIN a nonsteroidal anti-inflammatory drug (p.894) and drug used to treat gout (p.380)

INDORAMIN an alpha-blocker antihypertensive drug (p.897) and drug for prostate disorders (p.938)

INFACOL a brand name for dimeticone

INFADROPS a brand name for paracetamol

INNOHEP a brand name for tinzaparin

INNOVACE a brand name for enalapril

INNOZIDE a brand name for enalapril

INOSINE PRANOBEX an antiviral drug (p.886)

INOSITOL a substance related to the vitamin B complex

INOVEN a brand name for ibuprofen

INSULATARD a brand name for insulin

INSULIN a drug for diabetes mellitus (p.931)

INSULIN LISPRO a type of insulin

INTAL a brand name for sodium cromoglicate

INTEGRILIN a brand name for eptifibatide

INTERFERON ALFA, BETA, AND GAMMA a group of antiviral (p.886) and anticancer drugs (p.907)

INTRALGIN a brand-name topical non-steroidal anti-inflammatory drug (p.894)

INTRON-A a brand name for interferon alfa

INVIRASE a brand name for saquinavir

IODINE a mineral (p.929) preparation for skin infections and infestations (p.892), and drug for hyperthyroidism (p.932)

IONAMIN a brand name for phentermine

IONAX a brand-name treatment for acne (p.340)

IONIL T a brand-name dandruff (p.358) shampoo containing benzalkonium chloride, coal tar, and salicylic acid

IOPIDINE a brand name for apraclonidine

IPECACUANHA a drug used to induce vomiting (*see* DRUG OVERDOSE AND ACCIDENTAL INGESTION, p.321) and as an expectorant (*see* COUGH REMEDIES, p.909)

IPRATROPIUM BROMIDE an anticholinergic bronchodilator drug (p.910)

IRBESARTAN an angiotensin II blocker antihypertensive drug (p.897)

IRINOTECAN a cytotoxic anticancer drug (p.907)

IRON a mineral (p.929)

ISMELIN a brand name for guanethidine

ISMO a brand name for isosorbide mononitrate

ISOCARBOXAZID a monoamine oxidase inhibitor (MAOI) antidepressant (p.916)

ISOCONAZOLE an antifungal drug (p.889)

ISOFLURANE an inhaled general anaesthetic (p.914)

ISOGEL brand name for ispaghula

ISOKET a brand name for isosorbide dinitrate

ISOMETHEPTENE MUCATE an antimigraine drug (p.913)

ISONIAZID an antituberculous drug (p.886)

ISOPHANE INSULIN a type of insulin

ISOPTO ALKALINE a brand name for hypromellose

ISOPTO ATROPINE a brand-name drug acting on the eye (p.919) containing atropine and hypromellose

ISOPTO CARBACHOL a brand name for carbachol

ISOPTO CARPINE a brand-name drug for glaucoma (p.920) containing pilocarpine and hypromellose

ISOPTO FRIN brand-name eye drops (*see* DRUGS ACTING ON THE EYE, p.919) containing phenylephrine and hypromellose

ISOPTO PLAIN a brand name for hypromellose

ISORDIL a brand name for isosorbide dinitrate

ISOSORBIDE DINITRATE a nitrate drug (p.899) used to treat angina (p.407)

ISOSORBIDE MONONITRATE a nitrate drug (p.899) used to treat angina (p.407)

ISOTRATE a brand name for isosorbide mononitrate

ISOTRETINOIN a retinoid drug (p.890) used to treat acne (p.340)

ISOTREX a brand name for isotretinoin

ISPAGHULA a bulk-forming agent used as an antidiarrhoeal drug (p.924) and also as a laxative (p.924)

ISRADIPINE a calcium channel blocker drug (p.900)

ISTIN a brand name for amlodipine

ITRACONAZOLE an antifungal drug (p.889)

IVERMECTIN an anthelmintic drug (p.889)

J

JECTOFER a brand name for iron

JOY-RIDES a brand name for hyoscine

K

KABIKINASE a brand name for streptokinase

KALSPARE a brand-name diuretic drug (p.902) containing triamterene and chlortalidone

KALTEN a brand-name diuretic drug (p.902) containing amiloride, hydrochlorothiazide, and atenolol

KAMILLOSAN a brand-name emollient (*see* EMOLLIENTS AND BARRIER PREPARATIONS, p.890)

KANAMYCIN an aminoglycoside antibiotic (p.885)

KAOLIN an antidiarrhoeal drug (p.924)

KAPAKE a brand name for paracetamol

KARVOL a brand name for menthol

KAY-CEE-L a brand name for potassium

KEFADOL a brand name for cefamandole

KEFLEX a brand name for cefalexin

KEFZOL a brand name for cefazolin

KELFIZINE W a brand name for sulfametopyrazine

KEMADRIN a brand name for procyclidine

KEMICETINE a brand name for chloramphenicol

KENALOG a brand name for triamcinolone

KENTENE a brand name for piroxicam

KERAL a brand name for dexketoprofen

KERLONE a brand name for betaxolol

KETAMINE a general anaesthetic (p.914)

KETOCID a brand name for ketoprofen

KETOCONAZOLE an antifungal drug (p.889)

KETOPROFEN a nonsteroidal anti-inflammatory drug (p.894)

KETOROLAC a nonsteroidal anti-inflammatory drug (p.894) and nonopioid painkiller (p.912)

KETOTIFEN an antihistamine (p.906)

KETOVAIL a brand name for ketoprofen

KETOVITE a brand-name multivitamin supplement (*see* VITAMINS, p.927)

KLARICID a brand name for clarithromycin

KLEAN-PREP a brand-name osmotic laxative (p.924)

KLIOFEM a brand-name drug for menopausal problems (p.737) containing estradiol and norethisterone

KLOREF a brand-name potassium supplement (*see* MINERALS, p.929)

KOLANTICON a brand-name drug for irritable bowel syndrome (p.655) containing aluminium hydroxide, magnesium oxide, dicycloverine (dicyclomine), and dimeticone

KONAKION a brand name for phytomenadione

KONSYL a brand name for ispaghula

KWELLS a brand name for hyoscine

KYTRIL a brand name for granisetron

L

LABETALOL a beta-blocker drug (p.898)

LABOSEPT a brand-name throat antiseptic containing dequalinium

LACIDIPINE a calcium channel blocker drug (p.900)

LACRI-LUBE a brand-name ointment for dry eyes (*see* DRUGS ACTING ON THE EYE, p.919)

LACTIC ACID a moisturizing ingredient used in preparations for warts (p.354) and in emollients (*see* EMOLLIENTS AND BARRIER PREPARATIONS, p.890) and suppositories

LACTITOL an osmotic laxative (p.924)

LACTUGAL a brand name for lactulose

LACTULOSE an osmotic laxative (p.924)

LADROPEN a brand name for flucloxacillin

LAMICTAL a brand name for lamotrigine

LAMISIL a brand name for terbinafine

LAMIVUDINE an antiviral drug used to treat HIV infection (*see* DRUGS FOR HIV INFECTION AND AIDS, p.887)

LAMOTRIGINE an anticonvulsant drug (p.914)

LAMPRENE a brand name for clofazimine

LANOXIN a brand name for digoxin

LANOXIN-PG a brand name for digoxin

LANREOTIDE an anticancer drug (p.907)

LANSOPRAZOLE an ulcer-healing drug (p.923)

LARAFEN a brand name for ketoprofen

LARAPAM a brand name for piroxicam

LARIAM a brand name for mefloquine

LASIKAL a brand-name diuretic drug (p.902) containing furosemide (frusemide) and potassium

LASILACTONE a brand-name diuretic drug (p.902) containing furosemide (frusemide) and spironolactone

LASIX a brand name for furosemide (frusemide)

LASMA a brand name for theophylline

LASONIL a brand name for heparinoid

LASORIDE a brand-name diuretic drug (p.902) containing amiloride and furosemide (frusemide)

LASSAR'S PASTE a skin preparation used to treat psoriasis (p.332) containing dithranol, zinc oxide, and salicylic acid

LATANOPROST a drug for glaucoma (p.920)

LAXOBERAL a brand name for sodium picosulfate

LAXOSE a brand name for lactulose

LEDCLAIR a brand name for sodium calcium edetate

LEDERFEN a brand name for fenbufen

LEDERFOLIN a brand name for folinic acid

LEDERMYCIN a brand name for demeclocycline

LEDERSPAN a brand name for triamcinolone

LEMSIP a brand-name cold and flu remedy (p.910) containing paracetamol, phenylephrine, chlorphenamine (chlorpheniramine), and caffeine

LENIUM a brand-name dandruff (p.358) shampoo containing selenium sulphide

LENOGRASTIM a drug that stimulates the production of white blood cells

LENTARD MC a brand name for insulin

LENTARON a brand name for formestane

LENTIZOL a brand name for amitriptyline

LEPIRUDIN an anticoagulant (*see* DRUGS THAT PREVENT BLOOD CLOTTING, p.904)

LERCANIDIPINE a calcium channel blocker drug (p.900)

LESCOL a brand name for fluvastatin

LETROZOLE a hormonal anticancer drug (p.907)

LEUCOVORIN *see* calcium folinate

LEUKERAN a brand name for chlorambucil

LEUPRORELIN a gonadorelin analogue (*see* SEX HORMONES AND RELATED DRUGS, p.933, and DRUGS FOR INFERTILITY, p.936)

LEVAMISOLE an anthelmintic drug (p.889)

LEVOBUNOLOL a beta-blocker drug for glaucoma (p.920)

LEVOCABASTINE an antihistamine (p.906)

LEVODOPA a drug for parkinsonism (*see* PARKINSON'S DISEASE AND PARKINSONISM, p.539)

LEVOFLOXACIN a quinolone antibiotic (p.885)

LEVOMEPROMAZINE (methotrimeprazine) an antipsychotic drug (p.917)

LEVONELLE a brand-name postcoital contraceptive (*see* CONTRACEPTION, p.69) containing levonorgestrel

LEVONORGESTREL a progestogen (*see* CONTRACEPTION, p.69, SEX HORMONES AND RELATED DRUGS, p.933, and HORMONE REPLACEMENT THERAPY, p.937)

LEVOTHYROXINE (thyroxine) a thyroid hormone (*see* DRUGS FOR HYPOTHYROIDISM, p.932)

LIBRIUM a brand name for chlordiazepoxide

LIDOCAINE (lignocaine) a local anaesthetic (p.914) and antiarrhythmic drug (p.898)

LIGNOCAINE *see* lidocaine

LINDANE a topical antiparasitic drug (*see* PREPARATIONS FOR SKIN INFECTIONS AND INFESTATIONS, p.892)

LIORESAL a brand name for baclofen

LIOTHYRONINE a thyroid hormone (*see* DRUGS FOR HYPOTHYROIDISM, p.932)

LIPANTIL a brand name for fenofibrate

LIPITOR a brand name for atorvastatin

LIPOSTAT a brand name for pravastatin

LIQUID PARAFFIN an emollient (*see* EMOLLIENTS AND BARRIER PREPARATIONS. p.890) and laxative (p.924)

LIQUIFILM TEARS brand-name eye drops (*see* DRUGS ACTING ON THE EYE, p.919) containing polyvinyl alcohol

LISINOPRIL an ACE inhibitor drug (p.900)

LISKONUM a brand name for lithium

LISURIDE a drug for parkinsonism (*see* PARKINSON'S DISEASE AND PARKINSONISM, p.539)

LITAREX a brand name for lithium

LITHIUM a mood-stabilizing drug (p.918)

LIVIAL a brand name for tibolone

LIVOSTIN a brand name for levocabastine

LOCERYL a brand name for amorolfine

LOCOID a brand name for hydrocortisone

LOCORTEN-VIOFORM brand-name ear drops (*see* DRUGS ACTING ON THE EAR, p.921) containing clioquinol and flumetasone

LODINE SR a brand name for etodolac

LODOXAMIDE an antiallergy drug (p.905)

LOESTRIN a brand-name oral contraceptive (*see* CONTRACEPTION, p.69) containing ethinylestradiol and norethisterone

LOFEPRAMINE a tricyclic antidepressant (*see* ANTIDEPRESSANT DRUGS, p.916)

LOFEXIDINE a drug used to treat opioid withdrawal symptoms (*see* DRUG DEPENDENCE, p.564)

LOGYNON a brand-name oral contraceptive (*see* CONTRACEPTION, p.69) containing ethinylestradiol and levonorgestrel

LOMEXIN a brand name for fenticonazole

LOMOTIL a brand-name antidiarrhoeal drug (p.924) containing atropine and diphenoxylate

LOMUSTINE a cytotoxic anticancer drug (p.907)

LONITEN a brand name for minoxidil

LOPERAGEN a brand name for loperamide

LOPERAMIDE an antidiarrhoeal drug (p.924)

LOPID a brand name for gemfibrozil

LOPRAZOLAM a benzodiazepine sleeping drug (p.915)

LOPRESOR a brand name for metoprolol

LORATADINE an antihistamine (p.906)

LORAZEPAM a benzodiazepine anticonvulsant drug (p.914) and antianxiety drug (p.916)

LORMETAZEPAM a benzodiazepine sleeping drug (p.915)

LOSARTAN an antihypertensive drug (p.897)

LOSEC a brand name for omeprazole

LOTRIDERM a brand-name topical corticosteroid (p.892) containing clotrimazole and betamethasone

LOXAPAC a brand name for loxapine

LOXAPINE an antipsychotic drug (p.917)

LUBORANT a brand name for artificial saliva

LUDIOMIL a brand name for maprotiline

LUGOL'S SOLUTION an iodine solution used as a drug for hyperthyroidism (p.932)

LUSTRAL a brand name for sertraline

LUTEINIZING HORMONE (LH) a drug for infertility (p.936)

LYCLEAR a brand name for permethrin

LYMECYCLINE a tetracycline antibiotic (p.885)

M

MAALOX a brand-name antacid (p.923) containing aluminium hydroxide and magnesium hydroxide

MAALOX PLUS a brand-name antacid (p.923) containing aluminium hydroxide, magnesium hydroxide, and dimeticone

MACROBID a brand name for nitrofurantoin

MACRODANTIN a brand name for nitrofurantoin

MADOPAR a brand name for co-beneldopa

MAGNAPEN a brand-name penicillin antibiotic (p.885) containing ampicillin and flucloxacillin

MAGNESIUM a mineral (p.929)

MAGNESIUM ALGINATE an antifoaming agent

MAGNESIUM CARBONATE an antacid (p.923)

MAGNESIUM CITRATE a laxative (p.924)

MAGNESIUM HYDROXIDE an antacid (p.923) and laxative (p.924)

MAGNESIUM OXIDE an antacid (p.923)

MAGNESIUM SALTS an osmotic laxative (p.924)

MAGNESIUM TRISILICATE an antacid (p.923)

MALARONE a brand-name antimalarial drug (p.888) containing proguanil and atovaquone

MALATHION an antiparasitic drug (*see* PREPARATIONS FOR SKIN INFECTIONS AND INFESTATIONS, p.892)

MALOPRIM a brand-name antimalarial drug (p.888) containing dapsone and pyrimethamine

MANERIX a brand name for moclobemide

MANEVAC a brand-name stimulant laxative (p,924) containing senna and ispaghula

MANNITOL an osmotic diuretic drug (p.902)

MAPROTILINE an antidepressant drug (p.916)

MARCAIN a brand name for bupivacaine

MAREVAN a brand name for warfarin

MARVELON a brand-name oral contraceptive (*see* CONTRACEPTION, p.69) containing ethinylestradiol and desogestrel

MAXALT a brand name for rizatriptan

MAXEPA a brand-name lipid-lowering drug (p.935) containing concentrated fish oils

MAXIDEX brand-name eye drops (*see* DRUGS ACTING ON THE EYE, p.919) containing dexamethasone and hypromellose

MAXITROL brand-name eye preparations (*see* DRUGS ACTING ON THE EYE, p.919) containing dexamethasone, neomycin, and polymyxin B

MAXIVENT a brand name for salbutamol

MAXOLON a brand name for metoclopramide

MAXTREX a brand name for methotrexate

MCR-50 a brand name for isosorbide mononitrate

MEBENDAZOLE an anthelmintic drug (p.889)

MEBEVERINE an antispasmodic drug (p.926)

MECLOZINE an antiemetic drug (p.922) and antihistamine (p.906)

MECYSTEINE a mucolytic drug used as a cough remedy (p.909)

MEDIJEL a brand-name pain-relieving gel for mouth ulcers (p.632) containing lidocaine (lignocaine)

MEDINEX a brand name for diphenhydramine

MEDINOL a brand name for paracetamol

MEDISED a brand-name painkiller (p.912) and cough remedy (p.909) containing paracetamol and promethazine

MEDRONE a brand name for methylprednisolone

MEDROXYPROGESTERONE a progestogen (*see* SEX HORMONES AND RELATED DRUGS, p.933, and HORMONE REPLACEMENT THERAPY, p.937) and hormonal anticancer drug (p.907)

MEFENAMIC ACID a nonsteroidal anti-inflammatory drug (p.894)

MEFLOQUINE an antimalarial drug (p.888)

MEFOXIN a brand name for cefoxitin

MEFRUSIDE a thiazide-like diuretic (p.902)

MEGACE a brand name for megestrol

MEGESTROL a progestogen (*see* SEX HORMONES AND RELATED DRUGS, p.933) and hormonal anticancer drug (p.907)

MELATONIN a hormone used as a sleeping drug (p.915)

MELLERIL a brand name for thioridazine

MELOXICAM a nonsteroidal anti-inflammatory drug (p.894) and nonopioid painkiller (p.912)

MELPHALAN a cytotoxic anticancer drug (p.907)

MENADIOL another name for vitamin K

MENOREST a brand name for estradiol

MENOTROPHIN a drug for infertility (p.936)

MENTHOL an alcohol derived from mint oils used as an inhalation and topical antipruritic drug (p.891)

MEPACRINE HYDROCHLORIDE an antiprotozoal drug (p.888)

MEPERIDINE an opioid painkiller (p.912)

MEPIVACAINE a local anaesthetic (p.914)

MEPROBAMATE a nonbenzodiazepine antianxiety drug (p.916)

MEPTAZINOL an opioid painkiller (p.912)

MEQUITAZINE an antihistamine (p.906)

MERBENTYl a brand name for dicycloverine (dicyclomine)

MERCAPTOPURINE a cytotoxic anticancer drug (p.907)

MERCILON a brand-name oral contraceptive (*see* CONTRACEPTION, p.69) containing ethinylestradiol and desogestrel

MEROCAINE a brand-name throat antiseptic containing benzocaine and cetylpyridinium

MEROCET a brand name for cetylpyridinium

MESALAZINE an aminosalicylate drug (p.924) used to treat ulcerative colitis (p.659)

MESNA a drug used to protect the urinary tract from damage caused by some anticancer drugs (p.907)

MESTEROLONE a male sex hormone (*see* SEX HORMONES AND RELATED DRUGS, p.933)

MESTINON a brand name for pyridostigmine

MESTRANOL an oestrogen (*see* SEX HORMONES AND RELATED DRUGS, p.933, and HORMONE REPLACEMENT THERAPY, p.937)

METARAMINOL a drug used to treat hypotension (p.414)

METENIX-5 a brand name for metolazone

METFORMIN an oral drug for diabetes mellitus (p.931)

METHADONE an opioid painkiller (p.912), also used to treat heroin dependence (*see* DRUG DEPENDENCE, p.564)

METHADOSE a brand name for methadone

METHENAMINE a drug used to suppress urinary tract infections

METHEX a brand name for methadone

METHIONINE a drug used to treat paracetamol overdose (*see* DRUG OVERDOSE AND ACCIDENTAL INGESTION, p.321)

METHOCARBAMOL a muscle relaxant (p.896)

METHOTREXATE a cytotoxic anticancer drug (p.907) and antirheumatic drug (p.895), also used to treat psoriasis (p.332)

METHOTRIMEPRAZINE *see* levomepromazine

METHOXAMINE a drug used to treat hypotension (p.414)

METHOXSALEN a drug used to treat psoriasis (p.332)

METHYLCELLULOSE a substance used in artificial tears (*see* DRUGS ACTING ON THE EYE, p.919), bulk-forming laxative (p.924), and antidiarrhoeal drug (p.924)

METHYLDOPA an antihypertensive (p.897)

METHYLPHENIDATE a central nervous system stimulant drug (p.918)

METHYLPHENOBARBITAL an anticonvulsant drug (p.914)

METHYLPREDNISOLONE a corticosteroid (p.930)

METHYL SALICYLATE a topical painkiller (p.912)

METHYSERGIDE an antimigraine drug (p.913)

METIPRANOLOL a beta-blocker drug (p.898) and drug for glaucoma (p.920)

METIROSINE a drug used to treat adrenal tumours (p.684)

METOCLOPRAMIDE a gastrointestinal motility stimulant (*see* ANTISPASMODIC DRUGS AND MOTILITY STIMULANTS, p.926) and antiemetic drug (p.922)

METOLAZONE a thiazide-like diuretic (p.902)

METOPIRONE a brand name for metyrapone

METOPROLOL a beta-blocker drug (p.898)

METOSYN a brand name for fluocinonide

METRODIN a brand name for urofollitropin

METROGEL a brand name for topical metronidazole

METRONIDAZOLE an antibiotic (p.885) and antiprotozoal drug (p.888)

METYRAPONE a drug used to diagnose and treat Cushing's syndrome (p.684)

MEXILETINE an antiarrhythmic drug (p.898)

MIANSERIN an antidepressant drug (p.916)

MICONAZOLE an antifungal drug (p.889)

MICROGYNON 30 a brand-name oral contraceptive (*see* CONTRACEPTION, p.69) containing ethinylestradiol and levonorgestrel

MICRONOR a brand name for norethisterone

MICROVAL a brand name for levonorgestrel

MICTRAL a brand-name drug for urinary tract infections containing nalidixic acid and sodium bicarbonate

MIDAZOLAM a benzodiazepine (*see* ANTIANXIETY DRUGS, p.916) used as premedication (*see* HAVING MAJOR SURGERY, p.943)

MIDRID a brand-name antimigraine drug (p.913) containing paracetamol and isometheptene mucate

MIFEPRISTONE a drug used during labour (*see* DRUGS FOR LABOUR, p.938)

MIGRALEVE a brand-name antimigraine drug (p.913) containing codeine, paracetamol, and buclizine

MIGRANAL a brand name for dihydroergotamine

MIGRAVESS a brand-name antimigraine drug (p.913) containing aspirin and metoclopramide

MIGRIL a brand-name antimigraine drug (p.913) containing ergotamine, caffeine, and cyclizine

MILK OF MAGNESIA a brand name for magnesium hydroxide

MILPAR a brand-name laxative (p.924) containing magnesium hydroxide and liquid paraffin

MILRINONE a drug used to treat chronic heart failure (p.413)

MINIHEP a brand name for heparin

MINIMS ATROPINE a brand name for atropine

MINIMS CHLORAMPHENICOL a brand name for chloramphenicol

MINIMS CYCLOPENTOLATE a brand name for cyclopentolate

MINIMS GENTAMICIN a brand name for gentamicin

MINIMS PHENYLEPHRINE a brand name for phenylephrine

MINIMS PILOCARPINE a brand name for pilocarpine

MINIMS PREDNISOLONE a brand name for prednisolone

MINITRAN a brand name for glyceryl trinitrate

MINOCYCLINE a tetracycline antibiotic (p.885)

MINOXIDIL an antihypertensive drug (p.897) and drug for male-pattern baldness (p.359)

MINTEC a brand name for peppermint oil

MINTEZOL a brand name for tiabendazole

MINULET a brand-name oral contraceptive (*see* CONTRACEPTION, p.69) containing ethinylestradiol and gestodene

MIRAPEXIN a brand name for pramipexole

MIRENA an intrauterine contraceptive device (*see* CONTRACEPTION, p.69) containing levonorgestrel

MIRTAZAPINE an antidepressant drug (p.916)

MISOPROSTOL an ulcer-healing drug (p.923)

MISTAMINE a brand name for mizolastine

MITOBRONITOL an anticancer drug (p.907)

MITOMYCIN a cytotoxic anticancer drug (p.907)

MITOXANTRONE (mitozantrone) a cytotoxic anticancer drug (p.907)

MITOZANTRONE *see* mitoxantrone

MIVACURIUM a muscle relaxant used in general anaesthesia (*see* HAVING MAJOR SURGERY, p.943)

MIXTARD a brand name for insulin

MIZOLASTINE an antihistamine (p.906)

MOBIC a brand name for meloxicam

MOBIFLEX a brand name for tenoxicam

MOCLOBEMIDE a monoamine oxidase inhibitor (MAOI) antidepressant (p.916)

MODAFINIL a drug used to treat narcolepsy (p.526)

MODALIM a brand name for ciprofibrate

MODAPLATE a brand name for dipyridamole

MODRASONE a brand name for alclometasone

MODRENAL a brand name for trilostane

MODUCREN a brand-name antihypertensive drug (p.897) containing amiloride, hydrochlorothiazide, and timolol

MODURET-25 a brand-name antihypertensive drug (p.897) containing amiloride and hydrochlorothiazide

MODURETIC a brand-name antihypertensive drug (p.897) containing amiloride and hydrochlorothiazide

MOEXIPRIL an ACE inhibitor drug (p.900)

MOGADON a brand name for nitrazepam

MOLGRAMOSTIM a drug that stimulates the production of white blood cells

MOLIPAXIN a brand name for trazodone

MOLYBDENUM a mineral

MOMETASONE a topical corticosteroid (p.892)

MONIT a brand name for isosorbide mononitrate

MONO-CEDOCARD a brand name for isosorbide mononitrate

MONOCLATE-P a brand name for factor VIII

MONOCOR a brand name for bisoprolol

MONOPARIN a brand name for heparin

MONOSULFIRAM a drug used to treat scabies (p.355)

MONOTRIM a brand name for trimethoprim

MONOVENT a brand name for terbutaline

MONOZIDE a brand-name antihypertensive drug (p.897) containing bisoprolol and hydrochlorothiazide

MONPHYTOL a brand-name topical antifungal drug (p.889)

MONTELUKAST a leukotriene antagonist (*see* ANTIALLERGY DRUGS, p.905)

MORACIZINE an antiarrhythmic drug (p.898)

MORPHINE an opioid painkiller (p.912)

MOTENS a brand name for lacidipine

MOTIFENE a brand name for diclofenac

MOTILIUM a brand name for domperidone

MOTIPRESS a brand name for fluphenazine

MOTIVAL a brand name for fluphenazine

MOTRIN a brand name for ibuprofen

MOVELAT a brand-name topical non-steroidal anti-inflammatory drug (p.894)

MOVICOl an brand-name osmotic laxative (p.924)

MOXISYLYTE (thymoxamine) a drug used treat Raynaud's syndrome (*see* RAYNAUD'S PHENOMENON AND RAYNAUD'S DISEASE, p.436) and impotence (p.770)

MOXONIDINE a centrally acting antihypertensive drug (p.897)

MST CONTINUS a brand name for morphine

MUCAINE a brand-name antacid (p.923) containing aluminium hydroxide, magnesium hydroxide, and oxetacaine

MUCODYNE a brand name for carbocisteine

MUCOGEL a brand-name antacid (p.923) containing aluminium hydroxide and magnesium hydroxide

MU-CRON TABLETS a brand-name nonopioid painkiller (p.912) and decongestant (p.909) containing phenylpropanolamine and paracetamol

MULTIPARIN a brand name for heparin

MUPIROCIN a preparation for skin infections and infestations (p.892)

MUSTINE *see* chlormethine

MXL a brand name for morphine sulphate

MYCIL GOLD a brand name for clotrimazole

MYCOBUTIN a brand name for rifabutin

MYCOPHENOLATE MOFETIL an immunosuppressant drug (p.906)

MYCOTA a brand name for undecanoate acid

MYDRILATE a brand name for cyclopentolate

MYOCRISIN a brand name for sodium aurothiomalate

MYSOLINE a brand name for primidone

N

NABILONE an antiemetic drug (p.922)

NABUMETONE a nonsteroidal anti-inflammatory drug (p.894)

NADOLOL a beta-blocker drug (p.898)

NAFARELIN a hypothalamic hormone (*see* SEX HORMONES AND RELATED DRUGS, p.933) and gonadorelin analogue (*see* DRUGS FOR INFERTILITY, p.936)

NAFTIDROFURYL a vasodilator

NALBUPHINE an opioid painkiller (p.912)

NALCROM a brand name for sodium cromoglicate

NALIDIXIC ACID a quinolone antibiotic (p.885)

NALOREX a brand name for naltrexone

NALOXONE an antidote for opioid poisoning (*see* DRUG OVERDOSE AND ACCIDENTAL INGESTION, p.321)

NALTREXONE a drug used to treat opioid withdrawal (*see* DRUG DEPENDENCE, p.564)

NAPRATEC a brand-name antirheumatic drug (p.895) containing naproxen and misoprostol

NAPROSYN a brand name for naproxen

NAPROXEN a nonsteroidal anti-inflammatory drug (p.894)

NARAMIG a brand name for naratriptan

NARATRIPTAN an antimigraine drug (p.913)

NARDIL a brand name for phenelzine

NARPHEN a brand name for phenazocine

NASONEX a brand name for mometasone

NATRILIX a brand name for indapamide

NAVIDREX a brand name for cyclopenthiazide

NAVISPARE a brand-name diuretic (p.902) containing cyclopenthiazide and amiloride

NEBCIN a brand name for tobramycin

NEBILET a brand name for nebivolol

NEBIVOLOL a beta-blocker (p.898) and antihypertensive drug (p.897)

NEDOCROMIL SODIUM a mast cell stabilizer (*see* ANTIALLERGY DRUGS, p.905)

NEFAZODONE an antidepressant drug (p.916)

NEFOPAM a nonopioid painkiller (p.912)

NEGRAM a brand name for nalidixic acid

NELFINAVIR an antiviral drug used to treat HIV infection (*see* DRUGS FOR HIV INFECTION AND AIDS, p.887)

NEO-BENDROMAX a brand name for bendroflumethiazide (bendrofluazide)

NEOGEST a brand name for norgestrel

NEO-MERCAZOLE a brand name for carbimazole

NEOMYCIN an aminoglycoside antibiotic (p.885)

NEO-NACLEX a brand name for bendroflumethiazide (bendrofluazide)

NEO-NACLEX-K a brand-name diuretic drug (p.902) containing bendroflumethiazide (bendrofluazide) and potassium

NEORAL a brand name for cyclosporin

NEORECORMON a brand name for epoetin

NEOSPORIN a brand-name antibiotic (p.885) containing gramicidin, neomycin, and polymyxin B

NEOSTIGMINE a parasympathomimetic drug used to treat myasthenia gravis (p.549) and urinary retention (*see* DRUGS THAT AFFECT BLADDER CONTROL, p.939)

NEOTIGASON a brand name for acitretin

NEPHRIL a brand name for polythiazide

NERICUR a brand name for benzoyl peroxide

NERISONE a brand name for diflucortolone

NETILLIN a brand name for netilmicin

NETILMICIN an aminoglycoside antibiotic (p.885)

NEUPOGEN a brand name for filgrastim

NEURONTIN a brand name for gabapentin

NEUTREXIN a brand name for trimetrexate

NEVIRAPINE an antiviral drug used to treat HIV infection (*see* DRUGS FOR HIV INFECTION AND AIDS, p.887)

NIACIN a member of the vitamin B complex, a vasodilator, and a lipid-lowering drug (p.935)

NIACINAMIDE a form of niacin

NICARDIPINE a calcium channel blocker drug (p.900)

NICLOSAMIDE an anthelmintic drug (p.889)

NICORANDIL a drug used to treat angina (p.407)

NICORETTE a brand-name preparation containing nicotine, used to help people to stop smoking

NICOTINAMIDE another name for niacinamide

NICOTINE the addictive component of tobacco

NICOTINELL a brand-name preparation containing nicotine, used to help people to stop smoking

NICOTINIC ACID *see* niacin

NICOTINYL ALCOHOL *see* niacin

NICOUMALONE *see* acenocoumarol

NIFEDIPINE a calcium channel blocker (p.900) and antimigraine drug (p.913)

NIFEREX a brand name for polysaccharide-iron complex, a form of iron

NIGHT NURSE a brand-name cold remedy (*see* COLD AND FLU REMEDIES, p.910) containing paracetamol and promethazine

NIMODIPINE a calcium channel blocker drug (p.900)

NINDAXA a brand name for indapamide

NIPENT a brand name for pentostatin

NISOLDIPINE a calcium channel blocker drug (p.900)

NITRAZEPAM a benzodiazepine sleeping drug (p.915)

NITRO-DUR a brand name for glyceryl trinitrate

NITROFURANTOIN an antibiotic (p.885)

NITROLINGUAL a brand name for glyceryl trinitrate

NITROPRUSSIDE an antihypertensive (p.897)

NITROUS OXIDE a general anaesthetic (p.914)

NIVAQUINE a brand name for chloroquine

NIVEMYCIN a brand name for neomycin

NIZATIDINE an ulcer-healing drug (p.923)

NIZORAL a brand name for ketoconazole

NOLVADEX a brand name for tamoxifen

NOLVADEX FORTE a brand name for tamoxifen

NONOXINOL '9' a spermicide (*see* CONTRACEPTION, p.69)

NONTOCOG ALFA synthetic factor IX

NOOTROPIL a brand name for piracetam

NORADRENALINE *see* norepinephrine

NORDITROPIN a brand name for somatropin

NOREPINEPHRINE (noradrenaline) a drug used to raise blood pressure during shock (p.414)

NORETHISTERONE a female sex hormone (*see* SEX HORMONES AND RELATED DRUGS, p.933, and HORMONE REPLACEMENT THERAPY, p.937) and an oral contraceptive (*see* CONTRACEPTION, p.69)

NORFLOXACIN a quinolone antibiotic (p.885)

NORGALAX a brand name for docusate

NORGESTIMATE a progestogen used in oral contraceptives (*see* CONTRACEPTION, p.69)

NORGESTON a brand name for levonorgestrel

NORGESTREL a progestogen (*see* SEX HORMONES AND RELATED DRUGS, p.933, and HORMONE REPLACEMENT THERAPY, p.937)

NORIDAY a brand name for norethisterone

NORIMIN a brand-name oral contraceptive (*see* CONTRACEPTION, p.69) containing ethinylestradiol and norethisterone

NORIMODE a brand name for loperamide

NORINYL-1 a brand-name oral contraceptive (*see* CONTRACEPTION, p.69) containing norethisterone and mestranol

NORISTERAT a brand name for norethisterone

NORMACOL PLUS a brand-name laxative (p.924) containing frangula and sterculia

NORMAX a brand-name laxative (p.924) containing dantron and docusate

NORMOSANG a brand name for haem arginate, a treatment for porphyria (p.693)

NORPLANT a brand name for levonorgestrel

NORTRIPTYLINE a tricyclic antidepressant (p.916)

NORVIR a brand name for ritonavir

NOVONORM a brand name for repaglinide

NUBAIN a brand name for nalbuphine

NUELIN a brand name for theophylline

NULACIN a brand-name antacid (p.923) containing calcium carbonate, magnesium carbonate, magnesium trisilicate, and magnesium oxide

NUPERCAINAL a brand name for cinchocaine

NUROFEN a brand name for ibuprofen

NUROFEN PLUS a brand-name painkiller (p.912) containing ibuprofen and codeine

NU-SEALS ASPIRIN a brand name for aspirin

NUTRAPLUS a brand name for urea

NUTRIZYM GR a brand name for pancreatin

NUVELLE a brand-name preparation for menopausal problems (p.737) containing estradiol and levonorgestrel

NYCOPREN a brand name for naproxen

NYLAX a brand-name stimulant laxative (p.924)

NYSTADERMAL a brand-name topical corticosteroid (p.892) containing nystatin and triamcinolone

NYSTAFORM a brand-name antifungal drug (p.889) containing nystatin and chlorhexidine

NYSTAFORM-HC a brand-name topical corticosteroid (p.892) containing hydrocortisone, nystatin, and chlorhexidine

NYSTAMONT a brand name for nystatin

NYSTAN a brand name for nystatin

NYSTATIN an antifungal drug (p.889)

NYTOL a brand name for diphenhydramine

O

OCCLUSAL a brand name for salicylic acid

OCTOCOG ALFA synthetic factor VIII

OCTOXINOL a spermicide (*see* CONTRACEPTION, p.69)

OCTREOTIDE a synthetic hypothalamic hormone used to relieve symptoms of certain cancers (*see* ANTICANCER DRUGS, p.907)

OCUFEN a brand name for flurbiprofen

OCUSERT PILO a brand name for pilocarpine

ODRIK a brand name for trandolapril

OESTRIFEN a brand name for tamoxifen

OESTROGEL a brand name for estradiol

OESTROGEN a female hormone (*see* SEX HORMONES AND RELATED DRUGS, p.933)

OILATUM EMOLLIENT a brand-name bath additive containing liquid paraffin (*see* EMOLLIENTS AND BARRIER PREPARATIONS, p.890)

OILATUM GEL a brand-name shower gel containing liquid paraffin (*see* EMOLLIENTS AND BARRIER PREPARATIONS, p.890)

OLANZAPINE an antipsychotic drug (p.917)

OLBETAM a brand name for acipimox

OLSALAZINE an aminosalicylate drug (p.924)

OMEPRAZOLE an ulcer-healing drug (p.923)

ONCOVIN a brand name for vincristine

ONDANSETRON an antiemetic drug (p.922)

ONE-ALPHA a brand name for alfacalcidol

OPILON a brand name for moxisylyte (thymoxamine)

OPTICROM a brand name for sodium cromoglicate

OPTIMINE a brand name for azatadine

OPTREX EYE LOTION a brand-name eye preparation containing witch hazel

ORABASE a brand-name preparation for mouth ulcers (p.632)

ORABET a brand name for metformin

ORALDENE a brand-name for hexetidine

ORAMORPH a brand name for morphine

ORAP a brand name for pimozide

ORCIPRENALINE a sympathomimetic bronchodilator drug (p.910)

ORELOX a brand name for cefpodoxime

ORIMETEN a brand name for aminoglutethimide

ORLEPT a brand name for sodium valproate

ORLISTAT a drug used to treat obesity (p.631)

OROVITE a brand name for pyridoxine

ORPHENADRINE a muscle relaxant (p.896) and drug used to treat parkinsonism (*see* PARKINSON'S DISEASE AND PARKINSONISM, p.539)

ORTHO-CREME a brand name for nonoxinol '9'

ORTHOFORMS a brand name for nonoxinol '9'

ORTHO-GYNEST a brand name for estriol

ORUDIS a brand name for ketoprofen

ORUVAIL a brand name for ketoprofen

OSMOLAX a brand name for lactulose

OSSOPAN a brand name for hydroxyapatite

OTOMIZE a brand-name ear preparation (*see* DRUGS ACTING ON THE EAR, p.921) containing dexamethasone and neomycin

OTOSPORIN a brand-name ear preparation (*see* DRUGS ACTING ON THE EAR, p.921) containing hydrocortisone, neomycin, and polymyxin B

OTRIVINE a brand name for xylometazoline

OTRIVINE-ANTISTIN a brand-name eye preparation (*see* DRUGS ACTING ON THE EYE, p.919) containing antazoline and xylometazoline

OVESTIN a brand name for estriol

OVEX a brand name for mebendazole

OVRAN a brand-name oral contraceptive (*see* CONTRACEPTION, p.69) containing ethinylestradiol and levonorgestrel

OVRANETTE a brand-name oral contraceptive (*see* CONTRACEPTION, p.69) containing ethinylestradiol and levonorgestrel

OVYSMEN a brand-name oral contraceptive (*see* CONTRACEPTION, p.69) containing ethinylestradiol and norethisterone

OXAZEPAM a benzodiazepine antianxiety drug (p.916)

OXERUTIN a drug used to treat peripheral vascular disorders (pp.430–439)

OXETACAINE a local anaesthetic (p.914) used with antacids (p.923) to treat reflux oesophagitis

OXITROPIUM a bronchodilator drug (p.910)

OXIVENT a brand name for oxitropium

OXPENTIFYLLINE *see* pentoxifylline

OXPRENOLOL a beta-blocker drug (p.898)

OXYBENZONE a sunscreen (*see* SUNSCREENS AND SUNBLOCKS, p.893)

OXYBUPROCAINE a local anaesthetic (p.914)

OXYBUTYNIN an anticholinergic drug (*see* DRUGS THAT AFFECT BLADDER CONTROL, p.939)

OXYCODONE an opioid painkiller (p.912)

OXYMETAZOLINE a topical decongestant (p.909)

OXYMYCIN a brand name for oxytetracycline

OXYPERTINE an antipsychotic drug (p.917)

OXYTETRACYCLINE a tetracycline antibiotic (p.885)

OXYTOCIN a uterine stimulant (*see* DRUGS FOR LABOUR, p.938)

P

PACLITAXEL a cytotoxic anticancer drug (p.907)

PALDESIC a brand name for paracetamol

PALFIUM a brand name for dextromoramide

PALUDRINE a brand name for proguanil

PAMIDRONATE a drug for bone disorders (p.896)

PANADEINE a brand-name painkiller (p.912) containing paracetamol and codeine

PANADOL a brand name for paracetamol

PANADOL EXTRA a brand-name painkiller (p.912) containing paracetamol and caffeine

PANADOL ULTRA a brand-name painkiller (p.912) containing paracetamol and codeine

PANALEVE a brand name for paracetamol

PANCREATIN a preparation of the pancreatic enzymes amylase, protease, and lipase

PANCREX a brand name for pancreatin

PANCURONIUM a muscle relaxant used in general anaesthesia (*see* HAVING MAJOR SURGERY, p.943)

PANOXYL a brand name for benzoyl peroxide

PANTHENOL a member of the vitamin B complex

PANTOPRAZOLE an ulcer-healing drug (p.923)

PANTOTHENIC ACID a member of the vitamin B complex

PAPAVERETUM an opioid painkiller (p.912)

PAPAVERINE a smooth muscle relaxant (*see* ANTISPASMODIC DRUGS AND MOTILITY STIMULANTS, p.926)

PAPULEX a brand name for nicotinamide

PARACETAMOL a nonopioid painkiller (p.912)

PARACODOL a brand-name painkiller (p.912) containing codeine and paracetamol

PARADOTE a brand-name painkiller (p.912) containing paracetamol and methionine

PARAKE a brand-name painkiller (p.912) containing codeine and paracetamol

PARALDEHYDE an anticonvulsant drug (p.914)

PARAMAX a brand-name antimigraine drug (p.913) containing paracetamol and metoclopramide

PARAMOL a brand-name painkiller (p.912) containing paracetamol and dihydrocodeine

PARAPLATIN a brand name for carboplatin

PARIET a brand name for rabeprazole

PARLODEL a brand name for bromocriptine

PARMID a brand name for metoclopramide

PAROMOMYCIN an antiprotozoal (p.888)

PAROXETINE a selective serotonin reuptake inhibitor (SSRI) antidepressant (p.916)

PARVOLEX a brand name for acetylcysteine

PAVACOL-D a brand name for pholcodine

PENBRITIN a brand name for ampicillin

PENCICLOVIR an antiviral drug (p.886)

PENICILLAMINE an antirheumatic (p.895)

PENICILLIN an antibiotic (p.885)

PENICILLIN V another name for phenoxymethylpenicillin

PENTACARINAT a brand name for pentamidine

PENTAMIDINE an antiprotozoal drug (p.888)

PENTASA a brand name for mesalazine

PENTAZOCINE an opioid painkiller (p.912)

PENTOSTATIN an anticancer drug (p.907)

PENTOXIFYLLINE (oxpentifylline) a drug used to treat peripheral vascular disorders (pp.430–439)

PEPCID a brand name for famotidine

PEPPERMINT OIL an antispasmodic drug (p.926) and flavouring agent

PEPTIMAX a brand name for cimetidine

PEPTO-BISMOL a brand-name antidiarrhoeal drug (p.924) and antacid (p.923) containing bismuth

PERCUTOL a brand name for glyceryl trinitrate

PERDIX a brand name for moexipril

PERFAN a brand name for enoximone

PERGOLIDE a drug used to treat Parkinson's disease (*see* PARKINSON'S DISEASE AND PARKINSONISM, p.539)

PERGONAL a brand name for menotrophin

PERIACTIN a brand name for cyproheptadine

PERICYAZINE an antipsychotic drug (p.917)

PERINAL a brand-name drug used to treat haemorrhoids (p.668) containing hydrocortisone and lidocaine (lignocaine)

PERINDOPRIL an ACE inhibitor drug (p.900)

PERMETHRIN a topical antiparasitic drug (*see* PREPARATIONS FOR SKIN INFECTIONS AND INFESTATIONS, p.892)

PEROXYL a brand name for hydrogen peroxide

PERPHENAZINE an antipsychotic drug (p.917) and antiemetic drug (p.922)

PERSANTIN a brand name for dipyridamole

PERU BALSAM an antiseptic for haemorrhoids (p.668)

PETHIDINE an opioid painkiller (p.912)

PEVARYL a brand name for econazole

PHENAZOCINE an opioid painkiller (p.912)

PHENELZINE a monoamine oxidase inhibitor (MAOI) antidepressant (p.916)

PHENERGAN a brand name for promethazine

PHENINDIONE an oral anticoagulant (*see* DRUGS THAT PREVENT BLOOD CLOTTING, p.904)

PHENIRAMINE an antihistamine (p.906)

PHENOBARBITAL a barbiturate sleeping drug (p.915) and anticonvulsant drug (p.914)

PHENOL an antiseptic used in throat lozenges and sprays

PHENOTHRIN a topical antiparasitic drug used to treat head lice (p.831) and pubic lice (p.768)

PHENOXYBENZAMINE a drug used to treat phaeochromocytoma (p.686)

PHENOXYMETHYLPENICILLIN a penicillin antibiotic (p.885)

PHENSIC a brand-name painkiller (p.912) containing aspirin and caffeine

PHENTERMINE a central nervous system stimulant drug (p.918) that has been used as an appetite suppressant

PHENTOLAMINE an antihypertensive drug (p.897)

PHENYLBUTAZONE a nonsteroidal anti-inflammatory drug (p.894)

PHENYLEPHRINE a decongestant (p.909), mydriatic drug (*see* DRUGS ACTING ON THE EYE, p.919), and drug used to treat shock (p.414)

PHENYLPROPANOLAMINE a decongestant (p.909)

PHENYTOIN an anticonvulsant drug (p.914)

PHISO-MED a brand name for chlorhexidine

PHOLCODINE a cough remedy (p.909)

PHOSPHORUS a mineral (p.929)

PHYLLOCONTIN CONTINUS a brand name for aminophylline

PHYSEPTONE a brand name for methadone

PHYSIOTENS a brand name for moxonidine

PHYTEX a brand-name antifungal drug (p.889) containing salicylic acid

PHYTOMENADIONE a form of vitamin K

PICOLAX a brand-name laxative (p.924) containing sodium picosulfate and magnesium citrate

PILOCARPINE a miotic drug (*see* DRUGS FOR GLAUCOMA, p.920)

PIMOZIDE an antipsychotic drug (p.917)

PINDOLOL a beta-blocker drug (p.898)

PIPERACILLIN a penicillin antibiotic (p.885)

PIPERAZINE an anthelmintic drug (p.889)

PIPERONAL a repellent (*see* PREPARATIONS FOR SKIN INFECTIONS AND INFESTATIONS, p.892) used to treat head lice (p.831)

PIPOTIAZINE PALMITATE an antipsychotic drug (p.917)

PIPRIL a brand name for piperacillin

PIRACETAM an anticonvulsant drug (p.914)

PIRENZEPINE an ulcer-healing drug (p.923)

PIROXICAM a nonsteroidal anti-inflammatory drug (p.894), also used to treat gout (p.380)

PIROZIP a brand name for piroxicam

PIZOTIFEN an antimigraine drug (p.913)

PLAVIX a brand name for clopidogrel

PLENDIL a brand name for felodipine

PODOPHYLLIN a topical treatment for genital warts (p.768)

PODOPHYLLOTOXIN a topical treatment for genital warts (p.768)

PODOPHYLLUM a topical treatment for warts (p.354)

POLOXAMER a stimulant laxative (p.924)

POLYFAX a brand-name antibiotic (p.885) containing bacitracin and polymyxin B

POLYMYXIN B an antibiotic (p.885)

POLYNOXYLIN an antifungal drug (p.889) and antibiotic (p.885)

POLYSTYRENE SULPHONATE a drug to remove excess potassium from the blood

POLYTAR a brand name for coal tar

POLYTHIAZIDE a thiazide diuretic (p.902)

POLYTRIM a brand-name antibiotic (p.885) containing trimethoprim and polymyxin B

POLYVINYL ALCOHOL a substance used in artificial tears (*see* DRUGS ACTING ON THE EYE, p.919)

PONSTAN a brand name for mefenamic acid

PORACTANT ALFA a drug used to mature the lungs of premature babies with respiratory distress syndrome (*see* PROBLEMS OF THE PREMATURE BABY, p.816)

PORK INSULATARD a brand name for insulin

PORK MIXTARD a brand name for insulin

POSALFILIN a brand-name treatment for warts (p.354) containing podophyllum and salicylic acid

POTASSIUM a mineral

POTASSIUM BICARBONATE an antacid (p.923)

POTASSIUM CHLORIDE a form of potassium

POTASSIUM CITRATE a drug that reduces the acidity of urine, also used to treat cystitis (p.709)

POTASSIUM CLAVULANATE a preparation of clavulanic acid

POTASSIUM HYDROXYQUINOLONE SULPHATE an agent with antibacterial, antifungal, and deodorant properties

POTASSIUM IODIDE a drug for hyperthyroidism (p.932), also used as an expectorant (*see* COUGH REMEDIES, p.909)

POTASSIUM PERMANGANATE an astringent antiseptic (*see* PREPARATIONS FOR SKIN INFECTIONS AND INFESTATIONS, p.892) and deodorant

POVIDONE-IODINE a topical antiseptic (*see* PREPARATIONS FOR SKIN INFECTIONS AND INFESTATIONS, p.892)

PRAGMATAR a brand-name preparation for dandruff (p.358), eczema (p.333), and psoriasis (p.332), containing coal tar, salicylic acid, and sulphur

PRALIDOXIME MESYLATE an antidote to poisoning by organophosphates (*see* DRUG OVERDOSE AND ACCIDENTAL INGESTION, p.321)

PRAMIPEXOLE a drug for parkinsonism (*see* PARKINSON'S DISEASE AND PARKINSONISM, p.539)

PRAMOCAINE a local anaesthetic (p.914) used to relieve itching and burning

PRAVASTATIN a lipid-lowering agent (p.935)

PRAXILENE a brand name for naftidrofuryl

PRAZIQUANTEL an anthelmintic drug (p.889) used to treat tapeworm infestation

PRAZOSIN an alpha-blocker antihypertensive drug (p.897) and drug for prostate disorders (p.938)

PRECORTISYL a brand name for prednisolone

PREDENEMA a brand name for prednisolone

PREDFOAM a brand name for prednisolone

PREDNESOL a brand name for prednisolone

PREDNISOLONE a corticosteroid (p.930)

PREDSOL a brand name for prednisolone

PREDSOL-N a brand name for prednisolone and neomycin

PREGADAY a brand name for folic acid and iron

PREGNYL a brand name for human chorionic gonadotrophin

PREMARIN a brand name for conjugated oestrogens used in hormone replacement therapy (p.937)

PREMIQUE a brand-name preparation for menopausal problems (p.737) containing conjugated oestrogens and medroxyprogesterone

PREMPAK-C a brand-name preparation for menopausal problems (p.737) containing conjugated oestrogens and norgestrel

PREPADINE a brand name for dosulepin (dothiepin)

PRESCAL a brand name for isradipine

PRESERVEX a brand name for aceclofenac

PRESTIM a brand-name antihypertensive drug (p.897) containing timolol and bendroflumethiazide (bendrofluazide)

PRIADEL a brand name for lithium

PRILOCAINE a local anaesthetic (p.914)

PRIMALAN a brand name for mequitazine

PRIMAQUINE an antimalarial drug (p.888)

PRIMIDONE an anticonvulsant drug (p.914)

PRIMOLUT N a brand name for norethisterone

PRIMOTESTON DEPOT a brand name for testosterone

PRIMPERAN a brand name for metoclopramide

PRIODERM a brand name for malathion

PRIPSEN a brand-name anthelmintic drug (p.889) containing piperazine with senna

PRO-BANTHINE a brand name for propantheline

PROBENECID a drug used to prevent attacks of gout (p.380)

PROCAINAMIDE an antiarrhythmic drug (p.898)

PROCAINE a local anaesthetic (p.914)

PROCAINE BENZYLPENICILLIN (procaine penicillin) a penicillin antibiotic (p.885)

PROCAINE PENICILLIN *see* procaine benzylpenicillin

PROCARBAZINE an anticancer drug (p.907)

PROCHLORPERAZINE a phenothiazine antiemetic drug (p.922) and antipsychotic drug (p.917)

PROCTOFOAM HC a brand-name topical corticosteroid (p.892) containing pramocaine and hydrocortisone

PROCTOSEDYL a brand-name drug used to treat haemorrhoids (p.668) containing hydrocortisone and cinchocaine

PROCYCLIDINE an anticholinergic drug used to treat parkinsonism (*see* PARKINSON'S DISEASE AND PARKINSONISM, p.539)

PROFASI a brand name for chorionic gonadotrophin

PROFLEX a brand name for ibuprofen

PROGESTERONE a female sex hormone (*see* SEX HORMONES AND RELATED DRUGS, p.933)

PROGUANIL an antimalarial drug (p.888)

PROGYNOVA a brand name for estradiol

PROGYNOVA TS a brand name for estradiol

PROLUTON DEPOT a brand name for hydroxyprogesterone

PROMAZINE an antipsychotic drug (p.917)

PROMETHAZINE an antihistamine (p.906) and antiemetic drug (p.922)

PROMINAL a brand name for methylphenobarbital

PROPADERM a brand name for beclometasone

PROPAFENONE an antiarrhythmic drug (p.898)

PROPAIN a brand-name painkiller (p.912) containing codeine, diphenhydramine, paracetamol, and caffeine

PROPAMIDINE ISETHIONATE an antibiotic (p.885) used to treat eye infections (*see* DRUGS ACTING ON THE EYE, p.919)

PROPANIX a brand name for propranolol

PROPANTHELINE an anticholinergic antispasmodic drug (p.926), also used to treat urinary incontinence (*see* DRUGS THAT AFFECT BLADDER CONTROL, p.939)

PROPINE a brand name for dipivefrine

PROPIVERINE HYDROCHLORIDE a drug used to treat urinary incontinence (*see* DRUGS THAT AFFECT BLADDER CONTROL, p.939)

PRO-PLUS a brand name for caffeine

PROPOFOL a general anaesthetic (p.914)

PROPRANOLOL a beta-blocker drug (p.898)

PROPYLTHIOURACIL a drug for hyperthyroidism (p.932)

PROSCAR a brand name for finasteride

PROSTAGLANDIN a naturally occurring fatty acid that acts in a similar way to a hormone

PROTAMINE an antidote to heparin overdose

PROTHIADEN a brand name for dosulepin (dothiepin)

PROTIRELIN a drug used to assess thyroid function

PROTIUM a brand name for pantoprazole

PROTRIPTYLINE a tricyclic antidepressant (p.916)

PROVERA a brand name for medroxyprogesterone

PROVIGIL a brand name for modafinil

PRO-VIRON a brand name for mesterolone

PROXYMETACAINE a local anaesthetic (p.914)

PROZAC a brand name for fluoxetine

PROZIERE a brand name for prochlorperazine

PSEUDOEPHEDRINE a sympathomimetic decongestant (p.909)

PSORIN a brand-name preparation for psoriasis (p.332) containing dithranol, coal tar, and salicylic acid

PULMICORT a brand name for budesonide

PULMOZYME a brand name for dornase alfa

PUMACTANT a drug used to mature the lungs of premature babies with respiratory distress syndrome (*see* PROBLEMS OF THE PREMATURE BABY, p.816)

PURI-NETHOL a brand name for mercaptopurine

PYLORID a brand name for ranitidine bismuth citrate

PYRALVEX an anti-inflammatory drug used to treat mouth ulcers (p.632)

PYRAZINAMIDE an antituberculous drug (p.886)

PYRIDOSTIGMINE a drug used to treat myasthenia gravis (p.549)

PYRIDOXINE another name for vitamin B_6

PYRIMETHAMINE an antimalarial drug (p.888)

PYRITHIONE ZINC a drug used to treat dandruff (p.358)

Q

QUELLADA M a brand name for malathion

QUESTRAN a brand name for colestyramine

QUETIAPINE an antipsychotic drug (p.917)

QUINAGOLIDE a drug for infertility (p.936)

QUINAPRIL an ACE inhibitor drug (p.900)

QUINIDINE an antiarrhythmic drug (p.898)

QUININE an antimalarial drug (p.888) and muscle relaxant (p.896)

QUINOCORT a brand-name topical corticosteroid (p.892) containing hydrocortisone and potassium hydroxyquinoline sulphate

QUINODERM a brand-name preparation used to treat acne (p.340) containing benzoyl peroxide and potassium hydroxyquinoline sulphate

QUINOPED a brand-name antifungal drug (p.889) containing benzoyl peroxide and potassium hydroxyquinoline sulphate

R

RABEPRAZOLE SODIUM an ulcer-healing drug (p.923)

RADIAN-B a brand-name topical preparation for muscle aches and sprains

RALOXIFENE a drug used to prevent osteoporosis in postmenopausal women (*see* DRUGS FOR BONE DISORDERS, p.896)

RALTITREXED an anticancer drug (p.907)

RAMIPRIL an ACE inhibitor drug (p.900)

RANITIDINE an ulcer-healing drug (p.923)

RANITIDINE BISMUTH CITRATE an ulcer-healing drug (p.923)

RAPILYSIN a brand name for reteplase

RAPITARD MC a brand name for insulin

RAPITIL a brand name for nedocromil sodium

RAPPELL a brand name for piperonal

RAZOXANE a cytotoxic anticancer drug (p.907)

REBOXETINE an antidepressant drug (p.916)

REDOXON a brand name for vitamin C

REFOLINON a brand name for folinic acid

REGAINE a brand name for minoxidil, used to treat male-pattern baldness

REGULAN a brand name for ispaghula

REGULOSE a brand of lactulose

REHIDRAT a brand-name oral rehydration solution (p.926)

RELAXIT a brand-name laxative (p.924)

RELENZA a brand name for zanamivir

RELIFEX a brand name for nabumetone

REMEDEINE a brand-name painkiller (p.912) containing paracetamol and dihydrocodeine

REMIFENTANIL an opioid painkiller (p.912) used in general anaesthesia (*see* HAVING MAJOR SURGERY, p.943)

RENNIE DIGESTIF a brand-name antacid (p.923) containing calcium carbonate and magnesium carbonate

REPAGLINIDE a drug for diabetes mellitus (p.931)

REPROTEROL a bronchodilator drug (p.910)

REQUIP a brand name for ropinirole

RESOLVE a brand-name painkiller (p.912) and antacid (p.923)

RESORCINOL a drug used mainly to treat acne (p.340)

RESPACAL a brand name for tulobuterol

RESTANDOL a brand name for testosterone

RETEPLASE a thrombolytic drug (p.904)

RETIN-A a brand name for tretinoin

RETINOIC ACID a form of vitamin A and another name for tretinoin

RETINOIDS a form of vitamin A

RETINOL a form of vitamin A

RETINOVA a brand name for tretinoin

RETROVIR a brand name for zidovudine (AZT)

REVANIL a brand name for lisuride

RHEUMACIN LA a brand name for indometacin

RHEUMOX a brand name for azapropazone

RHINOCORT a brand name for budesonide

RHINOLAST a brand name for azelastine

RHUMALGAN a brand name for diclofenac

RIBAVIRIN (formerly tribavirin) an antiviral drug (p.886)

RIBOFLAVIN another name for vitamin B_2

RIDAURA a brand name for auranofin

RIDERIL a brand name for thioridazine

RIFABUTIN an antituberculous drug (p.886)

RIFADIN a brand name for rifampicin

RIFAMPICIN an antituberculous drug (p.886)

RIFATER a brand-name antituberculous drug (p.886) containing rifampicin, isoniazid, and pyrazinamide

RIFINAH a brand-name antituberculous drug (p.886) containing rifampicin and isoniazid

RILUTEK a brand name for riluzole

RILUZOLE a drug used to treat one form of motor neuron disease (p.540)

RIMACTANE a brand name for rifampicin

RIMOXALLIN a brand name for amoxicillin

RINATEC a brand name for ipratropium bromide

RISPERDAL a brand name for risperidone

RISPERIDONE an antipsychotic drug (p.917)

RITALIN a brand name for methylphenidate

RITODRINE a uterine muscle relaxant (*see* DRUGS FOR LABOUR, p.938)

RITONAVIR an antiviral drug used to treat HIV infection (*see* DRUGS FOR HIV INFECTION AND AIDS, p.887)

RITUXIMAB an anticancer drug (p.907)

RIVASTIGMINE a drug used to treat Alzheimer's disease (p.536)

RIVOTRIL a brand name for clonazepam

RIZATRIPTAN an antimigraine drug (p.913)

ROACCUTANE a brand name for isotretinoin

ROBAXIN a brand name for methocarbamol

ROBINUL-NEOSTIGMINE a brand name for neostigmine methylsulphate and glycopyrronium bromide

ROBITUSSIN DRY COUGH a brand name for guaifenesin

ROCALTROL a brand name for calcitriol

ROCURONIUM a muscle relaxant used in general anaesthesia (*see* HAVING MAJOR SURGERY, p.943)

ROFECOXIB a nonsteroidal anti-inflammatory drug (p.894)

ROFERON-A a brand name for interferon alfa

ROHYPNOL a brand name for flunitrazepam

ROMMIX a brand name for erythromycin

RONICOL a brand name for nicotinyl alcohol

ROPINIROLE a drug for parkinsonism (*see* PARKINSON'S DISEASE AND PARKINSONISM, p.539)

ROPIVACAINE a local anaesthetic (p.914) used for epidural anaesthesia

ROSIGLITAZONE a drug for diabetes mellitus (p.931)

ROTER a brand-name antacid (p.923) containing magnesium carbonate, sodium bicarbonate, frangula, and bismuth

ROWACHOL a brand-name preparation used to treat gallstones (p.651)

ROWATINEX a brand-name preparation used to treat kidney stones (p.701)

ROZEX a brand name for metronidazole

RYNACROM a brand name for sodium cromoglicate

RYNACROM COMPOUND a brand-name drug used to treat allergic rhinitis (p.466) containing sodium cromoglicate and xylometazoline

RYTHMODAN a brand name for disopyramide

S

SABRIL a brand name for vigabatrin

SAIZEN a brand name for somatropin

SALACTOL a brand-name treatment for warts (p.354) containing salicylic acid, lactic acid, and collodion

SALAGEN a brand name for pilocarpine

SALAMOL a brand name for salbutamol

SALATAC a brand-name treatment for warts (p.354) containing salicylic acid, lactic acid, and collodion

SALAZOPYRIN a brand name for sulfasalazine

SALBULIN a brand name for salbutamol

SALBUTAMOL a bronchodilator (p.910), also used in labour (*see* DRUGS FOR LABOUR, p.938)

SALCATONIN *see* calcitonin, salmon

SALICYLIC ACID a drug used to treat acne (p.340), dandruff (p.358), psoriasis (p.332), and warts (p.354)

SALIVACE a brand name for artificial saliva

SALIVA ORTHANA a brand name for artificial saliva

SALIVEZE a brand name for artificial saliva

SALIVIX a brand name for artificial saliva

SALMETEROL a sympathomimetic bronchodilator drug (p.910)

SALOFALK a brand name for mesalazine

SALURIC a brand name for chlorothiazide

SALZONE a brand name for paracetamol

SANDIMMUN a brand name for cyclosporin

SANDOCAL a brand name for calcium

SANDO-K a brand name for potassium

SANDOSTATIN a brand name for octreotide

SANOMIGRAN a brand name for pizotifen

SAQUINAVIR an antiviral drug used to treat HIV infection (*see* DRUGS FOR HIV INFECTION AND AIDS, p.887)

SAVENTRINE a brand name for isoprenaline

SAVLON a brand-name skin antiseptic (*see* PREPARATIONS FOR SKIN INFECTIONS AND INFESTATIONS, p.892) containing chlorhexidine and cetrimide

SCHERIPROCT a brand-name drug used to treat haemorrhoids (p.668) containing prednisolone and cinchocaine

SCOPODERM TTS a brand-name antiemetic drug (p.922) containing hyoscine

SEA-LEGS a brand name for meclozine

SECOBARBITAL a barbiturate sleeping drug (p.915)

SECONAL SODIUM a brand name for secobarbital

SECTRAL a brand name for acebutolol

SECURON SR a brand name for verapamil

SELEGILINE a drug used to treat severe parkinsonism (*see* PARKINSON'S DISEASE AND PARKINSONISM, p.539)

SELENIUM a mineral

SELENIUM SULPHIDE an antifungal drug (p.889) used to treat dandruff (p.358) and skin inflammation

SELSUN a brand-name dandruff shampoo (p.358) containing selenium sulphide

SEMPREX a brand name for acrivastine

SENNA a stimulant laxative (p.924)

SENOKOT a brand name for senna

SEPTANEST a brand name for articaine

SEPTRIN a brand name for co-trimoxazole

SERC a brand name for betahistine

SERDOLECT a brand name for sertindole

SERENACE a brand name for haloperidol

SEREVENT a brand name for salmeterol

SERMORELIN an agent used in the diagnosis of growth disorders

SEROPHENE a brand name for clomifene

SEROXAT a brand name for paroxetine

SERTINDOLE an antipsychotic drug (p.917)

SERTRALINE a selective serotonin reuptake inhibitor (SSRI) antidepressant (p.916)

SETLERS a brand-name antacid (p.923) containing calcium carbonate and magnesium hydroxide

SEVOFLURANE a general anaesthetic (p.914)

SEVREDOL a brand name for morphine

SILDENAFIL a drug for impotence (p.770)

SILVER NITRATE an antiseptic (*see* PREPARATIONS FOR SKIN INFECTIONS AND INFESTATIONS, p.892), an astringent, and a caustic substance

SILVER SULFADIAZINE a topical antibiotic (*see* PREPARATIONS FOR SKIN INFECTIONS AND INFESTATIONS, p.892) used to prevent infection in burns (p.318)

SIMECO a brand-name antacid (p.923) containing aluminium hydroxide, dimeticone, magnesium carbonate, and magnesium hydroxide

SIMPLENE a brand name for epinephrine (adrenaline)

SIMVASTATIN a lipid-lowering drug (p.935)

SINEMET a brand-name drug for parkinsonism (*see* PARKINSON'S DISEASE AND PARKINSONISM, p.539) containing levodopa and carbidopa

SINEQUAN a brand name for doxepin

SINGULAIR a brand name for montelukast

SINTHROME a brand name for acenocoumarol (nicoumalone)

SINUTAB a brand-name decongestant (p.909) containing paracetamol and phenylpropanolamine

SIOPEL a brand-name barrier cream (*see* BARRIER PREPARATIONS AND EMOLLIENTS, p.890) containing cetrimide and dimeticone

SKELID a brand name for tiludronic acid

SLO-INDO a brand name for indometacin

SLO-PHYLLIN a brand name for theophylline

SLOW-FE a brand name for ferrous sulphate

SLOW-K a brand name for potassium

SLOW-SODIUM a brand name for sodium chloride

SLOZEM a brand name for diltiazem

SNO PHENICOL a brand name for chloramphenicol

SNO TEARS a brand name for polyvinyl alcohol

SODA MINT TABLETS a preparation of sodium bicarbonate

SODIUM a mineral

SODIUM ACID PHOSPHATE a form of phosphorus used in laxatives (p.924) and to make urine more acidic

SODIUM AUROTHIOMALATE a gold-based antirheumatic drug (p.895)

SODIUM BICARBONATE an antacid (p.923), also used to soften earwax (*see* DRUGS ACTING ON THE EAR, p.921)

SODIUM CALCIUM EDETATE an antidote for poisoning by lead and other heavy metals (*see* DRUG OVERDOSE AND ACCIDENTAL INGESTION, p.321)

SODIUM CELLULOSE PHOSPHATE an agent used to reduce levels of calcium in the blood

SODIUM CHLORIDE common salt

SODIUM CITRATE a form of sodium used to to treat mild cystitis (p.709) and as a laxative (p.924)

SODIUM CLODRONATE a drug for bone disorders (p.896)

SODIUM CROMOGLICATE a mast cell stabilizer (*see* ANTI-ALLERGY DRUGS, p.905)

SODIUM FEREDETATE a form of iron

SODIUM FLUORIDE a mineral used to prevent dental caries (p.609)

SODIUM FUSIDATE an antibiotic (p.885)

SODIUM NITROPRUSSIDE an antihypertensive drug (p.897)

SODIUM PERBORATE an antiseptic (*see* PREPARATIONS FOR SKIN INFECTIONS AND INFESTATIONS, p.892)

SODIUM PICOSULFATE a stimulant laxative (p.924)

SODIUM STIBOGLUCONATE an antiprotozoal drug (p.888)

SODIUM TETRADECYL SULPHATE a drug used to treat varicose veins (p.438)

SODIUM VALPROATE an anticonvulsant (p.914), antimigraine(p.913), and mood-stabilizing drug (p.918)

SOFRADEX a brand-name topical preparation for eye or ear inflammation containing dexamethasone, framycetin, and gramicidin

SOLARCAINE a brand-name local anaesthetic (p.914) containing benzocaine and triclosan

SOLIAN a brand name for amisulpride

SOLPADEINE a brand-name painkiller (p.912) containing codeine, paracetamol, and caffeine

SOLPADOL a brand-name painkiller (p.912) containing paracetamol and codeine

SOLU-CORTEF a brand name for hydrocortisone

SOLU-MEDRONE a brand name for methylprednisolone

SOLVAZINC a brand name for zinc

SOMATROPIN a synthetic growth hormone (*see* PITUITARY DRUGS, p.934)

SOMATULINE a brand name for lanreotide

SOMINEX a brand-name sleeping drug (p.915) containing promethazine

SONERYL a brand name for butobarbital

SORBICHEW a brand name for isosorbide dinitrate

SORBID SA a brand name for isosorbide dinitrate

SORBITOL a sweetening agent, also used as a moisturizer in skin creams

SORBITRATE a brand name for isosorbide dinitrate

SOTACOR a brand name for sotalol

SOTALOL a beta-blocker drug (p.898)

SPASMONAL a brand name for alverine citrate

SPECTINOMYCIN an antibiotic (p.885)

SPECTRABAN a brand-name sunscreen (*see* SUNSCREENS AND SUNBLOCKS, p.893)

SPIRO-CO a brand-name diuretic drug (p.902) containing spironolactone and hydroflumethiazide

SPIROCTAN-M a brand name for canrenoate

SPIROLONE a brand name for spironolactone

SPIRONOLACTONE a potassium-sparing diuretic drug (p.902)

SPIROSPARE a brand name for spironolactone

SPORANOX a brand name for itraconazole

SPRILON a brand-name skin preparation (*see* EMOLLIENTS AND BARRIER PREPARATIONS, p.890) containing dimeticone and zinc oxide

STARIL a brand name for fosinopril

STAVUDINE an antiviral drug used to treat HIV infection (*see* DRUGS FOR HIV INFECTION AND AIDS, p.887)

STELAZINE a brand name for trifluoperazine

STEMETIL a brand name for prochlorperazine

STERCULIA a bulk-forming agent used as an antidiarrhoeal drug (p.924) and laxative (p.924)

STER-ZAC a brand name for triclosan

STESOLID a brand name for diazepam

STIEDEX a brand name for desoximetasone

STIEMYCIN a brand name for erythromycin

STILBOESTROL *see* diethylstilbestrol

STILNOCT a brand name for zolpidem

STIMLOR a brand name for naftidrofuryl

STREPSILS a brand-name antiseptic preparation for mouth and throat infections

STREPTASE a brand name for streptokinase

STREPTOKINASE a thrombolytic drug (p.904)

STREPTOMYCIN an antituberculous (p.886) and aminoglycoside antibiotic drug (p.885)

STUGERON a brand name for cinnarizine

SUCRALFATE an ulcer-healing drug (p.923)

SUDAFED a brand-name cold remedy (*see* COLD AND FLU REMEDIES, p.910) containing pseudoephedrine

SUDOCREM a brand-name skin preparation (*see* EMOLLIENTS AND BARRIER PREPARATIONS, p.890) containing benzyl benzoate and zinc oxide

SULCONAZOLE an antifungal drug (p.889)

SULEO-M a brand name for malathion

SULFACETAMIDE a sulphonamide antibiotic (p.885)

SULFADIAZINE a sulphonamide antibiotic (p.885)

SULFADIMIDINE a sulphonamide antibiotic (p.885)

SULFADOXINE an antimalarial drug (p.888) used with pyrimethamine

SULFAMETHOXAZOLE a sulphonamide antibiotic (p.885)

SULFAMETOPYRAZINE a sulphonamide antibiotic (p.885)

SULFASALAZINE an aminosalicylate (p.924) and antirheumatic drug (p.895)

SULFATHIAZOLE a sulphonamide antibiotic (p.885)

SULFINPYRAZONE a drug used to prevent attacks of gout (p.380)

SULINDAC a nonsteroidal anti-inflammatory drug (p.894)

SULPAREX a brand name for sulpiride

SULPHUR an ingredient in preparations used to treat acne (p.340) and dandruff (p.358)

SULPIRIDE an antipsychotic drug (p.917)

SULPITIL a brand name for sulpiride

SUMATRIPTAN an antimigraine drug (p.913)

SUPRANE a brand name for desflurane

SUPRAX a brand name for cefixime

SUPRECUR a brand name for buserelin

SUPREFACT a brand name for buserelin

SURGAM a brand name for tiaprofenic acid

SURMONTIL a brand name for trimipramine

SUSCARD a brand name for glyceryl trinitrate

SUSTAC a brand name for glyceryl trinitrate

SUSTANON a brand name for testosterone

SUSTIVA a brand name for efavirenz

SUXAMETHONIUM a muscle relaxant used in general anaesthesia (*see* HAVING MAJOR SURGERY, p.943)

SYNALAR a brand name for fluocinolone

SYNAREL a brand name for nafarelin

SYNDOL a brand-name painkiller (p.912) containing codeine, paracetamol, caffeine, and doxylamine

SYNFLEX a brand name for naproxen

SYNTARIS a brand name for flunisolide

SYNTOCINON a brand name for oxytocin

SYSCOR MR a brand name for nisoldipine

SYTRON a brand name for sodium feredetate

T

TACALCITOL a drug for psoriasis (p.332)

TACROLIMUS an immunosuppressant drug (p.906) used to prevent rejection of organ transplants

TAGAMET a brand name for cimetidine

TAMBOCOR a brand name for flecainide

TAMOFEN a brand name for tamoxifen

TAMOXIFEN an antioestrogen (*see* SEX HORMONES AND RELATED DRUGS, p.933) and a hormonal anticancer drug (p.907)

TAMPOVAGAN a brand-name topical oestrogen used in hormone replacement therapy (p.937) containing diethylstilboestrol and lactic acid

TAMSULOSIN an alpha-blocker drug for prostate disorders (p.938) and a drug that affects bladder control (p.939)

TANATRIL a brand name for imidapril

TARIVID a brand name for ofloxacin

TAVANIC a brand name for levofloxacin

TAVEGIL a brand name for clemastine

TAZAROTENE a retinoid drug (p.890) used to treat psoriasis (p.332)

TAZOBACTAM a drug given with penicillin to make it more effective

TCP LIQUID a brand-name antiseptic (*see* PREPARATIONS FOR SKIN INFECTIONS AND INFESTATIONS, p.892) containing phenol, chlorophenol, and 2-iodophenol

TEARS NATURALE a brand-name for hydroxypropyl methylcellulose

TEGRETOL a brand name for carbamazepine

TEICOPLANIN an antibiotic (p.885)

TELFAST a brand name for fexofenadine

TEMAZEPAM a benzodiazepine sleeping drug (p.915)

TEMODAL a brand name for temozolomide

TEMOZOLOMIDE an anticancer drug (p.907)

TENCHLOR a brand-name antihypertensive drug (p.897) containing atenolol and chlortalidone

TENIF a brand-name antihypertensive drug (p.897) containing atenolol and nifedipine

TENKICIN a brand name for phenoxymethylpenicillin

TENORET-50 a brand-name antihypertensive drug (p.897) containing atenolol and chlortalidone

TENORETIC a brand-name antihypertensive drug (p.897) containing atenolol and chlortalidone

TENORMIN a brand name for atenolol

TENOXICAM a nonsteroidal anti-inflammatory drug (p.894)

TENSIPINE MR a brand name for nifedipine

TENSIUM a brand name for diazepam

TEOPTIC a brand name for carteolol

TERAZOSIN an alpha-blocker antihypertensive (p.897), drug for prostate disorders (p.938), and drug that affects bladder control (p.939)

TERBINAFINE an antifungal drug (p.889)

TERBUTALINE a sympathomimetic bronchodilator (p.910) and uterine muscle relaxant (*see* DRUGS FOR LABOUR, p.938)

TERFENADINE an antihistamine (p.906)

TERFINAX a brand name for terfenadine

TERLIPRESSIN a drug similar to vasopressin, used to stop bleeding from the oesophagus

TERRA-CORTRIL a brand-name topical corticosteroid (p.892) containing hydrocortisone and oxytetracycline

TERRAMYCIN a brand name for oxytetracycline

TERTROXIN a brand name for liothyronine

TESTOSTERONE a male sex hormone (*see* SEX HORMONES AND RELATED DRUGS, p.933)

TETRABENAZINE a drug used to treat tremor

TETRACAINE (amethocaine) a local anaesthetic (p.914)

TETRACOSACTIDE a drug similar to corticotropin, used to assess adrenal-gland function

TETRACYCLINE an antibiotic (p.885) and antimalarial drug (p.888)

T-GEL a brand name for coal tar

THALIDOMIDE a drug used to treat Hansen's disease (p.302)

THEO-DUR a brand name for theophylline

THEOPHYLLINE a xanthine bronchodilator drug (p.910)

THIAMINE another name for vitamin B_1

THIOPENTAL a general anaesthetic (p.914)

THIORIDAZINE an antipsychotic drug (p.917)

THIOTEPA a cytotoxic anticancer drug (p.907)

THYMOXAMINE *see* moxisylyte

THYROID HORMONES synthetic hormones used to treat hypothyroidism (p.932)

THYROXINE *see* levothyroxine

TIABENDAZOLE an anthelmintic drug (p.889)

TIAGABINE an anticonvulsant drug (p.914)

TIAPROFENIC ACID a nonsteroidal anti-inflammatory drug (p.894)

TIBOLONE a female sex hormone (*see* SEX HORMONES AND RELATED DRUGS, p.933), a drug for bone disorders (p.896), and a drug used in hormone replacement therapy (p.937)

TICARCILLIN a penicillin antibiotic (p.885)

TICLID a brand name for ticlopidine

TICLOPIDINE an antiplatelet drug (*see* DRUGS THAT PREVENT BLOOD CLOTTING, p.904)

TILADE a brand name for nedocromil sodium

TILDIEM a brand name for diltiazem

TILORYTH a brand name for erythromycin

TILUDRONIC ACID a drug for bone disorders (p.896)

TIMECEF a brand name for cefodizime

TIMODINE a brand-name topical corticosteroid (p.892) containing hydrocortisone, nystatin, benzalkonium chloride, and dimeticone

TIMOLOL a beta-blocker drug (p.898) and drug for glaucoma (p.920)

TIMOPTOL a brand name for timolol

TIMPRON a brand name for naproxen

TINADERM-M a brand-name antifungal drug (p.889) containing nystatin and tolnaftate

TINIDAZOLE an antibiotic (p.885) and antiprotozoal drug (p.888)

TINZAPARIN a type of heparin

TIOCONAZOLE an antifungal drug (p.889)

TIOGUANINE a cytotoxic anticancer drug (p.907)

TIROFIBAN a drug that prevents myocardial infarction (p.410)

TISSUE PLASMINOGEN ACTIVATOR a thrombolytic drug (p.904)

TITRALAC a brand-name drug used to remove excess phosphate from the blood

TIXYLIX a brand-name cough remedy (p.909) containing pholcodine and promethazine

TOBRAMYCIN an aminoglycoside antibiotic (p.885)

TOCOPHEROL a form of vitamin E

TOCOPHERYL a form of vitamin E

TOFRANIL a brand name for imipramine

TOLANASE a brand name for tolazamide

TOLAZAMIDE an oral drug for diabetes mellitus (p.931)

TOLBUTAMIDE an oral drug for diabetes mellitus (p.931)

TOLFENAMIC ACID an antimigraine drug (p.913)

TOLNAFTATE an antifungal drug (p.889)

TOLTERODINE an anticholinergic drug (*see* DRUGS THAT AFFECT BLADDER CONTROL, p.939) used to treat urinary incontinence (p.710)

TOPAL a brand-name antacid (p.923) containing aluminium hydroxide, magnesium carbonate, and alginic acid

TOPAMAX a brand name for topiramate

TOPIRAMATE an anticonvulsant drug (p.914)

TOPOTECAN an anticancer drug (p.907)

TORADOL a brand name for ketorolac

TORASEMIDE a loop diuretic drug (p.902)

TOREM a brand name for torasemide

TOREMIFENE an anticancer drug (p.907)

TRAMADOL an opioid painkiller (p.912)

TRAMAZOLINE a decongestant (p.909)

TRAMIL a brand-name painkiller (p.912) containing paracetamol and caffeine

TRAMIL 500 a brand name for paracetamol

TRANDATE a brand name for labetalol

TRANDOLAPRIL an ACE inhibitor drug (p.900)

TRANEXAMIC ACID an antifibrinolytic drug (*see* DRUGS THAT PROMOTE BLOOD CLOTTING, p.903)

TRANSIDERM-NITRO a brand name for glyceryl trinitrate

TRANSVASIN a brand name for topical treatments for muscle and joint pain

TRANXENE a brand name for clorazepate

TRANYLCYPROMINE a monoamine oxidase inhibitor (MAOI) antidepressant (p.916)

TRASICOR a brand name for oxprenolol

TRAVOGYN a brand name for isoconazole

TRAXAM a brand name for felbinac

TRAZODONE an antidepressant drug (p.916)

TRENTAL a brand name for pentoxifylline (oxpentifylline)

TREOSULFAN an anticancer drug (p.907)

TRETINOIN a retinoid drug (p.890) used to treat acne (p.340)

TRI-ADCORTYL a brand-name topical corticosteroid (p.892) containing nystatin, triamcinolone, gramicidin, and neomycin

TRIADENE a brand-name oral contraceptive (*see* CONTRACEPTION, p.69) containing ethinylestradiol and gestodene

TRIAMAXCO a brand-name diuretic drug (p.902) containing triamterene and hydrochlorothiazide

TRIAMCINOLONE a corticosteroid (p.930)

TRIAMTERENE a potassium-sparing diuretic drug (p.902)

TRIBAVIRIN *see* ribavirin

TRICLOFOS a sleeping drug (p.915)

TRICLOSAN an antiseptic (*see* PREPARATIONS FOR SKIN INFECTIONS AND INFESTATIONS, p.892)

TRIDESTRA a brand-name preparation for menopausal problems (p.737) containing estradiol and medroxyprogesterone

TRIENTINE a drug used to treat Wilson's disease, a metabolic disorder

TRIFLUOPERAZINE a phenothiazine antipsychotic drug (p.917) and antiemetic drug (p.922)

TRIFYBA a brand name for a bulk-forming laxative (p.924) containing bran

TRIHEXYPHENIDYL (benzhexol) an anticholinergic drug used to treat parkinsonism (*see* PARKINSON'S DISEASE AND PARKINSONISM, p.539)

TRI-IODOTHYRONINE *see* liothyronine

TRILOSTANE an adrenal antagonist used to treat Cushing's syndrome (p.684) and breast cancer (p.759)

TRILUDAN a brand name for terfenadine

TRIMEPRAZINE *see* alimemazine

TREMETAPHAN a drug used to lower blood pressure below normal during surgery (*see* HAVING MAJOR SURGERY, p.943)

TRIMETHOPRIM an antibiotic (p.885)

TRIMETREXATE a drug used to treat *Pneumocystis carinii* pneumonia in people with AIDS (*see* HIV INFECTION AND AIDS, p.297)

TRI-MINULET a brand-name oral contraceptive (*see* CONTRACEPTION, p.69) containing ethinylestradiol and gestodene

TRIMIPRAMINE a tricyclic antidepressant (p.916)

TRIMOGAL a brand name for trimethoprim

TRIMOVATE a brand-name topical corticosteroid (p.892) containing clobetasone, nystatin, and oxytetracycline

TRINORDIOL a brand-name oral contraceptive (*see* CONTRACEPTION, p.69) containing ethinylestradiol and levonorgestrel

TRINOVUM a brand-name oral contraceptive (*see* CONTRACEPTION, p.69) containing ethinylestradiol and norethisterone

TRIOGESIC a brand-name cold remedy (*see* COLD AND FLU REMEDIES, p.910) containing paracetamol and phenylpropanolamine

TRIOMINIC a brand-name cough remedy (p.909) containing phenylpropanolamine and pheniramine

TRIPOTASSIUM DICITRATOBISMUTHATE an ulcer-healing drug (p.923)

TRIPRIMIX a brand name for trimethoprim

TRIPROLIDINE an antihistamine (p.906)

TRIPTAFEN a brand-name antidepressant (p.916) containing amitriptyline and perphenazine

TRIPTORELIN an anticancer drug (p.907)

TRISEQUENS a brand-name preparation for menopausal problems (p.737) containing estradiol and norethisterone

TRISODIUM EDETATE a drug to remove excess calcium from the blood

TRITACE a brand name for ramipril

TROBICIN a brand name for spectinomycin

TROPERGEN a brand-name antidiarrhoeal drug (p.924) containing diphenoxylate and atropine

TROPICAMIDE a mydriatic drug used in eye examinations (*see* DRUGS ACTING ON THE EYE, p.919)

TROPISETRON an antiemetic drug (p.922)

TROSYL a brand name for tioconazole

TRUSOPT a brand name for dorzolamide

TRYPTIZOL a brand name for amitriptyline

TRYPTOPHAN an antidepressant drug (p.916)

TUINAL a brand-name sleeping drug (p.915) containing amobarbital and secobarbital

TULOBUTEROL a bronchodilator (p.910)

TYLEX a brand-name painkiller (p.912) containing codeine and paracetamol

TYROZETS a brand-name throat antiseptic containing benzocaine and tyrothricin

U

UBRETID a brand name for distigmine

UCERAX a brand name for hydroxyzine

UKIDAN a brand name for urokinase

ULTEC a brand name for cimetidine

ULTRALANUM PLAIN a brand name for fluocortolone

ULTRAPROCT a brand-name drug used to treat haemorrhoids (p.668) containing cinchocaine and fluocortolone

UNDECENOIC ACID an antifungal drug (p.889) used to treat athlete's foot (p.353)

UNIFLU a brand-name cold and flu remedy (p.910) containing codeine, diphenhydramine, paracetamol, phenylephrine, and caffeine

UNIGEST a brand-name antacid (p.923) containing aluminium hydrochloride and dimeticone

UNIHEP a brand name for heparin

UNIPARIN a brand name for heparin

UNIPHYLLIN CONTINUS a brand name for theophylline

UNIROID HC a brand-name drug used to treat haemorrhoids (p.668) containing cinchocaine and hydrocortisone

UNIVER a brand name for verapamil

UREA a topical treatment used to moisturize dry skin and soften earwax (*see* DRUGS ACTING ON THE EAR, p.921)

URIBEN a brand name for nalidixic acid

URISPAS a brand name for flavoxate

UROFOLLITROPIN a drug for infertility (p.936)

UROKINASE a thrombolytic drug (p.904)

URSODEOXYCHOLIC ACID a drug used to treat gallstones (p.651)

URSOFALK a brand name for ursodeoxycholic acid

UTINOR a brand name for norfloxacin

UTOVLAN a brand name for norethisterone

V

VAGIFEM a brand name for estradiol

VAGINYL a brand name for metronidazole

VALACICLOVIR an antiviral drug (p.886)

VALCLAIR a brand name for diazepam

VALIUM a brand name for diazepam

VALLERGAN a brand name for alimemazine (trimeprazine)

VALOID a brand name for cyclizine

VALPROIC ACID an anticonvulsant drug (p.914)

VALSARTAN an antihypertensive drug (p.897)

VALTREX a brand name for valaciclovir

VANCOCIN a brand name for vancomycin

VANCOMYCIN an antibiotic (p.885)

VAQTA a brand-name vaccine (*see* VACCINES AND IMMUNOGLOBULINS, p.883) used to protect against viral hepatitis A

VARIDASE a brand-name preparation used to treat leg ulcers (p.350)

VASCACE a brand name for cilazapril

VASODILATOR a drug that is used to widen blood vessels and increase blood flow

VASOGEN a brand-name barrier cream (*see* EMOLLIENTS AND BARRIER PREPARATIONS, p.890) containing calamine, dimeticone, and zinc oxide

VASOPRESSIN a pituitary hormone (*see* PITUITARY DRUGS, p.934)

VECTAVIR a brand name for penciclovir

VECURONIUM a muscle relaxant used in general anaesthesia (*see* HAVING MAJOR SURGERY, p.943)

VEGANIN a brand-name painkiller (p.912) containing aspirin, paracetamol, and codeine

VELBE a brand name for vinblastine

VELOSEF a brand name for cefradine

VELOSULIN a brand name for insulin

VENLAFAXINE an antidepressant drug (p.916)

VENOFER a brand-name iron supplement (*see* MINERALS, p.929)

VENTMAX SR a brand name for salbutamol

VENTODISKS a brand name for salbutamol

VENTOLIN a brand name for salbutamol

VERACUR a brand name for formaldehyde

VERAPAMIL a calcium channel blocker drug (p.900) and antiarrhythmic drug (p.898)

VERMOX a brand name for mebendazole

VERRUGON a brand name for salicylic acid

VESAGEX a brand-name antiseptic (*see* PREPARATIONS FOR SKIN INFECTIONS AND INFESTATIONS, p.892) containing cetrimide

VESANOID a brand name for tretinoin

VIAGRA a brand name for sildenafil

VIAZEM XL a brand name for diltiazem

VIBRAMYCIN a brand name for doxycycline

VICKS COLD CARE a brand-name cold remedy (*see* COLD AND FLU REMEDIES, p.910) containing paracetamol, dextromethorphan, and phenylpropanolamine

VICKS MEDINITE a brand-name cold remedy (*see* COLD AND FLU REMEDIES, p.910) containing paracetamol, dextromethorphan, and pseudoephedrine

VIDENE a brand name for povidone-iodine

VIDEX (ddI) a brand name for didanosine

VIGABATRIN an anticonvulsant drug (p.914)

VIGRANON B a brand name for vitamin B complex

VILOXAZINE a tricyclic antidepressant (p.916)

VINBLASTINE a cytotoxic anticancer drug (p.907)

VINCRISTINE a cytotoxic anticancer drug (p.907)

VINDESINE a cytotoxic anticancer drug (p.907)

VINORELBINE a cytotoxic anticancer drug (p.907)

VIOFORM–HYDROCORTISONE a brand-name topical corticosteroid (p.892) containing hydrocortisone and clioquinol

VIOXX a brand name for rofecoxib

VIRACEPT a brand name for nelfinavir

VIRAFERON a brand name for interferon alfa

VIRAMUNE a brand name for nevirapine

VIRAZID a brand name for tribavirin

VIRIDAL a brand name for alprostadil

VIRORMONE a brand name for testosterone

VISCLAIR a brand name for mecysteine

VISCOTEARS a brand-name artificial tears preparation (*see* DRUGS ACTING ON THE EYE, p.919)

VISKALDIX a brand-name antihypertensive drug (p.897) containing pindolol and clopamide

VISKEN a brand name for pindolol

VISTA-METHASONE a brand name for betamethasone

VISTIDE a brand name for cidofovir

VITAMIN A a vitamin (p.927)

VITAMIN B COMPLEX a group of vitamins (p.927)

VITAMIN B_1 a vitamin (p.927)

VITAMIN B_3 a vitamin (p.927)

VITAMIN B_6 a vitamin (p.927)

VITAMIN B_{12} a vitamin (p.927)

VITAMIN C a vitamin (p.927)

VITAMIN D a vitamin (p.927)

VITAMIN E a vitamin (p.927)

VITAMIN H a member of the vitamin B complex

VITAMIN K a vitamin (p.927)

VIVALAN a brand name for viloxazine

VIVAPRYL a brand name for selegiline

VOLMAX a brand name for salbutamol

VOLRAMAN a brand name for diclofenac

VOLTAROL a brand name for diclofenac

W

WARFARIN an oral anticoagulant (*see* DRUGS THAT PREVENT BLOOD CLOTTING, p.904)

WARTICON a brand name for podophyllotoxin

WASPEZE a brand-name topical antihistamine (p.906) used to treat insect bites and stings

WAXSOL a brand name for docusate

WELLDORM ELIXIR a brand name for chloral hydrate

WELLDORM TABLETS a brand name for cloral betaine

WELLFERON a brand name for interferon

WELLVONE a brand name for atovaquone

WITCH HAZEL an astringent used in topical and rectal preparations

WOODWARD'S GRIPE WATER a brand-name preparation for wind pain in infants containing sodium bicarbonate and dill

X

XALATAN a brand name for latanoprost

XAMOTEROL a drug for mild chronic heart failure (p.413)

XANAX a brand name for alprazolam

XATRAL a brand name for alfuzosin

XENICAL a brand name for orlistat

XIPAMIDE a thiazide-like diuretic (p.902)

XYLOCAINE a brand name for lidocaine (lignocaine)

XYLOMETAZOLINE a decongestant (p.909)

XYLOPROCT a brand-name preparation used to treat haemorrhoids (p.668) containing hydrocortisone, aluminium acetate, lidocaine (lignocaine), and zinc oxide

Y

YOMESAN a brand name for niclosamide

YUTOPAR a brand name for ritodrine

Z

ZADITEN a brand name for ketotifen

ZAFIRLUKAST a leukotriene antagonist (*see* ANTIALLERGY DRUGS, p.905)

ZALCITABINE (ddC) an antiviral drug used to treat HIV infection (*see* DRUGS FOR HIV INFECTION AND AIDS, p.887)

ZAMADOL a brand name for tramadol

ZANAMIVIR an antiviral drug (p.886)

ZANIDIP a brand name for lercanidipine

ZANTAC a brand name for ranitidine

ZARONTIN a brand name for ethosuximide

ZENAPAX a brand name for daclizumab

ZERIT a brand name for stavudine

ZESTORETIC a brand-name antihypertensive drug (p.897) containing lisinopril and hydrochlorothiazide

ZESTRIL a brand name for lisinopril

ZIDOVUDINE (AZT) an antiviral drug used to treat HIV infection (*see* DRUGS FOR HIV INFECTION AND AIDS, p.887)

ZIMOVANE a brand name for zopiclone

ZINACEF a brand name for cefuroxime

ZINAMIDE a brand name for pyrazinamide

ZINC a mineral (p.929)

ZINCOMED a brand name for zinc

ZINC OXIDE an astringent and soothing agent (*see* EMOLLIENTS AND BARRIER PREPARATIONS, p.890)

ZINC PYRITHIONE an antimicrobial with antibacterial and antifungal properties, used to treat dandruff (p.358)

ZINC SULPHATE a form of zinc

ZINERYT a brand-name preparation used to treat acne (p.340) containing erythromycin and zinc

ZINNAT a brand name for cefuroxime

ZIRTEK a brand name for cetirizine

ZISPIN a brand name for mirtazapine

ZITA a brand name for cimetidine

ZITHROMAX a brand name for azithromycin

ZOCOR a brand name for simvastatin

ZOFRAN a brand name for ondansetron

ZOLADEX a brand name for goserelin

ZOLEPTIL a brand name for zotepine

ZOLMITRIPTAN an antimigraine drug (p.913)

ZOLPIDEM a sleeping drug (p.915)

ZOMACTON a brand name for somatropin

ZOMIG a brand name for zolmitriptan

ZOPICLONE a sleeping drug (p.915)

ZOTEPINE an antipsychotic drug (p.917)

ZOVIRAX a brand name for aciclovir

Z SPAN a brand name for zinc

ZUCLOPENTHIXOL an antipsychotic (p.917)

ZUMENON a brand name for estradiol

ZYDOL a brand name for tramadol

ZYLORIC a brand name for allopurinol

ZYPREXA a brand name for olanzapine

USEFUL ONLINE SITES AND ADDRESSES

To make informed decisions about your health, you need to have as much information as possible. Recently, many more easily accessible resources have become available to increase your awareness of health issues, enable you to make the best use of the health-care system, and deal effectively with health professionals.

Hundreds of associations and organizations throughout the UK are dedicated to helping people deal with medical and emotional conditions. Sources of information range from government agencies such as the Department of Health to nonprofit organizations such as the Red Cross. Only a limited sample could be included in this list. Most listings are the headquarters of national groups and organizations. Information on a wide range of such organizations is usually available from libraries as well as from your local hospital and your own GP or health clinic.

The sources are listed under broad headings and are in alphabetical order within these categories. The name of each organization is followed by its online and postal addresses, telephone numbers, and e-mail address if available. Most organizations provide information about resources for the management of specific conditions. Many have support groups to help people with a medical or emotional condition, or they can provide information about local groups in your area. Online sites are given for the UK self-help groups and for some of the most useful US sites. Most online sites provide links to related sites.

No responsibility for information provided by the organizations listed or for the content of their online sites can be accepted by the British Medical Association (BMA). The inclusion of a site in this listing does not indicate endorsement by the BMA, and you are advised always to consult your doctor for specific information on personal health matters.

GENERAL INFORMATION

BBC Education: The Health Site
Online: www.bbc.co.uk//education/health

BBC Online Health and Fitness
Online: www.bbc.co.uk/health

British Medical Association
Online: www.bma.org.uk
BMA House
Tavistock Square
London WC1H 9JP
Tel: (020) 7387 4499
E-mail: smanley@bma.org.uk

Centers for Disease Control and Prevention (US)
Online: www.cdc.gov

Department of Health
Online: www.doh.gov.uk
Richmond House
79 Whitehall
London SW1A 2NS
Tel: (020) 7210 4850

eBMJ (Electronic British Medical Journal)
Online: www.bmj.com

Eurohealth
Online: www.eurohealth.org

Food and Drug Administration (US)
Online: www.fda.gov

Health Education Authority
Online: www.hea.org.uk

Health Education Board for Scotland
Online: www.hebs.scot.nhs.uk

Healthnet
Online: www.healthnet.org.uk

Health Information Service
Tel: 0800 665544

Medic Alert Foundation
Online: www.medicalert.co.uk
1 Bridge Wharf
156 Caledonian Road
London N1 9UU
Tel: (020) 7833 3034

Medicines Control Agency
Online: www.open.gov.uk/mca
Market Towers
1 Nine Elms Lane
London SW8 5NQ
Tel: (020) 7273 0000
E-mail: info@mca.gov.uk

National Institutes of Health (US)
Online: www.nih.gov

NHS Direct Online
Online: www.nhsdirect.nhs.uk

Office of Rare Diseases (US)
Online: rarediseases.info.nih.gov/ord

Patient UK
Online: www.patient.co.uk
E-mail: info@patient.co.uk

Royal College of General Practitioners
Online: www.rcgp.org.uk
14 Princes Gate
Hyde Park
London SW7 1PU
Tel: (020) 7581 3232
E-mail: info@rcgp.org.uk

Self Help UK
Online: www.self-help.org.uk

UK Healthcare Centre
Online: www.healthcentre.org.uk

Wired for Health
Online: www.wiredforhealth.gov.uk

World Health Organization
Online: www.who.int

AGING

Age Concern
Online: www.ace.org.uk
1268 London Road
London SW16 4ER
Tel: (020) 8765 7200
E-mail: ace@ace.org.uk

Centre for Policy on Ageing
Online: www.cpa.org.uk
25–31 Ironmonger Row
London EC1V 3QP
Tel: (020) 7253 1787
E-mail: cpa@cpa.org.uk

Help the Aged
Online: www.helptheaged.org.uk
St. James's Walk
London EC1R 0BE
Tel: (020) 7253 0253
E-mail: info@helptheaged.org.uk

See also ALZHEIMER'S DISEASE, HOME CARE

AIDS

See HIV INFECTION AND AIDS

ALCOHOL-RELATED PROBLEMS

Addiction Recovery Foundation
Online: easyweb.easynet.co.uk/acw
122A Wilton Road
London SW1V 1JZ
Tel: (020) 7233 5333
E-mail: acw@easynet.co.uk

Al-Anon Family Groups
Online: www.hexnet.co.uk/alanon
61 Great Dover Street
London SE1 4YF
Helpline: (020) 7403 0888
E-mail: alanonuk@aol.com

Alcohol Concern
Online: www.alcoholconcern.org.uk
Waterbridge House
32–36 Loman Street
London SE1 0EE
Tel: (020) 7928 7377
E-mail: ac@ccon.dircon.co.uk

Alcoholics Anonymous
Online: www.alcoholics-anonymous.org.uk
PO Box 1
Stonebow House
Stonebow Road
York YO1 2NJ
Helpline: (020) 7833 0022
Tel: (01904) 644026

Drinkline
Helpline: 0800 917 8282

Drinksense
Online: www.gurney.co.uk/drinksense
79A Eastfield Road
Peterborough PE1 4AS
Tel: (01733) 347105
E-mail: drinksense@netcom.co.uk

Institute of Alcohol Studies
Online: www.ias.org.uk
1 The Quay
St. Ives
Cambridgeshire PE17 4AR
Tel: (01480) 466766
E-mail: info@ias.org.uk

National Association for Children of Alcoholics
PO Box 64
Fishponds
Bristol BS16 2UH
Helpline: 0800 289061
Tel: (0117) 957 3432

See also COUNSELLING AND PSYCHOLOGICAL THERAPIES, CRISIS SUPPORT, DRUG-RELATED PROBLEMS, LIVER DISORDERS

ALLERGY AND ASTHMA

Anaphylaxis Campaign
Online: www.anaphylaxis.org.uk
PO Box 149
Fleet
Hampshire GU13 9XU
Tel: (01252) 542029

Asthma and Allergy Foundation of America (US)
Online: www.aafa.org

Asthma and Allergy Information and Research
Online: www.users.globalnet.co.uk/~aair
Leicester General Hospital
Leicester LE5 4PW
Tel: (0116) 270 7557
E-mail: aair@globalnet.co.uk

British Allergy Foundation
Online: www.allergyfoundation.com
30 Bellegrove Road
Welling
Kent DA16 3PY
Helpline: (0189) 516500
Tel: (020) 8303 8525

European Federation of Asthma and Allergy Associations
Online: www.efanet.org

National Asthma Campaign
Online: www.asthma.org.uk
Providence House
Providence Place
London N1 0NT
Helpline: 0845 701 0203
Tel: (020) 7226 2260

See also IMMUNE DISORDERS, LUNG DISEASE, SKIN DISORDERS

ALZHEIMER'S DISEASE

Alzheimer Scotland – Action on Dementia
Online: www.alzscot.org
22 Drumsheugh Gardens
Edinburgh EH3 7RN
Tel: (0131) 243 1453
E-mail: alzheimer@alzscot.org

Alzheimer's Disease Society
Online: www.alzheimers.org.uk
10 Greencoat Place
London SW1P 1PH
Helpline: 0845 300 0336
Tel: (020) 7306 0606
E-mail: info@alzheimers.org.uk

See also AGING, HOME CARE

ARTHRITIS

Arthritis Care
Online: www.arthritiscare.org.uk
18 Stephenson Way
London NW1 2HD
Tel: (020) 7916 1500
E-mail: info@arc.org.uk

Arthritis Link
Online: www.arthritislink.com

Arthritis Research Campaign
Online: www.arc.org.uk
Copeman House
St Mary's Court
St Mary's Gate
Chesterfield
Derbyshire S41 7TD
Tel: (01246) 558033
E-mail: info@arc.org.uk

See also MUSCULOSKELETAL DISORDERS, RHEUMATIC DISORDERS

BACK PAIN

BackCare
Online: www.backpain.org
16 Elmtree Road
Teddington
Middlesex TW11 8ST
Tel: (020) 8977 5474
E-mail: back_pain@compuserve.com

See also COMPLEMENTARY THERAPIES, MUSCULOSKELETAL DISORDERS

BIRTH DEFECTS

Association for Spina Bifida and Hydrocephalus
Online: www.asbah.demon.co.uk
42 Park Road
Peterborough PE1 2UQ
Tel: (01733) 555988
E-mail: postmaster@asbah.demon.co.uk

Association of Birth Defect Children (US)
Online: www.birthdefects.org

Birth Defects Foundation
Online: www.birthdefects.co.uk
Martindale
Hawks Green
Cannock
Staffordshire WS11 2XN
Tel: (01543) 468888
E-mail: enquiries@birthdefects.co.uk

Spina Bifida Association of America (US)
Online: www.sbaa.org

See also GENETIC DISORDERS

BLINDNESS

See EYE AND VISION PROBLEMS

BLOOD DISORDERS

Anthony Nolan Bone Marrow Trust
Online: www.anthonynolan.com
Unit 2
Heathgate Buildings
75–87 Agincourt Road
London NW3 2NT
Tel: (020) 7284 1234

Haemophilia Society
Online: www.haemophilia.org.uk
385 Euston Road
London NW1 3AU
Helpline: 0800 018 6068
Tel: (020) 7380 0600
E-mail: info@haemophilia.org.uk

Leukaemia CARE
Online: www.leukaemiacare.org
14 Kingfisher Court
Venny Bridge
Pinhoe
Exeter
Devon EX4 8JN
Tel: 0345 673203
E-mail: support@leukaemiacare.org

Leukaemia Research Fund
Online: www.leukaemia.demon.co.uk
43 Great Ormond Street
London WC1N 3JJ
Tel: (020) 7405 0101
E-mail: info@leukaemia-research.org.uk

National Heart, Lung, and Blood Institute Information Center (US)
Online: www.nhlbi.nih.gov

Patient UK
Online: www.patient.co.uk
E-mail: info@patient.co.uk

Sickle Cell Society
Online: www.sicklecellsociety.org
54 Station Road
Harlesden
London NW10 4UA
Tel: (020) 8961 4006/7795

UK Thalassaemia Society
Online: www.ukts.org
19 The Broadway
Southgate Circus
London N14 6PH
Tel: (020) 8882 0011
E-mail: office@ukts.org

See also CANCER, GENETIC DISORDERS

BRAIN TUMOURS

American Brain Tumor Association (US)
Online: www.abta.org

Brain Tumour Action
30 Woodburn Terrace
Edinburgh EH10 4SS
Tel: (0131) 466 0236

Brain Tumour Foundation
PO Box 162
New Malden
Surrey KT3 3YN
Tel: (020) 8336 2020

British Brain Tumour Association
2 Oakfield Road
Hightown
Merseyside L38 9GQ
Tel: (0151) 929 3229

National Brain Tumor Foundation (US)
Online: www.braintumor.org

See also NEUROLOGICAL DISORDERS

BREAST CANCER

Action Against Breast Cancer
Online: www.aabc.org.uk
C2
Culham Science Centre
Oxfordshire OX14 3DB
Tel: (01865) 407384
E-mail: info@aabc.org.uk

Breakthrough Breast Cancer
Online: www.breakthrough.org.uk
6th Floor
Kingsway House
103 Kingsway
London WC2B 6QX
Tel: (020) 7405 5111
E-mail: info@breakthrough.org.uk

Breast Cancer Campaign
Online: www.bcc-uk.org
29–33 Scrutton Street
London EC2A 4HU
Tel: (020) 7749 3700

Breast Cancer Care
Online: www.breastcancercare.org.uk
210 New Kings Road
London SW6 4NZ
Helpline: 0808 800 6000
Tel: (020) 7384 2984
E-mail: bcc@breastcancercare.org.uk

UK Breast Cancer Awareness Campaign
Online: hosted.aware.easynet.co.uk

See also WOMEN'S HEALTH

CANCER

American Cancer Society (US)
Online: www.cancer.org

CancerBACUP
Online: www.cancerbacup.org.uk
3 Bath Place
Rivington Street
London EC2A 3DR
Tel: (020) 7696 9003
E-mail: info@cancerbacup.org

Cancer Care Society
Online: www.cancercaresoc.demon.co.uk
11 The Cornmarket
Romsey
Hampshire SO51 8GB
Tel: (01794) 830300
E-mail: info@cancercaresoc.demon.co.uk

Cancer Research Campaign
Online: www.crc.org.uk
10 Cambridge Terrace
London NW1 4JL
Tel: (020) 7224 1333
E-mail: crcinformation@crc.org.uk

Imperial Cancer Research Fund
Online: www.icnet.uk
PO Box 123
Lincoln's Inn Fields
London WC2 3PX
Tel: (020) 7242 0200

Institute of Cancer Research
Online: www.icr.ac.uk
D Block
15 Cotswold Road
Sutton
Surrey SM2 5NG
Tel: (020) 8643 8901
E-mail: lindy@icr.ac.uk

Macmillan Cancer Relief
Online: www.macmillan.org.uk
15–19 Britten Street
London SW3 3TZ
Helpline: 0845 601 6161
Tel: (020) 7351 7811
E-mail: information_line@macmillan.org.uk

Marie Curie Cancer Care
Online: www.mariecurie.org.uk
28 Belgrave Square
London SW1X 8QG
Tel: (020) 7201 2342
E-mail: info@mariecurie.org.uk

Oncolink (US)
Online: cancer.med.upenn.edu

See also BLOOD DISORDERS, BRAIN TUMOURS, BREAST CANCER, CHILDREN'S HEALTH, LUNG DISORDERS, DIGESTIVE DISORDERS, MEN'S HEALTH, PAIN RELIEF, PROSTATE DISORDERS, SKIN DISORDERS, WOMEN'S HEALTH

CHILD ABUSE AND NEGLECT

Childline
Online: www.childline.org.uk
Freepost 1111
London N1 0BR
Helpline: 0800 1111
Tel: (020) 7239 1000

The Children's Society
Online: www.the-childrens-society.org.uk
Edward Rudolf House
Margery Street
London WC1X 0JL
Tel: (020) 7841 4436
E-mail: info@the-childrens-society.org.uk

National Children's Bureau
Online: www.ncb.org.uk
8 Wakley Street
London EC1V 7QE
Tel: (020) 7843 6000

NCH Action for Children
Online: www.nchafc.org.uk
85 Highbury Park
London N5 1UD
Tel: (020) 7226 2033
E-mail: webcontact@mail.nchafc.org.uk

NSPCC
Online: www.nspcc.org.uk
42 Curtain Road
London EC2A 3HN
Helpline: 0800 800500
Textphone: 0800 056 0566
Tel: (020) 7825 2500

Parentline
Online: www.parentline.co.uk
Endway House
Endway
Hadleigh
Essex SS7 2AN
Helpline: 0808 800 2222
Textphone: 0800 783 6783
E-mail: helpline@parentline.co.uk

See also COUNSELLING AND PSYCHOLOGICAL THERAPIES, CRISIS SUPPORT

CHILDREN'S HEALTH

Action Research
Online: www.actionresearch.co.uk
Vincent House
North Parade
Horsham
West Sussex RH12 2DP
Tel: (01403) 210406

Cancer and Leukaemia in Childhood
Online: www.clic.uk.com
12–13 King Square
Bristol BS2 8JH
Tel: (0117) 924 8844

The Child Growth Foundation
Online: www.cgf.org.uk
2 Mayfield Avenue
Chiswick
London
Tel: (020) 8994 7625/8995 0257

Children's Liver Disease Foundation
Online: www.childliverdisease.org
36 Great Charles Street
Birmingham B3 3JY
Tel: (0121) 212 3839

Children with AIDS Charity
Online: www.cwac.org
9 Denbigh Street
London SW1V 2HF
Tel: (020) 7233 5966

Contact a Family
Online: www.cafamily.org.uk
c/o Contact a Family
170 Tottenham Court Road
London W1P 0HA
Tel: (020) 7383 3555

Great Ormond Street Hospital for Children NHS Trust
Online: ich.bpmf.ac.uk
Great Ormond Street
London WC1N 3JH
Tel: (020) 7405 9200

Institute of Child Health
Online: www.ich.ucl.ac.uk
30 Guilford Street
London WC1N 1EH
Tel: (020) 7242 9789
E-mail: kidsdocs@aap.org

National Asthma Campaign
Online: www.asthma.org.uk
Providence House
Providence Place
London N1 0NT
Helpline: 0845 701 0203
Tel: (020) 7226 2260

National Autistic Society
Online: www.oneworld.org/autism_uk
393 City Road
London EC1V 1NG
Helpline: (020) 7903 3555
Tel: (020) 7833 2299

National Children's Bureau
Online: www.ncb.org.uk
8 Wakley Street
London EC1V 7QE
Tel: (020) 7843 6000

Patient UK
Online: www.patient.co.uk
E-mail: info@patient.co.uk

UKparents
Online: www.ukparents.co.uk

See also BIRTH DEFECTS, CHILD ABUSE AND NEGLECT, CYSTIC FIBROSIS, GENETIC DISORDERS, INFECTIONS, LEARNING DISABILITIES

COMPLEMENTARY THERAPIES

British Chiropractic Association
Blagrave House
17 Blagrave Street
Reading
Berks RG1 1QB
Tel: (0118) 950 5950
E-mail: britchiro@aol.com

British Medical Acupuncture Society
Online: www.medical-acupuncture.co.uk
Newton House
Newton Lane
Whitley
Warrington
Cheshire WA4 4JA
Tel: (01925) 730727

British Osteopathic Association
Online: www.osteopathy.org
Langham House East
Luton
Bedfordshire LU1 2NA
Tel. (01582) 488455

UK Homoeopathic Medical Association
6 Livingstone Road
Gravesend
Kent DA12 5DZ
Tel: (01474) 560336

CONTRACEPTION

See FAMILY PLANNING

COUNSELLING AND PSYCHOLOGICAL THERAPIES

Association for Psychological Therapies
Online: www.apt.uk.com
PO Box 3
Thurnby
Leicester LE7 9QN
Tel: (0116) 241 9934

British Association for Counselling
Online: www.counselling.co.uk
1 Regent Place
Rugby
Warwickshire CV21 2PJ
Tel: (01788) 550899
E-mail: bac@bac.co.uk

British Psychological Society
Online: www.bps.org.uk
St Andrews House
48 Princess Road East
Leicester LE1 7DR
Tel: (0116) 254 9568
E-mail: enquiry@bps.org.uk

RELATE
Online: www.relate.org.uk
Herbert Gray College
Little Church Street
Rugby
Warwickshire CV21 3AP
Tel: (01788) 573241
E-mail: enquiries@national.relate.org.uk

The Samaritans
Online: www.samaritans.org.uk
10 The Grove
Slough
Berkshire SL1 1QP
Helpline: 0345 909090
Tel: (01753) 216500
E-mail: jo@samaritans.org

See also CRISIS SUPPORT

CRISIS SUPPORT

National Association of Citizens Advice Bureaux
Online: www.nacab.org.uk
E-mail: adviceguide@nacab.org.uk

The Samaritans
Online: www.samaritans.org.uk
10 The Grove
Slough
Berkshire SL1 1QP
Helpline: 0345 909090
Tel: (01753) 216500
E-mail: jo@samaritans.org

Victim Support
Online: www.victimsupport.com
Cranmer House
39 Brixton Road
London SW9 6DZ
Tel: (020) 7735 9166
E-mail: info@victimsupport.com

See also ALCOHOL-RELATED PROBLEMS, CHILD ABUSE AND NEGLECT, DEATH AND BEREAVEMENT, DRUG-RELATED PROBLEMS, HIV INFECTION AND AIDS

CYSTIC FIBROSIS

Cystic Fibrosis Resource Centre
Online: www.cysticfibrosis.co.uk/cystic.htm
E-mail: patientinfo.shl@solvay.com

Cystic Fibrosis Trust
Online: www.cftrust.org.uk
Alexandra House
5 Blyth Road
Bromley
Kent BR1 3RS
Tel: (020) 8464 7211
E-mail: emailenquiries@cftrust.org.uk

See also GENETIC DISORDERS, LUNG DISEASE

DEAFNESS

See HEARING DISORDERS

DEATH AND BEREAVEMENT

CRUSE Bereavement Care
CRUSE House
126 Sheen Road
Richmond
Surrey TW9 1UR
Tel: (020) 8940 4818

Growth House, Inc. (US)
Online: www.growthhouse.org

Hospice Information Service
St. Christopher's Hospice
51 Lawrie Park Road
Sydenham
London SE26 6DZ
Tel: (020) 8778 9252
E-mail: his@stchris.ftech.co.uk

National Association of Widows
54–57 Allison Street
Digbeth
Birmingham
West Midlands B5 5TH
Tel: (0121) 643 8348

Stillbirth and Neonatal Death Society
28 Portland Place
London W1N 4DE
Helpline: (020) 7436 5881
Tel: (020) 7436 7940

See also COUNSELLING AND PSYCHOLOGICAL THERAPIES, CRISIS SUPPORT

DENTISTRY

British Dental Association
Online: www.bda-dentistry.org.uk
64 Wimpole Street
London W1M 8AL
Tel: (020) 7935 0875
E-mail: infocentre@bda-dentistry.org.uk

British Dental Health Foundation
Online: www.dentalhealth.org.uk
Eastlands Court
St. Peter's Road
Rugby CV21 3QP
Helpline: 0870 333 1188
Tel: (01788) 546365
E-mail: feedback@dentalhealth.org.uk

DerWeb (Dental Education Resources on the Web)
Online: www.derweb.ac.uk

Fear of Dentists
Online: www.fod.org.uk
PO Box 5005
Derby DE1 9FS
Tel: (07050) 683618
E-mail: andy@fod.org.uk

DEPRESSION

Depression Alliance
Online: www.depressionalliance.org
35 Westminster Bridge Road
London SE1 7JB
Tel: (020) 7633 0557

See also COUNSELLING AND PSYCHOLOGICAL THERAPIES, MENTAL HEALTH PROBLEMS

DIABETES

British Diabetic Association
Online: www.diabetes.org.uk
10 Queen Anne Street
London W1M 0BD
Helpline: (020) 7636 6112
Tel: (020) 7323 1531

Insulin Dependent Diabetes Trust
Online: www.traders.co.uk/insulintrust
PO Box 294
Northampton NN3 2BN
Tel: (01604) 721325

Juvenile Diabetes Foundation
Online: www.jdf.org.uk
25 Gosfield Street
London W1P 8EB
Tel: (020) 7436 3112
E-mail: info@jdf.org.uk

DIET

See NUTRITION

DIGESTIVE DISORDERS

British Colostomy Association
Online: www.bcass.org.uk
15 Station Road
Reading
Berkshire RG1 1LG
Helpline: 0800 328 4257
E-mail: sue@bcass.org.uk

British Nutrition Foundation
Online: www.nutrition.org.uk
52–54 High Holborn
London WC1V 6RQ
Tel: (020) 7404 6504

British Society of Gastroenterology
Online: www.bsg.org.uk
3 St Andrews Place
London NW1 4LB
Tel: (020) 7387 3534
E-mail: bsg@mailbox.ulcc.ac.uk

The Coeliac Society
Online: www.coeliac.co.uk
PO Box 220
High Wycombe
Bucks HP11 2HY
Tel: (01494) 437278
E-mail: admin@coeliac.co.uk

Colon Cancer Concern
Online: www.coloncancer.org.uk
4 Rickett Street
London SW6 1RU
Helpline: (020) 7381 4711
Tel: (020) 7381 9711

Digestive Disorders Foundation
Online: www.digestivedisorders.org.uk
3 St Andrews Place
London NW1 4LB
Tel: (020) 7486 0341
E-mail: ddf@digestivedisorders.org.uk

International Foundation for Functional Gastrointestinal Disorders (US)
Online: www.iffgd.org

National Association for Colitis and Crohn's Disease
Online: www.nacc.org.uk
4 Beaumont House
Sutton Road
St Albans
Herts AL1 5HH
Tel: (01727) 844296
E-mail: nacc@nacc.org.uk

See also CANCER, LIVER DISORDERS

DISABILITY

Disability Net
Online: www.disabilitynet.co.uk
Suite 5D
North Mill
Bridgefoot
Belper
Derbyshire DE56 1YD
Tel: (01773) 824343
E-mail: paul@disabilitynet.co.uk

Disabled Living Foundation
380–384 Harrow Road
London W9 2HU
Tel: (020) 7289 6111
E-mail: dlfinfo@dlf.org.uk

John Grooms Association for Disabled People
50 Scrutton Street
London EC2A 4PH
Tel: (020) 7452 2000

MENCAP Royal Society for Mentally Handicapped Children and Adults
Online: www.mencap.org.uk
MENCAP National Centre
123 Golden Lane
London EC1Y 0RT
Tel: (020) 7454 0454
E-mail: info@mencap.org.uk

RADAR
Online: www.radar.org.uk
12 City Forum
250 City Road
London EC1V 8AF
Tel: (020) 7250 3222
Minicom: (020) 7250 4119

See also EYE AND VISION DISORDERS, HEARING DISORDERS, LEARNING DISABILITIES, REHABILITATION

DOWN'S SYNDROME

Down's Syndrome Association
Online: www.downs-syndrome.org.uk
155 Mitcham Road
London SW17 9PG
Tel: (020) 8682 4001

Down's Syndrome Educational Trust
Online: www.downsnet.org
The Sarah Duffen Centre
Belmont Street
Southsea
Hampshire PO5 1NA
Tel: (023) 9282 4261

Scottish Down's Syndrome Association
Online: www.sdsa.org.uk
158/160 Balgreen Road
Edinburgh EH11 3AU
Tel: (0131) 313 4225

See also GENETIC DISORDERS, LEARNING DISABILITIES

DRUG INFORMATION

Food and Drug Administration (US)
Online: www.fda.gov

Medicines Control Agency
Online: www.open.gov.uk/mca
Market Towers
1 Nine Elms Lane
London SW8 5NQ
Tel: (020) 7273 0000
E-mail: info@mca.gov.uk

PharmWeb
Online: www.pharmweb.net

DRUG-RELATED PROBLEMS

Cascade
Online: www.cascade.u-net.com
Keepers Lodge
Chelmsley Road
Chelmsley Wood
Solihull
West Midlands B37 7UA
Tel: (0121) 788 3436
E-mail: cascade@cascade.u-net.com

National Drugs Helpline
Tel: 0800 776600

SCODA (Standing Conference on Drug Abuse)
Online: www.ncvo-vol.org.uk/scoda.htm
32–36 Loman Street
London SE1 0EE
Tel: (020) 7928 9500
E-mail: info@scoda.demon.co.uk

United Nations International Drug Control Programme
Online: www.undcp.org

See also ALCOHOL-RELATED PROBLEMS, COUNSELLING AND PSYCHOLOGICAL THERAPIES, CRISIS SUPPORT

EAR, NOSE, AND THROAT DISORDERS

American Academy of Otolaryngology–Head and Neck Surgery (US)
Online: www.entnet.org

British Snoring and Sleep Apnoea Association
Online: www.britishsnoring.demon.co.uk
1 Duncroft Close
Reigate
Surrey RH2 9DE
Tel: (01249) 701010
Fax: (01737) 248744

See also HEARING DISORDERS

EATING DISORDERS

Anorexia and Bulimia Nervosa Association
Women's Health Centre
Tottenham Town Hall
Approach Road
London N15 4RS
Tel: (020) 8885 3936

Eating Disorders Association
Online: www.gurney.co.uk/eda
1st Floor
Wensum House
103 Prince of Wales Road
Norwich NR1 1DW
Helpline: (01603) 621414
Youth helpline: (01603) 765050
E-mail: eda@netcom.co.uk

Northern Ireland Eating Disorders
22 Ashmont Grove
Belfast BT4 2FP
Tel: (01232) 618299

Overeaters Anonymous
PO Box 19
Stretford
Manchester M32 9EB
Tel: (0161) 7629 3485

See also NUTRITION

ENDOCRINE DISORDERS

See HORMONAL AND METABOLIC DISORDERS

EPILEPSY

British Epilepsy Association
Online: www.epilepsy.org.uk
New Anstey House
Gate Way Drive
Leeds LS19 7XY
Helpline: 0808 800 5050
Tel: (0113) 210 8800
E-mail: epilepsy@bea.org.uk

Epilepsy Association of Scotland
Online: www.epilepsyscotland.org.uk
48 Govan Road
Glasgow G51 1JL
Helpline: (0141) 427 5225
Tel: (0141) 427 4911
E-mail: admin@epilepsyscotland.org.uk

Epilepsy International
Online: www.epiworld.com

National Society for Epilepsy
Chalfont St. Peter
Buckinghamshire SL9 0RJ
Tel: (01494) 601300

See also NEUROLOGICAL DISORDERS

EXERCISE

Active for Life
Online: www.active.org.uk

BBC Online Health and Fitness
Online: www.bbc.co.uk/health/fightingfat

Fitness Scotland
Caledonia House
South Gyle
Edinburgh EH12 9DQ
Tel: (0131) 317 7243

Health-club.net
Online: www.health-club.net

Keep Fit Association
Online: www.keepfit.org.uk
Francis House
Francis Street
London SW1P 1DE
Tel: (020) 7233 8898
E-mail: kfa@keepfit.org.uk

Sport England
Online: www.english.sports.gov.uk
16 Upper Woburn Place
London WC1H 0QP
Tel: (020) 7273 1500
E-mail: info@english.sports.gov.uk

See also GENERAL INFORMATION, MUSCULOSKELETAL DISORDERS, SAFETY AND HEALTH

EYE AND VISION DISORDERS

Action for Blind People
Online: www.demon.co.uk/afbp
14–16 Verney Road
London SE16 3DZ
Tel: (020) 7732 8771

Association for Macular Diseases (US)
Online: www.macula.org

College of Optometrists
Online: www.college-optometrists.org
42 Craven Street
London WC2N 5NG
Tel: (020) 7839 6000

Fight for Sight
Online: www.users.globalnet.co.uk/~ffs
Institute of Ophthalmology
Bath Street
London EC1V 9EL
Tel: (020) 7608 4000

Guide Dogs for the Blind Association
Online: www.gdba.org.uk
Hillfields
Burghfield Common
Reading RG7 3YG
Tel: (0118) 983 5555

International Glaucoma Association
Online: www.iga.org.uk
King's College Hospital
Denmark Hill
London SE5 9RS
Helpline: (020) 7346 5929
Tel: (020) 7737 3265

Royal College of Ophthalmologists
Online: www.rcophth.ac.uk
17 Cornwall Terrace
London NW1 4QW
Tel: (020) 7935 0702

Royal National Institute for the Blind
Online: www.rnib.org.uk
224 Great Portland Street
London W1N 6AA
Helpline: 0845 766 9999
Tel: (020) 7388 1266
Textphone: 0800 515152

FAMILY PLANNING

British Pregnancy Advisory Service
Online: www.bpas.demon.co.uk
Austy Manor
Wootton Warren
Solihull
West Midlands B95 6BX
Helpline: 0845 730 4030
Tel: (01564) 793225

Family Planning Association
Online: www.fpa.org.uk
2–12 Pentonwille Road
London N1 9FP
Helpline: (020) 7837 4044
Tel: (020) 7837 5432

FertilityUK
Online: www.fertilityuk.org
Clitherow House
1 Blythe Mews
Blythe Road
London W14 0NW
Tel: (020) 7371 1341
E-mail: admin@fertilityuk.org

International Planned Parenthood Federation
Online: www.ippf.org
Inner Circle
Regent's Park
London NW1 4NS
Tel: (020) 7487 7900
Email: info@ippf.org

Marie Stopes International
Online: www.mariestopes.org.uk
153 Cleveland Street
London W1P 5PG
Tel: (020) 7574 7400
Email: services@stopes.org.uk

National Abortion Campaign
Online: www.gn.apc.org/nac
The Print House
18 Ashwin Street
London E8 3DL
Tel: (020) 7923 4976
Email: nac@gn.apc.org

See also INFERTILITY, PREGNANCY AND CHILDBIRTH

FIRST AID

British Red Cross Society
Online: www.redcross.org.uk
9 Grosvenor Crescent
London SW1X 7EJ
Tel: (020) 7235 5454

First Aid Skills For Life (US)
Online: firstaid.ie.eu.org

St. Andrew's Ambulance Association
Online: www.firstaid.org.uk
St. Andrew's House
48 Milton Street
Glasgow G4 0HR
Tel: (0141) 332 4031

St. John Ambulance
Online: www.st-john-ambulance.org.uk
63 York Street
London W1H 1PS
Tel: (020) 7258 3456

GENETIC DISORDERS

Alliance of Genetic Support Groups (US)
Online: www.geneticalliance.org

Birth Defects Foundation
Online: www.birthdefects.co.uk
Martindale
Hawks Green
Cannock
Staffordshire WS11 2XN
Tel: (01543) 468888
E-mail: enquiries@birthdefects.co.uk

Climb (Research Trust for Metabolic Diseases in Children)
Online: www.rtmdc.org.uk
The Quadrangle
Crewe Hall
Weston Road
Crewe
Cheshire CW1 6UR
Tel: (01270) 250221

Contact a Family
Online: www.cafamily.org.uk
c/o Contact a Family
170 Tottenham Court Road
London W1P 0HA
Tel: (020) 7383 3555
E-mail: info@cafamily.org.uk

Office of Rare Diseases (US)
Online: rarediseases.info.nih.gov/ord

See also BIRTH DEFECTS, CYSTIC FIBROSIS, DOWN'S SYNDROME, HORMONAL AND METABOLIC DISORDERS

HEADACHE

Migraine Action Association
Online: www.migraine.org.uk
178A High Road
Byfleet
Surrey KT14 7ED
Tel: (01932) 352468
E-mail: info@migraine.org.uk

Migraine Trust
Online: www.migrainetrust.org
45 Great Ormond Street
London WC1N 3HZ
Tel: (020) 7831 4818
E-mail: migrainetrust@compuserve.com

National Headache Foundation (US)
Online: www.headaches.org

See also NEUROLOGICAL DISORDERS

HEAD INJURY

Brain Injury Association (US)
Online: www.biausa.org

British Brain and Spine Foundation
Online: www.bbsf.org.uk
7 Winchester House
Kennington Park
Cranmer Road
London SW9 6EJ
Helpline: 0800 328 5758
Tel: (020) 7793 5900
E-mail: info@bbsf.org.uk

See also DISABILITY, FIRST AID, NEUROLOGICAL DISORDERS, REHABILITATION

HEALTH CARE CHOICES

National Association for Patient Participation
Online: www.napp.org.uk
PO Box 999
Nuneaton
Warwickshire
Tel/Fax: (0151) 630 5786
E-mail: john.barlow@napp.org.uk

Private Healthcare UK
Online: www.privatehealth.co.uk
Acumen Solutions
Concept House
271 High Street
Berkhamsted
Hertfordshire HP4 1AA
Tel: (01442) 385000

Royal College of General Practitioners
Online: www.rcgp.org.uk
14 Princes Gate
Hyde Park
London SW7 1PU
Tel: (020) 7581 3232
E-mail: info@rcgp.org.uk

See also GENERAL INFORMATION

HEARING DISORDERS

British Deaf Association
Online: www.bda.org.uk
1–3 Worship Street
London EC2A 2AB
Tel: (020) 7588 3520
Minicom: (020) 7588 3529
E-mail: info@bda.org.uk

British Tinnitus Association
Online: www.tinnitus.org.uk
4th Floor
White Building
Fitzalan Square
Sheffield S1 2AZ
Tel: 0800 018 0527
E-mail: bta@tinnitus.org.uk

Deafness Research Foundation (US)
Online: www.drf.org

Hearing Concern
Online: web.ukonline.co.uk/hearing.concern
7–11 Armstrong Road
London W3 7JL
Tel: (020) 8743 1110

Royal Association in Aid of Deaf People
Online: www.royaldeaf.org.uk
Walsingham Road
Colchester
Essex CO2 7BP
Tel: (01206) 509509
Textphone: (01206) 577090

Royal National Institute for Deaf People
Online: www.rnid.org.uk
PO Box 16464
London EC1Y 8TT
Helpline: 0870 605 0123
Textphone: 0870 603 3007
E-mail: helpline@rnid.org.uk

See also EAR, NOSE, AND THROAT DISORDERS

HEART AND CIRCULATION DISORDERS

British Heart Foundation
Online: www.bhf.org.uk
14 Fitzhardinge Street
London W1H 4DH
Heartline: 0990 200656
Tel: (020) 7935 0185

High Blood Pressure Foundation
Online: www.hbpf.org.uk
Department of Medical Sciences
Western General Hospital
Edinburgh EH4 2XU
Tel: (0131) 332 9211
E-mail: hbpf@hbpf.org.uk

NHS Direct Online
Online: www.nhsdirect.nhs.uk

Northern Ireland Chest, Heart, and Stroke Association
Online: www.nichsa.com
21 Dublin Road
Belfast BT2 7HB
Tel: (02890) 320184
Helpline: 0345 697299

Patient UK
Online: www.patient.co.uk
E-mail: info@patient.co.uk

The Stroke Association
Online: www.stroke.org.uk
Stroke House
Whitecross Street
London EC1Y 8JJ
Tel: (020) 7566 0300

HIV INFECTION AND AIDS

AIDSmap
Online: www.aidsmap.com

AVERT
Online: www.avert.org
4 Brighton Road
Horsham
West Sussex RH13 5BA
Tel: (01403) 210202
E-mail: avert@dial.pipex.com

Body Positive
Online: www.bodypositive.org.uk
14 Greek Street
London W1V 5LE
Tel: (020) 7287 8010

Children with AIDS Charity
Online: www.cwac.org
9 Denbigh Street
London SW1V 2HF
Tel: (020) 7233 5966

Crusaid
Online: www.crusaid.org.uk
73 Collier Street
London N1 9BE
Tel: (020) 7833 3939

Terrence Higgins Trust
Online: www.tht.org.uk
52–54 Grays Inn Road
London WC1X 8JU
Tel: (020) 7831 0330
E-mail: info@tht.org.uk

See also INFECTIOUS DISEASES

HOME CARE

Carers National Association
20–25 Glasshouse Yard
London EC1A 4JS
Helpline: 0345 573369
Tel: (020) 7490 8818

Contact a Family
Online: www.cafamily.org.uk
170 Tottenham Court Road
London W1P 0HA
Tel: (020) 7383 3555
E-mail: info@cafamily.org.uk

Princess Royal Trust for Carers
Online: www.carers.org
16 Byward Street
London EC3R 5BA
Tel: (020) 7480 7788

HORMONAL AND METABOLIC DISORDERS

American Thyroid Association (US)
Online: www.thyroid.org

Child Growth Foundation
Online: www.cgf.org.uk
2 Mayfield Avenue
Chiswick
London W4 1PW
Tel: (020) 8994 7625/8995 0257

Climb (Research Trust for Metabolic Diseases in Children)
Online: www.rtmdc.org.uk
The Quadrangle
Crewe Hall
Weston Road
Crewe
Cheshire CW1 6UR
Tel: (01270) 250221

Contact a Family
Online: www.cafamily.org.uk
c/o Contact a Family
170 Tottenham Court Road
London W1P 0HA
Tel: (020) 7383 3555
E-mail: info@cafamily.org.uk

Endocrine Web (US)
Online: www.endocrineweb.com

National Adrenal Diseases Foundation (US)
Online: www.medhelp.org/nadf

National Society for Phenylketonuria
Online: web.ukonline.co.uk/nspku
7 Lingey Lane
Wardley
Gateshead
Tyne & Wear NE10 8BR
Tel: 0845 603 9136
E-mail: nspku@ukonline.co.uk

See also DIABETES

IMMUNE DISORDERS

Arthritis Research Campaign
Online: www.arc.org.uk
Copeman House
St. Mary's Court
St. Mary's Gate
Chesterfield
Derbyshire S41 7TD
Tel: (01246) 558033
E-mail: info@arc.org.uk

British Sjögren's Syndrome Association
Online: ourworld.compuserve.com/homepages/bssassociation
Unit 1
Manor Workshops
West End
Nailsea
Bristol BS19 2DD
Tel: (01275) 854215

DEBRA (epidermolysis bullosa)
Online: www.debra.org.uk
DEBRA House
13 Wellington Business Park
Dules's Ride
Growthorne
Berks RG11 6LS
Tel: (01344) 771961

Dermatomyositis and Polymyositis Support Group
Online: dialspace.dial.pipex.com/town/avenue/ye72
146 Newtown Road
Woolston
Southampton
Hampshire SO2 9HR
Tel: (023) 8044 9708

Lupus UK
Online: www.geocities.com/hotsprings/2911
1 Eastern Road
Romford
Essex RM1 3NH
Tel: (01708) 731251

Lymphoma Association
Online: www.lymphoma.org.uk
PO Box 386
Aylesbury
Buckinghamshire HP20 2GA
Helpline: 0808 808 5555

Primary Immunodeficiency Association
Online: www.pia.org.uk
Alliance House
12 Caxton Street
London SW1H 0QS
Helpline: 0845 603 9158
Tel: (020) 7976 7640

Raynaud's and Scleroderma Association
112 Crewe Road
Alsager
Cheshire ST7 2JA
Tel: (01270) 872776

See also ALLERGY AND ASTHMA, HIV INFECTION and AIDS

INCONTINENCE

The Continence Foundation
Online: www.vois.org.uk/cf
307 Hatton Square
16 Baldwins Gardens
London EC1N 7RJ
Helpline: (020) 7831 9831
Tel: (020) 7404 6875

National Association for Continence (US)
Online: www.nafc.org

See also URINARY SYSTEM DISORDERS

INFECTIOUS DISEASES

Centers for Disease Control and Prevention (US)
Online: www.cdc.gov

Medical Advisory Service for Travellers Abroad
Online: www.masta.org
Traveller's Health Line: (0906) 822 4100

Public Health Laboratory Service
Online: www.phls.co.uk
61 Colindale Avenue
London NW9 5DF
Tel: (020) 8200 1295

World Health Organization
Online: www.who.int

See also CHILDREN'S HEALTH, DIGESTIVE DISORDERS, HIV INFECTION AND AIDS, SEXUALLY TRANSMITTED INFECTIONS, TRAVEL HEALTH

INFERTILITY

Human Fertilisation and Embryology Authority
Online: www.hfea.org.uk
Paxton House
30 Artillery Lane
London E1 7LS
Tel: (020) 7377 5077

ISSUE, The National Fertility Association
Online: www.issue.co.uk
114 Lichfield Street
Walsall
West Midlands WS1 1SZ
Tel: (01922) 722888

See also FAMILY PLANNING, PREGNANCY AND CHILDBIRTH

INFLAMMATORY BOWEL DISEASE

See DIGESTIVE DISORDERS

INJURIES

British Red Cross Society
Online: www.redcross.org.uk
9 Grosvenor Crescent
London SW1X 7EJ
Tel: (020) 7235 5454

Changing Faces
Online: www.changingfaces.co.uk
1 & 2 Junction Mews
London W2 1PN
Tel: (020) 7706 4232
E-mail: info@changingfaces.co.uk

Royal Society for the Prevention of Accidents
Online: www.rospa.co.uk
353 Bristol Road
Edgbaston
Birmingham B5 7ST
Tel: (0121) 248 2000
E-mail: help@rospa.co.uk

St. Andrew's Ambulance Association
Online: www.firstaid.org.uk
St. Andrew's House
48 Milton Street
Glasgow G4 0HR
Tel: (0141) 332 4031

St. John Ambulance
Online: www.st-john-ambulance.org.uk
63 York Street
London W1H 1PS
Tel: (020) 7258 3456

See also DISABILITY, FIRST AID, SAFETY AND HEALTH

KIDNEY DISORDERS

See URINARY SYSTEM DISORDERS

LEARNING DISABILITIES

British Dyslexia Association
Online: www.bda-dyslexia.org.uk
98 London Road
Reading RG1 5AU
Helpline: (0118) 966 8271
Tel: (0118) 966 2677
E-mail: info@dyslexiahelp-bda.demon.co.uk

Dyspraxia Foundation
Online: www.emmbrook.demon.co.uk/dysprax/homepage.htm
8 West Alley
Hitchin
Hertfordshire SG5 1EG
Helpline: (01462) 454986

Leonard Cheshire
Online: www.leonard-cheshire.org
30 Millbank
London SW1P 4QD
Tel: (020) 7802 8200
E-mail: info@london.leonard-cheshire.org.uk

MENCAP Royal Society for Mentally Handicapped Children and Adults
Online: www.mencap.org.uk
MENCAP National Centre
123 Golden Lane
London EC1Y 0RT
Tel: (020) 7454 0454
E-mail: info@mencap.org.uk

See also CHILDREN'S HEALTH, DISABILITY, HEAD INJURY, SPEECH AND LANGUAGE DISORDERS

LIVER DISORDERS

American Liver Foundation (US)
Online: www.liverfoundation.org

British Liver Trust
Online: www.britishlivertrust.org.uk
Ransomes Europark
Ipswich
Suffolk IP3 9QG
Helpline: 0808 800 1000
Tel: (01473) 276326
E-mail: bsg@mailbox.ulcc.ac.uk

PBC Foundation
Online: www.nhtech.demon.co.uk/pbc
The Dean
Longniddry
East Lothian EH32 0PN
Tel: (01875) 853552
E-mail: pbcfoundation@msn.com

See also ALCOHOL-RELATED PROBLEMS, CHILDREN'S HEALTH

LUNG DISORDERS

Alpha1-Support UK
Online: www.alpha1.org.uk

British Lung Foundation
Online: www.lunguk.org
78 Hatton Garden
London EC1N 8LD
Tel: (020) 7831 5831
E-mail: blf_user@gpiag-asthma.org

National Heart, Lung, and Blood Institute Information Center (US)
Online: www.nhlbi.nih.gov

Pulmonary Hypertension Association, Inc. (US)
Online: www.phassociation.org

See also ALLERGY AND ASTHMA, CANCER, CYSTIC FIBROSIS

MEN'S HEALTH

Consumer Health Information Campaign
Online: www.chic.org.uk/menzone
Helpline: 0845 606 1611

Everyman, Action Against Male Cancer
Online: www.icr.ac.uk/everyman
The Institute of Cancer Research
Freepost LON 922
London SW7 3YY
Tel: 0800 731 9468
E-mail: everyman@icr.ac.uk

Impotence, Your Questions Answered
Online: www.impotence-help.co.uk

BBC Online Health and Fitness
Online: www.bbc.co.uk/health/mens

Men's Health Line
Helpline: (020) 8995 4448

Orchid Cancer Appeal
Online: www.orchid-cancer.org.uk
9 Grace Close
Hainault
Essex IG6 3DW
Tel: (020) 8501 3027
E-mail: colin@orchid-cancer-appeal.co.uk

See also PROSTATE DISORDERS, SEXUAL PROBLEMS

MENTAL HEALTH PROBLEMS

Addiction Recovery Foundation
Online: easyweb.easynet.co.uk/~acw
122A Wilton Road
London SW1V 1JZ
Tel: (020) 7233 5333
E-mail: acw@easynet.co.uk

CANDID (Counselling and Diagnosis in Dementia)
Online: 193.62.68.10:80/candid
The National Hospital for Neurology and Neurosurgery
Queen Square
London WC1N 3BG
Helpline: (020) 7829 8772

Careline
Helpline: (020) 8514 1177

Dementia Web
Online: dementia.ion.ucl.ac.uk

Gamblers Anonymous
Online: www.gamblersanonymous.org
PO Box 88
London SW10 0EU
Tel: (020) 7384 3040
E-mail: isomain@gamblersanonymous.org

Gamcare
Online: www.gamcare.org.uk
Suite 1
25–27 Catherine Place
London SW1E 6DU
Helpline: 0845 600 0133
Tel: (020) 7233 8988
E-mail: director@gamcare.org.uk

Manic Depression Fellowship
8–10 High Street
Kingston upon Thames
Surrey KT1 1EY
Tel (020) 8974 6550

Mental Health Foundation
Online: www.mentalhealth.org.uk
UK Office
20/21 Cornwall Terrace
London NW1 4QL
Tel: (020) 7535 7400
E-mail: mhf@mentalhealth.org.uk

MIND
Online: www.mind.org.uk
15–19 Broadway
London E15 4BQ
Helpline: 0345 660163 (National)/(020) 8522 1728 (Greater London only)

National Autistic Society
Online: www.oneworld.org/autism_uk
393 City Road
London EC1V 1NG
Tel: (020) 7833 2299
E-mail: nas@nas.org.uk

National Phobics Society
Online: www.good.co.uk/national-phobics-society
Zion CHRC
Royce Road
Hulme
Manchester M15 5FQ
Tel: (0161) 227 9898
E-mail: natphobsoc@good.co.uk

National Schizophrenia Fellowship
Online: www.nsf.org.uk
30 Tabernacle Street
London EC2A 4DD
Tel: (020) 7330 9100
E-mail: info@london.nsf.org.uk

Royal College of Psychiatrists
Online: www.rcpsych.ac.uk
17 Belgrave Square
London SW1X 8PG
Tel: (020) 7235 2351
E-mail: dhart@rcpsych.ac.uk

SANE
Online: mkn.co.uk/help/extra/charity/sane/index
1st Floor
Cityside House
40 Adler Street
London E1 1EE
Helpline: 0345 678000

Stress UK
Online: www.stress.org.uk

See also ALCOHOL-RELATED PROBLEMS, ALZHEIMER'S DISEASE, COUNSELLING AND PSYCHOLOGICAL THERAPIES, CRISIS SUPPORT, DEPRESSION, DRUG-RELATED PROBLEMS, EATING DISORDERS, STRESS

MUSCULOSKELETAL DISORDERS

Arthritis Research Campaign
Online: www.arc.org.uk
Copeman House
St Mary's Court
St Mary's Gate
Chesterfield
Derbyshire S41 7TD
Tel: (01246) 558033

RSI-UK (repetitive strain injury)
Online: www.rsi-uk.org.uk

WorldOrtho
Online: www.worldortho.com

See also ARTHRITIS, BACK PAIN, OSTEOPOROSIS, RHEUMATIC DISORDERS

NEUROLOGICAL DISORDERS

Action for ME (myalgic encephalomyelitis)
Online: www.afme.org.uk
PO Box 1302
Wells
Somerset BA5 1YE
Tel: 01749 670799

British Brain and Spine Foundation
Online: www.bbsf.org.uk
7 Winchester House
Kennington Park
Cranmer Road
London SW9 6EJ
Helpline: 0800 328 5758
Tel: (020) 7793 5900/5939

Glaxo Neurological Centre
Online: www.glaxocentre.merseyside.org

Guillain-Barré Syndrome Support Group
Online: www.gbs.org.uk
LCC Offices
Eastgate
Sleaford
Lincolnshire NG34 7EB
Tel: (01529) 304615

Motor Neurone Disease Association
Online: www.businessconnections.com/mnd
PO Box 246
Northampton NN1 2PR
Helpline: 0845 762 6262
Tel: (01604) 250 5050

Multiple Sclerosis Society
Online: www.mssociety.org.uk
25 Effie Road
London SW6 1EE
Helpline: 0808 800 8000
Tel: (020) 7610 7171

Muscular Dystrophy Campaign
Online: www.muscular-dystrophy.org
7–11 Prescott Place
London SW4 6BS
Tel: (020) 7720 8055

Myasthenia Gravis Association
Online: www.crabby.demon.co.uk/mga
Keynes House
Chester Park
Alfreton Road
Derby DE21 4AS
Helpline: 0800 919922
Tel: (01332) 290219

Neurofibromatosis Association
Online:www.nfa.zetnet.co.uk
82 London Road
Kingston upon Thames
Surrey KT2 6PX
Tel: (020) 8547 1636

Office of Rare Diseases (US)
Online: rarediseases.info.nih.gov/ord

See also BRAIN TUMOURS, HEADACHE, HEAD INJURY, REHABILITATION, STROKE

NUTRITION

BBC Online Health and Fitness
Online: www.bbc.co.uk/health/fightingfat

British Nutrition Foundation
Online: www.nutrition.org.uk
52–54 High Holborn
London WC1V 6RQ
Tel: (020) 7404 6504

Healthnet
Online: www.healthnet.org.uk

Health Supplement Information Service
Online: www.hsis.org

See also EATING DISORDERS, GENERAL INFORMATION

OSTEOPOROSIS

National Osteoporosis Society
Online: www.nos.org.uk
PO Box 10
Radstock
Bath BA3 3YB
Helpline: (01761) 472721
Tel: (01761) 471771
E-mail: info@nos.org.uk

Osteoporosis and Related Bone Diseases National Resource Center (US)
Online: www.osteo.org

See also MUSCULOSKELETAL DISORDERS

PAEDIATRICS

See CHILDREN'S HEALTH

PAIN RELIEF

American Pain Society (US)
Online: www.ampainsoc.org

Pain Concern
Helpline: 0345 413772

Pain Relief Foundation
Online: www.liv.ac.uk/pri
Rice Lane
Liverpool L9 1AE
Tel: (0151) 523 1486

PARKINSON'S DISEASE

Parkinson's Disease Foundation (US)
Online: www.parkinsons-foundation.org

Parkinson's Disease Society
215 Vauxhall Bridge Road
London SW1V 1EJ
Helpline: 0808 800 0303
Tel: (020) 7931 8080

See also NEUROLOGICAL DISORDERS

PREGNANCY AND CHILDBIRTH

Breastfeeding Network
Online: www.breastfeeding.co.uk
PO Box 11126
Paisley PA2 8YB
Helpline: 0870 900 8787
Tel: (0141) 884 2472
E-mail: broadfoot@btinternet.com

Miscarriage Association
Online: www.the-ma.org.uk
Clayton Hospital
Northgate
Wakefield WF1 3JS
Helpline: (01924) 200799
Tel: (01924) 200795
E-mail: admin@the-ma.org.uk

National Childbirth Trust
Online: www.nct-online.org
Alexandra House
Oldham Terrace
London W3 6NH
Tel: (020) 8992 8637

Stillbirth and Neonatal Death Society
28 Portland Place
London W1N 4DE
Helpline: (020) 7436 5881
Tel: (020) 7436 7940

TAMBA (Twins and Multiple Births Association)
Online: www.surreyweb.org.uk/tamba
309 Chester Road
Little Sutton
South Wirral L66 1TH
Helpline: (01732) 868000
Tel: 0870 121 4000

UKparents
Online: www.ukparents.co.uk

See also FAMILY PLANNING, INFERTILITY, WOMEN'S HEALTH

PROSTATE DISORDERS

Prostate Cancer Charity
Online: www.prostate-cancer.org.uk
Du Cane Road
London W12 0NN
Helpline: (020) 8383 1948
Tel: (020) 8383 8124
E-mail: info@prostate-cancer.org.uk

Prostate Help Association
Online: www.personal.u-net.com/~pha
PHA(W)
Langworth
Lincoln LN3 5DF
E-mail: philip@pha.u-net.com

See also MEN'S HEALTH, URINARY SYSTEM DISORDERS

REHABILITATION

emPOWER
Online: www.empowernet.org
Rehabilitation Centre
Roehampton Lane
London SW15 5PR
Tel: (020) 8788 1777

Limbless Association
Online: www.limbless-association.org
Rehabilitation Centre
Roehampton Lane
London SW15 5PR
Tel: (020) 8788 1777

RADAR
Online: www.radar.org.uk
12 City Forum
250 City Road
London EC1V 8AF
Tel: (020) 7250 3222
Minicom: (020) 7250 4119

See also DISABILITY, SPEECH AND LANGUAGE DISORDERS

RHEUMATIC DISORDERS

American College of Rheumatology (US)
Online: www.rheumatology.org

British Society for Rheumatology
Online: www.rheumatology.org.uk
41 Eagle Street
London WC1R 4AR
Tel: (020) 7242 3313

See also ARTHRITIS, MUSCULOSKELETAL DISORDERS

SAFETY AND HEALTH

Child Accident Prevention Trust
18–20 Farringdon Lane
London EC1R 3HA
Tel: (020) 7608 3828

Health and Safety Executive
Online: www.open.gov.uk/hse
Health and Safety Laboratory
Broad Lane
Sheffield S3 7HQ
Tel: (0114) 289 2333

Institute for Occupational Safety and Health
Online: www.iosh.co.uk
The Grange
Highfield Drive
Wigston
Leicestershire LE18 1NN
Tel: (01162) 573100

Royal Society for the Prevention of Accidents
Online: www.rospa.org.uk
353 Bristol Road
Edgbaston
Birmingham B5 7ST
Tel: (0121) 248 2000

SEXUALLY TRANSMITTED INFECTIONS

American Social Health Association (US)
Online: www.ashastd.org

Health Education Authority
Online: www.lovelife.hea.org.uk

See also HIV INFECTION AND AIDS, INFECTIOUS DISEASES, MEN'S HEALTH, WOMEN'S HEALTH

SEXUAL PROBLEMS

British Association for Sexual and Relationship Therapy
Online: www.basmt.org.uk
PO Box 13686
London SW20 9ZH
Tel: (020) 8543 2707
E-mail: info@basmt.org.uk

The Gender Trust
Online: www.gentrust.freeserve.co.uk
PO Box 3192
Brighton BN1 3WR
Helpline: 07000 790347
E-mail: gentrust@mistral.co.uk

Healthnet
Online: www.healthnet.org.uk

London Lesbian and Gay Switchboard
Online: www.llgs.org.uk
LLGS
PO Box 7324
London N1 9QS
Tel: (020) 7837 7324

See also COUNSELLING AND PSYCHOLOGICAL THERAPIES

SKIN DISORDERS

Acne Support Group
Online: www.m2w3.com/acne
PO Box 230
Hayes
Middlesex UB4 0UT
Tel: (020) 8561 6868

British Association of Dermatologists
Online: www.bad.org.uk
19 Fitzroy Square
London W1P 5HQ
Tel: (020) 7383 0266

National Eczema Society
Online: www.eczema.org
163 Eversholt Street
London NW1 1BU
Tel: (020) 7388 4097

Patient UK
Online: www.patient.co.uk
E-mail: info@patient.co.uk

Psoriasis Association
7 Milton Street
Northampton NN2 7JG
Tel: (01604) 711129

Skin Cancer Foundation (US)
Online: www.skincancer.org

Skin Care Campaign
Online: www.skincarecampaign.org

The Skin Site (US)
Online: www.capederm.com

SLEEP DISORDERS

American Sleep Disorders Association (US)
Online: www.asda.org

British Snoring and Sleep Apnoea Association
Online: www.britishsnoring.demon.co.uk
1 Duncroft Close
Reigate
Surrey RH2 9DE
Tel: (01249) 701010
Fax: (01737) 248744
E-mail: helpline@britishsnoring.co.uk

Narcolepsy Association UK
Online: www.narcolepsy.org.uk
Craven House
1st Floor
121 Kingsway
London WC2B 6PA
Tel: (020) 7721 8904

National Sleep Foundation (US)
Online: www.sleepfoundation.org

See also EAR, NOSE, AND THROAT DISORDERS

SMOKING

Action on Smoking and Health
Online: www.ash.org.uk
102 Clifton Street
London EC2A 4HW
Tel: (020) 7739 5902
E-mail: action.smoking.health@dial.pipex.com

Lifesaver
Online: www.lifesaver.co.uk

Quit
Online: www.healthnet.org.uk/quit
Victory House
170 Tottenham Court Road
London W1P 0HA
Helpline: 0800 002200
Tel: (020) 7388 5775

See also LUNG DISEASE

SPEECH AND LANGUAGE DISORDERS

American Speech–Language–Hearing Association (US)
Online: www.asha.org

Association for All Speech-Impaired Children
Online: www.afasic.org.uk
69–85 Old Street
London EC1V 9HX
Helpline: 0845 355 5577
Tel: (020) 7841 8900
E-mail: info@afasic.org.uk

British Stammering Association
Online: www.stammer.demon.co.uk
15 Old Ford Road
London E2 9PJ
Helpline: 0845 603 2001
Tel: (020) 8983 1003
E-mail: mail@stammer.demon.co.uk

National Aphasia Association (US)
Online: www.aphasia.org

National Stuttering Association (US)
Online: www.nsastutter.org

Stuttering Foundation of America (US)
Online: www.stuttersfa.org

STRESS

Healthnet
Online: www.healthnet.org.uk

International Stress Management Association
Online: www.isma.org
Division of Psychology
South Bank University
103 Borough Road
London SE1 0AA
Tel: 07000 780430

Stress UK
Online: www.stress.org.uk

See also COUNSELLING AND PSYCHOLOGICAL THERAPIES, MENTAL HEALTH PROBLEMS

STROKE

Northern Ireland Chest, Heart, and Stroke Association
Online: www.nichsa.com
21 Dublin Road
Belfast BT2 7HB
Tel: (02890) 320184
Helpline: 0345 697299

The Stroke Association
Online: www.stroke.org.uk
123 Whitecross Street
London EC1Y 8JJ
Tel: (020) 7566 0300

See also DISABILITY, NEUROLOGICAL DISORDERS, REHABILITATION, SPEECH AND LANGUAGE DISORDERS

SURGERY

American College of Surgeons
Online: www.facs.org

Royal College of Surgeons
Online: www.rcseng.ac.uk
35/43 Lincoln's Inn Fields
London WC2A 3PN
Tel: (020) 7405 3474

TRAVEL HEALTH

Department of Health
Online: www.doh.gov.uk
Richmond House
79 Whitehall
London SW1A 2NS
Tel: (020) 7210 4850

International Association for Medical Assistance to Travellers (US)
Online: www.sentex.net/~iamat

Medical Advisory Services for Travellers Abroad
Online: www.masta.org
Traveller's Health Line: (0906) 822 4100

URINARY SYSTEM DISORDERS

American Foundation for Urologic Disease (US)
Online: www.afud.org

British Kidney Patient Association
Oakhanger Place
Bordon
Hampshire GU35 9JZ
Tel: (01420) 472021

Continence Foundation
Online: www.vois.org.uk/cf
307 Hatton Square
16 Baldwins Gardens
London EC1N 7RJ
Tel: (020) 7404 6875
E-mail: continence.foundation@dial.pipex.com

Interstitial Cystitis Support Group
Online: www.interstitialcystitis.co.uk
76 High Street
Stony Stratford
Buckinghamshire MK11 1AH
Tel: (01908) 569 0169
E-mail: info@interstitialcystitis.co.uk

National Kidney Research Fund
Online: www.nkrf.org.uk
3 Archers Court
Stukeley Road
Huntingdon PE18 6XG
Helpline: 0845 300 1499
Tel: (01480) 454828

Urostomy Association
Buckland
Beaumont Park
Danbury
Essex CM3 4DE
Tel: (01245) 224294

National Kidney and Urological Diseases Information Clearing House (US)
Online: www.niddk.nih.gov/health/kidney.nkudic.htm

See also INCONTINENCE

WOMEN'S HEALTH

National Association for Premenstrual Syndrome
Online: www.pms.org. uk
50 Westminster Palace Gardens
Artillery Row
London SW1P 1RL
Helpline: (01732) 760012

National Endometriosis Society
Online: www.endo.org.uk
7 Swift's Court
High Street
Seal
Kent TN15 0EG
Helpline: (020) 7222 2776
Tel: (01732) 760011

Ovacome
Online: www.ovacome.org.uk
St. Bartholomew's Hospital
London EC1A 7BE
Tel: (07071) 781861
E-mail: gdq53@dial.pipex.com

Women's Health
52 Featherstone Street
London EC1Y 8RT
Helpline: (020) 7251 6580
Tel: (020) 7251 6333
E-mail: womenshealth@pop3.poptel:org.uk

Women's Health Concern
93–99 Upper Richmond Road
London SW15 2TG
Tel: (020) 8780 3007

Women's Nationwide Cancer Control Campaign
Online: www.wnccc.org. uk
128–130 Curtain Road
London EC2A 3AR
Tel: (020) 7729 4688
E-mail: info@wnccc.org.uk

See also BREAST CANCER, FAMILY PLANNING, INFERTILITY, PREGNANCY AND CHILDBIRTH

INDEX

A page number in *italic typeface* indicates a separate illustration, an illustrated box, or a table. Index entries entirely in *italic typeface* are the names of useful organizations and refer to entries in the Useful Online Sites and Addresses section.

A

Abacavir 1000
abciximab 1000
ABC of resuscitation, first aid *978*
abdomen
  abdominal examination during physical examination 219–220
  swollen abdomen, symptoms chart 156
abdominal hernia 661–662
abdominal hysterectomy *747*
abdominal pain, symptoms charts 152–155, 192–193, 208–209
abdominal thrusts, first aid for choking *980*
abducent nerve, nervous system structure and functions *511*
Abidec 1000
abnormalities
  abnormality of breast size 757
  abnormal nipples 757–758
  abnormal presentation, during labour and childbirth 800–801
  abnormal vaginal bleeding 737
  abnormal vaginal discharge, symptoms chart 194
  chromosomal *see* chromosome disorders; genetic tests
  nail 360–361
  puberty *see* abnormal puberty
abnormal puberty
  effect on height 869
  in females 739–740
  in males 728–729
ABO blood group system and blood typing 227, *441*
abortion
  spontaneous abortion *see* miscarriage
  termination of pregnancy *789*
abscesses
  anal abscess 669
  brain abscess 529
  breast abscess 754, 809
  dental abscess 611–612
  peritonsillar abscess 479
absent-mindedness *see* forgetfulness and/or confusion
absent periods
  menstrual problem *see* amenorrhoea
  symptoms chart 186–187
absorption of nutrients *see* digestion; metabolism
acamprosate 1000
acarbose 1000
  drugs for diabetes mellitus 931–932
acceptance, death and dying 965
accessing hospital care 956–958
accidents
  injuries in the home *77*
  prevention *see* safety statistics 314, 316
  see also environmental disorders; first aid; injuries; poisoning
Accolate 1000
accommodation
  accommodation errors in vision *see* refractive errors
  eye structure and functions *568*
Accupro 1000
Accuretic 1000
ACE inhibitor drugs *see* angiotensin converting enzyme (ACE) inhibitor drugs
acebutolol 1000
  beta-blocker drugs 898–899
aceclofenac 1000
acemetacin 1000
acenocoumarol 1000
Acepril 1000
acetazolamide 1000
  diuretic drugs 902
  drugs for glaucoma 920–921
acetomenaphthone 1000
acetylcholine 1000
  acetylcholine/dopamine imbalance in Parkinson's disease and parkinsonism 539
acetylcysteine 1000
Acezide 1000
achalasia 637–638
Achilles tendon disorders *see* ruptured tendons; tendinitis and tenosynovitis
achondroplasia *273*, 833
aciclovir 1000
  antiviral drugs 886–887
  drugs acting on the eye 919–920
  preparations for skin infections and infestations 892–893
acid reflux *see* gastro-oesophageal reflux (GOR)
acids *see* amino acids; fatty acids; folic acid; stomach acids
Aci-Jel 1000
acipimox 1000
Acitak 1000
acitretin 1000
  retinoid drugs 890–891
aclarubicin 1000
acne 340–341
  retinoid drugs 890–891
Acnecide 1000
Acne Support Group 1036
Acnidazil 1000
Acnisal 1000
acoustic nerve *see* vestibulocochlear nerve
acoustic neuroma 605
acquired immunodeficiency disorders
  acquired immunodeficiency 460–461
  acquired immunodeficiency syndrome *see* HIV infection and AIDS
acrivastine 1000
  antihistamines 906
acromegaly 677
Actal 1000
ACTH *see* adrenocorticotrophic hormone (ACTH)
Actifed Compound 1000
Actifed Expectorant 1000
Actinac 1000
actinic keratosis *see* solar keratosis
actinomycin D 1000
Action Against Breast Cancer 1028
Action for Blind People 1031
Action for ME 1035
Action Research 1028
Action on Smoking and Health 1037
activated charcoal 1000
active immunization 883, *884*
Active for Life 1031
Acular 1000
Acupan 1000
acupressure bands
  for nausea and vomiting
  symptom relief in the terminally ill 965
acupuncture *955*, 973
acute bronchitis 486–487
acute gastritis 640
acute glaucoma 575–576
acute glomerulonephritis 699–700
acute heart failure 412
  angiotensin converting enzyme (ACE) inhibitor drugs 900–901
  digitalis drugs 901–902
  diuretic drugs 902
acute hepatitis 644–645
  travel immunizations *86*
  vaccines and immunoglobulins 883–884
acute kidney failure 705, 706
acute laryngitis 479–480
acute leukaemia 454–455
acute liver failure 650–651
acute lymphoblastic leukaemia (ALL) 454–455
acute myeloid leukaemia (AML) 454–455
acute necrotizing ulcerative gingivitis (ANUG) 617–618
acute otitis media in children 860
acute pancreatitis 652–653
acute polyhydramnios 795
acute prostatitis 724
acute respiratory distress syndrome (ARDS) 506–507
acute sarcoidosis 498–499
acute subdural haemorrhage 535
acute urinary retention 713
acute urticaria 468
Adalat 1000
Adalat Retard 1000
adapalene 1000
Adcortyl 1000
ADD *see* attention deficit disorder (ADD)
addiction *see* dependency
Addiction Recovery Foundation 1026, 1034
Addison's disease 686
adenine, nucleotide base in DNA *265*
adenocarcinoma
  kidney cancer 704–705
  primary lung cancer 503–505
adenoidectomy and tonsillectomy *843*
adenoids
  enlarged adenoids 842–843
  removal *see* adenoidectomy and tonsillectomy
  respiratory system structure and functions 470, *471*
adenosine 1000
  antiarrhythmic drugs 898
adhesive tape, rejoining tissue after surgery *948*
adipocytes *see* fat cells
adipose tissue, surrounding internal organs *675*
Adizem-XL 1000
admission to hospital 956–958
adolescence
  health in adolescents 31–32
  sex education 32, 67
  stage in child growth and development 810, *815*
  see also puberty
adrenal gland disorders 684
  Addison's disease 686
  adrenal tumours 684
  congenital adrenal hyperplasia, in babies and children 866
  Cushing's syndrome 684–685
  hyperaldosteronism 685–686
  neuroblastoma in children 278, 850
  phaeochromocytoma 686
adrenal glands
  disorders *see* adrenal gland disorders
  hormones produced by the adrenal glands *673*
  location on kidneys *671*, *673*, *695*
  role in blood pressure control *401*, 670
  role in fight or flight response 670, *673*
  role in stem cell production control *440*
  stimulation by adrenocorticotrophic hormone (ACTH) *672*
  structure and functions 670, *671*, *673*
adrenaline *see* epinephrine
adrenal tumours 684
adrenocorticotrophic hormone (ACTH), production and functions *672*
adsorbents, antidiarrhoeal drugs 924
adult health *see* health at different ages
adult teeth *see* secondary teeth
AeroBec 1000
aerobic exercise *60*
Aerocrom 1000
Aerolin 1000
aerosols, recreational drug effects and risks *66*
Afrazine 1000
agammaglobulinaemia
  congenital immunodeficiency 827
Age Concern 1026
age factors
  in accident and serious injury statistics 314
  age and lifestyle factors in susceptibility to disease 27, 46, 261–262
  in breast cancer 759, *760*
  in cancer and cancer diagnosis 274, 279

in decline in basal metabolic rate (BMR) *674*
in female infertility 775
in health needs *see* health at different ages
in high-risk pregnancies 786
in presbyacusis 601
in presbyopia 589
in screening tests required 43
age spots *see* lentigo
aging
effect on health needs *see* health at different ages
effect on organs and body systems 20, *22–23*
effect on skin 328
useful online sites and addresses 1026
agonists, how they work *878*
agoraphobia 552–553
AIDS *see* HIV infection and AIDS
aids and equipment
in ambulances *957*
for arthritis *375*
artificial voice aids and devices, use in speech therapy 963
children's car seats *29*
digital meters for home blood glucose monitoring *689*
doctor's basic equipment *216*
emergency medical travel kit 85
first-aid kits *976*
glasses and contact lenses *588*
hearing aids *601*
in intensive care units *958*
lifejackets *81*
in medical laboratories *225*
in occupational therapy 963
pad and buzzer system for treating bedwetting *872*
safe use of exercise equipment 59
smoke detectors *79*
in special care baby units *959*
sphygmomanometer, use in blood pressure measurement *404*
stair safety gates *30*
sunglasses 81
surgical instruments *941*
thermometers *88*
tools and barbecues, garden safety 80
vehicle safety equipment *29*, *84*
for visualizing internal organs *see* imaging techniques; viewing techniques
walking aid *962*
work stations *82*
see also drug delivery systems; speculum
AIDSmap 1033
Ailax 1000
Airomir 1000
air pollution monitoring, home safety 79
air sacs *see* alveoli
airways
Airway, Breathing, Circulation *see* ABC of resuscitation
airway opening, first aid measure *978*
airway opening in spinal injuries, first aid measure *982*
effect of asthma *483*
effects of growth and aging *22–23*
see also bronchi; bronchioles; trachea
Akineton 1000
Aknemin 1000
Al-Anon Family Groups 1027
albendazole 1000
anthelmintic drugs 889
albinism *273*, 868–869
alclometasone 1000
topical corticosteroids 892
alcohol and alcohol-related problems 62–63
alcohol dependence 564–565
alcoholic hepatitis, alcohol-related liver disease 646–647
alcohol-related liver disease 646–647
assessing your alcohol consumption *63*
effect on blood glucose levels in people with diabetes mellitus *690*
effect on fetus 34
lifestyle choices *17*, *47*
units of alcohol and recommended daily limits *62*
useful online sites and addresses 1026–1027
Alcohol Concern 1027
Alcoholics Anonymous 1027
Aldactide 1000
Aldactone 1000
Aldara 1000
aldesleukin 1000
Aldomet 1001
aldosterone
deficiency disorder *see* congenital adrenal hyperplasia
overproduction disorder *see* hyperaldosteronism
production and functions *401*, *673*
alendronate 1001
drugs for bone disorders 896
alexitol 1001
alfacalcidol 1001
AlfaD 1001
alfentanil 1001
alfuzosin 1001
drugs that affect bladder control 939
drugs for prostate disorders 938–939
Algesal 1001
Algicon 1001
alginic acid, antacids 923
alimemazine 1001
Alka-Seltzer 1001
Alkeran 1001
ALL *see* acute lymphoblastic leukaemia (ALL)
allantoin 1001
Allegron 1001
alleles, forms of genes 264
Aller-eze 1001
allergen extracts, antiallergy drugs 905
allergens
common allergens causing allergic rhinitis 466–467
role in allergic reactions *445*, 466
allergic conjunctivitis 570–571
allergic reactions *see* allergies and allergic reactions
allergic rhinitis 466–467
allergies and allergic reactions *445*, 466
allergic conjunctivitis 570–571
allergic reaction mechanism *445*, 466
allergic rhinitis 466–467
anaphylaxis 469, 905, *987*
angioedema 469
antiallergy drugs 905
antihistamines 906
atopic eczema 333, 334
blepharitis 583–584
condom allergies 69
contact dermatitis 333, 335
cows' milk protein allergy in children 864
decongestants 909
dermatitis herpetiformis 336
desensitization treatment with allergen extracts 905
drug allergy 467–468
drug-induced rashes 338
eczema in children 829–830
extrinsic allergic alveolitis 502–503
food allergy 467
glossitis 633
patch testing *335*
perennial allergic rhinitis 466–467
seasonal allergic rhinitis 466–467
skin prick test *468*
urticaria 468
useful online sites and addresses 1027
see also asthma; intolerances
Alliance of Genetic Support Groups 1032
allopurinol 1001
Alomide 1001
alopecia 358–359
alpha$_1$-antitrypsin deficiency 489
Alpha1-Support UK 1034
alpha-blocker drugs
antihypertensive drugs 897–898
drugs that affect bladder control 939
drugs for prostate disorders 938–939
Alphaderm 1001
Alphagan 1001
Alphaparin 1001
alpha-thalassaemia 449
alpha-tocopheryl acetate 1001
Alphavase 1001
Alphosyl 1001
alprazolam 1001
alprostadil 1001
impotence treatment 771
Altacite Plus 1001
alteplase 1001
thrombolytic drugs 904–905
altitude sickness 324–325
altretamine 1001
Alu-Cap 1001
Aludrox 1001
aluminium acetate 1001
drugs acting on the ear 921
aluminium chloride 1001
aluminium hydroxide 1001
antacids 923
Alvedon 1001
alveoli
abnormally dilated *see* bulla
disorders *see* alveoli disorders
respiratory system structure and functions *471*, *473*
alveoli disorders
extrinsic allergic alveolitis 502–503
fibrosing alveolitis 497–498
pneumonia 490–491
pneumothorax 496–497
respiratory failure 507
Alvercol 1001
alverine 1001
antispasmodic drugs and motility stimulants 926
Alzheimer Scotland – Action on Dementia 1027
Alzheimer's disease 536–537
Alzheimer's Disease Society 1027
amantadine 1001
antiviral drugs 886–887
Amaryl 1001
AmBisome 1001
amblyopia 858
ambulances and paramedics *955*, *957*
ambulatory ECG *416*
amenorrhoea 735
American Academy of Otolaryngology–Head and Neck Surgery 1031
American Brain Tumor Association 1028
American Cancer Society 1028
American College of Rheumatology 1036
American College of Surgeons 1037
American Foundation for Urologic Disease 1037
American Liver Foundation 1034
American Pain Society 1035
American Sleep Disorders Association 1036
American Social Health Association 1036
American Speech–Language–Hearing Association 1037
American Thyroid Association 1033
amethocaine *see* tetracaine
Ametop 1001
Amias 1001
amifostine 1001
amikacin 1001
antibiotics 885–886
amiloride 1001
diuretic drugs 902
Amilospare 1001
amino acid 1001
amino acids
production by digestive system and use in metabolism *625*, *674–675*
protein creation from amino acids, role of DNA *266*
aminobenzoic acid 1001
sunscreens and sunblocks 893
aminoglutethimide 1001
anticancer drugs 907–908
aminoglycosides
antibiotics 885–886
aminophylline 1001
bronchodilator drugs 910–911

- aminosalicylate drugs 924
- amiodarone 1001
  - antiarrhythmic drugs 898
- amisulpride 1001
- amitriptyline 1001
  - antidepressant drugs 916–917
  - antimigraine drugs 913
- Amix 1001
- AML *see* acute myeloid leukaemia (AML)
- amlodipine 1001
  - calcium channel blocker drugs 900
- ammonium chloride 1001
- amniocentesis, antenatal genetic test *787*
- amniotic fluid
  - collecting samples for analysis *see* amniocentesis
  - excessive *see* polyhydramnios
  - in pregnancy *779*
  - premature loss *see* premature rupture of membranes
- amniotic sac
  - in pregnancy and childbirth *779*, *782*
  - premature rupture of the membranes 797
  - rupture in induction of labour *797*
- amobarbital 1001
  - amobarbital sodium, sleeping drugs 915–916
- amoebiasis 306
- amorolfine 1001
- amoxapine 1001
- amoxicillin 1001
  - antibiotics 885–886
- Amoxil 1001
- amphetamines
  - recreational drug effects and risks *66*
- Amphocil 1001
- amphotericin 1001
  - antifungal drugs 889
- ampicillin 1001
  - antibiotics 885-886
- ampullae, breast structure and functions *733*
- amsacrine 1001
- Amsidine 1001
- amyloidosis 693
- amyotrophic lateral sclerosis *see* motor neuron disease
- Amytal 1001
- anabolism, metabolic process *674–675*
- Anacal 1001
- Anadin 500 1001
- Anadin Extra 1001
- Anadin Paracetamol 1001
- anaemias 446–451
  - anaemia 446
  - aplastic anaemia 450–451
  - haemolytic anaemia 450
  - iron-deficiency anaemia 447
  - megaloblastic anaemia 448
  - sickle-cell disease 448–449
  - thalassaemia 449–450
- anaesthesia
  - epidural anaesthesia in labour *801*, 914
  - general anaesthesia and general anaesthetics 914, *944*
  - local anaesthesia and local anaesthetics 914, *942*
  - for major surgery 944
  - regional anaesthesia 914, *945*
  - spinal anaesthesia 914, *945*
- Anaflex 1001
- Anafranil 1001
- Anafranil SR 1001
- anal disorders
  - anal abscess 669
  - anal cancer 669
  - anal fissure 669
  - anal itching 669
  - anal and rectal problems, symptoms chart 157
  - external haemorrhoids 668
  - haemorrhoids 668
  - prolapsing haemorrhoids 668
  - threadworm infestation 310
- anaphylaxis 469, 905
  - first aid for anaphylactic shock *469*, 905, *987*
- *Anaphylaxis Campaign* 1027
- anastrozole 1001
- Anbesol 1001
- Andrews Antacid 1001
- Androcur 1001
- androgenic alopecia *see* male-pattern baldness
- androgens *see* male sex hormones
- Anethaine 1001
- aneurysms
  - aortic aneurysm 430–431
  - berry aneurysm rupture causing subarachnoid haemorrhage 534
  - dissecting aneurysm 430–431
- Angettes-75 1001
- Angilol 1001
- angina 407–409
  - drug treatment *see* beta-blocker drugs; nitrate drugs
- angioedema 469
- angiogenesis, by cancerous tumours *277*
- angiogenesis inhibition, biological therapy for cancer 282
- angiography and angiograms *243*, 246
  - cerebral angiography *533*
  - coronary angiography *408*
  - femoral angiography *433*
  - fluorescein angiography *580*
- Angiopine MR 1001
- angiotensin, role in blood pressure control *401*
- angiotensin converting enzyme (ACE) inhibitor drugs 900–901
  - antihypertensive drugs 897–898
- angiotensin II blocker drugs, antihypertensive drugs 897–898
- Angiozem 1001
- Angitil SR 1001
- Anhydrol Forte 1001
- animal bites
  - cause of rabies 296
  - first aid *995*
- animals, disorders transmitted by
  - brucellosis 300–301
  - Ebola fever, viral haemorrhagic fever 295
  - hantavirus infection, viral haemorrhagic fever 295
  - hydatid disease 313
  - Lassa fever, viral haemorrhagic fever 295
  - leptospirosis 81, 302–303
  - Marburg fever, viral haemorrhagic fever 295
  - plague 303–304
  - Q fever 304
  - rabies *86*, 296, 883
  - ringworm 352–353
  - risks from pets 82
  - tapeworm infestation 313
  - toxocariasis 82, 310–31
  - toxoplasmosis 82, 307–308, 817
  - viral haemorrhagic fevers 295
  - *see also* bites and stings
- anion-exchange resins, lipid-lowering drugs 935
- anistreplase 1001
  - thrombolytic drugs 904–905
- ankles, swollen *see* swollen ankles
- ankylosing spondylitis 378–379
- annulospiral sensory endings, type of muscle proprioceptor *513*
- Anodesyn 1001
- *Anorexia and Bulimia Nervosa Association* 1031
- anorexia nervosa 562–563
- anorgasmia *see* failure of orgasm
- Anquil 1001
- Antabuse 1001
- antacids 923
- antagonists
  - how they work *878*
- antazoline 1001
  - antipruritic drugs 891–892
- antenatal exercises *34*
- antenatal genetic tests *787*
  - amniocentesis *787*
  - chorionic villus sampling *787*
- antenatal tests and investigations
  - amniocentesis, antenatal genetic test *787*
  - antenatal genetic tests *787*
  - blood tests *786*
  - chorionic villus sampling, antenatal genetic test *787*
  - fetal monitoring *803*
  - routine tests *786*
  - ultrasound scanning in pregnancy *793*
  - urine tests *786*
- Antepsin 1001
- anterior lobe of the pituitary gland, structure and functions *672*
- anterior uveitis 574–575
- anthelmintic drugs 889
- Anthisan 1001
- *Anthony Nolan Bone Marrow Trust* 1027
- antiallergy drugs 905
- antiandrogens
  - drugs for prostate disorders 938–939
  - sex hormones and related drugs 933–934
- antianxiety drugs 916
- antiarrhythmic drugs 898
- antibiotics 885–886
  - antibiotic delivery system for intravenous antibiotics *825*
  - antibiotic resistance in bacteria *286*
  - antibiotic resistance in bacteria, tests for drug sensitivity 234–235
  - antituberculous drugs 886
  - drugs acting on the ear 921
  - preparations for skin infections and infestations 892–893
- antibodies
  - biological therapy for cancer 282
  - in breast milk *28*
  - in colostrum *783*
  - measurement in immune function tests 228
  - Rh antibodies in Rhesus incompatibility in pregnancy 795–796
  - role in allergic reactions *445*, 466
  - role in immune system 440, *441*, *445*
  - role in immunization 883, *884*
  - tests for antigens and antibodies 235
- antibody immune response, body's defences *445*
- anticancer drugs 907–908
  - *see also* chemotherapy
- anticholinergic drugs
  - antispasmodic drugs and motility stimulants 926
  - bronchodilator drugs 910–911
  - drugs that affect bladder control 939
- anticoagulants, drugs that prevent blood clotting 904
- anticonvulsant drugs 914–915
- antidepressant drugs 916–917
- antidiarrhoeal drugs 924
- anti-D immunoglobulin 1001
  - vaccines and immunoglobulins 883–884
- antidiuretic hormone (ADH) *see* vasopressin
- antiemetic drugs 922
  - drugs acting on the ear 921
- antifibrinolytic drugs, drugs that promote blood clotting 903
- antifungal drugs 889
  - drugs acting on the ear 921
  - preparations for skin infections and infestations 892–893
- antigenic drift and shift, viruses *285*
- antigens
  - in blood groups *441*
  - human leukocyte antigens (HLAs), role in multifactorial gene disorders 273
  - on microorganisms *285*, *445*
  - tests for antigens and antibodies 235
- antihaemophilic factor (Factor VIII) 1001
  - drugs that promote blood clotting 903
- antihistamines 906
  - antiallergy drugs 905
  - antiemetic drugs 922
  - antipruritic drugs 891–892
  - sleeping drugs 915–916
- antihypertensive drugs 897–898
- anti-infective drugs
  - drugs acting on the eye 919–920
  - *see also* antibiotics; antifungal drugs; antiprotozoal drugs; antiviral drugs
- anti-inflammatory drugs
  - aminosalicylate drugs 924
  - antirheumatic drugs 895–896
  - drugs acting on the ear 921

drugs acting on the eye 919–920
nonsteroidal anti-inflammatory drugs (NSAIDs) 894, *895*
see also corticosteroids
antimalarial drugs 888–889
antimigraine drugs 913
anti-oestrogens
drugs for infertility 936–937
sex hormones and related drugs 933–934
antiparasitic drugs, preparations for skin infections and infestations 892–893
antiplatelet drugs, drugs that prevent blood clotting 904
Antipressan 1001
antiprotozoal drugs 888
antimalarial drugs 888–889
antipruritic drugs 891–892
antipsychotic drugs 917–918
antiretroviral drugs, drugs for HIV infection and AIDS 887–888
antirheumatic drugs 895–896
antiseptics
preparations for skin infections and infestations 892–893
antisocial personality disorder 561
antispasmodic drugs and motility stimulants 926
antithyroid drugs
drugs for hyperthyroidism 932–933
how they work *933*
antituberculous drugs 886
antiviral drugs 886–887
drugs for HIV infection and AIDS 887–888
preparations for skin infections and infestations 892–893
Antizol 1001
Anturan 1001
ANUG *see* acute necrotizing ulcerative gingivitis (ANUG)
Anugesic-HC 1001
anus
digestive system structure and functions 620, *621*, *623*
disorders *see* anal disorders
Anusol-HC 1001
anxiety and anxiety-related disorders
agoraphobia 552–553
antianxiety drugs 916
anxiety disorders 551–552
anxiety, symptoms chart 124
claustrophobia 552
complex phobias 552–553
hypnotherapy 974–975
insomnia 554, 915–916
mental problems due to physical illness 558
obsessive–compulsive disorder 553–554
panic attacks and panic disorder 551–552
persistent anxiety state 551–552
post-traumatic stress disorder (PTSD) 553
simple phobias 552–553
social phobias 552–553
in the terminally ill 965, *966*
see also psychological therapies; stress
anxiolytics *see* antianxiety drugs
anxious or fearful personality disorders 561–562
aorta
connection to the kidneys 694, *695*
disorders *see* aortic aneurysm; coarctation of the aorta
location and role in cardiovascular system 396, *397–400*
aortic aneurysm 430–431
aortic incompetence 422–423
aortic stenosis 423
aortic valve
disorders *see* aortic incompetence; aortic stenosis
heart structure *398*
replacement *422*
aplastic anaemia 450–451
apomorphine 1001
APP 1001
appendicitis 664
appendicular skeleton *363*
appendix
digestive system structure *621*
inflamed *see* appendicitis
appetite *620*
loss of appetite, eating problems in children 852
apraclonidine 1002
drugs for glaucoma 920–921
Aprinox 1002
aprotinin 1002
drugs that promote blood clotting 903
Aprovel 1002
Apsolol 1002
Apstil 1002
AquaBan 1002
Aquadrate 1002
aqueous cream
emollients and barrier preparations 890
aqueous humour, eye structure and functions *567*
arachnoid
bleeding between dura mater and arachnoid *see* subdural haemorrhage
bleeding between pia mater and arachnoid *see* subarachnoid haemorrhage
brain and spinal cord structure *509*
arachnoid granulation, brain structure and functions *510*
ARDS *see* acute respiratory distress syndrome (ARDS)
Aredia 1002
areola
breast structure and functions *733*
during pregnancy *780*
argipressin 1002
Aricept 1002
Aridil 1002
arm disorders
lymphangitis 458–459
lymphoedema 459
painful arm or hand, symptoms chart 174
slings, first aid *998*
upper limb fractures, first aid *992*
see also fractures; hand disorders
arms
arm stretches, warming up and cooling down in your exercise routine *61*
disorders *see* arm disorders
fetal development during pregnancy *780*
roles of biceps and triceps muscles *362*
Arpimycin 1002
arrector pili muscle, in skin *329*, *331*
Arret 1002
arrhythmias 415–416
atrial fibrillation 417–418
cardioversion *420*
complete heart block 418
drug treatment *see* antiarrhythmic drugs; beta-blocker drugs
sick sinus syndrome 419
supraventricular tachycardia (SVT) 416–417
ventricular fibrillation, cause of cardiac arrest 419–420
arterial leg ulcers 350
arteries
arterial blood colour *442*
arterial blood samples, collection for testing 221, *501*
blood pressure levels *401*
disorders *see* artery disorders
effects of serious injuries *315*
in the heart (coronary arteries) *398*
location of major arteries in the body *397*
in the placenta and umbilical cord during pregnancy *781*
pressure points, use in first aid for bleeding *986*
structure and functions 396, *397–401*
in urinary system 694, *695*, *696*
see also individual arteries by name, e.g. renal artery
arterioles, role in blood circulation *397*, *400*
arteriovenous malformation, cause of subarachnoid haemorrhage 534
artery disorders
aortic aneurysm 430–431
atherosclerosis 402–403
berry aneurysm rupture causing subarachnoid haemorrhage 534
Buerger's disease 436
cerebral haemorrhage, cause of stroke 532
coarctation of the aorta, congenital heart disease in babies and children 837
coronary artery disease 405–407, *408*
patent ductus arteriosus, congenital heart disease in babies and children 837
polyarteritis nodosa 465
pulmonary hypertension 505–506
Raynaud's phenomenon and Raynaud's disease 436
stroke 532–534
subarachnoid haemorrhage 534–535
surgery *see* cardiovascular system surgery
temporal arteritis 464–465
tests and investigations *see* cardiovascular system tests and investigations
transient ischaemic attacks 531–532
see also embolism; thrombosis
arthritis
ankylosing spondylitis 378–379
antirheumatic drugs 895–896
cervical spondylosis 376
gout 380
joint aspiration *380*
juvenile chronic arthritis (JCA) 835
living with arthritis *375*
osteoarthritis 374–376
pauciarticular arthritis 835
polyarticular arthritis 835
pseudogout 381
reactive arthritis 379
rheumatoid arthritis 377–378
septic arthritis 381
systemic arthritis 835
types 374
useful online sites and addresses 1027
Arthritis Care 1027
Arthritis Link 1027
Arthritis Research Campaign 1027, 1033, 1035
Arthrofen 1002
arthroscopy *386*
Arthrosin 1002
Arthrotec 1002
Arthroxen 1002
articaine 1002
articular cartilage *364*, *812*
artificial insemination *775*
artificial joints *377*
artificial respiration, first aid *982–983*
use in choking in unconscious adults and children *981*
artificial tears, drugs acting on the eye 919–920
artificial teeth *see* crowns and replacement teeth
Arythmol 1002
Asacol 1002
asbestosis, asbestos-related disease 501–502
asbestos-related diseases 501–502
Ascabiol 1002
ascariasis 311
ascorbic acid 1002
Asendis 1002
asexual reproduction, bacteria 762
Asilone 1002
Asmaven 1002
asparaginase 1002
Aspav 1002
Asperger's disorder, autism spectrum disorder 852
aspergillosis 309
aspergillus fungi *287*
cause of aspergillosis 309
asphyxiation 326
result of serious injury to the trachea *315*
aspiration
aspiration of a breast lump *756*

aspiration (continued)
- bone marrow aspiration and biopsy *451*
- joint aspiration *380*
- needle aspiration of the thyroid gland *682*

aspiration pneumonia 491
aspirin 1002
- antimigraine drugs 913
- aspirin with codeine, painkillers 912–913
- cold and flu remedies 910
- drugs that prevent blood clotting 904
- nonsteroidal anti-inflammatory drugs (NSAIDs) 894
- painkillers 912–913

Aspro Clear 1002
assertiveness training, behaviour therapy technique 969
assisted conception *776*
- intracytoplasmic sperm injection (ICSI), for male infertility 777
- *see also* artificial insemination

assisted delivery, labour and childbirth *805*
Association for All Speech-Impaired Children 1037
association areas, role in information processing in the brain *515*
Association of Birth Defect Children 1027
Association for Macular Diseases 1031
Association for Psychological Therapies 1029
Association for Spina Bifida and Hydrocephalus 1027
asteatotic eczema 334
asthma 483–486
- asthma in children 839–840
- drug treatment *see* asthma drugs
- living with asthma *486*
- monitoring using peak flow meter *484*
- occupational asthma 83, 484, 499
- useful online sites and addresses 1027

Asthma and Allergy Foundation of America 1027
Asthma and Allergy Information and Research 1027
asthma drugs
- bronchodilator drugs 910–911
- for children *839*, 840
- corticosteroids for respiratory disease 911
- inhalers for children *839*
- inhalers and inhaler use *485*, *839*, *881*, 910
- nebulizer use *485*, 840, 910
- preventers 485, 840
- quick-relief (reliever) drugs 485, 840
- spacer devices *485*, *839*, 910

astigmatism 588–589
asystole, cause of cardiac arrest 420
Atenix 1002
atenolol 1002
- antianxiety drugs 916
- beta-blocker drugs 898–899

atherosclerosis 402–403
athlete's foot 353
Ativan 1002
atopic eczema 333, 334
atorvastatin 1002
- lipid-lowering drugs 935

atovaquone 1002
- antiprotozoal drugs 888

atracurium 1002
atria
- disorders *see* atrial fibrillation; atrioseptal defect
- in fetal heart *810*
- heart structure and functions 396, *396*, *398–399*

atrial fibrillation 417–418
atrial systole, heartbeat phase *399*
atrioseptal defect, congenital heart disease in babies and children 836–837
atrioventricular node, role in heartbeat cycle *399*
atrophic gastritis 640
atropine 1002
- bronchodilator drugs 910–911
- drugs acting on the eye 919–920

Atrovent 1002
attempted suicide and suicide 556–557
- suicidal thoughts, symptoms chart 122–123

attention deficit disorder (ADD) 855
Audicort 1002
audiometry, hearing test *600*
auditory cortex/auditory association cortex, location and role in information processing in the brain *515*, *594*
auditory nerve *see* cochlear nerve
auditory ossicles
- disorders *see* otosclerosis
- ear structure and functions *593*, *594*

auranofin 1002
- antirheumatic drugs 895–896

auras
- epilepsy auras 525
- migraine auras 519

Aureocort 1002
Aureomycin 1002
aurothiomalate 1002
auscultation, basic examination technique *220*
autism spectrum disorders 852–853
autoantibodies, measurement in immune function tests 228
autoimmune disorders 460, 461
- Addison's disease 686
- atrophic gastritis 640
- autoantibodies measurement, in immune function tests 228
- Behçet's syndrome 465
- chronic hepatitis 645–646, 907
- chronic–progressive multiple sclerosis (MS) 541–542
- discoid lupus erythematosus (DLE) 347
- drug treatments *see* immunosuppressants
- fibrosing alveolitis 497–498
- Graves' disease, cause of hyperthyroidism 679–680
- Hashimoto's thyroiditis 680, 681
- juvenile chronic arthritis (JCA) 835
- multiple sclerosis (MS) 541–542
- myasthenia gravis 549
- pauciarticular arthritis 835
- polyarteritis nodosa 465
- polyarticular arthritis 835
- polymyalgia rheumatica 464
- polymyositis and dermatomyositis 463–464
- primary biliary cirrhosis 647–648
- relapsing–remitting multiple sclerosis (MS) 541–542
- rheumatoid arthritis 377–378
- scleroderma 462–463
- Sjögren's syndrome 463
- systemic arthritis 835
- systemic lupus erythematosus (SLE) 461–462
- temporal arteritis 464–465
- useful online sites and addresses 1033
- uveitis 574–575
- vitiligo 342–343
- *see also* diabetes mellitus

automatic bodily functions and responses *see* involuntary responses
autonomic nerve neuropathies 544
autonomic nervous system and autonomic responses
- fight or flight response 670, *673*
- nervous system structure and functions *508*, *514*
- neuropathies *see* autonomic nerve neuropathies
- role in blood pressure control *401*

autosomal dominant disorders 272
- achondroplasia *273*, 833
- familial adenomatous polyposis (FAP), polyps in the colon 661, 666
- Huntington's disease 538
- inherited hyperlipidaemias *273*, 692, 935
- Marfan's syndrome *273*, 824
- multiple endocrine neoplasia (MEN) 683
- neurofibromatosis *273*, 827
- polycystic kidney disease *273*, 704
- porphyria *273*, 693
- tests and investigations *see* genetic tests
- von Willebrand's disease *273*, 452

autosomal recessive disorders 272
- albinism *273*, 868–869
- alpha$_1$-antitrypsin deficiency 489
- carriers 272
- cystic fibrosis 272, *273*, 824–825, *962*
- galactosaemia 868
- haemochromatosis *273*, 692–693
- juvenile polycystic kidney disease *273*, 704
- phenylketonuria 241, *273*, 867–868
- sickle-cell disease 26, *273*, 448–449
- Tay–Sachs disease 26, *273*, 868
- tests and investigations *see* genetic tests
- thalassaemia *273*, 449–450
- *see also* congenital immunodeficiency

autosomes
- autosomal abnormalities and disorders 270–271
- Down's syndrome, caused by autosomal abnormality *787*, 821–822
- types of chromosome 264, *265*, 270

AVERT 1033
Avloclor 1002
avoidant personality disorder 561
Avomine 1002
avulsed tooth 616
avulsion fractures 392
axial skeleton *363*
Axid 1002
axons *see* nerve fibres
Axsain 1002
Azactam 1002
Azamune 1002
azapropazone 1002
azatadine 1002
- antihistamines 906

azathioprine 1002
- antirheumatic drugs 895–896
- immunosuppressants 906–907

azelaic acid 1002
azelastine 1002
azidothymidine 1002
azithromycin 1002
- antibiotics 885–886

azlocillin 1002
AZT 1002
- *see also* zidovudine (AZT)

aztreonam 1002

B

babies and infants
- before birth *see* embryo; fetus
- car seats *29*
- diet 27, *28*
- disorders *see* babies and infants, problems and disorders
- drug treatments for 881, 882, *882*
- feeding *see* bottle-feeding; breast-feeding; weaning
- first aid *see* first aid for babies and infants
- growth charts *40–41*
- head circumference charts *40*
- health checkups 41
- health in infants 27–29
- heel prick blood test, screening for metabolic disorders *44*, *867*
- length charts *41*
- newborn *see* newborn babies
- physical appearance, growth and development 810, *811–814*
- positioning for sleep *820*
- premature *see* premature babies
- psychological health 28–29
- routine immunizations programme 45

screening for metabolic disorders *867*
symptoms charts *see* children's symptoms charts
tooth care 27
weight charts *41*
babies and infants, problems and disorders
atrioseptal defect, congenital heart disease 836–837
birthmarks 828
brain and spinal cord tumours in children 850
bronchiolitis 841
chordee, associated with hypospadias 870
cleft lip and palate 862
clubfoot 833
coarctation of the aorta, congenital heart disease 837
colic 819
congenital blindness 856–857
congenital deafness 859–860
congenital heart disease 836–837
congenital hip dysplasia 832
congenital infections 817
conjunctivitis 570
cows' milk protein allergy 864
cradle cap 829
croup 841–842
dacryocystitis 585
drug treatments 881, 882, *882*
eczema in children 829–830
endocrine and metabolic disorders *see* congenital adrenal hyperplasia; growth disorders; inborn errors of metabolism
excessive crying 819
Fallot's tetralogy, congenital heart disease 837
febrile convulsions 849, *989*
feeding problems in babies 819
fever reduction *289*
gastro-oesophageal reflux (GOR) in infants 863
haemangiomas, birthmarks 828
heat exhaustion and heatstroke 322–323
hormone disorders *see* congenital adrenal hyperplasia; growth disorders; inborn errors of metabolism
hydrocephalus 845–846
hypoplastic left heart syndrome, congenital heart disease 837
hypospadias 870
hypothermia 323–324
Kawasaki disease 837–838
metabolic disorders *see* congenital adrenal hyperplasia; growth disorders; inborn errors of metabolism
Mongolian blue spots, birthmarks 828
myelomeningocele, neural tube defect *845*
nappy rash 829
neonatal jaundice 817–818
neural tube defects 844–845
neuroblastoma 278, 850
oral thrush 862–863
patent ductus arteriosus, congenital heart disease 837
pigmented naevi, birthmarks 828
port-wine stains, birthmarks 828
positional clubfoot 833
problems of the premature baby 816–817
pyloric stenosis in infants 863
respiratory distress syndrome, in premature babies 816
routine immunizations 45
sleeping problems in babies 818
special care baby units *959*
spina bifida, neural tube defect 844–845
stork marks, birthmarks 828
strawberry haemangiomas, birthmarks 828
structural clubfoot 833
sudden infant death syndrome (SIDS) 28, 820
teething 819–820
testis, undescended 870
umbilical hernia 662
undescended testis 870
valve defects, congenital heart disease 837
ventriculoseptal defect, congenital heart disease 836–837
watery eye 585
see also childhood disorders; chromosome disorders
baby blues, depression after childbirth 807–808
bacilli, type of bacteria *286*
bacitracin 1002
back
backbone *see* spine
back-strengthening exercises *383*
disorders *see* back pain; spine disorders
BackCare 1027
back pain
backache in pregnancy *780, 785*
back pain prevention *382–383*
coccydynia 372
lower back pain 381–384
manipulative therapies *955*, 973–974
symptoms chart 170–171
useful online sites and addresses 1027
baclofen 1002
muscle relaxants 896
Baclospas 1002
bacteria
asexual reproduction 762
body's defences against *444–445*
in digestive system *623, 625*, 885
infections caused by bacteria *see* bacterial infections
infectious organisms size comparison *284*
Legionella pneumophilia 284, 490
role of harmless bacteria in body's defences *444*
structure and functions *286*
bacterial infections 299
acute otitis media in children 860
bacterial conjunctivitis 570–571
bacterial cystitis 709–710
bacterial pneumonia 490–491
bacterial stomatitis 633
bacterial vaginosis 753
bartholinitis 753
blepharitis 583–584
boils 351
botulism 301–302
brain abscess 529
brucellosis 300–301
cause of febrile convulsions in children 849
cause of lymphadenopathy 458
cause of lymphangitis 458
cause of reactive arthritis 379
cellulitis 352
chlamydial pelvic infection 765–766
cholecystitis 652
cholera 301
chronic gastritis 640
congenital infections, in newborn babies 817
dacryocystitis 585
diphtheria *45*, 300, 883
drug treatments *see* antibiotics
endemic typhus 304
epidemic typhus 304
epiglottitis 842
folliculitis 352
food poisoning 629–630
gastroenteritis 85, 628–629
gonorrhoea 764–765
Hansen's disease 302
Helicobacter pylori infection 639–640
impetigo 351–352
infective endocarditis 426–427
labyrinthitis 604
Legionnaires' disease 490
leptospirosis 81, 302–303
listeriosis 301, 817
Lyme disease 303,
mastitis 809
meningitis *see* bacterial meningitis
meningococcal meningitis 527–528
nongonococcal urethritis (NGU) 765
osteomyelitis 372
otitis externa 596
otitis media 597
paronychia 361
peritonitis 665
pertussis *45*, 492–493, 883
pharyngitis and tonsillitis 479, 843
plague 303–304
pneumonia 490–491
prevention *see* food poisoning; immunization; travel health
prostatitis 724
pyelonephritis 698–699, 871
Q fever 304
rheumatic fever 429
Rocky Mountain spotted fever 304
scarlet fever 300
scrub typhus 304
septicaemia 299
septic arthritis 381
styes 583
syphilis 766, 817
tuberculosis (TB) 491–492
tests for and on causative microorganisms 234–235
tetanus *45*, 302, 883
toxic shock syndrome 300
trachoma 572
typhoid and paratyphoid *86*, 301, 883
typhus 304
urinary tract infections in children 871
wet gangrene 435
bacterial meningitis 527–528
bacterial meningitis in children 848–849
travel immunizations *86*
Bactroban 1002
balance
disorders *see* balance disorders
role of inner ear structures 592, *593, 595*
role of proprioceptors *513*
role of vestibular and vestibulocochlear nerves *511*
balance disorders
labyrinthitis 604
motion sickness 85, 604
vertigo 603–604
balanitis 722–723
baldness
alopecia 358–359
male-pattern 359
ball-and-socket joints *364–365*
balloon angioplasty *see* coronary angioplasty
balloon valvuloplasty, for mitral stenosis 424
balsalazide 1002
aminosalicylate drugs 924
Bambec 1002
bambuterol 1002
bronchodilator drugs 910–911
bandages and dressings, first aid uses *976, 996–998*
banding haemorrhoids *668*
Baratol 1002
barbecue safety 80
barium (barium sulphate)
barium enema 246
barium swallow (barium meal) 246, *637*
double-contrast radiography 246–247
baroreceptors, role in blood pressure control *401*
barotrauma 598
Barrett's oesophagus, caused by gastro-oesophageal reflux (GOR) 636
barrier mechanisms, body's defences *444*
barrier methods of contraception 69, *70*
barrier preparations and emollients 890
bartholinitis 753
Bartholin's cysts, caused by bartholinitis 753
Bartholin's glands
disorders *see* bartholinitis; Bartholin's cysts
female reproductive system structure and functions *731*
basal cell carcinoma 344–345
basal cells, skin structure *330*

basal ganglia
  brain structure and functions *510, 514–515*
  disorders *see* Parkinson's disease and parkinsonism
basal metabolic rate (BMR) 52, 54, *674*
bases, nucleotide bases in DNA 264, *265–266, 269*
base triplets, in DNA *266*
basic hormone tests 232
basic viewing techniques 254
basilar membrane, ear structure and functions *594*
basiliximab 1002
basophils, white blood cell type *441*
Baxan 1002
Baycaron 1002
Bazuka 1002
BBC Education: The Health Site 1026
BBC Online Health and Fitness 1026, 1031, 1035
B-cells (B-lymphocytes), role in antibody immune response *445*
BCG, vaccines and immunoglobulins 883–884
Becker muscular dystrophy 826
Beclazone 1002
Becloforte 1002
beclometasone 1002
  corticosteroids 930–931
  corticosteroids for respiratory disease 911
  topical corticosteroids 892
Becodisks 1002
Beconase 1002
Becosym 1002
Becotide Rotacaps 1002
bedsores *see* pressure sores
bedwetting 872, 939
Beechams Powders 1002
Beechams Powders Capsules 1002
behaviour
  behavioural problems in children *see* developmental and psychological disorders in children
  hypnotherapy to change behaviour patterns 974–975
  social behaviour and play, developmental milestones during childhood *814*
behaviour therapy 969
  see also psychological therapies
Behçet's syndrome 465
being overweight *see* weight problems
belladonna 1002
Bell's palsy 548
bendrofluazide *see* bendroflumethiazide
bendroflumethiazide 1002
  diuretic drugs 902
bends, the *see* decompression sickness
Benemid 1002
benign prostatic hyperplasia *see* enlarged prostate gland
benign tumours *see* noncancerous tumours
Benoral 1002
benorilate 1002
benperidol 1002
benserazide 1002
Benylin 1002
benzalkonium chloride 1002
Benzamycin 1002
benzhexol *see* trihexyphenidyl 1024
benzocaine 1002
  antipruritic drugs 891–892
  local anaesthetics 914
benzodiazepines
  antianxiety drugs 916
  anticonvulsant drugs 914–915
  sleeping drugs 915–916
benzoyl peroxide 1002
benzthiazide 1002
benztropine 1002
benzydamine 1002
benzyl benzoate 1002
  preparations for skin infections and infestations 892–893
benzylpenicillin 1002
beractant 1002
bereavement and grieving 37, 76, 967
  grieving process 76
  useful online sites and addresses 1029
Berkolol 1002
Berkozide 1002
Berotec 1002
berry aneurysms, rupture causing subarachnoid haemorrhage 534
Beta-Adalat 1002
beta-adrenergic blocking agents *see* beta-blocker drugs
beta-blocker drugs 898–899
  antianxiety drugs 916
  antiarrhythmic drugs 898
  antihypertensive drugs 897–898
  drugs for glaucoma 920–921
Betacap 1002
Beta-Cardone 1002
betacarotene 1003
Betadine 1003
Betaferon 1003
Betagan 1003
betahistine 1003
Betaloc 1003
betamethasone 1003
  corticosteroids 930–931
  drugs acting on the ear 921
  drugs acting on the eye 919–920
  locally acting corticosteroids 895
  topical corticosteroids 892
Beta-Prograne 1003
beta-thalassaemia 449
betaxolol 1003
  drugs for glaucoma 920–921
bethanechol 1003
Betnesol 1003
Betnovate 1003
Betnovate-C 1003
Betnovate-N 1003
Betnovate-Rectal 1003
Betoptic 1003
Bettamousse 1003
bezafibrate 1003
  lipid-lowering drugs 935
bicalutamide 1003
  drugs for prostate disorders 938–939
  sex hormones and related drugs 933–934
biceps muscles *362, 366*
bile duct
  common bile duct, digestive system structure and functions *624*
  disorders *see* bile duct disorders
bile duct disorders
  bile duct obstruction, cause of jaundice 643
  blockage by gallstones 651
  blockage by gallstones causing cholecystitis 652
  endoscopic retrograde cholangiopancreatography (ERCP) *653*
  primary biliary cirrhosis 647–648
  sclerosing cholangitis, cause of cirrhosis 648
bile, production and role in digestive system *621, 624, 625*
bilharzia *see* schistosomiasis
bilirubin
  role in jaundice 643, 817–818
  tests for, routine blood chemistry 230
binge-eating, in bulimia 563
BiNovum 1003
biochemical analyser, use in chemical tests *230*
biochemical markers, tests for gene products or biochemical markers 241
biochemical (body chemical) tests *see* chemical tests
biofeedback 975
biological therapies, cancer 282
biopsies
  bone marrow aspiration and biopsy *451*
  cancer staging *279*
  cone biopsy, for cervical dysplasia *751*
  endometrial sampling *738*
  kidney biopsy *701*
  liver biopsy *647*
  prostate gland biopsy *726*
  skin biopsy *344*
  tissue samples, collection for testing 223
Bioral 1003
biotin 1003
biperiden 1003
bipolar affective disorder 557
  antipsychotic drugs 917–918
  mood-stabilizing drugs 918
bird fanciers' lung, extrinsic allergic alveolitis 502
birth *see* labour and childbirth
birth canal *see* vagina
birth control *see* contraception
Birth Defects Foundation 1027, 1032
birth defects, useful online sites and addresses 1027
birthmarks 828
  laser treatment removal *951*
bisacodyl 1003
  laxatives 924–925
bisexuality 762
Bismag 1003
bismuth 1003
  ulcer-healing drugs 923–924
BiSoDol 1003
bisoprolol 1003
  beta-blocker drugs 898–899
bisphosphonates, drugs for bone disorders 896
bites and stings
  animal bites, cause of rabies 296
  animal and human bites, first aid *995*
  diseases transmitted by flea bites *see* endemic typhus; plague
  diseases transmitted by mosquito bites *see* dengue fever; malaria; yellow fever
  diseases transmitted by tick bites *see* Lyme disease; Rocky Mountain spotted fever
  first aid 327, *994–995*
  human and animal bites, first aid *995*
  insect stings, first aid *995*
  poisonous bites and stings 327
  poisonous bites and stings, first aid *994*
  prevention 85, 86, 327
  tick bites, first aid *995*
bite-wing X-rays *609*
biting and chewing
  role in digestion 620, *622*
  teeth and jaw structure and functions 606, *607*
blackhead formation, in acne 340–341
black lung *see* coalworkers' pneumoconiosis
bladder
  bladder catheterization *713*
  compression during pregnancy *779*
  disorders *see* bladder and urethra disorders
  urinary system structure and functions 694, *695, 697*
bladder stones 714
  lithotripsy *702*
bladder and urethra disorders 709
  acute urinary retention 713
  bacterial cystitis 709–710
  bladder catheterization *713*
  bladder tumours 715
  chronic urinary retention 713
  cystitis 709–710
  cystoscopy *715*
  drugs that affect bladder control 939
  fistula, caused by diverticular disease 664
  incontinence *see* urinary incontinence
  interstitial cystitis 709–710
  intravenous urography (IVU) 246, *695, 699*
  nongonococcal urethritis (NGU) 765
  radiation cystitis 710
  urethral stricture 714
  urethral syndrome 710
  urinary retention 713, 939
  urination problems, symptoms charts 165–169
  urodynamic studies *711*
  useful online sites and addresses 1037
  see also bladder stones
blastomas
  nephroblastoma *see* Wilms' tumour

  neuroblastoma 278, 850
  retinoblastoma 858–859
bleeding
  abnormal vaginal bleeding 737
  abnormal vaginal bleeding, symptoms chart 190–191
  bleeding from the digestive tract 630
  bleeding in pregnancy, symptoms chart 190
  blood behind cornea *see* hyphaema
  blood in faeces, symptoms chart 160
  blood in semen, symptoms chart 182
  bloodstained discharge, nipple discharge 758
  blood in vomit, symptoms chart 148
  bruises 357
  coughing up blood, symptoms chart 142
  drugs that promote blood clotting 903
  first aid *986*
  inside cancerous tumours *275*
  inside skull *315*
  menstrual periods *see* menstruation and menstrual cycle
  nosebleeds 474–475
  postmenopausal bleeding 738–739
  severe bleeding, first aid *986*
  vaginal bleeding, abnormal 737
  vaginal bleeding outside menstruation, symptoms chart 190–191
  vaginal bleeding in pregnancy 791
  see also bleeding disorders; haemorrhages; viral haemorrhagic fevers
bleeding disorders 451–453
  drugs that promote blood clotting 903
  haemophilia and Christmas disease 452
  thrombocytopenia 453
  useful online sites and addresses 1027–1028
  von Willebrand's disease 452
  see also viral haemorrhagic fevers
Blemix 1003
bleomycin 1003
  anticancer drugs 907–908
blepharitis 583–584
blindness 591
  colour *see* colour blindness
  congenital blindness 856–857
  useful online sites and addresses 1031
blind spot
  disorders *see* papilloedema
  eye structure and functions *567*
blistering diseases 336
blisters 357
  blistering diseases 336
  chickenpox 290
  cold sores 354
  genital herpes 767–768
  hand, foot, and mouth disease 831
  herpes simplex infections 291
  herpes zoster 290–291
  impetigo 351–352
blockages *see* obstructions and blockages
blood
  blood filtration in the kidneys 694, *696–697*
  blood groups *441*
  blood products, drugs that promote blood clotting 903
  blood typing 227
  blood volume and its distribution 396, *400*, *441*, 694
  cancer spread in *277*
  cells *see* blood cells
  cholesterol levels *see* blood cholesterol levels
  circulation *see* circulation of the blood
  clots *see* blood clots
  colour *442*
  composition and function 440, *441–442*, *444–445*
  disorders *see* blood disorders
  glucose levels *see* blood glucose levels
  poisoning *see* septicaemia
  pressure *see* blood pressure
  Rhesus (Rh) proteins *see* Rhesus (Rh) blood group system
  tests and investigations *see* blood flow scans; blood tests
  transfusions *see* blood transfusions
  vessels *see* blood vessels
  see also bleeding; transport by the blood
blood cells
  blood cell tests 226–227
  disorders *see* blood disorders
  formation in bone marrow *440*
  platelets, formation and function 440, *441–442*, 446
  red blood cells, formation and function 440, *441–442*, 446
  types and functions 440, *441* *445*, 446
  white *see* white blood cells
blood cholesterol levels
  blood cholesterol tests *44*, 231–232
  disorders caused by high blood cholesterol levels *see* atherosclerosis; inherited hyperlipidaemias
  effect of diet and effect on health 50–51
  high (hypercholesterolaemia) 691–692
  lipid-lowering drugs 935
  optimal levels 692
blood clots
  blood clotting disorders *see* bleeding disorders; hypercoagulability
  cause of retinal vein occlusion 578
  drugs that prevent blood clotting 904
  formation *442*
  inside skull, effect of serious injuries *315*
  role in deep vein thrombosis 437–438
  role in multi-infarct dementia 537
  role in myocardial infarction 410, *410*
  role in pulmonary embolism 495
  role in stroke 532–533
  role in subdural haemorrhage 535
  role in superficial thrombophlebitis 439
  role in thrombosis and embolism 431–432
  role in transient ischaemic attacks 531
  thrombolytic drugs 904–905
  see also haematomas
blood clotting tests 227–228
blood disorders 446
  cancers *see* leukaemias; multiple myeloma
  clotting disorders *see* bleeding disorders; hypercoagulability
  drugs for blood disorders 903–905
  haemolytic jaundice 643
  jaundice 643–644
  neonatal jaundice 817–818
  polycythaemia 457
  septicaemia 299
  useful online sites and addresses 1027–1028
  see also anaemias; bleeding
blood flow scans
  carotid Doppler scanning *531*
  Doppler ultrasound scanning *243*, 251, *432*
  radionuclide lung scanning *494*
blood gases measurement *501*
blood glucose levels
  disorders affecting blood glucose levels *see* diabetes mellitus; hypoglycaemia
  effect of exercise *690*
  home monitoring *689*, 931
  hormone regulation *671*, *674*
  measurement using routine urine chemistry tests 231
blood poisoning *see* septicaemia
blood pressure
  blood pressure measurement *44*, *404*
  blood pressure monitoring for people with diabetes mellitus *690*
  control mechanisms 396, *401*, 694
  diastolic *401*
  disorders *see* blood pressure disorders
  high *see* hypertension
  low *see* hypotension
  systolic *401*
  variation during heartbeats *399*
blood pressure disorders
  antihypertensive drugs 897–898
  hypertension (high blood pressure) 403–405
  hypotension (low blood pressure) 414
  portal hypertension and varices 648–649
  postural hypotension 414
  in pregnancy *see* pre-eclampsia (pre-eclamptic toxaemia) and eclampsia
  pulmonary hypertension 505–506
  shock 414
blood products, drugs that promote blood clotting 903
blood tests
  blood cell tests 226–227
  blood cholesterol tests *44*, 231–232
  blood clotting tests 227–228
  blood gases measurement *501*
  blood smear, blood cell test *212*, 227
  blood typing 227
  C-reactive protein measurements, test for inflammation 233
  during pregnancy *786*
  erythrocyte sedimentation test, test for inflammation 233
  full blood count, blood cell test 226–227
  heel prick blood test, screening for metabolic disorders in newborn babies *44*, *867*
  home blood glucose monitoring *689*
  hormone tests 232
  immune function tests 228
  preoperative blood tests 943
  routine blood chemistry 229–230
  samples collection 221–223, *456*, *501*, *689*
  tests for inflammation 232–233
  tests for microorganisms 234–235
  tumour marker tests 233
  see also genetic tests
blood transfusions *447*
  blood group importance *441*
  blood typing 227
blood vessels
  angiogenesis by cancerous tumours *277*
  arterioles, role in blood circulation *397*, *400*
  in bones *363*, *364*, 368
  cancerous tumour damage *275*, *277*
  contrast X-rays *see* angiography and angiograms
  damage repair by blood clots *442*
  disorders *see* artery disorders; bleeding; peripheral vascular disorders; vein disorders
  effect of inflammatory response *444*
  effects of growth and aging *22–23*
  in the eye *567*, *568*
  location of major blood vessels in the body *397*
  in male reproductive system *717*
  nourishing noncancerous tumours *275*
  peripheral vascular system 430
  in the placenta and umbilical cord during pregnancy *781*
  portal system supplying pituitary gland *672*
  role in thermoregulation *331*

blood vessels (continued)
  structure and functions 396, *397–401*
  in teeth and gums 606, *607*
  in urinary system *694, 695–697*
  venules, role in blood circulation *397, 400*
  see also arteries; capillaries; sinusoids; veins
blue naevi, type of mole 343
BMI *see* body mass index (BMI)
BMR *see* basal metabolic rate (BMR)
Bocasan 1003
body fat
  distribution, health risks indicator 53
  subcutaneous *see* subcutaneous fat
body fluids
  retention *see* fluid retention
  samples collection for testing 223
  synovial fluid, in joints *364*
  see also amniotic fluid; cerebrospinal fluid (CSF); lymph (fluid); sweat
body hair
  pilonidal sinus 360
  pubic, facial, and body hair development during puberty *716, 730, 815*
body mass index (BMI) 53–54
Body Positive 1033
body proportions at different ages *812*
body ringworm 352–353
body systems 258–260
  effects of growth and aging 20, *22–23*
  see also individual body systems by name, e.g. nervous system
body temperature
  high *see* fever (high body temperature
  measuring with a thermometer *88*
  role in natural methods of contraception *71*
  thermoregulation *331*
boils 351
bolus of food, swallowing *622*
bone cancer
  bone marrow cancer *see* leukaemias; multiple myeloma
  bone metastases *279*, 373
  palliative surgery for fracture prevention *282*
  primary bone cancer 373
bone densitometry *369*
bone density loss *see* osteoporosis
bone disorders 368
  achondroplasia 833
  cancer *see* bone cancer
  coccydynia 372
  drugs for bone disorders 896
  kyphosis and lordosis 371
  noncancerous bone tumours 372–373
  Osgood–Schlatter disease in children 834
  osteomalacia and rickets 370
  osteomyelitis 372
  osteoporosis 368–369, *733*, 896
  otosclerosis 598
  Paget's disease of the bone 370–371, 896
  Perthes' disease in children 833–834
  scoliosis 371
  sports injuries 391–392
  see also bone marrow disorders; fractures
bone marrow
  bone marrow aspiration and biopsy *451*
  bone marrow transplant *454*
  disorders *see* bone marrow disorders
  role in blood cell formation 362, *440*
bone marrow disorders
  aplastic anaemia 450
  cancer *see* leukaemias; multiple myeloma
  polycythaemia 457
bone metastases *279*, 373
Bonefos 1003
bones
  compact *see* compact bone
  diaphyses and epiphyses during bone development *812*
  disorders *see* bone disorders
  effects of exercise 55, *56*
  effects of growth and aging *22–23*
  growth and development in babies and children *811, 812*
  location of major bones of the skeleton and skull *363*
  long *see* long bones
  in the middle ear *593, 594*
  ossification *812*
  repair and healing *364*
  routine blood chemistry tests for bone minerals 230
  skeleton *363*
  spongy *see* spongy bone
  structure and functions 362, *363–364*, 368
  see also individual bones by name, e.g. femur
Bonjela 1003
Bonjela pastilles 1003
booster immunization 45, 884
Boots Nirolex Lozenges 1003
borderline personality disorder 561
bottle-feeding *28*, 35
botulinum toxin 1003
  cause of botulism 301–302
  muscle relaxants 896
botulism 301–302
bovine spongiform encephalopathy (BSE), cause of new variant Creutzfeldt–Jakob disease 540
bowel disorders, inflammatory *see* Crohn's disease; ulcerative colitis
bowel movement disorders *see* constipation; diarrhoea; encopresis
bow legs, minor leg and foot problems in children 834
braces, use in orthodontic treatment *614*
brachial plexus, spinal nerves structure *511*
brachial pulse in infants, first aid circulation check *978*
Bradosol 1003
bradycardias
  type of arrhythmia 415
brain
  brain maps of information and sensory processing areas *515*
  brain tissue *see* grey matter; white matter
  disorders *see* brain and spinal cord disorders
  drugs acting on the brain and nervous system 912–918
  effects of growth and aging *22–23*
  effects of serious injuries *315*
  growth and development in babies and children *812, 813*
  nervous system structure and functions 508, *509–515*
  role in hearing and balance 592, *594–595*
  role in vision *515*, 566, *568–569*
brain abscess 529
brain attack *see* stroke
brain death 523
Brain Injury Association 1032
brain and spinal cord disorders
  acute subdural haemorrhage 535
  arteriovenous malformation, cause of subarachnoid haemorrhage 534
  berry aneurysm rupture causing subarachnoid haemorrhage 534
  brain abscess 529
  brain death 523
  carotid Doppler scanning *531*
  cerebral angiography *533*
  cerebral embolism, cause of stroke 533–534
  cerebral haemorrhage, cause of stroke 533–534
  cerebral palsy, in babies and children 846–847
  cerebral thrombosis, cause of stroke 532–534
  chronic subdural haemorrhage 535
  coma 522–523
  electroencephalography (EEG) *525*
  hydrocephalus, in babies and children 845–846
  injuries *see* head injuries; spinal injuries
  myelomeningocele, neural tube defect in babies and children *845*
  narcolepsy 526–527, 918
  neural tube defects, in babies and children 844–845
  persistent vegetative state 523
  rehabilitation *see* rehabilitation and rehabilitation therapies
  Reye's syndrome in children 849
  spina bifida, neural tube defect in babies and children 844–845
  stroke 532–534
  subarachnoid haemorrhage 534–535
  subdural haemorrhage 535
  transient ischaemic attacks 531–532
  tumours *see* brain tumours
  viral encephalitis *86*, 528–529
  whiplash, spinal injury 524
  see also degenerative disorders; dementia; epilepsy; headaches; meningitis
brain stem, nervous system structure and functions *510, 511, 514*
Brain Tumour Action 1028
Brain Tumour Foundation 1028
brain tumours 530
  brain and spinal cord tumours in children 850
  useful online sites and addresses 1028
  see also acoustic neuroma; pituitary tumours
bran
  antidiarrhoeal drugs 924
  laxatives 924–925
brand names and generic names, drugs 1000
Brasivol 1003
breakbone fever *see* dengue fever
Breakthrough Breast Cancer 1028
breast cancer 759–761
  age and risk of breast cancer *760*
  aspiration of a breast lump *756*
  lumpectomy 760, *761*
  mammography *44, 759*
  mastectomy 760, *761*
  quadrantectomy 760
  tumours 758
  useful online sites and addresses 1028
Breast Cancer Campaign 1028
Breast Cancer Care 1028
breast disorders 754
  abnormality of breast size 757
  abnormal nipples 757–758
  aspiration of a breast lump *756*
  breast abscess 754, 809
  breast cysts 755, *756*
  breast engorgement 808
  breast pain 756
  breast problems in females, symptoms chart 184–185
  breast reduction *757*
  cancer *see* breast cancer
  cracked nipples 808, *809*
  cyclical breast pain 756
  fibroadenoma 754–755
  galactorrhoea, nipple discharge 758
  lumps *see* breast lumps
  mammography *44, 759*
  mastitis 809
  nipple discharge 758
  nipple inversion, abnormal nipples 757–758
  Paget's disease of the breast, breast cancer 758, 759, 760
breast enlargement in males *see* gynaecomastia
breast-feeding *28*, 34–35
  cause of breast problems and disorders 808–809
  feeding problems in babies 819
  passing mother's drug intake on to the baby 881
  positioning baby on the nipple for breast-feeding *809*
  see also breast milk production

Breastfeeding Network, 1035
breast lumps 754
aspiration of a breast lump *756*
breast abscess 754, 809
breast cancer 759–761
breast cysts 755, *756*
fibroadenoma 754–755
lumpectomy, for breast cancer 760, *761*
mammography *44, 759*
mastectomy, for breast cancer 760, *761*
quadrantectomy, for breast cancer 760
breast milk production *733,* 778, *783*
causing breast engorgement 808
causing nipple discharge in second trimester of pregnancy *780*
effect of mother's drug intake 881
inadequate drainage, cause of mastitis 809
see also breast-feeding
breast pain 756
breasts
breast reduction *757*
colostrum and colostrum production *783*
development during puberty *730, 815*
disorders in females *see* breast disorders
disorders in males *see* gynaecomastia
during pregnancy 778, *780*
female reproductive system structure and functions 730, *733*
milk production *see* breast milk production
role in sexual arousal 730, *733, 762*
self-examination *755*
breathing
Airway, Breathing, Circulation *see* ABC of resuscitation
artificial respiration, first aid *982–983*
assistance using home oxygen therapy *507, 966*
breathing assistance for the terminally ill 965, *966*
breathing rate, checking children's *89, 205*
breathing and respiration, respiratory system functions 470, *471, 472–473*
breathing techniques, relaxation exercises *75*
disorders *see* respiratory system disorders
effect on the lungs of a baby's first breath *810, 811*
rebreathing technique for coping with panic attacks *552*
role of inhalation in venous return of blood *400*
breech presentation and birth, abnormal fetal presentation 800–801
bretylium 1003
antiarrhythmic drugs 898
Brevinor 1003
Bricanyl 1003
bridges, replacement teeth *615*
brimonidine 1003
drugs for glaucoma 920–921
Britaject 1003
British Allergy Foundation 1027
British Association for Counselling 1029
British Association of Dermatologists 1036
British Association for Sexual and Relationship Therapy 1036
British Brain and Spine Foundation 1032, 1035
British Brain Tumour Association 1028
British Chiropractic Association 1029
British Colostomy Association 1030
British Deaf Association 1032
British Dental Association 1030
British Dental Health Foundation 1030
British Diabetic Association 1030
British Dyslexia Association 1034
British Epilepsy Association 1031
British Heart Foundation 1032
British Kidney Patient Association 1037
British Liver Trust 1034
British Lung Foundation 1034
British Medical Acupuncture Society 1029
British Medical Association 1026
British Nutrition Foundation 1030, 1035
British Osteopathic Association 1029
British Pregnancy Advisory Service 1031
British Psychological Society 1029
British Red Cross Society 1032, 1034
British Sjögren's Syndrome Association 1033
British Snoring and Sleep Apnoea Association 1031, 1036
British Society of Gastroenterology 1030
British Society for Rheumatology 1036
British Stammering Association 1037
British Tinnitus Association 1032
Britlofex 1003
broad-spectrum antibiotics 885–886
Broca's area, location and role in information processing in the brain *515*
Broflex 1003
Brolene 1003
bromazepam 1003
bromocriptine 1003
pituitary drugs 934–935
brompheniramine 1003
antihistamines 906
bronchi
bronchoscopy *504*
disorders *see* asthma; bronchiectasis; bronchitis
effects of bronchodilator drugs *910*
respiratory system structure *471*
bronchiectasis 496
bronchioles
inflamed *see* bronchiolitis
respiratory system structure *471, 473*
bronchiolitis 841
bronchitis
acute bronchitis 486–487
chronic bronchitis with emphysema *see* chronic obstructive pulmonary disease (COPD)
Bronchodil 1003
bronchodilator drugs 910–911
bronchoscopy *504*
brow presentation, abnormal fetal presentation 801
brucellosis 300–301
Brufen 1003
bruises 357
brushing and flossing teeth 608, *610,* 617
BSE *see* bovine spongiform encephalopathy (BSE)
bubonic plague 303–304
buccal route, drug delivery route *879*
Buccastem 1003
buclizine 1003
budesonide 1003
corticosteroids for respiratory disease 911
Buerger's disease 436
bulimia 563
bulk-forming agents
antidiarrhoeal drugs 924
how they work *925*
laxatives 924–925
bulla, ruptured bulla causing pneumothorax 497
bumetanide 1003
diuretic drugs 902
bunions 387
bupivacaine 1003
local anaesthetics 914
buprenorphine 1003
Burinex 1003
Burinex A 1003
Burinex K 1003
Burkitt's lymphoma, caused by Epstein–Barr virus (EBV) 279, 459
BurnEze 1003
burns *315,* 316, 317–318
electrical injuries 316, 318–319
first aid 317, *988*
sunburn 80, 356, 357
bursitis 387
Buscopan 1003
buserelin 1003
drugs for infertility 936–937
sex hormones and related drugs 933–934
buspirone 1003
antianxiety drugs 916
busulfan 1003
anticancer drugs 907–908
Butacote 1003
butobarbital 1003
buzzer and pad system, treating bedwetting *872*
bypass grafts
coronary artery bypass graft *411*
femoral artery bypass graft *434*
mammary artery bypass graft *411*
saphenous vein bypass graft *411*

C

cabergoline 1003
pituitary drugs 934–935
Cacit 1003
CAD *see* coronary artery disease (CAD)
caecum, digestive system structure and functions *621, 623*
caesarean section *802*
café au lait spots, neurofibromatosis symptom *827*
Cafergot 1003
caffeine 1003
central nervous system (CNS) stimulant drugs 918
Calabren 1003
Caladryl 1003
calamine 1003
calamine lotion, antipruritic drugs 891–892
Calcicard CR 1003
calciferol 1003
drugs for bone disorders 896
Calcijex 1003
Calciparine 1003
calcipotriol 1003
calcitonin 1003
drugs for bone disorders 896
production and functions *673*
calcitonin, salmon 1003
calcitriol 1003
drugs for bone disorders 896
calcium 1003
in bladder stones 714
in bone cells *363*
disorders affecting blood calcium levels *see* hyperparathyroidism; hypoparathyroidism
drugs for bone disorders 896
feedback mechanism regulating body calcium levels *670, 673*
in kidney stones 701
mineral supplements 929
osteoporosis prevention 368–369, 896, 929
routine blood chemistry tests for calcium and other bone minerals 230
routine urine chemistry tests for calcium 231
in salivary gland stones 635
sources in diet and effects on health *51*
in tooth enamel 606
calcium acetate 1003
calcium carbonate 1003
antacids 923
drugs for bone disorders 896
calcium channel blocker drugs 900
antiarrhythmic drugs 898
antihypertensive drugs 897–898
calcium chloride 1003
calcium folinate 1003
calcium gluconate 1003
Calcium Resonium 1003
Calcort 1003
Calgel 1003
Calimal 1003
calluses and corns 349
callus, role in bone repair *364*
Calmurid HC 1003

calories
calorie intake in reducing diets 54
nutritional information on food labels *52*
units of energy 52
see also food energy
Calpol 1003
calyces, kidney structure and functions *696*
CAM 1003
Camcolit 1003
camphor 1003
Campral EC 1003
Campto 1003
campylobacter infections
food poisoning 629
Guillain–Barré syndrome 550
cancer 274–283
adult cancers 279
affecting people with HIV infection and AIDS 298, 346–347
affecting specific parts of the body *see* cancers in specific body areas
cells *see* cancerous cells
in children *see* cancer in children
cure rates and survival rates 283
genetic basis 274, *276*, 278–279
spread (metastasis) *275*, *277*, *279*
surviving cancer 283
tests and investigations *see* cancer tests and investigations
treatment *see* cancer treatments
tumours *see* cancerous tumours
useful online sites and addresses 1028
CancerBACUP 1028
Cancer Care Society 1028
cancer in children 278–279
acute leukaemia 454–455
brain and spinal cord tumours in children 850
neuroblastoma 278, 850
retinoblastoma 858–859
Wilms' tumour, kidney cancer 705, 872
Cancer and Leukaemia in Childhood 1028
cancerous cells
immune system defences against 440, *445*, 458
structure, formation, and spread 274, *275–277*, *279*
cancerous tumours
affecting specific parts of the body *see* cancers in specific body areas
secondary tumours *see* metastases (secondary tumours)
staging *279*
structure, formation, and spread *275–277*, *279*
tests and investigations *see* cancer tests and investigations
treatment *see* cancer treatments
tumour growth rates *276*
Cancer Research Campaign 1028
cancers in specific body areas
adenocarcinoma, kidney cancer 704–705
adrenal tumours 684
anal cancer 669
bladder tumours 715
blood cancers *see* leukaemias
bone marrow cancers *see* leukaemias; multiple myeloma
bones *see* bone cancer
brain and spinal cord tumours in children 850
brain tumours 530
breast cancer 759–761
cancer of the cervix *281*, 750–751
cancer of the larynx 481
cancer of the nasopharynx 480–481
cancer of the oesophagus 638
cancer of the ovary 744–745
cancer of the penis 723
cancer of the testis 719–720
cancer of the uterus *281*, 748
cancer of the vulva and vagina 753
choriocarcinoma in females 748
choriocarcinoma in males, cancer of the testis 719
colorectal cancer 665–667
embryonal carcinoma, cancer of the testis 719
follicular thyroid cancer 681–682
hereditary nonpolyposis colorectal cancer (HNPCC) 666
kidney cancer 704–705, 872
liver *see* liver cancer
lungs *see* lung cancer
lymphatic system *see* lymphomas
medullary thyroid cancer 681–682
mouth cancer 634–635
Paget's disease of the breast, breast cancer 758, 759, 760
pancreatic cancer 654
papillary thyroid cancer 681–682
phaeochromocytoma, in the adrenal glands 686
pituitary tumours 676
prostate cancer *281*, 726–727
retinoblastoma, in children's eyes 858–859
salivary gland tumours 635–636
seminoma, cancer of the testis 719–720
skin *see* skin cancer
spleen *see* lymphomas
stomach cancer 642
teratoma, cancer of the testis 719
thyroid cancer 681–682
thyroid nodules 681
transitional cell carcinoma, kidney cancer 704–705
Wilms' tumour, kidney cancer in children 705, 872
cancer tests and investigations
aspiration of a breast lump *756*
barium enema *243*, 246
barium swallow (barium meal) 246, *637*
cell tests 236–237
cervical smear test *44*, *749*
colposcopy *750*
faecal occult blood test *44*, 233
mammography *44*, *759*
screening tests for prostate cancer 726
sigmoidoscopy *661*
staging *279*
tumour marker tests 233
see also biopsies; endoscopy; self-examination
cancer treatments
angiogenesis inhibition 282
antibodies 282
biological therapies 282
bone marrow transplant *454*
breast cancer surgery 760, *761*
cancer vaccines 282
cervical dysplasia treatment *751*
colectomy *665*
colostomy *666*
drug treatment *see* chemotherapy
external radiotherapy *281*
gene therapy 282
hormonal therapies 281–282, 907–908
interferon drugs 282, 907–908
internal radiotherapy *281*
lumpectomy, for breast cancer 760, *761*
mastectomy, for breast cancer 760, *761*
pain relief *283*
palliative surgery *282*
quadrantectomy, for breast cancer 760
radical prostatectomy *727*
radioactive implants and seeds *281*
radiotherapy 281
supportive care 282
surgery 274, 280
candesartan 1003
antihypertensive drugs 897–898
CANDID (Counselling and Diagnosis in Dementia) 1034
Candida albicans infections
candidiasis 309
caused by antibiotics 885
drug treatment *see* antifungal drugs
glossitis 633
nongonococcal urethritis (NGU) 765
oral thrush in babies and children 862–863
stomatitis 632–633
vaginal thrush 752–753
vulvovaginitis 752
candidiasis 309
Canesten 1003
Canesten HC 1003
canines, tooth structure *606*, *607*
canrenoate 1003
Capastat 1004
capillaries
capillary blood samples, collection for testing 221,
in glomeruli in the kidneys 694, *696–697*
role in gas exchange in respiratory system *473*
structure and functions in cardiovascular system *397*, *398*, *400*
Capozide 1004
capreomycin 1004
antituberculous drugs 886
Caprin 1004
capsaicin 1004
capsid, virus structure *285*
capsomer, virus structure *285*
capsules
bacteria structure *286*
fibrous capsules in joints *364*
fibrous capsules around noncancerous tumours *275*
glomerular capsule, kidney structure and functions *696*, *697*
lymph node structure *443*
renal capsule, kidney structure and functions *696*
captopril 1004
ACE inhibitor drugs 900–901
Carace 1004
carbachol 1004
drugs for glaucoma 920–921
Carbalax 1004
carbamazepine 1004
anticonvulsant drugs 914–915
mood-stabilizing drugs 918
carbaryl 1004
Carbellon 1004
carbenoxolone 1004
carbidopa 1004
carbimazole 1004
drugs for hyperthyroidism 932–933
carbocisteine 1004
Carbo-Dome 1004
carbohydrates 50
chemical breakdown during digestion *625*, *674–675*
complex carbohydrates in diet for people with diabetes mellitus 689, *690*
nutritional information on food labels *52*
carbon dioxide
blood gases measurement *501*
oxygen/carbon dioxide gas exchange 470, *471*, *473*
rebreathing carbon dioxide technique for coping with panic attacks *552*
role in breathing regulation *472*
waste product in blood 440, *442*, 470, *473*
carbonic anhydrase inhibitors, drugs for glaucoma 920–921
carbon monoxide (CO) poisoning 77
carboplatin 1004
anticancer drugs 907–908
carboprost 1004
drugs for labour 938
carcinogens
cause of cancer *274*, 279
effect on genes 274
effect on oncogenes *276*
in tobacco smoke 64
carcinomas
adenocarcinoma, kidney cancer 704
adenocarcinoma, primary lung cancer 503–505
basal cell carcinoma 344–345
choriocarcinoma in females 748
choriocarcinoma in males, cancer of the testis 719
embryonal carcinoma, cancer of the testis 719

large cell carcinoma, primary lung cancer 503–505
small cell carcinoma, primary lung cancer 503–505
squamous cell carcinoma 345
squamous cell carcinoma, primary lung cancer 503–505
transitional cell carcinoma, kidney cancer 704–705
Cardene 1004
cardiac arrest 419–420
cardioversion *420*
cardiac arrhythmias *see* arrhythmias
cardiac bulge, embryo growth and development *780*
cardiac electrophysiological studies *417*
cardiac glycosides, digitalis drugs 901–902
cardiac muscle *see* heart muscle
cardiac pacemakers *419*, *940*
Cardilate MR 1004
Cardinol 1004
cardiomyopathy
dilated 427–428
hypertrophic 428
cardiopulmonary resuscitation (CPR), first aid *984–985*
cardioselective beta-blockers 898–899
cardiotocography *see* fetal monitoring
cardiovascular system
disorders *see* cardiovascular system disorders
effects of growth and aging *22–23*
effects of smoking 64
peripheral vascular system 430
role of exercise in cardiovascular health 55, *56*
structure and functions 396, *397–401*
cardiovascular system disorders
blood vessel disorders *see* artery disorders; bleeding; peripheral vascular disorders; vein disorders
in children *see* cardiovascular system disorders in children
drugs for cardiovascular disorders 897–902, 904–905
major 402–420
surgery *see* cardiovascular system surgery
tests and investigations *see* cardiovascular system tests and investigations
useful online sites and addresses 1032
see also blood disorders; blood pressure disorders; heart disorders
cardiovascular system disorders in children
atrioseptal defect, congenital heart disease 836–837
coarctation of the aorta, congenital heart disease 837
congenital heart disease 836–837
Fallot's tetralogy, congenital heart disease 837
Henoch–Schönlein purpura 339, 838–839
hypoplastic left heart syndrome, congenital heart disease 837
Kawasaki disease 837–838
patent ductus arteriosus, congenital heart disease 837
valve defects, congenital heart disease 837
ventriculoseptal defect, congenital heart disease 836–837
cardiovascular system surgery
balloon valvuloplasty, for mitral stenosis 424
cardiac pacemakers *419*, *940*
coronary angioplasty *409*
coronary artery bypass graft *411*
division of perforating veins *439*
femoral artery bypass graft *434*
heart–lung machines *953*
heart transplants *427*
heart valve replacement *422*
mammary artery bypass graft *411*
radiofrequency ablation *417*
saphenous vein bypass graft *411*
varicose vein treatment *439*
cardiovascular system tests and investigations
ambulatory ECG *416*
blood pressure measurement *44*, *404*
cardiac electrophysiological studies *417*
echocardiography *425*
electrocardiography (ECG) *406*, *407*, *416*
exercise testing *407*
see also angiography and angiograms; blood flow scans; blood tests
cardioversion *420*
Cardura 1004
care of the dying 954, 964–967
care of a terminally ill child 965
death and bereavement, useful online sites and addresses 1029
living wills 964
palliative surgery for people with cancer *282*
practical procedures after death 967
symptom relief 965, *966*
see also bereavement and grieving
Careline 1034
Carers National Association 1033
care of the sick 877, 954, 956
for the dying/terminally ill *see* care of the dying
emergency care *see* emergencies and emergency care
health care *see* health care providers
at home *see* home care
in hospital *see* hospital care
location choice 954
outpatient and day care treatment 956–957
see also therapies
carisoprodol 1004
carmustine 1004
carnitine 1004
Carnitor 1004
carotid Doppler scanning *531*
carotid pulse (neck pulse)
checking pulse recovery time after exercise *59*
first aid circulation check *978*
carpal tunnel syndrome 547
carriers, gene disorders 26, *269*, *272*, *273*
cars and driving
after major surgery 946
children's car seats *29*
correct driving position *382*
lifestyle choices *47*
road and vehicle safety 83, *84*
carteolol 1004
drugs for glaucoma 920–921
cartilage
articular cartilage *364*, *812*
disorders *see* cartilage disorders; joint and ligament disorders
epiglottis, respiratory system structure and functions 470, *471*, *622*
joint structure 362, *364*, *374*
in the pinna of the ear *593*
replacement by bone in babies and children *811*, *812*
cartilage disorders
deviated nasal septum 476
epiglottitis 842
outer-ear injury 596
torn knee cartilage 395
carvedilol 1004
Carylderm 1004
Cascade 1030
cascara 1004
cast immobilization, fracture treatment *393*
castor oil 1004
catabolism, metabolic process *674–675*
cataplexy, associated with narcolepsy 526
Catapres 1004
cataracts 573
cause of congenital blindness 856–857
cataract surgery *573*
Catarrh-Ex 1004
categories of disease *261*
catheterization
bladder catheterization *713*
skin-tunnelled catheters *456*
catheters, skin-tunnelled *456*
cauliflower ear, result of outer-ear injury 596
Caverject 1004
cavities in teeth *see* dental caries
CD4 lymphocytes, effect of HIV infection and AIDS 297, 887
Cedocard 1004
cefaclor 1004
antibiotics 885–886
cefadroxil 1004
cefalexin 1004
antibiotics 885–886
cefamandole 1004
cefazolin 1004
antibiotics 885–886
cefixime 1004
antibiotics 885–886
cefodizime 1004
cefotaxime 1004
cefoxitin 1004
antibiotics 885–886
cefpirome 1004
cefpodoxime 1004
cefprozil 1004
cefradine 1004
Cefrom 1004
ceftazidime 1004
ceftriaxone 1004
cefuroxime 1004
antibiotics 885–886
Celance 1004
Celectol 1004
Celevac 1004
celiprolol 1004
Cellcept 1004
cell division *266–267*
cancerous cells *276*
fertilized eggs *21*, *778*
meiosis *266–267*, 270
mitosis *266–267*
cell membranes
barrier to absorption of large food molecules 620, *625*
protozoa structure *287*
cell receptors
drug action on cell receptors *878*
virus action on cell receptors *285*
cells 258, *259*
bacterial invasion *286*
basal cells, in skin *330*
blood *see* blood cells
bone cells *363*
cancer *see* cancerous cells
cell and tissue samples, collection for testing 223
chondrocytes, in articular cartilage *364*
cones *see* rods and cones
division *see* cell division
effect of carcinogens 274
endocrine (hormone-secreting) cells 670, *671*
fat cells *675*
fibroblasts, role in skin repair *330*
genetic material in cells *see* chromosomes; DNA; genes
goblet cells, in mucous membranes *329*, *444*
granular cells, in skin *330*
hair cells, in the ear *594–595*
hepatocytes, in the liver *675*
islets of Langerhans, in the pancreas *674*
light-sensitive *see* rods and cones
mast cells, destruction in allergic reactions *445*, 466
metabolic activity in body cells *674–675*
morula, cell cluster in early pregnancy *778*
muscle fibres *366*, *367*
myocardial cells, in the heart 396
nerve *see* nerve cells
osteocytes, in bones *363*
pigmented skin cells *see* melanocytes
plasma cells, role in antibody immune response *445*
prickle cells, in skin *330*
protozoa-infected *287*
in the retina *see* rods and cones
rods *see* rods and cones

cells (continued)
sex cells, female *see* eggs
sex cells, male *see* sperm and sperm production
single-celled organisms *see* bacteria; protozoa; yeasts
skin and hair cells *329, 330*
stem cells, role in blood cell formation *440*
surface layer cells, in skin *329, 330*
tumour *see* tumour cells
virus reproduction in cells *285*
zygotes, in early pregnancy *778*
see also individual cell structures by name, e.g. mitochondria
cell tests 236–237
blood cell tests 226–227
cellular immune response, body's defences *445*
cellulitis 352
cell walls
bacteria structure *286*
fungi structure *287*
cementum, tooth structure *607*
Centers for Disease Control and Prevention 1026, 1033
centrally acting drugs, antihypertensive drugs 897–898
central nervous system (CNS)
central nervous system (CNS) stimulant drugs 918
disorders *see* brain and spinal cord disorders
structure and functions 508, *509–515*
central region of the brain *510*
central sleep apnoea 478
central vein, liver structure and functions *624*
Centre for Policy on Ageing 1026
centromere, chromosome region *265, 267*
cephalosporins, antibiotics 885–886
Ceporex 1004
cerebellum, brain structure and functions *509, 510, 514*
cerebral angiography *533*
cerebral cortex
brain structure and functions *510, 514, 515*
role in vision *see* visual cortex
stimulation by sounds *594*
cerebral embolism, cause of stroke 532–534
cerebral haemorrhage, cause of stroke 532–534
cerebral palsy 846–847
cerebral thrombosis, cause of stroke 532–534
cerebrospinal fluid (CSF)
build-up in the brain *see* hydrocephalus
lumbar puncture *527*
nervous system structure *509, 510*
Cerebrovase 1004
cerebrum, brain structure and functions *510, 515*
Cerezyme 1004
certoparin 1004
Cerumol 1004
cervical cap, barrier contraceptive 69, *70*
cervical disorders
cancer of the cervix *281*, 750–751
cervical dysplasia 749–750, *751*
cervical erosion 749
cervical incompetence, in pregnancy 794
chlamydial pelvic infection 765–766
uterine polyps *745*, 746
cervical mucus
destroying sperm, cause of female infertility 775, 776
mucus plug, functions in pregnancy and childbirth *779, 781, 782*
cervical nerves, nervous system structure and functions *511*
cervical smear test *44, 749*
results *213*
cervical spine *364*
cervical spondylosis 376
cervix
covered by placenta *see* placenta praevia
disorders *see* cervical disorders
female reproductive system structure and functions *731*
mucus *see* cervical mucus
in pregnancy and childbirth *731, 779, 782*
surgical removal *see* hysterectomy
tests and investigations *see* cervical smear test; colposcopy
cetirizine 1004
antihistamines 906
cetrimide 1004
cetrorelix 1004
Cetrotide 1004
cetylpyridinium 1004
chalazion 584
chambers of the heart 396, *398, 399*
in the fetal heart *810*
hole in septum between chambers *see* septal defects
see also atria; ventricles
chancre, symptom of syphilis 766
Changing Faces 1034
checkups *see* health checkups
chemical messengers *see* hormones; neurotransmitters
chemicals
in the eye, first aid *993*
in the garden, safe use 80
chemical signals in the nervous system *see* neurotransmitters
chemical tests 229
basic hormone tests 232
biochemical analysis of blood or urine *230*
blood cholesterol tests *44*, 231–232
C-reactive protein measurements, test for inflammation 233
dipstick testing of urine *231*
erythrocyte sedimentation test, test for inflammation 233
faecal occult blood test *44*, 233
home pregnancy tests *232*
hormone stimulation tests 232
hormone tests 232
routine urine chemistry 230–231
tests for inflammation 232–233
tumour marker tests 233
chemotherapy 274, 280
administration through skin-tunnelled catheter *456*
anticancer drugs 907–908
how it works *908*
chest clapping, chest physiotherapy *962*
chest compressions in cardiopulmonary resuscitation, first aid *984–985*
chest drain *497*
chest pain, symptoms chart 162–163
chest physiotherapy 962
chest stretch, warming up and cooling down in your exercise routine *60*
chest thrusts, first aid for choking *980*
chest X-ray 244, *244, 490*
radiation dose *246*
chewing and biting
role in digestion 620, *622*
teeth and jaw, structure and functions 606, *607*
chickenpox 290
vaccines and immunoglobulins 883–884
chilblains 350
child abuse and neglect, useful online sites and addresses 1028
Child Accident Prevention Trust 1036
childbirth *see* labour and childbirth
child development
developmental milestones *814*
disorders *see* developmental and psychological disorders in children
physical, mental and social development from birth to adolescence 810, *811–815*
sexual development *see* puberty
teeth development *606*
understanding of death and dying 76, 964
Child Growth Foundation, The 1028, 1033
childhood disorders
behavioural problems *see* developmental and psychological disorders in children
cancer *see* cancer in children
of cardiovascular system *see* cardiovascular system disorders in children
developmental disorders *see* developmental and psychological disorders in children
of digestive system *see* digestive system disorders in children
drug treatments 881, 882, *882*
of the ear *see* ear disorders in children
endocrine and metabolic disorders *see* congenital adrenal hyperplasia; growth disorders; inborn errors of metabolism
of the eye *see* eye disorders in children
gene disorders *see* gene disorders in children
hormone disorders *see* congenital adrenal hyperplasia; growth disorders; inborn errors of metabolism
infections *see* infections and infestations in children
metabolic disorders *see* congenital adrenal hyperplasia; growth disorders; inborn errors of metabolism
of musculoskeletal system *see* musculoskeletal disorders in children
of nervous system *see* nervous system disorders in children
paediatrics, useful online sites and addresses 1028, 1035
psychological disorders *see* developmental and psychological disorders in children
of respiratory system *see* respiratory system disorders in children
routine immunizations 45
skin disorders *see* skin and hair conditions and disorders in children
symptoms charts *see* children's symptoms charts
terminal illnesses *see* care of the dying
of urinary system *see* urinary and reproductive system disorders in children
see also babies and infants, problems and disorders; chromosome disorders
Childline 1028
children
accident and serious injury statistics 314
breathing rate assessment *89, 205*
car seats *29*
children's health, useful online sites and addresses 1028–1029
children's wards, hospital care for children 959
development *see* child development
diet 29, 30, 31, 210
disorders *see* childhood disorders
drug treatments for 881, 882, *882*
exercise requirements 30
first aid *see* first aid for children
genetic inheritance and genetic makeup *268–269*
growth charts *42–43*
health checkups 41–43
health in preschool and school-age children 29–31
height charts *43*
measuring children's height *42*
orthodontic treatment *614*
psychological health 30, 31, 72–73
road safety 83

routine immunizations 45
safety inside and outside the home 30, 31, 77–81
symptoms charts *see* children's symptoms charts
tooth care 29, 30
weight charts *43*
see also adolescence
Children with AIDS Charity 1029, 1033
Children's Liver Disease Foundation 1028
Children's Society, The 1028
children's symptoms charts
abdominal pain 208–209
breathing problems 204–205
coughing 206–207
diarrhoea 200–201
fever 202–203
vomiting 198–199
weight problems 210
children's wards, hospital care for children 959
Chimax 1004
chiropractic *see* manipulative therapies
chlamydial infections
chlamydial pelvic infection 765–766
nongonococcal urethritis 765
trachoma 572
Chloractil 1004
chloral hydrate 1004
sleeping drugs 915–916
chlorambucil 1004
anticancer drugs 907–908
chloramphenicol 1004
antibiotics 885–886
drugs acting on the ear 921
drugs acting on the eye 919–920
chlordiazepoxide 1004
antianxiety drugs 916
chlorhexidine 1004
preparations for skin infections and infestations 892–893
chlormethine 1004
Chloromycetin 1004
chloroquine 1004
antimalarial drugs 888–889
chlorothiazide 1004
diuretic drugs 902
chloroxylenol 1004
chlorphenamine 1004
antihistamines 906
chlorpheniramine *see* chlorphenamine
chlorpromazine 1004
antipsychotic drugs 917–918
chlorpropamide 1004
drugs for diabetes mellitus 931–932
chlortalidone 1004
chlortetracycline 1004
choking, first aid *980–981*
cholecystitis 652
cholera 301
cholesterol
blood levels *see* blood cholesterol levels
cholesterol content of packaged foods, nutritional information on food labels *52*
cholesterol stones, gallstones 651
high-density (HDLs) and low-density (LDLs) lipoproteins 231, 692
choline salicylate 1004
choline theophyllinate 1004
chondrocytes, articular cartilage cells *364*
chondromalacia 386
choosing a doctor 39
chordae tendineae, heart structure *398*
chordee, associated with hypospadias 870
choriocarcinoma
in females 748
in males, cancer of the testis 719
chorion, role in fetal nourishment during pregnancy *781*
chorionic gonadotrophin, human 1004
see also human chorionic gonadotrophin (HCG)
chorionic villi
chorionic villus sampling, antenatal genetic test *787*
role in fetal nourishment during pregnancy *781*
choroid, eye structure and functions *567*
choroid plexus, brain structure and functions *510*
Christmas disease *see* haemophilia and Christmas disease
chromium 1004
chromosome disorders 270–271
Down's syndrome 270, *787*, 821–822
Klinefelter's syndrome 271, 822–823
mosaicism 271
tests and investigations *see* genetic tests
Turner's syndrome *238*, 271, 823
useful online sites and addresses 1032
chromosomes
disorders *see* chromosome disorders
genetic material from egg and sperm combining at fertilization *21*, 264, *268*,
structure and functions *21*, 264, *265*, *267–269*
see also genetic tests
chronic fatigue syndrome (chronic fatigue and immune dysfunction syndrome) 520
chronic gastritis 640
chronic glaucoma 576–577
chronic glomerulonephritis 699–700
chronic granulomatous disease, congenital immunodeficiency 826–827
chronic heart failure 413
ACE (angiotensin converting enzyme) inhibitor drugs 900–901
digitalis drugs 901–902
diuretic drugs 902
chronic hepatitis 645–646
interferon drugs 907
chronic kidney failure 705, 706–708
chronic laryngitis 479–480
chronic liver failure 650–651
chronic lymphocytic leukaemia (CLL) 455
chronic myeloid leukaemia (CML) 455–456
chronic obstructive pulmonary disease (COPD) 487–489
bronchodilator drugs 910–911
corticosteroids for respiratory disease 911
chronic pancreatitis 653–654
chronic periodontitis 618
chronic polyhydramnios 795
chronic pre-existing disorders in pregnancy 788
chronic–progressive multiple sclerosis (MS) 541–542
chronic prostatitis 724
chronic sarcoidosis 498–499
chronic secretory otitis media 860–861
chronic subdural haemorrhage 535
chronic urinary retention 713
chronic urticaria 468
churning of food in stomach, digestive system function 620, *622*
chyme, production in and passage through digestive system 620, *622*, *623*
ciclosporin 1006
antirheumatic drugs 895–896
immunosuppressants 906–907
cidofovir 1004
cilastatin 1004
cilazapril 1004
angiotensin converting enzyme (ACE) inhibitor drugs 900–901
Cilest 1004
cilia in respiratory system
effect of tobacco smoke 64
role in body's defences *444*, 470
role in sense of smell *513*
ciliary body, eye structure and functions *567*, *568*
cimetidine 1004
ulcer-healing drugs 923–924
Cinaziere 1004
cinchocaine 1004
cinnarizine 1004
Cinobac 1004
cinoxacin 1004
Cipramil 1004
ciprofibrate 1004
ciprofloxacin 1004
antibiotics 885–886
drugs acting on the eye 919–920
Ciproxin 1004
circulation of the blood
Airway, Breathing, Circulation *see* ABC of resuscitation
checking by taking pulse, first aid *978*
checking circulation after bandaging, first aid *996*
checking during physical examination 219
effects of exercise 396, 440
fetal circulation, changes after birth *810*
maternal and fetal circulations in pregnancy *779*, *781*
through cardiovascular system 396, *397–401*
through the liver *440*, *624*
through urinary system 694, *695–697*
circulatory disorders *see* cardiovascular system disorders
circulatory system *see* cardiovascular system
circumcision *722*
cirrhosis 647–648
cisatracurium 1004
cisplatin 1004
anticancer drugs 907–908
citalopram 1004
antidepressant drugs 916–917
Citramag 1004
CJD *see* Creutzfeldt–Jakob disease (CJD)
cladribine 1005
clarithromycin 1005
antibiotics 885–886
Clarityn 1005
classic psychoanalysis 968
claustrophobia 552
clavulanic acid 1005
cleaning teeth and gums 608, *610*
cleft lip and palate 862
clemastine 1005
antihistamines 906
Clexane 1005
Climagest 1005
Climaval 1005
Climb (Research Trust for Metabolic Diseases in Children) 1032, 1033
Climesse 1005
clindamycin 1005
antibiotics 885–886
Clinitar 1005
Clinoril 1005
clioquinol 1005
drugs acting on the ear 921
clitoris, female reproductive system structure and functions *731*, *762*, *763*
CLL *see* chronic lymphocytic leukaemia (CLL)
clobazam 1005
clobetasol 1005
topical corticosteroids 892
clobetasone 1005
Cloburate 1005
clodronate 1005
clofazimine 1005
clomethiazole 1005
Clomid 1005
clomifene 1005
drugs for infertility 936–937
sex hormones and related drugs 933–934
clomipramine 1005
antidepressant drugs 916–917
clonazepam 1005
anticonvulsant drugs 914–915
clonidine 1005
antihypertensive drugs 897–898
antimigraine drugs 913
clopamide 1005
clopidogrel 1005
Clopixol 1005
cloral betaine 1005
clorazepate 1005
closed fractures 392

closed reduction, fracture treatment 392
Clotam 1005
clotrimazole 1005
antifungal drugs 889
drugs acting on the ear 921
preparations for skin infections and infestations 892–893
clots, blood *see* blood clots
clotting factors
disorders *see* bleeding disorders; hypercoagulability
role in blood clotting *442*
clozapine 1005
antipsychotic drugs 917–918
Clozaril 1005
clubbing, nail abnormality 360
clubfoot 833
cluster headaches 519–520
CML *see* chronic myeloid leukaemia (CML)
CMV infection *see* cytomegalovirus (CMV) infection
CNS *see* central nervous system (CNS)
CO poisoning *see* carbon monoxide (CO) poisoning
coagulation cascade, role in blood clotting *442*
coal tar 1005
coalworkers' pneumoconiosis 499–500
co-amilofruse 1005
co-amilozide 1005
co-amoxiclav 1005
antibiotics 885–886
coarctation of the aorta, congenital heart disease 837
Cobadex 1005
cobalamin, vitamin supplements 928
co-beneldopa 1005
Co-Betaloc 1005
cocaine
medical use 1005
recreational drug effects and risks 65, *66*
co-careldopa 1005
cocci, type of bacteria *286*
coccydynia 372
coccygeal nerves, nervous system structure and functions *511*
coccyx
location in spine *364*
pain in *see* coccydynia
cochlea, ear structure and functions *592, 593, 594*
cochlear duct, ear structure and functions *593, 594*
cochlear implants *603*
cochlear nerve, ear structure and functions *593, 594*
co-codamol 1005
co-codaprin 1005
Codafen Continus 1005
Codalax 1005
co-danthramer 1005
co-danthrusate 1005
codeine 1005
antimigraine drugs 913
aspirin with codeine, painkillers 912–913
codeine phosphate, antidiarrhoeal drugs 924
cough remedies 909–910
painkillers 912–913
paracetamol with codeine, painkillers 912–913
co-dergocrine mesylate 1005
Codis 1005
co-dydramol 1005
Coeliac Society, The 1030
co-fluampicil 1005
co-flumactone 1005
Cogentin 1005
cognitive therapy 970
coitus *see* sexual intercourse
Colazide 1005
colchicine 1005
cold cream 1005
cold and heat treatments, role in physiotherapy 961
colds
cold and flu remedies 910
common cold 288–289
cough remedies 909–910
cold sores 354
colecalciferol 1005
colectomy *665*
colestipol 1005
lipid-lowering drugs 935
colestyramine 1005
lipid-lowering drugs 935
colfosceril palmitate 1005
colic 819
Colifoam 1005
colistimethate 1005
colistin 1005
collagen
in articular cartilage *364*
in bones *362*
in heart valve cusps *399*
collapsed lung *315*
College of Optometrists 1031
collodion 1005
Colofac 1005
Colomycin 1005
colon
digestive system structure and functions *620, 621, 623, 625*
disorders *see* colon disorders
Colon Cancer Concern 1030
colon disorders
barium enema *243*, 246
colectomy *665*
colonoscopy *661*
colorectal cancer 665–667
colostomy *666*
Crohn's disease 658–659, 924
diverticular disease 663–664
double-contrast radiography 246–247
familial adenomatous polyposis (FAP), polyps in the colon 661, 666
hereditary nonpolyposis colorectal cancer (HNPCC) 666
partial colectomy *665*
permanent colostomy *666*
polyps in the colon 660–661
pseudomembranous colitis, caused by antibiotics 885
sigmoidoscopy *661*
temporary colostomy *666*
toxic megacolon, caused by ulcerative colitis 660
ulcerative colitis 659–660, 924
colonoscopy *661*
colorectal cancer 665–667
colostomy *666*
colostrum and colostrum production in the breasts *783*
colour blindness *269, 273*, 591
colour vision
disorders *see* colour blindness
role of cones in the retina 566, *569*
Colpermin 1005
colposcopy *750*
coma 522–523
co-magaldrox 1005
combination painkillers 912–913
combined contraceptive pill 69, *71*
Combivent 1005
Combivir 1005
co-methiamol 1005
comminuted fractures 392
common bile duct, digestive system structure and functions *624*
common cold 288–289
cold and flu remedies 910
cough remedies 909–910
common peroneal nerves, nervous system structure *509*
common warts 354–355
compact bone
role in bone repair *364*
structure 362, *362, 363*
complementary therapies 954, *955*, 972
acupuncture *955*, 973
biofeedback 975
choices 972
homeopathy 974
hypnotherapy 974–975
manipulative therapies *955*, 973–974
symptoms relief for the terminally ill *966*
useful online sites and addresses 1029
complete heart block 418
complex carbohydrates 50–51
chemical breakdown during digestion *625, 674–675*
in diet for people with diabetes mellitus 689, *690*
complex information and activities, processing by the brain 508, *515*
complex partial seizures, epilepsy 525, 526
complex phobias 552–553
complications
after major surgery 946
diabetic *see* complications of diabetes mellitus
complications of diabetes mellitus
diabetic kidney disease 705
diabetic neuropathy 545
diabetic retinopathy 579–580
diabetic small vessel disease, diabetic vascular disease 432–434
diabetic vascular disease 432–434
effect of smoking on risk of developing complications *690*
hypoglycaemia 691
ketoacidosis 688
compound fractures *see* open fractures
compound presentation, abnormal fetal presentation 801
Compound W 1005
compression fractures 392
compulsive disorders
obsessive–compulsive disorder 553–554
obsessive–compulsive personality disorder 562
see also dependency; psychological therapies
compulsive gambling 565
computerized tomography (CT) scanning *243*, 247–248
radiation doses, comparison with other imaging techniques *246*
spiral CT scanning 242, 248
Comtess 1005
Concavit 1005
concealed placental abruption 799
conception
assisted *see* artificial insemination; assisted conception
health before conception 33
infertility and problems conceiving 774–777
self-help techniques for maximizing chances of conception *774*
see also fertilization and implantation (embedding)
Concordin 1005
condoms
contraceptive use 69, *70*
female 69, *70*
safe sex use 68, 85, *765*
conduct disorder 855
conducting fibres, heart structure and functions *399*
conductive hearing loss 599, *600*
Condyline 1005
cone biopsy, for cervical dysplasia *751*
cones *see* rods and cones
confusion and/or forgetfulness, symptoms chart 120–121
congenital adrenal hyperplasia 866
congenital blindness 857–857
congenital deafness 859–860
congenital disorders
alpha$_1$-antitrypsin deficiency 489
aortic incompetence 422–423
aortic stenosis 423
arteriovenous malformation, cause of subarachnoid haemorrhage 534
atrioseptal defect, congenital heart disease 836–837
blistering diseases 336
cataracts, cause of congenital blindness 856–857
coarctation of the aorta, congenital heart disease 837
congenital adrenal hyperplasia 866
congenital blindness 856–857
congenital deafness 859–860
congenital glaucoma, cause of congenital blindness 856–857
congenital heart disease 836–837
congenital hip dysplasia 832
congenital infections, in newborn babies 817

cytomegalovirus (CMV) infection, congenital infection 817
Fallot's tetralogy, congenital heart disease 837
hepatitis, congenital infection 817
herpes simplex infections, congenital infection 817
HIV infection, congenital infections 817
hypertrophic cardiomyopathy 428
hypoplastic left heart syndrome, congenital heart disease 837
immunodeficiency *see* congenital immunodeficiency
listeriosis, congenital infection 817
patent ductus arteriosus, congenital heart disease 837
septal defects, congenital heart disease 836–837
sickle-cell disease *273*, 448–449
streptococcal infections, congenital infection 817
syphilis, congenital infection 817
thalassaemia *273*, 449–450
toxoplasmosis, congenital infection 82, 307–308, 817
valve defects, congenital heart disease 837
ventriculoseptal defect, congenital heart disease 836–837
see also chromosome disorders; gene disorders; inborn errors of metabolism
congenital glaucoma, cause of congenital blindness 856–85
congenital heart disease 836–837
congenital hip dysplasia 832
congenital immunodeficiency 826–827
agammaglobulinaemia 827
chronic granulomatous disease 827
severe combined immunodeficiency (SCID) 827
congenital infections, in newborn babies 817
conical cornea *see* keratoconus
conjugated oestrogens 1005
drugs for bone disorders 896
hormone replacement therapy (HRT) 937–938
conjugation, bacterial *286*
conjunctiva
disorders *see* conjunctivitis; subconjunctival haemorrhage
eye structure and functions *567*
conjunctivitis 570–571
connective tissue disorders *see* scleroderma; systemic lupus erythematosus (SLE)
Conotrane 1005
conscious activities and responses *see* voluntary movements and responses
consciousness, loss of *see* unconsciousness
constipation 628
cause of encopresis in children 852
in children 865
laxatives 924–925
in pregnancy 784, *785*
symptoms chart 160–161
in the terminally ill 965
constriction, pupil of the eye *see* dilation and constriction of the pupil of the eye
constrictive pericarditis 428–429
consulting your doctor 39, 212, 216–220
about exercise 58
health checkups 40–42
Consumer Health Information Campaign 1034
Contac 400 1005
Contac Cough Caps 1005
contact dermatitis 333, 335
Contact a Family 1029, 1032, 1033
contact lenses
for astigmatism 589
cause of corneal abrasion 571
causing eye pain or irritation 132
contact lens care *588*
for myopia and hypermetropia *588*
unsuitable eyedrops *919*
Contimin 1005
Continence Foundation, The 1033, 1037
contraception 69–71
after pregnancy 35
barrier methods 69, *70*
emergency contraception 70
hormonal *see* hormonal contraceptives
intrauterine device (IUD) 69–70, *71*
mechanical methods 69–70, *71*
natural methods 70, *71*
surgical *see* sterilization surgery
sympto-thermal method, natural method of contraception *71*
useful online sites and addresses 1031–1032
contraceptive pill
cause of spotting 191
combined and progestogen-only pills 69, *71*
effect of vomiting 69, 149
contractions
heart's pumping action 396, *399*
muscle *see* muscle contractions
uterine contractions in labour and childbirth *782–783*, 938
contrast media, use in imaging techniques *see* contrast X-rays
contrast X-rays *213*, 242, *243*, 245–247
barium enema 246
barium swallow (barium meal) 246, *637*
double-contrast radiograph 246–247
endoscopic retrograde cholangiopancreatography (ERCP) *653*
hysterosalpingography, female infertility investigation 776
intravenous urography (IVU) 246, *695*, *699*
radiation doses, comparison with other imaging techniques *246*
urodynamic studies *711*
see also angiography and angiograms
convalescence after major surgery 946
Convulex 1005
convulsions *see* seizures and convulsions
cooling down and warming up in your exercise routine *60–61*
COPD *see* chronic obstructive pulmonary disease (COPD)
co-phenotrope 1005
copper 1005
co-prenozide 1005
co-proxamol 1005
copying (replication) of genes and DNA 264, *266*
Coracten 1005
Cordarone X 1005
Cordilox 1005
cord prolapse
caused by premature rupture of the membranes 797
causing fetal distress 804
Corgard 1005
Corgaretic 1005
Corlan 1005
cornea
conical *see* keratoconus
disorders *see* corneal disorders
eye structure and functions 566, *567–568*
slit-lamp examination *574*
surgical reshaping for refractive errors *589*
corneal disorders
astigmatism 588–589
corneal abrasion 571
corneal ulcers 571–572
hyphaema 572
keratoconus 572–573
trachoma 572
corns and calluses 349
coronary angiography *408*
coronary angioplasty *409*
coronary arteries, heart structure and functions *398*
coronary artery bypass graft *411*
coronary artery disease (CAD) 405–407, *408*
coronary heart disease *see* coronary artery disease (CAD)
coronary *see* myocardial infarction
coronary veins, heart structure and functions *398*
Coro-Nitro 1005
corpus callosum, brain structure and functions *510*
corpus luteum, female reproductive system structure and functions *732*
Corsodyl 1005
cortex
adrenal gland structure *673*
brain structure *see* cerebral cortex
hair structure *329*
kidney structure *695*, *696*
Corti, organ of *see* organ of Corti
corticosteroid hormones
cause of Addison's disease 686
cause of Cushing's syndrome 684–685
production and functions *440*, *672*, *673*
use as drugs *see* corticosteroids
corticosteroids 930–931
antiallergy drugs 905
corticosteroids for respiratory disease 911
immunosuppressants 906–907
locally acting corticosteroids 895
topical *see* topical corticosteroids
corticotropin 1006
cortisol 1006
cortisone 1006
corticosteroids 930–931
Cortisyl 1006
Cosalgesic 1006
co-simalcite 1006
cosmetic surgery 952
Cosopt 1006
cot death *see* sudden infant death syndrome (SIDS)
co-tenidone 1006
co-triamterzide 1006
co-trimoxazole 1006
antibiotics 885–886
antiprotozoal drugs 888–889
cough 482–483
coughing, symptoms chart 142–143, 206–207
coughing in children, symptoms chart 206–207
coughing up blood, symptoms chart 142
cough reflex *473*
cough remedies 909–910
counselling 971
genetic counselling 26, *272*
in sex therapy *773*
supportive care for people with cancer 282
useful online sites and addresses 1029
Coversyl 1006
cows' milk protein allergy 864
Coxsackie virus infection, cause of hand, foot, and mouth disease 831
Cozaar-Comp 1006
CPR *see* cardiopulmonary resuscitation (CPR)
crabs *see* pubic lice
crack, recreational drug effects and risks *66*
cradle cap 829
cramps, muscle 388
cranial diabetes insipidus 678
cranial nerves
abducent nerve *511*
cochlear nerve *593*, *594*
glossopharyngeal nerve *511*
hypoglossal nerve *511*
oculomotor nerve *511*
olfactory nerve *511*
spinal accessory nerve *511*
structure and functions *509*, *511*
trigeminal nerve *511*
trochlear nerve *511*
vagus nerve *509*, *511*
vestibular nerve *593*, *595*
vestibulocochlear nerve *511*
see also facial nerve; optic nerve
cranium, growth and development in babies and children *813*

C-reactive protein measurements, test for inflammation 233
Cream of Magnesia 1006
creams *see* ointments, creams, and gels
creatine kinase, blood tests for 230, 241
creatinine, tests for
  routine blood chemistry 229
  routine urine chemistry 231
Cremalgin 1006
Creon 1006
Creutzfeldt–Jakob disease (CJD) 540
crisantaspase 1006
crisis support, useful online sites and addresses 1029
cristae
  ear structure and functions *595*
  mitochondrion structure *675*
Crixivan 1006
Crohn's disease 658–659
  aminosalicylate drugs 924
Cromogen 1006
cromoglicate 1006
crotamiton 1006
croup 841–842
crown, tooth structure 606, *607*
crowns and replacement teeth *615*
Crusaid 1033
CRUSE Bereavement Care 1029
crush injuries *315*, 316–317
crying
  colic in babies 819
  excessive crying in babies 819
cryptococcosis 308–309
cryptosporidiosis 307
Crystapen 1006
CSF *see* cerebrospinal fluid (CSF)
CT scanning see computerized tomography (CT) scanning
culture and tests for drug sensitivity 234–235
cumulative trauma disorder *see* repetitive strain injury (RSI)
Cupanol 1006
Cuplex 1006
Cuprofen 1006
cupulae, ear structure and functions *595*
Curatoderm 1006
curvature of the spine, abnormal *see* kyphosis and lordosis; scoliosis
Cushing's syndrome 684–685
cusps
  heart valve structure *398*, *399*
  in replacement heart valves *422*
  role in heart valve stenosis and regurgitation 421
  tooth structure *607*
cuticle
  hair structure *329*
  nail structure *328*, *331*
Cutivate 1006
cuts and scrapes 356
cyanocobalamin 1006
cyclical breast pain 756
Cyclimorph 1006
cyclizine 1006
  antiemetic drugs 922
Cyclogest 1006
cyclopenthiazide 1006
cyclopentolate 1006
  drugs acting on the eye 919–920
cyclophosphamide 1006
  anticancer drugs 907–908
  antirheumatic drugs 895–896
  immunosuppressants 906–907
Cyclo-Progynova 1006
cycloserine 1006
  antituberculous drugs 886
Cymalon 1006
Cymevene 1006
cyproheptadine 1006
  antihistamines 906
  antimigraine drugs 913
Cyprostat 1006
cyproterone
  drugs for prostate disorders 938–939
cyproterone acetate 1006
  sex hormones and related drugs 933–934
cystadenoma, ovarian cysts 743
cystic fibrosis 272, *273*, 824–825
  chest physiotherapy *962*
  useful online sites and addresses 1029
Cystic Fibrosis Resource Centre 1029
Cystic Fibrosis Trust 1029
cystitis 709–710
cystocele, prolapse of the uterus and vagina 747
Cystoleve 1006
Cystopurin 1006
cystoscopy *715*
Cystrin 1006
cysts
  Bartholin's cysts, caused by bartholinitis 753
  breast cysts 755, *756*
  cystadenoma, ovarian cysts 743
  dermoid cysts, ovarian cysts 743
  epididymal cysts 718
  follicular cysts, ovarian cysts 743
  ganglion 390
  kidney cysts 703
  ovarian cysts 743–744
  polycystic kidney disease 704
  polycystic ovary syndrome 744
  sebaceous cysts 348–349
  thyroid nodules 681
cytarabine 1006
  anticancer drugs 907–908
cytology *see* cell tests
cytomegalovirus (CMV) infection 292
  congenital infections, in newborn babies 817
  vaccines and immunoglobulins 883–884
cytoplasm
  bacteria structure *286*
  cell structure *265*, *266*
  fungi structure *287*
  protozoa structure *287*
cytosine, nucleotide base in DNA *265*
Cytotec 1006
cytotoxic drugs
  anticancer drugs 907–908
  cytotoxic immunosuppressants 906–907

D

dacarbazine 1006
  anticancer drugs 907–908
daclizumab 1006
dacryocystitis 585
dactinomycin 1006
dairy products and milk
  intolerance, allergies, and metabolism disorders *see* cows' milk protein allergy; galactosaemia; lactose intolerance
Daktacort 1006
Daktarin 1006
Dalacin C 1006
Dalivit 1006
Dalmane 1006
dalteparin 1006
  drugs that prevent blood clotting 904
danaparoid 1006
  drugs that prevent blood clotting 904
danazol 1006
  sex hormones and related drugs 933–934
dandruff 358
  seborrhoeic dermatitis 333, 335–336
Daneral-SA 1006
Danol 1006
Dantrium 1006
dantrolene 1006
  muscle relaxants 896
dantron 1006
  laxatives 924–925
dapsone 1006
  pyrimethamine with dapsone, antimalarial drugs 888–889
Daraprim 1006
daunorubicin 1006
Day Nurse 1006
day care *see* outpatient and day care treatment
dB *see* decibels (dB)
DDAVP 1006
ddC *see* zalcitabine (ddC)
ddI *see* didanosine (ddI)
deafness *see* hearing disorders
Deafness Research Foundation 1032
death
  brain death 523
  death and bereavement, useful online sites and addresses 1029
  loss and bereavement 76
  organ donation after death 967
  practical procedures after a death 967
  rates *see* death rates
  registering a death 967
  stillbirth 805
  sudden infant death syndrome (SIDS) 28, 820
  see also care of the dying
death rates
  accidents and serious injuries 314, 316
  cancer 278, *346*
  coronary artery disease (CAD) 405
  malignant melanoma *346*
  primary lung cancer *503*
DEBRA (epidermolysis bullosa) 1033
debrisoquine 1006
Decadron 1006
De-capeptyl SR 1006
decibels (dB), sound intensity measurement 592
deciduous teeth *see* primary teeth
decompression sickness 325
decongestants 909
  cold and flu remedies 910
decreased sex drive 769
deep vein thrombosis 437–438
defaecation *623*
  see also faeces
defibrillation *see* cardioversion
defibrillators
  defibrillator pacemakers *419*
  use in cardioversion *420*
deflazacort 1006
degenerative disorders
  category of disease 260, *261*
  chronic–progressive multiple sclerosis (MS) 541–542
  Creutzfeldt–Jakob disease (CJD) 540
  Huntington's disease 538
  motor neuron disease 540–541
  multiple sclerosis (MS) 541–542
  Parkinson's disease and parkinsonism 539–540
  relapsing–remitting multiple sclerosis (MS) 541–542
  therapies *see* rehabilitation and rehabilitation therapies
  see also dementia
dehydration
  caused by diarrhoea, symptoms chart 158
  dehydration prevention 627
  oral rehydration solutions 926
delayed first stage of labour 801–802
delayed puberty
  in females 739–740
  in males 728–729
Delfen 1006
delivery *see* labour and childbirth
Deltacortril Enteric 1006
Deltastab 1006
delusional disorders 561
demeclocycline 1006
dementia 535–536
  Alzheimer's disease 536–537
  multi-infarct dementia 537–538
  Wernicke–Korsakoff syndrome 538
  see also Creutzfeldt–Jakob disease (CJD); Huntington's disease
Dementia Web 1034
demix 1006
demyelination, in multiple sclerosis (MS) 541
dendrites, nerve cells structure *512*
dengue fever 296
De-Nol 1006
dental abscess 611–612
dental caries 609–611
dental checkups *609*
dental disorders *see* gum disorders; tooth disorders
dental floss or dental tape, use in tooth and gum care 608, *610*

dental treatments
bridges *615*
crowns and replacement teeth *615*
dental checkups *609*
dental implants *615*
dental X-rays *see* bite-wing X-rays
dentistry, useful online sites and addresses 1030
dentures *615*
orthodontic treatment *614*
root canal treatment *612*
tooth filling *611*
dentine
damaged, caused by fractured tooth 614–615
tooth structure 606, *607*
Dentomycin 1006
dentures, replacement teeth *615*
deoxygenated blood
circulation through cardiovascular system 396, *400*
fetal circulation *810*
role in gas exchange in respiratory system *471*, *473*
deoxyribonucleic acid *see* DNA
Department of Health 1026
Department of Health: Health Advice for Travellers 1037
dependency
alcohol dependence 564–565
compulsive gambling 565
drug dependence 66, 564, 880–881
dependent personality disorder 561–562
Depixol 1006
Depo-Medrone 1006
Deponit 1006
Depo-Provera 1006
Depostat 1006
depot injections
antipsychotic drugs 918
hormonal contraceptives 69, *71*
depression 554–556
antidepressant drugs 916–917
after childbirth 807–808
feeling depressed, symptoms chart 122–123
manic depression *see* bipolar affective disorder
mental problems due to physical illness 558
in the terminally ill 965
useful online sites and addresses 1030
see also psychological therapies
Depression Alliance 1030
Dequacaine 1006
Dequadin 1006
dequalinium 1006
Derbac-M 1006
Dermacort 1006
dermatitis
contact dermatitis 333, 335
dermatitis herpetiformis blistering disease 336
seborrhoeic dermatitis 333, 335–336
see also eczema
dermatomyositis and polymyositis 463–464
Dermatomyositis and Polymyositis Support Group 1033
Dermidex 1006
dermis
effect of burns 317
skin structure *329*
dermoid cysts, ovarian cysts 743
Dermovate 1006
Dermovate-NN 1006
DerWeb (Dental Education Resources on the Web) 1030
desensitization
desensitization and flooding, behaviour therapy techniques 969
treatment with allergen extracts for allergies and allergic reactions 905
desferrioxamine 1006
desflurane 1006
desirudin 1006
desmopressin 1006
drugs that affect bladder control 939
pituitary drugs 934–935
desogestrel 1006
desoximetasone 1006
topical corticosteroids 892
Destolit 1006
detached retina *see* retinal detachment
Deteclo 1006
Detrunorm 1006
Detrusitol 1006
Dettol 1007
development
babies and infants, growth and development 810, *811–814*
children *see* child development
fetal growth and development during pregnancy 778, *779–781*
developmental delay 853–854
bedwetting 872, 939
encopresis 852
developmental and psychological disorders in children 851
appetite loss, eating problems in children 852
Asperger's disorder, autism spectrum disorder 852
attention deficit disorder (ADD) 855
autism spectrum disorders 852–853
bedwetting 872, 939
conduct disorder 855
developmental delay 853–854
dyslexia, specific learning difficulty 854
eating problems in children 852
encopresis 852
food refusal, eating problems in children 852
generalized learning disabilities 854
nightmares and night terrors, sleeping problems in children 851
pica, eating problems in children 852
play therapy, type of speech therapy *955*, 963
sleeping problems in children 851
sleepwalking, sleeping problems in children 851
specific learning difficulties 854
speech and language difficulties 854–855
useful online sites and addresses 1028, 1029, 1034
see also occupational therapy; speech therapy
deviated nasal septum 476
dexamethasone 1007
corticosteroids 930–931
drugs acting on the ear 921
drugs acting on the eye 919–920
locally acting corticosteroids 895
dexamfetamine 1007
central nervous system stimulant drugs 918
Dexa-Rhinaspray Duo 1007
Dexedrine 1007
dexketoprofen 1007
dextromethorphan 1007
cough remedies 909–910
dextromoramide 1007
dextropropoxyphene 1007
dextropropoxyphene with paracetamol
painkillers 912
DF 118 1007
DHC Continus 1007
Diabetamide 1007
diabetes insipidus 678
drugs for diabetes insipidus, pituitary drugs 934–935
diabetes mellitus 687–691
complications *see* complications of diabetes mellitus
drugs for diabetes mellitus 931–932
gestational diabetes (diabetes developing in pregnancy) 687, 788–789
home blood glucose monitoring *689*, 931
insulin injection treatment *688*, 689, 931
living with diabetes *690*
pre-existing diabetes and pregnancy 788
recommended diet 689, *690*
type 1 diabetes 687–691
type 2 diabetes 687–691
useful online sites and addresses 1030, 1033
diabetic kidney disease 705
diabetic neuropathy 545
diabetic retinopathy 579–580
diabetic vascular disease 432–434
Diabinese 1007
diagnosis and the diagnostic method 212–215
see also tests and investigations
Dialar 1007
dialysis *707*
Diamicron 1007
diamorphine 1007
Diamox 1007
Dianette 1007
diaphragm, barrier contraceptive 69, *70*
diaphragm (muscle)
location and role in breathing *471*, *472*
role in hiccups 483
diaphyses, bone structure and development *812*
Diarphen 1007
Diarrest 1007
diarrhoea 627
antidiarrhoeal drugs 924
dehydration prevention 158, *627*, 926
diarrhoea in children, symptoms chart 200–201
symptoms chart 158–159
in the terminally ill 967
traveller's diarrhoea from food poisoning or gastroenteritis 85, 629
vomiting and diarrhoea in children 864
Diasorb 1007
diastole, heartbeat phase *399*
diastolic blood pressure *401*
Diazemuls 1007
diazepam 1007
antianxiety drugs 916
anticonvulsant drugs 914–915
muscle relaxants 896
diazoxide 1007
antihypertensive drugs 897–898
diclofenac 1007
nonsteroidal anti-inflammatory drugs (NSAIDs) 894
painkillers 912–913
Dicloflex 1007
Diclomax Retard 1007
dicobalt edetate 1007
Diconal 1007
dicyclomine *see* dicycloverine
dicycloverine 1007
antispasmodic drugs and motility stimulants 926
Dicynene 1007
didanosine (ddI) 1007
drugs for HIV infection and AIDS 887–888
Didronel PMO 1007
dienestrol 1007
hormone replacement therapy (HRT) 937–938
diet
adolescents 31
assessing your diet *48*
for babies and infants 27, *28*
balanced diet 49–52
for children 29, 30, 210
for diabetes mellitus 689, *690*
dietary disorders *see* metabolic disorders; nutritional deficiencies; weight problems
effect on health 48
effect on teeth *610*
energy from diet *see* food energy
food groups *49*
food processing in the body *see* digestion; metabolism
healthy eating 48–52
lifestyle choices *17*, *47*
nutritional information on food labels *52*
nutrition, useful online sites and addresses 1030, 1035
in old age 37
for older adults 35
possible cause of stomach cancer 642
for pregnant women 33–34, *785*

diet (continued)
- slimming diets 54
- variety of diets accommodated by digestive system 620
- for weaning infants *28*
- for weight gain 54
- *see also* carbohydrates; cholesterol; fats; food; minerals; protein in the diet; vitamins

diethylamine salicylate 1007
diethylcarbamazine 1007
- anthelmintic drugs 889

diethylstilbestrol 1007
- anticancer drugs 907–908
- drugs for prostate disorders 938–939

diethyltoluamide 1007
Differin 1007
difficulty sleeping, symptoms chart 100–101
difficulty speaking, symptoms chart 119
difficulty swallowing, symptoms chart 147
Difflam 1007
diffuse pleural thickening, asbestos-related disease 501–502
Diflucan 1007
diflucortolone 1007
diflunisal 1007
- nonsteroidal anti-inflammatory drugs (NSAIDs) 894

digestion 620, *621–625*, *674–675*
- role of the pancreas *621*, *624*, *674*
- *see also* metabolism

Digestive Disorders Foundation 1030
digestive enzymes
- deficiency disorders *see* enzyme deficiencies
- production in the pancreas *624*, *674*
- production and role in digestive system 620, *621–625*

digestive juices, production and role in digestive system 620, *621–625*
digestive system
- bacteria in digestive system *623*, *625*, 885
- disorders *see* digestive system disorders
- effects of growth and aging *22–23*
- structure and functions 620, *621–625*
- *see also* digestion

digestive system disorders
- abdominal pain, symptoms charts 152–155
- bowel movement disorders *see* constipation; diarrhoea; encopresis *see* digestive system disorders in children
- dehydration prevention 158, *627*, 926
- dietary *see* metabolic disorders; nutritional deficiencies; weight problems
- drugs for digestive disorders 922–926
- from food contamination *see* food poisoning
- gastroenteritis 85, 628–629
- indigestion 626, *627*, 923
- nonulcer dyspepsia 626–627
- recurrent abdominal pain, symptoms charts 154–155
- surgery *see* digestive system surgery
- swollen abdomen, symptoms chart 156
- symptoms charts 148–161
- tests and investigations *see* digestive system tests and investigations
- useful online sites and addresses 1030
- vomiting and nausea *see* nausea; vomiting
- *see also* digestive tract disorders; gallbladder disorders; liver disorders; pancreas disorders

digestive system disorders in children 862
- abdominal pain in children, symptoms chart 208–209
- cleft lip and palate 862
- constipation in children 865
- cows' milk protein allergy 864
- encopresis 852
- gastro-oesophageal reflux (GOR) in infants 863
- intussusception 864–865
- oral thrush 862–863
- pyloric stenosis in infants 863
- rectal prolapse 667–668
- vomiting and diarrhoea 864

digestive system surgery
- banding haemorrhoids *668*
- colectomy *665*
- colostomy *666*
- hernia repair *662*
- liver transplant *650*
- partial colectomy *665*
- permanent colostomy *666*
- pouch operation, for ulcerative colitis 660
- temporary colostomy *666*

digestive system tests and investigations
- barium enema *243*, 246
- barium swallow (barium meal) 246, *637*
- colonoscopy *661*
- double-contrast radiography 246–247
- endoscopic retrograde cholangiopancreatography (ERCP) *653*
- liver biopsy *647*
- oesophageal manometry, for achalasia 638
- sigmoidoscopy *661*
- upper digestive tract endoscopy *641*

digestive tract
- digestive system structure and functions 620, *621–623*, *625*
- disorders *see* digestive tract disorders

digestive tract disorders
- bleeding from the digestive tract 630
- *see also* anal disorders; intestinal disorders; mouth and tongue disorders; oesophageal disorders; stomach and duodenum disorders

Digibind 1007
digitalis drugs 901–902
- antiarrhythmic drugs 898

digitoxin 1007
- digitalis drugs 901–902

digoxin 1007
- antiarrhythmic drugs 898
- digitalis drugs 901–902

dihydrocodeine 1007
dihydrocodeine with paracetamol
- painkillers 912

dihydroergotamine 1007
dihydrotachysterol 1007
Dijex 1007
dilated cardiomyopathy 427–428
dilation and constriction of the pupil of the eye *568*
- autonomic system response *514*

diloxanide furoate 1007
- antiprotozoal drugs 888

diltiazem 1007
- calcium channel blocker drugs 900

Dilzem 1007
dimenhydrinate 1007
- antiemetic drugs 922

dimercaprol 1007
dimercaptosuccinic acid (DMSA) scanning *871*
dimeticone 1007
- emollients and barrier preparations 890

Dimetriose 1007
Dimotane 1007
Dimotapp 1007
Dindevan 1007
dinoprost 1007
dinoprostone 1007
- drugs for labour 938

Diocalm 1007
Diocalm Ultra 1007
Dioctyl 1007
Dioderm 1007
Dioralyte 1007
Diovol 1007
dioxybenzone
- sunscreens and sunblocks 893

Dipentum 1007
diphenhydramine 1007
- antihistamines 906

diphenoxylate 1007
- antidiarrhoeal drugs 924

diphenylpyraline 1007
diphtheria 300
- routine immunizations *45*
- travel immunizations *86*

diphtheria/tetanus/pertussis (DTP)
- vaccines and immunoglobulins 883–884

dipipanone 1007
dipivefrine 1007
- drugs for glaucoma 920–921

Diprobase 1007
Diprosalic 1007
Diprosone 1007
dipstick testing of urine *231*
dipyridamole 1007
direct smooth-muscle relaxants, antispasmodic drugs and motility stimulants 926
direct tests for abnormal genes 239–241
Dirythmin SA 1007

disability
- useful online sites and addresses 1030
- *see also* rehabilitation and rehabilitation therapies

Disability Net 1030
Disabled Living Foundation 1030
discharge from hospital 959
discharges
- abnormal vaginal discharge, symptoms chart 194
- in chlamydial pelvic infection 765
- in genital herpes 767
- in gonorrhoea 764
- nipple discharge 758
- in nongonococcal urethritis (NGU) 765
- in trichomoniasis 767

discoid eczema *see* nummular eczema
discoid lupus erythematosus (DLE) 347
discoloured teeth 612–613
discrimination, against cancer survivors 283
discs, intervertebral
- prolapsed or herniated disc (slipped disc) 384–385
- structure *364*

diseases
- care and treatment *see* care and caring; therapies; treatments
- categories *261*
- changing patterns of and landmarks in disease 262–263
- diagnostic method and landmarks in disease detection 212–215
- diagnostic tests *see* tests and investigations
- disease prevention at different ages *see* health at different ages
- disease process 260
- role of age and lifestyle in susceptibility to disease 27, 46, 261–262
- role of inheritance in susceptibility to disease *21*, 24–26
- *see also* individual diseases and disorders by category (e.g. bacterial infections) or by name (e.g. rheumatoid arthritis)

Disipal 1007
dislocated joints 394
disopyramide 1007
- antiarrhythmic drugs 898

disorders *see* diseases; and individual disorders by category (e.g. bacterial infections) or by name (e.g. rheumatoid arthritis)
Disprin 1007
Disprin Extra 1007
Disprol 1007
dissecting aneurysm 430–431
Distaclor MR 1007
distal convoluted tubule, kidney structure and functions *696*, *697*
Distalgesic 1007
Distamine 1007
distigmine 1007

disturbed or impaired vision, symptoms chart 134–135
disulfiram 1007
dithranol 1007
Dithrocream 1007
Ditropan 1007
Diumide-K Continus 1007
diuretic drugs 902
  antihypertensive drugs 897–898
Diurexan 1007
diverticula, in diverticular disease 663–664
diverticular disease 663–664
Dixarit 1008
dizziness *see* faintness; vertigo
DLE *see* discoid lupus erythematosus (DLE)
DMSA scanning *see* dimercapto-succinic acid (DMSA) scanning
DNA
  in bacteria *286*
  during cell division *266–267*
  genetic material from egg and sperm combining at fertilization *21*, 264, *268*, 762
  mitochondrial DNA *265*
  mutations *269*
  polymerase chain reaction (PCR) copying, for genetic tests 239
  replication (copying) of genes and DNA 264, *266*
  structure and functions 264,*265–266*
  use in tests for abnormal genes 239–241
  in viruses *285*
dobutamine 1008
docetaxel 1008
doctors
  consulting *see* consulting your doctor
  doctor's surgery *217*
  finding and choosing a doctor 39
docusate 1008
  drugs acting on the ear 921
  laxatives 924–925
Dolmatil 1008
Dolobid 1008
Doloxene 1008
Domical 1008
dominant genes and dominant inheritance *268*
  disorders *see* autosomal dominant disorders
dominant hemisphere, role in information processing in the brain *515*
domperidone 1008
donepezil 1008
dopamine 1008
  action blocked by antipsychotic drugs 918
  underproduction in Parkinson's disease and parkinsonism 539
dopexamine 1008
Doppler ultrasound scanning *243*, 251, *432*
  carotid Doppler scanning *531*
Doralese 1008
dorzolamide 1008
  drugs for glaucoma 920–921
Dostinex 1008
dosulepin 1008
Dothapax 1008
dothiepin *see* dosulepin 1008
double helix structure of DNA 264, *265*
double vision 589–590
doubling time, cancerous tumours *276*
Dovonex 1008
Down's syndrome 270, *787*, 821–822
  useful online sites and addresses 1030
Down's Syndrome Association 1030
Down's Syndrome Educational Trust 1030
doxapram 1008
doxazosin 1008
  antihypertensive drugs 897–898
  drugs for prostate disorders 938–939
  drugs that affect bladder control 939
doxepin 1008
doxorubicin 1008
  anticancer drugs 907–908
doxycycline 1008
  antibiotics 885–886
  antimalarial drugs 888–889
doxylamine 1008
Dozic 1008
drainage angle, eye structure and functions *575*, *577*
Dramamine 1008
Drapolene 1008
dressing and undressing, home care *954*
dressings and bandages, first aid uses *976*, *996–998*
Driclor 1008
Drinkline 1027
Drinksense 1027
Dristan Nasal Spray 1008
driving *see* cars and driving
Drogenil 1008
Droleptan 1008
droperidol 1008
  antiemetic drugs 922
  antipsychotic drugs 917–918
drowning and near-drowning 81, 314, 325–326
drug delivery systems
  antibiotic delivery system for intravenous antibiotics *825*
  for asthma treatments *485*, *839*, 840, 910
  drug delivery routes *879*
  drug preparations *881*
  eardrops *881*, *921*
  eyedrops *881*, *919*
  insulin pens, for diabetes mellitus treatment *688*
  insulin pumps, for diabetes mellitus treatment 931
  skin patches *879*, *937*
  skin-tunnelled catheters *456*
  sublingual sprays *900*
  syringe drivers/pumps, for analgesia/pain relief *283*, *966*
  see also injections; ointments, creams, and gels
drug groups
  ACE inhibitors *see* angiotensin converting enzyme (ACE) inhibitor drugs
  allergen extracts, antiallergy drugs 905
  alpha-blockers *see* alpha-blocker drugs
  aminosalicylate drugs 924
  anaesthetics *see* anaesthesia
  angiotensin II blocker drugs, antihypertensive drugs 897–898
  anion-exchange resins, lipid-lowering drugs 935
  antacids 923
  anthelmintic drugs 889
  antiallergy drugs 905
  antianxiety drugs 916
  antiarrhythmic drugs 898
  anticancer drugs 907–908
  anticholinergic drugs, antispasmodic drugs and motility stimulants 926
  anticonvulsant drugs 914–915
  antidepressant drugs 916–917
  antidiarrhoeal drugs 924
  antiemetics *see* antiemetic drugs
  antifibrinolytic drugs, drugs that promote blood clotting 903
  antifungal drugs 889
  antihypertensive drugs 897–898
  anti-infective *see* anti-infective drugs
  anti-inflammatories *see* anti-inflammatory drugs
  antimalarial drugs 888–889
  antimigraine drugs 913
  antiparasitic drugs, preparations for skin infections and infestations 892–893
  antiplatelet drugs, drugs that prevent blood clotting 904
  antiprotozoal drugs 888
  antipruritic drugs 891–892
  antipsychotic drugs 917–918
  antiretroviral drugs, drugs for HIV infection and AIDS 887–888
  antirheumatic drugs 895–896
  antispasmodic drugs and motility stimulants 926
  antithyroid drugs, drugs for hyperthyroidism 932–933
  antituberculous drugs 886
  antivirals *see* antiviral drugs
  artificial tears, drugs acting on the eye 919–920
  beta-blockers *see* beta-blocker drugs
  bisphosphonates, drugs for bone disorders 896
  blood products, drugs that promote blood clotting 903
  bronchodilator drugs 910–911
  calcium channel blockers *see* calcium channel blocker drugs
  carbonic anhydrase inhibitors, drugs for glaucoma 920–921
  cardiac glycosides, digitalis drugs 901–902
  centrally acting drugs, antihypertensive drugs 897–898
  central nervous system (CNS) stimulant drugs 918
  for coughs and colds *see* cold and flu remedies; cough remedies; decongestants
  cytotoxic *see* cytotoxic drugs
  digitalis *see* digitalis drugs
  direct smooth-muscle relaxants, antispasmodic drugs and motility stimulants 926
  diuretics *see* diuretic drugs
  drugs acting on the brain and nervous system 912–918
  drugs acting on the ear 921
  drugs acting on the endocrine system 930–935
  drugs acting on the eye 919–920
  drugs acting on the immune system 905–907
  drugs acting on the skin 890–893
  drugs that affect bladder control 939
  drugs for asthma *see* asthma drugs
  drugs for bone disorders 896
  drugs for cardiovascular disorders 897–902
  drugs for diabetes insipidus, pituitary drugs 934–935
  drugs for diabetes mellitus 931–932
  drugs for digestive disorders 922–926
  drugs for glaucoma 920–921
  drugs for HIV infection and AIDS 887–888
  drugs for hyperthyroidism 932–933
  drugs for hypothyroidism 932
  drugs for infections and infestations 883–889
  drugs for infertility 936–937
  drugs for labour 938
  drugs for mental health disorders 915–918
  drugs for musculoskeletal disorders 894–896
  drugs that prevent blood clotting 904
  drugs that promote blood clotting 903
  drugs for prostate disorders 938–939
  drugs for respiratory disorders 909–911
  earwax softeners, drugs acting on the ear 921
  emollients and barrier preparations 890
  expectorants, cough remedies 909–910
  fibrates, lipid-lowering drugs 935
  gold-based drugs, antirheumatic drugs 895–896
  H_2 blockers, ulcer-healing drugs 923–924
  interferons *see* interferon drugs
  laxatives 924–925
  lipid-lowering drugs 935
  loop diuretic drugs, diuretic drugs 902
  mast cell stabilizers, antiallergy drugs 905
  miotics, drugs for glaucoma 920–921
  monoamine oxidase inhibitors (MAOIs), antidepressant drugs 916–917

drug groups (continued)
mood-stabilizing drugs 918
mucolytic drugs, cough remedies 909–910
muscle relaxants 896
mydriatics, drugs acting on the eye 919–920
nitrate drugs 899–900
nonsteroidal anti-inflammatory drugs (NSAIDs) 894, *895*
nutritional supplements *see* minerals; vitamins
opioids *see* opioid drugs
oral rehydration solutions 926
pain-relieving drugs *see* painkillers
phenothiazines, antiemetic drugs 922
pituitary drugs 934–935
potassium-sparing diuretic drugs, diuretic drugs 902
preparations for skin infections and infestations 892–893
prolactin inhibitors, pituitary drugs 934–935
protease inhibitors, drugs for HIV infection and AIDS 887–888
proton pump inhibitors, ulcer-healing drugs 923–924
retinoid drugs 890–891
reverse transcriptase inhibitors, drugs for HIV infection and AIDS 887–888
selective serotonin reuptake inhibitors (SSRIs), antidepressant drugs 916–917
serotonin antagonists, antiemetic drugs 922
sex hormones and related drugs 933–934
sleeping drugs 915–916
statins, lipid-lowering drugs 935
sulphonylurea drugs, drugs for diabetes mellitus 931–932
sunscreens and sunblocks 893
sympathomimetics, bronchodilator drugs 910–911
thiazide drugs, diuretic drugs 902
thrombolytic drugs 904–905
tricyclics, antidepressant drugs 916–917
ulcer-healing drugs 923–924
uterine muscle relaxant drugs, drugs for labour 938
uterine stimulant drugs, drugs for labour 938
vaccines and immunoglobulins 883–884
xanthines, bronchodilator drugs 910–911
see also antibiotics; antihistamines; benzodiazepines; corticosteroids; immunosuppressants
drug-related problems and disorders
drug allergy 467–468
drug dependence 66, 564, 880–881
drug-induced acne 340
drug-induced rashes 338
drug overdose and accidental ingestion 321–322
swallowed poisons, first aid *994*
useful online sites and addresses 1030–31
drugs that prevent blood clotting 904
drugs
action on cell receptors *878*
brand and generic names 1000
delivery systems *see* drug delivery systems
development and landmarks in development 876–877
drug delivery routes *879*
drug preparations *881*
effects on fetus 34, 881
effects on your body 880–881
effects of vomiting on oral medications 149
groups *see* drug groups
in home care 960
how they work and are used 878
managing your medication 881–882
metabolism *879*
problems and disorders *see* drug-related problems and disorders
recreational *see* recreational drugs
role in weight control 54
side effects *see* side effects of drugs
storage 882
tolerance 880
useful online sites and addresses 1030
when travelling 85
see also individual drugs by generic or brand names
drugs for infertility 936–937
dry eye *see* keratoconjunctivitis sicca
dry gangrene 435
dry macular degeneration 580–581
dry mouth and tongue, in the terminally ill *966*
Dryptal 1008
dry socket 619
DTP *see* diphtheria/tetanus/pertussis (DTP)
Duchenne muscular dystrophy 826
ducts
bile *see* bile duct
cochlear duct, ear structure and functions *593, 594*
ductus arteriosus, in the fetal heart *810*, 837
ejaculatory duct, male reproductive system structure and functions 716, *717, 763*
lymph ducts, location and functions *443*
milk *see* milk ducts
nasolacrimal duct, in tear apparatus *566*
pancreatic, digestive system structure and functions *624, 674*
renal pelvis, kidney structure and functions *695, 696*
sweat ducts and pores, skin structure *329*
urine-collecting ducts, kidney structure and functions *696, 697*
ductus arteriosus
failure to close after birth *see* patent ductus arteriosus
in the fetal heart *810*
Dulco-Lax 1008
duodenal ulcer, type of peptic ulcer 640–642
duodenum
digestive system structure and functions *621, 622–625*
disorders *see* stomach and duodenum disorders
hormone production *624, 671*
Duofilm 1008
Duovent 1008
Duphalac 1008
Duphaston 1008
Dupuytren's contracture 390
Duragel 1008
dura mater
bleeding between dura mater and arachnoid *see* subdural haemorrhage
brain and spinal cord structure *509*
Durogesic 1008
dust inhalation disorders *see* occupational lung diseases; perennial allergic rhinitis
Dutonin 1008
Dyazide 1008
dydrogesterone 1008
dying *see* care of the dying; death
dyshidrotic eczema 334
dyslexia, specific learning difficulty 854
Dysman 1008
dysmenorrhoea 736
Dyspamet 1008
dyspareunia *see* painful intercourse
dyspepsia, nonulcer 626–627
dysplasia
cervical dysplasia 749–750, *751*
congenital hip dysplasia 832
dysplastic naevi, type of mole 343
Dyspraxia Foundation 1034
Dytac 1008
Dytide 1008

E

earache, symptoms chart 138
ear canal
disorders *see* otitis externa; wax blockage
ear structure and functions *592, 593, 594*
otoscopy *597*
ear disorders
acoustic neuroma 605
barotrauma 598
in children *see* ear disorders in children
drugs acting on the ear 921
earache, symptoms chart 138
labyrinthitis 604
Ménière's disease 604–605
otitis externa 596
otitis media 597
otosclerosis 598
otoscopy *597*
outer-ear injury 596
ruptured eardrum 597–598
useful online sites and addresses 1031
vertigo 603–604
wax blockage 597, 921
see also hearing disorders
ear disorders in children
acute otitis media in children 860
chronic secretory otitis media 860–861
congenital deafness 859–860
protruding ears 861
tests and investigations *see* hearing tests
eardrops *881, 921*
eardrum
ear structure and functions *592, 593, 594*
otoscopy *597*
ruptured 597–598
Earex 1008
early postpartum haemorrhage 806–807
early (precocious) puberty
effect on height 869
in females 739–740
in males 728–729
ears
auditory ossicles (bones in the middle ear) *593*
disorders *see* ear disorders
effects of growth and aging *22–23*
fetal development during pregnancy *780*
otoscopy *597*
structure and functions 592, *593–595*
earwax
cause of wax blockage 597
earwax softeners, drugs acting on the ear 921
eating *see* diet
eating disorders
anorexia nervosa 562–563
bulimia 563
eating problems in children 852
useful online sites and addresses 1031
see also psychological therapies
Eating Disorders Association 1031
Eating Disorders Northern Ireland 1031
eBMJ (Electronic British Medical Journal 1026
Ebola fever, viral haemorrhagic fever 295
Ebufac 1008
EBV *see* Epstein–Barr virus
eccentric or odd personality disorders 561
eccrine sweat glands, skin structure *329*
ECG *see* electrocardiography (ECG)
echocardiography *425*
eclampsia *see* pre-eclampsia and eclampsia
E. coli infections *see Escherichia coli* infections
Econacort 1008
econazole 1008
antifungal drugs 889
preparations for skin infections and infestations 892–893

Economycin 1008
Ecostatin 1008
ecothiopate 1008
ecstasy, recreational drug effects and risks 65, *66*
ECT (electroconvulsive therapy), for depression 556
ectopic beats 415
ectopic pregnancy 790–791
ectropion 584–585
eczema 333
  asteatotic eczema 334
  atopic eczema 333, 334
  dyshidrotic eczema 334
  eczema in children 829–830
  nummular eczema 334
  see also dermatitis
Edronax 1008
edrophonium 1008
EEG *see* electroencephalography (EEG)
Efalith 1008
Efamast 1008
efavirenz 1008
  drugs for HIV infection and AIDS 887–888
Efcortelan 1008
Efcortesol 1008
Effercitrate 1008
effusion
  pericardial effusion, result of pericarditis 428, *429*
  pleural effusion 494–495
eformoterol *see* formoterol
egg follicles, female reproductive system structure and functions 730, *731–732*
eggs
  chromosome content 264, *267*, *268*
  female reproductive system structure and functions 730, *731–732*
  fertilization *see* fertilization and implantation (embedding)
  meiosis (cell division) in sperm and eggs *267*, 270
  mutations in eggs and sperm *269*
  use in assisted conception *776*
  see also ovulation
eicosapentaenoic acid (epa) 1008
ejaculation and orgasm
  male reproductive system structure and functions 716, *762*, *763*
  orgasm phase, sexual response *762*
  premature ejaculation 771–772
  retrograde ejaculation after prostatectomy, cause of male infertility 777
ejaculatory duct, male reproductive system structure and functions 716, *717*, *763*
Elantan 1008
Elavil 1008
elbows
  elbow joint, hinge joint example *365*
  elbow and knee bandages, first aid *997*
  tennis elbow and golfer's elbow 389–390
elderly people
  falls, prevention 77
  health in old age 37
  risks of drug interactions and side effects 881
electrical impulses and signals in the ear *593*, *594*
electrical impulses and signals in the eye 566, *568–569*
electrical impulses and signals in the heart 396, *399*
  disorders *see* heart rate and rhythm disorders
  tests and investigations *see* cardiac electrophysiological studies; electrocardiography (ECG)
electrical impulses and signals in the nervous system disorders *see* epilepsy
  nerve cells, structure and functions 508, *512*
  tests and investigations *see* electroencephalography (EEG); nerve and muscle electrical tests
electrical injuries 316, 318–319
electrical nerve stimulation, transcutaneous *see* TENS
electrical stimulation, role in physiotherapy 961
electrocardiography (ECG) *406*, *407*, *416*
electroconvulsive therapy (ECT), for depression 556
electroencephalography (EEG) *525*
Electrolade 1008
electrolytes
  routine blood chemistry tests for electrolytes 229
electromyography (EMG) *544*
electron microscopy for infectious agents 234
electrophysiological studies, cardiac *417*
Elleste Duet 1008
Elleste Solo 1008
ellipsoidal joints *364–365*
Elocon 1008
Eltroxin 1008
Eludril 1008
Elyzol 1008
embedded object plus severe bleeding, first aid *986*
embolism
  cerebral embolism, cause of stroke 533–534
  drugs that prevent blood clotting 904
  pulmonary embolism 495
  thrombolytic drugs 904–905
  thrombosis and embolism 431–432
embolus *see* blood clots; embolism
embryo, growth and development in early pregnancy 778, *780*
embryonal carcinoma, cancer of the testis 719
Emcor 1008
emergencies and emergency care
  ambulances and paramedics *955*, *957*
  emergency action priorities 976, *977*
  emergency cardioversion *420*
  emergency care *955*
  emergency contraception 70
  emergency medical travel kit 85
  intensive care and intensive care units *955*, *958*, 959
  see also first aid
Emeside 1008
Emflex 1008
EMG *see* electromyography (EMG)
Eminase 1008
Emla 1008
emollients and barrier preparations 890
  emollients, antipruritic drugs 891–892
emotional or erratic personality disorders 561
emotional and/or psychological problems *see* developmental and psychological disorders in children; mental health disorders; sexual problems
emphysema with chronic bronchitis *see* chronic obstructive pulmonary disease (COPD)
emPOWER 1036
enalapril 1008
enamel
  broken, fractured tooth 614–615
  tooth structure 606, *607*
encephalitis *see* viral encephalitis
encopresis 852
En-De-Kay 1008
endemic typhus 304
endocardium
  disorders *see* infective endocarditis
  heart structure *398*, *399*
endocrine (hormone-secreting) cells 670, *671*
endocrine disorders *see* hormonal disorders; metabolic disorders
endocrine system 670
  drugs acting on the endocrine system 930–935
  see also glands; hormone functions; hormone production; hormones
Endocrine Web 1033
endometrial sampling *738*
endometriosis 742–743
endometrium
  disorders *see* cancer of the uterus; endometriosis
  female reproductive system structure and functions *732*
  tests and investigations *see* endometrial sampling; laparoscopy
endoplasmic reticulum, protozoa structure *287*
endoscopic and minimally invasive surgery 940, 948–950
endoscopy *214*, 242, 255–256
  arthroscopy *386*
  bronchoscopy *504*
  colonoscopy *661*
  cystoscopy *715*
  endoscopic and minimally invasive surgery 940, 948–950
  endoscopic retrograde cholangiopancreatography (ERCP) *653*
  endoscopy of the nose and throat *476*
  hysteroscopy *745*
  knee arthroscopy *386*
  laparoscopy *742*
  sigmoidoscopy *661*
  upper digestive tract endoscopy *641*
Endoxana 1008
end-stage kidney failure 705, 708
enemas
  barium enema *243*, 246
  for constipation 628
  rectal drug delivery route *879*
energy production from food *see* food energy
enflurane 1008
  general anaesthetics 914
engagement of the head of the fetus, during pregnancy *781*
enlarged adenoids 842–843
enlarged prostate gland 725–726
ENO's 1008
enoxaparin 1008
  drugs that prevent blood clotting 904
enoximone 1008
entacapone 1008
Entocort CR 1008
entropion 584
enuresis *see* bedwetting
envelopes, virus structure *285*
environmental disorders 314, 321
  altitude sickness 324–325
  asphyxiation 326
  barotrauma 598
  decompression sickness 325
  drowning and near-drowning 81, 314, 325–326
  frostbite 324
  heat exhaustion and heatstroke 322–323
  hypothermia 314, 323–324
  motion sickness 85, 604
  poisonous bites and stings 327
  see also occupational lung diseases
environmental factors
  effect on skin 328
  in infections 284
  see also carcinogens
environmental temperature
  effect of humidity *322*
  effect of wind (windchill factor) *323*
environmental tobacco smoke (ETS) and passive smoking 64–65
enzyme deficiencies
  alpha$_1$-antitrypsin deficiency 489
  congenital adrenal hyperplasia in babies and children 866
  lactose intolerance 657–658
  see also inborn errors of metabolism
enzymes
  blood tests for creatine kinase 230, 241
  deficiency disorders *see* enzyme deficiencies
  production and role in digestive system 620, *621–625*, *674*
  routine blood chemistry tests for enzymes 229–230

eosinophils, white blood cell type *441*
Epanutin 1008
ephedrine 1008
  cold and flu remedies 910
  decongestants 909
epidemic typhus 304
epidermis
  effect of burns 317
  skin structure 328, *329*, *330*
epididymal cysts 718
epididymis
  disorders *see* epididymal cysts; epididymo-orchitis
  male reproductive system structure and functions 716, *717*
epididymo-orchitis 718–719
epidural anaesthesia in labour *801*, 914
epigastric hernia 662
epiglottis
  inflamed *see* epiglottitis
  respiratory system structure and functions 470, *471*, *622*
epiglottitis 842
epilepsy 524–526
  anticonvulsant drugs 914–915
  first aid *989*
  status epilepticus 525, 526
  useful online sites and addresses 1031
Epilepsy Association of Scotland 1031
Epilepsy International 1031
Epilim 1008
epinephrine 1008
  antiallergy drugs 905
  injectable epinephrine as emergency treatment for anaphylaxis or angioedema *469*, 905, *987*
  overproduction due to phaeochromocytoma 686
  production blocked by beta-blocker drugs 899
  production and functions *673*
EpiPen 1008
epiphyses, bone structure and development *812*
epirubicin 1008
episiotomy *804*
epithelial tissue, site of cancerous tumours *275*
Epivir 1008
epoetin 1008
Epogam 1008
epoprostenol 1008
Eppy 1008
Eprex 1008
Epstein–Barr virus (EBV)
  cause of acute hepatitis 644
  cause of Burkitt's lymphoma in children 279, 459
  cause of infectious mononucleosis 291–292
eptifibatide 1008
Equagesic 1008
equipment and aids *see* aids and equipment
ERCP (endoscopic retrograde cholangiopancreatography) *653*
erectile dysfunction *see* impotence
erectile tissue, in penis *717*
erection of the penis 762, *763*
  erection problems *see* impotence; priapism
ergocalciferol 1008
  drugs for bone disorders 896
ergometrine 1008
  drugs for labour 938
ergotamine 1008
  antimigraine drugs 913
erosion, cervical 749
erratic or emotional personality disorders 561
eruption
  eruption failure *see* impacted teeth
  teeth development *606*
  teething in babies 819–820
Erwinase 1009
Erycen 1009
Erymax 1009
erythema multiforme 337
erythema nodosum 348
Erythrocin 1009
erythrocyte sedimentation test, test for inflammation 233
erythromycin 1009
  antibiotics 885–886
Erythroped 1009
erythropoietin 1009
  production and functions in body *440*, *671*
Escherichia coli infections
  bacterial cystitis 709–710
  food poisoning 629
  gastroenteritis 628–629
Eskamel 1009
Eskornade 1009
esmolol 1009
Estracombi 1009
Estraderm TTS 1009
estradiol 1009
  hormone replacement therapy (HRT) 937–938
  sex hormones and related drugs 933–934
estramustine 1009
Estrapak 1009
estriol 1009
estrone 1009
  hormone replacement therapy (HRT) 937–938
estropipate 1009
  hormone replacement therapy (HRT) 937–938
etacrynic acid 1009
etamsylate 1009
ethambutol 1009
  antituberculous drugs 886
ethinylestradiol 1009
  hormone replacement therapy (HRT) 937–938
  sex hormones and related drugs 933–934
ethmoid sinuses *470*
ethoheptazine 1009
ethosuximide 1009
  anticonvulsant drugs 914–915
etidronate 1009
  drugs for bone disorders 896
etodolac 1009
  nonsteroidal anti–inflammatory drugs (NSAIDs) 894
  painkillers 912–913
etomidate 1009
  general anaesthetics 914
etoposide 1009
  anticancer drugs 907–908
ETS *see* environmental tobacco smoke (ETS)
etynodiol 1009
Eucardic 1009
Euglucon 1009
Eugynon-30 1009
Eurax 1009
Eurax-Hydrocortisone 1009
Eurohealth 1026
European Federation of Asthma and Allergy Associations 1027
eustachian tubes, ear structure and functions *592*, *593*, *594*
Everyman, Action Against Male Cancer 1034
Evista 1009
Evorel 1009
examination techniques, basic *220*
excessive crying in babies 819
excessive hair 359–360
excessive sweating, symptoms chart 104–105
Exelderm 1009
Exelon 1009
exercise 55–61
  for adolescents 31
  aerobic exercise *60*
  for arthritis relief *375*
  back-strengthening exercises *383*
  cause of muscle cramp 388
  for children 30
  choices for fitness *58*
  effect on basal metabolic rate (BMR) 54, *674*
  effect on blood circulation 396, 440
  effect on blood glucose levels *690*
  effect on bones 55, *56*
  effect on cardiovascular health 55, *56*
  effect on heart rate 59, *399*
  effect on joints *56*, 57
  effect on lungs and respiratory health 55, *56*
  effect on musculoskeletal health 55–57
  effect on psychological health *56*, 57
  exercise testing, for cardiovascular disorders *407*
  exercise therapy in physiotherapy 961
  fitness assessment *57*, 58–59
  health benefits 55–57
  lifestyle choices *17*, *47*
  for muscle strength *56*, 57
  in old age *37*
  for older adults 35
  for osteoporosis prevention 368, 369
  overexertion dangers 60
  pelvic floor exercises 712
  in pregnancy *34*
  pulse recovery time *59*
  regular exercise programmes 57–59
  relaxation exercises *17*, *75*
  role in weight control 54
  safety 59–60
  speech therapy exercises 963
  target heart rate 59
  useful online sites and addresses 1031
  warming up and cooling down in your exercise routine *60–61*
exhaling, breathing mechanism *472*
Ex-Lax 1009
Exocin 1009
exophthalamos 582
expectorants, cough remedies 909–910
Expulin 1009
Expulin Decongestant 1009
external fetal monitoring 803
external fixation, fracture treatment *393*
external haemorrhoids 668
external radiotherapy, cancer *281*
Exterol 1009
extrinsic allergic alveolitis 502–503
eyeballs
  disorders caused by shape of the eyeball affecting focusing *see* refractive errors
  eye structure and functions *567*
  protruding *see* exophthalamos
eyebrows and eyelashes, functions *331*
eye disorders 570
  acute glaucoma 575–576, 920–921
  allergic conjunctivitis 570–571
  anterior uveitis 574–575
  bacterial conjunctivitis 570–571
  cataracts 573
  chemicals in the eye, first aid *993*
  in children *see* eye disorders in children
  chronic glaucoma 576–577, 920–921
  conjunctivitis 570–571
  corneal abrasion 571
  corneal ulcers 571–572
  diabetic retinopathy 579–580
  drugs acting on the eye 919–921
  dry macular degeneration 580–581
  exophthalamos 582
  eye injuries 582
  eye wounds, first aid *993*
  floaters 577
  foreign body in the eye, first aid *993*
  glaucoma 575, 920–921
  hyphaema 572
  keratoconus 572–573
  macular degeneration 580–581
  optic neuritis 581
  painful or irritated eye, symptoms chart 132–133
  papilloedema 581–582
  posterior uveitis 574–575
  retinal detachment 578–579
  retinal vein occlusion 578
  retinitis pigmentosa 581
  retinopathy 579
  sarcoidosis 498–499
  scleritis 574
  secondary glaucoma 575
  subconjunctival haemorrhage 571
  surgery *see* eye surgery

tests and investigations *see* eye and vision tests and investigations
trachoma 572
useful online sites and addresses 1031
uveitis 574–575
viral conjunctivitis 570–571
vitreous haemorrhage 578
wet macular degeneration 580–581
see also eyelid and tear system disorders; vision disorders
eye disorders in children 856
amblyopia 858
cataracts, cause of congenital blindness 856–857
congenital blindness 856–857
congenital glaucoma, cause of congenital blindness 856–857
conjunctivitis 570
retinoblastoma 858–859
strabismus 857–858
vision tests in children *857*
watery eye 585
eyedrops *881*, *919*
eyelids
disorders *see* eyelid and tear system disorders
eye structure and functions 566, 583
of newborn babies *811*
eyelid and tear system disorders 583
blepharitis 583–584
chalazion 584
dacryocystitis 585
ectropion 584–585
entropion 584
keratoconjunctivitis sicca 585
ptosis 584
Sjögren's syndrome 463
styes 583
watery eye 585
xerophthalmia 585
eye ointments *920*
eyes
autonomic nervous system responses *see* dilation and constriction of the pupil of the eye
disorders *see* eye disorders
effects of growth and aging *22–23*
fetal development during pregnancy *780*
inspection during physical examination *219*
of newborn babies *811*
role in body's defences *444*, *566*
structure and functions 566, *567–569*
surgery *see* eye surgery
tests and investigations *see* eye and vision tests and investigations
using eyedrops *919*
see also vision
eye surgery
cataract surgery *573*
laser-assisted in-situ keratomileusis (LASIK) *589*
laser iridotomy *576*
laser surgery for diabetic retinopathy *579*
photoreactive keratectomy (PRK) *589*
radial keratotomy (RK) *589*
for refractive errors *589*
trabeculectomy *577*
eye and vision tests and investigations
eye examinations for people with diabetes mellitus *690*
fluorescein angiography *580*
letter matching test in children *857*
ophthalmoscopy *578*
retinoscopy in babies and children *857*
slit-lamp examination *574*
tonometry *576*
vision tests in children *857*
vision tests for visual acuity *587*
visual field test *590*
eye wounds, first aid *993*

F

face
disorders *see* facial disorders
facial hair development during puberty *716*, *815*
facial hair in women 740
fetal facial features, development during pregnancy *780–781*
face presentation, abnormal fetal presentation 801
facet joints, in the spine *364*
facial disorders
acne 340–341, 890–891
Bell's palsy 548
facial pain, symptoms chart 118
facial palsy 548
impetigo 351–352
myasthenia gravis 549
nervous tics 550
rosacea 341–342
trigeminal neuralgia 546
facial nerve
disorders *see* facial palsy
nervous system structure and functions *509*, *511*
facial pain, symptoms chart 118
facial palsy 548
factitious disorder, Munchausen's syndrome 558
factor VIIa 1009
factor VIII 1009
drugs that promote blood clotting 903
factor VIII/factor IX deficiencies *see* haemophilia and Christmas disease
factor IX 1009
factor IX complex, drugs that promote blood clotting 903
factor VIII/factor IX deficiencies *see* haemophilia and Christmas disease
faecal occult blood test *44*, 233
faecal samples 222
faecal softeners, laxatives 924–925
faeces
blood in faeces, symptoms chart 160
bowel movement disorders *see* constipation; diarrhoea; encopresis
faecal occult blood test *44*, 233
faecal samples, collection for testing 222
production in and elimination by the digestive system 620, *621*, *623*, *625*
failure of orgasm 770
faintness
feeling faint and passing out, symptoms chart 108–109
feeling faint in pregnancy *785*
falciparum malaria 305–306
fallopian tubes
cutting and tying *see* female sterilization
damaged, cause of female infertility 775
egg fertilization in 730, *763*, *778*
embryo development in *see* ectopic pregnancy
female reproductive system structure and functions 730, *731–732*
surgical removal *see* hysterectomy
Fallot's tetralogy, congenital heart disease 837
falls
accident and serious injury statistics 314
prevention 77
false negative and false positive results, tests and investigations 44, 213
famciclovir 1009
antiviral drugs 886–887
familial adenomatous polyposis (FAP), polyps in the colon 661, 666
family history, importance in medical history 24–26, 218
family planning
useful online sites and addresses 1031–1032
see also contraception
Family Planning Association 1031
family trees, medical 24–26
famotidine 1009
ulcer-healing drugs 923–924
Famvir 1009
Fansidar 1009
FAP *see* familial adenomatous polyposis (FAP)
Farlutal 1009
farmer's lung, extrinsic allergic alveolitis 502
fascicles
muscle structure *366*
nervous system structure *509*
Fasigyn 1009
fat
body fat distribution, health risks indicator 53
in the diet *see* fats
subcutaneous *see* subcutaneous fat
fat cells, structure and functions *675*
fats 50–51
chemical breakdown during digestion *625*, *674–675*
healthy choices *50*
nutritional content on food labels *52*
fatty acids, production by digestive system and use in metabolism *625*, *674–675*
fatty liver, alcohol-related liver disease 646–647
Faverin 1009
Fear of Dentists 1030
febrile convulsions 849
first aid *989*
Fectrim 1009
feedback mechanism, hormone secretion *670*
feeding problems in babies 819
feeling depressed, symptoms chart 122–123
feeling unwell, symptoms chart 92–93
feet
disorders *see* foot and toe disorders
foot care for people with diabetes mellitus *690*
foot and hand bandages, first aid *997*
foot massage, symptoms relief for the terminally ill *966*
joint movement range 362
of newborn babies *811*
plane joints in *365*
Fefol 1009
felbinac 1009
Feldene 1009
felodipine 1009
female condoms 69, *70*
female hormonal problems and disorders 734
abnormal puberty in females 739–740
breast cancer 759–761
cyclical breast pain 756
decreased sex drive 67, 769
delayed puberty, in females 739–740
galactorrhoea, nipple discharge 758
hypogonadism in females 739
infertility *see* female infertility
menopausal problems *733*, 737–738
polycystic ovary syndrome 744
precocious puberty, in females 739–740
primary hypogonadism, in females 739
secondary hypogonadism, in females 739
virilization 740
see also menstrual problems
female infertility 775–777
treatments *see* infertility treatments
female reproductive system
disorders *see* female reproductive system disorders
during pregnancy *see* pregnancy
effects of growth and aging *22–23*
structure and functions 730, *731–733*
symptoms charts 184–197
tests and investigations *see* female reproductive system tests and investigations
see also sexual intercourse

female reproductive system disorders
abnormal vaginal bleeding 737
abnormal vaginal bleeding, symptoms chart 190–191
bacterial vaginosis 753
bartholinitis 753
breast disorders *see* breast disorders in females
cancer of the cervix *281*, 750–751
cancer of the ovary 744–745
cancer of the uterus *281*, 748
cancer of the vulva and vagina 753
cervical dysplasia 749–750, *751*
cervical erosion 749
chlamydial pelvic infection 765–766
choriocarcinoma 748
cystadenoma, ovarian cysts 743
cystocele, prolapse of the uterus and vagina 747
dermoid cysts, ovarian cysts 743
endometriosis 742–743
fibroids 745–746
fistula, caused by diverticular disease 664
follicular cysts, ovarian cysts 743
genital ambiguities caused by congenital adrenal hyperplasia 866
genital irritation in women, symptoms chart 195
lower abdominal pain in women, symptoms chart 192–193
ovarian cysts 743–744
painful intercourse in females 772–773
pelvic inflammatory disease (PID) 741
polycystic ovary syndrome 744
postmenopausal bleeding 738–739
prolapse of the uterus and vagina 747
rectocele, prolapse of the uterus and vagina 747
retroverted uterus 746
surgery *see* female reproductive system surgery
tests and investigations *see* female reproductive system tests and investigations
Turner's syndrome *238*, 271, 823
uterine polyps *745*, 746
vaginal bleeding, abnormal 737
vaginal bleeding outside menstruation, symptoms chart 190–191
vaginal thrush 752–753
vaginismus 773
vulvovaginitis 752
see also breast disorders in females; female hormonal problems and disorders; sexually transmitted infections (STIs)
female reproductive system surgery
abdominal hysterectomy *747*
breast cancer surgery 760, *761*
breast reduction *757*
for cervical dysplasia *751*
colposcopy *750*
female sterilization 70, *743*
hysterectomy *747*
hysteroscopy *745*
laparoscopy *742*
lumpectomy, for breast cancer 760, *761*
mastectomy, for breast cancer 760, *761*
quadrantectomy, for breast cancer 760
female reproductive system tests and investigations
aspiration of a breast lump *756*
breast self-examination *755*
cervical smear test *44*, *749*
colposcopy *750*
endometrial sampling *738*
hysteroscopy *745*
laparoscopy *742*
mammography *44*, *759*
pelvic examination during physical examination 220
females
breast self-examination *755*
excessive hair 359–360
female/male differences in lower urinary tract *694*, *695*
fertility 730
hirsutism 359–360, 740
puberty *730*, *815*
reproductive system *see* female reproductive system
sex hormones *see* female sex hormones
sexual assault 320
sexual problems *see* female sexual problems
urethra location in urinary and reproductive systems *694*, *695*, *731*
women's health, useful online sites and addresses 1037
female sex hormones
disorders *see* female hormonal problems and disorders
level changes after childbirth causing depression 807
level changes in pregnancy causing common complaints of pregnancy 784
levels during the menopause *see* menopause
production and role in female reproductive system 730, *731–733*
role in puberty *see* puberty
sex hormones and related drugs 933–934
see also oestrogen; progesterone
female sexual problems
decreased sex drive 67, 769
failure of orgasm 770
painful intercourse in women 772–773
vaginismus 773
female sterilization 70, *743*
Femapak 1009
Femara 1009
Fematrix 1009
Femeron 1009
Femigraine 1009
Feminax 1009
Femodene 1009
femoral angiography *433*
femoral artery bypass graft *434*
femoral hernia 662
femoral nerves, nervous system structure *509*
Femoston 1009
FemSeven 1009
Femulen 1009
femur
childhood disorders *see* Perthes' disease; slipped femoral epiphysis
fracture treatment *393*
location in skeleton *363*
lower limb fractures, first aid 992
Fenbid 1009
fenbufen 1009
Fenbuzip 1009
fenofibrate 1009
lipid-lowering drugs 935
Fenoket 1009
fenoprofen 1009
nonsteroidal anti-inflammatory drugs (NSAIDs) 894
painkillers 912–913
Fenopron 1009
fenoterol 1009
Fentamox 1009
fentanyl 1009
painkillers 912–913
Fentazin 1009
fenticonazole 1009
Feospan 1009
Ferfolic SV 1009
ferric ammonium citrate 1009
Ferrograd 1009
Ferrograd C 1009
Ferrograd Folic 1009
ferrous fumarate 1009
ferrous gluconate 1009
ferrous glycine sulphate 1009
ferrous sulphate 1009
Fersaday 1009
Fersamal 1009
fertility 762
females 730
males 716
problems *see* infertility
Fertility UK 1031
fertilization and implantation (embedding)
in female reproductive system 730, 762, *763*, *778*
genetic material from egg and sperm combining at fertilization *21*, 264, *268*, 762, *763*
problems *see* infertility
fetal distress 804
fetal monitoring *803*
fetus
abnormal presentation 800–801
disorders *see* fetal distress; intra-uterine growth retardation; stillbirth
during labour and childbirth *782–783*
effects of alcohol, tobacco, and drugs 34, 881
engagement of the head *781*
failure to grow *see* intra-uterine growth retardation
fetal health checks *see* antenatal tests and investigations
growth and development during pregnancy *21*, 778, *779–781*
heart before and after birth *810*
heart rate monitoring *see* fetal monitoring
nourishment and blood supply during pregnancy *779*, *781*
fever (high body temperature)
bringing down a fever *289*
cause of febrile convulsions in children 849
fever in children, symptoms chart 202–203
fever, symptoms charts 102–103, 128–129, 202–20
rash with fever, symptoms chart 128–129
fever blisters *see* cold sores
fexofenadine 1009
fibrates, lipid-lowering drugs 935
fibre (dietary fibre) 50
function in digestion *625*
passage through digestive tract *623*
possible effect on colorectal cancer 666
role in preventing constipation 628
fibres
muscle fibres *366*, *367*, *513*
nerve *see* nerve fibres
optical fibres, use in flexible endoscopes 255
fibrin
dissolved by thrombolytic drugs *905*
role in blood clotting *442*
fibrinogen, role in blood clotting *441*, *442*
fibrinolysin 1009
fibrinolytics *see* thrombolytic drugs
fibroadenoma 754–755
fibroblasts, role in skin repair *330*
fibroids 745–746
fibromyalgia 389
fibrosing alveolitis 497–498
fibrosis *see* fibrosing alveolitis 497–498
fibrous capsules
in joints *364*
around noncancerous tumours *275*
Fibro-vein 1009
fight or flight response, role of adrenal glands 670, *673*
Fight for Sight 1031
figure-eight bandaging for elbows and knees, first aid *997*
Filair 1009
filamentous fungi, structure *287*
filariasis, tropical worm infestation 312
filgrastim 1009
fillings, tooth *611*
filtration of the blood, in the kidneys 694, *696–697*
fimbriae, female reproductive system structure and functions *731*
finasteride 1009
drugs that affect bladder control 939
drugs for prostate disorders 938–939
sex hormones and related drugs 933–934

fingers
  disorders *see* hand disorders
  fetal development *780*
  finger joints, hinge joint example *365*
  finger and toe bandages, first aid *998*
fingertip units, for applying ointments, creams, and gels *891*
firearm injuries *see* gunshot injuries
fire prevention and smoke detection
  barbecue safety 80
  home safety 79
first aid 976
  ABC of resuscitation *978*
  actions at an emergency, priorities 976, *977*
  altitude sickness 324
  anaphylaxis (anaphylactic shock) *469*, 905, *987*
  animal and human bites *995*
  artificial respiration *982–983*
  asphyxiation 326
  babies and infants *see* first aid for babies and infants
  bites and stings 327, *994–995*
  bleeding *986*
  burns 317–318, *988*
  cardiopulmonary resuscitation (CPR) *984–985*
  checking circulation after bandaging *996*
  chemicals in the eye *993*
  children *see* first aid for children
  choking *980–981*
  courses 976
  dressings and bandages *976*, *996–998*
  drowning and near-drowning 81, 326
  elbow and knee bandages *997*
  electrical injuries 319
  embedded object plus severe bleeding *986*
  eye damage *993*
  eye wounds *993*
  febrile convulsions *989*
  figure-eight bandaging for elbows and knees *997*
  finger and toe bandages *998*
  foreign body in the eye *993*
  foreign body plus severe bleeding *986*
  fractures *992*
  frostbite 324
  gunshot injuries 320
  head injuries *991*
  heat exhaustion and heatstroke 322
  home first aid kit *976*
  human and animal bites *995*
  hypothermia 324
  insect stings *995*
  kit *976*
  log roll technique *990*
  lower limb fractures *992*
  major seizures *989*
  minor burns and scald 317–318, *988*
  mouth-to-mouth and mouth-to-nose artificial respiration *982*
  poisoning 321, *994*
  poisonous bites and stings 327, *994*
  pressure points *986*
  priorities and actions at an emergency 976, *977*
  rebreathing technique for coping with panic attacks *552*
  recovery positions *979*
  roller bandages *976*, *996–997*
  scalds and minor burns 317–318, *988*
  seizures *989*
  severe bleeding *986*
  severe burns 317–318, *988*
  shock *987*
  slings *998*
  spinal injuries *990*
  sprains and strains *991*
  stab injuries 319
  sterile dressings *996*
  stings and bites 327, *994–995*
  swallowed poisons 321, *994*
  tick bites *995*
  training 976
  triangular bandages as slings *998*
  tubular gauze dressings for fingers or toes *998*
  upper limb fractures *992*
  useful online sites and addresses 1032
  see also emergencies and emergency care; injuries
first aid for babies and infants
  airway opening *978*
  artificial respiration *983*
  cardiopulmonary resuscitation (CPR) *985*
  checking brachial pulse *978*
  choking *980–981*
  febrile convulsions *989*
  fever reduction *289*
  recovery position *979*
first aid for children
  artificial respiration *982*
  cardiopulmonary resuscitation (CPR) *985*
  choking *980–981*
  febrile convulsions *989*
  fever reduction *289*
  recovery position *979*
First Aid Skills for Life 1032
first-degree burns 317
first stage of labour *782*
  delayed 801–802
first trimester of pregnancy *780*
fish oils, lipid-lowering drugs 935
fistula, caused by diverticular disease 664
fitness
  assessment *57*, 58–59
  see also exercise
Fitness Scotland 1031
fixation, fracture treatment *393*
fixed joints *364–365*
flagella
  bacteria structure *286*
  protozoa structure *287*
Flagyl 1009
Flamatrol 1009
Flamazine 1009
flaps *see* leaflets
flat feet, minor leg and foot problems in children 834
flat warts 355
flatworms *287*
  flatworm infestations 312–313
flavoxate 1010
  drugs that affect bladder control 939
fleas, diseases transmitted by
  endemic typhus 304
  plague 303–304
flecainide 1010
  antiarrhythmic drugs 898
flexibility, spine *364*
flexible endoscopy 242, 255–256, *255*
  bronchoscopy *504*
  colonoscopy *661*
  cystoscopy *715*
  endoscopic retrograde cholangiopancreatography (ERCP) *653*
  endoscopy of the nose and throat *476*
  sigmoidoscopy *661*
  upper digestive tract endoscopy *641*
Flexin Continus 1010
Flixonase 1010
floaters 577
Flomax MR 1010
flooding and desensitization, behaviour therapy techniques 969
floppy mitral valve *see* mitral valve prolapse
Florinef 1010
flossing and brushing teeth 608, *610*, 617
Floxapen 1010
flu *see* influenza
Fluanxol 1010
flucloxacillin 1010
  antibiotics 885–886
fluconazole 1010
  antifungal drugs 889
flucytosine 1010
  antifungal drugs 889
fludarabine 1010
fludrocortisone 1010
  corticosteroids 930–931
fludroxycortide 1010
fluid retention
  in chronic heart failure *413*
  in pre-eclampsia and eclampsia 794
  role of diuretic drugs 902
fluids *see* body fluids; water
flukes *287*
  cause of schistosomiasis 81, 312–313
flumazenil 1010
flumetasone 1010
flunisolide 1010
flunitrazepam 1010
fluocinolone 1010
  corticosteroids 930–93
  topical corticosteroids 892
fluocinonide 1010
  topical corticosteroids 892
fluocortolone 1010
Fluor-a-day 1010
fluorescein 1010
fluorescein angiography *580*
fluoride 1010
  excess fluoride as cause of discoloured teeth 613
  fluoridation of water and toothpaste, role in reduction of tooth disorders 606, 608, 609–610, 929
  fluoride supplements to strengthen teeth *610*
  mineral supplements 929
Fluorigard 1010
fluorometholone 1010
fluorosis, cause of discoloured teeth 613
fluorouracil 1010
  anticancer drugs 907–908
fluoxetine 1010
  antidepressant drugs 916–917
flupentixol 1010
fluphenazine 1010
  antipsychotic drugs 917–918
flurandrenolone *see* fludroxycortide1010
flurazepam 1010
  sleeping drugs 915–916
flurbiprofen 1010
  nonsteroidal anti-inflammatory drugs (NSAIDs) 894
Flurex 1010
flushes, hot *see* hot flushes
flutamide 1010
  anticancer drugs 907–908
  drugs for prostate disorders 938–939
  sex hormones and related drugs 933–934
fluticasone 1010
  corticosteroids 930–931
  corticosteroids for respiratory disease 911
  topical corticosteroids 892
fluvastatin 1010
  lipid-lowering drugs 935
fluvoxamine 1010
  antidepressant drugs 916–917
focusing
  disorders *see* refractive errors
  eye structure and functions 566, *567–569*
folate sodium 1010
folic acid 1010
  deficiency disorders *see* folic acid deficiency disorders
  sources in diet and effects on health *51*
  supplements before and during pregnancy 33, 844, 845, 928
  vitamin supplements 928
folic acid deficiency disorders
  glossitis 633
  megaloblastic anaemia 448
  neural tube defects 844–845
  stomatitis 633
folinic acid 1010
follicles, egg *see* egg follicles
follicle-stimulating hormone (FSH) 1010
  effect of drugs for infertility on production 936–937
  effect of sex hormones and related drugs on production 933, 934
  increased production during the menopause *733*, 737–738
  production in pituitary gland and role in female reproductive system *672*, 730, *732–733*
  role in puberty *815*
follicular cysts, type of ovarian cysts 743
follicular thyroid cancer 681–682

folliculitis 352
follitropin alfa 1010
 drugs for infertility 936–937
follitropin beta 1010
fomepizole 1010
fontanelles
 during skull growth and development in babies and children *813*
 in newborn baby's skull *811*
food
 energy from food *see* food energy
 food allergy 467
 food groups *49*
 food hygiene, home safety *79*
 food intolerance 657
 food labels *52*
 food processing in the body *see* digestion; metabolism
 food refusal, eating problems in children 852
 poisoning *see* food poisoning
 see also carbohydrates; cholesterol; diet; fats; minerals; protein in the diet; vitamins
Food and Drug Administration 1026, 1030
food energy
 daily requirements, effects of growth and aging *22–23*
 energy production from food, metabolic process 440, *674–675*
 nutritional information on food labels *52*
food poisoning 629–630
 amoebiasis 306
 botulism 301–302
 cryptosporidiosis 307
 gastroenteritis 85, 628–629
 giardiasis 307
 listeriosis 301, 817
 prevention, food hygiene *79*
 salmonellosis 629
 typhoid and paratyphoid *86*, 301, 883
foot and toe disorders
 athlete's foot 353
 bunions 387
 chilblains 350
 clubfoot, in babies and children 833
 corns 349
 flat feet, minor leg and foot problems in children 834
 gangrene 435
 gout 380
 ingrown toenails 361
 in-toeing and out-toeing, in children 834–835
 minor leg and foot problems in children 834–835
 mosaic warts 354
 plantar warts 354
 positional clubfoot, in babies and children 833
 Raynaud's phenomenon and Raynaud's disease 436
 structural clubfoot, in babies and children 833
 useful online sites and addresses 1036
 warts 354–355
 see also nail disorders
footling breech presentation, abnormal fetal presentation 800–801
foramen ovale, opening in fetal heart *810*
forceps delivery, assisted delivery technique *805*
foreign bodies
 in the airway *see* choking
 in the eye, first aid *993*
 plus severe bleeding, first aid *986*
foreskin
 disorders *see* balanitis; chordee; phimosis
 male reproductive system structure *717*
 surgical removal *see* circumcision
forgetfulness and/or confusion, symptoms chart 120–121
formestane 1010
formoterol 1010
 bronchodilator drugs 910–911
formula and bottle-feeding *28*, 35
Fortagesic 1010
Fortral 1010
Fortum 1010
foscarnet 1010
 antiviral drugs 886–887
Foscavir 1010
fosfestrol 1010
fosinopril 1010
 angiotensin converting enzyme (ACE) inhibitor drugs 900–901
fovea, eye structure and functions *567*, *568*, *569*
fractures *315*, *364*, 392–394
 first aid *992*
 fractured tooth 614–615
 fracture treatments *393*
 palliative surgery for bone fracture prevention in cancer *282*
 skull fractures, head injuries *315*, 521–522
 X-rays 244–245
fragile X syndrome *273*, 822
Fragmin 1010
framycetin 1010
frangula 1010
frank breech presentation, abnormal fetal presentation 800
Franol 1010
freckles 343
free bases (units of DNA) *265–266*, *269*
free nerve endings, sensory receptors in skin *329*, *513*
frequency, of sound 592
frequent urination, symptoms chart 166–167
fresh frozen plasma
 drugs that promote blood clotting 903
Frisium 1010
Froben 1010
frontal lobe, brain structure *510*
frontal sinus *470*
Froop 1010
frostbite 324
frozen shoulder 385–386
Fru-Co 1010
Frumil 1010
frusemide *see* furosemide
Frusene 1010
FSH *see* follicle-stimulating hormone (FSH)
Fucibet 1010
Fucidin 1010
Fucidin H 1010
Fucithalmic 1010
full blood count, blood cell tests 226–227
Full Marks 1010
functional obstruction, intestinal obstruction 663
funeral arrangements 967
fungal infections 305
 aspergillosis 309
 athlete's foot 353
 body ringworm 352–353
 candidiasis 309
 cryptococcosis 308–309
 drug treatments *see* antifungal drugs
 glossitis 633
 nongonococcal urethritis (NGU) 765
 oral thrush in babies and children 862–863
 otitis externa 596
 pityriasis versicolor 353
 pneumocystis infection 298, 308
 pneumonia 490–491
 ringworm 352–353
 risk from pets 82
 scalp ringworm 352–353
 sporotrichosis 309
 stomatitis 633
 vaginal thrush 752–753
 vulvovaginitis 752
fungi
 aspergillus *287*, 309
 fungus balls, in aspergillosis 309
 infections *see* fungal infections
 infectious organisms size comparison *284*
 structure *287*
Fungilin 1010
Fungizone 1010
Furadantin 1010
Furamide 1010
furosemide 1010
 diuretic drugs 902
fusidic acid 1010
 antibiotics 885–886
Fybogel *see* ispaghula
Fynnon Calcium Aspirin 1010

G

gabapentin 1010
 anticonvulsant drugs 914–915
Gabitril 1010
gait training, role in physiotherapy 962
galactorrhoea, nipple discharge 758
galactosaemia *273*, 868
Galcodine 1010
Galenphol 1010
Galfer 1010
Galfer FA 1010
gallamine 1010
gallbladder
 digestive system structure and functions *621*, *624*
 disorders *see* gallbladder disorders
gallbladder disorders
 cholecystitis 652
 gallstones 651
 jaundice 643–644
 see also bile duct disorders
gallstones 651
 lithotripsy *702*
Galpseud 1010
Gamanil 1010
Gamblers Anonymous 1034
gambling, compulsive 565
Gamcare 1034
gamete intrafallopian transfer (GIFT), assisted conception technique *776*
gamma globulin 1010
gamma rays, use in scanning *see* radionuclide scanning
gamolenic acid 1010
ganciclovir 1010
 antiviral drugs 886–887
Ganda 1010
ganglion (disorder) 390
ganglion (nerve structure)
 spinal nerves structure *511*
 see also basal ganglia
gangrene 435
Garamycin 1010
garden safety 80
Gardenal 1010
gas exchange 470, *471*, *473*
gas-permeable contact lenses *588*
gastric glands, location and role in digestive tract *622*
gastric juice, production and role in digestive system *621*, *622*, *625*
gastric pits, location and role in digestive tract *622*
gastric ulcer, type of peptic ulcer 640–642
gastrin, production and functions *671*
gastritis 640
Gastrobid Continus 1010
Gastrocote 1010
gastroenteritis 85, 628–629
Gastroflux 1010
Gastromax 1010
gastro-oesophageal reflux (GOR) 636–637
 antacids 923
 cause of Barrett's oesophagus 636
 in infants 863
 in pregnancy 784, *785*
Gaviscon 1010
Gelcosal 1010
Gelcotar 1010
gels *see* ointments, creams, and gels
gemcitabine 1010
gemeprost 1010
gemfibrozil 1010
 lipid-lowering drugs 935
gender determination, role of sex chromosomes *268*
Gender Trust, The 1036
gene disorders 271–273
 carriers 26, *269*, 272, *273*
 caused by single genes *see* single gene disorders
 in children *see* gene disorders in children
 genetic counselling 26, *272*
 tests and investigations *see* genetic tests

useful online sites and addresses 1032
see also chromosome disorders
gene disorders in children
achondroplasia *273*, 833
Becker muscular dystrophy 826
cystic fibrosis 272, *273*, 824–825, *962*
Duchenne muscular dystrophy 826
fragile X syndrome *273*, 822
juvenile periodontitis 618
juvenile polycystic kidney disease 704
Marfan's syndrome *273*, 824
muscular dystrophy *273*, 826
neurofibromatosis *273*, 827
sickle-cell disease *273*, 448–449
tests and investigations *see* genetic tests
Tourette's syndrome, nervous tics in 550
see also congenital immunodeficiency; inborn errors of metabolism
gene probes
for abnormal genes *240*
for microorganisms 235
gene therapy, cancer 282
general anaesthesia and general anaesthetics 914, *944*
generalized learning disabilities 854
see also Down's syndrome; fragile X syndrome
generalized seizures, epilepsy 525
general medical wards
hospital care 958–959
postoperative care and monitoring 945
general skin problems, symptoms chart 126–127
generic names and brand names, drugs 1000
genes
in bacteria *286*
disorders *see* gene disorders
gene tests *see* genetic tests
genetic material from egg and sperm combining at fertilization *21*, 264, *268*, 762
oncogenes *276*
probes *see* gene probes
role in cancer 274, *276*, 278–279
role of inheritance in susceptibility to disease *21*, 24–26
structure and functions 20, 264, *265–269*
genetic counselling 26, *272*
genetic disorders *see* gene disorders
genetic fingerprinting, for microorganisms 235
genetic material
in bacteria *286*
from egg and sperm combining at fertilization *21*, 264, *268*, 762
in protozoa *287*
in viruses *285*
see also chromosomes; DNA; genes
genetic tests 20, 26
antenatal *see* antenatal genetic tests
chromosome staining, tests for abnormal chromosomes 239
direct tests for abnormal genes 239–241
gene probes for abnormal genes *240*
gene probes for microorganisms 235
gene tests for microorganisms 235
genetic fingerprinting for microorganisms 235
indirect tests for abnormal genes 241
linkage analysis, indirect test for abnormal genes 241
tests for abnormal chromosomes 238–239
tests for abnormal genes 239–241
tests for gene products or biochemical markers 241
genital herpes 767–768
genital irritation in women, symptoms chart 195
genitals
female genitals *see* vulva
male genitals *717*
newborn baby's genitals *811*
genital tract, role in body's defences *444*
genital ulcers, Behçet's syndrome 465
genital warts 768
genome, human genome and Human Genome Project *264*
Genotropin 1010
gentamicin 1010
antibiotics 885–886
drugs acting on the ear 921
drugs acting on the eye 919–920
Genticin 1011
Gentisone HC 1011
German measles *see* rubella
germs *see* microorganisms
Gestalt therapy, person-centred therapy 970
gestational diabetes (diabetes developing in pregnancy) 687, 788–789
gestodene 1011
Gestone 1011
gestonorone 1011
gestrinone 1011
GH *see* growth hormone (GH)
giant-cell arteritis *see* temporal arteritis
giardiasis 307
GIFT *see* gamete intrafallopian transfer (GIFT)
gigantism, growth disorder 869
gingiva *see* gums
gingival hyperplasia 619
gingivitis 617–618
gland disorders
adrenal glands *see* adrenal gland disorders
Bartholin's glands *see* bartholinitis; Bartholin's cysts
basic hormone tests 232
cystic fibrosis 272, 273, 824–825, *962*
drugs for gland disorders 930–934, 938–939
hormone stimulation tests 232
hormone tests 232
lobules (milk–producing glands) in breasts *see* breast engorgement; breast lumps; mastitis; nipple discharge
lymph nodes *see* lymph node disorders
multiple endocrine neoplasia (MEN) 683
parathyroid glands *see* parathyroid gland disorders
pituitary gland *see* pituitary gland disorders
prostate gland *see* prostate disorders
salivary glands *see* salivary gland disorders
sebaceous glands *see* boil
Sjögren's syndrome 463
tear glands *see* eyelid and tear system disorders
thyroid gland *see* thyroid gland disorders
useful online sites and addresses 1033
Glandosane 1011
glands
adrenal *see* adrenal glands
Bartholin's *see* Bartholin's glands
in digestive system 620, *621–625*
eccrine sweat glands, skin structure *329*
gastric, location and role in digestive tract *622*
lacrimal *see* tear glands
lymph *see* lymph nodes
milk-producing *see* lobules (milk-producing glands) in breasts
parathyroid glands 670, *671*, *673*
pineal gland *671*
pituitary *see* pituitary gland
prostate *see* prostate gland
salivary, digestive system structure and functions 620, *621*, *622*
sebaceous *see* sebaceous glands
seminal vesicles, male reproductive system structure and functions 716, *717*, *763*
sweat glands, skin structure *329*, *331*
swollen *see* lymphadenopathy
tear *see* tear glands
thymus *see* thymus gland
thyroid gland 670, *671*, *673*
see also liver; ovaries; pancreas; testes
glandular fever *see* infectious mononucleosis
glans penis, male reproductive system structure *717*
glasses
bifocals and progressive lenses for presbyopia correction 589
for refractive errors correction *588*
sunglasses 81
glaucoma 575
acute glaucoma 575–576
chronic glaucoma 576–577
drugs for glaucoma 920–921
secondary glaucoma 575
Glaxo Neurological Centre 1035
glibenclamide 1011
drugs for diabetes mellitus 931–932
gliclazide 1011
glimepiride 1011
drugs for diabetes mellitus 931–932
glipizide 1011
drugs for diabetes mellitus 931–932
gliquidone 1011
glomerular capsule, kidney structure and functions *696*, *697*
glomerular filtrate, production in the kidneys *696*, *697*
glomeruli
disorders *see* diabetic kidney disease; glomerulonephritis; nephrotic syndrome
kidney structure and functions 694, *696–697*
glomerulonephritis 699–700
glossitis 633
glossopharyngeal nerve, nervous system structure and functions *511*
GlucaGen 1011
glucagon 1011
injectable glucagon as treatment for hypoglycaemia 691, 931
production and functions *671*, *674*
Glucobay 1011
Glucophage 1011
glucose
glucose metabolism *674–675*
levels in blood *see* blood glucose levels
production by digestive system and use in metabolism *674–675*
reabsorption in the renal tubules of the kidneys 694, *697*
routine urine chemistry tests for glucose 231
transport by the blood 440
glue, recreational drug effects and risks *66*
Glurenorm 1011
glutaraldehyde 1011
Glutarol 1011
gluten intolerance *see* coeliac disease
glycerol 1011
laxatives 924–925
production during digestion *625*, *675*
glyceryl trinitrate 1011
nitrate drugs 899–900
glycogen, storage in muscles and liver *670*, *675*
glycopyrronium bromide 1011
Glytrin 1011
goblet cells, mucous membrane structure *329*, *444*
goitre 680–681
gold 1011
gold-based drugs, antirheumatic drugs 895–896
Golden Eye 1011
golfer's elbow and tennis elbow 389–390
gonadorelin 1011
drugs for infertility 936–937
sex hormones and related drugs 933–934

gonadorelin analogues
drugs for infertility 936–937
drugs for prostate disorders 938–939
sex hormones and related drugs 933–934
gonadotrophin, human chorionic 1011
gonadotrophins
drugs for infertility 936–937
see also follicle-stimulating hormone (FSH); human chorionic gonadotrophin (HCG); luteinizing hormone (LH)
gonorrhoea 764–765
goose pimples, role in thermoregulation *331*
GOR *see* gastro-oesophageal reflux (GOR)
goserelin 1011
anticancer drugs 907–908
drugs for infertility 936–937
drugs for prostate disorders 938–939
sex hormones and related drugs 933–934
gout 380
grafts
bypass *see* bypass grafts
skin grafting *318*
gramicidin 1011
Graneodin 1011
granisetron 1011
antiemetic drugs 922
granular cells, skin structure *330*
Graves' disease, cause of hyperthyroidism 679–680
Great Ormond Street Hospital for Children NHS Trust 1029
greenstick fractures 392
Gregoderm 1011
grey matter, brain and spinal cord structure *510, 511*
grieving *see* bereavement and grieving
griseofulvin 1011
antifungal drugs 889
Grisovin 1011
grommets *861*
group therapy 970–971
growth
baby and child growth and development from birth to adolescence 810, *811–815*
disorders *see* growth disorders
embryo growth and development in early pregnancy 778, *780*
factors affecting growth *813*, 869
fetal growth and development during pregnancy 778, *779–781*
growth and aging, effect on body systems *22–23*
growth charts for babies *40–41*
growth charts for children *42–43*
growth spurt during puberty *812, 813*
skin and hair *330*
growth disorders 869
achondroplasia 273, 833
acromegaly 677
gigantism 869
Klinefelter's syndrome 271, 822–823
Turner's syndrome *238*, 271, 823
growth hormone (GH) 1011
growth hormone antagonists, pituitary drugs 934–935
overproduction disorders *see* acromegaly; gigantism
pituitary drugs 934–935
production and functions *440, 672*
Growth House, Inc 1029
growth plates, in developing bones *812*
growth retardation, intra-uterine, in pregnancy 796
GTN 300 mcg 1011
guaifenesin 1011
cough remedies 909–910
guanethidine 1011
guanine, nucleotide base in DNA *265*
Guanor Expectorant 1011
Guarem 1011
guar gum 1011
Guide Dogs for the Blind Association 1031
Guillain-Barré syndrome 550
Guillain-Barré Syndrome Support Group 1035
gum disease *see* mild gingivitis
gum disorders 617
acute necrotizing ulcerative gingivitis (ANUG) 617–618
chronic adult periodontitis 618
dry socket 619
gingival hyperplasia 619
gingivitis 617–618
juvenile periodontitis 618
periapical periodontitis 618
periodontitis 618
receding gums 619
see also tooth disorders
gums
disorders *see* gum disorders
inspection during physical examination *219*
oral hygiene 608, *610*, 617
structure 606, *607*
gunshot injuries 314, *315*, 319–320
guttate psoriasis 332, *333*
gynaecomastia 729
Gyno-Daktarin 1011
Gynol II 1011
Gyno-Pevaryl 1011

H

H_2 blockers, ulcer-healing drugs 923–924
Haelan 1011
haemangiomas, birthmarks 828
haematomas
in outer-ear injury 596
role in subdural haemorrhage 535
see also blood clots
haemochromatosis *273*, 692–693
haemodialysis *707*
haemoglobin
disorders *see* anaemias
role in oxygen transport by the blood *442*, 470, *473*
haemolytic anaemia 450
haemolytic jaundice 643
haemophilia and Christmas disease *273*, 452
Haemophilia Society 1027
Haemophilus influenzae type b (Hib) infections
bacterial meningitis in children 848–849
epiglottitis 842
routine immunizations *45*
vaccines and immunoglobulins 883–884
haemorrhages
cerebral haemorrhage, cause of stroke 533–534
postpartum haemorrhage 806–807
splinter haemorrhages, effect of infective endocarditis *426*
subarachnoid haemorrhage 534–535
subconjunctival haemorrhage 571
subdural haemorrhage 535
vitreous haemorrhage 578
see also viral haemorrhagic fevers
haemorrhoids 668
hair
disorders *see* hair disorders
effects of growth and aging *22–23*
excessive 359–360
functions *331*
growth *330*
hairs in respiratory system *see* cilia in respiratory system
hair transplant *359*
inspection during physical examination *219*
lanugo hair on premature babies *811*
loss *see* alopecia; male-pattern baldness
pubic, facial, and body hair development during puberty *716, 730, 815*
structure *329, 330*
hair bulbs *329, 330*
hair cells in the ear, structure and functions *594–595*
hair disorders 358
alopecia 358–359
dandruff 358
excessive hair 359–360
hair and scalp problems, symptoms chart 130–131
hair transplants for baldness *359*
head lice 831
hirsutism, type of excessive hair growth in females 359–360, 740
hypertrichosis, type of excessive hair growth 359–360
male-pattern baldness 359
see also scalp disorders
hair follicles *329, 330*
infected *see* boils; folliculitis; pityriasis versicolor
inflamed *see* folliculitis; sebaceous cysts
hairy leukoplakia 634
Halciderm Topical 1011
halcinonide 1011
topical corticosteroids 892
Haldol 1011
halibut liver oil 1011
hallucinogens, recreational drug effects and risks 65, *66*
hallux valgus, cause of bunions 387
halo naevus, type of mole 343
haloperidol 1011
antipsychotic drugs 917–918
halothane 1011
general anaesthetics 914
Halycitrol 1011
hand–arm syndrome 436–437
hand disorders
calluses 349
carpal tunnel syndrome 547
chilblains 350
common warts 354–355
Dupuytren's contracture 390
effects of serious injuries *315*
flat warts 355
ganglion 390
hand–arm syndrome 436–437
hand eczema, management *334*
painful arm or hand, symptoms chart 174
Raynaud's phenomenon and Raynaud's disease 436
warts 354–355
see also nail disorders
hand and foot bandages, first aid *997*
hand, foot, and mouth disease 831
hands
disorders *see* hand disorders
fetal development during pregnancy *780*
hand bone growth and development *812*
of newborn babies *811*
Hansen's disease 302
hantavirus infection, viral haemorrhagic fever 295
hard drugs, recreational drugs category 65
Harmogen 1011
Hashimoto's thyroiditis 680, 681
Hay-Crom 1011
hay fever *see* seasonal allergic rhinitis
Haymine 1011
HCG *see* human chorionic gonadotrophin (HCG)
HDLs *see* high-density lipoproteins (HDLs)
head
delivery of the head during childbirth *782–783*
fetal head engagement during pregnancy *781*
head circumference charts for babies and infants *40*
head movement and position detection by the inner ear 592, *595*
injuries *see* head injuries
proportional size of head to rest of body at different ages *812*
headaches
cluster headaches 519–520
headache 518
headache in children 847
headache symptoms chart 110–111

temporal arteritis 464–465
tension headaches 518
tension headaches in children 847
useful online sites and addresses 1032
see also migraine
head injuries *315*, 521–522
first aid *991*
subdural haemorrhage 535
useful online sites and addresses 1032
head lice 831
health 16–19
checkups *see* health checkups
at different ages *see* health at different ages
effects of lifestyle *see* lifestyle
health and safety landmarks *18–19*
health and safety, useful online sites and addresses 1036
health and safety at work 82–83
provision of health care *see* health care providers
when travelling *see* travel health
health care providers 38–39
childhood immunizations 45
health care choices, useful online sites and addresses 1032
insurance 38–39
see also doctors; hospital care
health checkups 40–42
dental checkups *609*
eyes and vision *see* eye and vision tests and investigations
for people with diabetes mellitus *690*
in pregnancy *see* antenatal tests and investigations
see also screening and screening tests
Health-club.net 1031
health at different ages 20, 27
in adolescents 31–32
in adults 32–33
in infants 27–29
at the menopause 36
in old age 37
in older adults 35–36
in pregnancy and after childbirth 33–35
in preschool children 29–30
in school-age children 30–31
when considering conception 33
Health Education Authority 1026, 1036
Health Education Board for Scotland 1026
Health Information Service 1026
Healthnet 1026, 1035, 1036, 1037
health risks due to lifestyle, assessment *46*
Health and Safety Executive 1036
Health Supplement Information Service 1035
hearing
disorders *see* hearing disorders
hearing and language, developmental milestones during childhood *814*
information processing of sound in the brain *515*, 592, *594*
mechanism of hearing *594*
protecting your hearing *602*
role of cochlear and vestibulocochlear nerves *511*, *593*, *594*
tests and investigations *see* hearing tests
hearing aids *601*
Hearing Concern 1032
hearing disorders
acoustic neuroma 605
chronic secretory otitis media in children 860–861
cochlear implants *603*
conductive hearing loss 599, *600*
congenital deafness 859–860
grommet insertion *861*
hearing aids *601*
hearing loss 599, *600*
hearing loss, symptoms chart 136–137
labyrinthitis 604
Ménière's disease 604–605
noise-induced hearing loss 601–602
presbyacusis 601
sensorineural hearing loss 599, *600*
stapedotomy *598*
tests and investigations *see* hearing tests
tinnitus 602
useful online sites and addresses 1032
see also ear disorders
hearing tests *600*
audiometry *600*
hearing tests in children *859*
McCormick toy discrimination test, in children *859*
oto-acoustic emission test, in children *859*
Rinne test *600*
speech discrimination test, in children *859*
tuning fork tests *600*
tympanometry *600*
Weber test *600*
heart
autonomic nervous system responses *514*
chambers of the heart 396, *398*, *399*
disorders *see* heart disorders
effects of exercise 55, *56*
effects of growth and aging *22–23*
effects of serious injuries *315*
murmurs *see* heart murmurs
muscle *see* heart muscle
natriuretic hormone production *401*, *671*
pumping (beating) action 396, *399*, *400*
rate *see* heart rate
structural changes at birth *810*, *811*
structure and functions 396, *398–401*
valves *see* heart valves
heart attack *see* myocardial infarction
heartbeats 396, *399*
palpitations, symptoms chart 164
heart block, complete 418
heartburn *see* gastro-oesophageal reflux (GOR)
heart cycle *399*
heart disorders
acute heart failure 412
angina 407–409, 899–900
atrioseptal defect, congenital heart disease in babies and children 836–837
chronic heart failure 413
coarctation of the aorta, congenital heart disease in babies and children 837
congenital heart disease in babies and children 836–837
constrictive pericarditis 428–429
coronary artery disease (CAD) 405–407, *408*
drugs for cardiovascular disorders 897–902, 904–905
effects of Kawasaki disease 837–838
effects of rheumatic fever 429
Fallot's tetralogy, congenital heart disease in babies and children 837
heart rate disorders *see* heart rate and rhythm disorders
heart rhythm disorders *see* heart rate and rhythm disorders
hypoplastic left heart syndrome, congenital heart disease in babies and children 837
infective endocarditis 426
muscle disorders *see* heart muscle disorders
myocardial infarction 410–412
patent ductus arteriosus, congenital heart disease in babies and children 837
pericarditis 428–429
pulmonary hypertension 505–506
septal defects, congenital heart disease in babies and children 836–837
surgery *see* cardiovascular system surgery
tests and investigations *see* cardiovascular system tests and investigations
useful online sites and addresses 1032
valve disorders *see* heart valve disorders
ventriculoseptal defect, congenital heart disease in babies and children 836–837
heart failure
acute 412
angiotensin converting enzyme (ACE) inhibitor drugs 900–901
chronic 413
digitalis drugs 901–902
diuretic drugs 902
heart–lung machines *953*
heart murmurs
checked during physical examination 219
symptom of heart valve disorders 421, 424, 426
heart muscle 362, *367*, *398*
disorders *see* heart muscle disorders
myocardium 396, *398*
heart muscle disorders 421
dilated cardiomyopathy 427–428
effects of rheumatic fever 429
hypertrophic cardiomyopathy 428
myocardial infarction 410–412
myocarditis 426–427
routine blood chemistry tests for heart muscle damage 230
heart rate 396, 415
disorders *see* heart rate and rhythm disorders
effect of exercise 59, *399*
effect of pregnancy *780*
fetal heart rate monitoring *803*
target heart rate during exercise 59
heart rate and rhythm disorders 415
arrhythmias 415–416
atrial fibrillation 417–418
cardiac arrest 419–420
cardiac pacemakers *419*, *940*
cardioversion treatment *420*
complete heart block 418
drug treatment *see* antiarrhythmic drugs; beta-blocker drugs
ectopic beats 415
sick sinus syndrome 419
supraventricular tachycardia (SVT) 416–417
heart transplants *427*
heart valve disorders 421–422
aortic incompetence 422–423
aortic stenosis 423
effects of rheumatic fever 429
heart valve replacement *422*
hypoplastic left heart syndrome, congenital heart disease in babies and children 837
infective endocarditis 426
mitral incompetence 423–424
mitral stenosis 424
mitral valve prolapse 425–426
valve defects, congenital heart disease in babies and children 837
valve incompetence *421*
valve stenosis *421*
heart valves *398*, *399*
disorders *see* heart valve disorders
heart valve replacement *422*
human tissue and mechanical replacements *422*
heat and cold treatments, role in physiotherapy 961
heat exhaustion and heatstroke 322–323
heavy periods
menstrual problem *see* menorrhagia
symptoms chart 189
Hedex 1011
Hedex Extra 1011
heel prick blood test, screening for metabolic disorders in newborn babies *44*, *867*
height
effects of abnormal puberty 869
height charts for children *43*
height/weight chart for adults *53*

height (continued)
  length charts for babies and infants *41*
  measuring children's height *42*
  problems *see* growth disorders
Heliclear 1011
Helicobacter pylori infection 639–640
  duodenal ulcer, type of peptic ulcer 640–642
  gastric ulcer, type of peptic ulcer 640–642
  gastritis 640
  peptic ulcer 640–642
helix structure of DNA 264, *265*
helminth infestations *see* worm infestations
Help the Aged 1026
Heminevrin 1011
hemispheres
  division of cerebrum in brain *510*
  dominant hemisphere, role in information processing in the brain *515*
Henoch–Schönlein purpura 339, 838–839
heparin 1011
  drugs that prevent blood clotting 904
heparinoid 1011
hepatic artery, in liver *624*
hepatitis
  acute hepatitis *86*, 644–645
  alcoholic hepatitis, alcohol-related liver disease 646–647
  chronic hepatitis 645–646, 907
  congenital infections, in newborn babies 817
  travel immunizations *86*
  vaccines and immunoglobulins 883–884
hepatocytes, type of liver cell *624*, *675*
Hep-Flush 1011
hereditary disorders *see* chromosome disorders; gene disorders
hereditary nonpolyposis colorectal cancer (HNPCC) 666
hernias 661–662
  abdominal hernia 661–662
  epigastric hernia 662
  femoral hernia 662
  hernia repair surgery *662*
  hiatus hernia 636, 662
  incisional hernia 662
  inguinal hernia 662
  paraumbilical hernia 662
  strangulated hernia 661–662
  umbilical hernia 662
herniated disc *see* prolapsed or herniated disc (slipped disc)
heroin, recreational drug effects and risks 65, *66*
herpes simplex infections 291
  antiviral drugs 886–887
  cold sores 354
  congenital infections, in newborn babies 817
  corneal ulcers 571–572
  genital herpes 767–768
  glossitis 633
  nongonococcal urethritis (NGU) 765
  viral encephalitis *86*, 528–529
  viral stomatitis 633
herpes zoster 290–291
heterosexuality 762
hexachlorophene 1011
Hexalen 1011
hexamine 1011
hexetidine 1011
Hexopal 1011
hiatus hernia 636, 662
Hib infections *see Haemophilus influenzae* type b (Hib) infections
Hibitane 1011
hiccups 483
High Blood Pressure Foundation 1032
high-density lipoproteins (HDLs) 231, 691–692
higher brain *see* cerebral cortex
high-risk pregnancies 786–787
hinge joints *364–365*
  in the jaws *607*
Hioxyl 1011
hip joints
  congenital hip dysplasia, in babies and children 832
  hip replacement *377*
  movement range 362
  slipped femoral epiphysis in children 834
  type of ball-and-socket joint *365*
Hiprex 1011
hirsutism, type of excessive hair growth 359–360, 740
Hirudoid 1011
Histafen 1011
Histalix 1011
histamine
  drugs blocking histamine release *see* antiallergy drugs; antihistamines
  role in allergic reactions *445*, 466
histrionic personality disorder 561
hives *see* urticaria
Hivid 1011
HIV infection and AIDS 297–298
  congenital infections, in newborn babies 817
  drugs for HIV infection and AIDS 887–888
  safe sex measure to prevent transmission 68, 85, 765
  useful online sites and addresses 1033
HLAs *see* human leukocyte antigens (HLAs)
HMOs *see* health maintenance organizations (HMOs)
HNPCC *see* hereditary nonpolyposis colorectal cancer (HNPCC)
hoarseness and/or voice loss, symptoms chart 140–141
Hodgkin's lymphoma 459
hole in the heart *see* septal defects
Holter monitor, use in ambulatory ECG *416*
homatropine 1011
home care *954*, 960
  caring for someone with dementia *536*
  moving into long-term care 960
  outpatient and day care treatment 956
  useful online sites and addresses 1033
  see also care of the dying
home first aid kits *976*
homeopathy 974
home oxygen therapy *507*, *966*
home pregnancy tests *232*
home safety and health *47*, 77–80
homosexuality 762
hookworm infestation 311–312
hormonal contraceptives 69, *71*
  cause of spotting 191
  emergency contraception 70
  injections 69, *71*
  see also contraceptive pill
hormonal disorders *see* female hormonal problems and disorders; gland disorders; male hormonal problems and disorders; metabolic disorders
hormone functions 670, *671–674*
  blood glucose levels, regulation and control *671*, *674*
  blood pressure control 396, *401*, *671*, 694
  body calcium levels, regulation *670*, *671*, *673*
  digestive system, regulation and control 620, *624*
  fight or flight response 670, *673*
  pregnancy and childbirth control 778, *783*
  stem cell production control *440*
  urine concentration in the kidneys, regulation and control *401*, 670, *672*
hormone production
  in the adrenal glands *see* adrenal glands
  in the duodenum *624*, *671*
  in the heart *401*, *671*
  in the hypothalamus (releasing factors) *671*, *672*
  in the intestines 620, *671*
  in the kidneys *401*, 670, *671*, 694
  in the ovaries *671*, 730, *731–733*
  in the pancreas 670, *671*, *674*
  in the parathyroid glands 670, *671*, *673*
  in the pineal gland *671*
  in the pituitary gland *see* pituitary gland
  in the placenta *232*, *671*
  in the stomach 620, *671*
  in the testes *671*, 716
  in the thymus gland *671*
  in the thyroid gland 670, *671*, *673*
hormone replacement therapy (HRT) 36, 937–938
hormones 670, *671–674*
  adrenocorticotrophic hormone (ACTH) *672*
  aldosterone *401*, *673*
  angiotensin, role in blood pressure control *401*
  antidiuretic hormone (ADH) *401*
    see also vasopressin
  basic hormone tests 232
  calcitonin *673*
  cortisol *673*
  disorders *see* female hormonal problems and disorders; gland disorders; male hormonal problems and disorders; metabolic disorders
  erythropoietin *440*, *671*
  feedback mechanism *670*
  FSH *see* follicle-stimulating hormone (FSH)
  functions *see* hormone functions
  gastrin *671*
  GH *see* growth hormone (GH)
  home pregnancy tests *232*
  hormone stimulation tests 232
  hormone tests 232
  hormone transport by the blood 670
  LH *see* luteinizing hormone (LH)
  melatonin *671*
  natriuretic hormone *401*, *671*
  pancreatic hormones *see* glucagon; insulin
  parathyroid hormone (PTH) *670*, *671*, *673*
  production *see* hormone production
  prolactin *672*
  renin, role in blood pressure control *401*
  sex hormones *see* female sex hormones; male sex hormones
  T_3 *673*
  thyroid hormones *440*, 670, *671*, *673*
  thyroid-stimulating hormone (TSH) 670, *672*
  thyroxine (T_4) *673*
  in treatments *see* hormone therapies and hormone drugs
  see also corticosteroid hormones; epinephrine; gonadotrophins; norepinephrine; oxytocin; testosterone
hormone stimulation tests 232
hormone therapies and hormone drugs
  contraceptives *see* hormonal contraceptives
  for diabetes mellitus *see* insulin
  drugs for hypothyroidism 932
  drugs for infertility 936–937
  hormone replacement therapy at the menopause 36, 937–938
  hormones and hormone antagonists, anticancer drugs 281–282, 907–908
  pituitary drugs 934–935
  sex hormones and related drugs 933–934
  see also corticosteroids; epinephrine; oestrogen
Hospice Information Service 1029
hospital care 957
  accessing hospital care 956
  for babies and children, in children's wards and special care baby units 959
  intensive care and intensive care units *955*, *958*, 959
  leaving hospital 959
  outpatient and day care treatment 956
  see also care of the dying; surgery
hot flushes, symptom of the menopause *733*, 738
HPV infections *see* human papillomavirus infections

H. pylori infection *see Helicobacter pylori* infection
HRT *see* hormone replacement therapy (HRT)
HSV infections *see* herpes simplex infections
Humalog 1011
Human Actrapid 1011
human and animal bites, first aid *995*
  insect stings, first aid *995*
  poisonous bites and stings 327
    first aid *994*
    prevention 86, 327
  tick bites, first aid *995*
human chorionic gonadotrophin (HCG) 1011
  detected by pregnancy tests *232*
Human Fertilization and Embryology Authority 1033
human genome and Human Genome Project *264*
human immunodeficiency virus infection *see* HIV infection and AIDS
Human Insulatard 1011
human leukocyte antigens (HLAs), role in multifactorial gene disorders 273
human menopausal gonadotrophin 1011
Human Mixtard 1011
Human Monotard 1011
human papillomavirus (HPV) infections
  association with cancer of the cervix 69, 751
  association with cervical dysplasia 750
  cause of genital warts 768
  cause of warts 354
Human Ultratard 1011
Human Velosulin 1011
Humatrope 1011
humidity, effect on environmental temperature *322*
hump and sag, back-strengthening exercise *383*
Humulin 1011
hunger *620*
Huntington's disease (Huntington's chorea) *273*, 538
Hyalase 1011
hyaluronidase 1011
hydatid disease 313
hydatidiform mole *see* molar pregnancy
hydralazine 1011
  antihypertensive drugs 897–898
hydrocele 721
hydrocephalus 845–846
hydrochloric acid in stomach *see* stomach acids
hydrochlorothiazide 1011
  diuretic drugs 902
hydrocortisone 1011
  antiallergy drugs 905
  antipruritic drugs 891–892
  corticosteroids 930–931
  corticosteroids for respiratory disease 911
  drugs acting on the ear 921
  locally acting corticosteroids 895
  topical corticosteroids 892
Hydrocortistab 1011
Hydrocortone 1011
hydroflumethiazide 1011
hydrogenated fats 51
hydrogen peroxide 1011
hydromorphone 1011
hydronephrosis 703
HydroSaluric 1011
hydrotalcite 1011
hydrotherapy, role in physiotherapy 961
hydroxocobalamin 1012
hydroxyapatite 1012
hydroxycarbamide 1012
  anticancer drugs 907–908
hydroxychloroquine 1012
  antirheumatic drugs 895–896
hydroxyethylcellulose
  drugs acting on the eye 919–920
hydroxyprogesterone 1012
hydroxyurea *see* hydroxycarbamide
hydroxyzine 1012
  antiemetic drugs 922
hygiene
  food hygiene *79*
  oral hygiene 608, *610*, 617
Hygroton 1012
hyoscine 1012
  antispasmodic drugs and motility stimulants 926
  drugs acting on the ear 921
hyoscine hydrobromide
  antiemetic drugs 922
hyperaldosteronism 685–686
hypercholesterolaemia 691–692
hypercoagulability 453
hyperemesis 789
hyperhidrosis 342
hyperlipidaemias, inherited 692, 935
hypermetropia 586–588
  glasses and contact lenses for hypermetropia correction *588*
hyperparathyroidism 682–683
hyperplasia
  benign prostatic hyperplasia *see* enlarged prostate gland
  gingival hyperplasia 619
hypertension 403–405
  antihypertensive drugs 897–898
  portal hypertension and varices 648–649
  pulmonary hypertension 505–506
hyperthyroidism 679–680
  caused by thyroiditis 681
  caused by thyroid nodules 681
  drugs for hyperthyroidism 932–933
hypertrichosis, type of excessive hair growth 359–360
hypertrophic cardiomyopathy 428
hyphae, fungi structure *287*
hyphaema 572
hypnotherapy 974–975
hypochondriasis 559
hypoglossal nerve, nervous system structure and functions *511*
hypoglycaemia 691, 931
hypogonadism
  hypogonadism in females 739
  hypogonadism in males 729
hypoparathyroidism 683
hypopituitarism 678
hypoplastic left heart syndrome, congenital heart disease 837
hypospadias 870
Hypotears 1012
hypotension 414
hypothalamus
  control of pituitary gland 670, *671, 672*
  functions *510*
  location in brain *510*
  role in blood pressure control *401*
hypothermia 314, 323–324
hypothyroidism 680
  caused by thyroiditis 680, 681
  drugs for hypothyroidism 932
  heel prick blood test, screening for hypothyroidism in newborn babies *44, 867*
Hypovase 1012
hypromellose 1012
  drugs acting on the eye 919–920
Hypurin 1012
hysterectomy *747*
hysterosalpingography, female infertility investigation 776
hysteroscopy *745*
Hytrin 1012

I

Ibugel 1012
Ibuleve 1012
ibuprofen 1012
  cold and flu remedies 910
  nonsteroidal anti-inflammatory drugs (NSAIDs) 894
  painkillers 912–913
Ibuspray 1012
ichthammol 1012
ICSI *see* intracytoplasmic sperm injection (ICSI)
idarubicin 1012
identical twins, multiple pregnancy 762, *779*, 792
idoxuridine 1012
  antiviral drugs 886–887
ifosfamide 1012
IgA deficiency *see* immunoglobulin A (IgA) deficiency
Ikorel 1012
ileum, digestive system structure and functions *621, 623, 625*
illness
  mental illness *see* mental health disorders
  preventing illness at different ages *see* health at different ages
  terminal illnesses *see* care of the dying; death
  see also diseases
Ilosone 1012
Ilube 1012
imaging techniques *213*, 242, *243*, 244
  cancer staging *279*
  radiation doses comparison *246*
  see also scans and scanning techniques; X-rays
Imbrilon 1012
Imdur 1012
imidapril 1012
imiglucerase 1012
Imigran 1012
imipenem 1012
imipramine 1012
  antidepressant drugs 916–917
  drugs that affect bladder control 939
imiquimod 1012
immobilization, fracture treatment *393*
Immukin 1012
immune function tests 228
immune globulin, vaccines and immunoglobulins 883–884
immune system
  disorders *see* immune system disorders
  drugs acting on the immune system 905–907
  structure and functions 440, *441–445*
immune system disorders
  allergies *see* allergies and allergic reactions
  immune function tests 228
  immunodeficiency disorders *see* acquired immunodeficiency disorders; congenital immunodeficiency
  useful online sites and addresses 1033
  see also autoimmune disorders
immunization 45, 288
  active and passive immunization 883, *884*
  booster doses *45*, 884
  routine immunizations *45*
  travel immunizations 85, *86*
  vaccines and immunoglobulins 883–884
immunodeficiency disorders *see* acquired immunodeficiency disorders; congenital immunodeficiency
immunoglobulin 1012
immunoglobulins
  immunoglobulin A (IgA) deficiency, acquired immunodeficiency disorder 461
  vaccines and immunoglobulins 883–884
Immunoprin 1012
immunosuppressants 906–907
  antirheumatic drugs 895–896
Imodium 1012
impacted teeth 613
impaired or disturbed vision, symptoms chart 134–135
Imperial Cancer Research Fund 1028
impetigo 351–352
implantation *see* fertilization and implantation (embedding)
implants
  cochlear implants *603*
  dental implants, replacement teeth *615*
  hormonal contraceptive implants and injections 69, *71*
  hormone replacement therapy (HRT) 937
  penile implant, impotence treatment 771

implants (continued)
  radioactive implants and seeds, cancer treatment *281*
  transoesophageal implants, use in speech therapy 963
impotence 770–771
  symptoms chart 180
Impotence, Your Questions Answered 1034
Imuran 1012
inborn errors of metabolism 867
  albinism *273*, 868–869
  galactosaemia *273*, 868
  heel prick blood test, screening for metabolic disorders in newborn babies *44*, *867*
  lactose intolerance 657–658
  phenylketonuria 241, *273*, 867–868
  Tay–Sachs disease *273*, 868
incisional hernia 662
incisors, tooth structure *606*, *607*
incontinence, urinary *see* urinary incontinence
incus, ear structure and functions *593*, *594*
indapamide 1012
  diuretic drugs 902
Inderal 1012
Inderal-LA 1012
Inderetic 1012
Inderex 1012
indigestion 626
  antacids 923
  preventing indigestion *627*
indinavir 1012
  drugs for HIV infection and AIDS 887–888
indirect tests for abnormal genes 241
Indocid 1012
Indolar 1012
indometacin 1012
  nonsteroidal anti-inflammatory drugs (NSAIDs) 894
  painkillers 912–913
indoramin 1012
induction of labour *797*
  uterine stimulant drugs, drugs for labour 938
inevitable miscarriage 792
Infacol 1012
Infadrops 1012
infants *see* babies and infants
infections
  affecting the heart *see* infective endocarditis; myocarditis; pericarditis; rheumatic fever
  bacterial *see* bacterial infections
  bone *see* osteomyelitis
  in children *see* infections and infestations in children
  congenital infections, in newborn babies 817
  Creutzfeldt–Jakob disease (CJD) 540
  drug treatments *see* anti-infective drugs
  fungal *see* fungal infections
  infectious diseases, useful online sites and addresses 1033
  joint *see* septic arthritis
  opportunistic infections in HIV infection and AIDS 298, 308
  prevention *see* food hygiene; immunization; travel health
  protozoal *see* protozoal infections
  sexually transmitted *see* sexually transmitted infections (STIs)
  skin 351–355
  tests for microorganisms 234–235
  transmission, control and organisms responsible 284–287, 351
  viral *see* viral infections
  see also individual infections by name, e.g. measles
infections and infestations in children
  acute otitis media in children 860
  ascariasis 311
  bronchiolitis 841
  cause of febrile convulsions in children 849
  chickenpox 290
  croup 841–842
  diphtheria *45*, 300, 883
  drug treatment *see* anthelmintic drugs; anti-infective drugs
  epiglottitis 842
  fever reduction *289*
  head lice 831
  hookworm infestation 311–312
  hydatid disease 313
  impetigo 351–352
  measles *45*, 293, 883–884
  meningitis in children 848–849
  molluscum contagiosum 355
  mumps *45*, 293–294, 883–884
  otitis media 597
  parvovirus infection 294–295
  pertussis *45*, 492–493, 883
  routine immunizations programme *45*
  rubella *45*, 294, 883–884
  scalp ringworm 352–353
  scarlet fever 300
  threadworm infestation 310
  urinary tract infections in children 871
infectious mononucleosis 291–292
infectious organisms *see* microorganisms
infective endocarditis 426
inferior vena cava
  connection to the kidneys *695*, *696*
  connection to the liver *624*
  location and role in cardiovascular system *397–400*
infertility 774
  treatments *see* infertility treatments
  useful online sites and addresses 1033
infertility treatments
  artificial insemination *775*
  assisted conception *776*
  drugs for infertility 936–937
  gamete intrafallopian transfer (GIFT), assisted conception technique *776*
  intracytoplasmic sperm injection (ICSI), for male infertility 777
  in-vitro fertilization (IVF), assisted conception technique *776*
  zygote intrafallopian transfer (ZIFT), assisted conception technique *776*
infestations *see* infections and infestations in children; skin infections and infestations; worm infestations
inflammation
  chemical tests for 232–233
  drug treatments *see* anti-inflammatory drugs
inflammatory bowel disorders *see* Crohn's disease; ulcerative colitis
inflammatory response
  in allergic reactions *445*
  body's defences *444*
influenza 289–290
  cold and flu remedies 910
  immunizations 45
  vaccines and immunoglobulins 883–884
ingrown toenails 361
inguinal hernia 662
inhaled anaesthetics, general anaesthetics 914
inhaling
  breathing mechanism *472*
  role in venous return of blood *400*
inhaling steam, self-help treatment *475*
inheritance 20, *21*, 264, *265–269*
  genetic material *see* chromosomes; DNA; genes
  inherited disorders *see* chromosome disorders; gene disorders; and individual articles on specific disorders
  role of inheritance in susceptibility to disease *21*, 24–26, 43–44
inherited hyperlipidaemias *273*, 692, 935
injected anaesthetics, general anaesthetics 914
injected anticoagulants, drugs that prevent blood clotting 904
injections
  depot injections, antipsychotic drugs 918
  hormonal contraceptives 69, *71*
  injections in haemorrhoid treatment 668
  injection therapy, varicose vein treatment *439*
  insulin injection treatment for diabetes mellitus *688*, 689, 931
  intravenous and intramuscular drug delivery routes *879*
  vitamin K injections for newborn babies 903, 928
injuries
  accidental, in the home *77*
  avulsed tooth 616
  burns 317–318
  crush injuries *315*, 316–317
  effect on body *315*
  electrical injuries 318–319
  eye injuries 582
  eye wounds, first aid *993*
  fractured tooth 614–615
  fractures *315*, *364*, 392–394
  gunshot injuries 314, *315*, 319–320
  head *see* head injuries
  musculoskeletal *see* musculoskeletal injuries
  needlestick injuries 356
  outer-ear injury 596
  peripheral nerve injuries 548–549
  repetitive strain injury (RSI) 82, 389
  serious injuries 314, *315*, 316–320
  sexual assault 320
  skin *see* skin injuries
  spinal *see* spinal injuries
  sports injuries 391–392
  stab injuries *315*, 319
  statistics 314, 316
  useful online sites and addresses 1034
  whiplash, spinal injury 524
  see also first aid
inner-ear disorders
  labyrinthitis 604
  Ménière's disease 604–605
  motion sickness 85, 604
  vertigo 603–604
inner ear, structure and functions 592, *593–595*
Innohep 1012
Innovace 1012
Innozide 1012
inosine pranobex 1012
inositol 1012
Inoven 1012
inpatient care *see* hospital care
insect stings, first aid *995*
insemination, artificial *775*
insoluble fibre 50
insomnia 554
  sleeping drugs 915–916
inspection, during physical examination *219*
Institute of Alcohol Studies 1027
Institute of Cancer Research 1028
Institute of Child Health 1029
Institute for Occupational Safety and Health 1036
insufficient tear production *see* keratoconjunctivitis sicca
Insulatard 1012
insulin 1012
  insulin injection treatment for diabetes mellitus *688*, 689, 931
  insulin pumps for diabetes mellitus 689, 931
  production in the pancreas and role in regulating body glucose levels *671*, *674*
  underproduction disorder or response failure *see* diabetes mellitus
insulin-dependent diabetes mellitus *see* type 1 diabetes
Insulin Dependent Diabetes Trust 1030
insulin lispro 1012
insurance, health care 38–39
Intal 1012
Integrilin 1012
intensity of sound 592
  levels causing noise-induced hearing loss *601*

intensive care units *955*, *958*, 959
intercostal muscles, location and role in breathing *471*, *472*
intercourse *see* sexual intercourse
interferon alfa 1012
  anticancer drugs 907–908
  antiviral drugs 886–887
  interferon drugs 907
interferon beta 1012
  interferon drugs 907
interferon drugs 907
  biological therapy for cancer 282, 907–908
  drugs for HIV infection and AIDS 887–888
interferon gamma 1012
internal fetal monitoring *803*
internal fixation, fracture treatment *393*
internal haemorrhoids 668
internal radiotherapy, cancer *281*
International Association for Medical Assistance to Travellers 1037
International Foundation for Functional Gastrointestinal Disorders 1030
International Glaucoma Association 1031
International Planned Parenthood Federation 1031
International Stress Management Association 1037
interstitial cystitis 709–710
Interstitial Cystitis Support Group 1037
intervertebral discs
  prolapsed or herniated disc (slipped disc) 384–385
  structure *364*
intestinal disorders 655
  abdominal hernia 661–662
  appendicitis 664
  banding haemorrhoids *668*
  barium enema *243*, 246
  bowel movement disorders *see* constipation; diarrhoea; encopresis
  cholera 301
  coeliac disease 658
  colectomy *665*
  colonoscopy *661*
  colorectal cancer 665–667
  colostomy *666*
  Crohn's disease 658–659, 924
  diverticular disease 663–664
  double-contrast radiography 246–247
  drugs for intestinal disorders 924–926
  in duodenum *see* stomach and duodenum disorders
  epigastric hernia 662
  familial adenomatous polyposis (FAP), polyps in the colon 661, 666
  femoral hernia 662
  food intolerance 657
  functional obstruction, intestinal obstruction 663
  gastroenteritis 85, 628–629
  haemorrhoids 668
  hereditary nonpolyposis colorectal cancer (HNPCC) 666
  hernia repair surgery *662*
  hernias 661–662
  incisional hernia 662
  inguinal hernia 662
  internal haemorrhoids 668
  intestinal obstruction 663
  intussusception in children 864–865
  irritable bowel syndrome 655–656
  lactose intolerance 657–658
  malabsorption 656–657
  mechanical obstruction, intestinal obstruction 663
  paraumbilical hernia 662
  partial colectomy *665*
  permanent colostomy *666*
  polyps in the colon 660–661
  proctitis 667
  prolapsing haemorrhoids 668
  pseudomembranous colitis, caused by antibiotics 885
  rectal prolapse 667–668
  sigmoidoscopy *661*
  strangulated hernia 661–662
  tapeworm infestation 313
  temporary colostomy *666*
  toxic megacolon, caused by ulcerative colitis 660
  ulcerative colitis 659–660, 924
  umbilical hernia 662
  useful online sites and addresses 1030
  see also food poisoning
intestinal junction, digestive tract structure *623*
intestinal obstruction 663
intestines
  compression during pregnancy *779*, *781*
  digestive system structure and functions 620, *621–623*, *625*
  disorders *see* intestinal disorders
  effects of serious injuries *315*
  hormone production 620, *671*
  Peyer's patches, lymphatic system structure *443*
  role in body's defences *444*
in-toeing and out-toeing, minor leg and foot problems in children 834–835
intolerances
  food intolerance 657
  lactose intolerance 657–658
intoxicants
  recreational drug effects and risks 65, *66*
  see also alcohol and alcohol-related problems
intracytoplasmic sperm injection (ICSI), for male infertility 777
Intralgin 1012
intramuscular route, drug delivery route *879*
intrauterine device (IUD), contraceptive 69–70, *71*
intra-uterine growth retardation 796
intravenous route, drug delivery route *879*
intravenous urography (IVU) 246, *695*, *699*
Intron-A 1012
intussusception 864–865
inverted nipples *see* nipple inversion
investigations *see* tests and investigations
Invirase 1012
in-vitro fertilization (IVF), assisted conception technique *776*
involuntary movements
  of diaphragm *see* hiccups
  effects of cerebral palsy 846–847
  nervous tics 550
  pelvic floor muscle spasms *see* vaginismus
  twitching and tremor, symptoms chart 116–117
involuntary responses
  nervous system control 508, *514*
  see also reflexes
iodine 1012
  iodine deficiency, cause of hypothyroidism 680
  iodine dyes in contrast X-rays 246
  mineral supplements 929
  radioiodine, drugs for hyperthyroidism 932–933
Ionamin 1012
Ionax 1012
Ionil T 1012
Iopidine 1012
ipecacuanha 1012
ipratropium bromide 1012
  bronchodilator drugs 910–911
irbesartan 1012
  antihypertensive drugs 897–898
irinotecan 1012
  anticancer drugs 907–908
iris
  disorders *see* anterior uveitis
  eye structure and functions *566*, *567–568*
  slit-lamp examination *574*
iritis *see* anterior uveitis
iron 1012
  deficiency disorders *see* iron deficiency disorders
  excessive accumulation of iron in the body *see* haemochromatosis
  mineral supplements 929
  sources in diet and effects on health *51*
iron deficiency disorders
  glossitis 633
  iron-deficiency anaemia 447
  stomatitis 632–633
irregular periods 734
irreversible pulpitis 611
irritable bowel syndrome 655–656
  living with irritable bowel syndrome *656*
irritated or painful eye, symptoms chart 132–133
ischaemia, lower limb 434–435
ischaemic disease, category of disease 260, *261*
islets of Langerhans, pancreas structure and functions *674*
Ismelin 1012
Ismo 1012
isocarboxazid 1012
isoconazole 1012
isoflurane 1012
  general anaesthetics 914
Isogel 1012
Isoket 1012
isometheptene mucate 1012
isoniazid 1012
  antituberculous drugs 886
isophane insulin 1012
Isopto Alkaline 1012
Isopto Atropine 1012
Isopto Carbachol 1012
Isopto Carpine 1012
Isopto Frin 1012
Isopto Plain 1012
Isordil 1012
isosorbide dinitrate 1012
  nitrate drugs 899–900
isosorbide mononitrate 1012
  nitrate drugs 899–900
Isotrate 1012
isotretinoin 1012
  retinoid drugs 890–891
Isotrex 1012
ispaghula 1012
  antidiarrhoeal drugs 924
  laxatives 924–925
  lipid-lowering drugs 935
isradipine 1012
ISSUE, The National Fertility Association 1033
Istin 1012
itching 339
  anal itching 669
  antipruritic drugs 891–892
  genital irritation in women, symptoms chart 195
  symptoms chart 125
itraconazole 1012
  antifungal drugs 889
IUD *see* intrauterine device (IUD)
ivermectin 1012
  anthelmintic drugs 889
IVF *see* in-vitro fertilization (IVF)
IVU *see* intravenous urography (IVU)

J

Japanese B encephalitis
  travel immunizations *86*
jaundice 643–644
  haemolytic jaundice 643
  neonatal jaundice 817–818
jawbone 606, *607*
jaw injuries, artificial respiration for casualties with jaw injuries, first aid *982*
jaws
  of newborn babies *811*
  strength and movement range 606, *607*
JCA *see* juvenile chronic arthritis (JCA)
Jectofer 1013
jejunum, digestive system structure and functions *621*, *623*, *625*
jet lag, when travelling 85
John Grooms Association for Disabled People 1030
joint aspiration *380*
joint and ligament disorders 374
  arthroscopy *386*
  bunions 387
  bursitis 387
  chondromalacia 386
  dislocated joints 394

joint and ligament disorders (continued)
drug treatments *see* antirheumatic drugs; locally acting corticosteroids; nonsteroidal anti-inflammatory drugs (NSAIDs)
frozen shoulder 385–386
hip replacement *377*
joint aspiration *380*
joint replacement *377*
knee arthroscopy *386*
knee joint aspiration *380*
knee joint replacement *377*
ligament injuries 394
lower back pain 381–384
painful joints, symptoms chart 176–177
prolapsed or herniated disc 384–385
scleroderma 462–463
shoulder joint replacement *377*
spondylolithesis 385
sports injuries 391–392
sprains and strains, first aid *991*
temporomandibular joint disorder 616
torn knee cartilage 395
see also arthritis; physiotherapy
joint replacement *377*
joints
ball-and-socket joints *364–365*
between vertebrae *364–365*
disorders *see* joint and ligament disorders
effects of exercise *56*, 57
effects of growth and aging *22–23*
ellipsoidal joints *364–365*
facet joints in the spine *364*
fixed joints *364–365*
hinge joints *364–365*, *607*
inspection and examination during physical examination *219*, 220
investigations into *see* arthroscopy; joint aspiration
pivot joints *364–365*
plane joints *364–365*
saddle joints *364–365*
semi-movable joints *364–365*
structure and functions 362, *364–365*, 374
synovial joints *364–365*
temporomandibular joint, in the jaw *607*
Joy-rides 1013
juvenile chronic arthritis (JCA) 835
Juvenile Diabetes Foundation 1030
juvenile periodontitis 618
juvenile polycystic kidney disease *273*, 704

K

Kabikinase 1013
Kalspare 1013
Kalten 1013
Kamillosan 1013
kanamycin 1013
kaolin 1013
antidiarrhoeal drugs 924
Kapake 1013
Kaposi's sarcoma 346–347
Karvol 1013
karyotype, Turner's syndrome *238*, *271*
Kawasaki disease 837–838
Kay-Cee-L 1013
Keep Fit Association 1031
Kefadol 1013
Keflex 1013
Kefzol 1013
Kelfizine W 1013
keloids 349
Kemadrin 1013
Kemicetine 1013
Kenalog 1013
Kentene 1013
Keral 1013
keratin
effects of acitretin treatment 890–891
overproduction in acne 340
in skin, hair, and nails 328, *331*
keratoconjunctivitis sicca 585
keratoconus 572–573
keratoses
seborrhoeic keratosis 348
solar keratosis 347
Kerlone 1013
ketamine 1013
general anaesthetics 914
ketoacidosis, symptom and complication of diabetes mellitus 688
Ketocid 1013
ketoconazole 1013
antifungal drugs 889
preparations for skin infections and infestations 892–893
ketoprofen 1013
nonsteroidal anti-inflammatory drugs (NSAIDs) 894
painkillers 912–913
ketorolac 1013
nonsteroidal anti-inflammatory drugs (NSAIDs) 894
painkillers 912–913
ketotifen 1013
Ketovail 1013
Ketovite 1013
kidney biopsy *701*
kidney cancer 704–705, 872
kidney cysts 703
kidney disorders 698
acute glomerulonephritis 699–700
adenocarcinoma, kidney cancer 704–705
caused by urinary tract infections in children 871
chronic glomerulonephritis 699–700
diabetes insipidus 678, 934–935
diabetic kidney disease 705
dialysis *707*
dimercaptosuccinic acid (DMSA) scanning *871*
effects on drug treatments 881
failure *see* kidney failure
glomerulonephritis 699–700
haemodialysis *707*
hydronephrosis 703
intravenous urography (IVU) 246, *695*, *699*
juvenile polycystic kidney disease 704
kidney biopsy *701*
kidney cancer 704–705, 872
kidney cysts 703
kidney scarring, caused by urinary tract infections in children 871
kidney stones 701–703
kidney transplant *708*
lithotripsy *702*
nephrotic syndrome 700–701
peritoneal dialysis *707*
polycystic kidney disease 704
pyelonephritis 698–699, 871
transitional cell carcinoma, kidney cancer 704–705
useful online sites and addresses 1037
Wilms' tumour, kidney cancer in children 705, 872
kidney failure 705
acute kidney failure 705, 706
chronic kidney failure 705, 706–708
dialysis *707*
end-stage kidney failure 705, 708
kidney transplant *708*
kidney machines, use in haemodialysis *707*
kidneys
disorders *see* kidney disorders
effects of serious injuries *315*
hormone production *401*, 670, *671*, 694
role in blood pressure control *401*, 694
urinary system structure and functions 694, *695–697*
kidney stones 701–703
lithotripsy *702*
prevention *703*
kidney transplant *708*
killer T-cells, role in cellular immune response *445*
kilocalories
units of energy 52
see also food energy
kissing disease *see* infectious mononucleosis
kits
emergency medical travel kit 85
first aid *976*
Klaricid 1013
Klean-prep 1013
Klinefelter's syndrome 271, 822–823
Kliofem 1013
Kloref 1013
knee arthroscopy *386*
knee disorders
chondromalacia 386
knock-knees, minor leg and foot problems in children 834
Osgood–Schlatter disease in children 834
torn knee cartilage 395
knee and elbow bandages, first aid *997*
knee joints
hinge joint example *365*
knee joint aspiration *380*
knee joint replacement *377*
knife wounds *see* stab injuries
knock-knees, minor leg and foot problems in children 834
koilonychia *see* spoon-shaped nails
Kolanticon 1013
Konakion 1013
Konsyl 1013
Koplik spots, measles symptom *293*
Kwells 1013
kyphosis and lordosis 371
Kytril 1013

L

labetalol 1013
beta-blocker drugs 898–899
labia
during sexual arousal and sexual intercourse *762*, *763*
female reproductive system structure and functions 730, *731*
laboratories, medical *225*
Labosept 1013
labour and childbirth *782–783*
assisted delivery *805*
caesarean section *802*
drugs for labour 938
epidural anaesthesia in labour *801*, 914
episiotomy *804*
fetal monitoring *803*
first signs *782*
forceps delivery *805*
health in pregnancy and after childbirth 33–35
induction of labour *797*, 938
preparing for childbirth 34
problems after childbirth 35, 806
problems during labour *see* labour problems
useful online sites and addresses 1035–1036
vacuum suction delivery *805*
labour problems 800
abnormal presentation 800–801
assisted delivery *805*
breech presentation and birth, abnormal fetal presentation 800–801
brow presentation, abnormal fetal presentation 801
compound presentation, abnormal fetal presentation 801
delayed first stage of labour 801–802
episiotomy *804*
face presentation, abnormal fetal presentation 801
fetal distress 804
footling breech presentation, abnormal fetal presentation 800–801
forceps delivery *805*
frank breech presentation, abnormal fetal presentation 800
induction of labour *797*, 938
oblique presentation, abnormal fetal presentation 801
occipitoposterior presentation, abnormal fetal presentation 800

premature labour 798, 938
problems during delivery 802–804
shoulder presentation, abnormal fetal presentation 801
stillbirth 805
umbilical cord prolapse *see* cord prolapse
vacuum suction delivery *805*
labyrinth, ear structure and functions 604
labyrinthitis 604
lacidipine 1013
Lacri-Lube 1013
lacrimal glands *see* tear glands
lactation *see* breast milk production
lactic acid 1013
lactitol 1013
lactose intolerance 657–658
Lactugal 1013
lactulose 1013
laxatives 924–925
lacunae, in bones *363*
Ladropen 1013
Lamictal 1013
Lamisil 1013
lamivudine 1013
drugs for HIV infection and AIDS 887–888
lamotrigine 1013
anticonvulsant drugs 914–915
Lamprene 1013
landmarks
landmarks in disease *262–263*
landmarks in disease detection *214–215*
landmarks in health and safety *18–19*
landmarks in treatment *876–877*
Langerhans, islets of *see* islets of Langerhans
language *see* voice, speech, and language
Lanoxin 1013
Lanoxin-PG 1013
lanreotide 1013
pituitary drugs 934–935
lansoprazole 1013
ulcer-healing drugs 923–924
lanugo hair, on premature babies *811*
laparoscopy *742*
Larafen 1013
Larapam 1013
large cell carcinoma, primary lung cancer 503–505
large intestine
digestive system structure and functions 620, *621*, *623*, *625*
disorders *see* intestinal disorders
Lariam 1013
laryngitis 479–480
laryngopharynx, respiratory system structure *471*
larynx
cancer of the larynx 481
laryngitis 479–480
respiratory system structure *471*
tests and investigations *see* endoscopy of the nose and throat; mirror laryngoscopy
voice and speech production 470, *473*
laser-assisted in-situ keratomileusis (LASIK), surgical treatment for refractive errors *589*
laser treatments 940, 951–952
for cervical dysplasia *751*
laser-assisted in-situ keratomileusis (LASIK), refractive errors treatment *589*
laser iridotomy, acute glaucoma treatment *576*
laser surgery for diabetic retinopathy *579*
photoreactive keratectomy (PRK), refractive errors treatment *589*
on the skin *951*
LASIK *see* laser-assisted in-situ keratomileusis (LASIK)
Lasikal 1013
Lasilactone 1013
Lasix 1013
Lasma 1013
Lasonil 1013
Lasoride 1013
Lassa fever, viral haemorrhagic fever 295
Lassar's Paste 1013
latanoprost 1013
drugs for glaucoma 920–921
late postpartum haemorrhage 806–807
lateral ventricles, brain structure *510*
laxatives 924–925
Laxoberal 1013
Laxose 1013
LDLs *see* low-density lipoproteins (LDLs)
lead poisoning 77, 79
learning difficulties
useful online sites and addresses 1034
see generalized learning disabilities; specific learning difficulties
Ledclair 1013
Lederfen 1013
Lederfolin 1013
Ledermycin 1013
Lederspan 1013
leg disorders
bow legs, minor leg and foot problems in children 834
gangrene 435
knock-knees, minor leg and foot problems in children 834
leg ulcers 350
lower limb ischaemia 434–435
lymphangitis 458–459
lymphoedema 459
minor leg and foot problems in children 834–835
painful leg, symptoms chart 175
sciatica 546–547
sciatica in pregnancy *785*
superficial thrombophlebitis 439
varicose veins 438–439
in pregnancy 438, 784, *785*
see also foot and toe disorders; fractures
Legionella pneumophilia bacteria *284*
cause of Legionnaires' disease 490
Legionnaires' disease 490
leg stretches, warming up and cooling down in your exercise routine *61*
leg ulcers 350
leisure activities, lifestyle choices *47*
Lemsip 1013
length charts for babies and infants *41*
Lenium 1013
lenograstim 1013
lens of the eye
disorders *see* cataracts; refractive errors
eye structure and functions 566, *567–568*
slit-lamp examination *574*
Lentard MC 1013
Lentaron 1013
lentigo maligna, type of malignant melanoma 346
lentigo, type of freckle 343
Lentizol 1013
Leonard Cheshire 1034
lepirudin 1013
leprosy *see* Hansen's disease
leptospirosis 81, 302–303
lercanidipine 1013
Lescol 1013
letrozole 1013
letter matching test, vision test in children *857*
Leucovorin 1013
Leukaemia CARE 1027
Leukaemia Research Fund 1027
leukaemias 453–456
acute leukaemia 454–455
acute lymphoblastic leukaemia (ALL) 454–455
acute myeloid leukaemia (AML) 454–455
chronic lymphocytic leukaemia (CLL) 455
chronic myeloid leukaemia (CML) 455–456
leukaemia 453–454
Leukeran 1013
leukotriene antagonists, antiallergy drugs 905
leuprorelin 1013
anticancer drugs 907–908
drugs for infertility 936–937
drugs for prostate disorders 938–939
sex hormones and related drugs 933–934
levamisole 1013
levobunolol 1013
drugs for glaucoma 920–921
levocabastine 1013
levodopa 1013
levofloxacin 1013
antibiotics 885–886
levomepromazine 1013
levonelle 1013
levonorgestrel 1013
hormone replacement therapy (HRT) 937–938
sex hormones and related drugs 933–934
levothyroxine 1013
drugs for hypothyroidism 932
LH *see* luteinizing hormone (LH)
libido, loss of *see* decreased sex drive
Librium 1013
lice
epidemic typhus transmission 304
head lice 831
pubic lice 768
lichen planus 336–337
oral lichen planus 634
lidocaine 1013
antiarrhythmic drugs 898
antipruritic drugs 891–892
local anaesthetics 914
life events, stress ratings *74*
life expectancy 16–17, *20*
lifejackets *81*
Lifesaver 1037
lifestyle
changes at the menopause 36
choices 18–19, 46, *47*
health risks assessment *46*
importance in medical history 218
role in susceptibility to disease 27, 46, 261–262
see also individual aspects of lifestyle, e.g. diet
lifting an object correctly *382*
ligaments
disorders *see* joint and ligament disorders
from ovaries to uterus in female reproductive system *731*, *732*
periodontal ligaments in the jaw 606, *607*
role in joints 362, *364*, 374
in the spine *364*
suspensory ligament in the eye *567*
light-headedness *see* faintness; vertigo
light rays
focusing errors by the eye *see* refractive errors
focusing and processing by the eye 566, *567–569*
lignocaine *see* lidocaine
Limbless Association 1036
limbs
fetal development during pregnancy *780*
limb disorders *see* arm disorders; leg disorders
lindane 1013
preparations for skin infections and infestations 892–893
linear movements, detection by the inner ear *595*
lining of the uterus *see* endometrium
linkage analysis, indirect test for abnormal genes 241
Lioresal 1013
liothyronine 1013
drugs for hypothyroidism 932
Lipantil 1013
lipid-lowering drugs 935
Lipitor 1013
lipoproteins, high-density (HDLs) and low-density (LDLs) 231, 691–692
Lipostat 1013

liquid paraffin 1014
  laxatives 924–925
Liquifilm Tears 1014
lisinopril 1014
  angiotensin-converting enzyme (ACE) inhibitor drugs 900–901
Liskonum 1014
listeriosis 301
  congenital infections, in newborn babies 817
lisuride 1014
Litarex 1014
lithium 1014
  mood-stabilizing drugs 918
lithotripsy *702*
liver
  autonomic nervous system responses *514*
  blood circulation through the liver *440, 624*
  digestive system structures and functions 620, *621, 624–625*
  disorders *see* liver disorders
  effects of serious injuries *315*
  glycogen storage *675*
  of newborn babies *811*
  role in drug metabolism *879*
  role in metabolism *624, 625, 675*
liver biopsy *647*
liver cancer *277*, 649
  liver metastases 649–650
liver cell damage, cause of jaundice 643
liver disorders 643
  acute hepatitis *86*, 644–645, 883
  acute liver failure 650–651
  alcoholic hepatitis, alcohol-related liver disease 646–647
  alcohol-related liver disease 646–647
  alpha$_1$-antitrypsin deficiency 489
  chronic hepatitis 645–646, 907
  chronic liver failure 650–651
  cirrhosis 646, 647–648
  effects on drug treatments 881
  fatty liver, alcohol-related liver disease 646–647
  haemolytic jaundice 643
  jaundice 643–644
  liver biopsy *647*
  liver cancer *277*, 649
  liver cell damage, cause of jaundice 643
  liver failure 650–651
  liver metastases 649–650
  liver transplant *650*
  neonatal jaundice 817–818
  portal hypertension and varices 648–649
  primary biliary cirrhosis 647–648
  Reye's syndrome in children 849
  routine blood chemistry tests for liver damage 229–230
  sclerosing cholangitis, cause of cirrhosis 648
  useful online sites and addresses 1034
liver failure 650–651
liver lobules, structure and functions *624*
liver metastases 649–650
liver spots *see* lentigo
liver transplant *650*
Livial 1014
living wills 964
Livostin 1014
lobes of the brain *510*
lobes of the pituitary gland, structure and functions *672*
lobules (milk-producing glands), in breasts *733, 780, 783*
  disorders *see* breast engorgement; breast lumps; mastitis; nipple discharge
lobules, liver *see* liver lobules
local anaesthesia and local anaesthetics 914, *942*
  local anaesthetics, antipruritic drugs 891–892
locally-acting corticosteroids 895
Loceryl 1014
lockjaw *see* tetanus
Locoid 1014
Locorten-Vioform 1014
Lodine SR 1014
lodoxamide 1014
Loestrin 1014
lofepramine 1014
lofexidine 1014
log roll technique, first aid for spinal injuries *990*
Logynon 1014
Lomexin 1014
Lomotil 1014
lomustine 1014
London Lesbian and Gay Switchboard 1036
long bones
  diaphyses and epiphyses during bone development *812*
  growth and development in babies and children *811, 812*
  repair and healing *364*
  structure *363*
longer acting insulins, drugs for diabetes mellitus 931
longsightedness *see* hypermetropia
Loniten 1014
loop diuretic drugs, diuretic drugs 902
loop of Henle, kidney structure and functions *696, 697*
Loperagen 1014
loperamide 1014
  antidiarrhoeal drugs 924
Lopid 1014
loprazolam 1014
Lopresor 1014
loratadine 1014
  antihistamines 906
lorazepam 1014
  antianxiety drugs 916
  anticonvulsant drugs 914–915
lordosis and kyphosis 371
lormetazepam 1014
losartan 1014
  antihypertensive drugs 897–898
Losec 1014
loss and bereavement *see* bereavement and grieving
loss of consciousness *see* unconsciousness
loss of weight *see* weight problems
Lotriderm 1014
loudness *see* intensity of sound
low-density lipoproteins (LDLs) 231, 691–692
lower abdominal pain in women, symptoms chart 192–193
lower back pain 381–384
lower back stretch
  back-strengthening exercise *383*
  warming up and cooling down in your exercise routine *60–61*
lower jaw (mandible), location and movement range *363, 607*
lower limb fractures, first aid *992*
lower limb ischaemia 434–435
lower oesophageal sphincter, digestive tract structure and functions *622*
Loxapac 1014
loxapine 1014
  antipsychotic drugs 917–918
LSD *see* lysergic acid diethylamide
Luborant 1014
Ludiomil 1014
Lugol's solution 1014
lumbar nerves, nervous system structure and functions *511*
lumbar puncture *527*
lumbar spine *364*
lumpectomy 760, *761*
lumps *see* breast lumps; swelling and swellings
lung cancer *274*
  adenocarcinoma, primary lung cancer 503–505
  lung metastases 505
  mesothelioma, asbestos-related disease 501–502
  primary lung cancer 503–505
  small cell carcinoma, primary lung cancer 503–505
  squamous cell carcinoma, primary lung cancer 503–505
lung disorders 482
  acute bronchitis 486–487
  acute respiratory distress syndrome (ARDS) 506–507
  acute sarcoidosis 498–499
  alpha$_1$-antitrypsin deficiency 489
  aspergillosis 309
  aspiration pneumonia 491
  bacterial pneumonia 490–491
  bronchiectasis 496
  cancer *see* lung cancer
  chronic sarcoidosis 498–499
  collapsed lung *315*
  COPD *see* chronic obstructive pulmonary disease (COPD)
  cough 482–483
  extrinsic allergic alveolitis 502–503
  fibrosing alveolitis 497–498
  hiccups 483
  Legionnaires' disease 490
  lung oedema in acute heart failure *412*
  pertussis *45*, 492–493, 883
  pleural effusion 494–495
  pleurisy 493
  pneumocystis infection 308
  pneumonia 490–491
  pneumothorax 496–497
  pulmonary embolism 495
  pulmonary hypertension 505–506
  respiratory distress syndrome, in premature babies 816
  respiratory failure 507
  sarcoidosis 498–499
  TB *see* tuberculosis (TB)
  tests and investigations *see* respiratory system tests and investigations
  useful online sites and addresses 1034
  ventilation disorders, respiratory failure 507
  viral pneumonia 490–491
  see also asthma; occupational lung diseases
lung function tests *488*
lungs
  autonomic nervous system responses *514*
  blood circulation to the lungs *396, 400*
  compression in pregnancy *781*
  disorders *see* lung disorders
  effect of a baby's first breath *810, 811*
  effects of exercise 55, *56*
  effects of growth and aging *22–23*
  effects of serious injuries *315*
  effects of smoking 64
  examination during physical examination 219
  oxygen/carbon dioxide gas exchange 470, *471, 473*
  respiratory system structure and functions 470, *471–473*
lung volume tests *488*
lunula, nail structure *328*
lupus
  discoid lupus erythematosus (DLE) 347
  systemic lupus erythematosus (SLE) 461–462
Lupus UK 1033
Lustral 1014
luteinizing hormone (LH)
  effect of drugs for infertility on production 936–937
  effect of sex hormones and related drugs on production 933, 934
  production in pituitary gland *672*
  role in female reproductive system 730, *732*
  role in puberty *815*
luteinizing hormone 1014
Lyclear 1014
Lyme disease 303
  lymphadenopathy 458
lymecycline 1014
lymph (fluid)
  cancer spread in *277*
  movement through lymphatic system *443*, 458
lymphangitis 458–459
lymphatic system
  disorders *see* lymphatic system disorders
  structure and functions 440, *443*
lymphatic system disorders 458
  cancer spread in lymphatic system *277, 279*

enlarged adenoids in children 842–843
lymphangitis 458–459
lymphoedema 459
pharyngitis and tonsillitis 479, 843
see also lymph node disorders
lymphatic tissue, structure *443*
lymph ducts, location and functions *443*
lymph node disorders
cancer *see* lymphomas
infectious mononucleosis 291–292
lymphadenopathy 458
sarcoidosis 498–499
lymph nodes
disorders *see* lymph node disorders
penetration by cancerous cells *277, 279*
removal in breast cancer surgery 760, *761*
structure and functions *443*, 458
swollen *see* lymphadenopathy
lymphocytes
CD4 lymphocytes, effect of HIV infection and AIDS 297, 887
disorders *see* acute lymphoblastic leukaemia; chronic lymphocytic leukaemia
measurement in immune function tests 228
white blood cell types and functions *441, 443, 445*
lymphoedema 459
Lymphoma Association, The 1033
lymphomas 459
Burkitt's lymphoma, caused by Epstein–Barr virus (EBV) 279, 459
Hodgkin's lymphoma 459
non-Hodgkin's lymphomas 459
lymph vessels
disorders *see* lymphangitis; lymphoedema
penetration by cancerous cells *275, 277*
in small intestine lining *623*
structure and functions *443*
lysergic acid diethylamide (LSD), recreational drug effects and risks 65, *66*

M

Maalox 1014
Maalox Plus 1014
Macmillan Cancer Relief 1028
Macrobid 1014
Macrodantin 1014
macrolides, antibiotics 885–886
macrophages, white blood cell types and functions *440, 443*
macula (in the retina)
disorders *see* macular degeneration
eye structure and functions *568*
maculae (in the vestibule), ear structure and functions *595*
macular degeneration 580–581
Madopar 1014
magaldrate, antacids 923
magnesium 1014
drugs for labour 938
mineral supplements 929
magnesium alginate 1014
magnesium carbonate 1014
magnesium citrate 1014
magnesium hydroxide 1014
antacids 923
magnesium oxide 1014
magnesium salts 1014
laxatives 924–925
magnesium trisilicate 1014
magnetic resonance imaging (MRI) scans *213, 243*, 248–250
major calyces, kidney structure and functions *696*
major seizures, first aid *989*
major surgery, what to expect 943–946
malabsorption 656–657
malaria 85, 305–306
antimalarial drugs 888–889
Malarone 1014
malathion 1014
preparations for skin infections and infestations 892–893
male condoms
contraceptive use 69, *70*
safe sex use 68, 85, 765
male hormonal disorders
abnormal puberty in males 728–729
decreased sex drive 67, 769
delayed puberty in males 728–729
gynaecomastia 729
hypogonadism in males 729
male infertility 777
male-pattern baldness 359
precocious puberty in males 728–729
male infertility 777
treatments *see* infertility treatments
male-pattern baldness 359
male reproductive system
disorders *see* male reproductive system disorders
effects of growth and aging *22–23*
examination during physical examination 220
structure and functions 716, *717*
see also sexual intercourse
male reproductive system disorders
balanitis 722–723
cancer of the penis 723
cancer of the testis 719–720
choriocarcinoma, cancer of the testis 719
embryonal carcinoma, cancer of the testis 719
epididymal cysts 718
epididymo-orchitis 718–719
hydrocele 721
nongonococcal urethritis (NGU) 765
painful intercourse in men 772
Peyronie's disease 723
phimosis 721–722
priapism 723
problems with the penis, symptoms chart 182–183
seminoma, cancer of the testis 719–720
teratoma, cancer of the testis 719
testes and scrotum problems, symptoms chart 181
torsion of the testis 719
undescended testis in babies and children 870
varicocele 720–721
see also male hormonal disorders; prostate disorders; sexually transmitted infections (STIs)
males
circumcision *722*
fertility 716
male/female differences in lower urinary tract *694, 695*
men's health, useful online sites and addresses 1034
puberty *716, 815*
reproductive system *see* male reproductive system
sex hormones *see* male sex hormones
sexual problems *see* male sexual problems
sterilization surgery *see* vasectomy
testes self-examination *720*
male sex hormones
cause of polycystic ovary syndrome 744
cause of virilization in females 740
disorders *see* male hormonal problems and disorders
overproduction causing congenital adrenal hyperplasia 866
production in adrenal glands *673*
production and role in male reproductive system *671, 672*, 716
role in puberty *see* puberty
sex hormones and related drugs 933–934
underproduction caused by Klinefelter's syndrome 822–823
male sexual problems
decreased sex drive 67, 769
failure of orgasm 770
impotence 770–771
impotence, symptoms chart 180
painful intercourse in men 772
premature ejaculation 771–772
male urethra
in hypospadias 870
male reproductive system structure and functions 716, *717, 763*
urinary system structure and functions 694, *695*
malignant melanoma 343, 346, *346*
malignant tumours *see* cancerous tumours
malleus, ear structure and functions *593, 594*
malocclusion 613–614
Maloprim 1014
mammary artery bypass graft *411*
mammography *44, 759*
mandible (lower jaw), location and movement range *363, 607*
Manerix 1014
Manevac 1014
mania *see* bipolar affective disorder
manic depression *see* bipolar affective disorder
Manic Depression Fellowship 1034
manipulative therapies *955*, 973–974
mannitol 1014
diuretic drugs 902
drugs for glaucoma 920–921
manual dexterity, developmental milestones during childhood *814*
MAOIs *see* monoamine oxidase inhibitors (MAOIs)
maprotiline 1014
antidepressant drugs 916–917
Marburg fever, viral haemorrhagic fever 295
Marcain 1014
Marevan 1014
Marfan's syndrome *273*, 824
Marie Curie Cancer Care 1028
Marie Stopes International 1031
marijuana, recreational drugs effects and risks 65, *66*
marker tests
linkage analysis using DNA markers, indirect test for abnormal genes 241
tumour marker tests 233
Marvelon 1014
massage
for relaxation in pregnancy *34*
role in physiotherapy 961
role in symptoms relief for the terminally ill *966*
mast cells, destruction in allergic reactions *445*, 466
mast cell stabilizers, antiallergy drugs 905
mastectomy 760, *761*
master gland *see* pituitary gland
mastitis 809
maternal arteries and veins, nourishing the fetus in pregnancy *781*
Maxalt 1014
Maxepa 1014
Maxidex 1014
maxilla (upper jaw) *607*
maxillary sinus *470*
Maxitrol 1014
Maxivent 1014
Maxolon 1014
Maxtrex 1014
McCormick speech discrimination test, hearing test in children *859*
MCR-50 1014
ME *see* myalgic encephalomyelitis (ME)
measles 293
German measles *see* rubella
measles/mumps/rubella (MMR) vaccine
routine immunizations *45*
vaccines and immunoglobulins 883–884
mebendazole 1014
anthelmintic drugs 889
mebeverine 1014
antispasmodic drugs and motility stimulants 926

mechanical obstruction, intestinal obstruction 663
meclozine 1014
antiemetic drugs 922
mecysteine 1014
median nerves
compressed *see* carpal tunnel syndrome
nervous system structure *509, 547*
Medic Alert Foundation 1026
Medical Advisory Service for Travellers Abroad 1033, 1037
medical checkups *see* health checkups
medical family trees 24–26
medical history 212, 216, 218
family medical history and medical family trees 24–26
sexual history 68
medical laboratories *225*
medical wards
hospital care 957–959
postoperative care and monitoring 945
medications *see* drugs
Medicines Control Agency 1026, 1030
Medijel 1014
Medinex 1014
Medinol 1014
Medised 1014
Medrone 1014
medroxyprogesterone 1014
anticancer drugs 907–908
hormone replacement therapy (HRT) 937–938
sex hormones and related drugs 933–934
medulla
adrenal gland structure *673*
brain structure *510*
hair structure *329*
kidney structure and functions *695, 696*
medullary thyroid cancer 681–682
mefenamic acid 1014
nonsteroidal anti-inflammatory drugs (NSAIDs) 894
painkillers 912–913
mefloquine 1014
antimalarial drugs 888–889
Mefoxin 1014
mefruside 1014
Megace 1014
megaloblastic anaemia 448
megestrol 1014
meiosis, cell division *266–267*, 270
Meissner's ending (corpuscle), sensory receptors in skin *329, 513*
melanin
inadequate production *see* albinism
loss from skin *see* vitiligo
overproduction *see* freckles
in skin *331*
see also melanocytes
melanocytes
damaged, in malignant melanoma 346
overproduction, causing moles 343
see also melanin
melanoma, malignant *see* malignant melanoma
melatonin 1014
production and functions *671*
Melleril 1014
meloxicam 1014
melphalan 1014
anticancer drugs 907–908
membrane rupture in pregnancy and labour
induction of labour *797*
premature rupture of membranes 797
membranes
amniotic *see* amniotic sac
basilar membrane, in the ear *594*
brain and spinal cord protective membranes *see* meninges
cell *see* cell membranes
chorion, role in fetal nourishment during pregnancy *781*
conjunctiva, in the eye *567*
in the ear *593, 594, 595*
eardrum *592, 593, 594*
in the eye *567*
gelatinous membrane of the macula, in the inner ear *595*
mesentery, in digestive system *621, 623*
mucous *see* mucous membranes (mucosa)
omentum, in digestive system *621*
oval window, in the ear *593, 594*
pericardium, in the heart *398*
periosteum, in bones *363*
peritoneal *see* peritoneum
plasma membrane, in bacteria *286*
pleural *see* pleura
round window, in the ear *593, 594*
serosa, in intestines *623*
submucosa, in intestines *623*
synovial, in joints *364*
tectorial membrane, in the ear *594*
vestibular membrane, in the ear *594*
memory B-cells, role in antibody immune response *445*
memory T-cells, role in cellular immune response *445*
men *see* males; *see also* index entries beginning with the word "male"
MEN *see* multiple endocrine neoplasia (MEN)
menadiol 1014
MENCAP Royal Society for Mentally Handicapped Children and Adults 1030, 1034
Ménière's disease 604–605
meninges
arachnoid *509*
bleeding between *see* subarachnoid haemorrhage; subdural haemorrhage
dura mater *509*
inflamed *see* meningitis
nervous system structure *509, 510, 511*
pia mater *509*
meningitis 527–528
bacterial meningitis 527–528
bacterial meningitis in children 848–849
meningitis in children 848–849
meningococcal meningitis 527–528
meningococcal meningitis in children 848–849
routine immunizations *45*
travel immunizations *86*
viral meningitis 527–528
viral meningitis in children 848–849
meningococcus C
vaccines and immunoglobulins 883–884
menisci, damaged *see* torn knee cartilage
menopausal problems *733*, 737–738
postmenopausal bleeding 738–739
see also osteoporosis
menopause
changes in female reproductive system 730, *733*
health at the menopause 36
hormone replacement therapy (HRT) 36, 937–938
possibility of pregnancy during the menopause 186
problems *see* menopausal problems
Menorest 1014
menorrhagia 735
menotrophin 1014
drugs for infertility 936–937
Men's Health Line 1034
men's health, useful online sites and addresses 1034
menstrual cycle *see* menstruation and menstrual cycle
menstrual problems 734
absent periods, symptoms chart 186–187
amenorrhoea 735
dysmenorrhoea 736
heavy periods, symptoms chart 189
irregular periods 734
menorrhagia 735
painful periods, symptoms chart 188
period pain *see* dysmenorrhoea
premenstrual syndrome (PMS) 736–737
primary amenorrhoea 735
primary dysmenorrhoea 736
secondary amenorrhoea 735
secondary dysmenorrhoea 736
symptoms charts 186–189
menstruation and menstrual cycle
disorders *see* menstrual problems
effect of hormonal and mechanical contraceptive methods 69–70
female reproductive system structure and functions 730, *731–733*
mental health disorders 551
agoraphobia 552–553
alcohol dependence 564–565
anorexia nervosa 562–563
anxiety disorders 551–552
anxiety, symptoms chart 124
attempted suicide and suicide 122, 556–557
bipolar affective disorder 557, 917–918
bulimia 563
claustrophobia 552
complex phobias 552–553
compulsive gambling 565
delusional disorders 561
depression 554–556
depression after childbirth 807–808
drug dependence 66, 564, 880–881
drugs for mental health disorders 915–918
factitious disorder, Munchausen's syndrome 558
feeling depressed, symptoms chart 122–123
hypnotherapy 974–975
hypochondriasis 559
insomnia 554, 915–916
mental problems due to physical illness 558
Munchausen's syndrome 558–559
obsessive–compulsive disorder 553–554
panic attacks, anxiety disorder 551–552
persistent anxiety state 551–552
personality disorders 561–562
phobias 552–553
postpartum psychosis, depression after childbirth 807–808
post-traumatic stress disorder (PTSD) 553
psychological assessment *554*
schizophrenia 560, 917–918
simple phobias 552–553
social phobias 552–553
somatization 559
useful online sites and addresses 1034–1035
see also occupational therapy; psychological therapies
Mental Health Foundation 1034
menthol 1014
mepacrine hydrochloride 1014
meperidine 1014
painkillers 912–913
mepivacaine 1014
mepracrine hydrochloride
antiprotozoal drugs 888
meprobamate 1014
meptazinol 1014
mepyramine
antipruritic drugs 891–892
mequitazine 1014
Merbentyl 1014
mercaptopurine 1014
anticancer drugs 907–908
Mercilon 1015
Merkel's discs, sensory receptors in skin *513*
Merocaine 1015
Merocet 1015
mesalazine 1015
aminosalicylate drugs 924
mesentery, digestive system structure and functions *621, 623*
meshed graft *318*
mesna 1015
mesosomes, bacteria structure *286*
mesothelioma, asbestos-related disease 501–502

messenger RNA (mRNA), functions *266*
mesterolone 1015
sex hormones and related drugs 933–934
Mestinon 1015
mestranol 1015
hormone replacement therapy (HRT) 937–938
sex hormones and related drugs 933–934
metabolic disorders 687
amyloidosis 693
haemochromatosis 692–693
heel prick blood test, screening for metabolic disorders in newborn babies *44, 867*
hypercholesterolaemia 691–692
hypoglycaemia 691, 931
inherited hyperlipidaemias 692, 935
porphyria 693
useful online sites and addresses 1033
see also diabetes mellitus; enzyme deficiencies; inborn errors of metabolism
metabolism 670, *674–675*
basal metabolic rate (BMR) 52, 54, *674*
disorders *see* metabolic disorders
drug metabolism *879*
metaraminol 1015
metastases (secondary tumours) *277, 279*
bone metastases *279*, 373
liver metastases 649–650
lung metastases 505
metastasis (spread), cancer *275, 277, 279*
metastatic bone cancer *see* bone metastases
metastatic liver cancer *see* liver metastases
Metenix-5 1015
metered-dose inhalers, use in asthma treatment *485, 881*, 910
metformin 1015
drugs for diabetes mellitus 931–932
methadone 1015
painkillers 912–913
Methadose 1015
methenamine 1015
Methex 1015
methionine 1015
methocarbamol 1015
methotrexate 1015
anticancer drugs 907–908
antirheumatic drugs 895–896
immunosuppressants 906–907
methotrimeprazine *see* levomepromazine 1013
methoxamine 1015
methoxsalen 1015
methylcellulose 1015
antidiarrhoeal drugs 924
laxatives 924–925
methyldopa 1015
antihypertensive drugs 897–898
methylphenidate 1015
central nervous system (CNS) stimulant drugs 918
methylphenobarbital 1015
methylprednisolone 1015
corticosteroids 930–931
locally acting corticosteroids 895
methyl salicylate 1015
methysergide 1015
antimigraine drugs 913
metipranolol 1015
drugs for glaucoma 920–921
metirosine 1015
metoclopramide 1015
antiemetic drugs 922
antispasmodic drugs and motility stimulants 926
metolazone 1015
diuretic drugs 902
Metopirone 1015
metoprolol 1015
beta-blocker drugs 898–899
Metosyn 1015
Metrodin 1015
Metrogel 1015
metronidazole 1015
antibiotics 885–886
antiprotozoal drugs 888
metyrapone 1015
mexiletine 1015
antiarrhythmic drugs 898
mianserin 1015
miconazole 1015
antifungal drugs 889
preparations for skin infections and infestations 892–893
microdiscectomy *385*
Microgynon 30 1015
Micronor 1015
microorganisms
body's defences against *444–445*
comparative sizes *284*
tests for microorganisms 234–235
microscopy
cell tests 236–237
for infectious agents 234
tissue tests 236, 237
microsurgery 940, 950–951
Microval 1015
microvilli, in the small intestine *623*
Mictral 1015
midazolam 1015
midbrain, brain structure *510*
middle-ear disorders
acute otitis media in children 860
barotrauma 598
chronic secretory otitis media in children 860–861
otitis media 597
otosclerosis 598
ruptured eardrum 597–598
middle ear, ear structure and functions *592, 593, 594*
Midrid 1015
mifepristone 1015
migraine 518–519
antimigraine drugs 913
migraine in children 847–848
Migraine Action Association 1032
Migraine Trust 1032
Migraleve 1015
Migranal 1015
migration and spread, cancerous cells *275, 277, 279*
Migravess 1015
Migril 1015
mild cervical dysplasia 749, *750, 751*
mild gingivitis 617–618
milk and dairy products
intolerance, allergies, and metabolic disorders *see* cows' milk protein allergy; galactosaemia; lactose intolerance
milk ducts, in breasts *733*
blocked *see* mastitis
Milk of Magnesia 1015
milk-producing glands in breasts *see* lobules (milk-producing glands) in breasts
milk production in breasts *see* breast milk production
milk teeth *see* primary teeth
Milpar 1015
milrinone 1015
MIND 1035
mineral deficiency disorders
glossitis 633
hypothyroidism caused by iodine deficiency 680
iron-deficiency anaemia 447
stomatitis 632–633
minerals 51
absorption by the body *625*
in bones 362
deficiency disorders *see* mineral deficiency disorders
mineral supplements 929
nutritional information on food labels *52*
requirements during pregnancy 33
routine blood chemistry tests for minerals 230
sources and effects *51*
Minihep 1015
minimally invasive and endoscopic surgery 940, 948–950
Minims Atropine 1015
Minims Chloramphenicol 1015
Minims Cyclopentolate 1015
Minims Gentamicin 1015
Minims Phenylephrine 1015
Minims Pilocarpine 1015
Minims Prednisolone 1015
Minitran 1015
minocycline 1015
antibiotics 885–886
minor calyces, kidney structure and functions *696*
minor leg and foot problems in children 834–835
minor surgery, what to expect 942–943
minor tranquillizers *see* antianxiety drugs
minoxidil 1015
antihypertensive drugs 897–898
Mintec 1015
Mintezol 1015
Minulet 1015
miotics, drugs for glaucoma 920–921
Mirapexin 1015
Mirena 1015
mirror laryngoscopy *481*
mirtazapine 1015
miscarriage 791–792
Miscarriage Association 1036
misoprostol 1015
ulcer-healing drugs 923–924
missed miscarriage 792
missing teeth 615–616
Mistamine 1015
mites
mite infestation *see* scabies
scrub typhus transmission 304
mitobronitol 1015
mitochondria
in body cells *259, 265, 675*
DNA content *265*
fungi structure *287*
in heart muscle cells 396, *398*
protozoa structure *287*
mitochondrial DNA *265*
mitomycin 1015
mitosis, cell division *266–267*
mitoxantrone 1015
mitozantrone *see* mitoxantrone 1015
mitral incompetence 423–424
mitral stenosis 424
mitral valve
disorders *see* mitral incompetence; mitral stenosis; mitral valve prolapse
floppy *see* mitral valve prolapse
heart structure *398*
mitral valve prolapse 425–426
mivacurium 1015
Mixtard 1015
mizolastine 1015
MMR vaccine *see* measles/mumps/rubella (MMR) vaccine
Mobic 1015
Mobiflex 1015
mobility, improving *see* exercise; occupational therapy; physical therapy
moclobemide 1015
modafinil 1015
Modalim 1015
Modaplate 1015
moderate cervical dysplasia 749, *751*
Modrasone 1015
Modrenal 1015
Moducren 1015
Moduret-25 1015
Moduretic 1015
moexipril 1015
angiotensin-converting enzyme (ACE) inhibitor drugs 900–901
Mogadon 1015
molar pregnancy 790
molars, tooth structure *606, 607*
moles 343, 828
molgramostim 1015
Molipaxin 1015
molluscum contagiosum 355
molybdenum 1015
mometasone 1015
Mongolian blue spots, birthmarks 828
Monit 1015
monitoring, postoperative 945
monoamine oxidase inhibitors (MAOIs), antidepressant drugs 916–917
Mono-Cedocard 1016
Monoclate-P 1016

Monocor 1016
monocytes, white blood cell type *441*
Monoparin 1016
monosulfiram 1016
Monotrim 1016
monounsaturated fats *50*, 51
Monovent 1016
Monozide 1016
Monphytol 1016
montelukast 1016
mood-stabilizing drugs 918
moracizine 1016
  antiarrhythmic drugs 898
morning sickness, common complaint of normal pregnancy 784
morphine 1016
  painkillers 912–913
morula, cell cluster in early pregnancy *778*
mosaicism, chromosome disorder 271
mosaic warts 354
mosquitoes, diseases transmitted by
  dengue fever 296
  malaria 305–306
  precautions against, when travelling 85
  yellow fever *86*, 296
Motens 1016
Motifene 1016
motility stimulant drugs, antispasmodic drugs and motility stimulants 926
Motilium 1016
motion sickness 85, 604
Motipress 1016
Motival 1016
motor cortex, location and role in information processing in the brain *515*
motor map of brain *515*
motor nerve neuropathies 544
motor nerves
  disorders *see* motor nerve neuropathies; motor neuron disease
  motor nerve roots in spinal cord *511*
  role of motor nerve impulses in voluntary and involuntary responses *514*
motor neuron disease 540–541
Motor Neurone Disease Association 1035
Motrin 1016
mouth
  digestive system structure and functions 620, *621–622*, *625*
  disorders *see* mouth and tongue disorders
  inspection during physical examination *219*
  mouth care for the terminally ill *966*
  role in body's defences *444*
mouth cancer 634–635
mouth-to-mouth and mouth-to-nose artificial respiration, first aid *982*
mouth and tongue disorders 632
  bacterial stomatitis 633
  candidiasis 309
  cleft lip and palate 862
  dry mouth and tongue in the terminally ill *966*
  glossitis 633
  hairy leukoplakia 634
  mouth cancer 634–635
  mouth ulcers 632
  mouth ulcers in Behçet's syndrome 465
  oral leukoplakia 634
  oral lichen planus 634
  oral thrush in babies and children 862–863
  stomatitis 632–633
  trench mouth *see* acute necrotizing ulcerative gingivitis (ANUG)
  viral stomatitis 633
  see also gum disorders; salivary gland disorders; tooth disorders
mouth ulcers 632
Movelat 1016
movements
  detection by the inner ear 592, *593*, *595*
  fetal movements during pregnancy *780*
  involuntary *see* involuntary movements
  voluntary *see* voluntary movements and responses
Movicol 1016
moxisylyte 1016
moxonidine 1016
  antihypertensive drugs 897–898
MRI scans *see* magnetic resonance imaging (MRI) scans
mRNA *see* messenger RNA (mRNA)
MS *see* multiple sclerosis (MS)
MST Continus 1016
Mucaine 1016
Mucodyne 1016
Mucogel 1016
mucolytic drugs, cough remedies 909–910
mucous membranes (mucosa)
  damage caused by high-risk sexual activities 68
  digestive system structure and functions *622*, *623*
  structure and role in body's defences *259*, *329*, *444*
Mu-Cron Tablets 1016
mucus
  cervical *see* cervical mucus
  chest physiotherapy to prevent mucus from accumulating 962
  overproduction in smokers 64
  production in mucous membranes (mucosa) *259*, *329*, *444*
  production and role in digestive tract mucosa *622*, *623*, *625*
  production and role in the sinuses *470*
  role in body's defences *444*
  role in respiratory system 470, *471*
multifactorial gene disorders 273
multi-infarct dementia 537–538
Multiparin 1016
multiple endocrine neoplasia (MEN) 683
multiple myeloma 456–457
multiple pregnancy *779*, 792–793
multiple sclerosis (MS) 541–542
  chronic–progressive multiple sclerosis 541–542
  relapsing–remitting multiple sclerosis 541–542
Multiple Sclerosis Society 1035
mumps 293–294
  immunization *see* measles/mumps/rubella (MMR)
Munchausen's syndrome 558–559
mupirocin 1016
  preparations for skin infections and infestations 892–893
murine typhus *see* endemic typhus
muscle contractions *362*, *366–367*
  in digestive tract *see* peristalsis and peristaltic wave
  effect of muscle relaxants 896
  involuntary *see* involuntary movements
  role in venous return *400*
muscle cramp 388
muscle and nerve electrical tests *544*
muscle relaxants 896
muscles
  arrector pili, in skin *329*, *331*
  in the bladder *695*, *697*
  cardiac muscle *see* heart muscle
  contractions *see* muscle contractions
  disorders *see* heart muscle disorders; muscle and tendon disorders; musculoskeletal injuries
  effects of growth and aging *22–23*
  exercise for muscle strength *56*, 57
  in the eye *568*
  glycogen storage in muscles *670*, *675*
  heart *see* heart muscle
  location of major muscles in the body *366–367*
  muscle fibres *366*, *367*, *513*
  muscle layer in the digestive tract *622–623*
  muscle proprioceptors, role in sense of balance *513*
  muscle relaxation exercises *75*
  nerve–muscle junctions *514*
  role in movement *362*
  skeletal muscles 362, *366–367*
  smooth muscle 362, *367*
  structure and functions 362, *366–367*
  see also individual muscles by name, e.g. diaphragm
muscle and tendon disorders 388
  Becker muscular dystrophy 826
  Duchenne muscular dystrophy 826
  Dupuytren's contracture 390
  electromyography (EMG) *544*
  fibromyalgia 389
  ganglion 390
  Guillain–Barré syndrome 550
  muscle cramp 388
  muscle relaxant drugs 896
  muscle strains and tears 395
  muscular dystrophy *273*, 826
  myasthenia gravis 549
  nervous tics 550
  in the oesophagus *see* achalasia
  Osgood–Schlatter disease in children 834
  polymyalgia rheumatica 464
  polymyositis and dermatomyositis 463–464
  ptosis 584
  repetitive strain injury (RSI) 82, 389
  routine blood chemistry tests for muscle damage 230
  ruptured tendons 395
  sports injuries 391–392
  sprains and strains, first aid *991*
  tennis elbow and golfer's elbow 389–390
  tenosynovitis and tendinitis 390
  torticollis 388
  see also heart muscle disorders; musculoskeletal injuries; physiotherapy
muscle tension or tone 362
muscular dystrophy *273*, 826
Muscular Dystrophy Campaign 1035
musculoskeletal disorders in children 832
  achondroplasia *273*, 833
  bow legs, minor leg and foot problems in children 834
  clubfoot 833
  congenital hip dysplasia 832
  flat feet, minor leg and foot problems in children 834
  juvenile chronic arthritis (JCA) 835
  knock-knees, minor leg and foot problems in children 834
  minor leg and foot problems 834–835
  noncancerous bone tumours 372–373
  Osgood–Schlatter disease 834
  pauciarticular arthritis 835
  Perthes' disease 833–834
  polyarticular arthritis 835
  positional clubfoot 833
  rickets 370
  slipped femoral epiphysis 834
  structural clubfoot 833
  systemic arthritis 835
  see also physiotherapy
musculoskeletal disorders, useful online sites and addresses 1035
musculoskeletal injuries 391
  dislocated joints 394
  fractures 392–394
  ligament injuries 394
  muscle strains and tears 395
  ruptured tendons 395
  sprains and strains, first aid *991*
  torn knee cartilage 395
  see also physiotherapy
musculoskeletal system
  disorders *see* bone disorders; joint and ligament disorders; muscle and tendon disorders; musculoskeletal injuries
  disorders in children *see* musculoskeletal disorders in children

drugs affecting 894–898
effects of growth and aging *22–23*
role of exercise in musculoskeletal health 55–57
structure and functions 362, *363–367*
surgery *see* musculoskeletal system surgery
musculoskeletal system surgery
arthroscopy *386*
bunion surgery *387*
external fixation of fractures *393*
fracture treatments *393*
hip replacement *377*
internal fixation of fractures *393*
joint replacement *377*
knee arthroscopy *386*
knee joint replacement *377*
microdiscectomy *385*
shoulder joint replacement *377*
mustine *see* chlormethine 1004
mutations in DNA *269*
MXL 1016
myalgic encephalomyelitis (ME) *see* chronic fatigue syndrome
myasthenia gravis 549
Myasthenia Gravis Association 1035
Mycil Gold 1016
Mycobutin 1016
mycophenolate mofetil 1016
Mycota 1016
mydriatics, drugs acting on the eye 919–920
Mydrilate 1016
myelin sheaths
development in nerves of babies and children *813*
disorders *see* multiple sclerosis (MS)
nerve cell structure *509, 512*
myelomeningocele, neural tube defect *845*
myocardial cells, in the heart 396
myocardial infarction 410–412
antiplatelet drugs, drugs that prevent blood clotting 904
thrombolytic drugs 904–905
myocarditis 426–427
myocardium
disorders *see* myocardial infarction; myocarditis
heart structure 396, *398*
Myocrisin 1016
myofibrils, muscle structure *366*
myofilaments, muscle structure *366*
myopia 586
glasses and contact lenses for myopia correction *588*
Mysoline 1016

N

nabilone 1016
nabumetone 1016
nonsteroidal anti-inflammatory drugs (NSAIDs) 894
nadolol 1016
beta-blocker drugs 898–899
naevi
blue naevi, type of mole 343
dysplastic naevi, type of mole 343
halo naevi, type of mole 343
pigmented naevi, birthmarks 828
spider naevi, symptom of liver failure *650*
strawberry naevi, birthmarks 828
nafarelin 1016
drugs for infertility 936–937
sex hormones and related drugs 933–934
naftidrofuryl 1016
nail abnormalities 360–361
nail bed, nail structure *328*
nail disorders
ingrown toenails 361
nail abnormalities 360–361
nail separation 360
paronychia 361
nail matrix, nail structure *328*
nails
inspection during physical examination *219*
structure *328, 331*
nail separation 360
nalbuphine 1016
Nalcrom 1016
nalidixic acid 1016
Nalorex 1016
naloxone 1016
naltrexone 1016
nappy rash 829
managing nappy rash *829*
Napratec 1016
Naprosyn 1016
naproxen 1016
nonsteroidal anti-inflammatory drugs (NSAIDs) 894
painkillers 912–913
Naramig 1016
naratriptan 1016
narcissistic personality disorder 561
narcolepsy 526–527
central nervous system (CNS) stimulant drugs 918
Narcolepsy Association UK 1036
narcotic painkillers *see* opioid painkillers
Nardil 1016
Narphen 1016
narrow-angle glaucoma *see* acute glaucoma
narrow-spectrum antibiotics 885–886
nasal cavity
connecting passageways to ears and throat *592*
respiratory system structure *471*
nasal polyps 476–477
nasal route, drug delivery route *879*
nasal septum, deviated 476
nasolacrimal duct, in tear apparatus *566*
Nasonex 1016
nasopharyngeal cancer *see* cancer of the nasopharynx
nasopharynx, respiratory system structure *471*
National Abortion Campaign 1032
National Adrenal Diseases Foundation 1033
National Aphasia Association 1037
National Association for Children of Alcoholics 1027
National Association of Citizens Advice Bureaux 1029
National Association for Colitis and Crohn's Disease 1030
National Association for Continence 1033
National Association for Patient Participation 1032
National Association for Premenstrual Syndrome 1037
National Association of Widows 1029
National Asthma Campaign 1027, 1029
National Autistic Society 1029, 1035
National Brain Tumor Foundation 1028
National Childbirth Trust 1036
National Children's Bureau 1028, 1029
National Drugs Helpline 1030
National Eczema Society 1036
National Endometriosis Society 1037
National Headache Foundation 1032
National Heart, Lung, and Blood Institute Information Center 1027, 1034
National Institutes of Health 1026
National Kidney Research Fund 1037
National Kidney and Urological Diseases Information Clearing House 1037
National Osteoporosis Society 1035
National Phobics Society 1035
National Schizophrenia Fellowship 1035
National Sleep Foundation 1037
National Society for Epilepsy 1031
National Society for Phenylketonuria 1033
National Stuttering Association 1037
Natrilix 1016
natriuretic hormone, production and functions *401, 671*
natural methods of contraception 70, *71*
nausea
antiemetic drugs 922
in pregnancy *see* morning sickness
symptoms relief in the terminally ill 965, *966*
navel
formation in newborn baby *811*
hernias near or behind navel *see* paraumbilical hernia; umbilical hernia
Navidrex 1016
Navispare 1016
NCH Action for Children 1028
near-vision test *587*
Nebcin 1016
Nebilet 1016
nebivolol 1016
nebulizers, use in asthma treatment *485*, 840, 910
neck
disorders *see* neck disorders
neck stretch, warming up and cooling down in your exercise routine *60*
pivot joint in *365*
neck disorders
cervical spondylosis 376
neck pain or stiffness, symptoms chart 172–173
neck sprain or neck strain *see* whiplash
torticollis 388
neck pulse (carotid pulse)
checking pulse recovery time after exercise *59*
first aid circulation check *978*
nedocromil sodium 1016
antiallergy drugs 905
drugs acting on the eye 919–920
needle aspiration of the thyroid gland *682*
needlestick injury 356
nefazodone 1016
antidepressant drugs 916–917
nefopam 1016
Negram 1016
nelfinavir 1016
drugs for HIV infection and AIDS 887–888
Neo-Bendromax 1016
Neogest 1016
Neo-Mercazole 1016
neomycin 1016
antibiotics 885–886
drugs acting on the ear 921
drugs acting on the eye 919–920
preparations for skin infections and infestations 892–893
Neo-NaClex 1016
Neo-NaClex-K 1016
neonatal jaundice 817–818
Neoral 1016
NeoRecormon 1016
Neosporin 1016
neostigmine 1016
Neotigason 1016
Nephril 1016
nephritis *see* glomerulonephritis; pyelonephritis
nephroblastoma *see* Wilms' tumour
nephrogenic diabetes insipidus 678
nephrons, kidney structure and functions 694, *696–697*
nephrotic syndrome 700–701
Nericur 1016
Nerisone 1016
nerve cells
neuroglia *512*
neurons structure and functions 508, *510, 512*
structure and functions *512*
target cells *512*
nerve conduction studies *544*
nerve endings or nerve receptors *see* sensory receptors
nerve fascicles, nervous system structure *509*
nerve fibres
in cancerous tumours *275*
in corpus callosum *510*
development in babies and children *813*
in spinal cord *511*
structure and functions 508, *509, 512*
nerve and muscle electrical tests *544*
nerve roots, spinal nerves structure and functions *511*

nerves
- autonomic nerves *514*
- cranial *see* cranial nerves
- development in babies and children *813*
- disorders *see* nervous system disorders
- effects of growth and aging *22–23*
- motor *see* motor nerves
- nerve–muscle junctions *514*
- parasympathetic nerves *514*
- peripheral *see* peripheral nerves
- spinal *see* spinal nerves
- structure and functions 508, *509*, *511–514*
- sympathetic nerves *514*
- in teeth and gums 606, *607*

nervous system
- development in babies and children *813*
- disorders *see* nervous system disorders
- drugs acting on the brain and nervous system 912–918
- effects of growth and aging *22–23*
- examination during physical examination 220
- role in blood pressure control 396, *401*, *514*
- role in digestive system regulation and control 620, *622*
- role in urination control *697*
- structure and functions 508, *509–515*

nervous system disorders 516
- in children *see* nervous system disorders in children
- chronic fatigue syndrome 520
- Hansen's disease 302
- optic neuritis 581
- poliomyelitis *45*, 295, 883–884
- rabies *86*, 296, 883
- tests and investigations *see* nervous system tests and investigation
- useful online sites and addresses 1035
- *see also* brain and spinal cord disorders; headaches; pain; peripheral nervous system disorders

nervous system disorders in children 844
- brain and spinal cord tumours in children 850
- cerebral palsy 846–847
- epilepsy 524–526
- febrile convulsions 849, *989*
- headache in children 847
- hydrocephalus 845–846
- meningitis in children 848–849
- migraine in children 847–848
- myelomeningocele, neural tube defect *845*
- nervous tics 550
- neural tube defects 844–845
- neuroblastoma 278, 850
- Reye's syndrome 849
- spina bifida, neural tube defect 844–845
- Tourette's syndrome, nervous tics in 550

nervous system tests and investigations
- carotid Doppler scanning *531*
- cerebral angiography *533*
- electroencephalography (EEG) *525*
- electromyography (EMG) *544*
- lumbar puncture *527*
- nerve conduction studies *544*
- nerve and muscle electrical tests *544*
- visual evoked response test *542*

nervous tics 550

Netillin 1016

netilmicin 1016

Neupogen 1016

neural networks and pathways, development in babies and children *813*

neural tube defects 844–845

neuritis, optic neuritis 581

neuroblastoma 278, 850

neurofibromatosis *273*, 827

Neurofibromatosis Association 1035

neuroglia, type of nerve cell *512*

neurons
- in the brain and spinal cord *510*, *512*
- nerve cells structure and functions 508, *512*
- in newborn baby's brain *813*

Neurontin 1016

neuropathies
- autonomic nerve neuropathies 544
- diabetic neuropathy 545
- motor nerve neuropathies 544
- nutritional neuropathies 545–546
- peripheral neuropathies 543–545
- sensory nerve neuropathies 543–544

neurotransmitters *512*
- *see also* dopamine

Neutrexin 1016

neutrophils, white blood cell type *441*

nevirapine 1016
- drugs for HIV infection and AIDS 887–888

newborn babies
- congenital infections 817
- heel prick blood test, screening for metabolic disorders in newborn babies *44*, *867*
- neonatal jaundice 817–818
- physical appearance, growth and development 810, *811–813*
- special care baby units *959*
- vitamin K injections 903, 928
- *see also* babies and infants; premature babies

NGU *see* nongonococcal urethritis (NGU) 765

NHS Direct Online 1026, 1032

niacin 1016
- vitamin sources in diet and effects on health *51*
- vitamin supplements 927–928

niacinamide 1016

nicardipine 1016
- calcium channel blocker drugs 900

niclosamide 1016

nicorandil 1016

Nicorette 1016

nicotinamide 1016

nicotine 1016

Nicotinell 1016

nicotinic acid 1016
- lipid-lowering drugs 935

nicotinyl alcohol 1016

nicoumalone *see* acenocoumarol 1000

nifedipine 1016

Niferex 1016

nightmares and night terrors, sleeping problems in children 851

Night Nurse 1016

night vision, role of rods in the retina *569*

nimodipine 1016

Nindaxa 1016

Nipent 1016

nipple discharge 758
- during pregnancy *780*
- galactorrhoea 758

nipple disorders
- abnormal nipples 757–758
- cracked nipples 808, *809*
- discharge *see* nipple discharge
- nipple inversion, abnormal nipples 757–758

nipples
- breast structure and functions *733*
- disorders *see* nipple disorders
- during pregnancy *780*
- positioning baby on the nipple for breast-feeding *809*

nisoldipine 1016

nit combs, use in treating head lice *831*

nitrate drugs 899–900

nitrazepam 1016
- sleeping drugs 915–916

Nitro-Dur 1016

nitrofurantoin 1016

Nitrolingual 1017

nitroprusside 1017

nitrous oxide 1017
- general anaesthetics 914

nits *see* lice

Nivaquine 1017

Nivemycin 1017

nizatidine 1017
- ulcer-healing drugs 923–924

Nizoral 1017

nodes
- lymph *see* lymph nodes of Ranvier, nerve cells structure and functions *512*, *813*

nodules
- in erythema nodosum 348
- thyroid nodules 681
- vocal cord nodules 480

noise-induced hearing loss 601–602

Nolvadex 1017

Nolvadex Forte 1017

noncancerous tumours
- acoustic neuroma 605
- adrenal tumours 684
- bladder tumours 715
- brain tumours 530
- fibroadenoma 754–755
- fibroids 745–746
- lipomas *275*
- molar pregnancy 790
- multiple endocrine neoplasia (MEN) 683
- neurofibromatosis 827
- noncancerous bone tumours 372–373
- parathyroid tumours, cause of hyperparathyroidism 682–683
- phaeochromocytoma 686
- pituitary tumours 676
- prolactinoma 677
- salivary gland tumours 635–636
- structure *275*
- thyroid nodules 681
- vocal cord nodules 480

nongonococcal urethritis (NGU) 765

non-Hodgkin's lymphomas 459

nonidentical twins, multiple pregnancy *779*, 792

non-insulin-dependent diabetes mellitus *see* type 2 diabetes

non-narcotic painkillers *see* nonopioid painkillers

nonopioid painkillers 912–913

nonoxinol '9' 1017

nonsteroidal anti-inflammatory drugs (NSAIDs) 894, *895*

nontocog alfa 1017

nonulcer dyspepsia 626–627

Nootropil 1017

noradrenaline *see* norepinephrine

Norditropin 1017

norepinephrine 1017
- overproduction due to phaeochromocytoma 686
- production blocked by beta-blocker drugs 899
- production and functions *673*

norethisterone 1017
- hormone replacement therapy (HRT) 937–938

norfloxacin 1017

Norgalax 1017

norgestimate 1017

Norgeston 1017

norgestrel 1017
- hormone replacement therapy (HRT) 937–938
- sex hormones and related drugs 933–934

Noriday 1017

Norimin 1017

Norimode 1017

Norinyl 1017

Noristerat 1017

Normacol Plus 1017

normal immunoglobulin
- vaccines and immunoglobulins 883–884

Normax 1017

Normosang 1017

Norplant 1017

Northern Ireland Chest, Heart, and Stroke Association 1032, 1037

nortriptyline 1017

Norvir 1017

Norwalk virus 628, *629*, 630

nose
- connecting passageways to ears and throat *592*
- disorders *see* nose disorders

drug delivery into the nose *879*
endoscopy of the nose and throat *476*
nasal cavity, respiratory system structure *471*
nose disorders 474
allergic rhinitis 466–467
common cold 288–289
decongestants 909
deviated nasal septum 476
nasal polyps 476–477
nosebleeds 474–475
rhinophyma, effect of rosacea 341, 342
sinusitis 475
steam inhalation *475*
useful online sites and addresses 1031
NovoNorm 1017
NSAIDs *see* nonsteroidal anti-inflammatory drugs (NSAIDs)
NSPCC 1028
Nubain 1017
nucleoids, bacteria structure *286*
nucleotide bases, in DNA 264, *265–266*, *269*
nucleus
cancerous cells *275*
cell structure *265*
fungi structure *287*
protozoa structure *287*
Nuelin 1017
Nulacin 1017
numbness and/or tingling, symptoms chart 114–115
numerical chromosome abnormalities, cause of chromosome disorders 270–271
nummular eczema 334
Nupercainal 1017
Nurofen 1017
Nurofen Plus 1017
nursing care
at home *see* home care
in hospital *see* hospital care
Nu-Seals Aspirin 1017
Nutraplus 1017
nutrients
in the diet *see* diet
fetal nutrient supply during pregnancy *779*, *781*
inadequate absorption by the intestines *see* malabsorption
nutrient acquisition by cancerous tumours *277*
nutrient acquisition by noncancerous tumours *275*
nutrient transport by the blood 620, *623–625*, *675*
see also digestion; metabolism
nutrition *see* diet; nutrients
nutritional deficiencies 630–631
see also mineral deficiency disorders; vitamin deficiency disorders
nutritional neuropathies 545–546
Nutrizym GR 1017
Nuvelle 1017
Nycopren 1017
Nylax 1017
Nystadermal 1017
Nystaform 1017
Nystaform-HC 1017
Nystamont 1017
Nystan 1017
nystatin 1017
antifungal drugs 889
preparations for skin infections and infestations 892–893
Nytol 1017

obesity 631
oblique presentation, abnormal fetal presentation 801
obsessive–compulsive disorder 553–554
obsessive–compulsive personality disorder 562
obstructions and blockages
bile duct obstructions and blockages 643, 651, 652
blockage of the urinary tract *see* hydronephrosis
functional obstruction, intestinal obstruction 663
intestinal obstruction 663
intussusception in children 864–865
mechanical obstruction, intestinal obstruction 663
wax blockage of the ear 597, 921
obstructive pulmonary disease, chronic *see* chronic obstructive pulmonary disease (COPD)
obstructive sleep apnoea (OSA) 478
occipital cortex *see* visual cortex
occipital lobe, brain structure *510*
occipitoposterior presentation, abnormal fetal presentation 800
Occlusal 1017
occupational disorders
carpal tunnel syndrome 547
hand–arm syndrome 436–437
lung diseases *see* occupational lung diseases
occupational acne 340
repetitive strain injury (RSI) 82, 389
screening in hazardous occupations 44
see also contact dermatitis; eczema; lower back pain
occupational lung diseases 83, 499
asbestosis, asbestos-related disease 501–502
asbestos-related diseases 501–502
coalworkers' pneumoconiosis 499–500
diffuse pleural thickening, asbestos-related disease 501–502
extrinsic allergic alveolitis 502–503
mesothelioma, asbestos-related disease 501–502
occupational asthma 83, 484, 499
progressive massive fibrosis (PMF), complication of coalworkers' pneumoconiosis 499–500
silicosis 500
simple pneumoconiosis 499–500
occupational therapy 954, *955*, 962–963
octocog alfa 1017
octoxinol 1017
octreotide 1017
anticancer drugs 907–908
pituitary drugs 934–935
Ocufen 1017
oculomotor nerve, nervous system structure and functions *511*
Ocusert Pilo 1017
odd or eccentric personality disorders 561
Odrik 1017
oedema
angioedema 469
lung oedema in acute heart failure *412*
lymphoedema 459
papilloedema 581–582
oesophageal disorders
achalasia 637–638
barium swallow, contrast X-ray technique 246, *637*
Barrett's oesophagus, caused by gastro-oesophageal reflux (GOR) 636
cancer of the oesophagus 638
GOR *see* gastro-oesophageal reflux (GOR)
oesophageal manometry, for achalasia 638
oesophageal stricture 636, *637*
oesophageal varices, caused by portal hypertension 648–649
upper digestive tract endoscopy *641*
oesophageal manometry, test for achalasia 638
oesophageal sphincter
disorders *see* achalasia; gastro-oesophageal reflux (GOR)
lower oesophageal sphincter, digestive tract structure and functions *622*
oesophageal stents, use in palliative surgery for cancer *282*
oesophagus
digestive system structure and functions 620, *621*, *622*
disorders *see* oesophageal disorders
Oestrifen 1017
Oestrogel 1017
oestrogen 1017
cause of gynaecomastia in males 729
conjugated *see* conjugated oestrogens
drugs for prostate disorders 938–939
in hormonal contraceptives 69, *71*
in HRT *see* hormone replacement therapy (HRT)
level changes during the menopause *733*, 737–738
level changes during puberty *815*
oestrogens and compounds with oestrogen-like effects, drugs for bone disorders 896
production controlled by pituitary hormones *672*, 730, *732–733*
production and role in female reproductive system *671*, 730, *732–733*
Office of Rare Diseases 1026, 1032, 1035
Oilatum Emollient 1017
Oilatum Gel 1017
oils (medical use)
castor oil 1004
fish oils, lipid-lowering drugs 935
see also olive oil; peppermint oil
oils in the diet *see* fats
ointments, creams, and gels
drug preparations *881*
emollients and barrier preparations 890
eye ointments *920*
how to apply *891*, *920*
olanzapine 1017
antipsychotic drugs 917–918
Olbetam 1017
old age *see* elderly people
olfactory bulb and olfactory centres, role in sense of smell *513*
olfactory nerve, nervous system structure and functions *511*
olfactory receptors, type of sensory receptor *513*
olive oil
drugs acting on the ear 921
olsalazine 1017
aminosalicylate drugs 924
omentum, digestive system structure and functions *621*
omeprazole 1017
ulcer-healing drugs 923–924
oncogenes, functions and role in cancer process *276*
Oncolink 1028
Oncovin 1017
ondansetron 1017
antiemetic drugs 922
One-Alpha 1017
onychogryphosis *see* thickening, nail abnormality
onycholysis *see* nail separation
open-angle glaucoma *see* chronic glaucoma
open fractures 392
open reduction, fracture treatment 392
open surgery 947–948
operating theatres *941*, 945
operations *see* surgery
ophthalmoscopy *578*
Opilon 1017
opioid drugs
antidiarrhoeal drugs 924
heroin, recreational drug effects and risks 65, *66*
opioid painkillers 912–913
opportunistic infections in HIV infection and AIDS 298, 308
optical fibres, use in flexible endoscopes 255
optic chiasm, location in visual pathway between eyes and brain *569*

optic disc *see* blind spot
optic nerve
disorders *see* optic neuritis; papilloedema
eye structure and functions 566, *567–569*
function measurement *see* visual evoked response test
nervous system structure and functions *509*, *511*
optic neuritis 581
Opticrom 1017
optic tracts, location in visual pathway between eyes and brain *569*
Optimine 1017
Optrex Eye Lotion 1017
Orabase 1017
Orabet 1017
oral anticoagulants, drugs that prevent blood clotting 904
oral contraceptives *see* contraceptive pill
Oraldene 1017
oral hygiene, tooth and gum care 608, *610*, 617
oral leukoplakia 634
oral lichen planus 634
oral rehydration solutions 926
oral route, drug delivery route *879*
oral thrush 862–863
Oramorph 1017
Orap 1017
Orchid Cancer Appeal 1034
orchitis *see* epididymo-orchitis
orciprenaline 1017
Orelox 1017
organ of Corti, ear structure and functions *592*, *593*, *594*
organs
effects of growth and aging 20, *22–23*
organ donation 967
organ transplants *see* transplant surgery
visualizing internal organs *see* imaging techniques; viewing techniques
organ systems in the body 258–260
see also individual body systems by name, e.g. nervous system
orgasm *762*, *763*
failure of orgasm 770
orgasm and ejaculation in males *see* ejaculation and orgasm
Orimeten 1017
Orlept 1017
orlistat 1017
oropharynx, respiratory system structure *471*
Orovite 1017
orphenadrine 1017
Ortho-Creme 1017
orthodontic treatment *614*
Orthoforms 1017
Ortho-Gynest 1017
Orudis 1017
Oruvail 1017
OSA *see* obstructive sleep apnoea (OSA)
Osgood–Schlatter disease 834
Osmolax 1017
osmotic laxatives 924–925
ossification, bone development in babies and children *812*
Ossopan 1017
osteitis deformans *see* Paget's disease of the bone
osteoarthritis 374–376
cervical spondylosis 376
osteocytes, type of bone cell *363*
osteomalacia and rickets 370
osteomyelitis 372
osteons, bone structure *362*
osteopathy *see* manipulative therapies
osteoporosis 368–369, *733*
calcium and vitamin D for osteoporosis prevention 368–369, 896, 929
drugs for bone disorders 896
useful online sites and addresses 1035
Osteoporosis and Related Bone Diseases National Resource Center 1035
otitis externa 596
otitis media 597
acute otitis media in children 860
chronic secretory otitis media in children 860–861
oto-acoustic emission test, hearing test in children *859*
Otomize 1017
otosclerosis 598
otoscopy *597*
Otosporin 1017
Otrivine 1017
Otrivine-Antistin 1017
outer-ear disorders
otitis externa 596
outer-ear injury 596
ruptured eardrum 597–598
wax blockage 597, 921
outer ear, ear structure and functions *592*, *593*
outpatient and day care treatment 956
out-toeing and in-toeing, minor leg and foot problems in children 834–835
ova *see* eggs
Ovacome 1037
oval window, ear structure and functions *593*, *594*
ovarian cancer *see* cancer of the ovary
ovarian cysts 743–744
ovaries
disorders *see* ovary disorders
during puberty *815*
female reproductive system structure and functions 730, *731–733*, 762
hormone production *671*, 730, *731–733*
surgical removal *see* hysterectomy
ovary disorders
cancer of the ovary 744–745
cystadenoma, ovarian cysts 743
dermoid cysts, ovarian cysts 743
follicular cysts, ovarian cysts 743
ovarian cysts 743–744
polycystic ovary syndrome 744
see also female hormonal problems and disorders
Overeaters Anonymous 1031
overexertion, dangers of 60
overuse injury *see* repetitive strain injury (RSI)
Ovestin 1017
Ovex 1017
Ovran 1017
Ovranette 1017
ovulation
female reproductive system structure and functions 730, *732–733*, *815*
ovulation problems, cause of female infertility 775
Ovysmen 1017
oxazepam 1017
antianxiety drugs 916
oxerutin 1017
oxetacaine 1017
oxitropium 1017
Oxivent 1017
oxpentifylline *see* pentoxifylline 1018
oxprenolol 1018
beta-blocker drugs 898–899
oxybenzone 1018
sunscreens and sunblocks 893
oxybuprocaine 1018
oxybutynin 1018
drugs that affect bladder control 939
oxycodone 1018
oxygen
blood gases measurement *501*
fetal oxygen supply in pregnancy *779*, *781*
home oxygen therapy *507*, *966*
low blood levels *see* respiratory failure
oxygen/carbon dioxide gas exchange 470, *471*, *473*
oxygenated blood
circulation through cardiovascular system 396, *398*, *400*
fetal circulation before and after birth *810*
role in gas exchange in respiratory system 470, *471*, *473*
oxygen transport by the blood
role of haemoglobin and oxyhaemoglobin *442*, 470, *473*
role of red blood cells 440, *441*, *442*
oxyhaemoglobin, role in oxygen transport by the blood *442*
oxymetazoline 1018
cold and flu remedies 910
decongestants 909
Oxymycin 1018
oxypertine 1018
oxytetracycline 1018
antibiotics 885–886
oxytocin 1018
drugs for labour 938
production and functions *672*

P

pacemakers
cardiac pacemakers and their insertion *419*
sinoatrial node in the heart 396, *399*
Pacinian corpuscles, sensory receptors in skin *331*, *513*
packaged foods, nutritional information on food labels *52*
paclitaxel 1018
anticancer drugs 907–908
pad and buzzer system, overcoming bedwetting *872*
padimate O
sunscreens and sunblocks 893
Paget's disease of the bone 370–371
drugs for bone disorders 896
Paget's disease of the breast, breast cancer *758*, 759, 760
pain 516–517
angina 407–409, 899–900
back *see* back pain
breast pain 756
coccydynia 372
cyclical breast pain 756
dysmenorrhoea 736
indigestion 626, 923
nonulcer dyspepsia 626–627
painful intercourse in men 772
painful intercourse in women 772–773
period pain (dysmenorrhoea) 736
relief *see* pain relief
sciatica 546–547
sciatica in pregnancy *785*
symptoms charts *see* pain symptoms charts
toothache 608–609
trigeminal neuralgia 546
Pain Concern 1035
painkillers 912–913
antimigraine drugs 913
cold and flu remedies 910
nonsteroidal anti-inflammatory drugs (NSAIDs) 894, *895*
pain relief for cancer *283*
pain relief for the terminally ill 965, *966*
pain relief
acupuncture *955*, 973
arthritis *375*
cancer *283*
postoperative 945–946
for the terminally ill 965, *966*
transcutaneous electrical nerve stimulation (TENS) *517*
useful online sites and addresses 1035
see also anaesthesia; painkillers; physiotherapy
Pain Relief Foundation 1035
pain symptoms charts
abdominal pain 152–155, 192–193
abdominal pain in children 208–209
back pain 170–171
chest pain 162–163
earache 138
facial pain 118

lower abdominal pain in women 192–193
neck pain or stiffness 172–173
painful arm or hand 174
painful intercourse in women 196–197
painful or irritated eye 132–133
painful joints 176–177
painful leg 175
painful periods 188
painful urination 168–169
recurrent abdominal pain 154–155
palate
cleft lip and palate 862
soft *see* soft palate
Paldesic 1018
Palfium 1018
palliative care *see* care of the dying
palliative surgery, cancer *282*
palpation, basic examination technique *220*
palpitations, symptoms chart 164
Paludrine 1018
pamidronate 1018
Panadeine 1018
Panadol 1018
Panadol Extra 1018
Panadol Ultra 1018
Panaleve 1018
pancreas
digestive enzyme production *624, 674*
disorders *see* pancreas disorders
hormone production 670, *671, 674*
pancreas or insulin-secreting cells transplant, for type 1 diabetes 689
role in digestive system 620, *621, 624*
structure and location *621, 624, 674*
pancreas disorders
acute pancreatitis 652–653
chronic pancreatitis 653–654
endoscopic retrograde cholangiopancreatography (ERCP) *653*
jaundice 643–644
pancreatic cancer 654
see also diabetes mellitus
pancreatic ducts, digestive system structure and functions *624, 674*
pancreatic hormones *see* glucagon; insulin
pancreatic juice, role in digestion *624, 625*
pancreatin 1018
Pancrex 1018
pancuronium 1018
panic attacks and panic disorder, anxiety disorder 551–552
Panoxyl 1018
panthenol 1018
pantoprazole 1018
pantothenic acid 1018
papaveretum 1018
papaverine 1018
papillae, skin and hair structure *329, 330*
papillary thyroid cancer 681–682
papilloedema 581–582
papillomas, bladder tumours 715
Papulex 1018
para-aminobenzoic acid sunscreens and sunblocks 893
paracetamol 1018
antimigraine drugs 913
cold and flu remedies 910
dihydrocodeine with paracetamol, painkillers 912–913
painkillers 912–913
paracetamol with codeine, painkillers 912–913
propoxyphene with paracetamol, painkillers 912–913
Paracodol 1018
Paradote 1018
Parake 1018
paraldehyde 1018
Paramax 1018
paramedics and ambulances *955, 957*
Paramol 1018
paranoid personality disorder 561
Paraplatin 1018
parasitic infections and infestations *see* fungal infections; infestations; protozoal infections
parasympathetic nerves and parasympathetic responses, autonomic nervous system structure and functions *514*
parathyroid gland disorders 679
hyperparathyroidism 682–683
hypoparathyroidism 683
parathyroid tumours, cause of hyperparathyroidism 682–683
parathyroid glands 670, *671, 673*
disorders *see* parathyroid gland disorders
parathyroid hormone (PTH)
overproduction disorder *see* hyperparathyroidism
role in regulating body calcium levels *670, 671, 673*
underproduction disorder *see* hypoparathyroidism
paratyphoid *see* typhoid and paratyphoid
paraumbilical hernia 662
Parentline 1028
Pariet 1018
parietal lobe, brain structure *510*
Parkinson's Disease Foundation 1035
Parkinson's disease and parkinsonism 539–540
useful online sites and addresses 1035
Parkinson's Disease Society 1035
Parlodel 1018
Parmid 1018
paromomycin 1018
paronychia 361
parotid glands
disorders *see* salivary gland disorders
salivary glands location *622*
paroxetine 1018
antidepressant drugs 916–917
partial colectomy *665*
partial prostatectomy *725*
partial seizures, epilepsy 525–526
Parvolex 1018
parvovirus infection 294–295
passing out and feeling faint, symptoms chart 108–109
passive–aggressive personality disorder 561
passive immunization 883, *884*
passive smoking 64–65
patch testing *335*
patellofemoral pain syndrome *see* chondromalacia
patent ductus arteriosus, congenital heart disease 837
pathological gambling *see* compulsive gambling
Patient UK 1026, 1027, 1029, 1032, 1036
pauciarticular arthritis 835
Pavacol-D 1018
PBC Foundation 1034
PCP *see* phencyclidine (PCP)
PCR copying of DNA *see* polymerase chain reaction (PCR) copying of DNA
peak flow meters, use in monitoring asthma *484*
pellicles, protozoa structure *287*
pelvic examination, during physical examination 220
pelvic floor exercises *712*
pelvic floor muscles
involuntary spasms *see* vaginismus
strengthening with pelvic floor exercises *712*
weakness causing stress incontinence 711, *712*
pelvic inflammatory disease (PID) 741
pelvic tilts
antenatal exercises *34*
back-strengthening exercise *383*
pelvis
fractured *315*
location in skeleton *363*
of newborn babies *811*
pemphigoid, blistering disease 336
pemphigus, blistering disease 336
Penbritin 1018
penciclovir 1018
preparations for skin infections and infestations 892–893
penicillamine 1018
antirheumatic drugs 895–896
penicillin 1018
penicillins
antibiotics 885–886
how penicillins work *885*
penicillin V 1018
penis
disorders *see* penis disorders
during sexual arousal and sexual intercourse 716, 762, *763*
male reproductive system structure and functions 716, *717*
penile implant, impotence treatment 771
penis disorders
balanitis 722–723
cancer of the penis 723
chordee, associated with hypospadias in babies and children 870
hypospadias, in babies and children 870
Peyronie's disease 723
phimosis 721–722
priapism 723
problems with the penis, symptoms chart 182–183
see also impotence
Pentacarinat 1018
pentamidine 1018
antiprotozoal drugs 888
Pentasa 1018
pentazocine 1018
painkillers 912–913
pentostatin 1018
pentoxifylline 1018
Pepcid 1018
peppermint oil 1018
antispasmodic drugs and motility stimulants 926
peptic ulcer 640–642
antacids 923
ulcer-healing drugs 923–924
Peptimax 1018
Peptol-Bismo 1018
percussion, basic examination technique *220*
Percutol 1018
Perdix 1018
perennial allergic rhinitis 466–467
Perfan 1018
perforating veins, division of *439*
pergolide 1018
Pergonal 1018
Periactin 1018
periapical periodontitis 618
pericardial effusion, result of pericarditis 428, *429*
pericarditis 428–429
pericardium
heart structure *398*
inflamed *see* pericarditis
pericyazine 1018
perimetry *see* visual field test
perimysium, muscle structure *366*
Perinal 1018
perindopril 1018
angiotensin converting enzyme (ACE) inhibitor drugs 900–901
period pain *see* dysmenorrhoea
period problems *see* menstrual problems
periodontal ligaments, attaching teeth to gums and jawbone 606, *607*
periodontitis 618
periods, menstrual *see* menstruation and menstrual cycle
periosteum, bone structure *363*
peripheral nerves
common peroneal nerves *509*
disorders *see* peripheral nervous system disorders
femoral nerves *509*
median nerves *509, 547*
radial nerves *509*
sciatic nerves *509, 546*
in teeth and gums 606, *607*
tibial nerves *509*
ulnar nerves *509*
see also cranial nerves; spinal nerves
peripheral nervous system (PNS)
disorders *see* peripheral nervous system disorders
structure and functions 508, *509, 511–513*
see also peripheral nerves

peripheral nervous system
disorders 543
autonomic nerve neuropathies 544
Bell's palsy 548
carpal tunnel syndrome 547
diabetic neuropathy 545
electromyography (EMG) *544*
facial palsy 548
Guillain–Barré syndrome 550
motor nerve neuropathies 544
myasthenia gravis 549
nerve conduction studies *544*
nerve and muscle electrical tests *544*
nervous tics 550
nutritional neuropathies 545–546
peripheral nerve injuries 548–549
peripheral neuropathies 543–545
sciatica 546–547
sciatica in pregnancy *785*
sensory nerve neuropathies 543–544
Tourette's syndrome, nervous tics in 550
trigeminal neuralgia 546
peripheral vascular disorders 430
aortic aneurysm 430–431
Buerger's disease 436
deep vein thrombosis 437–438
diabetic vascular disease 432–434
femoral artery bypass graft treatment *434*
gangrene 435
hand–arm syndrome 436–437
Henoch–Schönlein purpura, in children 339, 838–839
lower limb ischaemia 434–435
purpura 339
Raynaud's phenomenon and Raynaud's disease 436
senile purpura 339
spider naevi, symptom of liver failure *650*
superficial thrombophlebitis 439
thrombosis and embolism 431–432
varicocele 720–721
varicose veins 438–439
varicose veins in pregnancy 438, *785*
peripheral vascular system 430
peristalsis and peristaltic wave *622*, *623*
peritoneal dialysis *707*
peritoneum (peritoneal membrane)
inflamed *see* peritonitis
location and functions *621*, *695*
use in peritoneal dialysis *707*
peritonitis 665
peritonsillar abscess 479
permanent colostomy *666*
permanent teeth *see* secondary teeth
permethrin 1018
preparations for skin infections and infestations 892–893
pernio *see* chilblains
Peroxyl 1018
perphenazine 1018
antiemetic drugs 922
Persantin 1018
persistent anxiety disorder *see* persistent anxiety state
persistent anxiety state 551–552
persistent vegetative state 523
personality disorders 561–562
person-centred therapy 970
perspiration *see* sweat
Perthes' disease 833–834
pertussis 492–493
routine immunizations *45*
Peru balsam 1018
petechiae and purpuric spots, purpura symptoms 339
pethidine 1018
petit mal seizures, epilepsy 525
petroleum jelly
emollients and barrier preparations 890
petrol, recreational drug effects and risks *66*
PET scanning *see* positron emission tomography (PET) scanning
pets and health *47*, 82
Pevaryl 1018
Peyer's patches, lymphatic system structure *443*
Peyronie's disease 723
phaeochromocytoma 686
phagocytes, role in body's defences *444*, *445*
PharmWeb 1030
pharyngitis and tonsillitis 479, 843
pharynx (throat)
connecting passageways to ears and nose *592*
digestive system structure and functions *621*
disorders *see* throat disorders
respiratory system structure and functions 470, *471*
tests and investigations *see* endoscopy of the nose and throat; indirect laryngoscopy; throat swabs
phenazocine 1018
phencyclidine (PCP), recreational drug effects and risks *66*
phenelzine 1018
antidepressant drugs 916–917
Phenergan 1018
phenindione 1018
pheniramine 1018
phenobarbital 1018
anticonvulsant drugs 914–915
phenol 1018
phenothiazines, antiemetic drugs 922
phenothrin 1018
phenoxybenzamine 1018
phenoxymethylpenicillin 1018
antibiotics 885–886
Phensic 1018
phentermine 1018
phentolamine 1018
phenylalanine metabolism disorder *see* phenylketonuria
phenylbutazone 1018
phenylephrine 1018
cold and flu remedies 910
decongestants 909
drugs acting on the eye 919–920
phenylketonuria 241, *273*, 867–868
heel prick blood test, screening for phenylketonuria in newborn babies *44*, *867*
phenylpropanolamine 1018
cold and flu remedies 910
decongestants 909
phenytoin 1018
anticonvulsant drugs 914–915
phimosis 721–722
pHiso-Med 1018
phobias 552–553
behaviour therapy 969
desensitization and flooding, behaviour therapy techniques 969
hypnotherapy 974–975
pholcodine 1018
cough remedies 909–910
phoropters, use in vision tests *587*
phosphates
laxatives 924–925
phosphorus 1018
mineral supplements 929
photoreactive keratectomy (PRK), surgical treatment for refractive errors *589*
photosensitivity 338
phototherapy, for neonatal jaundice *818*
Phyllocontin Continus 1018
Physeptone 1018
physical examination 41–42, 216, 219–220
physical skills, developmental milestones during childhood *814*
Physiotens 1018
physiotherapy 954, *955*, 961–962
back-strengthening exercises *383*
transcutaneous electrical nerve stimulation (TENS), use in pain relief *517*
Phytex 1018
phytomenadione 1018
drugs that promote blood clotting 903
pia mater
bleeding between pia mater and arachnoid *see* subarachnoid haemorrhage
brain and spinal cord structure *509*
pica, eating problems in children 852
Picolax 1018
PID *see* pelvic inflammatory disease (PID)
pigmented naevi, birthmarks 828
pigment loss from skin *see* vitiligo
pigments
pigment stones, gallstones 651
see also bilirubin; melanin
piles *see* haemorrhoids
pili, bacteria structure *286*
pilocarpine 1018
drugs for glaucoma 920–921
pilonidal sinus 360
pimozide 1018
antipsychotic drugs 917–918
pimples
acne 340–341
folliculitis 352
molluscum contagiosum 355
rosacea 341
see also rashes; spots
pinch grafts *318*
pindolol 1018
pineal gland, location and functions *671*
pink eye *see* conjunctivitis
pinna
ear structure and functions *592*, *593*
injured *see* outer-ear injury
pinning, fracture treatment *393*
piperacillin 1018
piperazine 1018
piperonal 1018
pipotiazine palmitate 1019
Pipril 1019
piracetam 1019
pirenzepine 1019
piroxicam 1019
nonsteroidal anti-inflammatory drugs (NSAIDs) 894
painkillers 912–913
Pirozip 1019
pitch, of sound 592
pitting, nail abnormality 360
pituitary drugs 934–935
pituitary gland
disorders *see* pituitary gland disorders
hormones produced by the pituitary gland *672*
increased follicle-stimulating hormone (FSH) production during the menopause *733*, 737–738
location, structure and functions *510*, 670, *671*, *672*
role in blood pressure control *401*
role in puberty *716*, 730, *815*
role in stem cell production control *440*
pituitary gland disorders 676
acromegaly 677
cause of hypothyroidism 680
cranial diabetes insipidus 678
diabetes insipidus 678, 934–935
gigantism, growth disorder 869
hypopituitarism 678
nephrogenic diabetes insipidus 678
pituitary drugs 934–935
pituitary tumours 676
prolactinoma 677
pituitary tumours 676
cause of acromegaly 677
cause of cranial diabetes insipidus 678
cause of gigantism 869
cause of hypopituitarism 678
cause of hypothyroidism 680
prolactinoma 677
pityriasis rosea 337–338
pityriasis versicolor 353
pivot joints *364–365*
pizotifen 1019
placenta
delivery during childbirth *783*
disorders *see* placental disorders
functions during pregnancy *779*, *781*, *810*
hormone production *232*, *671*
placental disorders
cause of fetal distress 804
choriocarcinoma 748
concealed placental abruption 799
molar pregnancy 790
placental abruption 799

placenta praevia 798–799
revealed placental abruption 799
placenta praevia 798–799
plague 303–304
plain X-rays *see* X-rays
plane joints *364–365*
plantar warts 354–355
plants, poisonous 80
plaque, dental 606, 610, 617
plaque psoriasis 332
plasma
blood components, structure and functions 440, *441*
decreased volume disorder *see* stress polycythaemia
fresh frozen plasma 903
role in oxygen/carbon dioxide gas exchange in respiratory system 470, *473*
plasma cells
abnormal production *see* multiple myeloma
role in antibody immune response *445*
plasma membrane, bacteria structure *286*
plasmids, bacteria structure *286*
plastic surgery 952
breast reduction *757*
laser treatment on the skin *951*
skin grafting *318*
plateau phase, sexual response *762*
platelets
blood components, formation and functions 440, *441–442*, 446
reduced platelet levels *see* thrombocytopenia
Plavix 1019
play
McCormick toy discrimination test, hearing test in children *859*
play and social behaviour, developmental milestones during childhood *814*
play therapy, use in speech therapy for children *955*, 963
Plendil 1019
pleura
disorders *see* pleural disorders
respiratory system structure *471*
pleural disorders
diffuse pleural thickening, asbestos-related disease 501–502
mesothelioma, asbestos-related disease 501–502
pleural effusion 494–495
pleurisy 493
pneumothorax 496–497
plexuses, spinal nerves structure *511*
PMF *see* progressive massive fibrosis (PMF)
PMS *see* premenstrual syndrome (PMS)
pneumococcus, vaccines and immunoglobulins 883–884
pneumoconiosis, coalworkers' pneumoconiosis 499–500
pneumocystis infection 308
pneumonia 490–491
aspiration pneumonia 491
bacterial pneumonia 490–491
Legionnaires' disease 490
pneumocystis infection 308
viral pneumonia 490–491
pneumonic plague 304
pneumonitis *see* extrinsic allergic alveolitis
pneumothorax 496–497
PNS *see* peripheral nervous system
podophyllin 1019
podophyllotoxin 1019
podophyllum 1019
poisoning 321–322
avoiding poisoning in the home 77
avoiding poisonous plants 80
blood poisoning *see* septicaemia
carbon monoxide (CO) poisoning 77
drug overdose and accidental ingestion 321–322
lead poisoning 77, 79
poisonous bites and stings 327
poisonous bites and stings, first aid *994*
statistics 314
swallowed poisons, first aid 321, *994*
see also food poisoning
poliomyelitis (polio) 295
routine immunizations *45*
vaccines and immunoglobulins 883–884
pollen allergy *see* seasonal allergic rhinitis
poloxamer 1019
polyarteritis nodosa 465
polyarticular arthritis 835
polycystic kidney disease *273*, 704
polycystic ovary syndrome 744
polycythaemia 457
polycythaemia vera *see* primary polycythaemia
Polyfax 1019
polyhydramnios 795
polymerase chain reaction (PCR)
copying of DNA, for genetic tests 239
polymyalgia rheumatica 464
polymyositis and dermatomyositis 463–464
polymyxin B 1019
drugs acting on the eye 919–920
polynoxylin 1019
polyps
familial adenomatous polyposis (FAP), polyps in the colon 661, 666
nasal polyps 476–477
polyps in the colon 660–661
uterine polyps *745*, 746
polystyrene sulphonate 1019
Polytar 1019
polythiazide 1019
Polytrim 1019
polyunsaturated fats *50*, 51
polyvinyl alcohol 1019
drugs acting on the eye 919–920
pons, brain structure *510*
Ponstan 1019
poor bladder control, symptoms chart 165
Poractant alfa 1019
Pork Insulatard 1019
Pork Mixtard 1019
porphyria *273*, 693
portal hypertension and varices 648–649
portal system of blood vessels supplying pituitary gland *672*
portal vein
disorders *see* portal hypertension and varices
role in blood circulation *400*, *624*
port-wine stains, birthmarks 828
Posalfilin 1019
positional clubfoot 833
positions and positioning
correct driving position *382*
correct sitting position *382*
positioning babies for sleep *820*
positioning baby on the nipple for breast-feeding *809*
recovery positions, first aid *979*
see also posture
positive pressure ventilation *478*
positron emission tomography (PET) scanning *213*, 253
posterior lobe of the pituitary gland, structure and functions *672*
posterior uveitis 574–575
post-extraction alveolitis *see* dry socket
postherpetic neuralgia, caused by herpes zoster 290, 291
postmenopausal bleeding 738–739
postoperative care and monitoring 945
postpartum depression *see* depression after childbirth
postpartum haemorrhage 806–807
postpartum psychosis, depression after childbirth 807–808
postpartum thyroiditis 681
post-traumatic stress disorder (PTSD) 553
postural hypotension 414
posture
correct *382*
disorders caused by postural problems *see* lordosis and kyphosis; lower back pain
effects of cerebral palsy 846–847
in pregnancy *785*
role of skeletal muscles 362
see also positions and positioning
post-viral fatigue syndrome *see* chronic fatigue syndrome
potassium 1019
potassium bicarbonate 1019
potassium chloride 1019
potassium citrate 1019
potassium clavulanate 1019
potassium hydroxyquinolone sulphate 1019
potassium iodide 1019
potassium permanganate 1019
potassium-sparing diuretic drugs, diuretic drugs 902
pouch operation, for ulcerative colitis 660
povidone-iodine 1019
Pragmatar 1019
pralidoxime mesylate 1019
pramipexole 1019
pramocaine 1019
pravastatin 1019
lipid-lowering drugs 935
Praxilene 1019
praziquantel 1019
anthelmintic drugs 889
prazosin 1019
antihypertensive drugs 897–898
precocious puberty *see* early (precocious) puberty
Precortisyl 1019
Predenema 1019
Predfoam 1019
Prednesol 1019
prednisolone 1019
corticosteroids 930–931
corticosteroids for respiratory disease 911
drugs acting on the ear 921
drugs acting on the eye 919–920
immunosuppressants 906–907
locally acting corticosteroids 895
Predsol 1019
Predsol-N 1019
pre-eclampsia (pre-eclamptic toxaemia) and eclampsia 794–795
prefrontal cortex, location and role in information processing in the brain *515*
Pregaday 1019
pregnancy 778, *779–781*
coping with pregnancy 33–35, *785*
diet during pregnancy 33–34, *785*
exercise and relaxation *34*
female reproductive system changes during pregnancy *779*, *780–781*
folic acid supplements for prevention of neural tube defects in babies and children 33, 844, 845, 928
health in pregnancy and after childbirth 33–35
home pregnancy tests *232*
labour and childbirth *782–783*
milk production *see* breast milk production
multiple pregnancy *779*, 792–793
possible pregnancy as reason for absent periods 186
prevention *see* contraception
problems after childbirth 35, 806–809
problems during labour *see* labour problems
problems during pregnancy *see* pregnancy problems and disorders
termination of pregnancy *789*
tests and investigations *see* antenatal tests and investigations
useful online sites and addresses 1035–1036
vitamin and mineral requirements 33
pregnancy problems and disorders
abdominal pain in pregnancy, symptoms chart 192

pregnancy problems and disorders (continued)
  acute polyhydramnios 795
  bleeding in pregnancy, symptoms chart 190
  cervical incompetence 794
  choriocarcinoma 748
  chronic polyhydramnios 795
  common complaints of normal pregnancy 784, *785*
  concealed placental abruption 799
  ectopic pregnancy 790–791
  fetal distress 804
  gestational diabetes (diabetes developing in pregnancy) 687, 788–789
  high-risk pregnancy 786–787
  hyperemesis 789
  intra-uterine growth retardation 796
  miscarriage 791–792
  molar pregnancy 790
  morning sickness, common complaint of normal pregnancy 784
  multiple pregnancy and its problems 792–793
  placental abruption 799
  placenta praevia 798–799
  polyhydramnios 795
  pre-eclampsia and eclampsia 794–795
  pre-existing diseases in pregnancy 786–787, 788
  premature labour 798, 938
  premature rupture of membranes 797
  revealed placental abruption 799
  Rhesus (Rh) incompatibility 795–796
  stillbirth 805
  vaginal bleeding in pregnancy 791
  vaginal bleeding in pregnancy, symptoms chart 190
Pregnyl 1019
Premarin 1019
premature babies
  hydrocephalus 845–846
  immunization 45
  lanugo hair *811*
  neonatal jaundice 817–818
  patent ductus arteriosus, congenital heart disease 837
  problems of the premature baby 816–817
  special care baby unit *959*
premature ejaculation 771–772
premature labour 798
  uterine muscle relaxant drugs, drugs for labour 938
premature rupture of membranes 797
premedication
  before major surgery 944
premenstrual syndrome (PMS) 736–737
Premique 1019
premolars, tooth structure *606, 607*
premotor cortex, location and role in information processing in the brain *515*
Prempak-C 1019
preoperative assessment, before major surgery 943
Prepadine 1019
preparations for major surgery 944
presbyacusis 601
presbyopia 589
Prescal 1019
presentation of fetus in pregnancy
  abnormal 800–801
  normal *779, 781, 782–783*
Preservex 1019
pressure
  applying pressure as first aid for bleeding *986*
  blood *see* blood pressure
  detection by Pacinian corpuscles in skin *331, 513*
  pressure changes, cause of barotrauma 598
pressure points, use in first aid for bleeding *986*
pressure sores 350
Prestim 1019
preventer drugs for asthma 485, 840
Priadel 1019
priapism 723
prickle cells, skin structure *330*
prickly heat 342
prilocaine 1019
Primalan 1019
primaquine 1019
  antimalarial drugs 888–889
primary amenorrhoea 735
primary amyloidosis 693
primary areas, role in information processing in the brain *515*
primary auditory cortex, location and role in information processing in the brain *515*
primary biliary cirrhosis 647–648
primary bone cancer 373
primary dysmenorrhoea 736
primary hypogonadism, in females 739
Primary Immunodeficiency Association 1033
primary lung cancer 503–505
primary polycythaemia 457
primary sensory cortex, location and role in information processing in the brain *515*
primary stage syphilis 766
primary teeth *606*
primary visual cortex, location and role in information processing in the brain *515*
primidone 1019
  anticonvulsant drugs 914–915
Primolut N 1019
Primoteston Depot 1019
Primperan 1019
Princess Royal Trust for Carers 1033
Prioderm 1019
prion infections, Creutzfeldt–Jakob disease (CJD) 540
Pripsen 1019
Private Healthcare UK 1032
PRK *see* photoreactive keratectomy (PRK)
Pro-Banthine 1019
probenecid 1019
problems with the penis, symptoms chart 182–183
procainamide 1019
  antiarrhythmic drugs 898
procaine 1019
procaine benzylpenicillin 1019
procaine penicillin *see* procaine benzylpenicillin 1019
procarbazine 1019
  anticancer drugs 907–908
prochlorperazine 1019
  antiemetic drugs 922
  drugs acting on the ear 921
proctitis 667
Proctofoam HC 1019
Proctosedyl 1019
procyclidine 1019
Profasi 1019
Proflex 1019
progesterone 1019
  in HRT *see* hormone replacement therapy (HRT)
  production and role in female reproductive system *671*, 730, *732–733*
  role in puberty *815*
  synthetic *see* progestogens
progestogens
  in hormonal contraceptives 69, *71*, 933
  in HRT *see* hormone replacement therapy (HRT)
  sex hormones and related drugs 933
progressive massive fibrosis (PMF), complication of coalworkers' pneumoconiosis 499–500
proguanil 1019
  antimalarial drugs 888–889
Progynova 1019
Progynova TS 1019
prolactin
  overproduction disorder *see* prolactinoma
  production and functions *672*
prolactin inhibitors, pituitary drugs 934–935
prolactinoma 677
prolapsed or herniated disc (slipped disc) 384–385
prolapse of the mitral valve *see* mitral valve prolapse
prolapse of the rectum *see* rectal prolapse
prolapse of the umbilical cord
  caused by premature rupture of the membranes 797
  causing fetal distress 804
prolapse of the uterus and vagina 747
prolapsing haemorrhoids 668
Proluton Depot 1019
promazine 1019
  antipsychotic drugs 917–918
promethazine 1019
  antiemetic drugs 922
  antihistamines 906
Prominal 1019
Propaderm 1019
propafenone 1019
  antiarrhythmic drugs 898
Propain 1019
propamidine isethionate 1019
Propanix 1019
propantheline 1019
  antispasmodic drugs and motility stimulants 926
  drugs that affect bladder control 939
Propine 1019
propiverine hydrochloride 1019
Pro-Plus 1020
propofol 1020
  general anaesthetics 914
proportions of body at different ages *812*
propranolol 1020
  antianxiety drugs 916
  antimigraine drugs 913
  beta-blocker drugs 898–899
proprioceptors, types of sensory receptors *513*
propylthiouracil 1020
  drugs for hyperthyroidism 932–933
Proscar 1020
prostaglandin 1020
  production blocked by nonsteroidal anti-inflammatory drugs (NSAIDs) *895*
  prostaglandin pessaries, for induction of labour *797*, 938
prostate cancer *281*, 726–727
Prostate Cancer Charity 1036
prostatectomy
  partial *725*
  radical *727*
prostate disorders 724
  acute prostatitis 724
  chronic prostatitis 724
  drugs for prostate disorders 938–939
  enlarged prostate gland 725–726
  partial prostatectomy *725*
  prostate cancer *281*, 726–727
  prostatitis 724
  radical prostatectomy *727*
  useful online sites and addresses 1036
prostate gland
  disorders *see* prostate disorders
  male reproductive system structure and functions 716, *717, 763*
  prostate gland biopsy *726*
  urinary system structure and functions *694, 695*
Prostate Help Association 1036
prostatitis 724
protamine 1020
protease inhibitors, drugs for HIV infection and AIDS 887–888
protein in the diet 50
  chemical breakdown during digestion *625, 674–675*
  nutritional information on food labels *52*
proteins
  excessive accumulation of abnormal proteins in the body *see* amyloidosis
  fibrinogen, role in blood clotting *441, 442*
  in food *see* protein in the diet
  functions *266*
  gene products, tests for 241

protein-building instructions in genetic material (genes/DNA) 20, 264, *265–266*
Rhesus (Rh) proteins *see* Rhesus (Rh) blood group system
routine blood chemistry tests for proteins 230
routine urine chemistry tests for proteins 231
tests for inflammatory proteins 232–233
virus surface proteins and protein shells *285*
see also antibodies; antigens; clotting factors; enzymes
Prothiaden 1020
protirelin 1020
Protium 1020
proton pump inhibitors, ulcer-healing drugs 923–924
protozoa
infections caused by protozoa *see* protozoal infections
infectious organisms size comparison *284*
structure *287*
protozoal infections 305
amoebiasis 306
cryptosporidiosis 307
drug treatments *see* antimalarial drugs; antiprotozoal drugs
food poisoning 629–630
giardiasis 307
malaria 305–306
nongonococcal urethritis (NGU) 765
pneumocystis infection 308
toxoplasmosis 82, 307–308, 817
trichomoniasis 767
vulvovaginitis 752
protriptyline 1020
protruding ears 861
Provera 1020
Provigil 1020
Pro-Viron 1020
proximal convoluted tubule, kidney structure and functions *696, 697*
proxymetacaine 1020
Prozac 1020
Proziere 1020
pruritus *see* itching
pruritus ani *see* anal itching
pseudoephedrine 1020
cold and flu remedies 910
decongestants 909
pseudogout 381
pseudomembranous colitis, caused by antibiotics 885
psoriasis 332–333
retinoid drugs 890–891
Psoriasis Association 1036
Psorin 1020
psychiatric disorders *see* mental health disorders
psychoanalytic-based psychotherapy 968–969
psychological assessment, use in mental health disorders diagnosis *554*
psychological health 72–73
adolescents 32
adults 33
assessing your psychological health *72*
babies and infants 28–29
effects of exercise *56*, 57
in old age 37
older adults 36
preschool children 30, 72–73
psychological and/or emotional problems *see* developmental and psychological disorders in children; mental health disorders; sexual problems
school-age children 31, 72–73
see also bereavement and grieving; sleep; stress
psychological therapies 954, *955*, 968
assertiveness training, behaviour therapy technique 969
behaviour therapy 969
classical psychoanalysis 968
cognitive therapy 970
counselling 971
desensitization and flooding, behaviour therapy techniques 969
Gestalt therapy, person-centred therapy 970
group therapy 970–971
person-centred therapy 970
psychoanalytic-based psychotherapy 968–969
response prevention, behaviour therapy technique 969
supportive care for people with cancer 282
supportive group therapy 971
useful online sites and addresses 1029
see also counselling
psychotherapy *see* psychological therapies
PTH *see* parathyroid hormone (PTH)
ptosis 584
PTSD *see* post-traumatic stress disorder (PTSD)
puberty 810, *815*
abnormal *see* abnormal puberty
delayed *see* delayed puberty
diet during puberty and adolescence 31
early *see* early (precocious) puberty
in females *730, 815*
growth spurt during puberty *813*
in males *716, 815*
see also adolescence
pubic hair
infestations *see* pubic lice
pubic, facial, and body hair development during puberty *716, 730, 815*
pubic lice 768
Public Health Laboratory Service 1033
Pulmicort 1020
pulmonary artery, location and role in cardiovascular system *397–400*
pulmonary circulation, blood circulation 396, *400*
pulmonary embolism 495
pulmonary hypertension 505–506
Pulmonary Hypertension Association, Inc. 1034
pulmonary valve, heart structure *398, 399*
pulmonary veins, location and role in cardiovascular system *397–400*
Pulmozyme 1020
pulp and pulp chamber
inflamed *see* pulpitis
tooth structure 606, *607*
pulpitis 611
pulse
checking brachial pulse in infants, first aid *978*
checking pulse during physical examination 219
checking neck (carotid) pulse, after exercise *59*
checking neck (carotid) pulse, first aid *978*
definition 396
pulse recovery time after exercise *59*
see also heart rate
pulse oximeters, use in blood gases measurement *501*
pumactant 1020
pupil of the eye, eye structure and functions *567, 568*
Puri-Nethol 1020
purpura 339
Henoch–Schönlein purpura, in children 339, 838–839
senile purpura 339
pustular psoriasis 333
pyelonephritis 698–699, 871
pyloric sphincter, digestive system structure and functions *621, 622*
pyloric stenosis in infants 863
Pylorid 1020
Pyralvex 1020
pyrazinamide 1020
antituberculous drugs 886
pyridostigmine 1020
pyridoxine 1020
vitamin supplements 928
pyrimethamine 1020
pyrimethamine with dapsone, antimalarial drugs 888–889
pyrimethamine with sulfadiazine, antiprotozoal drugs 888
pyrimethamine with sulfadoxine, antimalarial drugs 888–889
pyrithione zinc 1020

Q

Q fever 304
quadrantectomy, breast cancer surgery 760
Quellada M 1020
Questran 1020
quetiapine 1020
quick-relief drugs (relievers) for asthma 485, 840
quinagolide 1020
quinapril 1020
angiotensin converting enzyme (ACE) inhibitor drugs 900–901
quinidine 1020
antiarrhythmic drugs 898
quinine 1020
antimalarial drugs 888–889
muscle relaxants 896
Quinocort 1020
Quinoderm 1020
quinolones, antibiotics 885–886
Quinoped 1020
Quit 1037

R

rabeprazole sodium 1020
rabies 296
travel immunizations *86*
vaccines and immunoglobulins 883–884
RADAR 1030, 1036
radial keratotomy (RK), surgical treatment for refractive errors *589*
radial nerves, nervous system structure *509*
Radian-B 1020
radiation
cause of cancer *274*
radiation cystitis caused by radiotherapy 710
radiation doses from imaging techniques, comparison *246*
radiotherapy for cancer 281
radon protection, home safety 79
use in imaging techniques *see* computerized tomography (CT) scanning; radionuclide scanning; X-rays
radical prostatectomy *727*
radioactive implants and seeds, cancer treatment *281*
radiofrequency ablation *417*
radioiodine, drugs for hyperthyroidism 932–933
radionuclide scanning *243*, 251–252
blood flow scans, radionuclide lung scanning *494*
dimercaptosuccinic acid (DMSA) scanning *871*
positron emission tomography (PET) scanning *213*, 253
radiation doses, compared with other imaging techniques *246*
radionuclide lung scanning *494*
single-photon-emission computerized tomography (SPECT) scanning *243*, 253
ventilation scan, radionuclide lung scanning *494*
radon protection, home safety 79
raloxifene 1020
drugs for bone disorders 896
raltitrexed 1020
ramipril 1020
angiotensin converting enzyme (ACE) inhibitor drugs 900–901
ranitidine 1020
ulcer-healing drugs 923–924
ranitidine bismuth citrate 1020
rape *see* sexual assault
Rapilysin 1020
Rapitard MC 1020
Rapitil 1020

Rappell 1020
rash-causing disorders
acne 340–341, 890–891
chickenpox (varicella) 290, 883
dermatomyositis 463–464
discoid lupus erythematosus (DLE) 347
erythema multiforme 337
Henoch–Schönlein purpura 339, 838–839
herpes zoster 290–291
lichen planus 336–337
Lyme disease 303, 883
measles *45*, 293, 883–884
meningococcal (bacterial) meningitis 527–528, 848–849
parvovirus infection 294–295
pityriasis rosea 337–338
polyarteritis nodosa 465
prickly heat 342
Rocky Mountain spotted fever 304
roseola infantum 830–831
rubella *45*, 294, 883–884
scabies 355
scarlet fever 300
systemic lupus erythematosus (SLE) 461–462
urticaria 468
rashes
disorders causing rashes *see* rash-causing disorders
drug-induced rashes 338
general skin problems, symptoms chart 126–127
nappy rash 829
rash with fever, symptoms chart 128–129
red rash assessment *129*
see also pimples; spots
Raynaud's phenomenon and Raynaud's disease 436
Raynaud's and Scleroderma Association 1033
razoxane 1020
reactive arthritis 379
reboxetine 1020
rebreathing technique, coping with panic attacks *552*
receding gums 619
receptors
cell *see* cell receptors
sensory *see* sensory receptors
recessive genes and recessive inheritance *268–269*
disorders *see* autosomal recessive disorders; X-linked disorders
recovery positions, first aid *979*
recreational drugs 65–66
see also drug-related problems and disorders
rectal examination, during physical examination 220
rectal prolapse 667–668
rectal route, drug delivery route *879*
rectocele, prolapse of the uterus and vagina 747
rectum
digestive system structure and functions *621, 623, 625*
disorders *see* rectum disorders
rectal drug delivery route *879*
rectal examination during physical examination 220
rectum disorders
anal and rectal problems, symptoms chart 157
banding haemorrhoids *668*
colectomy *665*
colorectal cancer 665–667
colostomy *666*
external haemorrhoids 668
haemorrhoids 668
hereditary nonpolyposis colorectal cancer (HNPCC) 666
internal haemorrhoids 668
proctitis 667
prolapsing haemorrhoids 668
rectal prolapse 667–668
sigmoidoscopy *661*
ulcerative colitis 659–660, 924
recurrent abdominal pain, symptoms chart 154–155
recurrent vomiting, symptoms chart 150–151
red blood cells
disorders *see* anaemias; haemolytic jaundice; polycythaemia
erythrocyte sedimentation test, test for inflammation 233
formation and function 440, *441–442*, 446
red–green colour blindness 591
Redoxon 1020
reduction, fracture treatment 392, *393*
reflexes
cough reflex *473*
involuntary responses by the nervous system *514*
in newborn babies 810, *811*
reflux
gastro-oesophageal *see* gastro-oesophageal reflux (GOR)
urinary reflux, leading to urinary tract infections in children 871
Refolinon 1020
refractive errors 586
astigmatism 588–589
correction with glasses and contact lenses *588*
hypermetropia 586–588
myopia 586
presbyopia 589
surgical treatments *589*
Regaine 1020
regional anaesthesia 914, *945*
Regulan 1020
Regulose 1020
rehabilitation and rehabilitation therapies 954, 961
at home 960
occupational therapy 954, *955*, 962–963
physical *see* physiotherapy
speech therapy *955*, 963
useful online sites and addresses 1036
Rehidrat 1020
Reiter's syndrome, reactive arthritis 379
relapsing–remitting multiple sclerosis (MS) 541–542
RELATE 1029
relaxants, recreational drug effects and risks 65, *66*
relaxation
biofeedback 975
controlled breathing techniques *75*
hypnotherapy 974–975
in pregnancy *34*
relaxation exercises *17, 75*
Relaxit 1020
releasing factors, production in hypothalamus *671, 672*
Relenza 1020
reliability of tests and investigations 44, 213
reliever drugs for asthma 485, 840
Relifex 1020
Remedeine 1020
remedies, homeopathic 974
remifentanil 1020
renal artery, connection to the kidneys *695, 696*
renal capsule, kidney structure and functions *696*
renal pelvis, kidney structure and functions *695, 696*
renal pyramids, kidney structure and functions *696*
renal tubules, kidney structure and functions 694, *696–697*
renal vein
connection to the kidneys *695, 696*
location *397*
renin, role in blood pressure control *401*
Rennie Digestif 1020
repaglinide 1020
drugs for diabetes mellitus 931–932
repetitive strain injury (RSI) 82, 389
replacement teeth and crowns *615*
replication (copying) of genes and DNA 264, *266*
reproduction
asexual reproduction, bacteria 762
human *see* female reproductive system; male reproductive system; pregnancy; sexual intercourse
viruses *285*
reproductive system
female *see* female reproductive system
male *see* male reproductive system
reproterol 1020
Requip 1020
resolution phase, sexual response *762*
Resolve 1020
resorcinol 1020
Respacal 1020
respiration and breathing
artificial respiration, first aid *982–983*
respiratory system functions 470, *471, 472–473*
respiratory centre in brain, role in breathing control *472*
respiratory distress syndrome, in premature babies 816–817
respiratory failure 507
respiratory system
disorders *see* respiratory system disorders
effects of growth and aging *22–23*
effects of smoking 64
role in body's defences *444*, 470, *471*
role of exercise in respiratory health 55, *56*
structure and functions 470, *471–473*
symptoms charts *see* respiratory system symptoms charts
respiratory system disorders
allergic rhinitis 466–467
in children *see* respiratory system disorders in children
common cold 288–289
drugs for respiratory disorders 909–911
flu *see* influenza
home oxygen therapy *507, 966*
pneumocystis infection 308
sleep apnoea 477–478
snoring 477
steam inhalation *475*
symptoms charts *see* respiratory system symptoms charts
tests and investigations *see* respiratory system tests and investigations
useful online sites and addresses 1034
see also lung disorders; nose disorders; throat disorders
respiratory system disorders in children
asthma in children 839–840
bronchiolitis 841
croup 841–842
enlarged adenoids 842–843
epiglottitis 842
nosebleeds 474–475
respiratory distress syndrome, in premature babies 816–817
tonsillitis 479, 843
respiratory system symptoms charts
breathing problems in children 204–205
coughing 142–143
coughing in children 206–207
coughing up blood 142
shortness of breath 144–145
wheezing 146
respiratory system tests and investigations
asthma monitoring using peak flow meter *484*
blood gases measurement *501*
bronchoscopy *504*
children's breathing rate assessment *89, 205*
endoscopy of the nose and throat *476*
gas transfer test *488*
lung function tests *488*
lung volume tests *488*
mirror laryngoscopy *481*
pulse oximeter use in blood gases measurement *501*
radionuclide lung scanning *494*
sleep studies *477*

spirometry *488*
X-rays *see* chest X-ray
response prevention, behaviour therapy technique 969
Restandol 1020
rest, ice, compression, elevation (RICE), first aid for sprains and strains *991*
resuscitation, first aid
ABC of resuscitation *978*
artificial respiration *982–983*
cardiopulmonary resuscitation (CPR) *984–985*
retention of urine *see* urinary retention
reteplase 1020
Retin-A 1020
retina
damage caused by hypertension 404, *405*
disorders *see* retinal disorders
effects of toxoplasmosis *308*
eye structure and functions 566, *567–569*
fluorescein angiography *580*
retinal disorders
colour blindness *269*, 591
diabetic retinopathy 579–580
fluorescein angiography *580*
macular degeneration 580–581
papilloedema 581–582
retinal detachment 578–579
retinal vein occlusion 578
retinitis pigmentosa *273*, 581
retinoblastoma, in babies and children 858–859
retinopathy 579
tunnel vision, visual field defect 590–591
retinoic acid 1020
retinoid drugs 890–891
retinoids 1020
retinol 1020
retinopathy 579
diabetic retinopathy 579–580
retinoscopy, vision test in babies and children *857*
Retinova 1020
retrograde ejaculation after partial prostatectomy, cause of male infertility *725*, 777
retroverted uterus 746
Retrovir 1020
Revanil 1020
revealed placental abruption 799
reverse transcriptase inhibitors, drugs for HIV infection and AIDS 887–888
reversible pulpitis 611
Reye's syndrome 849
Rhesus (Rh) blood group system *441*
blood typing 227
Rhesus (Rh) incompatibility, in pregnancy 795–796
Rheumacin LA 1020
rheumatic disorders, useful online sites and addresses 1036
rheumatic fever 429
rheumatoid arthritis 377–378
antirheumatic drugs 895–896
juvenile chronic arthritis (JCA) 835
pauciarticular arthritis 835
polyarticular arthritis 835
systemic arthritis 835
Rheumox 1020
Rhinocort 1020
Rhinolast 1020
rhinophyma, effect of rosacea 341, 342
Rhumalgan 1020
ribavirin 1020
antiviral drugs 886–887
riboflavin 1020
vitamin sources in diet and effects on health *51*
ribosomes
bacteria structure *286*
DNA structure *266*
ribs, location and role in breathing *363*, *471*, *472*
RICE *see* rest, ice, compression, elevation (RICE)
rickets and osteomalacia 370
rickettsial infections
endemic typhus 304
Q fever 304
Rocky Mountain spotted fever 304
scrub typhus 304
typhus 304
Ridaura 1020
Rideril 1020
ridges, nail abnormality 360
rifabutin 1020
antituberculous drugs 886
Rifadin 1020
rifampicin 1020
antituberculous drugs 886
Rifater 1020
Rifinah 1020
rigid contact lenses *588*
for astigmatism 589
rigid endoscopy 242, 256
arthroscopy *386*
bronchoscopy *504*
cystoscopy *715*
hysteroscopy *745*
knee arthroscopy *386*
laparoscopy *742*
Rilutek 1020
riluzole 1020
Rimactane 1020
Rimoxallin 1020
Rinatec 1020
ringworm 352–353
Rinne test, hearing test *600*
risks assessment, health risks *46*
Risperdal 1020
risperidone 1020
antipsychotic drugs 917–918
Ritalin 1020
ritodrine 1020
drugs for labour 938
ritonavir 1020
drugs for HIV infection and AIDS 887–888
rituximab 1020
anticancer drugs 907–908
rivastigmine 1020
Rivotril 1020
rizatriptan 1020
RK *see* radial keratotomy (RK)
RNA
messenger RNA (mRNA), functions *266*
in viruses *285*
Roaccutane 1020
road safety 83, *84*
Robinul-Neostigmine 1020
Robitussin Dry Cough 1020
Rocaltrol 1021
Rocky Mountain spotted fever 304
rocuronium 1021
rods and cones
cone disorders *see* colour blindness
eye structure and functions 566, *567–569*
rofecoxib 1021
Roferon-A 1021
Rohypnol 1021
roller bandages, first aid uses *976*, *996–997*
Rommix 1021
root canal treatment *612*
root, tooth structure 606, *607*
ropinirole 1021
ropivacaine 1021
rosiglitazone 1021
drugs for diabetes mellitus 932
rosacea 341–342
roseola infantum 830–831
rotational movements, detection by the inner ear *595*
rotaviruses *284*
cause of gastroenteritis 628
Roter 1021
round window, ear structure and functions *593*, *594*
roundworms
roundworm infestations 310–312
structure *287*
routine blood chemistry 229–230
routine urine chemistry 230–231
Rowachol 1021
Rowatinex 1021
Royal Association in Aid of Deaf People 1032
Royal College of General Practitioners 1026, 1032
Royal College of Ophthalmologists 1031
Royal College of Psychiatrists 1035
Royal College of Surgeons 1037
Royal National Institute for the Blind 1031
Royal National Institute for Deaf People 1032
Royal Society for the Prevention of Accidents 1034, 1036
Rozex 1021
RSI *see* repetitive strain injury (RSI)
RSI-UK 1035
rubella 294
immunization *see* measles/mumps/rubella (MMR)
rugae, folds in empty stomach *622*
ruptured aneurysms
berry aneurysm rupture causing subarachnoid haemorrhage 534
ruptured aortic aneurysm 431
ruptured eardrum 597–598
ruptured membranes in pregnancy and labour
induction of labour *797*
premature rupture of the membranes 797
ruptured spleen *315*
ruptured tendons 395
ruptured varices 648–649
ruptures, involving digestive tract *see* hernias
Rynacrom 1021
Rynacrom Compound 1021
Rythmodan 1021

S

Sabril 1021
sacral nerves, nervous system structure and functions *511*
sacrum, location in spine *364*
saddle joints *364–365*
safe sex measures to prevent sexually transmitted infections (STIs) 68, 85, 765
safety
adolescents 32
air pollution monitoring 79
babies and infants 28
barbecue safety 80
children's car seats *29*
child safety inside and outside the home 30, 31, 77–81
drug and medication safety 881–882
exercising safely 59–60
fire prevention and smoke detection 79
food hygiene *79*
garden safety 80
health and safety landmarks *18–19*
health and safety, useful online sites and addresses 1036
home safety and health *47*, 77–80
in old age 37
pets and health 82
protecting your hearing *602*
radon protection 79
road safety 83, *84*
safe sex measures to prevent sexually transmitted infections (STIs) 68, 85, 765
stair safety gates *30*
in the sun *see* sunlight and sunbathing
water safety 81
work health and safety 82–83
see also accidents; injuries
St Andrew's Ambulance Association 1032, 1034
St John Ambulance 1032, 1034
Saizen 1021
Salactol 1021
Salagen 1021
Salamol 1021
Salatac 1021
Salazopyrin 1021
Salbulin 1021
salbutamol 1021
bronchodilator drugs 910–911
drugs for labour 938
salcatonin *see* calcitonin 1003
salicylic acid 1021
saliva
digestive system structure and functions 620, *621*, *622*, *625*
role in body's defences *444*

Salivace 1021
Saliva Orthana 1021
salivary gland disorders
  mumps, affecting parotid glands *45*, 293–294, 883–884
  salivary gland stones 635
  salivary gland tumours 635–636
  Sjögren's syndrome 463
salivary glands
  digestive system structure and functions 620, *621*, *622*
  disorders *see* salivary gland disorders
salivary gland stones 635
salivary gland tumours 635–636
Saliveze 1021
Salivix 1021
salmeterol 1021
  bronchodilator drugs 910–911
salmonellosis, food poisoning 629
Salofalk 1021
salt-losing crisis, in congenital adrenal hyperplasia 866
Saluric 1021
Salzone 1021
Samaritans, The 1029
samples collection for testing
  amniotic fluid, by amniocentesis *787*
  blood samples 221–222, *456*, *501*, *689*
  body fluid samples 223
  cell and tissue samples 223
  cerebrospinal fluid (CSF), by lumbar puncture *527*
  cervical cells, by cervical smear test *749*
  endometrial sampling, for tissue testing *738*
  faecal samples 222
  semen, for semen analysis 777
  sweat, by sweat testing for cystic fibrosis *824*
  throat swabs *223*
  urine samples 222
  see also aspiration; biopsies
samples testing 224
  blood *see* blood tests
  for body chemicals (biochemicals) *see* chemical tests
  cell tests 236–237
  genetic tests 238–241
  in medical laboratories *225*
  tests for abnormal chromosomes 238–239
  tests for abnormal genes 239–241
  tests for gene products or biochemical markers 241
  tests for microorganisms 234–235
  tissue tests 237
  urine *see* urine tests
Sandimmun 1021
Sandocal 1021
Sando-K 1021
Sandostatin 1021
SANE 1035
San Joaquin fever *see* coccidioidomycosis
Sanomigran 1021
saphenous vein bypass graft *411*
saquinavir 1021
  drugs for HIV infection and AIDS 887–888
sarcoidosis 498–499
sarcoma, Kaposi's *see* Kaposi's sarcoma
saturated fats *50*, 51
Saventrine 1021
Savlon 1021
scabies 355
scalds and minor burns, first aid 317, *988*
scalp disorders
  dandruff 358
  hair and scalp problems, symptoms chart 130–131
  scalp injuries 521
  scalp ringworm 352–353
  seborrhoeic dermatitis 333, 335–336
scans and scanning techniques
  blood flow *see* blood flow scans
  CT scanning *see* computerized tomography (CT) scanning
  magnetic resonance imaging (MRI) scans *213*, *243*, 248–250
  radionuclide *see* radionuclide scanning
  ultrasound *see* ultrasound scanning
scarlet fever 300
scars and scar formation
  keloids 349
  skin repair process *330*
Schering PC4 1021
Scheriproct 1021
schistosomiasis 81, 312–313
schizoid personality disorder 561
schizophrenia 560
  antipsychotic drugs 917–918
schizotypal personality disorder 561
sciatica 546–547
  in pregnancy *785*
sciatic nerves
  compressed *see* sciatica
  nervous system structure *509*, *546*
SCID *see* severe combined immunodeficiency (SCID)
sclera
  eye structure and functions *567*
  inflamed *see* scleritis
scleritis 574
scleroderma 462–463
sclerosing cholangitis, cause of cirrhosis 648
SCODA (Standing Conference on Drug Abuse) 1031
scoliosis 371
Scopoderm TTS 1021
scorpion stings *see* poisonous bites and stings 327
  poisonous bites and stings, first aid *994*
Scottish Down's Syndrome Association 1030
scrapes and cuts 356
screening and screening tests 42–45, 212, 214–215
  antenatal *see* antenatal tests and investigations
  blood cholesterol tests *44*, 231–232
  blood pressure measurement *44*, *404*
  cervical smear tests *44*, *749*
  common screening tests *44*
  for complications of diabetes mellitus *690*
  dental checkups *609*
  eyes and vision *see* eye and vision tests and investigations
  faecal occult blood test *44*, 233
  for gene disorders *see* genetic tests
  hearing tests in children *859*
  heel prick blood test in babies *44*, *867*
  mammography *44*, *759*
  for metabolic disorders *867*
  for prostate cancer 726
  reliability of test results 44
  sigmoidoscopy *661*
  using blood samples *see* blood tests
  using urine samples *see* urine tests
  see also self-examination
scrotum
  disorders *see* testes and scrotum disorders
  male reproductive system structure and functions 716, 717
scrub typhus 304
scurvy, caused by vitamin C deficiency 928
Sea-Legs 1021
seasonal allergic rhinitis 466–467
sebaceous cysts 348–349
sebaceous glands
  infected *see* boils
  skin structure *329*, *330*
seborrhoeic dermatitis 333, 335–336
seborrhoeic keratosis 348
sebum
  function and production in skin 328, *329*, *331*, *444*
  overproduction in acne 340
secobarbital 1021
Seconal Sodium 1021
secondary amenorrhoea 735
secondary amyloidosis 693
secondary bone cancer *see* bone metastases
secondary dysmenorrhoea 736
secondary glaucoma 575
secondary hyperparathyroidism 682–683
secondary hypogonadism, in females 739
secondary liver cancer *see* liver metastases
secondary lung cancer (lung metastases) 505
secondary polycythaemia 457
secondary stage syphilis 766
secondary teeth *606*
secondary tumours *see* metastases
second-degree burns 317
second stage of labour *782–783*
  problems during delivery 802–804
second trimester of pregnancy *780*
Sectral 1021
Securon SR 1021
seizures and convulsions
  anticonvulsant drugs 914–915
  first aid *989*
  see also epilepsy; febrile convulsions
selective serotonin reuptake inhibitors (SSRIs), antidepressant drugs 916–917
selegiline 1021
selenium 1021
selenium sulphide 1021
self-examination 44
  breasts *755*
  testes *720*
  urine appearance *169*
Self Help UK 1026
Selsun 1021
semen and semen production
  blood in semen, symptoms chart 182
  male reproductive system structure and functions 716, *717*, *763*
  semen analysis *777*
semicircular canals, ear structure and functions *593*, *595*
semi-movable joints *364–365*
seminal vesicles, male reproductive system structure and functions 716, *717*, *763*
seminiferous tubules, male reproductive system structure and functions *717*, *815*
seminoma, cancer of the testis 719–720
Semprex 1021
senile dementia *see* dementia
senile purpura 339
senna 1021
  laxatives 924–925
Senokot 1021
sensate focus technique, sex therapy *773*
senses *see* balance; hearing; smell; taste; touch; vision
sensorineural hearing loss 599, *600*
sensory cortex/sensory association cortex, location and role in information processing in the brain *515*
sensory nerve neuropathies 543–544
sensory nerves
  disorders *see* sensory nerve neuropathies
  role of sensory nerve impulses in voluntary and involuntary responses *514*
  sensory nerve roots in spinal cord *511*
sensory receptors
  baroreceptors, role in blood pressure control *401*
  nervous system structure and functions *513*
  organ of Corti, in the ear *592*, *593*, *594*
  in skin *329*, *331*, *513*
septal defects, congenital heart disease in babies and children 836–837
Septanest 1021
septicaemia 299
septic arthritis 381

Septrin 1021
septum
fungi structure *287*
heart structure *398*
hole in heart septum *see* septal defects
nasal septum, deviated 476
Serc 1021
Serdolect 1021
Serenace 1021
Serevent 1021
sermorelin 1021
Serophene 1021
serosa, digestive tract structure and functions *623*
serotonin antagonists, antiemetic drugs 922
serotonin reuptake inhibitors, selective *see* selective serotonin reuptake inhibitors (SSRIs)
Seroxat 1021
sertindole 1021
antipsychotic drugs 917–918
sertraline 1021
antidepressant drugs 916–917
Setlers 1021
severe cervical dysplasia 749, 750, *751*
severe combined immunodeficiency (SCID), congenital immunodeficiency 827
Sevoflurane 1021
Sevredol 1021
sex cells
female *see* eggs
male *see* sperm and sperm production
sex chromosome abnormalities and disorders
causes and inheritance *269*, 270–271
Klinefelter's syndrome 271, 822–823
tests and investigations *see* genetic tests
Turner's syndrome *238*, 271, 823
see also X-linked disorders
sex chromosomes 264, *265*
disorders *see* sex chromosome abnormalities and disorders
role in gender determination *268*, 270
sex drive 762
decreased 67, 769
effect of pregnancy 34
sex education 32, 67
sex hormones *see* female sex hormones; male sex hormones
sex therapy *773*
sexual arousal and sexual response 762, *763*
sexual assault 320
sexual history 68
sexual intercourse 762, *763*
after major surgery 946
communicating your sexual needs 67, 770
during and after pregnancy 34, 35
problems *see* sexual problems
rape *see* sexual assault
safe sex measures to prevent sexually transmitted infections (STIs) 68, 85, 765
sexual history 68
sexual relationships 67
see also contraception; female reproductive system; male reproductive system; sexually transmitted infections (STIs)
sexuality and sexual behaviour 67–68, 762
sexually transmitted infections (STIs) 85, 764
cause of pelvic inflammatory disease (PID) 741
chlamydial pelvic infection 765–766
genital herpes 767–768
genital warts 768
gonorrhoea 764–765
HIV infection and AIDS 297–298
molluscum contagiosum 355
nongonococcal urethritis (NGU) 765
prevention *765*
pubic lice 768
safe sex measures to prevent spread of STIs 68, 85, 765
syphilis 766, 817
trichomoniasis 767
useful online sites and addresses 1036
sexual needs, communicating 67, 770
sexual problems 67
decreased sex drive 67, 769
failure of orgasm 770
impotence 770–771
impotence, symptoms chart 180
painful intercourse in men 772
painful intercourse in women 772–773
painful intercourse in women, symptoms chart 196–197
premature ejaculation 771–772
squeeze technique *771*
sex therapy for *773*
useful online sites and addresses 1036
vaginismus 773
sexual reproduction, human *see* female reproductive system; male reproductive system; pregnancy; sexual intercourse
shinbone *see* tibia
shin disorders, erythema nodosum 348
shingles *see* herpes zoster
shock 414
anaphylactic *see* anaphylaxis
electric *see* cardioversion; electrical injuries
first aid *987*
shock waves, use in lithotripsy *702*
short-acting insulins, drugs for diabetes mellitus 931
shortness of breath
symptoms chart 144–145
symptoms relief for the terminally ill 965, *966*
shortsightedness *see* myopia
shoulder presentation, abnormal fetal presentation 801
shoulders
ball-and-socket joint in *365*
frozen shoulder 385–386
joint movement range 362
shoulder joint replacement *377*
show, sign that labour is about to start *782*
shunt for hydrocephalus *845*
sick building syndrome 82
sickle-cell disease *273*, 448–449
Sickle Cell Society 1027
sick sinus syndrome 419
side effects of drugs 880, 882
see also individual articles on specific drug groups
side stretch, warming up and cooling down in your exercise routine *61*
SIDS *see* sudden infant death syndrome (SIDS)
sight *see* vision
sigmoidoscopy *661*
sildenafil 1021
impotence treatment 771
silicosis 500
silver nitrate 1021
silver sulfadiazine 1021
Simeco 1021
simple fractures *see* closed fractures
simple interrupted stitches, rejoining tissue after surgery *948*
simple partial seizures, epilepsy 525–526
simple phobias 552–553
simple pneumoconiosis 499–500
Simplene 1021
simvastatin 1021
lipid-lowering drugs 935
Sinemet 1021
Sinequan 1021
single-celled organisms *see* bacteria; protozoa; yeasts
single gene disorders 271–273
achondroplasia *273*, 833
alpha$_1$-antitrypsin deficiency 489
Becker muscular dystrophy 826
colour blindness *269*, *273*, 591
cystic fibrosis 272, *273*, 824–825, *962*
Duchenne muscular dystrophy 826
familial adenomatous polyposis (FAP), polyps in the colon 661, 666
genetic counselling 26, *272*
haemochromatosis *273*, 692–693
haemophilia and Christmas disease *273*, 452
hereditary nonpolyposis colorectal cancer (HNPCC) 666
Huntington's disease *273*, 538
inherited hyperlipidaemias *273*, 692, 935
juvenile polycystic kidney disease *273*, 704
Marfan's syndrome *273*, 824
multiple endocrine neoplasia (MEN) 683
muscular dystrophy *273*, 826
nephrogenic diabetes insipidus 678
neurofibromatosis *273*, 827
polycystic kidney disease *273*, 704
porphyria *273*, 693
primary amyloidosis 693
retinitis pigmentosa *273*, 581
sickle-cell disease *273*, 448–449
tests and investigations *see* genetic tests
thalassaemia *273*, 449–450
von Willebrand's disease *273*, 452
see also congenital immunodeficiency; inborn errors of metabolism
single-photon-emission computerized tomography (SPECT) scanning *243*, 253
Singulair 1021
sinoatrial node
disorders *see* sick sinus syndrome; supraventricular tachycardia (SVT)
heart structure 396, *399*
Sinthrome 1021
sinuses (blood vessels), venous sinus in the brain *510*
sinuses (facial) *470*
inflamed *see* sinusitis
sinusitis 475
decongestants 909
sinusoids
blood vessels in bone marrow *440*
blood vessels in liver *624*
Sinutab 1021
Siopel 1021
sitting position, correct *382*
Sjögren's syndrome 463
skeletal muscles 362, *366–367*
skeleton *363*
Skelid 1021
skin
disorders *see* skin conditions and disorders
effect of environment 328
effects of growth and aging *22–23*
effect of sunlight *47*, 80, 328
functions 328, *331*, *444*
growth and repair *330*
inspection during physical examination *219*
pigmented cells *see* melanocytes
sensory receptors *329*, *331*, *513*
skin care for the terminally ill 965
structure *329*, *330*
subcutaneous and transdermal drug delivery routes *879*
vernix on skin of newborn babies *811*
skin cancer 80, 344–347
basal cell carcinoma 344–345
Kaposi's sarcoma 346–347
malignant melanoma 343, *346*
squamous cell carcinoma 345
Skin Cancer Foundation 1036
Skin Care Campaign 1036
skin grafting *318*
skin and hair conditions and disorders
acne 340–341, 890–891
atopic eczema 333, 334
birthmarks 828
blistering diseases 336
calluses and corns 349
cancer *see* skin cancer
chilblains 350

skin and hair conditions and disorders (continued)
in children *see* skin conditions and disorders in children
contact dermatitis 333, 335
dandruff 358
dermatitis herpetiformis, blistering disease 336
discoid lupus erythematosus (DLE) 347
drugs acting on the skin 890–893
eczema 333
erythema multiforme 337
erythema nodosum 348
freckles 343
generalized skin conditions 332–339
general skin problems, symptoms chart 126–127
haemangiomas, birthmarks 828
hyperhidrosis 342
infections and infestations *see* skin infections and infestations
injuries *see* skin injuries
itching 339
keloids 349
laser treatment on the skin *951*
leg ulcers 350
lichen planus 336–337
localized skin conditions 340–350
moles 343, 828
naevi 343, 828
pemphigoid, blistering disease 336
pemphigus, blistering disease 336
photosensitivity 338
pigmented naevi, birthmarks 828
pilonidal sinus 360
pityriasis rosea 337–338
port-wine stains, birthmarks 828
pressure sores 350
prickly heat 342
psoriasis 332–333, 890–891
purpura 339
rhinophyma, effect of rosacea 341, 342
rosacea 341–342
sarcoidosis 498–499
scalp *see* scalp disorders
scleroderma 462–463
sebaceous cysts 348–349
seborrhoeic dermatitis 333, 335–336
seborrhoeic keratosis 348
senile purpura 339
skin infections 351–355
skin tags 348
solar keratosis 347
stretch marks 349
symptoms charts 125–129
useful online sites and addresses 1036
vitiligo 342–343
see also rashes
skin and hair conditions and disorders in children 828
birthmarks 828
cradle cap 829
eczema in children 829–830
guttate psoriasis 332, *333*
haemangiomas, birthmarks 828
hand, foot, and mouth disease 831
Henoch–Schönlein purpura 339, 838–839
Mongolian blue spots, birthmarks 828
nappy rash 829
pigmented naevi, birthmarks 828
port-wine stains, birthmarks 828
roseola infantum 830–831
stork marks, birthmarks 828
strawberry naevi (haemangiomas), birthmarks 828
skin infections and infestations
athlete's foot 353
boils 351
cellulitis 352
cold sores 354
common warts 354–355
flat warts 355
folliculitis 352
Hansen's disease 302
impetigo 351–352
mite infestation *see* scabies
molluscum contagiosum 355
mosaic warts 354
paronychia 361
pityriasis versicolor 353
plantar warts 354
preparations for skin infections and infestations 892–893
pubic lice 768
ringworm 352–353
scabies 355
sporotrichosis 309
warts 354–355
skin injuries
blisters 357
bruises 357
burns 317–318
cuts and scrapes 356
effects of serious injuries *315*
needlestick injury 356
skin repair after injury *330*
sunburn 80, 356, 357
skin patches for transdermal drug delivery *879*, *937*
skin prick test *468*
Skin Site, The 1036
skin tags 348
skin tests
patch testing *335*
red rash assessment *129*
skin biopsy *344*
skin prick test *468*
skin-tunnelled catheters *456*
skull
appearance in multiple myeloma *457*
appearance in thalassaemia *449*
fixed joints *see* sutures (seams)
growth and development in babies and children *813*
of newborn babies *811*
role in protecting brain and eyes *509*, *567*
sinuses *470*
skull fractures, head injuries *315*, 521–522
structure and location of main skull bones *363*
SLE (systemic lupus erythematosus) 461–462
sleep 73–74
disorders *see* sleep problems and disorders
lifestyle choices *47*
positioning baby for sleep *820*
sleeping drugs 915–916
sleep studies *477*
sleep problems and disorders 74
central sleep apnoea 478
difficulty sleeping, symptoms chart 100–101
insomnia 554
narcolepsy 526–527, 918
nightmares and night terrors, sleeping problems in children 851
obstructive sleep apnoea (OSA) 478
in pregnancy *785*
sleep apnoea 477–478
sleeping drugs 915–916
sleeping problems in babies 818
sleeping problems in children 851
sleepwalking, sleeping problems in children 851
snoring 477
useful online sites and addresses 1036–1037
sleep studies *477*
slimming diets 54
slings, first aid uses *998*
slipped disc *see* prolapsed or herniated disc
slipped femoral epiphysis 834
slit-lamp examination *574*
Slo-Indo 1021
Slo-Phyllin 1021
Slow-Fe 1021
Slow-K 1021
Slow-Sodium 1021
Slozem 1021
small cell carcinoma, primary lung cancer 503–505
small intestine
digestive system structure and functions 620, *621–623*, *625*
disorders *see* intestinal disorders
small vessel disease, diabetic vascular disease 432–434
smell
role of olfactory nerve *511*
role of sensory receptors *513*
smoke detection *see* fire prevention and smoke detection
smoking *see* tobacco and smoking
smooth muscle 362, *367*
direct smooth-muscle relaxants, antispasmodic drugs and motility stimulants 926
snake bites *see* poisonous bites and stings
poisonous bites and stings, first aid *994*
Snellen chart, use in vision tests *587*
Sno Phenicol 1021
snoring 477
Sno Tears 1021
social behaviour and play, developmental milestones during childhood *814*
social phobias 552–553
soda mint tablets 1021
sodium 1021
sodium acid phosphate 1021
sodium aurothiomalate 1021
antirheumatic drugs 895–896
sodium bicarbonate 1021
antacids 923
drugs acting on the ear 921
sodium calcium edetate 1021
sodium cellulose phosphate 1021
sodium chloride 1021
sodium citrate 1021
laxatives 924–925
sodium clodronate 1022
sodium content of packaged foods, nutritional information on food labels *52*
sodium cromoglicate 1022
drugs acting on the eye 919–920
sodium feredetate 1022
sodium fluoride 1022
sodium fusidate 1022
sodium nitroprusside 1022
sodium perborate 1022
sodium picosulfate 1022
laxatives 924–925
sodium stibogluconate 1022
antiprotozoal drugs 888
sodium tetradecyl sulphate 1022
sodium valproate 1022
anticonvulsant drugs 914–915
antimigraine drugs 913
mood-stabilizing drugs 918
Sofradex 1022
soft contact lenses *588*
for astigmatism 589
cause of corneal abrasion 571
soft drugs, recreational drugs 65
soft palate, movement during swallowing *622*
soiling in children *see* encopresis
Solarcaine 1022
solar keratosis 347
Solian 1022
Solpadeine 1022
Solpadol 1022
soluble fibre 50
Solu-Cortef 1022
Solu-Medrone 1022
Solvazinc 1022
somatization 559
somatropin 1022
pituitary drugs 934–935
Somatuline 1022
Sominex 1022
Soneryl 1022
soothing preparations, antipruritic drugs 891–892
Sorbichew 1022
Sorbid SA 1022
sorbitol 1022
Sorbitrate 1022
sore throat 479
symptoms chart 139
Sotacor 1022
sotalol 1022
beta-blocker drugs 898–899
sound
information processing in the brain *515*, 592, *594*
pitch, frequency and intensity 592
see also hearing
spacer devices, use in asthma treatment *485*, *839*, 910

Spasmonal 1022
spasms
antispasmodic drugs and motility stimulants, for spasms in the intestine 926
muscle *see* muscle cramp; torticollis
special care baby units *959*
specific immune responses, body's defences *445*
specific learning disabilities 854
useful online sites and addresses 1034
SPECT scanning *see* single-photon-emission computerized tomography (SPECT) scanning
spectinomycin 1022
Spectraban 1022
speculum
use in artificial insemination *775*
use in cervical smear test *749*
use in colposcopy *750*
use in endometrial sampling *738*
use in viewing techniques 254
speech *see* voice, speech, and language
speech discrimination tests, hearing test in children *859*
speech therapy *955*, 963
sperm and sperm production
chromosome content of sperm cells 264, *267*, *268*
male reproductive system structure and functions 716, *717*, 762, *763*
meiosis (cell division) in sperm and eggs *267*, 270
mutations in eggs and sperm *269*
problems, cause of male infertility 777
sperm count and semen analysis *777*
sperm use in infertility treatments *see* artificial insemination; assisted conception
see also fertilization and implantation (embedding)
spermatic cord
male reproductive system structure *717*
twisted *see* torsion of the testis
spermatoceles *see* epididymal cysts
spermatozoa *see* sperm and sperm production
SPFs *see* sunscreens, sunblocks, and sun protection factors (SPFs)
sphenoid sinus *470*
sphincters
lower oesophageal sphincter, digestive tract structure and functions *622*
oesophageal sphincter disorders *see* achalasia; gastro-oesophageal reflux (GOR)
pyloric sphincter, digestive system structure and functions *621*, *622*
sphincter muscles, in the bladder *697*
sphygmomanometer, use in blood pressure measurement *404*
spider bites *see* poisonous bites and stings 327
poisonous bites and stings, first aid *994*
spider naevi, symptom of liver failure *650*
Spina Bifida Association of America 1027
spina bifida, neural tube defect 844–845
spinal accessory nerve, nervous system structure and functions *511*
spinal anaesthesia 914, *945*
spinal cord
disorders *see* brain and spinal cord disorders
nervous system structure and functions 508, *509–512*, *514*
spinal cord tissue *see* grey matter; white matter
spinal injuries 524
airway opening technique, first aid *982*
first aid *990*
spinal nerves
cervical nerves *511*
coccygeal nerves *511*
lumbar nerves *511*
sacral nerves *511*
structure and functions *509*, *511*
thoracic nerves *511*
spinal reflexes, involuntary responses by the nervous system *514*
spine
bone densitometry *369*
disorders *see* spine disorders
effects of serious injuries *315*
flexibility *364*
semi-movable joints in 362, *364–365*
structure and functions *364*, *509*
spine disorders
ankylosing spondylitis 378–379
cervical spondylosis 376
injuries *see* spinal injuries
kyphosis and lordosis 371
manipulative therapies *955*, 973–974
microdiscectomy *385*
prolapsed or herniated disc 384–385
scoliosis 371
spondylolithesis 385
see also brain and spinal cord disorders
spiral CT scanning 242, 248
spiral fractures 392
spirilla, type of bacteria *286*
spirochetes, type of bacteria *286*
Spiro-Co 1022
Spiroctan-M 1022
Spirolone 1022
spirometry *488*
spironolactone 1022
diuretic drugs 902
Spirospare 1022
spleen
cancer *see* lymphomas
effects of serious injuries *315*
location and role in lymphatic system *443*
ruptured *315*
splinter haemorrhages, effect of infective endocarditis *426*
split personality *see* schizophrenia
spondylolisthesis 385
spongy bone
role in bone repair *364*
structure 362, *362*, *363*
spongy erectile tissue, in penis *717*
spontaneous abortion *see* miscarriage
spoon-shaped nails, nail abnormality 360
Sporanox 1022
spores, fungal *287*
sporotrichosis 309
Sport England 1031
sports injuries 391–392
spots
age spots *see* lentigo
café au lait spots, neurofibromatosis symptom *827*
Koplik spots, measles symptom *293*
Mongolian blue spots, birthmarks 828
purpuric spots and petechiae, purpura symptoms 339
white spots, nail abnormality 360
see also pimples; rashes
sprains
neck sprain *see* whiplash
sprains and strains, first aid *991*
spray endings, type of muscle proprioceptor *513*
spread (metastasis), cancer *275*, *277*, *279*
Sprilon 1022
sprue *see* coeliac disease
squamous cell carcinoma 345
primary lung cancer 503–505
squeeze technique, premature ejaculation self-help technique *771*
SSRIs *see* selective serotonin reuptake inhibitors (SSRIs)
stab injuries *315*, 319
staghorn kidney stones 701, *702*
staging cancer *279*
stair safety gates *30*
standing correctly *382*
in pregnancy *785*
stapedotomy *598*
stapes
disorders *see* otosclerosis
ear structure and functions *593*, *594*
staphylococcal infections
bacterial pneumonia 490–491
food poisoning 629
mastitis 809
pneumonia 490
styes 583
toxic shock syndrome 300
staples, rejoining tissue after surgery *948*
starches *see* complex carbohydrates
Staril 1022
statins, lipid-lowering drugs 935
status epilepticus, epilepsy 525, 526
stavudine 1022
drugs for HIV infection and AIDS 887–888
STDs *see* sexually transmitted infections (STIs)
steam inhalation *475*
Stelazine 1022
stem cells, role in blood cell formation *440*
Stemetil 1022
stenosis
in heart valves *see* valve stenosis
pyloric stenosis in infants 863
stents
use in coronary angioplasty *409*
use in palliative surgery for cancer *282*, 654
sterculia 1022
stereoscopic vision *569*
sterile dressings, first aid uses *996*
sterilization surgery
female sterilization 70, *743*
male sterilization 70, *721*
Ster-Zac 1022
Stesolid 1022
Stiedex 1022
Stiemycin 1022
stilboestrol 1022
stillbirth 805
Stillbirth and Neonatal Death Society 1029, 1036
Still's disease *see* systemic juvenile chronic arthritis
Stilnoct 1022
Stimlor 1022
stimulant drugs
antispasmodic drugs and motility stimulants 926
central nervous system (CNS) stimulant drugs 918
recreational drug effects and risks 65, *66*
stimulant laxatives 924–925
uterine stimulant drugs, drugs for labour 938
stimuli, nervous system's responses to stimuli 328, 508, *513–514*
stings *see* bites and stings
stitches, rejoining tissue after surgery *948*
stomach
acids *see* stomach acids
autonomic nervous system responses *514*
digestive system structure and functions 620, *621–622*, *625*
disorders *see* stomach and duodenum disorders
hormone production 620, *671*
stomach acids
neutralized by antacids 923
production and role in digestive system 620, *622*, *625*
role in body's defences *444*
stomach cancer 642
stomach and duodenum disorders 639
acute gastritis 640
atrophic gastritis 640
chronic gastritis 640
drug treatments *see* antacids; antiemetic drugs; ulcer-healing drugs
duodenal ulcer, type of peptic ulcer 640–642
gastric ulcer, type of peptic ulcer 640–642

stomach and duodenum disorders (continued)
  gastritis 640
  gastroenteritis 85, 628–629
  gastro-oesophageal reflux (GOR) 636–637
  gastro-oesophageal reflux (GOR) in infants 863
  gastro-oesophageal reflux (GOR) in pregnancy 784
  Helicobacter pylori infection 639–640, 932
  indigestion 626, *627*, 923
  nonulcer dyspepsia 626–627
  peptic ulcer 640–642
  pyloric stenosis in infants 863
  stomach cancer 642
  upper digestive tract endoscopy *641*
stoma, created by colostomy surgery *666*
stomatitis 632–633
  of gums *see* gingivitis
  of tongue *see* glossitis
stones
  bladder stones 714
  cholesterol stones, gallstones 651
  gallstones 651
  kidney stones 701–703
  lithotripsy *702*
  pigment stones, gallstones 651
  salivary gland stones 635
  staghorn kidney stones 701, *702*
stools *see* faeces
stork marks, birthmarks 828
strabismus 857–858
strains
  muscle strains and tears 395
  neck strain *see* whiplash
  repetitive strain injury 82, 389
  sprains and strains, first aid *991*
strangulated hernia 661–662
strawberry naevi, birthmarks 828
Strepsils 1022
Streptase 1022
streptococcal infections
  bacterial meningitis 527
  bacterial meningitis in children 848–849
  bacterial pneumonia 490–491
  congenital infections, in newborn babies 817
  rheumatic fever 429
  scarlet fever 300
  toxic shock syndrome 300
streptokinase 1022
  thrombolytic drugs 904–905
streptomycin 1022
  antibiotics 885–886
  antituberculous drugs 886
stress *17*, 74–76
  biofeedback to overcome stress 975
  fight or flight response to stress or danger 670, *673*
  hypnotherapy to overcome stress 974–975
  post-traumatic stress disorder (PTSD) 553
  stress headaches *see* tension headaches
  stress ratings of life events *74*
  useful online sites and addresses 1037
  see also anxiety and anxiety-related disorders; relaxation
stress fractures 392
stress incontinence 711–712
stress polycythaemia 457
Stress UK 1035, 1037
stretch marks (striae) 349
  in Cushing's syndrome *685*
stretches
  back-strengthening exercises *383*
  warming up and cooling down in your exercise routine *60–61*
strictures
  oesophageal stricture 636, *637*
  urethral stricture 714
stroke 532–534
  useful online sites and addresses 1037
Stroke Association, The 1032, 1037
strongyloidiasis, tropical worm infestation 312
structural chromosomal abnormalities, cause of chromosome disorders 271
struts *see* trabeculae
Stugeron 1022
Stuttering Foundation of America 1037
styes 583
subarachnoid haemorrhage 534–535
subarachnoid space
  bleeding into *see* subarachnoid haemorrhage
  nervous system structure *509, 510*
subclavian vein, location and role in lymphatic system *443*
subconjunctival haemorrhage 571
subcutaneous fat
  function 328, *331*
  skin structure *329*
subcutaneous route, drug delivery route *879*
subcuticular stitches, rejoining tissue after surgery *948*
subdural haemorrhage 535
sublingual glands, salivary glands location *622*
sublingual route
  drug delivery route *879*
  using sublingual sprays *900*
submandibular glands, salivary glands location *622*
submucosa, digestive tract structure and functions *623*
sucralfate 1022
  ulcer-healing drugs 923–924
suction termination of pregnancy *789*
Sudafed 1022
sudden infant death syndrome (SIDS) 28, 820
Sudocrem 1022
suffocation
  statistics 314
  see also asphyxiation
sugars
  in the diet 49
  digestion and metabolism disorders *see* diabetes mellitus; galactosaemia; lactose intolerance
  production of simple sugars by digestive system and use in metabolism *625, 675*
  sugar content of packaged foods, information on food labels *52*
  see also glucose
suicide *see* attempted suicide and suicide
sulconazole 1022
  antifungal drugs 889
Suleo-M 1022
sulfacetamide 1022
sulfadiazine 1022
  antibiotics 885–886
  pyrimethamine with sulfadiazine, antiprotozoal drugs 888
sulfadimidine 1022
sulfadoxine 1022
  pyrimethamine with sulfadoxine, antimalarial drugs 888–889
sulfamethoxazole 1022
sulfametopyrazine 1022
sulfasalazine 1022
  aminosalicylate drugs 924
  antirheumatic drugs 895–896
sulfathiazole 1022
sulfinpyrazone 1022
sulindac 1022
  nonsteroidal anti-inflammatory drugs (NSAIDs) 894
Sulparex 1022
sulphonamides, antibiotics 885–886
sulphonylurea drugs
  drugs for diabetes mellitus 931–932
  how they work *931*
sulphur 1022
sulpiride 1022
Sulpitil 1022
sumatriptan 1022
  antimigraine drugs 913
sunlight and sunbathing
  cause of cancer 80, *274*, 344
  cause of freckles 343
  cause of solar keratosis 347
  cause of sunburn 80, 356, *357*
  effect on skin *47*, 80, 328
  lifestyle choices *47*
  photosensitivity to sunlight 338
  safety precautions 80–81
  sunglasses 81
  sunscreens, sunblocks, and sun protection factors (SPFs) 80–81, 893
  UVA and UVB components of sunlight 80, 893
superficial thrombophlebitis 439
superior vena cava, location and role in cardiovascular system *397–400*
supportive care, cancer 282
supportive group therapy 971
suppositories *879*
  prostaglandin suppositories/pessaries, for induction of labour *797*, 938
Suprane 1022
suprapubic catheterization, of the bladder *713*
supraventricular tachycardia (SVT) 416–417
Suprax 1022
Suprecur 1022
Suprefact 1022
surface layer cells, skin structure *329, 330*
surface proteins, on viruses *285*
Surgam 1022
surgeries, doctors' *217*
surgery 940
  advances and landmarks in surgery 876–877
  cardiovascular system *see* cardiovascular system surgery
  convalescence after major surgery 946
  cosmetic surgery 952
  digestive system *see* digestive system surgery
  ear surgery *see* cochlear implants; stapedotomy; grommet insertion
  endoscopic surgery 940, 948–950
  eye *see* eye surgery
  female reproductive system *see* female reproductive system surgery
  heart *see* cardiovascular system surgery
  heart–lung machines *953*
  for hydrocephalus *see* shunt for hydrocephalus
  for infertility *see* assisted conception
  laser *see* laser treatments
  major surgery 943–946
  male reproductive system surgery *see* circumcision; penile prosthesis implant; vasectomy
  microsurgery 950–951
  minimally invasive surgery *949*
  minor surgery 942–943
  musculoskeletal system *see* musculoskeletal system surgery
  open surgery 947–948
  operating theatres *941*
  in outpatient and day care treatment 956
  plastic *see* plastic surgery
  postoperative care and monitoring 945–946
  postoperative rehabilitation *see* rehabilitation and rehabilitation therapies
  in pregnancy, labour, and childbirth *see* caesarean section; episiotomy; termination of pregnancy
  preparations on the day of major surgery 944
  prostate gland surgery *see* prostatectomy
  rejoining tissue after surgery *948*
  role in weight control 54
  surgical advances 940
  on the throat *see* tonsillectomy and adenoidectomy
  transplant *see* transplant surgery
  undergoing surgery *940*
  useful online sites and addresses 1037
  see also anaesthesia
Surmontil 1022
survival rates, cancer 283
Suscard 1022
susceptibility to disease 261–262
  role of inheritance *21*, 24–26

suspensory ligament, eye structure and functions *567*
Sustac 1022
Sustanon 1022
Sustiva 1022
sutures (seams)
  during skull growth and development in babies and children *813*
  fixed joints in skull *364–365*
  in newborn baby's skull *811*
suxamethonium 1022
SVT *see* supraventricular tachycardia (SVT)
swallowing
  barium swallow, contrast X-ray technique 246, *637*
  digestive system function *622*
  oral drug delivery route *879*
  swallowed poisons, first aid 321, *994*
  swallowing difficulties, symptoms chart 147
sweat
  excessive sweating in hyperhidrosis 342
  excessive sweating, symptoms chart 104–105
  excessive sweating when travelling in hot climates 85–86
  production in skin *329, 331*
  role in body's defences *444*
  role in thermoregulation *331*
  sweat testing, for cystic fibrosis *824*
sweat ducts and pores, skin structure *329*
sweat glands, skin structure *329, 331*
swelling and swellings
  ankles *see* swollen ankles
  in the eyelid *see* chalazion
  lumps and swellings, symptoms chart 106–107
  swollen abdomen, symptoms charts 156
  swollen glands *see* lymphadenopathy
  in the testes *see* hydrocele
  see also oedema
swimmer's ear *see* otitis externa
swollen abdomen, symptoms chart 156
swollen ankles
  common complaints in pregnancy 784, *785*
  symptoms chart 178–179
swollen glands *see* lymphadenopathy
sympathetic nerves and responses, autonomic nervous system structure and functions *514*
sympathomimetics, bronchodilator drugs 910–911
symptoms
  assessing and understanding 88–89
  charts *see* symptoms charts
  symptoms relief as aim of treatment 874
  symptoms relief for the terminally ill 965, *966*
symptoms charts 88
  abdominal pain 152–156, 192–193, 208–209
  abdominal swelling 156
  abnormal vaginal bleeding 190–191
  abnormal vaginal discharge 194
  absent periods 186–187
  anal and rectal problems 157
  ankle swelling 178–179
  anxiety 124
  arm or hand pain 174
  back pain 170–171
  being overweight 98–99, 210
  bladder control problems 165
  bleeding in pregnancy 190
  bleeding from the vagina outside menstruation 190–191
  blood in faeces 160
  blood in semen 182
  blood in vomit 148
  breast problems in females 184–185
  breathing and respiratory problems 142–146, 204–205
  chest pain 162–163
  children's *see* children's symptoms charts
  confusion and/or forgetfulness 120–121
  constipation 160–161
  coughing 142–143, 206–207
  coughing up blood 142
  dehydration caused by diarrhoea 158
  depressed feelings 122–123
  diarrhoea 158–159, 200–201
  difficulty sleeping 100–101
  difficulty speaking 119
  difficulty swallowing 147
  digestive system disorders 148–161
  disturbed or impaired vision 134–135
  earache 138
  excessive sweating 104–105
  eye problems 132–133
  facial pain 118
  feeling depressed 122–123
  feeling faint and passing out 108–109
  feeling unwell 92–93
  female reproductive system 184–197
  fever 102–103, 202–203
  fever with rash 128–129
  forgetfulness and/or confusion 120–121
  frequent urination 166–167
  general skin problems 126–127
  genital irritation in women 195
  hair and scalp problems 130–131
  hand or arm pain 174
  headache 110–111
  hearing loss 136–137
  heavy periods 189
  hoarseness and/or voice loss 140–141
  impaired or disturbed vision 134–135
  impotence 180
  intercourse difficulties 180, 196–197
  irritated or painful eye 132–133
  itching 125
  joint pain 176–177
  leg pain 175
  loss of weight 96–97, 210
  lower abdominal pain in women 192–193
  lumps and swellings 106–107
  male reproductive system 180–183
  menstrual problems 186–189
  neck pain or stiffness 172–173
  numbness and/or tingling 114–115
  pain *see* pain symptoms charts
  painful arm or hand 174
  painful intercourse in women 196–197
  painful or irritated eye 132–133
  painful joints 176–177
  painful leg 175
  painful periods 188
  painful urination 168–169
  palpitations 164
  passing out and feeling faint 108–109
  penis problems 182–183
  period problems 186–189
  poor bladder control 165
  problems with the penis 182–183
  rash with fever 128–129
  rectal and anal problems 157
  recurrent abdominal pain 154–155
  recurrent vomiting 150–151
  respiratory and breathing problems 142–146, 204–205
  scalp and hair problems 130–131
  scrotum and testes problems 181
  sexual difficulties 180, 196–197
  shortness of breath 134–145
  sight problems 134–135
  skin problems 125–129
  sleeping difficulties 100–101
  sore throat 139
  speech problems 119, 140–141
  swallowing difficulties 147
  sweating excessively 104–105
  swellings and lumps 106–107
  swollen abdomen 156
  swollen ankles 178–179
  testes and scrotum problems 181
  throat problems 139, 147
  tingling and/or numbness 114–115
  tiredness 94–95
  twitching and tremor 116–117
  urination problems 165–169
  vaginal bleeding outside menstruation 190–191
  vaginal discharge, abnormal 194
  vertigo 112–113
  visual problems 134–135
  voice problems 119, 140–141
  vomiting 148–151, 198–199
  weight problems 96–99, 210
  wheezing 146
sympto-thermal method, natural method of contraception *71*
Synalar 1022
synapses, nerve cells structure and functions *512*
synaptic end bulbs, nerve cells structure and functions *512*
Synarel 1022
Syndol 1022
Synflex 1022
synovial fluid, in joints *364*
synovial joints *364–365*
synovial membrane, in joints *364*
Syntaris 1022
Syntocinon 1022
syphilis 766
  congenital infections, in newborn babies 817
syringe drivers/pumps, for analgesia/pain relief *283, 966*
Syscor MR 1022
systemic arthritis 835
systemic circulation 396, *400*
systemic lupus erythematosus (SLE) 461–462
systemic sclerosis *see* scleroderma
systolic blood pressure *401*
Sytron 1022

T

T_3 *see* thyroid hormone (T_3)
T_4 *see* thyroxine (T_4)
tacalcitol 1022
tachycardias
  atrial fibrillation 417–418
  supraventricular tachycardia (SVT) 416–417
  type of arrhythmia 415
  ventricular fibrillation, cause of cardiac arrest 419–420
tacrolimus 1022
  immunosuppressants 906–907
Tagamet 1022
talipes *see* clubfoot
TAMBA (Twins and Multiple Births Association) 1036
Tambocor 1022
Tamofen 1022
tamoxifen 1022
  anticancer drugs 907–908
  breast cancer treatment 761
  sex hormones and related drugs 933–934
Tampovagan 1022
tamsulosin 1022
  drugs that affect bladder control 939
  drugs for prostate disorders 938–939
Tanatril 1022
tapeworm infestation 313
target cells, type of nerve cell *512*
target heart rate during exercise 59
Tarivid 1022
taste
  role of cranial nerves *511*
  role of sensory receptors *513*
taste buds structure and functions *513*
Tavanic 1022
Tavegil 1022
Tay–Sachs disease *273*, 868
tazarotene 1022
tazobactam 1022
TB *see* tuberculosis (TB)
T-cells (T-lymphocytes)
  production control by thymus gland *671*
  role in cellular immune response *445*

TCP Liquid 1023
tear glands *566*, 583
  disorders *see* eyelid and tear system disorders
tears (eye secretion)
  artificial tears, drugs acting on the eye 919–920
  production disorders *see* eyelid and tear system disorders
  production and functions *566*, 583
  role in body's defences *444*, *566*, 583
  tear apparatus *566*
tears (injury)
  ligament injuries 394
  muscle strains and tears 395
  ruptured tendons 395
  torn knee cartilage 395
Tears Naturale 1023
tectorial membrane, ear structure and functions *594*
teeth
  artificial *see* crowns and replacement teeth
  dental checkups *609*
  discoloured 612–613
  dislodged or knocked out *see* avulsed tooth
  disorders *see* tooth disorders
  effects of growth and aging *22–23*
  missing 615–616
  of newborn babies *811*
  oral hygiene 608, *610*, 617
  role in digestion 620, *622*
  structure, functions, and development 606, *607*
  tooth care for babies and infants 27
  tooth care for children 29, 30
  tooth care for older adults 35
teething 819–820
Tegretol 1023
teicoplanin 1023
Telfast 1023
temazepam 1023
  sleeping drugs 915–916
Temodal 1023
temozolomide 1023
  anticancer drugs 907–908
temperature *see* body temperature; environmental temperature
temporal arteritis 464–465
temporal lobe, brain structure *510*
temporary colostomy *666*
temporomandibular joint disorder 616
temporomandibular joint, in the jaw *607*
Tenchlor 1023
tendinitis and tenosynovitis 390
tendons
  connecting muscles to bones *366*, 388
  disorders *see* muscle and tendon disorders
Tenif 1023
Tenkicin 1023
tennis elbow and golfer's elbow 389–390
Tenoret-50 1023
Tenoretic 1023
Tenormin 1023
tenosynovitis and tendinitis 390
tenoxicam 1023
TENS *see* transcutaneous electrical nerve stimulation (TENS)
tension headaches 518
  in children 847
tension, muscle 362
Tensipine MR 1023
Tensium 1023
Teoptic 1023
teratoma, cancer of the testis 719
terazosin 1023
  antihypertensive drugs 897–898
  drugs that affect bladder control 939
  drugs for prostate disorders 938–939
terbinafine 1023
  antifungal drugs 889
  preparations for skin infections and infestations 892–893
terbutaline 1023
  bronchodilator drugs 910–911
  drugs for labour 938
terfenadine 1023
  antihistamines 906
Terfinax 1023
terlipressin 1023
terminal illnesses *see* care of the dying; death
termination of pregnancy *789*
Terra-Cortril 1023
Terramycin 1023
Terrence Higgins Trust 1033
tertiary stage syphilis 766
Tertroxin 1023
testes
  disorders *see* testes and scrotum disorders
  during puberty *716*, *815*
  hormone production *671*, 717
  male reproductive system structure and functions 716, *717*, *762*, *763*
  self-examination *720*
testes and scrotum disorders
  cancer of the testis 719–720
  choriocarcinoma, cancer of the testis 719
  embryonal carcinoma, cancer of the testis 719
  epididymal cysts 718
  epididymo-orchitis 718–719
  hydrocele 721
  hypogonadism in males 729
  seminoma, cancer of the testis 719–720
  teratoma, cancer of the testis 719
  testes and scrotum problems, symptoms chart 181
  torsion of the testis 719
  undescended testis, in babies and children 870
  varicocele 720–721
testicular cancer *see* cancer of the testis
testosterone 1023
  production disorders *see* male hormonal problems and disorders
  production and role in male reproductive system *671*, *672*, 716, *717*
  rise in levels during puberty *716*, *815*
  sex hormones and related drugs 933–934
  see also male sex hormones
tests and investigations 212–215
  antenatal *see* antenatal tests and investigations
  before major surgery 943
  cancer *see* cancer tests and investigations
  cardiovascular system *see* cardiovascular system tests and investigations
  digestive system *see* digestive system tests and investigations in doctor's surgery 216–220
  eyes *see* eye and vision tests and investigations
  female reproductive system *see* female reproductive system tests and investigations
  of hearing *see* hearing tests
  mental health *see* psychological assessment
  nervous system *see* nervous system tests and investigations
  in outpatient and day care treatment 956
  reliability 44, 213
  respiratory system *see* respiratory system tests and investigations
  on samples *see* samples collection for testing; samples testing
  skin *see* skin tests
  sleep *see* sleep studies
  urinary system *see* urinary system tests and investigations
  vision *see* eye and vision tests and investigations
  see also imaging techniques; screening; viewing techniques
tetanus 302
  routine immunizations *45*
  vaccines and immunoglobulins 883–884
tetrabenazine 1023
tetracaine 1023
  antipruritic drugs 891–892
  local anaesthetics 914
tetracosactide 1023
tetracycline 1023
  antibiotics 885–886
  antimalarial drugs 888–889
tetralogy of Fallot *see* Fallot's tetralogy
T-Gel 1023
thalamus, brain structure and functions *510*
thalassaemia *273*, 449–450
thalidomide 1023
Theo-Dur 1023
theophylline 1023
  bronchodilator drugs 910–911
therapies
  choices 954, *955*
  complementary or alternative *see* complementary therapies
  occupational therapy 954, *955*, 962–963
  physical *see* physiotherapy
  psychological *see* psychological therapies
  rehabilitation *see* rehabilitation and rehabilitation therapies
  sex therapy *773*
  speech therapy *955*, 963
  see also care and caring; treatments
thermometers *88*
thermoregulation *331*
thiamine 1023
  vitamin sources in diet and effects on health *51*
  vitamin supplements 927
thiazide drugs, diuretic drugs 902
thickening, nail abnormality 360
thighbone *see* femur
thigh stretches, warming up and cooling down in your exercise routine *61*
thiopental 1023
  general anaesthetics 914
thioridazine 1023
  antipsychotic drugs 917–918
thiotepa 1023
third-degree burns 317
third stage of labour *783*
third trimester of pregnancy *781*
thirst prevention, symptoms relief for the terminally ill 965
thoracic nerves, nervous system structure and functions *511*
thoracic spine *364*
threadworm infestation 310
threatened miscarriage 792
throat
  connecting passageways to ears and nose *592*
  digestive system structure and functions *621*, *622*
  disorders *see* throat disorders
  endoscopy of the nose and throat *476*
  pharynx structure and functions 470, *471*
  throat swabs *223*
throat disorders
  acute laryngitis 479–480
  allergic rhinitis 466–467
  cancer of the larynx 481
  cancer of the nasopharynx 480–481
  candidiasis 309
  chronic laryngitis 479–480
  common cold 288–289
  difficulty swallowing, symptoms chart 147
  diphtheria *45*, 300, 883
  endoscopy of the nose and throat *476*
  infectious mononucleosis 291–292
  laryngitis 479–480
  mirror laryngoscopy *481*
  peritonsillar abscess 479
  pharyngitis and tonsillitis 479, 843
  scarlet fever 300
  sore throat 479
  sore throat, symptoms chart 139
  steam inhalation *475*
  throat swabs *223*
  tonsillectomy and adenoidectomy *843*
  useful online sites and addresses 1031
  vocal cord nodules 480

throat swabs *223*
thrombocytopenia 453
thrombolytic drugs 904–905
thrombophlebitis, superficial 439
thrombosis
cerebral thrombosis, cause of stroke 532–534
deep vein thrombosis 437–438
drugs that prevent blood clotting 904
thrombolytic drugs 904–905
thrombosis and embolism 431–432
thrombus *see* blood clots; thrombosis
thrush
antifungal drugs 889
oral thrush 862–863
vaginal thrush 752–753
see also Candida albicans infections
thumb, saddle joint in *365*
thymine, nucleotide base in DNA *265*
thymoxamine see moxisylyte 1016
thymus gland
location and role in lymphatic system *443, 671*
in newborn babies *810, 811*
thyroid cancer 681–682
thyroid gland 670, *671, 673*
disorders *see* thyroid gland disorders
needle aspiration of the thyroid gland *682*
thyroid gland disorders 679
drugs for thyroid gland disorders 932–933
follicular thyroid cancer 681–682
goitre 680–681
Graves' disease, cause of hyperthyroidism 679–680
Hashimoto's thyroiditis 680, 681
hormone tests 232
hypothyroidism 680, 932
medullary thyroid cancer 681–682
needle aspiration of the thyroid gland *682*
papillary thyroid cancer 681–682
postpartum thyroiditis 681
thyroid nodules 681–682
thyroiditis 681
thyroid tumours 681
viral thyroiditis 681
see also hyperthyroidism
thyroid hormone (T_3), production and functions *673*
thyroid hormones 1023
drugs for hypothyroidism 932
overproduction disorder *see* hyperthyroidism
production and functions *440*, 670, *671, 673*
underproduction disorder *see* hypothyroidism
thyroiditis 681
thyroid nodules 681
thyroid-stimulating hormone (TSH)
hormone tests for TSH 232
production and functions 670, *672*
underproduction, cause of hypothyroidism 680
thyroxine (T_4)
hormone tests for thyroxine 232
production and functions *673*
thyroxine see levothyroxine
tiabendazole 1023
anthelmintic drugs 889
tiagabine 1023
tiaprofenic acid 1023
tibia
fracture treatment *393*
inflamed tibia during childhood *see* Osgood–Schlatter disease
location in skeleton *363*
tibial nerves, nervous system structure *509*
tibolone 1023
drugs for bone disorders 896
hormone replacement therapy 937–938
sex hormones and related drugs 933–934
ticarcillin 1023
tick bites
first aid *995*
preventing *303*
ticks, diseases transmitted by
Lyme disease 303
Rocky Mountain spotted fever 304
Ticlid 1023
ticlopidine 1023
drugs that prevent blood clotting 904
tics, nervous 550
Tilade 1023
Tildiem 1023
Tiloryth 1023
tiludronic acid 1023
Timecef 1023
Timodine 1023
timolol 1023
beta-blocker drugs 898–899
drugs for glaucoma 920–921
Timoptol 1023
Timpron 1023
Tinaderm-M 1023
tinea capitis *see* scalp ringworm
tinea corporis *see* body ringworm
tinea pedis *see* athlete's foot
tinea versicolor *see* pityriasis versicolor
tingling and/or numbness, symptoms chart 114–115
tinidazole 1023
antiprotozoal drugs 888
tinnitus 602, 603
tinzaparin 1023
tioconazole 1023
preparations for skin infections and infestations 892–893
tioguanine 1023
anticancer drugs 907–908
tiredness
chronic fatigue syndrome 520
in pregnancy *785*
symptoms chart 94–95
tirofiban 1023
tissue
adipose tissue, surrounding internal organs *675*
brain tissue *see* grey matter; white matter
cancerous tumour infiltration *275*
connective tissue disorders *see* scleroderma; systemic lupus erythematosus (SLE)
effect of noncancerous tumours *275*
epithelial tissue, site of cancerous tumours *275*
lymphatic tissue *443*
rejoining tissue after surgery *948*
role in human body *259*
samples collection for testing *see* biopsies
spinal cord tissue *see* grey matter; white matter
spongy erectile tissue, in penis *717*
tissue tests 237
see also membranes
tissue plasminogen activator 1023
titanium dioxide
sunscreens and sunblocks 893
Titralac 1023
Tixylix 1023
tizanidine
muscle relaxants 896
tobacco and smoking 63–65
cause of cancer 64, *274*
correlation between cigarette consumption and deaths from lung cancer *503*
effects on cardiovascular system 64
effects on complications of diabetes mellitus *690*
effects on fetus 34
effects on respiratory system 64
environmental tobacco smoke (ETS) and passive smoking 64–65
hypnotherapy, aid to stopping smoking 975
stopping smoking *17*, 65
useful online sites and addresses 1037
tobramycin 1023
antibiotics 885–886
tocopherol 1023
tocopheryl 1023
toenails, ingrown 361
toes
disorders *see* foot and toe disorders
effects of serious injuries *315, 320*
toe or finger bandages, first aid *998*
Tofranil 1023
Tolanase 1023
tolazamide 1023
tolbutamide 1023
drugs for diabetes mellitus 931–932
tolfenamic acid 1023
tolnaftate 1023
tolterodine 1023
drugs that affect bladder control 939
tomography *see* computerized tomography (CT) scanning; positron emission tomography (PET) scanning; single-photon-emission computerized tomography (SPECT) scanning
tone, muscle 362
tongue
digestive system structure and functions 620, *621, 622*
disorders *see* mouth and tongue disorders
taste buds location and functions *513*
tonic–clonic seizures, epilepsy 525
tonometry, test for glaucoma *576*
tonsillectomy and adenoidectomy *843*
tonsils
disorders *see* infectious mononucleosis; pharyngitis and tonsillitis
removal *see* tonsillectomy and adenoidectomy
respiratory system structure and functions 470, *471*
tool safety in the garden 80
tooth disorders 608
avulsed tooth 616
dental abscess 611–612
dental caries (tooth decay) 609–611
dental checkups *609*
discoloured teeth 612–613
fractured tooth 614–615
impacted teeth 613
irreversible pulpitis 611
malocclusion 613–614
missing teeth 615–616
pulpitis 611
reversible pulpitis 611
teething, in babies 819–820
temporomandibular joint disorder 616
toothache 608–609
treatments *see* dental treatments
see also gum disorders
tooth filling *611*
Topal 1023
Topamax 1023
topical corticosteroids 892
antipruritic drugs 891–892
topical preparations for skin infections and infestations 892–893
topiramate 1023
anticonvulsant drugs 914–915
topotecan 1023
Toradol 1023
torasemide 1023
diuretic drugs 902
Torem 1023
toremifene 1023
toric lenses, soft contact lenses for astigmatism 589
torn knee cartilage 395
torsion of the testis 719
torticollis 388
total incontinence 710–711
touch
information processing in brain *515*
role of sensory receptors in skin 328, *513*
Tourette's syndrome, nervous tics in 550
toxaemia, pre-eclamptic *see* pre-eclampsia and eclampsia
toxic megacolon, caused by ulcerative colitis 660

toxic shock syndrome 300
toxins
  botulin toxin treatment for achalasia 638
  botulinum toxin 1003
  cause of botulism 301–302
  cause of food poisoning 629
  cause of tetanus 302
  cause of toxic shock syndrome 300
  production by bacteria *286*
  use in vaccines 883
toxocariasis 82, 310–311
toxoplasmosis 82, 307–308
  congenital infections, in newborn babies 817
trabeculae, bone structure 362
trabeculectomy, chronic glaucoma treatment *577*
trachea
  during swallowing *622*
  effects of serious injuries *315*
  respiratory system structure and functions 470, *471*
tracheoesophageal implants, use in speech therapy 963
trachoma 572
traction, fracture treatment *393*
traffic accident statistics 314, 316
training
  biofeedback *975*
  first aid 976
tramadol 1023
  painkillers 912–913
tramazoline 1023
Tramil 500 1023
Trandate 1023
trandolapril 1023
  angoitensin converting enzyme (ACE) inhibitor drugs 900–901
tranexamic acid 1023
  drugs that promote blood clotting 903
tranquillizers, minor *see* antianxiety drugs
transcutaneous electrical nerve stimulation (TENS), use in pain relief *517*
transdermal route, drug delivery route *879*
transducer, use in ultrasound scanning 250–251
transfats (hydrogenated fats) 51
Transiderm-Nitro 1023
transient ischaemic attacks 531–532
transitional cell carcinoma, kidney cancer 704–705
translocation between chromosomes, structural chromosomal abnormality causing chromosome disorders 271
transplant surgery 940, 952–953
  bone marrow transplant *454*
  hair transplant *359*
  heart transplant *427*
  immunosuppressants 906–907
  kidney transplant *708*
  liver transplant *650*
  organ donation after death 967
  pancreas or insulin-secreting cells transplant, for type 1 diabetes 689
transport by the blood
  drug treatments *879*
  fetal nourishment and blood supply during pregnancy *779*, *781*
  glucose transport 440
  hormone transport 670
  nutrient transport from the digestive system 620, *623–625*, *675*
  oxygen transport *see* oxygen transport by the blood
  waste products transport 396, 440, *473*
transurethral prostatectomy *see* partial prostatectomy
Transvasin 1023
transverse fractures 392
Tranxene 1023
tranylcypromine 1023
  antidepressant drugs 916–917
Trasicor 1023
travel health 85–86
  immunizations 85, *86*
  useful online sites and addresses 1037
traveller's diarrhoea, from food poisoning or gastroenteritis 85, 627
Travogyn 1023
Traxam 1023
trazodone 1023
  antidepressant drugs 916–917
treatments
  advances, improvements, and landmarks in treatments 875–877
  aims of treatment and treatment planning 874–875
  dental *see* dental treatments
  emergency *see* emergencies and emergency care; first aid
  living wills and treatments for the terminally ill 964
  for specific disorders *see* individual articles on disorders
  surgical *see* surgery
  transfusions *see* blood transfusions
  see also therapies
tremor (persistent trembling) and twitching, symptoms chart 116–117
trench mouth *see* acute necrotizing ulcerative gingivitis (ANUG)
Trental 1023
treosulfan 1023
tretinoin 1023
  retinoid drugs 890–891
Tri-Adcortyl 1023
Triadene 1023
TriamaxCo 1023
triamcinolone 1023
  corticosteroids 930–931
  drugs acting on the ear 921
  locally acting corticosteroids 895
  topical corticosteroids 892
triamterene 1023
  diuretic drugs 902
triangular bandages as slings, first aid *998*
tribavirin 1024
triceps muscles *362*, *367*
trichinosis, tropical worm infestation 312
trichomonas infections
  nongonococcal urethritis (NGU) 765
  trichomoniasis 767
  vulvovaginitis 752
trichomoniasis 767
trichuriasis, tropical worm infestation 312
triclofos 1024
triclosan 1024
  preparations for skin infections and infestations 892–893
tricuspid valve, heart structure *398*
tricyclics, antidepressant drugs 916–917
Tridestra 1024
trientine 1024
trifluoperazine 1024
  antiemetic drugs 922
  antipsychotic drugs 917–918
Trifyba 1024
trigeminal nerve, nervous system structure and functions *511*
trigeminal neuralgia 546
trihexyphenidyl 1024
tri-iodothyronine 1024
trilostane 1024
Triludan 1024
trimeprazine *see* alimemazine 1001
trimesters of pregnancy *780–781*
trimethoprim 1024
  antibiotics 885–886
trimetrexate 1024
Tri-Minulet 1024
trimipramine 1024
Trimogal 1024
Trimovate 1024
Trinordiol 1024
TriNovum 1024
Triogesic 1024
Triominic 1024
triplets
  base triplets in DNA *266*
  multiple pregnancy 792–793
tripotassium dicitratobismuthate 1024
Triprimix 1024
triprolidine 1024
Triptafen 1024
triptorelin 1024
  sex hormones and related drugs 933–934
Trisequens 1024
trisodium edetate 1024
trisomy 21 *see* Down's syndrome
Tritace 1024
Trobicin 1024
trochlear nerve, nervous system structure and functions *511*
Tropergen 1024
tropical diseases
  amoebiasis 306
  ascariasis 311
  cholera 301
  dengue fever 296
  Ebola fever, viral haemorrhagic fever 295
  filariasis, tropical worm infestation 312
  hantavirus infection, viral haemorrhagic fever 295
  hookworm infestation 311–312
  Lassa fever, viral haemorrhagic fever 295
  malaria 305–306
  Marburg fever, viral haemorrhagic fever 295
  prevention *see* immunization
  rabies *86*, 296, 883
  schistosomiasis 81, 312–313
  strongyloidiasis, tropical worm infestation 312
  trichinosis, tropical worm infestation 312
  trichuriasis, tropical worm infestation 312
  tropical worm infestations 312
  viral haemorrhagic fevers 295
  yellow fever *86*, 296
tropicamide 1024
tropisetron 1024
Trosyl 1024
true polycythaemia *see* primary polycythaemia
trunk stretches, warming up and cooling down in your exercise routine *61*
Trusopt 1024
Tryptizol 1024
tryptophan 1024
TSH *see* thyroid-stimulating hormone (TSH)
tubal ligation *see* female sterilization 70, *743*
tuberculosis (TB) 491–492
  antituberculous drugs 886
  BCG, vaccines and immunoglobulins 883–884
  routine immunizations *45*
tubular gauze dressings for fingers or toes, first aid *998*
Tuinal 1024
tulobuterol 1024
tumour cells
  cancerous 274, *275–277*, *279*
  noncancerous *275*
tumour growth rates *276*
tumour marker tests 233
tumours
  cancerous (malignant) *see* cancerous tumours
  noncancerous (benign) *see* noncancerous tumours
tuning fork tests, hearing tests *600*
tunnel vision, visual field defect 590–591
Turner's syndrome *238*, 271, 823
twins, multiple pregnancy 762, *779*, 792–793
twitching and tremor, symptoms chart 116–117
Tylex 1024
tympanic canal, ear structure and functions *593*, *594*
tympanometry, hearing test *600*
type 1 diabetes 687–691
type 2 diabetes 687–691
typhoid and paratyphoid 301
  travel immunizations *86*
  vaccines and immunoglobulins 883–884
typhus 304
Tyrozets 1024

U

Ubretid 1024
Ucerax 1024
UK Breast Cancer Awareness Campaign 1028
UK Healthcare Centre 1026
UK Homoeopathic Medical Association 1029
Ukidan 1024
UKparents 1029, 1036
UK Thalassaemia Society 1028
ulcerative colitis 659–660
  aminosalicylate drugs 924
ulcer-healing drugs, for peptic ulcers 923–924
ulcers and ulceration
  Behçet's syndrome 465
  caused by cancerous tumours *275*
  corneal ulcers 571–572
  duodenal ulcer, type of peptic ulcer 640–642
  gastric ulcer, type of peptic ulcer 640–642
  leg ulcers 350
  mouth ulcers 632
  peptic ulcer 640–642
  pressure sores 350
  ulcerative colitis 659–660, 924
  ulcer-healing drugs, for peptic ulcers 923–924
ulnar nerves, nervous system structure *509*
Ultec 1024
Ultralanum Plain 1024
Ultraproct 1024
ultrasound scanning *243*, 250–251
  carotid Doppler scanning *531*
  Doppler ultrasound scanning *243*, 251, *432*
  echocardiography *425*
  fetal heartbeat detection in fetal monitoring *803*
  ultrasound guidance in antenatal genetic tests *787*
  ultrasound scanning in pregnancy *793*
ultrasound therapy, role in physiotherapy 961–962
umbilical arteries and veins, nourishing the fetus in pregnancy *781*
umbilical cord
  during childbirth *783*
  functions during pregnancy *779*, *781*
  in the newborn baby *811*
  prolapse caused by premature rupture of the membranes 797
  prolapse causing fetal distress 797, 804
umbilical hernia 662
unconsciousness
  choking in unconscious adults and children, first aid *981*
  coma 522–523
  feeling faint and passing out, symptoms chart 108–109
  first aid 108, *983*
  persistent vegetative state 523
  recovery position, first aid *979*
undecenoic acid 1024
underweight *see* weight problems
undescended testis 870
undressing and dressing, home care *954*
Uniflu 1024
Unigest 1024
Unihep 1024
Uniparin 1024
Uniphyllin Continus 1024
Uniroid HC 1024
United Nations International Drug Control Programme 1031
Univer 1024
unsaturated fats *50*, 51
upper body stretches, warming up and cooling down in your exercise routine *60*
upper digestive tract endoscopy *641*
upper limb fractures, first aid *992*
urea 1024
  routine blood chemistry tests for urea 229
  waste product in urine 694, *697*
ureters, urinary system structure and functions 694, *695–697*
urethra
  disorders *see* bladder and urethra disorders
  female urethra, location in urinary and reproductive systems *694*, *695*, *731*
  in males *see* male urethra
  urinary system structure and functions 694, *695*, *697*
urethral catheterization, of the bladder *713*
urethral stricture 714
urethral syndrome, nonbacterial cystitis 710
urge incontinence 710, 712
Uriben 1024
uric acid
  increased levels in blood, caused by thiazide diuretics 902
  in kidney stones 701
  role in gout 380
urinary incontinence 710–711
  drugs for urinary incontinence 939
  overflow incontinence 710
  pelvic floor exercises 712
  poor bladder control, symptoms chart 165
  stress incontinence 711–712
  total incontinence 710–711
  urge incontinence 712
  urodynamic studies *711*
  useful online sites and addresses 1033
urinary reflux, leading to urinary tract infections in children 871
urinary and reproductive system disorders in children 870
  bedwetting 872, 939
  chordee, associated with hypospadias, in babies and children 870
  hydronephrosis 703
  hypospadias 870
  juvenile polycystic kidney disease 704
  kidney scarring, caused by urinary tract infections 871
  urinary reflux, leading to urinary tract infections in children 871
  urinary tract infections in children 871
  Wilms' tumour, kidney cancer 705, 872
urinary retention 713
  drugs for urinary retention 939
  inability to pass urine, symptoms chart 165
urinary system
  disorders *see* bladder and urethra disorders; kidney disorders
  disorders in children *see* urinary system disorders in children
  effects of growth and aging *22–23*
  role in body's defences *444*
  structure and functions 694, *695–697*
  tests and investigations *see* urinary system tests and investigations
  useful online sites and addresses 1037
urinary system tests and investigations
  cystoscopy *715*
  dimercaptosuccinic acid (DMSA) scanning *871*
  intravenous urography (IVU) 246, *695*, *699*
  kidney biopsy *701*
  routine blood chemistry tests for kidney damage 229
  urodynamic studies *711*
  see also urine tests
urinary tract *see* urinary system
urination
  control mechanism *697*
  disorders *see* bedwetting; bladder and urethra disorders; kidney disorders
urination problems symptoms charts
  frequent urination 166–167
  inability to pass urine 165
  painful urination 168–169
  poor bladder control 165
urine
  appearance assessment *169*
  formation in and excretion from urinary system 694, *695–697*
  production increased by diuretic drugs 902
  role in body's defences *444*
  tests and investigations *see* urine tests
urine-collecting ducts, kidney structure and functions *696*, *697*
urine tests
  dipstick testing of urine *231*
  during pregnancy *786*
  home pregnancy tests *232*
  hormone tests 232
  routine urine chemistry 230–231
  samples collection 222
  tests for microorganisms 234–235
  tumour marker tests 233
  urine appearance *169*
Urispas 1024
urodynamic studies *711*
urofollitropin 1024
  drugs for infertility 936–937
urokinase 1024
  thrombolytic drugs 904–905
Urostomy Association 1037
ursodeoxycholic acid 1024
Ursofalk 1024
urticaria 468
uterine muscle relaxant drugs, drugs for labour 938
uterine polyps *745*, 746
uterine stimulant drugs, drugs for labour *797*, 938
uterus
  contractions during labour and childbirth *782–783*, 938
  disorders *see* uterus disorders
  during sexual intercourse *763*
  expansion during pregnancy *731*, *779*, *780–781*
  female reproductive system structure and functions 730, *731–732*
  lining *see* endometrium
  shrinkage after childbirth *783*
  surgical removal *see* hysterectomy
uterus disorders
  cancer of the uterus *281*, 748
  choriocarcinoma 748
  fibroids 745–746
  prolapse of the uterus and vagina 747
  retroverted uterus 746
  uterine polyps *745*, 746
Utinor 1024
Utovlan 1024
UVA and UVB light, components of sunlight 80–81, 893
uveal tract, eye structure 574
uveitis 574–575

V

vaccines and immunoglobulins 883–884
  cancer vaccines 282
  see also immunization
vacuum constriction device, impotence treatment 771
vacuum suction delivery, assisted delivery technique *805*
Vagifem 1024
vagina
  disorders *see* vaginal disorders
  dryness at the menopause *733*, 738
  during sexual arousal and sexual intercourse *731*, *762*, *763*
  female reproductive system structure and functions 730, *731*
  in pregnancy and childbirth *731*, *779*, *782–783*
vaginal bleeding
  abnormal vaginal bleeding 737
  abnormal vaginal bleeding, symptoms chart 190–191
  periods *see* menstruation and menstrual cycle
  postmenopausal bleeding 738–739

vaginal bleeding (continued)
vaginal bleeding in pregnancy 791
vaginal bleeding in pregnancy, symptoms chart 190
vaginal disorders
abnormal vaginal discharge, symptoms chart 194
bacterial vaginosis 753
bleeding *see* vaginal bleeding
cancer of the vulva and vagina 753
candidiasis 309
cystocele, prolapse of the uterus and vagina 747
prolapse of the uterus and vagina 747
rectocele, prolapse of the uterus and vagina 747
vaginal dryness, cause of painful intercourse in women 772–773
vaginal thrush 752–753, 889
vaginismus 773
vulvovaginitis 752
Vaginyl 1024
vagus nerve, nervous system structure and functions *509*, *511*
valaciclovir 1024
antiviral drugs 886–887
Valclair 1024
Valium 1024
anticonvulsant drugs 914–915
antimigraine drugs 913
mood-stabilizing drugs 918
Vallergan 1024
Valoid 1024
valproic acid 1024
valsartan 1024
antihypertensive drugs 897–898
Valtrex 1024
valve defects, congenital heart disease 837
valve disorders
heart *see* heart valve disorders
in veins *see* varicose veins
valve incompetence
aortic incompetence 422–423
in heart valves *421*
mitral incompetence 423–424
valves
in digestive system *621*, *622*, *623*
heart *see* heart valves
in lymphatic system *443*
in veins *397*, *400*
valve stenosis
aortic stenosis 423
heart valves *421*
mitral stenosis 424
Vancocin 1024
vancomycin 1024
antibiotics 885–886
Vaqta 1024
varicella-zoster
vaccines and immunoglobulins 883–884
see also chickenpox
varicose veins 438–439
portal hypertension and varices 648–649
in pregnancy 438, 784, *785*
varicocele 720–721
Varidase 1024
Vascace 1024
vas deferens, male reproductive system structure and functions 716, *717*, *721*, *763*
vasectomy 70, *721*
vasodilators 1024
see also antihypertensive drugs
Vasogen 1024
vasopressin 1024
pituitary drugs 934–935
role in controlling urine concentration in the kidneys *401*, 670, *672*
underproduction disorder or response failure *see* diabetes insipidus
Vectavir 1024
vecuronium 1024
Veganin 1024
vegetative state, persistent 523
vehicle safety 83, *84*
children's car seats *29*
see also cars and driving
vein disorders
deep vein thrombosis 437–438
portal hypertension and varices 648–649
retinal vein occlusion 578
subdural haemorrhage 535
superficial thrombophlebitis 439
tests and investigations *see* cardiovascular system tests and investigations
thrombosis and embolism 431–432
varicocele 720–721
varicose veins 438–439
varicose veins in pregnancy 438, 784, *785*
veins
blood pressure levels *400*
disorders *see* vein disorders
in the heart *398*
location of major veins in the body *397*
in the placenta and umbilical cord during pregnancy *781*
structure and functions 396, *397*, *400*
in the urinary system *695*, *696*
venous blood colour *442*
venous blood samples, collection for testing 221, *222*
see also individual veins by name
Velbe 1024
Velosef 1024
Velosulin 1024
venae cavae *see* inferior vena cava; superior vena cava
venlafaxine 1024
antidepressant drugs 916–917
Venofer 1024
venous leg ulcers 350
venous return, blood circulation *400*
venous sinus, blood vessel in the brain *510*
ventilation disorders, respiratory failure 507
ventilation scan, radionuclide lung scanning *494*
Ventmax SR 1024
Ventodisks 1024
Ventolin 1024
ventricles
brain structure *510*
heart structure and functions 396, *396*, *398–399*
hole in septum between heart ventricles *see* ventriculoseptal defect
ventricular fibrillation, cause of cardiac arrest 419–420
ventricular systole, heartbeat phase *399*
ventriculoseptal defect, congenital heart disease 836–837
venules, role in blood circulation *397*, *400*
Veracur 1024
verapamil 1024
antiarrhythmic drugs 898
antimigraine drugs 913
calcium channel blocker drugs 900
Vermox 1024
vernix, on skin of newborn babies *811*
verruca plana *see* flat warts
verrucas *see* warts
Verrugon 1024
vertebrae
effects of serious injuries *315*
structure and functions *364*, *509*
vertebral column *see* spine
vertigo 603–604
symptoms chart 112–113
Vesagex 1025
Vesanoid 1025
vestibular apparatus, ear structure and functions *595*
vestibular canal, ear structure and functions *593*, *594*
vestibular membrane, ear structure and functions *594*
vestibular nerve, ear structure and functions *593*, *595*
vestibule, ear structure and functions *593*, *595*
vestibulocochlear nerve
nervous system structure and functions *511*
noncancerous tumour *see* acoustic neuroma
Viagra 1025
Viazem XL 1025
Vibramycin 1025
vibration white finger *see* hand–arm syndrome
Vicks Cold Care 1025
Vicks Medinite 1025
Victim Support 1029
Videne 1025
Videx 1025
viewing techniques 242, 254
basic viewing techniques 254
colposcopy *750*
dental checkups *609*
mirror laryngoscopy *481*
ophthalmoscopy *578*
otoscopy *597*
retinoscopy in babies and children *857*
slit-lamp examination *574*
using flexible or rigid endoscopes *see* endoscopy
vigabatrin 1025
Vigranon B 1025
villi
chorionic *see* chorionic villi
in the small intestine 620, *623*
viloxazine 1025
vinblastine 1025
vincristine 1025
anticancer drugs 907–908
vindesine 1025
vinorelbine 1025
Vioform–hydrocortisone 1025
Vioxx 1025
Viracept 1025
Viraferon 1025
viral infections 288
acute bronchitis 486–487
acute hepatitis 644–645, 883
bronchiolitis 841
cause of febrile convulsions in children 849
cause of lymphadenopathy 458
chickenpox (varicella) 290, 883
chronic hepatitis 645–646, 907
cold sores 354
common cold 288–289
common warts 354–355
congenital infections, in newborn babies 817
croup 841–842
cytomegalovirus (CMV) infection 292, 817, 883
dengue fever 296
drug treatments *see* antiviral drugs
Ebola fever, viral haemorrhagic fever 295
flat warts 355
flu *see* influenza
food poisoning 629–630
gastroenteritis 85, 628–629
genital herpes 767–768
genital warts 768
glossitis 633
hand, foot, and mouth disease 831
hantavirus infection, viral haemorrhagic fever 295
hepatitis *86*, 644–646, 883
herpes simplex infections 291
herpes zoster 290–291
HIV infection and AIDS 297–298
human papillomavirus (HPV) infections 69, 354, 750, 751, 768
immunization against 45, 288
infectious mononucleosis 291–292
labyrinthitis 604
Lassa fever, viral haemorrhagic fever 295
Marburg fever, viral haemorrhagic fever 295
measles *45*, 293, 883–884
molluscum contagiosum 355
mosaic warts 354
mumps *45*, 293–294, 883–884
otitis externa 596
otitis media 597
parvovirus infection 294–295
pharyngitis and tonsillitis 479, 843
plantar warts 354–355
poliomyelitis *45*, 295, 883–884
prevention *see* food hygiene; immunization; travel health

rabies *86*, 296, 883
roseola infantum 830–831
rubella *45*, 294, 883–884
tests for responsible microorganisms 234–235
viral conjunctivitis 570–571
viral encephalitis *86*, 528–529
viral haemorrhagic fevers 295
viral meningitis 527–528
viral meningitis in children 848–849
viral pneumonia 490–491
viral stomatitis 633
viral thyroiditis 681
warts 354–355
yellow fever *86*, 296
Viramune 1025
Virazid 1025
Viridal 1025
virilization 740
Virormone 1025
viruses
cause of cancer 278, 279
cellular immune response against *445*
Epstein–Barr *see* Epstein–Barr virus (EBV)
hepatitis viruses 644–645
infections caused by viruses *see* viral infections
infectious organisms size comparison *284*
Norwalk virus 628, *629*, 630
structure and functions *285*
see also rotaviruses
Visclair 1025
Viscotears 1025
vision 566, *567–569*
disorders *see* vision disorders
information processing in the brain *515*, 566, *569*
role of optic nerves *511*, 566, *567–569*
tests and investigations *see* eye and vision tests and investigations
vision and manual dexterity, developmental milestones during childhood *814*
vision disorders 586
amblyopia in children 858
astigmatism 588–589
blindness 591
colour blindness *269*, 591
congenital blindness 856–857
disturbed or impaired vision, symptoms chart 134–135
double vision 589–590
hypermetropia 586–588
myopia 586
presbyopia 589
red–green colour blindness 591
strabismus in children 857–858
surgical treatments *see* eye surgery
tests and investigations *see* eye and vision tests and investigations
tunnel vision, visual field defect 590–591
useful online sites and addresses 1031
visual field defects 590–591
see also eye disorders; eyelid and tear system disorders
visiting your doctor *see* consulting your doctor
Viskaldix 1025
Visken 1025
Vista-Methasone 1025
Vistide 1025
visual acuity
role of light-sensitive cells in the retina of the eye 566
vision tests for *587*
visual association cortex, location and role in information processing in the brain *515*
visual cortex
role in vision *515*, 566, *569*
visual evoked response test *542*
visual field defects 590–591
visual field test *590*
visual signal *see* electrical impulses and signals in the eye
vitamin A 51, 1025
deficiency disorder *see* xerophthalmia
drugs derived from vitamin A *see* retinoid drugs
sources and effects *51*
vitamin supplements 927
vitamin B_1 1025
deficiency disorder *see* Wernicke–Korsakoff syndrome
sources and effects *51*
vitamin supplements 927
vitamin B_2
sources and effects *51*
vitamin B_3 1025
sources and effects *51*
vitamin supplements 927–928
vitamin B_6 1025
sources and effects *51*
vitamin supplements 928
vitamin B_{12} 1025
deficiency disorder *see* megaloblastic anaemia
sources and effects *51*
vitamin supplements 928
vitamin B complex 1025
vitamin C 1025
sources and effects *51*
vitamin supplements 928
vitamin D 51, 1025
deficiency disorder *see* osteomalacia and rickets
drugs for bone disorders 896
sources and effects *51*
vitamin supplements 928
vitamin deficiency disorders
glossitis 633
megaloblastic anaemia 448
neural tube defects 844–845
nutritional neuropathies 545–546
osteomalacia and rickets 370
stomatitis 632–633
Wernicke–Korsakoff syndrome 538
xerophthalmia 585
vitamin E 51, 1025
sources and effects *51*
vitamin supplements 928
vitamin H 1025
vitamin K 51, 1025
drugs that promote blood clotting 903
injections for newborn babies 903, 928
sources and effects *51*
vitamin supplements 928
vitamins 51
absorption by the body *625*
deficiency disorders *see* vitamin deficiency disorders
folic acid and other vitamin requirements before and during pregnancy 33, 844, 845, 928
nutritional information on food labels *52*
role of vitamin D in osteoporosis prevention 368–369, 896
sources and effects *51*
vitamin supplements 927–928
vitiligo 342–343
vitreous haemorrhage 578
vitreous humour
bleeding into *see* vitreous haemorrhage
eye structure and functions *567*
specks in *see* floaters
Vivalan 1025
Vivapryl 1025
vocal cord nodules 480
vocal cords, voice and speech production 470, *473*
voice box *see* larynx
voice, speech, and language
difficulty speaking, symptoms chart 119
hearing and language, developmental milestones during childhood *814*
hoarseness and/or voice loss, symptoms chart 140–141
information processing in the brain *515*, *594*
speech discrimination tests, hearing test in children *859*
speech and language difficulties in children 854–855
speech and language disorders, useful online sites and addresses 1037
speech and language information processing in the brain *515*, *594*
speech therapy *955*, 963
voice and speech production by the larynx and vocal cords 470, *473*
Volmax 1025
Volraman 1025
Voltarol 1025
voluntary movements and responses
role of musculoskeletal system 362
role of nervous system 508, *509–511*, *514–515*
see also biting and chewing
vomiting
antiemetic drugs 922
blood in vomit, symptoms chart 148
dehydration prevention 158, *627*, 926
effect on oral medications 149
in pregnancy *see* hyperemesis; morning sickness
recurrent vomiting, symptoms chart 150–151
self-induced, in bulimia 563
symptoms charts 148–151
symptoms relief in the terminally ill 965
vomiting in children, symptoms chart 198–199
vomiting and diarrhoea in children 864
von Willebrand's disease *273*, 452
vulva
disorders *see* bartholinitis; cancer of the vulva and vagina; vulvovaginitis
female reproductive system structure and functions 730, *731*
vulvovaginitis 752

W

waist measurement, health risks indicator *53*
walking aids *962*
warfarin 1025
drugs that prevent blood clotting 904
warming up and cooling down in your exercise routine *60–61*
Warticon 1025
warts 354–355
common warts 354–355
flat warts 355
genital warts 768
mosaic warts 354
plantar warts 354–355
seborrhoeic *see* seborrhoeic keratosis
WaspEze 1025
waste products
carbon dioxide in the blood 440, *442*, 470, *473*
fetal waste products in pregnancy *779*, *781*
processing in urinary system 694, *696–697*
transport by blood 396, 440, *473*
see also creatinine; faeces; uric acid; urine
water (drink/body fluid)
absorption in the large intestine 620, *623*, 625
daily fluid intake 52
in faeces *625*
fluoridation of water, role in reduction of tooth disorders 606, 608, 609–610
processing in and excretion from urinary system 694, *697*
when travelling 85
water (freshwater/seawater areas)
drowning and near-drowning 81, 314, 325–326
water safety 81
water on the brain *see* hydrocephalus
watery eye 585
wax blockage 597
earwax softeners, drugs acting on the ear 921
Waxsol 1025

weaning *28*
Weber test, hearing test *600*
weight
height/weight chart for adults *53*
ideal weight and body mass index (BMI) 53–54
problems *see* weight problems
weight charts for babies and infants *41*
weight charts for children *43*
weight control 53–54
weight problems
being overweight, symptoms chart 98–99
being overweight/underweight, factors in high-risk pregnancies 786
causes and remedies 53–54
loss of weight, symptoms chart 96–97
obesity 631
overweight, causes and remedies 53–54
underweight, causes and remedies 53, 54
see also eating disorders
Weil's disease, form of leptospirosis 302–303
Welldorm Elixir 1025
Welldorm Tablets 1025
Wellferon 1025
Wellvone 1025
Wernicke–Korsakoff syndrome 538
Wernicke's area, location and role in information processing in the brain *515*
wet gangrene 435
wet macular degeneration 580–581
wheezing, symptoms chart 146
whiplash, spinal injury 524
whipworm infestation *see* trichuriasis
white blood cells
basophils *441*
B-cells (B-lymphocytes) *445*
CD4 lymphocytes 297, 887
destroying cancer cells *274*
disorders *see* leukaemias
eosinophils *441*
formation in bone marrow *440*
in lymphatic system *443*
lymphocytes *441, 443, 445*
macrophages *443*
monocytes *441*
neutrophils *441*
phagocytes, role in body's defences *444, 445*
roles in body's defences *444–445*
T-cells (T-lymphocytes) *445, 671*
types and functions 440, *441, 444–445*
white of the eye *see* sclera
white matter, brain and spinal cord structure *510, 511*
white spots, nail abnormality 360
whooping cough *see* pertussis
Wilms' tumour, kidney cancer in children 705, 872
wind, effect on environmental temperature (windchill factor) *323*
windpipe *see* trachea
Wired for Health 1026
wire stitches, rejoining tissue after surgery *948*
wisdom teeth
eruption pattern *606*
impacted *see* impacted teeth
witch hazel 1025
withdrawal symptoms, drug dependence 564, 881
womb *see* uterus
women *see* females; *see also* index entries beginning with the word "female"
Women's Health 1037
Women's Health Concern 1037
women's health, useful online sites and addresses 1037
Women's Nationwide Cancer Control Campaign 1037
Woodward's Gripe Water 1025
work
lifestyle choices *47*
returning to work after surgery 946
safety and health at work 82–83
sick building syndrome 82
work-related disorders *see* occupational disorders
work stations *82*
World Health Organization 1026, 1033
WorldOrtho 1035
worm infestations
anthelmintic drugs 889
ascariasis 311
filariasis, tropical worm infestation 312
hookworm infestation 311–312
hydatid disease 313
schistosomiasis 81, 312–313
strongyloidiasis, tropical worm infestation 312
tapeworm infestation 313
threadworm infestation 310
toxocariasis 82, 310–311
trichinosis, tropical worm infestation 312
trichuriasis, tropical worm infestation 312
tropical worm infestations 312
worms
infectious organisms size comparison *284*
infestations *see* worm infestations
structure *287*
wounds *see* injuries
wrist disorders
carpal tunnel syndrome 547
ganglion 390
wrists
disorders *see* wrist disorders
ellipsoidal joint in *365*
movement range 362
plane joint in *365*
wryneck *see* torticollis

X

Xalatan 1025
xamoterol 1025
Xanax 1025
xanthines, bronchodilator drugs 910–911
Xatral 1025
X chromosome
disorders *see* fragile X syndrome; Klinefelter's syndrome; Turner's syndrome; X-linked disorders
role in inheritance *264, 268–269*
Xenical 1025
xerophthalmia 585
xipamide 1025
X-linked disorders *264, 269,* 272, *273*
Becker muscular dystrophy 826
carriers 26, *269,* 272, *273*
colour blindness *269, 273,* 591
Duchenne muscular dystrophy 826
fragile X syndrome *273,* 822
haemophilia and Christmas disease *273,* 452
muscular dystrophy *273,* 826
nephrogenic diabetes insipidus 678
retinitis pigmentosa 581
tests and investigations *see* genetic tests
X-rays *213, 243,* 244–245
bite-wing X-rays, of teeth *609*
bone densitometry *369*
chest X-ray 244, *490*
contrast *see* contrast X-rays
mammography, of breasts *44, 759*
radiation doses, compared with other imaging techniques *246*
see also computerized tomography (CT) scanning
Xylocaine 1025
xylometazoline 1025
cold and flu remedies 910
decongestants 909
Xyloproct 1025

Y

Y chromosome, role in inheritance *268–269*
yeasts
role in dandruff 358
role in paronychia 361
role in seborrhoeic dermatitis 335
structure *287*
see also Candida albicans infections
yellow fever 296
travel immunizations *86*
vaccines and immunoglobulins 883–884
yellowing, nail abnormality 360
Yomesan 1025
Yutopar 1025

Z

Zaditen 1025
zafirlukast 1025
zalcitabine (ddC) 1025
drugs for HIV infection and AIDS 887–888
Zamadol 1025
zanamivir 1025
antiviral drugs 886–887
Zanidip 1025
Zantac 1025
Zarontin 1025
Zenapax 1025
Zerit 1025
Zestoretic 1025
Zestril 1025
zidovudine (AZT) 1025
drugs for HIV infection and AIDS 887–888
ZIFT *see* zygote intrafallopian transfer (ZIFT)
Zimovane 1025
Zinacef 1025
Zinamide 1025
zinc 1025
mineral supplements 929
zinc ointment
emollients and barrier preparations 890
Zincomed 1025
zinc oxide 1025
sunscreens and sunblocks 893
zinc pyrithione 1025
zinc sulphate 1025
Zineryt 1025
Zinnat 1025
Zirtek 1025
Zispin 1025
Zita 1025
Zithromax 1025
Zocor 1025
Zofran 1025
Zoladex 1025
Zoleptil 1025
zolmitriptan 1025
zolpidem 1025
sleeping drugs 915–916
Zomacton 1025
Zomig 1025
zopiclone 1025
sleeping drugs 915–916
zotepine 1025
Zovirax 1025
zuclopenthixol 1025
Zumenon 1025
Zydol 1025
zygote intrafallopian transfer (ZIFT), assisted conception technique *776*
zygotes
formation and division in early pregnancy *21, 778*
zygote intrafallopian transfer (ZIFT), assisted conception technique *776*
Zyloric 1025
Zyprexa 1025

ACKNOWLEDGMENTS

Dorling Kindersley would like to thank the individuals and organizations listed below for their assistance in the following capacities:

ADDITIONAL EDITORIAL ASSISTANCE

Susan Aldridge, Kathryn Allen, Robert Dinwiddie, Janet Fricker, Irene Gashurov, Alrica Goldstein, Cathy Meeus, Ruth Midgley, William Mills, Barbara Minton, Melanie Paton, Elizabeth Payne, Barbara Ravage, Ashley Ren, Ray Rogers, Clare Stewart, June Thompson, Anna Wahrman, Olivia Wrenhurst

EXPERT MEDICAL ADVICE

Sue Bateman MB ChB FRCOG DObst, Obstetrics and Ultrasound Department, St. Peter's Hospital, Chertsey; Valerie Dawe; Department of Clinical Neurophysiology, The Royal Free Hospital NHS Trust, London; Department of Clinical Neurophysiology, University College London Hospital NHS Trust; Anthony C. de Souza FRCS, Cardiology Department, Royal Brompton Hospital, London; Karen Ferguson, Department of Surgery, The Royal Free Hospital NHS Trust, London; Penelope Hooper; Ken Lang; Alan Lawford and Malcolm Nudd, Benenden Hospital, Benenden; Elizabeth Liebson MD; Janet Page BSc MB BS MRCP FRCR, Radiology Department, Redhill Hospital, Redhill; John Perry; Paul Pracy MB BS FRCPS; Ann Shaw CNM FMP MSN; Susan Whichello, Radiography Department, King's College Hospital, London; Mary H. Windels MD

ADDITIONAL DESIGN ASSISTANCE

Carla de Abreu, Paul Jackson, Mark Johnson-Davis, Philip Ormerod, Picthall and Gunzi, Eleanor Rose, Schermuly Design Company, Ina Stradins, Matthew Swift, Shadric Toop

ADDITIONAL ILLUSTRATORS

Paul Banville, Joanna Cameron, Gary Cross, John Egan, Simone End, Mick Gillah, Mark Iley, Jason Little, Brian Pearce, Peter Ruane, Les Smith, Philip Wilson, Deborah Woodward

PHOTOGRAPHERS

Andy Crawford, Steve Gorton, Gary Ombler, Tim Ridley

OTHER PHOTOGRAPHY

Steve Bartholomew, Jo Foord, Dave King, Susanna Price, Jules Selmes, Debi Treloar

LOAN OF EQUIPMENT

ALK (UK); Heather Auty, Cochlear Implant Ltd.; Roseanne Aitken, Oxford Instruments Medical Systems Division; Robert Bosch Ltd.; Central Medical Equipment Ltd.; Department of Clinical Neurophysiology, University College London Hospital NHS Trust; Dukes Avenue Practice; Peter Edwards, Birmingham Optical; Keep Able Ltd.; London Laser Clinic; Mothercare UK Ltd.; PC Worth Ltd.; Porter Nash Medical Showroom; growth charts on pages 40–43 are based on information and charts supplied by the Child Growth Foundation and are subject to copyright; data for the graph on page 65 was derived from *The Health Benefits of Smoking Cessation*, US Department of Health and Human Services, Centers for Disease Control, DHHS Publication No. (CDC) 90-8416, 1990.

MODELS

Peter Adams, C. Adebusuti, Francesca Agati, Zamir Akram, Danielle Allan, Richard Allen, Susan Alston, Evi Antoniou, Rebecca Ashford, Bert Audubert, Simone Aughterlony, Andrew Baguley, Bridget Bakokodie, Tricia Banham, Austin Barlow, John C. Barrett, Maria Bergman, Lisa Bissell, Adam Blaug, Clare Borg, Lucy Bottomley, Tirzah Bottomley, Laurence Bouvard, Natasha Bowden, Jacqui Boydon, Catherine Brennan, Alison Briegel, Lisa Brighten, Ashley Brown, Garfield Brown, Dominica Buckton, Tom Busch, Bibi Campbell, Steve Capon, Alesandra Caporale, Nefertiti Carnegie, Daniel Carter, Jane Cartwright, Julie Clarke, Sean Clarke, Adam Cockerton, Sam Cocking, Ciro Coleman, Declan Collins, Madeline Collins, Siobhan Contreras, Jonah Coombes, Kevin Cooper, Lilly Cooper, Alan Copeland, Carol Copeland, Barbara Cordell, Caitlin Cordell, Catherine Cordell, Liam Cordell, Ryan Cordell, Sam Cosking, Will Cox, Julia Crane, Andy Crawford, Grace Crawford, Sarah Crean, Mark Cronin, Jessica Currie, Nigel Currie, Laverne Daley, Tariq Daley, Jeff Daniel, Undra Dashdavaa, Katherine Davidson, Lucy de Keller, Nora Dennis, Terence Dennis, N. J. Deschamps, Flavio Dias, R. S. Dudoo, Maree Duffy, Barbara Egervary, Tony Elgie, Belinda Ellington, Fred English, Mehmet Ergan, Michael Esswood, Steve Etienne, Carole Evans, Julian Evans, Nadia Faris, Jane Farrell, Eric Ferretti, Mary Ferretti, Yvonne Fisher, Larry Francis, Ephraim Frank Otigbah, Annie Fraser, Jane Garioni, Laura Gartry, Hilda Gilbert, Timor Golan-Weyl, Anthony Grant, Sharon Green, Daniel Greendale, Culver Greenidge, Robin Grey, John Gunnery, Maudie Gunzi, Hainsley Guthrie, Charlotte Halfhide, Sarah Halfhide, Carmen Hanlan, Alfie Harrison, Christine Henry, B. M. Hewson, A. W. Hewson, Nigel Hill, Richard Hill, Kit Hillier, Lorraine Hilton, Jignesh Hirani, Manjula Hirani, Chris Hirst, Michael Hoey, Alfred Hoffman, Leila Hoffman, Anthony Howes, Tracey Hughes, Isaac Hughes-Batley, Lewis Hughes-Batley, Richard Hurdle, Faron Isaac, Robert Isaacs, Nora J. Dennis, Ouseynou Jagne, Beverly James, Kaye James, James Jeanes, Jane Jeanes, Thomas Jeanes, Cornell John, Christine Lloyd Jones, Marcia McKoy Jones, Roland John-Leopoldie, Cheryl Johnson, Fiona Johnson, John Johnson, Andy Jones, Mahesh Kanani, Hayley Kay, Taryn Kay, L. Keller, Cameron Kelleher, Peter Kelleher, Susan Kelleher, Mark Kennell, Alison Kerl, Amanda Kernot, Claudia Keston, Aline Kleinubing, Deborah Knight, Mahan Krinde, Krishna Kunari, Jane Law, Lisa Law, Roland John Leopoldie, Sarah Layesh-Melamed, Simon Lewandowski, William Liam, Kate Liasis, Leon Liasis, Nina Loving, Doreen Lum, Joanna Lyn Thompson, Denise Mack, Janey Madlani, Lee Mannion, Bryan Marsh, Maija Marsh, Jason Martin, Bobby Maru, David Mathison, Mary Matson, Nicole McClean, Maria McKenzie, Suzanne McLean, Phyllis McMahon, Karen McSween, Jeremy Melling, Hannah Mellows, Paul Mellows, Fiona Mentzel, Hilary Michel, Tony Mills, Olive Mitchell, Catherine Mobley, Alan Montgomery, Lee Moone, Robert Morrison, Teresa Munoz, Nicki Mylonas, Faron Naai, Terry Nelson, Charlotte Nettey, Julie Nettey, Nicole Nnonah, Eva Nowojenska, James O'Connor, Scarlett O'Hara, Akudo Okereafor, Roli Okorodudu, Simon Oon, Chris Orr, E. F. Otilbah, Lucinda Page, Gemma Papineau, Katie Paine, Ann Parkes, Derek Parkes, Nella Passarella, Josephine Peer, Sarah Peers, Flora Pereira, Cecilia Peries, Anthony Perry, Daniela Pettena, Joycelyn Phillips, Carol Pieters, Hamilton Pieters, Marcus Pieters, Sheila Power, Erick Rainey, Rebecca Rainsford, Alan Rawlings, Giles Rees, Valerie Renay, John Robey, Erroline Rose, Stuart Rose, Dawn Rowley, Rosie Ruddock, Sam Russell, Sol Rymer, H. Sajjan, Ruth Samuel, Paul Samuels, Rita Sanyaolu, Titi Sanyaolu, Mai Sasaki, Callum Savage, Angela Seaton, Tony de Sergio, Isaach Shaahu, Marianne Sharp, Hannah Vidal-Simon, Phyllis Slegg, Anthony Smalling, Ronella Smalling, Edwin So, Sally Somers, Susan Stowers, Itsuko Sugawara, Cara Sweeney, Sheila Tait, Kaz Takabatake, Flavia Taylor, Peter Taylor, Ann Theato, Graeme Thomas, Jack Thomas, Joanna Thomas, Ian Tilley, Jenny-Ann Topham, C. Turnbull, Andrew Turvill, D. Venerdiano, Richard Vidal, Ahmani Vidal-Simon, Philippe Von Lanthen, Teo-wa Vuong, Alison Waines, Aidan Walls, Rosie Walls, Tim Webster, Chris Wells, Alexander Williams, Henderson Williams, John Williams, Miranda Wilson, Seretta Wilson, Stefan Wilson, Syanice Wilson, Harsha Yogasundram, Matt Yoxall, Dominic Zwemmer

PICTURE CREDITS

The publisher would like to thank the following for permission to reproduce images:

Courtesy of Dr. R. N. Allan, Q.E.H., University Hospital, Birmingham: 658 r, l; **Courtesy of Miss Sue Bateman, Obstetric Ultrasound Department, St. Peter's Hospital, Chertsey:** 793 b; **Baxter, USA, Carpentier-Edwards, ® S. A. V. ®, Bioprosthesis:** 422 tr; **Biophoto Associates:** 367 t, c, b, 457 t, 694 tl, 701 b, 704, 726; **Courtesy of Dr. D. A. Burns, Leicester Royal Infirmary:** 332, 333, 334 t, 335 br, 336 tl, 349 b, 350, 355 b; **Courtesy of Professor Keith Cartwright, Public Health Laboratory, Gloucester Royal Hospital:** 527 b; **Courtesy of Dr. Erika Denton:** 243 tl, 251 b, 494 t, b, 531, 635 tr, 638, 653 r, 663 t, 739, 746, 759 br, 661, 660; **Courtesy of Mr J. M. Dixon, Edinburgh Breast Unit, Western General Hospital:** 755 tr, 760; **Courtesy of Professor Peter Ell, Institute of Nuclear Medicine, University College London Medical School:** 253 b, cb; **Courtesy ESL Healthcare, FLA:** 375 bc; **Courtesy of Dr. Roger C. Evans, The Emergency Unit, The Royal Infirmary, Cardiff:** 315 tl, br; **Courtesy of Dr. A. G. Fraser & Dr. A. Ionescu, University of Wales, College of Medicine, Cardiff:** 425 t, b; **Courtesy of Dr. Lorraine Gaunt, Director Regional Cytogenetics Unit/Central Manchester Healthcare Trust/St. Mary's Hospital:** 224 bl, 239; **Courtesy of Professor Gleeson, Guy's Hospital, London:** 592; **Courtesy of Donald R. Kauder, MD FACS:** 315 tl; 314; **Courtesy of Dr. Gordon, Anatomic Pathology Division of Department of Pathology and Laboratory Medicine, University of Pennsylvania Medical Center:** 682 r; **Great Ormond Street Hospital for Sick Children, Department of Medical Illustration:** 666, 838, 846 b, 850, 869; **Courtesy of Dr. C. Dyer & Dr. Owens** 811 tr, 833; **Courtesy of Professor Terry Hamblin, The Royal Bournemouth Hospital Medical Illustration Department:** 457 b; **Robert Harding Picture Library:** Ansell Horn/Phototake NYC 816; GJLP/CNRI/Phototake, NY 396 tl, 954 tl; **Courtesy of Mr T. Hillard, Poole Hospital, Dorset:** 733 cl, cr; **Courtesy of Mr Howard, Institute of Laryngoscopy, National Ear, Nose and Throat Hospital:** 480 t, 481; **© Photographic Unit, The Intitute of Psychiatry, London:** 563; **Courtesy of KeyMed (Medical & Industrial Equipment) Ltd., Southend-on-Sea:** 715 tc, r, 745 b; **Professor P. T. Khaw, Institute of Ophthalmology, Moorfields Eye Hospital:** 574 r; **Dr. Alex Leff, MRC Cyclotron Unit, Hammersmith Hospital, London:** 515; **The Leprosy Mission, Peterborough, England:** 302 tr, tl; **Professor Valerie Lund, Institute of Laryngology & Otology, University College London Medical School:** 242 br, 476 tr; **Professor William Wei, Queen Mary Hospital, Hong Kong:** 480b; **Courtesy of Dr. N. K. I. McIver, North Sea Medical Centre, Great Yarmouth:** 325; **Moorfields Eye Hospital, London, Department of Medical Illustration:** 580; **Courtesy of Dr. Keith Morris, Nottingham City Hospital:** 429; **© Mothercare:** 30; **National Blood Transfusion Service:** 227 tl, tr; **Oxford Medical Illustration OMI, John Radcliffe Hospital:** 304, 435, 848; **Courtesy of Dr. Janet Page, East Surrey Hospital & Community Healthcare Trust:** 12 bl, 244 b, 279 cr, 472 tl, tr; **Dr. N. R. Patel:** 372, 390, 729; **K. R. Patel, Queen Mary's University Hospital, Roehampton:** 738; **© Philips Medical:** 249 br; **Dr. Porter, University College London Hospital:** 449; **PowerStock Photolibrary/Zefa:** 375 cl; **Professor R. H. Rezneck, St. Bartholomew's Hospital, London:** 685 b; **Courtesy of Mr R. C. G. Russell:** 949 cl; **Science Photo Library:** 12 tl, c, cr, 21 br, 224 br, 237 b, 243 cbl, 244 t, 245 b, 246 t, 310, 343 b, 353, 365 b, 393 bl, bc, 399 br, 412, 413, 423, 438, 564, 584 t, 585, 634 tr, 699 r, 733 bl, 750 tl, tr, b, bc, 766 bl, 767 t, 775, 779; **Michael Abbey:** 299, 362 tl; **Department of Clinical Cytogenetics, Addenbrookes Hospital:** 238 b, 271; **Jonathan Ashton:** 236 b, 756 r; **Dr. Lewis Baxter:** 557; **Robert Becker/Custom Medical Stock Photo:** 440 b; **Dr. Beer-Gabel/CNRI 12:** br, 255b, 641 l, r; **Z. Binor/Custom Medical Stock Photo:** 742, 743; **Francis Leroy, Biocosmos:** 443 br; **Biology Media:** 444 br; **Biophoto Associates:** 11 cl, 20, 212 cr, 237 tr, 269, 279 bl, 444 t, ctr, 646, 787; **Chris Bjornberg:** 285, 534; **Simon Brown:** 365 tr; **BSIP Dr. T. Prichard:** 250 b; **BSIP Estiot:** 629; **BSIP VEM:** 21 cr, 431 b, 606 tl, 613 b, 652, 695, 841; **John Burbidge:** 331 cr; **Dr. Jeremy Burgess:** 328 t; **Dr. Monty Buchsbaum, Peter Arnold Inc.:** 560; **Scott Camazine:** 419 cr, 875 t, 940; **Dr. L. Caro:** 286; **CDC:** 284 tl, 528 b; **Department of Nuclear Medicine, Charing Cross Hospital:** 213 br, 243 tr, 871 b; **CNRI/Clinique Ste Catherine:** 243 ctl; **CNRI:** 9 t, 212 tl, 213 cbl, 242 tl, 243 ctl, cbl, br, 252 t, 261 tl, 262, 264 cr, 265, 267 b, 281 t, 306 t, 307, 365 ctl, cbl, 373 b, 408, 444 cl, 475, 502 t, 508 tl, cr, 517 b, 532, 533 b, 567 bl, 592 br, 606 cr, 620 tl, 639, 659, 812 b, 878; **Custom Medical Stock:** 567 tr; **Mike Delvin:** 377 l; **Martin Dohrn:** 566 t; **John Durham:** 224 ccr, 225 b, 235, 444 bl, 874 cr; **Ralph Eagle:** 566 cr, 567 br; **Ken Eward:** 440 tl, 609 br; **Eye of Science:** 768; **Don Fawcett:** 670 tl; **Professor C. Ferlaud/CNRI:** 473 cr, 473 cl; **Sue Ford:** 216 tl, 360 cr, 573; **Cecil H. Fox:** 275, 620 cr; **Simon Fraser/Medical Physics, RVI, Newcastle-upon-Tyne:** 727; **Simon Fraser/Neuroradiology Department/ Newcastle General Hospital:** 365 cb, 533 t, 530; **Simon Fraser/Royal Victoria Infirmary, Newcastle-upon-Tyne:** 540; **Dr. Freiburger, Peter Arnold Inc.:** 371 t; **GCa, CNRI:** 247 t, 365 ctr, 649, 846 t, 373 t, 651; **G-I Associates/Custom Medical Stock Photo:** 261 cbr, 667; **GJLP-CNRI:** 315 cl, 384, 744; **Dr. Peter Gordon:** 614 t, b; **Eric Grave:** 224 ctr, 226 b, 261 tr, 313, 448, 513; **E. Gueho, CNRI:** 287 bl; **Phil Jude:** 331 bl; **Manfred Kage:** 331 cl, 444 bcr, 509, 607, 730 tl; **Keith/Custom Medical Stock Photo:** 21 cl, 811 bl; **James King-Holmes:** 777 tl, tr; **Mehau Kulyk:** 8 t, 10, 11 tl, 16 t, 21 bl, 243 bl, 277, 315 cr, 365 cbr, 368, 496 t, 511, 605, 676, 751 b, 778 tl, 874 tl; **David Leah:** 811 ctr, cr; **Dr. Andrejs Liepins:** 274 cr; **Lunagrafix:** 20, 46, 246 b, 397 tr; **Dr. P. Marazzi:** 261 cbl, br, 290, 292, 293 t, 294 t, 315 bl, 316, 336 cb, 345 t, 357 t, 376, 377 c, 387, 426, 437, 452, 458, 468 br, 479, 548, 582 cr, 613 t, 632, 636, 767 br, 809 b, 828, 830, 843, 858 tl, 862, 863; **Matt Meadows:** 248 b, 781; **Astrid & Hanns-Frieder Michler:** 331 br, 329 bl, 647 r, 720 tl, 781 b, 764, 500, 670 cr; **Moredun Animal Health Ltd.:** 287 tr; **Professor P. M. Motta & E. Vizza:** 730 cr, 732 br; **Professor P. M. Motta, G. Macchiarelli, & S. A. Nottola:** 732 bl; **Professor P. Motta & A. Caggiati, University "La Sapienza," Rome:** 624 tl; **Professor P. Motta, Correr, & Nottola, University "La Sapienza," Rome:** 470; **Professor P. Motta, Department of Anatomy, University "La Sapienza," Rome:** 362 cr, 363, 440 c, 442 b, 444 ctl, 473 bl, 595, 623, 675 tr, 694 cr, 733 tr, tl; **Professors P. Motta & T. Naguro:** 624 tr, 675 tl; **Professors P. Motta, K. R. Porter, & P. M. Andrews:** 331 tc, 444 cr; **Professors P. M. Motta & J. Van Blerkom:** 815 ct; **Sidney Moulds:** 625; **Larry Mulvehill:** 303; **Dr. Gopal Murti:** 234 b, 398 cl; **National Cancer Institute:** 312; **National Institute of Health:** 253 t, 536, 537; **NIBSC:** 297; **Dr. Yorgos Nikas:** 778 cr; **Ohio Nuclear Corporation:** 248 tl; **Dr. G. Oran:** 594 bl; **David Parker:** 352 b, 355 t, 357 b; **Paul Parker:** 578 b, 579 t, b, 582 tl; **Alfred Pasieka:** 68, 213 cbr, 242 bl, 243 ct, 622, 644; **Petit Format/CSI:** 763 b; **Petit Format/E. M. de Monasterio:** 569 cr; **Petit Format/Nestle:** 780 t, b; **Petit Format/Nestle/Steiner:** 510 t; **Petit Format/CSI:** 267 t; **Dr. M. Phelps & Dr. J. Mazziotta et al/Neurology:** 569 cl, 594 br; **D. Phillips:** 21 tl, 329 tr, 399t, 762; **Philippe Plailly:** 264 tl, 279 br, 398 br; **Parviz M. Pour:** 716 cr; **Chris Priest:** 251 tr; **Princess Margaret Rose Orthopaedic Hospital:** 377 br, 393 tl; **Quest:** 21 tr, 276, 396 cr, 675 b, 697, 815 cb; **John Radcliffe Hospital:** 465, 528 t, 635 b, 740, 808; **Ed Reschke, Peter Arnold Inc.:** 443 bl; **J. C. Revy:** 9 b, 224 tl, 258 tl, 369 ct; **Dr. H. C. Robinson:** 294 b; **Salisbury District Hospital:** 642, 812 c; **Department of Clinical Radiology, Salisbury District Hospital:** 432 t, 432 b, 498, 502 b, 505, 522, 541, 705, 745 t, 792; **Francoise Sauze:** 308, 817; **David Scharf:** 311 t, 466; **Dr. K. F. R. Schiller:** 621; **Victor de Schwanberg:** 331 ctr; **Science Source:** 716 tl; **Secchi, Lecaque, Roussel, UCLAF, CNRI:** 512, 514, 696, 717, 815 b; **Dr. Gary Settles:** 288, 473 br; **St. Bartholomew's Hospital:** 553, 793 t; **St. Stephen's Hospital:** 320; **Sinclair Stammers:** 287 br, 311 t, 365 cl; **Dr. Linda Stannard, UCT:** 284 cr; **Volker Steger/Siemens:** 274 tl; **James Stevenson:** 64 tl, tr, 463; **Andrew Syred:** 720 tr, 815 t; **Sheila Terry:** 331 ctl; **Alexander Tsiaras:** 256 t; **Dr. E. Walker:** 213 t, 702 t; **M. I. Walker:** 364; **Garry Watson:** 643; **Richard Wehr/ Custom Medical Stock Photo:** 8 b, 88 tl; **Wellcome Department of Cognitive Neurology:** 555; **Western Opthalmic Hospital:** 571 b, 581, 583; **Hattie Young:** 822; **Dr. D. Singh, Institute of Orthopaedics, Royal National Orthpaedic Hospital, London:** 377 tr; **St. John's Institute of Dermatology, London:** 337 t, 342, 346, 352 t, 360 b; **Courtesy of Dr. Tony de Souza, Royal Brompton National Heart & Lung Hospital, London:** 875 clb; **Tony Stone Images:** Bob Torrez 58; Philip Watson 16 b, 776; **Courtesy of Dr. Peter Stradling c/o Dr. John Stradling, Osler Chest Unit, Churchill Hospital, Oxford:** 214 cr, 504 b; **Courtesy of Professor Roy Taylor, Royal Victoria Infirmary, Newcastle-upon-Tyne:** 261 ctr; **M. I. Walker, Microworld Services:** 329 br, 598 bl, 749 b; **Dr. Jean Watkins:** 293 b, 758; **The Wellcome Trust MPL:** 254 cb, 261 bl, 291, 300, 306 b, 317, 327, 338, 339 tr, b, 345 b, 347 t, 348, 371 b, 378, 380 t, b, 388, 405, 409, 419 cl, 422 br, 424, 433 bl, br, 436, 439 t, 451 b, 459, 461, 462, 464, 468 t, 469 t, 492, 495, 496 b, 529, 545, 549, 558, 562, 571 t, 584 b, 592 bl, 593, 596, 597 r, 618 t, b, 633, 634 bl, 637 r, 648, 650, 663 b, 677, 680, 685 t, 714, 766 tr, 810, 811 tl, 823, 827, 829, 831 t, 832, 835 t, b, 839 t, 856 b, 858 br, 861, 951 br, bl; **Dr. Ian Williams/ Medical Slide Library:** 337 b, 343 t; & V. Ankrett 341 br, 347 b, 393 tr, 570; **Courtesy of Professor A. Wright, Institute of Laryngology and Otology, Royal Free and University College Medical School, London:** 950 br; **Dr. Mike Wyndham Medical Picture Collection:** 251 tl, 261 ctl, 309, 348, 349 t, 490, 499, 755 tl, 860

Every effort has been made to acknowledge those individuals, organizations, and corporations that have helped with this book and to trace copyright holders. Dorling Kindersley apologizes in advance if any omission has been made. If an omission comes to light, the company will be pleased to insert the appropriate acknowledgment in any subsequent editions of this book.